11. **CONTRAINDICATIONS** Conditions, disease states, or patient populations in which use of the drug should be avoided.

12. **WARNINGS/PRECAUTIONS** Conditions related to the use of the drug and disease states or patient populations where caution is advised.

13. **ADVERSE REACTIONS** Side effects and adverse reactions listed in the FDA-approved labeling that occur with greater frequency (generally at a rate of ≥3%) or that are deemed significant in the clinical judgment of the editors. Refer to the full FDA-approved labeling for a complete list of adverse reactions.

14. **DRUG INTERACTIONS** Effects and implications of other drugs and food on the drug based on FDA-approved labeling.

PATIENT CONSIDERATIONS

15. **ASSESSMENT** Specific parameters and lab tests that the patient must be assessed for or undergo prior to starting treatment with the drug.

16. **MONITORING** Information used for monitoring patients currently treated with the drug; may include specific lab tests and drug-related or condition-specific information.

17. **COUNSELING** Important treatment information to discuss with the patient.

18. **STORAGE** Instructions for safe storage and disposal of the drug.

1 Not all fields described here are included in every monograph. Drug monographs in this handbook contain concise information. For more detailed information, please see the full FDA-approved labeling or visit PDR.net® for a complete drug summary and other listings.

2 Abbreviations used within monographs are defined in the *Abbreviations, Acronyms, and Symbols* table on page R1 of the Resource Information Tables.

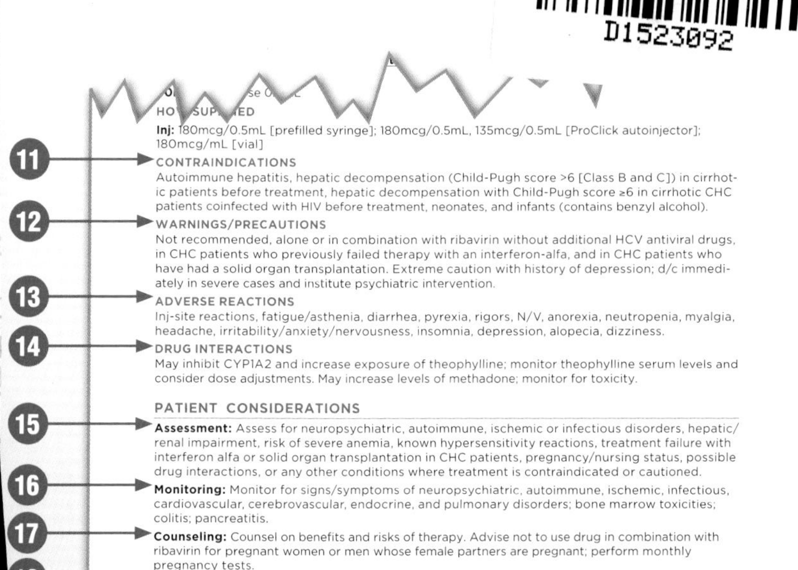

HO SUP ED

Inj: 180mcg/0.5mL [prefilled syringe]; 180mcg/0.5mL, 135mcg/0.5mL [ProClick autoinjector]; 180mcg/mL [vial]

11 CONTRAINDICATIONS

Autoimmune hepatitis, hepatic decompensation (Child-Pugh score >6 [Class B and C]) in cirrhotic patients before treatment, hepatic decompensation with Child-Pugh score ≥6 in cirrhotic CHC patients coinfected with HIV before treatment, neonates, and infants (contains benzyl alcohol).

12 WARNINGS/PRECAUTIONS

Not recommended, alone or in combination with ribavirin without additional HCV antiviral drugs, in CHC patients who previously failed therapy with an interferon-alfa, and in CHC patients who have had a solid organ transplantation. Extreme caution with history of depression; d/c immediately in severe cases and institute psychiatric intervention.

13 ADVERSE REACTIONS

Inj-site reactions, fatigue/asthenia, diarrhea, pyrexia, rigors, N/V, anorexia, neutropenia, myalgia, headache, irritability/anxiety/nervousness, insomnia, depression, alopecia, dizziness.

14 DRUG INTERACTIONS

May inhibit CYP1A2 and increase exposure of theophylline; monitor theophylline serum levels and consider dose adjustments. May increase levels of methadone; monitor for toxicity.

PATIENT CONSIDERATIONS

15 **Assessment:** Assess for neuropsychiatric, autoimmune, ischemic or infectious disorders, hepatic/renal impairment, risk of severe anemia, known hypersensitivity reactions, treatment failure with interferon alfa or solid organ transplantation in CHC patients, pregnancy/nursing status, possible drug interactions, or any other conditions where treatment is contraindicated or cautioned.

16 **Monitoring:** Monitor for signs/symptoms of neuropsychiatric, autoimmune, ischemic, infectious, cardiovascular, cerebrovascular, endocrine, and pulmonary disorders; bone marrow toxicities; colitis; pancreatitis.

17 **Counseling:** Counsel on benefits and risks of therapy. Advise not to use drug in combination with ribavirin for pregnant women or men whose female partners are pregnant; perform monthly pregnancy tests.

18 STORAGE: 2-8°C (36-46°F). Do not leave out of the refrigerator for >24 hrs. Do not freeze or shake. Protect from light.

For more drug summaries, visit PDR.net 1

(Continued)

*FDA/DEA CLASS

OTC: Available over-the-counter.

RX: Requires a prescription.

CII: High potential for abuse. Use may lead to severe physical or psychological dependence.

CIII: Potential for abuse less than the drugs or other substances in CII. Use may lead to low-to-moderate physical dependence or high psychological dependence.

CIV: Low potential for abuse relative to drugs or other substances in CIII. Use may lead to limited physical or psychological dependence relative to the drugs or other substances in CIII.

CV: Low potential for abuse relative to drugs or other substances in CIV. Use may lead to limited physical or psychological dependence relative to the drugs or other substances in CIV.

2017
EDITION

PDR®
Drug Information Handbook

THE INFORMATION STANDARD
FOR PROFESSIONALS IN HEALTHCARE

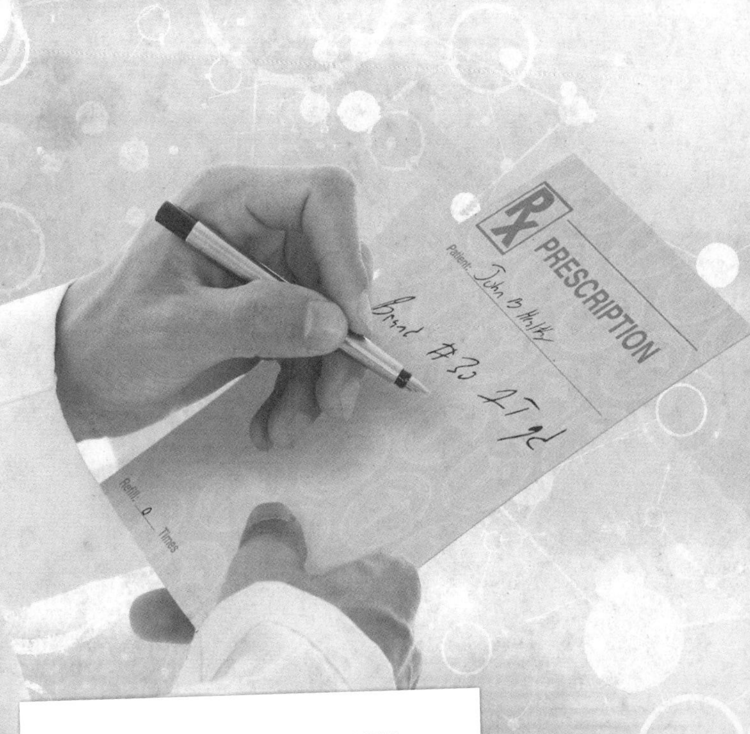

PDR® Drug Information Handbook

ISBN: 978-1-56363-837-4

Printed in Canada

Contents

Foreword

The inaugural edition of the *2017 PDR® Drug Information Handbook* is a comprehensive reference for pharmacotherapy information. Following in the esteemed, seventy-year tradition of the highly trusted *Physicians' Desk Reference®*, it is an excellent source for fast access to clear and concise drug information. Staying knowledgeable about safe pharmacotherapy is critical for pharmacists, physicians, physician assistants, and other professionals in healthcare. With information for thousands of drugs, all based on current FDA-approved labels, the *2017 PDR Drug Information Handbook* can help any member of a healthcare team improve medication safety and enhance patient care.

Specialized resource information tables, a compendium of succinct monographs on the most commonly prescribed drugs, detailed and carefully curated appendix content, an exclusive visual identification guide, and two highly useful indices are all included in the debut edition of the *2017 PDR Drug Information Handbook.* The concise drug monographs are thorough and functional. Each one efficiently covers a drug's brand and generic names, pharmacological class, boxed warning, indications/dosage, dosing considerations, administration information, how supplied details, contraindications, relevant warnings and precautions, key adverse reactions, drug interactions, and details on safe storage and handling instructions. Mindful of the importance of effective patient education and overcoming barriers to adherence, every monograph also has a unique section devoted to patient considerations, encompassing assessment, monitoring, and counseling information.

Presented in a streamlined, two-column format, each alphabetically ordered drug monograph shares the most useful information for adult and pediatric patients. Ease of access to vital labeling details improves the ability to educate patients, encouraging compliance and better health outcomes. The robust appendix of drug information tables adds another dimension of pharmacotherapy insight. Critical, quick-reference charts detail topics such as: diabetes treatment options, antiviral treatments, oral and systemic antibiotic treatment options, a comprehensive list of easily confused drug names (from ISMP), a compilation of drugs that should not be used during pregnancy, and a full reference list for pharmacogenomic biomarkers, patient subgroups, and effects.

The *2017 PDR Drug Information Handbook* is an essential volume for a wide range of clinicians, pharmacy staff, students, and others in the healthcare industry. For readers, PDR also recommends downloading *mobile*PDR®, which is the only medical information app with a drug comparison function. Additionally, PDR.net® provides online access to authoritative drug information, including select FDA-approved labeling. PDR's products and publications offer flexible access to dependable and current drug information.

Resource Information Tables

The following section provides quick access to select informational tools for professionals in healthcare. This resource content includes symbols and commonly abbreviated terms found throughout this handbook, as well as useful calculations, formulas, and normal lab values.

ABBREVIATIONS, ACRONYMS, AND SYMBOLS

ABBREVIATIONS	DESCRIPTIONS
- (eg, 6-8)	to (eg, 6 to 8)
/	per
<	less than
>	greater than
≤	less than or equal to
≥	greater than or equal to
α	alpha
β	beta
µL	microliter
µm	micrometer
µM	micromolar
µmol	micromole
5-FU	5-fluorouracil
5-HT	5-hydroxytryptamine (serotonin)
aa	of each
ABECB	acute bacterial exacerbation of chronic bronchitis
ac	before meals
ACE inhibitor	angiotensin converting enzyme inhibitor
ACTH	adrenocorticotropic hormone
ad	right ear
ADHD	attention-deficit hyperactivity disorder
A-fib	atrial fibrillation
A-flutter	atrial flutter
AIDS	acquired immunodeficiency syndrome
ALK	anaplastic lymphoma kinase
ALT	alanine transaminase (SGPT)
am or AM	morning
AMI	acute myocardial infarction
ANA	antinuclear antibody
ANC	absolute neutrophil count
APAP	acetaminophen
Apo B	apolipoprotein B
ARB	angiotensin II receptor blocker
as	left ear
ASA	aspirin
AST	aspartate transaminase (SGOT)
au	each ear

(Continued)

ABBREVIATIONS	DESCRIPTIONS
AUC	area under the curve
AV	atrioventricular
BCG	bacillus Calmette-Guerin
BCRP	breast cancer resistance protein
bid	twice daily
BMI	body mass index
BP	blood pressure
BPH	benign prostatic hypertrophy
bpm	beats per minute
BSA	body surface area
BUN	blood urea nitrogen
Ca^{2+}	calcium
CABG	coronary artery bypass graft
CAD	coronary artery disease
cAMP	cyclic-3',5'-adenosine monophosphate
cap	capsule or gelcap
CAP	community-acquired pneumonia
CBC	complete blood count
CCB	calcium channel blocker
CF	cystic fibrosis
cGMP	cyclic guanosine monophosphate
CHF	congestive heart failure
CK	creatine kinase
Cl^-	chloride
cm	centimeter
C_{max}	peak plasma concentration
CMV	cytomegalovirus
CNS	central nervous system
COMT inhibitor	catechol-O-methyl transferase inhibitor
COPD	chronic obstructive pulmonary disease
COX-2 inhibitor	cyclooxygenase-2 inhibitor
CPK	creatine phosphokinase
CR	controlled-release
CrCl	creatinine clearance
cre	cream
CRF	chronic renal failure
CSF	cerebrospinal fluid
cSSSI	complicated skin and skin structure infection
CTC	common toxicity criteria
CV	cardiovascular

ABBREVIATIONS	DESCRIPTIONS
CVA	cerebrovascular accident
CVD	cardiovascular disease
CYP450	cytochrome P450
D5	dextrose 5%
D5W	dextrose 5% in water
d/c or D/C	discontinue
DHEA	dehydroepiandrosterone
DM	diabetes mellitus
DMARD	disease modifying antirheumatic drug
DNA	deoxyribonucleic acid
DR	delayed-release
DVT	deep vein thrombosis
ECG	electrocardiogram
EDTA	edetate disodium
EEG	electroencephalogram
eg	for example
EGFR	epidermal growth factor receptor
EPS	extrapyramidal symptom
ER	extended-release
ESRD	end-stage renal disease
fl oz	fluid ounce
FPG	fasting plasma glucose
FSH	follicle-stimulating hormone
g	gram
G6PD	glucose-6-phosphate dehydrogenase
GABA	gamma-aminobutyric acid
GAD	general anxiety disorder
GERD	gastroesophageal reflux disease
GFR	glomerular filtration rate
GGT	gamma-glutamyl transpeptidase
GI	gastrointestinal
GnRH	gonadotropin-releasing hormone
GVHD	graft-versus-host disease
HbA1c	hemoglobin A1c
hCG	human chorionic gonadotropin
Hct	hematocrit
HCTZ	hydrochlorothiazide
HDL	high-density lipoprotein
HER2	human epidermal growth factor receptor 2
HF	heart failure

(Continued)

ABBREVIATIONS	DESCRIPTIONS
Hgb	hemoglobin
HIV	human immunodeficiency virus
HMG-CoA	3-hydroxy-3-methylglutaryl-coenzyme A
HR	heart rate
hr, hrs	hour, hours
hs	bedtime
HSV	herpes simplex virus
HTN	hypertension
IBD	inflammatory bowel disease
IBS	irritable bowel syndrome
ICH	intracranial hemorrhage
ICP	intracranial pressure
IgG	immunoglobulin G
IM	intramuscular/intramuscularly
INH	isoniazid
inh	inhalation
inj	injection
INR	international normalized ratio
IOP	intraocular pressure
IR	immediate-release
IU*	international unit
IUD	intrauterine device
IV	intravenous/intravenously
K^+	potassium
kg	kilogram
KIU	kallikrein inhibitor unit
L	liter
lb, lbs	pound, pounds
LD	loading dose
LDL	low-density lipoprotein
LFT	liver function test
LH	luteinizing hormone
LHRH	luteinizing-hormone releasing hormone
lot	lotion
loz	lozenge
LVEF	left ventricular ejection fraction
LVH	left ventricular hypertrophy
M	molar
MAC	*Mycobacterium avium* complex
maint	maintenance

ABBREVIATIONS	DESCRIPTIONS
MAOI	monoamine oxidase inhibitor
max	maximum
mcg	microgram
mEq	milliequivalent
mg	milligram
Mg^{2+}	magnesium
MI	myocardial infarction
min	minute (usually as mL/min)
mL	milliliter
mm	millimeter
mM	millimolar
MRI	magnetic resonance imaging
MS*	multiple sclerosis
msec	millisecond
MTX	methotrexate
N/A	not applicable or not available
Na^{+}	sodium
NaCl	sodium chloride
NG	nasogastric
NKA	no known allergies
NMS	neuroleptic malignant syndrome
NPO	nothing by mouth
NSAID	nonsteroidal anti-inflammatory drug
NV or N/V	nausea and vomiting
NYHA Class	New York Heart Association Class
OA	osteoarthritis
OCD	obsessive-compulsive disorder
od	right eye
oint	ointment
os	left eye
OTC	over-the-counter
ou	each eye
oz	ounce
P	phosphorus
PAT	paroxysmal atrial tachycardia
pc	after meals
PCN	penicillin
PCP	*Pneumocystis carinii* pneumonia
PD	Parkinson's disease
PDE-5 inhibitor	phosphodiesterase-5 inhibitor

(Continued)

ABBREVIATIONS	DESCRIPTIONS
PE	pulmonary embolism
P-gp	P-glycoprotein
PID	pelvic inflammatory disease
pkt, pkts	packet, packets
pm or PM	evening
po or PO	orally
PONV	postoperative nausea and vomiting
postop	postoperative/postoperatively
PPI	proton pump inhibitor
pr	rectally
preop	preoperative/preoperatively
prn or PRN	as needed
PSA	prostate-specific antigen
PSVT	paroxysmal supraventricular tachycardia
PT	prothrombin time
PTSD	post-traumatic stress disorder
PTT	partial thromboplastin time
PTU	propylthiouracil
PUD	peptic ulcer disease
PVD	peripheral vascular disease
q4h, q6h, q8h, etc.	every four hours, every six hours, every eight hours, etc.
qam	once every morning
qd*	once daily
qh	every hour
qhs	every night at bedtime/before retiring
qid	four times daily
qod*	every other day
qpm	once every evening
qs	a sufficient quantity
qs ad	a sufficient quantity to make
RA	rheumatoid arthritis
RAAS	renin-angiotensin-aldosterone system
RAS	renin-angiotensin system
RBC	red blood cell
RDS	respiratory distress syndrome
REM	rapid eye movement
RNA	ribonucleic acid
Rx	prescription
SA	sinoatrial

ABBREVIATIONS	DESCRIPTIONS
SAH	subarachnoid hemorrhage
SBP	systolic blood pressure
sec	second
SGOT	serum glutamic-oxaloacetic transaminase (AST)
SGPT	serum glutamic-pyruvic transaminase (ALT)
SIADH	syndrome of inappropriate antidiuretic hormone secretion
SJS	Stevens-Johnson syndrome
SL	sublingual/sublingually
SLE	systemic lupus erythematosus
SNRI	serotonin and norepinephrine reuptake inhibitor
SOB	shortness of breath
sol	solution
SQ, SC	subcutaneous/subcutaneously
SR	sustained-release
SrCr	serum creatinine
SSRI	selective serotonin reuptake inhibitor
SSSI	skin and skin structure infection
STD	sexually transmitted disease
sup or supp	suppository
sus	suspension
SVT	supraventricular tachycardia
SWFI	sterile water for injection
$T_{½}$	half-life
T3	triiodothyronine
T4	thyroxine
tab	tablet or caplet
tab, SL	sublingual tablet
TB	tuberculosis
TBG	thyroxine-binding globulin
tbl or tbsp	tablespoonful
TCA	tricyclic antidepressant
TD	tardive dyskinesia
TEN	toxic epidermal necrolysis
TFT	thyroid function test
TG	triglyceride
tid	three times daily
T_{max}	time to maximum concentration

(Continued)

ABBREVIATIONS	DESCRIPTIONS
TNF	tumor necrosis factor
total-C	total cholesterol
TPN	total parenteral nutrition
TSH	thyroid-stimulating hormone
tsp	teaspoonful
TTP	thrombotic thrombocytopenic purpura
U*	unit
UC	ulcerative colitis
ud	as directed
ULN	upper limit of normal
URTI/URI	upper respiratory tract infection
UTI	urinary tract infection
UV	ultraviolet
V_d	volume of distribution
VEGF	vascular endothelial growth factor
VLDL	very low density lipoprotein
VTE	venous thromboembolism
w/ or W/	with
w/in or W/IN	within
w/o or W/O	without
WBC	white blood cell
WHO	World Health Organization
X	times (eg, >2X ULN)
yr, yrs	year, years

*The Joint Commission cautions use of these abbreviations on orders and medication-related documentation that is handwritten (including free-text computer entry) or on pre-printed forms. Visit www.jointcommission.org for more information.

CALCULATIONS AND FORMULAS

METRIC MEASURES	
1 kilogram (kg)	1000 g
1 gram (g)	1000 mg
1 milligram (mg)	0.001 g
1 microgram (mcg or µg)	0.001 mg; 1×10^{-6} g
1 liter (L)	1000 mL
1 milliliter (mL)	0.001 L; 1 cubic centimeter (cc)
APOTHECARY MEASURES (AP)	
1 scruple	20 grains (gr)
1 dram	3 scruples; 27.3 gr
1 ounce (oz)	16 drams; 22 scruples; 437.5 gr
1 pound (lb)	16 oz; 256 drams; 350 scruples; 7000 gr
U.S. FLUID MEASURES	
1 fluid dram	60 minims
1 fluid ounce (fl oz)	8 fluid drams; 480 minims
1 pint (pt)	16 fl oz; 7680 minims
1 quart (qt)	2 pt; 32 fl oz
1 gallon (gal)	4 qt; 128 fl oz
AVOIRDUPOIS WEIGHT (AV)	
1 ounce	437.5 gr
1 pound	16 oz
CONVERSION FACTORS	
1 gram	15.4 gr
1 grain	64.8 mg
1 ounce (Av)	28.35 g; 437.5 gr
1 ounce (Ap)	31.1 g; 480 gr
1 pound (Av)	453.6 g
1 fluid ounce	29.57 mL
1 fluid dram	3.697 mL
1 minim	0.06 mL
COMMON MEASURES	
1 teaspoonful	5 mL; ⅙ fl oz
1 tablespoonful	15 mL; ½ fl oz
1 wineglassful	60 mL; 2 fl oz
1 teacupful	120 mL; 4 fl oz
1 gallon	3800 mL; 128 fl oz
1 quart	946 mL; 32 fl oz
1 pint	473 mL; 16 fl oz
8 fluid ounces	240 mL
4 fluid ounces	120 mL
2.2 lb	1 kg

DOSE EQUIVALENTS

WEIGHT (METRIC)	WEIGHT (APOTHECARY)
30 g	1 ounce
15 g	8.5 drams
10 g	5.6 drams
7.5 g	4.2 drams
6 g	92.6 grains
5 g	77.2 grains
4 g	60 grains; 1 dram
3 g	45 grains

(Continued)

DOSE EQUIVALENTS *(Continued)*	
WEIGHT (METRIC)	**WEIGHT (APOTHECARY)**
2 g	30 grains; ½ dram
1.5 g	22 grains
1 g	15 grains
750 mg	12 grains
600 mg	10 grains
500 mg	7½ grains
400 mg	6 grains
300 mg	5 grains
250 mg	4 grains
200 mg	3 grains
150 mg	2½ grains
125 mg	2 grains
100 mg	1½ grains
75 mg	1¼ grains
60 mg	1 grain
50 mg	¾ grain
40 mg	⅔ grain
30 mg	½ grain
25 mg	⅜ grain
20 mg	⅓ grain
15 mg	¼ grain
12 mg	⅕ grain
10 mg	⅙ grain
8 mg	⅛ grain
6 mg	1/10 grain
5 mg	1/12 grain
4 mg	1/15 grain
3 mg	1/20 grain
2 mg	1/30 grain
1.5 mg	1/40 grain
1.2 mg	1/50 grain
1 mg	1/60 grain
LIQUID MEASURES (METRIC)	**LIQUID MEASURES (APOTHECARY)**
1000 mL	1 quart
750 mL	1½ pints
500 mL	1 pint
230 mL	8 fluid ounces
200 mL	7 fluid ounces
100 mL	3½ fluid ounces
50 mL	1¾ fluid ounces
30 mL	1 fluid ounce
15 mL	4 fluid drams
10 mL	2½ fluid drams
8 mL	2 fluid drams
5 mL	1½ fluid drams
4 mL	1 fluid dram
3 mL	45 minims
2 mL	30 minims
1 mL	15 minims
0.75 mL	12 minims
0.6 mL	10 minims
0.5 mL	8 minims
0.3 mL	5 minims
0.25 mL	4 minims
0.2 mL	3 minims

DOSE EQUIVALENTS *(Continued)*	
LIQUID MEASURES (METRIC)	**LIQUID MEASURES (APOTHECARY)**
0.1 mL	1½ minims
0.06 mL	1 minim
0.05 mL	¾ minim
0.03 mL	½ minim

MOLES, MILLIGRAMS, & MILLIEQUIVALENTS

ELEMENT	ATOMIC WEIGHT (wt)	VALENCE
Calcium	40	2
Carbon	12	4
Chlorine	35.5	1
Hydrogen	1	1
Magnesium	24	2
Nitrogen	14	3
Oxygen	16	2
Phosphorus	31	2
Potassium	39	1
Sodium	23	1

CALCULATIONS

mEq = mg/atomic wt × valence = mmol × valence

mg = mEq × atomic wt/valence = mmol × atomic wt

mmol = mg/atomic wt = mEq/valence

Note: atomic wt = molecular wt

ACID-BASE ASSESSMENT

DEFINITIONS

PIO_2	Oxygen partial pressure of inspired gas (mmHg); 150 mmHg in room air at sea level
FiO_2	Fractional pressure of oxygen in inspired gas (0.21 in room air)
PAO_2	Alveolar oxygen partial pressure
$PACO_2$	Alveolar carbon dioxide partial pressure
PaO_2	Arterial oxygen partial pressure
$PaCO_2$	Arterial carbon dioxide partial pressure
P_{ATM}	Ambient barometric pressure (eg, 760 mmHg at sea level)
P_{H2O}	Partial pressure of water vapor (eg, usually 47 mmHg)
R	Respiratory quotient (typically 0.8, increases with high-carbohydrate diet, decreases with high-fat diet)

HENDERSON-HASSELBALCH EQUATION

$pH = 6.1 + \log [HCO_3^- / (0.03)(pCO_2)]$

ALVEOLAR GAS EQUATION

$$P_{AO2} = [F_{IO2} \times (P_{ATM} - P_{H2O})] - \frac{PaCO_2}{R}$$

(Continued)

ACID-BASE DISORDERS

DISORDER	pH	HCO_3^-	PCO_2	COMPENSATION
Metabolic acidosis	<7.35	Primary decrease	Compensatory decrease	1.2 mmHg decrease in PCO_2 for every 1 mmol/L decrease in HCO_3^- **OR** $PCO_2 = (1.5 \times HCO_3^-) + 8\ (\pm 2)$ **OR** $PCO_2 = HCO_3^- + 15$ **OR** PCO_2 = last 2 digits of pH × 100
Metabolic alkalosis	>7.45	Primary increase	Compensatory increase	0.6-0.75 mmHg increase in PCO_2 for every 1 mmol/L increase in HCO_3^-. PCO_2 should not rise above 55 mmHg in compensation.
Respiratory acidosis	<7.35	Compen-satory increase	Primary increase	***Acute:*** 1-2 mmol/L increase in HCO_3^- for every 10 mmHg increase in PCO_2. ***Chronic:*** 3-4 mmol/L increase in HCO_3^- for every 10 mmHg increase in PCO_2.
Respiratory alkalosis	>7.45	Compen-satory decrease	Primary decrease	***Acute:*** 1-2 mmol/L decrease in HCO_3^- for every 10 mmHg decrease in PCO_2. ***Chronic:*** 4-5 mmol/L decrease in HCO_3^- for every 10 mmHg decrease in PCO_2.

ACID-BASE EQUATION

H^+ (in mEq/L) = (24 × $PaCO_2$) divided by HCO_3^-

OTHER CALCULATIONS

ANION GAP

Anion gap = $Na^+ - (Cl^- + HCO_3^-)$ = Unmeasured Anions (UA) - Unmeasured Cations (UC)

OSMOLALITY

Definition:
Osmolality is a measure of the total number of particles in a solution.

U.S. units (sodium as mEq/L, BUN [blood urea nitrogen] and glucose as mg/dL)
Plasma osmolality (mOsm/kg) = 2[Na^+] + [(BUN)/2.8] + [(glucose)/18]

SI units (all variables in mmol/L):
Plasma osmolality (mOsm/kg) = 2[Na^+] + [urea] + [glucose]
Normal range plasma osmolality: 275 - 290 mOsm/kg

Corrected Sodium
Measured Na^+ + 0.016 (Serum glucose - 100), **OR**
Measured Na^+ + 0.024 (Serum glucose - 100)

Total Serum Calcium Corrected for Albumin Level
[(Normal albumin - patient's albumin) × 0.8] + patient's measured total calcium

Free Water Deficit

$$0.6 \times \text{body weight (kg)}\ \frac{[(\text{Current } Na^+)]}{140} - 1$$

Bicarbonate Deficit
[0.4 × weight (kg)] × (HCO_3^- desired - HCO_3^- measured)

CHILD-PUGH SCORE

The Child-Pugh classification is used to assess the prognosis of chronic liver disease, mainly cirrhosis. Child-Pugh is also used to determine the required strength of treatment and the necessity of liver transplantation.

Score:
The score employs five clinical measures of liver disease. Each measure is scored 1-3, with 3 indicating the most severe derangement.

Measure	1 point	2 points	3 points	Units
Bilirubin (total)	<2	2-3	>3	mg/dL
Serum albumin	>3.5	2.8-3.5	<2.8	g/dL
INR†	<1.7	1.71-2.3	>2.3	no unit
Ascites	None	Mild (or controlled by diuretics)	Moderate despite diuretic treatment	no unit

CHILD-PUGH SCORE *(Continued)*				
Measure	**1 point**	**2 points**	**3 points**	**Units**
Hepatic encephalopathy	None	Grade I-II (or suppressed with medication)	Grade III-IV (or refractory)	no unit

†Some older reference works substitute PT prolongation for INR.

Interpretation:
Chronic liver disease is classified into Child-Pugh class A to C, employing the added score from above.

Points	Class	One-year survival	Two-year survival
5-6	A	100%	85%
7-9	B	80%	60%
10-15	C	45%	35%

CREATININE CLEARANCE

Clinically, creatinine clearance is a useful measure for estimating the glomerular filtration rate (GFR) of the kidneys.

Factors	Abbreviations
Creatinine clearance	Cl_{Cr}
Plasma creatinine concentration	P_{Cr}
Serum creatinine concentration	S_{Cr}
Urine creatinine concentration	U_{Cr}
Urine flow rate	V

Calculations:

$$Cl_{Cr} = \frac{U_{Cr} \times V}{P_{Cr}}$$

Example:
Patient with P_{Cr} 1 mg/dL, U_{Cr} 60 mg/dL, and V of 0.5 dL/hr.

$$Cl_{Cr} = \frac{60 \text{ mg/dL} \times 0.5 \text{ dL/hr}}{1 \text{ mg/dL}} = 30 \text{ dL/hr}$$

Cockroft-Gault formula: Estimates creatinine clearance (mL/min).

Male:

$$Cl_{Cr} = \frac{(140 - \text{age}) \times \text{mass (kg)}}{72 \times S_{Cr} \text{ (mg/dL)}}$$

Example:
Male patient, 67 years of age, weight 75 kg, and S_{Cr} 1 mg/dL.

$$Cl_{Cr} = \frac{(140 - 67) \times 75}{72 \times 1} = 76 \text{ mL/min}$$

Female:

$$Cl_{Cr} = \frac{(140 - \text{age}) \times \text{mass (kg)} \times 0.85}{72 \times S_{Cr} \text{ (mg/dL)}}$$

Example:
Female patient, 67 years of age, weight 75 kg, and S_{Cr} 1 mg/dL.

$$Cl_{Cr} = \frac{(140 - 67) \times 75 \times 0.85}{72 \times 1} = 64.6 \text{ mL/min}$$

Note: Using actual body weight (ABW) in obese patients can significantly overestimate creatinine clearance. Adjusted ideal body weight (IBW) can provide a more approximate estimate. Adjusted IBW = IBW + 0.4 (ABW - IBW).

BASAL ENERGY EXPENDITURE (BEE)

Basal energy expenditure: the amount of energy required to maintain the body's normal metabolic activity (eg, respiration, maintenance of body temperature).
W = weight (kg), H = height (cm), A = age (years)

Male:
BEE = 66.67 + 13.75W + 5H - 6.76A

Female:
BEE = 655.1 + 9.56W + 1.85H - 4.68A

(Continued)

BODY MASS INDEX (BMI)

$$BMI = \frac{weight\ (kg)}{[height\ (m)]^2}$$

BODY SURFACE AREA (BSA)

$$BSA\ (m^2) = \sqrt{\frac{height\ (in) \times weight\ (lb)}{3131}}$$

OR

$$BSA\ (m^2) = \sqrt{\frac{height\ (cm) \times weight\ (kg)}{3600}}$$

IDEAL BODY WEIGHT (IBW)

Adults (18 years and older; IBW is in kg; height is in inches):
For adults ≥5 feet:
IBW (male) = 50 + [2.3 × (height - 60)]
IBW (female) = 45.5 + [2.3 × (height - 60)]

Children (IBW is in kg; height is in cm):
For children 1-18 years old and with a height <5 feet:

$$IBW\ (kg) = \frac{(height^2 \times 1.65)}{1000}$$

POUNDS/KILOGRAMS CONVERSION

1 POUND = 0.45359 KILOGRAM				1 KILOGRAM = 2.2 POUNDS			
lb	kg	lb	kg	lb	kg	lb	kg
1	0.45	105	47.63	210	95.25	315	142.88
5	2.27	110	49.89	215	97.52	320	145.15
10	4.54	115	52.16	220	99.79	325	147.42
15	6.80	120	54.43	225	102.06	330	149.68
20	9.07	125	56.70	230	104.33	335	151.95
25	11.34	130	58.97	235	106.59	340	154.22
30	13.61	135	61.23	240	108.86	345	156.49
35	15.88	140	63.50	245	111.13	350	158.76
40	18.14	145	65.77	250	113.40	355	161.02
45	20.41	150	68.04	255	115.67	360	163.29
50	22.68	155	70.31	260	117.93	365	165.56
55	24.95	160	72.57	265	120.20	370	167.83
60	27.22	165	74.84	270	122.47	375	170.10
65	29.48	170	77.11	275	124.74	380	172.36
70	31.75	175	79.38	280	127.01	385	174.63
75	34.02	180	81.65	285	129.27	390	176.90
80	36.29	185	83.91	290	131.54	395	179.17
85	38.56	190	86.18	295	133.81	400	181.44
90	40.82	195	88.45	300	136.08	405	183.70
95	43.09	200	90.72	305	138.34	410	185.97
100	45.36	205	92.99	310	140.61	415	188.24

TEMPERATURE CONVERSION

FAHRENHEIT TO CELSIUS = (°F - 32) × 5/9 = °C				CELSIUS TO FAHRENHEIT = (°C × 9/5) + 32 = °F			
°F	°C	°F	°C	°C	°F	°C	°F
0.0	-17.8	50.0	10.0	0.0	32.0	38.0	100.4
5.0	-15.0	55.0	12.8	5.0	41.0	39.0	102.2
10.0	-12.2	60.0	15.6	10.0	50.0	40.0	104.0

TEMPERATURE CONVERSION *(Continued)*							
FAHRENHEIT TO CELSIUS = (°F - 32) × $^5/_9$ = °C				**CELSIUS TO FAHRENHEIT = (°C × $^9/_5$) + 32 = °F**			
°F	**°C**	**°F**	**°C**	**°C**	**°F**	**°C**	**°F**
15.0	-9.4	65.0	18.3	15.0	59.0	41.0	105.8
20.0	-6.7	70.0	21.1	20.0	68.0	42.0	107.6
25.0	-3.9	75.0	23.9	25.0	77.0	43.0	109.4
30.0	-1.1	80.0	26.7	30.0	86.0	44.0	111.2
35.0	1.7	85.0	29.4	35.0	95.0	45.0	113.0
40.0	4.4	90.0	32.2	36.0	96.8	46.0	114.8
45.0	7.2	91.0	32.8	37.0	98.6	47.0	116.6
92.0	33.3	101.0	38.3	48.0	118.4	59.0	138.2
93.0	33.9	102.0	38.9	49.0	120.2	60.0	140.0
94.0	34.4	103.0	39.4	50.0	122.0	65.0	149.0
95.0	35.0	104.0	40.0	51.0	123.8	70.0	158.0
96.0	35.6	105.0	40.6	52.0	125.6	75.0	167.0
97.0	36.1	106.0	41.1	53.0	127.4	80.0	176.0
98.0	36.7	107.0	41.7	54.0	129.2	85.0	185.0
98.6	37.0	108.0	42.2	55.0	131.0	90.0	194.0
99.0	37.2	109.0	42.8	56.0	132.8	95.0	203.0
100.0	37.8	110.0	43.3	57.0	134.6	100.0	212.0
				58.0	136.4	105.0	221.0

PEDIATRIC DOSAGE ESTIMATION FORMULAS

The following formulas can be used to estimate the approximate pediatric dosage of a medication. These formulas are based on the adult dose and either the child's age or weight. These formulas should be used with caution, as the response to any drug is not always directly proportional to the age or weight of the child relative to the usual adult dose. Dosage will also vary based on the formula used. Care should be taken when using any of these methods to calculate the child's dosage. Some products have FDA-approved pediatric indications and dosages; always refer to the full prescribing information first before calculating a pediatric dosage.

BASED ON WEIGHT

Clark's Rule:
[weight (lb)/150] × adult dose = approximate child's dose
Example: If the child's weight is 15 kg (33 lb) and the adult dose is 50 mg then the child's dose is 11 mg.
(33/150) × 50 mg = 11 mg

BASED ON AGE

Dilling's Rule:
[age (years)/20] × adult dose = approximate child's dose
Example: If the child's age is 8 years and the adult dose is 50 mg then the child's dose is 20 mg.
(8/20) × 50 mg = 20 mg

Cowling's Rule:
$$\frac{\text{[age at next birthday (years)]}}{24} \times \text{adult dose} = \text{approximate child's dose}$$
Example: If the child is going to turn 8 years old in a few months and the adult dose is 50 mg then the child's dose is 16.7 mg.
(8/24) × 50 mg = 16.7 mg

Young's Rule:
$$\frac{\text{[age (years)]}}{\text{age} + 12} \times \text{adult dose} = \text{approximate child's dose}$$
Example: If the child's age is 8 years and the adult dose is 50 mg then the child's dose is 20 mg.
[8/(8 + 12)] × 50 mg = 20 mg

Fried's Rule (younger than 1 year):
$$\frac{\text{[age (months)]}}{150} \times \text{adult dose} = \text{approximate infant's dose}$$
Example: If the child's age is 10 months and the adult dose is 50 mg then the child's dose is 3.3 mg.
(10/150) × 50 mg = 3.33 mg

Normal Laboratory Values: Blood, Plasma, and Serum

TEST	SPECIMEN	CONVENTIONAL UNITS	SI UNITS
Acetoacetate	Plasma	< 1 mg/dL	< 0.1 mmol/L
Acetylcholinesterase (ACE), RBC	Blood	26.7–49.2 U/g Hb	—
Acid phosphatase	Serum	0.5–5.5 U/L	0–0.9 µkat/L
Activated partial thromboplastin time (aPTT)	Plasma	25–35 sec	—
Adrenocorticotropic hormone (ACTH)	Serum	9–52 pg/mL	2–11 pmol/L
Albumin	Serum	3.5–5.5 g/dL	35–55 g/L
Aldosterone:			
Standing	Serum	7–20 ng/dL	194–554 pmol/L
Supine	Serum	2–5 ng/dL	55–138 pmol/L
Alkaline phosphatase (ALP)	Serum	36–92 U/L	0.5–1.5 µkat/L
Alpha$_1$-antitrypsin (AAT)	Serum	83–199 mg/dL	—
Alpha fetoprotein (AFP)	Serum	0–20 ng/dL	0–20 pg/L
δ-Aminolevulinic acid (ALA)	Serum	15–23 µg/L	1.14–1.75 µmol/L
Aminotransferase, alanine (ALT)	Serum	0–35 U/L	0–0.58 µkat/L
Aminotransferase, aspartate (AST)	Serum	0–35 U/L	0–0.58 µkat/L
Ammonia	Plasma	40–80 µg/dL	23–47 µmol/L
Amylase	Serum	0–130 U/L	0–2.17 µkat/L
Antibodies to extractable nuclear antigen (AENA)	Serum	< 20.0 units	—
Anti–cyclic citrullinated peptide (anti-CCP) antibodies	Serum	≤ 5.0 units	—
Antidiuretic hormone (ADH; arginine vasopressin)	Plasma	< 1.7 pg/mL	< 1.57 pmol/L
Anti–double-stranded DNA (dsDNA) antibodies, IgG	Serum	< 25 IU	—
Antimitochondrial M2 antibodies	Serum	< 0.1 units	—
Antineutrophil cytoplasmic antibodies (cANCA)	Serum	Negative	—
Antinuclear antibodies (ANA)	Serum	≤ 1.0 units	—
Anti–smooth muscle antibodies (ASMA) titer	Serum	≤ 1:80	—
Antistreptolysin O titer	Serum	< 150 units	—
Antithyroid microsomal antibody titer	Serum	< 1:100	—
α$_1$-Antitrypsin (AAT)	Serum	83–199 mg/dL	15.3–36.6 µmol/L
Apolipoproteins:			
A-I, females	Serum	98–210 mg/dL	0.98–2.1 g/L
A-I, males	Serum	88–180 mg/dL	0.88–1.8 g/L
B-100, females	Serum	44–148 mg/dL	0.44–1.48 g/L
B-100, males	Serum	55–151 mg/dL	0.55–1.51 g/L

(Continued)

TEST	SPECIMEN	CONVENTIONAL UNITS	SI UNITS
Bicarbonate	Serum	23–28 mEq/L	23–28 mmol/L
Bilirubin:			
Direct	Serum	0–0.3 mg/dL	0–5.1 µmol/L
Total	Serum	0.3–1.2 mg/dL	5.1–20.5 µmol/L
Blood volume:			
Plasma, females	Blood	28–43 mL/kg body wt	0.028–0.043 L/kg body wt
Plasma, males	Blood	25–44 mL/kg body wt	0.025–0.044 L/kg body wt
RBCs, females	Blood	20–30 mL/kg body wt	0.02–0.03 L/kg body wt
RBCs, males	Blood	25–35 mL/kg body wt	0.025–0.035 L/kg body wt
Brain (B-type) natriuretic peptide (BNP)	Plasma	< 100 pg/mL	—
Calcitonin, age ≥ 16 yr:			
Females	Serum	< 8 pg/mL	—
Males	Serum	< 16 pg/mL	—
Calcium	Serum	9–10.5 mg/dL	2.2–2.6 mmol/L
Cancer antigen (CA):			
CA 125	Serum	< 35 U/mL	—
CA 15-3	Serum	< 30 U/mL	—
Carbon dioxide (CO_2) content	Serum	23–28 mEq/L	23–28 mmol/L
Carbon dioxide partial pressure (PCO_2)	Blood	35–45 mm Hg	—
Carboxyhemoglobin	Plasma	0.5–5%	—
Carcinoembryonic antigen (CEA)	Serum	< 2 ng/mL	< 2 µg/L
Carotene	Serum	75–300 µg/L	1.4–5.6 µmol/L
CD4:CD8 ratio	Blood	1–4	—
CD4+ T-cell count	Blood	640–1175/µL	0.64–1.18 x 10^9/L
CD8+ T-cell count	Blood	335–875/µL	0.34–0.88 x 10^9/L
Ceruloplasmin	Serum	25–43 mg/dL	250–430 mg/L
Chloride	Serum	98–106 mEq/L	98–106 mmol/L
Cholesterol, desirable level:			
High-density lipoprotein (HDL-C)	Plasma	≥ 40 mg/dL	≥ 1.04 mmol/L
Low-density lipoprotein (LDL-C)	Plasma	≤ 130 mg/dL	≤ 3.36 mmol/L
Total (TC)	Plasma	150–199 mg/dL	3.88–5.15 mmol/L
Coagulation factors:			
Factor I	Plasma	150–300 mg/dL	1.5–3.5 g/L
Factor II	Plasma	60–150% of normal	—
Factor IX	Plasma	60–150% of normal	—
Factor V	Plasma	60–150% of normal	—
Factor VII	Plasma	60–150% of normal	—
Factor VIII	Plasma	60–150% of normal	—
Factor X	Plasma	60–150% of normal	—
Factor XI	Plasma	60–150% of normal	—
Factor XII	Plasma	60–150% of normal	—
Complement:			
C3	Serum	55–120 mg/dL	0.55–1.20 g/L
C4	Serum	20–59 mg/dL	0.20–0.59 g/L
Total	Serum	37–55 U/mL	37–55 kU/L
Copper	Serum	70–155 µg/L	11–24.3 µmol/L

TEST	SPECIMEN	CONVENTIONAL UNITS	SI UNITS
Cortisol:			
1 h after cosyntropin	Serum	> 18 µg/dL and usually ≥ 8 µg/dL above baseline	> 498 nmol/L and usually ≥ 221 nmol/L above baseline
At 5 PM	Serum	3–13 µg/dL	83–359 nmol/L
At 8 AM	Serum	8–20 µg/dL	251–552 nmol/L
After overnight suppression test	Serum	< 5 µg/dL	< 138 nmol/L
C-peptide	Serum	0.9–4.3 ng/mL	297–1419 pmol/L
C-reactive protein (CRP)	Serum	< 0.5 mg/dL	< 0.005 g/L
C-reactive protein, highly sensitive (hsCRP)	Serum	< 1.1 mg/L	< 0.0011 g/L
Creatine kinase (CK)	Serum	30–170 U/L	0.5–2.83 µkat/L
Creatinine	Serum	0.7–1.3 mg/dL	61.9–115 µmol/L
D-Dimer	Plasma	≤ 300 ng/mL	≤ 300 µg/L
Dehydroepiandrosterone sulfate (DHEA-S):			
Females	Plasma	0.6–3.3 mg/mL	1.6–8.9 µmol/L
Males	Plasma	1.3–5.5 mg/mL	3.5–14.9 µmol/L
δ-Aminolevulinic acid (ALA)	Serum	15–23 µg/L	1.14–1.75 µmol/L
11-Deoxycortisol (DOC):			
After metyrapone	Plasma	> 7 µg/dL	> 203 nmol/L
Basal	Plasma	< 5 µg/dL	< 145 nmol/L
D-Xylose level 2 h after ingestion of 25 g of D-xylose	Serum	> 20 mg/dL	> 1.3 nmol/L
Epinephrine, supine	Plasma	< 75 ng/L	< 410 pmol/L
Erythrocyte sedimentation rate (ESR):			
Females	Blood	0–20 mm/h	0–20 mm/h
Males	Blood	0–15 mm/h	0–20 mm/h
Erythropoietin	Serum	4.0–18.5 mIU/mL	4.0–18.5 IU/L
Estradiol, females:			
Day 1–10 of menstrual cycle	Serum	14–27 pg/mL	50–100 pmol/L
Day 11–20 of menstrual cycle	Serum	14–54 pg/mL	50–200 pmol/L
Day 21–30 of menstrual cycle	Serum	19–40 pg/mL	70–150 pmol/L
Estradiol, males	Serum	10–30 pg/mL	37–110 pmol/L
Ferritin	Serum	15–200 ng/mL	15–200 µg/L
α-Fetoprotein (AFP)	Serum	0–20 ng/dL	0–20 pg/L
Fibrinogen	Plasma	150–350 mg/dL	1.5–3.5 g/L
Folate (folic acid):			
RBC	Blood	160–855 ng/mL	362–1937 nmol/L
Serum	Serum	2.5–20 ng/mL	5.7–45.3 nmol/L
Follicle-stimulating hormone (FSH), females:			
Follicular or luteal phase	Serum	5–20 mU/mL	5–20 U/L
Midcycle peak	Serum	30–50 mU/mL	30–50 U/L
Postmenopausal	Serum	> 35 mU/mL	> 35 U/L
Follicle-stimulating hormone (FSH), adult males	Serum	5–15 mU/mL	5–15 U/L
Fructosamine	Plasma	200–285 mol/L	—

(Continued)

TEST	SPECIMEN	CONVENTIONAL UNITS	SI UNITS
Gamma-glutamyl transpeptidase (GGT)	Serum	8–78 U/L	—
Gastrin	Serum	0–180 pg/mL	0–180 ng/L
Globulins:	Serum	2.5–3.5 g/dL	25–35 g/L
α_1-Globulins	Serum	0.2–0.4 g/dL	2–4 g/L
α_2-Globulins	Serum	0.5–0.9 g/dL	5–9 g/L
β-Globulins	Serum	0.6–1.1 g/dL	6–11 g/L
γ-Globulins	Serum	0.7–1.7 g/dL	7–17 g/L
β_2-Microglobulin	Serum	0.7–1.8 μg/mL	—
Glucose:			
2-h postprandial	Plasma	< 140 mg/dL	< 7.8 mmol/L
Fasting	Plasma	70–105 mg/dL	3.9–5.8 mmol/L
Glucose-6-phosphate dehydrogenase (G6PD)	Blood	5–15 U/g Hb	0.32–0.97 mU/mol Hb
γ-Glutamyl transpeptidase (GGT)	Serum	8–78 U/L	—
Growth hormone:			
After oral glucose	Plasma	< 2 ng/mL	< 2 μg/L
In response to provocative stimuli	Plasma	> 7 ng/mL	> 7 μg/L
Haptoglobin	Serum	30–200 mg/dL	300–2000 mg/L
Hematocrit:			
Females	Blood	36–47%	—
Males	Blood	41–51%	—
Hemoglobin:			
Females	Blood	12–16 g/dL	120–160 g/L
Males	Blood	14–17 g/dL	140–170 g/L
Hemoglobin A_{1c}	Blood	4.7–8.5%	—
Hemoglobin electrophoresis, adults:			
Hb A_1	Blood	95–98%	—
Hb A_2	Blood	2–3%	—
Hb C	Blood	0%	—
Hb F	Blood	0.8–2.0%	—
Hb S	Blood	0%	—
Hemoglobin electrophoresis, Hb F in children:			
Neonate	Blood	50–80%	—
1–6 mo	Blood	8%	—
> 6 mo	Blood	1–2%	—
Homocysteine:			
Females	Plasma	0.40–1.89 mg/L	3–14 μmol/L
Males	Plasma	0.54–2.16 mg/L	4–16 μmol/L
Human chorionic gonadotropin (hCG), quantitative	Serum	< 5 mIU/mL	—

TEST	SPECIMEN	CONVENTIONAL UNITS	SI UNITS
Immunoglobulins:			
IgA	Serum	70–300 mg/dL	0.7–3.0 g/L
IgD	Serum	< 8 mg/dL	< 80 mg/L
IgE	Serum	0.01–0.04 mg/dL	0.1–0.4 mg/L
IgG	Serum	640–1430 mg/dL	6.4–14.3 g/L
IgG_1	Serum	280–1020 mg/dL	2.8–10.2 g/L
IgG_2	Serum	60–790 mg/dL	0.6–7.9 g/L
IgG_3	Serum	14–240 mg/dL	0.14–2.4 g/L
IgG_4	Serum	11–330 mg/dL	0.11–3.3 g/L
IgM	Serum	20–140 mg/dL	0.2–1.4 g/L
Insulin, fasting	Serum	1.4–14 µIU/mL	10–104 pmol/L
International normalized ratio (INR):			
Therapeutic range (standard intensity therapy)	Plasma	2.0–3.0	—
Therapeutic range in patients at higher risk (eg, patients with prosthetic heart valves)	Plasma	2.5–3.5	—
Therapeutic range in patients with lupus anticoagulant	Plasma	3.0–3.5	—
Iron	Serum	60–160 µg/dL	11–29 µmol/L
Iron-binding capacity, total (TIBC)	Serum	250–460 µg/dL	45–82 µmol/L
Lactate dehydrogenase (LDH)	Serum	60–160 U/L	1–1.67 µkat/L
Lactic acid, venous	Blood	6–16 mg/dL	0.67–1.8 mmol/L
Lactose tolerance test	Plasma	> 15 mg/dL increase in plasma glucose level	> 0.83 mmol/L increase in plasma glucose level
Lead	Blood	< 40 µg/dL	< 1.9 µmol/L
Leukocyte alkaline phosphatase (LAP) score	Peripheral blood smear	13–130/100/polymorphonuclear (PMN) leukocyte neutrophils and bands	—
Lipase	Serum	< 95 U/L	< 1.58 µkat/L
Lipoprotein (a) [Lp(a)]	Serum	≤ 30 mg/dL	< 1.1 µmol/L
Luteinizing hormone (LH), females:			
Follicular or luteal phase	Serum	5–22 mU/mL	5–22 U/L
Midcycle peak	Serum	30–250 mU/mL	30–250 U/L
Postmenopausal	Serum	> 30 mU/mL	> 30 U/L
Luteinizing hormone, males	Serum	3–15 mU/mL	3–15 U/L
Magnesium	Serum	1.5–2.4 mg/dL	0.62–0.99 mmol/L
Manganese	Serum	0.3–0.9 ng/mL	5.5–16.4 nmol/L
Mean corpuscular hemoglobin (MCH)	Blood	28–32 pg	—
Mean corpuscular hemoglobin concentration (MCHC)	Blood	32–36 g/dL	320–360 g/L
Mean corpuscular volume (MCV)	Blood	80–100 fL	—
Metanephrines, fractionated:			
Metanephrines, free	Plasma	< 0.50 nmol/L	—
Normetanephrines, free	Plasma	< 0.90 nmol/L	—
Methemoglobin	Blood	< 1.0%	—
Methylmalonic acid (MMA)	Serum	150–370 nmol/L	—

(Continued)

TEST	SPECIMEN	CONVENTIONAL UNITS	SI UNITS
Myeloperoxidase (MPO) antibodies	Serum	< 6.0 U/mL	—
Myoglobin:			
Females	Serum	25–58 μg/L	1.4–3.5 nmol/L
Males	Serum	28–72 μg/L	1.6–4.1 nmol/L
Norepinephrine, supine	Plasma	50–440 pg/mL	0.3–2.6 nmol/L
N-Terminal propeptide of BNP (NT-proBNP)	Plasma	< 125 pg/mL	—
5'-Nucleotidase (5'NT)	Serum	4–11.5 U/L	—
Osmolality	Plasma	275–295 mOsm/kg H_2O	275–295 mmol/kg H_2O
Osmotic fragility test	Blood	Increased fragility if hemolysis occurs in > 0.5% NaCl Decreased fragility if hemolysis is incomplete in 0.3% NaCl	—
Oxygen partial pressure (PO_2)	Blood	80–100 mm Hg	—
Parathyroid hormone (PTH)	Serum	10–65 pg/mL	10–65 ng/L
Parathyroid hormone–related peptide (PTHrP)	Plasma	< 2.0 pmol/L	—
Partial thromboplastin time, activated (aPTT)	Plasma	25–35 sec	—
pH	Blood	7.38–7.44	—
Phosphorus, inorganic	Serum	3.0–4.5 mg/dL	0.97–1.45 mmol/L
Platelet count	Blood	150–350 x 10^3/μL	150–350 x 10^9/L
Platelet life span, using chromium-51 (^{51}Cr)	—	8–12 days	—
Porphyrins	Plasma	≤ 1.0 μg/dL	—
Potassium	Serum	3.5–5 mEq/L	3.5–5 mmol/L
Prealbumin (transthyretin)	Serum	18–45 mg/dL	—
Progesterone:			
Follicular phase	Serum	< 1 ng/mL	< 0.03 nmol/L
Luteal phase	Serum	3–30 ng/mL	0.1–0.95 nmol/L
Prolactin:			
Females	Serum	< 20 μg/L	< 870 pmol/L
Males	Serum	< 15 μg/L	< 652 pmol/L
Prostate-specific antigen, total (PSA-T)	Serum	0–4 ng/mL	—
Prostate-specific antigen, ratio of free to total (PSA-F:PSA-T)	Serum	> 0.25	—
Protein C activity	Plasma	67–131%	—
Protein C resistance, activated ratio (APC-R)	Plasma	2.2–2.6	—
Protein S activity	Plasma	82–144%	—
Protein, total	Serum	6–7.8 g/dL	60–78 g/L
Prothrombin time (PT)	Plasma	11–13 sec	—
Pyruvate	Blood	0.08–0.16 mmol/L	—
RBC count	Blood	4.2–5.9 x 10^6 cells/μL	4.2–5.9 x 10^{12} cells/L
RBC survival rate, using ^{51}Cr	Blood	$T_{1/2}$ = 28 days	—

TEST	SPECIMEN	CONVENTIONAL UNITS	SI UNITS
Renin activity, plasma (PRA), upright, in males and females aged 18–39 yr:			
Sodium-depleted	Plasma	2.9–24 ng/mL/h	—
Sodium-repleted	Plasma	0.6 (or lower)–4.3 ng/mL/h	—
Reticulocyte count:			
Percentage	Blood	0.5–1.5%	—
Absolute	Blood	23–90 x 10^3/μL	23–90 x 10^9/L
Rheumatoid factor (RF)	Serum	< 40 U/mL	< 40 kU/L
Sodium	Serum	136–145 mEq/L	136–145 mmol/L
Testosterone, adults:			
Females	Serum	20–75 ng/dL	0.7–2.6 nmol/L
Males	Serum	300–1200 ng/dL	10–42 nmol/L
Thrombin time	Plasma	18.5–24 sec	—
Thyroid iodine-123 (^{123}I) uptake	—	5–30% of administered dose at 24 h	—
Thyroid-stimulating hormone (TSH)	Serum	0.5–5.0 μIU/mL	0.5–5.0 mIU/L
Thyroxine (T_4):			
Free	Serum	0.9–2.4 ng/dL	12–31 pmol/L
Free index	—	4–11 μg/dL	—
Total	Serum	5–12 μg/dL	64–155 nmol/L
Transferrin	Serum	212–360 mg/dL	2.1–3.6 g/L
Transferrin saturation	Serum	20–50%	—
Triglycerides (desirable level)	Serum	< 250 mg/dL	< 2.82 mmol/L
Triiodothyronine (T_3):			
Uptake	Serum	25–35%	—
Total	Serum	70–195 ng/dL	1.1–3.0 nmol/L
Troponin I	Plasma	< 0.1 ng/mL	< 0.1 μg/L
Troponin T	Serum	≤ 0.03 ng/mL	≤ 0.03 μg/L
Urea nitrogen (BUN)	Serum	8–20 mg/dL	2.9–7.1 mmol/L
Uric acid	Serum	2.5–8 mg/dL	0.15–0.47 mmol/L
Vitamin B_{12}	Serum	200–800 pg/mL	148–590 pmol/L
Vitamin C (ascorbic acid):			
Leukocyte	Blood	< 20 mg/dL	< 1136 μmol/L
Total	Blood	0.4–1.5 mg/dL	23–85 μmol/L
Vitamin D:			
1,25-Dihydroxycholecalciferol (calcitriol)	Serum	25–65 pg/mL	65–169 pmol/L
25-Hydroxycholecalciferol	Serum	15–80 ng/mL	37–200 nmol/L
WBC count	Blood	3.9–10.7 x 10^3 cells/μL	3.9–10.7 x 10^9 cells/L
Zinc	Serum	66–110 μg/dL	10.1–16.8 μmol/L

μkat = microkatal; pkat = picokatal.

From the Merck Manual Professional Version (Known as the Merck Manual in the US and Canada and the MSD Manual in the rest of the world), edited by Robert Porter. Copyright 2016 by Merck Sharp & Dohme Corp., a subsidiary of Merck & Co, Inc., Kenilworth, NJ. Available at http://www.merckmanuals.com/professional. Accessed January 25, 2016.

ABILIFY – aripiprazole

RX

Class: Atypical antipsychotic

Elderly patients w/ dementia-related psychosis treated w/ antipsychotic drugs are at an increased risk of death. Not approved for treatment of patients w/ dementia-related psychosis. Antidepressants increased the risk of suicidal thoughts and behavior in children, adolescents, and young adults in short-term studies. Monitor closely for worsening, and for emergence of suicidal thoughts and behaviors in patients who are started on antidepressant therapy.

OTHER BRAND NAMES

Abilify Discmelt

ADULT DOSAGE

Schizophrenia

Initial/Target: 10mg or 15mg qd
Titrate: Should not increase dose before 2 weeks
Range: 10-30mg/day

Bipolar I Disorder

Manic and Mixed Episodes:
Monotherapy:
Initial/Target: 15mg qd
Titrate: May increase to 30mg/day based on clinical response
Max: 30mg/day

Adjunct to Lithium or Valproate:
Initial: 10-15mg qd
Target: 15mg/day
Titrate: May increase to 30mg/day based on clinical response
Max: 30mg/day

Major Depressive Disorder

Adjunct to Antidepressants:
Initial: 2-5mg/day
Titrate: Dose adjustments of up to 5mg/day should occur gradually at intervals of ≥1 week
Range: 2-15mg/day

Agitation

Agitation Associated w/ Schizophrenia or Bipolar Mania:
Inj:
9.75mg IM
Range: 5.25-15mg
A lower dose of 5.25mg may be considered when clinical factors warrant. If agitation warranting a 2nd dose persists following the initial dose, cumulative doses of up to a total of 30mg/day may be given
Max: 30mg/day or more frequently than q2h

If ongoing treatment is clinically indicated, replace w/ oral aripiprazole in a range of 10-30mg/day as soon as possible

PEDIATRIC DOSAGE

Schizophrenia

13-17 Years:
Initial: 2mg/day
Titrate: May increase to 5mg/day after 2 days and to the target dose of 10mg/day after 2 additional days
Administer subsequent dose increases in 5mg increments
Max: 30mg/day

Bipolar I Disorder

Monotherapy or Adjunct to Lithium/Valproate for Manic and Mixed Episodes:
10-17 Years:
Initial: 2mg/day
Titrate: May increase to 5mg/day after 2 days and to the target dose of 10mg/day after 2 additional days
Administer subsequent dose increases, if needed, in 5mg increments

Autistic Disorder

Irritability Associated w/ Autistic Disorder:
6-17 Years:
Initial: 2mg/day
Titrate: Increase to 5mg/day, w/ subsequent increases to 10 or 15mg/day, if needed
Dose adjustments of up to 5mg/day should occur gradually at intervals of ≥1 week
Range: 5-15mg/day

Tourette's Disorder

6-18 Years:
Range: 5-20mg/day
<50kg:
Initial: 2mg/day w/ a target dose of 5mg/day after 2 days
Titrate: Increase to 10mg/day in patients who do not achieve optimal control of tics
Dose adjustments should occur gradually at intervals of ≥1 week
≥50kg:
Initial: 2mg/day for 2 days
Titrate: Increase to 5mg/day for 5 days w/ a target dose of 10mg/day on Day 8; increase up to 20mg/day for patients who do not achieve optimal control of tics
Dose adjustments should occur gradually in increments of 5mg/day at intervals of ≥1 week

DOSING CONSIDERATIONS

Concomitant Medications
Strong CYP2D6 or CYP3A4 Inhibitors:
Administer 1/2 of usual dose

Strong CYP2D6 and CYP3A4 Inhibitors:
Administer 1/4 of the usual dose

Strong CYP3A4 Inducers:
Double usual dose over 1-2 weeks; when coadministered inducer is withdrawn, reduce aripiprazole dose to original level over 1-2 weeks

Combination of Strong, Moderate, and Weak Inhibitors of CYP3A4 and CYP2D6:
Reduce to 1/4 of usual dose initially, then adjust to achieve a favorable clinical response

Other Important Considerations

Known CYP2D6 Poor Metabolizers:
Administer 1/2 of usual dose

Known CYP2D6 Poor Metabolizers Taking Concomitant Strong CYP3A4 Inhibitors:
Administer 1/4 of usual dose

ADMINISTRATION

Oral/IM route

PO

Administer w/o regard to meals.
Oral sol can be substituted for tabs on a mg-per-mg basis up to 25mg dose level.
Patients receiving 30mg tabs should receive 25mg of the sol.

Inj

Inject slowly, deep into the muscle mass.

HOW SUPPLIED

Inj: 7.5mg/mL [1.3mL]; **Sol:** 1mg/mL [150mL]; **Tab:** 2mg, 5mg, 10mg, 15mg, 20mg, 30mg; **Tab, Disintegrating:** (Discmelt) 10mg, 15mg

CONTRAINDICATIONS

History of a hypersensitivity reaction to aripiprazole.

WARNINGS/PRECAUTIONS

Neuroleptic malignant syndrome (NMS) reported; d/c immediately, institute symptomatic treatment, and monitor. May cause tardive dyskinesia (TD), especially in the elderly; d/c if this occurs. Hyperglycemia, in some cases extreme and associated w/ ketoacidosis or hyperosmolar coma or death, reported. Dyslipidemia and weight gain reported. May cause orthostatic hypotension; caution w/ known cardiovascular disease (history of MI or ischemic heart disease, heart failure, or conduction abnormalities), cerebrovascular disease, or conditions that would predispose patients to hypotension (dehydration, hypovolemia). Leukopenia, neutropenia, and agranulocytosis reported; consider discontinuation at 1st sign of a clinically significant decline in WBC counts in the absence of other causative factors. D/C therapy and follow WBC counts until recovery in patients w/ severe neutropenia (ANC <1000/mm^3). Caution w/ history of seizures or w/ conditions that lower seizure threshold. May impair physical/mental abilities. May disrupt body's ability to reduce core body temperature; caution when exposed to conditions that may contribute to an elevation in core body temperature (eg, exercising strenuously, exposure to extreme heat, receiving concomitant medication w/ anticholinergic activity, or being subject to dehydration). May cause esophageal dysmotility and aspiration; caution in patients at risk for aspiration pneumonia.

ADVERSE REACTIONS

Adults: N/V, constipation, headache, dizziness, akathisia, anxiety, insomnia, restlessness.
Pediatrics: Somnolence, headache, N/V, extrapyramidal disorder, fatigue, increased appetite, insomnia, nasopharyngitis, weight increased.

DRUG INTERACTIONS

See Dosing Considerations. Strong CYP3A4 inhibitors (eg, itraconazole, clarithromycin) or strong CYP2D6 inhibitors (eg, quinidine, fluoxetine, paroxetine) may increase exposure. Strong CYP3A4 inducers (eg, carbamazepine, rifampin) may decrease exposure. May potentiate the effect of certain antihypertensive agents; monitor BP and adjust dose accordingly. Greater sedation and orthostatic hypotension observed w/ lorazepam; monitor sedation and BP and adjust dose accordingly in patients on concomitant therapy w/ benzodiazepines.

PATIENT CONSIDERATIONS

Assessment: Assess for dementia-related psychosis, drug hypersensitivity, any other conditions where treatment is cautioned, pregnancy/nursing status, and possible drug interactions. Obtain baseline FPG in patients w/ diabetes mellitus (DM) or at risk for DM. Obtain baseline CBC if at risk for leukopenia/neutropenia.

Monitoring: Monitor for clinical worsening of depression, suicidality, unusual changes in behavior, NMS, TD, hyperglycemia, dyslipidemia, orthostatic hypotension, seizures/convulsions, esophageal dysmotility, aspiration, weight gain, and other adverse reactions. Monitor CBC frequently during the 1st few months of therapy in patients w/ a history of a clinically significant low WBC count/ANC or drug-induced leukopenia/neutropenia. Monitor for fever or other signs/symptoms of infection in patients w/ neutropenia. Monitor for worsening of glucose control in patients w/ DM and FPG in patients at risk for DM periodically during therapy. Periodically reassess patient to determine the continued need for maintenance treatment.

Counseling: Inform about the risks and benefits of treatment. Instruct patients, families, and caregivers to be alert for the emergence of anxiety, agitation, panic attacks, insomnia, irritability, hostility, aggressiveness, impulsivity, akathisia, hypomania, mania, other unusual changes in behavior, worsening of depression, and suicidal ideation; advise to contact physician if these symptoms occur. Instruct to use caution when operating hazardous machinery. Counsel to avoid overheating and dehydration. Advise to notify physician if patient is taking or plans to take any prescription or OTC drugs. Instruct to not breastfeed during therapy. (Discmelt) Inform phenylketonurics that product contains phenylalanine. Instruct to not open blister until ready to administer. Instruct not push the tab through the foil because this could damage the tab. Advise that immediately upon opening the blister, using dry hands, remove the tab and place the entire tab on the tongue. Inform that tab disintegration occurs rapidly in saliva. Instruct that drug is to be taken w/o liquid, but that if needed, can be taken w/ liquid. Advise not to split the tab. (Sol) Inform that sol contains sucrose and fructose.

STORAGE: 25°C (77°F); excursions permitted to 15-30°C (59-86°F). **Sol:** May be used for up to 6 months after opening. **Inj:** Protect from light.

ABILIFY MAINTENA — aripiprazole

RX

Class: Atypical antipsychotic

Elderly patients w/ dementia-related psychosis treated w/ antipsychotic drugs are at an increased risk of death. Not approved for the treatment of patients w/ dementia-related psychosis.

ADULT DOSAGE

Schizophrenia

Initial/Maint: 400mg monthly (no sooner than 26 days after the previous inj); establish tolerability w/ oral aripiprazole prior to initiating treatment in aripiprazole-naive patients

After the 1st inj, administer oral aripiprazole (10-20mg) for 14 consecutive days, or if already stable on another oral antipsychotic (and known to tolerate aripiprazole), continue treatment w/ the antipsychotic for 14 consecutive days

Missed Dose

2nd or 3rd Doses are Missed:
>4 Weeks and <5 Weeks Since Last Inj: Administer inj as soon as possible
>5 Weeks Since Last Inj: Restart concomitant oral aripiprazole for 14 days w/ next administered inj

4th or Subsequent Doses are Missed:
>4 Weeks and <6 Weeks Since Last Inj: Administer inj as soon as possible
>6 Weeks Since Last Inj: Restart concomitant oral aripiprazole for 14 days w/ next administered inj

PEDIATRIC DOSAGE

Pediatric use may not have been established

DOSING CONSIDERATIONS

Concomitant Medications

Concomitant Use for >14 Days:

Patients Taking 300mg:
Strong CYP2D6 or CYP3A4 Inhibitors: 200mg
CYP2D6 and CYP3A4 Inhibitors: 160mg
CYP3A4 Inducers: Avoid use

Patients Taking 400mg:
Strong CYP2D6 or CYP3A4 Inhibitors: 300mg
CYP2D6 and CYP3A4 Inhibitors: 200mg
CYP3A4 Inducers: Avoid use

Adverse Reactions

If adverse reactions occur w/ the 400mg dose, consider reducing dose to 300mg once monthly

Other Important Considerations

CYP2D6 Poor Metabolizers: 300mg
CYP2D6 Poor Metabolizers Taking Concomitant CYP3A4 Inhibitors: 200mg

ADMINISTRATION

IM route

For deep IM deltoid or gluteal inj by healthcare professionals only; do not administer by any other route. Use 23-gauge, 1-inch needle for deltoid administration in non-obese patients; use 22-gauge, 1.5-inch needle for gluteal administration in non-obese patients or deltoid administration in obese patients; use 21-gauge, 2-inch needle for gluteal administration in obese patients.
Inject immediately following reconstitution.
Inject slowly; do not massage inj site.
Rotate inj sites between the 2 deltoid or gluteal muscles.
To obtain 200mg and 160mg dosage adjustments, use 300mg or 400mg strength vials.

Preparation

Prefilled Dual Chamber Syringe:

1. Reconstitute at room temperature.
2. Push plunger rod slightly to engage threads, then rotate plunger rod until the rod stops rotating to release diluent. Middle stopper will be at the indicator line after plunger rod is at a complete stop.
3. Vertically shake syringe vigorously for 20 sec until drug is uniformly milky white; reconstituted sus is a uniform, homogenous sus that is opaque and milky white.
4. Attach appropriate needle; hold syringe upright and advance plunger rod slowly to expel air until sus fills needle base.

Vial:

1. Reconstitute at room temperature.
2. Reconstitute 400mg vial w/ 1.9mL sterile water for inj (SWFI) and 300mg vial w/ 1.5mL SWFI.
3. Shake vigorously for 30 sec until sus appears uniform; reconstituted sus is a uniform, homogenous sus that is opaque and milky white.
4. If not injected immediately after reconstitution, keep vial at room temperature and shake vigorously for at least 60 sec to re-suspend prior to inj.
5. Inject 2mL for 400mg dose (400mg vial only), 1.5mL for 300mg dose, 1mL for 200mg dose, and 0.8mg for 160mg dose.

Refer to PI for further preparation and administration instructions.

HOW SUPPLIED

Inj, Extended-Release: 300mg, 400mg [vial, prefilled dual chamber syringe]

CONTRAINDICATIONS

Known hypersensitivity to aripiprazole.

WARNINGS/PRECAUTIONS

Do not substitute w/ other aripiprazole formulation. Neuroleptic malignant syndrome (NMS) may occur; d/c immediately and institute symptomatic treatment and medical monitoring. May cause tardive dyskinesia (TD), especially in the elderly; consider discontinuation if this occurs. Hyperglycemia, in some cases extreme and associated w/ ketoacidosis or hyperosmolar coma or death, reported w/ atypical antipsychotics. Dyslipidemia and weight gain reported w/ atypical antipsychotics. May cause orthostatic hypotension. Leukopenia, neutropenia, and agranulocytosis reported; consider discontinuation at 1st sign of clinically significant decline in WBC counts w/o causative factors in patients w/ history of clinically significant low WBC count/ANC or drug-induced leukopenia/neutropenia. D/C therapy and follow WBC counts until recovery in patients w/ severe neutropenia (ANC <1000/mm^3). Caution w/ history of seizures or w/ conditions that lower seizure threshold. May impair mental/physical abilities. May disrupt body's ability to reduce core body temperature. May cause esophageal dysmotility and aspiration; caution in patients at risk for aspiration pneumonia.

ADVERSE REACTIONS

Increased weight, akathisia, injection-site pain, sedation.

DRUG INTERACTIONS

See Dosing Considerations. Concomitant oral aripiprazole w/ strong CYP3A4/CYP2D6 inhibitors increased concentration of aripiprazole. Concomitant oral aripiprazole and carbamazepine decreased concentration of aripiprazole. May enhance effect of certain antihypertensives; monitor BP and adjust dose accordingly. Greater sedation and orthostatic hypotension observed w/ oral aripiprazole and lorazepam; monitor sedation and BP and adjust dose accordingly w/ benzodiazepines.

PATIENT CONSIDERATIONS

Assessment: Assess for history of dementia-related psychosis, diabetes mellitus (DM), drug hypersensitivity, any other conditions where treatment is cautioned, pregnancy/nursing status, and possible drug interactions. Obtain baseline FPG in patients at risk for DM. Obtain baseline CBC if at risk for leukopenia/neutropenia.

Monitoring: Monitor for NMS, TD, hyperglycemia, orthostatic hypotension, seizures, weight gain, dyslipidemia, esophageal dysmotility, aspiration, and other adverse reactions. Monitor CBC frequently during the 1st few months of therapy in patients w/ a history of a clinically significant low WBC count/ANC or drug-induced leukopenia/neutropenia. Monitor for fever or other symptoms/signs of infection in patients w/ neutropenia. Monitor for worsening of glucose control in patients w/ DM and FPG in patients at risk for DM. Periodically reassess need for continued treatment.

Counseling: Inform of the risks/benefits of therapy. Inform about NMS; advise to contact healthcare provider or report to emergency room if signs/symptoms develop. Instruct to notify healthcare provider if any movements that cannot be controlled in the face, tongue, or other body part develop. Inform about risk of metabolic changes, symptoms of hyperglycemia/DM, and the need for specific monitoring. Inform about risk of orthostatic hypotension and syncope especially early in treatment and at times of treatment reinitiation or dosage increases. Advise patients w/ preexisting low WBC count or history of drug-induced leukopenia/neutropenia to have their CBC monitored. Advise to use caution when operating hazardous machinery. Instruct to avoid overheating and dehydration. Instruct to notify healthcare provider of any changes to prescription or OTC drugs.

STORAGE: Prefilled Dual Chamber Syringe: <30°C (86°F). Do not freeze. Protect from light. **Vial:** 25°C (77°F); excursions permitted to 15-30°C (59-86°F).

ABSORICA – isotretinoin RX

Class: Retinoid

Not for use by females who are or may become pregnant. Severe birth defects, including death, have been documented. Increased risk of spontaneous abortion and premature births reported. D/C immediately if pregnancy occurs during treatment and refer to an obstetrician-gynecologist experienced in reproductive toxicity for further evaluation and counseling. Available only through a restricted program under a Risk Evaluation and Mitigation Strategy called iPLEDGE. Prescribers, patients, pharmacies, and distributors must enroll and be registered in the program.

ADULT DOSAGE

Severe Recalcitrant Nodular Acne

Unresponsive to Conventional Therapy, Including Systemic Antibiotics:
0.5-1mg/kg/day given in 2 divided doses for 15-20 weeks
Titrate: May adjust dose according to response of disease and/or appearance of clinical side effects

Very Severe Disease w/ Scarring or Primarily Manifested on Trunk:
May adjust dose up to 2mg/kg/day, as tolerated

May d/c if total nodule count has been reduced by >70% prior to completing 15-20 weeks of treatment

After a period of ≥2 months off therapy, and if warranted by persistent or recurring severe nodular acne, a 2nd course of therapy may be initiated; the optimal interval before retreatment has not been defined for patients who have not completed skeletal growth

PEDIATRIC DOSAGE

Severe Recalcitrant Nodular Acne

Unresponsive to Conventional Therapy, Including Systemic Antibiotics:
≥12 Years:
0.5-1mg/kg/day given in 2 divided doses for 15-20 weeks
Titrate: May adjust dose according to response of disease and/or appearance of clinical side effects

May d/c if total nodule count has been reduced by >70% prior to completing 15-20 weeks of treatment

After a period of ≥2 months off therapy, and if warranted by persistent or recurring severe nodular acne, a 2nd course of therapy may be initiated; the optimal interval before retreatment has not been defined for patients who have not completed skeletal growth

ADMINISTRATION

Oral route

Take w/o regard to meals.
Swallow caps w/ a full glass of liquid.

HOW SUPPLIED

Cap: 10mg, 20mg, 25mg, 30mg, 35mg, 40mg

CONTRAINDICATIONS

Pregnancy, hypersensitivity to this product (or Vitamin A) or to any of its components.

WARNINGS/PRECAUTIONS

Avoid long-term use. 25mg capsule contains tartrazine, which may cause allergic-type reactions (including bronchial asthma) in certain susceptible persons. Do not donate blood during therapy and for 1 month following discontinuation of therapy. Micro-dosed progesterone preparations are an inadequate method of contraception during therapy. May cause depression, psychosis, suicidal ideation/attempts, suicide, and aggressive and/or violent behaviors; d/c if symptoms occur. Associated w/ pseudotumor cerebri (benign intracranial HTN). Erythema multiforme and severe skin reactions (eg, Stevens-Johnson syndrome, toxic epidermal necrolysis) reported; closely monitor for severe skin reactions and consider discontinuation of therapy if warranted. Acute pancreatitis reported; d/c if hypertriglyceridemia cannot be controlled at an acceptable level or if symptoms of pancreatitis occur. Hypersensitivity reactions reported; d/c therapy and institute appropriate management if a severe allergic reaction occurs. Increased TG levels, increased cholesterol levels, decreased HDL levels, impaired hearing, hepatotoxicity, inflammatory bowel disease, premature epiphyseal closure, skeletal hyperostosis, dry eye, decreased night vision, corneal opacities, and impaired glucose control reported. D/C if symptoms of pseudotumor cerebri and papilledema are present, significant decrease in WBC count, tinnitus or hearing impairment, visual impairment, abdominal pain, rectal bleeding, severe diarrhea, or if liver enzyme levels do not normalize or if hepatitis is suspected. May have a negative effect on bone mineral density; caution w/ history of childhood osteoporosis conditions, osteomalacia, other bone metabolism disorders, or anorexia nervosa. Anaphylactic reactions and other allergic reactions reported; d/c and institute appropriate management if a severe allergic reaction occurs. Increased CPK levels and rhabdomyolysis reported. Osteoporosis, osteopenia, bone fractures, and/or delayed fracture healing reported; increased risk in patients participating in sports w/ repetitive impact.

ADVERSE REACTIONS

Cheilitis, hypertriglyceridemia, fatigue, irritability, pain, allergic reactions, vascular thrombotic disease, stroke, decreased appetite, weight fluctuation, chapped lips, N/V, nasopharyngitis, anemia, colitis.

DRUG INTERACTIONS

Avoid use w/ tetracyclines or vitamin supplements containing vitamin A. Caution w/ drugs that cause drug-induced osteoporosis/osteomalacia and/or affect vitamin D metabolism (eg, systemic corticosteroids, any anticonvulsant).

PATIENT CONSIDERATIONS

Assessment: Assess that females have had 2 negative urine or serum pregnancy tests separated by at least 19 days, and are on 2 forms of effective contraception. Assess for hypersensitivity to the drug or vitamin A, history of psychiatric disorder, depression, risk of hyperlipidemia, pregnancy/nursing status, and possible drug interactions. Obtain blood lipids and LFTs.

Monitoring: Monitor for signs/symptoms of psychiatric disorders, pseudotumor cerebri, lipid abnormalities, acute pancreatitis, hearing/visual impairment, inflammatory bowel disease (regional ileitis), hepatotoxicity, premature epiphyseal closure, hyperostosis, musculoskeletal symptoms/abnormalities, hypersensitivity reactions, and other adverse reactions. Monitor lipid levels and LFTs (weekly or biweekly), glucose levels, and CPK levels until response is established. Monitor that females remain on 2 forms of contraception during and for 1 month following discontinuation of therapy.

Counseling: Instruct to read the iPLEDGE and sign the Patient Information/Informed Consent form. Inform male patients and female patients not of childbearing potential about the risks and benefits of the drug. Inform females of childbearing potential that 2 forms of contraception are required starting 1 month prior to initiation, during treatment, and for 1 month following discontinuation. Inform that monthly pregnancy tests are required before new prescription is issued. Instruct patients to d/c therapy if signs/symptoms of pseudotumor cerebri (eg, papilledema, headache, N/V) occur. Counsel not to share drug w/ anyone and not to donate blood during therapy and 1 month following discontinuation. Inform that transient exacerbation (flare) of acne may occur. Instruct to notify physician if depression, mood disturbances, psychosis, or aggression occurs. Instruct to avoid wax epilation and skin resurfacing procedures during and for at least 6 months thereafter. Instruct to avoid prolonged UV rays or sunlight exposure. Inform that dry eye, corneal opacities, and decreased night vision may be experienced, and decreased tolerance to contact lenses during and after therapy may occur. Inform that musculoskeletal symptoms, transient chest pain, back pain in pediatric patients, arthralgias, neutropenia, agranulocytosis, anaphylactic/allergic/severe skin reactions, and inflammatory bowel disease may occur. Inform adolescent patients who participate in sports w/ repetitive impact that medication may increase their risk of spondylolisthesis or hip growth plate injuries.

STORAGE: 20-25°C (68-77°F); excursions permitted to 15-30°C (59-86°F). Protect from light.

ABSTRAL – fentanyl

CII

Class: Opioid analgesic

Fatal respiratory depression may occur. Contraindicated in the management of acute or postoperative pain (eg, headache/migraine) and in opioid-nontolerant patients. Keep out of reach of children. Concomitant use with CYP3A4 inhibitors may increase plasma levels, and may cause fatal respiratory depression. Do not convert patients on a mcg-per-mcg basis from any other fentanyl products to Abstral or substitute for any fentanyl products; may result in fatal overdose. Contains fentanyl with abuse liability similar to other opioid analgesics. Available only through a restricted program called Transmucosal Immediate Release Fentanyl (TIRF) Risk Evaluation Mitigation Strategy (REMS) Access program due to risk of misuse, abuse, addiction, and overdose. Outpatients, healthcare professionals who prescribe to outpatients, pharmacies, and distributors must enroll in this program.

ADULT DOSAGE

Pain

Management of breakthrough pain in cancer patients already receiving and are tolerant to opioid therapy for their underlying persistent cancer pain

Initial: 100mcg

Adequate Analgesia Obtained w/in 30 Min of Initial Dose: Continue to treat subsequent episodes of breakthrough pain with this dose

Adequate Analgesia Not Obtained After Initial Dose: Use 2nd dose (30 min after initial dose)

Titrate:

Continue dose escalation in a stepwise manner over consecutive breakthrough episodes until adequate analgesia with tolerable side effects is achieved.

Increase dose by 100mcg multiples up to 400mcg prn.

If adequate analgesia is not obtained w/ 400mcg dose, titrate to 600mcg.

If adequate analgesia is not obtained w/ a 600mcg dose, titrate to 800mcg.

During titration, patients may use multiples of 100mcg tabs and/or 200mcg tabs for any single dose.

May repeat the same dose if adequate analgesia is not obtained 30 min after use.

May use rescue medication if adequate analgesia not achieved.

Do not use more than 4 tabs at one time.

Maint:

Once an appropriate dose for pain management has been established, use only one tab of the appropriate strength per dose

Do not use more than 2 doses to treat an episode of breakthrough pain and wait at least 2 hrs before treating another episode

Conversions

Conversion from Actiq to Abstral:

200mcg: 100mcg

400mcg: 200mcg

600mcg: 200mcg

800mcg: 200mcg

1200mcg: 200mcg

1600mcg: 400mcg

PEDIATRIC DOSAGE

Pediatric use may not have been established

DOSING CONSIDERATIONS

Discontinuation

Patients Who No Longer Require Opioid Therapy: Consider discontinuing w/ a gradual downward titration of other opioids

Patients Who No Longer Require Treatment for Breakthrough Pain: D/C immediately

ADMINISTRATION

SL route

Allow tabs to completely dissolve in the SL cavity; do not chew, suck, or swallow

Do not eat or drink until tab is completely dissolved

In patients who have dry mouth, water may be used to moisten buccal mucosa before taking dose

HOW SUPPLIED

Tab, SL: 100mcg, 200mcg, 300mcg, 400mcg, 600mcg, 800mcg

CONTRAINDICATIONS

Opioid-nontolerant patients, management of acute or postoperative pain (eg, headache/migraine, dental pain, or use in emergency room), known intolerance or hypersensitivity to any of its components or the drug fentanyl.

WARNINGS/PRECAUTIONS

May cause anaphylaxis and hypersensitivity reactions. Increased risk of respiratory depression in patients with underlying respiratory disorders and in elderly/debilitated. May impair mental/physical abilities. Caution with chronic obstructive pulmonary disease or preexisting medical conditions predisposing to hypoventilation; may further decrease respiratory drive to the point of respiratory failure. Extreme caution in patients who may be susceptible to intracranial effects of CO_2 retention (eg, with evidence of increased intracranial pressure or impaired consciousness). May obscure clinical course of head injuries. Caution with bradyarrhythmias. Caution with hepatic/renal impairment.

ADVERSE REACTIONS

Respiratory depression, nausea, somnolence, dizziness, headache, constipation, stomatitis, dry mouth, dysgeusia, fatigue, dyspnea, hyperhidrosis, bradycardia, asthenia, anxiety.

DRUG INTERACTIONS

See Boxed Warning. May produce increased depressant effects with other CNS depressants (eg, other opioids, sedatives or hypnotics, general anesthetics, phenothiazines, tranquilizers, skeletal muscle relaxants, sedating antihistamines, and alcoholic beverages); adjust dose if warranted. CYP3A4 inducers (eg, barbiturates, carbamazepine, efavirenz, glucocorticoids, modafinil, nevirapine, oxcarbazepine, phenobarbital, phenytoin, pioglitazone, rifabutin, rifampin, St. John's wort, troglitazone) may decrease levels and efficacy. Not recommended with MAOIs or within 14 days of discontinuation of MAOIs. Respiratory depression is more likely to occur when given with other drugs that depress respiration.

PATIENT CONSIDERATIONS

Assessment: Assess for degree of opioid tolerance, previous opioid dose, level of pain intensity, type of pain, patient's general condition and medical status, and for any other conditions where treatment is contraindicated or cautioned. Assess for hypersensitivity to the drug, renal/hepatic function, pregnancy/nursing status, and possible drug interactions.

Monitoring: Monitor for signs/symptoms of respiratory depression, bradycardia, impairment of mental/physical abilities, drug abuse/addiction, hypersensitivity reactions, and other adverse reactions.

Counseling: Inform outpatients to enroll in the TIRF REMS Access program. Counsel that therapy may be fatal in children, in individuals for whom it is not prescribed, and who are not opioid tolerant. Counsel on proper administration and disposal. Advise to take drug as prescribed and avoid sharing it with anyone else. Instruct not to take medication for acute or postoperative pain, pain from injuries, headache, migraine, or any other short-term pain. Instruct to notify physician if breakthrough pain is not alleviated or worsens after taking the drug. Inform that drug may impair mental/physical abilities; caution against performing activities that require high level of attention (eg, driving/using heavy machinery). Advise not to combine with alcohol, sleep aids, or tranquilizers except if ordered by the physician. Instruct to notify physician if pregnant or planning to become pregnant.

STORAGE: 20-25°C (68-77°F); excursions permitted between 15-30°C (59-86°F). Protect from moisture.

ACANYA — benzoyl peroxide/clindamycin phosphate **RX**

Class: Antibacterial/keratolytic

ADULT DOSAGE

Acne Vulgaris

Apply a pea-sized amount to face qd

PEDIATRIC DOSAGE

Acne Vulgaris

≥12 Years:

Apply a pea-sized amount to face qd

ADMINISTRATION

Topical route

HOW SUPPLIED

Gel: (Clindamycin-Benzoyl Peroxide) 1.2%-2.5% [50g]

CONTRAINDICATIONS

Previous hypersensitivity to clindamycin, benzoyl peroxide, any components of the formulation, or lincomycin. History of regional enteritis, ulcerative colitis, or antibiotic-associated colitis.

WARNINGS/PRECAUTIONS

Not for oral, ophthalmic, or intravaginal use. Diarrhea, bloody diarrhea, and colitis (including pseudomembranous colitis) reported; d/c if significant diarrhea occurs. Minimize sun exposure including use of tanning beds or sun lamps, following application.

ADVERSE REACTIONS

Erythema, scaling, itching, burning, stinging.

DRUG INTERACTIONS

Caution with topical acne therapy; possible cumulative irritancy effect may occur, especially with the use of peeling, desquamating, or abrasive agents. Caution with other neuromuscular blocking agents. Antiperistaltic agents (eg, opiates, diphenoxylate with atropine) may prolong and/or worsen severe colitis. Avoid with topical or oral erythromycin-containing products.

PATIENT CONSIDERATIONS

Assessment: Assess for history of hypersensitivity to drug/lincomycin, regional enteritis, ulcerative colitis, antibiotic-associated colitis, pregnancy/nursing status, and possible drug interactions.

Monitoring: Monitor for local skin reactions, diarrhea, bloody diarrhea, colitis, and other adverse reactions.

Counseling: Instruct to d/c use and contact physician immediately if allergic reactions (eg, severe swelling, SOB) develop. Inform that medication may cause irritation (eg, erythema, scaling, itching, burning), especially when used with other topical acne therapies. Instruct to limit excessive/prolonged exposure to sunlight by wearing a hat or other clothing and using sunscreen. Inform that medication may bleach hair or colored fabric.

STORAGE: Prior to Dispensing: 2-8°C (36-46°F). After Dispensing: Room temperature up to 25°C (77°F). Do not freeze.

AccuNeb – albuterol sulfate

RX

Class: $Beta_2$ agonist

PEDIATRIC DOSAGE

Bronchospasm

2-12 Years w/ Asthma:

Initial: 0.63mg or 1.25mg tid-qid prn

6-12 Years w/ More Severe Asthma (Baseline FEV_1 <60% Predicted), Weight >40kg, or 11-12 Years:

May achieve better initial response w/ 1.25mg dose

ADMINISTRATION

Inh route

Administer using a jet nebulizer connected to an air compressor w/ adequate air flow, equipped w/ a mouthpiece or suitable face mask

Use the entire contents of one unit-dose vial (3mL of 1.25mg or 0.63mg inh sol)

Adjust nebulizer flow rate to deliver over 5 to 15 min

HOW SUPPLIED

Sol, Inhalation: 0.63mg/3mL, 1.25mg/3mL

CONTRAINDICATIONS

History of hypersensitivity to any of its components.

WARNINGS/PRECAUTIONS

Can produce paradoxical bronchospasm; d/c if this occurs. Consider adding anti-inflammatory agents (eg, corticosteroids) to adequately control asthma. Reevaluate patient and treatment regimen if deterioration of asthma observed. Can produce clinically significant cardiovascular (CV) effect (eg, ECG changes); caution with CV disorders (eg, coronary insufficiency, cardiac arrhythmias, HTN). Immediate hypersensitivity reactions reported. Aggravation of preexisting diabetes mellitus (DM) and ketoacidosis reported with large doses of IV albuterol. May cause hypokalemia. Has not been studied with acute attacks of bronchospasm.

ADVERSE REACTIONS

Asthma exacerbation, otitis media, allergic reaction, gastroenteritis, cold symptoms.

DRUG INTERACTIONS

Avoid other short-acting sympathomimetic aerosol bronchodilators and epinephrine. Extreme caution with MAOIs or TCAs, or within 2 weeks of discontinuation of such agents; action of albuterol may be potentiated. May decrease serum levels of digoxin; monitor levels. May worsen ECG changes and/or hypokalemia caused by non-K sparing diuretics (eg, loop/thiazide); caution is advised. Pulmonary effect blocked by β-blockers; caution with cardioselective β-blockers.

PATIENT CONSIDERATIONS

Assessment: Assess for previous hypersensitivity to the drug, CV disorders, HTN, DM, pregnancy/nursing status, and possible drug interactions.

Monitoring: Monitor for signs/symptoms of CV effects (measured by pulse rate and BP), worsening of symptoms, paradoxical bronchospasm, deterioration of asthma, hypokalemia, and hypersensitivity reactions.

Counseling: Instruct not to use more frequently than recommended. Advise not to increase dose or frequency without consulting physician. Counsel to seek medical attention if symptoms worsen, if therapy becomes less effective, or if there is need to use the drug more frequently than usual. Inform of the common effects (eg, palpitations, chest pain, rapid HR, tremor, nervousness). Advise not to use if the contents of vial change color or become cloudy. Inform that drug compatibility, clinical efficacy, and safety, when mixed with other drugs in nebulizer, have not been established.

STORAGE: 2-25°C (36-77°F). Protect from light and excessive heat. Store in protective foil pouch at all times. Once removed, use within 1 week. Discard if sol not colorless.

ACCUPRIL – quinapril hydrochloride

RX

Class: ACE inhibitor

D/C if pregnancy is detected. Drugs that act directly on the renin-angiotensin system (RAS) can cause injury/death to the developing fetus.

ADULT DOSAGE

Hypertension

Monotherapy:
Initial: 10mg or 20mg qd
Titrate: May adjust dosage at intervals of at least 2 weeks

Most patients have required doses of 20, 40, or 80mg/day, given as a single dose or in 2 equally divided doses

Concomitant Diuretics:
May add a diuretic if BP is uncontrolled w/ monotherapy
In patients currently treated w/ a diuretic, d/c diuretic, if possible, 2-3 days before beginning treatment w/ quinapril, to reduce likelihood of hypotension; may then resume diuretic if BP is not controlled w/ monotherapy
Initial: 5mg qd if diuretic therapy cannot be discontinued

Heart Failure

Adjunctive therapy when added to conventional therapy, including diuretics and/or digitalis

Initial: 5mg bid
Titrate: Adjust weekly
Usual: 20-40mg/day given in 2 equally divided doses

PEDIATRIC DOSAGE

Pediatric use may not have been established

DOSING CONSIDERATIONS

Renal Impairment

HTN:
CrCl >60mL/min:
Max Initial: 10mg/day
CrCl 30-60mL/min:
Max Initial: 5mg/day
CrCl 10-30mL/min:
Max Initial: 2.5mg/day

Heart Failure (HF) and Renal Impairment or Hyponatremia:
CrCl >30mL/min:
Initial: 5mg/day
CrCl 10-30mL/min:
Initial: 2.5mg/day
Titrate: May increase dose at weekly intervals

Elderly

≥65 Years:
HTN:
Initial: 10mg qd

ADMINISTRATION

Oral route

HOW SUPPLIED

Tab: 5mg*, 10mg, 20mg, 40mg *scored

CONTRAINDICATIONS

Hypersensitivity to quinapril HCl, history of ACE inhibitor-associated angioedema. Coadministration w/ aliskiren in patients w/ diabetes.

WARNINGS/PRECAUTIONS

Less effect on BP and higher incidence of angioedema in blacks than nonblacks. Head/neck angioedema reported; d/c and administer appropriate therapy if laryngeal stridor or angioedema of the face, tongue, or glottis occurs. Intestinal angioedema reported; monitor for abdominal pain. Patients w/ history of angioedema unrelated to ACE inhibitor therapy may be at increased risk of angioedema during therapy. Anaphylactoid reactions reported during desensitization w/ hymenoptera venom, dialysis w/ high-flux membranes, and LDL apheresis w/ dextran sulfate absorption. Associated w/ syndrome that starts w/ cholestatic jaundice and progresses to fulminant hepatic necrosis and, sometimes, death (rare); d/c if jaundice or marked hepatic enzyme elevations occur. Excessive hypotension sometimes associated w/ oliguria, azotemia, and (rarely) acute renal failure and/or death may occur. Risk factors for excessive hypotension include HF, hyponatremia, high-dose diuretic therapy, recent intensive diuresis, dialysis, or severe volume and/or salt depletion; eliminate or reduce the diuretic dose or cautiously increase salt intake (except w/ HF) prior to therapy and monitor closely. If symptomatic hypotension develops, reduce dose or d/c therapy or concomitant diuretic. May cause agranulocytosis and bone marrow depression; consider periodic monitoring of WBC counts in patients w/ collagen vascular disease and/or renal disease. May cause renal function changes. May be associated w/ oliguria and/or progressive azotemia and rarely acute renal failure and/or death in patients w/ severe HF whose renal function may depend on the activity of the renin-angiotensin-aldosterone system. May increase BUN and SrCr levels in hypertensive patients w/ unilateral/bilateral renal artery stenosis; monitor renal function during the 1st few weeks of therapy. Minor/transient increases in BUN/SrCr reported in patients w/ no apparent renal vascular disease, when therapy was given concomitantly w/ a diuretic; dose reduction and/or discontinuation of any diuretic and/or quinapril may be required. Hyperkalemia reported; risk factors include renal insufficiency and diabetes mellitus (DM). Persistent nonproductive cough reported. Hypotension may occur w/ surgery or during anesthesia. Caution in elderly.

ADVERSE REACTIONS

Headache, dizziness, cough.

DRUG INTERACTIONS

See Contraindications. Excessive reduction of BP may occur after initiation of treatment in patients on diuretics, especially those on recently instituted diuretic therapy; d/c the diuretic or cautiously increase salt intake prior to initiation of treatment. If not possible to d/c the diuretic, reduce starting dose of quinapril. Coadministration w/ other drugs that raise serum K^+ levels may result in hyperkalemia; monitor serum K^+ in such patients. Reduces tetracycline absorption (possibly due to Mg^{2+} content in quinapril) during simultaneous administration; consider this interaction w/ concomitant tetracycline or other drugs that interact w/ Mg^{2+}. May increase serum lithium levels and symptoms of lithium toxicity; use caution and monitor serum lithium levels. If a diuretic is also used, may increase the risk of lithium toxicity. Nitritoid reactions reported rarely w/ injectable gold (eg, sodium aurothiomalate). NSAIDs, including selective COX-2 inhibitors, may result in deterioration of renal function, including possible acute renal failure in patients who are elderly, volume-depleted, or w/ compromised renal function; monitor renal function periodically during coadministration. NSAIDs may attenuate the antihypertensive effect. Coadministration w/ mTOR inhibitors (eg, temsirolimus) may increase risk for angioedema. Dual blockade of the RAS is associated w/ increased risks of hypotension, hyperkalemia, and changes in renal function (including acute renal failure); avoid combined use of RAS inhibitors. Closely monitor BP, renal function, and electrolytes w/ other agents that also affect the RAS. Avoid concomitant use of aliskiren in patients w/ renal impairment (GFR <60mL/min). Hypotension risk and increased BUN and SrCr w/ diuretics.

PATIENT CONSIDERATIONS

Assessment: Assess for history of angioedema, hypersensitivity to drug, volume/salt depletion, collagen vascular disease, DM, renal artery stenosis, ischemic heart disease, cerebrovascular disease, renal function, pregnancy/nursing status, and possible drug interactions.

Monitoring: Monitor for signs/symptoms of hypotension, anaphylactoid or hypersensitivity reactions, head/neck/intestinal angioedema, agranulocytosis, neutropenia, bone marrow depression, cholestatic jaundice, fulminant hepatic necrosis, and hyperkalemia. Monitor BP and renal function. Monitor WBC count periodically in patients w/ collagen vascular disease and/or renal disease.

Counseling: Inform about the consequences of exposure to therapy during pregnancy; discuss treatment options w/ women planning to become pregnant. Instruct to report pregnancies to physician as soon as possible. Instruct to d/c therapy and immediately report signs/symptoms of angioedema. Caution about lightheadedness, especially during the 1st few days of therapy and advise to report to physician. Instruct to d/c and consult physician if syncope occurs. Caution that inadequate fluid intake or excessive perspiration, diarrhea, or vomiting may lead to an excessive fall in BP, w/ the same consequences of lightheadedness and syncope. Instruct to inform physician about therapy if planning to undergo surgery/anesthesia. Instruct not to use K^+ supplements or salt substitutes containing K^+ w/o consulting physician. Advise to report any symptoms of infection.

STORAGE: 15-30°C (59-86°F). Protect from light.

ACCURETIC – hydrochlorothiazide/quinapril hydrochloride

RX

Class: ACE inhibitor/thiazide diuretic

D/C if pregnancy is detected. Drugs that act directly on the renin-angiotensin system (RAS) can cause injury/death to the developing fetus.

ADULT DOSAGE

Hypertension

BP Uncontrolled w/ Quinapril Monotherapy:
10mg/12.5mg or 20mg/12.5mg qd. Further increases of either or both components depends on clinical response; may increase HCTZ after 2-3 weeks

BP Controlled w/ HCTZ 25mg/day w/ Significant K^+ Loss:
10mg/12.5mg or 20mg/12.5mg qd

Replacement Therapy:
Patients adequately treated w/ 20mg quinapril and 25mg HCTZ w/o significant electrolyte disturbances may switch to 20mg/25mg qd

Not for initial therapy; begin combination therapy only after a patient fails to achieve desired effect w/ monotherapy

PEDIATRIC DOSAGE

Pediatric use may not have been established

DOSING CONSIDERATIONS

Renal Impairment

CrCl ≤30mL/min: Not recommended; loop diuretics preferred

Elderly

Start at lower end of dosing range

ADMINISTRATION

Oral route

HOW SUPPLIED

Tab: (Quinapril/HCTZ) 10mg/12.5mg*, 20mg/12.5mg*, 20mg/25mg *scored

CONTRAINDICATIONS

Anuria, hypersensitivity to other sulfonamide-derived drugs, hypersensitivity to quinapril or hydrochlorothiazide, history of ACE inhibitor-associated angioedema. Coadministration w/ aliskiren in patients w/ diabetes.

WARNINGS/PRECAUTIONS

Not for initial therapy of HTN. May cause symptomatic hypotension; reduce dose or d/c if symptomatic hypotension occurs. Correct volume/salt depletion prior to therapy. Monitor patients at risk of excessive hypotension closely for the first 2 weeks of treatment and whenever dose of quinapril or diuretic is increased. Caution w/ ischemic heart or cerebrovascular disease in whom an excessive fall in BP could result in MI or cerebrovascular accident. Caution w/ impaired hepatic function or progressive liver disease; may precipitate hepatic coma. **Quinapril:** Higher incidence of angioedema and less effect on BP in blacks than nonblacks. Head/neck angioedema reported; d/c immediately and administer appropriate therapy if laryngeal stridor or angioedema of the face/tongue/glottis occurs. Intestinal angioedema reported; monitor for abdominal pain. Patients w/ history of angioedema unrelated to ACE inhibitor therapy may be at increased risk of angioedema during therapy. Anaphylactoid reactions reported during desensitization w/ hymenoptera venom, dialysis w/ high-flux membranes, and LDL apheresis w/ dextran sulfate absorption. Associated w/ syndrome that starts w/ cholestatic jaundice and progresses to fulminant hepatic necrosis, and sometimes death (rare); d/c if jaundice or marked hepatic enzyme elevation occurs. May cause changes in renal function. May be associated w/ oliguria and/or progressive azotemia and rarely w/ acute renal failure and/or death in patients w/ severe CHF whose renal function may depend on the activity of the renin-angiotensin-aldosterone system. May increase BUN and SrCr in patients w/ unilateral renal artery stenosis; monitor renal function during 1st few weeks of therapy. May increase BUN/SrCr in patients w/o preexisting renal vascular disease; may require dose reduction. May cause agranulocytosis and bone marrow depression; consider periodic monitoring of WBC counts in patients w/ collagen vascular disease and/or renal disease. Hyperkalemia reported; risk factors include renal insufficiency and diabetes mellitus. Persistent nonproductive cough reported. Hypotension may occur w/ surgery or during anesthesia. **HCTZ:** Antihypertensive effects may be enhanced in postsympathectomy patients. May precipitate azotemia w/ renal disease. May exacerbate/activate systemic lupus erythematosus (SLE). May cause idiosyncratic reaction, resulting in acute transient myopia and acute angle-closure glaucoma; d/c as rapidly as possible. May cause hyponatremia, hypokalemia, hyperkalemia, and hypomagnesemia. May alter glucose tolerance and raise serum levels of cholesterol, TG, and Ca^{2+}. May raise serum uric acid level and may cause/exacerbate hyperuricemia and precipitate gout in susceptible patients. May decrease protein-bound iodine levels w/o signs of thyroid disturbance. Interrupt treatment for a few days prior to carrying out parathyroid function tests.

ADVERSE REACTIONS

Headache, dizziness, cough, fatigue.

DRUG INTERACTIONS

See Contraindications. Coadministration w/ other drugs that raise serum K^+ levels may result in hyperkalemia; monitor serum K^+ in such patients. May increase lithium levels and risk of toxicity; use caution and monitor lithium levels. Avoid w/ aliskiren in patients w/ renal impairment (GFR <60mL/min). Coadministration w/ mTOR inhibitors (eg, temsirolimus) may increase risk for angioedema. **Quinapril:** Dual blockade of the RAS is associated w/ increased risk of hypotension, hyperkalemia, and changes in renal function (including acute renal failure); in general, avoid combined use of RAS inhibitors. Closely monitor BP, renal function, and electrolytes w/ concomitant agents that also affect the RAS. Reduces tetracycline absorption (possibly due to Mg^{2+} content in quinapril); consider this interaction if coadministering w/ tetracycline or other drugs that interact w/ Mg^{2+}. Nitritoid reactions reported rarely w/ injectable gold (eg, sodium aurothiomalate). NSAIDs, including selective COX-2 inhibitors, may result in deterioration of renal function, including possible acute renal failure, in patients who are elderly, volume depleted, or w/ compromised renal function. NSAIDs may attenuate the antihypertensive effects. **HCTZ:** Thiazide-induced electrolyte disturbances (eg, hypokalemia, hypomagnesemia) increase the risk of digoxin toxicity, which may lead to fatal arrhythmic events. May potentiate orthostatic hypotension w/ alcohol, barbiturates, and narcotics. Dose adjustment of the antidiabetic drug (oral agents and insulin) may be required. Cholestyramine and colestipol resins impair absorption. Corticosteroids and ACTH may intensify electrolyte depletion, particularly hypokalemia. May decrease response to pressor amines (eg, norepinephrine). May increase responsiveness to nondepolarizing skeletal muscle relaxants (eg, tubocurarine). NSAIDs may reduce diuretic, natriuretic, and antihypertensive effects of thiazide diuretics. May potentiate action of other antihypertensives, especially ganglionic or peripheral adrenergic-blocking drugs.

PATIENT CONSIDERATIONS

Assessment: Assess for hypersensitivity to drug or sulfonamides, anuria, history of angioedema, volume/salt depletion, heart failure, SLE, any other conditions where treatment is contraindicated or cautioned, pregnancy/nursing status, and possible drug interactions. Assess renal/hepatic function and electrolyte levels.

Monitoring: Monitor for angioedema, agranulocytosis, hyperkalemia, anaphylactoid reactions, hypotension, jaundice, hypersensitivity/idiosyncratic reactions, SLE, gout, myopia, and angle-closure glaucoma. Periodically monitor WBC counts in patients w/ collagen vascular disease and/or renal disease. Monitor serum electrolytes, BP, LFTs, BUN, SrCr, uric acid levels, and cholesterol/TG levels. Monitor Ca^{2+} levels in patients w/ hypercalcemia.

Counseling: Inform females of childbearing age of the consequences of exposure during pregnancy and of the treatment options for women planning to become pregnant. Instruct to report pregnancy to the physician as soon as possible. Instruct to d/c therapy and immediately report signs/symptoms of angioedema. Caution about lightheadedness, especially during the 1st days of therapy and advise to report to physician. Instruct to d/c and consult physician if syncope occurs. Caution that inadequate fluid intake or excessive perspiration, diarrhea, or vomiting may lead to an excessive fall in BP, resulting in lightheadedness or syncope. Instruct to inform physician about therapy if planning to undergo surgery/anesthesia. Instruct to avoid K^+ supplements or salt substitutes containing K^+ w/o consulting physician. Instruct to report any symptoms of infection.

STORAGE: 20-25°C (68-77°F).

ACEON – perindopril erbumine

RX

Class: ACE inhibitor

D/C if pregnancy is detected. Drugs that act directly on the renin-angiotensin system (RAS) can cause injury/death to the developing fetus.

ADULT DOSAGE

Hypertension

Initial: 4mg qd
Titrate: May titrate prn to max of 16mg/day
Maint: 4-8mg/day given in 1 or 2 divided doses

Stable Coronary Artery Disease

Initial: 4mg qd for 2 weeks
Maint: Increase as tolerated to 8mg qd

PEDIATRIC DOSAGE

Pediatric use may not have been established

DOSING CONSIDERATIONS

Concomitant Medications

Concomitant Diuretics:
Consider reducing diuretic dose prior to start of treatment

Renal Impairment

CrCl <30mL/min: Not recommended

CrCl ≥30mL/min:
Initial: 2mg/day
Max: 8mg/day

Elderly

HTN:
Initial: 4mg/day given in 1 or 2 divided doses
Monitor BP and titrate carefully w/ doses >8mg

>70 Years:
Stable CAD:
Initial: 2mg qd in the 1st week, followed by 4mg qd in the 2nd week
Maint: 8mg qd if tolerated

ADMINISTRATION

Oral route

HOW SUPPLIED

Tab: 2mg*, 4mg*, 8mg* *scored

CONTRAINDICATIONS

Known hypersensitivity (eg, angioedema) to this product or to any other ACE inhibitor, hereditary or idiopathic angioedema. Coadministration w/ aliskiren in patients w/ diabetes.

WARNINGS/PRECAUTIONS

Higher incidence of angioedema in blacks than nonblacks. Angioedema of the face, extremities, lips, tongue, glottis, or larynx reported; d/c and administer appropriate therapy. Intestinal angioedema reported; monitor for abdominal pain. Symptomatic hypotension may occur and is most likely in patients w/ volume/salt depletion. Closely monitor patients at risk for excessive hypotension, especially during the first 2 weeks of treatment and whenever dose is increased. May cause agranulocytosis and bone marrow depression, most frequently in renal impairment patients, especially w/ collagen vascular disease (eg, systemic lupus erythematosus [SLE] or scleroderma). May cause changes in renal function. Oliguria, progressive azotemia, and (rarely) acute renal failure and death may occur in patients w/ severe CHF. May increase BUN and SrCr in patients w/ renal artery stenosis. May cause hyperkalemia; risk factors include renal insufficiency and diabetes mellitus (DM). Persistent nonproductive cough reported. Rarely, associated w/ syndrome that starts w/ cholestatic jaundice and progresses to fulminant necrosis and sometimes death; d/c if jaundice or marked elevations of hepatic enzymes develop. Hypotension may occur w/ major surgery or during anesthesia.

ADVERSE REACTIONS

Cough, headache, asthenia, dizziness, hypotension.

DRUG INTERACTIONS

See Contraindications and Dosing Considerations. Dual blockade of the RAS is associated w/ increased risks of hypotension, hyperkalemia, and changes in renal function (including acute renal failure); avoid combined use of RAS inhibitors, or closely monitor BP, renal function, and electrolytes w/ concomitant agents that affect the RAS. Avoid w/ aliskiren in patients w/ renal impairment (GFR <60mL/min). Hypotension risk, increased BUN and SrCr, and reduced perindoprilat bioavailability w/ diuretics. Increased risk of hyperkalemia w/ K^+-sparing diuretics, drugs that increase serum K^+ (eg, indomethacin, heparin, cyclosporine), K^+ supplements and/or K^+-containing salt substitutes. May increase lithium levels and risk of toxicity; monitor lithium levels. Nitritoid reactions reported w/ injectable gold (sodium aurothiomalate). Caution w/ digoxin. Coadministration w/ NSAIDs, including selective COX-2 inhibitors, may attenuate antihypertensive effect of ACE inhibitors and may further deteriorate renal function.

PATIENT CONSIDERATIONS

Assessment: Assess for hereditary or idiopathic angioedema, volume and/or salt depletion, CHF, renal artery stenosis, ischemic heart disease, cerebrovascular disease, hepatic/renal impairment, DM, collagen vascular disease (eg, SLE), previous hypersensitivity to the drug, pregnancy/nursing status, and possible drug interactions.

Monitoring: Monitor for signs/symptoms of anaphylactoid reactions, head/neck/intestinal angioedema, hypotension, agranulocytosis, bone marrow depression, cholestatic jaundice, fulminant hepatic necrosis, hepatic failure, hyperkalemia, persistent nonproductive cough, hypersensitivity reactions, and neutropenia. Monitor hepatic/renal function, BP, and K^+ levels.

Counseling: Inform of pregnancy risks and discuss treatment options w/ women planning to become pregnant; advise to report pregnancy to physician as soon as possible. Instruct to d/c and immediately report to physician if any signs/symptoms of angioedema develop. Counsel to report any signs of infection (eg, sore throat, fever).

STORAGE: 20-25°C (68-77°F). Protect from moisture.

ACETAMINOPHEN AND CODEINE TABLETS – acetaminophen/codeine phosphate CIII

Class: Opioid analgesic

Associated with cases of acute liver failure, at times resulting in liver transplant and death. Most cases of liver injury are associated with acetaminophen (APAP) use at doses >4000mg/day, and often involve >1 APAP-containing product. Respiratory depression and death reported in children who received codeine following tonsillectomy and/or adenoidectomy and had evidence of being ultra-rapid metabolizers of codeine due to a CYP2D6 polymorphism.

OTHER BRAND NAMES

Tylenol with Codeine

ADULT DOSAGE

Mild to Moderately Severe Pain

Usual Range (Single Dose): 15mg-60mg codeine; 300mg-1000mg acetaminophen (APAP); may repeat doses up to q4h

Max: 360mg/24 hrs codeine; 4000mg/24 hrs APAP

PEDIATRIC DOSAGE

Pediatric use may not have been established

ADMINISTRATION

Oral route

HOW SUPPLIED

Tab: (APAP/Codeine) 300mg/15mg; (Tylenol with Codeine) 300mg/30mg, 300mg/60mg

CONTRAINDICATIONS

Postoperative pain management in children who have undergone tonsillectomy and/or adenoidectomy. Previously exhibited hypersensitivity to codeine or acetaminophen.

WARNINGS/PRECAUTIONS

Increased risk of acute liver failure in patients with underlying liver disease. May cause serious skin reactions (eg, acute generalized exanthematous pustulosis, Stevens-Johnson syndrome, toxic epidermal necrolysis), which can be fatal; d/c at the 1st appearance of skin rash or any other sign of hypersensitivity. Deaths reported in nursing infants exposed to high levels of morphine because their mothers were ultra-rapid metabolizers of codeine. Ultra-rapid metabolizers, due to specific CYP2D6 genotype (gene duplications denoted as *1/*1xN or *1/*2xN), may have life-threatening or fatal respiratory depression or experience signs of overdose (eg, extreme sleepiness, confusion, shallow breathing). Choose lowest effective dose for the shortest period of time. Hypersensitivity and anaphylaxis reported; d/c if signs/symptoms occur. Respiratory-depressant effects and capacity for elevating CSF pressure may be markedly enhanced in the presence of head injury or other intracranial lesions. May obscure diagnosis or clinical course of head injuries and acute abdominal conditions. Habit-forming and potentially abusable; extended use is not recommended. Caution with severe renal/hepatic impairment, head injuries, elevated intracranial pressure, acute abdominal conditions, hypothyroidism, urethral stricture, Addison's disease, prostatic hypertrophy, and in the elderly or debilitated. May increase serum amylase levels. Lab test interactions may occur. Avoid during labor if delivery of a premature infant is anticipated. (Tylenol with Codeine) Contains sodium metabisulfite; may cause allergic-type reactions in certain susceptible people.

ADVERSE REACTIONS

Acute liver failure, drowsiness, lightheadedness, dizziness, sedation, SOB, N/V.

DRUG INTERACTIONS

Increased risk of acute liver failure with alcohol ingestion. May enhance effects of other narcotic analgesics, alcohol, general anesthetics, tranquilizers (eg, chlordiazepoxide), sedative-hypnotics, or other CNS depressants; may increase CNS depression.

PATIENT CONSIDERATIONS

Assessment: Assess for hypersensitivity to drug, hepatic/renal impairment, head injury, intracranial lesions, acute abdominal conditions, any other conditions where treatment is contraindicated or cautioned, pregnancy/nursing status, and possible drug interactions.

Monitoring: Monitor for signs/symptoms of hepatotoxicity, respiratory depression, skin reactions, hypersensitivity, anaphylaxis, elevation in CSF pressure, drug abuse, tolerance, dependence, and other adverse reactions. Monitor effects of therapy with serial LFTs and/or renal function tests in patients with severe hepatic/renal disease. Closely monitor newborn infants for signs of respiratory depression if the mother received the drug during labor.

Counseling: Instruct to d/c therapy and contact physician immediately if signs of allergy develop. Instruct to look for APAP on package labels and not to use >1 APAP-containing product. Instruct to seek medical attention immediately upon ingestion of >4000mg/day APAP, even if patient is feeling well. Advise that drug may impair mental/physical abilities. Instruct to avoid performing potentially hazardous tasks (eg, driving, operating machinery), drinking alcohol, or taking other CNS depressants while on therapy. Inform that drug may be habit-forming; instruct to take ud.

STORAGE: 20-25°C (68-77°F).

ACIPHEX – rabeprazole sodium RX

Class: Proton pump inhibitor (PPI)

OTHER BRAND NAMES

Aciphex Sprinkle

ADULT DOSAGE

***Helicobacter pylori* Eradication**

Treatment of *H. pylori* infection and duodenal ulcer disease (active or history w/in past 5 yrs) for *H. pylori* eradication to reduce the risk of duodenal ulcer recurrence

20mg tab + clarithromycin 500mg + amoxicillin 1000mg, all bid w/ am and pm meals for 7 days

Pathological Hypersecretory Conditions

Treatment of pathological hypersecretory conditions, including Zollinger-Ellison syndrome

Initial: 60mg qd or in divided doses
Titrate: Adjust to individual needs and continue for as long as clinically indicated

Doses up to 100mg qd and 60mg bid have been administered. Some have been treated for up to 1 yr

Gastroesophageal Reflux Disease

Healing of Erosive or Ulcerative GERD:
20mg tab qd for 4-8 weeks; consider an additional 8 weeks if not healed after 8 weeks of treatment

Maint of Healing of Erosive or Ulcerative GERD:
20mg tab qd; controlled studies do not extend beyond 12 months

Symptomatic GERD:
Treatment of daytime and nighttime heartburn and other symptoms associated w/ GERD

20mg tab qd for 4 weeks; consider an additional course of treatment if symptoms do not resolve completely after 4 weeks

Duodenal Ulcers

Healing and Symptomatic Relief of Duodenal Ulcers:
20mg tab qd after am meal for up to 4 weeks; some patients may need additional therapy to achieve healing

PEDIATRIC DOSAGE

Gastroesophageal Reflux Disease

Treatment of GERD:
Cap:
1-11 Years:
<15kg: 5mg qd for up to 12 weeks w/ the option to increase to 10mg if inadequate response
≥15kg: 10mg qd for up to 12 weeks

Treatment of Symptomatic GERD:
Tab:
≥12 Years:
20mg qd for up to 8 weeks

ADMINISTRATION

Oral route

Tab

Swallow whole; do not chew, crush, or split
May be taken w/ or w/o food

Cap
Take 30 min ac
Open cap and sprinkle entire contents on a small amount of soft food (eg, applesauce, fruit or vegetable based baby food, yogurt) or empty contents into a small amount of liquid (eg, infant formula, apple juice, pediatric electrolyte sol); do not chew or crush granules
Take whole dose w/in 15 min of preparation
Food or liquid should be at or below room temperature; do not store mixture for future use

HOW SUPPLIED

Cap, Delayed-Release (Sprinkle): 5mg, 10mg; **Tab, Delayed-Release:** 20mg

CONTRAINDICATIONS

Known hypersensitivity to rabeprazole, substituted benzimidazoles, or to any component of the formulation.

WARNINGS/PRECAUTIONS

Symptomatic response does not preclude the presence of gastric malignancy. Acute interstitial nephritis reported; d/c if this develops. Cyanocobalamin (vitamin B12) deficiency may occur with daily long-term treatment (eg, >3 yrs) with any acid-suppressing medications. May increase risk of *Clostridium difficile*-associated diarrhea (CDAD), especially in hospitalized patients. May increase risk of osteoporosis-related fractures of the hip, wrist, or spine, especially with high-dose and long-term therapy. Use lowest dose and shortest duration appropriate to the condition being treated. Hypomagnesemia reported and may require Mg^{2+} replacement and discontinuation of therapy; consider monitoring Mg^{2+} levels prior to and periodically during therapy with prolonged treatment. Caution with severe hepatic impairment.

ADVERSE REACTIONS

Headache, flatulence, pain, pharyngitis, diarrhea, N/V, abdominal pain.

DRUG INTERACTIONS

May reduce absorption of drugs where gastric pH is an important determinant of their bioavailability; ketoconazole, atazanavir, iron salts, erlotinib, and mycophenolate mofetil (MMF) absorption can decrease, while digoxin absorption can increase. May substantially decrease atazanavir levels and reduce its therapeutic effect; concomitant use is not recommended. Caution in transplant patients receiving MMF. May inhibit cyclosporine metabolism. Increased INR and PT reported with warfarin. Combination with amoxicillin and clarithromycin may increase levels of rabeprazole and 14-hydroxyclarithromycin. May elevate and prolong levels of methotrexate (MTX) and/or its metabolite, possibly leading to MTX toxicities; consider temporary withdrawal of therapy with high-dose MTX. Caution with digoxin or with drugs that may cause hypomagnesemia (eg, diuretics).

PATIENT CONSIDERATIONS

Assessment: Assess for hypersensitivity to the drug, hepatic impairment, risk for osteoporosis-related fractures, pregnancy/nursing status, and possible drug interactions. Obtain baseline Mg^{2+} levels.

Monitoring: Monitor for signs/symptoms of acute interstitial nephritis, cyanocobalamin deficiency, CDAD, bone fractures, hypersensitivity reactions, and other adverse reactions. Monitor Mg^{2+} levels periodically. Monitor INR and PT when given with warfarin.

Counseling: Instruct to take ud. Advise to immediately report and seek care for diarrhea that does not improve.

STORAGE: 25°C (77°F); excursions permitted to 15-30°C (59-86°F). Protect from moisture.

ACTICLATE – doxycycline hyclate

Class: Tetracyclines

RX

ADULT DOSAGE

General Dosing

Usual: 100mg q12h on 1st day
Maint: 100mg qd or 50mg q12h

More Severe Infections (eg, Chronic UTIs): 100mg q12h

Streptococcal Infections: Continue therapy for 10 days

***Chlamydia trachomatis* Infections**

Uncomplicated Urethral/Endocervical/Rectal Infections:
100mg bid for 7 days

PEDIATRIC DOSAGE

General Dosing

>8 Years:
<45kg:
Usual: 4.4mg/kg divided into 2 doses on the 1st day
Maint: 2.2mg/kg qd or divided into 2 doses
More Severe Infections: May give up to 4.4mg/kg

>45kg:
Usual: 100mg q12h on 1st day
Maint: 100mg qd or 50mg q12h

Gonococcal Infections

Uncomplicated Gonococcal Infections (Except Anorectal Infections in Men):
100mg bid for 7 days or as an alternate single visit dose of 300mg stat followed in 1 hr by a second 300mg

Nongonococcal Urethritis

Caused by *Chlamydia trachomatis* and *Ureaplasma urealyticum*:
100mg bid for 7 days

Syphilis

Patients Allergic to Penicillin:
Early Syphilis: 100mg bid for 2 weeks
>1-Year Duration: 100mg bid for 4 weeks

Acute Epididymo-Orchitis

Caused by *Neisseria gonorrhoeae/Chlamydia trachomatis*:
100mg bid for at least 10 days

Malaria

Prophylaxis:
Usual: 100mg qd, beginning 1 or 2 days before travel, continuing daily during travel and for 4 weeks after departure from malarious area

Inhalational Anthrax (Postexposure)

Usual: 100mg bid for 60 days

Other Indications

The following infections caused by susceptible microorganisms: Rocky Mountain spotted fever, typhus fever and the typhus group, Q fever, rickettsialpox, tick fevers, lymphogranuloma venereum, granuloma inguinale, chancroid, respiratory tract infections, psittacosis (ornithosis), relapsing fever, plague, tularemia, cholera, *Campylobacter fetus* infections, brucellosis (in conjunction w/ streptomycin), bartonellosis, UTIs, trachoma, and inclusion conjunctivitis

Infections caused by susceptible strains of *Escherichia coli*, *Enterobacter aerogenes*, *Shigella* species, and *Acinetobacter* species

When penicillin is contraindicated, treatment of the following infections caused by susceptible microorganisms: yaws, listeriosis, Vincent's infection, actinomycosis, and infections caused by *Clostridium* species

Adjunct to amebicides in acute intestinal amebiasis

Adjunctive therapy in severe acne

Streptococcal Infections: Continue therapy for 10 days

Malaria

>8 Years:
Prophylaxis:
Usual: 2mg/kg qd up to 100mg qd, beginning 1 or 2 days before travel, continuing daily during travel and for 4 weeks after departure from malarious area

Inhalational Anthrax (Postexposure)

<45kg:
2.2mg/kg bid for 60 days

≥45kg:
100mg bid for 60 days

ADMINISTRATION

Oral route

Administer w/ adequate amounts of fluid
May be given w/ food or milk if gastric irritation occurs

HOW SUPPLIED

Tab: 75mg, 150mg* *scored

CONTRAINDICATIONS

Hypersensitivity to any of the tetracyclines.

WARNINGS/PRECAUTIONS

May cause permanent discoloration of the teeth (yellow-gray-brown) if used during tooth development (last 1/2 of pregnancy, infancy, and childhood to 8 yrs of age); do not use in this age group, except for anthrax. Enamel hypoplasia reported. *Clostridium difficile*-associated diarrhea (CDAD) reported; d/c if CDAD is suspected or confirmed. Photosensitivity, manifested by an exaggerated sunburn reaction, reported; d/c at the 1st evidence of skin erythema. May result in bacterial resistance if used in the absence of proven or suspected bacterial infection, or a prophylactic indication; take appropriate measures if superinfection develops. Associated with intracranial HTN (pseudotumor cerebri); increased risk in women of childbearing age who are overweight or have a history of intracranial HTN. If visual disturbance occurs, prompt ophthalmologic evaluation is warranted. Intracranial pressure can remain elevated for weeks after drug cessation; monitor patients until they stabilize. May decrease fibula growth rate in prematures. May cause fetal harm. May cause an increase in BUN. When used for malaria prophylaxis, patient may still transmit the infection to mosquitoes outside endemic areas. False elevations of urinary catecholamines may occur due to interference with the fluorescence test.

ADVERSE REACTIONS

Anorexia, N/V, diarrhea, glossitis, hepatotoxicity, maculopapular and erythematous rashes, Stevens-Johnson syndrome, toxic epidermal necrolysis, urticaria, angioneurotic edema, anaphylaxis, hemolytic anemia, thrombocytopenia, neutropenia.

DRUG INTERACTIONS

Avoid concomitant use with isotretinoin; may also cause pseudotumor cerebri. May depress plasma prothrombin activity; may require downward adjustment of anticoagulant dose. May interfere with bactericidal action of PCN; avoid concurrent use. Impaired absorption with bismuth subsalicylate, antacids containing aluminum, Ca^{2+}, or Mg^{2+}, and iron-containing preparations. May render oral contraceptives less effective. Decreased $T_{1/2}$ with barbiturates, carbamazepine, and phenytoin. Fatal renal toxicity reported with methoxyflurane.

PATIENT CONSIDERATIONS

Assessment: Assess for hypersensitivity to drug or any tetracyclines, risk for intracranial HTN, pregnancy/nursing status, and possible drug interactions. Perform culture and susceptibility testing.

Monitoring: Monitor for CDAD, photosensitivity, skin erythema, superinfection, intracranial HTN, visual disturbance, and other adverse reactions. In long-term therapy, perform periodic lab evaluation of organ systems, including hematopoietic, renal, and hepatic studies.

Counseling: Apprise of the potential hazard to fetus if used during pregnancy. Inform that therapy does not guarantee protection against malaria; advise to use measures that help avoid contact with mosquitoes. Advise to avoid excessive sunlight or artificial UV light and to d/c therapy if phototoxicity (eg, skin eruptions) occurs; advise to consider use of sunscreen or sunblock. Inform that absorption of drug is reduced when taken with bismuth subsalicylate, antacids containing aluminum, Ca^{2+}, or Mg^{2+}, iron-containing preparations, and with foods, especially those that contain Ca^{2+}. Inform that drug may increase the incidence of vaginal candidiasis. Inform that diarrhea may be experienced and instruct to immediately contact physician if watery and bloody stools (with or without stomach cramps and fever) occur, even as late as ≥2 months after the last dose. Counsel that therapy should only be used to treat bacterial, not viral infections. Instruct to take exactly ud even if the patient feels better early in the course of therapy. Inform that skipping doses or not completing the full course of therapy may decrease effectiveness of treatment and increase bacterial resistance.

STORAGE: 20-25°C (68-77°F); excursions permitted to 15-30°C (59-86°F). Protect from light and moisture.

ACTIQ – fentanyl citrate

CII

Class: Opioid analgesic

Fatal respiratory depression may occur. Contraindicated in the management of acute or postoperative pain (eg, headache/migraine) and in opioid-nontolerant patients. Death reported upon accidental ingestion in children; keep out of reach of children. Concomitant use with CYP3A4 inhibitors may increase plasma levels, and may cause fatal respiratory depression. Do not convert patients on a mcg-per-mcg basis from any other fentanyl products to Actiq. Do not substitute for any other fentanyl products; may result in fatal overdose. Contains fentanyl with abuse liability similar to other opioid analgesics. Available only through a restricted program called Transmucosal Immediate Release Fentanyl (TIRF) Risk Evaluation Mitigation Strategy (REMS) Access program due to risk of misuse, abuse, addiction, and overdose. Outpatients, healthcare professionals who prescribe to outpatients, pharmacies, and distributors must enroll in the program.

ADULT DOSAGE

Cancer Pain

Breakthrough pain in patients already receiving and tolerant to around-the-clock opioid therapy

Initial: 200mcg; dispense no more than 6 units initially

Titrate:

If signs of excessive opioid effects appear before unit is consumed, remove dosage unit, dispose properly, and decrease subsequent doses

PEDIATRIC DOSAGE

Cancer Pain

Breakthrough pain in patients already receiving and tolerant to around-the-clock opioid therapy

≥16 Years:

Initial: 200mcg; dispense no more than 6 units initially

Titrate:

If signs of excessive opioid effects appear before unit is consumed, remove dosage unit,

If breakthrough pain is not relieved 15 min after completion of previous dose, give only 1 additional dose of the same strength

Maint: Once titrated to an effective dose, use only 1 unit of the appropriate strength per breakthrough pain episode; limit to ≤4 units/day

Max: 2 doses/breakthrough pain episode; wait ≥4 hrs before treating another breakthrough pain episode

Increase dose only when a single administration of current dose fails to adequately treat breakthrough pain episode for several consecutive episodes

If >4 breakthrough pain episodes/day are experienced, reevaluate maint dose (around-the-clock) used for persistent pain

dispose properly, and decrease subsequent doses

If breakthrough pain is not relieved 15 min after completion of previous dose, give only 1 additional dose of the same strength

Maint: Once titrated to an effective dose, use only 1 unit of the appropriate strength per breakthrough pain episode; limit to ≤4 units/day

Max: 2 doses/breakthrough pain episode; wait ≥4 hrs before treating another breakthrough pain episode

Increase dose only when a single administration of current dose fails to adequately treat breakthrough pain episode for several consecutive episodes

If >4 breakthrough pain episodes/day are experienced, reevaluate maint dose (around-the-clock) used for persistent pain

DOSING CONSIDERATIONS

Discontinuation

Gradually titrate dose downward

ADMINISTRATION

Oral route

Place unit in mouth between cheek and lower gum, occasionally moving the drug matrix from one side to the other using the handle

Do not suck or chew

Consume unit over a 15-min period

HOW SUPPLIED

Loz: 200mcg, 400mcg, 600mcg, 800mcg, 1200mcg, 1600mcg

CONTRAINDICATIONS

Opioid-nontolerant patients, management of acute or postoperative pain including headache/migraine and dental pain, known intolerance or hypersensitivity to any of its components or the drug fentanyl.

WARNINGS/PRECAUTIONS

Increased risk of respiratory depression in patients with underlying respiratory disorders and in elderly/debilitated. May impair mental/physical abilities. Caution with chronic obstructive pulmonary disease or preexisting medical conditions predisposing to respiratory depression; may further decrease respiratory drive to the point of respiratory failure. Extreme caution in patients who may be susceptible to the intracranial effects of CO_2 retention (eg, with evidence of increased intracranial pressure or impaired consciousness). May obscure clinical course of head injuries. Caution with bradyarrhythmias. Anaphylaxis and hypersensitivity reported. Avoid use during labor and delivery. Caution with renal/hepatic impairment.

ADVERSE REACTIONS

Respiratory depression, circulatory depression, hypotension, shock, N/V, headache, constipation, dizziness, dyspnea, anxiety, somnolence, asthenia, confusion, depression.

DRUG INTERACTIONS

See Boxed Warning. Respiratory depression is more likely to occur when given with other drugs that depress respiration. Increased depressant effects with other CNS depressants (eg, other opioids, sedatives, hypnotics, general anesthetics, phenothiazines, tranquilizers, skeletal muscle relaxants, sedating antihistamines, alcoholic beverages); adjust dose if warranted. Avoid with grapefruit and grapefruit juice. CYP3A4 inducers may decrease levels. Not recommended with MAOIs or within 14 days of discontinuation of MAOIs.

PATIENT CONSIDERATIONS

Assessment: Assess for degree of opioid tolerance, previous opioid dose, level of pain intensity, type of pain, patient's general condition and medical status, and any other conditions where treatment is contraindicated or cautioned. Assess for hypersensitivity to the drug, renal/hepatic function, pregnancy/nursing status, and possible drug interactions.

Monitoring: Monitor for signs/symptoms of respiratory depression, impairment of mental/physical abilities, bradycardia, anaphylaxis/hypersensitivity, abuse/addiction, and other adverse reactions.

Counseling: Advise to enroll in TIRF REMS Access program. Instruct to keep drug out of reach of children. Advise to take drug as prescribed and avoid sharing it with anyone else. Instruct to notify physician if breakthrough pain is not alleviated or worsens after taking the drug. Inform that drug may impair mental/physical abilities; caution against performing activities that require high level of attention (eg, driving/using heavy machinery). Advise not to combine with alcohol, sleep aids, or tranquilizers, except if ordered by the physician. Instruct to notify physician if pregnant or planning to become pregnant. Inform that frequent consumption may increase risk of dental decay; advise to consult dentist to ensure appropriate oral hygiene. Inform diabetics that drug contains approximately 2g sugar/U. Inform of proper storage, administration, and disposal.

STORAGE: 20-25°C (68-77°F); excursions permitted between 15-30°C (59-86°F). Protect from freezing and moisture.

ACTONEL – risedronate sodium

RX

Class: Bisphosphonate

ADULT DOSAGE

Osteoporosis

Treatment/Prevention of Postmenopausal Osteoporosis:
Usual: 5mg qd, or 35mg once a week, or 75mg taken on 2 consecutive days for a total of 2 tabs/month, or 150mg once a month

Osteoporosis in Men:
Usual: 35mg once a week

Treatment/Prevention of Glucocorticoid-Induced Osteoporosis:
Usual: 5mg qd

Paget's Disease

Treatment in Men/Women:
Usual: 30mg qd for 2 months

May consider retreatment (following post-treatment observation of at least 2 months) if relapse occurs, or if treatment fails to normalize serum alkaline phosphatase; dose and duration of therapy are the same as for initial treatment

Missed Dose

35mg Once a Week is Missed:
Take 1 tab on the am after remembering and return to taking 1 tab once a week as originally scheduled on chosen day; do not take 2 tabs on same day

One or Both 75mg Tabs (Taken on 2 Consecutive Days/Month) are Missed:
If Next Month's Scheduled Doses are >7 Days Away:
If both tabs are missed, take one 75mg tab in the am after the day it is remembered, then take the other tab on the next consecutive am. If only one 75mg tab is missed, take the missed tab in the am after the day it is remembered. Return to taking 75mg on 2 consecutive days/month as originally scheduled. Do not take more than two 75mg tabs w/in 7 days
If Next Month's Scheduled Doses are w/in 7 Days:
Wait until the next month's scheduled doses and then continue taking 75mg on 2 consecutive days/month as originally scheduled

150mg Once a Month is Missed:
If Next Month's Scheduled Dose is >7 Days Away:
Take missed tab in the am after the day it is remembered, then return to taking 150mg once a month as originally scheduled; do not take more than one 150mg tab w/in 7 days

PEDIATRIC DOSAGE

Pediatric use may not have been established

If Next Month's Scheduled Doses are w/in 7 Days: Wait until the next month's scheduled dose and then continue taking 150mg once a month as originally scheduled	

DOSING CONSIDERATIONS

Renal Impairment

Severe (CrCl <30mL/min): Not recommended

ADMINISTRATION

Oral route

Take at least 30 min before the 1st food or drink of the day other than water, and before taking any oral medication or supplementation

Swallow tabs whole w/ a full glass of plain water (6-8 oz); avoid lying down for 30 min after taking medication

Do not chew or suck tab

Avoid water w/ supplements (including mineral water)

Take Ca^{2+} supplements, antacids, Mg^{2+}-based supplements/laxatives, and iron preparations at a different time of the day

HOW SUPPLIED

Tab: 5mg, 30mg, 35mg, 75mg, 150mg

CONTRAINDICATIONS

Esophageal abnormalities that delay esophageal emptying (eg, stricture or achalasia), inability to stand or sit upright for at least 30 min, hypocalcemia, known hypersensitivity to risedronate sodium or any of its excipients.

WARNINGS/PRECAUTIONS

Consider discontinuation after 3-5 yrs of use in patients at low risk for fracture; periodically reevaluate risk for fracture in patients who d/c therapy. Contains same active ingredient as Atelvia; do not treat w/ Actonel if on concomitant therapy w/ Atelvia. May cause local irritation of the upper GI mucosa; caution w/ active upper GI problems (eg, Barrett's esophagus, dysphagia, esophageal diseases, gastritis, duodenitis, ulcers). Esophageal reactions (eg, esophagitis, esophageal ulcers/erosions) reported; d/c if dysphagia, odynophagia, retrosternal pain, or new/worsening heartburn develops. Use therapy under appropriate supervision in patients who cannot comply w/ dosing instructions due to mental disability. Gastric and duodenal ulcers reported. Hypocalcemia reported; treat hypocalcemia and other disturbances of bone and mineral metabolism before starting therapy, and ensure adequate Ca^{2+} and vitamin D intake. Osteonecrosis of the jaw (ONJ) reported; risk may increase w/ duration of exposure to drug. For patients requiring invasive dental procedures, discontinuation of treatment may reduce risk for ONJ. Consider discontinuation if ONJ develops. Severe and occasionally incapacitating bone, joint, and/or muscle pain reported; consider discontinuation if severe symptoms develop. Atypical, low-energy, or low-trauma fractures of the femoral shaft reported; evaluate any patient w/ a history of bisphosphonate exposure who presents w/ thigh/groin pain to rule out an incomplete femur fracture, and consider interruption of therapy. Ascertain sex steroid hormonal status and consider appropriate replacement before initiating therapy for the treatment and prevention of glucocorticoid-induced osteoporosis. May interfere w/ the use of bone-imaging agents.

ADVERSE REACTIONS

Back pain, arthralgia, abdominal pain, dyspepsia, acute phase reaction, allergic reaction, arthritis, diarrhea, headache, infection, UTI, bronchitis, HTN, nausea, rash.

DRUG INTERACTIONS

Coadministration w/ Ca^{2+} supplements, antacids, or oral medications containing divalent cations will interfere w/ absorption.

PATIENT CONSIDERATIONS

Assessment: Assess for esophageal abnormalities, ability to stand or sit upright for at least 30 min, active upper GI problems, mental disability, hypocalcemia, disturbances of bone and mineral metabolism, risk for ONJ, renal impairment, drug hypersensitivity, any other conditions where treatment is contraindicated or cautioned, pregnancy/nursing status, and possible drug interactions. For glucocorticoid-induced osteoporosis treatment/prevention, assess sex steroid hormonal status.

Monitoring: Monitor for signs/symptoms of ONJ, atypical femoral fracture, esophageal reactions, hypocalcemia, musculoskeletal pain, and other adverse events. Periodically reevaluate the need for continued therapy.

Counseling: Instruct to pay particular attention to dosing instructions and counsel about missed dose instructions. Advise to take at least 30 min before 1st food or drink of the day other than water. Instruct to take while in an upright position w/ a full glass of plain water (6-8 oz) and to avoid lying down for 30 min after taking the drug. Advise to consult physician before continuing treatment if symptoms of esophageal disease develop. Instruct to take supplemental Ca^{2+} and vitamin D if dietary intake is inadequate; instruct to take Ca^{2+} supplements or Ca^{2+}-, aluminum-, and Mg^{2+}-containing medications at a different time of the day. Counsel to consider weight-bearing exercise along w/ the modification of certain behavioral factors (eg, excessive cigarette smoking and/or alcohol consumption) if these factors exist. Instruct to inform physician about medication history. Advise to consult physician any time they have a medical problem they think may be from treatment.

STORAGE: 20-25°C (68-77°F).

ACTOPLUS MET XR – metformin hydrochloride/pioglitazone RX

Class: Biguanide/thiazolidinedione (glitazone)

Thiazolidinediones, including pioglitazone, cause or exacerbate congestive heart failure (CHF) in some patients. After initiation and dose increases, monitor carefully for signs and symptoms of heart failure (HF); manage accordingly and consider discontinuation or dose reduction if HF develops. Not recommended with symptomatic HF. Contraindicated with established NYHA Class III or IV HF. Lactic acidosis may occur due to metformin accumulation; risk increases with conditions such as sepsis, dehydration, excess alcohol intake, hepatic/renal impairment, and acute CHF. If acidosis is suspected, d/c therapy and hospitalize patient immediately.

OTHER BRAND NAMES

Actoplus Met

ADULT DOSAGE

Type 2 Diabetes Mellitus

Initial:
Tab: 15mg/500mg bid or 15mg/850mg qd
Tab, Extended-Release (ER): 15mg/1000mg or 30mg/1000mg qd

NYHA Class I or II CHF:
Tab: 15mg/500mg or 15mg/850mg qd
Tab, ER: 15mg/1000mg or 30mg/1000mg qd

Inadequately Controlled on Metformin Monotherapy:
Tab: 15mg/500mg bid or 15mg/850mg qd or bid, depending on metformin dose already being taken
Tab, ER: 15mg/1000mg bid or 30mg/1000mg qd, depending on metformin dose already being taken

Inadequately Controlled on Pioglitazone Monotherapy:
Tab: 15mg/500mg bid or 15mg/850mg qd
Tab, ER: 15mg/1000mg bid or 30mg/1000mg qd

Switching from Combination Therapy of Pioglitazone plus Metformin as Separate Tabs:
Tab/Tab, ER: Take at doses that are as close as possible to the dose of pioglitazone and metformin already being taken

Titrate:
Gradually adjust, as needed, after assessing adequacy of response and tolerability

Max:
Tab: (45mg/2550mg)/day
Tab, ER: (45mg/2000mg)/day

Metformin doses >2000mg may be better tolerated given tid

PEDIATRIC DOSAGE

Pediatric use may not have been established

DOSING CONSIDERATIONS

Concomitant Medications

Insulin Secretagogue (eg, Sulfonylurea):
Reduce dose of insulin secretagogue if hypoglycemia occurs

Insulin:
Decrease insulin dose by 10-25% if hypoglycemia occurs; further insulin dose adjustments should be individualized based on glycemic response

Strong CYP2C8 Inhibitors (eg, Gemfibrozil):
Max:
Tab: (15mg/850mg)/day
Tab, ER: (15mg/1000mg)/day

Elderly
Do not titrate to max dose

ADMINISTRATION

Oral route

Take w/ meals

Tab, ER
Swallow whole; do not chew, cut, or crush

HOW SUPPLIED

(Pioglitazone/Metformin) Tab, ER (XR): 15mg/1000mg, 30mg/1000mg; **(Actoplus Met) Tab:** 15mg/500mg, 15mg/850mg

CONTRAINDICATIONS

NYHA Class III or IV HF; renal impairment (eg, SrCr ≥1.5mg/dL [males], ≥1.4mg/dL [females], or abnormal CrCl); metabolic acidosis, including diabetic ketoacidosis; known hypersensitivity to pioglitazone, metformin, or any other component of this medication.

WARNINGS/PRECAUTIONS

Not for use in type 1 DM or for treatment of diabetic ketoacidosis. Dose-related edema reported; caution in patients with edema or at risk for CHF. Fatal and nonfatal hepatic failure reported; caution with abnormal LFTs. Measure LFTs promptly in patients who report symptoms that may indicate liver injury. D/C if ALT >3X ULN; do not restart if cause of abnormal LFTs not established or if ALT remains >3X ULN with total bilirubin >2X ULN without alternative etiologies. May use with caution in patients with lesser ALT or bilirubin elevations and with an alternate probable cause. Avoid with clinical or lab evidence of hepatic disease. Increased incidence of bone fracture reported in females. Not for use in patients with active bladder cancer; consider benefits versus risks in patients with a prior history of bladder cancer. Caution in patients susceptible to hypoglycemic effects, such as elderly, debilitated/malnourished patients, and those with adrenal/pituitary insufficiency, or alcohol intoxication. Macular edema reported; promptly refer to an ophthalmologist if visual symptoms occur. May result in ovulation in some premenopausal anovulatory women, which may increase risk for pregnancy; adequate contraception is recommended. Assess renal function before initiation of therapy and at least annually thereafter; d/c with evidence of renal impairment. D/C at the time of or prior to radiologic studies involving the use of intravascular iodinated contrast materials, withhold for 48 hrs subsequent to the procedure, and reinstitute only if renal function is normal. D/C in hypoxic states (eg, acute CHF, shock, acute myocardial infarction). Temporarily suspend for any surgical procedure (except minor procedures not associated with restricted food and fluid intake); restart when oral intake is resumed and renal function is normal. May decrease serum vitamin B12 levels; monitor hematologic parameters annually. Caution in elderly.

ADVERSE REACTIONS

Lactic acidosis, CHF, diarrhea, headache, edema, upper respiratory tract infection, weight gain.

DRUG INTERACTIONS

See Dosage. Risk for hypoglycemia with insulin or other antidiabetic medications (particularly insulin secretagogues [eg, sulfonylureas]); may require a reduction in the dose of the concomitant antidiabetic medication. May be difficult to recognize hypoglycemia with β-adrenergic blocking drugs. Caution with drugs that may affect renal function or result in significant hemodynamic change or may interfere with the disposition of metformin (eg, cationic drugs eliminated by renal tubular secretion). Alcohol potentiates the effect of metformin on lactate metabolism; avoid excessive alcohol intake. Increased exposure and $T_{1/2}$ with strong CYP2C8 inhibitors (eg, gemfibrozil). CYP2C8 inducers (eg, rifampin) may decrease exposure; if a CYP2C8 inducer is started or stopped during treatment, changes in diabetes treatment may be needed based on clinical response. Topiramate or other carbonic anhydrase inhibitors (eg, zonisamide, acetazolamide, dichlorphenamide) may induce metabolic acidosis; use with caution. Cationic drugs that are eliminated by renal tubular secretion (eg, cimetidine, amiloride, digoxin, morphine, procainamide) may potentially produce an interaction; monitor and adjust dose of therapy and/or the interfering drug. Observe for loss of blood glucose control with thiazides and other diuretics, corticosteroids, phenothiazines, thyroid products, estrogens, oral contraceptives, phenytoin, nicotinic acid, sympathomimetics, calcium channel blockers, and isoniazid; observe for hypoglycemia when such drugs are withdrawn during therapy. Pioglitazone: May cause dose-related fluid retention when used with other antidiabetic medications, most commonly with insulin.

PATIENT CONSIDERATIONS

Assessment: Assess for HF or risk of HF, metabolic acidosis, risk factors for lactic acidosis, previous hypersensitivity to the drug, type of DM, diabetic ketoacidosis, edema, bone health, active/

history of bladder cancer, inadequate vitamin B12 or Ca^{2+} intake/absorption, any other conditions where treatment is cautioned, pregnancy/nursing status, and possible drug interactions. Assess if patient is planning to undergo any surgical procedure or radiologic studies involving the use of intravascular iodinated contrast materials. Obtain baseline LFTs, renal function, FPG and HbA1c levels, and hematologic parameters.

Monitoring: Monitor for signs/symptoms of HF, liver injury, lactic acidosis, edema, fractures, visual symptoms, hypoxic states, and other adverse reactions. Monitor renal function, especially in elderly, at least annually. Monitor hematologic parameters annually. Perform routine serum vitamin B12 measurements at 2- to 3-yr intervals in patients predisposed to developing subnormal vitamin B12 levels. Monitor FPG and HbA1c. Periodically monitor LFTs in patients with liver disease.

Counseling: Advise on the importance of adherence to dietary instructions and regular testing of blood glucose, HbA1c, renal function, and hematologic parameters. Advise to seek medical advice promptly during periods of stress, as medication requirements may change. Instruct to promptly report any signs/symptoms of bladder cancer or HF. Inform of the risk of lactic acidosis; instruct to d/c therapy immediately and notify physician if unexplained hyperventilation, myalgia, GI symptoms, malaise, unusual somnolence, or other nonspecific symptoms occur. Counsel against excessive alcohol intake while on therapy. Instruct to d/c use and seek medical advice promptly if signs/symptoms of hepatotoxicity occur. Counsel premenopausal women to use adequate contraception during treatment. Inform that hypoglycemia can occur; explain the risks, symptoms, and appropriate management. Instruct to take drug as prescribed and that any change in dosing should only be done if directed by physician. (Tab, ER) Inform that the inactive ingredients may occasionally be eliminated in the feces as a soft mass that may resemble the original tab.

STORAGE: 25°C (77°F); excursions permitted to 15-30°C (59-86°F). Protect from moisture and humidity.

ACTOS – pioglitazone

RX

Class: Thiazolidinedione (glitazone)

Thiazolidinediones cause or exacerbate congestive heart failure (CHF) in some patients. After initiation and dose increases, monitor carefully for signs and symptoms of heart failure (HF) and manage accordingly; consider discontinuation or dose reduction. Not recommended in patients with symptomatic HF. Contraindicated with established NYHA Class III or IV HF.

ADULT DOSAGE

Type 2 Diabetes Mellitus

W/O CHF:
Initial: 15mg or 30mg qd
Titrate: In increments of 15mg
Max: 45mg qd

W/ CHF (NYHA Class I or II):
Initial: 15mg qd
Titrate: In increments of 15mg
Max: 45mg qd

PEDIATRIC DOSAGE

Pediatric use may not have been established

DOSING CONSIDERATIONS

Concomitant Medications

Insulin Secretagogue:
Reduce dose of insulin secretagogue if hypoglycemia occurs

Insulin:
Decrease insulin dose by 10-25% if hypoglycemia occurs

Gemfibrozil/Other Strong CYP2C8 Inhibitors:
Max: 15mg qd

ADMINISTRATION

Oral route

Take w/o regard to meals

HOW SUPPLIED

Tab: 15mg, 30mg, 45mg

CONTRAINDICATIONS

Established NYHA Class III or IV HF, known hypersensitivity to pioglitazone or any other component of this medication.

WARNINGS/PRECAUTIONS

Not for use in treatment of type 1 DM or diabetic ketoacidosis. Fatal and nonfatal hepatic failure reported. May use with caution in patients with lesser ALT elevations or bilirubin and with an alternate probable cause. Obtain LFTs prior to initiation; caution with liver disease/abnormal LFTs. D/C if ALT >3X ULN; do not restart if cause of abnormal LFTs not established or if ALT remains >3X ULN with total bilirubin >2X ULN without alternative etiologies. Not for use in patients with active bladder cancer; consider benefits versus risks in patients with a prior history of bladder cancer. New onset or worsening of edema reported; caution in patients with edema and in patients at risk for CHF. Increased incidence of bone fractures reported in females. Macular edema reported; refer to an ophthalmologist if visual symptoms develop. Ovulation in premenopausal anovulatory patients may occur; use adequate contraception.

ADVERSE REACTIONS

CHF, URTI, hypoglycemia, edema, headache, cardiac failure, pain in extremity, sinusitis, back pain, myalgia, pharyngitis, chest pain.

DRUG INTERACTIONS

Increased exposure and $T_{1/2}$ with CYP2C8 inhibitors (eg, gemfibrozil). Decreased exposure with CYP2C8 inducers (eg, rifampin). Risk of fluid retention and hypoglycemia with insulin and other antidiabetic medications (eg, insulin secretagogues such as sulfonylureas).

PATIENT CONSIDERATIONS

Assessment: Assess for previous hypersensitivity, HF, edema, risk factors for developing HF, liver disease, bone health, active/history of bladder cancer, pregnancy/nursing status, and possible drug interactions. Obtain baseline LFTs.

Monitoring: Monitor for signs and symptoms of HF, edema, weight gain, hematological changes (eg, decreases in Hgb, Hct), liver injury, macular edema, bone fractures, ovulation in premenopausal anovulatory women, and other adverse reactions. Perform periodic measurements of FPG and HbA1c. Periodically monitor LFTs in patients with liver disease. Perform periodic eye exams.

Counseling: Advise to adhere to dietary instructions and have blood glucose and glycosylated Hgb levels tested regularly. Instruct to seek medical advice promptly during periods of stress and report rapid increase in weight or edema, SOB, or other symptoms of HF to physician. Instruct to d/c and consult physician if unexplained N/V, abdominal pain, anorexia, fatigue, or dark urine occurs. Advise to report any signs of macroscopic hematuria or other symptoms such as dysuria or urinary urgency. Advise to take qd with or without meals. If dose is missed, advise to not double the dose the following day. Inform about the risk of hypoglycemia when using with insulin or other antidiabetic medications. Inform that therapy may result in ovulation in some premenopausal anovulatory women; recommend adequate contraception for all premenopausal women.

STORAGE: 25°C (77°F); excursions permitted to 15-30°C (59-86°F). Protect from light, moisture, and humidity.

ACULAR LS – ketorolac tromethamine

RX

Class: NSAID

ADULT DOSAGE

Corneal Refractive Surgery

Reduction of Ocular Pain and Burning/Stinging:

1 drop qid in the operated eye prn for up to 4 days following surgery

PEDIATRIC DOSAGE

Corneal Refractive Surgery

Reduction of Ocular Pain and Burning/Stinging:

≥3 Years:

1 drop qid in the operated eye prn for up to 4 days following surgery

ADMINISTRATION

Ocular route

HOW SUPPLIED

Sol: 0.4% [5mL]

CONTRAINDICATIONS

Previously demonstrated hypersensitivity to any of the ingredients in the formulation.

WARNINGS/PRECAUTIONS

Potential cross-sensitivity to acetylsalicylic acid, phenylacetic acid derivatives, and other NSAIDs; caution with previous sensitivities to these drugs. May increase bleeding of ocular tissues (including hyphemas) in conjunction with ocular surgery; caution with known bleeding tendencies. May slow/delay healing or result in keratitis. Continued use may result in epithelial breakdown, corneal thinning, erosion, ulceration, or perforation; d/c if corneal epithelium breakdown occurs and closely monitor for corneal health. Caution with complicated ocular surgeries, corneal denervation, corneal epithelial defects, diabetes mellitus (DM), ocular surface diseases (eg, dry eye syndrome), rheumatoid arthritis (RA), or repeat ocular surgeries within a short period of time. Use for >24 hrs prior to surgery or beyond 14 days postsurgery may increase risk for occurrence and severity of corneal adverse events. Avoid in late pregnancy.

ADVERSE REACTIONS
Transient stinging/burning, allergic reactions, corneal edema, iritis, ocular inflammation/irritation/pain, superficial keratitis, superficial ocular infections.

DRUG INTERACTIONS
Concomitant use of topical NSAIDs and topical steroids may increase potential for healing problems. Caution with other medications that may prolong bleeding time.

PATIENT CONSIDERATIONS

Assessment: Assess for drug hypersensitivity, cross-sensitivity reactions, bleeding tendencies, complicated ocular surgeries, corneal denervation, corneal epithelial defects, DM, ocular surface diseases, RA, and possible drug interactions.

Monitoring: Monitor for bleeding of ocular tissues, healing problems, keratitis, corneal epithelial breakdown, and corneal thinning/erosion/ulceration/perforation.

Counseling: Advise not to use while wearing contact lenses.

STORAGE: 15-25°C (59-77°F).

ACZONE – dapsone

Class: Sulfone

RX

ADULT DOSAGE

Acne Vulgaris

Apply a pea-sized amount of gel in a thin layer to the affected areas bid

If no improvement seen after 12 weeks, reassess treatment

PEDIATRIC DOSAGE

Acne Vulgaris

≥12 Years:

Apply a pea-sized amount of gel in a thin layer to the affected areas bid

If no improvement seen after 12 weeks, reassess treatment

ADMINISTRATION
Topical route

Apply the gel after skin is gently washed and patted dry; rub in gently and completely. Wash hands after application.

HOW SUPPLIED
Gel: 5% [30g, 60g, 90g]

WARNINGS/PRECAUTIONS
Cases of methemoglobinemia reported; avoid use in patients w/ congenital or idiopathic methemoglobinemia. D/C and seek immediate medical attention in the event of cyanosis. Laboratory changes suggestive of hemolysis reported in some patients w/ G6PD deficiency; d/c if signs/symptoms suggestive of hemolytic anemia occur. Peripheral neuropathy (motor loss, muscle weakness) and skin reactions (toxic epidermal necrolysis, erythema multiforme, morbilliform/scarlatiniform reactions, bullous/exfoliative dermatitis, erythema nodosum, urticaria) reported w/ oral dapsone.

ADVERSE REACTIONS
Oiliness/peeling, dryness, erythema.

DRUG INTERACTIONS
Avoid w/ patients taking oral dapsone or antimalarial medications due to potential for hemolytic reactions. Trimethoprim/sulfamethoxazole may increase levels. Trimethoprim/sulfamethoxazole may increase likelihood of hemolysis in patients w/ G6PD deficiency. Topical benzoyl peroxide reported to cause a temporary local yellow or orange discoloration of the skin and facial hair. Folic acid antagonists (eg, pyrimethamine) may increase hematologic reactions w/ oral dapsone treatment. Coadministration of oral dapsone w/ certain medications (eg, rifampin, anticonvulsants, St. John's wort) may increase dapsone hydroxylamine formation, a metabolite of dapsone associated w/ hemolysis. Concomitant use w/ drugs that induce methemoglobinemia (eg, sulfonamides, acetaminophen, acetanilide, benzocaine, chloroquine, nitrates and nitrites, phenobarbital, phenytoin) may increase risk for developing methemoglobinemia.

PATIENT CONSIDERATIONS

Assessment: Assess for congenital or idiopathic methemoglobinemia, G6PD deficiency, previous allergic reactions to the drug, pregnancy/nursing status, and for possible drug interactions.

Monitoring: Monitor for signs/symptoms of methemoglobinemia, hemolytic anemia, skin reactions, and other adverse reactions. Monitor for response to treatment; reevaluate if no improvement is seen after 12 weeks of therapy.

Counseling: Advise to seek immediate medical attention for cyanosis. Instruct to use externally and ud. Inform that drug is not for oral, ophthalmic or intravaginal use. Instruct to notify physician if any signs of adverse reactions occur.

STORAGE: 20-25°C (68-77°F); excursions permitted to 15-30°C (59-86°F). Protect from freezing.

ADALAT CC – nifedipine

RX

Class: Calcium channel blocker (CCB) (dihydropyridine)

OTHER BRAND NAMES
Nifediac CC, Afeditab CR

ADULT DOSAGE

Hypertension

Initial: 30mg qd
Titrate: Increase dose over a 7- to 14-day period based on therapeutic efficacy and safety
Maint: 30-60mg qd
Max: 90mg qd

PEDIATRIC DOSAGE

Pediatric use may not have been established

DOSING CONSIDERATIONS

Elderly
Start at low end of dosing range

Discontinuation
Decrease dose gradually w/ close physician supervision

ADMINISTRATION
Oral route

Take PO on empty stomach
Swallow tab whole; do not chew, crush, or divide

HOW SUPPLIED
Tab, Extended-Release: (Adalat CC) 30mg, 60mg, 90mg, (Afeditab CR) 30mg, 60mg, (Nifediac CC) 30mg, 60mg, 90mg

CONTRAINDICATIONS
Known hypersensitivity to nifedipine or any component of the tablet. (Adalat CC) Cardiogenic shock and concomitant use with strong P450 inducers (eg, rifampin).

WARNINGS/PRECAUTIONS
May cause hypotension; monitor BP initially or with titration. May increase frequency, duration, and/or severity of angina or acute myocardial infarction (MI) upon starting or at time of dose increase, particularly with severe obstructive coronary artery disease (CAD). May develop congestive heart failure (CHF), especially with tight aortic stenosis or β-blockers. Peripheral edema may occur; rule out peripheral edema caused by left ventricular dysfunction if HTN is complicated by CHF. Transient elevations of enzymes (eg, alkaline phosphatase, CPK, LDH, SGOT, SGPT), cholestasis with/without jaundice, and allergic hepatitis reported rarely. May decrease platelet aggregation and increase bleeding time. Lab test interactions may occur. Reversible elevations in BUN and SrCr reported rarely in patients with chronic renal insufficiency. Caution with renal/hepatic impairment and in elderly. Adalat CC: Reduced clearance in cirrhosis; initiate lowest dose possible. Contains lactose; avoid with hereditary galactose intolerance problems, Lapp lactase deficiency, and glucose-galactose malabsorption. Nifediac CC: Contains tartrazine, which may cause allergic-type reactions in certain susceptible persons (eg, patients with aspirin hypersensitivity).

ADVERSE REACTIONS
Peripheral edema, headache, flushing, heat sensation, dizziness, fatigue, asthenia, nausea, constipation.

DRUG INTERACTIONS
See Contraindications. β-blockers may increase risk of CHF, severe hypotension, or angina exacerbation; avoid abrupt β-blocker withdrawal. Severe hypotension and/or increased fluid volume may occur with β-blockers and fentanyl or other narcotic analgesics. May increase plasma levels of digoxin; monitor digoxin levels when initiating, adjusting, and discontinuing therapy. May increase PT with coumarin anticoagulants. Monitor with other medications known to lower BP. Enhanced hypotensive effect with benazepril and timolol. Avoid with grapefruit juice; stop grapefruit juice intake at least 3 days prior to therapy. Increased exposure with CYP3A inhibitors (eg, ketoconazole, itraconazole, fluconazole, erythromycin, clarithromycin, nefazodone, fluoxetine, diltiazem, verapamil, cimetidine, quinupristin/dalfopristin, amprenavir, atazanavir, delavirdine, fosamprenavir, indinavir, nelfinavir, ritonavir, saquinavir), valproic acid, and doxazosin; monitor BP and consider dose reduction. Increased levels with quinidine; monitor HR and adjust dose if necessary. Monitor blood glucose levels and consider

dose adjustment with acarbose. May increase plasma levels of metformin. May increase exposure of tacrolimus; monitor blood levels and consider dose reduction. May decrease doxazosin levels; monitor BP and reduce dose. May inhibit metabolism of CYP3A substrates. Afeditab CR/Nifediac CC: Decreased exposure with CYP3A4 inducers (eg, rifampin, rifapentine, phenytoin, phenobarbitone, carbamazepine, St. John's wort); monitor BP and consider dose adjustment. Adalat CC: May increase the BP-lowering effects of diuretics, PDE-5 inhibitors, and α-methyldopa. Magnesium sulfate IV in pregnant women may cause excessive fall in BP. Increased plasma concentrations with cisapride.

PATIENT CONSIDERATIONS

Assessment: Assess for previous hypersensitivity to the drug, CHF, severe obstructive CAD, aortic stenosis, hepatic/renal impairment, pregnancy/nursing status, and possible drug interactions. (Adalat CC) Assess for cirrhosis, hereditary galactose intolerance problems, Lapp lactase deficiency, and glucose-galactose malabsorption. (Nifediac CC) Assess for susceptibility for tartrazine hypersensitivity (eg, aspirin hypersensitivity).

Monitoring: Monitor for excessive hypotension, increased frequency, duration and/or severity of angina and/or acute MI (especially during initiation and dose titration), CHF, peripheral edema, cholestasis with/without jaundice, and allergic hepatitis. Monitor BP, LFTs, BUN, SrCr, and increased bleeding time.

Counseling: Inform about potential benefits/risks of therapy. Instruct to notify physician if pregnant/nursing or if any adverse reactions occur. (Afeditab CR) Advise patients that empty matrix "ghost" tab may pass via colostomy or in the stool and this should not be a concern.

STORAGE: Adalat CC/Afeditab CR: <30°C (86°F). Nifediac CC: 25°C (77°F); excursions permitted to 15-30°C (59-86°F). Protect from light and moisture.

ADDERALL – amphetamine aspartate monohydrate/amphetamine sulfate/dextroamphetamine saccharate/dextroamphetamine sulfate CII

Class: CNS stimulant

High potential for abuse; prolonged use may lead to drug dependence and must be avoided. Misuse of amphetamine may cause sudden death and serious cardiovascular (CV) adverse events.

ADULT DOSAGE

Narcolepsy

Initial: 10mg/day
Titrate: May increase in increments of 10mg at weekly intervals until optimal response is obtained
Usual: 5-60mg/day in divided doses

Give 1st dose on awakening; additional doses (1 or 2) at intervals of 4-6 hrs

Attention-Deficit Hyperactivity Disorder

Refer to pediatric dosing

PEDIATRIC DOSAGE

Narcolepsy

Usual: 5-60mg/day in divided doses

6-12 Years:
Initial: 5mg/day
Titrate: May increase in increments of 5mg at weekly intervals until optimal response is obtained

≥12 Years:
Initial: 10mg/day
Titrate: May increase in increments of 10mg at weekly intervals until optimal response is obtained

Give 1st dose on awakening; additional doses (1 or 2) at intervals of 4-6 hrs

Attention-Deficit Hyperactivity Disorder

3-5 Years:
Initial: 2.5mg/day
Titrate: May increase in increments of 2.5mg at weekly intervals until optimal response is obtained

≥6 Years:
Initial: 5mg qd or bid
Titrate: May increase in increments of 5mg at weekly intervals until optimal response is obtained. Only in rare cases will it be necessary to exceed a total of 40mg/day

Give 1st dose on awakening; additional doses (1 or 2) at intervals of 4-6 hrs

Interrupt occasionally to determine the need for continued therapy

DOSING CONSIDERATIONS

Adverse Reactions

Narcolepsy Patients:

Reduce dose if bothersome adverse reactions appear (eg, insomnia or anorexia)

ADMINISTRATION

Oral route

Give 1st dose on awakening; avoid late pm doses due to potential for insomnia.

HOW SUPPLIED

Tab: 5mg*, 7.5mg*, 10mg*, 12.5mg*, 15mg*, 20mg*, 30mg* *scored

CONTRAINDICATIONS

Advanced arteriosclerosis, symptomatic CV disease, moderate to severe HTN, hyperthyroidism, known hypersensitivity or idiosyncrasy to the sympathomimetic amines, glaucoma, agitated states, history of drug abuse, during or w/in 14 days of MAOI use.

WARNINGS/PRECAUTIONS

Sudden death reported in children and adolescents w/ structural cardiac abnormalities or other serious heart problems. Sudden death, stroke, and MI reported in adults. Avoid use in patients w/ serious structural cardiac abnormalities, cardiomyopathy, serious heart rhythm abnormalities, coronary artery disease, or other serious cardiac problems. May cause modest increase in average BP and HR. Perform prompt cardiac evaluation when symptoms suggestive of cardiac disease develop. May exacerbate symptoms of behavior disturbance and thought disorder in patients w/ preexisting psychotic disorder. Caution in patients w/ comorbid bipolar disorder; may induce mixed/manic episodes. May cause treatment-emergent psychotic/manic symptoms in children and adolescents w/o prior history of psychotic illness or mania; consider discontinuation if such symptoms occur. Aggressive behavior or hostility reported in children and adolescents w/ ADHD. May cause long-term suppression of growth in children; may need to interrupt treatment if patients are not growing or gaining weight as expected. May lower convulsive threshold; d/c if seizures develop. Associated w/ peripheral vasculopathy, including Raynaud's phenomenon. Difficulties w/ accommodation and blurring of vision reported. May exacerbate motor and phonic tics and Tourette's syndrome. May cause a significant elevation in plasma corticosteroid levels or interfere w/ urinary steroid determinations.

ADVERSE REACTIONS

Palpitations, tachycardia, BP elevation, psychotic episodes, tremor, blurred vision, mydriasis, dry mouth, unpleasant taste, anorexia, urticaria, rash, libido changes, alopecia, rhabdomyolysis.

DRUG INTERACTIONS

See Contraindications. GI alkalinizing agents (eg, sodium bicarbonate, antacids) and urinary alkalinizing agents (eg, acetazolamide, some thiazides) may increase blood levels and potentiate effects; avoid w/ GI alkalinizing agents. GI acidifying agents (eg, guanethidine, reserpine, glutamic acid HCl) and urinary acidifying agents (eg, ammonium chloride, sodium acid phosphate) may lower blood levels and efficacy. May inhibit adrenergic blockers. May enhance activity of TCAs or sympathomimetic agents; caution w/ other sympathomimetic drugs. Increased d-amphetamine levels in the brain w/ desipramine or protriptyline and possibly other tricyclics. May counteract sedative effect of antihistamines. May antagonize the hypotensive effects of antihypertensives. Chlorpromazine and haloperidol may inhibit the central stimulant effects. Lithium carbonate may inhibit the anorectic and stimulatory effects. May delay intestinal absorption of ethosuximide, phenobarbital, and phenytoin; may produce a synergistic anticonvulsant action if coadministered w/ phenobarbital or phenytoin. May potentiate analgesic effect of meperidine. May enhance the adrenergic effect of norepinephrine. Use in cases of propoxyphene overdose may potentiate CNS stimulation and cause fatal convulsions. Monitor for changes in clinical effect when coadministered w/ proton pump inhibitors. May inhibit the hypotensive effect of veratrum alkaloids.

PATIENT CONSIDERATIONS

Assessment: Assess for advanced arteriosclerosis, symptomatic CV disease, moderate to severe HTN, hyperthyroidism, hypersensitivity or idiosyncrasy to sympathomimetic amines, glaucoma, agitation, history of drug abuse, psychiatric history, history of seizure, tics or Tourette's syndrome, pregnancy/nursing status, and possible drug interactions. Prior to treatment, adequately screen patients to determine risk for bipolar disorder.

Monitoring: Monitor for CV abnormalities, exacerbations of behavior disturbances and thought disorder, psychotic or manic symptoms, aggressive behavior, hostility, seizures, visual disturbances, exacerbation of motor and phonic tics and Tourette's syndrome, and other adverse reactions. Monitor BP and HR. Monitor growth and weight in children. Periodically reevaluate long-term usefulness of therapy. Observe carefully for signs and symptoms of peripheral vasculopathy; further clinical evaluation (eg, rheumatology referral) may be appropriate for certain patients.

Counseling: Inform about benefits and risks of treatment, appropriate use, and about the potential for abuse/dependence. Instruct to use caution when engaging in potentially hazardous activities (eg, operating machinery or vehicles). Inform about the risk of peripheral vasculopathy, including Raynaud's phenomenon; instruct to report to physician any new numbness, pain, skin color change, or sensitivity to temperature in fingers or toes, and to call physician immediately if any signs of unexplained wounds appear on fingers or toes while on therapy.

STORAGE: 20-25°C (68-77°F).

ADDERALL XR – amphetamine aspartate monohydrate/amphetamine sulfate/dextroamphetamine saccharate/dextroamphetamine sulfate CII

Class: CNS stimulant

High potential for abuse; prolonged use may lead to drug dependence. Misuse may cause sudden death and serious cardiovascular (CV) adverse reactions.

ADULT DOSAGE

Attention-Deficit Hyperactivity Disorder

Amphetamine-Naive/Switching from Another Medication: 20mg qam

Switching from Amphetamine Immediate-Release: Give the same total daily dose, qd

Titrate at weekly intervals as indicated

PEDIATRIC DOSAGE

Attention-Deficit Hyperactivity Disorder

Amphetamine-Naive/Switching from Another Medication:

6-12 Years:

Initial: 10mg qam or 5mg qam when lower initial dose is appropriate

Titrate: Adjust daily dosage in increments of 5mg or 10mg at weekly intervals

Max: 30mg/day

13-17 Years:

Initial: 10mg qam

Titrate: May increase to 20mg/day after 1 week if symptoms are not controlled

Switching from Amphetamine Immediate-Release:

≥6 Years:

Give the same total daily dose, qd

Titrate at weekly intervals as indicated

ADMINISTRATION

Oral route

Give upon awakening; avoid pm doses due to potential for insomnia

Take w/ or w/o food

Take caps whole or sprinkle entire contents on applesauce. Consume sprinkled applesauce immediately w/o chewing the sprinkled beads

Do not divide the dose of a single cap or take anything <1 cap/day

HOW SUPPLIED

Cap, Extended-Release: 5mg, 10mg, 15mg, 20mg, 25mg, 30mg

CONTRAINDICATIONS

Advanced arteriosclerosis, symptomatic CV disease, moderate to severe HTN, hyperthyroidism, known hypersensitivity or idiosyncrasy to the sympathomimetic amines (eg, anaphylaxis, angioedema, serious skin rashes), glaucoma, agitated states, history of drug abuse, during or w/in 14 days following MAOI use.

WARNINGS/PRECAUTIONS

Sudden death, stroke, and MI reported in adults. Sudden death reported in children and adolescents w/ structural cardiac abnormalities or other serious heart problems. Avoid use in patients w/ known serious structural cardiac and heart rhythm abnormalities, cardiomyopathy, coronary artery disease, or other serious cardiac problems. May cause modest increase in BP and HR. May exacerbate symptoms of behavior disturbance and thought disorder in patients w/ preexisting psychotic disorder. Caution in patients w/ comorbid bipolar disorder; may cause induction of mixed/manic episode. May cause treatment-emergent psychotic/manic symptoms in children and adolescents w/o a prior history of psychotic illness or mania; consider discontinuation if such symptoms occur. Aggressive behavior or hostility reported; monitor for appearance or worsening. May cause long-term suppression of growth in children; may need to d/c if patients are not growing or gaining weight as expected. May lower convulsive threshold; d/c if seizures develop. Associated w/ peripheral vasculopathy, including Raynaud's phenomenon. Difficulties w/ accommodation and blurring of vision reported. Exacerbation of motor and phonic tics and Tourette's syndrome reported. May significantly elevate plasma corticosteroid levels or interfere w/ urinary steroid determinations. Where possible, interrupt occasionally to determine the need for continued therapy.

ADVERSE REACTIONS
Dry mouth, loss of appetite, insomnia, headache, abdominal pain, weight loss, agitation, anxiety, N/V, dizziness, tachycardia, nervousness, asthenia, diarrhea, UTI.

DRUG INTERACTIONS
See Contraindications. Avoid w/ GI alkalinizing agents (eg, sodium bicarbonate, antacids). Urinary alkalinizing agents (eg, acetazolamide, some thiazides) may increase blood levels and potentiate effects. GI acidifying agents (eg, guanethidine, reserpine, ascorbic acid) and urinary acidifying agents (eg, ammonium chloride, sodium acid phosphate, methenamine salts) may lower blood levels and efficacy. May reduce CV effects of adrenergic blockers. May counteract sedative effects of antihistamines. May antagonize effects of antihypertensives. May inhibit hypotensive effect of veratrum alkaloids. May delay intestinal absorption of phenobarbital, phenytoin, and ethosuximide. May enhance activity of TCAs or sympathomimetic agents. Increased d-amphetamine levels in the brain w/ desipramine or protriptyline and possibly other tricyclics. May potentiate analgesic effect of meperidine. May enhance the adrenergic effect of norepinephrine. Chlorpromazine and haloperidol may inhibit central stimulant effects. Lithium carbonate may inhibit anorectic and stimulatory effects. Norepinephrine may enhance the adrenergic effect. Use in cases of propoxyphene overdose may potentiate CNS stimulation and cause fatal convulsions. Monitor for changes in clinical effect when coadministered w/ proton pump inhibitors.

PATIENT CONSIDERATIONS

Assessment: Assess for advanced arteriosclerosis, symptomatic CV disease, moderate to severe HTN, hyperthyroidism, hypersensitivity or idiosyncrasy to sympathomimetic amines, glaucoma, agitation, history of drug abuse, psychiatric history, history of seizure, tics or Tourette's syndrome, hepatic/renal dysfunction, pregnancy/nursing status, and possible drug interactions.

Monitoring: Monitor for CV abnormalities, exacerbations of behavior disturbances and thought disorder, psychotic or manic symptoms, aggressive behavior, hostility, seizures, visual disturbances, exacerbation of motor and phonic tics and Tourette's syndrome, and other adverse reactions. Monitor BP and HR. Monitor height and weight in children. Observe carefully for signs and symptoms of peripheral vasculopathy; further clinical evaluation (eg, rheumatology referral) may be appropriate for certain patients.

Counseling: Inform about benefits and risks of treatment, appropriate use, and about the potential for abuse/dependence. Advise about serious CV risks. Inform that treatment-emergent psychotic or manic symptoms may occur. Instruct to report signs/symptoms of peripheral vasculopathy, including Raynaud's phenomenon. Advise parents or guardians of pediatric patients to monitor growth and weight during treatment. Advise to notify physician if pregnant or planning to become pregnant. Advise to avoid breastfeeding. Advise to use caution when engaging in potentially hazardous activities (eg, operating machinery or vehicles).

STORAGE: 25°C (77°F); excursions permitted to 15-30°C (59-86°F).

Addyi – flibanserin

RX

Class: Mixed 5-HT_{1A} agonist/5-HT_{2A} antagonist

Alcohol increases the risk of severe hypotension and syncope; alcohol use is contraindicated. Before prescribing, assess the likelihood of abstaining from alcohol, taking into account current/past drinking behavior, and other pertinent social and medical history. Available only through a restricted program under a Risk Evaluation and Mitigation Strategy (REMS) called the Addyi REMS Program. Contraindicated w/ concomitant moderate or strong CYP3A4 inhibitors and in patients w/ hepatic impairment due to increases in flibanserin concentrations and potential for severe hypotension and syncope.

ADULT DOSAGE

Hypoactive Sexual Desire Disorder

Treatment of premenopausal women w/ acquired, generalized hypoactive sexual desire disorder (HSDD), as characterized by low sexual desire that causes marked distress or interpersonal difficulty and is not caused by a coexisting medical or psychiatric condition, problems w/in the relationship, or the effects of a medication or other drug substance

100mg qhs; d/c after 8 weeks if no improvement in symptoms

Missed Dose

If dose is missed at hs; take next dose at hs on the next day; do not double the next dose

PEDIATRIC DOSAGE

Pediatric use may not have been established

DOSING CONSIDERATIONS

Concomitant Medication

If initiating flibanserin following moderate/strong CYP3A4 inhibitor use, start 2 weeks after last dose of the CYP3A4 inhibitor

If initiating a moderate or strong CYP3A4 inhibitor following flibanserin use, start moderate or strong CYP3A4 inhibitor 2 days after the last dose of flibanserin

ADMINISTRATION

Oral route

HOW SUPPLIED

Tab: 100mg

CONTRAINDICATIONS

Concomitant use w/ alcohol, moderate or strong CYP3A4 inhibitors, and in patients w/ hepatic impairment.

WARNINGS/PRECAUTIONS

Not for use in HSDD due to a coexisting medical or psychiatric condition, problems w/in the relationship, or the effects of a medication or other drug substance. May cause CNS depression (eg, somnolence, sedation), hypotension, and syncope; increased risk if taken during waking hrs. Patients should not drive or engage in activities requiring full alertness until ≥6 hrs after taking the drug and until they know how it affects them. Consider the benefits of use and the risks of hypotension and syncope in patients w/ preexisting conditions that predispose them to hypotension. Immediately lie supine if experiencing presyncope and promptly seek medical help if the symptoms do not resolve or if experiencing syncope. CYP2C19 poor metabolizers had increased flibanserin exposures; increase monitoring for adverse reactions.

ADVERSE REACTIONS

Dizziness, somnolence, nausea, fatigue, insomnia.

DRUG INTERACTIONS

See Boxed Warning/Dosing Considerations. If benefit of initiating a moderate/strong CYP3A4 inhibitor (eg, ketoconazole, clarithromycin, ciprofloxacin) w/in 2 days of stopping flibanserin outweighs risk, monitor patient for signs of hypotension and syncope. Concomitant use of multiple weak CYP3A4 inhibitors (eg, cimetidine, fluoxetine, ginkgo) may increase flibanserin concentrations. CNS depressants (eg, diphenhydramine, opioids, hypnotics) may increase the risk of CNS depression. Strong CYP2C19 inhibitors (eg, proton pump inhibitors, SSRIs, benzodiazepines) may increase flibanserin exposure. CYP3A4 inducers (eg, carbamazepine, phenobarbital, rifampin) decrease flibanserin exposure; concomitant use is not recommended. May increase concentrations of digoxin or other P-gp substrates (eg, sirolimus); increase monitoring of concentrations of drugs transported by P-gp that have a narrow therapeutic index.

PATIENT CONSIDERATIONS

Assessment: Assess for coexisting medical or psychiatric conditions, problems w/in the relationship, or effects of a medication or other drug substance that may be contributing to HSDD. Assess for alcohol use and likelihood of the patient abstaining from alcohol, taking into account the patient's current and past drinking behavior, and other pertinent social and medical history. Assess if patient is a poor CYP2C19 metabolizer. Assess for preexisting conditions that predispose to hypotension, hepatic impairment, pregnancy/nursing status, and for possible drug interactions.

Monitoring: Monitor for somnolence, sedation, hypotension, syncope, and other adverse reactions. Perform increased monitoring for adverse reactions in patients who are CYP2C19 poor metabolizers. Increase monitoring of concentrations of drugs transported by P-gp that have a narrow therapeutic index (eg, digoxin).

Counseling: Advise to take at hs and not any other time of the day. Inform that drug may cause severe hypotension and syncope, particularly w/ alcohol or w/ moderate and strong CYP3A4 inhibitors; inform that concomitant use is contraindicated. Notify about the importance of abstaining from alcohol and to consult w/ physician before starting a new prescription, nonprescription medication, or using other products that contain CYP3A4 inhibitors (eg, grapefruit juice, St. John's wort). Advise patients who experience presyncope or lightheadedness to lie down and to call for help if symptoms persist. Inform that drug may cause CNS depression and that risk is increased if taken during waking hrs; advise to avoid engaging in activities requiring full alertness until ≥6 hrs after taking the drug and until the patient knows how it affects her. Advise not to breastfeed.

STORAGE: Store at 25°C (77°F); excursions permitted to 15-30°C (59-86°F).

ADVAIR DISKUS – fluticasone propionate/salmeterol RX

Class: $Beta_2$ agonist/corticosteroid

Long-acting β_2-adrenergic agonists (LABAs), such as salmeterol, increase the risk of asthma-related death. LABAs may increase the risk of asthma-related hospitalization in pediatric and adolescent patients. Use only for patients not adequately controlled on a long-term asthma control medication (eg, inhaled corticosteroid) or whose disease severity clearly warrants initiation of treatment with both an inhaled corticosteroid and a LABA. Do not use if asthma is adequately controlled on low- or medium-dose inhaled corticosteroids.

ADULT DOSAGE

Asthma

1 inh bid, approx 12 hrs apart

Titrate: May replace current strength with a higher strength if response to initial dose after 2 weeks is inadequate

Max: 500/50 bid

Chronic Obstructive Pulmonary Disease

Maint Treatment of Airflow Obstruction:

1 inh of 250/50 bid, approx 12 hrs apart

PEDIATRIC DOSAGE

Asthma

4-11 Years:

1 inh of 100/50 bid, approx 12 hrs apart

≥12 Years:

1 inh bid, approx 12 hrs apart

Titrate: May replace current strength with a higher strength if response to initial dose after 2 weeks is inadequate

Max: 500/50 bid

ADMINISTRATION

Oral inh route

After inhalation, rinse mouth with water without swallowing

HOW SUPPLIED

Disk: (Fluticasone-Salmeterol) (100/50) 100mcg-50mcg/inh, (250/50) 250mcg-50mcg/inh, (500/50) 500mcg-50mcg/inh [14, 60 blisters]

CONTRAINDICATIONS

Primary treatment of status asthmaticus or other acute episodes of asthma or COPD where intensive measures are required. Milk protein hypersensitivity.

WARNINGS/PRECAUTIONS

Not indicated for acute bronchospasm relief. Do not initiate during rapidly deteriorating or potentially life-threatening episodes of asthma or COPD; serious acute respiratory events reported. D/C regular use of oral/inhaled short-acting β_2-agonists (SABAs) when beginning treatment. Do not use more often or at higher doses than recommended; clinically significant cardiovascular (CV) effects and fatalities reported with excessive use. *Candida albicans* infections of mouth and pharynx reported; treat and if needed, interrupt therapy. Lower respiratory tract infections (eg, pneumonia) reported in patients with COPD. Increased susceptibility to infections. May lead to serious/fatal course of chickenpox or measles; avoid exposure and, if exposed, consider prophylaxis/treatment. Caution with active/quiescent tuberculosis (TB), systemic fungal, bacterial, viral, or parasitic infections, or ocular herpes simplex. Deaths due to adrenal insufficiency reported during and after transfer from systemic to inhaled corticosteroids; wean slowly from systemic corticosteroid use after transferring to therapy. Resume oral corticosteroids during periods of stress or a severe asthma attack in patients previously withdrawn from systemic corticosteroids. Transfer from systemic to inhaled corticosteroids may unmask allergic conditions previously suppressed by systemic therapy (eg, rhinitis, conjunctivitis, eczema). Monitor for systemic corticosteroid effects. Reduce dose slowly and consider other treatments if hypercorticism and adrenal suppression occur. May produce paradoxical bronchospasm; treat immediately with an inhaled, short acting bronchodilator; d/c and institute alternative therapy. Upper airway symptoms reported. Immediate hypersensitivity reactions, and CV and CNS effects may occur. Decreases in bone mineral density (BMD) reported with long-term use; caution with major risk factors for decreased bone mineral content, including chronic use of drugs that can reduce bone mass (eg, anticonvulsants, oral corticosteroids). Assess BMD prior to initiating therapy and periodically thereafter in patients with COPD; if significant reductions in BMD are seen and therapy is still considered medically important, use medicine to treat or prevent osteoporosis. May reduce growth velocity in pediatric patients; routinely monitor growth. Glaucoma, increased intraocular pressure (IOP), and cataracts reported with long-term use. Systemic eosinophilic conditions, and vasculitis consistent with Churg-Strauss syndrome may occur. Caution with CV disorders, convulsive disorders, thyrotoxicosis, diabetes mellitus (DM), ketoacidosis, hepatic disease, and in patients unusually responsive to sympathomimetic amines. Clinically significant changes in blood glucose and/or serum K^+ reported.

ADVERSE REACTIONS

Upper respiratory tract infection/inflammation, pharyngitis, hoarseness/dysphonia, bronchitis, cough, headache, N/V, sinusitis, throat irritation, viral respiratory infection, musculoskeletal pain, fever, dizziness.

DRUG INTERACTIONS

Do not use with other medicines containing LABA. Not recommended with strong CYP3A4 inhibitors (eg, ritonavir, clarithromycin, itraconazole); increased systemic corticosteroid and increased CV adverse effects may occur. Extreme caution with TCAs or MAOIs, or within 2 weeks of discontinuation of such agents; action on the vascular system may be potentiated. β-blockers may block pulmonary effects and produce severe bronchospasm; if such therapy is needed, consider cardioselective β-blockers and use with caution. Caution is advised when coadministered with non-K^+-sparing diuretics (eg, loop, thiazide).

PATIENT CONSIDERATIONS

Assessment: Assess for hypersensitivity to milk proteins, status asthmaticus, acute asthma/COPD episodes, rapidly deteriorating asthma/COPD, active/quiescent TB, systemic infections, ocular herpes simplex, risk factors for decreased bone mineral content, CV disorders, convulsive disorders, thyrotoxicosis, DM, ketoacidosis, history of increased IOP, glaucoma, and/or cataracts, hepatic disease, pregnancy/nursing status, and possible drug interactions. Assess BMD in patients with COPD.

Monitoring: Monitor for deteriorating disease, localized oropharyngeal *C. albicans* infections, pneumonia, infections, systemic corticosteroid effects (eg, hypercorticism, adrenal suppression), paradoxical bronchospasm, upper airway symptoms, immediate hypersensitivity reactions, CV and CNS effects, glaucoma, cataracts, increased IOP, eosinophilic conditions, changes in blood glucose and/or serum K^+, and other adverse reactions. Periodically monitor BMD in patients with COPD. Monitor growth of pediatric patients routinely. Closely monitor patients with hepatic disease.

Counseling: Counsel about the risks and benefits of therapy. Inform that drug is not meant to relieve acute asthma symptoms or exacerbations of COPD; advise to treat acute symptoms with an inhaled SABA (eg, albuterol). Instruct to seek medical attention immediately if experiencing a decrease in effectiveness of inhaled SABAs, a need for more inhalations than usual of inhaled SABAs, or a significant decrease in lung function. Advise not to d/c therapy without physician guidance and not to use other LABA. Instruct to contact physician if oropharyngeal candidiasis or symptoms of pneumonia develop. Advise to avoid exposure to chickenpox or measles, and, if exposed, to consult physician without delay. Inform about risk of immunosuppression, hypercorticism, adrenal suppression, reduction in BMD, reduced growth velocity in pediatric patients, ocular effects, and of adverse effects (eg, palpitations, chest pain, rapid HR, tremor, nervousness). Instruct to d/c therapy if immediate hypersensitivity reactions occur. Inform that the inhaler is not reusable and advise not to take the inhaler apart.

STORAGE: 20-25°C (68-77°F); excursions permitted from 15-30°C (59-86°F). Store in a dry place away from direct heat or sunlight. Store inside the unopened moisture-protective foil pouch and only remove from the pouch immediately before initial use. Discard 1 month after opening the foil pouch or when the counter reads "0," whichever comes 1st.

ADVAIR HFA – fluticasone propionate/salmeterol RX

Class: $Beta_2$ agonist/corticosteroid

Long-acting β_2-adrenergic agonists (LABAs), such as salmeterol, increase the risk of asthma-related death. LABAs may increase the risk of asthma-related hospitalization in pediatric and adolescent patients. Use only for patients not adequately controlled on a long-term asthma control medication (eg, inhaled corticosteroid) or whose disease severity clearly warrants initiation of treatment w/ both an inhaled corticosteroid and a LABA. Do not use if asthma is adequately controlled on low- or medium-dose inhaled corticosteroids.

ADULT DOSAGE

Asthma

2 inh bid, approx 12 hrs apart

Titrate: Replace w/ higher strength if response is inadequate after 2 weeks

Max: 2 inh of 230/21 bid

PEDIATRIC DOSAGE

Asthma

≥12 Years:

2 inh bid, approx 12 hrs apart

Titrate: Replace w/ higher strength if response is inadequate after 2 weeks

Max: 2 inh of 230/21 bid

DOSING CONSIDERATIONS

Elderly

Start at lower end of dosing range

ADMINISTRATION

Oral inh route

Rinse mouth w/ water (w/o swallowing) after inh.
Shake well for 5 sec before each spray.

Priming Instructions
Prime before using for the 1st time by releasing 4 sprays into the air away from the face; if the inhaler has not been used for >4 weeks or has been dropped, prime the inhaler by releasing 2 sprays into the air away from the face

HOW SUPPLIED
MDI: (Fluticasone/Salmeterol) (45/21) (45mcg/21mcg)/inh, (115/21) (115mcg/21mcg)/inh, (230/21) (230mcg/21mcg)/inh [60, 120 inhalations]

CONTRAINDICATIONS
Primary treatment of status asthmaticus or other acute episodes of asthma where intensive measures are required. Hypersensitivity to any of the ingredients.

WARNINGS/PRECAUTIONS
Not indicated for acute bronchospasm relief. Do not initiate during rapidly deteriorating or potentially life-threatening episodes of asthma. D/C regular use of oral/inhaled short-acting β_2-agonists (SABAs) when beginning treatment. May produce paradoxical bronchospasm; treat immediately, d/c Advair HFA, and institute alternative therapy. Upper airway symptoms reported. Immediate hypersensitivity reactions, including anaphylaxis, may occur. Fluticasone: *Candida albicans* infections of the mouth and pharynx reported; treat and, if needed, interrupt therapy w/ Advair HFA. Lower respiratory tract infections (eg, pneumonia) reported in patients w/ COPD. Increased susceptibility to infections. Chickenpox or measles may have a more serious/fatal course; avoid exposure and, if exposed, consider prophylaxis/treatment. Use w/ caution, if at all, in patients w/ active/quiescent tuberculosis (TB); systemic fungal, bacterial, viral, or parasitic infections; or ocular herpes simplex. Deaths due to adrenal insufficiency reported during and after transfer from systemic corticosteroids to inhaled corticosteroids. Patients who have been withdrawn from systemic corticosteroids should resume oral corticosteroids (in large doses) immediately during periods of stress or a severe asthma attack. Patients requiring oral corticosteroids should be weaned slowly from systemic corticosteroid use after transferring to therapy. Systemic corticosteroid effects (eg, hypercorticism and adrenal suppression) may occur in patients sensitive to these effects; if such effects occur, reduce therapy slowly and consider other treatments for management of asthma symptoms. Decreases in bone mineral density (BMD) reported w/ long-term use. May reduce growth velocity in pediatric patients. Glaucoma, increased IOP, and cataracts reported w/ long-term use. Systemic eosinophilic conditions may occur; some patients have clinical features of vasculitis consistent w/ Churg-Strauss syndrome. Salmeterol: Clinically significant cardiovascular (CV) effects and fatalities reported w/ excessive use. CNS effects (eg, seizures, angina, hypertension/hypotension) associated w/ excessive β-adrenergic stimulation. Caution w/ convulsive disorders, thyrotoxicosis, and in patients unusually responsive to sympathomimetic amines. Large doses of IV albuterol reported to aggravate preexisting diabetes mellitus (DM) and ketoacidosis. Clinically significant changes in blood glucose and/or serum K^+ reported infrequently.

ADVERSE REACTIONS
Upper respiratory tract infection or inflammation, headache, throat irritation, musculoskeletal pain, N/V, dizziness, viral GI infection, hoarseness/dysphonia, GI signs and symptoms.

DRUG INTERACTIONS
Do not use w/ other medicines containing LABAs. Not recommended w/ strong CYP3A4 inhibitors (eg, ritonavir [RTV], clarithromycin, itraconazole); increased systemic corticosteroid and increased CV adverse effects may occur. Fluticasone: RTV and ketoconazole may increase exposure and reduce cortisol levels. Salmeterol: Extreme caution w/ TCAs or MAOIs, or w/in 2 weeks of discontinuation of such agents; action on the vascular system may be potentiated. β-blockers may block pulmonary effects and also produce severe bronchospasm in patients w/ asthma; if such therapy is needed, consider cardioselective β-blockers and use w/ caution. Use caution when coadministered w/ non-K^+-sparing diuretics (eg, loop, thiazide).

PATIENT CONSIDERATIONS

Assessment: Assess for status asthmaticus, acute asthma episodes, rapidly deteriorating asthma, active/quiescent TB, systemic infections, ocular herpes simplex, risk factors for decreased bone mineral content, CV disorders, convulsive disorders, thyrotoxicosis, DM, ketoacidosis, history of increased IOP, glaucoma, and/or cataracts, hepatic disease, drug hypersensitivity, pregnancy/nursing status, and possible drug interactions.

Monitoring: Monitor for deteriorating asthma, localized oropharyngeal *C. albicans* infections, pneumonia, infections, systemic corticosteroid effects, paradoxical bronchospasm, upper airway symptoms, immediate hypersensitivity reactions, CV and CNS effects, decreases in BMD, glaucoma, cataracts, increased IOP, eosinophilic conditions, changes in blood glucose and/or serum K^+, and other adverse reactions. Monitor growth of pediatric patients routinely. Closely monitor patients w/ hepatic disease. Carefully monitor infants born of mothers receiving therapy during pregnancy for hypoadrenalism.

Counseling: Advise patients w/ asthma that LABAs increase the risk of asthma-related death and may increase the risk of asthma-related hospitalization in pediatric and adolescent patients. Inform that drug is not meant to relieve acute asthma symptoms and extra doses should not be used for that purpose; advise to treat acute symptoms w/ an inhaled SABA (eg, albuterol). Instruct to seek medical attention immediately if they experience decreasing effectiveness of inhaled SABA; a need for more inhalations than usual of inhaled SABA; or a significant decrease in lung function. Advise not to d/c therapy w/o physician guidance and not to use additional LABAs. Instruct to contact physician if oropharyngeal candidiasis or symptoms of pneumonia develop. Advise to rinse mouth w/ water w/o swallowing after inhalation. Advise to avoid exposure to chickenpox or measles, and, if exposed, to consult physician w/o delay. Inform about risk of immunosuppression, hypercorticism, adrenal suppression, reduction in BMD, reduced growth velocity, ocular effects, and other adverse effects (eg, palpitations, chest pain, rapid HR, tremor, nervousness). Advise to d/c therapy if immediate hypersensitivity reactions occur.

STORAGE: 20-25°C (68-77°F); excursions permitted from 15-30°C (59-86°F). Store w/ the mouthpiece down. Do not puncture, use/store near heat or open flame, or throw into fire/incinerator. Exposure to temperatures >49°C (120°F) may cause bursting. Discard when the counter reads "000."

ADVICOR – lovastatin/niacin RX

Class: HMG-CoA reductase inhibitor (statin)/nicotinic acid

ADULT DOSAGE

Primary Hypercholesterolemia/Mixed Dyslipidemia

Not Currently on Niacin ER:
Initial: 500mg-20mg qhs
Titrate: Increase by no more than 500mg qd (based on niacin ER component) every 4 weeks
Max: 2000mg-40mg qhs

Stable on Niacin ER:
May be directly switched to niacin-equivalent dose of Advicor

Should not be substituted for other modified-release (sustained-release or time-release) niacin preparations or other IR (crystalline) niacin preparations

If therapy is discontinued for an extended period (>7 days), reinstitution should begin with lowest dose

Advicor tab strengths are not interchangeable

Women may respond at lower niacin doses than men

PEDIATRIC DOSAGE

Pediatric use may not have been established

DOSING CONSIDERATIONS

Concomitant Medications

Danazol, Diltiazem, or Verapamil:
Lovastatin Content:
Initial: 10mg/day
Max: 20mg/day

Amiodarone:
Lovastatin Content:
Max: 40mg/day

Gemfibrozil:
Avoid lovastatin use w/ gemfibrozil

Renal Impairment

Severe (CrCl <30mL/min):
Carefully consider lovastatin dose increases >20mg/day; give cautiously if deemed necessary

ADMINISTRATION

Oral route

Take at hs w/ a low-fat snack
Take tab whole; do not break, crush, or chew
Avoid administration on an empty stomach and slowly increase niacin dose to reduce flushing, pruritus, and GI distress
May take ASA (up to 325mg) 30 min prior to treatment to reduce flushing

HOW SUPPLIED

Tab: (Niacin ER-Lovastatin) 500mg-20mg, 750mg-20mg, 1000mg-20mg, 1000mg-40mg

CONTRAINDICATIONS

Known hypersensitivity to Advicor or any component of this medication. Active liver disease or unexplained persistent elevations in serum transaminases, active peptic ulcer disease (PUD), arterial bleeding, pregnancy, women of childbearing age who may become pregnant, and nursing mothers. Concomitant administration with strong CYP3A4 inhibitors (eg, itraconazole, ketoconazole, posaconazole, HIV protease inhibitors, boceprevir, telaprevir, erythromycin, clarithromycin, telithromycin, nefazodone).

WARNINGS/PRECAUTIONS

Do not substitute for equivalent doses of immediate-release (IR) (crystalline) niacin or other modified-release (sustained-release or time-release) niacin preparations other than Niaspan. Severe hepatic toxicity, including fulminant hepatic necrosis, reported when substituting sustained-release niacin for IR niacin at equivalent doses. If switching from IR niacin, initiate with low doses (500mg qhs) and titrate to desired therapeutic response. Caution with renal impairment, or with substantial alcohol consumption and/or history of liver disease. Associated with abnormal LFTs; obtain LFTs prior to initiation and repeat as clinically indicated. Fatal and nonfatal hepatic failure (rare) reported; promptly interrupt therapy if serious liver injury with clinical symptoms and/or hyperbilirubinemia or jaundice occurs and do not restart if no alternate etiology found. Myopathy and/or rhabdomyolysis reported when lovastatin is used with lipid-altering doses (≥1g/day) of niacin; d/c if markedly elevated CPK levels occur or myopathy is diagnosed/suspected, and temporarily withhold in any patient experiencing acute or serious condition predisposing to development of renal failure secondary to rhabdomyolysis. Immune-mediated necrotizing myopathy (IMNM) reported. Closely observe patients with history of jaundice, hepatobiliary disease, or peptic ulcer. Increases in HbA1c and FPG levels reported; closely monitor diabetic/potentially diabetic patients, and adjust diet and/or hypoglycemic therapy if necessary. May increase PT and reduce platelet counts; carefully evaluate patients undergoing surgery. Associated with dose-related reductions in phosphorus (P) levels; periodically monitor P levels in patients at risk for hypophosphatemia. Caution with unstable angina or in the acute phase of MI, particularly when such patients are also receiving vasoactive drugs (eg, nitrates, calcium channel blockers, adrenergic blocking agents). Elevated uric acid levels reported; caution in patients predisposed to gout. Evaluate patients who develop endocrine dysfunction. Lab test interactions may occur.

ADVERSE REACTIONS

Flushing, infection, headache, pain, N/V, pruritus, flu syndrome, diarrhea, back pain, asthenia, rash, hyperglycemia, abdominal pain, myalgia, dyspepsia.

DRUG INTERACTIONS

See Contraindications and Dosage. Lovastatin: Due to the risk of myopathy, avoid with gemfibrozil, cyclosporine, and large quantities of grapefruit juice (>1 quart/day); caution with fibrates, colchicine, danazol, diltiazem, verapamil, and amiodarone. Voriconazole may increase concentrations and may increase risk of myopathy/rhabdomyolysis; consider dose adjustment of lovastatin. Ranolazine may increase risk of myopathy/rhabdomyolysis; consider dose adjustment of lovastatin. Caution with drugs (eg, spironolactone, cimetidine) that may decrease the levels or activity of endogenous steroid hormones. Determine PT before initiation and frequently during therapy with coumarin anticoagulants. Niacin ER: Avoid ingestion of alcohol, hot drinks, or spicy foods around the time of administration; may increase flushing and pruritus. May potentiate the effects of ganglionic blocking agents and vasoactive drugs, resulting in postural hypotension. ASA may decrease the metabolic clearance. Separate dosing from bile acid-binding resins (eg, colestipol, cholestyramine) by at least 4-6 hrs. Vitamins or other nutritional supplements containing large doses of niacin or related compounds (eg, nicotinamide) may potentiate adverse effects.

PATIENT CONSIDERATIONS

Assessment: Assess for history of/active liver disease or PUD, unexplained persistent hepatic transaminase elevations, arterial bleeding, history of jaundice or hepatobiliary disease, renal impairment, diabetes, risk for hypophosphatemia, any other conditions where treatment is contraindicated or cautioned, drug hypersensitivity, pregnancy/nursing status, and possible drug interactions. Assess lipid profile and LFTs.

Monitoring: Monitor for signs/symptoms of myopathy (including IMNM), rhabdomyolysis, liver/renal/endocrine dysfunction, decreases in platelet counts, increases in PT and uric acid levels, and other adverse reactions. Monitor LFTs, blood glucose, and CPK levels. Perform lipid determinations at intervals of ≥4 weeks. Periodically monitor P levels in patients at risk for hypophosphatemia. Check PT with coumarin anticoagulants.

Counseling: Instruct to report promptly any unexplained muscle pain, tenderness, or weakness, particularly if accompanied by malaise or fever or if muscle signs and symptoms persist after discontinuation. Instruct to report promptly any symptoms that may indicate liver injury (eg, fatigue, anorexia, right upper abdominal discomfort, dark urine, jaundice). Advise to carefully follow the prescribed dosing regimen. Inform that flushing may occur, but usually subsides after several weeks of consistent use of therapy. Instruct that if awakened by flushing, especially if taking antihypertensives, to rise slowly to minimize the potential for dizziness and/or syncope. Instruct to avoid ingestion of alcohol, hot beverages, or spicy foods around the time of administration to minimize flushing. Counsel to avoid administration with grapefruit juice. Instruct to contact physician prior to restarting therapy if therapy is discontinued for an extended length of time. Advise to notify physician if taking vitamins or other nutritional supplements containing niacin or related compounds, and if symptoms of dizziness occur. Instruct diabetic patients to notify physician of changes in blood glucose. Instruct to immediately d/c use and notify physician as soon as pregnancy is recognized.

STORAGE: 20-25°C (68-77°F).

AFINITOR – everolimus

RX

Class: Kinase inhibitor

OTHER BRAND NAMES

Afinitor Disperz

ADULT DOSAGE

Breast Cancer

Treatment of postmenopausal women w/ advanced hormone receptor (HR)-positive, HER2-negative breast cancer in combination w/ exemestane, after failure of treatment w/ letrozole or anastrozole

Tab:
10mg qd; continue until disease progression or unacceptable toxicity occurs

Advanced Pancreatic Neuroendocrine Tumors

Progressive Neuroendocrine Tumors of Pancreatic Origin w/ Unresectable, Locally Advanced or Metastatic Disease:
Tab:
10mg qd; continue until disease progression or unacceptable toxicity occurs

Advanced Renal Cell Carcinoma

After Failure of Treatment w/ Sunitinib or Sorafenib:
Tab:
10mg qd; continue until disease progression or unacceptable toxicity occurs

Renal Angiomyolipoma with Tuberous Sclerosis Complex

In Patients Not Requiring Immediate Surgery:
Tab:
10mg qd; continue until disease progression or unacceptable toxicity occurs

Subependymal Giant Cell Astrocytoma with Tuberous Sclerosis Complex

Requiring Therapeutic Intervention but Cannot Be Curatively Resected:
Tab/Tab for Oral Sus:
Initial: 4.5mg/m² qd
Adjust dose at 2-week intervals prn to achieve/maintain trough concentrations of 5-15ng/mL

Continue until disease progression or unacceptable toxicity occurs

Therapeutic Drug Monitoring:
Assess trough levels 2 weeks after initiation, a change in dose, a change in coadministration of CYP3A4/P-gp inducers/inhibitors, a change in hepatic function, or a change in dosage form.

PEDIATRIC DOSAGE

Subependymal Giant Cell Astrocytoma with Tuberous Sclerosis Complex

Requiring Therapeutic Intervention but Cannot Be Curatively Resected:
Tab/Tab for Oral Sus:
≥1 Year:
Initial: 4.5mg/m² qd
Adjust dose at 2-week intervals prn to achieve/maintain trough concentrations of 5-15ng/mL

Continue until disease progression or unacceptable toxicity occurs

Therapeutic Drug Monitoring:
Assess trough levels 2 weeks after initiation, a change in dose, a change in coadministration of CYP3A4/P-gp inducers/inhibitors, a change in hepatic function, or a change in dosage form.
Once a stable dose is attained, monitor trough levels every 3-6 months in patients w/ changing BSA or every 6-12 months in patients w/ stable BSA.

Titrate (Based on Trough Levels):
<5ng/mL: Increase daily dose by 2.5mg (tab) or 2mg (tab for oral sus)
>15ng/mL: Reduce daily dose by 2.5mg (tab) or 2mg (tab for oral sus)

If dose reduction is required for patients receiving the lowest available strength, administer qod

Once a stable dose is attained, monitor trough levels every 3-6 months in patients w/ changing BSA or every 6-12 months in patients w/ stable BSA.
Titrate (Based on Trough Levels):
<5ng/mL: Increase daily dose by 2.5mg (tab) or 2mg (tab for oral sus)
>15ng/mL: Reduce daily dose by 2.5mg (tab) or 2mg (tab for oral sus)

If dose reduction is required for patients receiving the lowest available strength, administer qod

DOSING CONSIDERATIONS

Concomitant Medications

Advanced HR-Positive, HER2-Negative Breast Cancer, Advanced Progressive Neuroendocrine Tumors of Pancreatic Origin (PNET), Advanced Renal Cell Carcinoma (RCC), Renal Angiomyolipoma w/ Tuberous Sclerosis Complex (TSC):

Strong CYP3A4/P-gp Inhibitors: Avoid use
Moderate CYP3A4/P-gp Inhibitors (If Coadministration Is Necessary):
- Reduce to 2.5mg qd; may increase to 5mg if tolerated
- 2-3 days after discontinuation of the moderate inhibitor, return to dose used prior to initiating the inhibitor

Avoid grapefruit, grapefruit juice, and other foods known to inhibit CYP450 and P-gp activity during treatment

Strong CYP3A4/P-gp Inducers: Avoid use
If Necessary:
- Consider doubling daily dose by increments of ≤5mg
- 3-5 days after discontinuation of the strong inducer, return to dose used prior to initiating the inducer

Avoid St. John's wort during treatment

Subependymal Giant Cell Astrocytoma (SEGA) w/ TSC:

Strong CYP3A4/P-gp Inhibitors: Avoid use
Moderate CYP3A4/P-gp Inhibitors (If Coadministration is Necessary):
Initial: 2.5mg/m^2 qd (reduce dose by approx 50%); administer qod if receiving the lowest available strength.
2-3 days after discontinuation of the moderate inhibitor, return to dose used prior to initiating the inhibitor
Avoid ingestion of foods or nutritional supplements (eg, grapefruit, grapefruit juice) known to inhibit CYP450 or P-gp activity

Strong CYP3A4/P-gp Inducers: Avoid use
If Necessary: Double the dose and assess tolerability
Initial: 9mg/m^2 qd
Return to dose used prior to initiating the inducer if the strong inducer is discontinued

Avoid ingestion of foods or nutritional supplements (eg, St. John's wort) known to induce CYP450 activity

Hepatic Impairment

Advanced HR-Positive, HER2-Negative Breast Cancer, Advanced PNET, Advanced RCC, Renal Angiomyolipoma w/ TSC:
Mild (Child-Pugh Class A): 7.5mg qd; reduce to 5mg qd if not tolerated
Moderate (Child-Pugh Class B): 5mg qd; reduce to 2.5mg qd if not tolerated
Severe (Child-Pugh Class C): 2.5mg qd if benefit outweighs the risk

SEGA w/ TSC:
Severe (Child-Pugh Class C):
Initial: 2.5mg/m^2 qd (reduce starting dose by approx 50%)

Adverse Reactions

Advanced HR-Positive, HER2-Negative Breast Cancer, Advanced PNET, Advanced RCC, Renal Angiomyolipoma w/ TSC:
If dose reduction is required, administer approx 50% lower than the previously administered daily dose

Noninfectious Pneumonitis:
Grade 1 (Asymptomatic, Radiographic Findings Only):
- Initiate appropriate monitoring

Grade 2 (Symptomatic, Not Interfering w/ Activities of Daily Living [ADL]):
- Consider interrupting therapy, rule out infection, and consider treatment w/ corticosteroids until symptoms improve to Grade ≤1
- Reinitiate at lower dose
- D/C if failure to recover w/in 4 weeks

Grade 3 (Symptomatic, Interfering w/ ADL; O_2 Indicated):
- Interrupt therapy until symptoms resolve to Grade ≤1, rule out infection, and consider treatment w/ corticosteroids
- Consider reinitiating at a lower dose
- Consider discontinuation if toxicity recurs at Grade 3

Grade 4 (Life-Threatening, Ventilator Support Indicated):
- D/C, rule out infection, and consider treatment w/ corticosteroids

Stomatitis:

Grade 1 (Minimal Symptoms, Normal Diet):
- Manage w/ nonalcoholic or salt water (0.9%) mouthwash several times a day

Grade 2 (Symptomatic but Can Eat and Swallow Modified Diet):
- Temporarily interrupt dose until recovery to Grade ≤1; reinitiate at the same dose
- If stomatitis recurs at Grade 2, interrupt dose until recovery to Grade ≤1; reinitiate at a lower dose
- Manage w/ topical analgesic mouth treatments (eg, benzocaine, butyl aminobenzoate, tetracaine, menthol, phenol) ± topical corticosteroids (eg, triamcinolone oral paste); avoid agents w/ alcohol, hydrogen peroxide, iodine, and thyme derivatives

Grade 3 (Symptomatic and Unable to Aliment or Hydrate Orally):
- Temporarily interrupt dose until recovery to Grade ≤1
- Reinitiate at a lower dose
- Manage w/ topical analgesic mouth treatments (eg, benzocaine, butyl aminobenzoate, tetracaine, menthol, phenol) ± topical corticosteroids (eg, triamcinolone oral paste); avoid agents w/ alcohol, hydrogen peroxide, iodine, and thyme derivatives

Grade 4 (Symptoms Associated w/ Life-Threatening Consequences):
- D/C and treat appropriately

Other Nonhematologic Toxicities (Excluding Metabolic Events):

Grade 1:
- If toxicity is tolerable, no dose adjustment required; initiate appropriate medical therapy and monitor

Grade 2:
- If toxicity is tolerable, no dose adjustment required; initiate appropriate medical therapy and monitor
- If toxicity becomes intolerable, temporarily interrupt dose until recovery to Grade ≤1; reinitiate at same dose
- If toxicity recurs at Grade 2, interrupt until recovery to Grade ≤1; reinitiate at lower dose

Grade 3:
- Temporarily interrupt dose until recovery to Grade ≤1
- Initiate appropriate therapy and monitor
- Consider reinitiating at a lower dose
- If toxicity recurs at Grade 3, consider discontinuation

Grade 4:
- D/C and treat appropriately

Metabolic Events (eg, Hyperglycemia, Dyslipidemia):

Grade 1:
- Initiate appropriate medical therapy and monitor

Grade 2:
- Manage w/ appropriate medical therapy and monitor

Grade 3:
- Temporarily interrupt dose
- Reinitiate at a lower dose
- Manage w/ appropriate therapy and monitor

Grade 4:
- D/C and treat appropriately

SEGA w/ TSC:
- Temporarily interrupt or permanently d/c for severe or intolerable adverse reactions
- If dose reduction is required when reinitiating therapy, reduce dose by 50%
- If dose reduction is required for patients receiving the lowest available strength, administer qod

ADMINISTRATION

Oral route

Take qd at the same time every day.
Take consistently either w/ or w/o food.
Do not combine the 2 dosage forms to achieve the desired total dose.
Do not break or crush.

Tab
Swallow whole w/ a glass of water.

Tab for Oral Sus
Wear gloves to avoid possible contact w/ drug when preparing sus for another person.
Administer as sus only.
Administer sus immediately after preparation and discard if not given w/in 60 min after preparation.
Prepare sus in water only.

Preparation Using an Oral Syringe:
1. Place prescribed dose into a 10mL syringe; do not exceed a total of 10mg/syringe and if higher doses are required, prepare an additional syringe.
2. Draw approx 5mL of water and 4mL of air into syringe.
3. Place the filled syringe into a container (tip up) for 3 min, until the tabs are in sus.
4. Gently invert the syringe 5X immediately prior to administration.
5. After administration of the prepared sus, draw approx 5mL of water and 4mL of air into the same syringe, and swirl the contents to suspend remaining particles; administer entire contents of the syringe.

Preparation Using a Small Drinking Glass:
1. Place prescribed dose into a small drinking glass (max size 100mL) containing approx 25mL of water; do not exceed a total of 10mg/glass and if higher doses are required, prepare an additional glass.
2. Allow 3 min for sus to occur.
3. Stir contents gently w/ a spoon, immediately prior to drinking.
4. After administration of the prepared sus, add 25mL of water and stir w/ the same spoon to resuspend remaining particles; administer entire contents of glass.

HOW SUPPLIED
Tab for Oral Sus: (Afinitor Disperz) 2mg, 3mg, 5mg; **Tab:** (Afinitor) 2.5mg, 5mg, 7.5mg, 10mg

CONTRAINDICATIONS
Hypersensitivity to the active substance, to other rapamycin derivatives, or to any of the excipients of this product.

WARNINGS/PRECAUTIONS
See Dosing Considerations. Not indicated for the treatment of functional carcinoid tumors in PNET. Noninfectious pneumonitis reported. Immunosuppressive properties may predispose patients to infections, including infections w/ opportunistic pathogens. Localized and systemic infections, including reactivation of hepatitis B, reported. Complete treatment of preexisting invasive fungal infections prior to therapy. Institute appropriate treatment if diagnosis of an infection is made and consider interruption or discontinuation of therapy. If a diagnosis of invasive systemic fungal infection is made, d/c therapy. *Pneumocystis jiroveci* pneumonia (PJP) reported; consider prophylaxis of PJP when concomitant use of corticosteroids or other immunosuppressive agents are required. Mouth ulcers, stomatitis, and oral mucositis reported. Cases of renal failure (including acute renal failure), some w/ fatal outcome, observed. May delay wound healing and increase the occurrence of wound-related complications (eg, wound dehiscence, wound infection, incisional hernia); use caution in the perisurgical period. Elevated SrCr, proteinuria, hyperglycemia, hyperlipidemia, hypertriglyceridemia, and decreased Hgb, lymphocytes, neutrophils, and platelets reported. Exposure is increased in patients w/ hepatic impairment. Avoid close contact w/ those who have received live vaccines during treatment. In pediatric patients w/ SEGA who do not require immediate treatment, complete the recommended childhood series of live virus vaccinations prior to therapy; an accelerated vaccination schedule may be appropriate. Can cause fetal harm; advise females of reproductive potential to avoid becoming pregnant and to use effective contraception during and for 8 weeks after ending treatment. Caution in elderly.

ADVERSE REACTIONS
Advanced HR-Positive, HER2-Negative Breast Cancer/Advanced PNET/Advanced RCC: Stomatitis, infections, rash, fatigue, diarrhea, edema, abdominal pain, nausea, fever, asthenia, cough, headache, decreased appetite.
Renal Angiomyolipoma w/ TSC: Stomatitis.
SEGA w/ TSC: Stomatitis, respiratory tract infection.

DRUG INTERACTIONS
See Dosing Considerations. ACE inhibitors may increase risk for angioedema. May increase levels of midazolam, octreotide, and exemestane. Avoid use of live vaccines while on therapy. More frequent monitoring is recommended when coadministered w/ other drugs that may induce hyperglycemia.

PATIENT CONSIDERATIONS
Assessment: Assess for hypersensitivity, preexisting fungal infections, pregnancy/nursing status, and possible drug interactions. Assess hepatic function and renal function, including measurement of BUN, urinary protein, or SrCr. Obtain FPG, lipid profile, and CBC prior to start of therapy. Assess vaccination history in pediatric patients w/ SEGA.

Monitoring: Monitor for signs/symptoms of hypersensitivity reactions, noninfectious pneumonitis, infections, mouth ulcers, stomatitis, oral mucositis, and other adverse reactions. Monitor FPG, lipid profile, CBC count, and renal function, including measurement of BUN, urinary protein, or SrCr, periodically. Routine therapeutic drug monitoring is recommended in SEGA w/ TSC.

Counseling: Inform that noninfectious pneumonitis or infections may develop; advise to report new or worsening respiratory symptoms or any signs or symptoms of infection. Inform patients that they are more susceptible to angioedema if concomitantly taking ACE inhibitors; advise to be aware of any signs/symptoms of angioedema and to seek prompt medical attention. Inform of the possibility of developing mouth ulcers, stomatitis, and oral mucositis; instruct to use topical treatments and mouthwashes (w/o alcohol, peroxide, iodine, or thyme) in such cases. Inform of the possibility of developing kidney failure and the need to monitor kidney function. Inform of the possibility of impaired wound healing or dehiscence during therapy. Inform of the need to monitor blood chemistry and hematology prior to therapy and periodically thereafter. Advise to notify healthcare provider of all concomitant medications, including OTC medications and dietary supplements. Advise to avoid the use of live vaccines and close contact w/ those who have received live vaccines. Advise of risk of fetal harm. Advise female patients of reproductive potential to use effective contraception during treatment and for 8 weeks after the last dose. Advise not to breastfeed during treatment and for 2 weeks after the last dose. Advise males and females of reproductive potential of the potential risk for impaired fertility. Instruct to follow the dosing instructions ud; inform that missed doses may be taken up to 6 hrs after scheduled time but that if >6 hrs have elapsed, dose should be skipped and resumed at next scheduled time. Advise to read and carefully follow the FDA-approved "Instructions for Use."

STORAGE: 25°C (77°F); excursions permitted between 15-30°C (59-86°F). Protect from light and moisture.

AFLURIA — influenza vaccine RX

Class: Vaccine

ADULT DOSAGE

Influenza

Active Immunization Against Virus Subtypes A and Type B:

1 dose of 0.5mL

PEDIATRIC DOSAGE

Influenza

Active Immunization Against Virus Subtypes A and Type B:

5-8 Years:
1 or 2 doses (at least 1 month apart) of 0.5mL, depending on vaccination history

≥9 Years:
1 dose of 0.5mL

ADMINISTRATION

IM route

Available by needle and syringe (≥5 years) or by PharmaJet Stratis Needle-Free Injection System (18-64 years)

Inject preferably in the deltoid muscle of the upper arm
Shake thoroughly before use and administer dose immediately
Administer in separate syringes and use a separate arm if to be given at the same time as another injectable vaccine(s)

Refer to PI for further administration instructions

HOW SUPPLIED

Inj: 0.5mL [prefilled syringe], 5mL [multidose vial]

CONTRAINDICATIONS

Known severe allergic reactions (eg, anaphylaxis) to any component of the vaccine including egg protein, or to a previous dose of any influenza vaccine.

WARNINGS/PRECAUTIONS

Increased rates of fever and febrile seizures reported in children predominantly <5 yrs of age; febrile events were also reported in children 5-8 yrs of age. Caution if Guillain-Barre syndrome (GBS) has occurred within 6 weeks of previous influenza vaccination. Appropriate medical treatment and supervision must be available to manage possible anaphylactic reactions. Immune response may be diminished if vaccine is administered to immunocompromised persons. May not protect all individuals.

ADVERSE REACTIONS

Inj-site reactions (pain, redness, swelling, tenderness, induration), headache, myalgia, irritability, malaise, N/V, fever, cough, diarrhea, oropharyngeal pain.

DRUG INTERACTIONS

Corticosteroid or immunosuppressive therapies may diminish immunological response to vaccine.

PATIENT CONSIDERATIONS

Assessment: Review vaccination history. Assess for known severe allergic reactions to any component of the vaccine (eg, egg protein) or to a previous influenza vaccine, development of GBS following a prior dose of influenza vaccine, immunosuppression, pregnancy/nursing status, and possible drug interactions.

Monitoring: Monitor for signs/symptoms of fever, febrile seizures, GBS, allergic reactions, and other adverse reactions.

Counseling: Inform of the potential benefits and risks of immunization. Inform that vaccine cannot cause influenza but produces antibodies that protect against influenza and that the full effect of the vaccine is achieved approximately 3 weeks after vaccination. Instruct to report any severe or unusual adverse reactions to physician. Instruct that annual revaccination is recommended.

STORAGE: 2-8°C (36-46°F). Do not freeze; discard if it has been frozen. Protect from light. Discard vial within 28 days once stopper has been pierced.

AGGRENOX – aspirin/dipyridamole

RX

Class: Antiplatelet agent

ADULT DOSAGE

Stroke

To reduce risk of stroke in patients who have had transient ischemia of the brain or completed ischemic stroke due to thrombosis

1 cap bid (1 in am and 1 in pm)

PEDIATRIC DOSAGE

Pediatric use may not have been established

DOSING CONSIDERATIONS

Adverse Reactions

Intolerable Headaches During Initial Treatment:

Switch to 1 cap at hs and low-dose aspirin (ASA) in am

Return to usual regimen as soon as possible, usually w/in 1 week

ADMINISTRATION

Oral route

Take PO w/ or w/o food.

Swallow whole; do not chew or crush.

HOW SUPPLIED

Cap: (ASA/Dipyridamole Extended-Release) 25mg/200mg

CONTRAINDICATIONS

NSAID allergy; syndrome of asthma, rhinitis, and nasal polyps; children or teenagers w/ viral infections; known hypersensitivity to any of the product components.

WARNINGS/PRECAUTIONS

May increase risk of bleeding. Intracranial hemorrhage reported. Risk of GI side effects (eg, stomach pain, heartburn, N/V, gross GI bleeding, dyspepsia); monitor for signs of ulceration and bleeding. May cause fetal harm; avoid in 3rd trimester of pregnancy. Not interchangeable w/ individual components of ASA and dipyridamole tabs. **ASA:** Avoid w/ history of active peptic ulcer disease (PUD) or w/ severe hepatic or severe renal (GFR <10mL/min) dysfunction. Bleeding risks reported w/ chronic, heavy alcohol use (≥3 alcoholic drinks/day). May not provide adequate treatment for cardiac indications for stroke/transient ischemic attack patients for whom ASA is indicated to prevent recurrent MI or angina pectoris. **Dipyridamole:** Elevations of hepatic enzymes and hepatic failure reported. Has a vasodilatory effect; may precipitate/aggravate chest pain in patients w/ underlying coronary artery disease (CAD). May exacerbate preexisting hypotension.

ADVERSE REACTIONS

Headache, dyspepsia, abdominal pain, N/V, diarrhea, fatigue, arthralgia, pain, back pain, GI bleeding, hemorrhage.

DRUG INTERACTIONS

Increased risk of bleeding w/ other drugs that increase the risk of bleeding (eg, anticoagulants, antiplatelet agents, heparin, fibrinolytics, NSAIDs). **Dipyridamole:** May increase plasma levels and cardiovascular (CV) effects of adenosine. May counteract effect of cholinesterase inhibitors, potentially aggravating myasthenia gravis. **ASA:** May decrease effects of ACE inhibitors and β-blockers. Concurrent use w/ acetazolamide may lead to high serum concentrations of acetazolamide (and toxicity). May displace warfarin from protein binding sites, leading to prolongation of both PT and bleeding time. May decrease total concentration of phenytoin. May increase serum valproic acid levels. May decrease effects of diuretics in renal or CV disease. May inhibit renal clearance of methotrexate, leading to bone marrow toxicity (especially in elderly/renally impaired). Decreased renal function w/ NSAIDs. May increase effectiveness of oral hypoglycemics. May antagonize uricosuric agents (probenecid and sulfinpyrazone).

PATIENT CONSIDERATIONS

Assessment: Assess for NSAID allergy, syndrome of asthma, rhinitis and nasal polyps, renal/hepatic dysfunction, history of active PUD, alcohol use, CAD, hypotension, hypersensitivity, pregnancy/nursing status, and possible drug interactions.

Monitoring: Monitor for signs/symptoms of allergic reactions, GI effects, elevated hepatic enzymes, hepatic failure, and bleeding.

Counseling: Inform of risk and signs/symptoms of bleeding (eg, occult bleeding). Instruct to notify physician of all medications and supplements being taken, especially drugs that may increase risk of bleeding. Counsel patients who consume ≥3 alcoholic drinks daily about the bleeding risks. Inform that transient headache may occur; instruct to notify physician if an intolerable headache develops. Inform about signs and symptoms of GI side effects and what steps to take if they occur. Advise that if a dose is missed, to take next dose on regular schedule and not to take a double dose. Inform of potential hazard to fetus if used during pregnancy; instruct to notify physician if patient is pregnant or becomes pregnant.

STORAGE: 25°C (77°F); excursions permitted to 15-30°C (59-86°F). Protect from excessive moisture.

AKYNZEO – netupitant/palonosetron

RX

Class: Substance P/neurokinin-1 (NK1) receptor antagonist and 5-HT_3 receptor antagonist

ADULT DOSAGE

Chemotherapy-Induced Nausea/Vomiting

Highly Emetogenic Chemotherapy (Including Cisplatin Based):
Day 1: 1 cap approx 1 hr prior to the start of chemotherapy w/ dexamethasone 12mg PO 30 min prior to chemotherapy
Days 2-4: Dexamethasone 8mg PO qd

Anthracyclines and Cyclophosphamide Based/Non-Highly Emetogenic Chemotherapy:
Day 1: 1 cap approx 1 hr prior to the start of chemotherapy w/ dexamethasone 12mg PO 30 min prior to chemotherapy
Days 2-4: Administration of dexamethasone is not necessary

PEDIATRIC DOSAGE

Pediatric use may not have been established

ADMINISTRATION

Oral route

Take w/ or w/o food

HOW SUPPLIED

Cap: (Netupitant-Palonosetron) 300mg-0.5mg

WARNINGS/PRECAUTIONS

Hypersensitivity reactions, including anaphylaxis, reported. Serotonin syndrome reported; d/c and initiate supportive treatment if symptoms occur. Avoid with severe hepatic/renal impairment and end-stage renal disease. Caution in elderly.

ADVERSE REACTIONS

Dyspepsia, fatigue, constipation, erythema, headache, asthenia.

DRUG INTERACTIONS

Serotonin syndrome reported with concomitant use of other serotonergic drugs (eg, SSRIs, SNRIs, MAOIs); d/c and initiate supportive treatment if symptoms occur. May increase levels of CYP3A4 substrates; use with caution. Increased exposure of dexamethasone. Increased exposure to midazolam; consider the potential effects of increased levels of midazolam or other benzodiazepines metabolized via CYP3A4 (alprazolam, triazolam). May increase exposure of chemotherapy agents metabolized by CYP3A4 (eg, docetaxel, imatinib, vinblastine); use with caution and monitor for chemotherapeutic-related adverse reactions. Strong CYP3A4 inducers may decrease efficacy; avoid with chronic strong CYP3A4 inducers (eg, rifampin). Strong CYP3A4 inhibitors (eg, ketoconazole) may increase exposure.

PATIENT CONSIDERATIONS

Assessment: Assess for hypersensitivity to drug, renal/hepatic impairment, pregnancy/nursing status, and possible drug interactions.

Monitoring: Monitor for hypersensitivity reactions, serotonin syndrome, and other adverse reactions.

Counseling: Instruct to seek immediate medical attention if any signs/symptoms of a hypersensitivity reaction or serotonin syndrome (eg, changes in mental status, autonomic instability, neuromuscular symptoms, with or without GI symptoms) occur.

STORAGE: 20-25°C (68-77°F); excursions permitted from 15-30°C (59-86°F).

ALDACTAZIDE – hydrochlorothiazide/spironolactone RX

Class: Aldosterone blocker/thiazide diuretic

Tumorigenic in chronic toxicity animal studies; avoid unnecessary use. Not for initial therapy of edema or HTN. Edema or HTN requires therapy titration, and treatment must be reevaluated as conditions in each patient warrant.

ADULT DOSAGE

Edema

For patients w/ congestive heart failure, cirrhosis of the liver accompanied by edema and/or ascites, nephrotic syndrome

Maint: 100mg of each component daily, as a single dose or in divided doses

Range: 25-200mg/day of each component depending on response to initial titration

Hypertension

Usual: 50-100mg of each component daily, as single dose or in divided doses

Other Indications

Edema during pregnancy due to pathologic causes

PEDIATRIC DOSAGE

Pediatric use may not have been established

ADMINISTRATION

Oral route

HOW SUPPLIED

Tab: (Spironolactone/HCTZ) 25mg/25mg, 50mg/50mg* *scored

CONTRAINDICATIONS

Anuria, acute renal insufficiency, significant impairment of renal excretory function, hypercalcemia, hyperkalemia, Addison's disease, allergy to thiazide diuretics or sulfonamide-derived drug hypersensitivity, acute or severe hepatic failure.

WARNINGS/PRECAUTIONS

Administration with conditions known to cause hyperkalemia may lead to severe hyperkalemia. Caution with hepatic dysfunction; alterations of fluid and electrolyte balance may precipitate hepatic coma. Somnolence and dizziness reported; may impair mental/physical abilities. HCTZ: Caution with severe renal disease; may precipitate azotemia. Sensitivity reactions with or without a history of allergy or bronchial asthma may occur. May exacerbate or activate systemic lupus erythematosus (SLE). Idiosyncratic reaction, resulting in acute transient myopia and acute angle-closure glaucoma may occur; d/c treatment as rapidly as possible and consider medical/surgical treatment if intraocular pressure remains uncontrolled. Hypokalemia, hyponatremia, and hypercalcemia may occur. May alter glucose tolerance and increase cholesterol and TG levels. May increase uric acid levels and cause or exacerbate hyperuricemia and precipitate gout in susceptible patients. Spironolactone: May cause hyperkalemia; increased risk in patients with renal insufficiency and diabetes mellitus (DM). Gynecomastia may occur. (Rare) Breast enlargement may persist when therapy is discontinued.

ADVERSE REACTIONS

Gastric bleeding, ulceration, gynecomastia, leukopenia, fever, urticaria, mental confusion, ataxia, renal dysfunction, electrolyte disturbances, weakness, irregular menses, toxic epidermal necrolysis, vertigo, muscle spasm.

DRUG INTERACTIONS

Avoid with K^+ supplements, K^+-sparing diuretics, or a diet rich in K^+; hyperkalemia may occur. Extreme caution with NSAIDs (eg, indomethacin), ACE inhibitors, angiotensin II receptor antagonists, aldosterone blockers, heparin, low molecular weight heparin, other drugs known to cause hyperkalemia, and salt substitutes containing K^+; severe hyperkalemia may occur. Alcohol, barbiturates, or narcotics may potentiate orthostatic hypotension. Dose adjustment of antidiabetic drugs (eg, oral agents, insulin) may be required. Intensified electrolyte depletion, particularly hypokalemia, may occur with corticosteroids and adrenocorticotropic hormone. Reduced vascular responsiveness to norepinephrine. Caution with regional or general anesthesia. Increased responsiveness to nondepolarizing skeletal muscle relaxants (eg, tubocurarine). Increased risk of lithium toxicity; avoid with lithium. NSAIDs may reduce the effects of therapy. HCTZ: May add to or potentiate the action of other antihypertensive drugs. Electrolyte disturbances (eg, hypokalemia, hypomagnesemia) may increase risk of digoxin toxicity. Spironolactone: May increase levels of digoxin; monitor digoxin levels and adjust dose accordingly. Hyperkalemic metabolic acidosis reported with cholestyramine.

PATIENT CONSIDERATIONS

Assessment: Assess for anuria, acute renal insufficiency, hypercalcemia, renal/hepatic impairment, risk factors for acute angle-closure glaucoma (eg, history of sulfonamide/penicillin allergy), hyperkalemia, SLE, DM, history of allergy or bronchial asthma, any other conditions where treatment is contraindicated or cautioned, pregnancy/nursing status, and possible drug interactions.

Monitoring: Monitor for signs/symptoms of serum electrolyte abnormalities, hyperkalemia, gynecomastia, exacerbation or activation of SLE, hyperuricemia or precipitation of gout, hypersensitivity reactions, idiosyncratic reactions, and other adverse reactions. Monitor serum electrolytes, TG, cholesterol, and Ca^{2+} levels, and renal/hepatic function.

Counseling: Instruct to avoid K^+ supplements and foods containing high levels of K^+, including salt substitutes. Inform of pregnancy risks. Advise to seek medical attention if signs/symptoms of serum electrolyte abnormalities, hypersensitivity reactions, or other adverse events occur.

STORAGE: <25°C (77°F).

ALDACTONE – spironolactone

RX

Class: Aldosterone blocker

Tumorigenic in chronic toxicity animal studies; avoid unnecessary use.

ADULT DOSAGE

Primary Hyperaldosteronism

As a Diagnostic Agent:
Long Test: 400mg/day for 3-4 weeks
Short Test: 400mg/day for 4 days
Short-Term Preoperative Treatment:
100-400mg/day
Unsuitable for Surgery/Long-Term Maint:
Lowest effective dose individualized for patient

Edema

Due to CHF, Hepatic Cirrhosis, or Nephrotic Syndrome:
Initial: 100mg/day given in either single or divided doses for at least 5 days
Range: 25-200mg/day
May adjust to optimal therapeutic or maintenance level in single or divided daily doses
May add 2nd diuretic that acts more proximally in the renal tubule if no adequate diuretic response after 5 days
Do not change spironolactone dose when other diuretic therapy is added

Hypertension

Initial: 50-100mg/day given in single or divided doses for at least 2 weeks
Adjust dose according to response

PEDIATRIC DOSAGE

Pediatric use may not have been established

Hypokalemia

Diuretic-Induced:
25-100mg/day

Severe Heart Failure

In Conjunction w/ Standard Therapy (Serum K^+ ≤5.0mEq/L, SrCr ≤2.5mg/dL):
Initial: 25mg qd
Titrate: If tolerated, may increase to 50mg qd as clinically indicated; may reduce to 25mg qod if not tolerated

---

ADMINISTRATION
Oral route

HOW SUPPLIED
Tab: 25mg, 50mg*, 100mg* *scored

CONTRAINDICATIONS
Anuria, acute renal insufficiency, significant impairment of renal excretory function, hyperkalemia, Addison's disease. Concomitant use of eplerenone.

WARNINGS/PRECAUTIONS
Administration in patients with conditions known to cause hyperkalemia may lead to severe hyperkalemia. Hyperkalemia may be fatal; monitor and manage serum K^+ in patients with severe HF. If hyperkalemia is suspected, obtain an ECG, monitor serum K^+, and d/c or interrupt treatment for serum K^+ >5mEq/L or SrCr >4mg/dL. Monitor for fluid/electrolyte balance (eg, hypomagnesemia, hyponatremia, hypochloremic alkalosis, hyperkalemia). Caution with hepatic impairment; may precipitate hepatic coma. Reversible hyperchloremic metabolic acidosis reported in patients with decompensated hepatic cirrhosis. Dilutional hyponatremia may occur in edematous patients in hot weather. May cause transient BUN elevation, especially with preexisting renal impairment. Mild acidosis and dose-related gynecomastia may occur. Somnolence and dizziness reported; may impair mental/physical abilities.

ADVERSE REACTIONS
Gastric bleeding, ulceration, inability to achieve or maintain erection, leukopenia, fever, urticaria, hyperkalemia, mental confusion, ataxia, renal dysfunction, irregular menses, postmenopausal bleeding, N/V, diarrhea, breast pain.

DRUG INTERACTIONS
See Contraindications. Concomitant administration of K^+ supplements, other K^+-sparing diuretics, ACE inhibitors, angiotensin II antagonists, aldosterone blockers, NSAIDs (eg, indomethacin), heparin and low molecular weight heparin, other drugs known to cause hyperkalemia, diet rich in K^+, or salt substitutes containing K^+, may lead to severe hyperkalemia; avoid with other K^+-sparing diuretics. Avoid using oral K^+ supplements in patients with serum K^+ >3.5mEq/L. Alcohol, barbiturates, or narcotics may potentiate orthostatic hypotension. Corticosteroids and adrenocorticotropic hormone may intensify electrolyte depletion, particularly hypokalemia. Reduced vascular responsiveness to norepinephrine, a pressor amine; caution with regional/general anesthesia. May increase responsiveness to nondepolarizing skeletal muscle relaxants (eg, tubocurarine). May increase digoxin levels and subsequent digitalis toxicity; may need to reduce maintenance and digitalization doses and carefully monitor. Avoid with lithium; may reduce clearance of lithium and cause lithium toxicity. NSAIDs may reduce the effects of therapy. Dilutional hyponatremia may be caused or aggravated with other diuretics. Hyperkalemic metabolic acidosis reported with cholestyramine.

PATIENT CONSIDERATIONS

Assessment: Assess for renal/hepatic impairment, hyperkalemia, Addison's disease or other conditions associated with hyperkalemia, anuria, any other conditions where treatment is contraindicated or cautioned, pregnancy/nursing status, and for possible drug interactions.

Monitoring: Monitor for signs/symptoms of fluid/electrolyte imbalance, dilutional hyponatremia, BUN elevation, hyperchloremic metabolic acidosis, somnolence, dizziness, gynecomastia, and other adverse reactions. Monitor serum electrolytes periodically at appropriate intervals particularly in the elderly and with significant renal/hepatic impairment. Monitor serum K^+ and SrCr one week after initiation or dose increase, monthly for the first 3 months, then quarterly for a yr, and then every 6 months with severe HF.

Counseling: Instruct to avoid K^+ supplements and foods containing high levels of K^+, including salt substitutes. Inform that somnolence and dizziness may occur; advise to use caution when driving or operating machinery, until response to initial treatment has been determined.

STORAGE: <25°C (77°F).

ALDARA – imiquimod

RX

Class: Immune response modifier

ADULT DOSAGE

Actinic Keratosis

Clinically Typical, Nonhyperkeratotic, Nonhypertrophic Actinic Keratoses on Face or Scalp:
Apply 2X/week (eg, Monday, Thursday) before hs for a full 16 weeks to defined treatment area (contiguous area 25cm^2 [eg, 5cm x 5cm]) on face (forehead or 1 cheek) or on scalp (but not both concurrently)
Max: 36 pkts for 16 weeks

Superficial Basal Cell Carcinomas

Biopsy-confirmed, primary carcinoma, w/ a max tumor diameter of 2cm, located on trunk (excluding anogenital skin), neck, or extremities (excluding hands and feet)

Tumor Diameter:
0.5-<1cm: 4mm cre droplet (10mg)
1-<1.5cm: 5mm cre droplet (25mg)
1.5-2cm: 7mm cre droplet (40mg)

Max: 36 pkts for 6 weeks

Apply before hs 5X/week for a full 6 weeks
Use only when surgical methods are medically less appropriate and follow-up can be assured

External Genital and Perianal Warts

Apply a thin layer 3X/week before hs until warts are totally cleared
Max: 16 weeks

PEDIATRIC DOSAGE

External Genital and Perianal Warts

≥12 Years:
Apply a thin layer before hs and rub in until no longer visible 3X/week until warts are totally cleared
Max: 16 weeks

ADMINISTRATION

Topical route

Prior to application, wash treatment area w/ mild soap and water and allow to dry thoroughly for at least 10 min
Wash hands before and after application
Use 1 pkt/application
Rub in until no longer visible
Wash off w/ mild soap and water
Do not occlude treatment area

Actinic Keratosis
Wash off after 8 hrs

Superficial Basal Cell Carcinoma
Apply a sufficient amount to cover treatment area including 1cm of skin surrounding tumor
Wash off after 8 hrs

External Genital and Perianal Warts/Condyloma Acuminata
Wash off after 6-10 hrs

HOW SUPPLIED

Cre: 5% [250mg, 12^s]

WARNINGS/PRECAUTIONS

Caution in patients with preexisting autoimmune conditions. Not recommended for treatment of BCC subtypes other than sBCC. Not for oral, ophthalmic, or intravaginal use. Not recommended until completely healed from any previous drug/surgical treatment or sunburn. Avoid contact with eyes, lips, and nostrils. Local skin reactions are common; a rest period of several days may be taken if required by patient's discomfort or severity of local skin reaction. Do not extend treatment beyond 16 weeks due to missed doses or rest periods. Non-occlusive dressings (eg, cotton gauze, cotton underwear) may be used in the management of skin reactions. Early clinical clearance cannot be adequately assessed until resolution of local skin reactions (eg, 12 weeks post-treatment). Consider biopsy or other alternative interventions if there is evidence of persistent tumor. Carefully reevaluate treatment and reconsider management with lesions that do not respond to treatment. Avoid or minimize exposure to sunlight (including sunlamps); sunburn susceptibility may be heightened. Caution in patients with considerable sun exposure (eg, due to occupation) and in those with inherent sensitivity to sunlight. Intense local inflammatory reactions (eg, skin weeping or erosion, severe vulvar swelling that can lead to urinary retention) may occur and may be accompanied or preceded by flu-like signs/symptoms. May exacerbate inflammatory skin conditions, including chronic graft versus host disease. Interruption of dosing should be considered if systemic/local inflammatory reactions occur.

ADVERSE REACTIONS

Application-site reaction, local skin reactions, URTI, sinusitis, headache, squamous cell carcinoma, diarrhea, back pain, rhinitis, lymphadenopathy, influenza-like symptoms.

PATIENT CONSIDERATIONS

Assessment: Assess for preexisting autoimmune conditions, immunosuppression, previous drug/surgical treatment, sunburn, inherent sensitivity to sunlight, and pregnancy/nursing status. For treatment of sBCC, perform biopsy to confirm diagnosis.

Monitoring: Monitor for local inflammatory reactions (eg, weeping or erosion, vulvar swelling), application-site reactions, systemic reactions (eg, flu-like symptoms), and other adverse reactions. For sBCC, monitor treatment site regularly; assess at 12 weeks post-treatment for clinical clearance.

Counseling: Instruct on proper application technique and to use ud. Instruct to avoid contact with eyes, lips, and nostrils. Instruct not to bandage or occlude treatment area. Inform that local skin reactions may occur; instruct to contact physician promptly if experiencing any sign/symptom at application site that restricts/prohibits daily activities or makes continued application difficult. For patients being treated for actinic keratosis and sBCC, encourage using sunscreen and minimizing or avoiding exposure to natural or artificial sunlight (tanning beds, UVA/B treatment) while on therapy. Inform that subclinical lesions may appear in treatment area and may subsequently resolve. For patients being treated for external genital warts, instruct to avoid sexual (genital, anal, oral) contact while cream is on the skin. Advise female patients to avoid vaginal application and caution when applying cream at the vaginal opening. Instruct uncircumcised males treating warts under the foreskin to retract foreskin and clean area daily. Inform that new warts may develop during therapy, as drug is not a cure. Inform that drug may also weaken condoms and vaginal diaphragms and that concurrent use is not recommended.

STORAGE: 4-25°C (39-77°F). Do not freeze. Discard unused and partially used pkts; do not reuse partially used pkts.

ALECENSA – alectinib

RX

Class: Kinase inhibitor

ADULT DOSAGE

Metastatic Non-Small Cell Lung Cancer

W/ anaplastic lymphoma kinase (ALK)-positive, metastatic non-small cell lung cancer (NSCLC) who have progressed on or are intolerant to crizotinib

600mg bid until disease progression or unacceptable toxicity

Missed Dose

If a dose is missed or vomiting occurs after taking a dose, take the next dose at the scheduled time

PEDIATRIC DOSAGE

Pediatric use may not have been established

DOSING CONSIDERATIONS

Adverse Reactions

Dose Reduction Schedule:
Starting Dose: 600mg bid
1st Dose Reduction: 450mg bid
2nd Dose Reduction: 300mg bid
D/C if patients are unable to tolerate the 300mg twice daily dose

ALT or AST >5X ULN w/ Total Bilirubin ≤2X ULN: Temporarily withhold until recovery to baseline or to ≤3X ULN, then resume at reduced dose as per dose reduction schedule
ALT or AST >3X ULN w/ Total Bilirubin >2X ULN in the Absence of Cholestasis or Hemolysis: Permanently d/c
Total Bilirubin Elevation of >3X ULN: Temporarily withhold until recovery to baseline or to ≤1.5X ULN, then resume at reduced dose as per dose reduction schedule

Any Grade Treatment-Related Interstitial Lung Disease (ILD)/Pneumonitis: Permanently d/c

Symptomatic Bradycardia: Withhold until recovery to asymptomatic bradycardia or to a HR ≥60 bpm
- If contributing concomitant medication is identified and discontinued, or its dose is adjusted, resume alectinib at previous dose upon recovery to asymptomatic bradycardia or to a HR ≥60 bpm
- If no contributing concomitant medication is identified, or if contributing concomitant medications are not discontinued or dose modified, resume alectinib at reduced dose as per dose reduction schedule upon recovery to asymptomatic bradycardia or to HR ≥60 bpm

Bradycardia (Life-Threatening Consequences, Urgent Intervention Indicated): Permanently d/c alectinib if no contributing concomitant medication is identified
- If contributing concomitant medication is identified and discontinued, or its dose is adjusted, resume alectinib at reduced dose upon recovery to asymptomatic bradycardia or to a HR ≥60 bpm w/ frequent monitoring as clinically indicated; permanently d/c in case of recurrence

Creatine Phosphokinase (CPK) Elevation>5X ULN: Temporarily withhold until recovery to baseline or to ≤2.5X ULN, then resume at same dose

CPK Elevation >10X ULN or 2nd Occurrence of CPK Elevation of >5X ULN: Temporarily withhold until recovery to baseline or ≤2.5X ULN, then resume at reduced dose as per dose reduction schedule

ADMINISTRATION

Oral route

Take w/ food.
Do not open or dissolve the contents of the capsule.

HOW SUPPLIED

Cap: 150mg

WARNINGS/PRECAUTIONS

See Dosing Considerations. Elevations of AST >5X ULN, ALT >5X ULN, and bilirubin >3X ULN reported; monitor LFTs including ALT, AST, and total bilirubin q2 weeks during the first 2 months of treatment, then periodically, w/ more frequent testing if transaminase/ bilirubin elevations occur. Severe ILD reported; promptly investigate for ILD/pneumonitis in any patient who presents w/ worsening of respiratory symptoms (eg, dyspnea, cough, fever). Immediately withhold treatment in patients diagnosed w/ ILD/pneumonitis and permanently d/c if no other potential causes of ILD/pneumonitis have been identified. Symptomatic bradycardia may occur; monitor HR and BP regularly. Myalgia or musculoskeletal pain and elevations of CPK levels reported. Assess CPK levels q2 weeks during 1st month of treatment and in patients reporting unexplained muscle pain, tenderness, or weakness. May cause fetal harm.

ADVERSE REACTIONS

Fatigue, constipation, edema, myalgia, cough, rash, N/V, headache, diarrhea, dyspnea, back pain, increased weight, vision disorder.

PATIENT CONSIDERATIONS

Assessment: Assess for hepatic impairment, pregnancy/nursing status, and possible drug interactions.

Monitoring: Monitor LFTs including ALT, AST, and total bilirubin q2 weeks during the first 2 months of treatment, then periodically w/ more frequent testing in patients who develop transaminase and bilirubin elevations. Monitor for worsening of respiratory symptoms indicative of ILD/pneumonitis (eg, dyspnea, cough, fever) and monitor for unexplained muscle pain, tenderness, or weakness. Assess CPK levels q2 weeks for the 1st month of treatment and as clinically indicated in patients reporting symptoms. Monitor HR and BP regularly.

Counseling: Advise about the signs/symptoms of bilirubin and hepatic transaminase elevations. Inform about the risks of severe ILD/pneumonitis. Instruct to report new or worsening respiratory symptoms, symptoms of bradycardia (eg, dizziness, lightheadedness, syncope), and to report about the use of any heart or BP medications. Advise of signs/symptoms of myalgia and instruct to report new or worsening symptoms of muscle pain or weakness. Advise to avoid prolonged sun exposure while taking this medication and for at least 7 days after discontinuation. Advise to use a broad spectrum UVA/UVB sunscreen and lip balm (SPF ≥50) to help protect against potential sunburn. Inform that therapy may cause fetal harm; advise females of reproductive potential to use effective contraception during treatment and for at least 1 week after the last dose. Advise male patients w/ female partners of reproductive potential to use effective contraception during treatment and for 3 months after the last dose. Advise women not to breastfeed during treatment and for 1 week after the last dose. Instruct to take alectinib twice a day w/ food, and to swallow whole. Advise that if a dose is missed or if the patient vomits after taking a dose, not to take an extra dose, but to take the next dose at the regular time.

STORAGE: ≤30°C (86°F); protect from light and moisture.

ALENDRONATE – alendronate sodium

RX

Class: Bisphosphonate

OTHER BRAND NAMES
Fosamax

ADULT DOSAGE

Osteoporosis

In Postmenopausal Women:
Treatment:
70mg tab/sol once weekly or 10mg tab qd
Prevention:
35mg tab once weekly or 5mg tab qd

Treatment to Increase Bone Mass in Men w/ Osteoporosis:
70mg tab/sol once weekly or 10mg tab qd

Treatment of Glucocorticoid-Induced Osteoporosis:
In men and women receiving glucocorticoids in a daily dosage equivalent to 7.5mg or greater of prednisone and who have low bone mineral density

5mg tab qd; 10mg tab qd for postmenopausal women not on estrogen

Paget's Disease

Treatment of Paget's Disease of Bone in Men and Women:
40mg tab qd for 6 months

Retreatment: Following a 6-month post-treatment evaluation period, may consider retreatment if relapse occurs (based on increases in serum alkaline phosphatase). May also consider retreatment if treatment fails to normalize serum alkaline phosphatase

Missed Dose

If once-weekly dose is missed, administer 1 dose on am after patient remembers; do not administer 2 doses on same day but return to 1 dose once a week, as originally scheduled on chosen day

PEDIATRIC DOSAGE

Pediatric use may not have been established

DOSING CONSIDERATIONS

Renal Impairment

CrCl <35mL/min: Not recommended

ADMINISTRATION

Oral route

Take upon arising for the day.
Swallow tabs w/ full glass of water (6-8 oz); do not chew or suck on the tab.
Oral sol should be followed by at least 2 oz of water.
Take at least 1/2 hr before the 1st food, beverage, or medication of the day w/ plain water only.
Do not lie down for at least 30 min and until after 1st food of the day.

HOW SUPPLIED

Oral Sol: 70mg [75mL]; **Tab:** 5mg, 10mg, 35mg, 40mg; (Fosamax) 70mg

CONTRAINDICATIONS

Esophageal abnormalities that delay esophageal emptying (eg, stricture, achalasia), inability to stand or sit upright for at least 30 min, hypocalcemia, hypersensitivity to any component of the medication. **Oral Sol:** Patients at increased risk of aspiration.

WARNINGS/PRECAUTIONS

May cause local irritation of the upper GI mucosa; caution w/ active upper GI problems (eg, Barrett's esophagus, dysphagia, other esophageal diseases, gastritis, duodenitis, ulcers). Esophageal reactions (eg, esophagitis, esophageal ulcers/erosions) reported; d/c and seek medical attention if dysphagia, odynophagia, retrosternal pain, or new/worsening heartburn develops. Use therapy under appropriate supervision in patients who cannot comply w/ dosing instructions due to mental disability. Gastric and duodenal ulcers reported. Treat hypocalcemia and other disorders affecting mineral metabolism (eg, vitamin D deficiency) prior to therapy. Asymptomatic decreases in serum Ca^{2+} and phosphate may occur; ensure adequate Ca^{2+} and vitamin D intake especially in patients w/ Paget's disease of bone and in patients taking glucocorticoids. Severe and occasionally incapacitating bone, joint, and/or muscle pain reported; d/c if severe symptoms develop. Osteonecrosis of the jaw (ONJ) reported; risk may increase w/ duration of exposure to drug. If invasive dental procedures are required, discontinuation of treatment may reduce risk for ONJ. Consider discontinuation if ONJ develops. Atypical, low-energy, or low-trauma fractures of the femoral shaft reported; evaluate any patient w/ a history of bisphosphonate exposure who presents w/ thigh/groin pain to rule out incomplete femur fracture, and consider interruption of therapy. **Tab:** Consider discontinuation after 3-5 yrs of use in patients at low risk for fracture; periodically reevaluate risk for fracture in patients who d/c therapy. Ascertain gonadal hormonal status and consider appropriate replacement before initiating therapy for glucocorticoid-induced osteoporosis.

ADVERSE REACTIONS

Nausea, abdominal pain, musculoskeletal pain, dyspepsia, constipation, diarrhea.

DRUG INTERACTIONS

Ca^{2+} supplements, antacids, or oral medications containing multivalent cations will interfere w/ absorption; wait at least 1/2 hr after taking alendronate before taking any other oral medications. Increased incidence of upper GI adverse events in patients receiving concomitant therapy w/ daily doses of alendronate >10mg and aspirin-containing products. NSAID use is associated w/ GI irritation; use w/ caution.

PATIENT CONSIDERATIONS

Assessment: Assess for esophageal abnormalities, ability to stand or sit upright for at least 30 min, hypocalcemia, risk for ONJ, active upper GI problems, mental disability, renal impairment, drug hypersensitivity, any other conditions where treatment is contraindicated or cautioned, pregnancy/nursing status, and possible drug interactions. **Tab:** For glucocorticoid-induced osteoporosis treatment, assess gonadal hormonal status and obtain bone mineral density.

Monitoring: Monitor for signs/symptoms of ONJ, atypical fractures, esophageal reactions, musculoskeletal pain, hypocalcemia, and other adverse reactions. Monitor serum Ca^{2+} levels. Periodically reevaluate the need for continued therapy. **Tab:** Monitor bone mineral density after 6-12 months of combined alendronate and glucocorticoid treatment. For Paget's disease treatment, monitor serum alkaline phosphatase periodically.

Counseling: Inform about benefits/risks of therapy. Instruct to follow all dosing instructions and inform that failure to follow them may increase risk of esophageal problems. Instruct to take upon arising for the day and at least 1/2 hr before the 1st food, beverage, or medication of the day w/ plain water only; advise to swallow tab w/ 6-8 oz of water and to follow oral sol by at least 2 oz of water. Advise to avoid lying down for at least 30 min after taking the drug and until after 1st food of the day. Instruct to take supplemental Ca^{2+} and vitamin D if daily dietary intake is inadequate. Advise to consider weight-bearing exercise along w/ the modification of certain behavioral factors (eg, cigarette smoking, excessive alcohol use), if these factors exist. Advise to d/c and consult physician if symptoms of esophageal disease develop. Instruct that if a once-weekly dose is missed, to take 1 dose the am after patient remembers and to return to taking the dose as originally scheduled on patient's chosen day; instruct not to take 2 doses on the same day.

STORAGE: **Oral Sol:** 25°C (77°F); excursions permitted to 15-30°C (59-86°F). Do not freeze. **Tab:** 20-25°C (68-77°F); (Fosamax) 15-30°C (59-86°F).

ALIMTA – pemetrexed disodium

RX

Class: Antifolate

ADULT DOSAGE

Nonsquamous Non-Small Cell Lung Cancer

Initial treatment of locally advanced or metastatic nonsquamous non-small cell lung cancer (NSCLC) in combination w/ cisplatin. Maint treatment of patients w/ locally advanced or metastatic nonsquamous NSCLC whose disease has not progressed after 4 cycles of platinum-based first-line chemotherapy. Single-agent for the treatment of patients w/ locally advanced or metastatic nonsquamous NSCLC after prior chemotherapy

PEDIATRIC DOSAGE

Pediatric use may not have been established

Combination w/ Cisplatin:
500mg/m^2 IV infused over 10 min on Day 1 of each 21-day cycle
Give cisplatin 75mg/m^2 infused over 2 hrs beginning 30 min after the end of administration

Single Agent:
500mg/m^2 IV infused over 10 min on Day 1 of each 21-day cycle

Malignant Pleural Mesothelioma

Patients whose disease is unresectable or who are otherwise not candidates for curative surgery in combination w/ cisplatin

Combination w/ Cisplatin:
500mg/m^2 IV infused over 10 min on Day 1 of each 21-day cycle
Give cisplatin 75mg/m^2 infused over 2 hrs beginning 30 min after the end of administration

Premedication

Initiate folic acid (400-1000mcg) PO qd beginning 7 days before the 1st dose; continue during the full course of therapy and for 21 days after the last dose of therapy
Administer vitamin B12 1mg IM 1 week prior to the 1st dose and every 3 cycles thereafter
Subsequent vitamin B12 inj may be given the same day as treatment
Give dexamethasone 4mg PO bid the day before, the day of, and the day after administration of therapy

DOSING CONSIDERATIONS

Adverse Reactions

As a Single Agent or in Combination:

Hematologic Toxicities:

Nadir ANC <500/mm³ and Nadir Platelets ≥50,000/mm³: 75% of previous dose (pemetrexed and cisplatin)
Nadir Platelets <50,000/mm³ w/o Bleeding Regardless of Nadir ANC: 75% of previous dose (pemetrexed and cisplatin)
Nadir Platelets <50,000/mm³ w/ Bleeding Regardless of Nadir ANC: 50% of previous dose (pemetrexed and cisplatin)

Nonhematologic Toxicities:

≥Grade 3 (Excluding Neurotoxicity): Withhold treatment until resolution to ≤pre-therapy value
Any Grade 3 or 4 Toxicities Except Mucositis: 75% of previous dose (pemetrexed and cisplatin)
Any Diarrhea Requiring Hospitalization (Irrespective of Grade) or Grade 3 or 4 Diarrhea: 75% of previous dose (pemetrexed and cisplatin)
Grade 3 or 4 Mucositis: 50% of previous pemetrexed dose, 100% of previous cisplatin dose

Neurotoxicity:

CTC Grade 1: 100% of previous pemetrexed and cisplatin dose
CTC Grade 2: 100% of previous pemetrexed dose, 50% of previous cisplatin dose

Discontinuation

For Any of the Following:

1. Experiences any hematologic or nonhematologic Grade 3 or 4 toxicity after 2 dose reductions
2. Grade 3 or 4 neurotoxicity is observed

ADMINISTRATION

IV route

Preparation

1. Calculate dose and determine the number of vials needed
2. Reconstitute each 100mg vial w/ 4.2mL of 0.9% NaCl (preservative free). Reconstitute each 500mg vial w/ 20mL of 0.9% NaCl (preservative free)
3. Gently swirl each vial until the powder is completely dissolved. The resulting sol is clear and ranges in color from colorless to yellow or green-yellow w/o adversely affecting product quality

4. An appropriate quantity of the reconstituted sol must be further diluted into a sol of 0.9% NaCl (preservative free), so that the total volume of sol is 100mL.
5. Administered as an IV infusion over 10 min

Compatibility and Stability

Compatible w/ standard polyvinyl chloride administration sets and IV sol bags
Stable for up to 24 hrs following initial reconstitution, when refrigerated

Handling Precautions

If sol contacts the skin, wash the skin immediately and thoroughly w/ soap and water
If sol contacts the mucous membranes, flush thoroughly w/ water

HOW SUPPLIED

Inj: 100mg, 500mg

CONTRAINDICATIONS

History of severe hypersensitivity reaction to pemetrexed.

WARNINGS/PRECAUTIONS

Not indicated for the treatment of patients with squamous cell NSCLC. Premedicate with folic acid and vitamin B12 to reduce hematologic/GI toxicity, and with dexamethasone. Do not substitute oral vitamin B12 for IM vitamin B12. Bone marrow suppression may occur; myelosuppression is usually the dose-limiting toxicity. Caution with renal/hepatic impairment and in elderly. Avoid in patients with CrCl <45mL/min. D/C if hematologic or nonhematologic Grade 3 or 4 toxicity after two dose reductions or immediately if Grade 3 or 4 neurotoxicity is observed. Do not start a cycle of treatment unless CrCl is ≥45mL/min, ANC is ≥1500 cells/mm^3, and platelet count is ≥100,000 cells/mm^3; obtain CBC and renal function tests at the beginning of each cycle and prn. May cause fetal harm; use effective contraception to prevent pregnancy.

ADVERSE REACTIONS

Anemia, anorexia, fatigue, leukopenia, N/V, stomatitis, neutropenia, rash/desquamation, thrombocytopenia, constipation, pharyngitis, diarrhea.

DRUG INTERACTIONS

Reduced clearance with ibuprofen. In patients with mild to moderate renal insufficiency (CrCl 45-79mL/min), caution with NSAIDs; avoid NSAIDs with short $T_{1/2}$ (eg, diclofenac, indomethacin) for 2 days before, the day of, and 2 days following therapy. Interrupt dosing of NSAIDs with longer $T_{1/2}$ (eg, meloxicam, nabumetone) for at least 5 days before, the day of, and 2 days following therapy. If concomitant NSAID administration is necessary, monitor for toxicity. Delayed clearance with nephrotoxic or tubularly secreted drugs (eg, probenecid).

PATIENT CONSIDERATIONS

Assessment: Assess for drug hypersensitivity, renal/hepatic impairment, pregnancy/nursing status, and possible drug interactions. Obtain CBC and renal function tests at the beginning of each cycle.

Monitoring: Monitor for signs and symptoms of hematologic/nonhematologic toxicities, bone marrow suppression (eg, neutropenia, thrombocytopenia, anemia), GI toxicity, neurotoxicity, and other adverse events. Monitor CBC with platelet counts and for nadir and recovery. Perform renal and hepatic function tests periodically.

Counseling: Inform about benefits and risks of therapy. Instruct on the need for folic acid and vitamin B12 supplementation to reduce treatment-related hematological and GI toxicities, and of the need for corticosteroids to reduce treatment-related dermatologic toxicity. Inform about risks of low blood cell counts and instruct to contact physician immediately if signs of infection (eg, fever, bleeding or symptoms of anemia) occur. Instruct to contact physician if persistent vomiting, diarrhea, or signs of dehydration appear. Instruct to inform physician of all concomitant prescription or OTC medications (eg, NSAIDs). Inform female patients of the potential hazard to fetus; advise to avoid pregnancy and to use effective contraceptive measures to prevent pregnancy during treatment.

STORAGE: Unreconstituted: 25°C (77°F); excursions permitted to 15-30°C (59-86°F). Reconstituted and Infusion Sol: Stable at 2-8°C (36-46°F) for up to 24 hrs.

ALOPRIM – allopurinol sodium RX

Class: Xanthine oxidase inhibitor

ADULT DOSAGE

Chemotherapy-Induced Hyperuricemia

Management of patients w/ leukemia, lymphoma, and solid tumor malignancies who are receiving cancer therapy that causes elevations of serum and urinary uric acid levels and who cannot tolerate oral therapy

PEDIATRIC DOSAGE

Chemotherapy-Induced Hyperuricemia

Management of patients w/ leukemia, lymphoma, and solid tumor malignancies who are receiving cancer therapy that causes elevations of serum and urinary uric acid levels and who cannot tolerate oral therapy

Usual: 200-400mg/m²/day, as a single infusion or in equally divided infusions at 6-, 8-, or 12-hr intervals
Max: 600mg/day

Whenever possible, initiate therapy 24-48 hrs before the start of chemotherapy known to cause tumor cell lysis (including adrenocortical steroids)

Initial: 200mg/m²/day, as a single infusion or in equally divided infusions at 6-, 8-, or 12-hr intervals

Whenever possible, initiate therapy 24-48 hrs before the start of chemotherapy known to cause tumor cell lysis (including adrenocortical steroids)

DOSING CONSIDERATIONS

Renal Impairment
CrCl 10-20mL/min: 200mg/day
CrCl 3-10mL/min: 100mg/day
CrCl <3mL/min: 100mg/day at extended intervals

Elderly
Start at lower end of dosing range

ADMINISTRATION

IV route

Hydration
Fluid intake sufficient to yield a daily urinary output of ≥2L in adults and the maint of a neutral or, preferably, slightly alkaline urine are desirable

Preparation of Sol
1. Dissolve the contents of each 30mL vial w/ 25mL of sterile water for inj; reconstitution yields a concentrated sol w/ a pH of 11.1-11.8
2. Dilute the sol to the desired concentration w/ 0.9% NaCl inj or D5 for inj; refer to PI for drugs that are physically incompatible in sol w/ allopurinol
3. A final concentration of ≤6mg/mL is recommended

Administration
Begin administration w/in 10 hrs after reconstitution
The rate of infusion depends on the volume of infusate
Do not mix w/ or administer through the same IV port w/ agents that are incompatible in sol w/ allopurinol

HOW SUPPLIED

Inj: 500mg

CONTRAINDICATIONS

Re-initiation in patients who developed a severe reaction to allopurinol.

WARNINGS/PRECAUTIONS

D/C at 1st appearance of skin rash or other signs of an allergic reaction. Hepatotoxicity and elevated serum alkaline phosphatase/transaminase reported with PO allopurinol. Bone marrow suppression reported. Evaluate liver function if anorexia, weight loss, or pruritus develops. Periodically monitor LFTs during early stages of therapy in patients with preexisting liver disease. May impair mental/physical abilities. Maintain sufficient fluid intake to yield a daily urinary output in adults of at least 2L and maintain neutral or slightly alkaline urine. Caution with renal impairment or concurrent illnesses affecting renal function (eg, HTN, diabetes mellitus); periodically monitor renal function. Caution in elderly.

ADVERSE REACTIONS

Rash, eosinophilia, local inj-site reaction, diarrhea, nausea, decreased renal function, generalized seizure.

DRUG INTERACTIONS

Inhibits oxidation of mercaptopurine and azathioprine; reduce mercaptopurine or azathioprine dose to 1/3-1/4 of usual dose when given with 300-600mg of allopurinol. May prolong $T_{1/2}$ of dicumarol; monitor PT with concomitant use. Inhibition of xanthine oxidase by oxypurinol may be decreased and urinary excretion of uric acid may be increased with concomitant uricosuric agents. May increase toxicity and occurrence of hypersensitivity reactions with concomitant thiazide diuretics in patients with decreased renal function; monitor renal function. May increase frequency of skin rash when used with ampicillin or amoxicillin. Bone marrow suppression may be enhanced with cyclophosphamide and other cytotoxic agents among patients with neoplastic disease, except leukemia. May increase risk of hypoglycemia in the presence of renal insufficiency with concomitant chlorpropamide. May increase cyclosporine levels; monitor cyclosporine levels and consider possible adjustment of cyclosporine dose.

PATIENT CONSIDERATIONS

Assessment: Assess for renal/hepatic disease, concurrent illnesses affecting renal function, previous severe reaction to the drug, pregnancy/nursing status, and possible drug interactions. Obtain serum uric acid level to provide correct dosage and schedule.

Monitoring: Monitor for signs/symptoms of hypersensitivity/allergic reactions, drowsiness, bone marrow suppression, and other adverse reactions. Monitor fluid intake, LFTs, renal function (BUN, SrCr, CrCl), and serum uric acid level.

Counseling: Inform of risks and benefits of therapy. Counsel that drug may impair mental/physical abilities. Advise to take sufficient fluid to yield urinary output of at least 2L/day in adults and inform of the need to maintain a neutral or, preferably, slightly alkaline urine. Instruct to report any adverse events to physician.

STORAGE: 20-25°C (68-77°F). Do not refrigerate reconstituted/diluted sol.

Aloxi – palonosetron hydrochloride

Class: 5-HT_3 receptor antagonist

RX

ADULT DOSAGE

Chemotherapy-Induced Nausea/Vomiting

Moderately Emetogenic Chemotherapy:
Prevention of acute and delayed N/V associated w/ initial and repeat courses

0.25mg IV as a single dose over 30 sec; begin approx 30 min before the start of chemotherapy

Highly Emetogenic Chemotherapy:
Prevention of acute N/V associated w/ initial and repeat courses

0.25mg IV as a single dose over 30 sec; begin approx 30 min before the start of chemotherapy

Postoperative Nausea/Vomiting

Prevention for Up to 24 Hrs Following Surgery:

0.075mg IV as single dose over 10 sec immediately before induction of anesthesia

PEDIATRIC DOSAGE

Chemotherapy-Induced Nausea/Vomiting

Prevention of Acute N/V Associated w/ Initial and Repeat Courses of Emetogenic Cancer Chemotherapy, Including Highly Emetogenic Cancer Chemotherapy:

1 Month-<17 Years:

20mcg/kg IV as a single dose over 15 min; begin approx 30 min before the start of chemotherapy

Max Dose: 1.5mg

ADMINISTRATION

IV route

Do not mix w/ other drugs
Flush infusion line w/ normal saline before and after administration

HOW SUPPLIED

Inj: 0.075mg/1.5mL, 0.25mg/5mL

CONTRAINDICATIONS

Known hypersensitivity to the drug or any of its components.

WARNINGS/PRECAUTIONS

Hypersensitivity reactions, including anaphylaxis, reported with or without known hypersensitivity to other 5-HT_3 receptor antagonists. Routine prophylaxis is not recommended in patients who demonstrate low risk of PONV. Therapy is recommended in patients where N/V must be avoided during the postoperative period. Serotonin syndrome reported; d/c treatment and initiate supportive treatment if symptoms occur.

ADVERSE REACTIONS

Headache, constipation, QT prolongation, bradycardia.

DRUG INTERACTIONS

Serotonin syndrome reported with concomitant use of serotonergic drugs (eg, SSRIs, SNRIs, MAOIs, mirtazapine, fentanyl).

PATIENT CONSIDERATIONS

Assessment: Assess for hypersensitivity to drug, risk/possibility of PONV, emetogenicity of cancer chemotherapy, pregnancy/nursing status, and possible drug interactions.

Monitoring: Monitor for hypersensitivity reactions, emergence of serotonin syndrome, and other adverse reactions.

Counseling: Inform of the benefits/risks of therapy. Advise to report to physician all medical conditions, including any pain, redness, or swelling in and around infusion site. Advise of the possibility of serotonin syndrome, especially with concomitant use of other serotonergic agents;

instruct to seek immediate medical attention if changes in mental status, autonomic instability, or neuromuscular symptoms with or without GI symptoms occur.

STORAGE: 20-25°C (68-77°F); excursions permitted to 15-30°C (59-86°F). Protect from light and freezing.

ALPHAGAN P – brimonidine tartrate

RX

Class: Selective $alpha_2$ agonist

ADULT DOSAGE

Elevated Intraocular Pressure

Reduction of Elevated IOP in Patients w/ Open-Angle Glaucoma or Ocular HTN:
Instill 1 drop in affected eye(s) tid (8 hrs apart)

PEDIATRIC DOSAGE

Elevated Intraocular Pressure

Reduction of Elevated IOP in Patients w/ Open-Angle Glaucoma or Ocular HTN:
≥2 Years:
Instill 1 drop in affected eye(s) tid (8 hrs apart)

ADMINISTRATION

Ocular route

Space by at least 5 min if using >1 topical ophthalmic drug

HOW SUPPLIED

Sol: 0.1%, 0.15% [5mL, 10mL, 15mL]

CONTRAINDICATIONS

Neonates and infants <2 yrs of age, hypersensitivity reaction to any component of this medication.

WARNINGS/PRECAUTIONS

May potentiate syndromes associated with vascular insufficiency. Caution with severe cardiovascular disease (CVD), depression, cerebral or coronary insufficiency, Raynaud's phenomenon, orthostatic hypotension, or thromboangiitis obliterans. Bacterial keratitis reported with multidose containers.

ADVERSE REACTIONS

Allergic conjunctivitis, conjunctival hyperemia, eye pruritus, burning sensation, conjunctival folliculosis, HTN, oral dryness, ocular allergic reaction, visual disturbance, somnolence, decreased alertness.

DRUG INTERACTIONS

May potentiate effect with CNS depressants (alcohol, barbiturates, opiates, sedatives, anesthetics). Caution with antihypertensives, cardiac glycosides, and TCAs. May increase systemic side effects (eg, hypotension) with MAOIs; caution is advised.

PATIENT CONSIDERATIONS

Assessment: Assess for hypersensitivity, severe CVD, depression, cerebral or coronary insufficiency, Raynaud's phenomenon, orthostatic hypotension, thromboangiitis obliterans, pregnancy/nursing, and possible drug interactions.

Monitoring: Monitor vascular insufficiency, bacterial keratitis, and other adverse reactions.

Counseling: Advise to avoid touching tip of applicator to eye or surrounding areas. Instruct patient to notify physician if they have ocular surgery or develop an intercurrent ocular condition (eg, trauma or infection). Inform patients that fatigue and/or drowsiness may occur; may impair physical or mental abilities. Instruct to space by at least 5 min if using >1 topical ophthalmic drug.

STORAGE: 15-25°C (59-77°F).

ALTACE – ramipril

RX

Class: ACE inhibitor

D/C when pregnancy is detected. Drugs that act directly on the renin-angiotensin system (RAS) can cause injury/death to the developing fetus.

ADULT DOSAGE

Hypertension

Not Receiving a Diuretic:
Initial: 2.5mg qd
Maint: 2.5-20mg/day as single dose or in 2 equally divided doses
May add a diuretic if BP is not controlled

PEDIATRIC DOSAGE

Pediatric use may not have been established

Risk Reduction of Myocardial Infarction, Stroke, Cardiovascular Death

High Risk Patients ≥55 Years:
Initial: 2.5mg qd for 1 week
Titrate: Increase to 5mg qd for next 3 weeks, then increase as tolerated
Maint: 10mg qd
May be given as a divided dose if patient is hypertensive or recently post-MI

Congestive Heart Failure Post-Myocardial Infarction

Stable patients w/ signs of CHF w/in 1st few days after sustaining acute MI
Initial: 2.5mg bid; may switch to 1.25mg bid if patient becomes hypotensive at this dose
Titrate: After 1 week at initial dose, increase dose, if tolerated, to target dose of 5mg bid, w/ dose increases being about 3 weeks apart
After initial dose, observe for at least 2 hrs and until BP has stabilized for at least an additional hr
Reduce dose of any concomitant diuretic, if possible, to decrease incidence of hypotension

DOSING CONSIDERATIONS

Renal Impairment
CrCl ≤40mL/min:
HTN:
Initial: 1.25mg qd
Max: 5mg/day

Heart Failure Post MI:
Initial: 1.25mg qd
Titrate: May increase to 1.25mg bid
Max: 2.5mg bid

Other Important Considerations
Renal Artery Stenosis/Volume Depletion (eg, Past and Current Diuretic Use):
Initial: 1.25mg qd

ADMINISTRATION

Oral route
Swallow caps whole.
May also open cap and sprinkle content on a small amount (about 4 oz) of applesauce or mix in 4 oz (120mL) of water or apple juice; consume mixture in its entirety.
May pre-prepare mixture and store for up to 24 hrs at room temperature or up to 48 hrs under refrigeration.

HOW SUPPLIED

Cap: 1.25mg, 2.5mg, 5mg, 10mg

CONTRAINDICATIONS

Hypersensitivity to this product or any other ACE inhibitor (eg, history of ACE inhibitor-associated angioedema), coadministration w/ aliskiren in patients w/ diabetes.

WARNINGS/PRECAUTIONS

Increased risk of angioedema in patients w/ history of angioedema unrelated to ACE inhibitor therapy. Head/neck angioedema reported; d/c and institute appropriate therapy if laryngeal stridor or angioedema of the face, tongue, or glottis occurs. Higher rate of angioedema in blacks than nonblacks. Intestinal angioedema reported; monitor for abdominal pain. Anaphylactoid reactions reported during desensitization w/ hymenoptera venom, dialysis w/ high-flux membranes, and LDL apheresis w/ dextran sulfate absorption. Rarely, associated w/ a syndrome that starts w/ cholestatic jaundice and progresses to fulminant hepatic necrosis and sometimes death; d/c if jaundice or marked hepatic enzyme elevations develop. May cause changes in renal function. May be associated w/ oliguria or progressive azotemia and rarely w/ acute renal failure or death, in patients w/ severe CHF whose renal function may depend on the activity of the RAS. Increases in BUN and SrCr may occur in hypertensive patients w/ unilateral or bilateral renal artery stenosis; monitor renal function during the 1st few weeks of therapy. Increases in BUN and SrCr reported in some hypertensive patients w/ no apparent preexisting renal vascular disease; dose reduction of ramipril and/or discontinuation of the diuretic may be required. Agranulocytosis, pancytopenia, bone marrow depression, and mild reductions in RBC count and Hgb content, blood cell or platelet counts may occur; consider monitoring WBCs in patients w/ collagen vascular disease (eg, systemic lupus erythematosus, scleroderma), especially w/ renal impairment. Symptomatic hypotension may occur and is most likely to occur in patients w/ volume and/or salt depletion; correct depletion prior to therapy. May cause excessive hypotension, which may be associated w/ oliguria or azotemia and rarely, w/ acute renal failure and death, in patients with CHF, w/ or w/o associated renal insufficiency; follow patients closely for the first 2 weeks of treatment and whenever the dose of therapy or diuretic is increased. Hypotension may occur w/ surgery or during anesthesia. Hyperkalemia reported; monitor serum K^+ in patients w/ risk factors (eg, renal insufficiency, diabetes mellitus). Persistent nonproductive cough reported.

ADVERSE REACTIONS

Hypotension, cough increased, dizziness, headache, asthenia, fatigue.

DRUG INTERACTIONS

See Contraindications. Dual blockade of the RAS is associated w/ increased risks of hypotension, hyperkalemia, and changes in renal function (including acute renal failure); avoid combined use of RAS inhibitors, or closely monitor BP, renal function, and electrolytes w/ other agents that also affect the RAS. Not recommended w/ telmisartan; increased risk of renal dysfunction. Avoid w/ aliskiren in patients w/ renal impairment (GFR <60mL/min). Initiation of therapy in patients on diuretics (especially those in whom diuretic therapy was recently instituted) may result in excessive reduction of BP. Decrease or d/c diuretic or increase the salt intake prior to initiation of therapy; if this is not possible, reduce the starting dose of ramipril. Increased risk of hyperkalemia w/ K^+-sparing diuretics, K^+ supplements, and/or K^+-containing salt substitutes; monitor serum K^+. Increased lithium levels and symptoms of lithium toxicity reported; frequently monitor serum lithium levels. Diuretics may further increase risk of lithium toxicity. Nitritoid reactions reported rarely w/ injectable gold (sodium aurothiomalate). NSAIDs, including selective COX-2 inhibitors, may result in deterioration of renal function, including possible acute renal failure in elderly, volume depleted or patients w/ compromised renal function. Antihypertensive effect may be attenuated by NSAIDs. Coadministration w/ mTOR inhibitors (eg, temsirolimus) may increase risk for angioedema. Increased BUN and SrCr w/ diuretics.

PATIENT CONSIDERATIONS

Assessment: Assess for history of angioedema, CHF, renal artery stenosis, collagen vascular disease, volume/salt depletion, risk factors for hyperkalemia, renal/hepatic impairment, hypersensitivity to drug, pregnancy/nursing status, and possible drug interactions.

Monitoring: Monitor for signs/symptoms of angioedema, anaphylactoid reactions, hyperkalemia, cough, jaundice, and other adverse reactions. Consider monitoring WBCs in patients w/ collagen vascular disease, especially w/ renal impairment. Monitor BP and renal/hepatic function.

Counseling: Instruct to d/c therapy and to immediately report any signs/symptoms of angioedema. Advise to promptly report any indication of infection. Instruct to report lightheadedness, especially during 1st days of therapy; advise to d/c and consult w/ a physician if syncope occurs. Inform that inadequate fluid intake or excessive perspiration, diarrhea, or vomiting may lead to an excessive fall in BP, w/ the same consequences of lightheadedness and possible syncope. Inform females of childbearing age about the consequences of exposure during pregnancy and discuss treatment options in women planning to become pregnant; instruct to report pregnancy to physician as soon as possible. Advise not to use salt substitutes containing K^+ w/o consulting physician.

STORAGE: 15-30°C (59-86°F).

ALTOPREV – lovastatin

RX

Class: HMG-CoA reductase inhibitor (statin)

ADULT DOSAGE

Hyperlipidemia/Mixed Dyslipidemia

Usual: 20-60mg/day given qhs

Prevention of Coronary Heart Disease

Dose based on current clinical practice

PEDIATRIC DOSAGE

Pediatric use may not have been established

DOSING CONSIDERATIONS

Concomitant Medications

Danazol, Diltiazem, Dronedarone, or Verapamil:
Max: 20mg/day

Amiodarone:
Max: 40mg/day

Renal Impairment

Severe (CrCl <30mL/min): Consider dosage increases >20mg/day only if the expected benefit exceeds the increased risk of myopathy/rhabdomyolysis

Elderly
Initial: 20mg qhs

ADMINISTRATION
Oral route

HOW SUPPLIED
Tab, Extended-Release: 20mg, 40mg, 60mg

CONTRAINDICATIONS
Concomitant strong CYP3A inhibitors and erythromycin, hypersensitivity to any component of this product. Active liver disease (eg, unexplained persistent elevations of hepatic transaminase levels), women who are or may become pregnant, nursing mothers.

WARNINGS/PRECAUTIONS
Myopathy (including immune-mediated necrotizing myopathy) and rhabdomyolysis with acute renal failure secondary to myoglobinuria reported; d/c if markedly elevated creatine kinase levels occur or myopathy is diagnosed/suspected and temporarily withhold in any patient experiencing an acute or serious condition predisposing to development of renal failure secondary to rhabdomyolysis. Increases in serum transaminases reported. Fatal and nonfatal hepatic failure rarely reported; promptly interrupt therapy if serious liver injury with clinical symptoms and/or hyperbilirubinemia or jaundice occurs and do not restart if no alternate etiology found. Caution in patients who consume substantial quantities of alcohol and/or have history of chronic liver disease. Increases in HbA1c and FPG levels reported. Evaluate patients who develop endocrine dysfunction. Caution in elderly.

ADVERSE REACTIONS
Infection, pain, headache, asthenia, myalgia, back pain, flu syndrome, arthralgia, sinusitis, diarrhea.

DRUG INTERACTIONS
See Contraindications and Dosage. Ranolazine may increase risk of myopathy/rhabdomyolysis; consider dose adjustment of lovastatin. Due to the risk of myopathy, avoid with gemfibrozil, cyclosporine, and grapefruit juice, and caution with other fibrates, lipid-lowering doses (≥1g/day) of niacin, colchicine, danazol, diltiazem, dronedarone, verapamil, or amiodarone. Determine PT before initiation and frequently enough during early therapy with anticoagulants; bleeding and/or increased PT reported with coumarin anticoagulants. Caution with drugs that may decrease the levels or activity of endogenous steroid hormones (eg, spironolactone, cimetidine).

PATIENT CONSIDERATIONS

Assessment: Assess for drug hypersensitivity, active/history of liver disease, alcohol consumption, renal impairment, pregnancy/nursing status, and possible drug interactions. Obtain baseline LFTs, lipid profile, and check PT with coumarin anticoagulants.

Monitoring: Monitor for signs/symptoms of myopathy, rhabdomyolysis, endocrine/renal dysfunction, and other adverse effects. Monitor LFTs. Monitor PT with coumarin anticoagulants.

Counseling: Instruct to promptly report any unexplained muscle pain, tenderness, or weakness, particularly if accompanied by malaise or fever or if muscle signs/symptoms persist after discontinuation. Inform about substances that should be avoided during therapy, and advise to discuss all medications, both prescription and OTC, with physician. Inform that liver enzyme tests should be performed before the initiation of therapy and if signs/symptoms of liver injury occur; advise to promptly report any symptoms that may indicate liver injury. Advise women of childbearing age to use an effective method of birth control, to stop taking the drug if they become pregnant, and not to breastfeed while on therapy.

STORAGE: 20-25°C (68-77°F); excursions permitted to 15-30°C (59-86°F). Avoid excessive heat and humidity.

AMBIEN — zolpidem tartrate

CIV

Class: Imidazopyridine hypnotic

ADULT DOSAGE
Insomnia
Difficulties w/ Sleep Initiation:
Initial:
Women: 5mg qhs
Men: 5mg or 10mg qhs
Titrate: May increase to 10mg if the 5mg dose is not effective
Max: 10mg qhs

PEDIATRIC DOSAGE
Pediatric use may not have been established

DOSING CONSIDERATIONS

Concomitant Medications

CNS Depressants: May need to adjust dose of zolpidem

Hepatic Impairment

5mg qhs

Elderly

Elderly/Debilitated: 5mg qhs

ADMINISTRATION

Oral route

Take immediately before hs w/ at least 7-8 hrs remaining before the planned time of awakening

Do not administer w/ or immediately after a meal

HOW SUPPLIED

Tab: 5mg, 10mg

CONTRAINDICATIONS

Known hypersensitivity to zolpidem.

WARNINGS/PRECAUTIONS

Increased risk of next-day psychomotor impairment if taken with less than a full night of sleep remaining (7-8 hrs). May impair mental/physical abilities. Initiate only after careful evaluation; failure of insomnia to remit after 7-10 days of treatment may indicate presence of a primary psychiatric and/or medical illness. Angioedema and anaphylaxis reported; do not rechallenge if such reactions develop. Abnormal thinking, behavior changes, and visual and auditory hallucinations reported. Complex behaviors (eg, sleep-driving) while not fully awake reported; consider discontinuation if a sleep-driving episode occurs. Amnesia, anxiety, and other neuropsychiatric symptoms may occur. Worsening of depression and suicidal thoughts and actions (including completed suicides) reported primarily in depressed patients; prescribe the lowest feasible number of tabs at a time. Caution with compromised respiratory function; prior to prescribing, consider the risk of respiratory depression in patients with respiratory impairment (eg, sleep apnea, myasthenia gravis). Withdrawal signs and symptoms reported following rapid dose decrease or abrupt discontinuation; monitor for tolerance, abuse, and dependence. May cause drowsiness and a decreased level of consciousness, which may lead to falls and consequently to severe injuries (eg, hip fractures, intracranial hemorrhage).

ADVERSE REACTIONS

Drowsiness, dizziness, headache, diarrhea, drugged feeling, lethargy, dry mouth, back pain, pharyngitis, sinusitis, allergy.

DRUG INTERACTIONS

See Dosage. Increased risk of CNS depression and complex behaviors with other CNS depressants (eg, benzodiazepines, opioids, TCAs, alcohol). Use with other sedative-hypnotics (eg, other zolpidem products) at hs or the middle of the night is not recommended. Increased risk of next-day psychomotor impairment with other CNS depressants or drugs that increase zolpidem levels. May decrease peak levels of imipramine. Additive effect of decreased alertness with imipramine or chlorpromazine. Additive adverse effect on psychomotor performance with chlorpromazine or alcohol. Sertraline and CYP3A inhibitors may increase exposure. Fluoxetine may increase $T_{1/2}$. Rifampin (a CYP3A4 inducer) may reduce exposure, pharmacodynamic effects, and efficacy. Ketoconazole (a potent CYP3A4 inhibitor) may increase pharmacodynamic effects; consider lower dose of zolpidem.

PATIENT CONSIDERATIONS

Assessment: Assess for physical and/or psychiatric disorder, depression, compromised respiratory function, sleep apnea, myasthenia gravis, hepatic impairment, history of drug/alcohol addiction or abuse, hypersensitivity to the drug, pregnancy/nursing status, and possible drug interactions.

Monitoring: Monitor for angioedema, anaphylaxis, emergence of any new behavioral signs/symptoms of concern, respiratory depression, withdrawal signs/symptoms, tolerance, abuse, dependence, drowsiness, decreased level of consciousness, and other adverse reactions.

Counseling: Inform about the benefits and risks of treatment. Instruct to take only as prescribed; advise to wait at least 8 hrs after dosing before driving or engaging in other activities requiring full mental alertness. Instruct to contact physician immediately if any adverse reactions (eg, severe anaphylactic/anaphylactoid reactions, sleep-driving, other complex behaviors, suicidal thoughts) develop. Advise not to use the drug if patient drank alcohol that pm or before bed. Instruct not to increase the dose and to inform physician if it is believed that the drug does not work.

STORAGE: 20-25°C (68-77°F).

AMBIEN CR – zolpidem tartrate

CIV

Class: Imidazopyridine hypnotic

ADULT DOSAGE

Insomnia

Difficulties w/ Sleep Onset and/or Sleep Maintenance:
Initial:
Women: 6.25mg qhs
Men: 6.25mg or 12.5mg qhs
Titrate: May increase to 12.5mg if the 6.25mg dose is not effective
Max: 12.5mg qhs

PEDIATRIC DOSAGE

Pediatric use may not have been established

DOSING CONSIDERATIONS

Concomitant Medications

CNS Depressants: May need to adjust dose of zolpidem

Hepatic Impairment

6.25mg qhs

Elderly

Elderly/Debilitated: 6.25mg qhs

ADMINISTRATION

Oral route

Swallow whole; do not divide, crush, or chew
Take immediately before hs w/ at least 7-8 hrs remaining before the planned time of awakening
Do not administer w/ or immediately after a meal

HOW SUPPLIED

Tab, Extended-Release: 6.25mg, 12.5mg

CONTRAINDICATIONS

Known hypersensitivity to zolpidem.

WARNINGS/PRECAUTIONS

May impair daytime function; monitor for excess depressant effects. May impair mental/physical abilities. Increased risk of next-day psychomotor impairment if taken with less than a full night of sleep remaining (7-8 hrs). Initiate only after careful evaluation; failure of insomnia to remit after 7-10 days of treatment may indicate presence of a primary psychiatric and/or medical illness. Angioedema and anaphylaxis reported; do not rechallenge if such reactions develop. Abnormal thinking, behavior changes, and visual and auditory hallucinations reported. Complex behaviors (eg, sleep-driving) while not fully awake reported; consider discontinuation if a sleep-driving episode occurs. Amnesia, anxiety, and other neuropsychiatric symptoms may occur. Worsening of depression and suicidal thoughts and actions (including completed suicides) reported primarily in depressed patients; prescribe the lowest feasible number of tabs at a time. Caution with compromised respiratory function; prior to prescribing, consider the risk of respiratory depression in patients with respiratory impairment (eg, sleep apnea, myasthenia gravis). Withdrawal signs and symptoms reported following rapid dose decrease or abrupt discontinuation; monitor for tolerance, abuse, and dependence. May cause drowsiness and a decreased level of consciousness, which may lead to falls and consequently to severe injuries (eg, hip fractures, intracranial hemorrhage).

ADVERSE REACTIONS

Headache, somnolence, dizziness, anxiety, nausea, influenza, hallucinations, back pain, myalgia, fatigue, disorientation, memory disorder, visual disturbance, nasopharyngitis.

DRUG INTERACTIONS

See Dosage. Additive effects with other CNS depressants (eg, benzodiazepines, opioids, TCAs, alcohol), including daytime use. Use with other sedative-hypnotics (eg, other zolpidem products) at hs or the middle of the night is not recommended. Increased risk of next-day psychomotor impairment with other CNS depressants or drugs that increase zolpidem levels. Increased risk of complex behaviors with alcohol and other CNS depressants. May decrease peak levels of imipramine. Additive effect of decreased alertness with imipramine or chlorpromazine. Additive adverse effect on psychomotor performance with chlorpromazine or alcohol. Sertraline and CYP3A inhibitors may increase exposure. Fluoxetine may increase $T_{1/2}$. Rifampin (a CYP3A4 inducer) may reduce exposure, pharmacodynamic effects, and efficacy. Ketoconazole (a potent CYP3A4 inhibitor) may increase pharmacodynamic effects; consider lower dose of zolpidem.

PATIENT CONSIDERATIONS

Assessment: Assess for physical and/or psychiatric disorder, depression, compromised respiratory function, sleep apnea, myasthenia gravis, hepatic impairment, history of drug/alcohol addiction or abuse, hypersensitivity to the drug, pregnancy/nursing status, and possible drug interactions.

Monitoring: Monitor for angioedema, anaphylaxis, emergence of any new behavioral signs/ symptoms of concern, respiratory depression, withdrawal signs/symptoms, tolerance, abuse, dependence, drowsiness, decreased level of consciousness, and other adverse reactions. Monitor for excess depressant effects.

Counseling: Inform about the benefits and risks of treatment. Instruct to take only as prescribed. Caution against driving and other activities requiring complete mental alertness the day after use. Instruct to contact physician immediately if any adverse reactions (eg, severe anaphylactic/ anaphylactoid reactions, sleep-driving, other complex behaviors, suicidal thoughts) develop. Advise not to use the drug if patient drank alcohol that pm or before bed. Instruct not to increase the dose and to inform physician if it is believed that the drug does not work.

STORAGE: 15-25°C (59-77°F); limited excursions permissible up to 30°C (86°F).

AmBisome – amphotericin B liposome RX

Class: Polyene antifungal

ADULT DOSAGE

Fungal Infections

Empirical therapy for presumed fungal infection in febrile, neutropenic patients

Initial: 3mg/kg/day IV

Systemic Infections

Aspergillus species, *Candida* species, and/or *Cryptococcus* species infections refractory to amphotericin B deoxycholate, or in patients where renal impairment or unacceptable toxicity precludes the use of amphotericin B deoxycholate

Initial: 3-5mg/kg/day IV

Cryptococcal Meningitis

HIV-Infected Patients:
Initial: 6mg/kg/day IV

Visceral Leishmaniasis

Immunocompetent Patients:
3mg/kg/day IV on Days 1-5, 14, 21; may repeat course if parasitic clearance is not achieved w/ recommended dose

Immunocompromised Patients:
4mg/kg/day IV on Days 1-5, 10, 17, 24, 31, 38

PEDIATRIC DOSAGE

Fungal Infections

Empirical therapy for presumed fungal infection in febrile, neutropenic patients

≥1 Month of Age:
Initial: 3mg/kg/day IV

Systemic Infections

Aspergillus species, *Candida* species, and/or *Cryptococcus* species infections refractory to amphotericin B deoxycholate, or in patients where renal impairment or unacceptable toxicity precludes the use of amphotericin B deoxycholate

≥1 Month of Age:
Initial: 3-5mg/kg/day IV

Cryptococcal Meningitis

HIV-Infected Patients:
Initial: 6mg/kg/day IV

Visceral Leishmaniasis

≥1 Month of Age:
Immunocompetent Patients:
3mg/kg/day IV on Days 1-5, 14, 21; may repeat course if parasitic clearance is not achieved w/ recommended dose

Immunocompromised Patients:
4mg/kg/day IV on Days 1-5, 10, 17, 24, 31, 38

ADMINISTRATION

IV route

Infuse over 120 min; may reduce to 60 min if well tolerated or increase duration if experiencing discomfort
An in-line membrane filter may be used provided the mean pore diameter of the filter is not <1.0 micron
Flush existing IV line w/ D5W prior to infusion; if not feasible, administer through a separate line

Preparation

Reconstitute w/ 12mL of sterile water for inj and shake vial vigorously for 30 sec
Do not reconstitute w/ saline or add saline to reconstituted sol or mix w/ other drugs
Calculate appropriate volume of reconstituted sol to be further diluted and withdraw amount into syringe
Attach provided 5-micron filter to syringe and inject contents through filter into appropriate amount of D5 inj diluent for a final concentration of 1-2mg/mL (lower concentrations [0.2-0.5mg/ mL] may be appropriate for infants and small children)
Use only 1 filter per vial and discard partially used vials

HOW SUPPLIED

Inj: 50mg

CONTRAINDICATIONS

Known hypersensitivity to amphotericin B deoxycholate or any other constituents of the product.

WARNINGS/PRECAUTIONS

Anaphylaxis reported; d/c immediately and do not give further infusions if severe anaphylactic reaction occurs. Should be administered by medically trained personnel; monitor closely during the initial dosing period. Significantly less toxic than amphotericin B deoxycholate. False elevations of serum phosphate seen with PHOSm assays.

ADVERSE REACTIONS

Hypokalemia, chills/rigors, SrCr elevation, anemia, N/V, diarrhea, hypomagnesemia, rash, dyspnea, bilirubinemia, BUN increased, headache, abdominal pain.

DRUG INTERACTIONS

Antineoplastic agents may enhance potential for renal toxicity, bronchospasm, and hypotension. Corticosteroids and adrenocorticotropic hormone may potentiate hypokalemia; closely monitor serum electrolytes and cardiac function. May induce hypokalemia and potentiate digitalis toxicity with digitalis glycosides; closely monitor serum K^+ levels. May increase flucytosine toxicity. Imidazoles (eg, ketoconazole, miconazole, clotrimazole, fluconazole) may induce fungal resistance; use with caution, especially in immunocompromised patients. Acute pulmonary toxicity reported with simultaneous leukocyte transfusions. Nephrotoxic drugs may enhance drug-induced renal toxicity; intensive monitoring of renal function is recommended. Amphotericin B-induced hypokalemia may enhance curariform effect of skeletal muscle relaxants (eg, tubocurarine); closely monitor serum K^+ levels.

PATIENT CONSIDERATIONS

Assessment: Assess for hypersensitivity, health status, pregnancy/nursing status, and possible drug interactions.

Monitoring: Monitor for severe anaphylactic and other adverse reactions. Monitor renal, hepatic and hematopoietic function, and serum electrolytes (particularly Mg^{2+} and K^+).

Counseling: Inform of risks and benefits of therapy. Advise to seek medical attention if any adverse reactions occur.

STORAGE: Unopened Vials: ≤25°C (77°F). Reconstituted Concentrate: 2-8°C (36-46°F) for up to 24 hrs. Do not freeze. Diluted Product: Inj should commence within 6 hrs of dilution with D5W.

AMERGE – naratriptan hydrochloride

RX

Class: 5-$HT_{1B/1D}$ agonist (triptans)

ADULT DOSAGE

Migraine

W/ or w/o Aura:

1mg or 2.5mg; may repeat once after 4 hrs if migraine returns or if patient has only partial response

Max: 5mg/24 hrs

Safety of treating an average of >4 migraine attacks in a 30-day period has not been established

PEDIATRIC DOSAGE

Pediatric use may not have been established

DOSING CONSIDERATIONS

Renal Impairment

Mild-Moderate:

Initial: 1mg

Max: 2.5mg/24 hrs

Hepatic Impairment

Mild or Moderate (Child-Pugh Grade A or B):

Initial: 1mg

Max: 2.5mg/24 hrs

Elderly

Start at lower end of dosing range

ADMINISTRATION

Oral route

HOW SUPPLIED

Tab: 1mg, 2.5mg

CONTRAINDICATIONS

Ischemic coronary artery disease (CAD) (angina pectoris, history of MI, documented silent ischemia), or coronary artery vasospasm, including Prinzmetal's angina; Wolff-Parkinson-White syndrome or arrhythmias associated w/ other cardiac accessory conduction pathway disorders; history of stroke or transient ischemic attack or history of hemiplegic or basilar migraine; peripheral vascular disease; ischemic bowel disease; uncontrolled HTN; recent use (eg, w/in 24 hrs) of another 5-HT_1 agonist, ergotamine-containing medication, ergot-type medication (eg, dihydroergotamine, methysergide); severe renal/hepatic impairment; hypersensitivity to naratriptan HCl.

WARNINGS/PRECAUTIONS

Rare reports of serious cardiac adverse reactions, including acute MI, occurring w/in a few hrs following administration. May cause coronary artery vasospasm (Prinzmetal's angina). Perform cardiovascular (CV) evaluation in triptan-naive patients w/ multiple CV risk factors; if CV evaluation is negative, consider administering 1st dose in a medically supervised setting, performing an ECG immediately following administration, and consider periodic CV evaluation w/ long-term intermittent use. Life-threatening disturbances of cardiac rhythm, including ventricular tachycardia and ventricular fibrillation leading to death, reported; d/c if these disturbances occur. Sensations of tightness, pain, and pressure in the chest, throat, neck, and jaw may occur after treatment and are usually noncardiac in origin; perform a cardiac evaluation if these patients are at high cardiac risk. Cerebral hemorrhage, subarachnoid hemorrhage, and stroke reported; d/c if a cerebrovascular event occurs. Exclude other potentially serious neurological conditions before treating headaches in patients not previously diagnosed as migraineurs and in migraineurs who present w/ symptoms atypical for migraine. May cause noncoronary vasospastic reactions (eg, peripheral vascular ischemia, GI vascular ischemia and infarction, splenic infarction, Raynaud's syndrome); rule out a vasospastic reaction in patients who experience signs/symptoms before administering additional doses. Transient and permanent blindness and significant partial vision loss reported. Overuse of acute migraine drugs may lead to exacerbation of headache; detoxification, including withdrawal of overused drugs, and treatment of withdrawal symptoms may be necessary. Serotonin syndrome may occur; d/c if suspected. Significant BP elevation, including hypertensive crisis w/ acute impairment of organ systems reported. Anaphylaxis/anaphylactoid/hypersensitivity reactions, including angioedema reported.

ADVERSE REACTIONS

Paresthesias, nausea, dizziness, drowsiness, malaise/fatigue, throat and neck symptoms.

DRUG INTERACTIONS

See Contraindications. Serotonin syndrome reported during coadministration of triptans and SSRIs, SNRIs, TCAs, and MAOIs.

PATIENT CONSIDERATIONS

Assessment: Confirm diagnosis of migraine before therapy. Assess for CAD, uncontrolled HTN, history of hemiplegic/basilar migraine, ECG changes, renal/hepatic impairment, or any conditions where treatment is cautioned or contraindicated. Assess for pregnancy/nursing status and for possible drug interactions. Exclude other potentially serious neurological conditions before therapy. Perform a CV evaluation in triptan-naive patients who have multiple CV risk factors (eg, increased age, diabetes, HTN, smoking, obesity, strong family history of CAD).

Monitoring: Monitor for serious cardiac adverse reactions, arrhythmias, cerebrovascular events, noncoronary vasospastic reactions, exacerbation of headache, serotonin syndrome, increase in BP, anaphylactic/anaphylactoid reactions, and other adverse reactions. Perform ECG immediately after administration of 1st dose in patients w/ multiple CV risk factors. Consider periodic cardiac evaluation in patients who have multiple CV risk factors and are long-term intermittent users.

Counseling: Inform that drug may cause serious CV effects; instruct to be alert for signs/symptoms of chest pain, SOB, irregular heartbeat, significant rise in BP, weakness, and slurring of speech, and ask for medical advice if any indicative sign/symptoms are observed. Inform that anaphylactic/anaphylactoid reactions may occur. Inform that use of drug w/in 24 hrs of another triptan or an ergot-type medication is contraindicated. Caution about the risk of serotonin syndrome, particularly during combined use w/ SSRIs, SNRIs, TCAs, and MAOIs. Inform that use of acute migraine drugs for ≥10 days/month may lead to an exacerbation of headache, and encourage to record headache frequency and drug use (eg, by keeping a headache diary). Inform that drug should not be used during pregnancy unless the potential benefit justifies the potential risk to the fetus. Advise to notify physician if breastfeeding or planning to breastfeed. Inform that treatment may cause somnolence and dizziness; instruct to evaluate the ability to perform complex tasks after drug administration.

STORAGE: 20-25°C (68-77°F).

AMIKACIN – amikacin sulfate

Class: Aminoglycoside

RX

Potential ototoxicity/nephrotoxicity associated w/ therapy; safety for treatment periods >14 days has not been established. Increased risk of nephrotoxicity in patients w/ impaired renal function and in those who receive high doses or prolonged therapy. Neurotoxicity can occur in patients w/ preexisting renal damage and in patients w/ normal renal function treated at higher doses and/or periods longer than those recommended. Increased risk of ototoxicity w/ renal damage. Increased risk of hearing loss w/ degree of exposure to either high peak or high trough serum concentrations. Total/partial irreversible bilateral deafness may occur after therapy has been discontinued. D/C therapy or adjust the dose upon evidence of ototoxicity or nephrotoxicity. Neuromuscular blockade and respiratory paralysis reported following parenteral inj, topical instillation, and following oral use of therapy; consider possibility of these phenomena if therapy is administered by any route, especially in patients taking anesthetics, neuromuscular blocking agents (eg, tubocurarine, succinylcholine, decamethonium), or massive transfusions of citrate-anticoagulated blood. If blockage occurs, Ca^{2+} salts may reverse these phenomena, but mechanical respiratory assistance may be necessary. Closely monitor renal and 8th nerve function. Monitor serum concentrations of amikacin to assure adequate levels and to avoid potentially toxic levels and prolonged peak concentrations >35mcg/mL. Examine urine for decreased specific gravity, increased protein excretion, and presence of cells/casts. Obtain serial audiograms in patients old enough to be tested. Avoid concurrent and/or sequential systemic, oral, or topical use of other neurotoxic/nephrotoxic products (eg, bacitracin, cisplatin, amphotericin B). Advanced age and dehydration may increase risk of toxicity. Avoid concurrent use w/ potent diuretics (eg, furosemide, ethacrynic acid).

OTHER BRAND NAMES

Amikin (Discontinued)

ADULT DOSAGE

General Dosing

15mg/kg/day IM/IV divided into 2 or 3 equal doses given at equally divided intervals
Max: 15mg/kg/day
Max for Heavier Weight Patients: 1.5g/day

Avoid peak levels >35mcg/mL and trough levels >10mcg/mL

Urinary Tract Infections

Uncomplicated:
250mg IM/IV bid

Avoid peak levels >35mcg/mL and trough levels >10mcg/mL

Treatment Duration

Usual: 7-10 days; d/c therapy if definite clinical response does not occur w/in 3-5 days

Reevaluate if considering therapy beyond 10 days in difficult and complicated infections

Other Indications

Treatment of the Following Infections Caused by Susceptible Microorganisms:
Serious infections due to gram-negative bacteria
Bacterial septicemia (including neonatal sepsis)
Serious respiratory tract infections
Serious bone and joint infections
Serious CNS infections (including meningitis)
Serious skin and soft tissue infections
Serious intra-abdominal infections (including peritonitis)
Burns and postoperative infections (including post-vascular surgery)
Serious complicated and recurrent UTIs
Staphylococcal infections

Infections caused by gentamicin- and/or tobramycin-resistant strains of gram-negative organisms, particularly *Proteus rettgeri, Providencia stuartii, Serratia marcescens*, and *Pseudomonas aeruginosa*

Certain severe infections in combination w/ a penicillin-type drug

PEDIATRIC DOSAGE

General Dosing

Newborns:
LD: 10mg/kg IM/IV
Maint: 7.5mg/kg IM/IV q12h

Older Infants and Children:
15mg/kg/day IM/IV divided into 2 or 3 equal doses given at equally divided intervals
Max: 15mg/kg/day
Max for Heavier Weight Patients: 1.5g/day

Avoid peak levels >35mcg/mL and trough levels >10mcg/mL

Treatment Duration

Usual: 7-10 days; d/c therapy if definite clinical response does not occur w/in 3-5 days

Reevaluate if considering therapy beyond 10 days in difficult and complicated infections

DOSING CONSIDERATIONS

Renal Impairment

Reduce dose or prolong intervals

Normal Dosage at Prolonged Intervals:

If CrCl is unavailable and patient's condition is stable, may calculate dosage interval in hrs by multiplying patient's SrCr by 9 (eg, if SrCr concentration is 2mg/100mL, recommended single dose (7.5mg/kg) should be administered q18h)

Reduced Dosage at Fixed Intervals:

Initial LD: 7.5mg/kg

Maint Dose q12h: (Observed CrCl [mL/min]/Normal CrCl [mL/min]) x Calculated LD (mg)

Alternatively, may determine reduced q12h dose (if steady state SrCr known) by dividing normal recommended dose by SrCr

ADMINISTRATION

IM/IV route

IV

Add contents of a 500mg vial to 100 or 200mL of sterile diluent (eg, 0.9% NaCl inj, D5 inj).
Administer over a period of 30-60 min; infuse over 1-2 hrs in infants.
Do not physically premix w/ other drugs; administer separately.

Stability:

Stable for 24 hrs at room temperature (at concentrations of 0.25 and 5mg/mL) in D5 inj, D5 and 0.2% or 0.45% NaCl inj, 0.9% NaCl inj, lactated Ringer's inj, Normosol M in D5 inj (or Plasma-Lyte 56 inj in D5W), and Normosol R in D5 inj (or Plasma-Lyte inj 148 in D5W).
At same concentrations, sol frozen and aged for 30 days at -15°C, thawed, and stored at 25°C had utility times of 24 hrs.
At same concentrations, sol aged for 60 days at 4°C and then stored at 25°C had utility times of 24 hrs.

HOW SUPPLIED

Inj: 250mg/mL [2mL, 4mL]

CONTRAINDICATIONS

History of hypersensitivity to amikacin, history of hypersensitivity or serious toxic reactions to aminoglycosides.

WARNINGS/PRECAUTIONS

May cause fetal harm. Not for uncomplicated initial episodes of UTI unless the causative organisms are not susceptible to antibiotics having less potential toxicity. Contains sodium metabisulfite; allergic-type reactions may occur more frequently in asthmatics. *Clostridium difficile*-associated diarrhea (CDAD) reported; may need to d/c if CDAD is suspected or confirmed. May result in overgrowth of nonsusceptible organisms; institute appropriate therapy if this occurs. Use in the absence of a proven or strongly suspected bacterial infection or prophylactic indication is unlikely to provide benefit and increases the risk of the development of drug-resistant bacteria. Irreversible deafness, renal failure, and death due to neuromuscular blockade reported following irrigation of surgical fields w/ an aminoglycoside preparation. If signs of renal irritation appear (eg, casts, white/red cells, albumin), increase hydration; if azotemia increases or if progressive decrease in urinary output occurs, d/c treatment. May aggravate muscle weakness; caution w/ muscular disorders (eg, myasthenia gravis, parkinsonism). Cross-allergenicity among aminoglycosides demonstrated. Caution in elderly and in premature and neonatal infants. Specimens of body fluids collected for assay should be properly handled.

ADVERSE REACTIONS

Ototoxicity, neurotoxicity, nephrotoxicity.

DRUG INTERACTIONS

See Boxed Warning. Increased nephrotoxicity w/ parenteral administration of aminoglycosides, antibiotics, and cephalosporins. Concomitant cephalosporins may falsely elevate creatinine determinations. Significant mutual inactivation may occur w/ β-lactam antibiotics.

PATIENT CONSIDERATIONS

Assessment: Obtain pretreatment body weight for calculation of correct dosage. Assess and document bacterial infection using culture and susceptibility techniques. Assess for history of hypersensitivity to drug, other aminoglycosides, or to sulfites. Assess for muscular disorders, pregnancy/nursing status, and possible drug interactions. Assess renal function.

Monitoring: Monitor for signs/symptoms of nephrotoxicity, neurotoxicity, ototoxicity, hypersensitivity reactions, neuromuscular blockade, respiratory paralysis, and other adverse reactions. Periodically monitor hydration status, BUN, SrCr, CrCl, 8th nerve function, and peak and trough concentrations. Perform urinalysis.

Counseling: Inform about potential risks/benefits of therapy. Inform that drug only treats bacterial, not viral, infections. Instruct to take exactly ud even if patient feels better early in the course of therapy. Inform that skipping doses or not completing the full course of therapy may decrease effectiveness and increase the likelihood of bacterial resistance. Inform that diarrhea may occur and to contact physician as soon as possible if watery/bloody stools (w/ or w/o stomach cramps, fever) develop even as late as ≥2 months after the last dose.

STORAGE: 20-25°C (68-77°F).

AMITIZA – lubiprostone

RX

Class: Chloride channel activator

ADULT DOSAGE

Chronic Idiopathic Constipation

24mcg bid

Opioid-Induced Constipation

Chronic Non-Cancer Pain:
24mcg bid

Irritable Bowel Syndrome with Constipation

Women:
8mcg bid

PEDIATRIC DOSAGE

Pediatric use may not have been established

DOSING CONSIDERATIONS

Hepatic Impairment

Chronic Idiopathic Constipation/Opioid-Induced Constipation (OIC):
Moderate (Child-Pugh Class B):
Initial: 16mcg bid
Severe (Child-Pugh Class C):
Initial: 8mcg bid
Titrate: If dose is tolerated but adequate response not obtained, may escalate to full dose w/ appropriate monitoring
Irritable Bowel Syndrome w/ Constipation:
Severe (Child-Pugh Class C):
Initial: 8mcg qd
Titrate: If dose is tolerated but adequate response not obtained, may escalate to full dose w/ appropriate monitoring

ADMINISTRATION

Oral route

Take w/ food and water
Swallow caps whole; do not break or chew

HOW SUPPLIED

Cap: 8mcg, 24mcg

CONTRAINDICATIONS

Known or suspected mechanical GI obstruction.

WARNINGS/PRECAUTIONS

Effectiveness not established in treatment of OIC in patients taking diphenylheptane opioids (eg, methadone). May cause nausea; give with food to reduce symptoms of nausea. Diarrhea may occur; avoid in patients with severe diarrhea and d/c therapy if severe diarrhea occurs. Dyspnea reported; resolves within a few hrs after dose but may recur with subsequent doses. Thoroughly evaluate patients with symptoms suggestive of mechanical GI obstruction prior to initiation of therapy.

ADVERSE REACTIONS

N/V, diarrhea, headache, abdominal pain/distention, flatulence, loose stools, dizziness, edema, dyspnea, abdominal discomfort.

DRUG INTERACTIONS

Diphenylheptane opioids (eg, methadone) may cause dose-dependent decrease in efficacy.

PATIENT CONSIDERATIONS

Assessment: Assess for known or suspected mechanical GI obstruction, severe diarrhea, pregnancy/nursing status, and possible drug interactions.

Monitoring: Monitor for nausea, dyspnea, severe diarrhea, and other adverse reactions. Periodically assess the need for continued therapy.

Counseling: Instruct to notify physician if experiencing severe nausea, diarrhea, or dyspnea during treatment. Inform that dyspnea may occur within an hr after 1st dose and resolves within 3 hrs, but may recur with repeat dosing. Advise lactating women to monitor their breastfed infants for diarrhea while on therapy.

STORAGE: 25°C (77°F); excursions permitted to 15-30°C (59-86°F). Protect from light and extreme temperatures.

AMITRIPTYLINE — amitriptyline hydrochloride

RX

Class: Tricyclic antidepressant (TCA)

Antidepressants increased the risk of suicidal thinking and behavior (suicidality) in children, adolescents, and young adults in short-term studies of major depressive disorder and other psychiatric disorders. Monitor and observe closely for clinical worsening, suicidality, or unusual changes in behavior in patients who are started on antidepressant therapy. Not approved for use in pediatric patients.

OTHER BRAND NAMES

Elavil (Discontinued)

ADULT DOSAGE

Depression

Outpatients:
Initial (Divided Dose): 75mg/day in divided doses
Titrate: May increase to 150mg/day; increases are made preferably in the late afternoon and/or hs doses

Initial (Single Dose): 50-100mg at hs
Titrate: May increase by 25mg or 50mg in the hs dose, to a total of 150mg/day

Hospitalized Patients:
Initial: 100mg/day
Titrate: May increase gradually to 200mg/day; some patients as much as 300mg/day

Maint: 50-100mg/day (40mg/day is sufficient in some patients); total daily dose may be given in a single dose, preferably at hs. Continue ≥3 months

PEDIATRIC DOSAGE

Depression

≥12 Years:
10mg tid w/ 20mg at hs

DOSING CONSIDERATIONS

Elderly
10mg tid w/ 20mg at hs

ADMINISTRATION

Oral route

HOW SUPPLIED

Tab: 10mg, 25mg, 50mg, 75mg, 100mg, 150mg

CONTRAINDICATIONS

Prior hypersensitivity to the product, use of an MAOI concomitantly, treatment w/in 14 days of discontinuing an MAOI, coadministration w/ cisapride, during the acute recovery phase following myocardial infarction (MI).

WARNINGS/PRECAUTIONS

Not approved for the treatment of bipolar depression. May precipitate a mixed/manic episode in patients at risk for bipolar disorder; screen for risk for bipolar disorder prior to initiating treatment. Caution w/ history of seizures, history of urinary retention, angle-closure glaucoma, or increased IOP. Caution w/ cardiovascular disorders (CVD), hyperthyroidism, liver dysfunction, and in elderly. Pupillary dilation that occurs following therapy may trigger an angle-closure attack in a patient w/ anatomically narrow angles who does not have a patent iridectomy. Dose may be reduced or a major tranquilizer (eg, perphenazine) may be administered concurrently if schizophrenic patients develop increased symptoms of psychosis (patients w/ paranoid symptomatology may have an exaggeration of such symptoms), or if depressed patients, particularly those w/ known manic-depressive illness, experience a shift to mania or hypomania. Hazards may be increased w/ electroshock therapy. D/C several days before elective surgery. May alter blood glucose levels.

ADVERSE REACTIONS

MI, stroke, coma, seizures, paralytic ileus, hyperpyrexia, skin rash, urticaria, bone marrow depression, N/V, epigastric distress, increased/decreased libido, alopecia, edema.

DRUG INTERACTIONS

See Contraindications. May block antihypertensive action of guanethidine or similarly acting compounds. Caution in patients receiving thyroid medication. May enhance the response to alcohol and the effects of barbiturates and other CNS depressants. Delirium reported w/ disulfiram. Drugs that inhibit CYP2D6 (eg, quinidine, cimetidine, many CYP2D6 substrates [other antidepressants, phenothiazines, propafenone, flecainide]) may increase plasma concentrations; may require lower doses for either TCA or the other drug, and monitoring of TCA plasma levels. Caution w/ SSRI coadministration and when switching between TCAs and SSRIs (eg, fluoxetine, sertraline, paroxetine); sufficient time must elapse before starting therapy when switching from fluoxetine (at least 5 weeks may be necessary). Close supervision and careful dose adjustment is required when given w/ anticholinergic agents or sympathomimetic drugs, including epinephrine combined w/ local anesthetics. Hyperpyrexia reported w/ anticholinergics or neuroleptics, particularly during hot weather. Paralytic ileus may occur w/ anticholinergic-type drugs. Caution w/ large doses of ethchlorvynol; transient delirium reported.

PATIENT CONSIDERATIONS

Assessment: Assess for acute recovery phase following MI, hypersensitivity to drug, risk for bipolar disorder, history of seizures or urinary retention, susceptibility to angle-closure glaucoma, increased IOP, CVD, hyperthyroidism, liver dysfunction, schizophrenia, paranoid symptomatology, manic-depressive illness, pregnancy/nursing status, and possible drug interactions.

Monitoring: Monitor for signs/symptoms of clinical worsening, suicidality, unusual changes in behavior, angle-closure glaucoma, increased psychosis symptoms, exaggeration of paranoid symptoms, hypomanic/manic episodes, changes in blood glucose levels, and other adverse reactions.

Counseling: Inform about benefits, risks, and appropriate use of therapy. Advise that drug may impair mental/physical abilities required for the performance of hazardous tasks (eg, operating machinery, driving). Caution about the risk of angle-closure glaucoma. Advise to monitor for unusual changes in behavior, worsening of depression, and suicidal ideation on a day-to-day basis, and to report such symptoms to physician.

STORAGE: 20-25°C (68-77°F). Protect from light.

AMOXICILLIN – amoxicillin

RX

Class: Semisynthetic ampicillin derivative

OTHER BRAND NAMES

Amoxil (Discontinued), Trimox (Discontinued)

ADULT DOSAGE

Helicobacter pylori Eradication

W/ (Active or 1-Year History) Duodenal Ulcer Disease:

Dual Therapy: 1g + 30mg lansoprazole, each q8h for 14 days

Triple Therapy: 1g + 30mg lansoprazole + 500mg clarithromycin, all q12h for 14 days

Ear/Nose/Throat Infection

Mild/Moderate: 500mg q12h or 250mg q8h

Severe: 875mg q12h or 500mg q8h

Genitourinary Tract Infections

Mild/Moderate: 500mg q12h or 250mg q8h

Severe: 875mg q12h or 500mg q8h

Skin and Skin Structure Infections

Mild/Moderate: 500mg q12h or 250mg q8h

Severe: 875mg q12h or 500mg q8h

Lower Respiratory Tract Infections

Mild/Moderate or Severe: 875mg q12h or 500mg q8h

Treatment Duration

Continue for a minimum of 48-72 hrs beyond the time the patient becomes asymptomatic or evidence of bacterial eradication has been obtained

***Streptococcus pyogenes* Infections:** Treat for at least 10 days

PEDIATRIC DOSAGE

Lower Respiratory Tract Infections

≤12 Weeks of Age:

Max: 30mg/kg/day divided q12h

>3 Months of Age:

<40kg: 45mg/kg/day divided q12h or 40mg/kg/day divided q8h

≥40kg: 875mg q12h or 500mg q8h

Ear/Nose/Throat Infection

≤12 Weeks of Age:

Max: 30mg/kg/day divided q12h

>3 Months of Age:

<40kg:

Mild/Moderate: 25mg/kg/day divided q12h or 20mg/kg/day divided q8h

Severe: 45mg/kg/day divided q12h or 40mg/kg/day divided q8h

≥40kg:

Mild/Moderate: 500mg q12h or 250mg q8h

Severe: 875mg q12h or 500mg q8h

Genitourinary Tract Infections

≤12 Weeks of Age:

Max: 30mg/kg/day divided q12h

>3 Months of Age:

<40kg:

Mild/Moderate: 25mg/kg/day divided q12h or 20mg/kg/day divided q8h

Severe: 45mg/kg/day divided q12h or 40mg/kg/day divided q8h

≥40kg:
Mild/Moderate: 500mg q12h or 250mg q8h
Severe: 875mg q12h or 500mg q8h

Skin and Skin Structure Infections

≤12 Weeks of Age:
Max: 30mg/kg/day divided q12h

>3 Months of Age:

<40kg:
Mild/Moderate: 25mg/kg/day divided q12h or 20mg/kg/day divided q8h
Severe: 45mg/kg/day divided q12h or 40mg/kg/day divided q8h

≥40kg:
Mild/Moderate: 500mg q12h or 250mg q8h
Severe: 875mg q12h or 500mg q8h

Treatment Duration

Continue for a minimum of 48-72 hrs beyond the time that patient becomes asymptomatic or evidence of bacterial eradication has been obtained

***S. pyogenes* Infections:** Treat for at least 10 days

DOSING CONSIDERATIONS

Renal Impairment

Adults:
GFR <30mL/min: Should not receive an 875mg dose
GFR 10-30mL/min: 250mg or 500mg q12h, depending on severity of infection
GFR <10mL/min: 250mg or 500mg q24h, depending on severity of infection
Hemodialysis: 250mg or 500mg q24h, depending on severity of infection; give an additional dose during and at end of dialysis

Other Important Considerations

Bacteria that are intermediate in their susceptibility to amoxicillin should follow the recommendations for severe infections

ADMINISTRATION

Oral route

Oral Sus

Can be added to formula, milk, fruit juice, water, ginger ale, or cold drinks; take immediately.
Shake well before use.
Discard any unused portion of the reconstituted sus after 14 days; refrigeration is preferable, but not required.

Reconstitution:
125mg/5mL: Reconstitute 80mL, 100mL, or 150mL bottle size w/ 62mL, 77mL, or 113mL of water, respectively.
200mg/5mL: Reconstitute 50mL, 75mL, or 100mL bottle size w/ 39mL, 57mL, or 75mL of water, respectively.
250mg/5mL: Reconstitute 80mL, 100mL, or 150mL bottle size w/ 47mL, 60mL, or 90mL of water, respectively.
400mg/5mL: Reconstitute 50mL, 75mL, or 100mL bottle size w/ 35mL, 51mL, or 67mL of water, respectively.
Add approximately 1/3 of the total amount of water to wet powder, then shake vigorously.
Add the remainder of the water and shake vigorously.
Place directly on tongue for swallowing.

HOW SUPPLIED

Cap: 250mg, 500mg; **Oral Sus:** 125mg/5mL [80mL, 100mL, 150mL], 200mg/5mL [50mL, 75mL, 100mL], 250mg/5mL [80mL, 100mL, 150mL], 400mg/5mL [50mL, 75mL, 100mL]; **Tab:** 500mg, 875mg*; **Tab, Chewable:** 125mg, 250mg *scored

CONTRAINDICATIONS

Serious hypersensitivity reaction to amoxicillin or to other β-lactam antibiotics.

WARNINGS/PRECAUTIONS

Serious and occasionally fatal hypersensitivity (anaphylactic) reactions reported; increased risk w/ a history of penicillin (PCN) hypersensitivity and/or history of sensitivity to multiple allergens. D/C and institute appropriate therapy if an allergic reaction occurs. *Clostridium difficile*-associated diarrhea (CDAD) reported; may need to d/c if CDAD is suspected or confirmed. Avoid use w/ mononucleosis; erythematous skin rash may develop in these patients. May result in bacterial resistance if used in the absence of a proven/suspected bacterial indication. Lab test interactions may occur. Caution in elderly; monitor renal function.

ADVERSE REACTIONS

N/V, diarrhea, rash.

DRUG INTERACTIONS

Decreased renal tubular secretion and increased/prolonged levels w/ probenecid. May reduce efficacy of combined oral estrogen/progesterone contraceptives. Chloramphenicol, macrolides, sulfonamides, and tetracyclines may interfere w/ bactericidal effects of PCN. PT prolongation (increased INR) reported w/ oral anticoagulants; dose adjustments of oral anticoagulants may be necessary. Increased incidence of rashes w/ allopurinol.

PATIENT CONSIDERATIONS

Assessment: Assess for history of allergic reaction to PCNs, cephalosporins, or other allergens, mononucleosis, renal function, pregnancy/nursing status, and possible drug interactions. Obtain culture and susceptibility information.

Monitoring: Monitor for serious anaphylactic reactions, erythematous skin rash, development of drug-resistant bacteria, and CDAD. Monitor renal function. Monitor PT and INR if coadministered w/ an oral anticoagulant.

Counseling: Inform that drug treats only bacterial, not viral, infections. Instruct to take exactly ud; inform that skipping doses or not completing the full course of therapy may decrease effectiveness and increase resistance. Instruct to notify physician as soon as possible if watery and bloody stools (w/ or w/o stomach cramps and fever) develop, even as late as ≥2 months after having last dose. Advise patients that drug may cause allergic reactions.

STORAGE: 20-25°C (68-77°F).

AMPHOTEC – amphotericin B cholesteryl sulfate complex RX

Class: Polyene antifungal

ADULT DOSAGE

Aspergillosis

Invasive aspergillosis in patients where renal impairment or unacceptable toxicity precludes the use of amphotericin B deoxycholate in effective doses, and in patients w/ invasive aspergillosis where prior amphotericin B deoxycholate therapy has failed

3-4mg/kg as required, qd, at infusion rate of 1mg/kg/hr

Test Dose:

Infuse small amount (eg, 10mL of the final preparation containing between 1.6-8.3mg) over 15-30 min immediately preceding the first dose; carefully observe for next 30 min

PEDIATRIC DOSAGE

Aspergillosis

Invasive aspergillosis in patients where renal impairment or unacceptable toxicity precludes the use of amphotericin B deoxycholate in effective doses, and in patients w/ invasive aspergillosis where prior amphotericin B deoxycholate therapy has failed

3-4mg/kg as required, qd, at infusion rate of 1mg/kg/hr

Test Dose:

Infuse small amount (eg, 10mL of the final preparation containing between 1.6-8.3mg) over 15-30 min immediately preceding the first dose; carefully observe for next 30 min

ADMINISTRATION

IV route

May shorten infusion time to a minimum of 2 hrs if no evidence of intolerance or infusion-related reactions

If acute reactions or intolerance to infusion volume occurs, may extend infusion time

Do not reconstitute w/ saline or dextrose sol, or admix reconstituted liquid w/ saline or electrolytes

Avoid addition of sol containing a bacteriostatic agent (eg, benzyl alcohol)

Do not mix infusion admixture w/ other drugs; if administered through existing IV line, flush w/ D5 for inj prior to and following infusion of therapy

Do not filter or use an in-line filter

Preparation

Reconstitute w/ 10mL or 20mL of sterile water for inj in 50mg or 100mg vial, respectively, using a sterile syringe and a 20-gauge needle

Further dilute reconstituted liquid to final concentration of 0.6mg/mL (range 0.16-0.83mg/mL) by adding appropriate reconstituted volume to D5 for inj infusion bag

HOW SUPPLIED

Inj: 50mg [20mL], 100mg [50mL]

CONTRAINDICATIONS

Documented hypersensitivity to any component of Amphotec, unless benefit outweighs risk.

WARNINGS/PRECAUTIONS

Anaphylaxis reported; administer epinephrine, oxygen, IV steroids, and airway management as indicated. D/C if severe respiratory distress occurs; do not give further infusions. Acute infusion-related reactions may occur 1-3 hrs after starting IV infusion; manage by pretreatment with antihistamines and corticosteroids and/or by reducing the rate of infusion and by prompt administration of antihistamines and corticosteroids. Avoid rapid IV infusion. Monitor renal and hepatic function, serum electrolytes, CBC, and PT as medically indicated.

ADVERSE REACTIONS

Chills, fever, tachycardia, N/V, increased creatinine, hypotension, HTN, headache, thrombocytopenia, hypokalemia, hypomagnesemia, hypoxia, abnormal LFTs, dyspnea.

DRUG INTERACTIONS

Caution with antineoplastic agents; may enhance potential for renal toxicity, bronchospasm, hypotension. Corticosteroids and corticotropin may potentiate hypokalemia; monitor serum electrolytes and cardiac function. Cyclosporine and tacrolimus may cause renal toxicity. Concurrent use with digitalis glycosides may induce hypokalemia and may potentiate digitalis toxicity of digitalis glycosides; closely monitor serum K^+ levels. May increase flucytosine toxicity; use with caution. Antagonism with imidazole derivatives (eg, miconazole, ketoconazole) reported. Nephrotoxic agents (eg, aminoglycosides, pentamidine) may enhance the potential for drug-induced renal toxicity; use with caution and intensively monitor renal function. Amphotericin B-induced hypokalemia may enhance curariform effect of skeletal muscle relaxants (eg, tubocurarine) due to hypokalemia; closely monitor serum K^+ levels.

PATIENT CONSIDERATIONS

Assessment: Assess for previous hypersensitivity to the drug, pregnancy/nursing status, and for possible drug interactions. Assess renal function.

Monitoring: Monitor for anaphylaxis, respiratory distress, and acute infusion-related reactions. Monitor renal and hepatic function, serum electrolytes, CBC, and PT. Monitor patients for 30 min after administering the test dose.

Counseling: Inform of risks and benefits of therapy. Advise to seek medical attention if any adverse reactions occur.

STORAGE: Unopened Vials: 15-30°C (59-86°F). Retain in carton until time of use. Reconstituted: 2-8°C (36-46°F). Use within 24 hrs. Do not freeze. Further Diluted with D5W for Inj: 2-8°C (36-46°F). Use within 24 hrs.

AMPICILLIN ORAL – ampicillin trihydrate RX

Class: Semisynthetic penicillin (PCN) derivative

ADULT DOSAGE

Genitourinary Tract Infections

Usual: 500mg qid in equally spaced doses; severe or chronic infections may require larger doses

Prolonged intensive therapy is needed for complications (eg, prostatitis, epididymitis)

Gonorrhea

Usual: 3.5g single dose w/ 1g probenecid; use no less than the recommended dosage

Gastrointestinal Infections

Usual: 500mg qid in equally spaced doses; severe or chronic infections may require larger doses

Respiratory Tract Infections

Usual: 250mg qid in equally spaced doses; severe or chronic infections may require larger doses

Treatment Duration

Except for single dose regimen of gonorrhea, continue therapy for a minimum of 48-72 hrs after patient becomes asymptomatic or evidence of bacterial eradication has been

PEDIATRIC DOSAGE

Genitourinary Tract Infections

≤20kg:
100mg/kg/day total, qid in equally divided and spaced doses

>20kg:
500mg qid in equally spaced doses

Severe or chronic infections may require larger doses

Prolonged intensive therapy is needed for complications (eg, prostatitis, epididymitis)

Gastrointestinal Infections

≤20kg:
100mg/kg/day total, qid in equally divided and spaced doses

>20kg:
500mg qid in equally spaced doses

Severe or chronic infections may require larger doses

Gonorrhea

>20kg:
3.5g single dose w/ 1g probenecid; use no less than the recommended dosage

obtained; stubborn infections may require treatment for several weeks

Hemolytic Strains of Streptococci: Treat for a minimum of 10 days

Other Indications

Meningitis

Respiratory Tract Infections

≤20kg:
Usual: 50mg/kg/day total, in equally divided and spaced doses tid-qid
Max: Do not exceed adult doses
>20kg:
250mg qid in equally spaced doses

Severe or chronic infections may require larger doses

Treatment Duration

Except for single dose regimen of gonorrhea, continue therapy for a minimum of 48-72 hrs after patient becomes asymptomatic or evidence of bacterial eradication has been obtained; stubborn infections may require treatment for several weeks

Hemolytic Strains of Streptococci: Treat for a minimum of 10 days

ADMINISTRATION

Oral route

Take at least 30 min ac or 2 hrs pc w/ a full glass of water.

Sus Preparation
125mg/5mL: Reconstitute 100mL and 200mL package sizes w/ 86mL and 170mL of water respectively.
250mg/5mL: Reconstitute 100mL and 200mL package sizes w/ 70mL and 139mL of water respectively.
Add water in 2 portions; shake well after each addition.

HOW SUPPLIED

Cap: 250mg, 500mg; **Sus:** 125mg/5mL, 250mg/5mL [100mL, 200mL]

CONTRAINDICATIONS

History of a previous hypersensitivity reaction to any of the penicillins, infections caused by penicillinase-producing organisms.

WARNINGS/PRECAUTIONS

Serious and fatal hypersensitivity reactions reported w/ PCN therapy; increased risk w/ history of sensitivity to multiple allergens. Anaphylactoid reactions require immediate treatment w/ appropriate management. Possible cross-sensitivity w/ cephalosporins. Pseudomembranous colitis reported; initiate therapeutic measures if diagnosed and consider discontinuation of treatment. May result in bacterial resistance w/ prolonged use or use in the absence of a proven or suspected bacterial infection or a prophylactic indication; take appropriate measures if superinfection develops. Give additional parenteral PCN in patients w/ gonorrhea who also have syphilis. Treatment does not preclude the need for surgical procedures, particularly in staphylococcal infections. Lab test interactions may occur.

ADVERSE REACTIONS

Glossitis, stomatitis, N/V, diarrhea, skin rash, pruritus, urticaria, erythema multiforme, agranulocytosis, anemia, eosinophilia, leukopenia, thrombocytopenia, thrombocytopenic purpura.

DRUG INTERACTIONS

Increased risk of rash w/ allopurinol. Bacteriostatic antibiotics (eg, chloramphenicol, erythromycins, sulfonamides, tetracyclines) may interfere w/ bactericidal activity. May increase breakthrough bleeding w/ oral contraceptives and decrease oral contraceptive effectiveness. Probenecid may increase levels and toxicity.

PATIENT CONSIDERATIONS

Assessment: Assess for previous hypersensitivity reactions to PCNs, cephalosporins, or other allergens; history of allergy; pregnancy/nursing status; syphilis; and possible drug interactions. Perform appropriate culture and susceptibility tests.

Monitoring: Monitor for hypersensitivity reactions, pseudomembranous colitis, and overgrowth of nonsusceptible organisms. Evaluate renal/hepatic/hematopoietic systems periodically w/ prolonged therapy. Upon completion, obtain cultures to determine organism eradication. Monitor for masked syphilis; perform follow-up serologic test for each month for 4 months for syphilis in patients w/o suspected lesions of syphilis.

Counseling: Instruct to notify physician of history of hypersensitivity to PCNs, cephalosporins, or other allergens. Advise diabetics to consult w/ physician prior to changing diet or dosage of diabetic medication. Instruct to take exactly ud; explain that skipping doses or not completing full course decreases effectiveness and increases bacterial resistance. Instruct to d/c and notify physician if side effects occur. Inform that therapy only treats bacterial, and not viral, infections.

STORAGE: Cap/Dry Powder: 20-25°C (68-77°F). **Sus:** Store reconstituted sus in the refrigerator; discard unused portion after 14 days.

AMRIX – cyclobenzaprine hydrochloride

RX

Class: Skeletal muscle relaxant (centrally acting)

ADULT DOSAGE

Muscle Spasms

Relief of Muscle Spasm Associated w/ Acute, Painful Musculoskeletal Conditions:

15mg qd; may require up to 30mg qd

Use for periods longer than 2 or 3 weeks is not recommended

PEDIATRIC DOSAGE

Pediatric use may not have been established

DOSING CONSIDERATIONS

Hepatic Impairment

Mild/Moderate/Severe: Not recommended

Elderly

Not recommended

ADMINISTRATION

Oral route

Take at approx the same time each day.

HOW SUPPLIED

Cap, Extended-Release: 15mg, 30mg

CONTRAINDICATIONS

Hypersensitivity to any component of this product, concomitant use of MAOIs or w/in 14 days after their discontinuation, during the acute recovery phase of MI, arrhythmias, heart block or conduction disturbances, CHF, hyperthyroidism.

WARNINGS/PRECAUTIONS

Not effective in the treatment of spasticity associated w/ cerebral or spinal cord disease or in children w/ cerebral palsy. May produce arrhythmias, sinus tachycardia, and conduction time prolongation leading to MI and stroke; consider discontinuation if clinically significant CNS symptoms develop. Caution w/ history of urinary retention, angle-closure glaucoma, and increased IOP.

ADVERSE REACTIONS

Dry mouth, dizziness, somnolence, fatigue, constipation, nausea, dyspepsia.

DRUG INTERACTIONS

See Contraindications. Serotonin syndrome reported when used w/ SSRIs, SNRIs, TCAs, tramadol, bupropion, meperidine, verapamil, or MAOIs; d/c immediately if this occurs. Observe carefully, particularly during treatment initiation or dose increases, if concomitant use w/ other serotonergic drugs is warranted. May enhance effects of alcohol, barbiturates, and other CNS depressants. Caution w/ anticholinergics. May block the antihypertensive action of guanethidine and similarly acting compounds. May enhance seizure risk w/ tramadol.

PATIENT CONSIDERATIONS

Assessment: Assess for arrhythmias, heart block or conduction disturbances, CHF, hyperthyroidism, acute recovery phase of MI, history of urinary retention, angle-closure glaucoma, increased IOP, hepatic impairment, drug hypersensitivity, pregnancy/nursing status, and possible drug interactions.

Monitoring: Monitor for arrhythmias, sinus tachycardia, conduction time prolongation, CNS symptoms, and other adverse reactions.

Counseling: Advise to d/c use and notify physician immediately if experiencing symptoms of an allergic reaction (eg, difficulty breathing, hives, swelling of face/tongue, itching), arrhythmias, or tachycardia. Caution about the risk of serotonin syndrome; instruct to seek medical care immediately if signs/symptoms occur. Inform that drug may enhance impairment effects of alcohol and other CNS depressants. Caution about operating an automobile or other hazardous machinery until accustomed to effects of medication.

STORAGE: 25°C (77°F); excursions permitted to 15-30°C (59-86°F).

AMTURNIDE – aliskiren/amlodipine/hydrochlorothiazide

RX

Class: Calcium channel blocker (CCB) (dihydropyridine)/renin inhibitor/thiazide diuretic

D/C when pregnancy is detected. Drugs that act directly on the renin-angiotensin system can cause injury/death to the developing fetus.

ADULT DOSAGE

Hypertension

Dose qd; may increase dose after 2 weeks of therapy

Max: 300mg/10mg/25mg

Add-On/Switch Therapy:

Use if not adequately controlled w/ any 2 of the following: aliskiren, dihydropyridine calcium channel blockers, and thiazide diuretics

W/ dose-limiting adverse reactions to any component on dual therapy, switch to triple therapy at a lower dose of that component

Replacement Therapy:

Switch from separate tabs to Amturnide containing the same component doses

PEDIATRIC DOSAGE

Pediatric use may not have been established

DOSING CONSIDERATIONS

Renal Impairment

Consider lower doses; safety and effectiveness in patients w/ severe renal impairment (CrCl <30mL/min) have not been established

Hepatic Impairment

Consider lower doses

Elderly

Consider starting w/ the lowest available dose of amlodipine; the lowest strength of Amturnide contains 5mg of amlodipine

ADMINISTRATION

Oral route

Establish a routine pattern for taking the drug, either w/ or w/o a meal; high-fat meals decrease absorption of aliskiren substantially.

HOW SUPPLIED

Tab: (Aliskiren/Amlodipine/Hydrochlorothiazide [HCTZ]) 150mg/5mg/12.5mg, 300mg/5mg/12.5mg, 300mg/5mg/25mg, 300mg/10mg/12.5mg, 300mg/10mg/25mg

CONTRAINDICATIONS

Anuria, known hypersensitivity to sulfonamide-derived drugs (eg, hydrochlorothiazide) or to any of the components. Concomitant use w/ ARBs or ACE inhibitors in patients w/ diabetes.

WARNINGS/PRECAUTIONS

Not indicated for initial therapy of HTN. Symptomatic hypotension may occur in patients w/ marked volume depletion or w/ salt depletion; correct volume/salt depletion prior to administration, or start treatment under close medical supervision. May cause changes in renal function, including acute renal failure; caution in patients whose renal function may depend in part on the activity of the renin-angiotensin-aldosterone system (RAAS) (eg, renal artery stenosis, severe heart failure [HF], post-MI, volume depletion). Consider withholding or discontinuing therapy if clinically significant decrease in renal function develops. May cause serum electrolyte abnormalities (eg, hyper/hypokalemia, hyponatremia, hypomagnesemia); correct hypokalemia and any coexisting hypomagnesemia prior to initiation. D/C if hypokalemia is accompanied by clinical signs (eg, muscular weakness, paresis, ECG alterations). **Aliskiren:** Hypersensitivity reactions and head/neck angioedema reported; d/c therapy immediately and do not readminister if anaphylactic reactions or angioedema develops. **Amlodipine:** May cause symptomatic hypotension, particularly in patients w/ severe aortic stenosis. May develop worsening of angina and acute MI after starting or increasing the dose, particularly w/ severe obstructive coronary artery disease (CAD). **HCTZ:** May cause hypersensitivity reactions and exacerbation or activation of systemic lupus erythematosus (SLE). Minor alterations of fluid and electrolyte balance may precipitate hepatic coma in patients w/ hepatic impairment or progressive liver disease. May cause idiosyncratic reaction, resulting in transient myopia and acute angle-closure glaucoma; d/c as rapidly as possible. May alter glucose tolerance, increase serum cholesterol/TG levels, and increase serum Ca^{2+}. May cause or exacerbate hyperuricemia and precipitate gout in susceptible patients.

ADVERSE REACTIONS

Peripheral edema, dizziness, headache.

DRUG INTERACTIONS

See Contraindications. **Aliskiren:** Cyclosporine or itraconazole may increase levels; avoid concomitant use w/ such drugs. NSAIDs, including selective COX-2 inhibitors, may deteriorate renal function and attenuate antihypertensive effect. Dual blockade of the RAAS is associated w/ increased risk of hypotension, hyperkalemia, and changes in renal function (including acute renal failure); in general, avoid combined use w/ ACE inhibitors or ARBs, particularly in patients w/ CrCl <60mL/min. Oral coadministration w/ furosemide reduced exposure to furosemide; monitor diuretic effects when coadministered. Risk of developing hyperkalemia w/ NSAIDs, K^+ supplements, or K^+-sparing diuretics. **Amlodipine:** May increase simvastatin exposure; limit simvastatin dose to 20mg/day. Increased systemic exposure w/ CYP3A inhibitors (moderate and strong) warranting dose reduction; monitor for symptoms of hypotension and edema w/ CYP3A4 inhibitors to determine the need for dose adjustment. Monitor BP when coadministered w/ CYP3A4 inducers. **HCTZ:** Dosage adjustment of antidiabetic drugs (insulin or oral agents) may be required. Space dosing ≥4 hrs before or 4-6 hrs after the administration of ion-exchange resins (eg, cholestyramine, colestipol). May increase risk of lithium toxicity; monitor serum lithium levels.

PATIENT CONSIDERATIONS

Assessment: Assess for diabetes, sulfonamide-derived drug hypersensitivity, hepatic/renal impairment, anuria, CAD, renal artery stenosis, HF, post-MI status, history of penicillin allergy, volume/salt depletion, SLE, severe aortic stenosis, bronchial asthma, pregnancy/nursing status, and possible drug interactions. Correct electrolyte imbalances prior to initiation of therapy.

Monitoring: Monitor for hypersensitivity/anaphylactic reactions, head/neck angioedema, airway obstruction, worsening of angina and MI, exacerbation of SLE, idiosyncratic reaction, transient myopia, acute angle-closure glaucoma, and other adverse reactions. Monitor BP, hepatic/renal function, serum uric acid, serum electrolytes, and glucose/cholesterol/TG levels.

Counseling: Advise female patients of childbearing age about consequences of exposure during pregnancy and discuss the treatment options w/ women planning to become pregnant. Advise to report pregnancy to physician as soon as possible. Caution that lightheadedness may occur, especially during the 1st days of therapy; instruct to contact physician if lightheadedness occurs. Advise to d/c treatment and to consult physician if syncope occurs. Caution that inadequate fluid intake, excessive perspiration, diarrhea, or vomiting can lead to excessive fall in BP. Advise to d/c and immediately report any signs/symptoms of severe allergic reaction or angioedema. Inform that angioedema, including laryngeal edema, may occur anytime during treatment. Instruct not to use K^+ supplements or salt substitutes containing K^+ w/o consulting physician.

STORAGE: 25°C (77°F); excursions permitted to 15-30°C (59-86°F). Protect from heat and moisture.

ANDROGEL – testosterone

CIII

Class: Androgen

Virilization reported in children secondarily exposed to testosterone gel. Children should avoid contact w/ unwashed or unclothed application sites in men using testosterone gel. Advise to strictly adhere to recommended instructions for use.

ADULT DOSAGE

Testosterone Replacement Therapy

Congenital/Acquired Primary Hypogonadism or Hypogonadotropic Hypogonadism in Males:

1%:

Initial: Apply 50mg (4 pump actuations, two 25mg pkts, or one 50mg pkt) qd in am (preferably at the same time every day)

Titrate: May increase to 75mg qd and then to 100mg qd if serum testosterone is below normal range

May decrease daily dose if serum testosterone exceeds normal range

D/C therapy if serum testosterone consistently exceeds the normal range at a daily dose of 50mg

Refer to PI for specific dosing guidelines using the multidose pump

PEDIATRIC DOSAGE

Pediatric use may not have been established

1.62%:
Initial: Apply 40.5mg (2 pump actuations or a single 40.5mg pkt) qd in am
Titrate: May adjust dose between a minimum of 20.25mg (1 pump actuation or a single 20.25mg pkt) and a max of 81mg (4 pump actuations or two 40.5mg pkts)
Titrate based on the predose am serum testosterone concentration from a single blood draw at approx 14 days and 28 days after starting treatment or following dose adjustment
Titration Based on Predose AM Serum Testosterone:
Serum Testosterone >750ng/dL: Decrease daily dose by 20.25mg (1 pump actuation or a single 20.25mg pkt)
Serum Testosterone 350-750ng/dL: Continue current dose
Serum Testosterone <350ng/dL: Increase daily dose by 20.25mg (1 pump actuation or a single 20.25mg pkt)

ADMINISTRATION
Topical route

Apply to clean, dry, healthy, intact skin
Refer to PI for additional administration and priming instructions

1%
Apply to right and left upper arms/shoulders and/or right and left abdomen; do not apply to any other parts of the body (eg, genitals, chest)
Avoid swimming or showering for at least 5 hrs after application

1.62%
Apply to upper arms and shoulders; do not apply to any other parts of the body (eg, abdomen, genitals)
Avoid swimming, showering, or washing the administration site for a minimum of 2 hrs after application

HOW SUPPLIED
Gel: 1% [2.5g pkt, 5g pkt (30^s); 75g pump (60 pumps)], 1.62% [1.25g pkt, 2.5g pkt (30^s); 88g pump (60 pumps)]

CONTRAINDICATIONS
Breast carcinoma or known/suspected prostate carcinoma in men; women who are or may become pregnant, or are breastfeeding.

WARNINGS/PRECAUTIONS
Topical testosterone products may have different doses, strengths, or application instructions that may result in different systemic exposure. Application site and dose are not interchangeable w/ other topical testosterone products. Patients w/ BPH treated w/ androgens, may be at increased risk for worsening of signs/symptoms of BPH. May increase risk for prostate cancer. Increases in Hct, reflective of increases in RBC mass, may require lowering or discontinuation of therapy; increase in RBC mass may increase risk for thromboembolic events. Venous thromboembolic events reported; d/c and initiate appropriate workup and management if a venous thromboembolic event is suspected. Suppression of spermatogenesis may occur w/ large doses. Edema w/ or w/o CHF may be a serious complication in patients w/ preexisting cardiac, renal, or hepatic disease. Gynecomastia may develop and persist. May potentiate sleep apnea. Changes in serum lipid profile may require dose adjustment or discontinuation of therapy. Caution in cancer patients at risk of hypercalcemia and associated hypercalciuria. May decrease levels of thyroxin-binding globulins, resulting in decreased total T4 serum concentrations and increased resin uptake of T3 and T4. Flammable; avoid fire, flame, or smoking until the gel has dried.

ADVERSE REACTIONS
(1.62%) Prostate specific antigen (PSA) increase. (1%) Acne, application-site reactions, prostatic/urinary/testicular disorders, abnormal lab tests, headache, emotional lability, gynecomastia, HTN, nervousness, asthenia, decreased libido.

DRUG INTERACTIONS
Changes in insulin sensitivity or glycemic control may occur; may decrease blood glucose and, therefore, may decrease insulin requirements in diabetic patients. Changes in anticoagulant activity may occur; frequently monitor INR and PT in patients taking anticoagulants, especially at initiation and termination of androgen therapy. Adrenocorticotropic hormone or corticosteroids may increase fluid retention; caution in patients w/ cardiac, renal, or hepatic disease.

PATIENT CONSIDERATIONS

Assessment: Assess for BPH, breast/prostate cancer, cardiac/renal/hepatic disease, risk factors for sleep apnea, cancer patients at risk for hypercalcemia, any conditions where treatment is contraindicated or cautioned, and possible drug interactions. Obtain baseline Hct and serum testosterone levels.

Monitoring: Monitor for prostate cancer, edema w/ or w/o CHF, venous thromboembolic events, gynecomastia, sleep apnea, worsening of signs/symptoms of BPH, and other adverse reactions. Perform periodic monitoring of Hgb, PSA, serum lipid profile, LFTs, and serum testosterone concentrations. In cancer patients at risk for hypercalcemia, regularly monitor serum Ca^{2+} levels. Reevaluate Hct 3-6 months after start of therapy, then annually. Frequently monitor PT/INR w/ anticoagulants. Assess serum testosterone concentrations periodically.

Counseling: Inform that men w/ known or suspected prostate/breast cancer should not use androgen therapy. Advise to report signs and symptoms of secondary exposure in children and women to the physician. Instruct women and children to avoid contact w/ unwashed or unclothed application sites of men. Instruct to apply ud and to wash hands w/ soap and water after application, cover application site w/ clothing after gel dries, and wash application site w/ soap and water prior to direct skin-to-skin contact w/ others. Counsel about possible adverse reactions. Advise to read Medication Guide before therapy and reread each time prescription is renewed. Inform that drug is flammable; instruct to avoid fire, flame, or smoking until the gel has dried. Advise not to share the medication w/ anyone. Inform patients about importance of adhering to all the recommended monitoring and instruct to report changes in their state of health and to wait 5 hrs (1%) or 2 hrs (1.62%) before swimming or bathing.

STORAGE: (1%) 25°C (77°F); excursions permitted to 15-30°C (59-86°F). (1.62%) 20-25°C (68-77°F); excursions permitted to 15-30°C (59-86°F).

ANGIOMAX – bivalirudin

RX

Class: Direct thrombin inhibitor (DTI)

ADULT DOSAGE

Percutaneous Transluminal Coronary Angioplasty/Percutaneous Coronary Intervention

Anticoagulant in patients w/ unstable angina undergoing percutaneous transluminal coronary angioplasty (PTCA). Anticoagulant in patients undergoing percutaneous coronary intervention (PCI) w/ provisional use of glycoprotein IIb/IIIa inhibitor (GPI). Indicated for patients w/, or at risk of, heparin induced thrombocytopenia (HIT) or heparin induced thrombocytopenia and thrombosis syndrome (HITTS) undergoing PCI

Give w/ aspirin (300-325mg/day)

Patients w/o HIT/HITTS:

0.75mg/kg IV bolus, then 1.75mg/kg/hr infusion for the duration of the PCI/PTCA procedure

An activated clotting time should be performed 5 min after the bolus dose and an additional bolus of 0.3mg/kg should be given if needed

Consider GPI administration in the event that any conditions listed in the REPLACE-2 clinical trial description is present; refer to PI

Patients w/ HIT/HITTS Undergoing PCI:

0.75mg/kg IV bolus, then 1.75mg/kg/hr infusion for the duration of the procedure

Ongoing Treatment Post-Procedure:

Continuation of infusion following PCI/PTCA for up to 4 hrs post-procedure is optional

After 4 hrs, an additional infusion may be initiated at a rate of 0.2mg/kg/hr (low-rate infusion), for up to 20 hrs, if needed

PEDIATRIC DOSAGE

Pediatric use may not have been established

DOSING CONSIDERATIONS

Renal Impairment

Reduction in bolus dose not needed

Severe (CrCl <30mL/min): Consider reducing infusion to 1mg/kg/hr

Hemodialysis: 0.25mg/kg/hr infusion

ADMINISTRATION

IV route

Reconstitution and Dilution

1. To each 250mg vial, add 5mL of sterile water for inj
2. Gently swirl until all material is dissolved
3. Further dilute in 50mL of D5W or 0.9% NaCl for inj for final concentration of 5mg/mL, or further dilute in 500mL of D5W or 0.9% NaCl for inj for final concentration of 0.5mg/mL

Incompatibilities

Alteplase, amiodarone HCl, amphotericin B, chlorpromazine HCl, diazepam, prochlorperazine edisylate, reteplase, streptokinase, and vancomycin HCl. Dobutamine compatibility varies w/ concentration; see PI

HOW SUPPLIED

Inj: 250mg

CONTRAINDICATIONS

Active major bleeding, hypersensitivity (eg, anaphylaxis) to bivalirudin or its components.

WARNINGS/PRECAUTIONS

Hemorrhage may occur at any site; caution with disease states associated with increased risk of bleeding. D/C with unexplained fall in BP or Hct. Associated with increased risk of thrombus formation, including fatal outcomes in gamma brachytherapy; maintain meticulous catheter technique, with frequent aspiration and flushing, paying special attention to minimize stasis condition within the catheter/vessels. May need to reduce infusion dose and monitor anticoagulant status in patients with renal impairment.

ADVERSE REACTIONS

Bleeding, back pain, pain, N/V, headache, hypotension, HTN, bradycardia, dyspepsia, insomnia, pelvic pain, anxiety, abdominal pain, fever, inj-site pain.

DRUG INTERACTIONS

Increased risk of major bleeding events with heparin, warfarin, thrombolytics, or GPIs.

PATIENT CONSIDERATIONS

Assessment: Assess for drug hypersensitivity, active major bleeding, renal impairment, disease states associated with increased risk of bleeding, pregnancy/nursing status, and for possible drug interactions.

Monitoring: Monitor for signs/symptoms of hemorrhage, thrombus formation in gamma brachytherapy, and other adverse reactions. For patients with renal impairment, monitor anticoagulant status.

Counseling: Advise to watch for any signs of bleeding/bruising and to report to physician if these occur. Advise to inform physician about the use of any other medications (eg, warfarin and heparin), including OTC medicines or herbal products, prior to therapy.

STORAGE: 20-25°C (68-77°F); excursions permitted to 15-30°C (59-86°F). Reconstituted: 2-8°C (36-46°F) for up to 24 hrs. Diluted concentration of between 0.5mg/mL and 5mg/mL is stable at room temperature for up to 24 hrs. Do not freeze.

ANORO ELLIPTA – umeclidinium/vilanterol RX

Class: Anticholinergic/beta$_2$ agonist

Long-acting β_2-adrenergic agonists (LABAs) increase the risk of asthma-related death. Not indicated for the treatment of asthma.

ADULT DOSAGE

Chronic Obstructive Pulmonary Disease

Long-Term Maint Treatment of Airflow Obstruction:

1 inh qd; do not use >1 time q24h

PEDIATRIC DOSAGE

Pediatric use may not have been established

ADMINISTRATION

Oral inh route

Take at the same time every day

HOW SUPPLIED

Powder, Inhalation: (Umeclidinium/Vilanterol) (62.5mcg/25mcg)/blister [7, 30 blisters]

CONTRAINDICATIONS

Severe hypersensitivity to milk proteins or hypersensitivity to umeclidinium, vilanterol, or any of the excipients.

WARNINGS/PRECAUTIONS

Not indicated for acute bronchospasm relief. Do not initiate during rapidly deteriorating or potentially life-threatening episodes of COPD. D/C regular use of oral/inhaled short acting β_2-agonist when beginning treatment. Do not use more often or at higher doses than recommended; clinically significant cardiovascular (CV) effects and fatalities reported with excessive use. May produce paradoxical bronchospasm; treat immediately with an inhaled, short acting bronchodilator; d/c and institute alternative therapy. Hypersensitivity reactions and CV effects may occur. Caution with CV disorders, convulsive disorders, thyrotoxicosis, diabetes mellitus (DM), ketoacidosis, narrow-angle glaucoma, urinary retention, and in patients unusually responsive to sympathomimetic amines. Monitor for signs and symptoms of acute narrow-angle glaucoma and urinary retention (especially in those with prostatic hyperplasia or bladder-neck obstruction). May produce significant hypokalemia or transient hyperglycemia.

ADVERSE REACTIONS

Pharyngitis, diarrhea, pain in extremity, sinusitis, lower respiratory tract infection, constipation, muscle spasms, neck pain, chest pain, productive cough, dry mouth, dyspepsia, abdominal pain, gastroesophageal reflux disease, vomiting.

DRUG INTERACTIONS

Do not use with other medicines containing LABAs. Caution with long-term ketoconazole and other strong CYP3A4 inhibitors (eg, ritonavir, clarithromycin, conivaptan); increased CV adverse effects may occur. Extreme caution with MAOIs, TCAs, or drugs known to prolong the QTc interval or within 2 weeks of discontinuation of such agents; effect on CV system may be potentiated. β-blockers may block pulmonary effects and produce severe bronchospasm in patients with COPD; if such therapy is needed, consider cardioselective β-blockers and use with caution. Caution is advised when coadministered with non-K^+-sparing diuretics (eg, loop, thiazide). Avoid with other anticholinergics; may increase anticholinergic adverse effects.

PATIENT CONSIDERATIONS

Assessment: Assess for hypersensitivity to milk proteins, COPD status, CV/convulsive disorders, thyrotoxicosis, DM, ketoacidosis, narrow-angle glaucoma, urinary retention, prostatic hyperplasia, bladder-neck obstruction, pregnancy/nursing status, and possible drug interactions.

Monitoring: Monitor for deteriorating disease, paradoxical bronchospasm, hypersensitivity reactions, CV effects, narrow-angle glaucoma, urinary retention, hypokalemia, hyperglycemia, and other adverse reactions.

Counseling: Inform that drug is not for treatment of asthma or to relieve acute symptoms of COPD. Advise that acute symptoms should be treated with a rescue inhaler (eg, albuterol). Instruct to seek medical attention immediately if experiencing worsening of symptoms, or a need for more inhalations than usual of the rescue inhaler. Advise not to d/c therapy without physician guidance and not to use an additional LABA. Instruct to d/c therapy if paradoxical bronchospasm occurs. Inform about adverse effects (eg, palpitations, chest pain, rapid HR, tremor, nervousness) and other risks (eg, narrow-angle glaucoma, urinary retention) associated with therapy; instruct to consult physician immediately if any signs/symptoms develop. Advise to contact physician if pregnancy occurs while on therapy. Inform that the inhaler is not reusable and advise not to take the inhaler apart.

STORAGE: 20-25°C (68-77°F); excursions permitted from 15-30°C (59-86°F). Store in a dry place away from direct heat or sunlight. Store inside the unopened moisture-protective foil tray and only remove from the tray immediately before initial use. Discard 6 weeks after opening the foil tray or when the counter reads "0" (after all blisters have been used), whichever comes 1st.

ANTIVERT — meclizine hydrochloride

RX

Class: Antihistamine

ADULT DOSAGE

Motion Sickness

25-50mg 1 hr prior to embarkation
Thereafter, may repeat dose q24h for the duration of the journey

Vertigo

25-100mg/day in divided doses, depending upon clinical response

PEDIATRIC DOSAGE

Motion Sickness

≥12 Years:
25-50mg 1 hr prior to embarkation
Thereafter, may repeat dose q24h for the duration of the journey

Vertigo

≥12 Years:
25-100mg/day in divided doses, depending upon clinical response

ADMINISTRATION
Oral route

HOW SUPPLIED
Tab: 12.5mg, 25mg, 50mg

CONTRAINDICATIONS
Previous hypersensitivity.

WARNINGS/PRECAUTIONS
Caution with asthma, glaucoma, enlargement of the prostate gland, hepatic/renal impairment, and in elderly. Drowsiness may occur. May impair physical/mental abilities.

ADVERSE REACTIONS
Anaphylactoid reaction, drowsiness, dry mouth, headache, fatigue, vomiting.

DRUG INTERACTIONS
Avoid alcohol use. Increased CNS depression with other CNS depressants (eg, alcohol, tranquilizers, sedatives). Possible interaction with CYP2D6 inhibitors.

PATIENT CONSIDERATIONS

Assessment: Assess for previous hypersensitivity to the drug, asthma, glaucoma, prostate gland enlargement, renal/hepatic impairment, pregnancy/nursing status, and possible drug interactions.

Monitoring: Monitor for drowsiness and other adverse reactions.

Counseling: Inform that drowsiness may occur; instruct to use caution when driving a vehicle or operating machinery. Advise to avoid alcohol use. Advise to notify physician if pregnant/nursing.

STORAGE: <30°C (86°F).

ANUSOL-HC SUPPOSITORY – hydrocortisone acetate RX

Class: Corticosteroid

OTHER BRAND NAMES
Anucort HC

ADULT DOSAGE

Colorectal Disorders

For use in inflamed hemorrhoids, post-irradiation (factitial) proctitis, as an adjunct in the treatment of chronic ulcerative colitis, cryptitis, other inflammatory conditions of the anorectum, and pruritus ani

Usual: 1 sup rectally bid (am and pm) for 2 weeks, in nonspecific proctitis. In more severe cases, 1 sup rectally tid or 2 sup rectally bid. In factitial proctitis, recommended therapy is 6-8 weeks or less, according to response

PEDIATRIC DOSAGE

Pediatric use may not have been established

ADMINISTRATION
Rectal route

HOW SUPPLIED
Sup: (Anusol-HC) 25mg [12^{s} 24^{s}]

CONTRAINDICATIONS
History of hypersensitivity to any of the components.

WARNINGS/PRECAUTIONS
D/C if irritation develops. D/C if infection develops that does not respond to appropriate therapy. May stain fabric. Only use after adequate proctologic exam.

ADVERSE REACTIONS
Burning, itching, irritation, dryness, folliculitis, hypopigmentation, allergic contact dermatitis, secondary infection.

PATIENT CONSIDERATIONS

Assessment: Proctologic examination should be done. Assess for drug hypersensitivity and presence of infection.

Monitoring: Monitor possible local adverse reactions including burning, itching, irritation, dryness, folliculitis, hypopigmentation, allergic contact dermatitis, and secondary infection.

Counseling: Advise that staining of fabric may occur with use of sup; precautionary measures recommended. If irritation develops, d/c therapy and institute appropriate therapy. Report adverse effects.

STORAGE: Store at 20-25°C (68-77°F). Store away from heat. Protect from freezing.

APIDRA – insulin glulisine (rDNA origin)

RX

Class: Insulin (rapid-acting)

OTHER BRAND NAMES
Apidra Solostar

ADULT DOSAGE

Diabetes Mellitus

Total Daily Insulin Requirement:
Usual: 0.5-1 U/kg/day; give SQ w/in 15 min ac or w/in 20 min after starting a meal

IV:
Use at concentrations of 0.05-1 U/mL in infusion systems using polyvinyl chloride bags

PEDIATRIC DOSAGE

Type 1 Diabetes Mellitus

≥4 Years:
Total Daily Insulin Requirement:
Usual: 0.5-1 U/kg/day; give SQ w/in 15 min ac or w/in 20 min after starting a meal

DOSING CONSIDERATIONS

Renal Impairment
May require dose reduction

Hepatic Impairment
May require dose reduction

ADMINISTRATION
SQ/IV route

SQ
Inject SQ in the abdominal wall, thigh, or upper arm; rotate inj sites w/in the same region
Use w/ an intermediate or long-acting insulin
Do not mix w/ insulin preparations other than NPH insulin; if mixed w/ NPH insulin, draw Apidra into syringe 1st, and inject mixture immediately after mixing

Continuous SQ Insulin Infusion by External Pump
Read the pump label to make sure the pump has been evaluated w/ Apidra
Administer by continuous SQ infusion in the abdominal wall by an external insulin pump; rotate infusion sites w/in the same region
Must have an alternative insulin delivery system in case of pump system failure
Do not mix w/ other insulins

IV
Do not mix w/ other insulins
Stable only in 0.9% NaCl

HOW SUPPLIED
Inj: 100 U/mL [3mL, SoloStar; 10mL, vial]

CONTRAINDICATIONS
During episodes of hypoglycemia, known hypersensitivity to Apidra or its excipients.

WARNINGS/PRECAUTIONS
Insulin pens must never be shared between patients; poses a risk for transmission of blood-borne pathogens. Any change in insulin regimen should be made cautiously and only under medical supervision. Changes in insulin strength, manufacturer, type, or method of administration may result in the need for a change in dosage or adjustment in concomitant oral antidiabetic treatment. Insulin requirements may be altered during stress, major illness, or w/ changes in exercise, meal patterns, or coadministered drugs. Hypoglycemia may occur and may impair ability to concentrate and react; caution in patients w/ hypoglycemia unawareness and in those predisposed to hypoglycemia. Severe, life-threatening, generalized allergy, including anaphylaxis, may occur. Hypokalemia may occur; caution in patients who may be at risk. May be administered IV under medical supervision w/ close monitoring of glucose and K^+ levels to avoid potentially fatal hypoglycemia and hypokalemia. Malfunction of insulin pump or infusion set, handling errors, or insulin degradation can rapidly lead to hyperglycemia, ketosis, and diabetic ketoacidosis; prompt identification/correction of the cause is necessary and interim SQ inj may be required. Train patients using CSII pump therapy how to administer by inj and have alternate insulin therapy available. Caution in elderly.

ADVERSE REACTIONS
Allergic reactions, infusion-site reactions, hypoglycemia, influenza, nasopharyngitis, URTI, arthralgia, HTN, headache, peripheral edema.

DRUG INTERACTIONS

Dose adjustment and close monitoring may be necessary w/ drugs that may increase blood-glucose-lowering effect and susceptibility to hypoglycemia (eg, oral antidiabetic products, pramlintide, ACE inhibitors), drugs that may reduce blood-glucose-lowering effect (eg, corticosteroids, danazol, niacin), or drugs that may either increase or decrease blood-glucose-lowering effect (eg, β-blockers, clonidine, lithium salts, alcohol). Pentamidine may cause hypoglycemia, sometimes followed by hyperglycemia. Hypoglycemic signs may be reduced or absent w/ antiadrenergic drugs (eg, β-blockers, clonidine, guanethidine, reserpine). Caution w/ K^+-lowering drugs and drugs sensitive to serum K^+ levels. Concomitant use w/ thiazolidinediones (TZDs) may cause dose-related fluid retention and heart failure (HF); observe for signs/symptoms of HF and consider dose reduction or discontinuation of TZDs if HF occurs.

PATIENT CONSIDERATIONS

Assessment: Assess for predisposition to hypoglycemia, risk of hypokalemia, hypersensitivity to drug or to any of its excipients, renal/hepatic impairment, pregnancy/nursing status, and possible drug interactions. Obtain baseline blood glucose and HbA1c levels.

Monitoring: Monitor for signs/symptoms of hypoglycemia, hypokalemia, allergic reactions, and other adverse reactions. Monitor blood glucose, HbA1c levels, and renal/hepatic function. Frequent glucose monitoring may be required w/ renal/hepatic impairment. Monitor glucose and K^+ levels frequently during IV administration.

Counseling: Advise never to share insulin pen w/ another person, even if needle is changed. Counsel on self-management procedures including glucose monitoring, proper inj technique, and management of hypo/hyperglycemia. Instruct on handling of special situations (eg, intercurrent conditions, inadequate or skipped dose, inadvertent administration of increased dose, inadequate food intake, skipped meals). Advise to inform physician if pregnant or contemplating pregnancy. Instruct to always check the label before each inj to avoid medication errors. Instruct on how to use an external infusion pump.

STORAGE: Unopened: 2-8°C (36-46°F). Do not freeze; discard if frozen. Protect from light. Must be used within 28 days if not stored in a refrigerator. Open (In-Use): <25°C (77°F). Discard after 28 days. Protect from direct heat and light. Do not refrigerate opened (in-use) SoloStar. Discard infusion sets and insulin in reservoir after 48 hrs of use or after exposure to temperatures >37°C (98.6°F). Prepared Infusion Bags: Room temperature for 48 hrs.

APRISO – mesalamine

RX

Class: 5-aminosalicylic acid derivative

ADULT DOSAGE

Ulcerative Colitis

Maint of Remission:
1.5g (4 caps) qam

PEDIATRIC DOSAGE

Pediatric use may not have been established

ADMINISTRATION

Oral route

HOW SUPPLIED

Cap, Extended Release: 0.375g

CONTRAINDICATIONS

Hypersensitivity to salicylates, aminosalicylates, or any of the components of this medication.

WARNINGS/PRECAUTIONS

Renal impairment, including minimal change nephropathy, acute and chronic interstitial nephritis, and, rarely, renal failure reported; caution with renal dysfunction or history of renal disease. Evaluate renal function prior to therapy and periodically thereafter. May cause acute intolerance syndrome (eg, acute abdominal pain, cramping, bloody diarrhea); d/c if suspected. Hepatic failure reported in patients with preexisting liver disease; caution with liver disease. Caution with sulfasalazine hypersensitivity and in elderly.

ADVERSE REACTIONS

Headache, diarrhea, upper abdominal pain, nausea, nasopharyngitis, influenza/influenza-like illness, sinusitis.

DRUG INTERACTIONS

Avoid with antacids.

PATIENT CONSIDERATIONS

Assessment: Assess for previous hypersensitivity to sulfasalazine or salicylates, history of or known renal/hepatic dysfunction, phenylketonuria, pregnancy/nursing status, and possible drug interactions. Evaluate renal function prior to initiation of therapy.

Monitoring: Monitor for renal impairment, hepatic failure, acute intolerance syndrome, and hypersensitivity reactions. Perform periodic monitoring of renal function and blood cell counts (in elderly).

Counseling: Inform patients with phenylketonuria that each cap contains aspartame. Instruct not to take with antacids. Instruct to contact a healthcare provider if symptoms of ulcerative colitis worsen.

STORAGE: 20-25°C (68-77°F); excursions permitted between 15-30°C (59-86°F).

ARANESP – darbepoetin alfa

RX

Class: Erythropoiesis stimulator

Increased risk of death, MI, stroke, venous thromboembolism (VTE), thrombosis of vascular access, and tumor progression or recurrence. Use the lowest dose sufficient to reduce/avoid the need for RBC transfusions. Chronic Kidney Disease (CKD): Greater risks for death, serious adverse cardiovascular (CV) reactions, and stroke when administered erythropoiesis-stimulating agents (ESAs) to target Hgb level of >11g/dL. Cancer: Shortened overall survival and/or increased risk of tumor progression or recurrence in patients w/ breast, non-small cell lung, head and neck, lymphoid, and cervical cancers. Must enroll in and comply w/ the ESA APPRISE Oncology Program to prescribe and/or dispense drug to patients. Use only for anemia from myelosuppressive chemotherapy. Not indicated for patients receiving myelosuppressive chemotherapy when anticipated outcome is cure. D/C following completion of chemotherapy course.

ADULT DOSAGE

Anemia Due to Chronic Kidney Disease

On Dialysis:
Initiate when Hgb is <10g/dL
Initial: 0.45mcg/kg IV/SQ weekly or 0.75mcg/kg IV/SQ once every 2 weeks
Titrate: Adjust dose based on Hgb levels. If Hgb approaches or exceeds 11g/dL, reduce or interrupt dose

Not on Dialysis:
Initiate when Hgb is <10g/dL, the rate of Hgb decline indicates likelihood of a RBC transfusion, and when reducing the risk of alloimmunization and/or other RBC transfusion-related risks is a goal
Initial: 0.45mcg/kg IV/SQ once every 4 weeks
Titrate: Adjust dose based on Hgb levels. If Hgb exceeds 10g/dL, reduce or interrupt dose and use lowest dose sufficient to reduce RBC transfusion

All Patients:
Titrate:
Do not increase dose more frequently than once every 4 weeks; decreases may occur more frequently
Rapid Increase in Hgb (>1g/dL in Any 2-Week Period): Reduce by ≥25% prn to reduce rapid responses
Hgb Has Not Increased by >1g/dL After 4 Weeks of Therapy: Increase by 25%
No Adequate Response Over a 12-Week Escalation Period: Further dose increase is unlikely to improve response and may increase risks. Use lowest dose to maintain Hgb level sufficient to reduce the need of RBC transfusion; d/c if responsiveness does not improve

Anemia Due to Chemotherapy

Initiate when Hgb is <10g/dL and if there is a minimum of 2 additional months of chemotherapy

Initial: 2.25mcg/kg SQ weekly or 500mcg SQ every 3 weeks until completion of chemotherapy course

PEDIATRIC DOSAGE

Anemia Due to Chronic Kidney Disease

Initiate when Hgb is <10g/dL
Initial: 0.45 mcg/kg IV/SQ weekly; patients not receiving dialysis may be initiated at a dose of 0.75mcg/kg once every 2 weeks
Titrate: If Hgb approaches or exceeds 12g/dL, reduce or interrupt dose

Conversion from Epoetin Alfa:
Administer less frequently than epoetin alfa; estimate the starting weekly dose based on weekly epoetin alfa dose at the time of substitution

Epoetin Alfa Dose (U/Week):
1500-2499: 6.25mcg/week
2500-4999: 10mcg/week
5000-10,999: 20mcg/week
11,000-17,999: 40mcg/week
18,000-33,999: 60mcg/week
34,000-89,999: 100mcg/week
≥90,000: 200mcg/week

Administer once weekly or every 2 weeks in patients who were receiving epoetin alfa 2-3X weekly or once weekly, respectively

Titrate:
Hgb Increases >1g/dL in Any 2-Week Period/ Hgb Reaches a Level Needed to Avoid RBC Transfusion: Reduce dose by 40%
Hgb Exceeds Level Needed to Avoid RBC Transfusion: Withhold until Hgb approaches a level where RBC transfusions may be required; reinitiate at a dose 40% below previous dose
Hgb Increases by <1g/dL and Remains <10g/dL After 6 Weeks of Therapy: Increase dose to 4.5mcg/kg/week (weekly schedule) or no dose adjustment (3-week schedule)
No Response in Hgb Levels/Still Require RBC Transfusions After 8 Weeks of Therapy/ Following Completion of Chemotherapy Course: D/C therapy

Conversions

Adults w/ CKD on Dialysis:
Conversion from Epoetin Alfa:
Administer less frequently than epoetin alfa; estimate the starting weekly dose based on weekly epoetin alfa dose at the time of substitution
Epoetin Alfa Dose (U/Week):
<1500: 6.25mcg/week
1500-2499: 6.25mcg/week
2500-4999: 12.5mcg/week
5000-10,999: 25mcg/week
11,000-17,999: 40mcg/week
18,000-33,999: 60mcg/week
34,000-89,999: 100mcg/week
≥90,000: 200mcg/week
Administer once weekly or every 2 weeks in patients who were receiving epoetin alfa 2-3X weekly or once weekly, respectively

ADMINISTRATION

IV/SQ route
IV route is recommended for hemodialysis patients.
Do not shake.
Do not use if it has been frozen or shaken.
Do not dilute and do not administer in conjunction w/ other drug sol.
Discard any unused portion in vials or prefilled syringes; do not re-enter vial.
Maintain route of administration when converting from epoetin alfa.

HOW SUPPLIED

Inj: 25mcg/mL, 40mcg/mL, 60mcg/mL, 100mcg/mL, 150mcg/0.75mL, 200mcg/mL, 300mcg/mL [single-dose vial]; 10mcg/0.4mL, 25mcg/0.42mL, 40mcg/0.4mL, 60mcg/0.3mL, 100mcg/0.5mL, 150mcg/0.3mL, 200mcg/0.4mL, 300mcg/0.6mL, 500mcg/mL [single-dose prefilled syringe]

CONTRAINDICATIONS

Uncontrolled HTN, pure red cell aplasia (PRCA) that begins after treatment w/ darbepoetin alfa or other erythropoietin protein drugs, serious allergic reactions to darbepoetin alfa.

WARNINGS/PRECAUTIONS

Not indicated for use in patients w/ cancer receiving hormonal agents, biologic products, or radiotherapy, unless also receiving concomitant myelosuppressive chemotherapy, or as a substitute for RBC transfusions in patients requiring immediate correction of anemia. Evaluate transferrin saturation and serum ferritin prior to and during treatment; administer supplemental iron when serum ferritin is <100mcg/L or serum transferrin saturation is <20%. Correct/exclude other causes of anemia (eg, vitamin deficiency, metabolic/chronic inflammatory conditions, bleeding) before initiating therapy. Caution in patients w/ coexistent CV disease and stroke. Not approved for reduction of RBC transfusions in patients scheduled for surgical procedures. Hypertensive encephalopathy and seizures reported in patients w/ CKD. Appropriately control HTN prior to initiation of and during treatment; reduce/withhold therapy if BP becomes difficult to control. Cases of PRCA and severe anemia, w/ or w/o other cytopenias that arise following development of neutralizing antibodies to erythropoietin reported. Withhold and evaluate for neutralizing antibodies to erythropoietin if severe anemia and low reticulocyte count develop; d/c permanently if PRCA develops, and do not switch to other ESAs. Serious allergic reactions may occur; immediately and permanently d/c treatment and administer appropriate therapy if a serious allergic/anaphylactic reaction occurs. Patients may require adjustments in dialysis prescriptions after initiation of therapy, or require increased anticoagulation w/ heparin to prevent clotting of extracorporeal circuit during hemodialysis. Needle cover of the prefilled syringe contains dry natural rubber (a derivative of latex), which may cause allergic reactions.

ADVERSE REACTIONS

MI, stroke, VTE, thrombosis of vascular access, tumor progression/recurrence, HTN, dyspnea, peripheral edema, cough, procedural hypotension, angina pectoris, fluid overload, rash/erythema.

PATIENT CONSIDERATIONS

Assessment: Assess for uncontrolled HTN, previous hypersensitivity to the drug, latex allergy, causes of anemia, pregnancy/nursing status, and other conditions where treatment is cautioned/contraindicated. Obtain baseline Hgb levels, transferrin saturation, and serum ferritin.

Monitoring: Monitor for signs/symptoms of an allergic reaction, CV/thromboembolic events, stroke, PRCA, severe anemia, progression/recurrence of tumor, HTN, and other adverse reactions. Monitor BP, transferrin saturation, and serum ferritin. Monitor closely for premonitory neurologic symptoms during the 1st several months following initiation of treatment. Following initiation of therapy and after each dose adjustment, monitor Hgb weekly until Hgb is stable and sufficient to minimize need for RBC transfusion, and then monitor Hgb less frequently, provided Hgb levels remain stable.

Counseling: Inform of the risks/benefits of therapy and of the increased risks of mortality, serious CV reactions, thromboembolic reactions, stroke, and tumor progression. Advise of the need to have regular lab tests for Hgb. Inform cancer patients that they must sign the patient-physician acknowledgment form prior to the start of each treatment course. Instruct to undergo regular BP monitoring, adhere to prescribed antihypertensive regimen, and follow recommended dietary restrictions. Advise to contact physician for new-onset neurologic symptoms or change in seizure frequency. Instruct regarding proper disposal and caution against reuse of needles, syringes, or unused portions of single-dose vials.

STORAGE: 2-8°C (36-46°F). Do not freeze. Protect from light.

ARAVA – leflunomide

Class: Pyrimidine synthesis inhibitor

RX

Contraindicated for use in pregnant women due to the potential for fetal harm; exclude pregnancy before start of treatment in females of reproductive potential. Advise females of reproductive potential to use effective contraception during treatment and during an accelerated drug elimination procedure after treatment. If patient becomes pregnant, d/c therapy and use an accelerated drug elimination procedure. Severe liver injury, including fatal liver failure, reported; contraindicated in patients w/ severe hepatic impairment. Concomitant use w/ other potentially hepatotoxic drugs may increase risk of liver injury. Not for use in patients w/ preexisting acute or chronic liver disease, or those w/ serum ALT >2X ULN before initiating treatment. Monitor ALT levels at least monthly for 6 months after starting therapy, and thereafter every 6-8 weeks. If leflunomide-induced liver injury is suspected, d/c treatment, start an accelerated drug elimination procedure, and monitor liver tests weekly until normalized.

ADULT DOSAGE

Rheumatoid Arthritis

Recommended Dose: 20mg qd

Max: 20mg qd

Consider dose reduction to 10mg qd if unable to tolerate 20mg qd

May initiate treatment w/ or w/o LD, depending on risk of drug-associated hepatotoxicity and drug-associated myelosuppression

Low Risk for Hepatotoxicity and Myelosuppression:

LD: 100mg qd for 3 days

Maint: 20mg qd

High Risk for Hepatotoxicity (eg, Concomitant Methotrexate [MTX]) or Myelosuppression (eg, Concomitant Immunosuppressants):

Recommended Dose: 20mg qd w/o LD

PEDIATRIC DOSAGE

Pediatric use may not have been established

DOSING CONSIDERATIONS

Hepatic Impairment

Not recommended

Discontinuation

Procedure for Accelerated Elimination of Leflunomide and its Active Metabolite:

Use of an accelerated drug elimination procedure will rapidly reduce plasma levels of leflunomide and its active metabolite, teriflunomide; w/o use of an accelerated drug elimination procedure, it may take up to 2 yrs to reach plasma teriflunomide levels of <0.02mg/L

Consider an accelerated elimination procedure at any time after discontinuation of leflunomide, and in particular, when a patient has experienced a severe adverse reaction (eg, hepatotoxicity, serious infection, bone marrow suppression, Stevens-Johnson syndrome, toxic epidermal necrolysis, peripheral neuropathy, interstitial lung disease [ILD]), suspected hypersensitivity, or has become pregnant; all women of childbearing potential should undergo an accelerated elimination procedure after stopping treatment

Elimination Can Be Accelerated by the Following Procedures:

1. Administer cholestyramine 8g PO tid for 11 days, or alternatively, administer 50g of activated charcoal powder (made into a sus) PO q12h for 11 days
2. Verify plasma teriflunomide levels of <0.02mg/L by 2 separate tests at least 14 days apart; if plasma teriflunomide levels are higher than 0.02mg/L, repeat cholestyramine and/or activated charcoal treatment

The duration of accelerated drug elimination treatment may be modified based on the clinical status and tolerability of the elimination procedure; may repeat procedure as needed, based on teriflunomide levels and clinical status

ADMINISTRATION

Oral route

HOW SUPPLIED

Tab: 10mg, 20mg, 100mg

CONTRAINDICATIONS

Pregnant women, severe hepatic impairment, patients being treated w/ teriflunomide. Known hypersensitivity to leflunomide or any of the other components in this medication.

WARNINGS/PRECAUTIONS

Interrupt therapy if ALT elevation >3X ULN occurs; if likely leflunomide-induced, perform the accelerated drug elimination procedure and monitor liver tests weekly until normalized. If leflunomide-induced liver injury is unlikely, may consider resumption of therapy. Use of the accelerated drug elimination procedure may result in return of disease activity if patient had been responding to treatment. Not recommended w/ severe immunodeficiency, bone marrow dysplasia, or severe, uncontrolled infections; consider interrupting therapy and initiating the accelerated drug elimination procedure if a serious infection occurs. May cause immunosuppression and increased susceptibility to infections, including opportunistic infections, especially *Pneumocystis jiroveci* pneumonia, tuberculosis (TB), and aspergillosis. Screen all patients for active and inactive (latent) TB infection prior to initiating therapy; treat patients testing positive in TB screening prior to therapy and monitor carefully during treatment w/ leflunomide for possible reactivation of the infection. Pancytopenia, agranulocytosis, and thrombocytopenia reported; monitor platelets, WBC count, and Hgb or Hct at baseline and monthly for 6 months following initiation of therapy and every 6-8 weeks thereafter. D/C therapy if evidence of bone marrow suppression occurs. Monitor for hematologic toxicity if switching to another antirheumatic agent w/ a known potential for hematologic suppression. Peripheral neuropathy, rare cases of Stevens-Johnson syndrome and toxic epidermal necrolysis, and drug reaction w/ eosinophilia and systemic symptoms (DRESS) reported; d/c therapy if any of these occur. Age >60 yrs and diabetes may increase risk for peripheral neuropathy. May increase risk of malignancy, particularly lymphoproliferative disorders. ILD and worsening of preexisting ILD reported. New onset or worsening of pulmonary symptoms (eg, cough, dyspnea), w/ or w/o associated fever, may be a reason for discontinuation of therapy and for further investigation as appropriate. BP elevation reported. Caution w/ renal impairment.

ADVERSE REACTIONS

Diarrhea, abnormal liver enzymes, alopecia, headache, N/V, rash, HTN, allergic reaction, bronchitis, abdominal/back/GI pain, asthenia, dizziness, rhinitis.

DRUG INTERACTIONS

See Boxed Warning and Contraindications. Concomitant use w/ rifampin increased levels of teriflunomide; caution if receiving both leflunomide and rifampin. May increase exposure of drugs metabolized by CYP2C8 (eg, paclitaxel, pioglitazone, repaglinide); monitor and adjust the dose of the concomitant drug as required. Closely monitor INR w/ warfarin; teriflunomide may decrease peak INR. Teriflunomide may increase exposures of ethinyl estradiol and levonorgestrel. May reduce exposure of drugs metabolized by CYP1A2 (eg, alosetron, duloxetine, theophylline); monitor and adjust the dose of the concomitant drug as required. May increase exposure of OAT3 substrates (eg, cefaclor, cimetidine, ciprofloxacin); monitor and adjust the dose of the concomitant drug as required. For a patient taking leflunomide, the dose of rosuvastatin should not exceed

10mg qd. For other substrates of BCRP (eg, mitoxantrone) and drugs in the OATP family (eg, MTX, rifampin), especially HMG-Co reductase inhibitors (eg, atorvastatin, nateglinide, pravastatin), consider reducing the dose of these drugs and monitor closely for signs/symptoms of increased exposures to the drugs while taking leflunomide. Vaccination w/ live vaccines is not recommended; consider long $T_{1/2}$ of the active metabolite when contemplating administration of live vaccine after stopping therapy. May increase risk of peripheral neuropathy w/ neurotoxic medications. If given concomitantly w/ MTX, follow the American College of Rheumatology guidelines for monitoring MTX liver toxicity w/ ALT, AST, and serum albumin testing.

PATIENT CONSIDERATIONS

Assessment: Assess for hypersensitivity to drug or any of the other components of the drug, severe immunodeficiency, bone marrow dysplasia, severe uncontrolled infections, hepatic/renal impairment, any other conditions where treatment is contraindicated or cautioned, pregnancy/nursing status, and possible drug interactions. Evaluate for active TB and screen for latent TB infection. Obtain baseline BP, platelet counts, WBC count, Hgb or Hct, and ALT levels. Perform pregnancy testing for females of reproductive potential to exclude pregnancy before the start of treatment.

Monitoring: Monitor for signs/symptoms of hepatotoxicity, immunosuppression, infections (including opportunistic infections), pancytopenia, agranulocytosis, thrombocytopenia, Stevens-Johnson syndrome, toxic epidermal necrolysis, DRESS, peripheral neuropathy, ILD, malignancy, and other adverse reactions. Monitor BP periodically. Monitor platelets, WBC count, Hgb or Hct monthly for 6 months following initiation of therapy and every 6-8 weeks thereafter; chronic monitoring should be monthly if used w/ concomitant MTX and/or other potential immunosuppressive agents. Monitor ALT levels monthly for 6 months after starting treatment and every 6-8 weeks thereafter. Monitor carefully after dose reduction and after stopping therapy. Monitor for hematologic toxicity when switching to another antirheumatic agent w/ known potential for hematologic suppression.

Counseling: Advise females of reproductive potential of the potential for fetal harm if drug is taken during pregnancy. Instruct to notify physician immediately if a pregnancy occurs or is suspected and to use effective contraception during treatment and until plasma concentration of the active metabolite is verified to be <0.02mg/L. Advise nursing women to d/c breastfeeding during treatment. Inform of the possibility of rare, serious skin reactions; instruct to promptly report if a skin rash or mucous membrane lesions develop. Advise of the potential hepatotoxic effects and of the need for monitoring liver enzymes; instruct to notify physician if symptoms such as unusual tiredness, abdominal pain, or jaundice develop. Advise that lowering of blood counts may develop; instruct to have frequent hematologic monitoring, particularly in patients who are receiving other concurrent immunosuppressive therapy or who have had a history of significant hematologic abnormality; instruct to notify physician if symptoms of pancytopenia (eg, easy bruising/bleeding, recurrent infections, fever, paleness, unusual tiredness) develop. Inform about the early warning signs of ILD and instruct to contact physician promptly if these symptoms appear/worsen during therapy.

STORAGE: 25°C (77°F); excursions permitted to 15-30°C (59-86°F). Protect from light.

ARICEPT — donepezil hydrochloride

RX

Class: Acetylcholinesterase (AChE) inhibitor

ADULT DOSAGE

Alzheimer's Disease

Treatment of Dementia of the Alzheimer's Type:

Mild to Moderate:
Initial: 5mg qhs
Max: 10mg/day

Moderate to Severe:
Initial: 5mg qhs
Max: 23mg/day

Do not administer 10mg/day dose until patients have been on 5mg/day for 4-6 weeks
Do not administer 23mg/day dose until patients have been on 10mg/day for at least 3 months

PEDIATRIC DOSAGE

Pediatric use may not have been established

ADMINISTRATION

Oral route

Take qhs.
Take w/ or w/o food.

23mg Tab

Do not split, crush, or chew.

ODT

Allow to dissolve on the tongue and follow w/ water.

HOW SUPPLIED

Tab: 5mg, 10mg, 23mg; **Tab, Disintegrating:** (ODT) 5mg, 10mg

CONTRAINDICATIONS

Known hypersensitivity to donepezil HCl or to piperidine derivatives.

WARNINGS/PRECAUTIONS

May exaggerate succinylcholine-type muscle relaxation during anesthesia. May have vagotonic effects on sinoatrial (SA) and atrioventricular (AV) nodes, manifesting as bradycardia or heart block. Syncopal episodes reported. May produce N/V and diarrhea; observe closely at initiation of treatment and after dose increases. May increase gastric acid secretion; monitor closely for symptoms of active or occult GI bleeding, especially in patients at increased risk for developing ulcers (eg, concurrent NSAID use). Weight loss reported. May cause bladder outflow obstruction and generalized convulsions. Caution w/ history of asthma or obstructive pulmonary disease.

ADVERSE REACTIONS

Diarrhea, anorexia, N/V, ecchymosis, insomnia, muscle cramps, fatigue, headache, dizziness, weight loss, abnormal dreams, infection, HTN, back pain.

DRUG INTERACTIONS

May interfere w/ activity of anticholinergic medications. Synergistic effect when given concurrently w/ succinylcholine, similar neuromuscular blocking agents, or cholinergic agonists (eg, bethanechol).

PATIENT CONSIDERATIONS

Assessment: Assess for hypersensitivity to the drug or to piperidine derivatives, underlying cardiac conduction abnormalities, risks for developing ulcers, history of asthma or obstructive pulmonary disease, pregnancy/nursing status, and possible drug interactions.

Monitoring: Monitor for vagotonic effects on SA and AV nodes, syncopal episodes, diarrhea, N/V, active/occult GI bleeding, weight loss, bladder outflow obstruction, generalized convulsions, and other possible adverse reactions.

Counseling: Instruct to take as prescribed. Advise that N/V, diarrhea, insomnia, muscle cramps, fatigue, and decreased appetite may occur.

STORAGE: 15-30°C (59-86°F).

ARIMIDEX – anastrozole

RX

Class: Nonsteroidal aromatase inhibitor

ADULT DOSAGE

Breast Cancer

In postmenopausal women for adjuvant treatment of hormone receptor-positive early breast cancer; 1st-line treatment of hormone receptor-positive or hormone receptor unknown locally advanced or metastatic breast cancer; and treatment of advanced breast cancer w/ disease progression following tamoxifen therapy

Advanced Breast Cancer:
1mg qd; continue until tumor progression

Adjuvant Treatment of Early Breast Cancer:
1mg qd; administered for 5 years in a clinical trial

PEDIATRIC DOSAGE

Pediatric use may not have been established

ADMINISTRATION

Oral route

Take w/ or w/o food

HOW SUPPLIED

Tab: 1mg

CONTRAINDICATIONS

Women who are or may become pregnant, premenopausal women, hypersensitivity reaction to the drug or to any of the excipients.

WARNINGS/PRECAUTIONS

Increased incidence of ischemic cardiovascular (CV) events in women with preexisting ischemic heart disease reported. Decreases in bone mineral density (BMD) may occur. Elevated serum cholesterol reported.

ADVERSE REACTIONS

Hot flashes, asthenia, arthritis, pain, pharyngitis, HTN, depression, N/V, rash, osteoporosis, fractures, headache, bone pain, peripheral edema.

DRUG INTERACTIONS

Tamoxifen may decrease levels; avoid concomitant use. Avoid with estrogen-containing therapies.

PATIENT CONSIDERATIONS

Assessment: Assess for hypersensitivity to drug, preexisting ischemic cardiac disease, premenopausal status, pregnancy/nursing status, and possible drug interactions.

Monitoring: Monitor for hypersensitivity reactions and other adverse reactions. Monitor BMD and serum cholesterol levels.

Counseling: Inform that drug may cause fetal harm and is not for use in premenopausal women; instruct to d/c therapy if patient becomes pregnant and to immediately contact physician. Instruct to seek medical attention immediately if serious allergic reactions occur. Inform patients with preexisting ischemic heart disease that an increased incidence of CV events has been observed; advise to seek medical attention immediately if new or worsening chest pain or SOB occurs. Inform that drug may lower estrogen level, which may lead to a loss of the mineral content of bones, possibly decreasing the bone strength, leading to an increased risk of fractures. Inform that an increased level of cholesterol might be seen while receiving therapy. Instruct to notify physician if tickling, tingling, or numbness is experienced. Advise not to take drug with tamoxifen.

STORAGE: 20-25°C (68-77°F).

ARISTADA — aripiprazole lauroxil RX

Class: Atypical antipsychotic

Elderly patients w/ dementia-related psychosis treated w/ antipsychotic drugs are at an increased risk of death. Not approved for the treatment of patients w/ dementia-related psychosis.

ADULT DOSAGE

Schizophrenia

Establish tolerability w/ oral aripiprazole prior to initiating treatment in patients who have never taken aripiprazole; it may take up to 2 weeks to fully assess tolerability

Dosing Frequency and Site of Inj:
441mg: Administer monthly in the deltoid or gluteal muscle
662mg: Administer monthly in the gluteal muscle
882mg: Administer monthly or every 6 weeks in the gluteal muscle

Dose Based on Oral Aripiprazole Total Daily Dose:
10mg/day PO: 441mg/month inj
15mg/day PO: 662mg/month inj
≥20mg/day PO: 882mg/month inj

In conjunction w/ the 1st Aristada inj, administer treatment w/ oral aripiprazole for 21 consecutive days

In the event of early dosing, an inj should not be given earlier than 14 days after the previous inj

PEDIATRIC DOSAGE

Pediatric use may not have been established

Missed Dose

Concomitant Oral Aripiprazole Supplementation Following Missed Doses:
441mg Monthly:
≤6 Weeks Since Last Inj: No oral aripiprazole required; administer next inj as soon as possible
>6 and ≤7 Weeks Since Last Inj: Supplement next inj dose w/ 7 days oral aripiprazole
>7 Weeks Since Last Inj: Supplement next inj dose w/ 21 days oral aripiprazole

662mg & 882mg Monthly or 882mg Every 6 Weeks:
≤8 Weeks Since Last Inj: No oral aripiprazole required; administer next inj as soon as possible
>8 and ≤12 Weeks Since Last Inj: Supplement next inj dose w/ 7 days oral aripiprazole
>12 Weeks Since Last Inj: Supplement next inj dose w/ 21 days oral aripiprazole

Supplement w/ the same dose of oral aripiprazole as when the patient began therapy

DOSING CONSIDERATIONS

Concomitant Medications

CYP450 Modulators (Added for >2 Weeks):
Strong CYP3A4 Inhibitor:
Reduce Aristada dose to the next lower strength. No adjustment is necessary in patients taking 441mg, if tolerated.
Poor Metabolizers of CYP2D6: Reduce dose to 441mg from 662mg or 882mg; no dosage adjustment is necessary in patients taking 441mg, if tolerated.

Strong CYP2D6 Inhibitor:
Reduce Aristada dose to the next lower strength. No adjustment is necessary in patients taking 441mg, if tolerated.
Poor Metabolizers of CYP2D6: No dose adjustment required.

Both Strong CYP3A4 Inhibitor and Strong CYP2D6 Inhibitor:
Avoid use for patients at 662mg or 882mg dose. No dosage adjustment is necessary in patients taking 441mg, if tolerated.

CYP3A4 Inducers:
No dose adjustment for 662mg and 882mg dose. Increase the 441mg dose to 662mg.

For the 882mg dose administered every 6 weeks, the next lower strength is 441mg administered every 4 weeks.

ADMINISTRATION

IM route

Inj Site and Associated Needle Length:
441mg Dose:
Deltoid: 21 gauge, 1 inch or 20 gauge, 1.5 inch
Gluteal: 20 gauge, 1.5 inch or 20 gauge, 2 inch

662mg Dose:
Gluteal: 20 gauge, 1.5 inch or 20 gauge, 2 inch

882mg Dose:
Gluteal: 20 gauge, 1.5 inch or 20 gauge, 2 inch

HOW SUPPLIED

Inj, Extended-Release: 441mg/1.6mL, 662mg/2.4mL, 882mg/3.2mL

CONTRAINDICATIONS

Known hypersensitivity reaction to aripiprazole.

WARNINGS/PRECAUTIONS

Neuroleptic malignant syndrome (NMS) may occur; d/c immediately and institute intensive symptomatic treatment and medical monitoring. If patient appears to require antipsychotic treatment after recovery from NMS, reintroduction of therapy should be closely monitored, since recurrences of NMS have been reported. May cause tardive dyskinesia (TD), especially in the elderly; consider discontinuation if signs/symptoms appear. Associated w/ metabolic changes (eg, hyperglycemia/diabetes mellitus [DM], dyslipidemia, weight gain). May cause orthostatic hypotension, w/ greatest risk at therapy initiation and during dose escalation;

consider using a lower starting dose and monitor orthostatic vital signs in patients at increased risk of adverse reactions related to orthostatic hypotension or at increased risk of developing complications from hypotension. Leukopenia, neutropenia, and agranulocytosis reported; frequently monitor CBC during the first few months of therapy in patients w/ a history of a clinically significant low WBC count/ANC or drug-induced leukopenia/neutropenia, and consider discontinuation at the 1st sign of a clinically significant decline in WBC counts w/o other causative factors. D/C therapy in patients w/ severe neutropenia (ANC <1000/mm^3) and follow their WBC count until recovery. Caution w/ history of seizures or w/ conditions that lower seizure threshold. May impair mental/physical abilities and disrupt body temperature regulation. May cause esophageal dysmotility and aspiration; caution in patients at risk for aspiration pneumonia.

ADVERSE REACTIONS

Akathisia.

DRUG INTERACTIONS

See Dosing Considerations. Use of oral aripiprazole w/ strong CYP3A4 inhibitors (eg, itraconazole, clarithromycin) or strong CYP2D6 inhibitors (eg, quinidine, fluoxetine, paroxetine) increased exposure of aripiprazole. Use of oral aripiprazole w/ carbamazepine, a strong CYP3A4 inducer, decreased exposure of aripiprazole. May enhance effect of certain antihypertensives; monitor BP and adjust dose accordingly. Intensity of sedation and orthostatic hypotension observed was greater w/ the combination of oral aripiprazole and lorazepam; monitor sedation and BP and adjust dose accordingly w/ concomitant benzodiazepines.

PATIENT CONSIDERATIONS

Assessment: Assess for dementia-related psychosis, DM, dehydration, hypovolemia, cardiovascular disease, cerebrovascular disease, seizures, risk for aspiration pneumonia, drug hypersensitivity, any other conditions where treatment is cautioned, pregnancy/nursing status, and possible drug interactions. Obtain baseline FPG in patients at risk for DM. Obtain baseline CBC in patients w/ a history of a clinically significant low WBC counts/ANC or drug-induced leukopenia/neutropenia.

Monitoring: Monitor for NMS, TD, hyperglycemia/DM, dyslipidemia, weight gain, orthostatic hypotension, leukopenia, neutropenia, agranulocytosis, seizures, disruption of body temperature regulation, esophageal dysmotility, aspiration, and other adverse reactions. Monitor for worsening of glucose control in patients w/ DM and FPG in patients at risk for DM. Monitor CBC frequently during the 1st few months of therapy in patients w/ a history of a clinically significant low WBC counts/ANC or drug-induced leukopenia/neutropenia. Monitor for fever or other symptoms/signs of infection in patients w/ clinically significant neutropenia. Periodically reassess need for continued treatment.

Counseling: Educate about NMS; advise to contact a healthcare provider or report to the emergency room if signs/symptoms develop. Instruct to notify healthcare provider if any movements that cannot be controlled in the face, tongue, or other body part develop. Educate about the risk of metabolic changes, how to recognize symptoms of hyperglycemia/DM, and the need for specific monitoring. Educate about the risk of orthostatic hypotension, particularly at the time of initiating treatment, reinitiating treatment, or increasing the dose. Advise patients w/ preexisting low WBC count or a history of drug-induced leukopenia/neutropenia to have their CBC monitored during treatment. Instruct to use caution when operating hazardous machinery. Instruct to avoid overheating and dehydration. Instruct to notify healthcare provider of any changes to prescription or OTC drugs. Advise that therapy may cause extrapyramidal and/or withdrawal symptoms in a neonate and to notify healthcare provider w/ a known or suspected pregnancy.

STORAGE: 20-25°C (68-77°F); excursions permitted between 15-30°C (59-86°F).

ARMOUR THYROID – thyroid

RX

Class: Thyroid replacement hormone

Do not use for the treatment of obesity or weight loss; doses within range of daily hormonal requirements are ineffective for weight reduction in euthyroid patients. Serious or life-threatening manifestations of toxicity may occur when given in larger doses, particularly when given in association with sympathomimetic amines.

ADULT DOSAGE

Hypothyroidism

Replacement/supplemental therapy in hypothyroidism of any etiology, except transient hypothyroidism during the recovery phase of subacute thyroiditis

PEDIATRIC DOSAGE

Hypothyroidism

Congenital:

0-6 Months of Age: 4.8-6mg/kg/day

6-12 Months of Age: 3.6-4.8mg/kg/day

Initial: 30mg/day; 15mg/day in patients w/ long-standing myxedema
Titrate: Increase by 15mg every 2-3 weeks
Readjust dose w/in the first 4 weeks
Maint: 60-120mg/day

Myxedema Coma: Resume oral therapy when clinical situation has been stabilized after IV administration and patient is able to take oral medications

Pituitary TSH Suppressant

Used to treat/prevent various types of euthyroid goiters (eg, thyroid nodules, subacute or chronic lymphocytic thyroiditis [Hashimoto's], multinodular goiter) and to manage thyroid cancer

Thyroid Suppression Therapy:
1.56mcg/kg/day T4 for 7-10 days

Thyroid Cancer:
Give larger doses than those used for replacement therapy

1-5 Years: 3-3.6mg/kg/day
6-12 Years: 2.4-3mg/kg/day
>12 Years: 1.2-1.8mg/kg/day

ADMINISTRATION
Oral route

HOW SUPPLIED
Tab: 15mg, 30mg, 60mg, 90mg, 120mg, 180mg*, 240mg, 300mg* *scored

CONTRAINDICATIONS
Uncorrected adrenal cortical insufficiency, untreated thyrotoxicosis, apparent hypersensitivity to any of the active or extraneous constituents of this medication.

WARNINGS/PRECAUTIONS
Use is unjustified for the treatment of male or female infertility unless accompanied by hypothyroidism. Caution with cardiovascular (CV) disorders (eg, angina pectoris) and elderly with risk of occult cardiac disease; initiate at low doses (eg, 15-30mg/day) and reduce dose if euthyroid state can only be reached at the expense of aggravation of CV disease. May aggravate diabetes mellitus (DM), diabetes insipidus (DI), and adrenal cortical insufficiency. Treatment of myxedema coma requires simultaneous administration of glucocorticoids. Excessive doses in infants may cause craniosynostosis. Caution with strong suspicion of thyroid gland autonomy. Androgens, corticosteroids, estrogens, iodine-containing preparations, and salicylates may interfere with lab tests.

DRUG INTERACTIONS
See Boxed Warning. Closely monitor PT in patients on oral anticoagulants; dose reduction of anticoagulant may be required. May increase insulin or oral hypoglycemic requirements. Impaired absorption with cholestyramine and colestipol; space dosing by 4-5 hrs. Estrogens may increase thyroxine-binding globulin and may decrease free T4; increase in thyroid dose may be needed.

PATIENT CONSIDERATIONS

Assessment: Assess for adrenal cortical insufficiency, thyrotoxicosis, previous hypersensitivity to the drug, CV disorders (eg, coronary artery disease, angina pectoris), DM, DI, myxedema coma, nursing status, and possible drug interactions.

Monitoring: Monitor response to treatment, urinary glucose levels in patients with DM, PT in patients receiving anticoagulants, and aggravation of diabetes or CV disease. Monitor thyroid function periodically.

Counseling: Inform that replacement therapy is to be taken essentially for life, except in transient hypothyroidism. Instruct to immediately report any signs/symptoms of thyroid hormone toxicity. Inform about the importance of frequent/close monitoring of PT and urinary glucose and the need for dose adjustment of antidiabetic and/or oral anticoagulant medication. Inform that partial hair loss may be seen in children in 1st few months of therapy. Inform that drug is not for treatment of obesity or weight loss.

STORAGE: 15-30°C (59-86°F). Protect from light and moisture.

ARNUITY ELLIPTA – fluticasone furoate

RX

Class: Corticosteroid

ADULT DOSAGE

Asthma

Prophylactic Maint Treatment:
Initial:
Not on an Inhaled Corticosteroid: 100mcg qd
All Other Patients: Dose based on previous asthma drug therapy and disease severity
Titrate: May replace w/ 200mcg in patients who do not respond to 100mcg after 2 weeks of therapy
Max: 200mcg/day

PEDIATRIC DOSAGE

Asthma

Prophylactic Maint Treatment:
≥12 Years:
Initial:
Not on an Inhaled Corticosteroid: 100mcg qd
All Other Patients: Dose based on previous asthma drug therapy and disease severity
Titrate: May replace w/ 200mcg in patients who do not respond to 100mcg after 2 weeks of therapy
Max: 200mcg/day

DOSING CONSIDERATIONS

Elderly

Start at lower end of dosing range

ADMINISTRATION

Oral inh route

Administer as 1 inh qd, at the same time every day; do not use >1X q24h
Rinse mouth w/ water w/o swallowing after each dose

HOW SUPPLIED

Powder, Inh: 100mcg/blister, 200mcg/blister [14, 30 inh]

CONTRAINDICATIONS

Primary treatment of status asthmaticus or other acute episodes of asthma where intensive measures are required, known severe hypersensitivity to milk proteins or have demonstrated hypersensitivity to fluticasone furoate or any of the excipients.

WARNINGS/PRECAUTIONS

Not indicated for acute bronchospasm relief. *Candida albicans* infections of mouth and pharynx reported; treat and, if needed, interrupt therapy. Increased susceptibility to infections. May lead to serious/fatal course of chickenpox or measles; avoid exposure and if exposed, consider prophylaxis/treatment. Use w/ caution, if at all, in patients w/ active/quiescent tuberculosis (TB); untreated systemic fungal, bacterial, viral, or parasitic infections; or ocular herpes simplex. Deaths due to adrenal insufficiency reported during and after transfer from systemic to inhaled corticosteroids; wean slowly from systemic corticosteroid use after transferring to therapy. Resume oral corticosteroids during periods of stress or a severe asthma attack in patients previously withdrawn from systemic corticosteroids. Transfer from systemic corticosteroids to therapy may unmask allergic conditions previously suppressed by systemic therapy (eg, rhinitis, conjunctivitis, eczema). Monitor for systemic corticosteroid effects; reduce dose slowly if hypercorticism and adrenal suppression occur. Bronchospasm may occur w/ an immediate increase in wheezing after dosing; treat immediately w/ an inhaled, short acting bronchodilator; d/c Arnuity Ellipta immediately, and institute alternative therapy. Hypersensitivity reactions may occur; d/c if such reactions occur. Decreases in bone mineral density (BMD) reported w/ long-term use; caution w/ major risk factors for decreased bone mineral content, including chronic use of drugs that can reduce bone mass (eg, anticonvulsants, oral corticosteroids). May reduce growth velocity in children and adolescents. Glaucoma, increased IOP, and cataracts reported w/ long-term use. Caution w/ moderate or severe hepatic impairment.

ADVERSE REACTIONS

Nasopharyngitis, bronchitis, URTI, headache, pharyngitis, sinusitis, toothache, viral gastroenteritis, oral candidiasis, oropharyngeal candidiasis/pain, influenza, back pain, dysphonia, rhinitis, throat irritation.

DRUG INTERACTIONS

Ketoconazole increases exposure. Caution w/ long-term ketoconazole and other known strong CYP3A4 inhibitors (eg, ritonavir, clarithromycin, itraconazole); increased systemic corticosteroid adverse effects may occur.

PATIENT CONSIDERATIONS

Assessment: Assess for status asthmaticus; acute episodes of asthma; hypersensitivity to drug or to milk proteins; active/quiescent TB; untreated systemic infections; ocular herpes simplex; risk factors for decreased bone mineral content; history of increased IOP, glaucoma, and/or cataracts; hepatic impairment; pregnancy/nursing status; and possible drug interactions.

Monitoring: Monitor for localized oropharyngeal infections w/ *C. albicans*, infections, systemic corticosteroid effects (eg, hypercorticism, adrenal suppression), paradoxical bronchospasm, hypersensitivity reactions, decreases in BMD, glaucoma, cataracts, increased IOP, and other adverse reactions. Monitor growth of children and adolescents routinely (eg, via stadiometry). Closely monitor patients w/ moderate to severe hepatic disease.

Counseling: Inform that drug is not meant to relieve acute asthma symptoms; advise to treat acute symptoms w/ an inhaled short-acting β_2-agonist (SABA). Instruct to seek medical attention immediately if experiencing worsening of symptoms, a significant decrease in lung function, or a need for more inhalations than usual of inhaled SABAs. Advise to use at regular intervals, not to increase the dose or frequency of therapy, and not to d/c or reduce therapy w/o physician guidance. Instruct to contact physician if oropharyngeal candidiasis develops, or if symptoms do not improve after 2 weeks. Advise to rinse mouth w/ water w/o swallowing after inhalation. Advise to avoid exposure to chickenpox or measles, and, if exposed, to consult physician w/o delay. Inform about risk of immunosuppression, hypercorticism, adrenal suppression, reduction in BMD, reduced growth velocity in pediatric patients, ocular effects, and hypersensitivity reactions, including anaphylaxis; instruct to d/c if hypersensitivity reactions occur. Inform that the inhaler is not reusable and advise not to take the inhaler apart.

STORAGE: 20-25°C (68-77°F); excursions permitted from 15-30°C (59-86°F). Store in a dry place away from direct heat or sunlight. Store inside the unopened moisture-protective foil tray and only remove from the tray immediately before initial use. Discard 6 weeks after opening the foil tray or when the counter reads "0" (after all blisters have been used), whichever comes 1st.

AROMASIN – exemestane

RX

Class: Aromatase inactivator

ADULT DOSAGE

Estrogen-Receptor Positive Early Breast Cancer

Adjuvant treatment of postmenopausal women who have received 2-3 years of tamoxifen and are switched to exemestane for completion of a total of 5 consecutive years of adjuvant hormonal therapy

Usual: 25mg qd

Advanced Breast Cancer

In postmenopausal women whose disease has progressed following tamoxifen therapy

Usual: 25mg qd

PEDIATRIC DOSAGE

Pediatric use may not have been established

DOSING CONSIDERATIONS

Concomitant Medications

Strong CYP3A4 Inducers: 50mg qd

ADMINISTRATION

Oral route

Take after a meal

HOW SUPPLIED

Tab: 25mg

CONTRAINDICATIONS

Women who are or may become pregnant, premenopausal women, known hypersensitivity to the drug or to any of the excipients.

WARNINGS/PRECAUTIONS

Lymphocytopenia (common toxicity criteria [CTC] Grade 3 or 4) reported with advanced breast cancer; most had a preexisting lower grade lymphopenia. Elevations of serum levels of AST, ALT, alkaline phosphatase, and gamma-glutamyl transferase >5X ULN (eg, ≥CTC Grade 3) have been rarely reported with advanced breast cancer, but appear mostly attributable to the underlying presence of liver and/or bone metastases. Elevations in bilirubin, alkaline phosphatase, and creatinine reported with early breast cancer. Reductions in bone mineral density (BMD) over time reported. During adjuvant treatment, assess BMD in women with osteoporosis or at risk of osteoporosis at the commencement of treatment. Monitor patients for BMD loss and treat as appropriate. Perform routine assessment of 25-hydroxy vitamin D levels prior to treatment; give vitamin D supplementation in women with vitamin D deficiency.

ADVERSE REACTIONS

Hot flushes, fatigue, arthralgia, headache, insomnia, increased sweating, HTN, dizziness, limb/back pain, nausea, depression, osteoarthritis, visual disturbances, alopecia.

DRUG INTERACTIONS

See Dosage. Avoid coadministration with estrogen-containing agents. CYP3A4 inducers (eg, rifampicin, phenytoin, carbamazepine, phenobarbital, St. John's wort) may significantly decrease exposure; dose modification is recommended with a strong CYP3A4 inducer.

PATIENT CONSIDERATIONS

Assessment: Assess for hypersensitivity, preexisting lower grade lymphopenia, liver and/or bone metastases, osteoporosis/at risk of osteoporosis, pregnancy/nursing status, and for possible drug interactions. Perform routine assessment of 25-hydroxy vitamin D levels prior to treatment. Assess BMD in women with osteoporosis/at risk of osteoporosis.

Monitoring: Monitor for hematological abnormalities, BMD loss, osteoporosis, and other adverse reactions. Monitor LFTs, creatinine, alkaline phosphatase, and bilirubin levels.

Counseling: Advise that drug is not for use in premenopausal women. Inform not to take concomitant estrogen-containing agents. Counsel that drug lowers estrogen level in the body, which may lead to reduction in BMD over time, and that the lower the BMD, the greater the risk of osteoporosis and fracture.

STORAGE: 25°C (77°F); excursions permitted to 15-30°C (59-86°F).

ARTHROTEC — diclofenac sodium/misoprostol

RX

Class: NSAID/prostaglandin E_1 analogue

Misoprostol can cause abortion, premature birth, or birth defects. Uterine rupture reported when used to induce labor or abortion beyond the 8th week of pregnancy. Not for use by pregnant women. Has an abortifacient property and must not be given to others. Use only in women of childbearing potential if at high risk for developing gastric or duodenal ulcers or complications with NSAID therapy, has had a (-) serum pregnancy test within 2 weeks of starting therapy, is capable of complying with effective contraceptive measures, has received both oral and written warnings of the hazards of misoprostol use, the risk of contraception failure, and the danger to other women of childbearing potential should the drug be taken by mistake, and will begin therapy only on the 2nd or 3rd day of next normal menstrual period. NSAIDs may increase risk of serious cardiovascular (CV) thrombotic events, myocardial infarction (MI), and stroke; increased risk with duration of use and with cardiovascular disease (CVD) or risk factors for CVD. Increased risk of serious GI adverse events, which may be fatal and may occur at any time during use without warning symptoms; elderly patients are at greater risk. Contraindicated for the treatment of perioperative pain in the setting of coronary artery bypass graft (CABG) surgery.

ADULT DOSAGE

Osteoarthritis

Treatment of signs/symptoms of osteoarthritis in patients at high risk of developing NSAID-induced gastric and duodenal ulcers and their complications

50mg/200mcg:
Usual: 1 tab tid

Patients Who Develop Intolerance:
50mg/200mcg:
Usual: 1 tab bid
75mg/200mcg:
Usual: 1 tab bid

Max:
Diclofenac: >150mg/day not recommended
Misoprostol: 200mcg/dose or 800mcg/day

Rheumatoid Arthritis

Treatment of the signs/symptoms of rheumatoid arthritis in patients at high risk of developing NSAID-induced gastric and duodenal ulcers and their complications

50mg/200mcg:
Usual: 1 tab tid or qid

Patients Who Develop Intolerance:
50mg/200mcg:
Usual: 1 tab bid
75mg/200mcg:
Usual: 1 tab bid

Max:
Diclofenac: >225mg/day not recommended
Misoprostol: 200mcg/dose or 800mcg/day

PEDIATRIC DOSAGE

Pediatric use may not have been established

DOSING CONSIDERATIONS

Elderly

May need to reduce dose

ADMINISTRATION

Oral route

HOW SUPPLIED

Tab: (Diclofenac/Misoprostol) 50mg/200mcg, 75mg/200mcg

CONTRAINDICATIONS

Pregnancy, hypersensitivity to diclofenac or to misoprostol or other prostaglandins, history of asthma, urticaria, or allergic-type reactions after taking aspirin (ASA) or other NSAIDs, active GI bleeding, perioperative pain in the setting of CABG surgery.

WARNINGS/PRECAUTIONS

Not recommended for patients who would not receive the appropriate dose of both ingredients. Use lowest effective dose for the shortest duration possible. May lead to onset of new HTN or worsening of preexisting HTN. Fluid retention and edema reported. Extreme caution with history of ulcer disease or GI bleeding, or risk factors for GI bleeding (eg, longer duration of NSAID therapy, smoking, older age, poor general health status); d/c if a serious GI event occurs. Renal papillary necrosis and other renal injury reported after long-term use. Renal toxicity reported in patients in whom renal prostaglandins have a compensatory role in the maintenance of renal perfusion; increased risk with renal/hepatic impairment, HF, and in elderly. Not recommended with advanced renal disease; monitor renal function closely if therapy must be initiated. May cause hepatotoxicity, elevation of LFTs, or severe hepatic reactions; d/c therapy immediately if abnormal LFTs persist/worsen, liver disease develops, or systemic manifestations occur. Anaphylactic reactions may occur; avoid in patients with ASA triad. May cause serious skin adverse events; d/c at 1st appearance of skin rash or any other signs of hypersensitivity. Avoid in late pregnancy; may cause premature closure of the ductus arteriosus. Not a substitute for corticosteroids or for the treatment of corticosteroid insufficiency. May mask signs of inflammation and fever. Anemia may occur. May inhibit platelet aggregation and prolong bleeding time. Aseptic meningitis with fever and coma may occur. Avoid with hepatic porphyria. Caution with preexisting asthma, in elderly, debilitated, or volume-depleted patients.

ADVERSE REACTIONS

Abdominal pain, diarrhea, dyspepsia, nausea, flatulence.

DRUG INTERACTIONS

Diclofenac: Avoid with other NSAIDs including COX-2 inhibitors. Not recommended with ASA; potential for increased adverse effects. May diminish the antihypertensive effect of ACE inhibitors. Elevated digoxin levels reported with concomitant use; monitor for possible digoxin toxicity. May increase risk of GI bleeding with oral corticosteroids, anticoagulants (eg, warfarin), smoking, and alcohol. Caution with concomitant drugs known to be potentially hepatotoxic (eg, antibiotics, antiepileptics). May alter a diabetic patient's response to insulin or oral hypoglycemics. May enhance methotrexate toxicity; use caution when coadministered. Possible increased risk of nephrotoxicity with tacrolimus. May increase cyclosporine nephrotoxicity; observe closely, particularly if renal function is impaired. May elevate lithium levels; monitor for lithium toxicity. May reduce the natriuretic effect of loop (eg, furosemide) and thiazide diuretics. Increased risk of renal toxicity with diuretics and ACE inhibitors. May increase serum K^+ levels with K^+-sparing diuretics. Caution with CYP2C9 inhibitors (eg, voriconazole); may enhance diclofenac toxicity. When concomitant use of CYP2C9 inhibitors is necessary, total daily diclofenac dose should not exceed the lowest recommended dose of 50mg-200mcg bid. Caution with CYP2C9 inducers (eg, rifampin); may lead to compromised efficacy due to a decrease in systemic exposure to diclofenac. Phenobarbital toxicity reported with chronic phenobarbital treatment following initiation of diclofenac therapy. May minimally interfere with protein binding of prednisolone. Antacids may delay absorption. Misoprostol: Antacids may reduce bioavailability. Mg^{2+}-containing antacids exacerbate misoprostol-associated diarrhea; coadministration is not recommended.

PATIENT CONSIDERATIONS

Assessment: Assess for history of asthma, urticaria, or allergic-type reactions with ASA or other NSAIDs, ASA triad, previous hypersensitivity to misoprostol, CVD, HTN, history of ulcer disease or GI bleeding, active GI bleeding, coagulation disorders, renal/hepatic impairment, any other conditions where treatment is contraindicated or cautioned, fluid status, nursing status, and possible drug interactions. In women of childbearing potential, assess pregnancy status.

Monitoring: Monitor for CV/GI events, anaphylactic/skin/hypersensitivity reactions, hematological effects, aseptic meningitis, porphyria, and other adverse reactions. Monitor BP, LFTs, renal function, CBC, and chemistry profile; monitor LFTs within 4-8 weeks of initiation. Monitor use of effective contraception in women of childbearing potential.

Counseling: Inform women of childbearing potential that they must not take medication if pregnant, and must use an effective contraception during therapy. Instruct not to give medication to anyone else. Inform that misoprostol may cause abortion (sometimes incomplete), premature labor, or birth defects if given to pregnant women. Instruct to contact physician if signs/symptoms of CV events, GI effects, or unexplained weight gain or edema occur. Instruct to d/c immediately and contact physician if signs/symptoms of skin reactions or hepatotoxicity occur. Instruct to seek immediate medical attention if an anaphylactic reaction occurs.

STORAGE: ≤25°C (77°F), in a dry area.

Asacol HD – mesalamine

RX

Class: 5-aminosalicylic acid derivative

ADULT DOSAGE

Ulcerative Colitis

Moderately Active:

Two 800mg tabs tid for 6 weeks

PEDIATRIC DOSAGE

Pediatric use may not have been established

ADMINISTRATION

Oral route

Swallow tab whole; do not cut, break, or chew

Take with or without food

HOW SUPPLIED

Tab, Delayed-Release: 800mg

CONTRAINDICATIONS

Known hypersensitivity to salicylates or aminosalicylates or to any of the ingredients of this medication.

WARNINGS/PRECAUTIONS

Renal impairment, including minimal change nephropathy, acute and chronic interstitial nephritis, and, rarely, renal failure reported; evaluate renal function prior to therapy and periodically thereafter. Has been associated with an acute intolerance syndrome that may be difficult to distinguish from an exacerbation of UC. Exacerbation of symptoms of colitis reported; symptoms usually abate when therapy is discontinued. Patients with sulfasalazine hypersensitivity may have similar reaction to therapy. Mesalamine-induced cardiac hypersensitivity reactions (myocarditis and pericarditis) reported; caution with conditions that predispose to the development of myocarditis or pericarditis. Hepatic failure reported in patients with preexisting liver disease; caution with liver disease. Organic or functional obstruction in the upper GI tract may cause prolonged gastric retention of the drug, which could delay the release of mesalamine in the colon. Caution in elderly.

ADVERSE REACTIONS

Headache.

DRUG INTERACTIONS

Known nephrotoxic agents, including NSAIDs, may increase the risk of renal reactions. Azathioprine or 6-mercaptopurine may increase the risk for blood disorders.

PATIENT CONSIDERATIONS

Assessment: Assess for hypersensitivity to sulfasalazine, salicylates, or aminosalicylates; conditions that predispose to the development of myocarditis or pericarditis; organic or functional obstruction in the upper GI tract; hepatic impairment; pregnancy/nursing status; and possible drug interactions. Evaluate renal function prior to initiation of therapy.

Monitoring: Monitor for acute intolerance syndrome, exacerbation of symptoms of colitis, myocarditis, pericarditis, hepatic failure, hypersensitivity reactions, and other adverse reactions. Perform periodic monitoring of renal function. Monitor blood cell counts in elderly patients.

Counseling: Instruct to swallow tabs whole and not to break, cut, or chew tabs. Advise to d/c previous oral mesalamine therapy and follow dosing instructions if switching therapy. Instruct to contact physician if intact, partially intact, and/or tab shells are seen in stool repeatedly. Advise pregnant and breastfeeding women, or women of childbearing potential that the medication contains dibutyl phthalate, which is excreted in breast milk and could possibly cause fetal malformations. Instruct to leave any desiccant pouches present in the bottle.

STORAGE: 20-25°C (68-77°F); excursions permitted 15-30°C (59-86°F). Protect from moisture.

ASMANEX – mometasone furoate

RX

Class: Corticosteroid

ADULT DOSAGE

Asthma

Maint Treatment of Asthma as Prophylactic Therapy:

Previous Therapy:

Bronchodilators Alone or Inhaled Corticosteroids:
Initial: 220mcg qpm
Titrate: Higher doses may provide additional control if inadequate response after 2 weeks of therapy; adjust to lowest effective dose once asthma stability is achieved
Max: 440mcg qpm or 220mcg bid

Oral Corticosteroids:
Initial: 440mcg bid
Titrate: Higher doses may provide additional control if inadequate response after 2 weeks of therapy; adjust to lowest effective dose once asthma stability is achieved
Max: 880mcg/day

PEDIATRIC DOSAGE

Asthma

Maint Treatment of Asthma as Prophylactic Therapy:

4-11 Years:
Initial/Max: 110mcg qpm

≥12 Years:
Previous Therapy:

Bronchodilators Alone or Inhaled Corticosteroids:
Initial: 220mcg qpm
Titrate: Higher doses may provide additional control if inadequate response after 2 weeks of therapy; adjust to lowest effective dose once asthma stability is achieved
Max: 440mcg qpm or 220mcg bid

Oral Corticosteroids:
Initial: 440mcg bid
Titrate: Higher doses may provide additional control if inadequate response after 2 weeks of therapy; adjust to lowest effective dose once asthma stability is achieved
Max: 880mcg/day

ADMINISTRATION

Orally inhaled powder

When administered qd, Asmanex should be taken only in the pm
Inhale rapidly and deeply
Rinse mouth after inh

HOW SUPPLIED

Powder, Inhalation: 110mcg/actuation, 220mcg/actuation

CONTRAINDICATIONS

Primary treatment of status asthmaticus or other acute episodes of asthma where intensive measures are required, known hypersensitivity to milk proteins or any ingredients of this medication.

WARNINGS/PRECAUTIONS

Not for the relief of acute bronchospasm. Localized *Candida albicans* infections of the mouth and pharynx reported; treat accordingly or interrupt therapy if needed. D/C if hypersensitivity reactions occur. Contains small amount of lactose that contains milk proteins; anaphylactic reactions with milk protein allergy reported. May increase susceptibility to infections; caution with active or quiescent tuberculosis (TB) infection, untreated systemic fungal, bacterial, viral, or parasitic infections, or ocular herpes simplex. Avoid exposure to chickenpox and measles. Deaths due to adrenal insufficiency have occurred with transfer from systemic to inhaled corticosteroids; wean slowly from systemic corticosteroid therapy. Resume oral corticosteroids immediately during periods of stress or severe asthma attack. Transferring from systemic corticosteroid may unmask allergic conditions (eg, rhinitis, conjunctivitis, eczema, arthritis, eosinophilic conditions). Monitor for systemic corticosteroid effects, such as hypercorticism and adrenal suppression; reduce dose slowly when the effects occur. Prolonged use may result in decrease of bone mineral density (BMD); caution in patients at risk (eg, prolonged immobilization, family history of osteoporosis, chronic use of drugs that reduce bone mass [eg, anticonvulsants, corticosteroids]). May cause reduction in growth velocity in pediatric patients; monitor growth routinely. Glaucoma, increased IOP, and cataracts reported. Bronchospasm may occur with an increase in wheezing after dosing; d/c treatment and institute alternative therapy.

ADVERSE REACTIONS

Headache, allergic rhinitis, pharyngitis, URTI, sinusitis, oral candidiasis, dysmenorrhea, musculoskeletal pain, back pain, dyspepsia, myalgia, abdominal pain, nausea.

DRUG INTERACTIONS

Ketoconazole may increase plasma levels.

PATIENT CONSIDERATIONS

Assessment: Assess for status asthmaticus, acute asthma episodes, known hypersensitivity to milk proteins or to any drug component, risk factors for decreased BMD, history of increased IOP/

glaucoma/cataracts, active or quiescent pulmonary TB, ocular herpes simplex, untreated systemic infections, chickenpox, measles, pregnancy/nursing status, and possible drug interactions.

Monitoring: Monitor for localized infections of mouth and pharynx with *C. albicans*, decreased BMD, asthma instability, growth in pediatrics routinely, development of glaucoma, increased IOP, cataracts, change in vision, hypercorticism, signs and symptoms of adrenal insufficiency, paradoxical bronchospasm, hypersensitivity reactions, and immunosuppression. Monitor for lung function, β-agonist use, and asthma symptoms during withdrawal of oral corticosteroids

Counseling: Advise that localized infection with *C. albicans* may occur in mouth and pharynx; instruct to rinse mouth after inhalation. Inform that therapy should not be used to treat status asthmaticus or to relieve acute asthma symptoms. Counsel to d/c if hypersensitivity reactions occur. Advise to avoid exposure to chickenpox or measles and to seek medical attention if exposed. Inform of potential worsening of existing TB, other infections, or ocular herpes simplex. Inform that drug may cause systemic corticosteroid effects of hypercorticism and adrenal suppression, may reduce BMD, and may cause reduction in growth rate (pediatrics). Advise to take ud, to use medication at regular intervals, and to contact physician if symptoms do not improve or if condition worsens. Instruct on proper administration procedures and on when to discard inhaler.

STORAGE: 25°C (77°F); excursions permitted to 15-30°C (59-86°F). Store in dry place. Discard inhaler 45 days after opening foil pouch or when dose counter reads "00," whichever comes 1st.

ASTELIN — azelastine hydrochloride

RX

Class: H_1 antagonist

ADULT DOSAGE

Vasomotor Rhinitis

Usual: 2 sprays/nostril bid

Seasonal Allergic Rhinitis

Usual: 1-2 sprays/nostril bid

PEDIATRIC DOSAGE

Vasomotor Rhinitis

≥12 Years:
Usual: 2 sprays/nostril bid

Seasonal Allergic Rhinitis

5-11 Years:
Usual: 1 spray/nostril bid

≥12 Years:
Usual: 1-2 sprays/nostril bid

DOSING CONSIDERATIONS

Elderly
Start at lower end of dosing range

ADMINISTRATION

Intranasal route

Priming
Prime before initial use by releasing 4 sprays or until a fine mist appears
When not used for ≥3 days, reprime w/ 2 sprays or until a fine mist appears

HOW SUPPLIED

Spray: 137mcg/spray [30mL]

WARNINGS/PRECAUTIONS

Occurrence of somnolence reported. May impair physical/mental abilities. Caution in elderly.

ADVERSE REACTIONS

Bitter taste, headache, somnolence, dysesthesia, rhinitis, cough, conjunctivitis, asthma, epistaxis, sinusitis, nasal burning, pharyngitis, paroxysmal sneezing.

DRUG INTERACTIONS

Avoid alcohol or other CNS depressants; additional reductions in alertness and CNS performance impairment may occur.

PATIENT CONSIDERATIONS

Assessment: Assess for pregnancy/nursing status and possible drug interactions.

Monitoring: Monitor for somnolence and other adverse reactions.

Counseling: Instruct to use only as prescribed. Caution patients against engaging in hazardous occupations requiring complete mental alertness and motor coordination (eg, driving a car or operating machinery). Instruct to avoid concurrent use with alcohol or other CNS depressants because additional reductions in alertness or CNS performance impairment may occur. Inform that therapy may lead to adverse reactions (eg, bitter taste, headache, somnolence). Instruct to consult physician if pregnant/nursing or planning to become pregnant. Instruct to keep out of reach of children and to seek medical help or call a poison control center immediately if a child accidentally ingests the medication.

STORAGE: 20-25°C (68-77°F). Store upright. Protect from freezing.

ATACAND – candesartan cilexetil

RX

Class: Angiotensin II receptor blocker (ARB)

D/C when pregnancy is detected. Drugs that act directly on the renin-angiotensin system (RAS) can cause injury/death to the developing fetus.

ADULT DOSAGE

Hypertension

Initial: 16mg qd as monotherapy in patients who are not volume depleted
Dose Range: 8-32mg/day given qd or bid

May add diuretic if BP not controlled and may be administered w/ other antihypertensive agents

Heart Failure

Heart Failure (HF) (NYHA Class II-IV) w/ Left Ventricular Systolic Dysfunction (Ejection Fraction ≤40%):

Initial: 4mg qd
Titrate: Double the dose at 2-week intervals, as tolerated, to the target dose of 32mg qd

PEDIATRIC DOSAGE

Hypertension

1 to <6 Years:
Initial: 0.20mg/kg (Sus)
Dose Range: 0.05-0.4mg/kg/day

6 to <17 Years:

<50kg:
Initial: 4-8mg
Dose Range: 2-16mg/day

>50kg:
Initial: 8-16mg
Dose Range: 4-32mg/day

May be administered qd or divided into 2 equal doses

DOSING CONSIDERATIONS

Renal Impairment
Pediatric Patients:
GFR <30mL/min/1.73m^2: Do not use; has not been studied in this population

Hepatic Impairment
Adults:
Moderate:
Initial: 8mg
Dosing recommendations cannot be provided for severe hepatic insufficiency

Other Important Considerations
Intravascular Volume Depletion in Pediatric Patients:
Consider initiating at a lower dose

ADMINISTRATION

Oral route

Take w/ or w/o food.
For children who cannot swallow tabs, oral sus may be substituted.

Oral Sus
Shake well before each use.
Store at room temperature (<30°C [86°F]); use w/in 30 days after opening.

Preparation of Oral Sus:
The number of tabs and volume of vehicle specified below will yield 160mL of a 1mg/mL sus.
1. Prepare the vehicle by adding equal volumes of Ora-Plus (80mL) and Ora-Sweet SF (80mL) or, alternatively, use Ora-Blend SF (160mL).
2. Add a small amount of vehicle to five 32mg tabs and grind into a smooth paste using a mortar and pestle.
3. Add the paste to a preparation vessel of suitable size.
4. Rinse the mortar and pestle clean using the vehicle and add this to the vessel. Repeat, if necessary.
5. Prepare the final volume by adding the remaining vehicle.
6. Mix thoroughly and dispense into suitably sized amber PET bottles.
7. Label w/ an expiration date of 100 days.

HOW SUPPLIED

Tab: 4mg*, 8mg*, 16mg*, 32mg* *scored

CONTRAINDICATIONS

Hypersensitivity to candesartan, coadministration w/ aliskiren in patients w/ diabetes.

WARNINGS/PRECAUTIONS

Symptomatic hypotension may occur; most likely in patients who have been volume- and/or salt-depleted (eg, prolonged diuretic therapy, dietary salt restriction, dialysis, diarrhea, vomiting); correct volume and/or salt depletion prior to therapy and temporary dose reduction of candesartan, diuretic, or both may be required. Hypotension may occur during major surgery and anesthesia. Renal function changes including acute renal failure may occur. Oliguria, progressive azotemia, or acute renal failure may occur in patients whose renal function is dependent on the RAS (eg, renal artery stenosis, chronic kidney disease, severe HF, volume depletion); consider withholding or discontinuing therapy if clinically significant decrease in renal function develops. May cause hyperkalemia.

ADVERSE REACTIONS

HTN: URTI, dizziness, back pain.

DRUG INTERACTIONS

See Contraindications. Dual blockade of the RAS w/ ARBs, ACE inhibitors, or aliskiren, is associated w/ increased risk of hypotension, hyperkalemia, and changes in renal function (eg, acute renal failure); closely monitor BP, renal function, and electrolytes w/ concomitant agents that also affect the RAS. Avoid concomitant aliskiren in patients w/ renal impairment (GFR <60mL/min). NSAIDs, (eg, selective COX-2 inhibitors), may deteriorate renal function in patients who are elderly, volume-depleted, or w/ compromised renal function; monitor renal function periodically. NSAIDs may attenuate antihypertensive effect of candesartan. Increased lithium levels and toxicity reported; monitor serum lithium levels. May result in hyperkalemia w/ K^+-sparing diuretics, K^+ supplements, K^+-containing salt substitutes, or other drugs that raise serum K^+ levels.

PATIENT CONSIDERATIONS

Assessment: Assess for hypersensitivity to drug, volume/salt depletion, diabetes, HF, hepatic/renal impairment, pregnancy/nursing status, and possible drug interactions.

Monitoring: Monitor for signs/symptoms of hypotension, renal function changes, and other adverse reactions. Monitor serum K^+ periodically and BP during dose escalation and periodically thereafter.

Counseling: Inform of risks/benefits of therapy. Inform of pregnancy risks; instruct to notify physician as soon as possible if pregnant.

STORAGE: 25°C (77°F); excursions permitted to 15-30°C (59-86°F).

ATACAND HCT – candesartan cilexetil/hydrochlorothiazide

RX

Class: Angiotensin II receptor blocker (ARB)/thiazide diuretic

D/C when pregnancy is detected. Drugs that act directly on the renin-angiotensin system (RAS) can cause injury/death to developing fetus.

ADULT DOSAGE

Hypertension

16-32mg candesartan/12.5-25mg hydrochlorothiazide (HCTZ) qd

Replacement Therapy:
May be substituted for its titrated components

Dose Titration by Clinical Effect:
BP Not Controlled on 25mg HCTZ QD: Can expect an incremental effect from Atacand HCT 16mg/12.5mg

BP Controlled on 25mg HCTZ but Experiencing Decreases in Serum K^+: Can expect the same or incremental BP effects from Atacand HCT 16mg/12.5mg and serum K^+ may improve

BP Not Controlled on 32mg Atacand: Can expect incremental BP effects from Atacand HCT 32mg/12.5mg and then 32mg/25mg

May be administered w/ other antihypertensive agents

PEDIATRIC DOSAGE

Pediatric use may not have been established

DOSING CONSIDERATIONS

Renal Impairment

CrCl <30mL/min: Dosing recommendations cannot be provided

Hepatic Impairment

Moderate to Severe: Not recommended for initiation

ADMINISTRATION

Oral route

Take w/ or w/o food.

HOW SUPPLIED

Tab: (Candesartan/HCTZ) 16mg/12.5mg*, 32mg/12.5mg*, 32mg/25mg* *scored

CONTRAINDICATIONS

Hypersensitivity to candesartan, HCTZ, or other sulfonamide-derived drugs; coadministration w/ aliskiren in patients w/ diabetes, anuria.

WARNINGS/PRECAUTIONS

See Dosing Considerations. Not for initial therapy. Symptomatic hypotension may occur in patients who have been volume- and/or salt-depleted (eg, prolonged diuretic therapy, dietary salt restriction, dialysis, diarrhea, vomiting); may require temporary dose reduction. Correct volume and/or salt depletion prior to therapy. May cause excessive hypotension leading to oliguria, azotemia, and (rarely) w/ acute renal failure and death in patients w/ heart failure (HF); monitor closely for the first 2 weeks of therapy and whenever dose is increased. Oliguria, progressive azotemia, or acute renal failure may occur in patients whose renal function is dependent on the RAS (eg, severe HF, renal artery stenosis, chronic kidney disease, volume depletion); consider withholding or discontinuing therapy if clinically significant decrease in renal function develops. **HCTZ:** May cause hypokalemia and hyponatremia. May cause idiosyncratic reaction, resulting in acute transient myopia and acute angle-closure glaucoma; d/c as rapidly as possible. May cause hypersensitivity reactions (w/ or w/o history of allergy or bronchial asthma), alter glucose tolerance, raise serum levels of cholesterol/TG/uric acid, cause/exacerbate hyperuricemia and precipitate gout, and exacerbate/activate systemic lupus erythematosus (SLE). May decrease urinary Ca^{2+} excretion and cause elevation of serum Ca^{2+}; avoid w/ hypercalcemia.

ADVERSE REACTIONS

URTI, back pain.

DRUG INTERACTIONS

See Contraindications. NSAIDs, including selective COX-2 inhibitors, may deteriorate renal function and attenuate the antihypertensive effect; monitor renal function periodically. Increased lithium levels and lithium toxicity reported; monitor serum lithium levels. **Candesartan:** Dual blockade of the RAS is associated w/ increased risk of hypotension, hyperkalemia, and changes in renal function (including acute renal failure); closely monitor BP, renal function, and electrolytes w/ concomitant agents that also affect the RAS. Coadministration w/ K^+-sparing diuretics, K^+ supplements, K^+-containing salt substitutes, or other drugs that raise serum K^+ levels may result in hyperkalemia; monitor serum K^+. Avoid w/ aliskiren in patients w/ renal impairment (GFR <60mL/min). **HCTZ:** Alcohol, barbiturates, or narcotics may potentiate orthostatic hypotension. Dose adjustment of antidiabetic drugs (oral agents and insulin) may be required. Hyperglycemic effect of diazoxide may be enhanced. Single doses of either cholestyramine or colestipol resins may impair absorption; administer therapy at least 4 hrs before or 4-6 hrs after administration of resins. May increase responsiveness to nondepolarizing skeletal muscle relaxants (eg, tubocurarine). Thiazide-induced hypokalemia or hypomagnesemia may predispose to digoxin toxicity. May decrease arterial responsiveness to noradrenaline, but not enough to preclude effectiveness of the pressor agent for therapeutic use. Hypokalemia may develop during concomitant use of steroids or ACTH. May reduce the renal excretion of cytotoxic medicinal products (eg, cyclophosphamide, methotrexate) and potentiate their myelosuppressive effects. Concomitant treatment w/ cyclosporine may increase the risk of hyperuricemia and gout-type complications.

PATIENT CONSIDERATIONS

Assessment: Assess for hypersensitivity to the drugs and their components, anuria, sulfonamide-derived drug hypersensitivity, history of penicillin allergy, volume/salt depletion, SLE, diabetes, HF, hepatic/renal impairment, renal artery stenosis, pregnancy/nursing status, and possible drug interactions.

Monitoring: Monitor for signs/symptoms of fluid/electrolyte imbalance, exacerbation or activation of SLE, hypotension, hypersensitivity reactions, idiosyncratic reaction, renal function changes, and other adverse reactions. Monitor BP and serum electrolytes periodically.

Counseling: Inform females of childbearing potential of the consequences of exposure during pregnancy and of the treatment options for women planning to become pregnant; instruct to notify physician as soon as possible if pregnant. Inform that lightheadedness may occur, especially during the 1st days of therapy; instruct to d/c therapy if syncope occurs and seek consult. Caution that inadequate fluid intake, excessive perspiration, diarrhea, or vomiting may lead to an excessive fall in BP, w/ the same consequences of lightheadedness and possible syncope. Instruct not to use K^+ supplements, salt substitutes containing K^+, or other drugs that may increase serum K^+ levels w/o consulting physician.

STORAGE: 25°C (77°F); excursions permitted to 15-30°C (59-86°F).

ATIVAN INJECTION – lorazepam

CIV

Class: Benzodiazepine

ADULT DOSAGE

Status Epilepticus

Usual: 4mg IV (given slowly at 2mg/min); may repeat 1 dose after 10-15 min if seizures recur or fail to cease

PEDIATRIC DOSAGE

Pediatric use may not have been established

Preanesthetic

To produce sedation, anxiety relief, and to decrease ability to recall events related to the day of surgery

Usual:

IM:

0.05mg/kg given at least 2 hrs prior to anticipated operative procedure

IV:

2mg or 0.044mg/kg IV (whichever is smaller) 15-20 min prior to anticipated operative procedure

Max (IM/IV): 4mg

DOSING CONSIDERATIONS

Concomitant Medications

Probenecid or Valproate: Reduce lorazepam dose by 50%

Oral Contraceptives: May be necessary to increase lorazepam dose

Elderly

Start at the low end of the dosing range

ADMINISTRATION

IM/IV route

Can be used w/ atropine sulfate, narcotic analgesics, other parenterally used analgesics, commonly used anesthetics, and muscle relaxants

IM

Inject undiluted deep in muscle mass

IV

Must be diluted w/ an equal volume of compatible sol (Sterile Water for Inj, NaCl Inj, D5 Inj)

Mix thoroughly by gently inverting container repeatedly until a homogenous solution results; do not shake vigorously

When properly diluted, the drug may be injected directly into a vein or into the tubing of an existing IV infusion

Rate of inj should not exceed 2.0mg/min

HOW SUPPLIED

Inj: 2mg/mL, 4mg/mL [1mL, 10mL]

CONTRAINDICATIONS

Known sensitivity to benzodiazepines or its vehicle (polyethylene glycol, propylene glycol, and benzyl alcohol), acute narrow-angle glaucoma, sleep apnea syndrome, severe respiratory insufficiency. Not for intra-arterial inj.

WARNINGS/PRECAUTIONS

May produce heavy sedation. Airway obstruction and respiratory depression may occur; ensure airway patency and monitor respiration. May impair mental/physical abilities. Avoid in patients with hepatic and/or renal failure; caution in patients with hepatic and/or renal impairment. May cause fetal damage during pregnancy. When used for peroral endoscopic procedures, adequate topical/regional anesthesia is recommended to minimize reflex activity. Extreme caution when administering inj to elderly, very ill, or to patients with limited pulmonary reserve; hypoventilation and/or hypoxic cardiac arrest may occur. Paradoxical reaction, propylene glycol toxicity (eg, lactic acidosis, hyperosmolality, hypotension) and polyethylene glycol toxicity (eg, acute tubular necrosis) reported; premature and low birth weight infants as well pediatric patients receiving high-doses may be at higher risk. Pediatric patients may exhibit sensitivity to benzyl alcohol; "gasping syndrome" associated with administration of IV sol containing benzyl alcohol in neonates. Repeated doses over a prolonged period may result in physical and psychological dependence and withdrawal symptoms following abrupt discontinuation.

ADVERSE REACTIONS

Respiratory depression/failure, hypotension, somnolence, headache, hypoventilation, inj-site reactions, paradoxical excitement.

DRUG INTERACTIONS

Additive CNS depression with other CNS depressants (eg, ethyl alcohol, phenothiazines, barbiturates, MAOIs, antidepressants). Increased sedation, hallucinations, and irrational behavior with scopolamine. Reduce dose by 50% when given in combination with valproate or probenecid due to decreased clearance. Increased clearance with oral contraceptives. Severe adverse effects with clozapine, loxapine, and haloperidol reported. Prolonged and profound effect with concomitant sedatives, tranquilizers, narcotic analgesics.

PATIENT CONSIDERATIONS

Assessment: Perform a comprehensive review of benefits/risks in status epilepticus. Assess for hypersensitivity to benzodiazepine or its vehicle, acute-angle glaucoma, preexisting respiratory impairment, hepatic/renal impairment, pregnancy/nursing status, and possible drug interactions.

Monitoring: Monitor for respiratory depression, airway obstruction, heavy sedation, drowsiness, excessive sleepiness, hypoglycemia and hyponatremia in status epilepticus, seizures, myoclonus, somnolence, inj-site reactions, and paradoxical reactions. Monitor for signs of toxicity to the vehicle's components (eg, lactic acidosis, hyperosmolarity, hypotension, acute tubular necrosis). Monitor for hypersensitivity reactions.

Counseling: Inform of risks/benefits. Advise to use caution with hazardous tasks. Instruct to not get out of bed unassisted. Advise to avoid alcoholic beverages for at least 24-48 hrs after receiving drug. Advise about potential for physical/psychological dependence and withdrawal symptoms.

STORAGE: Refrigerate; protect from light.

ATRIPLA – efavirenz/emtricitabine/tenofovir disoproxil fumarate RX

Class: Non-nucleoside reverse transcriptase inhibitor (NNRTI)/nucleoside analogue combination

Lactic acidosis and severe hepatomegaly w/ steatosis, including fatal cases, reported w/ the use of nucleoside analogues. Not approved for the treatment of chronic hepatitis B virus (HBV) infection and safety and efficacy have not been established in patients coinfected w/ HBV and HIV. Severe acute exacerbations of hepatitis B reported in patients coinfected w/ HBV upon discontinuation of emtricitabine or tenofovir disoproxil fumarate (TDF); closely monitor hepatic function for at least several months after stopping therapy. If appropriate, initiation of antihepatitis B therapy may be warranted.

ADULT DOSAGE

HIV-1 Infection

Alone/Combination w/ Other Antiretrovirals:
1 tab qd

PEDIATRIC DOSAGE

HIV-1 Infection

Alone/Combination w/ Other Antiretrovirals:
≥12 Years and ≥40kg:
1 tab qd

DOSING CONSIDERATIONS

Concomitant Medications

Rifampin:
≥50kg: Additional 200mg/day of efavirenz is recommended

Renal Impairment

Moderate or Severe (CrCl <50mL/min): Not recommended for use

Hepatic Impairment

Moderate or Severe: Not recommended for use

ADMINISTRATION

Oral route

Take on an empty stomach.

Bedtime dosing may improve tolerability of nervous system symptoms.

HOW SUPPLIED

Tab: (Efavirenz/Emtricitabine/TDF) 600mg/200mg/300mg

CONTRAINDICATIONS

Hypersensitivity to efavirenz. Coadministration w/ voriconazole.

WARNINGS/PRECAUTIONS

Hepatic failure reported; monitor liver enzymes w/ underlying hepatic diseases. In patients w/ persistent elevations of serum transaminases >5X ULN, weigh benefit of continued therapy against risks of significant liver toxicity. Immune reconstitution syndrome and autoimmune disorders (eg, Graves' disease, polymyositis, Guillain-Barre syndrome) in the setting of immune reconstitution reported. Redistribution/accumulation of body fat has been observed. Caution in elderly. **Efavirenz:** Serious psychiatric adverse events and CNS symptoms reported; if serious psychiatric adverse events occur, evaluate to assess if they are related to therapy and determine risks and benefits of continued therapy. May impair mental/physical abilities. May cause fetal harm if administered during 1st trimester of pregnancy; avoid pregnancy during use. Use adequate contraceptive measures for 12 weeks after discontinuation. Skin rash reported; d/c if severe rash associated w/ blistering, desquamation, mucosal involvement, or fever develops. Consider alternative therapy in patients who have had a life-threatening cutaneous reaction (eg, Stevens-Johnson syndrome). Consider appropriate antihistamine prophylaxis in pediatric patients before initiating therapy. Convulsions reported; caution w/ history of seizures. **TDF:** Obesity and prolonged nucleoside exposure may be risk factors for lactic acidosis and severe hepatomegaly w/ steatosis. Caution w/ known risk factors for liver disease. D/C if lactic acidosis or pronounced hepatotoxicity occurs. Renal impairment, including acute renal failure and Fanconi syndrome, reported. Decreased bone mineral density (BMD), increased biochemical markers of bone metabolism, and osteomalacia reported; consider assessment of BMD in patients w/ a history of pathologic bone fracture or other risk factors for osteoporosis or bone loss. Arthralgias and muscle pain/weakness reported in cases of proximal renal tubulopathy. Consider hypophosphatemia and osteomalacia secondary to proximal renal tubulopathy in patients at risk of renal dysfunction who present w/ persistent or worsening bone or muscle symptoms.

ADVERSE REACTIONS

Diarrhea, nausea, fatigue, headache, dizziness, depression, insomnia, abnormal dreams, rash.

DRUG INTERACTIONS

See Contraindications. Avoid w/ adefovir dipivoxil, drugs which contain the same active components as Atripla, atazanavir, drugs containing same component or lamivudine, other NNRTIs, boceprevir, posaconazole, or nephrotoxic agents (eg, high-dose or multiple NSAIDs). Potential additive CNS effects w/ alcohol or psychoactive drugs. May increase levels of didanosine and ritonavir (RTV). May decrease levels of amprenavir, indinavir, lopinavir, saquinavir, maraviroc, raltegravir, simeprevir, carbamazepine, anticonvulsants, bupropion, sertraline, itraconazole, ketoconazole, clarithromycin, rifabutin, diltiazem or other calcium channel blockers, atorvastatin, pravastatin, simvastatin, norelgestromin, levonorgestrel, etonogestrel, immunosuppressants, and methadone. May decrease levels of artemether, dihydroartemisinin, and/or lumefantrine resulting in a decrease antimalarial efficacy of artemether/lumefantrine; use w/ caution. **Efavirenz:** RTV may increase levels. Avoid w/ simeprevir. Carbamazepine, anticonvulsants, rifabutin, and rifampin may decrease levels. CYP3A substrates, inhibitors, or inducers may alter levels. May alter plasma levels of warfarin or drugs metabolized by CYP3A or CYP2B6. **TDF/Emtricitabine:** Coadministration of drugs that reduce renal function or compete for active tubular secretion (eg, acyclovir, adefovir dipivoxil, cidofovir, ganciclovir, valacyclovir, valganciclovir, aminoglycosides [eg, gentamicin], and high-dose or multiple NSAIDs) may increase levels of emtricitabine, TDF, and/or other renally eliminated drugs. Monitor closely for didanosine-associated adverse reactions w/ TDF. Atazanavir, darunavir w/ RTV, and lopinavir/RTV may increase TDF levels. An increase in absorption may be observed when TDF is coadministered w/ an inhibitor of P-gp or breast cancer resistance protein. Refer to PI for further information on drug interactions.

PATIENT CONSIDERATIONS

Assessment: Assess for obesity, prolonged nucleoside exposure, liver dysfunction or risk factors for liver disease, renal dysfunction, HBV infection, psychiatric history, history of injection drug use/seizures/cutaneous reaction, drug hypersensitivity, pregnancy/nursing status, and possible drug interactions. Assess BMD in patients w/ a history of pathological bone fracture or w/ other risk factors for osteoporosis or bone loss. Assess estimated CrCl, serum P, urine glucose and urine protein in patients at risk for renal dysfunction.

Monitoring: Monitor for signs/symptoms of lactic acidosis, severe hepatomegaly w/ steatosis, psychiatric/nervous system symptoms, new onset/worsening renal impairment, decreased BMD, increased biochemical markers for bone metabolism, osteomalacia, convulsions, immune reconstitution syndrome (eg, opportunistic infections), fat redistribution/accumulation, skin rash, and other adverse reactions. Monitor for acute exacerbations of hepatitis B in patients w/ coinfection upon discontinuation of therapy. Monitor LFTs. Monitor estimated CrCl, serum P, urine glucose, and urine protein periodically in patients at risk for renal dysfunction.

Counseling: Inform that therapy is not a cure for HIV-1 infection and illnesses associated w/ HIV-1 infection may still be experienced. Advise to practice safe sex, use latex or polyurethane condoms, not to share personal items (eg, toothbrush, razor blades), needles, or other inj equipment, and not to breastfeed. Inform that lactic acidosis, severe hepatomegaly w/ steatosis, and renal impairment have occurred. Instruct to avoid potentially hazardous tasks such as driving or operating machinery if CNS symptoms occur. Instruct to contact physician if severe psychiatric adverse experiences or a rash occur. Advise that fat redistribution/accumulation and decreases in BMD may occur. Advise to avoid pregnancy while on therapy and to use adequate contraceptive measures for 12 weeks after discontinuation; instruct that barrier contraception must always be used in combination w/ other methods of contraception. Advise to avoid potentially hazardous tasks if experiencing CNS/psychiatric symptoms or taking alcohol or psychoactive drugs. Advise that severe acute exacerbation of hepatitis B may occur if coinfected. Advise to report use of any prescription, nonprescription medication, vitamins, and herbal supplements.

STORAGE: 25°C (77°F); excursions permitted to 15-30°C (59-86°F).

ATROPINE INJECTION – atropine sulfate

RX

Class: Anticholinergic

ADULT DOSAGE

General Dosing

Temporary blockade of severe or life-threatening muscarinic effects

Antisialagogue or Other Antivagal Effects:
0.5-1mg; repeat in 1-2 hrs

Antidote for Organophosphorus or Muscarinic Mushroom Poisoning:
2-3mg; repeat in 20-30 min

Bradyasystolic Cardiac Arrest:
1mg; repeat in 3-5 min
Max: 3mg

Titrate based on HR, PR interval, BP, and symptoms

PEDIATRIC DOSAGE

General Dosing

Dosing in pediatric populations has not been well studied

Initial: 0.01-0.03mg/kg

DOSING CONSIDERATIONS

Elderly
Start at lower end of dosing range

ADMINISTRATION
IV (preferred)/IM/SQ/Endotracheal route

Endotracheal Administration
Dilute 1-2mg in no more than 10mL of sterile water or normal saline.

HOW SUPPLIED
Inj: 0.05mg/mL [5mL], 0.1mg/mL [5mL, 10mL]

WARNINGS/PRECAUTIONS
Restrict total dose to 2-3mg (maximum 0.03-0.04mg/kg) when recurrent use is essential in patients w/ coronary artery disease. May precipitate acute glaucoma, convert partial organic pyloric stenosis into complete obstruction, lead to complete urinary retention in patients w/ prostatic hypertrophy, or cause inspissation of bronchial secretions and formation of viscid plugs in patients w/ chronic lung disease.

ADVERSE REACTIONS
Dry mouth, blurred vision, photophobia, tachycardia.

DRUG INTERACTIONS
May decrease the absorption rate of mexiletine.

PATIENT CONSIDERATIONS

Assessment: Assess for glaucoma, pyloric stenosis, prostatic hypertrophy, chronic lung disease, pregnancy/nursing status, and possible drug interactions.

Monitoring: Monitor for acute glaucoma, conversion of partial organic pyloric stenosis into complete obstruction, complete urinary retention, inspissation of bronchial secretions, formation of viscid plugs, and other possible adverse effects.

Counseling: Inform about the risks and benefits of the treatment.

STORAGE: 20-25°C (68-77°F); excursions permitted between 15-30°C (59-86°F).

ATROVENT HFA – ipratropium bromide

RX

Class: Anticholinergic

ADULT DOSAGE

Chronic Obstructive Pulmonary Disease

Maint Treatment of Bronchospasm:
Initial: 2 inh qid; may take additional inh as required
Max: 12 inh/24 hrs

PEDIATRIC DOSAGE

Pediatric use may not have been established

ADMINISTRATION

Oral inh route

Priming

Prime inhaler before using for the 1st time or if inhaler has not been used for >3 days by releasing 2 test sprays into the air, away from the face

HOW SUPPLIED

MDI: 17mcg/inh [200 inhalations]

CONTRAINDICATIONS

Hypersensitivity to ipratropium bromide or other components in this medication, hypersensitivity to atropine or any of its derivatives.

WARNINGS/PRECAUTIONS

Not for initial treatment of acute episodes of bronchospasm. Hypersensitivity reactions and/or paradoxical bronchospasm may occur; d/c therapy and consider alternative treatment if these occur. May increase IOP, which may result in precipitation/worsening of narrow-angle glaucoma; caution with narrow-angle glaucoma. Avoid spraying in eyes. May cause urinary retention; caution with prostatic hyperplasia or bladder neck obstruction.

ADVERSE REACTIONS

Bronchitis, COPD exacerbation, sinusitis, UTI, influenza-like symptoms, dyspnea, back pain, dyspepsia, headache, dizziness, nausea, dry mouth.

DRUG INTERACTIONS

Avoid with other anticholinergic-containing drugs; may lead to an increase in anticholinergic adverse effects.

PATIENT CONSIDERATIONS

Assessment: Assess for hypersensitivity to drug or to atropine or any of its derivatives, narrow-angle glaucoma, prostatic hyperplasia, bladder neck obstruction, pregnancy/nursing status, and possible drug interactions.

Monitoring: Monitor for hypersensitivity reactions, paradoxical bronchospasm, increased IOP, urinary retention, and other adverse reactions.

Counseling: Inform that drug is not for initial treatment of acute episodes of bronchospasm where rescue therapy is required for rapid response. Instruct to d/c use if paradoxical bronchospasm occurs. Instruct to avoid spraying the aerosol into the eyes; advise to consult physician immediately if ocular effects develop. Inform that dizziness, accommodation disorder, mydriasis, and blurred vision may occur; caution about engaging in activities requiring balance and visual acuity (eg, driving, operating appliances/machinery). Advise to consult physician if experiencing difficulty with urination. Instruct to use consistently as prescribed throughout the course of therapy. Counsel not to increase the dose or frequency without consulting physician, and to seek immediate medical attention if treatment becomes less effective for symptomatic relief, symptoms become worse, and/or there is a need to use the product more frequently than usual. Advise on the use of medication in relation to other inhaled drugs.

STORAGE: 25°C (77°F); excursions permitted to 15-30°C (59-86°F). Do not puncture, use/store near heat or open flame, or throw into fire/incinerator. Exposure to temperatures >49°C (120°F) may cause bursting. Discard when indicator displays "0."

AUGMENTIN — amoxicillin/clavulanate potassium RX

Class: Aminopenicillin/beta lactamase inhibitor

ADULT DOSAGE

General Dosing

Usual: One 500mg tab q12h or one 250mg tab q8h

Severe Infections: One 875mg tab q12h or one 500mg tab q8h

Lower Respiratory Tract Infections

Usual: One 875mg tab q12h or one 500mg tab q8h

Other Indications

Skin and skin structure infections
UTIs
Acute bacterial otitis media
Sinusitis

PEDIATRIC DOSAGE

General Dosing

<12 Weeks of Age:

Usual: 30mg/kg/day divided q12h (125mg/5mL sus)

≥12 Weeks of Age:

Less Severe Infections:

25mg/kg/day q12h (200mg/5mL or 400mg/5mL sus; 200mg or 400mg chewable tab) or 20mg/kg/day q8h (125mg/5mL or 250mg/5mL sus; 125mg or 250mg chewable tab)

Severe Infections:

45mg/kg/day q12h (200mg/5mL or 400mg/5mL sus; 200mg or 400mg chewable tab) or 40mg/kg/day q8h (125mg/5mL or 250mg/5mL sus; 125mg or 250mg chewable tab)

≥40kg:
Use adult dose

Otitis Media

≥12 Weeks of Age:
45mg/kg/day q12h (200mg/5mL or 400mg/5mL sus; 200mg or 400mg chewable tab) or 40mg/kg/day q8h (125mg/5mL or 250mg/5mL sus; 125mg or 250mg chewable tab) for 10 days

Sinusitis

≥12 Weeks of Age:
45mg/kg/day q12h (200mg/5mL or 400mg/5mL sus; 200mg or 400mg chewable tab) or 40mg/kg/day q8h (125mg/5mL or 250mg/5mL sus; 125mg or 250mg chewable tab)

Lower Respiratory Tract Infections

≥12 Weeks of Age:
45mg/kg/day q12h (200mg/5mL or 400mg/5mL sus; 200mg or 400mg chewable tab) or 40mg/kg/day q8h (125mg/5mL or 250mg/5mL sus; 125mg or 250mg chewable tab)

DOSING CONSIDERATIONS

Renal Impairment

GFR <30mL/min: Do not give the 875mg dose
GFR 10-30mL/min: 500mg or 250mg q12h
GFR <10mL/min: 500mg or 250mg q24h
Hemodialysis: 500mg or 250mg q24h; give additional dose during and at the end of dialysis

ADMINISTRATION

Oral route

Doses are based on amoxicillin component
Take w/ or w/o food
Take at start of a meal to reduce GI intolerance

Sus

Shake well before use
Reconstituted sus must be stored under refrigeration and discarded after 10 days
Refer to PI for mixing directions

Adults:
May use 125mg/5mL or 250mg/5mL sus in place of 500mg tab
May use 200mg/5mL or 400mg/5mL sus in place of 875mg tab

HOW SUPPLIED

(Amoxicillin-Clavulanic Acid) Sus: 125mg-31.25mg/5mL, 250mg-62.5mg/5mL [75mL, 100mL, 150mL], 200mg-28.5mg/5mL, 400mg-57mg/5mL [50mL, 75mL, 100mL]; **Tab:** 250mg-125mg, 500mg-125mg, 875mg-125mg*; **Tab, Chewable:** 125mg-31.25mg, 200mg-28.5mg, 250mg-62.5mg, 400mg-57mg *scored

CONTRAINDICATIONS

History of amoxicillin/clavulanate-associated cholestatic jaundice/hepatic dysfunction.

WARNINGS/PRECAUTIONS

Serious and occasionally fatal hypersensitivity (anaphylactic) reactions reported; d/c if an allergic reaction occurs and institute appropriate therapy. Hepatic dysfunction, including hepatitis and cholestatic jaundice, may occur. *Clostridium difficile*-associated diarrhea (CDAD) reported; d/c if CDAD is suspected or confirmed. Avoid with mononucleosis. May result in bacterial resistance with prolonged use in the absence of a proven/suspected bacterial infection; take appropriate measures if superinfection develops. The 200mg and 400mg chewable tabs and 200mg/5mL and 400mg/5mL sus contain phenylalanine; avoid with phenylketonurics. The 250mg tab and 250mg chewable tab are not interchangeable due to unequal clavulanic acid amounts; do not use 250mg tab in pediatric patients until child weighs at least 40kg. Do not substitute two 250mg tabs for one 500mg tab. May decrease estrogen levels in pregnant women. Lab test interactions may occur. Caution in elderly.

ADVERSE REACTIONS
Diarrhea/loose stools, nausea, skin rashes, urticaria

DRUG INTERACTIONS
Probenecid may increase/prolong levels of amoxicillin; coadministration not recommended. Abnormal prolongation of PT (increased INR) reported with oral anticoagulants; may require oral anticoagulant dose adjustment. Allopurinol may increase incidence of rashes. May reduce efficacy of combined oral estrogen/progesterone contraceptives.

PATIENT CONSIDERATIONS

Assessment: Assess for history of serious hypersensitivity reactions to other β-lactam antibacterial drugs (eg, PCN, cephalosporins) or other allergens, history of amoxicillin/clavulanate-associated cholestatic jaundice/hepatic dysfunction, hepatic/renal impairment, mononucleosis, phenylketonuria, pregnancy/nursing status, and possible drug interactions.

Monitoring: Monitor for anaphylactic reactions, superinfection, skin rash, CDAD, and other adverse reactions. Periodically monitor renal (especially in elderly) and hepatic function. Monitor PT/INR with oral anticoagulants.

Counseling: Instruct to take each dose with a meal or snack to reduce possibility of GI upset. Counsel that drug only treats bacterial, not viral (eg, common cold), infections. Instruct to take ud; inform that skipping doses or not completing the full course of therapy may decrease effectiveness of the drug and increase resistance of bacteria. Advise to consult physician if severe diarrhea or watery/bloody stools occur (even as late as ≥2 months after treatment). Instruct to use a dosing spoon or medicine dropper when dosing a child with sus, and rinse measuring device after each use. Instruct to discard any unused medicine.

STORAGE: ≤25°C (77°F).

AUGMENTIN XR – amoxicillin/clavulanate potassium RX

Class: Aminopenicillin/beta lactamase inhibitor

ADULT DOSAGE

Acute Bacterial Sinusitis

2 tabs q12h for 10 days

Community-Acquired Pneumonia

2 tabs q12h for 7-10 days

PEDIATRIC DOSAGE

Acute Bacterial Sinusitis

≥40kg (Able to Swallow Tab):
2 tabs q12h for 10 days

Community-Acquired Pneumonia

≥40kg (Able to Swallow Tab):
2 tabs q12h for 7-10 days

DOSING CONSIDERATIONS

Hepatic Impairment
Caution and monitor hepatic function at regular intervals

ADMINISTRATION
Oral route

Take at the start of a meal; not recommended w/ a high-fat meal.

HOW SUPPLIED
Tab, Extended-Release: (Amoxicillin/Clavulanic Acid) 1000mg/62.5mg* *scored

CONTRAINDICATIONS
History of serious hypersensitivity reactions (eg, anaphylaxis or Stevens-Johnson syndrome) to amoxicillin, clavulanate, or to other beta-lactam antibacterial drugs (eg, penicillins and cephalosporins). Severe renal impairment (CrCl <30mL/min), hemodialysis, history of amoxicillin/clavulanate-associated cholestatic jaundice/hepatic dysfunction.

WARNINGS/PRECAUTIONS
Serious, occasionally fatal, hypersensitivity reactions reported with PCN therapy; d/c if allergic reaction occurs and institute appropriate therapy. *Clostridium difficile*-associated diarrhea (CDAD) reported; d/c if CDAD is suspected or confirmed. Caution with hepatic dysfunction. Avoid with mononucleosis. May result in bacterial resistance with prolonged use or use in the absence of a proven/suspected bacterial infection or a prophylactic indication; take appropriate measures if superinfection develops. May decrease estrogen levels in pregnant women. Lab test interactions may occur.

ADVERSE REACTIONS
Diarrhea, vaginal mycosis.

DRUG INTERACTIONS
Probenecid may increase/prolong levels; coadministration not recommended. Abnormal prolongation of PT (increased INR) reported with oral anticoagulants; may require anticoagulant

dose adjustment. Allopurinol may increase incidence of rashes. May reduce efficacy of oral contraceptives.

PATIENT CONSIDERATIONS

Assessment: Assess for history of serious hypersensitivity reactions to other β-lactam antibacterial drugs (eg, PCN, cephalosporins) or other allergens, history of amoxicillin/clavulanate-associated cholestatic jaundice/hepatic dysfunction, hepatic/renal impairment, mononucleosis, pregnancy/nursing status, and possible drug interactions.

Monitoring: Monitor for anaphylactic reactions, hepatic toxicity, superinfection, skin rash, diarrhea, CDAD, and other adverse reactions. Monitor PT/INR with oral anticoagulants. Monitor renal function in elderly. Monitor renal, hepatic, and hematopoietic functions with prolonged use.

Counseling: Instruct to take q12h with a meal or snack to reduce possibility of GI upset. Advise to consult physician if severe diarrhea or watery/bloody stools occur (even as late as ≥2 months after treatment). Instruct to take ud; skipping doses or not completing the full course of therapy may decrease effectiveness of the drug and increase resistance of bacteria. Instruct to discard any unused medicine.

STORAGE: ≤25°C (77°F).

Auvi-Q – epinephrine

RX

Class: Sympathomimetic catecholamine

ADULT DOSAGE

Allergic Reactions

Emergency treatment of allergic reactions (Type I) including anaphylaxis to allergens, as well as idiopathic anaphylaxis or exercise-induced anaphylaxis

15-30kg:
0.15mg IM/SQ

≥30kg:
0.3mg IM/SQ

Repeat inj may be necessary in patients with severe persistent anaphylaxis; >2 sequential doses should only be administered under direct medical supervision

PEDIATRIC DOSAGE

Allergic Reactions

Emergency treatment of allergic reactions (Type I) including anaphylaxis to allergens, as well as idiopathic anaphylaxis or exercise-induced anaphylaxis

15-30kg:
0.15mg IM/SQ

≥30kg:
0.3mg IM/SQ

Repeat inj may be necessary in patients with severe persistent anaphylaxis; >2 sequential doses should only be administered under direct medical supervision

ADMINISTRATION

IM/SQ route

Inject into the anterolateral aspect of the thigh, through clothing if necessary

HOW SUPPLIED

Inj: 0.15mg/0.15mL, 0.3mg/0.3mL

WARNINGS/PRECAUTIONS

Intended for immediate administration in patients who are determined to be at increased risk for anaphylaxis, including those with a history of anaphylactic reactions. Intended for immediate self-administration as emergency supportive therapy only and is not a substitute for immediate medical care. More than two sequential doses should only be administered under direct medical supervision. Do not inject IV. Large doses or accidental IV inj use may result in cerebral hemorrhage due to sharp rise in BP; rapidly acting vasodilators can counteract the marked pressor effect of epinephrine. Do not inject into buttock; may not provide effective treatment of anaphylaxis. Do not inject into digits, hands, or feet; may result in loss of blood flow to the affected area if accidentally injected into digits, hands, or feet. Contains sodium bisulfite; may cause allergic-type reactions, including anaphylactic symptoms or life-threatening or less severe asthmatic episodes in certain susceptible persons. Caution in patients with heart disease (eg, cardiac arrhythmias, coronary artery or organic heart disease, or HTN), hyperthyroidism, diabetes, elderly, and pregnant women. May temporarily worsen symptoms of Parkinson's disease.

ADVERSE REACTIONS

Anxiety, apprehensiveness, restlessness, tremor, weakness, dizziness, sweating, palpitations, pallor, N/V, headache, respiratory difficulties.

DRUG INTERACTIONS

May precipitate/aggravate angina pectoris as well as produce ventricular arrhythmias with drugs that may sensitize the heart to arrhythmias; use with caution. Monitor for cardiac arrhythmias with anti-arrhythmics, cardiac glycosides, and diuretics. Effects may be potentiated by TCAs, MAOIs, levothyroxine sodium, and certain antihistamines (notably, chlorpheniramine, tripelennamine, diphenhydramine). Cardiostimulating and bronchodilating effects antagonized by β-adrenergic blockers (eg, propranolol). Vasoconstricting and hypertensive effects antagonized by α-adrenergic blockers (eg, phentolamine). Ergot alkaloids may reverse pressor effects.

PATIENT CONSIDERATIONS

Assessment: Assess for risk of anaphylaxis, heart disease, HTN, diabetes mellitus (DM), hyperthyroidism, Parkinson's disease, pregnancy/nursing status, and for possible drug interactions.

Monitoring: Monitor for allergic-type reactions, angina pectoris, ventricular arrhythmias, cerebral hemorrhage, and for other adverse reactions. Monitor HR and BP.

Counseling: Advise that therapy may produce signs and symptoms that include increased HR, sensation of more forceful heartbeat, palpitations, sweating, N/V, difficulty breathing, pallor, dizziness, weakness or shakiness, headache, apprehension, nervousness, or anxiety; advise that these signs and symptoms usually subside rapidly, especially with rest, quiet, and recumbency. Inform that patients may develop more severe or persistent effects if they have HTN or hyperthyroidism. Inform that patients may experience angina if they have coronary artery disease. Advise that patients may develop increased blood glucose levels following administration if they have DM. Advise that may notice a temporary worsening of symptoms if patient has Parkinson's disease. Instruct to seek immediate medical care in case of accidental inj.

STORAGE: 20-25°C (68-77°F); excursions permitted to 15-30°C (59-86°F). Protect from light; store in the outer case provided. Do not refrigerate. Replace auto-injector if sol is discolored, cloudy, or contains particles.

AVALIDE – hydrochlorothiazide/irbesartan

RX

Class: Angiotensin II receptor blocker (ARB)/thiazide diuretic

D/C when pregnancy is detected. Drugs that act directly on the renin-angiotensin system (RAS) can cause injury/death to the developing fetus.

ADULT DOSAGE

Hypertension

Add-On Therapy:
Use if not controlled on monotherapy w/ irbesartan or HCTZ
150mg/12.5mg, 300mg/12.5mg, and 300mg/25mg

Replacement Therapy:
May be substituted for titrated components

Initial Therapy:
Usual: 150mg/12.5mg qd
Titrate: May increase after 1-2 weeks of therapy
Max: 300mg/25mg qd

PEDIATRIC DOSAGE

Pediatric use may not have been established

ADMINISTRATION

Oral route
Take w/ or w/o food

HOW SUPPLIED

Tab: (Irbesartan-HCTZ) 150mg/12.5mg, 300mg/12.5mg

CONTRAINDICATIONS

Hypersensitivity to any component of this product, anuria or sulfonamide-derived drug hypersensitivity, coadministration w/ aliskiren in patients w/ diabetes.

WARNINGS/PRECAUTIONS

Not for initial therapy with intravascular volume depletion. Not recommended with severe renal impairment (CrCl ≤30mL/min). Symptomatic hypotension may occur in intravascular volume- or Na^+-depleted patients (eg, patients treated vigorously with diuretics or on dialysis); correct volume depletion prior to therapy. Hypokalemia and hyperkalemia reported. Irbesartan: May increase BUN or SrCr levels in patients with renal artery stenosis. Oliguria and/or progressive azotemia and (rarely) acute renal failure and/or death may occur in patients whose renal function may depend on the renin-angiotensin-aldosterone system activity (eg, severe congestive heart failure [CHF]). HCTZ: May cause hypersensitivity reactions, exacerbation or activation of systemic lupus erythematosus (SLE), hyponatremia, hypomagnesemia, and hyperuricemia or precipitation of frank gout. May alter glucose tolerance and increase cholesterol, TG, and Ca^{2+} levels. D/C before testing for parathyroid function. May cause idiosyncratic reaction, resulting in transient myopia and acute angle-closure glaucoma; d/c as rapidly as possible. Enhanced effects in postsympathectomy patients. Caution with hepatic impairment or progressive liver disease; may precipitate hepatic coma. May precipitate azotemia in patients with renal disease.

ADVERSE REACTIONS

Dizziness, hypokalemia, fatigue, musculoskeletal pain, influenza, edema, N/V, headache.

DRUG INTERACTIONS

See Contraindications. NSAIDs, including selective COX-2 inhibitors, may decrease effects of diuretics and angiotensin II receptor antagonists and may deteriorate renal function. Increases in lithium concentrations and lithium toxicity reported; monitor lithium levels. Irbesartan: Dual blockade of the RAS is associated with increased risks of hypotension, hyperkalemia, and changes in renal function (including acute renal failure); avoid combined use of RAS inhibitors, or closely monitor BP, renal function, and electrolytes with concomitant agents that also affect the RAS. Avoid with aliskiren in patients with renal impairment (GFR <60mL/min). Concomitant use with K^+-sparing diuretics, K^+ supplements, or salt substitutes containing K^+ may increase serum K^+. HCTZ: Alcohol, barbiturates, and narcotics may potentiate orthostatic hypotension. Dosage adjustment of antidiabetic drugs (oral agents and insulin) may be required. Anionic exchange resins (eg, cholestyramine, colestipol) may impair absorption; take at least 1 hr before or 4 hrs after these medications. Additive effect or potentiation with other antihypertensive drugs. Corticosteroids and adrenocorticotropic hormone may intensify electrolyte depletion, particularly hypokalemia. May decrease response to pressor amines (eg, norepinephrine). May increase responsiveness to nondepolarizing skeletal muscle relaxants (eg, tubocurarine). Risk of symptomatic hyponatremia with carbamazepine; monitor electrolytes.

PATIENT CONSIDERATIONS

Assessment: Assess for hypersensitivity to drug and its components, anuria, sulfonamide-derived drug hypersensitivity, diabetes, volume/salt depletion, SLE, CHF, renal/hepatic impairment, renal artery stenosis, postsympathectomy status, pregnancy/nursing status, and possible drug interactions.

Monitoring: Monitor for hypersensitivity/idiosyncratic reactions, exacerbation/activation of SLE, hyperuricemia, precipitation of gout, myopia, angle-closure glaucoma, and other adverse reactions. Monitor BP, serum electrolytes, cholesterol and TG levels, and renal/hepatic function.

Counseling: Inform females of childbearing age about the consequences of exposure during pregnancy. Discuss treatment options with women planning to become pregnant. Instruct to report pregnancies to physician as soon as possible. Inform that lightheadedness may occur, especially during 1st days of use; instruct to d/c use and contact physician if fainting occurs. Inform that dehydration, which may occur with excessive sweating, diarrhea, vomiting, and not drinking enough liquids, may lower BP too much and lead to lightheadedness and possible fainting.

STORAGE: 25°C (77°F); excursions permitted to 15-30°C (59-86°F).

AVANDAMET — metformin hydrochloride/rosiglitazone maleate RX

Class: Biguanide/thiazolidinedione (glitazone)

Thiazolidinediones, including rosiglitazone, cause or exacerbate CHF in some patients. After initiation and dose increases, observe for signs and symptoms of heart failure (HF); manage accordingly and consider discontinuation or dose reduction if signs/symptoms develop. Not recommended in patients with symptomatic HF. Contraindicated with established NYHA Class III or IV HF. Lactic acidosis may occur due to metformin accumulation; risk increases with conditions such as sepsis, dehydration, excess alcohol intake, hepatic/renal impairment, and acute CHF. If acidosis is suspected, d/c therapy and hospitalize patient immediately.

ADULT DOSAGE

Type 2 Diabetes Mellitus

Initial: 2mg/500mg qd or bid; may consider a starting dose of 2mg/500mg bid w/ HbA1c >11% or FPG >270mg/dL

Titrate: May increase in increments of (2mg/500mg)/day given in divided doses if inadequately controlled after 4 weeks

Max: (8mg/2000mg)/day

Start the rosiglitazone component at the lowest recommended dose

Inadequately Controlled on Rosiglitazone or Metformin Monotherapy:

PEDIATRIC DOSAGE

Pediatric use may not have been established

Initial:
On Metformin 1000mg/day: 2mg/500mg bid
On Metformin 2000mg/day: 2mg/1000mg bid
On Rosiglitazone 4mg/day: 2mg/500mg bid
On Rosiglitazone 8mg/day: 4mg/500mg bid
Individualize therapy if on metformin 1000-2000mg/day

Titrate:
If additional glycemic control is needed, may increase daily dose by increments of 4mg rosiglitazone and/or 500mg metformin
After an increase in metformin dose, if inadequately controlled, titrate after 1-2 weeks
After an increase in rosiglitazone dose, if inadequately controlled, titrate after 8-12 weeks

Max: (8mg/2000mg)/day taken in divided doses bid

DOSING CONSIDERATIONS

Hepatic Impairment

Active Liver Disease/Increased Serum Transaminase Levels (ALT >2.5X ULN): Do not initiate therapy

Elderly

Elderly/Debilitated/Malnourished: Dose conservatively; do not titrate to max dose

ADMINISTRATION

Oral route

Take in divided doses w/ meals

HOW SUPPLIED

Tab: (Rosiglitazone/Metformin) 2mg/500mg, 4mg/500mg, 2mg/1000mg, 4mg/1000mg

CONTRAINDICATIONS

NYHA Class III or IV HF, renal disease or dysfunction (eg, SrCr ≥1.5mg/dL [males], ≥1.4mg/dL [females], abnormal CrCl), acute/chronic metabolic acidosis including diabetic ketoacidosis w/ or w/o coma, use in patients undergoing radiologic studies involving intravascular administration of iodinated contrast materials, history of a hypersensitivity reaction to rosiglitazone or any of the product's ingredients.

WARNINGS/PRECAUTIONS

Assess renal function before initiation of therapy and at least annually thereafter; d/c with evidence of renal impairment. Promptly withhold in the presence of any condition associated with hypoxemia, dehydration, or sepsis. Temporarily d/c at the time of or prior to radiologic studies involving the use of intravascular iodinated contrast materials, withhold for 48 hrs subsequent to the procedure, and reinstitute only if renal function is normal. Temporarily suspend for any surgical procedure (except minor procedures not associated with restricted food and fluid intake); restart when oral intake is resumed and renal function is normal. Evaluate patients previously well-controlled on therapy who develop laboratory abnormalities or clinical illness for evidence of ketoacidosis or lactic acidosis; d/c if acidosis occurs. Increased risk of cardiovascular events in patients with CHF NYHA Class I and II. Treatment initiation is not recommended for patients experiencing an acute coronary event; consider discontinuation during this acute phase. Increased risk for myocardial infarction (MI) reported. Caution in patients with edema or at risk for HF. Edema and dose-related weight gain reported. Macular edema reported; promptly refer to an ophthalmologist if visual symptoms develop. Increased incidence of bone fracture, particularly in females. Dose-related decreases in Hgb and Hct reported. May decrease serum vitamin B12 levels. Temporary loss of glycemic control may occur when exposed to stress (eg, fever, trauma, infection, surgery); may be necessary to withhold therapy and temporarily administer insulin. Caution in patients susceptible to hypoglycemic effects, such as elderly, debilitated/malnourished patients, and those with adrenal/pituitary insufficiency, or alcohol intoxication. May result in ovulation in some premenopausal anovulatory women, which may increase risk for pregnancy; adequate contraception is recommended. Review benefits of continued therapy if unexpected menstrual dysfunction occurs. Do not initiate in patients ≥80 yrs of age unless renal function is not reduced. Not recommended for use in pregnancy. Avoid with active liver disease or if ALT levels >2.5X ULN. Caution in patients with mild LFT elevations (ALT levels ≤2.5X ULN). If ALT levels increase to >3X ULN during therapy, recheck LFTs as soon as possible; d/c if ALT levels remain >3X ULN. Check LFTs if symptoms suggesting hepatic dysfunction develop; d/c if jaundice is observed.

ADVERSE REACTIONS

CHF, lactic acidosis, N/V, upper respiratory tract infection, headache, diarrhea, arthralgia, dyspepsia, dizziness, edema, nasopharyngitis, abdominal pain, loose stools, constipation, anemia.

DRUG INTERACTIONS

Caution with drugs that may affect renal function or result in significant hemodynamic change or may interfere with the disposition of metformin, such as cationic drugs eliminated by renal tubular secretion (eg, cimetidine, amiloride, digoxin, morphine, procainamide); monitor and adjust dose of Avandamet and/or the interfering drug. Alcohol potentiates the effects of metformin on lactate metabolism; avoid excessive alcohol intake. Increased risk of CHF with insulin; coadministration is not recommended. Hypoglycemia may occur with other hypoglycemic agents (eg, sulfonylureas, insulin) or ethanol; may need to reduce dose of the concomitant agent. May be difficult to recognize hypoglycemia with β-adrenergic blocking drugs. CYP2C8 inhibitors (eg, gemfibrozil) may increase exposure and CYP2C8 inducers (eg, rifampin) may decrease exposure; if an inhibitor or an inducer of CYP2C8 is started or stopped during treatment, changes in diabetes treatment may be needed based upon clinical response. Observe for loss of glycemic control with drugs that produce hyperglycemia.

PATIENT CONSIDERATIONS

Assessment: Assess for HF or risk of HF, metabolic acidosis, diabetic ketoacidosis, risk factors for lactic acidosis, previous hypersensitivity to the drug, presence of an acute coronary event, cardiac status, edema, bone health, inadequate vitamin B12 or Ca^{2+} intake/absorption, any other conditions where treatment is cautioned, pregnancy/nursing status, and possible drug interactions. Assess if patient is planning to undergo any surgical procedure, radiologic studies involving the use of intravascular iodinated contrast materials, or is under any form of stress. Assess baseline renal function, LFTs, FPG, and HbA1c levels, and hematologic parameters.

Monitoring: Monitor for signs/symptoms of HF, lactic acidosis, hypoxic states, MI, edema, weight gain, visual symptoms, fractures, menstrual dysfunction, and other adverse reactions. Monitor for changes in clinical status. Monitor renal function, especially in elderly, at least annually. Monitor hematologic parameters annually. Perform routine serum vitamin B12 measurements at 2- to 3-yr intervals in patients predisposed to developing subnormal vitamin B12 levels. Periodically monitor LFTs, FPG, and HbA1c levels.

Counseling: Inform of the risks and benefits of therapy. Inform of the risk of lactic acidosis; instruct to d/c therapy immediately and notify physician if unexplained hyperventilation, myalgia, malaise, unusual somnolence, or other nonspecific symptoms occur. Counsel against excessive alcohol intake. Advise on the importance of adherence to dietary instructions and regular testing of blood glucose, HbA1c, renal/hepatic function, and hematologic parameters. Instruct to immediately report any signs/symptoms of hepatotoxicity or HF to physician. Counsel premenopausal women to use adequate contraception during treatment.

STORAGE: 25°C (77°F); excursions permitted to 15-30°C (59-86°F).

AVANDARYL — glimepiride/rosiglitazone maleate RX

Class: Sulfonylurea/thiazolidinedione (glitazone)

Thiazolidinediones, including rosiglitazone, cause or exacerbate CHF in some patients. After initiation and dose increases, observe for signs and symptoms of heart failure (HF); manage accordingly and consider discontinuation or dose reduction if signs/symptoms develop. Not recommended in patients w/ symptomatic HF. Contraindicated w/ established NYHA Class III or IV HF.

ADULT DOSAGE

Type 2 Diabetes Mellitus

Initial: 4mg/1mg qd w/ 1st meal of the day; may consider 4mg/2mg for patients already treated w/ a sulfonylurea or rosiglitazone
Max: (8mg/4mg)/day

Start the rosiglitazone component at the lowest recommended dose; if hypoglycemia occurs, may consider dose reduction of glimepiride component

Switching from Combination Therapy of Rosiglitazone Plus Glimepiride as Separate Tablets:
Initial: Start at the dose of rosiglitazone and glimepiride already being taken

Conversions

Switching to Avandaryl in Patients Currently Treated w/ Rosiglitazone:
If not adequately controlled after 1-2 weeks, may increase glimepiride component of

PEDIATRIC DOSAGE

Pediatric use may not have been established

Avandaryl in no >2mg increments; afterwards, may titrate Avandaryl if not adequately controlled after 1-2 weeks

Switching to Avandaryl in Patients Currently Treated w/ Sulfonylurea:
If not adequately controlled after 8-12 weeks, may titrate rosiglitazone component of Avandaryl; afterwards, may titrate Avandaryl if not adequately controlled after 2-3 months

DOSING CONSIDERATIONS

Concomitant Medications

Colesevelam: Administer therapy at least 4 hrs prior to colesevelam

ADMINISTRATION

Oral route

Take w/ the 1st meal of the day

HOW SUPPLIED

Tab: (Rosiglitazone/Glimepiride) 4mg/1mg, 4mg/2mg, 4mg/4mg, 8mg/2mg, 8mg/4mg

CONTRAINDICATIONS

NYHA Class III or IV HF. History of a hypersensitivity reaction to rosiglitazone or glimepiride or any of the product's ingredients.

WARNINGS/PRECAUTIONS

Not for use in patients w/ type 1 DM or for the treatment of diabetic ketoacidosis. Treatment initiation is not recommended in patients experiencing an acute coronary event; consider discontinuation during this acute phase. May cause severe hypoglycemia; caution in patients susceptible to hypoglycemic action, such as elderly, debilitated, or malnourished patients, and those w/ adrenal, pituitary, renal, or hepatic insufficiency. Temporary loss of glycemic control may occur when exposed to stress (eg, fever, trauma, infection, surgery); may be necessary to withhold therapy and temporarily administer insulin. Should not be used during pregnancy. Rosiglitazone: Increased risk of CHF w/ insulin; coadministration is not recommended. Caution in patients w/ edema or at risk for HF. Edema and dose-related weight gain reported. Elevation of LFTs may occur; hepatic impairment and hepatitis reported. Do not initiate in patients w/ increased baseline LFTs (ALT levels >2.5X ULN). Caution in patients w/ mild LFT elevations (ALT levels ≤2.5X ULN). If ALT levels increase to >3X ULN during therapy, recheck LFTs as soon as possible; d/c if ALT levels remain >3X ULN. Check LFTs if symptoms suggesting hepatic dysfunction develop; d/c if jaundice is observed. Increased risk of cardiovascular (CV) events in patients w/ CHF NYHA Class I and II. Increased risk for MI reported. Macular edema reported; promptly refer to an ophthalmologist if visual symptoms develop. Increased incidence of bone fracture, particularly in females. Dose-related decreases in Hgb and Hct reported. May result in ovulation in some premenopausal anovulatory women, which may increase risk for pregnancy; adequate contraception is recommended. Review benefits of continued therapy if unexpected menstrual dysfunction occurs. Glimepiride: May be associated w/ increased CV mortality. Hypersensitivity reactions (eg, anaphylaxis, angioedema, Stevens-Johnson syndrome) reported; if suspected, promptly d/c therapy, assess for other potential causes for the reaction, and institute alternative treatment. May cause hemolytic anemia; caution w/ G6PD deficiency and consider the use of a non-sulfonylurea alternative.

ADVERSE REACTIONS

CHF, headache, hypoglycemia, nasopharyngitis, HTN, edema.

DRUG INTERACTIONS

See Dosing Considerations. May require dose adjustment and close monitoring for hypoglycemia or worsening glycemic control w/ drugs that may increase glucose-lowering effect (eg, ACE inhibitors, fibrates, somatostatin analogues, highly protein-bound drugs), drugs that may reduce glucose-lowering effect (eg, protease inhibitors, corticosteroids, oral contraceptives), or drugs that may either increase or decrease glucose-lowering effect (eg, β-blockers, clonidine, reserpine). Signs of hypoglycemia may be reduced or absent w/ sympatholytic drugs (eg, β-blockers, clonidine, guanethidine, reserpine). Glimepiride: Alcohol may also potentiate or weaken glucose-lowering action. Colesevelam may reduce levels. Potential interaction leading to severe hypoglycemia reported w/ oral miconazole. Potential interaction may occur w/ other drugs metabolized by CYP2C9 (eg, phenytoin, ibuprofen, mefenamic acid), and w/ CYP2C9 inhibitors (eg, fluconazole) or inducers (eg, rifampin). Rosiglitazone: CYP2C8 inhibitors (eg, gemfibrozil) may increase AUC and CYP2C8 inducers (eg, rifampin) may decrease AUC; if an inhibitor or an inducer of CYP2C8 is started or stopped during treatment, changes in diabetes treatment may be needed based upon clinical response. Refer to PI for additional drug interactions.

PATIENT CONSIDERATIONS

Assessment: Assess for HF or risk of HF, presence of acute coronary event, cardiac status, susceptibility to hypoglycemia, edema, bone health, G6PD deficiency, previous hypersensitivity to the drug or sulfonamide derivatives, pregnancy/nursing status, and possible drug interactions. Assess if patient is under any form of stress. Obtain baseline renal function, LFTs, FPG, and HbA1c levels.

Monitoring: Monitor for signs/symptoms of HF, MI, hypoglycemia, edema, weight gain, visual symptoms, fractures, hypersensitivity reactions, hematologic effects, menstrual dysfunction, and other adverse reactions. Periodically monitor LFTs, FPG, and HbA1c levels.

Counseling: Inform of the risks and benefits of therapy. Advise on the importance of adherence to dietary instructions and regular testing of blood glucose, HbA1c, and liver function. Inform about the risk of hypoglycemia, its symptoms and treatment, and conditions that predispose to its development. Instruct to immediately report to physician any symptoms of HF or hepatic dysfunction. Counsel premenopausal women to use adequate contraception during treatment.

STORAGE: 25°C (77°F); excursions permitted to 15-30°C (59-86°F).

AVANDIA – rosiglitazone maleate RX

Class: Thiazolidinedione (glitazone)

Thiazolidinediones, including rosiglitazone, cause or exacerbate congestive heart failure (CHF) in some patients. After initiation and dose increases, observe for signs and symptoms of heart failure (HF); manage accordingly and consider discontinuation or dose reduction if signs/symptoms develop. Not recommended in patients with symptomatic HF. Contraindicated with established NYHA Class III or IV HF.

ADULT DOSAGE

Type 2 Diabetes Mellitus

Initial: 4mg as qd dose or in 2 divided doses

Titrate: May increase to 8mg/day if response is inadequate after 8-12 weeks

Max: 8mg/day

PEDIATRIC DOSAGE

Pediatric use may not have been established

DOSING CONSIDERATIONS

Concomitant Medications

Other Hypoglycemic Agents: May need to reduce dose of the concomitant agent

Hepatic Impairment

Do not initiate therapy in patients w/ clinical evidence of active liver disease or increased serum transaminase levels (ALT >2.5X ULN at start of therapy)

ADMINISTRATION

Oral route

Take w/ or w/o food

HOW SUPPLIED

Tab: 2mg, 4mg, 8mg

CONTRAINDICATIONS

NYHA Class III or IV HF, history of a hypersensitivity reaction to rosiglitazone or any of the product's ingredients.

WARNINGS/PRECAUTIONS

Not for use in patients with type 1 DM or for the treatment of diabetic ketoacidosis. Increased risk of cardiovascular events in patients with CHF NYHA Class I and II. Treatment initiation is not recommended for patients experiencing an acute coronary event; consider discontinuation during this acute phase. Increased risk for myocardial infarction (MI) reported. Caution in patients with edema or at risk for HF. Edema and dose-related weight gain reported. Do not initiate in patients with active liver disease or increased baseline LFTs (ALT levels >2.5X ULN). Caution in patients with mild LFT elevations (ALT levels ≤2.5X ULN). If ALT levels increase to >3X ULN during therapy, recheck LFTs as soon as possible; d/c if ALT levels remain >3X ULN. Check LFTs if symptoms suggesting hepatic dysfunction develop; d/c if jaundice is observed. Macular edema reported; promptly refer to an ophthalmologist if visual symptoms develop. Increased incidence of bone fracture, particularly in females. Dose-related decreases in Hgb and Hct reported. May result in ovulation in some premenopausal anovulatory women, which may increase risk for pregnancy; adequate contraception is recommended. Review benefits of continued therapy if unexpected menstrual dysfunction occurs.

ADVERSE REACTIONS

CHF, upper respiratory tract infection, headache, back pain, hyperglycemia, fatigue, sinusitis, edema.

DRUG INTERACTIONS

See Dosage. Risk for hypoglycemia when given with other hypoglycemic agents; a reduction in the dose of concomitant agent may be necessary. CYP2C8 inhibitors (eg, gemfibrozil) may increase exposure and CYP2C8 inducers (eg, rifampin) may decrease exposure; if an inhibitor or an inducer of CYP2C8 is started or stopped during treatment, changes in diabetes treatment may be needed based upon clinical response. Increased risk of CHF with insulin; coadministration is not recommended.

PATIENT CONSIDERATIONS

Assessment: Assess for HF or risk factors for HF, presence of an acute coronary event, cardiac status, edema, drug hypersensitivity, pregnancy/nursing status, and possible drug interactions. Obtain baseline LFTs, FPG and HbA1c levels, and bone health.

Monitoring: Monitor for signs/symptoms of HF, MI, edema, weight gain, macular edema, fractures, hematologic effects, menstrual dysfunction, and other adverse reactions. Periodically monitor LFTs, FPG, and HbA1c levels.

Counseling: Inform of the risks and benefits of therapy. Advise on the importance of adherence to dietary instructions and regular testing of blood glucose, HbA1c, and liver function. Instruct to immediately report to physician any symptoms of HF or hepatic dysfunction. Inform about the risk of hypoglycemia, its symptoms and treatment, and conditions that predispose to its development when using in combination with other hypoglycemic agents. Counsel premenopausal women to use adequate contraception during treatment.

STORAGE: 25°C (77°F); excursions permitted to 15-30°C (59-86°F).

AVAPRO – irbesartan

RX

Class: Angiotensin II receptor blocker (ARB)

D/C when pregnancy is detected. Drugs that act directly on the renin-angiotensin system (RAS) can cause injury/death to the developing fetus.

ADULT DOSAGE

Hypertension

Initial: 150mg qd
Titrate: May increase to 300mg qd
Max: 300mg qd
A low dose diuretic may be added if BP is not controlled

Diabetic Nephropathy

Elevated SrCr/Proteinuria (>300mg/day) in Patients w/ Type 2 Diabetes and HTN:
Maint: 300mg qd

PEDIATRIC DOSAGE

Pediatric use may not have been established

DOSING CONSIDERATIONS

Other Important Considerations

Intravascular Volume and Salt Depleted Patients:
Initial: 75mg qd

ADMINISTRATION

Oral route

Take w/ or w/o food

HOW SUPPLIED

Tab: 75mg, 150mg, 300mg

CONTRAINDICATIONS

Hypersensitivity to any component of this product, coadministration w/ aliskiren in patients w/ diabetes.

WARNINGS/PRECAUTIONS

Symptomatic hypotension may occur in patients with intravascular volume or Na^+ depletion (eg, patients treated vigorously with diuretics or on dialysis); correct volume depletion prior to therapy or use low starting dose. Changes in renal function may occur. Oliguria and/or progressive azotemia and (rarely) acute renal failure and/or death may occur in patients whose renal function may depend on the renin-angiotensin-aldosterone system activity (eg, severe congestive heart failure [CHF]). May increase SrCr or BUN in patients with renal artery stenosis.

ADVERSE REACTIONS

Hyperkalemia, dizziness, orthostatic dizziness, orthostatic hypotension, fatigue, diarrhea.

DRUG INTERACTIONS

See Contraindications. Increases in serum lithium concentrations and lithium toxicity reported; monitor lithium levels. CYP2C9 substrates/inhibitors sulphenazole, tolbutamide, and nifedipine significantly inhibited metabolism in vitro. Concomitant use with K^+-sparing diuretics, K^+ supplements, or salt substitutes containing K^+ may increase serum K^+. NSAIDs, including selective

COX-2 inhibitors, may attenuate antihypertensive effect and may deteriorate renal function. Dual blockade of the RAS is associated with increased risks of hypotension, hyperkalemia, and changes in renal function (including acute renal failure); avoid combined use of RAS inhibitors, or closely monitor BP, renal function, and electrolytes with concomitant agents that also affect the RAS. Avoid with aliskiren in patients with renal impairment (GFR <60mL/min).

PATIENT CONSIDERATIONS

Assessment: Assess for hypersensitivity, volume/salt depletion, renal impairment, CHF, renal artery stenosis, diabetes, pregnancy/nursing status, and possible drug interactions.

Monitoring: Monitor for signs/symptoms of hypotension, renal dysfunction, and other adverse reactions.

Counseling: Inform about the consequences of exposure during pregnancy in females of childbearing age. Discuss treatment options with women planning to become pregnant. Instruct to report pregnancies to physician as soon as possible.

STORAGE: 25°C (77°F); excursions permitted to 15-30°C (59-86°F).

AVAR – sodium sulfacetamide/sulfur RX

Class: Sulfonamide/sulfur combination

OTHER BRAND NAMES

Avar-e LS, Avar-e, Avar LS

ADULT DOSAGE

Acne Vulgaris/Acne Rosacea

Cre:
Apply a thin layer to the affected area qd-tid or ud

Sol:
Wash affected areas qd-bid or ud

Foam:
Treat affected area qd-tid or ud

Seborrheic Dermatitis

Cre:
Apply a thin layer to the affected area qd-tid or ud

Sol:
Wash affected areas qd-bid or ud

Foam:
Treat affected area qd-tid or ud

PEDIATRIC DOSAGE

Acne Vulgaris/Acne Rosacea

≥12 Years:

Cre:
Apply a thin layer to the affected area qd-tid or ud

Sol:
Wash affected areas qd-bid or ud

Foam:
Treat affected area qd-tid or ud

Seborrheic Dermatitis

≥12 Years:

Cre:
Apply a thin layer to the affected area qd-tid or ud

Sol:
Wash affected areas qd-bid or ud

Foam:
Treat affected area qd-tid or ud

ADMINISTRATION

Topical route

Cre

Wash hands and cleanse affected area.
Massage cre completely and uniformly into skin.

Sol

Wet skin and liberally apply to areas to be cleansed.
Massage gently into skin for 10-20 sec working into a full lather, then rinse thoroughly and pat dry.
Rinse off sooner or use less frequently if drying occurs.

Foam

Shake well before use.
Clean affected skin thoroughly and pat dry before each application.
Dispense product into palm of hand, holding can upright.
Massage into the affected area and wait for 10 min.
Rinse thoroughly w/ water and pat dry.

HOW SUPPLIED

(Sodium Sulfacetamide/Sulfur) **Sol:** 10%/5% [227g]; (LS) 10%/2% [227g]; **Cre:** (E) 10%/5% [45g tube, 57g bottle]; (E LS) 10%/2% [45g tube, 57g bottle]; **Foam:** 9.5%/5% [100g]; (LS) 10%/2% [100g]

CONTRAINDICATIONS

Kidney disease, known hypersensitivity to sulfonamides, sulfur, or any other component of this preparation.

WARNINGS/PRECAUTIONS

Carefully supervise and use caution in patients who may be prone to hypersensitivity to topical sulfonamides; systemic toxic reactions (eg, agranulocytosis, acute hemolytic anemia, purpura hemorrhagica, drug fever, jaundice, contact dermatitis) indicate sulfonamide hypersensitivity. Caution if areas of denuded or abraded skin are involved. Stevens-Johnson syndrome (SJS) and drug induced systemic lupus erythematosus (SLE) reported. Carefully observe for possible local irritation or sensitization during long-term therapy. D/C and institute appropriate therapy if irritation develops. May cause reddening and scaling of the epidermis. (Foam) Nonsusceptible organisms, including fungi, may proliferate w/ the use of this preparation. D/C use if product produces signs of hypersensitivity or other untoward reaction. Systemic absorption is greater following application to larger, infected, abraded, denuded, or severely burned areas; under these circumstances, any of the adverse effects produced by the systemic administration of these agents could potentially occur, and appropriate observations and lab determinations should be performed.

ADVERSE REACTIONS

Local irritation.

DRUG INTERACTIONS

(Foam) Incompatible w/ silver preparations.

PATIENT CONSIDERATIONS

Assessment: Assess for hypersensitivity to sulfonamides or sulfur, kidney disease, and pregnancy/nursing status. Assess if affected areas involve denuded or abraded skin.

Monitoring: Monitor for hypersensitivity reactions, local irritation or sensitization, reddening and scaling of epidermis, SJS, drug-induced SLE, and other possible adverse reactions. Following application to large, infected, abraded, denuded or severely burned areas, perform appropriate observations and lab determinations.

Counseling: Advise to avoid contact w/ eyes, lips, and mucous membranes. Inform that reddening and scaling of epidermis may occur. Instruct to notify physician if any sensitivity/systemic toxic reaction (eg, agranulocytosis, acute hemolytic anemia, purpura hemorrhagica, drug fever, jaundice, contact dermatitis) occurs. Advise to use particular caution when applying to affected skin areas that are denuded or abraded. Advise to notify physician if irritation occurs. Advise to d/c if the condition worsens or if rash develops in the area being treated or elsewhere. Advise to promptly d/c and notify physician if any arthritis, fever or sores in the mouth develop.

STORAGE: Protect from freezing and excessive heat. (Sol) 25°C (77°F); excursions permitted to 15-30°C (59-86°F). (Cre, Foam) 20-25°C (68-77°F); excursions permitted between 15-30°C (59-86°F). Brief exposures up to 40°C (104°F) may be tolerated provided the mean kinetic temperature does not exceed 25°C (77°F); minimize such exposure. (Foam) Contents under pressure. Do not puncture or incinerate.

AVASTIN – bevacizumab

RX

Class: Vascular endothelial growth factor (VEGF) inhibitor

GI perforation reported; d/c w/ GI perforation. Increased incidence of wound-healing and surgical complications; d/c at least 28 days prior to elective surgery. Do not initiate for at least 28 days after surgery and until surgical wound is fully healed. D/C in patients w/ wound dehiscence. Severe or fatal hemorrhage, including hemoptysis, GI bleeding, CNS hemorrhage, epistaxis, and vaginal bleeding, may occur; do not administer to patients w/ serious hemorrhage or recent hemoptysis.

ADULT DOSAGE

Metastatic Colorectal Cancer

1st- or 2nd-line treatment in combination w/ IV 5-fluorouracil-based chemotherapy; 2nd-line treatment in combination w/ fluoropyrimidine-irinotecan- or fluoropyrimidine-oxaliplatin-based chemotherapy, in patients who have progressed on a 1st-line bevacizumab-containing regimen

In Combination w/ Bolus-IFL:
5mg/kg every 2 weeks

In Combination w/ FOLFOX4:
10mg/kg every 2 weeks

In Combination w/ Fluoropyrimidine-Irinotecan- or Fluoropyrimidine-Oxaliplatin-Based Chemotherapy:
5mg/kg every 2 weeks or 7.5mg/kg every 3 weeks

PEDIATRIC DOSAGE

Pediatric use may not have been established

Nonsquamous Non-Small Cell Lung Cancer

1st-line treatment of unresectable, locally advanced, recurrent, or metastatic nonsquamous non-small cell lung cancer in combination w/ carboplatin and paclitaxel

15mg/kg every 3 weeks

Glioblastoma

W/ progressive disease following prior therapy as a single agent

10mg/kg every 2 weeks

Metastatic Renal Cell Carcinoma

10mg/kg every 2 weeks w/ Interferon Alfa

Cervical Cancer

Treatment of persistent, recurrent, or metastatic carcinoma of the cervix in combination w/ paclitaxel and cisplatin or paclitaxel and topotecan

15mg/kg every 3 weeks

Ovarian, Fallopian Tube, or Peritoneal Cancer

Treatment of patients w/ platinum-resistant recurrent epithelial ovarian, fallopian tube, or primary peritoneal cancer who received no more than 2 prior chemotherapy regimens in combination w/ paclitaxel, pegylated liposomal doxorubicin, or topotecan

10mg/kg every 2 weeks w/ 1 of the following IV chemotherapy regimens: paclitaxel, pegylated liposomal doxorubicin, or topotecan (weekly); or 15mg/kg every 3 weeks in combination w/ topotecan (every 3 weeks)

DOSING CONSIDERATIONS

Discontinuation

D/C For:

1. GI perforations, fistula formation in the GI tract or involving an internal organ, intra-abdominal abscess
2. Wound dehiscence and wound healing complications requiring medical intervention
3. Serious hemorrhage (requiring medical intervention)
4. Severe arterial thromboembolic events
5. Life-threatening (Grade 4) venous thromboembolic events, including pulmonary embolism
6. Hypertensive crisis or hypertensive encephalopathy
7. Posterior reversible encephalopathy syndrome
8. Nephrotic syndrome

Temporarily Suspend For:

1. At least 4 weeks prior to elective surgery
2. Severe HTN not controlled w/ medical management
3. Moderate to severe proteinuria
4. Severe infusion reactions

ADMINISTRATION

IV route

Do not administer as an IV push/bolus; administer only as an IV infusion.
Do not initiate until ≥28 days following major surgery and after surgical incision has fully healed.
Give 1st infusion over 90 min.
Give 2nd infusion over 60 min if 1st infusion is tolerated.
Give all subsequent infusions over 30 min if infusion over 60 min is tolerated.

Preparation

Withdraw necessary amount and dilute in a total volume of 100mL of 0.9% NaCl inj.
Discard any unused portion left in a vial, as the product contains no preservatives.
Do not administer or mix w/ dextrose sol.

HOW SUPPLIED

Inj: 100mg/4mL, 400mg/16mL

WARNINGS/PRECAUTIONS

Not indicated for adjuvant treatment of colon cancer. Avoid use in patients w/ ovarian cancer w/ evidence of recto-sigmoid involvement by pelvic examination or bowel involvement on CT scan or clinical symptoms of bowel obstruction. GI fistula reported. Serious and sometimes fatal non-GI fistula formation involving tracheoesophageal (TE), bronchopleural, biliary, vaginal, renal, and bladder sites may occur; d/c permanently in patients w/ TE fistula or any Grade 4 fistula. Necrotizing fasciitis, usually secondary to wound-healing complications, GI perforation, or fistula formation, reported; d/c therapy if necrotizing fasciitis develops. Arterial thromboembolic events (ATEs) (eg, cerebral infarction, transient ischemic attacks, MI, angina) reported; increased risk w/ history of arterial thromboembolism, diabetes, or age >65 yrs. May increase risk of venous thromboembolic events (VTEs) in patients treated for persistent, recurrent, or metastatic cervical cancer. Increased incidence of severe HTN. Posterior reversible encephalopathy syndrome (PRES) reported. Increased incidence and severity of proteinuria; suspend therapy for ≥2g proteinuria/24 hrs and resume when proteinuria is <2g/24 hrs. Nephrotic syndrome may occur. Infusion reactions reported. May cause fetal harm. Increases the risk of ovarian failure.

ADVERSE REACTIONS

Epistaxis, headache, HTN, rhinitis, proteinuria, taste alteration, dry skin, rectal hemorrhage, lacrimation disorder, back pain, exfoliative dermatitis.

DRUG INTERACTIONS

May decrease paclitaxel exposure w/ paclitaxel/carboplatin.

PATIENT CONSIDERATIONS

Assessment: Assess for recent hemoptysis, serious hemorrhage, HTN, proteinuria, history of ATEs, diabetes, pregnancy/nursing status, and possible drug interactions. Assess for prior surgical history and for any scheduled elective surgeries. Assess for evidence of recto-sigmoid involvement in patients w/ ovarian cancer.

Monitoring: Monitor for GI perforation, fistula formation, wound-healing complications, hemorrhage, ATEs, VTEs, hypertensive crisis, hypertensive encephalopathy, PRES, nephrotic syndrome, severe infusion reactions, and other adverse reactions. Monitor BP every 2-3 weeks, treat w/ appropriate anti-hypertensive therapy, and monitor BP regularly; continue to monitor BP at regular intervals w/ drug-induced or -exacerbated HTN after drug discontinuation. Monitor for proteinuria by dipstick urine analysis for the development or worsening of proteinuria w/ serial urinalyses.

Counseling: Advise to undergo routine BP monitoring and to contact physician if BP is elevated. Instruct to immediately seek medical attention for unusual bleeding, high fever, rigors, sudden onset of worsening neurological function, persistent/severe abdominal pain, severe constipation, or vomiting. Inform of the increased risk of wound-healing complications, ovarian failure, and ATE. Advise females of reproductive potential to use effective contraception during treatment and for 6 months after therapy, and to inform physician of a known/suspected pregnancy. Advise nursing women that breastfeeding is not recommended during treatment.

STORAGE: 2-8°C (36-46°F). Protect from light. Do not freeze or shake. **Diluted Sol:** May be stored at 2-8°C (36-46°F) for up to 8 hrs. Store in original carton until time of use.

AVELOX – moxifloxacin hydrochloride

RX

Class: Fluoroquinolone

Fluoroquinolones are associated w/ an increased risk of tendinitis and tendon rupture in all ages. Risk is further increased in patients >60 yrs of age, patients taking corticosteroids, and w/ kidney, heart, or lung transplants. May exacerbate muscle weakness w/ myasthenia gravis; avoid in patients w/ known history of myasthenia gravis.

ADULT DOSAGE

Skin and Skin Structure Infections

Uncomplicated: 400mg PO/IV q24h for 7 days

Complicated: 400mg PO/IV q24h for 7-21 days

Intra-Abdominal Infections

Complicated: 400mg PO/IV q24h for 5-14 days

Acute Bacterial Sinusitis

400mg PO/IV q24h for 10 days

Acute Bacterial Exacerbation of Chronic Bronchitis

400mg PO/IV q24h for 5 days

Community-Acquired Pneumonia

400mg PO/IV q24h for 7-14 days

PEDIATRIC DOSAGE

Pediatric use may not have been established

Plague

400mg PO/IV q24h for 10-14 days

Conversions

Patients started w/ IV therapy may be switched to tabs when clinically indicated

ADMINISTRATION

Oral/IV route

Tab

W/ Multivalent Cations:

Administer at least 4 hrs before or 8 hrs after products containing Mg^{2+}, aluminum, iron or zinc, including antacids, sucralfate, multivitamins, and didanosine buffered tabs for oral sus or the pediatric powder for oral sol

W/ Food:

Take w/ or w/o food
Drink fluids liberally

IV

Administer by IV infusion only; avoid rapid or bolus IV infusion
Infuse IV over 60 min by direct infusion or through a Y-type IV infusion set

Drug and Diluent Compatibilities:

Do not add other IV substances, additives, or other medications to inj or infuse simultaneously through same IV line
Flush the line before and after infusion w/ an infusion sol compatible w/ the inj as well as w/ other drug(s) administered via this common line if the same IV line or a Y-type line is used for sequential infusion of other drugs, or if the "piggyback" method of administration is used

Compatible IV Sol:

0.9% NaCl inj
1M NaCl inj
D5 inj
Sterile Water for inj
D10 for inj
Lactated Ringer's for inj

HOW SUPPLIED

Inj: 400mg/250mL; **Tab:** 400mg

CONTRAINDICATIONS

History of hypersensitivity to moxifloxacin or any member of the quinolone class.

WARNINGS/PRECAUTIONS

D/C if pain, swelling, inflammation, or rupture of a tendon occurs. May prolong QT interval; avoid w/ known QT interval prolongation, ventricular arrhythmias including torsades de pointes, ongoing proarrhythmic conditions (eg, clinically significant bradycardia, acute myocardial ischemia), or uncorrected hypokalemia or hypomagnesemia. Elderly using IV formulation may be more susceptible to drug-associated QT prolongation. May lead to QT prolongation in patients w/ mild, moderate, or severe liver cirrhosis, or in patients w/ metabolic disturbances associated w/ hepatic insufficiency; monitor ECG in patients w/ liver cirrhosis. Serious anaphylactic reactions and other serious and sometimes fatal events reported; d/c immediately and institute supportive measures if skin rash, jaundice, or any other signs of hypersensitivity occur. Convulsions, increased intracranial pressure (eg, pseudotumor cerebri), and other CNS reactions reported; d/c and institute appropriate measures if CNS reactions (eg, dizziness, confusion, tremors) occur. Use therapy when the benefits of treatment exceed the risks w/ CNS disorders (eg, severe cerebral arteriosclerosis, epilepsy) or in the presence of other risk factors that may predispose to seizures or lower seizure threshold. *Clostridium difficile*-associated diarrhea (CDAD) reported; may need to d/c if CDAD is suspected or confirmed. Cases of sensory or sensorimotor axonal polyneuropathy, resulting in paresthesias, hypoesthesias, dysesthesias, and weakness reported; d/c immediately if symptoms of peripheral neuropathy occur. Blood glucose disturbances (eg, hypo/hyperglycemia) in diabetics reported; d/c therapy and immediately initiate appropriate therapy if hypoglycemic reaction occurs. May cause photosensitivity/phototoxicity reactions; d/c if phototoxicity occurs. Avoid excessive exposure to sun/UV light. May result in bacterial resistance if used in the absence of a proven/strongly suspected bacterial infection or a prophylactic indication.

ADVERSE REACTIONS

Tendinitis, tendon rupture, nausea, diarrhea, headache, dizziness.

DRUG INTERACTIONS

See Boxed Warning. Avoid w/ Class IA (eg, quinidine, procainamide), Class III (eg, amiodarone, sotalol) antiarrhythmics, or other drugs that prolong the QT interval (eg, cisapride, erythromycin, antipsychotics, TCAs). NSAIDs may increase risk of CNS stimulation and convulsions. May enhance anticoagulant effects of warfarin or its derivatives; monitor PT and INR. Disturbances of blood glucose in diabetic patients receiving a concomitant antidiabetic agent reported; monitor glucose levels. (Tab) Antacids containing Mg^{2+} or aluminum, sucralfate, metal cations (eg, iron), multivitamins containing iron or zinc, or formulations containing divalent and trivalent cations such as didanosine buffered tabs for oral sus or the pediatric powder for oral sol, may substantially interfere w/ absorption and lower systemic concentrations.

PATIENT CONSIDERATIONS

Assessment: Assess for risk factors for developing tendinitis and tendon rupture, history of myasthenia gravis, drug hypersensitivity, known QT interval prolongation, ventricular arrhythmias including torsades de pointes, uncorrected hypokalemia or hypomagnesemia, ongoing proarrhythmic conditions, liver cirrhosis, CNS disorders or risk factors that may predispose to seizures or lower seizure threshold, diabetes, hepatic impairment, pregnancy/nursing status, and possible drug interactions. Obtain baseline culture and susceptibility tests.

Monitoring: Monitor for ECG changes (eg, QT interval prolongation), signs/symptoms of anaphylactic reactions, CNS reactions, drug resistance, CDAD, peripheral neuropathy, tendon rupture, tendinitis, photosensitivity/phototoxicity reactions, and other adverse reactions. Monitor for muscle weakness in patients w/ myasthenia gravis. Monitor blood glucose levels in diabetic patients. Monitor PT and INR if administered w/ warfarin or its derivatives.

Counseling: Inform that drug treats only bacterial, not viral infections. Instruct to take exactly ud; skipping doses or not completing full course may decrease effectiveness and increase bacterial resistance. Instruct to notify physician if pain, swelling, or inflammation of a tendon, or weakness or inability to move joints occurs; advise to rest and refrain from exercise and to d/c therapy. Instruct to notify physician if experiencing worsening muscle weakness or breathing problems, palpitations or fainting spells, sunburn-like reaction or skin eruption, or if watery and bloody stools (even ≥2 months after last dose) develop. Advise to notify physician of all medications and supplements currently being used. Instruct to inform physician of any personal or family history of QT prolongation, proarrhythmic conditions, convulsions, or psychiatric illness. Instruct diabetic patients being treated w/ antidiabetic agents to d/c therapy and notify physician if hypoglycemia occurs. Instruct to d/c and notify physician if an allergic reaction, skin rash, or symptoms of peripheral neuropathy develop. Inform that drug may cause dizziness, lightheadedness, and vision disorders; instruct to use caution w/ activities requiring mental alertness or coordination. Advise to minimize or avoid exposure to natural or artificial light (eg, tanning beds or UVA/B treatment). Inform that efficacy studies of therapy could not be conducted in humans w/ plague for feasibility reasons and that approval for plague was based on efficacy studies conducted in animals.

STORAGE: 25°C (77°F); excursions permitted to 15-30°C (59-86°F). (Tab) Avoid high humidity. (Inj) Do not refrigerate.

AVIANE – ethinyl estradiol/levonorgestrel RX

Class: Estrogen/progestogen combination

Cigarette smoking increases the risk of serious cardiovascular side effects. This risk increases with age (>35 yrs of age) and with extent of smoking (≥15 cigarettes/day). Women who use oral contraceptives should be strongly advised not to smoke.

OTHER BRAND NAMES

Orsythia

ADULT DOSAGE

Contraception

1 tab qd for 28 days at the same time each day, then repeat

Start on 1st Sunday after onset of menses or on Day 1 of menses

Conversions

Switching from 21-Day Regimen Tabs:
Wait 7 days after last tab before starting therapy

Switching from 28-Day Regimen Tabs:
Start on the day after the last tab is taken; do not wait any days between packs

Switching from a Progestin-Only Pill:
May switch any day from progestin-only pill and begin therapy the next day; use a

PEDIATRIC DOSAGE

Contraception

Not indicated for use premenarche; refer to adult dosing

nonhormonal backup method for the first 7 days

Switching from an Implant/Inj:
Start on the day of implant removal or the day the next inj would be due; use a nonhormonal backup method for the first 7 days

DOSING CONSIDERATIONS

Other Important Considerations

Use After Pregnancy/Abortion/Miscarriage:
Initiate no earlier than 28 days postpartum in the nonlactating mother or after a 2nd trimester abortion; use a nonhormonal backup method for the first 7 days
May initiate immediately after a 1st trimester abortion/miscarriage; backup contraception is not needed

ADMINISTRATION

Oral route

Take exactly ud and at intervals not exceeding 24 hrs
If therapy is started later than Day 1 of 1st menstrual cycle or postpartum, use a nonhormonal backup method of birth control during the first 7 days of therapy

HOW SUPPLIED

Tab: (Ethinyl Estradiol [EE]-Levonorgestrel) 0.02mg-0.1mg

CONTRAINDICATIONS

Thrombophlebitis or history of deep vein thrombophlebitis, presence or history of thromboembolic disorders, presence or history of cerebrovascular or coronary artery disease, valvular heart disease with thrombogenic complications, thrombogenic rhythm disorders, hereditary or acquired thrombophilias, major surgery with prolonged immobilization, uncontrolled HTN, diabetes mellitus (DM) with vascular involvement, headaches with focal neurological symptoms, presence or history of breast cancer, carcinoma of the endometrium or other known or suspected estrogen-dependent neoplasia, undiagnosed abnormal genital bleeding, cholestatic jaundice of pregnancy or jaundice with prior pill use, hepatic adenomas/carcinomas or active liver disease, known/suspected pregnancy, hypersensitivity to any of the components of this product.

WARNINGS/PRECAUTIONS

Increased risk of MI, vascular disease, thromboembolism, stroke, hepatic neoplasia, and gallbladder disease. Increased risk of morbidity and mortality with certain inherited/acquired thrombophilias, HTN, hyperlipidemia, obesity, DM, and surgery or trauma with increased risk of thrombosis. If feasible, d/c at least 4 weeks prior to and for 2 weeks after elective surgery of a type associated with an increase in risk of thromboembolism, and during and following prolonged immobilization. Start use no earlier than four weeks after delivery in women who elect not to breastfeed or after a midtrimester pregnancy termination. May increase risk of breast cancer and cancer of the reproductive organs. Contact lens wearers who develop visual changes or changes in lens tolerance should be assessed by an ophthalmologist. Retinal thrombosis reported; d/c if unexplained partial/complete loss of vision; onset of proptosis or diplopia; papilledema; or retinal vascular lesions develop. Should not be used to induce withdrawal bleeding as a test for pregnancy, nor to treat threatened or habitual abortion during pregnancy. Rule out pregnancy if 2 consecutive periods are missed. May cause glucose intolerance; monitor prediabetic and diabetic patients. May elevate serum TG and LDL levels and may render the control of hyperlipidemias more difficult. Caution with history of depression; d/c if depression recurs to a serious degree. May cause increased BP and fluid retention; d/c if a significant BP elevation occurs. Onset/exacerbation of migraine, or recurrent, persistent, severe headache may develop; d/c if this occurs. Breakthrough bleeding and spotting reported; rule out malignancy or pregnancy. Post-pill amenorrhea or oligomenorrhea may occur. Ectopic and intrauterine pregnancy may occur in contraceptive failures. D/C if jaundice develops. Diarrhea and/or vomiting may reduce hormone absorption, resulting in decreased serum concentrations. May affect certain endocrine function tests, LFTs, and blood components.

ADVERSE REACTIONS

N/V, dizziness, spotting, amenorrhea, change in menstrual flow, mood changes, vaginal candidiasis, edema, weight changes, melasma, breast changes, changes in cervical erosion and secretion, allergic rash, change in appetite.

DRUG INTERACTIONS

May reduce contraceptive effectiveness, resulting in unintended pregnancy or breakthrough bleeding when used concomitantly with antibiotics, anticonvulsants, and other drugs that increase the metabolism of contraceptive steroids (eg, rifampin, barbiturates, dexamethasone); consider a backup nonhormonal method of birth control. Several cases of contraceptive failure and breakthrough bleeding reported with concomitant administration of antibiotics (eg, ampicillin and other penicillins, tetracyclines). Anti-HIV protease inhibitors may increase or decrease plasma levels. Herbal products containing St. John's wort (*Hypericum perforatum*) may induce hepatic enzymes (cytochrome P450) and P-gp transporter; may reduce effectiveness of contraceptive steroids and may also result in breakthrough bleeding. Atorvastatin may increase EE exposure. Ascorbic acid and acetaminophen (APAP) may increase bioavailability of EE. CYP3A4 inhibitors (eg, indinavir, ketoconazole, troleandomycin) may increase plasma hormone levels. Troleandomycin may increase risk of intrahepatic cholestasis. Increased plasma levels of cyclosporine, prednisolone and other corticosteroids, and theophylline have been reported. Decreased plasma concentrations of APAP and increased clearance of temazepam, salicylic acid, morphine, and clofibric acid reported.

PATIENT CONSIDERATIONS

Assessment: Assess for hypersensitivity to drug, thrombophlebitis or thromboembolic disorders, HTN, hyperlipidemia, diabetes, breast cancer, endometrial cancer or other estrogen-dependent neoplasia, undiagnosed abnormal genital bleeding, cholestatic jaundice of pregnancy or jaundice with prior pill use, pregnancy/nursing status, and for any other conditions where treatment is contraindicated/cautioned. Assess for possible drug interactions.

Monitoring: Monitor for MI, thromboembolism, stroke, hepatic neoplasia, and other adverse effects. Monitor BP with history of HTN, serum glucose levels in diabetic or prediabetic patients, lipid levels with hyperlipidemia, and for signs of worsening depression with previous history. Monitor liver function. Refer contact lens wearer to an ophthalmologist if visual changes or changes in lens tolerance develop. Monitor women with a strong family history of breast cancer or who have breast nodules. Perform periodic personal and family medical history and complete physical examination.

Counseling: Inform that the drug does not protect against transmission of HIV and other sexually transmitted diseases. Counsel about potential adverse effects. Advise to avoid smoking. Instruct to take exactly ud and at intervals not exceeding 24 hrs. Advise about risks of pregnancy if dose is missed; counsel to have a back up nonhormonal birth control method (eg, condoms, spermicide) at all times. Instruct that if one dose is missed, take as soon as possible and take next pill at regular scheduled time. Inform that spotting, light bleeding, or nausea may occur during the first 1-3 packs of pills; advise not to d/c medication and if symptoms persist, to notify physician. Instruct to d/c if pregnancy is confirmed/suspected.

STORAGE: 20-25°C (68-77°F).

AVINZA – morphine sulfate CII

Class: Opioid analgesic

Exposes users to risks of addiction, abuse, and misuse, leading to overdose and death; assess each patient's risk prior to prescribing, and monitor regularly for development of these behaviors/conditions. Serious, life-threatening, or fatal respiratory depression may occur; monitor during initiation or following a dose increase. Crushing, chewing, or dissolving can cause rapid release and absorption of a potentially fatal dose; instruct to swallow caps whole or sprinkle contents on applesauce. Accidental ingestion, especially by children, can result in fatal overdose. Prolonged use during pregnancy can result in neonatal opioid withdrawal syndrome; advise pregnant women of the risk and ensure availability of appropriate treatment. Avoid alcohol consumption or medications containing alcohol; may result in increased plasma levels and potentially fatal overdose of morphine.

ADULT DOSAGE

Severe Pain (Daily, Around-the-Clock Management)

1st Opioid Analgesic:
Initial: 30mg q24h
Titrate: Adjust dose in increments of ≥30mg every 3-4 days

Opioid Intolerant:
Initial: 30mg q24h

Titration/Maint:
Individually titrate to a dose that provides adequate analgesia and minimizes adverse reactions; dose adjustments may be dose every 3-4 days
Max Daily Dose: 1600mg/day

Breakthrough Pain:
May require a dose increase or may need rescue medication w/ an appropriate dose of an immediate-release analgesic

Conversions

From Other Opioids:
Initial: 30mg q24h; d/c all other around-the-clock opioids

PEDIATRIC DOSAGE

Pediatric use may not have been established

From Other Oral Morphine Formulations:
Administer total daily oral morphine dose once daily; do not give more frequently than q24h

From Parenteral Morphine:
Between 2-6mg of oral morphine may be required to provide analgesia equivalent to 1mg of parenteral morphine

From Other Non-Morphine Opioids (Parenteral or Oral):
Initial: 1/2 the estimated daily morphine requirement

DOSING CONSIDERATIONS

Discontinuation

Do not abruptly d/c; use a gradual downward titration of dose every 2-4 days to prevent signs/symptoms of withdrawal

ADMINISTRATION

Oral route

Take caps whole; do not crush, chew, or dissolve the pellets in the caps

Alternative Administration

Sprinkle over applesauce and consume immediately w/o chewing
Rinse mouth to ensure all pellets have been swallowed
Discard any unused portion of caps after contents have been sprinkled on applesauce

Do not administer through a NG or gastric tubes

HOW SUPPLIED

Cap, Extended-Release: 30mg, 45mg, 60mg, 75mg, 90mg, 120mg

CONTRAINDICATIONS

Significant respiratory depression, acute or severe bronchial asthma in an unmonitored setting or in the absence of resuscitative equipment, known/suspected paralytic ileus, hypersensitivity (eg, anaphylaxis) to morphine.

WARNINGS/PRECAUTIONS

Reserve use in patients for whom alternative treatment options are ineffective, not tolerated, or would be otherwise inadequate to provide sufficient management of pain. Should be prescribed only by healthcare professionals knowledgeable in the use of potent opioids for management of chronic pain. 90mg and 120mg caps are for use in opioid-tolerant patients only. Doses >1600mg/day contain a quantity of fumaric acid that may cause serious renal toxicity. Life-threatening respiratory depression is more likely to occur in elderly, cachectic, or debilitated patients. Consider alternative nonopioid analgesics in patients with significant chronic obstructive pulmonary disease (COPD) or cor pulmonale, and in patients having a substantially decreased respiratory reserve, hypoxia, hypercapnia, or preexisting respiratory depression. May cause severe hypotension, including orthostatic hypotension and syncope; increased risk in patients whose ability to maintain BP has already been compromised by a reduced blood volume or concurrent administration of certain CNS depressants. Avoid with circulatory shock, impaired consciousness, coma, or GI obstruction. Monitor patients who may be susceptible to intracranial effects of carbon dioxide retention (eg, those with evidence of increased intracranial pressure, brain tumors) for signs of sedation and respiratory depression, particularly when initiating therapy. May obscure clinical course in patients with head injury. May cause spasm of sphincter of Oddi and increases in serum amylase; monitor patients with biliary tract disease, including acute pancreatitis, for worsening symptoms. May aggravate convulsions and induce/aggravate seizures. May impair mental/physical abilities. Not recommended for use during and immediately prior to labor.

ADVERSE REACTIONS

Respiratory depression, constipation, N/V, somnolence, headache, peripheral edema, diarrhea, abdominal pain, infection, urinary tract infection, flu syndrome, back pain, rash, insomnia, depression, dyspnea.

DRUG INTERACTIONS

See Boxed Warning. Concomitant use with other CNS depressants (eg, sedatives, anxiolytics, neuroleptics) may increase risk of respiratory depression, profound sedation, hypotension, coma and death; if coadministration is required, consider dose reduction of one or both agents. Monitor use in elderly, cachectic, and debilitated patients when coadministered with other drugs that depress respiration. Mixed agonist/antagonists (eg, pentazocine, nalbuphine, butorphanol) and partial agonist (buprenorphine) analgesics may reduce analgesic effect or precipitate withdrawal symptoms; avoid coadministration. May enhance neuromuscular blocking action of skeletal muscle relaxants and produce an increased degree of respiratory depression. MAOIs may potentiate effects of morphine; avoid use with MAOIs or within 14 days of stopping such treatment. Cimetidine may potentiate morphine-induced respiratory depression. Confusion and severe respiratory depression in a patient undergoing hemodialysis reported with concurrent cimetidine. May reduce efficacy of diuretics and lead to acute urinary retention. Anticholinergics or other medications with anticholinergic activity may increase risk of urinary retention and/or severe constipation and lead to paralytic ileus. Absorption/exposure may be increased with p-glycoprotein inhibitors (eg, quinidine).

PATIENT CONSIDERATIONS

Assessment: Assess for abuse/addiction risk, pain intensity, prior opioid therapy, opioid tolerance, respiratory depression, drug hypersensitivity, pregnancy/nursing status, possible drug interactions, or any other condition where treatment is contraindicated or cautioned.

Monitoring: Monitor for respiratory depression (especially within first 24-72 hrs of initiation), hypotension, seizures/convulsions, and other adverse reactions. Monitor BP and serum amylase levels. Routinely monitor for signs of misuse, abuse, and addiction. Periodically reassess the continued need for therapy.

Counseling: Inform that use of drug can result in addiction, abuse, and misuse; instruct not to share with others and to take steps to protect from theft or misuse. Inform about risk of respiratory depression and advise to seek medical attention if breathing difficulties develop. Advise to store securely and dispose unused caps by flushing down the toilet. Inform female patients of reproductive potential that prolonged use during pregnancy may result in neonatal opioid withdrawal syndrome and instruct to inform physician if pregnant or planning to become pregnant. Inform that potentially serious additive effects may occur when used with alcohol or other CNS depressants, and not to use such drugs unless supervised by physician. Instruct about proper administration instructions. Inform that drug may cause orthostatic hypotension, syncope, and impair the ability to perform potentially hazardous activities; advise to not perform such tasks until patients know how they will react to medication. Advise of potential for severe constipation, including management instructions. Advise how to recognize anaphylaxis and when to seek medical attention.

STORAGE: 25°C (77°F); excursions permitted to 15-30°C (59-86°F). Protect from light and moisture.

AVODART — dutasteride RX

Class: Type I and II 5 alpha-reductase inhibitor (5-ARI) (2nd generation)

ADULT DOSAGE

Benign Prostatic Hyperplasia

Monotherapy:

1 cap (0.5mg) qd

W/ Tamsulosin:

1 cap (0.5mg) qd and tamsulosin 0.4mg qd

PEDIATRIC DOSAGE

Pediatric use may not have been established

ADMINISTRATION

Oral route

Swallow whole; do not chew or open.

Take w/ or w/o food.

HOW SUPPLIED

Cap: 0.5mg

CONTRAINDICATIONS

Pregnancy; women of childbearing potential; pediatric patients; previously demonstrated, clinically significant hypersensitivity (eg, serious skin reactions, angioedema) to dutasteride or other 5 alpha-reductase inhibitors.

WARNINGS/PRECAUTIONS

Not approved for the prevention of prostate cancer. May decrease serum prostate specific antigen (PSA) concentration during therapy or in the presence of prostate cancer; establish a new baseline PSA at least 3 months after starting treatment and monitor PSA periodically thereafter. Any confirmed increase from the lowest PSA value while on treatment may signal presence of prostate cancer. May increase risk of high-grade prostate cancer. Prior to initiating treatment, consider other urological conditions that may cause similar symptoms; BPH and prostate cancer may coexist. Risk to male fetus; caps should not be handled by pregnant women or women who could become pregnant. Avoid donating blood until at least 6 months after last dose. Reduced total sperm count, semen volume, and sperm motility reported.

ADVERSE REACTIONS

Impotence, decreased libido, breast disorders, ejaculation disorders.

DRUG INTERACTIONS
Caution w/ potent, chronic CYP3A4 inhibitors (eg, ritonavir).

PATIENT CONSIDERATIONS

Assessment: Assess for urological conditions that may cause similar symptoms, previous hypersensitivity to the drug, and for possible drug interactions.

Monitoring: Monitor for signs/symptoms of prostate cancer and other urological diseases. Obtain new PSA baseline at least 3 months after starting treatment and monitor PSA periodically thereafter.

Counseling: Inform of the importance of periodic PSA monitoring. Advise that therapy may increase risk of high-grade prostate cancer. Counsel that drug should not be handled by women who are pregnant or who could become pregnant, due to potential fetal risks; advise to wash area immediately w/ soap and water if contact is made. Instruct not to donate blood until at least 6 months after last dose.

STORAGE: 25°C (77°F); excursions permitted to 15-30°C (59-86°F).

AVYCAZ – avibactam/ceftazidime

RX

Class: Beta-lactamase inhibitor/cephalosporin

ADULT DOSAGE

Intra-Abdominal Infections

Complicated Infections:
2.5g (2g/0.5g) IV q8h for 5-14 days in combination w/ metronidazole

Urinary Tract Infections

Complicated Infections, Including Pyelonephritis:
2.5g (2g/0.5g) IV q8h for 7-14 days

PEDIATRIC DOSAGE

Pediatric use may not have been established

DOSING CONSIDERATIONS

Renal Impairment

CrCl 31-50mL/min: 1.25g (1g/0.25g) IV q8h
CrCl 16-30mL/min: 0.94g (0.75g/0.19g) IV q12h
CrCl 6-15mL/min: 0.94g (0.75g/0.19g) IV q24h
CrCl ≤5mL/min: 0.94g (0.75g/0.19g) IV q48h

Administer after hemodialysis on hemodialysis days
For patients w/ changing renal function, monitor CrCl at least daily and adjust the dose accordingly

ADMINISTRATION

IV route

Administer by IV infusion over 2 hrs.

Preparation of Sol for Administration

1. Constitute powder in the vial w/ 10mL of 1 of the following sol: sterile water for inj (SWFI); 0.9% NaCl inj; D5 inj; all combinations of dextrose inj and NaCl inj, containing up to 2.5% dextrose, and 0.45% NaCl; or lactated Ringer's inj.
2. Mix gently; constituted sol will have an approx ceftazidime level of 0.167g/mL and an approx avibactam level of 0.042g/mL. The constituted sol is not for direct injection; must be diluted before IV infusion.
3. Prepare the required dose for IV infusion by withdrawing the appropriate volume from the constituted vial; refer to PI for volume to withdraw.
4. Before infusion, dilute the withdrawn volume of the constituted sol further w/ the same diluent used for constitution of the powder (except SWFI), to achieve total volume between 50mL (0.04g/mL ceftazidime and 0.01g/mL avibactam) to 250mL (0.008g/mL ceftazidime and 0.002g/mL avibactam) in an infusion bag. If SWFI was used for constitution, use any of the other appropriate constitution diluents for dilution.
5. Mix gently and ensure contents are dissolved completely.

Drug Compatibility

The sol for administration at the range of diluted concentrations of ceftazidime 0.008g/mL and avibactam 0.002g/mL to ceftazidime 0.04g/mL and avibactam 0.01g/mL is compatible w/ the more commonly used IV infusion fluids in infusion bags such as:
1. 0.9% NaCl inj
2. D5 inj
3. All combinations of dextrose inj and NaCl inj, containing up to 2.5% dextrose, and 0.45% NaCl

4. Lactated Ringer's inj
5. Baxter Mini-Bag Plus containing 0.9% NaCl inj or D5 inj

Stability

Upon constitution w/ appropriate diluent, the constituted sol may be held for no longer than 30 min prior to transfer and dilution in a suitable infusion bag.

Following dilution of the constituted sol w/ the appropriate diluents, sol in the infusion bags are stable for 12 hrs when stored at room temperature; may also be refrigerated at 2-8°C (36-46°F) for up to 24 hrs; and then should be used w/in 12 hrs of subsequent storage at room temperature.

HOW SUPPLIED

Inj: (Ceftazidime/Avibactam) 2g/0.5g

CONTRAINDICATIONS

Known serious hypersensitivity to the components of Avycaz (ceftazidime and avibactam), avibactam-containing products, or other members of the cephalosporin class.

WARNINGS/PRECAUTIONS

Reserve use in patients who have limited or no alternative treatment options. Decreased clinical response in patients w/ baseline CrCl 30 to ≤50mL/min. Serious and occasionally fatal hypersensitivity (anaphylactic) reactions and serious skin reactions reported; d/c if an allergic reaction occurs. Cross-sensitivity among β-lactam antibacterials reported; caution in penicillin (PCN) or other β-lactam allergic patients. *Clostridium difficile*-associated diarrhea (CDAD) reported; may need to d/c if CDAD is suspected or confirmed. Seizures, nonconvulsive status epilepticus, encephalopathy, coma, asterixis, neuromuscular excitability, and myoclonia reported, particularly in the setting of renal impairment; adjust dosing based on CrCl. Use in the absence of a proven or strongly suspected bacterial infection is unlikely to provide benefit and increases the risk of development of drug-resistant bacteria. Caution in elderly. Lab test interactions may occur.

ADVERSE REACTIONS

N/V, constipation, anxiety, abdominal pain, dizziness, increased blood alkaline phosphatase, increased alanine aminotransferase.

DRUG INTERACTIONS

Not recommended w/ probenecid.

PATIENT CONSIDERATIONS

Assessment: Assess for hypersensitivity to drug, cephalosporins, PCNs, carbapenems, or other β-lactam antibiotics; renal impairment; pregnancy/nursing status; and possible drug interactions. Perform culture and susceptibility testing.

Monitoring: Monitor for signs/symptoms of hypersensitivity reactions, CDAD, seizures, nonconvulsive status epilepticus, encephalopathy, coma, asterixis, neuromuscular excitability, myoclonia, and other adverse reactions. Monitor CrCl at least daily w/ changing renal function.

Counseling: Advise that allergic reactions, including serious allergic reactions, may occur and require immediate treatment. Advise that diarrhea is a common problem caused by antibacterial drugs; instruct to contact physician if severe watery or bloody diarrhea develops. Inform that neurological adverse reactions may occur; instruct to inform physician immediately if any neurological signs and symptoms develop. Inform that therapy should only be used to treat bacterial, not viral, infections. Advise to take exactly ud; inform that skipping doses or not completing full course of therapy may decrease effectiveness of therapy and increase bacterial resistance.

STORAGE: 25°C (77°F); excursions permitted between 15-30°C (59-86°F). Protect from light.

AXIRON – testosterone CIII

Class: Androgen

Virilization reported in children secondarily exposed to topical testosterone. Children should avoid contact w/ unwashed or unclothed application sites in men using topical testosterone. Advise patients to strictly adhere to recommended instructions for use.

ADULT DOSAGE

Testosterone Replacement Therapy

Congenital/Acquired Primary Hypogonadism or Hypogonadotropic Hypogonadism in Males:

Initial: Apply 60mg (2 pump actuations) qam

Titrate: May adjust dose based on serum testosterone concentration from a single blood draw 2-8 hrs after application, and at least

PEDIATRIC DOSAGE

Pediatric use may not have been established

14 days after starting treatment or following dose adjustment
If Serum Testosterone Concentration <300ng/dL: May increase from 60mg to 90mg or from 90mg to 120mg
If Serum Testosterone Concentration >1050ng/dL: Decrease from 60mg to 30mg
D/C if serum testosterone concentration is consistently >1050ng/dL at lowest daily dose of 30mg

ADMINISTRATION

Topical route

Apply to clean, dry, intact skin of axilla, preferably at the same time each am
Do not apply to other parts of the body, including the scrotum, penis, abdomen, shoulders, or upper arms
Prime pump in upright position, depress actuator 3X prior to 1st use

Application
30mg Dose: Apply once to 1 axilla only
60mg Dose: Apply once to the left axilla and then once to the right axilla
90mg Dose: Apply once to the left and once to the right axilla, wait for the product to dry, and then apply once again to the left or right axilla
120mg: Apply once to the left and once to the right axilla, wait for the product to dry, and then apply once again to the left and right axilla

HOW SUPPLIED

Sol: 30mg/actuation [110mL]

CONTRAINDICATIONS

Breast carcinoma or known/suspected prostate carcinoma in men, women who are or may become pregnant, or are breastfeeding.

WARNINGS/PRECAUTIONS

Application site and dose are not interchangeable w/ other topical testosterone products. Monitor patients w/ BPH for worsening of signs and symptoms of BPH. May increase risk for prostate cancer. Risk of virilization in women due to secondary exposure. Increases in Hct/RBC mass may occur; if Hct elevates, lower dose or d/c therapy until Hct decreases to acceptable level. Increases in RBC mass may increase risk of thromboembolic events. Venous thromboembolic events (eg, deep vein thrombosis, pulmonary embolism) reported; d/c treatment and initiate appropriate workup and management if suspected. Increased risk of major adverse cardiovascular events (MACE) reported. Suppression of spermatogenesis may occur w/ large doses. Hepatic adverse effects reported w/ prolonged use of high doses of orally active 17-α-alkyl androgens and long-term therapy w/ IM testosterone enanthate. May promote retention of Na^+ and water. Edema w/ or w/o CHF may be a serious complication w/ preexisting cardiac/renal/hepatic disease. Gynecomastia may develop and persist. May potentiate sleep apnea, especially w/ risk factors such as obesity or chronic lung disease. Changes in serum lipid profile may require dose adjustment or discontinuation. Caution in cancer patients at risk of hypercalcemia and associated hypercalciuria. May decrease concentrations of thyroxine-binding globulins, resulting in decreased total T4 serum concentrations and increased resin uptake of T3 and T4. Flammable; avoid fire, flame, or smoking until applied dose has dried.

ADVERSE REACTIONS

Application-site irritation, application-site erythema, headache, Hct increase, diarrhea, vomiting, increases in prostate specific antigen.

DRUG INTERACTIONS

Changes in insulin sensitivity or glycemic control may occur; may decrease blood glucose and insulin requirements in diabetic patients. Changes in anticoagulant activity may occur; frequently monitor INR and PT in patients taking anticoagulants, especially at initiation and termination of androgen therapy. ACTH or corticosteroids may increase fluid retention; caution in patients w/ cardiac, renal, or hepatic disease.

PATIENT CONSIDERATIONS

Assessment: Assess for prostate cancer, breast carcinoma, BPH, cardiac/renal/hepatic disease, risk factors for sleep apnea, and any other conditions where treatment is contraindicated or cautioned, and possible drug interactions. Obtain baseline Hct, lipid, and serum testosterone levels. Confirm diagnosis of hypogonadism by measuring testosterone levels in am on at least 2 separate days prior to initiation.

Monitoring: Monitor for worsening of BPH, edema, gynecomastia, sleep apnea, venous thromboembolic events, MACE, and other adverse reactions. Perform periodic monitoring of serum lipid profile and serum testosterone levels. In cancer patients at risk for hypercalcemia, regularly monitor serum Ca^{2+} levels. Reevaluate Hct 3-6 months after start of therapy, then annually. Reevaluate for prostate cancer 3-6 months after initiation of treatment, and then in accordance w/ screening practices.

Counseling: Inform that men w/ known or suspected prostate/breast cancer should not use androgen therapy. Advise to report signs/symptoms of secondary exposure in children and in women. Inform that children and women should avoid contact w/ unwashed or unclothed application sites of men using topical testosterone. Instruct to apply only to axilla and not to any other part of the body, to wash hands immediately w/ soap and water after application, and to cover application site w/ clothing after waiting 3 min for the sol to dry. Instruct to wash application site w/ soap and water prior to any situation in which direct skin-to-skin contact is anticipated, and to immediately wash area of contact if unwashed/unclothed skin comes in direct contact w/ skin of another person. Inform of the potential adverse reactions. Instruct to prime the pump by depressing 3X prior to 1st use; advise that no priming is needed w/ subsequent uses of the pump. Instruct patient to allow the sol to dry after the 1st application before the 2nd. Instruct to apply to clean, dry skin at approx the same time each day. Inform that antiperspirant or deodorant may be used before applying the medication. Counsel to avoid swimming or washing application site until 2 hrs following application. Advise to avoid splashing in the eyes; instruct to flush thoroughly w/ water in case of contact and to seek medical advice if irritation persists.

STORAGE: 25°C (77°F); excursions permitted to 15-30°C (59-86°F). Discard used bottles and applicators in household trash in a manner that prevents accidental exposure of children or pets.

AZOPT — brinzolamide

RX

Class: Carbonic anhydrase inhibitor

ADULT DOSAGE

Elevated Intraocular Pressure

Ocular HTN/Open-Angle Glaucoma:

1 drop in the affected eye(s) tid

May be used concomitantly w/ other topical ophthalmic drugs to lower IOP

PEDIATRIC DOSAGE

Pediatric use may not have been established

DOSING CONSIDERATIONS

Concomitant Medications

Space dosing by at least 10 min if using >1 topical ophthalmic drug

ADMINISTRATION

Ocular route

Shake well before use.

HOW SUPPLIED

Ophthalmic Sus: 1% [10mL, 15mL]

CONTRAINDICATIONS

Hypersensitivity to any component of this product.

WARNINGS/PRECAUTIONS

Systemically absorbed. Fatalities occurred (rarely) due to severe reactions to sulfonamides including Stevens-Johnson syndrome, toxic epidermal necrolysis, fulminant hepatic necrosis, agranulocytosis, aplastic anemia, and other blood dyscrasias. Sensitization may recur when a sulfonamide is readministered irrespective of route. D/C if signs of serious reactions or hypersensitivity occur. Caution w/ low endothelial cell counts; increased potential for corneal edema. Not recommended w/ severe renal impairment (CrCl <30mL/min). Contains benzalkonium chloride, which may be absorbed by soft contact lenses; contact lenses should be removed during instillation, but may be reinserted 15 min after instillation.

ADVERSE REACTIONS

Blurred vision, bitter/sour/unusual taste.

DRUG INTERACTIONS

Potential additive systemic effects w/ oral carbonic anhydrase inhibitors; coadministration is not recommended. Acid-base alterations reported w/ high-dose salicylate therapy in patients treated w/ oral carbonic anhydrase inhibitors.

PATIENT CONSIDERATIONS

Assessment: Assess for hypersensitivity to drug or to sulfonamides, low endothelial cell counts, renal impairment, contact lens use, pregnancy/nursing status, and possible drug interactions.

Monitoring: Monitor for sulfonamide/hypersensitivity reactions, and other adverse reactions.

Counseling: Advise to d/c use and consult physician if serious or unusual ocular or systemic reactions or signs of hypersensitivity occur. Inform that vision may be temporarily blurred following administration; instruct to use caution in operating machinery or driving a motor vehicle. Instruct to avoid allowing the container tip to contact the eye or surrounding structures or other surfaces. Instruct to consult physician about the continued use of the present multidose container if undergoing ocular surgery or if an intercurrent ocular condition (eg, trauma, infection) develops. Instruct that if using >1 topical ophthalmic drug, to administer the drugs at least 10 min apart. Advise that contact lenses should be removed during instillation, but may be reinserted 15 min after instillation.

STORAGE: 4-30°C (39-86°F).

AZOR – amlodipine/olmesartan medoxomil RX

Class: Angiotensin II receptor blocker (ARB)/calcium channel blocker (CCB) (dihydropyridine)

D/C when pregnancy is detected. Drugs that act directly on the renin-angiotensin system (RAS) can cause death/injury to the developing fetus.

ADULT DOSAGE

Hypertension

Initial Therapy:
Initial: 5mg-20mg qd
Titrate: May increase dose after 1-2 weeks
Max: 10mg-40mg qd

Replacement Therapy:
May substitute for individually titrated components
When substituting for individual components, the dose of 1 or both components may be increased if BP is not adequately controlled

Add-On Therapy:
May be used to provide additional BP lowering when not adequately controlled on amlodipine (or another dihydropyridine calcium channel blocker) or olmesartan (or another ARB) alone

PEDIATRIC DOSAGE

Pediatric use may not have been established

DOSING CONSIDERATIONS

Hepatic Impairment
Initial Therapy: Not recommended

Elderly
≥75 Years:
Initial Therapy: Not recommended

ADMINISTRATION

Oral route

Take w/ or w/o food
May be administered w/ other antihypertensive agents

HOW SUPPLIED

Tab: (Amlodipine-Olmesartan) 5mg-20mg, 5mg-40mg, 10mg-20mg, 10mg-40mg

CONTRAINDICATIONS

Coadministration with aliskiren in patients with diabetes.

WARNINGS/PRECAUTIONS

Not recommended for use as initial therapy in patients ≥75 yrs of age or with hepatic impairment. May decrease Hct and Hgb levels. Amlodipine: Acute hypotension reported (rare); caution with severe aortic stenosis. May develop increased frequency, duration, or severity of angina or acute MI with dosage initiation or increase, particularly in patients with severe obstructive coronary artery disease (CAD). May cause hepatic enzyme elevation. Caution with severe hepatic impairment and in elderly. Olmesartan: Symptomatic hypotension, especially in patients with an activated RAS (eg, volume- and/or salt-depleted patients treated with high doses of diuretics), may occur after initiation of treatment; initiate treatment under close medical supervision. May cause changes in renal function. Oliguria or progressive azotemia and (rare) acute renal failure and/or death may occur in patients whose renal function may depend upon the activity of the RAS (eg, severe CHF). May increase BUN or SrCr levels in patients with renal artery stenosis. Sprue-like enteropathy with symptoms of severe, chronic diarrhea with substantial weight loss reported; exclude other etiologies if these symptoms develop, and consider discontinuation in cases where no other etiology is identified. Hyperkalemia may occur.

ADVERSE REACTIONS

Edema, headache, palpitation, dizziness, flushing.

DRUG INTERACTIONS

See Contraindications. Amlodipine: May increase simvastatin exposure; limit simvastatin dose to 20mg/day. Olmesartan: Dual blockade of the RAS is associated with increased risks of hypotension, hyperkalemia, and changes in renal function (including acute renal failure); avoid combined use of RAS inhibitors, or closely monitor BP, renal function, and electrolytes with concomitant agents that affect the RAS. Avoid with aliskiren in patients with renal impairment (GFR <60mL/min). NSAIDs, including selective COX-2 inhibitors, may deteriorate renal function and attenuate antihypertensive effect; monitor renal function periodically. Colesevelam may decrease levels; administer at least 4 hrs before colesevelam dose. Increases in serum lithium levels and lithium toxicity reported; monitor lithium levels.

PATIENT CONSIDERATIONS

Assessment: Assess for severe obstructive CAD, CHF, severe aortic stenosis, volume/salt depletion, diabetes, renal/hepatic impairment, pregnancy/nursing status, and possible drug interactions.

Monitoring: Monitor for signs/symptoms of hypotension, sprue-like enteropathy, and other adverse reactions. Monitor for symptoms of angina or MI, particularly in patients with severe obstructive CAD, after dosage initiation or increase. Monitor for decrease in Hct/Hgb, increase in SrCr, BUN, K^+ levels, and hepatic enzymes.

Counseling: Inform about the consequences of exposure during pregnancy and of the treatment options in women if planning to become pregnant; instruct to report pregnancy to the physician as soon as possible.

STORAGE: 25°C (77°F); excursions permitted to 15-30°C (59-86°F).

AZULFIDINE — sulfasalazine RX

Class: 5-aminosalicylic acid derivative/sulfapyridine

ADULT DOSAGE

Ulcerative Colitis

Treatment of mild to moderate ulcerative colitis (UC), adjunctive therapy in severe UC, and to prolong remission period between acute attacks of UC

Initial: 3-4g/day in evenly divided doses w/ intervals not >8 hrs; may initiate w/ a lower dose (eg, 1-2g/day) to reduce GI intolerance
Maint: 2g/day

When endoscopic examination confirms satisfactory improvement, reduce dose to a maint level; if diarrhea recurs, increase dose to previously effective level

Desensitization Regimen:
Initial: 50-250mg/day
Titrate: Double dose every 4-7 days until desired therapeutic level is achieved; d/c if sensitivity symptoms recur

PEDIATRIC DOSAGE

Ulcerative Colitis

Treatment of mild to moderate ulcerative colitis (UC), adjunctive therapy in severe UC, and to prolong remission period between acute attacks of UC

≥6 Years:
Initial: 40-60mg/kg/24 hrs divided into 3-6 doses
Maint: 30mg/kg/24 hrs divided into 4 doses

When endoscopic examination confirms satisfactory improvement, reduce dose to a maint level; if diarrhea recurs, increase dose to previously effective level

Desensitization Regimen:
Initial: 50-250mg/day
Titrate: Double dose every 4-7 days until desired therapeutic level is achieved; d/c if sensitivity symptoms recur

DOSING CONSIDERATIONS

Other Important Considerations

Gastric Intolerance:
If symptoms of gastric intolerance (eg, anorexia, N/V) occur after 1st few doses, may be alleviated by halving daily dose and subsequently increasing gradually over several days; if gastric intolerance continues, stop drug for 5-7 days, then reintroduce at a lower daily dose

ADMINISTRATION

Oral route

Take in evenly divided doses, preferably pc.

HOW SUPPLIED

Tab: 500mg* *scored

CONTRAINDICATIONS

Intestinal or urinary obstruction; porphyria; hypersensitivity to sulfasalazine, its metabolites, sulfonamides, or salicylates.

WARNINGS/PRECAUTIONS

Caution with hepatic/renal damage, blood dyscrasias, severe allergy, bronchial asthma, history of recurring/chronic infections, or with underlying conditions or concomitant drugs that may predispose patients to infections. Deaths reported from hypersensitivity reactions, agranulocytosis, aplastic anemia, other blood dyscrasias, renal and liver damage, irreversible neuromuscular and CNS changes, and fibrosing alveolitis. Perform CBC, including differential WBC count, and LFTs before starting therapy, every 2nd week for the first 3 months, monthly for the next 3 months, then every 3 months thereafter, and as clinically indicated; d/c while awaiting the results of blood tests. Monitor urinalysis and renal function periodically. Oligospermia and infertility reported in males. Serious infections (eg, fatal sepsis, pneumonia) reported. D/C if serious infection or toxic/hypersensitivity reactions develop. Closely monitor for signs and symptoms of infection during and after treatment; if a new infection develops, perform a prompt and complete diagnostic workup for infection and myelosuppression. Serious skin reactions, some fatal (eg, exfoliative dermatitis, Stevens-Johnson syndrome, toxic epidermal necrolysis), reported; d/c at 1st appearance of skin rash, mucosal lesions, or any other sign of hypersensitivity. Severe, life-threatening, systemic hypersensitivity reactions (eg, drug rash with eosinophilia and systemic symptoms) reported; evaluate immediately if signs/symptoms develop, and d/c if an alternative etiology cannot be established. Maintain adequate fluid intake to prevent crystalluria and stone formation. Closely monitor patients with G6PD deficiency for signs of hemolytic anemia. Do not attempt desensitization in patients who have a history of agranulocytosis, or who have experienced an anaphylactoid reaction with previous sulfasalazine (SSZ) therapy. Serum sulfapyridine (SP) levels >50mcg/mL appear to be associated with increased incidence of adverse reactions. Lab test interactions may occur.

ADVERSE REACTIONS

Anorexia, headache, N/V, gastric distress, reversible oligospermia.

DRUG INTERACTIONS

May reduce absorption of folic acid and digoxin.

PATIENT CONSIDERATIONS

Assessment: Assess for intestinal or urinary obstruction, porphyria, renal dysfunction, severe allergy, bronchial asthma, G6PD deficiency, pregnancy/nursing status, possible drug interactions, history of hypersensitivity to the drug, its metabolites, sulfonamides, or salicylates, history of recurring/chronic infections, and underlying conditions which may predispose patients to infections. Obtain CBC, including differential WBC count, and LFTs.

Monitoring: Monitor for GI intolerance, hypersensitivity/skin reactions, neuromuscular and CNS changes, fibrosing alveolitis, infection, signs of hemolytic anemia (in patients with G6PD deficiency), and other adverse reactions. Monitor CBC, including differential WBC count, and LFTs every 2nd week for the first 3 months, monthly for the next 3 months, then every 3 months thereafter, and as clinically indicated. Monitor urinalysis and renal function periodically, and serum SP levels. Monitor for diarrhea and/or bloody stools in infants fed milk from mothers taking SSZ. Monitor newborns for kernicterus.

Counseling: Inform of possible adverse reactions and need for careful medical supervision. Instruct to seek medical advice if sore throat, fever, pallor, purpura, or jaundice occurs. Inform that UC rarely remits completely and that risk of relapse can be reduced by continued administration at a maintenance dosage. Advise that orange-yellow discoloration of urine or skin may occur.

STORAGE: 25°C (77°F); excursions permitted to 15-30°C (59-86°F).

AZULFIDINE EN-TABS – sulfasalazine RX

Class: 5-aminosalicylic acid derivative/sulfapyridine

ADULT DOSAGE

Ulcerative Colitis

Treatment of mild to moderate ulcerative colitis (UC), adjunctive therapy in severe UC, and to prolong remission period between acute attacks of UC

Initial: 3-4g/day in evenly divided doses w/ intervals not >8 hrs; may initiate w/ a lower dose (eg, 1-2g/day) to reduce GI intolerance

Maint: 2g/day

When endoscopic exam confirms satisfactory improvement, reduce dose to a maint level; if

PEDIATRIC DOSAGE

Ulcerative Colitis

Treatment of mild to moderate ulcerative colitis (UC), adjunctive therapy in severe UC, and to prolong remission period between acute attacks of UC

≥6 Years:

Initial: 40-60mg/kg/24 hrs divided into 3-6 doses

Maint: 30mg/kg/24 hrs divided into 4 doses

When endoscopic exam confirms satisfactory improvement, reduce dose to a maint level; if diarrhea recurs, increase dose to previously effective levels

Indicated particularly in patients w/ UC who cannot take uncoated sulfasalazine tabs because of GI intolerance, and in whom there is evidence that this intolerance is not primarily the result of high blood levels of sulfapyridine and its metabolites

Desensitization Regimen:
Initial: 50-250mg/day
Titrate: Double dose every 4-7 days until desired therapeutic level is achieved; d/c if sensitivity recurs

Rheumatoid Arthritis

Treatment of Patients Who Have Responded Inadequately to Salicylates or Other NSAIDs:
Initial: 0.5-1g/day
Usual: 2g/day in 2 evenly divided doses; may consider increasing to 3g/day if clinical response after 12 weeks is inadequate

Suggested Dosing Schedule:
Week 1: 1 tab qpm
Week 2: 1 tab qam and 1 tab qpm
Week 3: 1 tab qam and 2 tabs qpm
Week 4: 2 tabs qam and 2 tabs qpm

Desensitization Regimen:
Initial: 50-250mg/day
Titrate: Double dose every 4-7 days until desired therapeutic level is achieved; d/c if sensitivity recurs

Concurrent treatment w/ analgesics and/or NSAIDs is recommended at least until effect is apparent

diarrhea recurs, increase dose to previously effective levels

Indicated particularly in patients w/ UC who cannot take uncoated sulfasalazine tabs because of GI intolerance, and in whom there is evidence that this intolerance is not primarily the result of high blood levels of sulfapyridine and its metabolites

Desensitization Regimen:
Initial: 50-250mg/day
Titrate: Double dose every 4-7 days until desired therapeutic level is achieved; d/c if sensitivity recurs

Juvenile Rheumatoid Arthritis

Treatment of Patients w/ Polyarticular-Course Juvenile Rheumatoid Arthritis Who Have Responded Inadequately to Salicylates or Other NSAIDs:
≥6 Years:
Usual: 30-50mg/kg/day in 2 evenly divided doses; begin w/ 1/4-1/3 of planned maint dose and increase weekly until reaching maint dose at 1 month
Max: 2g/day

Desensitization Regimen:
Initial: 50-250mg/day
Titrate: Double dose every 4-7 days until desired therapeutic level is achieved; d/c if sensitivity recurs

Concurrent treatment w/ analgesics and/or NSAIDs is recommended at least until effect is apparent

DOSING CONSIDERATIONS

Other Important Considerations
Gastric Intolerance:
If symptoms of gastric intolerance (eg, anorexia, N/V) occur after 1st few doses, may be alleviated by halving daily dose and subsequently increasing gradually over several days; if gastric intolerance continues, stop drug for 5-7 days, then reintroduce at a lower daily dose

ADMINISTRATION

Oral route

Take in evenly divided doses, preferably pc.
Swallow tabs whole.
Careful monitoring is recommended for doses >2g/day.

HOW SUPPLIED

Tab, Delayed-Release: 500mg

CONTRAINDICATIONS

Hypersensitivity to sulfasalazine, its metabolites, sulfonamides, or salicylates; intestinal or urinary obstruction; porphyria.

WARNINGS/PRECAUTIONS

Caution with hepatic/renal damage, blood dyscrasias, severe allergy, bronchial asthma, history of recurring/chronic infections, or with underlying conditions or concomitant drugs that may predispose patients to infections. Deaths reported from hypersensitivity reactions, agranulocytosis, aplastic anemia, other blood dyscrasias, renal and liver damage, irreversible neuromuscular and CNS changes, and fibrosing alveolitis. Perform CBC, including differential WBC count, and LFTs before starting therapy, every 2nd week for the first 3 months, monthly for the next 3 months, then every 3 months thereafter, and as clinically indicated; d/c while awaiting the results of blood tests. Monitor urinalysis and renal function periodically. Oligospermia and infertility reported in males. Serious infections (eg, fatal sepsis, pneumonia) reported. D/C if serious infection or toxic/hypersensitivity reactions develop. Closely monitor for signs and symptoms of infection during and after treatment; if a new infection develops, perform a prompt/complete diagnostic workup for infection and myelosuppression. Serious skin reactions, some fatal (eg, exfoliative dermatitis, Stevens-Johnson syndrome, toxic epidermal necrolysis), reported; d/c at 1st appearance of skin rash, mucosal lesions, or any other sign of hypersensitivity. Severe, life-threatening, systemic hypersensitivity reactions (eg, drug rash with eosinophilia and systemic symptoms) reported; evaluate immediately if signs/symptoms develop, and d/c if an alternative etiology cannot be established. Maintain adequate fluid intake to prevent crystalluria and stone formation. Closely monitor patients with G6PD deficiency for signs of hemolytic anemia. Do not attempt desensitization in patients who have a history of agranulocytosis, or have experienced an anaphylactoid reaction with previous sulfasalazine (SSZ) therapy. Serum sulfapyridine (SP) levels >50mcg/mL appear to be associated with increased incidence of adverse reactions. D/C immediately if tabs pass without disintegrating. Lab test interactions may occur.

ADVERSE REACTIONS
Anorexia, headache, N/V, gastric distress, reversible oligospermia, dyspepsia, rash, abdominal pain, fever, dizziness, stomatitis, pruritus, abnormal LFTs, leukopenia.

DRUG INTERACTIONS
May reduce absorption of folic acid and digoxin. Increased incidence of GI adverse events (especially nausea) with methotrexate.

PATIENT CONSIDERATIONS

Assessment: Assess for intestinal or urinary obstruction, porphyria, renal dysfunction, severe allergy, bronchial asthma, G6PD deficiency, pregnancy/nursing status, possible drug interactions, history of hypersensitivity to the drug, its metabolites, sulfonamides, or salicylates, history of recurring/chronic infections, and underlying conditions which may predispose patients to infections. Obtain CBC, including differential WBC count, and LFTs.

Monitoring: Monitor for GI intolerance, hypersensitivity/skin reactions, neuromuscular and CNS changes, fibrosing alveolitis, infection, signs of hemolytic anemia (in patients with G6PD deficiency), and other adverse reactions. Monitor CBC, including differential WBC count, and LFTs every 2nd week for the first 3 months, monthly for the next 3 months, then every 3 months thereafter, and as clinically indicated. Monitor urinalysis and renal function periodically, and serum SP levels. Monitor for tabs passing without disintegrating. Monitor for diarrhea and/or bloody stools in infants fed milk from mothers taking SSZ. Monitor newborns for kernicterus.

Counseling: Inform of possible adverse effects and need for careful medical supervision. Instruct to seek medical advice if sore throat, fever, pallor, purpura, or jaundice occurs. Advise that orange-yellow discoloration of urine or skin may occur. Inform that UC rarely remits completely and that risk of relapse can be substantially reduced by continued administration at a maintenance dosage. Inform that RA rarely remits; instruct to follow up with physician to determine the need for continued administration.

STORAGE: 25°C (77°F); excursions permitted to 15-30°C (59-86°F).

BACLOFEN – baclofen

RX

Class: GABA analogue

ADULT DOSAGE

Spasticity

Alleviation of signs and symptoms of spasticity resulting from multiple sclerosis. May be effective in spinal cord injuries and other spinal cord diseases

Initial: 5mg tid for 3 days
Titrate: May increase by 5mg tid every 3 days
Usual: 40-80mg/day
Max: 80mg/day (20mg qid)

PEDIATRIC DOSAGE

Spasticity

Alleviation of signs and symptoms of spasticity resulting from multiple sclerosis. May be effective in spinal cord injuries and other spinal cord diseases

≥12 Years:
Initial: 5mg tid for 3 days
Titrate: May increase by 5mg tid every 3 days
Usual: 40-80mg/day
Max: 80mg/day (20mg qid)

DOSING CONSIDERATIONS

Renal Impairment
Dose reduction may be necessary

ADMINISTRATION
Oral route

HOW SUPPLIED
Tab: 10mg*, 20mg* *scored

CONTRAINDICATIONS
Hypersensitivity to baclofen.

WARNINGS/PRECAUTIONS
Not recommended w/ stroke, cerebral palsy, and Parkinson's disease. Hallucinations and seizures reported w/ abrupt withdrawal; reduce dose slowly when therapy is discontinued except for serious

adverse reactions. Caution w/ impaired renal function. Should be used during pregnancy only if the benefit clearly justifies the potential risk to fetus. May impair physical/mental abilities. Caution where spasticity is utilized to sustain upright posture and balance in locomotion or to obtain increased function. Deterioration in seizure control and EEG reported; monitor clinical state and EEG at regular intervals in patients w/ epilepsy. Ovarian cysts reported in patients treated for up to 1 yr; in most cases these cysts disappeared spontaneously while patients continued therapy.

ADVERSE REACTIONS

Drowsiness, dizziness, weakness, fatigue, confusion, headache, insomnia, hypotension, nausea, constipation, urinary frequency.

DRUG INTERACTIONS

Additive CNS effects w/ alcohol and other CNS depressants.

PATIENT CONSIDERATIONS

Assessment: Assess for drug hypersensitivity, stroke, cerebral palsy, Parkinson's disease, epilepsy, renal impairment, pregnancy/nursing status, and possible drug interactions.

Monitoring: Monitor for hallucinations, seizures, ovarian cysts, and other adverse reactions. Monitor clinical state and EEG at regular intervals in patients w/ epilepsy.

Counseling: Instruct to take ud. Instruct to notify physician of any adverse effects. Caution against performing hazardous tasks (eg, operating machinery/driving). Instruct to notify physician if pregnant/nursing.

STORAGE: 20-25°C (68-77°F); excursions permitted to 15-30°C (59-86°F).

BACTROBAN TOPICAL – mupirocin RX

Class: Bacterial protein synthesis inhibitor

ADULT DOSAGE

Secondarily Infected Traumatic Skin Lesions

Lesions up to 10cm in length or 100cm^2 in area due to *Staphylococcus aureus* and *Streptococcus pyogenes*

Cre:

Apply a small amount to the affected area tid for 10 days; reevaluate if no clinical response w/in 3-5 days

Impetigo

Due to *S. aureus* and *S. pyogenes*

Oint:

Apply a small amount to the affected area tid for up to 10 days; reevaluate if no clinical response w/in 3-5 days

PEDIATRIC DOSAGE

Secondarily Infected Traumatic Skin Lesions

Lesions up to 10cm in length or 100cm^2 in area due to *S. aureus* and *S. pyogenes*

3 Months-16 Years:

Cre:

Apply a small amount to the affected area tid for 10 days; reevaluate if no clinical response w/in 3-5 days

Impetigo

Due to *S. aureus* and *S. pyogenes*

2 Months-16 Years:

Oint:

Apply a small amount to the affected area tid for up to 10 days; reevaluate if no clinical response w/in 3-5 days

DOSING CONSIDERATIONS

Concomitant Medications

Do not apply concurrently w/ any other lotions, creams, or ointments

ADMINISTRATION

Topical route

Apply w/ a cotton swab or gauze pad.
Cover treated area w/ gauze dressing if desired.

HOW SUPPLIED

Cre: 2% [15g, 30g]; **Oint:** 2% [22g]

CONTRAINDICATIONS

Known hypersensitivity to mupirocin or any of the excipients of cre/oint.

WARNINGS/PRECAUTIONS

Systemic allergic reactions reported. Avoid contact w/ eyes; rinse well w/ water in case of accidental contact. D/C and institute appropriate alternative therapy if sensitization or severe local irritation occurs. *Clostridium difficile*-associated diarrhea (CDAD) reported; may need to d/c if CDAD is suspected/confirmed. Prolonged use may result in overgrowth of nonsusceptible microorganisms, including fungi. Not for use on mucosal surfaces. **Oint:** Polyethylene glycol can be absorbed from open wounds and damaged skin and is excreted by the kidneys; avoid use in conditions where absorption of large quantities of polyethylene glycol is possible, especially if there is evidence of moderate or severe renal impairment. Avoid use w/ IV cannulae or at central IV sites; may promote fungal infections and antimicrobial resistance.

ADVERSE REACTIONS

Cre: Headache, burning at application site, nausea, rash.
Oint: Burning, stinging, pain, itching.

PATIENT CONSIDERATIONS

Assessment: Assess for hypersensitivity to the drug and pregnancy/nursing status.

Monitoring: Monitor for systemic allergic reactions, sensitization, severe local irritation, CDAD, and other adverse reactions.

Counseling: Instruct to use only ud. Inform that medication is for external use only. Instruct to avoid contact w/ eyes; advise to rinse thoroughly w/ water if product gets in the eyes. Advise not to use in the nose. Instruct to wash hands before and after applying the product. Inform that treated area can be covered w/ a gauze dressing if desired. Advise to d/c medication and contact physician if irritation, severe itching, or rash occurs. Instruct to report to physician or go to the nearest emergency room if severe allergic reactions (eg, swelling of the lips/face/tongue, wheezing) occur. Advise to notify physician if no improvement is seen in 3-5 days.

STORAGE: **Cre:** ≤25°C (77°F). Do not freeze. **Oint:** 20-25°C (68-77°F).

BELBUCA – buprenorphine

CIII

Class: Partial opioid agonist

Exposes patients and other users to risks of opioid addiction, abuse, and misuse, which can lead to overdose and death; assess each patient's risk prior to prescribing, and monitor regularly for development of these behaviors/conditions. Serious, life-threatening, or fatal respiratory depression may occur; monitor for respiratory depression, especially during initiation or following a dose increase. Misuse or abuse by chewing, swallowing, snorting, or injecting buprenorphine extracted from the buccal film will result in uncontrolled delivery of buprenorphine and pose a significant risk of overdose and death. Accidental exposure, especially in children, can result in a fatal overdose. Prolonged use during pregnancy can result in neonatal opioid withdrawal syndrome; advise of the risk and ensure availability of appropriate treatment if opioid use is required for a prolonged period in a pregnant woman.

ADULT DOSAGE

Severe Pain (Daily, Around-the-Clock Management)

Management of pain severe enough to require daily, around-the-clock, long-term opioid treatment and for which alternative treatment options are inadequate

Initial:

Opioid-Naive Patients: 75mcg qd or, if tolerated, q12h for at least 4 days, then increase to 150mcg q12h

Conversion from Other Opioids: See conversions section below

Titrate:

Increase in increments of 150mcg q12h, no more frequently than every 4 days

Doses up to 450mcg q12h were studied in opioid-naive patients

Max:

900mcg q12h

Consider an alternate analgesic if pain is not adequately managed on 900mcg

Conversions

From Other Opioids:

To reduce the risk of opioid withdrawal, taper to no more than 30mg oral morphine sulfate equivalents (MSEs) daily before beginning Belbuca. Following analgesic taper, base the starting dose on patient's daily opioid dose prior to taper; may require additional short-acting analgesics during the taper period and during titration

PEDIATRIC DOSAGE

Pediatric use may not have been established

B

Initial Belbuca Dose Based on Prior Daily Opioid Analgesic Dose Before Taper:
<30mg Oral MSEs: 75mcg qd or q12h
30-89mg Oral MSEs: 150mcg q12h
90-160mg Oral MSEs: 300mcg q12h
>160mg Oral MSEs: Consider alternate analgesic

Doses of 600mcg, 750mcg, and 900mcg are only for use following titration from lower doses of Belbuca

From Methadone:
The ratio between methadone and other opioid agonists may vary widely as a function of previous dose exposure. Methadone has a long $T_{1/2}$ and can accumulate in the plasma; monitor closely during conversion

DOSING CONSIDERATIONS

Hepatic Impairment

Severe (Child-Pugh Class C): Reduce initial and titration dose by 1/2 that of patients w/ normal liver function (from 150mcg to 75mcg)

Discontinuation

Use gradual downward titration; do not abruptly d/c

Other Important Considerations

Oral Mucositis: Reduce initial dose and titration incremental dose by 1/2 compared to patients w/o mucositis

ADMINISTRATION

Buccal route

Apply to the buccal mucosa q12h.
Avoid applying to areas of the mouth w/ any open sores or lesions.
Use the tongue to wet the inside of the cheek or rinse mouth w/ water to wet the area for placement.
Apply immediately after removal from the individually sealed package.
Place the yellow side of the film against the inside of the cheek.
Hold the entire film in place w/ clean, dry fingers for 5 sec and then leave in place on the inside of the cheek until fully dissolved.
Film will completely dissolve after application, usually w/in 30 min. Do not manipulate film w/ tongue or finger(s).
Avoid eating food and drinking liquids until the film has dissolved.
Dispose of unused film as soon as it is no longer needed; refer to PI for disposal instructions.

HOW SUPPLIED

Film, Buccal: 75mcg, 150mcg, 300mcg, 450mcg, 600mcg, 750mcg, 900mcg [60[s]]

CONTRAINDICATIONS

Significant respiratory depression, acute or severe bronchial asthma in an unmonitored setting or in the absence of resuscitative equipment, known/suspected GI obstruction (eg, paralytic ileus), hypersensitivity (eg, anaphylaxis) to buprenorphine.

WARNINGS/PRECAUTIONS

Reserve use in patients for whom alternative treatment options are ineffective, not tolerated, or would be otherwise inadequate to provide sufficient management of pain. Should be prescribed only by healthcare professionals who are knowledgeable in the use of potent opioids for the management of chronic pain. Life-threatening respiratory depression is more likely to occur in elderly, cachectic, or debilitated patients. Increased risk of decreased respiratory drive, including apnea, even at recommended doses in patients w/ significant COPD or cor pulmonale, and those w/ substantially decreased respiratory reserve, hypoxia, hypercapnia, or preexisting respiratory depression; monitor closely (especially when initiating/titrating therapy) or, alternatively, consider other nonopioid analgesics. QTc prolongation reported; caution in patients w/ hypokalemia, hypomagnesemia, or clinically unstable cardiac disease and periodically monitor ECG in these patients. Avoid use in patients w/ history of or immediate family w/ long QT syndrome. May cause severe hypotension, including orthostatic hypotension and syncope in ambulatory patients; increased risk in patients whose ability to maintain BP has already been compromised by a reduced blood volume or concurrent administration of certain CNS depressants. Avoid in patients w/ circulatory shock. Monitor patients who may be susceptible to intracranial effects of carbon dioxide retention (eg, those w/ evidence of increased intracranial pressure or brain tumors) for signs of sedation and respiratory depression, particularly when initiating therapy. May obscure clinical course in patients w/ a head injury. Avoid w/ impaired consciousness or coma. Cases of cytolytic hepatitis and hepatitis w/ jaundice reported in patients receiving SL buprenorphine for opioid dependence treatment. Obtain baseline liver enzyme levels in patients at increased risk of hepatotoxicity (eg, history of excessive alcohol intake, IV drug abuse, or liver disease), and monitor periodically during treatment. Monitor for signs/symptoms of toxicity or overdose in patients w/ moderate or severe hepatic impairment. Cases of acute and chronic hypersensitivity, bronchospasm, angioneurotic edema, and anaphylactic shock reported. May cause spasm of the sphincter of Oddi. May increase serum amylase; monitor patients w/ biliary tract disease, including acute pancreatitis, for worsening symptoms. May increase seizure frequency in patients w/ seizure disorders and the risk of seizures occurring in other clinical settings associated w/ seizures. Cancer patients w/ oral mucositis may absorb buprenorphine more rapidly than intended; monitor for signs/symptoms of toxicity/overdose caused by increased levels of buprenorphine. May impair mental/physical abilities. Caution in elderly.

ADVERSE REACTIONS

N/V, constipation, headache, dizziness, somnolence, fatigue, diarrhea, dry mouth, URTI.

DRUG INTERACTIONS

Hypotension, profound sedation, coma, or respiratory depression may occur if used concomitantly w/ alcohol or other CNS depressants (eg, sedatives, anxiolytics, hypnotics); consider dose reduction of one or both drugs. Closely monitor elderly, cachectic, and debilitated patients when therapy is coadministered w/ other drugs that depress respiration. Avoid w/ Class IA antiarrhythmics (eg, quinidine, procainamide, disopyramide) or Class III antiarrhythmics (eg, sotalol, amiodarone, dofetilide), or other medications that prolong the QT interval. Closely monitor w/ concomitant benzodiazepines; coma and death associated w/ the misuse/abuse of the combination of buprenorphine and benzodiazepines reported. CYP3A4 inhibitors may increase levels, resulting in increased/prolonged opioid effects, particularly when an inhibitor is added after a stable dose of therapy is achieved. If concomitant use of a CYP3A4 inhibitor is necessary, consider dose reduction of Belbuca and monitor for respiratory depression/sedation at frequent intervals; if a CYP3A4 inhibitor is discontinued, consider increasing Belbuca dose and monitor for signs of opioid withdrawal. CYP3A4 inducers may decrease levels, potentially resulting in decreased efficacy or onset of a withdrawal syndrome. If concomitant use of a CYP3A4 inducer is necessary, consider increasing Belbuca dose and monitor for signs of opioid withdrawal; if a CYP3A4 inducer is discontinued, consider Belbuca dose reduction and monitor for signs of respiratory depression. Avoid w/ mixed agonist/antagonist and partial agonist opioid analgesics (eg, butorphanol, nalbuphine, pentazocine); may reduce analgesic effect and/or precipitate withdrawal symptoms. May enhance neuromuscular blocking action of skeletal muscle relaxants and produce an increased degree of respiratory depression; monitor and decrease dose of therapy and/or the muscle relaxant as necessary. May reduce efficacy of diuretics; monitor for signs of diminished diuresis and/or effects on BP and increase diuretic dose prn. Concomitant use w/ anticholinergics may increase risk of urinary retention and/or severe constipation, which may lead to paralytic ileus; monitor for signs of urinary retention or reduced gastric motility. Monitor dose of patients on chronic treatment if NNRTIs are added to treatment regimen. Certain protease inhibitors w/ CYP3A4 inhibitory activity (atazanavir and atazanavir/ritonavir [RTV]) resulted in elevated levels of buprenorphine and norbuprenorphine; monitor patients taking atazanavir w/ and w/o RTV, and dose reduction of Belbuca may be warranted.

PATIENT CONSIDERATIONS

Assessment: Assess for hypersensitivity to therapy, risk of addiction/abuse/misuse, respiratory depression, mucositis, GI obstruction, circulatory shock, chronic pulmonary disease, long QT syndrome, impaired consciousness or coma, biliary tract disease, seizure disorders, hepatic impairment, other conditions where treatment is contraindicated or cautioned, pregnancy/nursing status, and possible drug interactions. Obtain baseline liver enzyme levels in patients at increased risk of hepatotoxicity.

Monitoring: Monitor for respiratory depression (especially w/in the first 24-72 hrs of initiating therapy and following dose increases), misuse/abuse, QTc prolongation, severe hypotension, hepatotoxicity, hypersensitivity, bronchospasm, angioneurotic edema, anaphylactic shock, spasm of the sphincter of Oddi, serum amylase increases, worsened seizure control in patients w/ history of seizure disorders, and other adverse reactions. Monitor cancer patients w/ oral mucositis for signs/symptoms of toxicity/overdose. Periodically monitor ECG in patients w/ hypokalemia, hypomagnesemia, or clinically unstable cardiac disease. Periodically monitor liver enzyme levels in patients at increased risk of hepatotoxicity. Periodically reassess the continued need for therapy.

Counseling: Advise about risks/benefits of therapy. Inform that use of therapy, even when taken as recommended, can result in addiction, abuse, and misuse; instruct not to share w/ others and to take steps to protect from theft or misuse. Inform of the risk of life-threatening respiratory depression; advise how to recognize respiratory depression and instruct to seek medical attention if breathing difficulties develop. Inform that accidental exposure, especially in children, may result in respiratory depression or death; instruct to store securely and to dispose of unused product by opening unused packages and flushing the film down the toilet. Inform about interaction w/ alcohol, other CNS depressants, and benzodiazepines. Inform that therapy may cause orthostatic hypotension and syncope; instruct how to recognize symptoms of low BP and how to reduce risk of serious consequences should hypotension occur (eg, sit or lie down, carefully rise from a sitting or lying position). Advise of the risk for severe constipation and anaphylaxis. Inform that therapy may impair ability to perform potentially hazardous activities (eg, driving a car or operating heavy machinery); advise not to perform such tasks until effects of medication are known. Inform of risk of neonatal opioid withdrawal syndrome, and inform that therapy may cause fetal harm; instruct to inform healthcare provider of a known or suspected pregnancy. Inform that breastfeeding is not recommended during treatment. Inform about important administration and disposal instructions.

STORAGE: 25°C (77°F); excursions permitted to 15-30°C (59-86°F).

BELEODAQ – belinostat

RX

Class: Histone deacetylase (HDAC) inhibitor

ADULT DOSAGE

Peripheral T-Cell Lymphoma

Relapsed or Refractory:

1000mg/m² IV infusion over 30 min qd on Days 1-5 of a 21-day cycle

May repeat cycles every 21 days until disease progression or unacceptable toxicity

Dosing Based on Genotype Consideration

Patients Homozygous for the UGT1A1*28 Allele:

Reduce starting dose to 750mg/m²

PEDIATRIC DOSAGE

Pediatric use may not have been established

DOSING CONSIDERATIONS

Adverse Reactions

Hematologic Toxicities:

Nadir ANC <0.5 x 10^9/L (Any Platelet Count): Decrease dose by 25% (750mg/m²)

Platelet Count <25 x 10^9/L (Any Nadir ANC): Decrease dose by 25% (750mg/m²)

Recurrent Nadir ANC <0.5 x 10^9/L and/or Recurrent Platelet Count <25 x 10^9/L After 2 Dosage Reductions: D/C therapy

Nonhematologic Toxicities:

Any CTCAE Grade 3 or 4 Adverse Reaction: Decrease dose by 25% (750mg/m²); for N/V, and diarrhea, only dose modify if the duration is >7 days w/ supportive management

Recurrence of CTCAE Grade 3 or 4 Adverse Reaction After 2 Dosage Reductions: D/C therapy

ADMINISTRATION

IV route

Reconstitution and Infusion Instructions

1. Add 9mL of sterile water for inj into the vial w/ a suitable syringe to achieve a concentration of 50mg/mL
2. Swirl the contents of the vial until there are no visible particles in the resulting sol
3. Withdraw the volume needed for the required dosage (based on the 50mg/mL concentration and the patient's BSA) and transfer to an infusion bag containing 250mL of 0.9% NaCl inj
4. Connect the infusion bag containing drug sol to an infusion set w/ a 0.22µm in-line filter for administration
5. Infuse over 30 min; may extend to 45 min if infusion-site pain or other symptoms potentially attributable to the infusion occur

HOW SUPPLIED

Inj: 500mg

WARNINGS/PRECAUTIONS

May cause thrombocytopenia, leukopenia (neutropenia and lymphopenia), and/or anemia. Serious and sometimes fatal infections, including pneumonia and sepsis, reported; do not administer to patients with an active infection. Patients with a history of extensive or intensive chemotherapy may be at higher risk of life-threatening infections. May cause fatal hepatotoxicity and LFT abnormalities. Tumor lysis syndrome (TLS) reported; caution with advanced stage disease and/or high tumor burden. N/V and diarrhea reported and may require the use of antiemetic and antidiarrheal medications. May cause fetal harm.

ADVERSE REACTIONS

N/V, fatigue, pyrexia, anemia, constipation, diarrhea, dyspnea, rash, peripheral edema, cough, thrombocytopenia, pruritus, chills, increased blood lactate dehydrogenase, decreased appetite.

DRUG INTERACTIONS

Avoid with strong UGT1A1 inhibitors.

PATIENT CONSIDERATIONS

Assessment: Assess for active infection, history of extensive or intensive chemotherapy, advanced stage disease and/or high tumor burden, reduced UGT1A1 activity, pregnancy/nursing status, and possible drug interactions. Obtain baseline CBCs. Perform serum chemistry tests, including renal and hepatic functions, prior to the start of the 1st dose of each cycle.

Monitoring: Monitor for signs/symptoms of hematologic/hepatic/GI toxicity, infections, TLS, and other adverse reactions. Monitor CBCs weekly.

Counseling: Instruct to report symptoms of N/V, diarrhea, thrombocytopenia, leukopenia, anemia, and infection. Inform of the potential risk to the fetus and for women to avoid pregnancy while receiving therapy. Advise to understand the importance of monitoring LFT abnormalities and to immediately report potential symptoms of liver injury.

STORAGE: 20-25°C (68-77°F); excursions permitted between 15-30°C (59-86°F). Retain in original package until use. Reconstituted Sol: 15-25°C (59-77°F) for up to 12 hrs. Infusion Bag with Drug Sol: 15-25°C (59-77°F) for up to 36 hrs including infusion time.

BELSOMRA – suvorexant — CIV

Class: Orexin receptor antagonist

ADULT DOSAGE

Insomnia

Treatment of insomnia characterized by difficulties w/ sleep onset and/or sleep maintenance

10mg, taken no more than once per night and w/in 30 min of going to bed, w/ at least 7 hrs remaining before planned time of awakening

Titrate: May increase dose if 10mg is well tolerated but not effective

Max: 20mg qd

PEDIATRIC DOSAGE

Pediatric use may not have been established

DOSING CONSIDERATIONS

Concomitant Medications

Other CNS Depressants:

Dose adjustment of suvorexant and/or the other drug(s) may be necessary

Moderate CYP3A Inhibitors:

Recommended Dose: 5mg

Max: 10mg

Strong CYP3A Inhibitors:

Not recommended

Hepatic Impairment

Severe: Not recommended

ADMINISTRATION

Oral route

May be taken w/ or w/o food; however, for faster sleep onset, do not administer w/ or soon after a meal.

HOW SUPPLIED

Tab: 5mg, 10mg, 15mg, 20mg

CONTRAINDICATIONS

Narcolepsy.

WARNINGS/PRECAUTIONS

Exposure is increased in obese patients and in women. Particularly in obese women, the increased risk of exposure-related adverse effects should be considered before increasing the dose. May impair mental/physical abilities. Risk of next-day impairment, including impaired driving, is increased if taken w/ less than a full night of sleep remaining or if a higher than recommended dose is taken. Initiate only after careful evaluation of patient; failure of insomnia to remit after 7-10 days of treatment may indicate presence of a primary psychiatric and/or medical illness. Variety of cognitive and behavioral changes (eg, amnesia, anxiety, hallucinations) reported. Complex behaviors (eg, sleep-driving) may occur; strongly consider discontinuation for patients who report any complex sleep behavior. Worsening of depression and suicidal thoughts and actions (including completed suicides) reported in primarily depressed patients treated w/ sedative-hypnotics; immediately evaluate patients w/ suicidal ideation or any new behavioral sign/symptom. Increase in suicidal ideation was observed to be dose-dependent in patients taking suvorexant. Consider effects on respiratory function when prescribing to patients w/ compromised respiratory function. Sleep paralysis and hypnagogic/hypnopompic hallucinations, including vivid and disturbing perceptions by the patient, may occur. Symptoms similar to mild cataplexy may occur, w/ risk increasing w/ the dose. Has an abuse potential; carefully monitor patients w/ a history of abuse or addiction to alcohol or other drugs.

ADVERSE REACTIONS

Somnolence, headache, dizziness.

DRUG INTERACTIONS

See Dosing Considerations. Coadministration w/ other CNS depressants (eg, benzodiazepines, opioids, TCAs, alcohol) increases the risk of CNS depression, abnormal thinking, and behavioral changes. Avoid w/ alcohol. The risk of next-day impairment is increased if coadministered w/ other CNS depressants or other drugs that increase suvorexant levels. Not recommended w/ other drugs used to treat insomnia. Strong CYP3A inducers (eg, rifampin, carbamazepine, phenytoin) may substantially decrease exposure and reduce efficacy. Concomitant administration w/ digoxin slightly increased digoxin levels; monitor digoxin levels during coadministration.

PATIENT CONSIDERATIONS

Assessment: Assess for narcolepsy, physical and/or psychiatric disorders, depression, suicidal ideation, compromised respiratory function, severe hepatic impairment, history of abuse/addiction to alcohol or other drugs, pregnancy/nursing status, and possible drug interactions.

Monitoring: Monitor for somnolence, CNS depressant effects, next-day impairment, cognitive and behavioral changes, complex behaviors, worsening of depression/suicidal ideation, sleep paralysis, hypnagogic/hypnopompic hallucinations, cataplexy-like symptoms, abuse, and other adverse reactions.

Counseling: Caution against driving or engaging in other activities requiring full alertness w/in 8 hrs of taking suvorexant. Instruct to contact physician if sleep-driving or other complex behaviors occur. Advise to report any worsening of depression or suicidal thoughts immediately. Advise not to take suvorexant if patient drank alcohol that evening or before bed. Advise to take only when preparing for or getting into bed and only if patient can stay in bed for a full night before being active again. Advise to report all prescription and nonprescription medicines to the physician.

STORAGE: 20-25°C (68-77°F); excursions permitted to 15-30°C (59-86°F). Protect from light and moisture.

Belviq – lorcaserin hydrochloride

CIV

Class: Serotonin 2C receptor agonist

ADULT DOSAGE

Weight Loss

Adjunct to reduced-calorie diet and increased physical activity for chronic weight management in patients w/ initial BMI ≥30kg/m², or ≥27kg/m² in the presence of ≥1 weight-related comorbid condition

Usual: 10mg bid

Evaluate response to therapy by Week 12; d/c therapy if patient has not lost at least 5% of baseline weight

PEDIATRIC DOSAGE

Pediatric use may not have been established

ADMINISTRATION

Oral route

Take w/ or w/o food

HOW SUPPLIED

Tab: 10mg

CONTRAINDICATIONS

Pregnancy.

WARNINGS/PRECAUTIONS

Potentially life-threatening serotonin syndrome or neuroleptic malignant syndrome (NMS)-like reactions reported; monitor for emergence of serotonin syndrome or NMS-like signs/symptoms. Regurgitant cardiac valvular disease reported; evaluate and consider discontinuation of therapy if signs/symptoms of valvular heart disease develop. Caution with chronic heart failure (CHF). May impair mental/physical abilities. Monitor for emergence or worsening of depression, suicidal thoughts or behavior, and/or any unusual changes in mood or behavior; d/c in patients who experience suicidal thoughts or behaviors. Hypoglycemia reported; measure blood glucose levels prior to and during therapy in patients with type 2 diabetes. Caution in men who have conditions that might predispose them to priapism, or in men with anatomical deformation of the penis. Caution with bradycardia or history of heart block >1st degree, moderate renal impairment, and severe hepatic impairment. Not recommended with severe renal impairment or ESRD. Decrease in WBCs and RBCs reported; consider monitoring CBC periodically during therapy. May elevate prolactin levels. May increase risk for pulmonary HTN.

ADVERSE REACTIONS

Nasopharyngitis, headache, constipation, diarrhea, hypoglycemia, cough, dizziness, fatigue, back pain, N/V, dry mouth, URTI, peripheral edema, UTI, muscle spasms.

DRUG INTERACTIONS

Use extreme caution, particularly during initiation and dose increases, with drugs that may affect the serotonergic neurotransmitter system (eg, triptans, drugs that impair metabolism of serotonin including MAOIs [eg, linezolid], SSRIs, SNRIs, dextromethorphan, TCAs, bupropion, lithium, tramadol, tryptophan, St. John's wort, antipsychotics, other dopamine antagonists); d/c lorcaserin and any concomitant serotonergic or antidopaminergic agents immediately if serotonin syndrome occurs. Consider decreasing dose of non-glucose dependent antidiabetic medications in order to mitigate risk of hypoglycemia. Caution with CYP2D6 substrates. Avoid with serotonergic and dopaminergic drugs that are potent 5-HT_{2B} receptor agonists and are known to increase the risk for cardiac valvulopathy (eg, cabergoline). Caution with medications indicated for erectile dysfunction (eg, PDE-5 inhibitors).

PATIENT CONSIDERATIONS

Assessment: Assess for CHF, bradycardia or history of heart block >1st degree, renal/hepatic impairment, pregnancy/nursing status, and possible drug interactions. Assess for conditions in men that might predispose them to priapism and assess for anatomical deformities of the penis. Assess baseline body weight and CBC. Assess baseline blood glucose levels in patients with type 2 diabetes.

Monitoring: Monitor for signs/symptoms of serotonin syndrome or NMS-like reactions, valvular heart disease, emergence or worsening of depression, suicidal thoughts or behavior, any unusual changes in mood or behavior, and other adverse reactions. Monitor CBC periodically during therapy. Monitor blood glucose levels in patients with type 2 diabetes. Evaluate response to treatment by Week 12 of therapy.

Counseling: Inform about the risk and benefits of the drug. Inform that therapy is indicated for chronic weight management only in conjunction with a reduced-calorie diet and increased physical activity. Instruct to d/c therapy if patient has not achieved 5% weight loss by 12 weeks of therapy. Inform of the possibility of serotonin or NMS-like reactions. Instruct to use caution when operating hazardous machinery, including automobiles, until aware of the effects of the medication. Instruct not to increase the dose. Instruct to notify physician if signs/symptoms of valvular heart disease, emergence or worsening of depression, suicidal thoughts or behavior, or if any unusual changes in mood or behavior develop. Instruct men who have an erection lasting >4 hrs to immediately d/c and seek emergency medical attention. Advise to avoid pregnancy/breastfeeding while on therapy and to inform physician if planning to get pregnant/breastfeed. Instruct to inform physician about all medications, nutritional supplements, and vitamins that patient is taking while on therapy.

STORAGE: 25°C (77°F); excursions permitted to 15-30°C (59-86°F).

BENAZEPRIL — benazepril hydrochloride

RX

Class: ACE inhibitor

D/C when pregnancy is detected. Drugs that act directly on the renin-angiotensin system (RAS) can cause injury/death to the developing fetus.

OTHER BRAND NAMES

Lotensin

ADULT DOSAGE

Hypertension

Initial: 10mg qd; 5mg qd in patients on a diuretic

Maint: 20-40mg/day as single dose or in 2 equally divided doses. A dose of 80mg gives an increased response, but experience w/ this dose is limited

May add a low dose of diuretic if BP is not controlled

PEDIATRIC DOSAGE

Hypertension

≥6 Years:

Initial: 0.2mg/kg qd

Max: 0.6mg/kg qd (or 40mg/day)

DOSING CONSIDERATIONS

Renal Impairment

Adults:

GFR <30mL/min/1.73m² (SrCr >3mg/dL):
Initial: 5mg qd
Titrate: May increase until BP is controlled
Max: 40mg/day

Pediatric Patients:
GFR <30mL/min/1.73m²: Not recommended

ADMINISTRATION

Oral route

Preparation of Sus (for 150mL of a 2mg/mL Sus):

1. Add 75mL of Ora-Plus oral suspending vehicle to an amber polyethylene terephthalate (PET) bottle containing 15 benazepril 20mg tabs, and shake for at least 2 min.
2. Allow the sus to stand for a minimum of 1 hr.
3. After the standing time, shake the sus for a minimum of 1 additional min.
4. Add 75mL of Ora-Sweet oral syrup vehicle to the bottle and shake the sus to disperse the ingredients.
5. Store the sus at 2-8°C (36-46°F) for up to 30 days in the PET bottle.
6. Shake before each use.

HOW SUPPLIED

Tab: 5mg; (Lotensin) 10mg, 20mg, 40mg

CONTRAINDICATIONS

Hypersensitivity to benazepril or to any other ACE inhibitors, history of angioedema w/ or w/o previous ACE inhibitor treatment, coadministration w/ aliskiren in patients w/ diabetes.

WARNINGS/PRECAUTIONS

Head/neck angioedema reported; d/c and institute appropriate therapy immediately. Patients w/ a history of angioedema unrelated to ACE inhibitor therapy may be at increased risk of angioedema during therapy. Higher rate of angioedema in blacks than nonblacks. Intestinal angioedema reported. Anaphylactoid reactions reported during desensitization w/ hymenoptera venom, dialysis w/ high-flux membranes, and LDL apheresis w/ dextran sulfate absorption. May cause changes in renal function, including acute renal failure, especially in patients whose renal function may depend on the activity of the RAS; consider withholding or discontinuing therapy if a clinically significant decrease in renal function develops. May cause symptomatic hypotension, sometimes complicated by oliguria, progressive azotemia, acute renal failure, or death; closely monitor patients at risk of excessive hypotension for the first 2 weeks of treatment and whenever the dose of benazepril and/or diuretic is increased; correct by volume expansion if hypotension occurs. Avoid in patients who are hemodynamically unstable after acute MI. Hypotension may occur w/ major surgery or during anesthesia. May cause hyperkalemia; periodically monitor serum K^+ during therapy. Associated w/ a syndrome that starts w/ cholestatic jaundice and progresses to fulminant hepatic necrosis and (sometimes) death; d/c therapy if jaundice or marked hepatic enzymes elevations develop. Less antihypertensive effect in blacks than in nonblacks as monotherapy. Caution in elderly.

ADVERSE REACTIONS

Headache, dizziness.

DRUG INTERACTIONS

See Contraindications. Initiation of therapy in patients on diuretics (especially those in whom diuretic therapy was recently instituted) may result in excessive reduction of BP; d/c or decrease the dose of diuretic prior to initiation of treatment w/ benazepril to minimize the possibility of hypotensive effects. K^+-sparing diuretics (eg, spironolactone, amiloride, triamterene) may increase risk of hyperkalemia; frequently monitor serum K^+ if concomitant use of such agents is indicated. Attenuates K^+ loss caused by thiazide-type diuretics. Increased risk of hyperkalemia w/ K^+-containing salt substitutes or K^+ supplements. Concomitant administration w/ antidiabetic medicines (insulins, oral hypoglycemic agents) may increase risk of hypoglycemia. Coadministration of NSAIDs, including selective COX-2 inhibitors, in patients who are elderly, volume-depleted, or w/ compromised renal function, may result in deterioration of renal function, including possible acute renal failure; monitor renal function periodically in patients receiving concomitant therapy w/ NSAIDs. Antihypertensive effect may be attenuated by NSAIDs. Dual blockade of the RAS is associated w/ increased risks of hypotension, hyperkalemia, and changes in renal function (including acute renal failure); in general, avoid combined use of RAS inhibitors, or closely monitor BP, renal function, and electrolytes w/ concomitant agents that affect the RAS. Avoid w/ aliskiren in patients w/ renal impairment (GFR <60mL/min). Coadministration w/ mammalian target of rapamycin (mTOR) inhibitor (eg, temsirolimus, sirolimus, everolimus) therapy may increase risk for angioedema; monitor for signs of angioedema. Lithium toxicity reported; monitor serum lithium levels during concurrent use. Nitritoid reactions reported w/ injectable gold.

PATIENT CONSIDERATIONS

Assessment: Assess for history of angioedema w/ or w/o previous ACE inhibitor treatment, hypersensitivity to drug, risk factors for hyperkalemia, risk of excessive hypotension, renal impairment, pregnancy/nursing status, and possible drug interactions.

Monitoring: Monitor for angioedema, anaphylactoid reactions, hyperkalemia, and other adverse reactions. Monitor BP, LFTs, serum K^+, and renal function.

Counseling: Inform female patients of childbearing age about the consequences of exposure to benazepril during pregnancy and discuss treatment options w/ women planning to become pregnant; instruct to report pregnancies to physician as soon as possible. Advise to d/c therapy and to immediately report to physician signs/symptoms of angioedema. Instruct to report to physician lightheadedness, especially during the 1st few days of therapy; if syncope occurs, advise to d/c therapy until physician is consulted. Inform that excessive perspiration, dehydration, and other causes of volume depletion (eg, vomiting, diarrhea) may lead to an excessive fall in BP. Instruct not to use K^+ supplements or salt substitutes containing K^+ w/o consulting physician. Advise diabetic patients treated w/ oral antidiabetic agents or insulin to closely monitor for hypoglycemia, especially during the 1st month of combined use.

STORAGE: 20-25°C (68-77°F); excursions permitted to 15-30°C (59-86°F). Protect from moisture. **Lotensin:** ≤30°C (86°F). Protect from moisture.

BENICAR – olmesartan medoxomil

RX

Class: Angiotensin II receptor blocker (ARB)

D/C when pregnancy is detected. Drugs that act directly on the renin-angiotensin system (RAS) can cause injury/death to the developing fetus.

ADULT DOSAGE

Hypertension

Initial: 20mg qd
Titrate: May increase to 40mg qd after 2 weeks if needed
May add diuretic if BP is not controlled

PEDIATRIC DOSAGE

Hypertension

6-16 Years:
20-<35kg:
Initial: 10mg qd
Titrate: May increase to 20mg qd after 2 weeks if needed
Max: 20mg qd

≥35kg:
Initial: 20mg qd
Titrate: May increase to 40mg qd after 2 weeks if needed
Max: 40mg qd

DOSING CONSIDERATIONS

Other Important Considerations

Intravascular Volume Depleted Patients:
Consider a lower initial dose and monitor closely

ADMINISTRATION

Oral route

May be administered w/ or w/o food
May administer same dose as sus if unable to swallow tabs

Preparation of Sus (for 200mL of a 2mg/mL Sus):

1. Add 50mL of purified water to an amber polyethylene terephthalate bottle containing twenty Benicar 20mg tabs and allow to stand for a minimum of 5 min
2. Shake the container for at least 1 min and allow the sus to stand for at least 1 min
3. Repeat 1 min shaking and 1 min standing for 4 additional times
4. Add 100mL of Ora-Sweet and 50mL of Ora-Plus to the sus and shake well for at least 1 min
5. The sus should be refrigerated at 2-8°C (36-46°F) and can be stored for up to 4 weeks
6. Shake the sus well before each use and return promptly to the refrigerator

HOW SUPPLIED

Tab: 5mg, 20mg, 40mg

CONTRAINDICATIONS

Coadministration with aliskiren in patients with diabetes.

WARNINGS/PRECAUTIONS

Symptomatic hypotension may occur after treatment initiation in patients with an activated renin-angiotensin-aldosterone system (RAAS) (eg, volume- and/or salt-depleted patients [eg, those being treated with high doses of diuretics]). Changes in renal function may occur. Oliguria and/or progressive azotemia and (rare) acute renal failure and/or death may occur in patients whose renal function may depend on the RAAS activity (eg, severe CHF). May increase SrCr or BUN levels in patients with renal artery stenosis. Sprue-like enteropathy with symptoms of severe, chronic diarrhea with substantial weight loss reported; exclude other etiologies if these symptoms develop, and consider discontinuation in cases where no other etiology is identified.

ADVERSE REACTIONS

Dizziness.

DRUG INTERACTIONS

See Contraindications. NSAIDs, including selective COX-2 inhibitors, may attenuate antihypertensive effect and may deteriorate renal function. Dual blockade of the RAS is associated with increased risks of hypotension, hyperkalemia, and changes in renal function (including acute renal failure); avoid combined use of RAS inhibitors, or closely monitor BP, renal function, and electrolytes with concomitant agents that also affect the RAS. Avoid with aliskiren in patients with renal impairment (GFR <60mL/min). Reduced levels with colesevelam; administer at least 4 hrs before colesevelam dose. Increases in serum lithium concentrations and lithium toxicity reported; monitor lithium levels.

PATIENT CONSIDERATIONS

Assessment: Assess for diabetes, CHF, renal artery stenosis, and volume/salt depletion, renal function, pregnancy/nursing status, and for possible drug interactions.

Monitoring: Monitor for signs/symptoms of hypotension, renal dysfunction, sprue-like enteropathy, and other adverse reactions.

Counseling: Inform females of childbearing potential of the consequences of exposure to drug during pregnancy and of the treatment options for women planning to become pregnant. Instruct to report pregnancy to the physician as soon as possible.

STORAGE: (Tab) 20-25°C (68-77°F). (Sus) 2-8°C (36-46°F) for up to 4 weeks.

BENICAR HCT – hydrochlorothiazide/olmesartan medoxomil RX

Class: Angiotensin II receptor blocker (ARB)/thiazide diuretic

D/C when pregnancy is detected. Drugs that act directly on the renin-angiotensin system (RAS) can cause injury/death to the developing fetus.

ADULT DOSAGE

Hypertension

Uncontrolled BP on Olmesartan or HCTZ Alone:
Switch to once-daily combination therapy
Usual: 1 tab qd
Titrate: May adjust at intervals of 2-4 weeks
Max: 1 tab/day

Replacement Therapy:
May be substituted for its titrated components

PEDIATRIC DOSAGE

Pediatric use may not have been established

DOSING CONSIDERATIONS

Elderly

Start at lower end of dosing range

ADMINISTRATION

Oral route

HOW SUPPLIED

Tab: (Olmesartan/HCTZ) 20mg/12.5mg, 40mg/12.5mg, 40mg/25mg

CONTRAINDICATIONS

Hypersensitivity to any component of this product, anuria or sulfonamide-derived drug hypersensitivity, coadministration w/ aliskiren in patients w/ diabetes.

WARNINGS/PRECAUTIONS

Not indicated for initial therapy. Symptomatic hypotension may occur after treatment initiation in patients with an activated RAS (eg, volume- or salt-depleted patients [eg, those being treated with high doses of diuretics]). Sprue-like enteropathy with symptoms of severe, chronic diarrhea with substantial weight loss reported; exclude other etiologies if these symptoms develop, and consider discontinuation where no other etiology is identified. Hypo/hyperkalemia reported. Not recommended with severe renal impairment (CrCl ≤30mL/min). Oliguria and/or progressive azotemia and (rare) acute renal failure and/or death may occur in patients whose renal function may depend on the renin-angiotensin-aldosterone system activity (eg, severe CHF). May increase SrCr or BUN levels in patients with renal artery stenosis. Caution with severe renal disease; may precipitate azotemia. Caution in elderly. HCTZ: Caution with hepatic impairment or progressive liver disease; may precipitate hepatic coma. May cause hypersensitivity reactions (with or without a history of allergy or bronchial asthma), exacerbation or activation of systemic lupus erythematosus (SLE), hyperuricemia or precipitation of frank gout, hyperglycemia, hypomagnesemia, hypercalcemia, and manifestations of latent diabetes mellitus (DM). May cause idiosyncratic reaction, resulting in acute transient myopia and acute angle-closure glaucoma; d/c as rapidly as possible. Observe for signs of fluid or electrolyte imbalance (eg, hyponatremia, hypochloremic alkalosis, hypokalemia). Hypokalemia may sensitize/exaggerate the response of the heart to toxic effects of digitalis. D/C before testing for parathyroid function. Enhanced effects in postsympathectomy patients. D/C or withhold if progressive renal impairment becomes evident. Increased cholesterol and TG levels reported.

ADVERSE REACTIONS

Dizziness, URTI, hyperuricemia, nausea.

DRUG INTERACTIONS

See Contraindications. NSAIDs, including selective COX-2 inhibitors, may decrease antihypertensive effects and may deteriorate renal function. Increases in serum lithium concentrations and lithium toxicity reported; monitor lithium levels. Olmesartan: Dual blockade of the RAS is associated with increased risks of hypotension, hyperkalemia, and changes in renal function (including acute renal failure); avoid combined use of RAS inhibitors, or closely monitor BP, renal function, and electrolytes with concomitant agents that also affect the RAS. Avoid with aliskiren in patients with renal impairment (GFR <60mL/min). Reduced levels with colesevelam; administer at least 4 hrs before colesevelam dose. HCTZ: Alcohol, barbiturates, or narcotics may potentiate orthostatic hypotension. Dose adjustment of antidiabetic drugs (eg, oral agents and insulin) may be required. Additive effect or potentiation with other antihypertensives. Anionic exchange resins (eg, cholestyramine, colestipol) may impair absorption. Corticosteroids and adrenocorticotropic hormone may intensify electrolyte depletion, particularly hypokalemia. May decrease response to pressor amines (eg, norepinephrine). May increase responsiveness to nondepolarizing skeletal muscle relaxants (eg, tubocurarine).

PATIENT CONSIDERATIONS

Assessment: Assess for hypersensitivity to the drug and its components, anuria, sulfonamide-derived drug hypersensitivity, volume/salt depletion, SLE, DM, CHF, hepatic/renal impairment, postsympathectomy status, renal artery stenosis, pregnancy/nursing status, and possible drug interactions.

Monitoring: Monitor for signs/symptoms of fluid/electrolyte imbalance, sprue-like enteropathy, exacerbation/activation of SLE, idiosyncratic reaction, latent DM, hyperuricemia, precipitation of gout, hypersensitivity reactions, and other adverse reactions. Monitor BP, serum electrolytes, cholesterol, and TG levels, and renal/hepatic function.

Counseling: Inform females of childbearing potential of the consequences of exposure during pregnancy and of the treatment options for women planning to become pregnant. Instruct to report pregnancy to the physician as soon as possible. Counsel that lightheadedness may occur, especially during the 1st days of therapy; instruct to report to physician. Instruct to d/c therapy and consult physician if syncope occurs. Advise that inadequate fluid intake, excessive perspiration, diarrhea, or vomiting may lead to an excessive fall in BP, with the same consequences of lightheadedness and possible syncope.

STORAGE: 20-25°C (68-77°F).

BenzaClin – benzoyl peroxide/clindamycin

RX

Class: Antibacterial/keratolytic

ADULT DOSAGE

Acne Vulgaris

Apply bid (am and pm) or ud to affected areas

PEDIATRIC DOSAGE

Acne Vulgaris

≥12 Years:

Apply bid (am and pm) or ud to affected areas

ADMINISTRATION

Topical route

Prior to application, wash skin gently, then rinse w/ warm water and pat dry

Reconstitute before dispensing; refer to PI for reconstitution instructions

HOW SUPPLIED

Gel: (Clindamycin-Benzoyl Peroxide) 1%-5% [25g, jar; 35g, 50g, pump]

CONTRAINDICATIONS

Hypersensitivity to any of its components or to lincomycin, history of regional enteritis, ulcerative colitis (UC), or antibiotic-associated colitis.

WARNINGS/PRECAUTIONS

Severe colitis, which may result in death, reported following oral and parenteral clindamycin administration. Diarrhea, bloody diarrhea, and colitis (including pseudomembranous colitis) reported; d/c if significant diarrhea occurs. Not for ophthalmic use. May cause overgrowth of nonsusceptible organisms, including fungi; d/c use and take appropriate measures if this occurs. Avoid contact with eyes and mucous membranes.

ADVERSE REACTIONS

Dry skin, application-site reaction.

DRUG INTERACTIONS

Antiperistaltic agents (eg, opiates, diphenoxylate with atropine) may prolong and/or worsen colitis. Caution with concomitant topical acne therapy (eg, peeling, desquamating, or abrasive agents) because of possible cumulative irritancy effect. Do not use with erythromycin-containing products.

PATIENT CONSIDERATIONS

Assessment: Assess for hypersensitivity to drug or to lincomycin, history of regional enteritis, UC, or antibiotic-associated colitis, pregnancy/nursing status, and possible drug interactions.

Monitoring: Monitor for signs/symptoms of diarrhea, colitis, overgrowth of nonsusceptible organisms, and other adverse reactions. For colitis, perform stool culture and assay for *Clostridium difficile* toxin. Consider large bowel endoscopy in cases of severe diarrhea.

Counseling: Instruct to use externally ud and to avoid contact with eyes, and inside the nose, mouth, and all mucous membranes. Advise not to use for any disorder other than for which it was prescribed and not to use any other topical acne preparation unless otherwise directed by physician. Counsel to minimize or avoid exposure to natural or artificial sunlight (tanning beds or UVA/B treatment) while using medication; instruct to wear a wide-brimmed hat or other protective clothing, and use a sunscreen with SPF ≥15 to minimize exposure to sunlight. Instruct to report any signs of local adverse reactions to physician. Inform that drug may bleach hair or colored fabric.

STORAGE: Room temperature up to 25°C (77°F). Do not freeze. Discard product 3 months following reconstitution.

BENZAMYCIN – benzoyl peroxide/erythromycin

RX

Class: Antibacterial/keratolytic

ADULT DOSAGE

Acne Vulgaris

Apply bid (am and pm) or ud

PEDIATRIC DOSAGE

Acne Vulgaris

≥12 Years:

Apply bid (am and pm) or ud

ADMINISTRATION

Topical route

Wash and dry skin prior to administration

Requires thorough mixing immediately prior to each use

HOW SUPPLIED

Gel: (Benzoyl Peroxide-Erythromycin) 5%-3% [46.6g]

CONTRAINDICATIONS

Hypersensitivity to any of its components.

WARNINGS/PRECAUTIONS

D/C if severe irritation or overgrowth of nonsusceptible organisms (eg, fungi) occurs. Avoid eyes, mouth, and mucous membranes. Pseudomembranous colitis reported with nearly all antibacterial agents, including erythromycin.

ADVERSE REACTIONS

Dryness, urticaria.

DRUG INTERACTIONS

Additive irritation with peeling, desquamating, or abrasive agents. Lincomycin, chloramphenicol, and clindamycin antagonizes protein inhibition of erythromycin *in vitro*.

PATIENT CONSIDERATIONS

Assessment: Assess proper diagnosis of acne vulgaris. Assess use in patients who are using other concomitant topical acne therapies. Assess use in pregnant/nursing patients.

Monitoring: Monitor for occurrence of cumulative irritancy effect when using other concomitant topical acne agents. Monitor for development of severe skin irritation and for overgrowth of nonsusceptible organisms that is associated with antibiotic usage.

Counseling: Counsel to report to physician signs of local adverse reactions (eg, skin irritation, photosensitivity reaction). Advise not to use any other topical acne preparation unless directed by physician. Advise that contact with hair or fabrics may bleach them.

STORAGE: Prior to reconstitution: 15°-30°C (59°-86°F). After reconstitution: 2°-8°C (36°-46°F). Do not freeze. Keep tightly closed. Discard after 3 months.

BENZONATATE – benzonatate

RX

Class: Non-narcotic antitussive

OTHER BRAND NAMES

Tessalon

ADULT DOSAGE

Cough

Usual: 100mg or 200mg tid prn
Max: 600mg/day in 3 divided doses

PEDIATRIC DOSAGE

Cough

>10 Years:
Usual: 100mg or 200mg tid prn
Max: 600mg/day in 3 divided doses

ADMINISTRATION

Oral route

Swallow whole; do not break, chew, dissolve, cut, or crush

HOW SUPPLIED

Cap: 200mg; (Tessalon) 100mg

CONTRAINDICATIONS

Hypersensitivity to benzonatate or related compounds.

WARNINGS/PRECAUTIONS

Severe hypersensitivity reactions (eg, bronchospasm, laryngospasm, cardiovascular collapse) reported, possibly related to local anesthesia from sucking or chewing the cap instead of swallowing. Accidental ingestion resulting in death reported in children <10 yrs of age. May cause adverse CNS effects; caution with prior sensitivity to related agents, such as para-aminobenzoic acid (PABA) based anesthetics (eg, procaine, tetracaine).

ADVERSE REACTIONS

Hypersensitivity reactions, sedation, headache, dizziness, mental confusion, visual hallucinations, constipation, nausea, GI upset, pruritus, skin eruptions, nasal congestion, numbness of the chest, sensation of burning in the eyes, vague "chilly" sensation.

DRUG INTERACTIONS

Bizarre behavior (eg, mental confusion, visual hallucinations) reported when taken in combination with other prescribed drugs. May cause adverse CNS effects with concomitant medications.

PATIENT CONSIDERATIONS

Assessment: Assess for hypersensitivity to the drug or previous sensitivity to related compounds such as PABA based anesthetics, pregnancy/nursing status, and possible drug interactions.

Monitoring: Monitor for hypersensitivity reactions, CNS adverse effects, and other adverse reactions.

Counseling: Inform to take ud. Inform that release of benzonatate from the cap in the mouth can produce a temporary local anesthesia of the oral mucosa and choking may occur. Instruct to refrain from oral ingestion of food or liquids if numbness or tingling of the tongue, mouth, throat, or face occurs until numbness resolves. Advise to seek medical attention if symptoms worsen/persist. Inform that overdosage resulting in death may occur in adults; instruct not to exceed a single dose of 200mg and a total daily dosage of 600mg.

STORAGE: Protect from light. (200mg Cap) 20-25°C (68-77°F). (Tessalon) 25°C (77°F); excursions permitted to 15-30°C (59-86°F).

B

BENZTROPINE – benztropine mesylate

RX

Class: Anticholinergic

OTHER BRAND NAMES

Cogentin

ADULT DOSAGE

Parkinsonism

Adjunct in the Therapy of All Forms of Parkinsonism:
Initiate w/ a low dose
Titrate: May increase in increments of 0.5mg, to a max of 6mg, or until optimal results obtained, at 5- to 6-day intervals

Idiopathic Parkinsonism:
Initial: 0.5-1mg qhs; 4-6mg/day may be required in other patients

Postencephalitic Parkinsonism:
Initial: 2mg/day given in 1 or more doses; 0.5mg qhs and increase as necessary in highly sensitive patients

Postencephalitic and Idiopathic Parkinsonism:
Usual: 1-2mg/day
Range: 0.5-6mg/day

Inj:
Emergency Situations:
1-2mL
Dose can be repeated if the parkinsonian effect begins to return

Do not terminate other antiparkinsonian agents abruptly when therapy is started; gradually reduce or d/c other agents

Drug-Induced Extrapyramidal Reactions

Control of extrapyramidal disorders (except tardive dyskinesia) due to neuroleptic drugs (eg, phenothiazines)
Usual: 1-4mg qd or bid
1-2mg bid or tid for extrapyramidal disorders that develop soon after initiation of neuroleptic drugs

Tab:
D/C to determine continued need after 1 or 2 weeks
May reinstitute therapy if disorders recur

Acute Dystonic Reactions:
1-2mL IM/IV relieves the condition quickly
After the inj, 1-2mg tab bid usually prevents recurrence

PEDIATRIC DOSAGE

Parkinsonism

Adjunct in the Therapy of All Forms of Parkinsonism:
>3 Years:
Initiate w/ a low dose
Titrate: May increase in increments of 0.5mg, to a max of 6mg, or until optimal results obtained, at 5- to 6-day intervals

Idiopathic Parkinsonism:
Initial: 0.5-1mg qhs; 4-6mg/day may be required in other patients

Postencephalitic Parkinsonism:
Initial: 2mg/day given in 1 or more doses; 0.5mg qhs and increase as necessary in highly sensitive patients

Postencephalitic and Idiopathic Parkinsonism:
Usual: 1-2mg/day
Range: 0.5-6mg/day

Inj:
Emergency Situations:
1-2mL
Dose can be repeated if the parkinsonian effect begins to return

Do not terminate other antiparkinsonian agents abruptly when therapy is started; gradually reduce or d/c other agents

Drug-Induced Extrapyramidal Reactions

Control of extrapyramidal disorders (except tardive dyskinesia) due to neuroleptic drugs (eg, phenothiazines)

>3 Years:
Usual: 1-4mg qd or bid
1-2mg bid or tid for extrapyramidal disorders that develop soon after initiation of neuroleptic drugs

Tab:
D/C to determine continued need after 1 or 2 weeks
May reinstitute therapy if disorders recur

Acute Dystonic Reactions:
1-2mL IM/IV relieves the condition quickly
After the inj, 1-2mg tab bid usually prevents recurrence

DOSING CONSIDERATIONS

Concomitant Medications

Concomitant Carbidopa-Levodopa or Levodopa: May require periodic dose adjustment

Elderly

Start at lower end of dosing range, and increase dose prn w/ monitoring for the emergence of adverse events

ADMINISTRATION

IV/IM/Oral route

HOW SUPPLIED

Inj: (Cogentin) 1mg/mL [2mL, ampul]; **Tab:** 0.5mg*, 1mg*, 2mg* *scored

CONTRAINDICATIONS

Hypersensitivity to benztropine mesylate tablets or to any component of the tablets, pediatric patients <3 yrs of age.

WARNINGS/PRECAUTIONS

May impair mental/physical abilities. Caution with use during hot weather, especially when given with other atropine-like drugs to the chronically ill, alcoholics, those who have CNS disease, or those who do manual labor in a hot environment; severe anhidrosis and hyperthermia may occur; consider dose reduction. Continued supervision is advisable. Closely monitor patients with a tendency to tachycardia and those with prostatic hypertrophy. Dysuria may occur. Urinary retention reported. May cause weakness and inability to move particular muscle groups, especially in large doses; may require dose adjustment. Mental confusion and excitement may occur with large doses, or in susceptible patients. Visual hallucinations reported occasionally. In the treatment of extrapyramidal disorders due to neuroleptic drugs, may intensify mental symptoms in patients with mental disorders and precipitate toxic psychosis; monitor patients with mental disorders, especially at start of therapy or if dose is increased. Not recommended for use in patients with TD; may aggravate TD symptoms. Glaucoma may develop; avoid with angle-closure glaucoma. Certain drug-induced extrapyramidal disorders that develop slowly may not respond to therapy. Caution in pediatric patients >3 yrs of age.

ADVERSE REACTIONS

Tachycardia, paralytic ileus, constipation, N/V, dry mouth, toxic psychosis, blurred vision, dilated pupils, urinary retention, dysuria, allergic reaction, heat stroke, hyperthermia, fever.

DRUG INTERACTIONS

May cause GI complaints, fever, or heat intolerance with phenothiazines, haloperidol, or other drugs with anticholinergic/antidopaminergic activity. Paralytic ileus, hyperthermia, and heat stroke reported with phenothiazines and/or TCAs.

PATIENT CONSIDERATIONS

Assessment: Assess for drug hypersensitivity, exposure to hot weather, tachycardia, prostatic hypertrophy, mental disorders, TD, angle-closure glaucoma, chronic illness, alcohol consumption, CNS disease, pregnancy/nursing status, and for possible drug interactions.

Monitoring: Monitor for anhidrosis, hyperthermia, tachycardia, dysuria, urinary retention, weakness, inability to move muscles, mental confusion and excitement, toxic psychosis, visual hallucinations, glaucoma, and other adverse reactions. Monitor patients with mental disorders at start of therapy or if dose is increased.

Counseling: Inform of the risks/benefits of therapy. Advise to use with caution during hot weather. Inform that drug may impair mental/physical abilities; caution against performing hazardous tasks (eg, operating machinery/driving). Advise to report GI complaints, fever, or heat intolerance promptly.

STORAGE: (Inj) 20-25°C (68-77°F). (Tab) 15-30°C (59-86°F).

BESIVANCE – besifloxacin

Class: Fluoroquinolone

RX

ADULT DOSAGE

Bacterial Conjunctivitis

1 drop in affected eye(s) tid, 4-12 hrs apart for 7 days

PEDIATRIC DOSAGE

Bacterial Conjunctivitis

≥1 Year:
1 drop in affected eye(s) tid, 4-12 hrs apart for 7 days

ADMINISTRATION

Ocular route

Invert closed bottle and shake once before use

HOW SUPPLIED

Sus: 0.6% [5mL]

WARNINGS/PRECAUTIONS

For topical ophthalmic use only; should not be injected subconjunctivally, nor should it be introduced directly into the anterior chamber of the eye. May result in overgrowth of nonsusceptible organisms (eg, fungi) with prolonged use; d/c and institute alternative therapy if superinfection occurs. Avoid wearing contact lenses if signs or symptoms of bacterial conjunctivitis occur and avoid wearing contact lenses during the course of therapy.

ADVERSE REACTIONS

Conjunctival redness.

PATIENT CONSIDERATIONS

B

Assessment: Assess for previous hypersensitivity to the drug, use of contact lenses, and pregnancy/nursing status. Assess for proper diagnosis of causative organisms.

Monitoring: Monitor for superinfection; examine with magnification (eg, slit-lamp biomicroscopy) and fluorescein staining, where appropriate. Monitor for hypersensitivity reactions and other adverse reactions.

Counseling: Advise to avoid contaminating applicator tip with material from the eye, fingers, or other source. Advise to d/c use immediately and contact physician at first sign of a rash or allergic reaction. Instruct to use medication exactly ud. Inform that skipping doses or not completing the full course of therapy may decrease effectiveness and increase bacterial resistance. Advise to avoid wearing contact lenses if having signs or symptoms of bacterial conjunctivitis and avoid wearing during the course of therapy. Advise to thoroughly wash hands before use. Instruct to invert closed bottle and shake once before each use. Instruct to remove cap with bottle still in inverted position. Instruct to tilt head back, and with bottle inverted, gently squeeze bottle to instill 1 drop into the affected eye(s).

STORAGE: 15-25°C (59-77°F). Protect from light.

BETAPACE – sotalol hydrochloride

RX

Class: Beta blocker (group II/III antiarrhythmic)

To minimize risk of arrhythmia, for a minimum of 3 days, place patients initiated or reinitiated on therapy in a facility that can provide cardiac resuscitation and continuous ECG monitoring. Calculate CrCl prior to dosing. Not approved for A-fib or A-flutter; do not substitute for Betapace AF.

OTHER BRAND NAMES

Sorine

ADULT DOSAGE

Ventricular Arrhythmias

Documented Ventricular Arrhythmias (eg, Sustained Ventricular Tachycardia):
Initial: 80mg bid
Titrate: May increase after appropriate evaluation to 240 or 320mg/day (120-160mg bid); adjust dose gradually, allowing 3 days between dosing increments
Total Daily Dose: 160-320mg/day in 2 or 3 divided doses

Refractory Ventricular Arrhythmia:
480-640mg/day when benefit outweighs risk

Transferring to Betapace/Sorine:
Withdraw previous antiarrhythmic therapy for a minimum of 2-3 plasma half-lives before initiating therapy
After discontinuation of amiodarone, do not initiate therapy until QT interval is normalized

PEDIATRIC DOSAGE

Ventricular Arrhythmias

Documented Ventricular Arrhythmias (eg, Sustained Ventricular Tachycardia):
<2 Years:
Refer to PI for dosing chart
≥2 Years:
Initial: 30mg/m² tid (90mg/m² total daily dose)
Titrate: Allow at least 36 hrs between dose increments; guide titration by response, HR, and QTc
Max: 60mg/m²
Reduce dose or d/c if QTc >550 msec

Transferring to Betapace/Sorine:
Withdraw previous antiarrhythmic therapy for a minimum of 2-3 plasma half-lives before initiating therapy
After discontinuation of amiodarone, do not initiate therapy until QT interval is normalized

DOSING CONSIDERATIONS

Renal Impairment

Adults:
CrCl >60mL/min: Dose q12h
CrCl 30-59mL/min: Dose q24h
CrCl 10-29mL/min: Dose q36-48h
CrCl <10mL/min: Dose should be individualized

Pediatrics:
Lower doses or increase intervals between doses

ADMINISTRATION

Oral route

Preparation of Extemporaneous Oral Sol

1. Measure 120mL of simple syrup containing 0.1% sodium benzoate
2. Transfer the syrup to a 6-oz amber plastic (polyethylene terephthalate) prescription bottle

3. Add 5 sotalol 120mg tabs to the bottle. These tabs are added intact; it is not necessary to crush the tabs
4. Shake the bottle to wet the entire surface of the tabs. If the tabs have been crushed, shake the bottle until the endpoint is achieved
5. Allow the tabs to hydrate for at least 2 hrs. After at least 2 hrs have elapsed, shake the bottle intermittently over the course of at least another 2 hrs until the tabs are completely disintegrated
6. The procedure results in a sol containing 5mg/mL of sotalol HCl

HOW SUPPLIED

Tab: (Betapace) 80mg*, 120mg*, 160mg*; (Sorine) 80mg*, 120mg*, 160mg*, 240mg* *scored

CONTRAINDICATIONS

Bronchial asthma, sinus bradycardia, 2nd- and 3rd-degree atrioventricular (AV) block (unless a functioning pacemaker is present), congenital or acquired long QT syndromes, cardiogenic shock, uncontrolled CHF, previous evidence of hypersensitivity to sotalol.

WARNINGS/PRECAUTIONS

May provoke new or worsen ventricular arrhythmias (eg, sustained ventricular tachycardia or ventricular fibrillation). Torsades de pointes, QT interval prolongation, and new or worsened CHF reported. Anticipate proarrhythmic events upon initiation and every upward dose adjustment. Caution in patients w/ QTc >500 msec on-therapy and consider reducing dose or discontinuing therapy when QTc >550 msec. Avoid w/ uncorrected hypokalemia or hypomagnesemia. Give special attention to electrolyte and acid-base balance in patients w/ severe/prolonged diarrhea or w/ concomitant diuretic drugs. May cause further depression of myocardial contractility and precipitate more severe failure; caution w/ CHF controlled by digitalis and/or diuretics. Caution w/ left ventricular dysfunction, sick sinus syndrome associated w/ symptomatic arrhythmias, and renal impairment (especially w/ hemodialysis). Caution during the first 2 weeks post-MI; careful dose titration is especially important (eg, in patients w/ markedly impaired ventricular function). Exacerbation of angina pectoris, arrhythmias, and MI reported after abrupt discontinuation; reduce dose gradually over 1-2 weeks. May unmask latent coronary insufficiency in patients w/ arrhythmias. Avoid in patients w/ bronchospastic diseases; use lowest effective dose. Impaired ability of the heart to respond to reflex adrenergic stimuli may augment the risks of general anesthesia and surgical procedures; chronically administered therapy should not be routinely withdrawn prior to major surgery. Patients w/ a history of anaphylactic reaction to various allergens may have a more severe reaction on repeated challenge and may be unresponsive to usual doses of epinephrine. Caution in patients w/ diabetes (especially labile diabetes) or w/ a history of episodes of spontaneous hypoglycemia; may mask premonitory signs of acute hypoglycemia (eg, tachycardia). May mask certain clinical signs (eg, tachycardia) of hyperthyroidism.

ADVERSE REACTIONS

Torsades de pointes, dyspnea, fatigue, dizziness, bradycardia, chest pain, palpitation, asthenia, abnormal ECG, hypotension, headache, light-headedness, edema, N/V, pulmonary problems.

DRUG INTERACTIONS

Avoid w/ Class Ia (eg, disopyramide, quinidine, procainamide) and Class III (eg, amiodarone) antiarrhythmics. Additive Class II effects w/ other β-blockers. Proarrhythmic events were more common when concomitantly used w/ digoxin. May increase risk of bradycardia w/ digitalis glycosides. Possible additive effects on AV conduction or ventricular function and BP w/ calcium-blocking agents. May produce excessive reduction of resting sympathetic nervous tone w/ catecholamine-depleting drugs (eg, reserpine, guanethidine). Hyperglycemia may occur; may require dose adjustment of insulin or antidiabetic agents. β_2-agonists (eg, salbutamol, terbutaline, isoprenaline) may need dose increase. May potentiate rebound HTN w/ clonidine withdrawal. Avoid administration w/in 2 hrs of antacids containing aluminum oxide and magnesium hydroxide; may reduce levels. Caution w/ drugs that prolong QT interval (eg, Class I and III antiarrhythmics, phenothiazines, TCAs, astemizole, bepridil, certain oral macrolides, certain quinolone antibiotics).

PATIENT CONSIDERATIONS

Assessment: Assess for hypersensitivity to drug, bronchial asthma, sinus bradycardia, sick sinus syndrome, 2nd- and 3rd-degree AV block, pacemaker, long QT syndromes, cardiogenic shock, left ventricular dysfunction or uncontrolled CHF, recent MI, ischemic heart disease, hypokalemia or hypomagnesemia, bronchospastic disease, diabetes, episodes of hypoglycemia, upcoming major surgery, hyperthyroidism, renal impairment, any other conditions where treatment is contraindicated or cautioned, pregnancy/nursing status, and possible drug interactions.

Monitoring: Monitor for ECG changes, tachycardia, arrhythmias, depressed myocardial contractility, severe CHF, anaphylaxis, hypoglycemia, electrolyte imbalance, hyperthyroidism, and other adverse reactions.

Counseling: Inform of the benefits/risks of therapy. Advise not to d/c therapy w/o consulting physician. Instruct to report any adverse reactions to physician.

STORAGE: **Betapace:** 25°C (77°F); excursions permitted to 15-30°C (59-86°F). **Sorine:** 15-30°C (59-86°F). **Sus:** Stable for 3 months at 15-30°C (59-86°F) and ambient humidity.

B

BEXSERO – meningococcal group B vaccine RX

Class: Vaccine

ADULT DOSAGE

Meningococcal Vaccine

Active Immunization to Prevent Invasive Disease Caused by *Neisseria meningitidis* Serogroup B:

≤25 Years:

2 doses (0.5mL/dose) at least 1 month apart

Sufficient data not available on the safety and effectiveness of using interchangeably w/ other meningococcal group B vaccines to complete vaccination series

PEDIATRIC DOSAGE

Meningococcal Vaccine

Active Immunization to Prevent Invasive Disease Caused by *Neisseria meningitidis* Serogroup B:

≥10 Years:

2 doses (0.5mL/dose) at least 1 month apart

Sufficient data not available on the safety and effectiveness of using interchangeably w/ other meningococcal group B vaccines to complete vaccination series

ADMINISTRATION

IM route

Shake syringe immediately before use; do not use if vaccine cannot be resuspended

Administer into the deltoid muscle of upper arm

HOW SUPPLIED

Inj: 0.5mL

CONTRAINDICATIONS

Hypersensitivity, including severe allergic reaction, to any component of the vaccine, or after a previous dose of Bexsero.

WARNINGS/PRECAUTIONS

Appropriate observation and medical treatment should always be readily available in case of an anaphylactic event. Syncope may occur; procedures should be in place to avoid injury from falling. Tip caps of prefilled syringes contain natural rubber latex; may cause allergic reactions in latex sensitive individuals. May not protect all vaccine recipients. May not provide protection against all meningococcal serogroup B strains. Individuals w/ altered immunocompetence may have reduced immune responses to therapy.

ADVERSE REACTIONS

Inj-site pain, myalgia, erythema, fatigue, headache, induration, nausea, arthralgia.

PATIENT CONSIDERATIONS

Assessment: Assess for hypersensitivity, vaccination history, latex sensitivity, altered immunocompetence, and pregnancy/nursing status.

Monitoring: Monitor for allergic/anaphylactic reactions, syncope, and other adverse reactions. Monitor immune response to vaccine.

Counseling: Inform patients and parents/guardians about the importance of completing the immunization series. Instruct to report any adverse reactions to physician. Inform women who receive therapy while pregnant that they will need to be registered in the vaccine's pregnancy registry.

STORAGE: 2-8°C (36-46°F). Do not freeze; discard if the vaccine has been frozen. Protect from light.

BEYAZ – drospirenone/ethinyl estradiol/levomefolate calcium RX

Class: Estrogen/progestogen combination

Cigarette smoking increases the risk of serious cardiovascular (CV) events from combination oral contraceptive (COC) use. Risk increases w/ age (>35 yrs) and w/ the number of cigarettes smoked. Should not be used by women who are >35 yrs of age and smoke.

ADULT DOSAGE

Contraception

1 tab qd at the same time each day for 28 days, then repeat

Start either on 1st day of menses or on 1st Sunday after onset of menses

PEDIATRIC DOSAGE

Contraception

Not indicated for use premenarche; refer to adult dosing

Premenstrual Dysphoric Disorder

In Women Who Desire Oral Contraception:
1 tab qd at the same time each day for 28 days, then repeat

Start either on 1st day of menses or on 1st Sunday after onset of menses

Acne Vulgaris

Moderate Acne in Women Who Desire Oral Contraception:
1 tab qd at the same time each day for 28 days, then repeat

Start either on 1st day of menses or on 1st Sunday after onset of menses

Other Indications

May be used to raise folate levels for the purpose of reducing the risk of neural tube defect in a pregnancy conceived while taking the product or shortly after discontinuation

Conversions

Switching from a Different Birth Control Pill:
Start on the same day that a new pack of the previous oral contraceptive would have been started

Switching from a Method Other than a Birth Control Pill:
Transdermal Patch/Vaginal Ring/Inj: Start when the next application/inj would have been due
Intrauterine Contraceptive/Implant: Start on day of removal

Premenstrual Dysphoric Disorder

Not indicated for use premenarche; refer to adult dosing

Acne Vulgaris

Moderate Acne in Postpubertal Women ≥14 Years Who Desire Oral Contraception:
1 tab qd at the same time each day for 28 days, then repeat

Start either on 1st day of menses or on 1st Sunday after onset of menses

DOSING CONSIDERATIONS

Adverse Reactions

GI Disturbances: If vomiting occurs w/in 3-4 hrs after taking tab, may regard as missed tab

Other Important Considerations

Postpartum Women Who Elect Not to Breastfeed/After 2nd Trimester Abortion:
Start therapy no earlier than 4 weeks postpartum; if patient initiates therapy postpartum and has not yet had a period, use an additional method of contraception until patient has taken 7 consecutive days of therapy

ADMINISTRATION

Oral route

Take tabs in the order directed on the package, at the same time each day, preferably after pm meal or hs
Take w/o regard to meals
If 1st taken later than the 1st day of menstrual cycle, use a nonhormonal contraceptive as backup during the first 7 days

HOW SUPPLIED

Tab: (Drospirenone [DRSP]/Ethinyl Estradiol [EE]/Levomefolate calcium) 3mg/0.02mg/0.451mg; **Tab:** (Levomefolate calcium) 0.451mg

CONTRAINDICATIONS

Renal impairment, adrenal insufficiency, high risk of arterial/venous thrombotic disease (eg, smoking if >35 yrs of age, history/presence of deep vein thrombosis/pulmonary embolism, cerebrovascular disease, coronary artery disease, thrombogenic valvular or thrombogenic rhythm diseases of the heart [eg, subacute bacterial endocarditis w/ valvular disease, A-fib], inherited/acquired hypercoagulopathies, uncontrolled HTN, diabetes mellitus [DM] w/ vascular disease, headaches w/ focal neurological symptoms or migraine w/ or w/o aura if >35 yrs of age), undiagnosed abnormal uterine bleeding, history/presence of breast or other estrogen-/progestin-sensitive cancer, benign/malignant liver tumors, liver disease, pregnancy.

WARNINGS/PRECAUTIONS

May increase risk of venous thromboembolism (VTE) and arterial thromboses (eg, stroke, MI); d/c if arterial or venous thrombotic event occur. D/C if unexplained loss of vision, proptosis, diplopia, papilledema, or retinal vascular lesions occur; evaluate for retinal vein thrombosis immediately. If feasible, d/c at least 4 weeks before and through 2 weeks after major surgery or other surgeries known to have an elevated risk of thromboembolism. Potential for hyperkalemia in high-risk patients; contraindicated in patients predisposed to hyperkalemia. May increase risk of cervical cancer or intraepithelial neoplasia, and gallbladder disease. D/C if jaundice develops. May increase risk of hepatic adenomas and hepatocellular carcinoma. Cholestasis may occur w/ history of pregnancy-related cholestasis; women w/ a history of COC-related cholestasis may have the condition recur w/ subsequent COC use. Increased BP reported; d/c if BP rises significantly. May decrease glucose tolerance; monitor prediabetic and diabetic women. Consider alternative contraception for women w/ uncontrolled dyslipidemia. May increase risk of pancreatitis in women w/ hypertriglyceridemia or family history thereof. Evaluate the cause and d/c if indicated, if new headaches that are recurrent, persistent, or severe develop; increase in frequency/severity of migraines may be a reason for immediate discontinuation of therapy. Unscheduled bleeding and spotting may occur; rule out pregnancy or malignancy. Post-pill amenorrhea or oligomenorrhea may occur. Caution w/ history of depression; d/c if depression recurs to a serious degree. May change results of some lab tests (eg, coagulation factors, binding proteins). Folate may mask vitamin B12 deficiency. May induce/exacerbate angioedema in patients w/ hereditary angioedema. Chloasma may occur, especially w/ history of chloasma gravidarum; avoid sun or UV radiation exposure in women w/ a tendency to chloasma. Absorption may not be complete and additional contraceptive measures should be taken in case of severe vomiting or diarrhea; if vomiting occurs w/in 3-4 hrs after tab taking, regard this as a missed tab.

ADVERSE REACTIONS

Menstrual irregularities, N/V, headache/migraine, breast pain/tenderness, fatigue.

DRUG INTERACTIONS

Consider monitoring serum K^+ levels in high-risk patients who take a strong CYP3A4 inhibitor long-term and concomitantly. Potential for an increase in serum K^+ levels w/ use of other drugs that may increase serum K^+ levels (eg, ACE inhibitors, heparin, aldosterone antagonists, NSAIDs); monitor serum K^+ levels during 1st treatment cycle in women receiving daily, long-term treatment for chronic conditions/diseases. May reduce effectiveness or increase breakthrough bleeding when used w/ drugs or herbal products that induce certain enzymes, including CYP3A4 (eg, phenytoin, barbiturates, carbamazepine); use an alternative or backup method of contraception when using enzyme inducers and continue backup contraception for 28 days after discontinuation of the enzyme inducer. Atorvastatin may increase EE exposure; ascorbic acid and acetaminophen may increase EE levels. Moderate or strong CYP3A4 inhibitors (eg, itraconazole, verapamil, clarithromycin, diltiazem) may increase plasma levels of estrogen or progestin or both. Significant changes (increase/decrease) in plasma estrogen and progestin levels w/ HIV/hepatitis C virus protease inhibitors or non-nucleoside reverse transcriptase inhibitors. Pregnancy reported w/ antibiotics. May decrease levels of lamotrigine and reduce seizure control; may need to adjust dose of lamotrigine. May increase levels of CYP3A4 substrates (eg, midazolam), CYP2C19 substrates (eg, omeprazole, voriconazole), and CYP1A2 substrates (eg, theophylline, tizanidine). Increases thyroid-binding globulin levels; may need to increase dose of thyroid hormone in women on thyroid hormone replacement therapy. May decrease pharmacological effect of antifolate drugs (eg, antiepileptics [phenytoin], methotrexate, pyrimethamine). Reduced folate levels reported via inhibition of dihydrofolate reductase enzyme (eg, methotrexate, sulfasalazine), reduced folate absorption (eg, cholestyramine), or unknown mechanism (eg, antiepileptics [carbamazepine, phenytoin, primidone]).

PATIENT CONSIDERATIONS

Assessment: Assess for renal impairment, abnormal uterine bleeding, adrenal insufficiency, predisposition to hyperkalemia, pregnancy/nursing status, other conditions where treatment is cautioned or contraindicated, and for possible drug interactions.

Monitoring: Monitor for bleeding irregularities, thromboembolic disorders and other vascular problems, cervical cancer or intraepithelial neoplasia, retinal vein thrombosis or any other ophthalmic changes, jaundice, acute/chronic disturbances in liver function, new/worsening headaches or migraines, serious depression, cholestasis w/ history of pregnancy-related cholestasis, pancreatitis, and other adverse reactions. Monitor K^+ levels, thyroid function if receiving thyroid replacement therapy, glucose levels in diabetic and prediabetic women, and lipids levels w/ dyslipidemia. Check BP annually.

Counseling: Inform of risks/benefits of therapy. Explain that cigarette smoking increases the risk of serious CV events. Inform of the risk of VTE. Inform that drug does not protect against HIV infection and other STDs. Instruct to take ud and at the same time every day. Instruct on what to do if pills are missed or vomiting occurs w/in 3-4 hrs after taking tab. Advise to inform physician of preexisting medical conditions and of all concomitant medications and herbal supplements currently being taken. Instruct to d/c if pregnancy occurs during treatment. Instruct to use a backup or alternative method of contraception when enzyme inducers are used concomitantly. Inform that therapy may reduce breast milk production. Inform that amenorrhea may occur and pregnancy should be ruled out if amenorrhea occurs in ≥2 consecutive cycles. Counsel women who start therapy postpartum and have not yet had a period to use additional method of contraception until a pink tab has been taken for 7 consecutive days. Advise to report if taking folate supplements and to maintain folate supplementation upon discontinuation due to pregnancy.

STORAGE: 25°C (77°F); excursions permitted to 15-30°C (59-86°F).

BIAXIN – clarithromycin

RX

B

Class: Macrolide

OTHER BRAND NAMES
Biaxin XL

ADULT DOSAGE
Mycobacterial Infections
Tab/Sus:
Prophylaxis of Disseminated *Mycobacterium avium* Complex (MAC) in Patients w/ Advanced HIV Infection:
Usual: 500mg bid
Treatment of Disseminated Infection Due to MAC or *M. intracellulare*:
Usual: 500mg bid; continue therapy if clinical response is observed
D/C when the patient is considered at low risk of disseminated infection

Pharyngitis/Tonsillitis
Due to *Streptococcus pyogenes*:
Tab/Sus:
250mg q12h for 10 days

Acute Maxillary Sinusitis
Due to *Haemophilus influenzae*, *Moraxella catarrhalis*, or *Streptococcus pneumoniae*:
Tab/Sus:
500mg q12h for 14 days
XL Tab:
1000mg q24h for 14 days

Community-Acquired Pneumonia
Tab/Sus:
***Haemophilus influenzae*:**
250mg q12h for 7 days
***Streptococcus pneumoniae*, *Chlamydophila pneumoniae*, or *Mycoplasma pneumoniae*:**
250mg q12h for 7-14 days
XL Tab:
***H. influenzae*, *Haemophilus parainfluenzae*, *Moraxella catarrhalis*, *S. pneumoniae*, *C. pneumoniae*, or *M. pneumoniae*:**
1000mg q24h for 7 days

Skin and Skin Structure Infections
Uncomplicated Infections Due to *Staphylococcus aureus* or *Streptococcus pyogenes*:
Tab/Sus:
250mg q12h for 7-14 days

Helicobacter pylori Eradication
Tab:
Triple Therapy:
500mg + 1g amoxicillin + 20mg omeprazole, all q12h for 10 days; give additional 20mg omeprazole qd for 18 days for ulcer healing/symptom relief if an ulcer was present at the time of initiation
or
500mg + 1g amoxicillin + 30mg lansoprazole, all q12h for 10 or 14 days
Dual Therapy:
500mg q8h + 40mg omeprazole qam for 14 days; give additional 20mg omeprazole qd for 14 days for ulcer healing/symptom relief
or

PEDIATRIC DOSAGE
General Dosing
Pharyngitis/tonsillitis due to *Streptococcus pyogenes*; community-acquired pneumonia due to *Mycoplasma pneumoniae*, *S. pneumoniae*, or *Chlamydophila pneumoniae*; acute maxillary sinusitis or acute otitis media due to *Haemophilus influenzae*, *Moraxella catarrhalis*, or *S. pneumoniae*; or uncomplicated skin and skin structure infections due to *Staphylococcus aureus* or *S. pyogenes*
Tab/Sus:
≥6 Months of Age: 15mg/kg/day divided q12h for 10 days

Mycobacterial Infections
Tab/Sus:
≥20 Months of Age:
Prophylaxis of Disseminated Mycobacterium avium Complex (MAC) in Patients w/ Advanced HIV Infection:
Usual: 7.5mg/kg bid, up to 500mg bid
Treatment of Disseminated Infection Due to MAC or *M. intracellulare*:
Usual: 7.5mg/kg bid, up to 500mg bid; continue therapy if clinical response is observed
D/C when the patient is considered at low risk of disseminated infection

500mg q8h or q12h + 400mg ranitidine bismuth citrate q12h for 14 days; give additional 400mg ranitidine bismuth citrate bid for 14 days for ulcer healing/symptom relief

Acute Bacterial Exacerbation of Chronic Bronchitis

Tab/Sus:

***Moraxella catarrhalis* or *Streptococcus pneumoniae*:**
250mg q12h for 7-14 days

***Haemophilus influenzae*:**
500mg q12h for 7-14 days

***Haemophilus parainfluenzae*:**
500mg q12h for 7 days

XL Tab:

***H. influenzae, H. parainfluenzae, M. catarrhalis*, or *S. pneumoniae*:**
1000mg q24h for 7 days

DOSING CONSIDERATIONS

Concomitant Medications

Ranitidine Bismuth Citrate: Not recommended if CrCl <25mL/min or w/ history of acute porphyria

Renal Impairment

Severe (CrCl <30mL/min): Reduce dose by 50%

Concomitant Atazanavir or Ritonavir:
CrCl 30-60mL/min: Reduce dose by 50%
CrCl <30mL/min: Reduce dose by 75%

ADMINISTRATION

Oral route

Tab/Sus

Take w/ or w/o food; may be taken w/ milk

Sus

Shake well before each use
Reconstitute 50mL bottle sizes w/ 27mL of water and 100mL bottle sizes w/ 55mL of water
Add water in 2 portions and shake after each aliquot
Use w/in 14 days

XL Tab

Take w/ food
Swallow whole; do not chew, crush, or break

HOW SUPPLIED

Sus: 125mg/5mL, 250mg/5mL [50mL, 100mL]; **Tab:** 250mg, 500mg; **Tab, Extended-Release (XL):** 500mg

CONTRAINDICATIONS

Known hypersensitivity to clarithromycin or any of its excipients, erythromycin, or any of the macrolide antibiotics. History of cholestatic jaundice/hepatic dysfunction associated w/ prior use of clarithromycin. History of QT prolongation or ventricular cardiac arrhythmia, including torsades de pointes. Concomitant use w/ cisapride, pimozide, astemizole, terfenadine, ergotamine, or dihydroergotamine, and w/ HMG-CoA reductase inhibitors that are extensively metabolized by CYP3A4 (lovastatin or simvastatin). Concomitant use w/ colchicine in patients w/ renal/hepatic impairment.

WARNINGS/PRECAUTIONS

Avoid in pregnancy, except in clinical circumstances where no alternative therapy is appropriate. Hepatic dysfunction, including increased liver enzymes, and hepatocellular and/or cholestatic hepatitis, w/ or w/o jaundice, reported; d/c immediately if signs/symptoms of hepatitis occur. QT interval prolongation, arrhythmia (infrequent), and torsades de pointes reported; avoid w/ ongoing proarrhythmic conditions (eg, uncorrected hypokalemia, hypomagnesemia) and clinically significant bradycardia. *Clostridium difficile*-associated diarrhea (CDAD) reported; may need to d/c if CDAD is suspected or confirmed. D/C therapy immediately and initiate prompt treatment if severe acute hypersensitivity reactions (eg, Stevens-Johnson syndrome, toxic epidermal necrolysis, drug rash w/ eosinophilia and systemic symptoms, Henoch-Schonlein purpura) occur. May result in bacterial resistance w/ prolonged use in the absence of a proven/suspected bacterial infection or a prophylactic indication. Exacerbation of symptoms of myasthenia gravis and new onset of symptoms of myasthenic syndrome reported. Caution in elderly.

ADVERSE REACTIONS

Diarrhea, N/V, dysgeusia, abdominal pain.

DRUG INTERACTIONS

See Contraindications and Dosing Considerations. Avoid Class IA (quinidine, procainamide) or Class III (dofetilide, amiodarone, sotalol) antiarrhythmic agents. May increase serum theophylline, carbamazepine, omeprazole, and digoxin, drugs metabolized by CYP3A, colchicine, saquinavir, tolterodine, and itraconazole levels. Bradyarrhythmias and lactic acidosis observed w/ verapamil. Hypotension and acute kidney injury may occur w/ calcium channel blockers metabolized by CYP3A4 (eg, verapamil, amlodipine, diltiazem). Increased levels w/ fluconazole, itraconazole, and saquinavir. Avoid doses of >1000mg/day w/ protease inhibitors. May potentiate oral anticoagulant effects. Risk of serious hemorrhage and significant elevations in PT/INR w/ warfarin; monitor PT/INR frequently. Caution w/ other drugs known to be CYP3A enzyme substrates, especially if substrate has a narrow safety margin (eg, carbamazepine) and/or substrate is extensively metabolized by this enzyme. Decreased levels w/ CYP3A inducers (eg, efavirenz, rifampicin, rifapentine); consider alternative antibacterial treatment. May increase levels of rifabutin and increase risk of uveitis w/ rifabutin. Etravirine may decrease exposure; consider alternative for treatment of MAC. Concomitant use w/ phosphodiesterase inhibitors (sildenafil, tadalafil, vardenafil) is not recommended. Consider reduction of sildenafil dose. CNS effects, increased sedation, and prolongation of sedation reported w/ concomitant triazolobenzodiazepines (eg, triazolam, midazolam); monitor for additive CNS effects and consider appropriate dose adjustments. May increase AUC of midazolam; possible prolongation and intensity of effect should be anticipated. Occurrence of torsades de pointes w/ quinidine or disopyramide reported; monitor serum levels and for QT prolongation. Interactions may occur w/ cyclosporine, tacrolimus, alfentanil, rifabutin, methylprednisolone, cilostazol, bromocriptine, vinblastine, phenobarbital, St. John's wort, hexobarbital, phenytoin, and valproate. Significant hypoglycemia may occur w/ oral hypoglycemic agents (eg, nateglinide, pioglitazone, repaglinide) and/or insulin. Caution when prescribing w/ statins; if concomitant use w/ atorvastatin or pravastatin cannot be avoided, do not exceed 20mg/day of atorvastatin and 40mg/day of pravastatin. Consider use of a statin that is not dependent on CYP3A metabolism (eg, fluvastatin); prescribe the lowest registered dose if concomitant use cannot be avoided. (Tab) May decrease levels of zidovudine; separate zidovudine administration by at least 2 hrs.

PATIENT CONSIDERATIONS

Assessment: Assess for history of cholestatic jaundice/hepatic dysfunction associated w/ prior use of clarithromycin, hepatic/renal impairment, history of QT prolongation, ongoing proarrhythmic conditions, clinically significant bradycardia, ventricular cardiac arrhythmia, torsades de pointes, myasthenia gravis, history of acute porphyria, pregnancy/nursing status, possible drug interactions, and hypersensitivity to the drug, any of its ingredients, erythromycin, or any of the macrolide antibiotics.

Monitoring: Monitor for development of drug-resistant bacteria, CDAD, hepatitis, QT prolongation, severe acute hypersensitivity reactions, exacerbation of myasthenia gravis, new onset of symptoms of myasthenic syndrome, and other adverse reactions. Monitor LFTs and renal function. Frequently monitor INR/PT w/ oral anticoagulants.

Counseling: Inform about potential benefits/risks of therapy. Counsel that therapy should only be used to treat bacterial, not viral, infections. Instruct to take exactly ud; inform that skipping doses or not completing full course may decrease effectiveness and increase antibiotic resistance. Instruct to notify physician if watery/bloody diarrhea (w/ or w/o stomach cramps and fever) develops, even as late as ≥2 months after treatment. Instruct to notify physician if pregnant/nursing and of all medications currently being taken.

STORAGE: (250mg tab) 15-30°C (59-86°F). Protect from light. (500mg tab) 20-25°C (68-77°F). (Sus) <25°C (77°F). Do not refrigerate. (XL tab) 20-25°C (68-77°F); excursions permitted 15-30°C (59-86°F).

BLINCYTO – blinatumomab

RX

Class: CD19-directed CD3 T-cell engager

Cytokine release syndrome (CRS), which may be life-threatening or fatal, reported; interrupt or d/c therapy as recommended. Neurological toxicities, which may be severe, life-threatening, or fatal, reported; interrupt or d/c therapy as recommended.

ADULT DOSAGE

Acute Lymphoblastic Leukemia

Philadelphia Chromosome-Negative: Relapsed or Refractory B-Cell Precursor:

≥45kg:

Cycle 1: 9mcg/day on Days 1-7, and 28mcg/day on Days 8-28

PEDIATRIC DOSAGE

Acute Lymphoblastic Leukemia

Philadelphia Chromosome-Negative: Relapsed or Refractory B-Cell Precursor:

Limited experience in pediatric patients

Evaluated in a dose-escalation study of 41 pediatric patients with relapsed or refractory

B

Subsequent Cycles: 28mcg/day on Days 1-28

Single cycle of treatment consists of 4 weeks of continuous IV infusion followed by a 2-week treatment-free interval

Treatment course consists of up to 2 cycles for induction followed by 3 additional cycles for consolidation treatment (up to a total of 5 cycles)

B-precursor acute lymphoblastic leukemia (median age was 6 yrs [range: 2-17 yrs]). Administered at doses of 5-30mcg/m^2/day. Recommended phase 2 regimen was 5mcg/m^2/day on Days 1-7 and 15mcg/m^2/day on Days 8-28 for cycle 1, and 15mcg/m^2/day on Days 1-28 for subsequent cycles

Steady-state concentrations were comparable in adult and pediatric patients at the equivalent dose levels based on BSA-based regimens

DOSING CONSIDERATIONS

Adverse Reactions

If interruption after an adverse event is no longer than 7 days, continue same cycle to a total of 28 days of infusion inclusive of days before and after the interruption in that cycle. If an interruption due to an adverse event is >7 days, start a new cycle

Cytokine Release Syndrome:

Grade 3: Withhold until resolved, then restart at 9mcg/day. Escalate to 28mcg/day after 7 days if the toxicity does not recur

Grade 4: D/C permanently

Neurological Toxicity:

Seizure: D/C permanently if >1 seizure occurs

Grade 3: Withhold until no more than Grade 1 (mild) for at least 3 days, then restart at 9mcg/day. Escalate to 28mcg/day after 7 days if the toxicity does not recur. If the toxicity occurred at 9mcg/day, or if the toxicity takes >7 days to resolve, d/c permanently

Grade 4: D/C permanently

Other Clinically Relevant Adverse Reactions:

Grade 3: Withhold until no more than Grade 1 (mild), then restart at 9mcg/day. Escalate to 28mcg/day after 7 days if the toxicity does not recur. If the toxicity takes >14 days to resolve, d/c permanently

Grade 4: Consider discontinuing permanently

ADMINISTRATION

IV route

Premedicate with dexamethasone 20mg IV 1 hr prior to the 1st dose of each cycle, prior to a step dose (eg, Cycle 1 day 8), or when restarting an infusion after an interruption of ≥4 hrs

Administer as a continuous IV infusion at a constant flow rate using an infusion pump that is programmable, lockable, non-elastomeric, and has an alarm

Infusion bags should be infused over 24 hrs or 48 hrs

Infuse the total 240mL sol according to the instructions on the pharmacy label on the bag at 1 of the following constant infusion rates:

Infusion rate of 10mL/hr for a duration of 24 hrs, or 5mL/hr for a duration of 48 hrs

Refer to PI for further administration, reconstitution, and preparation instructions

HOW SUPPLIED

Inj: 35mcg

CONTRAINDICATIONS

Known hypersensitivity to blinatumomab or to any component of the product formulation.

WARNINGS/PRECAUTIONS

Hospitalization is recommended for the first 9 days of the 1st cycle and the first 2 days of the 2nd cycle. For all subsequent cycle starts and reinitiation (eg, if treatment is interrupted for ≥4 hrs), supervision by a healthcare professional or hospitalization is recommended. Infusion reactions may occur and may be clinically indistinguishable from manifestations of CRS. Disseminated intravascular coagulation (DIC), capillary leak syndrome (CLS), and hemophagocytic lymphohistiocytosis/macrophage activation syndrome (HLH/MAS) reported in the setting of CRS. Serious infections (eg, sepsis, pneumonia, bacteremia, opportunistic infections, catheter-site infections) reported; administer prophylactic antibiotics and employ surveillance testing during treatment as appropriate. Tumor lysis syndrome (TLS) reported; use appropriate prophylactic measures, including pretreatment nontoxic cytoreduction and on-treatment hydration; may require either temporary interruption or discontinuation of therapy. Neutropenia and febrile neutropenia, including life-threatening cases, reported; interrupt therapy if prolonged neutropenia occurs. Risk for loss of consciousness. Associated with transient elevations in liver enzymes; interrupt therapy if the transaminases rise to >5X ULN or if bilirubin rises to >3X ULN. Cranial magnetic resonance imaging changes showing leukoencephalopathy observed, especially in patients with prior treatment with cranial irradiation and antileukemic chemotherapy (including systemic high-dose methotrexate or intrathecal cytarabine); clinical significance of this is unknown. Preparation and administration errors reported; follow instructions strictly to minimize medication errors. Potential for immunogenicity. Caution in elderly.

ADVERSE REACTIONS
CRS, neurological toxicities, pyrexia, headache, peripheral edema, febrile neutropenia, nausea, hypokalemia, constipation, anemia, diarrhea, fatigue, bacterial infections, tremor, cough.

DRUG INTERACTIONS
May suppress CYP450 enzymes; highest risk during the first 9 days of the 1st cycle and the first 2 days of the 2nd cycle in patients receiving concomitant CYP450 substrates, particularly those with a narrow therapeutic index; monitor for toxicity (eg, warfarin) or drug concentrations (eg, cyclosporine) and adjust dose of concomitant drug PRN.

PATIENT CONSIDERATIONS

Assessment: Assess for known hypersensitivity to drug or to any component of the formulation, prior treatment with cranial irradiation and antileukemic chemotherapy, pregnancy/nursing status, and possible drug interactions. Obtain baseline WBC count, absolute neutrophil count (ANC), ALT, AST, gamma-glutamyl transferase (GGT), and total bilirubin.

Monitoring: Monitor for signs/symptoms of CRS, DIC, CLS, HLH/MAS, neurological toxicities, infections, TLS, loss of consciousness, and other adverse reactions. Monitor for neutropenia/febrile neutropenia; monitor lab parameters (eg, WBC count, ANC) during infusion. Monitor ALT, AST, GGT, and total blood bilirubin during therapy.

Counseling: Advise to contact physician for any signs/symptoms of CRS or infusion reactions, neurological toxicities, or infections (eg, pneumonia). Advise to refrain from driving and engaging in hazardous occupations/activities (eg, operating heavy/potentially dangerous machinery) while on therapy and inform that neurological events may be experienced. Inform that it is very important to keep area around the IV catheter clean to reduce the risk of infection. Advise to not adjust setting on the infusion pump; inform that any changes to pump function may result in dosing errors. Instruct to contact physician or nurse immediately if there is a problem with the infusion pump or the pump alarms.

STORAGE: 2-8°C (36-46°F). Protect from light until time of use. Do not freeze. May store lyophilized vial and IV sol stabilizer for a max of 8 hrs at room temperature. Reconstituted Vial: 23-27°C (73-81°F) for 4 hrs, or 2-8°C (36-46°F) for 24 hrs. Protect from light. Prepared IV Bag Containing Sol for Infusion: 23-27°C (73-81°F) for 48 hrs (storage time includes infusion time; if not administered within the time frames and temperatures indicated, discard and do not refrigerate again), or 2-8°C (36-46°F) for 8 days. Ship in packaging that has been validated to maintain temperature of the contents at 2-8°C (36-46°F). Do not freeze.

BONIVA – ibandronate; ibandronate sodium

RX

Class: Bisphosphonate

ADULT DOSAGE

Osteoporosis

Inj:
Treatment in Postmenopausal Women:
3mg IV over 15-30 sec every 3 months

Tab:
Treatment and Prevention in Postmenopausal Women:
150mg once monthly on the same date each month

Missed Dose

Inj:
If dose is missed, administer as soon as it can be rescheduled
Thereafter, schedule every 3 months from date of last inj

Tab:
If next scheduled ibandronate day is >7 days away, take one 150mg tab in am following date that it is remembered
If next scheduled ibandronate day is 1-7 days away, wait until subsequent month's scheduled ibandronate day to take tab
For both scenarios, return to original schedule by taking one 150mg tab every month on previous chosen day for subsequent doses

PEDIATRIC DOSAGE

Pediatric use may not have been established

B

DOSING CONSIDERATIONS

Renal Impairment

Severe (CrCl <30mL/min): Not recommended

ADMINISTRATION

IV/Oral route

Inj

Do not mix w/ Ca^{2+}-containing sol or other IV administered drugs.
Do not use prefilled syringes w/ particulate matter or discoloration.
Administer only w/ the enclosed needle.
Do not administer more frequently than once every 3 months.

Tab

Take at least 60 min before the 1st food or drink of the day other than water or before taking any oral medication or supplementation.
Swallow tabs whole; do not chew or suck.
Swallow tabs w/ full glass of plain water (6-8 oz) while standing or sitting in upright position; avoid lying down for 60 min after taking medication.
Do not eat, drink anything except plain water, or take other medications for at least 60 min after taking ibandronate.

HOW SUPPLIED

Inj: 3mg/3mL [prefilled syringe]; **Tab:** 150mg

CONTRAINDICATIONS

Hypocalcemia. (Tab) Esophageal abnormalities that delay esophageal emptying (eg, stricture or achalasia), inability to stand or sit upright for at least 60 min, known hypersensitivity to ibandronate sodium or to any of its excipients.

WARNINGS/PRECAUTIONS

Consider discontinuation after 3-5 yrs of use in patients at low-risk for fracture; periodically reevaluate risk for fracture in patients who d/c therapy. Hypocalcemia reported; treat hypocalcemia and other disturbances of bone and mineral metabolism before therapy. Osteonecrosis of the jaw (ONJ) reported; risk may increase w/ duration of exposure to drug or w/ concomitant administration of drugs associated w/ ONJ. Consider a dental examination w/ appropriate preventive dentistry prior to treatment in patients w/ a history of concomitant risk factors (eg, cancer, chemotherapy, angiogenesis inhibitors, radiotherapy, corticosteroids, poor oral hygiene) and if possible, avoid invasive dental procedures while on treatment. For patients requiring invasive dental procedures, discontinuation of treatment may reduce risk for ONJ. Consider discontinuation if ONJ develops. Severe and occasionally incapacitating bone, joint, and/or muscle pain reported; d/c if severe symptoms develop. Atypical, low-energy, or low-trauma fractures of the femoral shaft reported; evaluate any patient w/ a history of bisphosphonate exposure who presents w/ thigh/groin pain to rule out an incomplete femur fracture, and consider interruption of therapy. (Inj) Caution not to administer intra-arterially or paravenously as this could lead to tissue damage. Anaphylaxis reported; d/c and initiate appropriate treatment if anaphylactic or other severe hypersensitivity/allergic reactions occur. (Tab) May cause local irritation of the upper GI mucosa; caution w/ active upper GI problems (eg, Barrett's esophagus, dysphagia, esophageal diseases, gastritis, duodenitis, ulcers). Esophageal reactions (eg, esophagitis, esophageal ulcers/erosions) reported; d/c if dysphagia, odynophagia, retrosternal pain, or new/worsening heartburn develops. Use therapy under appropriate supervision in patients who cannot comply w/ dosing instructions due to mental disability. Gastric and duodenal ulcers reported.

ADVERSE REACTIONS

Influenza, nasopharyngitis, abdominal pain, dyspepsia, constipation, arthralgia, back pain, pain in extremity, headache, diarrhea, UTI, myalgia.

DRUG INTERACTIONS

May interfere w/ the use of bone-imaging agents. (Tab) Products containing Ca^{2+} and other multivalent cations (eg, aluminum, Mg^{2+}, iron) may interfere w/ absorption; do not take these products w/in 60 min of dosing. Caution w/ aspirin or NSAIDs due to GI irritation.

PATIENT CONSIDERATIONS

Assessment: Assess for hypocalcemia, disturbances of bone and mineral metabolism, risk for ONJ, renal impairment, drug hypersensitivity, any other conditions where treatment is contraindicated or cautioned, pregnancy/nursing status, and possible drug interactions. (Inj) Obtain SrCr before each dose. Perform routine oral exam, and consider appropriate preventive dentistry in patients w/ history of concomitant risk factors for ONJ. (Tab) Assess for esophageal abnormalities, ability to stand or sit upright for at least 60 min, active upper GI problems, and mental disability.

Monitoring: Monitor for signs/symptoms of ONJ, musculoskeletal pain, hypocalcemia, atypical femoral fracture, and other adverse reactions. Monitor renal function and periodically reevaluate the need for continued therapy. (Tab) Monitor for esophageal reactions. (Inj) Monitor for severe hypersensitivity/allergic reactions.

Counseling: Inform about benefits/risks of therapy. Instruct to take supplemental Ca^{2+} and vitamin D if dietary intake is inadequate. (Tab) Instruct to carefully follow dosing instructions and on what to do if doses are missed. Advise to d/c and seek medical attention if symptoms of esophageal irritation develop. Instruct on appropriate administration of drug.

STORAGE: 25°C (77°F); excursions permitted to 15-30°C (59-86°F).

Boostrix – tetanus toxoid, reduced diphtheria toxoid and acellular pertussis vaccine, adsorbed

RX

Class: Toxoid/vaccine combination

ADULT DOSAGE

Active Booster Immunization Against Tetanus, Diphtheria, and Pertussis

0.5mL IM single dose

Wound Management:

May be given as a tetanus prophylaxis if no previous dose of any tetanus toxoid, reduced diphtheria toxoid, and acellular pertussis vaccine, adsorbed (Tdap) has been administered

PEDIATRIC DOSAGE

Active Booster Immunization Against Tetanus, Diphtheria, and Pertussis

≥10 Years:

0.5mL IM single dose

Wound Management:

May be given as a tetanus prophylaxis if no previous dose of any tetanus toxoid, reduced diphtheria toxoid, and acellular pertussis vaccine, adsorbed (Tdap) has been administered

ADMINISTRATION

IM route

5 yrs should have elapsed since last dose of recommended series of diphtheria and tetanus toxoids and acellular pertussis vaccine adsorbed (DTaP) and/or tetanus and diphtheria toxoids adsorbed for adult use (Td) vaccine

Shake well before use
Inject into the deltoid muscle of the upper arm
Do not administer IV, intradermally, or SQ
Do not mix w/ any other vaccine in the same syringe or vial

HOW SUPPLIED

Inj: 0.5mL [vial, prefilled syringe]

CONTRAINDICATIONS

A severe allergic reaction (eg, anaphylaxis) after a previous dose of any tetanus toxoid-, diphtheria toxoid-, or pertussis antigen-containing vaccine or any component of this vaccine, encephalopathy (eg, coma, decreased level of consciousness, prolonged seizures) w/in 7 days of administration of a previous dose of a pertussis antigen-containing vaccine that is not attributable to another identifiable cause.

WARNINGS/PRECAUTIONS

Administer 5 yrs after last dose of recommended series of diphtheria and tetanus toxoids and acellular pertussis vaccine adsorbed and/or tetanus and diphtheria toxoids adsorbed for adult use vaccine. Tip caps of prefilled syringes may contain natural rubber latex; allergic reactions may occur in latex-sensitive individuals. May cause brachial neuritis and Guillain-Barre syndrome. Risk of Guillain-Barre syndrome may increase if Guillain-Barre syndrome occurred within 6 weeks of receipt of a prior tetanus toxoid-containing vaccine. Syncope may occur and can be accompanied by transient neurological signs (eg, visual disturbance, paresthesia, tonic-clonic limb movements). Defer vaccination in patients with progressive/unstable neurologic conditions (eg, cerebrovascular events, acute encephalopathic conditions). Avoid if experienced an Arthus-type hypersensitivity reaction following a prior dose of tetanus toxoid-containing vaccine unless at least 10 yrs have elapsed since last dose of tetanus toxoid-containing vaccine. Expected immune response may not be obtained in immunosuppressed persons. Review immunization history for possible vaccine sensitivity and previous vaccination-related adverse reactions; epinephrine and other appropriate agents should be immediately available for control of allergic reactions.

ADVERSE REACTIONS

Inj-site reactions (eg, pain, redness, swelling, increased arm circumference), headache, fatigue, fever, GI symptoms.

DRUG INTERACTIONS

Lower postvaccination geometric mean antibody concentrations (GMCs) to pertactin observed following concomitant administration with meningococcal conjugate vaccine as compared to Boostrix administered 1st. Lower GMCs for antibodies to the pertussis antigens filamentous hemagglutinin and pertactin observed when concomitantly administered with influenza virus

B

vaccine as compared with Boostrix alone. Immunosuppressive therapies, including irradiation, antimetabolites, alkylating agents, cytotoxic drugs, and corticosteroids (used in greater than physiologic doses), may reduce the immune response to vaccine.

PATIENT CONSIDERATIONS

Assessment: Assess for history of encephalopathy, latex hypersensitivity, development of Guillain-Barre syndrome following a prior vaccine containing tetanus toxoid, progressive/unstable neurologic conditions, immunosuppression, pregnancy/nursing status, and for possible drug interactions. Review immunization history for possible vaccine sensitivity and previous vaccination-related adverse reactions.

Monitoring: Monitor for signs and symptoms of Guillain-Barre syndrome, brachial neuritis, allergic reactions, syncope, neurological signs, and other adverse reactions. Monitor immune response.

Counseling: Inform about benefits/risks of immunization. Advise about the potential for adverse reactions. Instruct to notify physician if any adverse reactions occur, if pregnant, or planning to become pregnant. Encourage pregnant women receiving the vaccine to contact the pregnancy registry.

STORAGE: 2-8°C (36-46°F). Do not freeze; discard if has been frozen.

Botox Cosmetic — onabotulinumtoxinA

RX

Class: Acetylcholine release inhibitor

Distant spread of toxin effects (eg, asthenia, generalized muscle weakness, diplopia, ptosis, dysphagia, dysphonia, dysarthria, urinary incontinence, breathing difficulties) reported hrs to weeks after inj. Swallowing and breathing difficulties can be life threatening; reports of death. Risk of symptoms greatest in children treated for spasticity; may also occur in adults treated for spasticity and other conditions, particularly in patients who have an underlying condition that would predispose them to these symptoms. In unapproved uses, including spasticity in children, and in approved indications, cases of spread of effect have been reported at doses comparable to those used to treat cervical dystonia and upper limb spasticity and at lower doses.

ADULT DOSAGE

Correction of Moderate to Severe Facial Wrinkles and Folds

Glabellar Lines:

For temporary improvement in appearance of moderate to severe glabellar lines associated w/ corrugator and/or procerus muscle activity

Inject 4 U/0.1mL IM into each of 5 sites; 2 in each corrugator muscle and 1 in the procerus muscle, for a total dose of 20 U

Lateral Canthal Lines:

For temporary improvement in appearance of moderate to severe lateral canthal lines associated w/ orbicularis oculi activity

Inject 4 U/0.1mL into 3 sites/side (6 total inj points) in lateral orbicularis oculi muscle for a total of 24 U/0.6mL (12 U/side)

Max Cumulative Dose When Treating for ≥1 Indication: 360 U in a 3-month interval

For simultaneous treatment w/ glabellar lines, the dose is 24 U for lateral canthal lines and 20 U for glabellar lines, w/ a total dose of 44 U

PEDIATRIC DOSAGE

Pediatric use may not have been established

ADMINISTRATION

IM route

Dilution

2.5mL diluent added to 100 U vial results in 4 U/0.1mL.

1.25mL diluent added to 50 U vial results in 4 U/0.1mL.

Preparation

1. Prior to IM inj, reconstitute each vial w/ sterile, preservative-free 0.9% NaCl inj.
2. Draw up proper amount of diluent to obtain a reconstituted sol at a concentration of 4 U/0.1mL and a total treatment dose of 20 U in 0.5mL for glabellar lines and 24 U in 0.6mL for lateral canthal lines.
3. Slowly inject diluent into vial; discard vial if vacuum does not pull diluent into vial.
4. Gently mix by rotating vial.

Administration

Administer w/in 24 hrs after reconstitution; store at 2-8°C (36-46°F) during this time period.
Use a 30- to 33-gauge needle.

Glabellar Lines:

Avoid inj near the levator palpebrae superioris, particularly in patients w/ larger brow depressor complexes.
Lateral corrugator inj should be placed at least 1cm above the bony supraorbital ridge.
Do not inject toxin closer than 1cm above the central eyebrow.

Lateral Canthal Lines:

Inj should be given w/ needle bevel tip up and oriented away from the eye.
The 1st inj should be approximately 1.5-2.0cm temporal to the lateral canthus and just temporal to the orbital rim.

Refer to PI for diagrams depicting proper administration.

HOW SUPPLIED

Inj: 50 U, 100 U

CONTRAINDICATIONS

Infection at proposed inj site(s), known hypersensitivity to any botulinum toxin preparation or to any of the components in the formulation.

WARNINGS/PRECAUTIONS

Not interchangeable w/ other botulinum toxin products; cannot be compared nor converted into U of any other botulinum toxin products. Serious/fatal adverse reactions (eg, excessive weakness, dysphagia, aspiration pneumonia) reported in patients who received inj for unapproved uses. Serious and/or immediate hypersensitivity reactions reported; d/c further injections and institute appropriate medical therapy immediately. Caution w/ preexisting cardiovascular (CV) disease; adverse events involving CV system (eg, arrhythmia, MI) reported. Increased risk of clinically significant effects (eg, severe dysphagia, respiratory compromise) in patients w/ neuromuscular disorders; monitor patients w/ peripheral motor neuropathic diseases, amyotrophic lateral sclerosis, or neuromuscular junction disorders. May result in swallowing or breathing difficulties; increased risk of dysphagia in patients w/ smaller neck muscle mass and those who require bilateral inj into the sternocleidomastoid muscle for treatment of cervical dystonia. Caution w/ inflammation at the proposed inj site(s), ptosis, or when excessive weakness or atrophy is present in the targeted muscle(s). Reduced blinking from inj of orbicularis muscle may lead to corneal exposure, persistent epithelial defect, and corneal ulceration, especially in patients w/ VII nerve disorders; vigorously treat any epithelial defect. Inducing paralysis in one or more extraocular muscles may produce spatial disorientation, double vision, or past pointing; covering affected eye may alleviate symptoms. Contains albumin; carries an extremely remote risk for transmission of viral diseases and Creutzfeldt-Jakob disease.

ADVERSE REACTIONS

Eyelid ptosis.

DRUG INTERACTIONS

Potentiation of toxic effects may occur w/ aminoglycosides or other agents interfering w/ neuromuscular transmission (eg, curare-like compounds); use w/ caution. Use of anticholinergic drugs after administration may potentiate systemic anticholinergic effects. Excessive neuromuscular weakness may be exacerbated by administration of another botulinum toxin prior to the resolution of the effects of a previously administered botulinum toxin. Excessive weakness may be exaggerated by administration of muscle relaxant before or after administration of onabotulinumtoxinA.

PATIENT CONSIDERATIONS

Assessment: Assess for hypersensitivity to any botulinum toxin preparation or any components of the product, infection/inflammation at proposed inj site(s), ptosis, weakness/atrophy in targeted muscle(s), CV disease, neuromuscular disorders, preexisting swallowing/breathing difficulties, smaller neck muscle mass, patients w/ required bilateral inj into the sternocleidomastoid muscle, VII nerve disorders, pregnancy/nursing status, and possible drug interactions.

Monitoring: Monitor for spread of toxin effects, swallowing/speech/respiratory difficulties, hypersensitivity reactions, CV system adverse events, dysphagia, infections, epithelial defects, and other adverse reactions. Monitor patients w/ peripheral motor neuropathic diseases, amyotrophic lateral sclerosis, neuromuscular junction disorders, or compromised respiratory status.

Counseling: Advise to seek immediate medical attention if any unusual symptoms (eg, swallowing/speaking/breathing difficulty) develop, or if any existing symptom worsens. Instruct to avoid driving a car or engaging in other potentially hazardous activities if loss of strength, muscle weakness, blurred vision, or drooping eyelids occur.

STORAGE: 2-8°C (36-46°F).

B

BREO ELLIPTA – fluticasone furoate/vilanterol

RX

Class: $Beta_2$ agonist/corticosteroid

Long-acting β_2-adrenergic agonists (LABAs) increase the risk of asthma-related death. LABAs may increase the risk of asthma-related hospitalization in pediatric and adolescent patients. Use only for patients not adequately controlled on a long-term asthma control medication (eg, inhaled corticosteroid [ICS]) or whose disease severity clearly warrants initiation of treatment w/ both an ICS and a LABA. Once asthma control is achieved and maintained, assess the patient at regular intervals and step down therapy (eg, d/c Breo Ellipta) if possible w/o loss of asthma control and maintain the patient on a long-term asthma control medication. Do not use if asthma is adequately controlled on low- or medium-dose ICS.

ADULT DOSAGE

Chronic Obstructive Pulmonary Disease

Long-term maint treatment of airflow obstruction; also indicated to reduce COPD exacerbations in patients w/ history of exacerbations

1 inh of 100mcg/25mcg qd

Max: 1 inh of 100mcg/25mcg qd

If shortness of breath occurs in the period between doses, an inhaled, short-acting β_2-agonist (eg, albuterol) should be taken for immediate relief

Asthma

Initial: 1 inh of 100mcg/25mcg or 200mcg/25mcg qd

Previous Low- to Mid-Dose Corticosteroid-Containing Treatment: Consider 1 inh of 100mcg/25mcg qd

Previous Mid- to High-Dose Corticosteroid-Containing Treatment: Consider 1 inh of 200mcg/25mcg qd

Max: 1 inh of 200mcg/25mcg qd

If asthma symptoms arise in the period between doses, an inhaled, short-acting β_2-agonist (eg, albuterol) should be taken for immediate relief

PEDIATRIC DOSAGE

Pediatric use may not have been established

ADMINISTRATION

Oral inh route

After inh, patient should rinse mouth w/ water w/o swallowing.

Take at the same time every day; do not use >1 inh q24h.

HOW SUPPLIED

Powder, Inhalation: (Fluticasone/Vilanterol) (100mcg/25mcg)/blister, (200mcg/25mcg)/blister [14, 30 inh]

CONTRAINDICATIONS

Primary treatment of status asthmaticus or other acute episodes of COPD or asthma where intensive measures are required. Severe hypersensitivity to milk proteins or demonstrated hypersensitivity to fluticasone furoate, vilanterol, or any of the excipients.

WARNINGS/PRECAUTIONS

Not indicated for acute bronchospasm relief. Do not initiate during rapidly deteriorating or potentially life-threatening episodes of COPD or asthma. D/C regular use of oral/inhaled short-acting β_2-agonists when beginning treatment; use only for symptomatic relief of acute respiratory symptoms. Increased incidence of pneumonia reported in COPD patients receiving 100mcg/25mcg. May produce paradoxical bronchospasm; treat immediately, d/c Breo Ellipta, and institute alternative therapy. Hypersensitivity reactions may occur; d/c if such reactions occur. **Fluticasone:** *Candida albicans* infections of mouth and pharynx reported; treat and, if needed, interrupt therapy. Increased susceptibility to infections. Chickenpox or measles may have a more serious/fatal course; avoid exposure and, if exposed, consider prophylaxis/treatment. Use w/ caution, if at all, in patients w/ active/quiescent tuberculosis (TB); systemic fungal, bacterial, viral, or parasitic infections; or ocular herpes simplex. Deaths due to adrenal insufficiency reported in asthma patients during and after transfer from a systemic corticosteroid to an ICS. Patients who have been withdrawn from systemic corticosteroids should resume oral corticosteroids immediately during periods of stress, a severe COPD exacerbation, or a severe asthma attack. Patients requiring oral corticosteroids should be weaned slowly from systemic corticosteroid use after transferring to therapy. Systemic corticosteroid effects (eg, hypercorticism and adrenal suppression) may occur in patients sensitive to these effects; if such effects occur, reduce therapy slowly and consider other treatments for management of COPD or asthma symptoms. Decreases in bone mineral density (BMD) reported w/ long-term use. Assess BMD in COPD patients prior to initiating therapy and periodically thereafter; if significant reductions are seen and therapy is still considered medically important, consider using medicine to treat or prevent osteoporosis. Glaucoma, increased IOP, and cataracts reported w/ long-term use. Caution w/ moderate/severe hepatic impairment. May cause reduction in growth velocity in children and adolescents. **Vilanterol:** Clinically significant cardiovascular (CV) effects may occur (eg, increases in pulse rate, BP, cardiac arrhythmias); if such effects occur, therapy may need to be discontinued. Caution w/ CV disorders, convulsive disorders, thyrotoxicosis, and in patients unusually responsive to sympathomimetic amines. Doses of IV albuterol reported to aggravate preexisting diabetes mellitus (DM) and ketoacidosis. May produce significant hypokalemia or transient hyperglycemia.

ADVERSE REACTIONS

Nasopharyngitis, URTI, oral candidiasis, headache, sinusitis, cough, oropharyngeal pain, dysphonia, influenza, bronchitis.

DRUG INTERACTIONS

Do not use w/ another medicine containing a LABA; CV effects and fatalities reported w/ excessive use of inhaled sympathomimetic drugs. Caution w/ long-term ketoconazole and other strong CYP3A4 inhibitors (eg, ritonavir, clarithromycin, conivaptan); increased systemic corticosteroid and increased CV adverse effects may occur. **Vilanterol:** Extreme caution w/ MAOIs, TCAs, or drugs known to prolong the QTc interval or w/in 2 weeks of discontinuation of such agents; effect on CV system may be potentiated by these agents. β-blockers block pulmonary effects and may produce severe bronchospasm in COPD or asthma patients; if such therapy is needed, consider cardioselective β-blockers and use w/ caution. Caution is advised when coadministered w/ non-K^+-sparing diuretics; may acutely worsen ECG changes and/or hypokalemia that may result from non-K^+-sparing diuretics.

PATIENT CONSIDERATIONS

Assessment: Assess for hypersensitivity to drug or to milk proteins, COPD/asthma status, active/quiescent TB, systemic infections, ocular herpes simplex, CV disorders, risk factors for decreased bone mineral content, convulsive disorders, thyrotoxicosis, DM, ketoacidosis, history of increased IOP, glaucoma, and/or cataracts, hepatic impairment, pregnancy/nursing status, and possible drug interactions. Assess BMD.

Monitoring: Monitor for deteriorating disease, localized oropharyngeal *C. albicans* infections, pneumonia, infections, systemic corticosteroid effects, paradoxical bronchospasm, hypersensitivity reactions, CV effects, glaucoma, cataracts, increased IOP, hypokalemia, hyperglycemia, and other adverse reactions. Periodically monitor BMD.

Counseling: Advise patients w/ asthma that LABAs increase the risk of asthma-related death and may increase the risk of asthma-related hospitalization in pediatric and adolescent patients. Inform that drug is not meant to relieve acute symptoms of COPD or asthma and extra doses should not be used for that purpose; advise to treat acute symptoms w/ an inhaled, short-acting β_2-agonist (eg, albuterol). Instruct to seek medical attention immediately if they experience decreasing effectiveness of inhaled, short-acting β_2-agonist; a need for more inhalations than usual of inhaled, short-acting β_2-agonist; or a significant decrease in lung function. Advise not to d/c therapy w/o physician guidance and not to use additional LABAs. Instruct to contact physician if oropharyngeal candidiasis or symptoms of pneumonia develop. Advise to rinse mouth w/ water w/o swallowing after inhalation. Advise to avoid exposure to chickenpox or measles, and, if exposed, to consult physician w/o delay. Inform about risk of immunosuppression, hypercorticism, adrenal suppression, reduction in BMD, ocular effects, and adverse effects (eg, palpitations, chest pain, rapid HR, tremor, nervousness). Instruct to taper slowly from systemic corticosteroids if transferring to Breo Ellipta. Advise that hypersensitivity reactions may occur; instruct to d/c therapy if any occur. Inform that the inhaler is not reusable and advise not to take the inhaler apart.

STORAGE: 20-25°C (68-77°F); excursions permitted from 15-30°C (59-86°F). Store in a dry place away from direct heat or sunlight. Store inside the unopened moisture-protective foil tray and only remove from the tray immediately before initial use. Discard 6 weeks after opening the foil tray or when the counter reads "0" (after all blisters have been used), whichever comes 1st.

B

BREVIBLOC – esmolol hydrochloride

RX

Class: Selective $beta_1$ blocker

ADULT DOSAGE

Supraventricular Tachycardia/ Noncompensatory Sinus Tachycardia

Short-term use for rapid control of ventricular rate in patients w/ A-fib or A-flutter in perioperative, postoperative, or other emergent circumstances, and for noncompensatory sinus tachycardia

Administer by continuous IV infusion w/ or w/o LD
Additional LD and/or titration of maint infusion (step-wise dosing) may be necessary based on desired ventricular response

Step 1: Optional LD (500mcg/kg over 1 min), then 50mcg/kg/min for 4 min
Step 2: Optional LD if necessary, then 100mcg/kg/min for 4 min
Step 3: Optional LD if necessary, then 150mcg/kg/min for 4 min
Step 4: If necessary, increase dose to 200mcg/kg/min
Maint: 50-200mcg/kg/min; may continue maint infusions for up to 48 hrs
Max: 200mcg/kg/min

Intraoperative/Postoperative Tachycardia and/or Hypertension

Short-term treatment of tachycardia and HTN that occur during induction and tracheal intubation, during surgery, on emergence from anesthesia, and in the postoperative period

Immediate Control:
1mg/kg bolus over 30 sec followed by 150mcg/kg/min infusion, if necessary
Titrate: Adjust infusion rate as required to maintain desired HR and BP

Gradual Control:
500mcg/kg bolus over 1 min followed by maint infusion of 50mcg/kg/min for 4 min
Continue dosing as for supraventricular tachycardia, depending on response

Maint Infusion:
Tachycardia:
Max: 200mcg/kg/min
HTN:
May require higher maint infusion dosages (250-300mcg/kg/min)
Max: 300mcg/kg/min

Conversions

Transition to Alternative Drugs:
Reduce infusion rate by 50%, 30 min following 1st dose of alternative drug. After administration of 2nd dose of alternative drug, monitor response and if satisfactory control is maintained for 1st hr, d/c infusion

PEDIATRIC DOSAGE

Pediatric use may not have been established

DOSING CONSIDERATIONS

Elderly
Start at lower end of dosing range

ADMINISTRATION

IV route

Premixed Bag

Medication port is used solely for withdrawing initial bolus from the bag

Do not add any additional medications to the bag

Ready-to-Use Vial

May be used to administer LD by hand-held syringe while maint infusion is being prepared

Compatible IV Fluids

D5 inj
D5 in Lactated Ringer's inj
D5 in Ringer's inj
D5 and NaCl 0.45% inj
D5 and NaCl 0.9% inj
Lactated Ringer's inj
Potassium Chloride (40mEq/L) in D5 inj
NaCl 0.45% inj
NaCl 0.9% inj

Refer to PI for additional administration and preparation instructions

HOW SUPPLIED

Inj: 10mg/mL [10mL, vial; 250mL, premixed inj bag], 20mg/mL [100mL, double strength premixed inj bag]

CONTRAINDICATIONS

Severe sinus bradycardia, heart block >1st degree, sick sinus syndrome, decompensated heart failure (HF), cardiogenic shock, pulmonary HTN, IV administration of cardiodepressant calcium channel antagonists (eg, verapamil) and esmolol in close proximity (eg, while cardiac effects from the other are still present), hypersensitivity reactions, including anaphylaxis, to esmolol or any of the inactive ingredients of the product (cross-sensitivity between beta blockers is possible).

WARNINGS/PRECAUTIONS

Not for prevention of intraoperative/postoperative tachycardia and/or HTN. Dose-related hypotension, loss of consciousness, cardiac arrest, and death may occur; reduce dose or d/c in case of an unacceptable drop in BP. Bradycardia, including sinus pause, heart block, and severe bradycardia, may occur; patients w/ 1st-degree AV block, sinus node dysfunction, or conduction disorders may be at increased risk. Reduce dose or d/c if severe bradycardia develops. May cause cardiac failure and cardiogenic shock; d/c at 1st sign/symptom of impending cardiac failure and start supportive therapy. Monitor vital signs closely and titrate slowly in the treatment of patients whose BP is primarily driven by vasoconstriction associated w/ hypothermia. Should generally not be given to patients w/ reactive airways disease; titrate to lowest possible effective dose and d/c immediately in the event of bronchospasm. Caution in patients w/ hypoglycemia and in diabetics; may mask tachycardia occurring w/ hypoglycemia. Infusion-site reactions may develop; use an alternative infusion site and avoid extravasation if a local infusion-site reaction develops. Avoid infusions into small veins or through a butterfly-catheter. May exacerbate anginal attacks in patients w/ Prinzmetal's angina; do not use nonselective β-blockers. If used in the setting of pheochromocytoma, give in combination w/ an α-blocker, and only after α-blocker has been initiated; may cause a paradoxical increase in BP if administered alone. Can attenuate reflex tachycardia and increase risk of hypotension in hypovolemic patients. May aggravate peripheral circulatory disorders (eg, Raynaud's disease or syndrome, peripheral occlusive vascular disease). Severe exacerbations of angina, MI, and ventricular arrhythmias reported upon abrupt discontinuation in patients w/ CAD; observe for signs of myocardial ischemia when discontinued. Hyperkalemia reported; increased risk in patients w/ renal impairment. May cause hyperkalemic renal tubular acidosis. May mask clinical signs of hyperthyroidism (eg, tachycardia). May precipitate thyroid storm w/ abrupt withdrawal. Patients at risk of anaphylactic reactions may be more reactive to allergen exposure (accidental, diagnostic, or therapeutic). Caution in elderly.

ADVERSE REACTIONS

Hypotension, dizziness, somnolence, nausea, infusion-site reactions.

DRUG INTERACTIONS

See Contraindications. May exaggerate effects on BP, contractility, and impulse propagation w/ other drugs that can lower BP, reduce myocardial contractility, or interfere w/ sinus node function or electrical impulse propagation in the myocardium. Concomitant use w/ digoxin may increase the risk of bradycardia and may increase digoxin levels. May prolong effects of succinylcholine-induced neuromuscular blockade. May moderately prolong effects and recovery index of mivacurium. Increased risk of clonidine-, guanfacine-, moxonidine-withdrawal rebound HTN; d/c β-blocker gradually 1st if antihypertensive therapy needs to be interrupted or discontinued. In patients w/ depressed myocardial function, use w/ cardiodepressant calcium channel antagonists (eg, verapamil) can lead to fatal cardiac arrests. Sympathomimetic drugs having β-adrenergic agonist activity will counteract effects. Do not use to control tachycardia in patients receiving drugs that are vasoconstrictive and have positive inotropic effects (eg, dopamine, epinephrine, norepinephrine) because of risk of reducing cardiac contractility in presence of high systemic vascular resistance. May be unresponsive to usual doses of epinephrine used to treat anaphylactic/anaphylactoid reactions. May enhance the effect of antidiabetic agents.

PATIENT CONSIDERATIONS

Assessment: Assess for severe sinus bradycardia, heart block >1st degree, sick sinus syndrome, decompensated HF, cardiogenic shock, pulmonary HTN, hypersensitivity, or any other conditions where treatment is contraindicated or cautioned. Assess pregnancy/nursing status and for possible drug interactions. Obtain baseline BP, HR and rhythm, and serum electrolytes.

Monitoring: Monitor for hypotension, bradycardia, signs/symptoms of impending cardiac failure, bronchospasm, infusion-site reactions, and other adverse reactions. Monitor for signs of thyrotoxicosis when withdrawing therapy in patients w/ hyperthyroidism. Monitor BP, HR and rhythm, and serum electrolytes.

Counseling: Inform about benefits/risks of therapy. Instruct to report any adverse reactions to physician.

STORAGE: 25°C (77°F); excursions permitted to 15-30°C (59-86°F). Protect from freezing. Avoid excessive heat. Ready to Use Bag: Use w/in 24 hrs once drug has been withdrawn; discard any unused portion. Do not use plastic containers in series connections. Do not remove unit from overwrap until time of use.

BRIDION – sugammadex

RX

Class: Antidote

ADULT DOSAGE

Reversal of Neuromuscular Blockade

Reversal of Blockade Induced by Rocuronium Bromide and Vecuronium Bromide in Adults Undergoing Surgery:

Base doses/timing of administration on twitch responses and extent of spontaneous recovery that has occurred

Satisfactory recovery should be determined through assessment of skeletal muscle tone and respiratory measurements in addition to the response to peripheral nerve stimulation

Rocuronium + Vecuronium:
4mg/kg if spontaneous recovery of twitch response has reached 1-2 post-tetanic counts and there are no twitch responses to train-of-four (TOF) stimulation following rocuronium- or vecuronium-induced neuromuscular blockade
2mg/kg if spontaneous recovery has reached the reappearance of the second twitch in response to TOF stimulation following rocuronium- or vecuronium-induced neuromuscular blockade

Rocuronium Only:
16mg/kg if there is a clinical need to reverse neuromuscular blockade soon (approx 3 min) after administration of a single dose of 1.2mg/kg of rocuronium

Re-Administration of Neuromuscular Blocking Agents for Intubation Following Reversal

Re-Administration After Reversal w/ ≤4mg/kg of Sugammadex:
1.2mg/kg Rocuronium: Wait ≥5 min
0.6mg/kg Rocuronium or 0.1mg/kg Vecuronium: Wait ≥4 hrs. Wait 24 hrs w/ mild or moderate renal impairment. If shorter wait time is required, give a 1.2mg/kg rocuronium dose

When rocuronium 1.2mg/kg is administered w/in 30 min after reversal, onset of neuromuscular blockade may be delayed ≤4 min and duration may be shortened ≤15 min

For re-administration of rocuronium or administration of vecuronium after reversal of

PEDIATRIC DOSAGE

Pediatric use may not have been established

rocuronium w/ 16mg/kg sugammadex, wait 24 hrs

Use a nonsteroidal neuromuscular blocking agent if neuromuscular blockade is required before recommended waiting time has elapsed

DOSING CONSIDERATIONS

Renal Impairment

Severe/Dialysis: Not recommended

ADMINISTRATION

IV route

Administer as single bolus inj; may be given over 10 sec, into an existing IV line.
Ensure infusion line is adequately flushed (eg, w/ 0.9% NaCl) between administration of sugammadex and other drugs.

Compatibility

May inject into IV line of a running infusion w/ the following IV sol (do not mix w/ other products):
0.9% NaCl
D5
0.45% NaCl and 2.5% dextrose
D5 in 0.9% NaCl
isolyte P w/ D5
Ringer's lactate sol
Ringer's sol

Physically incompatible w/ verapamil, ondansetron, and ranitidine.

HOW SUPPLIED

Inj: 200mg/2mL, 500mg/5mL

CONTRAINDICATIONS

Hypersensitivity to sugammadex or any of its components.

WARNINGS/PRECAUTIONS

Serious hypersensitivity reactions, including anaphylaxis, reported. Marked bradycardia reported, some resulting in cardiac arrest; closely monitor for hemodynamic changes during and after reversal of neuromuscular blockade. Ventilatory support is mandatory until adequate spontaneous respiration is restored and the ability to maintain a patent airway is assured; should neuromuscular blockade persist after administration or recur following extubation, provide adequate ventilation. Delayed or minimal response to sugammadex reported in a small number of patients. Use of lower than recommended dose is not recommended; may lead to an increased risk of recurrence of neuromuscular blockade after initial reversal. Doses ≤16mg/kg reported to be associated w/ increases in aPTT and PT/INR; carefully monitor coagulation parameters in patients w/ known coagulopathies, being treated w/ therapeutic anticoagulation, receiving thromboprophylaxis drugs other than heparin and low molecular weight heparin (LMWH), or receiving thromboprophylaxis drugs and who then receive a dose of 16mg/kg sugammadex. Signs of light anesthesia noted occasionally when neuromuscular blockade was reversed intentionally in the middle of anesthesia. Do not use to reverse blockade induced by nonsteroidal neuromuscular blocking agents (eg, succinylcholine/benzylisoquinolinium compounds) and steroidal neuromuscular blocking agents other than rocuronium or vecuronium.

ADVERSE REACTIONS

N/V, pain, hypotension, headache.

DRUG INTERACTIONS

Certain drugs may become less effective due to a lowering of (free) plasma concentrations; consider re-administration of other drug, administration of a therapeutically equivalent drug, and/or non-pharmacological interventions. Administration of a bolus dose of sugammadex is equivalent to missing dose(s) of oral contraceptives containing an estrogen or progestogen; if an oral contraceptive is taken on same day that sugammadex is administered or non-oral hormonal contraception is being used, use additional, non-hormonal contraceptive method or back-up method of contraception for the next 7 days. May interfere w/ serum progesterone assay. Certain drugs may displace rocuronium or vecuronium from sugammadex; d/c drug causing displacement and provide adequate ventilation if required. Recovery of TOF ratio to 0.9 could be delayed in patients who have received toremifene on the same day of surgery. Drugs that potentiate neuromuscular blockade used postoperatively may cause recurrence of neuromuscular blockade; may require mechanical ventilation.

PATIENT CONSIDERATIONS

Assessment: Assess for drug hypersensitivity, renal impairment, known coagulopathies, pregnancy/nursing status, hormonal contraception use, and for other possible drug interactions.

Monitoring: Monitor twitch responses and the extent of spontaneous recovery that has occurred. Monitor patient to assure adequate ventilation and maintenance of a patent airway from the time of administration of sugammadex until complete recovery of neuromuscular function. Monitor for hemodynamic changes during and after neuromuscular blockade. Monitor for hypersensitivity reactions and for other adverse reactions. Monitor coagulation parameters in patients w/ known coagulopathies, being treated w/ therapeutic anticoagulation, receiving thromboprophylaxis drugs other than heparin and LMWH, or receiving thromboprophylaxis drugs and who then receive a dose of 16mg/kg sugammadex.

Counseling: Advise females of reproductive potential using hormonal contraceptives that concomitant use may reduce contraceptive effect. Instruct females to use an additional, non-hormonal method of contraception for the next 7 days following administration of sugammadex.

STORAGE: 25°C (77°F); excursions permitted to 15-30°C (59-86°F). Protect from light. When not protected from light, use w/in 5 days.

BRILINTA – ticagrelor

RX

Class: Antiplatelet agent

May cause significant, sometimes fatal, bleeding. Do not use in patients w/ active pathological bleeding or a history of intracranial hemorrhage. Do not start therapy in patients undergoing urgent CABG. If possible, manage bleeding w/o discontinuing therapy; stopping therapy increases the risk of subsequent cardiovascular (CV) events. Maintenance doses of aspirin (ASA) >100mg reduce the effectiveness of ticagrelor and should be avoided.

ADULT DOSAGE

Acute Coronary Syndrome

To reduce the rate of CV death, MI, and stroke in patients w/ acute coronary syndrome or a history of MI; also reduces the rate of stent thrombosis in patients who have been stented for treatment of acute coronary syndrome

LD: 180mg

Maint: 90mg bid during 1st year; 60mg bid after 1 year

Use w/ daily maint dose of ASA of 75-100mg

Missed Dose

If a dose is missed, take 1 tab (next dose) at its scheduled time

PEDIATRIC DOSAGE

Pediatric use may not have been established

DOSING CONSIDERATIONS

Hepatic Impairment

Severe: Avoid use

ADMINISTRATION

Oral route

Take w/ or w/o food.

If unable to swallow tab(s) whole, tab can be crushed, mixed w/ water, and drunk; the mixture can also be administered via a NG tube (≥CH8).

Do not administer w/ another oral P2Y12 platelet inhibitor.

HOW SUPPLIED

Tab: 60mg, 90mg

CONTRAINDICATIONS

History of intracranial hemorrhage, active pathological bleeding (eg, peptic ulcer, intracranial hemorrhage), hypersensitivity (eg, angioedema) to ticagrelor or any component of the product.

WARNINGS/PRECAUTIONS

Dyspnea reported. If new, prolonged, or worsened dyspnea is determined to be related to therapy, no specific treatment is required; continue therapy w/o interruption. In the case of intolerable dyspnea requiring discontinuation of therapy, consider another antiplatelet agent. Discontinuation of therapy increases risk of MI, stroke, and death; if therapy must be temporarily discontinued, restart it as soon as possible. When possible, interrupt therapy for 5 days prior to surgery that has major risk of bleeding; resume as soon as hemostasis is achieved.

ADVERSE REACTIONS

Bleeding, dyspnea, dizziness, nausea, diarrhea.

DRUG INTERACTIONS

See Boxed Warning. Strong CYP3A inhibitors substantially increase ticagrelor exposure and may increase adverse events; avoid w/ strong CYP3A inhibitors (eg, atazanavir, clarithromycin, ketoconazole). Strong CYP3A inducers substantially reduce ticagrelor exposure and may decrease efficacy; avoid w/ strong CYP3A inducers (eg, rifampin, phenytoin, carbamazepine). May increase concentrations of simvastatin and lovastatin (CYP3A4 substrates); avoid simvastatin and lovastatin doses >40mg. Inhibits P-gp transporter; monitor digoxin levels w/ initiation of or any change in ticagrelor therapy.

PATIENT CONSIDERATIONS

Assessment: Assess for history of intracranial hemorrhage, active pathological bleeding, risk factors for bleeding, severe hepatic impairment, hypersensitivity to drug, pregnancy/nursing status, and possible drug interactions.

Monitoring: Monitor for bleeding, dyspnea, and other adverse reactions.

Counseling: Advise that daily doses of ASA should not exceed 100mg and to avoid taking any other medications that contain ASA. Advise that patients may experience bleeding and bruising more easily and will take longer than usual to stop bleeding; instruct to report any unanticipated, prolonged, or excessive bleeding, or blood in the stool or urine. Advise to contact physician if unexpected shortness of breath occurs. Advise to inform physicians and dentists of ticagrelor therapy before any surgery or dental procedure.

STORAGE: 25°C (77°F); excursions permitted to 15-30°C (59-86°F).

BRINTELLIX – vortioxetine

RX

Class: Miscellaneous antidepressant

Antidepressants increased the risk of suicidal thoughts and behavior in children, adolescents, and young adults in short-term studies. Monitor closely for worsening and for emergence of suicidal thoughts and behaviors in patients who are started on antidepressant therapy. Not evaluated for use in pediatric patients.

ADULT DOSAGE

Major Depressive Disorder

Initial: 10mg/day
Titrate: Increase to 20mg/day, as tolerated. May consider decreasing dose to 5mg/day for patients who do not tolerate higher doses
Max: 20mg/day
Maint: Acute episodes of major depression should be followed by several months or longer of sustained therapy to decrease risk of recurrence

Dosing Considerations with MAOIs

Switching to/from an MAOI for Psychiatric Disorders:
Allow at least 14 days between discontinuation of an MAOI and initiation of treatment, and allow at least 21 days between discontinuation of treatment and initiation of an MAOI

Use w/ Other MAOIs (eg, Linezolid, IV Methylene Blue):
Do not start vortioxetine in a patient being treated w/ linezolid or IV methylene blue
In patients already receiving vortioxetine, if acceptable alternatives are not available and benefits outweigh risks, d/c vortioxetine and administer linezolid or IV methylene blue; monitor for serotonin syndrome for 21 days or until 24 hrs after the last dose of linezolid or IV methylene blue, whichever comes 1st. May resume vortioxetine therapy 24 hrs after the last dose of linezolid or IV methylene blue

PEDIATRIC DOSAGE

Pediatric use may not have been established

DOSING CONSIDERATIONS

Concomitant Medications

Use w/ Strong CYP2D6 Inhibitors:
Reduce vortioxetine dose by 1/2; increase dose to original level when CYP2D6 inhibitor is discontinued

B

Use w/ Strong CYP Inducers:
Consider increasing vortioxetine dose when a strong CYP inducer is coadministered for >14 days; max recommended dose should not exceed 3X original dose
Reduce dose to original level w/in 14 days, when the inducer is discontinued

Hepatic Impairment
Severe: Not recommended

Discontinuation
Decrease dose to 10mg/day for 1 week before full discontinuation of 15mg/day or 20mg/day

Other Important Considerations
CYP2D6 Poor Metabolizers:
Max: 10mg/day

ADMINISTRATION
Oral route

Take w/o regard to meals

HOW SUPPLIED
Tab: 5mg, 10mg, 15mg, 20mg

CONTRAINDICATIONS
Hypersensitivity to vortioxetine or any components of the formulation, use of an MAOI for psychiatric disorders either concomitantly or w/in 21 days of stopping treatment, treatment w/in 14 days of stopping an MAOI for psychiatric disorders, starting treatment in patients being treated w/ other MAOIs (eg, linezolid, IV methylene blue).

WARNINGS/PRECAUTIONS
May increase likelihood of precipitation of a mixed/manic episode in patients at risk for bipolar disorder. Screen patient to determine if at risk for bipolar disorder; not approved for treatment of bipolar depression. Serotonin syndrome reported; d/c immediately and initiate supportive symptomatic treatment. May increase risk of bleeding events. Activation of mania/hypomania reported. Pupillary dilation that occurs following use may trigger an angle-closure attack in a patient with anatomically narrow angles who does not have a patent iridectomy. Transient adverse reactions (eg, headache, muscle tension) reported following abrupt discontinuation of doses of 15mg/day or 20mg/day. Hyponatremia reported; caution in the elderly and in volume-depleted patients. D/C in patients with symptomatic hyponatremia and institute appropriate medical intervention. Not recommended with severe hepatic impairment.

ADVERSE REACTIONS
N/V, constipation, diarrhea, dry mouth, dizziness, flatulence, abnormal dreams, pruritus, sexual dysfunction.

DRUG INTERACTIONS
See Dosage and Contraindications. May cause serotonin syndrome when coadministered with other serotonergic drugs (eg, SSRIs, triptans, TCAs, fentanyl, lithium) and with drugs that impair metabolism of serotonin; d/c immediately if this occurs and initiate supportive symptomatic treatment. Increased risk of bleeding with ASA, NSAIDs, warfarin, and other anticoagulants; monitor patients receiving other drugs that interfere with hemostasis when vortioxetine is initiated or discontinued. Increased risk of hyponatremia with diuretics. Consider increasing vortioxetine dose when coadministered with a strong CYP inducer. Coadministration with another drug that is highly protein bound may increase free concentrations of the other drug.

PATIENT CONSIDERATIONS

Assessment: Assess for history or family history of bipolar disorder, mania, or hypomania. Assess for hypersensitivity to drug or any of its components, syndrome of inappropriate antidiuretic hormone secretion, volume depletion, susceptibility to angle-closure glaucoma, hepatic dysfunction, pregnancy/nursing status, and for possible drug interactions.

Monitoring: Monitor for clinical worsening, suicidality, unusual changes in behavior, serotonin syndrome, abnormal bleeding, activation of mania/hypomania, angle-closure glaucoma, hyponatremia, hypersensitivity reactions, and other adverse reactions. If discontinuing therapy (particularly if abrupt), monitor for discontinuation symptoms.

Counseling: Inform of risks, benefits, and appropriate use of therapy. Advise patients and caregivers to look for the emergence of suicidality, especially early during treatment and when the dose is adjusted up or down. Inform that if taking 15mg/day or 20mg/day, patient may experience headache, muscle tension, mood swings, sudden outburst of anger, dizziness, and runny nose if therapy is abruptly discontinued; advise not to d/c without notifying physician. Advise to inform physician if taking or planning to take any prescription or OTC drugs. Caution about risk of bleeding with NSAIDs, ASA, warfarin, or other drugs that affect hemostasis. Advise to look for signs of activation of mania/hypomania. Inform that drug may cause mild pupillary dilation, which in susceptible individuals may lead to an episode of angle-closure glaucoma. Inform of the greater risk of hyponatremia if treated with diuretics, if volume depleted, or if elderly. Inform that nausea is the most common adverse reaction, and is dose related. Instruct to notify physician if an allergic reaction occurs, if pregnant/planning to become pregnant, or if breastfeeding/planning to breastfeed.

STORAGE: 25°C (77°F); excursions permitted to 15-30°C (59-86°F).

BRISDELLE – paroxetine

RX

Class: Selective serotonin reuptake inhibitor (SSRI)

Antidepressants increase the risk of suicidal thoughts and behavior in pediatrics and young adults when used to treat major depressive disorder and other psychiatric disorders. Monitor closely for worsening and for emergence of suicidal thoughts and behaviors.

ADULT DOSAGE

Menopausal Vasomotor Symptoms

Moderate to Severe:
7.5mg qhs

Dosing Considerations with MAOIs

Use Before or After an MAOI:
Wait at least 14 days after discontinuation of an MAOI before initiating therapy, and allow at least 14 days after stopping therapy before starting an MAOI

PEDIATRIC DOSAGE

Pediatric use may not have been established

ADMINISTRATION

Oral route

Take w/ or w/o food.

HOW SUPPLIED

Cap: 7.5mg

CONTRAINDICATIONS

Concomitant use of an MAOI or w/in 14 days of stopping treatment, starting treatment in a patient being treated w/ linezolid or IV methylene blue. Concomitant use w/ thioridazine or pimozide, pregnancy, history of hypersensitivity to paroxetine or any of the other ingredients in this product.

WARNINGS/PRECAUTIONS

Not indicated for treatment of any psychiatric condition. Serotonin syndrome reported; d/c immediately and initiate supportive symptomatic treatment. May increase risk of bleeding events. Hyponatremia may occur; caution in elderly and volume-depleted patients. Bone fracture risk reported. May increase the likelihood of precipitation of a mixed/manic episode in patients at risk for bipolar disorder. Caution in patients with a history of seizures or with conditions that potentially lower the seizure threshold. Akathisia may develop; d/c if this occurs. Pupillary dilation that occurs following use may trigger an angle closure attack in a patient with anatomically narrow angles who does not have a patent iridectomy. May impair physical/mental abilities.

ADVERSE REACTIONS

Headache, fatigue/malaise/lethargy, N/V.

DRUG INTERACTIONS

See Contraindications. Increased risk of serotonin syndrome with other serotonergic drugs (eg, triptans, TCAs, fentanyl) and with drugs that impair metabolism of serotonin; d/c therapy and any concomitant serotonergic agents immediately if serotonin syndrome occurs and initiate supportive symptomatic treatment. Not recommended with tryptophan or other paroxetine products. May decrease effectiveness of tamoxifen; consider avoiding concomitant use. Increased risk of bleeding with aspirin, NSAIDs, warfarin, and other anticoagulants reported. Carefully monitor patients receiving warfarin therapy when paroxetine is initiated or discontinued. Increased risk of hyponatremia with diuretics. May increase levels of risperidone, atomoxetine, or theophylline; dosage of coadministered drug may need to be decreased. May increase levels and elimination $T_{1/2}$ of TCAs (eg, desipramine); may need to monitor levels and reduce dose of TCAs. May decrease digoxin levels; monitor digoxin levels and digoxin dosage may need to be increased. Caution with other drugs metabolized by CYP2D6 (eg, fluoxetine, risperidone, propafenone) and with CYP2D6 inhibitors (eg, quinidine). Increased levels with highly protein-bound drugs (eg, warfarin); monitor INR. Increased levels with cimetidine. Decreased exposure with phenobarbital or phenytoin. Decreased plasma levels with fosamprenavir/ritonavir.

PATIENT CONSIDERATIONS

Assessment: Assess for hypersensitivity to drug, history of seizures or conditions that potentially lower the seizure threshold, risk of bipolar disorder, volume depletion, susceptibility to angle-closure glaucoma, pregnancy/nursing status, and possible drug interactions.

Monitoring: Monitor for signs/symptoms of worsening and emergence of suicidal thoughts and behaviors, serotonin syndrome, abnormal bleeding, hyponatremia, bone fractures, mania/hypomania, seizures, akathisia, angle-closure glaucoma, and other adverse reactions.

Counseling: Advise patients, families, and caregivers to look for the emergence of suicidality, especially early during treatment, and to observe for signs of activation of mania/hypomania. Caution about the risk of serotonin syndrome and hypernatremia. Inform of the possibility for an increased risk of fracture. Advise to notify physician if patient becomes pregnant during therapy. Caution about the risk of angle closure glaucoma. Caution about operating hazardous machinery, including motor vehicles, until reasonably certain that therapy does not affect ability to engage in such activities. Advise to inform physician if taking or planning to take any prescription or OTC drugs, including herbal supplements.

STORAGE: 20-25°C (68-77°F); excursions permitted to 15-30°C (59-86°F). Protect from light and humidity.

Bromday – bromfenac

RX

Class: NSAID

ADULT DOSAGE

Ocular Pain and Inflammation

Instill 1 drop qd in affected eye(s), starting 1 day prior to cataract surgery, continued on day of surgery, and through first 14 days of postoperative period

PEDIATRIC DOSAGE

Pediatric use may not have been established

DOSING CONSIDERATIONS

Concomitant Medications

Space dosing ≥5 min apart with other topical ophthalmic medications

ADMINISTRATION

Ocular route

HOW SUPPLIED

Sol: 0.09% [1.7mL]

WARNINGS/PRECAUTIONS

Contains sodium sulfite; may cause allergic-type reactions (eg, anaphylactic symptoms, asthmatic episodes). Sulfite sensitivity is seen more frequently in asthmatics. May slow or delay healing. Potential cross-sensitivity to acetylsalicylic acid, phenylacetic acid derivatives, and other NSAIDs. Caution when treating individuals who previously exhibited sensitivity to these drugs. May increase bleeding of ocular tissues (eg, hyphemas) in conjunction with ocular surgery. Caution in patients with known bleeding tendencies. May result in keratitis. Continued use may lead to sight-threatening epithelial breakdown, corneal thinning, corneal erosion, corneal ulceration, or corneal perforation; d/c if corneal epithelium breakdown occurs. Caution in patients with complicated ocular surgeries, corneal denervation, corneal epithelial defects, diabetes mellitus (DM), ocular surface diseases (eg, dry eye syndrome), rheumatoid arthritis (RA), or repeat ocular surgeries within a short period of time. Increased risk for occurrence and severity of corneal adverse events if used >24 hrs prior to surgery or use beyond 14 days postsurgery. Avoid use with contact lenses. Avoid use during late pregnancy because of the known effects on the fetal cardiovascular system (closure of ductus arteriosus).

ADVERSE REACTIONS

Abnormal sensation in eye, conjunctival hyperemia, eye irritation (burning/stinging), eye pain, eye pruritus, eye redness, headache, iritis.

DRUG INTERACTIONS

Concomitant use of topical NSAIDs and topical steroids may increase potential for healing problems. Caution with other medications that may prolong bleeding time.

PATIENT CONSIDERATIONS

Assessment: Assess for hypersensitivity (eg, sodium sulfite) or cross-sensitivity (eg, aspirin) reactions, history of complicated or repeated ocular surgeries, corneal denervation, corneal epithelial defects, DM, ocular surface diseases (eg, dry eye syndrome), RA, bleeding tendencies, pregnancy/nursing status, and possible drug interactions.

Monitoring: Monitor for anaphylactic symptoms, severe asthma attacks, wound-healing problems, keratitis, corneal epithelial breakdown, corneal thinning/erosion/ulceration/perforation, increased bleeding time, and bleeding of ocular tissues (hyphemas) in conjunction with ocular surgery.

Counseling: Advise not to wear contact lenses during therapy. Advise of the possibility of slow or delayed healing that may occur while using this product. Advise not to touch the dropper tip to any surface, as this may contaminate the contents. If >1 topical ophthalmic medication is used, instruct to administer 5 min apart.

STORAGE: 15-25°C (59-77°F).

BROMFED DM – brompheniramine maleate/dextromethorphan hydrobromide/pseudoephedrine hydrochloride

RX

Class: Antihistamine/antitussive/decongestant

ADULT DOSAGE

Antihistamine/Cough Suppressant/Nasal Decongestant

Relief of coughs and upper respiratory symptoms, including nasal congestion, associated with allergy or the common cold

10mL (2 tsp) q4h
Max: 6 doses/24 hrs

PEDIATRIC DOSAGE

Antihistamine/Cough Suppressant/Nasal Decongestant

Relief of coughs and upper respiratory symptoms, including nasal congestion, associated with allergy or the common cold

6 Months to <2 Years:
Dosage to be established by physician

2 to <6 Years:
2.5mL (1/2 tsp) q4h
Max: 6 doses/24 hrs

6 to <12 Years:
5mL (1 tsp) q4h
Max: 6 doses/24 hrs

≥12 Years:
10mL (2 tsp) q4h
Max: 6 doses/24 hrs

ADMINISTRATION

Oral route

HOW SUPPLIED

Syrup: (Brompheniramine Maleate-Pseudoephedrine HCl-Dextromethorphan HBr) 2mg-30mg-10mg/5mL [118mL, 473mL]

CONTRAINDICATIONS

Hypersensitivity to any of the ingredients, severe HTN, severe coronary artery disease (CAD), lower respiratory tract conditions including asthma, newborn, premature infants, and nursing mothers. Coadministration with MAOIs.

WARNINGS/PRECAUTIONS

Overdosage may cause hallucinations, convulsions, and death, especially in infants and small children. May diminish mental alertness. May produce excitation in the young child. Caution with diabetes, HTN, heart or thyroid disease, history of bronchial asthma, narrow-angle glaucoma, or GI or urinary bladder neck obstruction.

ADVERSE REACTIONS

Sedation, dryness of mouth, nose and throat, thickening of bronchial secretions, dizziness.

DRUG INTERACTIONS

See Contraindications. Additive effects with alcohol and other CNS depressants (eg, hypnotics, sedatives, tranquilizers, antianxiety agents). May reduce effects of antihypertensive drugs.

PATIENT CONSIDERATIONS

Assessment: Assess for HTN, CAD, lower respiratory tract conditions, diabetes, heart/thyroid disease, history of bronchial asthma, narrow-angle glaucoma, GI or urinary bladder neck obstruction, drug hypersensitivity, pregnancy/nursing status, and possible drug interactions.

Monitoring: Monitor for excitation in the young child, diminished mental alertness, and other adverse reactions.

Counseling: Warn about engaging in activities requiring mental alertness (eg, driving a car, operating dangerous machinery). Advise to notify physician if taking any other medications, and if pregnant/breastfeeding.

STORAGE: 20-25°C (68-77°F). Keep tightly closed.

B

BUMETANIDE – bumetanide

RX

Class: Loop diuretic

May lead to profound diuresis with water and electrolyte depletion if given in excessive amounts; careful medical supervision required and dose and dosage schedule must be adjusted to individual patient's needs.

OTHER BRAND NAMES

Bumex (Discontinued)

ADULT DOSAGE

Edema

Associated w/ CHF, Hepatic/Renal Disease (Nephrotic Syndrome):

Tab:

Usual: 0.5-2mg/day as single dose; may give a 2nd or 3rd dose at 4- to 5-hr intervals if response is not adequate

Maint: Give on alternate days or for 3-4 days w/ rest periods of 1-2 days in between

Max: 10mg/day

Inj:

Initial: 0.5-1mg IV/IM (give IV over 1-2 min); may give a 2nd or 3rd dose at 2- to 3-hr intervals if response is insufficient

Max: 10mg/day

Initiate oral treatment as soon as possible

PEDIATRIC DOSAGE

Pediatric use may not have been established

DOSING CONSIDERATIONS

Hepatic Impairment

Tab: Give minimum dose, and if necessary, increase dose very carefully

Elderly

Tab/Inj: Start at lower end of dosing range

ADMINISTRATION

Oral/IV/IM route

Compatibility

5% dextrose sol; 0.9% NaCl; lactated Ringer's inj

HOW SUPPLIED

Inj: 0.25mg/mL [4mL, 10mL]; **Tab:** 0.5mg*, 1mg*, 2mg* *scored

CONTRAINDICATIONS

Anuria, hepatic coma, severe electrolyte depletion, hypersensitivity to this product.

WARNINGS/PRECAUTIONS

Excessive doses may cause dehydration, blood volume reduction, and circulatory collapse with possible vascular thrombosis and embolism, particularly in elderly. Hypokalemia may occur; caution with hepatic cirrhosis and ascites, states of aldosterone excess with normal renal function, K^+-losing nephropathy, certain diarrheal states, other states where hypokalemia represents added risks, or in patients receiving digitalis and diuretics for CHF. Sudden alterations of electrolyte balance may precipitate hepatic encephalopathy and coma in patients with hepatic cirrhosis and ascites; initiate therapy in hospital. Ototoxicity, thrombocytopenia, hypocalcemia, hypomagnesemia, and hyperuricemia may occur. May affect glucose metabolism; monitor glucose levels in patients with diabetes or suspected latent diabetes. Monitor for blood dyscrasias, hepatic damage, or idiosyncratic reactions. Caution with sulfonamide allergy. Reversible elevations of BUN and creatinine may occur; d/c if marked increase in BUN or creatinine occurs, or if oliguria develops in patients with progressive renal disease. Tab may be substituted at approximately a 1:40 ratio of bumetanide tabs to furosemide in patients allergic to furosemide.

ADVERSE REACTIONS

Muscle cramps, dizziness, hypotension, headache, nausea, encephalopathy, hyperuricemia, hypochloremia, hypokalemia, hyponatremia, hyperglycemia, azotemia, increased SrCr.

DRUG INTERACTIONS

Avoid with drugs known to have a nephrotoxic potential. Not recommended for use with indomethacin. High risk of lithium toxicity; avoid coadministration. Pretreatment with probenecid reduces effects; do not administer concurrently. May potentiate the effect of various antihypertensives; reduction in the dose of these drugs may be necessary. (Inj) Avoid with aminoglycosides (except in life-threatening situations).

PATIENT CONSIDERATIONS

Assessment: Assess for progressive renal disease, severe electrolyte depletion, anuria, diabetes or suspected latent diabetes, sulfonamide allergy, liver disease (hepatic coma), any other conditions where treatment is contraindicated or cautioned, pregnancy/nursing status, and possible drug interactions.

Monitoring: Monitor for ototoxicity, blood dyscrasias, liver damage or idiosyncratic reactions, hypersensitivity reactions, hyperuricemia, oliguria, thrombocytopenia, and other adverse reactions. Periodically monitor serum K^+, serum electrolytes, blood glucose, and renal function.

Counseling: Inform of the risks/benefits of therapy. Advise to seek medical attention if adverse reactions occur.

STORAGE: 20-25°C (68-77°F). Protect from light. (Inj) Excursions permitted to 15-30°C (59-86°F).

BUPRENEX — buprenorphine hydrochloride

CIII

Class: Partial opioid agonist

ADULT DOSAGE

Moderate to Severe Pain

Usual: 0.3mg IM/IV q6h prn; repeat once (up to 0.3mg) if needed, 30-60 min after initial dose

May use single doses up to 0.6mg IM if not in a high risk category

PEDIATRIC DOSAGE

Moderate to Severe Pain

2-12 Years:

2-6mcg/kg IM/IV q4-6h

≥13 Years:

Usual: 0.3mg IM/IV q6h prn; repeat once (up to 0.3mg) if needed, 30-60 min after initial dose

May use single doses up to 0.6mg IM if not in a high risk category

DOSING CONSIDERATIONS

Concomitant Medications

Reduce dose by approximately 50% in patients taking other CNS depressants

Other Important Considerations

High-Risk Patients (eg, Elderly, Debilitated, Presence of Respiratory Disease):

Reduce dose by approximately 50%

ADMINISTRATION

IM/IV route

Administer deep IM or slow IV route (over at least 2 min)

HOW SUPPLIED

Inj: 0.3mg/mL

CONTRAINDICATIONS

Hypersensitivity to the product.

WARNINGS/PRECAUTIONS

Clinically significant respiratory depression may occur; caution with compromised respiratory function. Naloxone may not be effective in reversing respiratory depression. May increase CSF pressure; caution with head injury, intracranial lesions, and other circumstances where cerebrospinal pressure may be increased. Can produce miosis and changes in level of consciousness. May impair mental or physical abilities; caution in ambulatory patients. May result in withdrawal effects in physically dependent patients. Caution in elderly, debilitated, and pediatric patients. Caution with hepatic/renal/pulmonary impairment, myxedema or hypothyroidism, adrenal cortical insufficiency, CNS depression or coma, toxic psychoses, prostatic hypertrophy or urethral stricture, acute alcoholism, delirium tremens, kyphoscoliosis, or biliary tract dysfunction.

ADVERSE REACTIONS

Sedation, N/V, dizziness, sweating, hypotension, headache, miosis, hypoventilation.

DRUG INTERACTIONS

Caution with MAOIs and CNS and respiratory depressants. Increased CNS depression with other narcotic analgesics, general anesthetics, antihistamines, benzodiazepines, phenothiazines, other tranquilizers, sedative-hypnotics, or other CNS depressants (eg, alcohol); reduce dose of one or both agents. Respiratory and cardiovascular collapse reported with diazepam. Suspected interaction with phenprocoumon resulting in purpura. Decreased clearance with CYP3A4 inhibitors (eg, macrolides, azole antifungals, protease inhibitors). Increased clearance with CYP3A4 inducers (eg, rifampin, carbamazepine, phenytoin).

PATIENT CONSIDERATIONS

Assessment: Assess for compromised respiratory function (eg, chronic obstructive pulmonary disease, hypoxia), head injury, intracranial lesions, hepatic/renal function, any condition where treatment is cautioned, pregnancy/nursing status, and possible drug interactions.

Monitoring: Monitor for signs/symptoms of respiratory depression, CNS depression, elevation of CSF pressure, increased intracholedochal pressure, drug abuse/dependence, and withdrawal effects.

Counseling: Counsel that effects (eg, drowsiness) may be potentiated by other centrally acting agents (eg, alcohol); advise not to drive/operate machinery under these circumstances. Advise that medication may lead to dependence. Counsel to not exceed prescribed dosage. Advise to notify physician of all medications currently being taken.

STORAGE: 20-25°C (68-77°F); excursions permitted between 15-30°C (59-86°F). Protect from prolonged exposure to light.

BUSPIRONE – buspirone hydrochloride

RX

Class: Atypical anxiolytic

OTHER BRAND NAMES

Buspar (Discontinued)

ADULT DOSAGE

Anxiety Disorders

Management of Disorders or Short-Term Relief of Symptoms:

Initial: 7.5mg bid

Titrate: May increase by 5mg/day at intervals of 2-3 days, prn

Usual: 20-30mg/day in divided doses

Max: 60mg/day

Periodically reassess usefulness of drug if used for extended periods

PEDIATRIC DOSAGE

Pediatric use may not have been established

DOSING CONSIDERATIONS

Renal Impairment

Severe: Not recommended

Hepatic Impairment

Severe: Not recommended

ADMINISTRATION

Oral route

Take in a consistent manner w/ regard to the timing of dosing; either always w/ or always w/o food

HOW SUPPLIED

Tab: 5mg*, 7.5mg*, 10mg*, 15mg*, 30mg* *scored

CONTRAINDICATIONS

Hypersensitivity to buspirone HCl.

WARNINGS/PRECAUTIONS

May impair mental/physical abilities. Does not exhibit cross-tolerance with benzodiazepines and other common sedatives/hypnotics; before starting therapy, withdraw gradually from prior treatment, especially in patients using a CNS depressant chronically. May cause acute and chronic changes in dopamine-mediated neurological function; syndrome of restlessness, appearing shortly after initiation, reported. May interfere with urinary metanephrine/catecholamine assay; d/c therapy for at least 48 hrs prior to undergoing urine collection for catecholamines. Not recommended with severe hepatic/renal impairment.

ADVERSE REACTIONS

Dizziness, nausea, headache, nervousness, lightheadedness, excitement, drowsiness, fatigue, insomnia, dry mouth.

DRUG INTERACTIONS

See Dosage. Elevated BP reported with MAOI; avoid concomitant use. Avoid with alcohol. Dizziness, headache, nausea, and increased nordiazepam reported with diazepam. May increase serum concentrations of haloperidol. ALT elevations reported with trazodone. Caution with CNS-active drugs. CYP3A4 inhibitors (eg, diltiazem, ketoconazole, ritonavir) may increase concentrations; may require dose adjustment. CYP3A4 inducers (eg, dexamethasone, phenytoin, rifampin), including potent inducers, may decrease concentrations; may require dose adjustment of buspirone. Avoid with large amounts of grapefruit juice. Nefazodone may decrease concentrations of metabolite 1-pyrimidinylpiperazine (1-PP). May increase levels of nefazodone. Cimetidine may increase C_{max} and T_{max}. Prolonged PT reported with warfarin. May displace less firmly bound drugs like digoxin.

PATIENT CONSIDERATIONS

Assessment: Assess for hypersensitivity to drug, hepatic/renal impairment, pregnancy/nursing status, and possible drug interactions.

Monitoring: Monitor for CNS effects, syndrome of restlessness, and other adverse reactions. Periodically reassess usefulness of drug if used for extended periods.

Counseling: Instruct to inform physician about any medications, prescription or nonprescription, alcohol, or drugs patient is taking or planning to take, and if patient is pregnant/breastfeeding, becomes pregnant, or is planning to become pregnant. Advise not to drive a car or operate potentially dangerous machinery until effects have been determined. Instruct to avoid drinking large amounts of grapefruit juice.

STORAGE: (5mg, 10mg, 15mg, 30mg) 20-25°C (68-77°F). (7.5mg) 25°C (77°F); excursions permitted between 15-30°C (59-86°F).

BUTRANS – buprenorphine

CIII

Class: Partial opioid agonist

Exposes users to risks of addiction, abuse, and misuse, which can lead to overdose and death; assess each patient's risk prior to prescribing, and monitor regularly for development of these behaviors/conditions. Serious, life-threatening, or fatal respiratory depression may occur; monitor during initiation or following a dose increase. Chewing, swallowing, snorting, or injecting buprenorphine extracted from the transdermal system will result in uncontrolled delivery and pose risk of overdose and death. Accidental exposure, especially in children, can result in a fatal overdose. Prolonged use during pregnancy can result in neonatal opioid withdrawal syndrome; advise pregnant women of the risk and ensure availability of appropriate treatment.

ADULT DOSAGE

Severe Pain (Daily, Around-the-Clock Management)

Long-Term Opioid Treatment for Which Alternative Treatment Options are Inadequate:

First Opioid Analgesic:

Initial: 5mcg/hr

Titrate: Individualize dose

Minimum Titration Interval: 72 hrs; may adjust dose every 3 days

Max: 20mcg/hr

Dose adjustments may be made in 5mcg/hr, 7.5mcg/hr, or 10mcg/hr increments by using no more than 2 patches of the 5mcg/hr, 7.5mcg/hr, or 10mcg/hr systems

Conversions

From Other Opioids to Buprenorphine Transdermal System:

D/C all other around-the-clock opioid drugs when therapy is initiated

Prior Total Daily Dose of Opioid <30mg of Oral Morphine Equivalents/Day:

Initiate treatment w/ 5mcg/hr at the next dosing interval

Prior Total Daily Dose of Opioid Between 30mg to 80mg of Oral Morphine Equivalents/Day:

Taper the patient's current around-the-clock opioids for up to 7 days to no more than 30mg of morphine or equivalent/day before beginning treatment

Then initiate treatment w/ 10mcg/hr at the next dosing interval

Patients may use short-acting analgesics prn until efficacy is attained

PEDIATRIC DOSAGE

Pediatric use may not have been established

B

Prior Total Daily Dose of Opioid >80mg of Oral Morphine Equivalents/Day:
20mcg/hr may not provide adequate analgesia for patients requiring >80mg/day oral morphine equivalents
Consider the use of an alternate analgesic

DOSING CONSIDERATIONS

Hepatic Impairment

Severe: Consider use of an alternate analgesic that may permit more flexibility w/ dosing

Discontinuation

Use gradual downward titration every 7 days
Consider introduction of an appropriate immediate-release opioid medication

ADMINISTRATION

Transdermal route

Each patch is intended to be worn for 7 days
Do not cut patch
Apply immediately after removal from individually sealed pouch
Apply to intact skin on upper outer arm, upper chest, upper back, or side of chest; rotate application site w/ a minimum of 21 days before reapplying to the same skin site
For use of 2 patches, remove current patch and apply the 2 new patches at the same time, adjacent to one another at a different application site
Refer to PI for further administration and disposal instructions

HOW SUPPLIED

Patch: 5mcg/hr, 7.5mcg/hr, 10mcg/hr, 15mcg/hr, 20mcg/hr

CONTRAINDICATIONS

Significant respiratory depression, acute or severe bronchial asthma in an unmonitored setting or in the absence of resuscitative equipment, known or suspected paralytic ileus. Hypersensitivity (eg, anaphylaxis) to buprenorphine.

WARNINGS/PRECAUTIONS

Reserve use in patients for whom alternative treatment options are ineffective, not tolerated, or would be otherwise inadequate to provide sufficient management of pain. Should only be prescribed by healthcare professionals who are knowledgeable in the use of potent opioids for management of chronic pain. Doses of 7.5, 10, 15, and 20mcg/hr are for opioid-experienced patients only. Life-threatening respiratory depression is more likely to occur in elderly, cachectic, or debilitated patients. Consider alternative nonopioid analgesics in patients with significant chronic obstructive pulmonary disease or cor pulmonale, and in patients who have a substantially decreased respiratory reserve, hypoxia, hypercapnia, or preexisting respiratory depression. QTc interval prolongation observed at dose of 40mcg/hr; caution with hypokalemia or clinically unstable cardiac disease. Avoid use with history/immediate family history of long QT syndrome. May cause severe hypotension, orthostatic hypotension, and syncope; increased risk in patients whose ability to maintain BP has already been compromised by a reduced blood volume or concurrent administration of certain CNS depressants. Monitor patients who may be susceptible to intracranial effects of carbon dioxide retention for signs of sedation and respiratory depression when initiating therapy. Therapy may obscure clinical course in patients with head injury. Avoid with impaired consciousness or coma. Obtain baseline liver enzyme levels and monitor periodically during treatment in patients at increased risk of hepatotoxicity (eg, history of excessive alcohol intake, IV drug abuse). Application-site skin reactions with signs of marked inflammation reported; d/c if severe application-site reactions develop. Cases of acute and chronic hypersensitivity, bronchospasm, angioneurotic edema, and anaphylactic shock reported. Potential for temperature-dependent increases in drug release, resulting in possible overdose and death; avoid exposure of application site and surrounding area to direct external heat sources. If fever or increased core body temperature due to strenuous exertion develops, monitor for side effects and adjust dose if signs of respiratory/CNS depression occur. Avoid with GI obstruction. May cause spasm of sphincter of Oddi and increase in serum amylase; monitor patients with biliary tract disease. May aggravate convulsions and induce/aggravate seizures. May impair mental/physical abilities. Not approved for management of addictive disorders. Not for use during and immediately prior to labor. Caution in elderly.

ADVERSE REACTIONS

Respiratory depression, N/V, dizziness, headache, application-site pruritus/irritation/erythema/rash, constipation, somnolence, dry mouth, fatigue, hyperhidrosis, peripheral edema.

DRUG INTERACTIONS

Respiratory depression, hypotension, profound sedation, or coma may occur with alcohol and other CNS depressants (eg, sedatives, anxiolytics, neuroleptics); if coadministration is required, consider dose reduction of one or both agents. Monitor use in elderly, cachectic, and debilitated patients when coadministered with other drugs that depress respiration. Monitor closely with benzodiazepines. CYP3A4 inhibitors may increase levels and prolong opioid effects; these effects could be more pronounced with concomitant use of CYP2D6 and 3A4 inhibitors; if coadministration is necessary, monitor for respiratory depression and sedation at frequent intervals and consider dose adjustments. CYP3A4 inducers may decrease levels and cause lack of efficacy or development of abstinence syndrome; if coadministration or discontinuation of a CYP3A4 inducer is necessary, monitor for signs of opioid withdrawal and consider dose adjustments. May enhance neuromuscular blocking action of skeletal muscle relaxants and increase respiratory depression. Avoid with Class IA antiarrhythmics (eg, quinidine, procainamide, disopyramide) or Class III antiarrhythmics (eg, sotalol, amiodarone, dofetilide). Anticholinergics or other drugs with anticholinergic activity may increase risk of urinary retention and/or severe constipation and lead to paralytic ileus.

PATIENT CONSIDERATIONS

Assessment: Assess for abuse/addiction risk, pain intensity, prior opioid therapy, opioid tolerance, respiratory depression, drug hypersensitivity, pregnancy/nursing status, possible drug interactions, or any other conditions where treatment is contraindicated or cautioned. Obtain baseline liver enzyme levels in patients at increased risk of hepatotoxicity.

Monitoring: Monitor for respiratory depression (especially within first 24-72 hrs of initiation), hypotension, application-site skin reactions, seizures/convulsions, and other adverse reactions. Monitor BP and serum amylase levels. Regularly monitor for signs of misuse, abuse, and addiction. Periodically reassess the continued need for therapy. Monitor liver enzyme levels periodically in patients at increased risk of hepatotoxicity.

Counseling: Inform that use of drug can result in addiction, abuse, and misuse; instruct not to share with others and to take steps to protect from theft or misuse. Inform patients about risk of respiratory depression. Advise to store securely and dispose unused patch by folding the patch in 1/2 and flushing down the toilet. Inform women of reproductive potential that prolonged use during pregnancy may result in neonatal opioid withdrawal syndrome and instruct to inform physician if pregnant or planning to become pregnant. Inform that potentially serious additive effects may occur when used with alcohol or CNS depressants, and not to use such drugs unless supervised by healthcare provider. Instruct about proper application, removal, and disposal instructions. Inform that drug may cause orthostatic hypotension, syncope, impair the ability to perform potentially hazardous activities; advise to not perform such tasks until patients know how they will react to medication. Advise of potential for severe constipation, including management instructions. Advise how to recognize anaphylaxis and when to seek medical attention.

STORAGE: 25°C (77°F); excursions permitted between 15-30°C (59-86°F).

BYDUREON – exenatide

RX

Class: Glucagon-like peptide-1 (GLP-1) receptor agonist

Causes an increased incidence in thyroid C-cell tumors at clinically relevant exposures in animal studies. It is unknown whether drug causes thyroid C-cell tumors (eg, medullary thyroid carcinoma [MTC]) in humans. Contraindicated in patients w/ a personal/family history of MTC and w/ multiple endocrine neoplasia syndrome type 2 (MEN 2). Counsel patients on the potential risk for MTC w/ exenatide use and inform them of symptoms of thyroid tumors (eg, mass in the neck, dysphagia, dyspnea, persistent hoarseness). Routine monitoring of serum calcitonin or using thyroid ultrasound is of uncertain value for detection of MTC in patients treated w/ exenatide.

ADULT DOSAGE

Type 2 Diabetes Mellitus

2mg/dose SQ once every 7 days, at any time of day

Changing Weekly Dosing Schedule:
May change the day of weekly administration if necessary as long as the last dose was given ≥3 days before

Conversions

Changing from Byetta to Bydureon:
Prior treatment w/ Byetta is not required when initiating Bydureon therapy
D/C Byetta if the decision is made to start Bydureon in a patient already taking Byetta
Patients changing from Byetta to Bydureon may experience transient (approx 2 weeks) elevations in blood glucose concentrations

PEDIATRIC DOSAGE

Pediatric use may not have been established

Missed Dose

If a dose is missed, administer it as soon as noticed, provided the next regularly scheduled dose is due at least 3 days later. Thereafter, may resume usual dosing schedule of once every 7 days (weekly)

If a dose is missed and the next regularly scheduled dose is due 1 or 2 days later, do not administer the missed dose and instead resume therapy w/ the next regularly scheduled dose

DOSING CONSIDERATIONS

Renal Impairment

Moderate (CrCl 30-50mL/min): Use w/ caution

Severe (CrCl <30mL/min) or ESRD: Not recommended

Patients w/ Renal Transplantation: Use w/ caution

Elderly

Caution when initiating treatment

ADMINISTRATION

SQ route

Administer at any time of day, w/ or w/o meals.
Inject in the abdomen, thigh, or upper arm region; use a different inj site each week when injecting in the same region.
Do not administer IV or IM.
Intended for patient self-administration.
Administer immediately after powder is suspended in diluent.
Refer to PI for further administration instructions.

HOW SUPPLIED

Inj, Extended-Release: 2mg [vial, pen]

CONTRAINDICATIONS

MEN 2, personal/family history of MTC, prior serious hypersensitivity reaction to exenatide or to any of its components.

WARNINGS/PRECAUTIONS

Not recommended as 1st-line therapy for patients who have inadequate glycemic control on diet and exercise. Not a substitute for insulin; do not use in type 1 DM or for treatment of diabetic ketoacidosis. Not studied and cannot be recommended w/ insulin. Acute pancreatitis, including fatal and nonfatal hemorrhagic or necrotizing pancreatitis, reported; d/c promptly if suspected, and do not restart therapy if confirmed. Consider other antidiabetic therapies in patients w/ history of pancreatitis. Patients w/ elevated calcitonin levels and those w/ thyroid nodules noted on physical examination or neck imaging should be further evaluated. Altered renal function, including increased SrCr, renal impairment, worsened chronic renal failure, and acute renal failure reported. Not recommended w/ severe GI disease. May develop antibodies; consider alternative antidiabetic therapy if there is worsening glycemic control or failure to achieve targeted glycemic control. Serious hypersensitivity reactions reported; d/c if a hypersensitivity reaction occurs. Serious inj-site reactions (eg, abscess, cellulitis, necrosis), w/ or w/o subcutaneous nodules reported; isolated cases required surgical intervention.

ADVERSE REACTIONS

Constipation, diarrhea, dyspepsia, headache, N/V, inj-site nodule, fatigue, decreased appetite, inj-site pruritus, viral gastroenteritis, GERD, inj-site erythema, inj-site hematoma.

DRUG INTERACTIONS

Increased risk of hypoglycemia w/ insulin secretagogues (eg, sulfonylureas) or insulin; may require a lower dose of the secretagogue or insulin. May reduce the rate of absorption of orally administered drugs; caution w/ oral medications. May increase INR w/ warfarin, sometimes associated w/ bleeding; monitor INR more frequently after initiation of exenatide. Should not be used w/ other drugs containing the same active ingredient (eg, Byetta).

PATIENT CONSIDERATIONS

Assessment: Assess for previous hypersensitivity reactions, MEN 2, personal/family history of MTC, history of pancreatitis, type of DM, diabetic ketoacidosis, renal impairment, severe GI disease, pregnancy/nursing status, and possible drug interactions. Assess glucose and HbA1c levels.

Monitoring: Monitor for signs/symptoms of thyroid tumor, pancreatitis, elevated serum calcitonin levels, hypoglycemia, GI events, immunogenicity, hypersensitivity reactions, inj-site reactions, and other adverse reactions. Monitor renal function, blood glucose levels, and HbA1c levels. Monitor INR more frequently after initiation of therapy in patients receiving warfarin.

Counseling: Counsel on potential risks/benefits of therapy and alternative modes of therapy. Inform of importance of adhering to dietary instructions, regular physical activity, periodic blood glucose monitoring and HbA1c testing, recognition/management of hypo/hyperglycemia, and assessment for diabetes complications. Advise to report symptoms of thyroid tumors (eg, lump in the neck, hoarseness, dysphagia, dyspnea) to physician. Inform of potential risk for pancreatitis, worsening of renal function, and serious hypersensitivity reactions. Instruct to d/c therapy promptly and contact physician if persistent severe abdominal pain and/or symptoms of a hypersensitivity reaction occur. Inform that serious inj-site reactions w/ or w/o subcutaneous nodules may occur; advise to seek medical advice if symptomatic nodules occur, or for any signs/symptoms of abscess, cellulitis, or necrosis. Instruct to never share a prefilled syringe/pen w/ another person, even if the needle is changed. Inform that therapy may result in nausea, particularly upon initiation of therapy. Advise that if a dose is missed, administer as soon as noticed, provided that the next regularly scheduled dose is due at least 3 days later. Instruct to then resume the usual dosing schedule thereafter. Inform that if a dose is missed and the next regularly scheduled dose is due in 1 or 2 days, to not administer the missed dose and instead resume w/ the next regularly scheduled dose. Advise to inform physician if pregnant/intending to become pregnant. Inform about the importance of proper storage, inj technique, and dosing.

STORAGE: 2-8°C (36-46°F). May store at room temperature not exceeding 25°C (77°F) for ≤4 weeks, if needed. Do not freeze; do not use if product has been frozen. Protect from light.

BYETTA – exenatide

RX

Class: Glucagon-like peptide-1 (GLP-1) receptor agonist

ADULT DOSAGE

Type 2 Diabetes Mellitus

Initial: 5mcg SQ bid, at any time w/in 60 min before am and pm meals (or before the 2 main meals of the day, approx 6 hrs or more apart)

Titrate: May increase to 10mcg bid after 1 month based on response

PEDIATRIC DOSAGE

Pediatric use may not have been established

DOSING CONSIDERATIONS

Renal Impairment

Moderate (CrCl 30-50mL/min): Caution when initiating or escalating doses from 5mcg to 10mcg
Severe (CrCl <30mL/min) or ESRD: Not recommended
Renal Transplantation: Use w/ caution

ADMINISTRATION

SQ route

Inject into thigh, abdomen, or upper arm
Do not mix w/ insulin
Do not transfer from the pen to a syringe or a vial

HOW SUPPLIED

Inj: 5mcg/dose, 10mcg/dose [60 doses]

CONTRAINDICATIONS

Prior serious hypersensitivity reaction to exenatide or to any of its components.

WARNINGS/PRECAUTIONS

Not a substitute for insulin; do not use in type 1 DM or for the treatment of diabetic ketoacidosis. Not studied and cannot be recommended w/ prandial insulin. Evaluate dose of insulin if used in combination; consider dose reduction in patients at risk of hypoglycemia. Do not share pens between patients, even if needle is changed; risk of transmission of blood-borne pathogens. Acute pancreatitis, including fatal and nonfatal hemorrhagic or necrotizing pancreatitis, reported; observe for signs/symptoms of pancreatitis after initiation of therapy and dose increases, d/c promptly if suspected, and do not restart therapy if confirmed. Consider other antidiabetic therapies in patients w/ history of pancreatitis. Altered renal function, including increased SrCr, renal impairment, worsened chronic renal failure, and acute renal failure, reported. Not recommended w/ severe GI disease. May develop antibodies; consider alternative antidiabetic therapy if there is worsening glycemic control or failure to achieve targeted glycemic control. Serious hypersensitivity reactions (eg, anaphylaxis, angioedema) reported; d/c if a hypersensitivity reaction occurs.

ADVERSE REACTIONS

Hypoglycemia, N/V, immunogenicity, dyspepsia, diarrhea, feeling jittery, dizziness, headache, constipation, asthenia, GERD, hyperhidrosis, abdominal distension, decreased appetite.

DRUG INTERACTIONS

Increased risk of hypoglycemia w/ a sulfonylurea or other glucose-independent insulin secretagogues (eg, meglitinides); may require a lower dose of the sulfonylurea. May reduce the extent and rate of absorption of orally administered drugs; caution w/ oral medications w/ narrow therapeutic index or that require rapid GI absorption. Oral medications that are dependent on threshold concentrations for efficacy (eg, contraceptives, antibiotics) should be taken at least 1 hr before inj. May increase INR w/ warfarin, sometimes associated w/ bleeding; monitor PT more frequently after initiation or alteration of therapy.

PATIENT CONSIDERATIONS

Assessment: Assess for history of hypersensitivity to drug or any product components, type of DM, diabetic ketoacidosis, history of pancreatitis, renal impairment, severe GI disease, pregnancy/nursing status, and possible drug interactions.

Monitoring: Monitor for signs/symptoms of hypoglycemia, pancreatitis, GI events, immunogenicity, hypersensitivity reactions, and other adverse reactions. Monitor renal function, blood glucose levels, and HbA1c levels. Monitor PT more frequently after initiation or alteration of therapy in patients receiving warfarin.

Counseling: Counsel on the potential risks/benefits of therapy and alternative modes of therapy. Inform of importance of proper storage of drug, inj technique, timing of dosage and concomitant oral drugs, adherence to meal planning, regular physical activity, periodic blood glucose monitoring and HbA1c testing, recognition/management of hypo/hyperglycemia, and assessment for diabetes complications. Advise to never share inj pen w/ another person, even if needle is changed. Inform that pen needles are purchased separately and advise on proper needle selection and disposal. Inform that if a dose is missed, treatment regimen should be resumed as prescribed w/ the next scheduled dose. Instruct to inform physician if pregnant or intending to become pregnant. Advise that treatment may result in reduction in appetite, food intake, and/or body weight, and that there is no need to modify the dosing regimen due to such effects. Inform that nausea, particularly upon initiation of therapy, may occur. Instruct to contact a physician if signs/symptoms of acute pancreatitis (eg, severe abdominal pain), renal dysfunction, or hypersensitivity reactions develop.

STORAGE: Prior to 1st Use: 2-8°C (36-46°F). After 1st Use: <25°C (77°F). Do not freeze. Do not use if it has been frozen. Protect from light. Discard pen 30 days after 1st use.

BYSTOLIC — nebivolol

RX

Class: Selective $beta_1$ blocker

ADULT DOSAGE

Hypertension

Initial: 5mg qd

Titrate: May increase at 2-week intervals

Max: 40mg

PEDIATRIC DOSAGE

Pediatric use may not have been established

DOSING CONSIDERATIONS

Renal Impairment

Severe (CrCl <30mL/min):

Initial: 2.5mg qd; titrate up slowly if needed

Hepatic Impairment

Moderate:

Initial: 2.5mg qd; titrate up slowly if needed

ADMINISTRATION

Oral route

Take w/ or w/o food

HOW SUPPLIED

Tab: 2.5mg, 5mg, 10mg, 20mg

CONTRAINDICATIONS

Severe bradycardia, heart block >1st degree, cardiogenic shock, decompensated cardiac failure, sick sinus syndrome (unless permanent pacemaker in place), severe hepatic impairment (Child-Pugh >B), hypersensitivity to any component of this product.

WARNINGS/PRECAUTIONS

Severe exacerbation of angina, myocardial infarction, and ventricular arrhythmias reported in patients with coronary artery disease (CAD) following abrupt discontinuation; taper over 1-2 weeks when possible. Restart therapy promptly, at least temporarily, if angina worsens or acute coronary insufficiency develops. Caution patients without overt CAD against interruption or abrupt discontinuation of therapy. Avoid with bronchospastic disease. Treatment should generally be continued throughout perioperative period. If therapy is to be continued perioperatively, monitor closely when anesthetic agents that depress myocardial function (eg, ether, cyclopropane, trichloroethylene) are used. If therapy is withdrawn prior to major surgery, impaired ability of the heart to respond to reflex adrenergic stimuli may augment the risks of general anesthesia and surgical procedures; difficulty in restarting and maintaining heartbeat reported. May mask manifestations of hypoglycemia/hyperthyroidism, particularly tachycardia; abrupt withdrawal may be followed by exacerbation of the symptoms of hyperthyroidism or may precipitate a thyroid storm. May precipitate/aggravate symptoms of arterial insufficiency with peripheral vascular disease (PVD). Patients with history of severe anaphylactic reactions to variety of allergens may be more reactive to repeated accidental/diagnostic/therapeutic challenge; may be unresponsive to usual doses of epinephrine. Initiate an α-blocker prior to use of any β-blocker in patients with known/suspected pheochromocytoma.

ADVERSE REACTIONS

Headache, fatigue, dizziness, diarrhea, nausea.

DRUG INTERACTIONS

Avoid with other β-blockers. D/C for several days before the gradual tapering of clonidine. Caution with CYP2D6 inhibitors (eg, quinidine, propafenone, paroxetine, fluoxetine); may need to reduce dose of nebivolol. May produce excessive reduction of sympathetic activity with catecholamine-depleting drugs (eg, reserpine, guanethidine). May increase risk of bradycardia with digitalis glycosides. May exacerbate effects of myocardial depressants/inhibitors of atrioventricular conduction (eg, antiarrhythmics, certain Ca^{2+} antagonists). May potentiate hypoglycemic effect of insulin and oral hypoglycemics. Significant negative inotropic and chronotropic effects may occur with verapamil and diltiazem type; monitor ECG and BP.

PATIENT CONSIDERATIONS

Assessment: Assess for CAD, bronchospastic disease, diabetes mellitus, hypoglycemia, hyperthyroidism, PVD, pheochromocytoma, hepatic/renal impairment, pregnancy/nursing status, any other conditions where treatment is contraindicated or cautioned, and possible drug interactions.

Monitoring: Monitor for precipitation/aggravation of arterial insufficiency, hypersensitivity, and other adverse reactions. Monitor ECG, BP, and serum glucose levels.

Counseling: Inform of the risks and benefits of therapy. Advise to take drug regularly and continuously, ud. Instruct to take only the next scheduled dose, without doubling it, if a dose is missed, and not to interrupt or d/c without consulting physician. Advise to consult physician if any difficulty in breathing occurs, or signs/symptoms of worsening congestive heart failure develop. Caution about operating automobiles, using machinery, or engaging in tasks requiring alertness. Caution patients subject to spontaneous hypoglycemia, or diabetic patients receiving insulin or oral hypoglycemics, that the drug may mask some of the manifestations of hypoglycemia, particularly tachycardia.

STORAGE: 20-25°C (68-77°F).

CADUET — amlodipine besylate/atorvastatin calcium

RX

Class: Calcium channel blocker (CCB)/HMG-CoA reductase inhibitor (statin)

ADULT DOSAGE

Hypertension

Treatment alone or in combination w/ other antihypertensive agents

Amlodipine:
Initial: 5mg qd
Max: 10mg qd

Adjust dose according to BP goals. In general, wait 7-14 days between titration steps; titration may proceed more rapidly if clinically warranted

Angina

Chronic stable angina or confirmed or suspected vasospastic (Prinzmetal's/variant) angina, alone or in combination w/ other antianginals

Amlodipine:
5-10mg qd

PEDIATRIC DOSAGE

Hypertension

Treatment alone or in combination w/ other antihypertensive agents

Amlodipine:
6-17 Years:
Usual: 2.5-5mg qd
Max: 5mg qd

Heterozygous Familial Hypercholesterolemia

As an adjunct to diet if after an adequate trial of diet therapy LDL remains ≥190mg/dL or LDL remains ≥160mg/dL and there is a positive family history of premature cardiovascular disease (CVD) or 2 or more other CVD risk factors are present in the pediatric patient

Atorvastatin:
Heterozygous Familial Hypercholesterolemia:
10-17 Years (Postmenarchal):

C

Coronary Artery Disease

Reduces the risk of hospitalization due to angina and reduces risk of coronary revascularization procedures in patients w/ recently documented coronary artery disease (CAD) by angiography and w/o heart failure or an ejection fraction <40%

Amlodipine:
5-10mg qd

Hyperlipidemia/Mixed Dyslipidemia

Adjunct to diet for treatment of primary hypercholesterolemia (heterozygous familial and nonfamilial) and mixed dyslipidemia (Types IIa and IIb); adjunct to diet for treatment of patients w/ elevated serum TG levels (Type IV); primary dysbetalipoproteinemia (Type III) inadequately responding to diet; adjunct to other lipid-lowering treatments or if treatments are unavailable, for treatment of homozygous familial hypercholesterolemia

Atorvastatin:
Hyperlipidemia (Heterozygous Familial and Nonfamilial) and Mixed Dyslipidemia (Fredrickson Types IIa and IIb):
Initial: 10 or 20mg qd; patients who require ≥45% reduction in LDL-C may be started at 40mg qd
Titrate: Analyze lipid levels w/in 2-4 weeks and adjust dose accordingly
Range: 10-80mg qd

Homozygous Familial Hypercholesterolemia:
Range: 10-80mg qd
Atorvastatin should be used as an adjunct to other lipid-lowering treatments (eg, LDL apheresis)

Risk Reduction of Myocardial Infarction, Stroke, Cardiovascular Death

Reduces the risk of MI, stroke, revascularization procedures, and angina in adults w/o clinically evident coronary heart disease (CHD), but w/ multiple risk factors for CHD; reduces the risk of MI and stroke in patients w/ type 2 diabetes, and w/o clinically evident CHD, but w/ multiple risk factors for CHD; reduces the risk of nonfatal MI, fatal and nonfatal stroke, revascularization procedures, hospitalization for CHF, and angina in patients w/ clinically evident CHD

Initial: 10mg/day
Max: 20mg/day
Dose adjustments should be made at intervals of ≥4 weeks

DOSING CONSIDERATIONS

Concomitant Medications

Antihypertensives: Start w/ 2.5mg qd amlodipine
Cyclosporine or HIV Protease Inhibitors (Tipranavir Plus Ritonavir [RTV]) or Telaprevir: Avoid therapy w/ atorvastatin
Lopinavir Plus RTV: Use lowest necessary dose of atorvastatin
Clarithromycin, Itraconazole, Fosamprenavir, or Combination of Saquinavir/Darunavir/ Fosamprenavir Plus RTV: Limit therapy w/ atorvastatin to 20mg and ensure lowest dose needed is employed
Nelfinavir or Boceprevir: Limit therapy w/ atorvastatin to 40mg and ensure lowest dose needed is employed

Hepatic Insufficiency

Initial: 2.5mg qd amlodipine

Elderly

Initial: 2.5mg qd amlodipine

Other Important Considerations
Small Adults or Fragile Patients:
Initial: 2.5mg qd amlodipine

ADMINISTRATION

Oral route

Take w/ or w/o food.

HOW SUPPLIED

Tab: (Amlodipine/Atorvastatin) 2.5mg/10mg, 2.5mg/20mg, 2.5mg/40mg, 5mg/10mg, 5mg/20mg, 5mg/40mg, 5mg/80mg, 10mg/10mg, 10mg/20mg, 10mg/40mg, 10mg/80mg

CONTRAINDICATIONS

Active liver disease, which may include unexplained persistent elevations in hepatic transaminases, women who are pregnant or may become pregnant, and nursing mothers.

WARNINGS/PRECAUTIONS

Amlodipine: Worsening angina and acute MI may develop after starting or increasing the dose, particularly w/ severe obstructive CAD. Symptomatic hypotension may occur, particularly in patients w/ severe aortic stenosis. **Atorvastatin:** Rare cases of rhabdomyolysis w/ acute renal failure secondary to myoglobinuria reported. Increased risk of rhabdomyolysis in patients w/ history of renal impairment; closely monitor for skeletal muscle effects. Myopathy (including immune-mediated necrotizing myopathy [IMNM]) reported; predisposing factor includes advanced age (≥65 yrs of age). D/C if markedly elevated creatine phosphokinase (CPK) levels occur or if myopathy is diagnosed or suspected. Withhold or d/c if an acute, serious condition suggestive of a myopathy occurs or if there is a risk factor predisposing to development of renal failure secondary to rhabdomyolysis. Persistent increases in serum transaminases reported; perform LFTs prior to initiation and repeat as clinically indicated. Fatal and nonfatal hepatic failure (rare) reported; promptly interrupt therapy if serious liver injury w/ clinical symptoms and/or hyperbilirubinemia or jaundice occurs and do not restart if no alternate etiology found. Increases in HbA1c and FPG levels reported. May blunt adrenal and/or gonadal steroid production. Increased risk of hemorrhagic stroke in patients w/ recent stroke or transient ischemic attack (TIA).

ADVERSE REACTIONS

Amlodipine: Dizziness, edema.
Atorvastatin: Nasopharyngitis, arthralgia, diarrhea, pain in extremity, UTI.

DRUG INTERACTIONS

See Dosing Considerations. **Amlodipine:** CYP3A inhibitors (moderate and strong) may increase systemic exposure to amlodipine and may require dose reduction; monitor for symptoms of hypotension and edema to determine the need for dose adjustment. Closely monitor BP if coadministered w/ CYP3A inducers. Monitor for hypotension when coadministered w/ sildenafil. May increase systemic exposure of cyclosporine or tacrolimus; monitor trough blood levels of cyclosporine and tacrolimus frequently and adjust dose when appropriate. **Atorvastatin:** Avoid w/ gemfibrozil and drugs that decrease levels or activity of endogenous steroid hormones (eg, ketoconazole, spironolactone, cimetidine). Increased risk of myopathy w/ fibric acid derivatives, erythromycin, strong CYP3A4 inhibitors, clarithromycin, combinations of HIV protease inhibitors, and azole antifungals; consider lower initial and maintenance doses of atorvastatin. Increased risk of myopathy w/ cyclosporine and telaprevir. Risk of skeletal muscle effects may be enhanced when used w/ niacin; consider a reduction in atorvastatin dose. Strong CYP3A4 inhibitors (eg, clarithromycin, several combinations of HIV protease inhibitors, telaprevir, itraconazole, boceprevir) and grapefruit juice may increase levels. CYP3A4 inducers (eg, efavirenz, rifampin) may decrease levels; simultaneous coadministration w/ rifampin is recommended. May increase digoxin levels; monitor appropriately. May increase exposure of norethindrone and ethinyl estradiol. Myopathy, including rhabdomyolysis, reported w/ colchicine; use w/ caution. OATP1B1 inhibitors (eg, cyclosporine) may increase bioavailability.

PATIENT CONSIDERATIONS

Assessment: Assess for active liver disease, unexplained and persistent elevations in serum transaminase levels, history of renal impairment, risk factors for developing renal failure secondary to rhabdomyolysis, recent stroke or TIA, CAD, aortic stenosis, hypersensitivity to the drug, pregnancy/nursing status, and possible drug interactions. Obtain baseline lipid profile (total-C, LDL, HDL, TG), liver function (eg, AST, ALT) parameters, and BP.

Monitoring: Monitor for signs/symptoms of rhabdomyolysis, myopathy (eg, IMNM), worsening angina, MI, and other adverse reactions. Monitor lipid profile, and CPK levels. Monitor LFTs as clinically indicated, and for increases in HbA1c and FPG levels. Monitor BP.

Counseling: Advise to adhere to medication, along w/ the National Cholesterol Education Program-recommended diet, a regular exercise program, and periodic fasting lipid panel testing. Inform of the substances that should not be taken concomitantly w/ the drug. Advise patients to inform other healthcare professionals that they are taking the drug. Inform of the risk of myopathy; instruct to report promptly any unexplained muscle pain, tenderness, or weakness, particularly if accompanied by malaise or fever, or if muscle signs and symptoms persist after discontinuation. Instruct to report promptly any symptoms that may indicate liver injury. Instruct women of childbearing potential to use effective contraceptive methods to prevent pregnancy and to d/c therapy and contact physician if pregnancy occurs. Instruct not to use the drug if breastfeeding.

STORAGE: 25°C (77°F); excursions permitted to 15-30°C (59-86°F).

CALAN – verapamil hydrochloride

RX

Class: Calcium channel blocker (CCB) (nondihydropyridine)

ADULT DOSAGE

Hypertension

Initial (Monotherapy): 80mg tid (240mg/day)
Range: 360-480mg/day; no evidence that dosages >360mg/day provided added effect
Titrate: Based upward titration on therapeutic efficacy, assessed at the end of the dosing interval

Angina

Angina at rest including vasospastic (Prinzmetal's variant) angina and unstable (crescendo, pre-infarction) angina/chronic stable angina (classic effort-associated angina)
Usual: 80-120mg tid
Titrate: Base upward titration on therapeutic efficacy and safety evaluated approx 8 hrs after dosing; may increase daily (eg, patients w/ unstable angina) or at weekly intervals until optimum response is obtained

Arrhythmias

In association w/ digitalis, for the control of ventricular rate at rest and during stress in patients w/ chronic A-flutter/A-fib
Range: 240-320mg/day in divided doses tid or qid

Paroxysmal Supraventricular Tachycardia

Prophylaxis (Non-Digitalized):
Range: 240-480mg/day in divided doses tid or qid
Max effects for any given dosage will be apparent during the first 48 hrs of therapy

PEDIATRIC DOSAGE

Pediatric use may not have been established

DOSING CONSIDERATIONS

Hepatic Impairment

Severe Dysfunction: Give 30% of normal dose

Other Important Considerations

Patients Who May Respond to Lower Doses (eg, Elderly, People of Small Stature):
HTN: Consider beginning titration at 40mg tid
Angina: 40mg tid may be warranted

ADMINISTRATION

Oral route

HOW SUPPLIED

Tab: 40mg, 80mg*, 120mg* *scored

CONTRAINDICATIONS

Severe left ventricular dysfunction, hypotension (systolic pressure <90mmHg) or cardiogenic shock, sick sinus syndrome or 2nd- or 3rd-degree atrioventricular (AV) block (except with functioning ventricular artificial pacemaker), A-fib/flutter and an accessory bypass tract (eg, Wolff-Parkinson-White, Lown-Ganong-Levine syndromes), hypersensitivity to verapamil HCl.

WARNINGS/PRECAUTIONS

Has negative inotropic effect; avoid with severe left ventricular dysfunction (eg, ejection fraction <30%) or moderate to severe symptoms of cardiac failure. Patients with milder ventricular dysfunction should, if possible, be controlled with optimum doses of digitalis and/or diuretics before treatment. May cause congestive heart failure (CHF), pulmonary edema, hypotension, asymptomatic 1st-degree AV block, transient bradycardia, and PR interval prolongation. Marked

1st-degree AV block or progressive development to 2nd- or 3rd-degree AV block requires dose reduction, or in rare instances, discontinuation and institution of appropriate therapy. Hepatocellular injury as well as elevated transaminases with or without concomitant elevations in alkaline phosphatase and bilirubin reported; monitor LFTs periodically. Sinus bradycardia, 2nd-degree AV block, pulmonary edema, severe hypotension, and sinus arrest reported in patients with hypertrophic cardiomyopathy. Caution with renal/hepatic impairment; monitor for abnormal PR interval prolongation or other signs of overdosage. 30% of normal dose should be given to patients with severe hepatic dysfunction. May decrease neuromuscular transmission in patients with Duchenne muscular dystrophy and may cause worsening of myasthenia gravis; may be necessary to decrease dose when administered to patients with attenuated neuromuscular transmission. Caution in elderly.

ADVERSE REACTIONS

Constipation, dizziness.

DRUG INTERACTIONS

CYP3A4 inhibitors (eg, erythromycin, ritonavir) and grapefruit juice may increase levels. CYP3A4 inducers (eg, rifampin) may decrease levels. May cause myopathy/rhabdomyolysis with HMG-CoA reductase inhibitors that are CYP3A4 substrates and may increase levels of such drugs; limit dose of simvastatin to 10mg/day and lovastatin to 40mg/day, and lower starting/maintenance doses of other CYP3A4 substrates (eg, atorvastatin) may be required. Increased bleeding times with aspirin. Additive negative effects on HR, AV conduction, and/or cardiac contractility with β-blockers; monitor closely and avoid with any degree of ventricular dysfunction. Combined therapy with propranolol should usually be avoided in patients with AV conduction abnormalities and those with depressed left ventricular function. May produce asymptomatic bradycardia with a wandering atrial pacemaker with timolol eye drops. Decreased metoprolol and propranolol clearance and variable effect with atenolol reported. Chronic treatment may increase digoxin levels, which may result in digitalis toxicity; reduce maintenance and digitalization doses and monitor carefully to avoid over-/under-digitalization. May reduce total body/extra renal clearance of digitoxin. Additive effects with other oral antihypertensives (eg, vasodilators, ACE inhibitors, diuretics); monitor appropriately. Coadministration with agents that attenuate α-adrenergic function (eg, prazosin) may excessively reduce BP. Avoid disopyramide within 48 hrs before or 24 hrs after administration. Coadministration with flecainide may result in additive negative inotropic effect and AV conduction prolongation. May counteract effects of quinidine on AV conduction and increase levels of quinidine; avoid concomitant use in patients with hypertrophic cardiomyopathy. Reduced or unchanged clearance with cimetidine. Increased sensitivity to effects of lithium (neurotoxicity) when used concomitantly; monitor carefully. May increase carbamazepine, theophylline, cyclosporine, and alcohol levels. Increased clearance with phenobarbital. Rifampin may reduce oral bioavailability. Titrate both verapamil and inhalation anesthetics carefully, in order to avoid excessive cardiovascular depression. May potentiate neuromuscular blockers (eg, curare-like and depolarizing); verapamil or both agents may need dose reduction. Hypotension and bradyarrhythmias reported with telithromycin. Sinus bradycardia resulting in hospitalization and pacemaker insertion reported with clonidine; monitor HR.

PATIENT CONSIDERATIONS

Assessment: Assess for known hypersensitivity to the drug, cardiac failure, severe left ventricular dysfunction, hypertrophic cardiomyopathy, hepatic/renal impairment, attenuated neuromuscular transmission (eg, Duchenne muscular dystrophy), any conditions where treatment is contraindicated or cautioned, pregnancy/nursing status, and possible drug interactions.

Monitoring: Monitor for CHF, hypotension, AV block, abnormal prolongation of the PR interval, transient bradycardia, and other adverse reactions. Monitor LFTs periodically.

Counseling: Inform of the risks/benefits of therapy. Advise to seek medical attention if any adverse reactions occur.

STORAGE: 15-25°C (59-77°F). Protect from light.

Calan SR – verapamil hydrochloride

RX

Class: Calcium channel blocker (CCB) (nondihydropyridine)

ADULT DOSAGE

Hypertension

Initial: 180mg qam

Titrate: If response is inadequate, increase to 240mg qam, then 180mg bid (am and pm) or 240mg qam plus 120mg qpm, then 240mg q12h

PEDIATRIC DOSAGE

Pediatric use may not have been established

Upward titration should be based on therapeutic efficacy and safety evaluated weekly and approx 24 hrs after the previous dose

Switching from IR Calan to Calan SR: Total daily dose in mg may remain the same

C

DOSING CONSIDERATIONS

Hepatic Impairment

Severe Dysfunction: Give 30% of normal dose

Other Important Considerations

Increased Response to Verapamil (eg, Elderly, Small Stature):

Initial: 120mg qam may be warranted

ADMINISTRATION

Oral route

Take w/ food

HOW SUPPLIED

Tab, Extended-Release: 120mg, 180mg*, 240mg* *scored

CONTRAINDICATIONS

Severe left ventricular dysfunction, hypotension (systolic pressure <90mmHg) or cardiogenic shock, sick sinus syndrome or 2nd- or 3rd-degree AV block (except with functioning artificial ventricular pacemaker), A-flutter/A-fib and an accessory bypass tract (eg, Wolff-Parkinson-White, Lown-Ganong-Levine syndromes), hypersensitivity to verapamil HCl.

WARNINGS/PRECAUTIONS

Has negative inotropic effect; avoid with severe left ventricular dysfunction (eg, ejection fraction <30%) or moderate to severe symptoms of cardiac failure. Patients with milder ventricular dysfunction should, if possible, be controlled with optimum doses of digitalis and/or diuretics before treatment. May cause hypotension, CHF, pulmonary edema, asymptomatic 1st-degree AV block, transient bradycardia, and PR-interval prolongation. Marked 1st-degree AV block or progressive development to 2nd- or 3rd-degree AV block requires dose reduction, or in rare instances, discontinuation and institution of appropriate therapy. Sinus bradycardia, pulmonary edema, severe hypotension, 2nd-degree AV block, and sinus arrest reported in patients with hypertrophic cardiomyopathy. Hepatocellular injury as well as elevated transaminases with or without concomitant elevations in alkaline phosphatase and bilirubin reported; monitor LFTs periodically. Caution with renal/hepatic impairment; monitor for abnormal PR interval prolongation or other signs of overdosage. 30% of normal dose should be given to patients with severe hepatic dysfunction. May decrease neuromuscular transmission in patients with Duchenne muscular dystrophy; may be necessary to decrease dose when administered to patients with attenuated neuromuscular transmission. Caution in elderly.

ADVERSE REACTIONS

Constipation, dizziness.

DRUG INTERACTIONS

May cause myopathy/rhabdomyolysis with HMG-CoA reductase inhibitors that are CYP3A4 substrates and may increase levels of such drugs; limit dose of simvastatin to 10mg/day or lovastatin to 40mg/day, and consider lower starting/maintenance doses of other CYP3A4 substrates (eg, atorvastatin). Additive negative effects on HR, AV conduction, and/or cardiac contractility with β-blockers; monitor closely and avoid with any degree of ventricular dysfunction. May produce asymptomatic bradycardia with a wandering atrial pacemaker with timolol eye drops. Decreased metoprolol and propranolol clearance and variable effect with atenolol reported. Additive effects with other oral antihypertensives (eg, vasodilators, ACE inhibitors, diuretics); monitor appropriately. Coadministration with agents that attenuate α-adrenergic function (eg, prazosin) may excessively reduce BP. May increase carbamazepine, theophylline, and cyclosporine levels. Chronic treatment may increase digoxin levels, which may result in digitalis toxicity; reduce maintenance and digitalization doses and monitor carefully to avoid over-/under-digitalization. May reduce total body/extrarenal clearance of digitoxin. Avoid disopyramide within 48 hrs before or 24 hrs after administration. Coadministration with flecainide may result in additive negative inotropic effect and AV conduction prolongation. May counteract effects of quinidine on AV conduction and increase levels of quinidine; avoid concomitant use in patients with hypertrophic cardiomyopathy. May increase ethanol concentrations that may prolong the intoxicating effects of alcohol. Increased sensitivity to effects of lithium (neurotoxicity) when used concomitantly; monitor carefully. Increased clearance with phenobarbital. Rifampin may reduce oral bioavailability. May potentiate neuromuscular blockers (eg, curare-like and depolarizing); verapamil or both agents may need dose reduction. Titrate both verapamil and inhalation anesthetics carefully to avoid excessive cardiovascular depression. Hypotension and bradyarrhythmias reported with telithromycin. Sinus bradycardia resulting in hospitalization and pacemaker insertion reported with clonidine; monitor HR. Reduced or unchanged clearance with cimetidine.

PATIENT CONSIDERATIONS

Assessment: Assess for known hypersensitivity to drug, severe left ventricular dysfunction, attenuated neuromuscular transmission (eg, Duchenne muscular dystrophy), cardiac failure, hypertrophic cardiomyopathy, hepatic/renal impairment, and for any other conditions where treatment is contraindicated or cautioned. Assess pregnancy/nursing status and for possible drug interactions.

Monitoring: Monitor for abnormal prolongation of PR-interval, hypotension, CHF, pulmonary edema, AV block, transient bradycardia, and other adverse reactions. Monitor LFTs periodically.

Counseling: Inform of the risks/benefits of therapy. Advise to seek medical attention if any adverse reactions occur.

STORAGE: 15-25°C (59-77°F). Protect from light and moisture.

CANCIDAS – caspofungin acetate

RX

Class: Echinocandin

ADULT DOSAGE

Aspergillosis

Invasive Aspergillosis, Refractory/Intolerant of Other Therapies:
LD: 70mg on Day 1
Maint: 50mg qd thereafter

Duration of treatment should be based upon severity of underlying disease, recovery from immunosuppression, and clinical response

Fungal Infections

Empirical Therapy in Febrile, Neutropenic Patients:
LD: 70mg on Day 1
Maint: 50mg qd thereafter; may increase to 70mg/day if 50mg dose is well tolerated but provides inadequate clinical response

Continue until resolution of neutropenia for empiric therapy; treat for a minimum of 14 days if a fungal infection is found and continue for at least 7 days after neutropenia and clinical symptoms are resolved

Candida Infections

Candidemia, Intra-Abdominal Abscesses, Peritonitis, and Pleural Space Infections:
LD: 70mg on Day 1
Maint: 50mg qd thereafter

Continue for at least 14 days after the last positive culture; may warrant a longer course of therapy pending resolution of neutropenia in patients who remain persistently neutropenic

Esophageal Candidiasis

50mg qd for 7-14 days after symptom resolution

Consider suppressive oral therapy in patients w/ HIV infections due to risk of relapse

PEDIATRIC DOSAGE

Fungal Infections

Empirical Therapy in Febrile, Neutropenic Patients:
3 Months-17 Years:
LD: 70mg/m^2 on Day 1
Maint: 50mg/m^2 qd thereafter; may increase to 70mg/m^2 qd if 50mg/m^2 dose is well tolerated but provides inadequate clinical response
Max: 70mg/day

Continue until resolution of neutropenia for empiric therapy; treat for a minimum of 14 days if a fungal infection is found and continue for at least 7 days after neutropenia and clinical symptoms are resolved

Candida Infections

Candidemia, Intra-Abdominal Abscesses, Peritonitis, and Pleural Space Infections:
3 Months-17 Years:
LD: 70mg/m^2 on Day 1
Maint: 50mg/m^2 qd thereafter; may increase to 70mg/m^2 qd if 50mg/m^2 dose is well tolerated but provides inadequate clinical response
Max: 70mg/day

Continue for at least 14 days after the last positive culture; may warrant a longer course of therapy pending resolution of neutropenia in patients who remain persistently neutropenic

Esophageal Candidiasis

3 Months-17 Years:
LD: 70mg/m^2 on Day 1
Maint: 50mg/m^2 qd thereafter; may increase to 70mg/m^2 qd if 50mg/m^2 dose is well tolerated but provides inadequate clinical response
Max: 70mg/day

Treat for 7-14 days after symptom resolution
Consider suppressive oral therapy in patients w/ HIV infections due to risk of relapse

Aspergillosis

Invasive Aspergillosis, Refractory/Intolerant of Other Therapies:
3 Months-17 Years:
LD: 70mg/m^2 on Day 1

Maint: 50mg/m^2 qd thereafter; may increase to 70mg/m^2 qd if 50mg/m^2 dose is well tolerated but provides inadequate clinical response
Max: 70mg/day
Duration of treatment should be based upon severity of underlying disease, recovery from immunosuppression, and clinical response

DOSING CONSIDERATIONS

Concomitant Medications
Adults:
Concomitant Rifampin: 70mg qd
Concomitant Nevirapine/Efavirenz/Carbamazepine/Dexamethasone/Phenytoin: May require dose increase to 70mg qd
Pediatrics:
Concomitant Inducers of Drug Clearance (eg, Rifampin, Efavirenz, Nevirapine): Consider 70mg/m^2 qd (not to exceed 70mg)

Hepatic Impairment
Adults:
Moderate Impairment (Child-Pugh Score 7-9):
Maint: 35mg qd; still administer 70mg LD on Day 1 if recommended

ADMINISTRATION

IV route
Not for IV bolus administration.
Give by slow IV infusion over approx 1 hr.
Do not mix or coinfuse w/ other medications or use diluents containing dextrose (α-D-glucose).

Preparation
Equilibrate product vials to room temperature.
Reconstitute 50mg or 70mg vials w/ 10.8mL of appropriate reconstitution diluent for a final concentration of 5mg/mL or 7mg/mL, respectively.
Transfer appropriate reconstituted volume to an IV bag/bottle containing 250mL of 0.9%, 0.45%, or 0.225% NaCl inj or lactated Ringer's inj.
Alternatively, reconstituted volume may be added to a reduced volume of 0.9%, 0.45%, or 0.225% NaCl inj or lactated Ringer's inj, not to exceed a final concentration of 0.5mg/mL.
Special Considerations for Pediatrics ≥3 Months of Age:
Reconstitute as above using the 70mg or 50mg vial, then remove volume of drug equal to calculated LD/maint dose.
For doses <50mg, use 50mg vials; for doses >50mg, use 70mg vials.

Reconstitution Diluents
0.9% NaCl
Sterile water for inj
Bacteriostatic water for inj w/ methylparaben and propylparaben
Bacteriostatic water for inj w/ 0.9% benzyl alcohol

HOW SUPPLIED

Inj: 50mg, 70mg

CONTRAINDICATIONS

Hypersensitivity (eg, anaphylaxis) to any component of this product.

WARNINGS/PRECAUTIONS

Anaphylaxis reported; d/c and administer appropriate treatment if this occurs. Possible histamine-mediated adverse reactions (eg, rash, facial swelling, angioedema) reported and may require discontinuation and/or administration of appropriate treatment. Limit concomitant use w/ cyclosporine to patients for whom potential benefit outweighs potential risk. Abnormal LFTs reported; monitor patients who develop abnormal LFTs for evidence of worsening hepatic function and evaluate risk/benefit of continuing therapy. Isolated cases of significant hepatic dysfunction, hepatitis, and hepatic failure reported w/ multiple concomitant medications in patients w/ serious underlying conditions.

ADVERSE REACTIONS

Pyrexia, chills, hypokalemia, hypotension, diarrhea, increased blood alkaline phosphatase, increased ALT/AST, N/V, abdominal pain, peripheral edema, headache, rash, increased blood bilirubin, septic shock, pneumonia.

DRUG INTERACTIONS

See Dosing Considerations. Increased exposure and transient increases in ALT and AST reported w/ concomitant cyclosporine. Reduced levels of tacrolimus; monitor tacrolimus blood concentrations and adjust tacrolimus dosage appropriately. Inducers of drug clearance (eg, efavirenz, nevirapine, phenytoin, rifampin, dexamethasone, carbamazepine) may decrease levels.

PATIENT CONSIDERATIONS

Assessment: Assess for drug hypersensitivity, hepatic function, pregnancy/nursing status, and possible drug interactions.

Monitoring: Monitor for anaphylaxis, histamine-mediated adverse reactions, resolution of neutropenia, and other adverse reactions. Monitor LFTs.

Counseling: Inform that anaphylactic reactions have been reported; instruct to report signs/symptoms of hypersensitivity to physician. Inform that there have been isolated reports of serious hepatic effects.

STORAGE: 2-8°C (36-46°F). **Reconstituted:** ≤25°C (77°F) for 1 hr prior to preparation of infusion sol. **Diluted:** ≤25°C (77°F) for 24 hrs or 2-8°C (36-46°F) for 48 hrs.

C

CAPTOPRIL – captopril

RX

Class: ACE inhibitor

D/C when pregnancy is detected. Drugs that act directly on the renin-angiotensin system (RAS) can cause injury and death to the developing fetus.

ADULT DOSAGE

Hypertension

D/C previous antihypertensive drug regimen for 1 week before starting captopril therapy, if possible

Initial: 25mg bid or tid

Titrate: May increase to 50mg bid or tid if satisfactory BP reduction is not achieved after 1 or 2 weeks. Add a modest dose of a thiazide diuretic (eg, hydrochlorothiazide, 25mg/day) if BP is not controlled after 1-2 weeks at 50mg tid and patient is not already receiving a diuretic; diuretic dose may be increased at 1- to 2-week intervals until its highest usual antihypertensive dose is reached. If further BP reduction is required, may increase captopril dose to 100mg bid or tid and then, if necessary, to 150mg bid or tid (while continuing the diuretic)

Usual Range: 25-150mg bid or tid

Max: 450mg/day

Severe HTN (eg, Accelerated or Malignant HTN):

When temporary discontinuation of current antihypertensive therapy is not practical or desirable, or when prompt titration to more normotensive blood pressure levels is indicated, continue the diuretic but d/c other current antihypertensive medication and promptly initiate captopril at 25mg bid or tid

Congestive Heart Failure

Initial: 25mg tid; 6.25mg or 12.5mg tid in patients w/ normal/low BP, who have been vigorously treated w/ diuretics and who may be hyponatremic and/or hypovolemic

Titrate: After a dose of 50mg tid is reached, delay further increases in dosage, where possible, for at least 2 weeks to determine if a satisfactory response occurs. Most patients studied have had a satisfactory clinical improvement at 50mg or 100mg tid

Max: 450mg/day

Captopril should generally be used in conjunction w/ a diuretic and digitalis

PEDIATRIC DOSAGE

Pediatric use may not have been established

Left Ventricular Dysfunction Post-Myocardial Infarction

May initiate therapy as early as 3 days following MI

Initial: 6.25mg single dose, then 12.5mg tid
Titrate: Increase to 25mg tid during the next several days, then to 50mg tid over next several weeks
Maint: 50mg tid

May be used in patients treated w/ other post-MI therapies (eg, thrombolytics, aspirin, beta blockers)

Diabetic Neuropathy

25mg tid

Other antihypertensives (eg, diuretics, beta blockers, centrally acting agents, or vasodilators) may be used in conjunction w/ captopril if additional therapy is required

DOSING CONSIDERATIONS

Renal Impairment

Patients may respond to smaller or less frequent doses

Significant Impairment:

Reduce initial daily dosage, and utilize smaller increments for titration, which should be quite slow (1- to 2-week intervals)

After desired effect is achieved, slowly back-titrate dose to determine the minimal effective dose

When concomitant diuretic therapy is required, administer a loop diuretic (eg, furosemide) rather than a thiazide diuretic

ADMINISTRATION

Oral route

Take 1 hr ac.

HOW SUPPLIED

Tab: 12.5mg*, 25mg*, 50mg*, 100mg* *scored

CONTRAINDICATIONS

Hypersensitivity to this product or any other ACE inhibitor (ACE inhibitor-associated angioedema). Coadministration w/ aliskiren in patients w/ diabetes.

WARNINGS/PRECAUTIONS

Head/neck angioedema reported; promptly institute appropriate therapy if this occurs. Intestinal angioedema reported; monitor for abdominal pain. Higher rate of angioedema in black patients than in nonblack patients. Anaphylactoid reactions reported during desensitization w/ hymenoptera venom, dialysis w/ high-flux membranes, and LDL apheresis w/ dextran sulfate absorption. Consider using a different type of dialysis membrane or a different class of medication in patients undergoing hemodialysis w/ high-flux dialysis membranes. Neutropenia/agranulocytosis reported; risk of neutropenia is dependent on the clinical status of the patient. In patients w/ collagen vascular disease or who are exposed to other drugs known to affect the white cells or immune response, particularly w/ impaired renal function, use captopril only after an assessment of benefit and risk, and then w/ caution. Perform WBC counts if infection is suspected. Withdraw therapy and closely follow patient's course if neutropenia (neutrophil count $<1000/mm^3$) is confirmed. Total urinary proteins >1g/day reported. Excessive hypotension may occur in patients w/ salt/volume depletion, heart failure (HF), or those undergoing renal dialysis; initiate therapy under very close medical supervision in these patients. Rarely, associated w/ a syndrome that starts w/ cholestatic jaundice and progresses to fulminant hepatic necrosis and sometimes death; d/c if jaundice or marked elevations of hepatic enzymes develop. May increase BUN/SrCr after reduction of BP or upon long-term HF treatment. Hyperkalemia and persistent nonproductive cough reported. Patients w/ aortic stenosis may be at particular risk of decreased coronary perfusion. Hypotension may occur w/ major surgery or during anesthesia. Lab test interactions may occur.

ADVERSE REACTIONS

Anemia, thrombocytopenia, pancytopenia, rash, diminution/loss of taste perception.

DRUG INTERACTIONS

Coadministration w/ mTOR (mammalian target of rapamycin) inhibitors (eg, temsirolimus, sirolimus, everolimus) may increase risk for angioedema. Dual blockade of the RAS is associated w/ increased risks of hypotension, hyperkalemia, and changes in renal function (including acute renal failure); avoid combined use of RAS inhibitors. Closely monitor BP, renal function, and electrolytes w/ concomitant agents that also block the RAS. Do not coadminister w/ aliskiren in patients w/

diabetes or renal impairment (GFR <60mL/min). Coadministration w/ NSAIDs, including selective COX-2 inhibitors, may cause deterioration of renal function, including possible acute renal failure, in patients who are elderly, volume-depleted, or w/ compromised renal function. NSAIDs may also attenuate antihypertensive effect. Precipitous BP reduction may occur w/ diuretics, usually w/in the 1st hr after the initial dose of captopril. Nitroglycerin, other nitrates, or drugs having vasodilator activity should, if possible, be discontinued before starting captopril; administer such agents cautiously, and perhaps at lower dosage if resumed during captopril therapy. Antihypertensive agents that cause renin release may augment effect of captopril (eg, diuretics [eg, thiazides] may activate renin-angiotensin-aldosterone system [RAAS]). Caution w/ agents affecting sympathetic activity (eg, ganglionic-blocking agents, adrenergic neuron-blocking agents); β-adrenergic blocking drugs may add further antihypertensive effect. Increased risk of hyperkalemia w/ K^+-sparing diuretics (eg, spironolactone, triamterene, amiloride), K^+ supplements, K^+-containing salt substitutes, or other drugs associated w/ increases in serum K^+; use w/ caution. Increased serum lithium levels and symptoms of lithium toxicity reported; coadminister w/ caution and frequently monitor serum lithium levels. Nitritoid reactions reported w/ injectable gold.

PATIENT CONSIDERATIONS

Assessment: Assess for hypersensitivity to drug, history of ACE inhibitor-associated angioedema, diabetes, collagen vascular disease, volume/salt depletion, HF, renal artery stenosis, risk factors for hyperkalemia, renal function, aortic stenosis, pregnancy/nursing status, and possible drug interactions. In patients w/ renal impairment, evaluate WBC and differential counts.

Monitoring: Monitor for angioedema, anaphylactoid reactions, neutropenia/agranulocytosis, hyperkalemia, and other adverse reactions. Monitor BP, LFTs, and renal function. In patients w/ renal impairment, evaluate WBC and differential counts at approx 2-week intervals for about 3 months, then periodically.

Counseling: Instruct to d/c therapy and to immediately report to physician any signs/symptoms of angioedema. Advise to report promptly any indication of infection (eg, sore throat, fever) or of progressive edema. Inform that excessive perspiration, dehydration, and other causes of volume depletion (eg, vomiting, diarrhea) may lead to excessive fall in BP; advise to consult w/ physician. Instruct not to use K^+-sparing diuretics, K^+ supplements, or K^+-containing salt substitutes w/o consulting physician. Warn against interruption or discontinuation of medication unless instructed by physician. Caution HF patients against rapid increases in physical activity. Inform female patients of childbearing age about the consequences of exposure to captopril during pregnancy and discuss treatment options w/ those planning to become pregnant; instruct to report pregnancies to physician as soon as possible.

STORAGE: 20-25°C (68-77°F). Protect from moisture.

CARAFATE – sucralfate

RX

Class: Duodenal ulcer adherent complex

ADULT DOSAGE

Active Duodenal Ulcer

1g qid on an empty stomach; continue for 4-8 weeks unless healing has been demonstrated by x-ray or endoscopic exam

Antacids may be prescribed prn for relief of pain but should not be taken w/in 1/2 hr before or after administration

Tab:

Maint: 1g bid

PEDIATRIC DOSAGE

Pediatric use may not have been established

DOSING CONSIDERATIONS

Elderly

Start at the lower end of dosing range

ADMINISTRATION

Oral route

Sus

Shake well before use

HOW SUPPLIED

Sus: 1g/10mL [14 fl oz]; **Tab:** 1g* *scored

CONTRAINDICATIONS

Hypersensitivity reactions to the active substance or to any of the excipients.

WARNINGS/PRECAUTIONS

DU is a chronic, recurrent disease; a successful course of treatment should not be expected to alter post healing frequency or severity of duodenal ulceration. May impair excretion of absorbed aluminum with chronic renal failure or those receiving dialysis; aluminum accumulation and toxicity (aluminum osteodystrophy, osteomalacia, encephalopathy) reported with renal impairment. Caution with chronic renal failure and in elderly. (Sus) Episodes of hyperglycemia reported in diabetic patients; may need to adjust dose of antidiabetic treatment during therapy. (Tab) Aspiration with accompanying respiratory complications reported; caution with known conditions that may impair swallowing (eg, recent or prolonged intubation, tracheostomy, prior history of aspiration, dysphagia), or any other conditions that may alter gag and cough reflexes, or diminish oropharyngeal coordination or motility.

ADVERSE REACTIONS

Constipation, diarrhea, N/V, pruritus, rash, dizziness, insomnia, back pain, headache, dry mouth, flatulence, gastric discomfort, indigestion, sleepiness, vertigo.

DRUG INTERACTIONS

Simultaneous administration may reduce the extent of absorption of single doses of cimetidine, digoxin, fluoroquinolone antibiotics, ketoconazole, l-thyroxine, phenytoin, quinidine, ranitidine, tetracycline, and theophylline; administer separately when alterations in bioavailability are felt to be critical and monitor patients appropriately. Subtherapeutic PT with concomitant warfarin reported. Concomitant use with other products that contain aluminum (eg, aluminum-containing antacids) may increase the total body burden of aluminum.

PATIENT CONSIDERATIONS

Assessment: Assess for drug hypersensitivity or to any of the excipients, chronic renal failure or receiving dialysis, pregnancy/nursing status, and possible drug interactions. (Sus) Assess for diabetes mellitus. (Tab) Assess for known conditions that may impair swallowing or any other conditions that may alter gag and cough reflexes, or diminish oropharyngeal coordination or motility.

Monitoring: Monitor for aluminum accumulation and toxicity in patients with renal impairment and other adverse reactions. Monitor renal function. (Sus) Monitor for episodes of hyperglycemia. (Tab) Monitor for aspiration with accompanying respiratory complications.

Counseling: Inform about the risks/benefits of treatment. Instruct to take exactly ud. Advise to contact physician if any side effects develop. Counsel about the possible drug interactions. Advise to notify physician if pregnant/nursing or planning to become pregnant.

STORAGE: (Sus) 20-25°C (68-77°F). Avoid freezing. (Tab) 15-30°C (59-86°F).

CARBAMAZEPINE – carbamazepine RX

Class: Carboxamide

Serious and sometimes fatal dermatologic reactions, including toxic epidermal necrolysis (TEN) and Stevens-Johnson syndrome (SJS) reported; increased risk w/ presence of HLA-B*1502 allele. Screen patients w/ ancestry in genetically at-risk populations for the presence of HLA-B*1502 prior to initiation of therapy. Avoid in patients testing positive for the allele unless benefits clearly outweigh risks. Aplastic anemia and agranulocytosis reported; obtain complete pretreatment hematological testing as a baseline and monitor closely if a patient exhibits low/decreased WBC or platelet counts during treatment. Consider discontinuation if evidence of significant bone marrow depression develops.

OTHER BRAND NAMES

Tegretol-XR, Epitol, Tegretol

ADULT DOSAGE

Trigeminal Neuralgia

Initial (Day 1): 100mg bid (tab/tab, extended-release [ER]) or 1/2 tsp qid (200mg/day) (sus)
Titrate: May increase by up to 200mg/day using increments of 100mg q12h (tab/tab, ER) or 50mg (1/2 tsp) qid (sus) prn
Maint: 400-800mg/day. Attempt to reduce dose to minimum effective level or even to d/c therapy at least once every 3 months
Max: 1200mg/day

Beneficial results have also been reported in glossopharyngeal neuralgia

PEDIATRIC DOSAGE

Epilepsy

Partial Seizures w/ Complex Symptomatology (Psychomotor, Temporal Lobe), Generalized Tonic-Clonic Seizures (Grand Mal), and Mixed Seizure Patterns of These, or Other Partial or Generalized Seizures:

<6 Years:
Initial: 10-20mg/kg/day bid or tid (tab) or qid (sus)
Titrate: Increase weekly to tid or qid (tab/sus)
Maint: Optimal clinical response is achieved at daily doses <35mg/kg; no recommendation regarding safety at doses >35mg/kg/24 hrs

Epilepsy

Partial Seizures w/ Complex Symptomatology (Psychomotor, Temporal Lobe), Generalized Tonic-Clonic Seizures (Grand Mal), and Mixed Seizure Patterns of These, or Other Partial or Generalized Seizures:

Initial: 200mg bid (tab/tab, ER) or 1 tsp qid (400mg/day) (sus)
Titrate: Increase at weekly intervals by adding up to 200mg/day bid (tab, ER) or tid or qid (all other formulations)
Maint: 800-1200mg/day
Max: 1200mg/day; doses up to 1600mg/day have been used in rare instances
Combination Therapy:
When added to existing anticonvulsant therapy, add gradually while other anticonvulsants are maintained or gradually decreased (except phenytoin, which may have to be increased)

Conversions

From Oral Carbamazepine Tabs to Carbamazepine Sus:
Patients should be converted by administering the same number of mg/day in smaller, more frequent doses (eg, bid tabs to tid sus)
From Carbamazepine Conventional Tabs to Carbamazepine ER Tabs:
The same total daily mg dose of carbamazepine ER tabs should be administered

6-12 Years:
Initial: 100mg bid (tab/tab, ER) or 1/2 tsp qid (200mg/day) (sus)
Titrate: Increase at weekly intervals by adding up to 100mg/day bid (tab, ER) or tid or qid (all other formulations)
Maint: 400-800mg/day
Max: 1000mg/day

>12 Years:
Initial: 200mg bid (tab/tab, ER) or 1 tsp qid (400mg/day) (sus)
Titrate: Increase at weekly intervals by adding up to 200mg/day bid (tab, ER) or tid or qid (all other formulations)
Maint: 800-1200mg/day
Max:
12-15 Years: 1000mg/day
>15 Years: 1200mg/day
Combination Therapy:
When added to existing anticonvulsant therapy, add gradually while other anticonvulsants are maintained or gradually decreased (except phenytoin, which may have to be increased)

Conversions

From Oral Carbamazepine Tabs to Carbamazepine Sus:
Patients should be converted by administering the same number of mg/day in smaller, more frequent doses (eg, bid tabs to tid sus)
From Carbamazepine Conventional Tab to Carbamazepine ER Tabs:
The same total daily mg dose of carbamazepine ER tabs should be administered

ADMINISTRATION

Oral route

Take w/ meals.
Sus will produce higher peak levels than the same dose given as the tab; start patients given sus on lower doses and increase slowly to avoid unwanted side effects.

Sus
Do not administer simultaneously w/ other liquid medications or diluents.
Shake well before using.

Tab, ER
Swallow whole; do not chew or crush.

HOW SUPPLIED

Tab, Chewable: 200mg*, (Tegretol) 100mg*; **Sus:** (Tegretol) 100mg/5mL [450mL]; **Tab:** (Tegretol, Epitol) 200mg*; **Tab, ER:** (Tegretol-XR) 100mg, 200mg, 400mg *scored

CONTRAINDICATIONS

History of previous bone marrow depression; hypersensitivity to the drug, or sensitivity to any of the tricyclic compounds (eg, amitriptyline, desipramine, imipramine, protriptyline, nortriptyline); coadministration w/ nefazodone; concomitant use w/ an MAOI or w/in 14 days after discontinuing an MAOI.

WARNINGS/PRECAUTIONS

D/C at 1st sign of rash; do not resume treatment and consider alternative therapy if signs/symptoms suggest SJS/TEN. Consider risks and benefits of therapy in patients known to be positive for HLA-A*3101. Patients w/ a history of adverse hematologic reaction to any drug may be particularly at risk of bone marrow depression. Drug reaction w/ eosinophilia and systemic symptoms (DRESS), also known as multiorgan hypersensitivity, reported; evaluate immediately if signs/symptoms (eg, fever, lymphadenopathy) are present and d/c if an alternative etiology cannot be established. Caution in patients w/ history of hypersensitivity reactions to anticonvulsants (eg, phenytoin, primidone, phenobarbital). Increased risk of suicidal thoughts or behavior reported. Has mild anticholinergic activity that may be associated w/ increased IOP; closely observe patients w/ increased IOP during therapy. Consider the possibility of activation of latent psychosis and, in elderly patients, of confusion or agitation. Avoid in patients w/ history of hepatic porphyria (eg, acute intermittent porphyria, variegate porphyria, porphyria cutanea tarda); acute attacks reported. Withdraw gradually to minimize potential of increased seizure frequency. Hyponatremia may occur and in many cases, appears to be caused by the syndrome of inappropriate antidiuretic hormone secretion; consider discontinuing therapy in patients w/ symptomatic hyponatremia. May cause fetal harm and symptoms representing neonatal withdrawal syndrome. Caution in patients w/ a mixed seizure disorder that includes atypical absence seizures; therapy associated w/ increased frequency of generalized convulsions in these patients. Caution in patients w/ history of cardiac conduction disturbance, cardiac/hepatic/renal damage, adverse hematologic or hypersensitivity reaction to other drugs, and interrupted courses of therapy w/ carbamazepine. Atrioventricular heart block (eg, 2nd- and 3rd-degree block) and hepatic effects (ranging from slight elevations in liver enzymes to rare cases of hepatic failure) reported. D/C if new or worsening clinical/lab evidence of liver dysfunction/hepatic damage, or active liver disease develops. Interference w/ some pregnancy tests, decreased values of thyroid function tests, renal dysfunction, and eye changes reported. Higher prevalence of teratogenic effects w/ the use of anticonvulsants in combination therapy; if therapy is to be continued, monotherapy may be preferable for pregnant women. **Sus/Tab, Chewable 200mg:** Contains sorbitol; avoid w/ rare hereditary problems of fructose intolerance. **Tab, ER:** Coating is not absorbed and is excreted in the feces; may be noticeable in the stool.

ADVERSE REACTIONS

Dizziness, drowsiness, unsteadiness, N/V.

DRUG INTERACTIONS

See Contraindications. Close monitoring of carbamazepine levels is indicated and dosage adjustment may be required when given w/ drugs that increase/decrease levels. CYP3A4 inhibitors (eg, azole antifungals, erythromycin, protease inhibitors) may increase levels. Coadministration of inhibitors of human microsomal epoxide hydrolase may result in increased carbamazepine-10,11 epoxide levels; adjust dose and/or monitor levels of carbamazepine when used w/ loxapine, quetiapine, or valproic acid. CYP3A4 inducers (eg, cisplatin, doxorubicin, rifampin) may decrease levels. May decrease levels of CYP1A2, 2B6, 2C9/19, and 3A4 substrates; monitoring of concentrations or dosage adjustment of the concomitant agents may be necessary. When added to aripiprazole therapy, double aripiprazole dose and if carbamazepine is later withdrawn, reduce aripiprazole dose. When used w/ tacrolimus, monitoring of tacrolimus levels and appropriate dosage adjustments are recommended. Avoid w/ temsirolimus; consider dose adjustment of temsirolimus if coadministration is a must. Avoid w/ lapatinib; gradually titrate up dose of lapatinib if carbamazepine is started in a patient already taking lapatinib and reduce lapatinib dose when carbamazepine is discontinued. Monitor concentrations of valproate when carbamazepine is introduced or withdrawn in patients using valproic acid. May cause, or would be expected to cause, decreased levels of the following drugs, for which monitoring of concentrations or dosage adjustment may be necessary: acetaminophen, albendazole, alprazolam, aprepitant, buprenorphine, bupropion, citalopram, clonazepam, clozapine, corticosteroids (eg, prednisolone, dexamethasone), cyclosporine, dicumarol, dihydropyridine calcium channel blockers (eg, felodipine), doxycycline, ethosuximide, everolimus, haloperidol, imatinib, itraconazole, lamotrigine, levothyroxine, methadone, methsuximide, mianserin, midazolam, olanzapine, oxcarbazepine, paliperidone, phensuximide, phenytoin, praziquantel, protease inhibitors, risperidone, sertraline, sirolimus, tadalafil, theophylline, tiagabine, topiramate, tramadol, trazodone, TCAs (eg, imipramine, amitriptyline, nortriptyline), valproate, warfarin, ziprasidone, zonisamide. May increase cyclophosphamide toxicity. May increase risk of neurotoxic side effects w/ lithium. Increased isoniazid-induced hepatotoxicity reported w/ isoniazid. Alterations of thyroid function reported w/ other anticonvulsant medications. May decrease levels of hormonal contraceptive products (eg, oral and levonorgestrel subdermal implant contraceptives) that may render contraceptives less effective; consider alternative or back-up method of contraception. Resistance to the neuromuscular blocking action of the nondepolarizing neuromuscular blocking agents (eg, pancuronium, vecuronium, rocuronium) reported w/ chronic carbamazepine administration; monitor closely for more rapid recovery from neuromuscular blockade than expected, and infusion rate requirements may be higher. Increased risk of developing hyponatremia w/ diuretics. **Sus:** Occurrence of stool precipitate reported w/ liquid chlorpromazine or thioridazine.

PATIENT CONSIDERATIONS

Assessment: Assess for hypersensitivity to the drug, known sensitivity to any of the tricyclic compounds, mixed seizure disorder, history of cardiac conduction disturbance, renal/hepatic impairment, any other conditions where treatment is contraindicated or cautioned, pregnancy/nursing status, and possible drug interactions. Perform detailed history and physical exam prior to treatment. Screen for HLA-B*1502 and HLA-A*3101 allele in suspected populations. Obtain baseline CBCs w/ platelets and reticulocytes and serum iron, LFTs, complete urinalysis, BUN determinations, and eye examination (including slit-lamp exam, funduscopy, and tonometry).

Monitoring: Monitor for signs/symptoms of dermatologic reactions, DRESS, bone marrow depression, aplastic anemia, agranulocytosis, increase in seizure frequency, emergence or worsening of depression, suicidal thoughts/behavior, unusual changes in mood/behavior, latent psychosis, confusion or agitation in elderly patients, hepatic effects, and other adverse reactions. Periodically monitor WBC and platelet counts, LFTs, serum drug levels, complete urinalysis, BUN determinations, and eye examinations.

Counseling: Inform of the early toxic signs and symptoms of a potential hematologic problem, as well as dermatologic, hypersensitivity, or hepatic reactions; advise to report to physician even if the signs and symptoms are mild or when occurring after extended use. Instruct to immediately contact physician if a skin reaction occurs. Inform about the increased risk of suicidal thoughts and behavior; advise to report behaviors of concern immediately and to be alert for the emergence/worsening of symptoms of depression, any unusual changes in mood or behavior, the emergence of suicidal thoughts, or behavior/thoughts about self-harm. Advise to report the use of any other prescription or nonprescription medications or herbal products. Instruct to exercise caution when taken w/ alcohol due to a possible additive sedative effect. Inform that drowsiness or dizziness may occur; caution against hazardous tasks. Encourage patients to enroll in the NAAED Pregnancy Registry.

STORAGE: **Tab, Chewable:** 20-25°C (68-77°F). Protect from light/moisture. (Tegretol) **Tab, Chewable:** ≤30°C (86°F). Protect from light/moisture. **Sus:** ≤30°C (86°F). **Tab:** ≤30°C (86°F). Protect from moisture. **Tab, ER:** 25°C (77°F); excursions permitted to 15-30°C (59-86°F). Protect from moisture. (Epitol) **Tab:** 20-25°C (68-77°F). Protect from moisture.

C

CARDENE IV – nicardipine hydrochloride

RX

Class: Calcium channel blocker (CCB) (dihydropyridine)

ADULT DOSAGE

Hypertension

Short-term treatment when oral therapy is not feasible or not desirable

Patients Not Receiving Oral Nicardipine:
Initial: 5mg/hr IV infusion
Titrate: May increase by 2.5mg/hr every 5 min (for rapid titration) to 15 min (for gradual titration) if desired BP reduction is not achieved
Max: 15mg/hr
Decrease infusion rate to 3mg/hr after BP goal is achieved w/ rapid titration

IV Dosage as a Substitute for Oral Nicardipine Therapy:
20mg PO q8h=0.5mg/hr IV infusion
30mg PO q8h=1.2mg/hr IV infusion
40mg PO q8h=2.2mg/hr IV infusion

Transition to Oral Antihypertensives:
Transfer to Oral Nicardipine: Give 1st dose 1 hr prior to discontinuation of infusion
Transfer to Oral Antihypertensive Other Than Nicardipine: Initiate therapy upon discontinuation of IV nicardipine

PEDIATRIC DOSAGE

Pediatric use may not have been established

DOSING CONSIDERATIONS

Renal Impairment
Titrate slowly

Hepatic Impairment
Impaired Function/Reduced Hepatic Blood Flow: Consider lower dosages and titrate slowly

Elderly
Use low initial doses

Other Important Considerations
Heart Failure: Titrate slowly

D/C infusion if there is concern of impending hypotension/tachycardia; may restart infusion at low doses (3-5mg/hr) when BP has stabilized and adjust to maintain desired BP

ADMINISTRATION

IV route

Administer by a central line or through a large peripheral vein; change infusion site q12h if administered via peripheral vein

Premixed Sol
No further dilution is required
Do not combine w/ any product in the same IV line or premixed container; do not add supplementary medication to the bag
Do not use plastic containers in series connections

C

Ampules
Administer by slow continuous infusion at a concentration of 0.1mg/mL
Dilute each ampule (25mg) w/ 240mL of compatible IV fluid (yielding 250mL of sol at a concentration of 0.1mg/mL); diluted sol is stable for 24 hrs at room temperature

IV Compatibilities:
Compatible and stable in glass or polyvinyl chloride containers for 24 hrs at controlled room temperature w/:
D5 inj
D5 and NaCl 0.45% inj
D5 and NaCl 0.9% inj
D5 w/ 40mEq K^+
NaCl 0.45% inj
NaCl 0.9% inj

IV Incompatibilities:
Sodium bicarbonate (5%) inj
Lactated Ringer's inj

HOW SUPPLIED
Inj: 2.5mg/mL [10mL, ampule]; 0.1mg/mL, 0.2mg/mL [200mL, premixed sol]

CONTRAINDICATIONS
Advanced aortic stenosis.

WARNINGS/PRECAUTIONS
May occasionally produce symptomatic hypotension or tachycardia. Avoid systemic hypotension when administering drug to patients who have sustained an acute cerebral infarction or hemorrhage. May induce or exacerbate angina in coronary artery disease (CAD) patients. Caution w/ heart failure (HF) or significant left ventricular dysfunction. To reduce possibility of venous thrombosis, phlebitis, local irritation, swelling, extravasation, and occurrence of vascular impairment, administer through large peripheral or central veins; change IV site q12h to minimize risk of peripheral venous irritation.

ADVERSE REACTIONS
Headache, hypotension, tachycardia, N/V.

DRUG INTERACTIONS
Titrate slowly when used in combination w/ β-blockers in patients w/ HF or significant left ventricular dysfunction due to possible negative inotropic effects. Increased nicardipine levels when oral nicardipine is given w/ cimetidine; frequently monitor response in patients receiving both drugs. Elevated cyclosporine levels reported w/ oral nicardipine; closely monitor cyclosporine levels and reduce cyclosporine dose accordingly.

PATIENT CONSIDERATIONS
Assessment: Assess for advanced aortic stenosis, HF, CAD, left ventricular dysfunction, acute cerebral infarction or hemorrhage, hepatic/renal impairment, pregnancy/nursing status, and possible drug interactions.

Monitoring: Monitor for symptomatic hypotension, tachycardia, induction or exacerbation of angina, and other adverse reactions. Monitor BP and HR during administration. Closely monitor responses w/ impaired liver function or reduced hepatic blood flow.

Counseling: Advise to seek medical attention if adverse reactions occur.

STORAGE: 20-25°C (68-77°F). Avoid excessive heat. Protect from light. Premixed Sol: Protect from freezing.

Cardizem CD – diltiazem hydrochloride
RX

Class: Calcium channel blocker (CCB) (nondihydropyridine)

OTHER BRAND NAMES
Cartia XT

ADULT DOSAGE
Hypertension

Initial (Monotherapy): 180-240mg qd
Titrate: Max antihypertensive effect usually observed by 14 days of chronic therapy; schedule dose adjustments accordingly
Usual Range: 240-360mg qd
Max: 480mg qd

PEDIATRIC DOSAGE
Pediatric use may not have been established

Angina

Chronic Stable Angina and Angina Due to Coronary Artery Spasm:
Initial: 120mg or 180mg qd
Titrate: Adjust to each patient's needs; may be carried out over a 7- to 14-day period when necessary
Max: 480mg qd

DOSING CONSIDERATIONS

Concomitant Medications

SL Nitroglycerin: May take as required to abort acute anginal attacks during therapy
Prophylactic Nitrate Therapy: May be coadministered w/ short- and long-acting nitrates
Other Antihypertensives: Diltiazem or the concomitant antihypertensives may need to be adjusted when adding 1 to the other

Elderly

Start at lower end of dosing range

ADMINISTRATION

Oral route

HOW SUPPLIED

Cap, Extended Release: (Cardizem CD, Cartia XT) 120mg, 180mg, 240mg, 300mg, (Cardizem CD) 360mg

CONTRAINDICATIONS

Sick sinus syndrome and 2nd- or 3rd-degree atrioventricular block (AV) block (except w/ functioning ventricular pacemaker), hypotension (<90mmHg systolic), demonstrated hypersensitivity to the drug, acute MI and pulmonary congestion documented by x-ray on admission.

WARNINGS/PRECAUTIONS

May cause abnormally slow HR(s) (particularly in patients w/ sick sinus syndrome) or 2nd- or 3rd-degree AV block. Periods of asystole (2-5 sec) reported in a patient w/ Prinzmetal's angina. Worsening of CHF reported in patients w/ preexisting impairment of ventricular function. Symptomatic hypotension may occur. Mild transaminase elevation w/ or w/o concomitant alkaline phosphatase and bilirubin elevation reported. Significant enzyme elevations and other phenomena consistent w/ acute hepatic injury reported in rare instances. Caution w/ renal/hepatic impairment. Dermatologic reactions (eg, erythema multiforme, exfoliative dermatitis) may occur; d/c if a dermatologic reaction persists.

ADVERSE REACTIONS

Dizziness, bradycardia, 1st-degree AV block, headache, edema.

DRUG INTERACTIONS

See Dosing Considerations. May increase levels of propranolol, carbamazepine, buspirone, and lovastatin. Increased levels w/ cimetidine. Monitor digoxin and cyclosporine levels. Depression of cardiac contractility, conductivity, automaticity, and vascular dilation potentiated w/ anesthetics. Additive cardiac conduction effects w/ digitalis or β-blockers. Potential additive effects w/ agents known to affect cardiac contractility and/or conduction; caution and careful titration warranted. May have significant impact on efficacy and side effect profile w/ CYP3A4 substrates, inducers, and inhibitors. Avoid w/ CYP3A4 inducers (eg, rifampin). Patients taking other drugs that are CYP3A4 substrates, especially patients with renal and/or hepatic impairment, may require dosage adjustment when starting or stopping concomitantly administered diltiazem. Sinus bradycardia resulting in hospitalization and pacemaker insertion reported w/ clonidine; monitor HR. Increased exposure of simvastatin; limit daily doses of simvastatin to 10mg and diltiazem to 240mg. Risk of myopathy and rhabdomyolysis w/ statins metabolized by CYP3A4 may be increased; when possible, use a non-CYP3A4 metabolized statin or consider dose adjustments for both diltiazem and the statin. May increase elimination of half-lives and levels of midazolam, triazolam, and quinidine.

PATIENT CONSIDERATIONS

Assessment: Assess for previous hypersensitivity to the drug, sick sinus syndrome, 2nd- or 3rd-degree AV block, presence of a functioning ventricular pacemaker, hypotension, acute MI and pulmonary congestion, ventricular dysfunction, hepatic/renal impairment, pregnancy/nursing status, and possible drug interactions.

Monitoring: Monitor for bradycardia, AV block, symptomatic hypotension, dermatological reactions, and other adverse reactions. Perform regular monitoring of liver and renal function.

Counseling: Counsel to report any adverse reactions to physician and to notify physician if pregnant or nursing.

STORAGE: Avoid excessive humidity. (Cardizem CD) 25°C (77°F); excursions permitted to 15-30°C (59-86°F). (Cartia XT) 20-25°C (68-77°F).

CARDIZEM LA – diltiazem hydrochloride

RX

Class: Calcium channel blocker (CCB) (nondihydropyridine)

C

ADULT DOSAGE

Hypertension

Initial: 180-240mg qd; some patients may respond to lower doses
Titrate: Adjust according to BP
Max: 540mg/day

Angina

Improve exercise tolerance in patients w/ chronic stable angina
Initial: 180mg qd
Titrate: Increase dose at intervals of 7-14-days if adequate response is not obtained
Max: 360mg

Conversions

Switching from Diltiazem Alone or in Combination w/ Other Medications: May switch to Cardizem LA qd at the nearest equivalent total daily dose. Higher doses may be needed in some patients based on clinical response

PEDIATRIC DOSAGE

Pediatric use may not have been established

DOSING CONSIDERATIONS

Elderly

Start at lower end of dosing range

ADMINISTRATION

Oral route

Take at approx the same time each day
Swallow tab whole; do not chew or crush

HOW SUPPLIED

Tab, Extended-Release: 120mg, 180mg, 240mg, 300mg, 360mg, 420mg

CONTRAINDICATIONS

Sick sinus syndrome and 2nd- or 3rd-degree atrioventricular (AV) block (except w/ functioning ventricular pacemaker), hypotension (<90mmHg systolic), demonstrated hypersensitivity to the drug, acute MI and pulmonary congestion.

WARNINGS/PRECAUTIONS

May cause abnormally slow HR(s) or 2nd- or 3rd-degree AV block. Patients w/ sick sinus syndrome are at increased risk of bradycardia. Periods of asystole (2-5 sec) reported in a patient w/ Prinzmetal's angina. Worsening of heart failure (HF) reported in patients w/ ventricular impairment. Significant elevations in liver enzymes (eg, alkaline phosphatase, lactate dehydrogenase, AST, ALT) and signs of acute hepatic injury reported; mild elevations of transaminases w/ and w/o concomitant elevation in alkaline phosphatase and bilirubin also observed. Stevens-Johnson syndrome (SJS), toxic epidermal necrolysis (TEN), erythema multiforme, and/or exfoliative dermatitis reported.

ADVERSE REACTIONS

Edema lower limb, dizziness, fatigue, bradycardia, 1st degree AV block.

DRUG INTERACTIONS

Use w/ other agents known to affect cardiac conduction or contractility may increase risk of bradycardia, AV block, and HF. β-blockers or digitalis may result in additive effects on cardiac conduction. Increased exposure of simvastatin; limit daily dose of simvastatin to 10mg and diltiazem to 240mg if coadministration is required. Avoid w/ rifampin.

PATIENT CONSIDERATIONS

Assessment: Assess for previous hypersensitivity to the drug, sick sinus syndrome, 2nd- or 3rd-degree AV block, presence of a functioning ventricular pacemaker, hypotension, acute MI and pulmonary congestion, ventricular impairment, pregnancy/nursing status, and possible drug interactions. Obtain baseline hepatic function.

Monitoring: Monitor for elevation of liver enzymes, signs of acute hepatic injury, SJS, TEN, erythema multiforme, exfoliative dermatitis, and other adverse reactions. Monitor effects on HR and cardiac conduction. Monitor for worsening of HF in patients w/ ventricular impairment.

Counseling: Advise to consult prescribing physician before taking/stopping any other medications (eg, OTC products, nutritional supplements [eg, St. John's wort]). Advise to contact physician immediately if possible adverse reactions (eg, bradycardia, arrhythmias, symptoms indicative of hypotension or HF, hepatic/skin reactions) develop. Advise to consult physician if pregnant/ planning to become pregnant.

STORAGE: 25°C (77°F); excursions permitted to 15-30°C (59-86°F). Avoid excessive humidity and temperatures >30°C (86°F).

C

CARDURA – doxazosin mesylate

RX

Class: $Alpha_1$ blocker (quinazoline)

ADULT DOSAGE

Hypertension

Initial: 1mg qd (am or pm)
Titrate: May increase to 2mg and thereafter if necessary to 4mg, 8mg, and 16mg qd depending on standing BP response

Benign Prostatic Hyperplasia

Initial: 1mg qd (am or pm)
Titrate: May increase to 2mg and thereafter to 4mg, and 8mg qd in 1- to 2-week intervals, depending on urodynamics and BPH symptomatology
Max: 8mg qd

PEDIATRIC DOSAGE

Pediatric use may not have been established

DOSING CONSIDERATIONS

Elderly

Start at lower end of dosing range

ADMINISTRATION

Oral route

HOW SUPPLIED

Tab: 1mg*, 2mg*, 4mg*, 8mg* *scored

CONTRAINDICATIONS

Known sensitivity to quinazolines (eg, prazosin, terazosin), doxazosin, or any inert ingredients.

WARNINGS/PRECAUTIONS

May cause syncope and orthostatic hypotension (eg, dizziness, lightheadedness, vertigo), especially with 1st dose, dose increase, or if therapy is interrupted for more than a few days; restart using initial dosing regimen if therapy was discontinued for several days. Rule out carcinoma of the prostate prior to therapy. Priapism (rare) and leukopenia/neutropenia reported. Intraoperative floppy iris syndrome (IFIS) observed during cataract surgery. Caution with hepatic impairment and in the elderly.

ADVERSE REACTIONS

Dizziness, headache, fatigue/malaise, somnolence, edema, nausea, rhinitis.

DRUG INTERACTIONS

Caution with additional antihypertensive agents and drugs known to influence hepatic metabolism. Additive BP-lowering effects and symptomatic hypotension with PDE-5 inhibitors.

PATIENT CONSIDERATIONS

Assessment: Assess for previous sensitivity to drug/quinazolines, hepatic impairment, prostate cancer, pregnancy/nursing status, and possible drug interactions.

Monitoring: Monitor for signs/symptoms of orthostatic hypotension, syncope, priapism, IFIS during cataract surgery, and other adverse reactions. Measure BP periodically, particularly 2-6 hrs after the 1st dose and with each increase in dose.

Counseling: Inform of the possibility of syncopal and orthostatic symptoms, especially at the initiation of therapy; urge to avoid driving or hazardous tasks for 24 hrs after the 1st dose, dose increase, and interruption of therapy when treatment is resumed. Caution to avoid situations where injury could result should syncope occur. Advise to sit or lie down when symptoms of low BP occur. Instruct to report to physician if dizziness, lightheadedness, or palpitations are bothersome. Advise of possibility of priapism and to seek immediate medical attention if this occurs. Counsel to inform surgeon of drug use prior to cataract surgery.

STORAGE: 25°C (77°F); excursions permitted to 15-30°C (59-86°F).

CARDURA XL – doxazosin mesylate

RX

Class: $Alpha_1$ blocker (quinazoline)

ADULT DOSAGE

Benign Prostatic Hyperplasia

Initial: 4mg qd w/ breakfast
Titrate: May increase to 8mg after 3-4 weeks based on symptomatic response and tolerability
Max: 8mg

If discontinued for several days, restart using 4mg qd dose

Conversions

Switching from Cardura Immediate-Release to Cardura XL:
Initial: 4mg qd; final pm dose of Cardura should not be taken prior to starting therapy w/ Cardura XL

PEDIATRIC DOSAGE

Pediatric use may not have been established

DOSING CONSIDERATIONS

Concomitant Medications

PDE-5 Inhibitors: Initiate PDE-5 inhibitor therapy at the lowest dose

Hepatic Impairment

Severe: Not recommended

ADMINISTRATION

Oral route

Swallow tab whole; do not chew, divide, cut, or crush

HOW SUPPLIED

Tab, Extended-Release: 4mg, 8mg

CONTRAINDICATIONS

Known hypersensitivity to doxazosin, other quinazolines (eg, prazosin, terazosin), or any inert ingredients.

WARNINGS/PRECAUTIONS

Postural hypotension w/ or w/o symptoms (eg, dizziness) and syncope may develop; caution w/ symptomatic hypotension or patients who have had a hypotensive response to other medications. Intraoperative floppy iris syndrome has been observed during cataract surgery in some patients on, or previously treated w/, α_1-blockers. Caution w/ preexisting severe GI narrowing (pathologic or iatrogenic). Prostate cancer causes many of the same symptoms associated w/ BPH; rule out prostate cancer prior to therapy. Caution w/ mild or moderate hepatic impairment. D/C if symptoms of worsening of or new onset of angina pectoris develop. Priapism reported (rarely); may lead to permanent impotence if not promptly treated.

ADVERSE REACTIONS

Dizziness, asthenia, headache, respiratory tract infection, abdominal pain, hypotension, somnolence, vertigo, dyspepsia, myalgia, UTI, postural hypotension, nausea, dyspnea.

DRUG INTERACTIONS

Caution w/ strong CYP3A4 inhibitors (eg, atazanavir, clarithromycin, itraconazole). Additive BP-lowering effects and symptomatic hypotension w/ PDE-5 inhibitors.

PATIENT CONSIDERATIONS

Assessment: Assess for hepatic impairment, symptomatic hypotension, history of hypotensive response to other medications, severe GI narrowing (chronic constipation), coronary insufficiency, and possible drug interactions. Rule out prostate cancer.

Monitoring: Monitor for signs/symptoms of postural hypotension, new onset or worsening of angina pectoris, and priapism.

Counseling: Instruct to take exactly ud. Advise that symptoms related to postural hypotension (eg, dizziness, syncope) may occur; caution about driving, operating machinery, or performing hazardous tasks, until drug's effect has been determined. Inform about the possibility of priapism. Explain that there is no need for concern if something that looks like a tab is occasionally noticed in the stool. Instruct to inform ophthalmologist of drug use prior to cataract surgery.

STORAGE: 25°C (77°F); excursions permitted to 15-30°C (59-86°F).

CASODEX – bicalutamide

RX

Class: Antiandrogen

ADULT DOSAGE

D_2 Metastatic Prostate Carcinoma

Combination w/ Luteinizing Hormone-Releasing Hormone (LHRH) Analogue:
50mg qd (am or pm) at the same time as LHRH analogue

Missed Dose

If a dose is missed, take the next dose at the scheduled time; do not take the missed dose and do not double the next dose

PEDIATRIC DOSAGE

Pediatric use may not have been established

ADMINISTRATION
Oral route

Take w/ or w/o food
Take at the same time each day

HOW SUPPLIED
Tab: 50mg

CONTRAINDICATIONS
Hypersensitivity reaction to the drug or any of the tab's components, women, pregnancy.

WARNINGS/PRECAUTIONS
Death or hospitalization due to severe liver injury (hepatic failure) reported. Hepatitis or marked increases in liver enzymes leading to discontinuation reported. Measure serum ALT immediately if signs/symptoms of liver dysfunction occur; d/c immediately w/ close follow-up of liver function if jaundice occurs or ALT rises >2X ULN. Reduction in glucose tolerance reported. Regularly assess serum prostate-specific antigen (PSA) to monitor response; evaluate for clinical progression if PSA levels rise during therapy. For patients w/ objective disease progression w/ an elevated PSA, consider a treatment period free of antiandrogen while continuing the LHRH analogue. Caution w/ moderate-severe hepatic impairment.

ADVERSE REACTIONS
Pain, hot flashes, asthenia, infection, back pain, constipation, nausea, diarrhea, anemia, peripheral edema, dizziness, dyspnea, rash, nocturia, hematuria.

DRUG INTERACTIONS
Can displace coumarin anticoagulants from binding sites; closely monitor PT and consider anticoagulant dose adjustment. Caution w/ CYP3A4 substrates. May increase levels of midazolam.

PATIENT CONSIDERATIONS

Assessment: Assess for drug hypersensitivity, diabetes, hepatic impairment, and possible drug interactions. Measure serum transaminase levels.

Monitoring: Measure serum transaminase levels at regular intervals for the first 4 months of treatment, then periodically thereafter. Measure serum ALT for signs/symptoms of liver dysfunction. Monitor LFTs in hepatically impaired patients on long-term therapy. Regularly monitor serum PSA levels. Monitor blood glucose levels.

Counseling: Advise not to interrupt or d/c medication w/o consulting physician. Inform that somnolence may occur; advise to use caution when driving or operating machinery. Advise to monitor blood glucose levels while on therapy. Inform that photosensitivity has been reported during treatment; advise to avoid direct exposure to excessive sunlight or UV-light exposure and to consider using sunscreen.

STORAGE: 20-25°C (68-77°F).

CATAFLAM – diclofenac potassium

RX

Class: NSAID

NSAIDs may cause an increased risk of serious cardiovascular (CV) thrombotic events, MI, stroke, and serious GI adverse events, including bleeding, ulceration, and perforation of the stomach or intestines. Contraindicated for the treatment of perioperative pain in the setting of CABG surgery.

ADULT DOSAGE

Osteoarthritis

100-150mg/day in divided doses, 50mg bid or tid

Rheumatoid Arthritis

150-200mg/day in divided doses, 50mg tid or qid

Mild to Moderate Pain

50mg tid; may give initial dose of 100mg followed by 50mg doses in some

Primary Dysmenorrhea

50mg tid; may give initial dose of 100mg followed by 50-mg doses in some

PEDIATRIC DOSAGE

Pediatric use may not have been established

ADMINISTRATION

Oral route

HOW SUPPLIED

Tab: 50mg

CONTRAINDICATIONS

Known hypersensitivity to diclofenac. Aspirin (ASA) or other NSAID allergy that precipitates asthma, urticaria, or allergic reactions. Treatment of perioperative pain in the setting of CABG surgery.

WARNINGS/PRECAUTIONS

May lead to onset of new HTN or worsening of preexisting HTN; monitor BP closely. Fluid retention and edema reported; caution in patients with fluid retention or heart failure (HF). Caution with history of ulcer disease or GI bleeding. Caution in patients with considerable dehydration. Renal papillary necrosis and other renal injury reported after long-term use. Caution with impaired renal function, HF, liver dysfunction, and the elderly. Not recommended for use with advanced renal disease; if therapy must be initiated, monitor renal function. May cause elevations of LFTs; d/c if liver disease develops or systemic manifestations occur. Anaphylactoid reactions may occur. May cause serious skin adverse events (eg, exfoliative dermatitis, Stevens-Johnson syndrome, toxic epidermal necrolysis). Avoid in late pregnancy; may cause premature closure of ductus arteriosus. Not a substitute for corticosteroids or for the treatment of corticosteroid insufficiency. Anemia may occur; with long-term use, monitor Hgb/Hct if signs or symptoms of anemia develop. May inhibit platelet aggregation and prolong bleeding time; monitor with coagulation disorders. Caution with asthma and avoid with ASA-sensitive asthma.

ADVERSE REACTIONS

Dyspepsia, constipation, diarrhea, GI ulceration/perforation, N/V, flatulence, abnormal renal function, anemia, dizziness, edema, elevated liver enzymes, headache, increased bleeding time, rash, tinnitus.

DRUG INTERACTIONS

Avoid use with ASA. May enhance methotrexate toxicity; caution when coadministering. May increase nephrotoxicity of cyclosporine; caution when coadministering. May diminish antihypertensive effect of ACE inhibitors. May reduce natriuretic effect of furosemide and thiazides; monitor for renal failure. May increase lithium levels; monitor for toxicity. Synergistic effects on GI bleeding with warfarin. Caution with hepatotoxic drugs (eg, antibiotics, antiepileptics). Increased risk of GI bleeding with concomitant oral corticosteroids, anticoagulants, or alcohol. ACE inhibitors and diuretics may increase the risk of overt renal decompensation.

PATIENT CONSIDERATIONS

Assessment: Assess for history of a hypersensitivity reaction to ASA or other NSAIDs, asthma, cardiovascular disease (CVD) (eg, preexisting HTN, congestive heart failure) or risk factors for CVD, risk factors for a GI event (eg, prior history of ulcer disease or GI disease, smoking), fluid retention, renal/hepatic dysfunction, coagulation disorders, pregnancy/nursing status, and for possible drug interactions. Assess baseline LFTs, renal function, and CBC.

Monitoring: Monitor for signs/symptoms of CV thrombotic events, new onset or worsening of preexisting HTN, GI events (eg, inflammation, bleeding, ulceration, perforation), fluid retention and edema, renal effects (eg, renal papillary necrosis), hepatic effects (eg, jaundice, liver necrosis, liver failure), anaphylactoid reactions, skin reactions (eg, exfoliative dermatitis, Stevens-Johnson syndrome, toxic epidermal necrolysis), hematological effects (eg, anemia, prolongation of bleeding time), and for bronchospasm. Monitor BP. Perform periodic monitoring of CBC, renal function, and LFTs.

Counseling: Instruct to seek medical attention for symptoms of hepatotoxicity (eg, nausea, fatigue, jaundice), anaphylactic reactions (eg, difficulty breathing, swelling of the face/throat), rash, CV events (eg, chest pain, SOB, weakness, slurring of speech), or if unexplained weight gain or edema occurs. Inform of risks if used during pregnancy.

STORAGE: Do not store at >30°C (86°F). Dispense in tight container.

CATAPRES – clonidine

RX

Class: Alpha-adrenergic agonist

C

OTHER BRAND NAMES

Catapres-TTS

ADULT DOSAGE

Hypertension

Tab:

Initial: 0.1mg bid (am and hs)
Maint: May increase by 0.1mg/day at weekly intervals prn until desired response is achieved
Range: 0.2-0.6mg/day in divided doses
Max: 2.4mg/day

Patch:

Initial: Apply 1 patch every 7 days; start w/ TTS-1
Titrate: If inadequate reduction in BP after 1-2 weeks, increase dosage by adding another TTS-1 or changing to a larger system

No usual additional efficacy w/ dose increase above 2 TTS-3

When substituting for PO clonidine or other antihypertensives, gradually reduce prior drug dose; effect of patch may not commence until 2-3 days after initial application

PEDIATRIC DOSAGE

Pediatric use may not have been established

DOSING CONSIDERATIONS

Renal Impairment

Patch/Tab:

May benefit from lower initial dose

Elderly

Tab:

May benefit from lower initial dose

ADMINISTRATION

Oral/Transdermal route

Patch

Apply to hairless area of intact skin of upper outer arm or chest once every 7 days
Apply each new patch on different skin site from previous location
If the system loosens during 7-day wearing, the adhesive cover should be applied directly over the system to ensure good adhesion

HOW SUPPLIED

Patch, Extended-Release (TTS): (TTS-1) 0.1mg, (TTS-2) 0.2mg, (TTS-3) 0.3mg; **Tab:** 0.1mg, 0.2mg, 0.3mg

CONTRAINDICATIONS

Known hypersensitivity to clonidine or to any other components of the medication.

WARNINGS/PRECAUTIONS

Sudden cessation of treatment may cause nervousness, agitation, headache, confusion, and tremor accompanied or followed by a rapid rise in BP and elevated catecholamine concentrations; if discontinuing therapy, reduce dose gradually over 2 to 4 days to avoid withdrawal symptoms. Rare instances of hypertensive encephalopathy, cerebrovascular accidents (CVAs), and death reported after withdrawal. Continuation of clonidine transdermal system or substitution to PO may cause generalized skin rash and elicit an allergic reaction if with localized contact sensitization or allergic reaction to clonidine transdermal system. Monitor BP during surgery; additional measures to control BP should be available. No therapeutic effect can be expected in HTN caused by pheochromocytoma. May worsen sinus node dysfunction and atrioventricular (AV) block, especially with other sympatholytic drugs; patients with conduction abnormalities and/or taking other sympatholytic drugs may develop severe bradycardia. (Tab) Continue administration to within 4 hrs of surgery and resume as soon as possible thereafter. (Patch) Loss of BP control reported (rare). Do not remove during surgery. Remove before defibrillation or cardioversion due to potential for altered electrical conductivity, and before undergoing an MRI due to the occurrence of skin burns.

ADVERSE REACTIONS

Dry mouth, drowsiness, dizziness, constipation, sedation.

C

DRUG INTERACTIONS
May potentiate CNS depressive effects of alcohol, barbiturates, or other sedating drugs. Hypotensive effect may be reduced by TCAs; may need to increase clonidine dose. Neuroleptics may induce or exacerbate orthostatic regulation disturbances (eg, orthostatic hypotension, dizziness, fatigue). Monitor HR with agents that affect sinus node function or AV nodal conduction (eg, digitalis, calcium channel blockers, β-blockers). D/C concurrent β-blockers several days before the gradual withdrawal of clonidine. Reports of sinus bradycardia and pacemaker insertion with diltiazem or verapamil. High IV doses of clonidine may increase the arrhythmogenic potential (QT prolongation, ventricular fibrillation) of high IV doses of haloperidol as observed in patients in a state of alcoholic delirium.

PATIENT CONSIDERATIONS

Assessment: Assess for pheochromocytoma, renal impairment, allergic reactions/contact sensitization, pregnancy/nursing status, and for possible drug interactions.

Monitoring: Monitor BP and renal function periodically. Monitor for withdrawal signs/symptoms (eg, hypertensive encephalopathy, CVA), presence of generalized skin rash, and allergic reactions.

Counseling: Caution patients against interrupting therapy without physician's advice and engaging in hazardous activities (eg, driving, operating appliances/machinery). Inform that sedative effect may be increased by concomitant use of alcohol, barbiturates, or other sedating drugs. Caution patients who wear contact lenses that drug may cause dryness of eyes. (Patch) Instruct to consult physician promptly about possible need to remove or replace patch if skin reactions develop. Inform that if patch begins to loosen, place adhesive cover directly over the patch to ensure adhesion for 7 days total. Advise to keep used and unused patch out of reach of children; instruct to fold in half with adhesive sides together and discard.

STORAGE: (Patch) Below 30°C (86°F). (Tab) 25°C (77°F); excursions permitted to 15-30°C (59-86°F).

CEFADROXIL – cefadroxil

RX

Class: Cephalosporin (1st generation)

OTHER BRAND NAMES
Duricef (Discontinued)

ADULT DOSAGE

Urinary Tract Infections

Uncomplicated Lower UTIs (eg, Cystitis):
Usual: 1 or 2g/day given qd or bid

Other UTIs:
Usual: 2g/day given bid

Skin and Skin Structure Infections

Usual: 1g/day given qd or bid

Tonsillitis and/or Pharyngitis

Caused by Group A β-Hemolytic Streptococci:
1g/day given qd or bid for 10 days

PEDIATRIC DOSAGE

Urinary Tract Infections

Usual: 30mg/kg/day in divided doses q12h

Skin and Skin Structure Infections

Impetigo:
Usual: 30mg/kg/day given qd or in equally divided doses q12h

Other SSSIs:
Usual: 30mg/kg/day in divided doses q12h

Tonsillitis and/or Pharyngitis

Usual: 30mg/kg/day given qd or in equally divided doses q12h

Streptococcal Infections

β-Hemolytic Infections:
Administer for at least 10 days

DOSING CONSIDERATIONS

Renal Impairment

Adults:
Initial: 1g
Maint:
CrCl 25-50mL/min: 500mg q12h
CrCl 10-25mL/min: 500mg q24h
CrCl 0-10mL/min: 500mg q36h

ADMINISTRATION
Oral route
Take w/o regard to meals

Sus

Suspend 50mL bottle size in a total of 34mL water, 75mL bottle size in a total of 51mL water, 100mL bottle size in a total of 67mL water; add water in two portions and shake well after each addition
Shake well before using

Refer to PI for daily dosage of oral sus

HOW SUPPLIED

Cap: 500mg; **Sus:** 250mg/5mL [50mL, 100mL], 500mg/5mL [50mL, 75mL, 100mL]; **Tab:** 1000mg*
*scored

CONTRAINDICATIONS

Known allergy to cephalosporins.

WARNINGS/PRECAUTIONS

Caution in penicillin (PCN)-sensitive patients; cross-sensitivity among β-lactam antibiotics may occur. D/C if an allergic reaction occurs. *Clostridium difficile*-associated diarrhea (CDAD) reported; may need to d/c if CDAD is suspected or confirmed. Caution w/ renal impairment (CrCl <50mL/min); monitor prior to and during therapy. May result in bacterial resistance if used in the absence of proven or suspected bacterial infection, or a prophylactic indication. May result in overgrowth of nonsusceptible organisms w/ prolonged use; take appropriate measures if superinfection develops. Caution w/ history of GI disease, particularly colitis. Lab test interactions may occur. D/C if seizures associated w/ drug therapy occur. Caution in elderly.

ADVERSE REACTIONS

Diarrhea, allergies, hepatic dysfunction, genital moniliasis, vaginitis, moderate transient neutropenia, fever, toxic epidermal necrolysis, abdominal pain, superinfection, renal dysfunction, toxic nephropathy, aplastic anemia, hemolytic anemia, hemorrhage.

PATIENT CONSIDERATIONS

Assessment: Assess for allergy to other cephalosporins, PCN, or to other drugs, renal impairment, history of GI disease, and pregnancy/nursing status. Initiate culture and susceptibility tests prior to therapy.

Monitoring: Monitor for signs/symptoms of an allergic reaction, CDAD, seizure, and superinfection. Carefully observe patients w/ known or suspected renal impairment.

Counseling: Inform that therapy only treats bacterial, not viral, infections. Instruct to take exactly ud; inform that skipping doses or not completing full course of therapy may decrease effectiveness and increase risk of bacterial resistance. Inform that diarrhea is a common problem that usually ends upon discontinuation. Instruct to notify physician as soon as possible if watery and bloody stools (w/ or w/o stomach cramps/fever) occur, even as late as ≥2 months after last dose.

STORAGE: (Cap/Tab) 20-25°C (68-77°F). (Sus) Before Reconstitution: 25°C (77°F); excursions permitted to 15-30°C (59-86°F). After Reconstitution: Store in refrigerator; discard unused portion after 14 days.

CEFDINIR – cefdinir

RX

Class: Cephalosporin (3rd generation)

OTHER BRAND NAMES

Omnicef (Discontinued)

ADULT DOSAGE

Community-Acquired Pneumonia

Cap:
300mg q12h for 10 days

Acute Bacterial Exacerbation of Chronic Bronchitis

Cap:
300mg q12h for 5-10 days or 600mg q24h for 10 days

Acute Maxillary Sinusitis

Cap:
300mg q12h or 600mg q24h for 10 days

Pharyngitis/Tonsillitis

Cap:
300mg q12h for 5-10 days or 600mg q24h for 10 days

PEDIATRIC DOSAGE

Skin and Skin Structure Infections

Uncomplicated:

Sus:
6 Months-12 Years:
7mg/kg q12h for 10 days
≥43kg: 600mg/day
Max: 600mg/day

Cap:
≥13 Years:
300mg q12h for 10 days

Acute Otitis Media

Sus:
6 Months-12 Years:
7mg/kg q12h for 5-10 days or 14mg/kg q24h for 10 days

C

Skin and Skin Structure Infections

Uncomplicated:
Cap:
300mg q12h for 10 days

≥43kg: 600mg/day
Max: 600mg/day

Community-Acquired Pneumonia

Cap:
≥13 Years:
300mg q12h for 10 days

Acute Bacterial Exacerbation of Chronic Bronchitis

Cap:
≥13 Years:
300mg q12h for 5-10 days or 600mg q24h for 10 days

Acute Maxillary Sinusitis

Sus:
6 Months-12 Years:
7mg/kg q12h or 14mg/kg q24h for 10 days
≥43kg: 600mg/day
Max: 600mg/day
Cap:
≥13 Years:
300mg q12h or 600mg q24h for 10 days

Pharyngitis/Tonsillitis

Sus:
6 Months-12 Years:
7mg/kg q12h for 5-10 days or 14mg/kg q24h for 10 days
≥43kg: 600mg/day
Max: 600mg/day
Cap:
≥13 Years:
300mg q12h for 5-10 days or 600mg q24h for 10 days

DOSING CONSIDERATIONS

Renal Impairment

Adults:
CrCl <30mL/min: 300mg qd
Hemodialysis:
Initial: 300mg or 7mg/kg qod; give 300mg or 7mg/kg at the end of each hemodialysis session
Subsequent Doses: 300mg or 7mg/kg qod

Pediatrics:
CrCl <30mL/min/1.73m²: 7mg/kg (up to 300mg) qd
Hemodialysis:
Initial: 300mg or 7mg/kg qod; give 300mg or 7mg/kg at the end of each hemodialysis session
Subsequent Doses: 300mg or 7mg/kg qod

ADMINISTRATION

Oral route

May take w/o regard to food.

Oral Sus

Shake well before use.
Reconstitute w/ 37mL of water (for final volume of 60mL) or 62mL of water (for final volume of 100mL); add water in 2 portions, shake well after each aliquot.
After mixing, store at room temperature (20-25°C [68-77°F]).
May use for 10 days and discard any unused portion.

HOW SUPPLIED

Cap: 300mg; **Oral Sus:** 125mg/5mL, 250mg/5mL [60mL, 100mL]

CONTRAINDICATIONS

Known allergy to cephalosporins.

WARNINGS/PRECAUTIONS

Caution in penicillin (PCN)-sensitive patients; cross-hypersensitivity among β-lactam antibiotics may occur. D/C use if an allergic reaction occurs. Serious acute hypersensitivity reactions may require the use of SQ epinephrine and other emergency measures. *Clostridium difficile*-associated diarrhea (CDAD) reported; may need to d/c if CDAD is suspected/confirmed. May result in bacterial resistance w/ prolonged use in the absence of a proven or suspected bacterial infection, or a prophylactic indication; take appropriate measures if superinfection develops. Caution in patients w/ a history of colitis. Reduce dose in patients w/ transient or persistent renal insufficiency (CrCl <30mL/min). Lab test interactions may occur.

C

ADVERSE REACTIONS

Cap: Diarrhea, vaginal moniliasis, nausea.
Oral Sus: Diarrhea, rash.

DRUG INTERACTIONS

Iron-fortified foods (except iron-fortified infant formula), iron supplements, and aluminum- or Mg^{2+}-containing antacids reduce absorption; take dose at least 2 hrs before or after these medications. Inhibited renal excretion w/ probenecid. Reddish stools reported w/ iron-containing products.

PATIENT CONSIDERATIONS

Assessment: Assess for allergy to other cephalosporins, PCN, or to other drugs, history of colitis, renal impairment, and for possible drug interactions. Assess for diabetes if planning to use sus formulation.

Monitoring: Monitor for signs/symptoms of hypersensitivity reactions, CDAD, and development of superinfection.

Counseling: Inform that therapy only treats bacterial, not viral, infections. Instruct to take ud; skipping doses or not completing full course may decrease drug effectiveness and increase risk of bacterial resistance. Instruct to take dose at least 2 hrs before or after antacid or iron supplements. Inform diabetic patients and caregivers that oral sus contains 2.86g of sucrose/tsp. Instruct to contact physician as soon as possible if watery and bloody stools (w/ or w/o stomach cramps and fever) develop even as late as ≥2 months after having taken the last dose.

STORAGE: **Cap/Unsuspended Powder:** 20-25°C (68-77°F). **Reconstituted Oral Sus:** Can be stored at controlled room temperature for 10 days.

CEFPROZIL – cefprozil

RX

Class: Cephalosporin (2nd generation)

ADULT DOSAGE

Pharyngitis/Tonsillitis

500mg q24h for 10 days; administer for >10 days for *Streptococcus pyogenes* infections

Acute Bacterial Sinusitis

250mg or 500mg q12h for 10 days; use the higher dose for moderate to severe infections

Lower Respiratory Tract Infections

Secondary Bacterial Infection of Acute Bronchitis/Acute Bacterial Exacerbation of Chronic Bronchitis:
500mg q12h for 10 days

Skin and Skin Structure Infections

Uncomplicated:
250mg or 500mg q12h or 500mg q24h for 10 days

PEDIATRIC DOSAGE

Acute Otitis Media

6 Months-12 Years:
15mg/kg q12h for 10 days

Do not exceed recommended adult doses

Acute Bacterial Sinusitis

6 Months-12 Years:
7.5mg/kg or 15mg/kg q12h for 10 days
≥13 Years:
250mg or 500mg q12h for 10 days; use the higher dose for moderate to severe infections

Do not exceed recommended adult doses

Pharyngitis/Tonsillitis

2-12 Years:
7.5mg/kg q12h for 10 days
≥13 Years:
500mg q24h for 10 days

Administer for >10 days for *Streptococcus pyogenes* infections
Do not exceed recommended adult doses

Skin and Skin Structure Infections

Uncomplicated:
2-12 Years:
20mg/kg q24h for 10 days
≥13 Years:
250mg or 500mg q12h or 500mg q24h for 10 days

Lower Respiratory Tract Infections

Acute Bacterial Exacerbation of Chronic Bronchitis/Secondary Bacterial Infection of Acute Bronchitis:
≥13 Years:
500mg q12h for 10 days

DOSING CONSIDERATIONS

Renal Impairment

CrCl 0-29mL/min: Give 50% of standard dose

ADMINISTRATION

C

Oral route

Shake sus well before use

Administer after completion of hemodialysis

Reconstitution

Final Concentration of 125mg/5mL:

Add 36mL, 54mL, or 72mL of water to the 50mL, 75mL, or 100mL bottle size respectively

Final Concentration of 250mg/5mL:

Add 36mL, 54mL, or 72mL of water to the 50mL, 75mL, or 100mL bottle size respectively

HOW SUPPLIED

Sus: 125mg/5mL, 250mg/5mL [50mL, 75mL, 100mL]; **Tab:** 250mg, 500mg

CONTRAINDICATIONS

Known allergy to cephalosporins.

WARNINGS/PRECAUTIONS

Caution with previous hypersensitivity to cephalosporins, penicillins (PCNs), or other drugs; cross-sensitivity may occur with history of PCN allergy. D/C if allergic reaction occurs. *Clostridium difficile*-associated diarrhea (CDAD) reported. May result in bacterial resistance with prolonged use or use in the absence of a proven/suspected bacterial infection or a prophylactic indication; take appropriate measures if superinfection develops. Caution with GI disease, particularly colitis. Caution with renal impairment and elderly. Lab test interactions may occur.

ADVERSE REACTIONS

Diarrhea, N/V, ALT/AST elevation, eosinophilia, genital pruritus, vaginitis, superinfection, diaper rash, dizziness, abdominal pain.

DRUG INTERACTIONS

Nephrotoxicity with aminoglycosides reported. Probenecid may increase plasma levels. Caution with potent diuretics.

PATIENT CONSIDERATIONS

Assessment: Assess for previous hypersensitivity reactions to PCNs/cephalosporins or other drugs, renal/hepatic function, GI disease, pregnancy/nursing status, and possible drug interactions. Perform appropriate culture and susceptibility studies to determine susceptible causative organisms.

Monitoring: Periodically monitor renal/hepatic/hematopoietic functions. Monitor for CDAD (may range from mild diarrhea to fatal colitis), development of superinfections or drug resistance, allergic reactions, and other adverse reactions.

Counseling: Inform that the oral sus contains phenylalanine. Inform that drug only treats bacterial, not viral, infections. Instruct to take ud and that skipping doses or not completing full course may decrease effectiveness and increase resistance. Inform about potential benefits/risks. Notify physician if watery/bloody stools (with/without stomach cramps/fever) occur even ≥2 months after therapy. Notify if pregnant/nursing.

STORAGE: Tab/Dry Powder: 20-25°C (68-77°F). Reconstituted Sus: Refrigerate after mixing and discard unused portion after 14 days.

CELEBREX — celecoxib

RX

Class: COX-2 inhibitor

May increase risk of serious cardiovascular (CV) thrombotic events, MI, and stroke, which can be fatal; increased risk with duration of use and with CV disease (CVD) or risk factors for CVD. Increased risk of serious GI adverse events (eg, bleeding, ulceration, perforation of stomach/intestines) that can be fatal and occur anytime during use, without warning symptoms; elderly patients are at a greater risk. Contraindicated for treatment of perioperative pain in the setting of CABG surgery.

ADULT DOSAGE

Osteoarthritis

200mg qd or 100mg bid

Rheumatoid Arthritis

100-200mg bid

Ankylosing Spondylitis

Usual: 200mg qd or 100mg bid

PEDIATRIC DOSAGE

Juvenile Rheumatoid Arthritis

≥2 Years:

10-25kg:

50mg bid

>25kg:

100mg bid

C

Titrate: May increase to 400mg/day if no effect is observed after 6 weeks; consider alternative treatment if no effect is observed after 6 weeks on 400mg/day

Acute Pain

Initial: 400mg initially, then 200mg if needed on 1st day
Maint: 200mg bid prn on subsequent days

Primary Dysmenorrhea

Initial: 400mg initially, then 200mg if needed on 1st day
Maint: 200mg bid prn on subsequent days

DOSING CONSIDERATIONS

Renal Impairment
Severe: Not recommended

Hepatic Impairment
Moderate (Child-Pugh Class B): Reduce daily dose by 50%
Severe: Not recommended

Elderly
<50kg:
Initial: Lowest recommended dose

Other Important Considerations
Poor Metabolizers of CYP2C9 Substrates:
Initial: Consider 1/2 the lowest recommended dose; consider alternative management in juvenile rheumatoid arthritis patients

ADMINISTRATION

Oral route

May be given w/o regard to timing of meals
For patients w/ difficulty swallowing caps, contents may be added to applesauce; entire cap contents should be emptied onto a level tsp of cool or room temperature applesauce and ingested immediately w/ water

HOW SUPPLIED

Cap: 50mg, 100mg, 200mg, 400mg

CONTRAINDICATIONS

Known hypersensitivity to celecoxib, aspirin (ASA), or other NSAIDs; demonstrated allergic-type reactions to sulfonamides; history of asthma, urticaria, or other allergic-type reactions w/ ASA or other NSAIDs; treatment of perioperative pain in the setting of CABG surgery; active GI bleeding.

WARNINGS/PRECAUTIONS

Use lowest effective dose for the shortest duration possible. Not recommended with severe hepatic impairment. May lead to onset of new HTN or worsening of preexisting HTN; caution with HTN, and monitor BP closely. Fluid retention and edema reported; caution with fluid retention or HF. Caution with history of ulcer disease, GI bleeding, and other risk factors for GI bleeding (eg, prolonged NSAID therapy, older age, poor general health status); monitor for GI ulceration/bleeding. May cause elevations of LFTs or severe hepatic reactions (eg, jaundice, fatal fulminant hepatitis, liver necrosis, hepatic failure); d/c if liver disease develops or systemic manifestations occur, or if abnormal LFTs persist/worsen. Renal injury reported with long-term use; increased risk with renal/hepatic impairment, HF, and in elderly. Not recommended with advanced renal disease; if therapy must be initiated, closely monitor renal function. D/C if abnormal renal tests persist/worsen. Anaphylactoid/anaphylactic reactions and angioedema reported. Caution with asthma and avoid with ASA-sensitive asthma and the ASA triad. May cause serious skin adverse events (eg, exfoliative dermatitis, Stevens-Johnson syndrome, toxic epidermal necrolysis); d/c at 1st appearance of skin rash or any other sign of hypersensitivity. Avoid in late pregnancy (starting at 30 weeks gestation); may cause premature closure of ductus arteriosus. Not a substitute for corticosteroids or for the treatment of corticosteroid insufficiency. Anemia reported; monitor Hgb/Hct if signs/symptoms of anemia or blood loss develop with long-term use. Caution in pediatric patients with systemic onset JRA due to risk of disseminated intravascular coagulation. Monitor CBC and chemistry profile periodically with long-term treatment. May mask signs of inflammation and fever. Caution with poor CYP2C9 metabolizers. Not a substitute for ASA for CV prophylaxis.

ADVERSE REACTIONS

CV thrombotic events, MI, stroke, GI adverse events, headache, HTN, diarrhea, fever, dyspepsia, URI, abdominal pain, N/V, cough, nasopharyngitis.

C

DRUG INTERACTIONS

Avoid with non-ASA NSAIDs. Caution with CYP2C9 inhibitors. Potential interaction with CYP2D6 substrates. Warfarin or similar agents may increase risk of bleeding complications; monitor anticoagulant activity. May increase lithium levels; monitor closely. ASA may increase rate of GI ulceration or other complications. May diminish the antihypertensive effect of ACE inhibitors and ARBs. Fluconazole may increase levels. May reduce the natriuretic effect of loop diuretics (eg, furosemide) and thiazides. Oral corticosteroids, anticoagulants, smoking, or alcohol may increase risk of GI bleeding. Risk of renal toxicity with diuretics, ACE inhibitors, and ARBs. Aluminum- and magnesium-containing antacids may reduce plasma concentrations.

PATIENT CONSIDERATIONS

Assessment: Assess for history of allergic-type reactions to sulfonamides, history of asthma, urticaria, other allergic-type reactions with ASA or other NSAIDs, active GI bleeding, CVD, risk factors for CVD, renal/hepatic impairment, HTN, history of ulcer disease or GI bleeding, risk factors for GI bleeding, asthma, ASA triad, other conditions where treatment is contraindicated or cautioned, pregnancy/nursing status, and possible drug interactions.

Monitoring: Monitor for signs/symptoms of CV thrombotic events, GI events, anaphylactoid/hypersensitivity reactions, and other adverse reactions. Monitor BP, renal function, LFTs, CBC, and chemistry profile periodically. Monitor for development of abnormal coagulation tests in patients with systemic onset JRA.

Counseling: Advise to seek medical attention if signs/symptoms of CV events (eg, chest pain, SOB, weakness, slurring of speech), GI ulceration/bleeding (eg, epigastric pain, dyspepsia, melena, hematemesis), hepatotoxicity (eg, nausea, fatigue, lethargy, pruritus, jaundice, right upper quadrant tenderness, and flu-like symptoms), skin/hypersensitivity reactions (eg, rash, blisters, fever, itching), unexplained weight gain or edema, or anaphylactoid reactions (eg, difficulty breathing, swelling of the face/throat) occur. Instruct to d/c the drug immediately if any type of rash or if signs/symptoms of hepatotoxicity occur. Instruct patients with preexisting asthma to seek immediate medical attention if asthma worsens after taking the medication. Inform that medication should be avoided in late pregnancy.

STORAGE: 25°C (77°F); excursions permitted to 15-30°C (59-86°F). Sprinkled contents on applesauce are stable for up to 6 hrs at 2-8°C (35-45°F).

CellCept – mycophenolate mofetil

RX

Class: Inosine monophosphate dehydrogenase (IMPDH) inhibitor

Use during pregnancy is associated w/ increased risks of 1st trimester pregnancy loss and congenital malformations; counsel females of reproductive potential regarding pregnancy prevention and planning. Immunosuppression may lead to increased susceptibility to infection and possible development of lymphoma. Should only be prescribed by physicians experienced in immunosuppressive therapy and management of organ transplant patients. Manage patients in facilities equipped and staffed w/ adequate lab and supportive medical resources.

ADULT DOSAGE

Renal Transplant

Prophylaxis of organ rejection in patients receiving allogeneic renal transplants; use concomitantly w/ cyclosporine and corticosteroids

1g PO/IV bid

Cardiac Transplant

Prophylaxis of organ rejection in patients receiving allogeneic cardiac transplants; use concomitantly w/ cyclosporine and corticosteroids

1.5g PO/IV bid

Hepatic Transplant

Prophylaxis of organ rejection in patients receiving allogeneic hepatic transplants; use concomitantly w/ cyclosporine and corticosteroids

1.5g PO bid or 1g IV bid

PEDIATRIC DOSAGE

Renal Transplant

Prophylaxis of organ rejection in patients receiving allogeneic renal transplants; use concomitantly w/ cyclosporine and corticosteroids

3 Months-18 Years:

Sus:

600mg/m^2 bid

Max Daily Dose: 2g/10mL

Cap:

BSA 1.25-1.5m^2: 750mg bid

Cap/Tab:

BSA >1.5m^2: 1g bid

DOSING CONSIDERATIONS

Renal Impairment

Renal Transplant:

Severe Chronic Renal Impairment (GFR <25mL/min) Outside the Immediate Post-Transplant Period: Avoid doses >1g bid

No dose adjustments needed in renal transplant patients experiencing delayed graft function postoperatively

Adverse Reactions

Neutropenia (ANC <1.3 x $10^3/\mu L$): Interrupt or reduce dose

ADMINISTRATION

Oral/IV route

Exercise caution in handling; refer to PI.

Oral

Give initial dose as soon as possible after transplant.
Administer on an empty stomach; may administer w/ food if necessary in stable renal transplant patients.
Do not crush tab; do not open or crush cap.
Sus may be given via NG tube (minimum size of 8 French).

IV

Administer w/in 24 hrs following transplant.
Administer by slow IV infusion over no less than 2 hrs by either peripheral or central vein.
May administer for up to 14 days; switch to oral therapy as soon as patient can tolerate oral medication.
Start administration w/in 4 hrs from reconstitution and dilution.
Do not mix or administer concurrently via same infusion catheter w/ other IV drugs or infusion admixtures.

Preparation

Sus:

1. Measure 94mL of water in a graduated cylinder.
2. Add approx 1/2 the total amount of water to bottle and shake closed bottle well for about 1 min.
3. Add remainder of water and shake closed bottle well for about 1 min.
4. Remove child-resistant cap and push bottle adapter into neck of bottle; close bottle w/ child-resistant cap tightly.

IV Reconstitution:

2 vials are needed to prepare a 1g dose; 3 vials are needed for a 1.5g dose.
Reconstitute contents of each vial by injecting 14mL of D5 inj; gently shake vials to dissolve.

IV Dilution:

For a 1g dose, further dilute contents of the 2 reconstituted vials into 140mL of D5 inj.
For a 1.5g dose, further dilute contents of the 3 reconstituted vials into 210mL of D5 inj.
Final concentration of both sol is 6mg/mL.

HOW SUPPLIED

Cap: 250mg; **Inj:** 500mg/20mL; **Sus:** 200mg/mL; **Tab:** 500mg

CONTRAINDICATIONS

Hypersensitivity to mycophenolate mofetil, mycophenolic acid, or any component of the medication. **Inj:** Allergy to Polysorbate 80.

WARNINGS/PRECAUTIONS

Do not administer IV sol by rapid or bolus inj. May increase risk of developing malignancies, particularly of the skin; limit exposure to sunlight and UV light in patients w/ increased risk for skin cancer. Polyomavirus-associated nephropathy (PVAN), JC virus-associated progressive multifocal leukoencephalopathy (PML), cytomegalovirus infections, and reactivation of hepatitis B virus (HBV) or hepatitis C virus (HCV) reported; consider dose reduction if new or reactivated viral infection develops. PVAN, especially due to BK virus infection, may lead to deteriorating renal function and renal graft loss. Consider PML in differential diagnosis in patients reporting neurological symptoms and consider consultation w/ a neurologist. Severe neutropenia reported; interrupt or reduce dose if neutropenia develops. Cases of pure red cell aplasia (PRCA) reported when used w/ other immunosuppressive agents. Acceptable birth control must be used during therapy and for 6 weeks after discontinuation. GI bleeding, ulceration, and perforation reported; caution w/ active serious digestive system disease. Avoid doses >1g bid in renal transplant patients w/ severe chronic renal impairment (GFR <25mL/min); caution w/ delayed renal graft function post-transplant. More reports of opportunistic/herpes virus infections in cardiac transplant patients in comparison w/ azathioprine. Avoid w/ rare hereditary deficiency of hypoxanthine-guanine phosphoribosyl-transferase (HGPRT) (eg, Lesch-Nyhan and Kelley-Seegmiller syndromes). Oral sus contains 0.56mg phenylalanine/mL; caution w/ phenylketonurics. Caution in elderly.

ADVERSE REACTIONS

Infection, diarrhea, leukopenia, sepsis, N/V, HTN, peripheral edema, abdominal pain, fever, headache, constipation, hyperglycemia, anemia, insomnia.

C

DRUG INTERACTIONS

Avoid w/ azathioprine, drugs that interfere w/ enterohepatic recirculation (eg, cholestyramine), and norfloxacin-metronidazole combination. Vaccinations may be less effective; avoid live, attenuated vaccines. Decreased exposure w/ rifampin; concomitant use not recommended unless benefit outweighs risk. Increased levels of both drugs w/ drugs that compete w/ renal tubular secretion (eg, acyclovir/valacyclovir, ganciclovir/valganciclovir, probenecid). Oral ciprofloxacin and amoxicillin plus clavulanic acid may decrease levels. Mean mycophenolic acid (MPA) exposure may be 30-50% greater when mycophenolate mofetil is administered w/o cyclosporine compared to when coadministered w/ cyclosporine. Expect changes in exposure when switching from cyclosporine A to an immunosuppressant that does not interfere w/ the enterohepatic cycle (eg, tacrolimus, belatacept). Telmisartan decreases levels. May decrease levels and effectiveness of hormonal contraceptives; use w/ caution and must use additional barrier contraceptive methods. Drugs that alter GI flora may reduce levels available for absorption. Decreased levels w/ proton pump inhibitors (eg, lansoprazole, pantoprazole), Mg^{2+}- and aluminum-containing antacids, and Ca^{2+} free phosphate binders (eg, sevelamer). Do not administer simultaneously w/ antacids containing aluminum and magnesium hydroxides. Do not administer Ca^{2+} free phosphate binders simultaneously; may give 2 hrs after intake. Combination immunosuppressant therapy should be used w/ caution.

PATIENT CONSIDERATIONS

Assessment: Assess for hypersensitivity to the drug or its components, hepatic/renal impairment, delayed renal graft function post-transplant, phenylketonuria, hereditary deficiency of HGPRT (eg, Lesch-Nyhan and Kelley-Seegmiller syndromes), active digestive disease, vaccination history, nursing status, and possible drug interactions. Assess pregnancy status using serum or urine test of at least 25 mIU/mL sensitivity, immediately before starting therapy.

Monitoring: Monitor for signs/symptoms of lymphomas, skin cancer, and other malignancies, infections, HCV/HBV reactivation, neutropenia, PRCA, GI bleeding/perforation/ulceration, and other adverse reactions. Monitor CBC weekly during the 1st month, twice monthly for the 2nd and 3rd months of therapy, and then monthly through the 1st yr. Monitor pregnancy status by obtaining pregnancy test 8-10 days after initiation of therapy and repeatedly during follow-up visits.

Counseling: Inform that use during pregnancy is associated w/ an increased risk of 1st trimester pregnancy loss and congenital malformations; discuss pregnancy testing, prevention (including acceptable contraception methods), and planning. Discuss appropriate alternative immunosuppressants w/ less potential for embryofetal toxicity if patient is considering pregnancy. Advise of complete dosage instructions and inform about increased risk of lymphoproliferative disease and certain other malignancies. Inform of the need for repeated appropriate lab tests during therapy. Instruct patients to report immediately any evidence of infection, unexpected bruising, bleeding, or any other manifestation of bone marrow depression. Advise not to breastfeed during therapy. Encourage to enroll in the pregnancy registry if patient becomes pregnant while on medication.

STORAGE: 25°C (77°F); excursions permitted to 15-30°C (59-86°F). Constituted Sus: Stable up to 60 days; may also be refrigerated at 2-8°C (36-46°F). Do not freeze.

CEPHALEXIN – cephalexin

RX

Class: Cephalosporin (1st generation)

OTHER BRAND NAMES

Keflex

ADULT DOSAGE

General Dosing

Usual: 250mg q6h; may administer a dose of 500mg q12h. Treat for 7-14 days

More Severe Infections:
May need larger doses, up to 4g/day in 2-4 equally divided doses

Other Indications

Treatment of the Following Infections Caused by Susceptible Microorganisms:
Respiratory tract infections
Otitis media
Skin and skin structure infections
Bone infections
Genitourinary tract infections, including acute prostatitis

PEDIATRIC DOSAGE

General Dosing

>1 Year:
Recommended Dose: 25-50mg/kg/day in equally divided doses for 7-14 days

Severe Infections:
May administer 50-100mg/kg/day in equally divided doses

β-Hemolytic Streptococcal Infections:
Administer for at least 10 days

≥15 Years:
Usual: 250mg q6h; may administer a dose of 500mg q12h. Treat for 7-14 days

More Severe Infections:
May need larger doses, up to 4g/day in 2-4 equally divided doses

	Otitis Media
	>1 Year: 75-100mg/kg/day given in equally divided doses

DOSING CONSIDERATIONS

Renal Impairment

Adults and Pediatric Patients ≥15 Years:
CrCl 30-59mL/min: No dose adjustment; max dose should not exceed 1g/day
CrCl 15-29mL/min: 250mg q8h or q12h
CrCl 5-14mL/min Not Yet on Dialysis: 250mg q24h
CrCl 1-4mL/min Not Yet on Dialysis: 250mg q48h or q60h

ADMINISTRATION

Oral route

Take w/o regard to meals.

Oral Sus

Shake well before using.
After mixing, store in refrigerator; may be kept for 14 days w/o significant loss of potency.

Directions for Mixing:
125mg/5mL: Add to the bottle a total of 71mL (for 100mL when mixed) or 140mL (for 200mL when mixed) of water in 2 portions. Shake well after each addition.
250mg/5mL: Add to the bottle a total of 71mL (for 100mL when mixed) or 140mL (for 200mL when mixed) of water in 2 portions. Shake well after each addition.

HOW SUPPLIED

Oral Sus: 125mg/5mL [100mL, 200mL], 250mg/5mL [100mL, 200mL]; **Tab:** 250mg*, 500mg*; **Cap** (Keflex): 250mg, 500mg, 750mg *scored

CONTRAINDICATIONS

Known hypersensitivity to cephalexin or other cephalosporins.

WARNINGS/PRECAUTIONS

Allergic reactions reported. Prior to therapy, inquire about hypersensitivity reactions to cephalexin, cephalosporins, penicillins (PCNs), or other drugs; cross-hypersensitivity among β-lactam antibacterials may occur in patients w/ history of PCN allergy. D/C therapy and institute appropriate treatment if an allergic reaction occurs. *Clostridium difficile*-associated diarrhea (CDAD) reported; may need to d/c if CDAD is suspected or confirmed. Positive direct Coombs' tests and acute intravascular hemolysis induced by cephalexin therapy reported; if anemia develops during or after therapy, perform a diagnostic work-up for drug-induced hemolytic anemia, d/c cephalexin, and institute appropriate therapy. May trigger seizures (particularly w/ renal impairment when dose is not reduced); d/c if seizures occur. May be associated w/ prolonged PT; patients w/ renal/hepatic impairment, poor nutritional state, or who are receiving a protracted course of antibacterial therapy and anticoagulant therapy may be at risk. May result in bacterial resistance w/ prolonged use or if used in the absence of a proven/suspected bacterial infection or a prophylactic indication; take appropriate measures if superinfection develops. Lab test interactions may occur. Caution in elderly.

ADVERSE REACTIONS

Diarrhea, N/V, dyspepsia, gastritis, abdominal pain.

DRUG INTERACTIONS

Increased metformin levels and decreased renal clearance of metformin; monitor patient carefully and adjust dose of metformin. Probenecid inhibits renal excretion; coadministration w/ probenecid is not recommended.

PATIENT CONSIDERATIONS

Assessment: Assess for previous hypersensitivity to cephalexin, cephalosporins, PCNs, or other drugs. Assess renal/hepatic function, pregnancy/nursing status, and possible drug interactions. Obtain baseline culture and susceptibility tests.

Monitoring: Monitor for signs/symptoms of hypersensitivity reactions, CDAD, superinfection, and other adverse reactions. Monitor PT and renal function when indicated. Perform culture and susceptibility tests.

Counseling: Advise that allergic reactions, including serious allergic reactions, may occur and that serious reactions require immediate treatment. Inform that drug only treats bacterial, not viral, infections. Instruct to take exactly ud; inform that skipping doses or not completing full course of therapy may decrease effectiveness and increase likelihood of bacterial resistance. Advise that diarrhea is a common problem caused by therapy and usually resolves when the drug is discontinued; instruct to contact physician if severe watery or bloody diarrhea (w/ or w/o stomach cramps and fever) develops even as late as ≥2 months after taking last dose.

STORAGE: 20-25°C (68-77°F). **Keflex:** 25°C (77°F); excursions permitted to 15-30°C (59-86°F).

Cerdelga – eliglustat

RX

Class: Glucosylceramide synthase inhibitor

C

ADULT DOSAGE

Type 1 Gaucher Disease

Long-term treatment of patients who are CYP2D6 extensive metabolizers (EMs), intermediate metabolizers (IMs), or poor metabolizers (PMs) as detected by an FDA-cleared test

Usual:

CYP2D6 EMs/IMs: 84mg bid
CYP2D6 PMs: 84mg qd

PEDIATRIC DOSAGE

Pediatric use may not have been established

DOSING CONSIDERATIONS

Concomitant Medications

Strong/Moderate CYP2D6 Inhibitors:
CYP2D6 EMs/IMs: Reduce dose to 84mg qd

Strong/Moderate CYP3A Inhibitors:
Grapefruit/Grapefruit Juice: Avoid
CYP2D6 EMs: Reduce dose to 84mg qd

Renal Impairment

Moderate to Severe Impairment/ESRD: Use not recommended

Hepatic Impairment

All Stages/Cirrhosis: Use not recommended

Other Important Considerations

Administer therapy 24 hrs after the last dose of the previous enzyme replacement therapy (eg, imiglucerase, velaglucerase alfa, taliglucerase alfa)

ADMINISTRATION

Oral route

Swallow caps whole, preferably w/ water; do not crush, dissolve, or open
May be taken w/ or w/o food

HOW SUPPLIED

Cap: 84mg

CONTRAINDICATIONS

EMs or IMs taking a strong or moderate CYP2D6 inhibitor concomitantly with a strong or moderate CYP3A inhibitor. IMs or PMs taking a strong CYP3A inhibitor.

WARNINGS/PRECAUTIONS

May cause increases in ECG intervals (PR, QTc, and QRS) at substantially elevated eliglustat plasma concentrations; not recommended in patients with preexisting cardiac disease (congestive heart failure, recent acute myocardial infarction, bradycardia, heart block, ventricular arrhythmia) or long QT syndrome. Not recommended with moderate to severe renal impairment, end-stage renal disease, and in all stages of hepatic impairment or cirrhosis. Patients who are CYP2D6 ultra-rapid metabolizers may not achieve adequate concentrations of eliglustat to achieve a therapeutic effect.

ADVERSE REACTIONS

Fatigue, headache, nausea, diarrhea, back pain, pain in extremities, upper abdominal pain, flatulence, oropharyngeal pain, dizziness, asthenia, cough, dyspepsia, gastroesophageal reflux disease, constipation.

DRUG INTERACTIONS

See Contraindications and Dosage. Avoid consumption of grapefruit or grapefruit juice. For patients currently treated with imiglucerase, velaglucerase alfa, or taliglucerase alfa, eliglustat may be administered 24 hrs after the last dose of the previous enzyme replacement therapy (ERT). Not recommended with class IA (eg, quinidine, procainamide) and class III (eg, amiodarone, sotalol) antiarrhythmic medications. CYP2D6 and CYP3A inhibitors may significantly increase exposure and result in prolongation of the PR, QTc, and/or QRS cardiac interval which could result in cardiac arrhythmias; not recommended with moderate CYP3A inhibitors (eg, fluconazole) in IMs and PMs, or weak CYP3A inhibitors (eg, ranitidine) in PMs. Strong CYP3A inducers (eg, rifampin, carbamazepine, St. John's wort) significantly decrease exposure; coadministration is not recommended in EMs, IMs, and PMs. May increase concentrations of P-glycoprotein (eg, digoxin, phenytoin, colchicine, dabigatran etexilate) or CYP2D6 (eg, metoprolol, nortriptyline, perphenazine) substrates; monitor therapeutic drug concentrations, as indicated, or consider reducing the dosage of the concomitant drug and titrate to clinical effect. Measure serum digoxin concentrations before initiating eliglustat, reduce digoxin dose by 30%, and continue monitoring.

PATIENT CONSIDERATIONS

Assessment: Assess for preexisting cardiac disease, long QT syndrome, renal/hepatic impairment, CYP2D6 metabolizer status, pregnancy/nursing status, and possible drug interactions.

Monitoring: Monitor for ECG changes and other adverse reactions.

Counseling: Advise to discuss all the medications being taken, including any herbal supplements or vitamins, with physician. Advise to inform physician if new symptoms (eg, palpitations, fainting, dizziness) develop. Instruct to avoid consumption of grapefruit or its juice. Inform patients currently treated with imiglucerase, velaglucerase alfa, or taliglucerase alfa, that drug may be administered 24 hrs after the last dose of the previous ERT.

STORAGE: 20-25°C (68-77°F); excursions permitted between 15-30°C (59-86°F).

CHANTIX – varenicline

RX

Class: Nicotinic acetylcholine receptor agonist

Serious neuropsychiatric events including, but not limited to, depression, suicidal ideation, suicide attempt, and completed suicide reported. Some reported cases might have been complicated by nicotine withdrawal symptoms in patients who stopped smoking. Monitor for neuropsychiatric symptoms, including changes in behavior, hostility, agitation, depressed mood, and suicide-related events. Worsening of preexisting psychiatric illness and completed suicide reported in some patients attempting to quit smoking while on therapy. Advise patients and caregivers that the patient should stop taking therapy and contact a healthcare provider immediately if agitation, hostility, depressed mood, changes in behavior or thinking, suicidal ideation, or suicidal behavior occurs. Weigh risks against benefits of use.

ADULT DOSAGE

Smoking Cessation Aid

Set quit date and start 1 week before quit date. Alternatively, may begin therapy and then quit smoking between Days 8 and 35 of treatment

Days 1-3: 0.5mg qd
Days 4-7: 0.5mg bid
Day 8-End of Treatment: 1mg bid
Treat for 12 weeks

If patient has successfully stopped smoking at end of 12 weeks, additional course of 12-week treatment is recommended to ensure long-term abstinence

If patient is motivated to quit and not successful in stopping smoking during prior therapy for reasons other than intolerability due to adverse events, or if relapse occurs after treatment, should make another attempt once factors contributing to failed attempt are identified and addressed

PEDIATRIC DOSAGE

Pediatric use may not have been established

DOSING CONSIDERATIONS

Renal Impairment

Severe (CrCl <30mL/min):
Initial: 0.5mg qd
Titrate: May titrate prn to a max dose of 0.5mg bid

ESRD w/ Hemodialysis:
Max: 0.5mg qd if tolerated

Adverse Reactions

Consider a temporary/permanent dose reduction in patients who cannot tolerate adverse effects

ADMINISTRATION

Oral route

Take pc and w/ a full glass of water
Provide patients w/ appropriate educational materials and counseling to support the quit attempt

HOW SUPPLIED

Tab: 0.5mg, 1mg

CONTRAINDICATIONS

Known history of serious hypersensitivity reactions or skin reactions to varenicline.

WARNINGS/PRECAUTIONS

Seizures reported; caution w/ history of seizures or other factors that can lower the seizure threshold. Somnolence, dizziness, loss of consciousness, and difficulty concentrating reported;

may impair physical/mental abilities. Cardiovascular (CV) events reported in patients w/ stable CV disease. Hypersensitivity reactions, including angioedema, and rare but serious skin reactions (eg, Stevens-Johnson syndrome, erythema multiforme) reported. Nausea reported; consider dose reduction for patients w/ intolerable nausea. Caution in elderly.

ADVERSE REACTIONS

N/V, headache, insomnia, somnolence, abnormal dreams, flatulence, constipation, dysgeusia, fatigue, upper respiratory tract disorder, abdominal pain, dyspepsia, dry mouth, sleep disorder, increased appetite.

DRUG INTERACTIONS

May increase intoxicating effects of alcohol. Nicotine replacement therapy (transdermal nicotine) may increase incidence of adverse events. Physiological changes resulting from smoking cessation may alter pharmacokinetics or pharmacodynamics of certain drugs (eg, theophylline, warfarin, insulin) for which dosage adjustment may be necessary.

PATIENT CONSIDERATIONS

Assessment: Assess for preexisting psychiatric illness, history of seizures or other factors that can lower the seizure threshold, CV disease, history of hypersensitivity to the drug, renal impairment, pregnancy/nursing status, and for possible drug interactions.

Monitoring: Monitor for neuropsychiatric symptoms or worsening of preexisting psychiatric illness, seizures, somnolence, dizziness, loss of consciousness, difficulty concentrating, CV events, skin reactions, hypersensitivity reactions, nausea, and other adverse reactions. Monitor renal function.

Counseling: Inform about risks and benefits of treatment. Instruct to set a date to quit smoking and initiate treatment 1 week before quit date. Encourage to continue to attempt to quit even w/ early lapses after quit day. Encourage patients who are motivated to quit and who did not succeed in stopping smoking during prior therapy for reasons other than intolerability due to adverse events, or who relapsed after treatment to make another attempt w/ therapy once factors contributing to the failed attempt have been identified and addressed. Provide educational materials and necessary counseling to support attempt at quitting smoking. Instruct to notify physician if persistent nausea or insomnia develops. Advise to d/c and notify physician if agitation, hostility, depressed mood, or changes in behavior/thinking develop. Advise to notify physician prior to treatment of any history of psychiatric illness. Inform that quitting smoking may be associated w/ nicotine withdrawal symptoms or exacerbation of preexisting psychiatric illness. Advise to inform physician of any history of seizures or other factors that can lower seizure threshold; instruct patient to d/c treatment and contact physician immediately if seizure is experienced. Instruct patient to reduce amount of alcohol they consume while on therapy until they know whether therapy affects their tolerance for alcohol. Advise to use caution when driving or operating machinery until patients know how quitting smoking and/or therapy may affect them. Advise to notify physician if symptoms of new or worsening CV events develop and to seek immediate medical attention if signs/symptoms of a MI or stroke are experienced. Instruct to d/c and seek immediate medical care if angioedema or a skin reaction occurs. Inform that vivid, unusual, or strange dreams may occur. If patient is pregnant, planning to become pregnant, or breastfeeding, advise about the risks of smoking, the potential risks of therapy, and the benefits of smoking cessation.

STORAGE: 25°C (77°F); excursions permitted to 15-30°C (59-86°F).

CHLORPROMAZINE — chlorpromazine hydrochloride

RX

Class: Typical antipsychotic

Elderly patients with dementia-related psychosis treated with antipsychotic drugs are at increased risk of death; most deaths appeared to be cardiovascular (eg, heart failure, sudden death) or infectious (eg, pneumonia) in nature. Not approved for the treatment of patients with dementia-related psychosis.

ADULT DOSAGE

Psychotic Disorders

Hospitalized Patients:

Acute Schizophrenic or Manic States:

Initial treatment should be w/ chlorpromazine inj until patient is controlled

IM:

Initial: 25mg; give additional 25-50mg inj in 1 hr, if necessary

Titrate: Increase gradually over several days up to 400mg q4-6h until controlled, then switch to PO

PO:

Generally, 500mg/day is sufficient; gradual increases to 2000mg/day or more may be necessary

PEDIATRIC DOSAGE

Behavioral Problems

6 Months-12 Years:

Outpatient:

Select route of administration according to severity of condition

PO:

1/4mg/lb q4-6h prn

IM:

1/4mg/lb q6-8h prn

Inpatient:

PO/IM:

Initial: Start low and may increase gradually to 50-100mg/day; ≥200mg/day in older children

C

Less Acutely Disturbed:
Initial: 25mg tid
Titrate: Increase gradually to effective dose
Usual: 400mg/day

More Severe Cases:
Initial: 25mg tid
Titrate: After 1-2 days, may increase by 20-50mg at semi-weekly intervals until calm and cooperative

Outpatients:
Usual: 10mg tid-qid or 25mg bid-tid

Prompt Control of Severe Symptoms:
Initial treatment should be w/ IM chlorpromazine; subsequent doses should be oral, 25-50 mg tid
IM:
Usual: 25mg; repeat in 1 hr, if necessary

Nausea/Vomiting

PO:
Usual: 10-25mg q4-6h prn; increase, if necessary

IM:
Usual: 25mg; give 25-50mg q3-4h prn if no hypotension occurs until vomiting stops, then switch to PO

Preoperative Medication

For Relief of Restlessness and Apprehension Before Surgery:

Presurgical Apprehension:
PO:
Usual: 25-50mg, given 2-3 hrs before operation

IM:
Usual: 12.5-25mg, given 1-2 hrs before operation

During Surgery:
IM:
Usual: 12.5mg; repeat in 1/2 hr, if necessary, if no hypotension occurs

IV:
Usual: 2mg per fractional inj, at 2-min intervals
Max: 25mg
Dilute to 1mg/mL (eg, 1mL [25mg] mixed w/ 24mL of saline)

Intractable Hiccups

Initial: 25-50mg PO tid-qid; if symptoms persist for 2-3 days, give 25-50mg IM; if symptoms still persist, give 25-50mg in 500-1000mL of saline as slow IV infusion w/ patient flat in bed

Porphyria

Acute Intermittent Porphyria:
PO:
Usual: 25-50mg tid-qid; maint therapy may be necessary in some patients

IM:
Usual: 25mg tid-qid until patient can take PO therapy

Tetanus

Adjunct Treatment:
IM:
Usual: 25-50mg tid-qid, usually in conjunction w/ barbiturates; determine total doses and frequency by patient's response

IV:
Usual: 25-50mg; dilute to at least 1mg/mL and administer at a rate of 1mg/min

Max:
PO:
500mg/day
IM:
Up to 5 Years (or 50 lbs): ≤40mg/day
5-12 Years (or 50-100 lbs): ≤75mg/day except in unmanageable cases

Nausea/Vomiting

6 Months-12 Years:
Adjust dosage/frequency according to severity of symptoms and patient response
PO:
1/4mg/lb q4-6h

IM:
1/4mg/lb q6-8h, prn

Max:
IM:
6 Months-5 Years (or 50 lbs): ≤40mg/day
5-12 Years (or 50-100 lbs): ≤75mg/day except in severe cases

Preoperative Medication

For Relief of Restlessness and Apprehension Before Surgery:
6 Months-12 Years:

Presurgical Apprehension:
PO:
Usual: 1/4mg/lb, given 2-3 hrs before operation

IM:
Usual: 1/4mg/lb, given 1-2 hrs before operation

During Surgery:
IM:
Usual: 1/8mg/lb; repeat in 1/2 hr, if necessary, if no hypotension occurs

IV:
Usual: 1mg per fractional inj, at 2-min intervals and not exceeding recommended IM dosage
Dilute to 1mg/mL (eg, 1mL [25mg] mixed w/ 24mL of saline)

Tetanus

Adjunct Treatment:
6 Months-12 Years:

IM/IV:
1/4mg/lb q6-8h
When given IV, dilute to at least 1mg/mL and administer at a rate of 1mg/2 min
Max:
≤50 lbs: ≤40mg/day
50-100 lbs: ≤75mg/day except in severe cases

DOSING CONSIDERATIONS

Elderly

Elderly/Debilitated:
Start at lower end of dosing range; increase gradually and monitor closely

ADMINISTRATION

Oral/IM/IV route

Inj

Inject slowly, deep into upper outer quadrant of buttock
Reserve parenteral administration for bedfast patients or for acute ambulatory cases, and keep patient lying down for at least 1/2 hr after inj
If irritation is a problem, dilute inj w/ saline or 2% procaine; do not mix w/ other agents in syringe
Avoid injecting undiluted inj into vein
Avoid getting sol on hands or clothing, because of possibility of contact dermatitis

HOW SUPPLIED

Inj: 25mg/mL [1mL, 2mL]; **Tab:** 10mg, 25mg, 50mg, 100mg, 200mg

CONTRAINDICATIONS

Known hypersensitivity to phenothiazines. Comatose states or the presence of large amounts of CNS depressants (eg, alcohol, barbiturates, narcotics).

WARNINGS/PRECAUTIONS

Extrapyramidal symptoms may be confused with CNS signs of undiagnosed primary disease responsible for vomiting; avoid in children/adolescents with signs of Reye's syndrome. Risk of tardive dyskinesia (TD), especially in elderly; consider d/c if signs/symptoms appear. Neuroleptic malignant syndrome (NMS) reported; d/c therapy and carefully monitor for recurrences if therapy is reintroduced. May impair mental/physical abilities. Neonates exposed during 3rd trimester of pregnancy are at risk for extrapyramidal and/or withdrawal symptoms. Leukopenia, neutropenia, and agranulocytosis reported. Monitor for fever or infection with neutropenia; d/c in patients with severe neutropenia (absolute neutrophil count $<1000/mm^3$). Caution with chronic respiratory disorders, acute respiratory infections (especially in children), glaucoma, cardiovascular, hepatic, or renal disease. May suppress cough reflex; aspiration of vomitus possible. Caution if exposed to extreme heat. May elevate prolactin levels. May produce α-adrenergic blockade. May mask signs and symptoms of overdosage of other drugs and obscure diagnosis and treatment of other conditions (eg, intestinal obstruction, brain tumor, Reye's syndrome). Avoid abrupt withdrawal of high-dose therapy. Evaluate patients with a history of long-term therapy on whether the maint dose could be lowered or d/c therapy to lessen likelihood of adverse reactions related to cumulative drug effect. May produce false-(+) phenylketonuria test results. (Inj) Contains sulfites.

ADVERSE REACTIONS

Drowsiness, jaundice, agranulocytosis, hypotensive effects, ECG changes, dystonia, motor restlessness, pseudo-parkinsonism, TD, anticholinergic effects, NMS, ocular changes, skin pigmentation, allergic reactions.

DRUG INTERACTIONS

See Contraindications. Monitor for neurological toxicity with lithium; d/c if signs occur. Prolongs and intensifies action of CNS depressants (eg, anesthetics, barbiturates, narcotics); administer about 1/4 to 1/2 the usual dose of such agents when used concomitantly. Caution with organophosphorus insecticides, atropine or related drugs. Avoid use of alcohol due to possible additive effects and hypotension. May counteract the antihypertensive effect of guanethidine and related compounds. Diminished effect of oral anticoagulants reported. May lower convulsive threshold; anticonvulsant dose adjustment may be needed. May interfere with phenytoin metabolism and precipitate phenytoin toxicity. Increased plasma levels of both agents with propranolol. Thiazide diuretics may potentiate orthostatic hypotension. Do not use with metrizamide; d/c at least 48 hrs before myelography and should not be resumed for at least 24 hrs after; do not administer for control of N/V prior to or after procedure with metrizamide. May obscure vomiting as a sign of toxicity of chemotherapeutic drugs. Certain pressor agents, such as epinephrine, may cause paradoxical further lowering of BP; do not use to control hypotension.

PATIENT CONSIDERATIONS

Assessment: Assess for Reye's syndrome in children and adolescents prior to initiation, mental status, renal/hepatic/cardiovascular function, glaucoma, respiratory disorders, bone marrow depression, use of large amounts of CNS depressants, heat exposure, hypersensitivity to drug, pregnancy/nursing status, and possible drug interactions.

Monitoring: Monitor for hypersensitivity reactions, TD, NMS, hypotension, leukopenia/neutropenia/agranulocytosis, fever, infection, and other adverse reactions. Monitor CBC frequently during the 1st few months of therapy.

Counseling: Counsel on risks/benefits of therapy. Instruct to immediately report signs of infection and to avoid exposure to extreme heat. Inform that drug may impair mental/physical abilities, especially during first few days of therapy; caution with activities requiring alertness (eg, operating vehicles or machinery). Advise to avoid alcohol and abrupt withdrawal of therapy.

STORAGE: (Inj) 20-25°C (68-77°F); excursions permitted to 15-30°C (59-86°F). Protect from light and freezing. (Tab) 20-25°C (68-77°F). Protect from moisture.

CHOLBAM – cholic acid

RX

Class: Bile acid

ADULT DOSAGE

Bile Acid Synthesis Disorders

Treatment of bile acid synthesis disorders due to single enzyme defects

Usual: 10-15mg/kg qd, or in 2 divided dose

Peroxisomal Disorders

Adjunctive treatment of peroxisomal disorders including Zellweger spectrum disorders in patients who exhibit manifestations of liver disease, steatorrhea, or complications from decreased fat soluble vitamin absorption

Usual: 10-15mg/kg qd, or in 2 divided doses

PEDIATRIC DOSAGE

Bile Acid Synthesis Disorders

Treatment of bile acid synthesis disorders due to single enzyme defects

≥3 Weeks of Age:

Usual: 10-15mg/kg qd, or in 2 divided doses

Peroxisomal Disorders

Adjunctive treatment of peroxisomal disorders including Zellweger spectrum disorders in patients who exhibit manifestations of liver disease, steatorrhea, or complications from decreased fat soluble vitamin absorption

≥3 Weeks of Age:

Usual: 10-15mg/kg qd, or in 2 divided doses

DOSING CONSIDERATIONS

Discontinuation

D/C if liver function does not improve w/in 3 months of the start of treatment or complete biliary obstruction develops

D/C at any time if there are persistent clinical or lab indicators of worsening liver function or cholestasis. Concurrent elevations of serum gamma glutamyltransferase and serum ALT may indicate overdose. Continue to monitor lab parameters of liver function and consider restarting dose when the parameters return to baseline

Other Important Considerations

Familial Hypertriglyceridemia:

Patients w/ newly diagnosed, or a family history of, familial hypertriglyceridemia may have a poor absorption of therapy from the intestine and require a 10% increase in the recommended dosage

Usual: 11-17mg/kg qd, or in 2 divided doses

Monitor clinical response including steatorrhea, and lab values including transaminases, bilirubin, and PT/INR to determine the adequacy of the dosage regimen

Administer the lowest dose of therapy that effectively maintains liver function

ADMINISTRATION

Oral route

Take w/ food

Take at least 1 hr before or 4-6 hrs (or at as great an interval as possible) after a bile acid binding resin or aluminum-based antacid

Do not crush or chew the caps

Refer to PI for number of caps needed to achieve dosage of 10mg/kg/day and 15mg/kg/day

Patients Unable to Swallow Caps

Caps can be opened and the contents mixed w/ either infant formula or expressed breast milk (for younger children), or soft food such as mashed potatoes or apple puree (for older children and adults) in order to mask any unpleasant taste:

1. Hold the cap over the prepared liquid/food, gently twist open, and allow the contents to fall into the liquid/food
2. Mix the entire cap contents w/ 1 or 2 tbsp (15-30mL) of infant formula, expressed breast milk, or soft food
3. Stir for 30 sec
4. Cap contents will remain as fine granules in the milk or food, and will not dissolve
5. Administer the mixture immediately

HOW SUPPLIED

Cap: 50mg, 250mg

WARNINGS/PRECAUTIONS

Should be initiated and monitored by an experienced hepatologist or pediatric gastroenterologist. Monitor liver function and d/c in patients who develop worsening of liver function while on treatment.

ADVERSE REACTIONS

Diarrhea, reflux esophagitis, malaise, jaundice, skin lesion, nausea, abdominal pain, intestinal polyp, UTI, peripheral neuropathy.

DRUG INTERACTIONS

Concomitant medications that inhibit canalicular membrane bile acid transporters such as bile salt efflux pump (eg, cyclosporine) may exacerbate accumulation of conjugated bile salts in the liver and result in clinical symptoms; avoid concomitant use, and if concomitant use is necessary, monitor serum transaminases and bilirubin. Bile acid binding resins (eg, cholestyramine, colestipol, colesevelam) adsorb and reduce bile acid absorption and may reduce efficacy of cholic acid; take cholic acid at least 1 hr before or 4-6 hrs (or at as great an interval as possible) after a bile acid binding resin. Aluminum-based antacids may reduce the bioavailability of cholic acid; take cholic acid at least 1 hr before or 4-6 hrs (or at as great an interval as possible) after an aluminum-based antacid.

PATIENT CONSIDERATIONS

Assessment: Assess for newly diagnosed or a family history of familial hypertriglyceridemia, hepatic impairment, pregnancy/nursing status, and possible drug interactions. Assess serum or urinary bile acid levels using mass spectrometry.

Monitoring: Monitor for worsening liver function or cholestasis, complete biliary obstruction, and other adverse reactions. Monitor serum AST/ALT/gamma-glutamyl transpeptidase, alkaline phosphatase, bilirubin, and INR every month for the first 3 months, every 3 months for the next 9 months, every 6 months during the subsequent 3 yrs, and annually thereafter. Monitor liver function more frequently during periods of rapid growth, concomitant disease, and pregnancy. Monitor clinical response to therapy.

Counseling: Advise the need to undergo lab testing periodically while on treatment to assess liver function. Advise that therapy may worsen liver impairment; instruct to immediately report to physician any symptoms associated w/ liver impairment (eg, skin or the whites of eyes turn yellow, urine turns dark or brown [tea colored], pain on the right side of stomach, bleeding or bruising occurs more easily than normal, increased lethargy). Instruct to take exactly ud. Advise that there is a pregnancy surveillance program that monitors pregnancy outcomes in women exposed to cholic acid during pregnancy.

STORAGE: 20-25°C (68-77°F); excursions permitted between 15-30°C (59-86°F).

Cialis – tadalafil

RX

Class: Phosphodiesterase-5 (PDE-5) inhibitor

ADULT DOSAGE

Erectile Dysfunction

PRN Use:
Initial: 10mg prior to sexual activity
Titrate: May increase to 20mg or decrease to 5mg, based on individual efficacy and tolerability
Max Dosing Frequency: Once daily

Once-Daily Use:
Initial: 2.5mg qd
Titrate: May increase to 5mg qd based on individual efficacy and tolerability

Benign Prostatic Hyperplasia

W/ or w/o Erectile Dysfunction (ED): 5mg qd

Initiated w/ Finasteride: 5mg qd for ≤26 weeks

PEDIATRIC DOSAGE

Pediatric use may not have been established

DOSING CONSIDERATIONS

Concomitant Medications

α-Blockers:
ED:
Initial: Use lowest recommended dose; should be stable on α-blocker therapy prior to initiating treatment
BPH:
Not recommended

Potent CYP3A4 Inhibitors (eg, Ketoconazole, Ritonavir):
PRN Use:

Max: 10mg/72 hrs
Once-Daily Use:
Max: 2.5mg

Renal Impairment
PRN Use:
CrCl 30-50mL/min:
Initial: 5mg qd
Max: 10mg/48 hrs
CrCl <30mL/min or Hemodialysis:
Max: 5mg/72 hrs

Once-Daily Use:
ED:
CrCl <30mL/min or Hemodialysis:
Not recommended
BPH or ED/BPH:
CrCl 30-50mL/min:
Initial: 2.5mg
Titrate: May increase to 5mg based on individual response
CrCl <30mL/min or Hemodialysis:
Not recommended

Hepatic Impairment
PRN Use:
Mild/Moderate (Child-Pugh Class A/B):
Max: 10mg qd
Severe (Child-Pugh Class C):
Not recommended

Once-Daily Use:
Mild/Moderate (Child-Pugh Class A/B): Use caution
Severe (Child-Pugh Class C): Not recommended

ADMINISTRATION

Oral route

May be taken w/o regard to food.
Do not split; entire dose should be taken.

Once-Daily Use
Take at approx the same time every day.

HOW SUPPLIED

Tab: 2.5mg, 5mg, 10mg, 20mg

CONTRAINDICATIONS

Any form of organic nitrate, either regularly and/or intermittently used. Known serious hypersensitivity to tadalafil. Concomitant guanylate cyclase (GC) stimulators (eg, riociguat).

WARNINGS/PRECAUTIONS

Cardiac risk associated w/ sexual activity; avoid in men for whom sexual activity is inadvisable due to underlying cardiovascular (CV) status. Caution in patients w/ left ventricular outflow obstruction (eg, aortic stenosis, idiopathic hypertrophic subaortic stenosis) and w/ severely impaired autonomic control of BP. Avoid w/ MI (w/in last 90 days), unstable angina or angina occurring during sexual intercourse, NYHA Class 2 or greater HF (in the last 6 months), uncontrolled arrhythmias, hypotension (<90/50mmHg), uncontrolled HTN, and stroke (w/in the last 6 months). Mild systemic vasodilatory properties may result in transient decreases in BP. Prolonged erections (>4 hrs) and priapism (painful erections >6 hrs in duration) reported; caution in patients who have conditions predisposing to priapism (eg, sickle cell anemia, multiple myeloma, leukemia), or w/ anatomical deformation of the penis (eg, angulation, cavernosal fibrosis, Peyronie's disease). Nonarteritic anterior ischemic optic neuropathy (NAION) reported; d/c if sudden loss of vision is experienced in one or both eyes. Caution in patients w/ underlying NAION risk factors, individuals who have experienced NAION, and individuals w/ "crowded" optic disc. Sudden decrease or loss of hearing reported, which may be accompanied by tinnitus and dizziness; d/c if this occurs. Avoid qd use in patients w/ CrCl <30mL/min or on hemodialysis. Avoid use w/ severe hepatic impairment (Child-Pugh Class C) and hereditary degenerative retinal disorders, including retinitis pigmentosa. Caution w/ mild to moderate hepatic impairment (Child-Pugh Class A/B), bleeding disorders, or significant active peptic ulceration. Consider other urological conditions that may cause similar symptoms prior to initiating treatment for BPH.

ADVERSE REACTIONS

Headache, dyspepsia, back pain, myalgia, nasal congestion, flushing, limb pain, nasopharyngitis, URTI, gastroenteritis, cough, GERD, HTN.

DRUG INTERACTIONS

See Contraindications and Dosing Considerations. Avoid concomitant use w/ other PDE-5 inhibitors, including Adcirca. Avoid concomitant use w/ nitrates w/in 48 hrs. Potential additive BP-lowering effects w/ α-blockers and selected antihypertensives (amlodipine, ARBs, bendrofluazide, enalapril, metoprolol). Concomitant use not recommended w/ α-blockers for the treatment of BPH. BP-lowering effects of each individual compound may be increased w/ alcohol. Antacids (eg, magnesium hydroxide/aluminum hydroxide) may reduce the apparent rate of absorption. CYP3A4 inhibitors (eg, ketoconazole, erythromycin, itraconazole, grapefruit juice), ritonavir, and other HIV protease inhibitors may increase exposure. CYP3A4 inducers (eg, rifampin, carbamazepine, phenytoin, phenobarbital) may decrease exposure. A small increase in HR reported w/ theophylline.

PATIENT CONSIDERATIONS

Assessment: Assess for previous hypersensitivity to drug, CV disease, hereditary degenerative retinal disorders, bleeding disorders, significant active peptic ulceration, anatomical deformation of the penis or presence of conditions that would predispose to priapism, underlying NAION risk factors, "crowded" optic disc, potential underlying causes of ED, other urological conditions, renal/hepatic impairment, pregnancy/nursing status, and possible drug interactions.

Monitoring: Monitor for hypersensitivity reactions, BP decrease, decrease/loss of hearing or vision, prolonged erection, priapism, and other adverse reactions.

Counseling: Instruct to seek emergency medical attention if erection persists >4 hrs. Advise of potential BP-lowering effect of α-blockers, antihypertensive medications, and alcohol. Inform of the potential cardiac risk of sexual activity in patients w/ preexisting CV disease; instruct patients who experience symptoms upon initiation of sexual activity to refrain from further sexual activity and seek immediate medical attention. Counsel about the protective measures necessary to guard against STDs (including HIV) that should be considered. Inform about contraindication w/ regular and/or intermittent use of organic nitrates and potential interactions w/ medications. Instruct to d/c and seek medical attention if sudden decrease or loss of vision or hearing occurs. Inform of the increased risk of NAION in individuals who have already experienced NAION in 1 eye and in patients w/ a "crowded" optic disc. Counsel to take 1 tab at least 30 min before anticipated sexual activity for prn use in men w/ ED, and at approx the same time every day w/o regard to timing of sexual activity for qd use in men w/ ED, BPH, or ED/BPH.

STORAGE: 25°C (77°F); excursions permitted to 15-30°C (59-86°F).

CIMETIDINE – cimetidine

RX

Class: H_2 blocker

OTHER BRAND NAMES

Tagamet (Discontinued)

ADULT DOSAGE

Duodenal Ulcers

Short-Term Treatment of Active Ulcer:
800mg qhs (preferred) or 300mg qid (w/ meals and qhs) or 400mg bid (qam and qhs) for 4-6 weeks

Maint Therapy After Healing of Active Ulcer:
400mg qhs

Concomitant antacids should be given prn for relief of pain; however, simultaneous administration not recommended

Gastric Ulcers

Short-Term Treatment of Active, Benign Ulcer:
800mg qhs (preferred) or 300mg qid (w/ meals and qhs) for 6 weeks

Gastroesophageal Reflux Disease

Erosive Esophagitis Diagnosed by Endoscopy:
800mg bid or 400mg qid for 12 weeks
Max: 12 weeks

Pathological Hypersecretory Conditions

Treatment of Pathological Hypersecretory Conditions (eg, Zollinger-Ellison Syndrome, Systemic Mastocytosis, Multiple Endocrine Adenomas):
Usual: 300mg qid (w/ meals and qhs)
Max: 2400mg/day
Continue as long as clinically indicated

PEDIATRIC DOSAGE

Duodenal Ulcers

≥16 Years:
Short-Term Treatment of Active Ulcer:
800mg qhs (preferred) or 300mg qid (w/ meals and qhs) or 400mg bid (qam and qhs) for 4-6 weeks

Maint Therapy After Healing of Active Ulcer:
400mg qhs

Concomitant antacids should be given prn for relief of pain; however, simultaneous administration not recommended

Gastric Ulcers

Short-Term Treatment of Active, Benign Ulcer:
≥16 Years:
800mg qhs or 300mg qid (w/ meals and qhs) for 6 weeks

Gastroesophageal Reflux Disease

Erosive Esophagitis Diagnosed by Endoscopy:
≥16 Years:
800mg bid or 400mg qid for 12 weeks
Max: 12 weeks

Pathological Hypersecretory Conditions

Treatment of Pathological Hypersecretory Conditions (eg, Zollinger-Ellison Syndrome, Systemic Mastocytosis, Multiple Endocrine Adenomas):

≥16 Years:
Usual: 300mg qid (w/ meals and qhs)
Max: 2400mg/day
Continue as long as clinically indicated

DOSING CONSIDERATIONS

Renal Impairment

Severe: 300mg q12h; may increase to q8h or further w/ caution if required
Hemodialysis: Adjust so that timing of scheduled dose coincides w/ end of hemodialysis

ADMINISTRATION

Oral route

HOW SUPPLIED

Sol: 300mg/5mL [237mL]; **Tab:** 200mg, 300mg, 400mg*, 800mg* *scored

CONTRAINDICATIONS

Known hypersensitivity to the product.

WARNINGS/PRECAUTIONS

Symptomatic response does not preclude the presence of gastric malignancy. Reversible confusional states observed on occasion, predominantly in severely ill patients; contributing factors include advancing age (≥50 yrs) and preexisting liver and/or renal disease. Increased possibility of a hyperinfection of strongyloidiasis in immunocompromised patients. Cardiac arrhythmias and hypotension reported (rare) following rapid administration of inj by IV bolus.

ADVERSE REACTIONS

Headache, reversible confusional states, reversible impotence, increased serum transaminase, gynecomastia.

DRUG INTERACTIONS

Increases blood levels of warfarin-type anticoagulants, phenytoin, propranolol, nifedipine, chlordiazepoxide, diazepam, certain TCAs, lidocaine, theophylline, and metronidazole. Closely monitor PT and adjust dose of warfarin anticoagulants. Adverse effects reported with phenytoin, lidocaine, and theophylline. May affect absorption of certain drugs due to alteration of pH (eg, ketoconazole); give at least 2 hrs before cimetidine. Antacids may interfere with absorption; simultaneous administration of oral cimetidine with antacids is not recommended.

PATIENT CONSIDERATIONS

Assessment: Assess for hypersensitivity to drug, immunosuppression, renal/hepatic impairment, pregnancy/nursing status, and possible drug interactions.

Monitoring: Monitor for hypersensitivity reactions and other adverse reactions.

Counseling: Inform that antacids may be given PRN for pain relief; however, concomitant use of antacids is not recommended. Instruct to contact physician if hypersensitivity or other adverse reactions develop.

STORAGE: 20-25°C (68-77°F). (Tab) Protect from light.

CIMZIA – certolizumab pegol

Class: Tumor necrosis factor (TNF) blocker

RX

Increased risk for developing serious infections (eg, active tuberculosis [TB], latent TB reactivation, invasive fungal infections, bacterial/viral and other opportunistic infections) leading to hospitalization or death, mostly w/ concomitant use w/ immunosuppressants (eg, methotrexate or corticosteroids). D/C if serious infection or sepsis develops. Active TB/reactivation of latent TB may present w/ disseminated or extrapulmonary disease; test for latent TB before and during therapy and initiate treatment for latent TB prior to therapy. Invasive fungal infections reported; consider empiric antifungal therapy in patients at risk who develop severe systemic illness. Consider risks and benefits prior to therapy in patients w/ chronic or recurrent infection. Monitor patients for development of infection during and after treatment, including development of TB in patients who tested (-) for latent TB infection prior to therapy. Lymphoma and other malignancies, some fatal, reported in children and adolescents.

ADULT DOSAGE

Crohn's Disease

Moderately to Severely Active Disease w/ Inadequate Response to Conventional Therapy:
Initial: 400mg (given as 2 SQ inj of 200mg) initially, and at Weeks 2 and 4
Maint: 400mg every 4 weeks

PEDIATRIC DOSAGE

Pediatric use may not have been established

Rheumatoid Arthritis

Moderately to Severely Active:
Recommended: 400mg (given as 2 SQ inj of 200mg) initially and at Weeks 2 and 4, followed by 200mg every other week
Maint: Consider 400mg every 4 weeks

Psoriatic Arthritis

Active:
Recommended: 400mg (given as 2 SQ inj of 200mg) initially and at Weeks 2 and 4, followed by 200mg every other week
Maint: Consider 400mg every 4 weeks

Ankylosing Spondylitis

Active:
Recommended: 400mg (given as 2 SQ inj of 200mg) initially and at Weeks 2 and 4, followed by 200mg every 2 weeks or 400mg every 4 weeks

DOSING CONSIDERATIONS

Concomitant Medications
Not recommended in combination w/ biological disease-modifying anti-rheumatic drugs (DMARDs) or other TNF blocker therapy

ADMINISTRATION

SQ route

Rotate inj sites; avoid areas where the skin is tender, bruised, red, or hard.
Once reconstituted, can store in the vials for up to 24 hrs between 2-8°C (36-46°F) prior to inj; do not freeze.

Lyophilized Powder for Inj
Preparation:
1. Bring to room temperature before reconstituting.
2. Reconstitute vial(s) w/ 1mL of sterile water for inj (SWFI) using 20-gauge needle provided.
3. Gently swirl each vial w/o shaking, assuring that all of the powder comes in contact w/ SWFI.
4. Leave the vial(s) undisturbed to fully reconstitute, which may take approx 30 min.
5. Final reconstituted sol contains 200mg/mL.

Administration:
1. Prior to injecting, reconstituted sol should be at room temperature (but not for >2 hrs prior to administration).
2. Withdraw reconstituted sol into a separate syringe for each vial using a new 20-gauge needle for each vial so that each syringe contains 1mL of sol (200mg of certolizumab pegol).
3. Replace 20-gauge needle(s) on syringes w/ a 23-gauge(s) for administration.
4. Inject full contents of syringe(s) SQ into thigh or abdomen; when a 400mg dose is needed (given as 2 SQ inj of 200mg), inj should occur at separate sites in the thigh or abdomen.

Prefilled Syringe
After proper training in SQ inj technique, a patient may self-inject w/ a prefilled syringe if appropriate.
Patients using prefilled syringes should be instructed to inject full amount in syringe (1mL), according to the directions provided in Instructions for Use booklet.

HOW SUPPLIED

Inj: 200mg/mL [prefilled syringe, vial]

WARNINGS/PRECAUTIONS

May be used as monotherapy or concomitantly w/ non-biological DMARDs. Do not initiate w/ an active infection. Increased risk of infection in elderly patients and in patients w/ comorbid conditions; consider the risks prior to therapy for those who have been exposed to TB, w/ a history of an opportunistic infection, who have resided or traveled in areas of endemic TB or mycoses, or w/ any underlying conditions predisposing to infection. Postmarketing cases of aggressive and fatal hepatosplenic T-cell lymphoma (HSTCL) reported; the majority of cases occurred in adolescent and young adult males w/ Crohn's disease or ulcerative colitis. Acute and chronic leukemia reported. Perform periodic skin examination, particularly in patients w/ risk factors for skin cancer. New onset and worsening of CHF reported; caution in patients w/ heart failure (HF) and monitor carefully. Hypersensitivity reactions reported (rare); d/c and institute appropriate therapy if such reactions occur. Hepatitis B virus (HBV) reactivation reported; if reactivation occurs, d/c and initiate antiviral therapy w/ appropriate supportive treatment. Monitor patients closely and exercise caution when considering resumption of therapy. Associated w/ rare cases of new onset or exacerbation of clinical symptoms and/or radiographic evidence of CNS and peripheral demyelinating disease; caution w/ preexisting or recent-onset central or peripheral nervous system demyelinating disorders. Rare cases of neurological disorders (eg, seizure disorder, optic neuritis, peripheral neuropathy) reported. Hematological reactions (eg, leukopenia, pancytopenia, thrombocytopenia) reported; caution in patients w/ ongoing, or a history of, significant hematologic abnormalities, and consider discontinuation in patients w/ confirmed significant hematologic abnormalities. May result in the formation of autoantibodies and rarely, in the development of a lupus-like syndrome; d/c if lupus-like syndrome develops. Lab test interactions may occur.

ADVERSE REACTIONS

URTIs, rash, UTIs.

DRUG INTERACTIONS

See Boxed Warning and Dosing Considerations. Avoid concurrent use w/ live (eg, attenuated) vaccines. Not recommended w/ anakinra, abatacept, rituximab, or natalizumab; may increase risk of serious infections. Carefully consider the potential risk of HSTCL w/ the combination of azathioprine or 6-mercaptopurine.

PATIENT CONSIDERATIONS

Assessment: Assess for active/chronic/recurrent infection (eg, TB, HBV), TB exposure, history of an opportunistic infection, recent travel to areas of endemic TB or endemic mycoses, underlying conditions that may predispose to infection, HF, presence or history of significant hematologic abnormalities, neurologic disorders, risk factors for skin cancer, pregnancy/nursing status, and possible drug interactions. Assess vaccination history in pediatric patients. Perform test for latent TB infection.

Monitoring: Monitor for sepsis, TB (active, reactivation, or latent), invasive fungal infections, bacterial/viral/other infections, lymphoma/other malignancies, new onset/worsening of CHF, active HBV infection, hematological events, hypersensitivity reactions, CNS demyelinating disorders, lupus-like syndrome, and other adverse reactions. Perform periodic skin examination, particularly in patients w/ risk factors for skin cancer and test for latent TB infection.

Counseling: Advise of potential risks and benefits of therapy. Inform that therapy may lower the ability of the immune system to fight infections; instruct to immediately contact physician if any signs/symptoms of an infection develop, including TB and HBV reactivation. Inform about the risks of lymphoma and other malignancies while on therapy. Advise to seek immediate medical attention if any symptoms of severe allergic reactions occur. Advise to report to physician signs of new or worsening medical conditions (eg, heart disease, neurological diseases, autoimmune disorders) and symptoms of cytopenia (eg, bruising, bleeding, persistent fever). Instruct about proper administration techniques.

STORAGE: 2-8°C (36-46°F). Do not freeze. Protect sol from light.

CIPRO XR – ciprofloxacin

RX

Class: Fluoroquinolone

Fluoroquinolones are associated w/ an increased risk of tendinitis and tendon rupture in all ages. Risk is further increased in patients >60 yrs of age, patients taking corticosteroids, and w/ kidney, heart, or lung transplants. May exacerbate muscle weakness w/ myasthenia gravis; avoid in patients w/ known history of myasthenia gravis.

ADULT DOSAGE

Urinary Tract Infections

Uncomplicated (Acute Cystitis):
500mg q24h for 3 days

Complicated UTI/Acute Uncomplicated Pyelonephritis:
1000mg q24h for 7-14 days

May switch from IV to Cipro XR at discretion of physician

PEDIATRIC DOSAGE

Pediatric use may not have been established

DOSING CONSIDERATIONS

Renal Impairment

Hemodialysis/Peritoneal Dialysis: Give after procedure is completed
Max: 500mg q24h
Continuous Ambulatory Peritoneal Dialysis:
Max: 500mg q24h

Complicated UTI/Acute Uncomplicated Pyelonephritis:
CrCl ≤30mL/min: Reduce dose from 1000mg to 500mg qd; use of 1000mg tab is not recommended in this population

ADMINISTRATION

Oral route

Swallow tab whole; do not split, crush, or chew
Take w/ or w/o food
Space Ca^{2+} intake (>800mg) by 2 hrs
Administer ≥2 hrs before or 6 hrs after antacids containing Mg^{2+} or aluminum, polymeric phosphate binders, sucralfate, didanosine, chewable/buffered tabs or pediatric powder, other highly buffered drugs, metal cations such as iron, and multivitamin preparations w/ zinc.

HOW SUPPLIED

Tab, Extended-Release: 500mg, 1000mg

CONTRAINDICATIONS

History of hypersensitivity to ciprofloxacin, any member of the quinolone class of antibacterials, or any of the product components. Concomitant administration w/ tizanidine.

WARNINGS/PRECAUTIONS

Caution w/ history of tendon disorders; d/c if patient experiences pain, swelling, inflammation, or rupture of tendon. Serious and occasionally fatal hypersensitivity (anaphylactic) reactions reported; d/c immediately at the 1st appearance of a skin rash, jaundice, or any other sign of hypersensitivity, and institute supportive measures. Severe hepatotoxicity, including hepatic necrosis, life-threatening hepatic failure, and fatal events, reported; d/c immediately if signs and symptoms of hepatitis occur. Convulsions, status epilepticus, increased intracranial pressure (including pseudotumor cerebri), toxic psychosis, and other CNS events reported; d/c and institute appropriate measures if CNS events occur. Caution w/ epilepsy and CNS disorders (eg, severe cerebral arteriosclerosis, history of convulsion, reduced cerebral blood flow) or other risk factors that may predispose to seizures or lower seizure threshold; d/c if seizures occur. *Clostridium difficile*-associated diarrhea (CDAD) reported; may need to d/c if CDAD is suspected or confirmed. Cases of sensory or sensorimotor axonal polyneuropathy resulting in paresthesias, hypoesthesias, dysesthesias, and weakness reported; d/c immediately if symptoms of peripheral neuropathy occur. May prolong QT interval; avoid w/ known QT interval prolongation and w/ risk factors for QT prolongation/torsades de pointes (eg, congenital long QT syndrome, uncorrected hypokalemia/hypomagnesemia, cardiac disease). Crystalluria reported; maintain hydration and avoid alkalinity of urine. May cause photosensitivity/phototoxicity reactions; d/c if phototoxicity occurs. Avoid excessive exposure to sun/UV light. May result in bacterial resistance if used in the absence of a proven or strongly suspected bacterial infection or a prophylactic indication. Has not been shown to be effective in the treatment of syphilis; antimicrobial agents used in high dose for short periods to treat gonorrhea may mask or delay symptoms of incubating syphilis. Caution in elderly. Not interchangeable w/ immediate-release tabs.

ADVERSE REACTIONS

Tendinitis, tendon rupture, nausea, headache.

DRUG INTERACTIONS

See Boxed Warning and Contraindications. Avoid concomitant administration w/ dairy products (eg, milk, yogurt), or Ca^{2+}-fortified products alone; absorption may be reduced. May increase levels of CYP1A2 substrates (eg, theophylline, methylxanthines, olanzapine), duloxetine, or sildenafil. Increased theophylline levels may increase the risk of developing CNS or other adverse reactions; if coadministration cannot be avoided, monitor theophylline levels and adjust dose. May inhibit the formation of paraxanthine after caffeine administration (or pentoxifylline-containing products); monitor for xanthine toxicity and adjust dose as necessary. Avoid use w/ duloxetine; monitor for duloxetine toxicity if coadministration is unavoidable. Monitor for clozapine- or ropinirole-related adverse reactions and adjust dose of clozapine or ropinirole during and shortly after coadministration. Monitor for sildenafil toxicity. Avoid w/ Class IA (eg, quinidine, procainamide) and Class III (eg, amiodarone, sotalol) antiarrhythmics, TCAs, macrolides, and antipsychotics; may further prolong the QT interval. Hypoglycemia reported w/ oral antidiabetic agents, mainly sulfonylureas (eg, glyburide, glimepiride); monitor blood glucose. May alter serum levels of phenytoin; monitor phenytoin therapy, including phenytoin levels during and shortly after coadministration. Transient SrCr elevations w/ cyclosporine; monitor renal function. May increase effects of oral anticoagulants; monitor PT and INR frequently during and shortly after coadministration. May increase levels and toxic reactions of methotrexate; carefully monitor w/ concomitant use. High-dose quinolones in combination w/ NSAIDs (not acetyl salicylic acid) may provoke convulsions. Antacids, sucralfate, multivitamins, and other multivalent cation-containing products (eg, Mg^{2+}/aluminum antacids, polymeric phosphate binders, chewable/buffered tab or pediatric powder) may decrease absorption, resulting in lower serum and urine levels lower than desired; administer ≥2 hrs before or 6 hrs after these drugs. Probenecid may increase levels. Caution w/ drugs that may lower seizure threshold.

PATIENT CONSIDERATIONS

Assessment: Assess for risk factors for developing tendinitis and tendon rupture, history of myasthenia gravis, drug hypersensitivity, epilepsy, CNS disorders or other risk factors that may predispose to seizures or lower seizure threshold, QT interval prolongation, renal/hepatic dysfunction, pregnancy/nursing status, and possible drug interactions. Obtain baseline culture and susceptibility tests. Perform serologic test for syphilis in patients w/ gonorrhea.

Monitoring: Monitor for tendinitis or tendon rupture, exacerbation of myasthenia gravis, signs/symptoms of hypersensitivity reactions, ECG changes, arrhythmias, CNS effects, CDAD, hepatotoxicity, peripheral neuropathy, crystalluria, photosensitivity/phototoxicity reactions, and other adverse reactions. Monitor PT and INR if coadministered w/ an oral anticoagulant (eg, warfarin). Monitor renal function. Perform periodic culture and susceptibility testing. Perform follow-up serologic test for syphilis 3 months after treatment.

Counseling: Inform that drug treats only bacterial, not viral, infections. Advise to take exactly ud; inform that skipping doses or not completing full course of therapy may decrease effectiveness and increase likelihood of drug resistance. Advise to drink fluids liberally. Counsel to avoid concomitant use w/ dairy products or Ca^{2+}-fortified juices alone. Advise to contact physician of any tendon disorder symptoms; instruct to d/c therapy and rest/refrain from exercise. Instruct to notify physician if experiencing symptoms of myasthenia gravis, photosensitivity/phototoxicity, or liver injury. Instruct to notify physician of any history of convulsions. Advise to assess reaction to therapy before engaging in activities that require mental alertness or coordination; instruct to notify physician if persistent headache w/ or w/o blurred vision occurs. Advise to contact physician as soon as possible if watery and bloody stools (w/ or w/o stomach cramps and fever) develop even as late as ≥2 months after last dose. Instruct to d/c and notify physician if hypersensitivity reactions or symptoms of peripheral neuropathy develop. Inform physician of any personal or family history of QT prolongation or proarrhythmic conditions and if symptoms of prolongation of the QT interval occur. Advise to seek medical help immediately if experiencing seizures, palpitations, or breathing difficulty. Counsel to minimize or avoid exposure to natural/artificial sunlight (tanning beds or UVA/B treatment). Instruct to contact physician if low blood sugar occurs.

STORAGE: 25°C (77°F); excursions permitted to 15-30°C (59-86°F).

CIPRODEX – ciprofloxacin/dexamethasone

RX

Class: Antibacterial/corticosteroid combination

ADULT DOSAGE

Acute Otitis Externa

4 drops into the affected ear bid for 7 days

PEDIATRIC DOSAGE

Acute Otitis Media

≥6 Months of Age w/ Tympanostomy Tubes:
4 drops into the affected ear bid for 7 days

Acute Otitis Externa

≥6 Months of Age:
4 drops into the affected ear bid for 7 days

ADMINISTRATION

Otic route

Shake well immediately before use.

Instructions

1. Warm sus by holding bottle in hand for 1 or 2 min to avoid dizziness, which may result from instillation of cold sus.
2. Lie w/ affected ear upward, and then instill drops.
3. For treatment of otitis media in patients w/ tympanostomy tubes, the tragus should be pumped 5X by pushing inward to facilitate penetration of the drops into the middle ear.
4. Maintain position for 60 sec and repeat, if necessary, for the opposite ear.

HOW SUPPLIED

Otic Sus: (Ciprofloxacin/Dexamethasone) 0.3%/0.1% [7.5mL]

CONTRAINDICATIONS

History of hypersensitivity to ciprofloxacin, other quinolones, or any components in this medication. Viral infections of the external canal (eg, herpes simplex infections) and fungal otic infections.

WARNINGS/PRECAUTIONS

For otic use only; not for ophthalmic use, or for injection. D/C at 1st appearance of skin rash or any other sign of hypersensitivity. Serious and occasionally fatal hypersensitivity (anaphylactic) reactions reported in patients receiving systemic quinolones. Prolonged use may result in overgrowth of nonsusceptible bacteria and fungi; perform culture testing if infection is not improved after 1 week and d/c and institute alternative therapy if such infections occur. If otorrhea persists after full course of therapy, or if ≥2 episodes of otorrhea occur w/in 6 months, evaluate further to exclude an underlying condition (eg, cholesteatoma, foreign body, tumor)

ADVERSE REACTIONS

Ear discomfort/pain/precipitate/pruritus/debris/congestion, irritability, taste perversion, superimposed ear infection, erythema.

PATIENT CONSIDERATIONS

Assessment: Assess for history of drug hypersensitivity, viral infection of the external canal (eg, herpes simplex infections), fungal otic infections, and pregnancy/nursing status.

Monitoring: Monitor for hypersensitivity reactions, skin rash, overgrowth of nonsusceptible bacteria and fungi, continued/recurrent otorrhea, and other adverse reactions. Perform culture testing if infection is not improved after 1 week of treatment.

Counseling: Inform that drug is for otic use only. Advise to avoid contaminating the tip w/ material from the ear, fingers, or other sources. Instruct to d/c immediately and consult physician if rash or allergic reaction occurs. Advise to warm bottle in hand for 1-2 min prior to use and to shake well immediately before using. Instruct to take ud, even if symptoms improve. Instruct to protect product from light and to discard unused portion after therapy is completed.

STORAGE: 20-25°C (68-77°F); excursions permitted to 15-30°C (59-86°F). Avoid freezing. Protect from light.

CIPROFLOXACIN ORAL – ciprofloxacin

RX

Class: Fluoroquinolone

Fluoroquinolones are associated w/ an increased risk of tendinitis and tendon rupture in all ages. Risk is further increased in patients >60 yrs of age, patients taking corticosteroids, and patients w/ kidney, heart, or lung transplants. May exacerbate muscle weakness w/ myasthenia gravis; avoid in patients w/ known history of myasthenia gravis.

OTHER BRAND NAMES

Cipro

ADULT DOSAGE

Urinary Tract Infections

250-500mg q12h for 7-14 days

Uncomplicated Cystitis

Acute:
250mg q12h for 3 days

Chronic Bacterial Prostatitis

500mg q12h for 28 days

Lower Respiratory Tract Infections

500-750mg q12h for 7-14 days

Acute Bacterial Sinusitis

500mg q12h for 10 days

Skin and Skin Structure Infections

500-750mg q12h for 7-14 days

Bone/Joint Infections

500-750mg q12h for 4-8 weeks

Intra-Abdominal Infections

Complicated:
500mg q12h for 7-14 days, in conjunction w/ metronidazole

Diarrhea

Infectious:
500mg q12h for 5-7 days

Typhoid Fever

500mg q12h for 10 days

Gonococcal Infections

Uncomplicated Urethral and Cervical:
250mg single dose

Inhalational Anthrax (Postexposure)

500mg q12h for 60 days

Begin as soon as possible after suspected or confirmed exposure

PEDIATRIC DOSAGE

Urinary Tract Infections

Complicated UTIs or Pyelonephritis:
1-17 Years:
10-20mg/kg q12h for 10-21 days
Max: 750mg/dose; not to be exceeded even if >51kg

Inhalational Anthrax (Postexposure)

15mg/kg q12h for 60 days
Max: 500mg/dose

Begin as soon as possible after suspected or confirmed exposure

Plague

15mg/kg q8-12h for 10-21 days
Max: 500mg/dose

Begin as soon as possible after suspected or confirmed exposure

Plague

500-750mg q12h for 14 days

Begin as soon as possible after suspected or confirmed exposure

Conversions

Switching from IV to Oral:
200mg IV q12h: 250mg tab q12h
400mg IV q12h: 500mg tab q12h
400mg IV q8h: 750mg tab q12h

DOSING CONSIDERATIONS

Renal Impairment

Adults:
CrCl 30-50mL/min: 250-500mg q12h
CrCl 5-29mL/min: 250-500mg q18h
Hemodialysis/Peritoneal Dialysis: 250-500mg q24h (after dialysis)
Severe Impairment w/ Severe Infection: Unit dose of 750mg may be administered at intervals noted above

ADMINISTRATION

Oral route

Take w/ or w/o food.

Administer ≥2 hrs before or 6 hrs after Mg^{2+}/aluminum antacids; polymeric phosphate binders or sucralfate; Videx (didanosine) chewable/buffered tabs or pediatric powder for oral sol; other highly buffered drugs; or other products containing Ca^{2+}, iron, or zinc.

Avoid concomitant administration w/ dairy products or Ca^{2+}-fortified juices alone; may take w/ a meal that contains these products.

Assure adequate hydration.

Reconstitution

Pour the microcapsules completely into the larger bottle of diluent; do not add water to the sus. Close the larger bottle completely and shake vigorously for about 15 sec.

May store reconstituted product below 30°C (86°F) for 14 days; protect from freezing.

HOW SUPPLIED

Sus: (Cipro) 250mg/5mL, 500mg/5mL [100mL]; **Tab:** 100mg, 750mg; (Cipro) 250mg, 500mg

CONTRAINDICATIONS

History of hypersensitivity to ciprofloxacin, any member of the quinolone class of antibacterials, or any of the product components. Concomitant administration w/ tizanidine.

WARNINGS/PRECAUTIONS

Not a drug of 1st choice in the treatment of presumed or confirmed pneumonia secondary to *Streptococcus pneumoniae*. Not a drug of 1st choice in the pediatric population due to an increased incidence of adverse events. Caution w/ history of tendon disorders; d/c if patient experiences pain, swelling, inflammation, or rupture of tendon. Serious and occasionally fatal hypersensitivity (anaphylactic) reactions reported; d/c immediately at the 1st appearance of a skin rash, jaundice, or any sign of hypersensitivity, and institute supportive measures. Severe hepatotoxicity, including hepatic necrosis, life-threatening hepatic failure, and fatal events, reported; d/c immediately if signs and symptoms of hepatitis occur. Convulsions, status epilepticus, increased intracranial pressure (including pseudotumor cerebri), toxic psychosis, and other CNS events reported; d/c and institute appropriate measures if CNS events occur. Caution w/ epilepsy and CNS disorders (eg, severe cerebral arteriosclerosis, history of convulsion, reduced cerebral blood flow), or other risk factors that may predispose to seizures or lower the seizure threshold; d/c if seizures occur. *Clostridium difficile*-associated diarrhea (CDAD) reported; may need to d/c if CDAD is suspected or confirmed. Cases of sensory or sensorimotor axonal polyneuropathy resulting in paresthesias, hypoesthesias, dysesthesias, and weakness reported; d/c immediately if symptoms of peripheral neuropathy occur. May prolong the QT interval; avoid w/ known QT interval prolongation and risk factors for QT prolongation/torsades de pointes (eg, congenital long QT syndrome, uncorrected electrolyte imbalance, cardiac disease). Increased incidence of adverse reactions related to joints and/or surrounding tissues observed in pediatric patients. Crystalluria reported; maintain hydration and avoid alkalinity of urine. May cause photosensitivity/phototoxicity reactions; d/c if phototoxicity occurs. Avoid excessive exposure to sun/UV light. May result in bacterial resistance if used in the absence of a proven or strongly suspected bacterial infection or a prophylactic indication. Has not been shown to be effective in the treatment of syphilis; antimicrobial agents used in high dose for short periods to treat gonorrhea may mask or delay symptoms of incubating syphilis. Caution in elderly.

ADVERSE REACTIONS

N/V, diarrhea, abnormal LFTs, rash.

DRUG INTERACTIONS

See Boxed Warning and Contraindications. Avoid concomitant administration w/ dairy products (eg, milk, yogurt), or Ca^{2+}-fortified juices alone; absorption may be reduced. May increase levels of CYP1A2 substrates (eg, theophylline, methylxanthines, olanzapine), duloxetine, or sildenafil. Use w/ caution and monitor for sildenafil toxicity. Avoid use w/ duloxetine; if unavoidable, monitor for duloxetine toxicity. Increased theophylline levels may increase the risk of developing CNS or other adverse reactions; if coadministration cannot be avoided, monitor theophylline levels and adjust dose. May inhibit the formation of paraxanthine after caffeine administration (or pentoxifylline containing products); monitor for xanthine toxicity and adjust dose as necessary. Monitor for clozapine- or ropinirole-related adverse reactions and adjust dose of clozapine or ropinirole during and shortly after coadministration. Avoid w/ Class IA (eg, quinidine, procainamide) and Class III (eg, amiodarone, sotalol) antiarrhythmics, TCAs, macrolides, antipsychotics, and any other drug known to prolong the QT interval; may further prolong the QT interval. Hypoglycemia reported w/ oral antidiabetic agents, mainly sulfonylureas (eg, glyburide, glimepiride); monitor blood glucose. May alter serum levels of phenytoin; monitor phenytoin therapy, including phenytoin levels during and shortly after coadministration. Transient SrCr elevations w/ cyclosporine; monitor renal function. May increase effects of oral anticoagulants; monitor PT and INR frequently during and shortly after coadministration. May increase levels and toxic reactions of methotrexate; carefully monitor w/ concomitant use. High-dose quinolones in combination w/ NSAIDs (not acetyl salicylic acid) may provoke convulsions. Antacids, sucralfate, multivitamins, and other multivalent cation-containing products (eg, Mg^{2+}/aluminum antacids, polymeric phosphate binders, Videx [didanosine] chewable/buffered tab or pediatric powder, products containing Ca^{2+}, iron, or zinc; dairy product) may decrease absorption, resulting in lower serum and urine levels than desired; administer ≥2 hrs before or 6 hrs after multivalent cation-containing products administration. Probenecid may increase levels; use w/ caution. Caution w/ drugs that may lower seizure threshold.

PATIENT CONSIDERATIONS

Assessment: Assess for risk factors for developing tendinitis and tendon rupture, history of myasthenia gravis, drug hypersensitivity, epilepsy, CNS disorders or other risk factors that may predispose to seizures or lower seizure threshold, QT interval prolongation, renal dysfunction, previous liver damage, pregnancy/nursing status, and possible drug interactions. Obtain baseline culture and susceptibility tests. Perform serologic test for syphilis in patients w/ gonorrhea.

Monitoring: Monitor for tendinitis or tendon rupture, exacerbation of myasthenia gravis, signs/symptoms of hypersensitivity reactions, QT prolongations, CNS effects, CDAD, hepatotoxicity, peripheral neuropathy, musculoskeletal disorders (pediatric patients), crystalluria, photosensitivity/phototoxicity reactions, and other adverse reactions. Monitor PT and INR if coadministered w/ an oral anticoagulant (eg, warfarin). Monitor renal function. Perform periodic culture and susceptibility testing. Perform follow-up serologic test for syphilis after 3 months in patients w/ gonorrhea.

Counseling: Inform that drug treats only bacterial, not viral, infections. Instruct to take exactly ud; inform that skipping doses or not completing full course of therapy may decrease effectiveness and increase bacterial resistance. Advise to drink fluids liberally. Instruct to avoid concomitant use w/ dairy products or Ca^{2+}-fortified juices alone, but explain that drug may be taken w/ a meal that contains these products. Advise to notify physician if tendon disorder symptoms occur; instruct to d/c therapy and rest/refrain from exercise. Instruct to notify physician if myasthenia gravis, liver injury, or photosensitivity/phototoxicity symptoms occur. Instruct to notify physician of any history of convulsions. Advise to assess reaction to therapy before engaging in activities that require mental alertness or coordination; instruct to notify physician if persistent headache w/ or w/o blurred vision occurs. Advise to contact physician as soon as possible if watery and bloody stools (w/ or w/o stomach cramps and fever) develop even as late as ≥2 months after last dose. Instruct to d/c and notify physician if hypersensitivity reactions or symptoms of peripheral neuropathy develop. Instruct to inform physician of any personal or family history of QT prolongation or proarrhythmic conditions and if symptoms of prolongation of the QT interval occur. Counsel caregiver to inform physician if child has joint-related problems prior to, during, or after therapy. Advise to seek medical help immediately if experiencing seizures, palpitations, or breathing difficulty. Instruct to minimize or avoid exposure to natural/artificial sunlight (tanning beds or UVA/B treatment). Instruct to contact physician if low blood sugar occurs. Inform that efficacy studies of ciprofloxacin could not be conducted in humans w/ plague and anthrax for feasibility reasons and that approval for these conditions was therefore based on efficacy studies conducted in animals.

STORAGE: Tab: 20-25°C (68-77°F). (Cipro) Excursions permitted to 15-30°C (59-86°F). **Microcapsules and Diluent:** <25°C (77°F); excursions permitted from 15-30°C (59-86°F). **Reconstituted Sus:** 25°C (77°F); excursions permitted from 15-30°C (59-86°F). Store reconstituted product for 14 days. Protect from freezing.

CITALOPRAM — citalopram hydrobromide

RX

Class: Selective serotonin reuptake inhibitor (SSRI)

Antidepressants increased the risk of suicidal thinking and behavior (suicidality) in children, adolescents, and young adults in short-term studies of major depressive disorder and other psychiatric disorders. Monitor and observe closely for clinical worsening, suicidality, or unusual changes in behavior. Not approved for use in pediatric patients.

OTHER BRAND NAMES

Celexa

ADULT DOSAGE

Depression

Initial Treatment:
Initial: 20mg qd
Titrate: Increase dose to 40mg/day at an interval of no less than 1 week
Max: 40mg/day

Maint Treatment:
Consider decreasing dose to 20mg/day if adverse reactions are bothersome

Periodically reevaluate long-term usefulness of drug if used for extended periods

Dosing Considerations with MAOIs

Switching to/from an MAOI for Psychiatric Disorders:
Allow at least 14 days between discontinuation of an MAOI and initiation of treatment, and allow at least 14 days between discontinuation of treatment and initiation of an MAOI

W/ Other MAOIs (eg, Linezolid, IV Methylene Blue):
Do not start citalopram in patient being treated w/ linezolid or IV methylene blue
In patients already receiving citalopram, if acceptable alternatives are not available and benefits outweigh risks, d/c citalopram and administer linezolid or IV methylene blue; monitor for serotonin syndrome for 2 weeks or until 24 hrs after the last dose of linezolid or IV methylene blue, whichever comes 1st. May resume citalopram therapy 24 hrs after the last dose of linezolid or IV methylene blue

PEDIATRIC DOSAGE

Pediatric use may not have been established

DOSING CONSIDERATIONS

Concomitant Medications

Cimetidine or Another CYP2C19 Inhibitor:
Max: 20mg/day

Hepatic Impairment

Max: 20mg/day

Elderly

>60 Years:
Max: 20mg/day

Discontinuation

Gradually reduce dose to d/c; if intolerable symptoms occur following a decrease in dose or upon discontinuation of treatment, may consider resuming previously prescribed dose or continue decreasing dose at a more gradual rate

Other Important Considerations

CYP2C19 Poor Metabolizers:
Max: 20mg/day

ADMINISTRATION

Oral route

Administer qd, in am or pm, w/ or w/o food.

HOW SUPPLIED

Sol: 10mg/5mL [240mL]; **Tab:** (Celexa) 10mg, 20mg*, 40mg* *scored

C

CONTRAINDICATIONS

Use of an MAOI for psychiatric disorders either concomitantly or w/in 14 days of stopping treatment. Treatment w/in 14 days of stopping an MAOI for psychiatric disorders. Starting treatment in a patient being treated w/ MAOIs (eg, linezolid, IV methylene blue). Concomitant use w/ pimozide. Hypersensitivity to citalopram or any of the inactive ingredients in the medication.

WARNINGS/PRECAUTIONS

Not approved for the treatment of bipolar depression. May cause dose-dependent QTc prolongation. Avoid in patients w/ congenital long QT syndrome, bradycardia, hypokalemia or hypomagnesemia, recent acute MI (AMI), or uncompensated HF; monitor ECG if therapy is needed. Correct hypokalemia and/or hypomagnesemia prior to initiation of therapy and monitor periodically. D/C therapy w/ persistent QTc measurements >500 msec. May precipitate mixed/manic episode in patients at risk for bipolar disorder; screen for risk for bipolar disorder prior to initiating treatment. Serotonin syndrome reported; d/c immediately and initiate supportive symptomatic treatment. Pupillary dilation that occurs following use may trigger an angle-closure attack in a patient w/ anatomically narrow angles who does not have a patent iridectomy. Adverse events reported upon discontinuation; gradually reduce dose. May increase risk of bleeding events. Hyponatremia may occur; caution in elderly and volume-depleted patients. Consider discontinuation in patients w/ symptomatic hyponatremia and institute appropriate medical intervention. Activation of mania/hypomania reported; caution w/ history of mania. Seizures reported; caution w/ history of seizure disorder. Caution w/ hepatic impairment, severe renal impairment, and in pregnancy (3rd trimester). May impair mental/physical abilities.

ADVERSE REACTIONS

N/V, dyspepsia, diarrhea, dry mouth, somnolence, insomnia, increased sweating, ejaculation disorder, fatigue, URTI, rhinitis, anxiety, anorexia, tremor, agitation.

DRUG INTERACTIONS

See Contraindications and Dosage. Avoid w/ alcohol and drugs that prolong the QTc interval (eg, Class 1A [eg, quinidine, procainamide] or Class III [eg, amiodarone, sotalol] antiarrhythmic medications, antipsychotic medications [eg, chlorpromazine, thioridazine], antibiotics [eg, gatifloxacin, moxifloxacin], pentamidine, levomethadyl acetate, methadone). Caution w/ other centrally acting drugs or TCAs (eg, imipramine). Risk of QT prolongation w/ CYP2C19 inhibitors (eg, cimetidine). May cause serotonin syndrome w/ other serotonergic drugs (eg, triptans, TCAs, fentanyl) and w/ drugs that impair metabolism of serotonin; d/c immediately if this occurs. Risk of bleeding may be increased w/ aspirin, NSAIDs, warfarin, and other drugs that affect coagulation. May increase PT w/ warfarin. Monitor lithium levels and adjust its dose appropriately. Rare reports of weakness, hyperreflexia, and incoordination w/ sumatriptan. Possible increased clearance w/ carbamazepine. May decrease levels of ketoconazole. May increase levels of metoprolol. Increased risk of hyponatremia w/ diuretics.

PATIENT CONSIDERATIONS

Assessment: Assess for drug hypersensitivity, risk for bipolar disorder, history of mania, history of seizures, susceptibility to angle-closure glaucoma, volume depletion, congenital long QT syndrome, hypokalemia, hypomagnesemia, bradycardia, recent AMI, uncompensated HF, hepatic/renal impairment, pregnancy/nursing status, and possible drug interactions. Obtain baseline serum K^+ and Mg^{2+} measurements for patients being considered for therapy who are at risk for significant electrolyte disturbances.

Monitoring: Monitor for signs/symptoms of clinical worsening, suicidality, unusual changes in behavior, serotonin syndrome, bleeding events, hyponatremia, seizures, angle-closure glaucoma, activation of mania/hypomania, discontinuation symptoms, and other adverse reactions. Monitor electrolytes in patients w/ diseases or conditions that cause hypokalemia or hypomagnesemia. Monitor ECG in patients w/ cardiac conditions/disorders and in patients on concomitant QTc interval prolonging agents. Periodically reevaluate long-term usefulness.

Counseling: Inform about risks, benefits, and appropriate use of therapy. Caution about operating hazardous machinery, including automobiles, until reasonably certain that therapy does not affect ability to engage in such activities. Inform about serotonin syndrome and bleeding risks. Caution about risk of angle-closure glaucoma. Instruct to avoid alcohol. Advise to notify physician if taking or planning to take any prescription or OTC drugs. Instruct to notify physician if pregnant, intending to become pregnant, or breastfeeding. Encourage to be alert to unusual changes in behavior, worsening of depression, and suicidal ideation, especially early during treatment and when dose is adjusted up/down; instruct to report such symptoms, especially if severe, abrupt in onset, or not part of presenting symptoms.

STORAGE: (Tab) 25°C (77°F); excursions permitted to 15-30°C (59-86°F). (Sol) 20-25°C (68-77°F); excursions permitted to 15-30°C (59-86°F).

CLARINEX-D – desloratadine/pseudoephedrine sulfate

RX

Class: H_1 antagonist/sympathomimetic amine

ADULT DOSAGE

Seasonal Allergic Rhinitis

Relief of Nasal and Non-Nasal Symptoms, Including Nasal Congestion:

12 Hour:

Usual/Max: 1 tab bid, approx 12 hrs apart

24 Hour:

Usual/Max: 1 tab qd

PEDIATRIC DOSAGE

Seasonal Allergic Rhinitis

Relief of Nasal and Non-Nasal Symptoms, Including Nasal Congestion:

≥12 Years:

12 Hour:

Usual/Max: 1 tab bid, approx 12 hrs apart

24 Hour:

Usual/Max: 1 tab qd

ADMINISTRATION

Oral route

Take w/ or w/o a meal

Swallow tab whole; do not break, chew, or crush

HOW SUPPLIED

Tab, Extended-Release: (Desloratadine/Pseudoephedrine) (12 Hour) 2.5mg/120mg, (24 Hour) 5mg/240mg

CONTRAINDICATIONS

Narrow-angle glaucoma, urinary retention, MAOI therapy or within 14 days of stopping an MAOI, severe HTN, or severe coronary artery disease (CAD). Hypersensitivity to any of its ingredients, or to loratadine.

WARNINGS/PRECAUTIONS

Can produce cardiovascular (CV) and CNS effects (eg, insomnia, dizziness, weakness, tremor, arrhythmias). CNS stimulation with convulsions or CV collapse with hypotension reported. Caution with CV disorders, diabetes, hyperthyroidism, prostatic hypertrophy, or increased intraocular pressure (IOP). Hypersensitivity reactions (eg, rash, pruritus, urticaria, edema, dyspnea, anaphylaxis) reported; d/c and consider alternative treatment if this occurs. Avoid in patients with hepatic/renal impairment. Caution in elderly patients.

ADVERSE REACTIONS

Dry mouth, headache, insomnia, fatigue, pharyngitis, somnolence, dizziness.

DRUG INTERACTIONS

See Contraindications. May reduce the antihypertensive effects of β-adrenergic blocking agents, methyldopa, and reserpine; use caution with these agents. Increased ectopic pacemaker activity may occur with concomitant digitalis; use caution with these agents.

PATIENT CONSIDERATIONS

Assessment: Assess for drug hypersensitivity, increased IOP, prostatic hypertrophy, CV disorders, diabetes, hyperthyroidism, narrow-angle glaucoma, urinary retention, HTN, CAD, hepatic/renal impairment, pregnancy/nursing status, and possible drug interactions.

Monitoring: Monitor for CV/CNS effects, hypersensitivity reactions, and other adverse reactions. Monitor for urinary retention and narrow-angle glaucoma in patients with prostatic hypertrophy or increased IOP.

Counseling: Inform that CV or CNS effects may occur. Advise not to increase the dose or dosing frequency. Advise not to use with other antihistamines and/or decongestants. Advise not to use with an MAOI or within 14 days of stopping an MAOI. Advise patients with severe HTN or severe CAD, narrow-angle glaucoma, or urinary retention not to use this drug.

STORAGE: 25°C (77°F); excursions permitted to 15-30°C (59-86°F). Heat sensitive; avoid exposure at or >30°C (86°F). Protect from excessive moisture and light.

CLEOCIN – clindamycin

RX

Class: Lincomycin derivative

***Clostridium difficile*-associated diarrhea (CDAD) reported and may range in severity from mild diarrhea to fatal colitis. Due to the association w/ severe colitis, which may be fatal, reserve use for serious infections where less toxic agents are inappropriate. Not for use w/ nonbacterial infections such as most URTIs. CDAD must be considered in all patients w/ diarrhea following antibiotic use. Careful medical history is necessary since CDAD has been reported to occur over 2 months after the administration of antibacterial agents. If CDAD is suspected or confirmed, ongoing antibiotic use not directed against *C. difficile* may need to be discontinued. Appropriate fluid and electrolyte management, protein supplementation, antibiotic treatment of *C. difficile*, and surgical evaluation should be instituted as clinically indicated.**

OTHER BRAND NAMES
Cleocin Pediatric

ADULT DOSAGE

Serious Infections

Respiratory tract/skin and skin structure/intra-abdominal/gynecological infections and septicemia; (IV) bone and joint infections and adjunctive therapy in the surgical treatment of chronic bone and joint infections

Cap:
150-300mg PO q6h
More Severe: 300-450mg PO q6h

Inj:
Aerobic Gram-Positive Cocci and More Susceptible Anaerobes:
600-1200mg/day IV/IM given in 2, 3, or 4 equal doses
More Severe (Particularly Due to *Bacteroides fragilis, Peptococcus* species, or *Clostridium* species other than *Clostridium perfringens*):
1200-2700mg/day IV/IM given in 2, 3, or 4 equal doses
More Serious/Life-Threatening:
May have to increase dose; as much as 4800mg/day IV have been given
Single IM inj >600mg are not recommended

Alternative Administration:
Administer 1st dose as a single rapid infusion, followed by continuous IV infusion as follows:
To Maintain Serum Clindamycin Levels >4mcg/mL:
Rapid Infusion Rate: 10mg/min for 30 min
Maint Infusion Rate: 0.75mg/min

To Maintain Serum Clindamycin Levels >5mcg/mL:
Rapid Infusion Rate: 15mg/min for 30 min
Maint Infusion Rate: 1mg/min

To Maintain Serum Clindamycin Levels >6mcg/mL:
Rapid Infusion Rate: 20mg/min for 30 min
Maint Infusion Rate: 1.25mg/min

β-Hemolytic Streptococcal Infection:
Continue treatment for at least 10 days

PEDIATRIC DOSAGE

Serious Infections

Cap:
8-16mg/kg/day (4-8mg/lb/day) PO divided into 3 or 4 equal doses
More Severe: 16-20mg/kg/day (8-10mg/lb/day) PO divided into 3 or 4 equal doses

Oral Sol:
8-12mg/kg/day (4-6mg/lb/day) PO divided into 3 or 4 equal doses
Severe: 13-16mg/kg/day (6.5-8mg/lb/day) PO divided into 3 or 4 equal doses
More Severe: 17-25mg/kg/day (8.5-12.5mg/lb/day) PO divided into 3 or 4 equal doses

≤10kg:
Minimum Dose: 1/2 tsp (37.5mg) tid

Inj:
Neonates (<1 Month):
15-20mg/kg/day given in 3-4 equal doses; lower dosage may be adequate for small prematures

1 Month-16 Years:
20-40mg/kg/day IV/IM given in 3 or 4 equal doses; use higher dose for more severe infections
Alternative Dosing:
350mg/m²/day for serious infections; 450mg/m²/day for more severe infections

β-Hemolytic Streptococcal Infection:
Continue treatment for at least 10 days

ADMINISTRATION
Oral/IM/IV route

Cap
Take w/ full glass of water to avoid esophageal irritation.

Oral Sol
Reconstitute 100mL bottles w/ 75mL of water.
Do not refrigerate the reconstituted sol; stable at room temperature for 2 weeks.
Reconstitution Instructions:
1. Add a large portion of water and shake vigorously.
2. Add the remainder of the water and shake until sol is uniform.

Inj
IM administration should be used undiluted.
IV administration should be diluted.

Dilution for IV Use and IV Infusion Rates:
Concentration of clindamycin in diluent should not exceed 18mg/mL.
Infusion rates should not exceed 30mg/min.
300mg Dose: Dilute w/ 50mL; infuse over 10 min
600mg Dose: Dilute w/ 50mL; infuse over 20 min
900mg Dose: Dilute w/ 50-100mL; infuse over 30 min
1200mg Dose: Dilute w/ 100mL; infuse over 40 min
Administration of >1200mg in a single 1-hr infusion is not recommended.

C

Physical Incompatibilities:
Ampicillin sodium, phenytoin sodium, barbiturates, aminophylline, calcium gluconate, and magnesium sulfate.

Do not add supplementary medication to Galaxy container.
Refer to PI for stability information regarding diluted sol and further directions for use.

HOW SUPPLIED

Cap: (HCl) 75mg, 150mg, 300mg; **Inj:** (Phosphate) 150mg/mL [2mL, 4mL, 6mL vial]; 150mg/mL [2mL, 4mL, 6mL ADD-Vantage vial]; 300mg/50mL, 600mg/50mL, 900mg/50mL [Galaxy plastic container]; (Pediatric) **Oral Sol:** (Palmitate HCl) 75mg/5mL [100mL]

CONTRAINDICATIONS

History of hypersensitivity to preparations containing clindamycin or lincomycin.

WARNINGS/PRECAUTIONS

D/C use if significant diarrhea occurs during therapy. Reserve use for penicillin (PCN)-allergic patients or other patients for whom a PCN is inappropriate. Severe hypersensitivity reactions, including severe skin reactions (eg, toxic epidermal necrolysis, drug reaction w/ eosinophilia and systemic symptoms [DRESS], and Stevens-Johnson syndrome), reported; permanently d/c treatment in case of such an event. May increase bacterial resistance if used in the absence of a proven/strongly suspected bacterial infection or a prophylactic indication; take appropriate measures if superinfection develops. Not for treatment of meningitis. Caution w/ severe liver disease, history of GI disease (eg, colitis), and in atopic or elderly patients. Indicated surgical procedures should be performed in conjunction w/ antibiotic therapy. **Cap (75mg, 150mg):** Contains tartrazine, which may cause allergic-type reactions (eg, bronchial asthma); caution w/ aspirin hypersensitivity. **Inj:** Do not inject IV undiluted as bolus; infuse over at least 10-60 min. Contains benzyl alcohol; benzyl alcohol preservative has been associated w/ serious adverse events, including "gasping syndrome" and death in pediatric patients. Premature infants and low birth weight infants may be more likely to develop benzyl alcohol toxicity.

ADVERSE REACTIONS

Abdominal pain, pseudomembranous colitis, N/V, maculopapular skin rash, pruritus, vaginitis, jaundice, abnormal LFTs, transient neutropenia, eosinophilia, DRESS, azotemia, oliguria, polyarthritis.

DRUG INTERACTIONS

May enhance the action of neuromuscular blockers; use w/ caution. Antagonism reported between clindamycin and erythromycin; avoid concurrent use.

PATIENT CONSIDERATIONS

Assessment: Assess for history of hypersensitivity to drug or lincomycin, aspirin hypersensitivity, history of GI disease, presence of meningitis, atopy, and possible drug interactions. Assess hepatic function and pregnancy/nursing status. Obtain baseline culture and susceptibility tests.

Monitoring: Monitor for CDAD, superinfection, allergic reactions, severe skin reactions, and other adverse reactions. Monitor for changes in bowel frequency in older patients w/ severe illness. If available, consider culture and susceptibility information when modifying antibacterial therapy. If on prolonged therapy, perform periodic LFTs, renal function tests, and blood counts. Perform periodic liver enzyme determinations in patients w/ severe liver disease.

Counseling: Inform about potential benefits/risks of therapy. Inform that therapy only treats bacterial, not viral, infections. Instruct to take exactly ud and inform that skipping doses or not completing full course may decrease effectiveness and increase likelihood of bacterial resistance. Instruct to contact physician if an allergic reaction develops. Inform that diarrhea is a common problem; instruct to contact physician if watery and bloody stools (w/ or w/o stomach cramps and fever) occur, even as late as ≥2 months after last dose of therapy. Advise to notify physician if pregnant/nursing.

STORAGE: 20-25°C (68-77°F). **Inj:** (Galaxy Container) 25°C (77°F); avoid temperatures >30°C (86°F).

CLEOCIN VAGINAL – clindamycin phosphate

RX

Class: Lincomycin derivative

ADULT DOSAGE

Bacterial Vaginosis

Cre:

Nonpregnant and Pregnant Women During 2nd and 3rd Trimesters:

1 applicatorful (5g) intravaginally qhs for 3 or 7 consecutive days in nonpregnant patients and for 7 consecutive days in pregnant patients

Sup:

Nonpregnant:

1 sup intravaginally qhs for 3 consecutive days

PEDIATRIC DOSAGE

Bacterial Vaginosis

Postmenarchal:

1 sup intravaginally qhs for 3 consecutive days

C

ADMINISTRATION

Intravaginal route

Instructions for Use

Cre:

1. Remove cap from cre tube; screw a plastic applicator on the threaded end of the tube.
2. Rolling tube from the bottom, squeeze gently and force the medication into the applicator; applicator is filled when the plunger reaches its predetermined stopping point.
3. Unscrew the applicator from the tube and replace the cap.
4. Firmly grasp the applicator barrel and insert into vagina as far as possible w/o causing discomfort while lying on your back.
5. Slowly push the plunger until it stops.
6. Carefully withdraw applicator from vagina, and discard applicator.

Sup:

W/ Applicator:

1. Remove the ovule from its packaging.
2. Pull back the plunger about an inch and place the ovule in the wider end of the applicator barrel.
3. Gently insert the end of the applicator into the vagina as far as it will go comfortably while lying on back w/ knees bent, or while standing w/ feet apart and knees bent.
4. While holding the barrel of the applicator in place, push the plunger in until it stops to release the ovule.
5. Remove the applicator from the vagina and lie down as soon as possible to minimize leakage.
6. Clean the applicator after each use; pull the 2 pieces apart and wash them w/ soap and warm water then rinse well and dry.

W/O Applicator:

1. Hold the ovule w/ thumb and a finger and insert it into the vagina.
2. Gently push the ovule into the vagina as far as it will comfortably go.
3. Lie down as soon as possible to minimize leakage.

HOW SUPPLIED

Cre: 2% [40g]; **Sup:** (Ovules) 100mg [3^{s}]

CONTRAINDICATIONS

History of hypersensitivity to clindamycin, lincomycin, or any components of the medication. History of regional enteritis, ulcerative colitis, or a history of antibiotic-associated colitis.

WARNINGS/PRECAUTIONS

Diarrhea, bloody diarrhea, and colitis (including pseudomembranous colitis) reported w/ oral, parenteral, and topical formulations; consider this diagnosis in patients who present w/ diarrhea subsequent to clindamycin administration. May cause overgrowth of nonsusceptible organisms in the vagina. Use only during the 1st trimester of pregnancy if clearly needed. **Cre:** Burning and irritation of the eye may occur w/ accidental contact.

ADVERSE REACTIONS

Cre: Vulvovaginal disorder, vulvovaginitis, vaginal moniliasis.
Sup: Vulvovaginal disorder.

DRUG INTERACTIONS

Systemic clindamycin may enhance the action of neuromuscular blocking agents; use w/ caution.

PATIENT CONSIDERATIONS

Assessment: Assess for clinical diagnosis of bacterial vaginosis, history of hypersensitivity to the drug or lincomycin, history of regional enteritis, ulcerative colitis, history of antibiotic-associated colitis, pregnancy/nursing status, and for possible drug interactions.

Monitoring: Monitor for signs/symptoms of diarrhea, colitis, overgrowth of nonsusceptible organisms, burning/irritation of the eye, and other adverse reactions.

Counseling: Instruct not to engage in vaginal intercourse, or use other vaginal products (eg, tampons, douches) during therapy. Inform that product contains mineral oil/oleaginous base that may weaken latex or rubber products (eg, condoms, vaginal contraceptive diaphragms); instruct not to use such products w/in 72 hrs following treatment.
Cre: Instruct to rinse the eye w/ copious amounts of cool tap water if accidental contact w/ the eye occurs.

STORAGE: **Cre:** 20-25°C (68-77°F). Protect from freezing. **Sup:** 25°C (77°F); excursions permitted to 15-30°C (59-86°F). Avoid heat >30°C (86°F). Avoid high humidity.

Cleviprex – clevidipine

RX

Class: Calcium channel blocker (CCB) (dihydropyridine)

ADULT DOSAGE

Hypertension

Oral Therapy Not Feasible/Desirable:

Initial: 1-2mg/hr
Titrate: May double the dose at 90-sec intervals initially; as BP approaches goal, increase in doses should be less than doubling and the time between dose adjustments should be lengthened to every 5-10 min
Maint: 4-6mg/hr
Max: 1000mL or 21mg/hr per 24 hrs

PEDIATRIC DOSAGE

Pediatric use may not have been established

DOSING CONSIDERATIONS

Elderly

Start at the lower end of dosing range

Discontinuation

Transition to PO Therapy:

D/C or titrate downward until PO therapy is established
Consider the lag time of onset of the PO agent's effect when PO antihypertensive is instituted
Continue BP monitoring until desired effect is reached

ADMINISTRATION

IV route

Compatible IV Sol

Water for Inj
0.9% NaCl Inj
Dextrose 5% Inj
Dextrose 5% in NaCl Inj
Dextrose 5% in Ringer's Lactate Inj
Lactated Ringer's Inj
10% amino acid

Administration Instructions

Use within 12 hrs once the stopper is punctured; discard any unused portion
Invert vial gently several times before use
Administer using an infusion device allowing calibrated infusion rates
Commercially available standard plastic cannulae may be used to administer infusion
Administer via central or peripheral line
Should not be diluted

HOW SUPPLIED

Inj: 0.5mg/mL [50mL, 100mL, 250mL]

CONTRAINDICATIONS

Allergies to soybeans, eggs, soy or egg products, severe aortic stenosis, defective lipid metabolism (eg, pathologic hyperlipemia, lipoid nephrosis, or acute pancreatitis if it is accompanied by hyperlipidemia).

WARNINGS/PRECAUTIONS

Systemic hypotension and reflex tachycardia may occur; decrease dose if either occurs. Lipid intake restrictions may be necessary with significant disorders of lipid metabolism; a reduction in the quantity of concurrently administered lipids may be necessary to compensate for the amount of lipid infused as part of the drug's formulation. May produce negative inotropic effects and exacerbation of heart failure (HF). Does not reduce HR and does not protect against the effects of abrupt β-blocker withdrawal. Monitor for the possibility of rebound HTN for at least 8 hrs after discontinuation of infusion in patients who receive prolonged infusions and are not transitioned to other antihypertensive therapies. Caution in elderly.

ADVERSE REACTIONS

Atrial fibrillation, acute renal failure, headache, N/V.

PATIENT CONSIDERATIONS

Assessment: Assess for allergies to soybeans, eggs or soy/egg products, defective lipid metabolism, β-blocker usage, and pregnancy/nursing status. Obtain baseline parameters for BP, HR, and lipid profile.

Monitoring: Monitor for hypotension, reflex tachycardia, rebound HTN, HF exacerbation, and other adverse reactions. Monitor BP and HR during infusion, and until vital signs are stable.

Counseling: Advise patients with underlying HTN that they require continued follow up for their medical condition, and, if applicable, to continue taking oral antihypertensive medication(s) ud. Instruct to report any signs of new hypertensive emergency (eg, neurological symptoms, visual changes, evidence of congestive HF) to a healthcare provider immediately.

STORAGE: 2-8°C (36-46°F). Do not freeze. Leave vials in cartons until use; may be transferred to 25°C (77°F) for a period not to exceed 2 months. Do not return to refrigerated storage after beginning room temperature storage. Discard any unused portion within 12 hrs of stopper puncture.

CLOBETASOL – clobetasol propionate RX

Class: Corticosteroid

ADULT DOSAGE

Inflammatory and Pruritic Manifestations of Corticosteroid-Responsive Dermatoses

Cre/Gel/Oint:

Apply a thin layer to affected skin areas bid and rub in gently and completely

Max: 50g/week; limit treatment to 2 consecutive weeks

D/C therapy when control is achieved; reassess diagnosis if no improvement is seen w/in 2 weeks

Moderate to Severe Dermatoses of the Scalp: Sol:

Apply to affected scalp areas bid (am and pm)

Max: 50mL/week; limit treatment to 2 consecutive weeks

PEDIATRIC DOSAGE

Inflammatory and Pruritic Manifestations of Corticosteroid-Responsive Dermatoses

≥12 Years:

Cre/Gel/Oint:

Apply a thin layer to affected skin areas bid and rub in gently and completely

Max: 50g/week; limit treatment to 2 consecutive weeks

D/C therapy when control is achieved; reassess diagnosis if no improvement is seen w/in 2 weeks

Moderate to Severe Dermatoses of the Scalp: Sol:

Apply to affected scalp areas bid (am and pm)

Max: 50mL/week; limit treatment to 2 consecutive weeks

ADMINISTRATION

Topical route

Avoid use w/ occlusive dressings

HOW SUPPLIED

Cre/Oint: 0.05% [15g, 30g, 45g, 60g]; **Gel:** 0.05% [15g, 30g, 60g]; **Sol:** 0.05% [50mL]

CONTRAINDICATIONS

History of hypersensitivity to any of the components of the preparations. (Sol) Primary infections of the scalp.

WARNINGS/PRECAUTIONS

Systemic absorption may produce reversible hypothalamic-pituitary-adrenal (HPA) axis suppression, manifestations of Cushing's syndrome, hyperglycemia, and glucosuria. Application of more potent corticosteroids, use over large surface areas, prolonged use, and the addition of occlusive dressings may augment systemic absorption. Evaluate periodically for evidence of HPA axis suppression when large dose is applied to large surface area or under occlusive dressings; if noted, withdraw treatment, reduce frequency of application, or substitute w/ a less potent steroid. Infrequently, signs/symptoms of steroid withdrawal may occur, requiring supplemental systemic corticosteroids. Pediatric patients may be more susceptible to systemic toxicity. D/C and institute appropriate therapy if irritation develops. Use appropriate antifungal or antibacterial agent if concomitant skin infections are present or develop; if favorable response does not occur promptly, d/c until infection is controlled. Not for use in rosacea and perioral dermatitis. Caution in elderly. (Cre/Gel/Oint) Allergic contact dermatitis may occur; confirm by patch testing. Do not use on the face, groin, or axillae. (Sol) Certain areas of the body (eg, face, groin, axillae) are more prone to atrophic changes than other areas of the body following therapy; monitor frequently if these areas are to be treated. Should not be used for acne treatment or as sole therapy in widespread plaque psoriasis. May cause eye irritation if sol contacts the eye; flush eye w/ a large volume of water immediately.

ADVERSE REACTIONS

Burning/stinging sensation, irritation, itching, folliculitis. (Sol) Scalp pustules, tingling.

PATIENT CONSIDERATIONS

Assessment: Assess for hypersensitivity to the drug, conditions that augment systemic absorption, concomitant skin infections, rosacea, perioral dermatitis, and pregnancy/nursing status. (Sol) Assess for primary infections of the scalp, acne, and widespread plaque psoriasis.

Monitoring: Monitor for signs/symptoms of HPA axis suppression, Cushing's syndrome, hyperglycemia, glucosuria, skin irritation, and other adverse reactions. Perform periodic monitoring of HPA axis suppression by using urinary free cortisol and adrenocorticotropic hormone stimulation tests.

Counseling: Instruct to use externally and ud, to avoid contact w/ eyes, and not to use for any disorder other than that for which it was prescribed. Counsel not to bandage, cover, or wrap treated skin area, unless directed by physician. Advise to report any signs of local adverse reactions to physician. (Cre/Gel/Oint) Instruct to inform physician of clobetasol use if contemplating surgery.

STORAGE: (Cre/Gel/Oint) 15-30°C (59-86°F). Do not refrigerate. (Sol) 20-25°C (68-77°F); excursions permitted to 15-30°C (59-86°F). Do not refrigerate or use near an open flame.

Clomid — clomiphene citrate

RX

Class: Ovulatory stimulant

OTHER BRAND NAMES

Serophene

ADULT DOSAGE

Ovulatory Dysfunction

Initial: 50mg qd for 5 days

If progestin-induced bleeding is planned, or if spontaneous uterine bleeding occurs prior to therapy, start on 5th day of cycle; may start at any time if w/o recent uterine bleeding

Titrate: Increase to 100mg qd for 5 days only in patients who do not ovulate in response to cyclic 50mg after the 1st course of therapy; may start as early as 30 days after 1st course

Max: 100mg/day for 5 days

Long-term cyclic therapy beyond a total of 6 cycles is not recommended

If ovulation does not occur after 3 courses of therapy or if 3 ovulatory responses occur but pregnancy is not achieved, further treatment is not recommended

If menses does not occur after an ovulatory response, reevaluate patient

PEDIATRIC DOSAGE

Pediatric use may not have been established

DOSING CONSIDERATIONS

Other Important Considerations

Polycystic Ovary Syndrome (PCOS)/Unusual Pituitary Gonadotropin Sensitivity:
Use lowest recommended dose and shortest treatment duration for the 1st course of therapy

ADMINISTRATION

Oral route

HOW SUPPLIED

Tab: 50mg* *scored

CONTRAINDICATIONS

Known hypersensitivity or allergy to clomiphene or to any of its components, pregnancy, liver disease or history of liver dysfunction, abnormal uterine bleeding of undetermined origin, ovarian cysts or enlargement not due to PCOS, uncontrolled thyroid or adrenal dysfunction or in the presence of an organic intracranial lesion (eg, pituitary tumor).

WARNINGS/PRECAUTIONS

Workup and treatment should be supervised by physician experienced in management of gynecologic or endocrine disorders. Visual symptoms (eg, blurring, spots, flashes), some occurring after discontinuation of therapy, reported; d/c treatment and perform complete ophthalmological evaluation promptly if visual symptoms develop. Visual disturbances may be irreversible, especially w/ increased dosage or duration of therapy. Ovarian hyperstimulation syndrome (OHSS), which may progress rapidly (w/in 24 hrs to several days) reported; monitor for abdominal pain/distention, N/V, diarrhea, weight gain, and for other warning signs. If conception results, rapid progression to severe form of the syndrome may occur. Use lowest effective dose consistent w/ expected clinical results to minimize the hazard of abnormal ovarian enlargement. If ovarian enlargement occurs, do not give additional therapy until the ovaries have returned to pretreatment size, and reduce the dosage or duration of the next course. Ovarian enlargement and cyst formation usually regresses spontaneously w/in a few days or weeks after discontinuing treatment; manage cystic enlargement conservatively unless surgical indication for laparotomy exists. Perform a thorough evaluation to rule out ovarian neoplasia if ovarian cysts do not regress spontaneously. Prolonged use may increase risk of borderline/invasive ovarian tumor. Perform pelvic exam prior to initiating therapy and before each subsequent course. Carefully evaluate to exclude pregnancy, ovarian enlargement, or ovarian cyst formation between each treatment cycle. Caution w/ uterine fibroids; potential for further enlargement.

ADVERSE REACTIONS

Ovarian enlargement, vasomotor flushes, abdominal-pelvic discomfort/distention/bloating.

PATIENT CONSIDERATIONS

Assessment: Assess for hypersensitivity to drug, ovarian cysts/enlargement, abnormal vaginal/uterine bleeding, presence of organic intracranial lesion, primary pituitary/ovarian failure, endometriosis/endometrial carcinoma, liver disease or history of liver dysfunction, impediments to pregnancy (eg, thyroid/adrenal disorders, hyperprolactinemia, male factor infertility), uterine fibroids, preexisting or family history of hyperlipidemia, and pregnancy/nursing status. Perform pelvic exam prior to treatment. Assess estrogen levels.

Monitoring: Monitor for signs/symptoms of visual symptoms (eg, blurring, spots, flashes), OHSS, ovarian neoplasia, and other adverse reactions. Monitor plasma TG levels periodically in patients w/ preexisting or family history of hyperlipidemia. Exclude pregnancy, ovarian enlargement, or ovarian cyst formation between each treatment cycle. Perform pelvic exam before each subsequent course.

Counseling: Advise that blurring or other visual symptoms may occur during or shortly after therapy and inform that in some instances, visual disturbances may be prolonged, and possibly irreversible, especially w/ increased dosage or duration of therapy. Advise that visual symptoms may render such activities as driving a car or operating machinery more hazardous than usual, particularly under conditions of variable lighting. Instruct to inform physician whenever any unusual visual symptoms occur and to d/c therapy. Advise that ovarian enlargement may occur during or shortly after therapy; instruct to inform physician if any abdominal/pelvic pain, weight gain, discomfort, or distention occurs after taking therapy. Inform that preexisting or family history of hyperlipidemia and use of higher than recommended dose and/or longer duration of treatment may increase risk of hypertriglyceridemia. Inform of the increased chance of multiple pregnancy (eg, bilateral tubal pregnancy, coexisting tubal and intrauterine pregnancy), and the potential complications/hazards of multiple pregnancy.

STORAGE: 15-30°C (59-86°F). Protect from heat, light, and excessive humidity.

CLONAZEPAM – clonazepam

CIV

Class: Benzodiazepine

OTHER BRAND NAMES

Klonopin

ADULT DOSAGE

Seizures

Treatment of Lennox-Gastaut syndrome (petit mal variant), akinetic, and myoclonic seizures. May be useful in patients w/ absence seizures (petit mal) who have failed to respond to succinimides

Initial: Not to exceed 1.5mg/day divided into 3 doses
Titrate: May increase in increments of 0.5-1mg every 3 days until seizures are controlled or until side effects preclude any further increase
Maint: Individualize dose
Max: 20mg/day

Panic Disorder

Initial: 0.25mg bid
Titrate: May increase to target dose of 1mg/day after 3 days; for some, may increase in increments of 0.125-0.25mg bid every 3 days until panic disorder is controlled or until side effects make further increases undesired
Max: 4mg/day

PEDIATRIC DOSAGE

Seizures

Treatment of Lennox-Gastaut syndrome (petit mal variant), akinetic, and myoclonic seizures. May be useful in patients w/ absence seizures (petit mal) who have failed to respond to succinimides

≤10 Years or ≤30kg:
Initial: 0.01-0.03mg/kg/day up to 0.05mg/kg/day given in 2 or 3 divided doses
Titrate: May increase by no more than 0.25-0.5mg every 3 days until daily maintenance dose is reached, unless seizures are controlled or until side effects preclude further increase
Maint: 0.1-0.2mg/kg/day divided into 3 doses. Whenever possible, divide daily dose into 3 equal doses; give the largest dose qhs if doses are not equally divided

ADMINISTRATION

Oral route

To reduce somnolence, may give 1 dose at hs.

Tab, Disintegrating

Peel back foil on blister; do not push tab through foil.
Using dry hands, remove tab and place it in mouth.

Tab

Swallow whole w/ water.

HOW SUPPLIED

Tab, Disintegrating: 0.125mg, 0.25mg, 0.5mg, 1mg, 2mg; (Klonopin) **Tab:** 0.5mg*, 1mg, 2mg *scored

CONTRAINDICATIONS

History of sensitivity to benzodiazepines, significant liver disease, acute narrow angle glaucoma.

WARNINGS/PRECAUTIONS

May be used with treated open angle glaucoma. May impair mental/physical abilities. May increase risk of suicidal thoughts/behavior. Caution with use in pregnancy and women of childbearing potential; may increase risk of congenital malformations. Avoid use during the 1st trimester of pregnancy. May increase incidence or precipitate the onset of generalized tonic-clonic seizures in patients in whom several different types of seizure disorders coexist; addition of appropriate anticonvulsants or increase in their dosages may be required. Withdrawal symptoms reported after discontinuation. Abrupt withdrawal of therapy may precipitate status epilepticus; gradual withdrawal is essential, and simultaneous substitution of another anticonvulsant may be indicated while therapy is being gradually withdrawn. May produce an increase in salivation; caution with chronic respiratory diseases. Caution with renal impairment, addiction-prone individuals, and in elderly. (Tab, Disintegrating) Contains phenylalanine.

ADVERSE REACTIONS

CNS depression, ataxia, drowsiness, abnormal coordination, depression, somnolence, behavior problems, dizziness, URTI, memory disturbance, dysmenorrhea, fatigue, influenza, nervousness, sinusitis.

DRUG INTERACTIONS

CYP450 inducers (eg, phenytoin, carbamazepine, phenobarbital), and propantheline may decrease levels. Caution with CYP3A inhibitors (eg, oral antifungals). Alcohol, narcotics, barbiturates, nonbarbiturate hypnotics, antianxiety agents, phenothiazines, thioxanthene and butyrophenone antipsychotics, MAOIs, TCAs, other anticonvulsant drugs, and other CNS depressant drugs may potentiate CNS-depressant effects. May produce absence status with valproic acid.

PATIENT CONSIDERATIONS

Assessment: Assess for drug/benzodiazepine hypersensitivity, significant liver disease, acute narrow angle glaucoma, mental depression, history of drug or alcohol addiction, renal/hepatic impairment, chronic respiratory diseases, pregnancy/nursing status, and possible drug interactions.

Monitoring: Monitor for CNS depression, emergence or worsening of depression, suicidal thoughts/behavior, unusual changes in mood or behavior, worsening of seizures, withdrawal symptoms upon discontinuation, and other adverse reactions. Periodically monitor blood counts and LFTs during long-term therapy.

Counseling: Instruct to take only as prescribed. Inform that therapy may produce psychological and physical dependence; instruct to consult physician before either increasing the dose or abruptly discontinuing the drug. Caution about operating hazardous machinery, including automobiles. Counsel that drug may increase risk of suicidal thoughts and behavior; advise of the need to be alert for the emergence/worsening of symptoms of depression, any unusual changes in mood or behavior, or the emergence of suicidal thoughts, behavior, or thoughts of self-harm and immediately report to physician behaviors of concern. Advise to notify physician if becomes pregnant or intends to become pregnant during therapy; encourage enrollment in the North American Antiepileptic Drug Pregnancy Registry. Advise not to breastfeed while on therapy. Advise to inform physician if taking, or planning to take, any prescription or OTC drugs and to avoid alcohol while on therapy. (Tab, Disintegrating) Inform that drug contains phenylalanine.

STORAGE: (Tab, Disintegrating) 20-25°C (68-77°F). (Tab) 25°C (77°F); excursions permitted to 15-30°C (59-86°F).

CLOZAPINE — clozapine

RX

Class: Atypical antipsychotic

Severe neutropenia, defined as an ANC <500/µL, reported; may lead to serious infection and death. Prior to initiating treatment, a baseline ANC must be ≥1500/µL for the general population, and ≥1000/µL for patients w/ documented benign ethnic neutropenia (BEN). Regularly monitor ANC during treatment. Available only through a restricted program under a Risk Evaluation Mitigation Strategy (REMS) called the Clozapine REMS program. Orthostatic hypotension, bradycardia, syncope, and cardiac arrest reported; risk is highest during the initial titration period, particularly w/ rapid dose escalation. Caution w/ cardiovascular (CV)/cerebrovascular disease or conditions predisposing to hypotension (eg, dehydration, use of antihypertensives). Seizures reported and risk is dose related; caution w/ history of seizures or other predisposing risk factors for seizure (eg, CNS pathology, medications that lower seizure threshold, alcohol abuse). Fatal myocarditis and cardiomyopathy reported; d/c and obtain cardiac evaluation upon suspicion of these reactions. Do not rechallenge patients w/ clozapine-related myocarditis or cardiomyopathy. Elderly patients w/ dementia-related psychosis treated w/ antipsychotic drugs are at an increased risk of death. Not approved for the treatment of dementia-related psychosis.

OTHER BRAND NAMES

Clozaril

C

ADULT DOSAGE

Schizophrenia

Treatment of severely ill patients w/ schizophrenia who fail to respond adequately to standard antipsychotic treatment. Reduction in risk of recurrent suicidal behavior in patients w/ schizophrenia or schizoaffective disorder who are judged to be at chronic risk for reexperiencing suicidal behavior

Initial: 12.5mg qd or bid
Titrate: May increase total daily dose in increments of 25-50mg/day, if well tolerated
Target Dose: 300-450mg/day (in divided doses) by the end of 2 weeks. Subsequently, may increase dose once weekly or twice weekly, in increments of up to 100mg
Max: 900mg/day

Patients responding to treatment should generally continue maint treatment on their effective dose beyond the acute episode

Reinitiation of Treatment:
When restarting in patients who have discontinued clozapine (≥2 days since last dose), reinitiate w/ 12.5mg qd or bid; if well tolerated, may increase to previous therapeutic dose more quickly than recommended for initial treatment

PEDIATRIC DOSAGE

Pediatric use may not have been established

DOSING CONSIDERATIONS

Concomitant Medications

Strong CYP1A2 Inhibitors:
During coadministration, use 1/3 of clozapine dose; when discontinuing comedication, increase clozapine dose based on clinical response

Moderate or Weak CYP1A2 Inhibitors:
During coadministration, monitor for adverse reactions and consider reducing clozapine dose if necessary; when discontinuing comedication, monitor for lack of effectiveness and consider increasing clozapine dose if necessary

CYP2D6 or CYP3A4 Inhibitors:
During coadministration, monitor for adverse reactions and consider reducing clozapine dose if necessary; when discontinuing comedication, monitor for lack of effectiveness and consider increasing clozapine dose if necessary

Strong CYP3A4 Inducers:
Concomitant use is not recommended; however, if the inducer is necessary, may need to increase clozapine dose and monitor for decreased effectiveness. When discontinuing comedication, reduce clozapine dose based on clinical response

Moderate or Weak CYP1A2 or CYP3A4 Inducers:
During coadministration, monitor for decreased effectiveness and consider increasing clozapine dose if necessary; when discontinuing comedication, monitor for adverse reactions and consider reducing clozapine dose if necessary

Renal Impairment
May need to reduce dose w/ significant renal impairment

Hepatic Impairment
May need to reduce dose w/ significant hepatic impairment

Discontinuation
Method of treatment discontinuation will vary depending on patient's last ANC:
1. If abrupt treatment discontinuation is necessary due to moderate-severe neutropenia, refer to PI for appropriate ANC monitoring based on the level of neutropenia
2. If termination of therapy is planned and there is no evidence of moderate-severe neutropenia, reduce dose gradually over 1-2 weeks
3. For abrupt discontinuation for a reason unrelated to neutropenia, continue existing ANC monitoring for general population patients until ANC is ≥1500/μL and for BEN patients until ANC is ≥1000/μL or above baseline
4. During the 2 weeks after discontinuation, additional ANC monitoring is required for any patient reporting onset of fever (temperature of ≥38.5°C [≥101.3°F])

Other Important Considerations

CYP2D6 Poor Metabolizers:
May need to reduce dose

ADMINISTRATION
Oral route

Administer in divided doses.
May be taken w/ or w/o food.

HOW SUPPLIED
Tab: 50mg*, 200mg*; (Clozaril) 25mg*, 100mg* *scored

CONTRAINDICATIONS
History of serious hypersensitivity to clozapine (eg, photosensitivity, vasculitis, erythema multiforme, or Stevens-Johnson syndrome) or any other component of the medication.

WARNINGS/PRECAUTIONS
Interrupt therapy as a precautionary measure in any patient who develops fever, defined as a temperature of ≥38.5°C (101.3°F), and obtain an ANC level; fever is often the 1st sign of neutropenic infection. In general, do not rechallenge patients who develop severe neutropenia w/ clozapine; for some patients, the risk of serious psychiatric illness from discontinuing treatment may be greater than the risk of rechallenge. Eosinophilia may occur and may be associated w/ myocarditis, pancreatitis, hepatitis, colitis, and nephritis. Evaluate promptly for signs/symptoms of systemic reactions if eosinophilia develops and d/c immediately if clozapine-related systemic disease is suspected. QT prolongation, torsades de pointes, and other life-threatening ventricular arrhythmias, cardiac arrest, and sudden death reported. D/C if QTc interval exceeds 500msec or symptoms consistent w/ torsades de pointes or other arrhythmias develop. Caution in patients at risk for significant electrolyte disturbance, particularly hypokalemia; correct electrolyte abnormalities before initiating treatment. Associated w/ metabolic changes (eg, hyperglycemia sometimes associated w/ ketoacidosis or hyperosmolar coma, dyslipidemia, weight gain) that may increase CV and cerebrovascular risk. Neuroleptic malignant syndrome (NMS) reported; d/c therapy immediately and institute symptomatic treatment. Transient fever may occur and may necessitate discontinuing treatment; carefully evaluate patients to rule out severe neutropenia or infection, and consider the possibility of NMS. Pulmonary embolism (PE), deep vein thrombosis (DVT), and tardive dyskinesia (TD) reported; consider discontinuation if TD occurs. Has potent anticholinergic effects; may result in CNS and peripheral anticholinergic toxicity. Caution w/ narrow-angle glaucoma, prostatic hypertrophy, or other conditions in which anticholinergic effects can lead to significant adverse reactions. May result in GI adverse reactions (eg, constipation, intestinal obstruction, fecal impaction, paralytic ileus). May impair mental/physical abilities. Consider dose reduction if sedation, or impairment of cognitive/motor performance occurs. Caution in patients w/ risk factors for cerebrovascular adverse reactions. If abrupt discontinuation is necessary, monitor carefully for the recurrence of psychotic symptoms and adverse reactions related to cholinergic rebound (eg, profuse sweating, headache, N/V, diarrhea). Caution in elderly. Refer to PI for treatment recommendations based on ANC monitoring for the general patient population and for patients w/ BEN.

ADVERSE REACTIONS
CNS reactions (eg, sedation, dizziness/vertigo, headache, tremor), CV reactions (eg, tachycardia, hypotension, syncope), autonomic nervous system reactions (eg, hypersalivation, sweating, dry mouth, visual disturbances), GI reactions (eg, constipation, nausea), fever.

DRUG INTERACTIONS
See Boxed Warning and Dosing Considerations. Caution w/ drugs that are inducers or inhibitors of CYP1A2, CYP3A4, and CYP2D6. CYP1A2 inhibitors (eg, fluvoxamine, ciprofloxacin, oral contraceptives), CYP2D6 or CYP3A4 inhibitors (eg, cimetidine, escitalopram, erythromycin) may increase levels, potentially resulting in adverse reactions. CYP1A2 inducers (eg, tobacco) or CYP3A4 inducers (eg, carbamazepine, phenytoin, St. John's wort) may decrease levels, resulting in decreased effectiveness. Caution w/ medications that prolong the QT interval (eg, ziprasidone, erythromycin, quinidine) or inhibit the metabolism of clozapine. Use caution when coadministering w/ other drugs metabolized by CYP2D6 (eg, phenothiazines, carbamazepine, propafenone) and may be necessary to use lower doses of such drugs; concomitant use may increase levels these CYP2D6 substrates. Caution w/ anticholinergic medications. NMS reported w/ CNS-active medications, including lithium. If used concurrently w/ an agent known to cause neutropenia (eg, some chemotherapeutic agents), consider monitoring more closely than the treatment guidelines.

PATIENT CONSIDERATIONS

Assessment: Assess for hypersensitivity to drug, history of seizures or other predisposing factors for seizure, risk factors for QT prolongation and serious CV reactions, narrow-angle glaucoma, prostatic hypertrophy, renal/hepatic impairment, any other conditions where treatment is cautioned, pregnancy/nursing status, and possible drug interactions. Obtain baseline ANC, lipid evaluations, ECG, and serum chemistry panel (K^+ and Mg^{2+}). Obtain baseline FPG in patients w/ diabetes mellitus (DM) or at risk for DM.

Monitoring: Monitor for signs/symptoms of severe neutropenia, orthostatic hypotension, bradycardia, syncope, cardiac arrest, seizures, myocarditis, cardiomyopathy, cognitive/motor impairment, eosinophilia, NMS, recurrence of psychosis and cholinergic rebound after abrupt discontinuation, metabolic changes (hyperglycemia, DM, dyslipidemia, weight gain), QT interval prolongation, fever, PE, DVT, TD, cerebrovascular adverse reactions, and other adverse reactions. Monitor serum electrolyte levels, glucose control in patients w/ DM and periodic FPG levels if at risk for hyperglycemia. Monitor ANC regularly to continue treatment; refer to PI for monitoring frequency.

Counseling: Inform about benefits/risks of therapy. Advise about risk of developing severe neutropenia and infection. Instruct to immediately report any sign/symptom of infection occurring at any time during therapy. Inform that drug is available only through a restricted program called the Clozapine REMS Program designed to ensure the required blood monitoring; advise of the importance of having blood tested ud. Inform about risks of orthostatic hypotension and syncope, especially during the period of initial dose titration; instruct to strictly follow the instructions of the physician for dosage and administration. Advise to consult physician immediately if patients feel faint, lose consciousness, or have signs/symptoms suggestive of bradycardia or arrhythmia. Inform about significant risk of seizure during therapy; caution about driving and any other potentially hazardous activity while taking treatment. Instruct to inform physician if taking clozapine before any new drug. Educate about the risk of metabolic changes and the need for specific monitoring. If dose was missed for >2 days, instruct not to restart medication at same dose but to contact physician for dosing instructions. Advise to notify physician if taking/planning to take any prescription or OTC drugs. Instruct to notify physician if pregnant/intending to become pregnant during therapy. Advise not to breastfeed if taking the drug.

STORAGE: 20-25°C (68-77°F). **Clozaril:** Should not exceed 30°C (86°F).

COLCRYS — colchicine

RX

Class: Miscellaneous gout agent

ADULT DOSAGE

Gout Flares

Prophylaxis:
>16 Years:
Usual: 0.6mg qd or bid
Max: 1.2mg/day

Treatment:
Usual: 1.2mg at the 1st sign of flare followed by 0.6mg 1 hr later
Max: 1.8mg over a 1-hr period
May administer for treatment of gout flare during prophylaxis at doses not to exceed 1.2mg at the 1st sign of the flare followed by 0.6mg 1 hr later; wait 12 hrs, then resume prophylactic dose

Familial Mediterranean Fever

Usual Range: 1.2-2.4mg/day in 1-2 divided doses
Titrate: Increase or decrease dose in 0.3mg increments based on disease control or intolerable side effects

PEDIATRIC DOSAGE

Familial Mediterranean Fever

4-6 Years: 0.3-1.8mg/day
6-12 Years: 0.9-1.8mg/day
>12 Years: 1.2-2.4mg/day
May be given qd or bid

DOSING CONSIDERATIONS

Concomitant Medications

Strong CYP3A4 Inhibitors:

Gout Flare Prophylaxis:
Original Dose 0.6mg BID: Adjust to 0.3mg qd
Original Dose 0.6mg QD: Adjust to 0.3mg qod

Gout Flare Treatment:
0.6mg for 1 dose, followed by 0.3mg 1 hr later; repeat dose no earlier than 3 days

Familial Mediterranean Fever:
Max: 0.6mg/day (may be given as 0.3mg bid)

Moderate CYP3A4 Inhibitors:

Gout Flare Prophylaxis:
Original Dose 0.6mg BID: Adjust to 0.3mg bid or 0.6mg qd
Original Dose 0.6mg QD: Adjust to 0.3mg qd

Gout Flare Treatment:
1.2mg for 1 dose; repeat dose no earlier than 3 days

Familial Mediterranean Fever:
Max: 1.2mg/day (may be given as 0.6mg bid)

P-gp Inhibitors:

Gout Flare Prophylaxis:
Original Dose 0.6mg BID: Adjust to 0.3mg qd
Original Dose 0.6mg QD: Adjust to 0.3mg qod

Gout Flare Treatment:
0.6mg for 1 dose; repeat dose no earlier than 3 days

Familial Mediterranean Fever:
Max: 0.6mg/day (may be given as 0.3mg bid)

Renal Impairment
Gout Flare Prophylaxis:
Severe Impairment:
Initial: 0.3mg/day
Titrate: Increase dose w/ close monitoring
Dialysis:
Initial: 0.3mg twice a week w/ close monitoring

Gout Flare Treatment:
Severe Impairment: Repeat treatment course no more than once every 2 weeks; consider alternate therapy if repeat treatment courses are required
Dialysis: Reduce to 0.6mg single dose; do not repeat treatment course more than once every 2 weeks

Familial Mediterranean Fever:
Mild (CrCl 50-80mL/min) to Moderate (CrCl 30-50mL/min): Consider reducing dose
Severe (CrCl <30mL/min)/Dialysis:
Initial: 0.3mg/day
Titrate: Increase dose w/ close monitoring

Hepatic Impairment
Gout Flare Prophylaxis:
Severe Impairment: Consider reducing dose

Gout Flare Treatment:
Severe Impairment: Repeat treatment course no more than once every 2 weeks; consider alternate therapy if repeat treatment courses are required

Familial Mediterranean Fever:
Severe Impairment: Consider reducing dose

ADMINISTRATION
Oral route

Take w/o regard to meals.

HOW SUPPLIED
Tab: 0.6mg* *scored

CONTRAINDICATIONS
Concomitant use w/ P-gp or strong CYP3A4 inhibitors (includes all protease inhibitors, except fosamprenavir) in patients w/ renal/hepatic impairment.

WARNINGS/PRECAUTIONS
Not an analgesic medication and should not be used to treat pain from other causes. Fatal overdoses (accidental/intentional), myelosuppression, leukopenia, granulocytopenia, thrombocytopenia, pancytopenia, and aplastic anemia reported. Drug-induced neuromuscular toxicity and rhabdomyolysis reported w/ chronic use; increased risk in elderly and in patients w/ renal dysfunction. Treatment of gout flare w/ Colcrys is not recommended in patients w/ renal/ hepatic impairment who are receiving Colcrys for prophylaxis. Caution w/ renal/hepatic impairment and in elderly.

ADVERSE REACTIONS
Diarrhea, pharyngolaryngeal pain, cramping, abdominal pain, N/V, fatigue.

DRUG INTERACTIONS
See Dosing Considerations and Contraindications. Significant increase in plasma levels reported w/ strong CYP3A4 inhibitors (eg, atazanavir, clarithromycin, itraconazole), moderate CYP3A4 inhibitors (eg, amprenavir, aprepitant, diltiazem, erythromycin), and P-gp inhibitors (eg, cyclosporine, ranolazine); see PI for dose adjustments. Fatal toxicity reported w/ clarithromycin and cyclosporine. Neuromuscular toxicity reported w/ diltiazem and verapamil. May potentiate the development of myopathy and rhabdomyolysis when used w/ HMG-CoA reductase inhibitors (eg, atorvastatin, simvastatin), gemfibrozil, and fibrates. May potentiate the development of myopathy when used w/ cyclosporine. Rhabdomyolysis reported w/ digoxin.

PATIENT CONSIDERATIONS

Assessment: Assess for renal/hepatic impairment, pregnancy/nursing status, and possible drug interactions.

Monitoring: Monitor for myelosuppression, leukopenia, granulocytopenia, thrombocytopenia, pancytopenia, aplastic anemia, neuromuscular toxicity, rhabdomyolysis, and other adverse reactions.

Counseling: Instruct to take medication ud. If a dose is missed for treatment of gout flare, instruct to take missed dose as soon as possible. If a dose is missed for treatment of gout flare during prophylaxis, instruct to take missed dose immediately, wait 12 hrs, and then resume previous schedule. If a dose is missed for prophylaxis w/o treatment of gout flares or familial Mediterranean fever, instruct to take next dose as soon as possible, then return to normal dosing schedule, and not to double the next dose. Inform that fatal overdoses were reported. Instruct to avoid grapefruit/grapefruit juice consumption during treatment. Inform that bone marrow depression w/ agranulocytosis, aplastic anemia, and thrombocytopenia may occur. Advise to notify physician of all medications currently being taken and to notify physician before starting any new medications, particularly antibiotics. Advise to d/c therapy and notify physician if experiencing muscle pain/weakness and/or tingling/numbness of fingers/toes.

STORAGE: 20-25°C (68-77°F). Protect from light.

COLESTID — colestipol hydrochloride RX

Class: Bile acid sequestrant

ADULT DOSAGE

Primary Hypercholesterolemia

Tab:
Initial: 2g qd-bid
Titrate: Increase by 2g qd or bid at 1- or 2-month intervals
Usual: 2-16g/day qd or in divided doses

Granules:
Initial: 1 pkt or 1 scoopful qd-bid
Titrate: May increase at an increment of 1 dose/day (1 pkt or 1 level tsp of granules) at 1- or 2-month intervals
Usual: 1-6 pkts or scoopfuls qd or in divided doses

Significant Rise in TG Levels:
Consider dose reduction, drug discontinuation, or combined/alternate therapy

PEDIATRIC DOSAGE

Pediatric use may not have been established

ADMINISTRATION

Oral route

Tab

Take 1 tab at a time and promptly swallow tabs whole using plenty of water or other appropriate liquid

Do not cut, crush, or chew

Granules

Always mix granules with water or other fluids before ingesting

Refer to PI for mixing and administration guide (with beverages/cereals/soups/fruits)

HOW SUPPLIED

Granules: 5g/pkt [30^s 90^s], 5g/scoopful [300g, 500g]; **Tab:** 1g

CONTRAINDICATIONS

Hypersensitivity to any of the components.

WARNINGS/PRECAUTIONS

Exclude secondary causes of hypercholesterolemia. May interfere with normal fat absorption. Chronic use may be associated with an increase bleeding tendency due to hypoprothrombinemia from vitamin K deficiency. May cause hypothyroidism. May produce or severely worsen preexisting constipation. Avoid constipation with symptomatic coronary artery disease. Constipation associated with colestipol may aggravate hemorrhoids. May produce hyperchloremic acidosis with prolonged use. (Granules) Flavored form contains phenylalanine. Avoid taking in dry form; always mix granules with water or other fluids before ingesting.

ADVERSE REACTIONS

Constipation, abdominal discomfort, indigestion/heartburn, musculoskeletal pain, headache, AST/ALT/alkaline phosphatase elevation, chest pain, rash, anorexia, fatigue, tachycardia, SOB.

C

DRUG INTERACTIONS
May interfere the absorption of folic acid, fat-soluble vitamins (eg, A, D, K), oral phosphate supplements, and hydrocortisone. May delay or reduce absorption of concomitant oral medication; take other drugs at least 1 hr before or 4 hrs after colestipol. Reduces absorption of chlorothiazide, tetracycline, furosemide, penicillin G, HCTZ, and gemfibrozil. Caution with digitalis preparations, propranolol. Reduce mycophenolic acid exposure and potentially reduce efficacy of mycophenolate mofetil.

PATIENT CONSIDERATIONS
Assessment: Assess for hypersensitivity to the drug, secondary causes of hypercholesterolemia (eg, hypothyroidism, poorly controlled diabetes mellitus, nephrotic syndrome, dysproteinemias, obstructive liver disease, alcoholism), preexisting constipation, pregnancy/nursing status, and possible drug interactions. Determine baseline lipid profile.

Monitoring: Monitor for signs/symptoms of vitamin K deficiency (eg, tendency for bleeding), constipation, hypothyroidism, hyperchloremic acidosis, and other adverse reactions. Monitor serum cholesterol, lipoprotein, and TG levels.

Counseling: Inform about benefits/risks of therapy. Instruct to take ud. Advise to take other medications at least 1 hr before or 4 hrs after taking colestipol. Instruct to report any adverse reactions to physician.

STORAGE: 20-25°C (68-77°F).

COMBIGAN – brimonidine tartrate/timolol maleate
RX

Class: Alpha$_2$ agonist/beta blocker

ADULT DOSAGE
Elevated Intraocular Pressure

Reduction of elevated IOP in patients w/ glaucoma or ocular HTN requiring adjunctive or replacement therapy due to inadequately controlled IOP

Instill 1 drop in affected eye(s) bid q12h

PEDIATRIC DOSAGE
Elevated Intraocular Pressure

Reduction of elevated IOP in patients w/ glaucoma or ocular HTN requiring adjunctive or replacement therapy due to inadequately controlled IOP

≥2 Years:

Instill 1 drop in affected eye(s) bid q12h

DOSING CONSIDERATIONS
Concomitant Medications

Space by at least 5 min if using >1 topical ophthalmic product

ADMINISTRATION
Ocular route

HOW SUPPLIED
Ophthalmic Sol: (Brimonidine/Timolol) 0.2%/0.5% [5mL, 10mL, 15mL]

CONTRAINDICATIONS
Reactive airway disease including bronchial asthma, history of bronchial asthma, severe COPD. Sinus bradycardia, 2nd- or 3rd-degree atrioventricular (AV) block, overt cardiac failure, cardiogenic shock. Neonates and infants (<2 yrs of age). History of hypersensitivity reaction to any component of the medication.

WARNINGS/PRECAUTIONS
May potentiate syndromes associated w/ vascular insufficiency; caution w/ depression, cerebral or coronary insufficiency, Raynaud's phenomenon, orthostatic hypotension, or thromboangiitis obliterans. Bacterial keratitis reported w/ use of multiple-dose containers of topical ophthalmic products. **Timolol:** May be absorbed systemically. Severe respiratory reactions and cardiac reactions including death due to bronchospasm in patients w/ asthma, and rarely death in association w/ cardiac failure, reported following systemic or ophthalmic administration of timolol. Ophthalmic β-blockers may impair compensatory tachycardia and increase risk of hypotension. May precipitate more severe failure in patients w/ diminished myocardial contractility. Continued depression of the myocardium w/ β-blocking agents over a period of time may lead to cardiac failure in patients w/o a history of cardiac failure; d/c at the 1st sign/symptom of cardiac failure. Avoid in patients w/ mild to moderate COPD (eg, chronic bronchitis, emphysema), bronchospastic disease, or a history of bronchospastic disease. May increase reactivity to allergens. May potentiate muscle weakness consistent w/ certain myasthenic symptoms (eg, diplopia, ptosis, generalized weakness). Increased muscle weakness in some patients w/ myasthenia gravis or myasthenic symptoms reported rarely w/ timolol. May mask signs/symptoms of acute hypoglycemia; caution in patients subject to spontaneous hypoglycemia and in diabetic patients (especially

those w/ labile diabetes) receiving insulin or hypoglycemic agents. May mask certain clinical signs of hyperthyroidism (eg, tachycardia); carefully manage patients suspected of developing thyrotoxicosis to avoid abrupt withdrawal that may precipitate a thyroid storm. May impair the ability of the heart to respond to β-adrenergically mediated reflex stimuli during surgery; gradual withdrawal of β-blocking agents is recommended in patients undergoing elective surgery. **Brimonidine:** Ocular hypersensitivity reactions reported.

ADVERSE REACTIONS

Allergic conjunctivitis, conjunctival folliculosis, conjunctival hyperemia, eye pruritus, ocular burning/stinging.

DRUG INTERACTIONS

May reduce BP; caution w/ antihypertensives and/or cardiac glycosides. Monitor for potentially additive effects, both systemic and on IOP w/ concomitant oral or IV β-blockers; concomitant use of 2 topical β-blocking agents is not recommended. Possibility of additive or potentiating effect w/ CNS depressants (eg, alcohol, barbiturates, opiates, sedatives, anesthetics). May affect the metabolism and uptake of circulating amines w/ TCAs and/or MAOIs; caution w/ TCAs and MAOIs. **Timolol:** Possible AV conduction disturbances, left ventricular failure, and hypotension may occur w/ oral or IV calcium antagonists; use w/ caution and avoid coadministration in patients w/ impaired cardiac function. Closely observe patients receiving catecholamine-depleting drugs (eg, reserpine) because of possible additive effects and the production of hypotension and/or marked bradycardia. Concomitant use of β-blockers w/ digitalis or calcium antagonists may have additive effects in prolonging AV conduction time. Potentiated systemic β-blockade (eg, decreased HR, depression) reported w/ concomitant CYP2D6 inhibitors (eg, quinidine, SSRIs).

PATIENT CONSIDERATIONS

Assessment: Assess for reactive airway disease, sinus bradycardia, AV block, cardiac failure, or any other conditions where treatment is contraindicated or cautioned. Assess pregnancy/nursing status, and for possible drug interactions.

Monitoring: Monitor for respiratory or cardiac reactions, potentiation of syndromes associated w/ vascular insufficiency, muscle weakness, increased reactivity to allergens, masking of signs/symptoms of hypoglycemia or hyperthyroidism, ocular hypersensitivity reactions, bacterial keratitis, and other adverse reactions.

Counseling: Inform that ocular infections may occur if handled improperly or if the tip of dispensing container contacts the eye or surrounding structures. Advise that serious damage to the eye and subsequent loss of vision may result from using contaminated sol or by inadvertent contact w/ dropper tip. Instruct to always replace cap after using. Advise not to use if sol changes color or becomes cloudy. Advise to immediately consult physician concerning continued use of multidose container if undergoing ocular surgery or if an intercurrent ocular condition (eg, trauma, infection) develops. Instruct to space dosing by at least 5 min apart if >1 topical ophthalmic drug is being used. Inform that drug contains benzalkonium chloride, which may be absorbed by soft contact lenses; instruct to remove contact lenses prior to administration and explain that lenses may be reinserted 15 min following administration. Inform that drug may cause fatigue and/or drowsiness in some patients; advise to use caution in engaging in hazardous activities because of the potential for a decrease in mental alertness.

STORAGE: 15-25°C (59-77°F). Protect from light.

CombiPatch – estradiol/norethindrone acetate **RX**

Class: Estrogen/progestogen combination

Should not be used for prevention of cardiovascular (CV) disease or dementia. Increased risk of MI, stroke, pulmonary embolism (PE), and deep vein thrombosis (DVT) in postmenopausal women (50-79 yrs of age) reported. Increased risk of developing probable dementia in postmenopausal women ≥65 yrs of age reported. Increased risk of invasive breast cancer reported. Increased risk of endometrial cancer in women w/ a uterus who use unopposed estrogens. Perform adequate diagnostic measures to rule out malignancy in postmenopausal women w/ undiagnosed persistent or recurrent abnormal vaginal bleeding. Should be prescribed at the lowest effective dose and for the shortest duration consistent w/ treatment goals and risks.

ADULT DOSAGE

Menopausal Vasomotor Symptoms

Moderate to Severe:

Initiation of Therapy:

Start at lowest dose. Women not currently using continuous estrogen or combination estrogen + progestin therapy may start therapy w/ CombiPatch at any time. However, women currently using continuous estrogen or combination estrogen + progestin therapy

PEDIATRIC DOSAGE

Pediatric use may not have been established

should complete current cycle of therapy prior to initiating CombiPatch therapy

Women often experience withdrawal bleeding at the completion of the cycle. The first day of this bleeding would be an appropriate time to begin CombiPatch therapy

Continuous Combined Regimen:
Wear a (0.05mg/0.14mg)/day patch for continuous uninterrupted treatment twice weekly on the lower abdomen; replace every 3-4 days (twice weekly) during a 28-day cycle

Use 0.05mg/0.25mg if a greater progestin dose is desired

Continuous Sequential Regimen:
CombiPatch can be applied as a sequential regimen in combination w/ an estradiol-only patch

Days 1-14: Wear a 0.05mg/day estradiol patch (Vivelle-Dot); replace every 3-4 days (twice weekly)

Days 15-28: Wear CombiPatch (0.05mg/0.14mg)/day patch continuously on the lower abdomen; replace every 3-4 days (twice weekly)

Use 0.05mg/0.25mg if a greater progestin dose is desired

Use the lowest effective dose for the shortest duration; reevaluate at 3- to 6-month intervals

Menopausal Vulvar/Vaginal Atrophy

Moderate to Severe:
Initiation of Therapy:
Start at lowest dose. Women not currently using continuous estrogen or combination estrogen + progestin therapy may start therapy w/ CombiPatch at any time. However, women currently using continuous estrogen or combination estrogen + progestin therapy should complete current cycle of therapy prior to initiating CombiPatch therapy

Women often experience withdrawal bleeding at the completion of the cycle. The first day of this bleeding would be an appropriate time to begin CombiPatch therapy

Continuous Combined Regimen:
Wear a (0.05mg/0.14mg)/day patch for continuous uninterrupted treatment twice weekly on the lower abdomen; replace every 3-4 days (twice weekly) during a 28-day cycle

Use 0.05mg/0.25mg if a greater progestin dose is desired

Continuous Sequential Regimen:
CombiPatch can be applied as a sequential regimen in combination w/ an estradiol-only patch

Days 1-14: Wear a 0.05mg/day estradiol patch (Vivelle-Dot); replace every 3-4 days (twice weekly)

Days 15-28: Wear CombiPatch (0.05mg/0.14mg)/day patch continuously on the lower abdomen; replace every 3-4 days (twice weekly)

Use 0.05mg/0.25mg if a greater progestin dose is desired

Use the lowest effective dose for the shortest duration; reevaluate at 3- to 6-month intervals

Hypoestrogenism

Due to Hypogonadism, Castration, or Primary Ovarian Failure:
Initiation of Therapy:
Start at lowest dose. Women not currently using continuous estrogen or combination estrogen + progestin therapy may start therapy w/ CombiPatch at any time. However, women currently using continuous estrogen or combination estrogen + progestin therapy should complete current cycle of therapy prior to initiating CombiPatch therapy

Women often experience withdrawal bleeding at the completion of the cycle. The first day of this bleeding would be an appropriate time to begin CombiPatch therapy

Continuous Combined Regimen:
Wear a (0.05mg/0.14mg)/day patch for continuous uninterrupted treatment twice weekly on the lower abdomen; replace every 3-4 days (twice weekly) during a 28-day cycle

Use 0.05mg/0.25mg if a greater progestin dose is desired

Continuous Sequential Regimen:
CombiPatch can be applied as a sequential regimen in combination w/ an estradiol-only patch

Days 1-14: Wear a 0.05mg/day estradiol patch (Vivelle-Dot); replace every 3-4 days (twice weekly)
Days 15-28: Wear CombiPatch (0.05mg/0.14mg)/day patch continuously on the lower abdomen; replace every 3-4 days (twice weekly)

Use 0.05mg/0.25mg if a greater progestin dose is desired

Use the lowest effective dose for the shortest duration; reevaluate at 3- to 6-month intervals

ADMINISTRATION

Transdermal route

Site Selection

Place on a smooth (fold-free), clean, dry area of the skin on the lower abdomen. Do not apply to or near the breasts. Area selected should not be oily, damaged, or irritated. Avoid application to the waistline, as tight clothing may rub the system off or modify drug delivery. Rotate site of application, w/ an interval of at least 1 week allowed between applications to the same site

Application

1. After opening the pouch, remove 1 side of the protective liner, taking care not to touch the adhesive part of the patch w/ the fingers
2. Immediately apply the patch to a smooth (fold-free) area of skin on the lower abdomen
3. Remove the 2nd side of the protective liner and press the patch firmly in place for at least 10 sec, making sure there is good contact, especially around the edges

If a patch falls off, reapply the same patch to another area of the lower abdomen. If necessary, a new patch may be applied, in which case, the original treatment schedule should be continued. Only 1 system should be worn at any 1 time during the 3- to 4-day dosing interval

Once in place, the patch should not be exposed to the sun for prolonged periods of time

Removal

Remove the patch carefully and slowly to avoid skin irritation. Should any adhesive remain on the skin after removal of the patch, allow the area to dry for 15 min, then gently rub the area w/ an oil-based cream or lotion to remove adhesive residue

HOW SUPPLIED

Patch: (Estradiol/Norethindrone Acetate) (0.05mg/0.14mg)/day, (0.05mg/0.25mg)/day [8[s]]

CONTRAINDICATIONS

Undiagnosed abnormal genital bleeding, known/suspected/history of breast cancer, known/suspected estrogen-dependent neoplasia, active/history of DVT/PE, active/history of arterial thromboembolic disease (eg, stroke, MI), known anaphylactic reaction/angioedema/hypersensitivity to CombiPatch, known liver impairment/disease, known protein C/protein S/antithrombin deficiency or other known thrombophilic disorders, known/suspected pregnancy.

WARNINGS/PRECAUTIONS

In some cases, hysterectomized women w/ a history of endometriosis may need a progestin. D/C immediately if stroke, DVT, PE, or MI occurs or is suspected. Manage risk factors for arterial vascular disease and/or venous thromboembolism appropriately. If feasible, d/c at least 4-6 weeks before surgery of the type associated w/ an increased risk of thromboembolism, or during periods of prolonged immobilization. May increase risk of ovarian cancer and gallbladder disease. May lead to severe hypercalcemia in patients w/ breast cancer and bone metastases; d/c and take appropriate measures if hypercalcemia occurs. Retinal vascular thrombosis reported in women; d/c pending exam if sudden partial/complete loss of vision or sudden onset of proptosis, diplopia, or migraine occurs. D/C permanently if exam reveals papilledema or retinal vascular lesions. Angioedema involving eye/eyelid, face, larynx, pharynx, tongue, and extremity w/ or w/o urticaria requiring medical intervention reported. Women who develop angioedema anytime during the course of treatment should not receive treatment again. May exacerbate symptoms of angioedema in women w/ hereditary angioedema. Cases of anaphylactic/anaphylactoid reactions, which developed anytime during the course of treatment and required emergency medical management reported; involvement of skin (hives, pruritus, swollen lips-tongue-face) and either respiratory tract (respiratory compromise) or GI tract (abdominal pain, vomiting) has been noted. May elevate BP and thyroid-binding globulin levels. May elevate plasma TGs in women w/ preexisting hypertriglyceridemia, leading to pancreatitis; consider discontinuation if pancreatitis occurs. Caution w/ history of cholestatic jaundice associated w/ past estrogen use or w/ pregnancy; d/c in case of recurrence. May cause fluid retention. Caution w/ hypoparathyroidism as estrogen-induced hypocalcemia may occur. May exacerbate endometriosis, asthma, diabetes mellitus, epilepsy, migraine, porphyria, systemic lupus erythematosus, and hepatic hemangiomas. May affect certain endocrine and blood components in lab tests.

ADVERSE REACTIONS

Abdominal pain, back pain, asthenia, flu syndrome, headache, application-site reaction, diarrhea, nausea, nervousness, pharyngitis, respiratory disorder, breast pain, dysmenorrhea, menstrual disorder, vaginitis.

DRUG INTERACTIONS

CYP3A4 inducers (eg, St. John's wort preparations, phenobarbital, phenylbutazone, rifabutin) may decrease levels and may decrease therapeutic effects and/or change uterine bleeding profile. CYP3A4 inhibitors (eg, erythromycin, clarithromycin, ketoconazole, nelfinavir) may increase levels, which may result in side effects. Women concomitantly receiving thyroid hormone replacement therapy and estrogens may require increased doses of their thyroid replacement therapy; monitor thyroid function.

PATIENT CONSIDERATIONS

Assessment: Assess for undiagnosed abnormal genital bleeding, presence/history of breast cancer, estrogen-dependent neoplasia, active/history of DVT/PE/arterial thromboembolic disease, liver impairment/disease, thrombophilic disorders, drug hypersensitivity, pregnancy/nursing status, any other conditions where treatment is contraindicated or cautioned, and possible drug interactions.

Monitoring: Monitor for signs/symptoms of CV disease, malignant neoplasms, dementia, gallbladder disease, hypercalcemia, visual abnormalities, BP and plasma TG elevations, pancreatitis, cholestatic jaundice, fluid retention, exacerbation of endometriosis and other conditions, angioedema, anaphylactic/anaphylactoid reactions, and other adverse reactions. Perform annual breast exam; schedule mammography based on age, risk factors, and prior mammogram results. Periodically reevaluate (every 3-6 months) to determine need for continued therapy. Perform adequate diagnostic measures (eg, endometrial sampling) to rule out malignancies in postmenopausal women w/ undiagnosed, persistent, or recurring abnormal genital bleeding. Regularly monitor thyroid function if on thyroid hormone replacement therapy.

Counseling: Inform of the importance of reporting abnormal vaginal bleeding to physician as soon as possible. Inform of possible serious adverse reactions of therapy (eg, CV disorders, malignant neoplasms, probable dementia) and of possible less serious, but common adverse reactions (eg, headache, breast pain and tenderness, nausea). Instruct to have yearly breast exams by a healthcare provider and to perform monthly breast self-exams. Advise that monthly withdrawal bleeding often occurs w/ the continuous sequential regimen.

STORAGE: Prior to Dispensing: 2-8°C (36-46°F). After Dispensing: 20-25°C (66-77°F) for up to 6 months. Store the systems in the sealed foil pouch. Do not store in areas where extreme temperatures may occur.

COMBIVENT RESPIMAT – albuterol/ipratropium bromide RX

Class: Anticholinergic/beta$_2$ agonist

C

ADULT DOSAGE	PEDIATRIC DOSAGE
Chronic Obstructive Pulmonary Disease **Bronchospasm Requiring a 2nd Bronchodilator:** **Usual:** 1 inh qid. May take additional inh as required **Max:** 6 inh/24 hrs	Pediatric use may not have been established

ADMINISTRATION

Oral inh route

Priming

-Prior to 1st use, insert cartridge into the inhaler and prime the unit; actuate the inhaler toward the ground until an aerosol cloud is visible and then repeat the process 3 more times.
-If not used for >3 days, actuate the inhaler once.
-If not used for >21 days, actuate the inhaler until an aerosol cloud is visible and then repeat the process 3 more times.

HOW SUPPLIED

Spray, Inhalation: (Albuterol/Ipratropium) (100mcg/20mcg)/actuation [60, 120 actuations]

CONTRAINDICATIONS

Hypersensitivity to any of the ingredients in the medication or to atropine or any of its derivatives.

WARNINGS/PRECAUTIONS

May produce paradoxical bronchospasm; d/c and institute alternative therapy if this occurs. Hypersensitivity reactions may occur; d/c and consider alternative treatment if such a reaction occurs. Albuterol: May produce significant cardiovascular (CV) effects (eg, ECG changes); may need to d/c if symptoms occur. Caution with CV disorders (eg, coronary insufficiency, cardiac arrhythmias, HTN). Fatalities reported with excessive use of inhaled sympathomimetic drugs in patients with asthma. Caution with convulsive disorders, hyperthyroidism, diabetes mellitus (DM), and in patients who are unusually responsive to sympathomimetic amines. May produce significant but usually transient hypokalemia. Ipratropium: May increase IOP and result in precipitation/worsening of narrow-angle glaucoma. May cause urinary retention; caution with prostatic hyperplasia or bladder-neck obstruction.

ADVERSE REACTIONS

Nasopharyngitis, cough, headache, bronchitis, URI, dyspnea.

DRUG INTERACTIONS

Potential for an additive interaction with other anticholinergic-containing drugs; avoid coadministration. Increased risk of adverse CV effects with other sympathomimetic agents; use with caution. β-blockers and albuterol inhibit the effect of each other; use β-blockers with caution in patients with hyperreactive airways. ECG changes and/or hypokalemia that may result from non-K^+-sparing diuretics (eg, loop or thiazide diuretics) may be acutely worsened; use with caution and consider monitoring K^+ levels. Administration with MAOIs or TCAs, or within 2 weeks of discontinuation of such agents may potentiate the action of albuterol on CV system; use with extreme caution and consider alternative therapy.

PATIENT CONSIDERATIONS

Assessment: Assess for hypersensitivity to drug or to atropine or any of its derivatives, CV disorders, narrow-angle glaucoma, prostatic hyperplasia, bladder-neck obstruction, convulsive disorders, hyperthyroidism, DM, pregnancy/nursing status, and possible drug interactions. Assess if unusually responsive to sympathomimetic amines.

Monitoring: Monitor for signs/symptoms of hypersensitivity reactions, paradoxical bronchospasm, CV effects (measured by pulse rate and BP), hypokalemia, unexpected development of severe acute asthmatic crisis, hypoxia, and other adverse reactions.

Counseling: Instruct to use caution to avoid spraying the product into eyes. Instruct to consult physician if ocular symptoms or difficulty with urination develops. Instruct to exercise caution when engaging in activities requiring balance and visual acuity (eg, driving a car, operating appliances/machinery). Instruct not to increase dose or frequency without consulting physician. Instruct to seek immediate medical attention if therapy lessens in effectiveness, symptoms worsen, and/or product is needed more frequently than usual. Counsel to take other inhaled drugs only ud by physician. Counsel to d/c if paradoxical bronchospasm occurs. Inform of possible adverse effects (eg, palpitations, chest pain, rapid HR, tremor, nervousness). Instruct to contact physician if pregnant/nursing.

STORAGE: 25°C (77°F); excursions permitted to 15-30°C (59-86°F). Avoid freezing.

COMPLERA – emtricitabine/rilpivirine/tenofovir disoproxil fumarate

RX

Class: Non-nucleoside reverse transcriptase inhibitor (NNRTI)/nucleoside analogue combination

Lactic acidosis and severe hepatomegaly w/ steatosis, including fatal cases, reported w/ the use of nucleoside analogues. Not approved for the treatment of chronic hepatitis B virus (HBV) infection. Severe acute exacerbations of hepatitis B reported in patients coinfected w/ HBV upon discontinuation of therapy; closely monitor hepatic function for at least several months. If appropriate, initiation of antihepatitis B therapy may be warranted.

ADULT DOSAGE

HIV-1 Infection

Antiretroviral Treatment-Naive w/ HIV-1 RNA ≤100,000 copies/mL at Initiation:
Usual: 1 tab qd

HIV-1 RNA <50 copies/mL on Stable Antiretroviral Treatment at Initiation:
Usual: 1 tab qd

PEDIATRIC DOSAGE

Pediatric use may not have been established

DOSING CONSIDERATIONS

Concomitant Medications

Rifabutin: Add 25mg of rilpivirine qd to therapy

Renal Impairment

Moderate or Severe (CrCl <50mL/min): Not recommended for use

ADMINISTRATION

Oral route

Take w/ food

HOW SUPPLIED

Tab: (Emtricitabine/Rilpivirine/Tenofovir Disoproxil Fumarate [TDF]) 200mg/25mg/300mg

CONTRAINDICATIONS

Coadministration w/ CYP3A inducers or agents that increase gastric pH causing decreased plasma concentrations, which may result in loss of virologic response and possible resistance (eg, carbamazepine, oxcarbazepine, phenobarbital, phenytoin, rifampin, rifapentine, proton pump inhibitors [eg, dexlansoprazole, esomeprazole, lansoprazole, omeprazole, pantoprazole, rabeprazole], systemic dexamethasone [more than a single dose], St. John's wort).

WARNINGS/PRECAUTIONS

When considering replacing the current regimen in virologically-suppressed adults, patients should have no history of virologic failure, have been stably suppressed for at least 6 months prior to switching therapy, currently be on the 1st or 2nd antiretroviral regimen prior to switching therapy, and have no current/past history of resistance to any of the 3 drug components. Additional monitoring of HIV-1 RNA and regimen tolerability is recommended after replacing therapy to assess for potential virologic failure or rebound. Immune reconstitution syndrome, autoimmune disorders (eg, Graves' disease, polymyositis, Guillain-Barre syndrome) in the setting of immune reconstitution, and redistribution/accumulation of body fat reported. Caution in elderly. Rilpivirine: Severe skin and hypersensitivity reactions reported, including cases of drug reaction w/ eosinophilia and systemic symptoms; d/c immediately and initiate appropriate therapy if signs/symptoms develop. Depressive disorders reported; immediate medical evaluation is recommended if severe depressive symptoms occur. Hepatic adverse events reported; increased risk for worsening/development of liver-associated test elevations in patients w/ underlying hepatitis B or C, or marked liver-associated test elevations prior to treatment. Consider liver-associated test monitoring for patients w/o preexisting hepatic dysfunction or other risk factors. TDF: Caution w/ known risk factors for liver disease. D/C if lactic acidosis or pronounced hepatotoxicity occurs. Renal impairment (eg, acute renal failure, Fanconi syndrome) reported. Decreased bone mineral density (BMD), increased biochemical markers of bone metabolism, and osteomalacia reported. Consider assessment of BMD in patients w/ history of pathologic bone fracture or other risk factors for osteoporosis or bone loss. Arthralgias and muscle pain/weakness reported in cases of proximal renal tubulopathy. Consider hypophosphatemia and osteomalacia secondary to proximal renal tubulopathy in patients at risk of renal dysfunction who present w/ persistent or worsening bone or muscle symptoms.

ADVERSE REACTIONS

Lactic acidosis, severe hepatomegaly w/ steatosis, nausea, headache, dizziness, depressive disorders, insomnia, abnormal dreams, rash, diarrhea, fatigue.

DRUG INTERACTIONS

See Dosing Considerations and Contraindications. Avoid w/ concurrent or recent use of nephrotoxic agents (eg, high dose or multiple NSAIDs), other antiretrovirals, adefovir dipivoxil, or drugs containing any of the same active components or lamivudine. Avoid w/ rilpivirine unless needed for dose adjustment (eg, w/ rifabutin). Rilpivirine: Caution w/ drugs that may reduce exposure or drugs w/ a known risk of torsades de pointes. Decreased levels, loss of virologic response, and possible resistance w/ CYP3A inducers or drugs increasing gastric pH (eg, antacids, H_2-receptor antagonists [H_2-RAs]). Administer antacids at least 2 hrs before or at least 4 hrs after dosing, and H_2-RAs at least 12 hrs before or at least 4 hrs after dosing. Decreased levels w/ rifabutin. CYP3A inhibitors, azole antifungals, clarithromycin, erythromycin, or telithromycin may increase levels. May decrease levels of ketoconazole and methadone. Emtricitabine and TDF: Drugs that reduce renal function or compete for active tubular secretion (eg, acyclovir, aminoglycosides [eg, gentamicin], high dose or multiple NSAIDs) may increase levels of emtricitabine, TDF, and/or other renally eliminated drugs. TDF: Cases of acute renal failure after initiation of high dose or multiple NSAIDs reported in HIV-infected patients w/ risk factors for renal dysfunction who appeared stable on TDF; consider alternatives to NSAIDs, if needed.

PATIENT CONSIDERATIONS

Assessment: Assess for history of virologic failure, current/past history of resistance to any of the drug components, obesity, prolonged nucleoside exposure, liver dysfunction or risk factors for liver disease, renal impairment, HBV infection, pregnancy/nursing status, and possible drug interactions. Assess BMD in patients w/ a history of pathological bone fracture or w/ other risk factors for osteoporosis/bone loss. Assess estimated CrCl, serum phosphorus (P), urine glucose, and urine protein in patients at risk for renal dysfunction.

Monitoring: Monitor for signs/symptoms of lactic acidosis, severe skin and hypersensitivity reactions, severe hepatomegaly w/ steatosis, depressive symptoms, hepatotoxicity, decreased BMD, increased biochemical markers for bone metabolism, osteomalacia, fat redistribution/accumulation, immune reconstitution syndrome (eg, opportunistic infections), autoimmune disorders, renal impairment, and other adverse reactions. Monitor patients coinfected w/ HBV and HIV-1 w/ clinical and lab follow-up for acute exacerbations of hepatitis B for at least several months upon discontinuation of therapy. Monitor estimated CrCl, serum P, urine glucose, and urine protein periodically in patients at risk for renal dysfunction. Additional monitoring of HIV-1 RNA and regimen tolerability is recommended after replacing therapy to assess for potential virologic failure or rebound.

Counseling: Inform that therapy is not a cure for HIV infection; advise that continuous therapy is necessary to control HIV infection and decrease HIV-related illnesses. Advise to practice safer sex and use latex or polyurethane condoms. Instruct to never reuse or share needles. Advise not to breastfeed. Counsel to take on a regular dosing schedule w/ food and avoid missing doses. Inform that a protein drink is not a substitute for food. Counsel on missed dose instructions. Instruct to contact physician if symptoms of lactic acidosis or severe hepatomegaly w/ steatosis, depression, or infection occurs. Inform that hepatotoxicity has been reported during treatment. Instruct to immediately stop taking therapy and seek medical attention if patient develops a rash associated w/ any of the following symptoms: fever; blisters; mucosal involvement; eye inflammation (conjunctivitis); severe allergic reaction causing swelling of the face, eyes, lips, mouth, tongue or throat; and any signs/symptoms of liver problems. Inform that laboratory tests will be performed and appropriate therapy will be initiated if severe rash occurs. Inform that fat redistribution/accumulation, renal impairment, and decreases in BMD may occur. Advise to inform physician if taking any other prescription/nonprescription medications or herbal products (eg, St. John's wort).

STORAGE: 25°C (77°F); excursions permitted to 15-30°C (59-86°F).

CONCERTA — methylphenidate hydrochloride CII

Class: CNS stimulant

Caution w/ history of drug dependence or alcoholism. Chronic abusive use may lead to marked tolerance and psychological dependence w/ varying degrees of abnormal behavior. Frank psychotic episodes may occur, especially w/ parenteral abuse. Careful supervision is required during withdrawal from abusive use since severe depression may occur. Withdrawal following chronic use may unmask symptoms of underlying disorder that may require follow-up.

ADULT DOSAGE

Attention-Deficit Hyperactivity Disorder

18-65 Years:

New to Methylphenidate:

Initial: 18mg or 36mg qam

Range: 18-72mg/day

Currently on Methylphenidate:

Initial:

18mg qam if previous dose 5mg bid-tid

36mg qam if previous dose 10mg bid-tid

PEDIATRIC DOSAGE

Attention-Deficit Hyperactivity Disorder

New to Methylphenidate:

6-12 Years:

Initial: 18mg qam

Range: 18-54mg/day

13-17 Years:

Initial: 18mg qam

Range: 18-72mg/day not to exceed 2mg/kg/day

54mg qam if previous dose 15mg bid-tid
72mg qam if previous dose 20mg bid-tid
Conversion dosage should not exceed 72mg/day

Titrate: May increase in 18mg increments at weekly intervals if optimal response is not achieved at a lower dose

Max: 72mg/day

Maint/Extended Treatment:
Periodically reevaluate the long-term usefulness of the drug

D/C if no improvement observed after appropriate dosage adjustment over 1 month

Currently on Methylphenidate:
≥6 Years:
Initial:
18mg qam if previous dose 5mg bid-tid
36mg qam if previous dose 10mg bid-tid
54mg qam if previous dose 15mg bid-tid
72mg qam if previous dose 20mg bid-tid
Conversion dosage should not exceed 72mg/day

Titrate: May increase in 18mg increments at weekly intervals if optimal response is not achieved at a lower dose

Max:
6-12 Years: 54mg/day
13-17 Years: 72mg/day

Maint/Extended Treatment:
Periodically reevaluate the long-term usefulness of the drug

D/C if no improvement observed after appropriate dosage adjustment over 1 month

DOSING CONSIDERATIONS

Adverse Reactions
Reduce dose or, if necessary, d/c if paradoxical aggravation of symptoms or other adverse events occur

ADMINISTRATION

Oral route

Take w/ or w/o food.
Swallow tab whole w/ the aid of liquids; do not chew, divide, or crush.

HOW SUPPLIED

Tab, Extended-Release: 18mg, 27mg, 36mg, 54mg

CONTRAINDICATIONS

Hypersensitivity to methylphenidate or other components of the medication; marked anxiety, tension, and agitation; glaucoma; motor tics or family history or diagnosis of Tourette's syndrome. Treatment w/ MAOIs or w/in a minimum of 14 days following discontinuation of an MAOI.

WARNINGS/PRECAUTIONS

Avoid w/ known serious structural cardiac abnormalities, cardiomyopathy, serious heart rhythm abnormalities, coronary artery disease, or other serious cardiac problems. Sudden death reported in children and adolescents w/ structural cardiac abnormalities or other serious heart problems. Sudden deaths, stroke, and MI reported in adults. May increase BP and HR; caution w/ conditions that might be compromised by increases in BP/HR (eg, preexisting HTN, heart failure, recent MI, ventricular arrhythmia). Prior to treatment, obtain medical history (including assessment for family history of sudden death or ventricular arrhythmia) and perform physical exam to assess for presence of cardiac disease. Promptly perform cardiac evaluation if symptoms of cardiac disease develop. May exacerbate symptoms of behavior disturbance and thought disorder in patients w/ preexisting psychotic disorder. Caution in patients w/ comorbid bipolar disorder; may induce mixed/manic episode. May cause treatment-emergent psychotic or manic symptoms (eg, hallucinations, delusional thinking, mania) in patients w/o prior history of psychotic illness or mania; consider discontinuation if such symptoms occur. Aggressive behavior or hostility reported. May lower convulsive threshold; d/c if seizures occur. Priapism reported; seek immediate medical attention if abnormally sustained or frequent and painful erections develop. Associated w/ peripheral vasculopathy (eg, Raynaud's phenomenon); carefully observe for digital changes. May cause long-term suppression of growth in children; monitor growth, and may need to interrupt treatment in patients not growing or gaining height or weight as expected. Difficulties w/ accommodation and blurring of vision reported. Tab is nondeformable and does not appreciably change in shape in the GI tract; avoid w/ preexisting severe GI narrowing (pathologic or iatrogenic).

ADVERSE REACTIONS

Decreased appetite, headache, dry mouth, nausea, insomnia, anxiety, dizziness, decreased weight, irritability, upper abdominal pain, hyperhidrosis, palpitations, tachycardia, depressed mood, nervousness.

DRUG INTERACTIONS

See Contraindications. Caution w/ vasopressor agents. May inhibit metabolism of coumarin anticoagulants, anticonvulsants (eg, phenobarbital, phenytoin, primidone), and some antidepressants (eg, TCAs, SSRIs); downward dose adjustment and monitoring of plasma drug concentrations (or coagulation times for coumarin) of these drugs may be necessary when initiating or discontinuing methylphenidate.

PATIENT CONSIDERATIONS

C

Assessment: Assess for hypersensitivity to the drug, marked anxiety, tension, agitation, glaucoma, motor tics, family history or diagnosis of Tourette's syndrome, cardiovascular conditions, history of drug dependence or alcoholism, psychotic disorder, comorbid bipolar disorder, severe GI narrowing, any other conditions where treatment is contraindicated or cautioned, pregnancy/nursing status, and possible drug interactions.

Monitoring: Monitor for changes in HR and BP, signs/symptoms of cardiac disease, exacerbation of behavior disturbance and thought disorder, psychosis, mania, appearance of or worsening of aggressive behavior or hostility, seizures, priapism, peripheral vasculopathy (eg, Raynaud's phenomenon), visual disturbances, and other adverse reactions. In pediatric patients, monitor growth. Perform periodic monitoring of CBC, differential, and platelet counts during prolonged therapy. Periodically reevaluate long-term usefulness of drug.

Counseling: Inform about risks, benefits, and appropriate use of the medication. Advise of the possibility of priapism; instruct to seek immediate medical attention in the event of priapism. Inform about the risk of peripheral vasculopathy (eg, Raynaud's phenomenon); instruct to report to physician any new numbness, pain, skin color change, sensitivity to temperature in fingers or toes, or any signs of unexplained wounds appearing on fingers/toes. Advise that the tab shell, along w/ insoluble core components, is eliminated from the body; inform not to be concerned if something that looks like a tab is noticed in the stool. Inform that therapy may impair mental/physical abilities; advise to use caution w/ hazardous tasks (eg, operating machinery, driving).

STORAGE: 25°C (77°F); excursions permitted to 15-30°C (59-86°F). Protect from humidity.

CONTRAVE — bupropion hydrochloride/naltrexone hydrochloride RX

Class: Aminoketone/opioid antagonist

Not approved for use in the treatment of major depressive disorder or other psychiatric disorders. Contains bupropion, the same active ingredient as some other antidepressants (including, but not limited to, Wellbutrin, Wellbutrin SR/XL, and Aplenzin). Antidepressants increased the risk of suicidal thoughts and behavior in children, adolescents, and young adults in short-term trials. Monitor closely for worsening and for the emergence of suicidal thoughts and behaviors. Not approved for use in pediatric patients. Serious neuropsychiatric reactions reported in patients taking bupropion for smoking cessation. Although not approved for smoking cessation, observe all patients for neuropsychiatric reactions.

ADULT DOSAGE

Chronic Weight Management

Adjunct to a reduced-calorie diet and increased physical activity in patients w/ BMI $\geq$30kg/m^2, or $\geq$27kg/m^2 in the presence of at least 1 weight related comorbid condition

Week 1: 1 tab qam
Week 2: 1 tab qam and 1 tab qpm
Week 3: 2 tabs qam and 1 tab qpm
Week 4 Onward/Maint: 2 tabs qam and 2 tabs qpm
Max: 32mg/360mg/day (2 tabs bid)

Evaluate response to therapy after 12 weeks at the maint dose; d/c if patient has not lost at least 5% of baseline weight

Dosing Considerations with MAOIs

Switching to or from an MAOI Antidepressant:
Allow at least 14 days to elapse between discontinuation of an MAOI and initiation of treatment, and conversely allow at least 14 days after discontinuing treatment before starting an MAOI

PEDIATRIC DOSAGE

Pediatric use may not have been established

DOSING CONSIDERATIONS

Concomitant Medications

CYP2B6 Inhibitors:
Max: 2 tabs/day (1 tab qam and qpm)

Renal Impairment

Moderate/Severe:
Max: 2 tabs/day (1 tab qam and qpm)

ESRD: Not recommended

Hepatic Impairment
Max: 1 tab qam

ADMINISTRATION

Oral route

Take no more than 2 tabs at 1 time.
May take w/ meals; avoid high-fat meals.
Swallow tab whole; do not cut, chew, or crush.

HOW SUPPLIED

Tab, Extended-Release: (Naltrexone/Bupropion) 8mg/90mg

CONTRAINDICATIONS

Uncontrolled HTN, seizure disorder or a history of seizures, use of other bupropion-containing products, bulimia or anorexia nervosa, chronic opioid or opiate agonist (eg, methadone) or partial agonists (eg, buprenorphine) use, acute opiate withdrawal, and pregnancy. Undergoing abrupt discontinuation of alcohol, benzodiazepines, barbiturates, and antiepileptic drugs (AEDs). Concomitant administration of MAOIs; allow at least 14 days to elapse between discontinuation of an MAOI and initiation of treatment. Starting treatment in a patient treated with reversible MAOIs (eg, linezolid, IV methylene blue). Known allergy to bupropion, naltrexone, or any other component of this medication.

WARNINGS/PRECAUTIONS

Dose-related risk of seizures; do not exceed 360mg of bupropion component (4 tabs/day in divided doses [bid]), and escalate dose gradually. D/C and do not restart if seizure occurs while on therapy. Caution with predisposing factors that may increase risk of seizure (eg, history of head trauma or prior seizure, severe stroke, arteriovenous malformation, CNS tumor/infection, metabolic disorders [eg, hypoglycemia, hyponatremia, severe hepatic impairment, hypoxia]). May cause an increase in systolic and/or diastolic BP as well as increase in resting HR. D/C treatment if anaphylactoid/anaphylactic reactions occur. Arthralgia, myalgia, fever with rash, and other symptoms suggestive of delayed hypersensitivity reported. Cases of hepatitis, clinically significant liver dysfunction, and transient, asymptomatic hepatic transaminase elevations reported; d/c in the event of symptoms and/or signs of acute hepatitis. May precipitate manic/mixed/hypomanic episodes; risk is increased in patients with or at risk for bipolar disorder. Pupillary dilation may occur and may trigger an angle-closure attack in a patient with anatomically narrow angles who does not have a patent iridectomy. Weight loss may increase risk of hypoglycemia in patients with type 2 DM treated with insulin and/or insulin secretagogues (eg, sulfonylureas, meglitinides); consider decreasing doses of antidiabetic medications that are non-glucose-dependent to mitigate the risk of hypoglycemia. Appropriate changes should be made to antidiabetic regimen if hypoglycemia develops after starting treatment. False (+) urine immunoassay screening tests for amphetamines reported. Not recommended in patients with ESRD. Caution in elderly (>65 yrs of age).

ADVERSE REACTIONS

N/V, constipation, headache, dizziness, insomnia, dry mouth, diarrhea, anxiety, hot flush, fatigue, tremor, upper abdominal pain, viral gastroenteritis, influenza, tinnitus.

DRUG INTERACTIONS

See Dosage and Contraindications. Increased risk for hypertensive reactions with other drugs that inhibit the reuptake of dopamine or norepinephrine, including MAOIs. In patients requiring intermittent opiate treatment, d/c therapy temporarily and do not increase opioid dose above standard dose; use with caution after chronic opioid use has been stopped for 7-10 days to prevent precipitation of withdrawal. Caution with CYP2D6 substrates (eg, SSRIs, haloperidol, metoprolol, propafenone); consider decreasing the dose of CYP2D6 substrate, particularly for drugs with a narrow therapeutic index. CYP2B6 inhibitors (eg, ticlopidine, clopidogrel) may increase bupropion exposure but decrease hydroxybupropion exposure. Ritonavir, lopinavir, or efavirenz may decrease bupropion and hydroxybupropion exposure; avoid concomitant use. Extreme caution with other drugs that lower the seizure threshold (eg, antipsychotics, TCAs, theophylline, systemic corticosteroids); use low initial doses and gradually increase dose. CNS toxicity reported with levodopa or amantadine; caution and monitor for adverse events when administered concomitantly. Minimize or avoid alcohol. Caution with excessive use of alcohol or sedatives, addiction to cocaine or stimulants, withdrawal from sedatives, and diabetics treated with insulin/oral diabetic medications; may increase risk of seizures. May increase levels of drugs transported by the renal organic cation transporter 2 (eg, amantadine, cimetidine, famotidine, metformin); use with caution and monitor for adverse effects.

PATIENT CONSIDERATIONS

Assessment: Assess for known allergy to drug, uncontrolled HTN, seizure disorder or conditions that may increase risk of seizure, bipolar disorder, susceptibility to angle-closure glaucoma, renal/hepatic impairment, any conditions where treatment is contraindicated or cautioned, pregnancy/nursing status, and possible drug interactions. Measure blood glucose levels in patients with type 2 DM. Obtain baseline BP and pulse.

Monitoring: Monitor for clinical worsening, suicidality, or unusual changes in behavior, seizures, neuropsychiatric signs/symptoms, increase in BP and HR, allergic reactions, angle-closure glaucoma, and other adverse reactions. Monitor blood glucose levels in patients with type 2 DM. Monitor hepatic/renal function, especially in the elderly.

Counseling: Inform of benefits/risks of therapy. Advise to take exactly as prescribed. Inform that drug contains the same ingredient found in certain antidepressants and smoking cessation products; instruct not to use in combination with other bupropion-containing products. Advise patients and caregivers of need for close observation for clinical worsening and suicidal risks; instruct to immediately report to physician any agitation, hostility, depressed mood, or changes in thinking or behavior that are not typical for them, or if suicidal ideation or behavior develops. Inform that drug may cause mild pupillary dilation, which in susceptible individuals, may lead to an episode of angle-closure glaucoma. Inform of the symptoms of hypersensitivity; instruct to d/c therapy if a severe allergic reaction occurs. Instruct to d/c and not restart if a seizure is experienced while on treatment. Inform that excessive use or abrupt discontinuation of alcohol, benzodiazepines, AEDs, or sedatives/hypnotics can increase the risk of seizure. Instruct to minimize or avoid alcohol. Advise patients that they may be more sensitive to lower doses of opioids if they previously used opioids, and may be at risk of accidental overdose should they use opioids after treatment is discontinued or temporarily interrupted. Advise patients that because naltrexone can block the effects of opioids, they will not perceive any effect if they attempt to self-administer any opioid drug in small doses while on therapy and that the attempt to administer large doses of any opioid or to bypass the blockade while on therapy may lead to serious injury, coma, or death. Advise patients not to take medication if they have any symptoms of opioid withdrawal. Advise patients to notify healthcare provider if they experience increased BP or HR. Instruct to notify physician if taking/planning to take any prescription or OTC drugs. Inform physician if pregnant, intending to become pregnant, or if breastfeeding during therapy. Advise diabetic patients on antidiabetic therapy to monitor their blood glucose levels and to report symptoms of hypoglycemia to physician. If a dose is missed, instruct to wait until the next scheduled dose to resume the regular dosing schedule.

STORAGE: 25°C (77°F); excursions permitted to 15-30°C (59-86°F).

COPAXONE — glatiramer acetate injection

RX

Class: Immunomodulatory agent

ADULT DOSAGE

Multiple Sclerosis

Relapsing Forms:

20mg/mL: Administer SQ qd
40mg/mL: Administer SQ 3X/week and at least 48 hrs apart

PEDIATRIC DOSAGE

Pediatric use may not have been established

ADMINISTRATION

SQ route

Allow to stand at room temperature for 20 min before administration
Areas for SQ self-inj include arms, abdomen, hips, and thighs

HOW SUPPLIED

Inj: 20mg/mL, 40mg/mL

CONTRAINDICATIONS

Known hypersensitivity to glatiramer acetate or mannitol.

WARNINGS/PRECAUTIONS

20mg/mL and 40mg/mL are not interchangeable. Immediate post-inj reaction (eg, flushing, chest pain, palpitations, anxiety, dyspnea, throat constriction, urticaria) reported. Transient chest pain reported. Localized lipoatrophy at inj sites and inj-site skin necrosis may occur; follow proper inj technique and rotate inj sites with each inj. May interfere with immune functions. Continued alteration of cellular immunity due to chronic treatment may result in untoward effects.

ADVERSE REACTIONS

Inj-site reactions, vasodilatation, rash, dyspnea, chest pain, nasopharyngitis, infection, asthenia, pain, N/V, influenza, anxiety, back pain, palpitations, edema.

PATIENT CONSIDERATIONS

Assessment: Assess for hypersensitivity to drug or mannitol, and pregnancy/nursing status.

Monitoring: Monitor for immediate post-inj reactions, chest pain, lipoatrophy, inj-site skin necrosis, and other adverse reactions.

Counseling: Advise to inform physician if pregnant, planning to become pregnant, or breastfeeding. Inform that drug may cause an immediate post-inj reaction and that symptoms are generally transient and self-limited and do not require specific treatment; inform that these symptoms may occur early or may have their onset several months after treatment initiation. Inform that transient chest pain (either as part of the immediate post-inj reaction or in isolation) may occur; advise to seek medical attention if chest pain of unusual duration or intensity occurs. Instruct to follow proper inj technique and to rotate inj areas and sites with each inj to help minimize localized lipoatrophy and inj-site necrosis. Inform that 20mg/mL and 40mg/mL are not interchangeable. Caution to use aseptic technique. Caution against the reuse of needles or syringes. Inform of safe disposal procedures.

STORAGE: 2-8°C (36-46°F). If needed, may store at 15-30°C (59-86°F) for up to 1 month, but refrigeration is preferred; avoid exposure to higher temperatures or intense light. Do not freeze; discard if frozen.

CORDARONE – amiodarone hydrochloride

RX

Class: Class III antiarrhythmic

Use only in patients w/ the indicated life-threatening arrhythmias because of potentially fatal toxicities, including pulmonary toxicity (hypersensitivity pneumonitis or interstitial/alveolar pneumonitis). Liver injury is common, usually mild, and evidenced only by abnormal liver enzymes. Overt liver disease may occur, and has been fatal. May exacerbate arrhythmia. Significant heart block or sinus bradycardia reported. Patients must be hospitalized while LD is given, and a response generally requires at least 1 week, usually 2 or more. Maintenance-dose selection is difficult and may require dosage decrease or discontinuation of treatment.

ADULT DOSAGE

Ventricular Tachycardia

Documented, life-threatening recurrent hemodynamically unstable ventricular arrhythmia that has not responded to documented adequate doses of other available antiarrhythmics or when alternative agents could not be tolerated

LD: 800-1600mg/day for 1-3 weeks; give in divided doses w/ meals for total daily dose ≥1000mg or if GI intolerance occurs
Titrate: After control is achieved or w/ prominent side effects, reduce to 600-800mg/day for 1 month
Maint: 400mg/day; up to 600mg/day
Use lowest effective dose

Ventricular Fibrillation

Documented, life-threatening recurrent ventricular arrhythmia that has not responded to documented adequate doses of other available antiarrhythmics or when alternative agents could not be tolerated

LD: 800-1600mg/day for 1-3 weeks; give in divided doses w/ meals for total daily dose ≥1000mg or if GI intolerance occurs
Titrate: After control is achieved or w/ prominent side effects, reduce to 600-800mg/day for 1 month
Maint: 400mg/day; up to 600mg/day
Use lowest effective dose

PEDIATRIC DOSAGE

Pediatric use may not have been established

DOSING CONSIDERATIONS

Elderly

Start at the lower end of dosing range

Other Important Considerations

Avoid grapefruit juice

ADMINISTRATION

Oral route

Give LD in the hospital.
Administer consistently w/ regard to meals.
May be administered as a single dose, or in patients w/ severe GI intolerance, as a bid dose.

HOW SUPPLIED
Tab: 200mg* *scored

CONTRAINDICATIONS
Cardiogenic shock; severe sinus-node dysfunction, causing marked sinus bradycardia; 2nd- or 3rd-degree atrioventricular (AV) block; when episodes of bradycardia have caused syncope (except when used w/ a pacemaker). Known hypersensitivity to amiodarone or any components of the medications, including iodine.

WARNINGS/PRECAUTIONS
D/C and institute steroid therapy if hypersensitivity pneumonitis occurs. Reduce dose or d/c if interstitial/alveolar pneumonitis occurs and institute appropriate treatment. The risk of arrhythmia exacerbation may be increased when other risk factors are present (eg, electrolytic disorders). Correct hypokalemia, hypomagnesemia, or hypocalcemia whenever possible before initiating therapy; monitor electrolyte and acid-base balance in patients experiencing severe/prolonged diarrhea. Chronic administration w/ implanted defibrillators/pacemakers may affect pacing and defibrillating thresholds. Amiodarone-induced hyperthyroidism may result in thyrotoxicosis and/or the possibility of arrhythmia breakthrough or aggravation. D/C or reduce dose if LFTs are >3X normal or double in patients w/ elevated baseline. Optic neuropathy and/or optic neuritis, usually resulting in visual impairment, reported. May cause fetal harm in pregnancy and neonatal hypo/hyperthyroidism. May develop reversible corneal microdeposits (eg, visual halos, blurred vision), photosensitivity, and peripheral neuropathy (rare). May cause hypo/hyperthyroidism and myxedema coma; monitor particularly in elderly and w/ history of thyroid nodules, goiter, or other thyroid dysfunction. Thyroid nodules/cancer reported. Hypotension reported upon discontinuation of cardiopulmonary bypass during open-heart surgery (rare). Adult respiratory distress syndrome (ARDS) reported w/ either cardiac or noncardiac surgery. Lab test interactions may occur. May be contraindicated w/ corneal refractive laser surgery devices. Caution w/ severe left ventricular dysfunction.

ADVERSE REACTIONS
Pulmonary toxicity, arrhythmia exacerbation, liver injury, overt liver disease, heart block/sinus bradycardia, malaise, fatigue, involuntary movements, peripheral neuropathy, constipation, poor coordination and gait, N/V, anorexia, photosensitivity.

DRUG INTERACTIONS
See Dosing Considerations. Risk of interactions exists not only w/ concomitant medication, but also w/ drugs administered after discontinuation of therapy due to long and variable $T_{1/2}$. The risk of arrhythmia exacerbation may be increased w/ concomitant antiarrhythmics or other interacting drugs. Monitor electrolyte and acid-base balance w/ concomitant diuretics and laxatives, systemic corticosteroids, amphotericin B (IV), or other drugs affecting electrolyte levels. Avoid concomitant use of drugs that prolong the QT interval (eg, Class I and III antiarrhythmics, lithium, certain phenothiazines); increases risk of torsades de pointes. Concomitant use of drugs w/ depressant effects on the sinus and AV node (eg, digoxin, β-blockers, verapamil, diltiazem, clonidine) can potentiate the electrophysiologic and hemodynamic effects of therapy; monitor HR. May increase sensitivity to myocardial depressant and conduction effects of halogenated inhalation anesthetics. Drugs/substances that inhibit CYP3A (eg, certain protease inhibitors, loratadine, cimetidine, trazodone) may decrease metabolism and increase serum concentrations of therapy. Grapefruit juice may increase levels. Concomitant use of CYP3A inducers (eg, rifampin, St. John's wort) may lead to decreased serum concentrations and loss of efficacy; consider serial measurement of amiodarone serum concentration during concomitant use of drugs affecting CYP3A activity. Reduced serum levels and $T_{1/2}$ w/ cholestyramine. Inhibits P-gp, CYP1A2, CYP2C9, CYP2D6, and CYP3A and may increase levels of their substrates. Rhabdomyolysis/myopathy reported w/ HMG-CoA reductase inhibitors that are CYP3A substrates; limit simvastatin dose to 20mg/day and lovastatin dose to 40mg/day. Lower initial/maintenance doses of other CYP3A substrates (eg, atorvastatin) may be required. Elevated SrCr reported w/ cyclosporine; monitor cyclosporine drug levels and renal function in patients taking both drugs. May increase levels of cyclosporine, quinidine, and procainamide. May inhibit metabolism of quinidine, procainamide, and flecainide. Initiate any added antiarrhythmic drug at a lower than usual dose w/ monitoring. May increase levels of digoxin; d/c or reduce dose by approx 50% upon amiodarone initiation. May inhibit metabolism of lidocaine, resulting in increased lidocaine levels; sinus bradycardia and seizure reported in patients receiving concomitant lidocaine. Reduce warfarin dose by 1/3-1/2 and monitor PT closely. Ineffective inhibition of platelet aggregation reported w/ clopidogrel. May result in elevated serum levels of dabigatran etexilate. Fentanyl may cause hypotension, bradycardia, and decreased cardiac output. Increased steady-state levels of phenytoin reported; monitor phenytoin levels. May impair metabolism of dextromethorphan, leading to increased serum levels w/ chronic (>2 weeks) amiodarone treatment. Antithyroid drugs' action may be delayed in amiodarone-induced thyrotoxicosis. Radioactive iodine is contraindicated w/ amiodarone-induced hyperthyroidism.

PATIENT CONSIDERATIONS

Assessment: Assess for cardiogenic shock, severe sinus node dysfunction causing marked sinus bradycardia, 2nd- or 3rd-degree AV block, life-threatening arrhythmias, renal/hepatic impairment, thyroid dysfunction, hypersensitivity to the drug (including iodine), pregnancy/nursing status, and possible drug interactions. Assess pacing and defibrillation thresholds in patients w/ implanted defibrillators or pacemakers. Obtain chest x-ray, pulmonary function tests (including diffusion capacity), and physical exam. Correct hypokalemia, hypomagnesemia, or hypocalcemia whenever possible.

Monitoring: Monitor for pulmonary toxicities, worsened arrhythmia, sinus bradycardia, heart block, photosensitivity, and other adverse reactions. Perform history, physical exam, and chest x-ray every 3-6 months. Monitor LFTs and thyroid function tests. Monitor pacing and defibrillation thresholds in patients w/ implanted defibrillators or pacemakers. Peri/postoperative monitoring for patients undergoing general anesthesia and for patients w/ ARDS recommended. Perform regular ophthalmic examination, including funduscopy and slit-lamp examination.

Counseling: Inform about benefits and risks of therapy. Advise to report any adverse reactions to physician. Counsel to take ud and not to take w/ grapefruit juice. Advise to avoid prolonged sunlight exposure and to use sun-barrier cre or protective clothing. Advise that corneal refractive laser surgery is contraindicated w/ therapy. Instruct to notify physician if pregnant/nursing.

STORAGE: 20-25°C (68-77°F). Protect from light.

Coreg CR – carvedilol

RX

Class: $Alpha_1$/beta blocker

OTHER BRAND NAMES

Coreg

ADULT DOSAGE

Heart Failure

Tab, Immediate-Release (IR):
Initial: 3.125mg bid for 2 weeks
Titrate: If tolerated, may increase dose to 6.25mg, 12.5mg, and 25mg bid over successive intervals of at least 2 weeks
Max: 50mg bid in patients w/ mild to moderate heart failure (HF) weighing >85kg

Cap, Extended-Release (ER):
Initial: 10mg qd for 2 weeks
Titrate: If tolerated, may increase dose to 20mg, 40mg, and 80mg qd over successive intervals of at least 2 weeks

Left Ventricular Dysfunction Post-Myocardial Infarction

Tab, IR:
Initial: 6.25mg bid
Titrate: Increase after 3-10 days, based on tolerability, to 12.5mg bid, then again to target dose of 25mg bid
May use lower starting dose and/or slower titration

Cap, ER:
Initial: 20mg qd
Titrate: Increase after 3-10 days, based on tolerability, to 40mg qd, then again to target dose of 80mg qd
May use lower starting dose and/or slower titration

Hypertension

Tab, IR:
Initial: 6.25mg bid
Titrate: If needed, based on blood pressure control, may increase to 12.5mg bid, then to 25mg bid over intervals of 7-14 days
Max: 50mg/day

Cap, ER:
Initial: 20mg qd
Titrate: If needed, based on blood pressure control, may increase to 40mg qd, then to 80mg qd, over intervals of 7-14 days
Max: 80mg/day

PEDIATRIC DOSAGE

Pediatric use may not have been established

Conversions

Daily Dose of IR Tabs to ER Caps:
6.25mg (3.125mg BID): 10mg qd
12.5mg (6.25mg BID): 20mg qd
25mg (12.5mg BID): 40mg qd
50mg (25mg BID): 80mg qd

Elderly/Patients at Increased Risk of Hypotension, Dizziness, or Syncope:
Initial:
Switching from 12.5mg bid IR Tabs: 20mg qd
Switching from 25mg bid IR Tabs: 40mg qd
Titrate: Increase doses, as appropriate, after an interval of at least 2 weeks

DOSING CONSIDERATIONS

Hepatic Impairment

Not for use in severe hepatic impairment

ADMINISTRATION

Oral route

Take w/ food.

Cap, ER

Take in am.
Swallow caps whole.
Cap may be opened and beads sprinkled over a spoonful of applesauce and consumed immediately, and may not be stored for future use.
Applesauce should not be warm.
Do not crush, chew, or divide cap and/or its contents.

HOW SUPPLIED

Cap, ER (CR): (Phosphate) 10mg, 20mg, 40mg, 80mg; **Tab:** 3.125mg, 6.25mg, 12.5mg, 25mg

CONTRAINDICATIONS

Bronchial asthma or related bronchospastic conditions, 2nd- or 3rd-degree atrioventricular (AV) block, sick sinus syndrome, severe bradycardia (w/o permanent pacemaker), cardiogenic shock, decompensated HF requiring IV inotropic therapy, severe hepatic impairment, history of serious hypersensitivity reaction (eg, Stevens-Johnson syndrome, anaphylactic reaction, angioedema) to carvedilol or any components of the medication.

WARNINGS/PRECAUTIONS

Minimize fluid retention prior to initiation of treatment. Severe exacerbation of angina and occurrence of MI and ventricular arrhythmias reported in angina patients following abrupt discontinuation; d/c therapy over 1-2 weeks whenever possible. If angina worsens or acute coronary insufficiency develops, promptly reinstitute therapy, at least temporarily. Avoid abrupt discontinuation even in patients treated only for HTN or HF. Bradycardia reported; reduce dose if HR drops <55 BPM. Hypotension, postural hypotension, and syncope reported; highest risk during the first 30 days of dosing. May impair mental/physical abilities. Worsening HF or fluid retention may occur during up-titration; if such symptoms occur, increase dose of diuretics. If deemed necessary, use w/ caution in patients w/ bronchospastic disease who do not respond to, or cannot tolerate, other antihypertensives. May mask signs of hypoglycemia and hyperthyroidism (eg, tachycardia). May exacerbate symptoms of hyperthyroidism or precipitate thyroid storm w/ abrupt withdrawal. May lead to worsening hyperglycemia in HF patients w/ diabetes. May precipitate or aggravate symptoms of arterial insufficiency in patients w/ peripheral vascular disease. Rarely, use in patients w/ HF resulted in deterioration of renal function; d/c or reduce dosage if worsening of renal function occurs. Chronically administered therapy should not be routinely withdrawn prior to major surgery; may augment risks of general anesthesia and surgical procedures. Caution w/ pheochromocytoma and Prinzmetal's variant angina. Patients w/ history of severe anaphylactic reaction to a variety of allergens may be more reactive to repeated challenge and may be unresponsive to usual doses of epinephrine. Intraoperative floppy iris syndrome observed during cataract surgery.

ADVERSE REACTIONS

Bradycardia, fatigue, hypotension, dizziness, headache, diarrhea, N/V, hyperglycemia, weight increase, increased cough, asthenia.

DRUG INTERACTIONS

Potent CYP2D6 inhibitors (eg, quinidine, fluoxetine, propafenone) may increase levels. Monitor closely for signs of hypotension and/or severe bradycardia w/ drugs that can deplete catecholamines (eg, reserpine, MAOIs). Potentiated BP- and HR-lowering effects w/ clonidine; when coadministration is to be terminated, d/c therapy several days before clonidine is withdrawn. May increase cyclosporine levels; monitor concentrations and adjust dose of cyclosporine as appropriate. Increased risk of bradycardia w/ digitalis glycosides. May increase digoxin levels; monitor digoxin. Rifampin may reduce levels. Cimetidine may increase exposure. Amiodarone and its metabolite desethyl amiodarone, CYP2C9 inhibitors, and P-gp inhibitors may increase levels. Amiodarone or other CYP2C9 inhibitors (eg, fluconazole) may enhance β-blocking properties; monitor for signs of bradycardia or heart block. Conduction disturbance reported w/ diltiazem; monitor ECG and BP w/ calcium channel blockers of the verapamil or diltiazem type. May enhance blood glucose-reducing effect of insulin and oral hypoglycemics; regularly monitor blood glucose. If treatment is to be continued perioperatively, use caution when anesthetic agents that depress myocardial function (eg, ether, cyclopropane, trichloroethylene) are used. Additive effects and exaggerated orthostatic component w/ diuretics.

PATIENT CONSIDERATIONS

Assessment: Assess for bronchial asthma, 2nd- or 3rd-degree AV block, sick sinus syndrome, severe bradycardia, cardiogenic shock, hepatic/renal impairment, angina, fluid retention, diabetes, hyperthyroidism, any other conditions where treatment is contraindicated or cautioned, pregnancy/nursing status, and possible drug interactions.

Monitoring: Monitor for bradycardia, worsening HF/fluid retention, masking of signs of hypoglycemia/hyperthyroidism, and other adverse reactions. Monitor BP. Monitor blood glucose during dose initiation, adjustment, or discontinuation. Monitor renal function during up-titration in patients w/ risk factors for renal function deterioration.

Counseling: Instruct not to interrupt or d/c therapy w/o consulting physician. Instruct patients w/ HF to consult physician if signs/symptoms of worsening HF occur. Inform that a drop in BP when standing, resulting in dizziness and, rarely, fainting, may occur; advise to sit or lie down when these symptoms occur. Advise to avoid driving or hazardous tasks if experiencing dizziness or fatigue, and to notify physician if dizziness or faintness occurs. Inform contact lens wearers that decreased lacrimation may be experienced, and diabetic patients to report any changes in blood sugar levels.

STORAGE: **Cap, ER:** 25°C (77°F); excursions permitted to 15-30°C (59-86°F). **Tab:** <30°C (86°F). Protect from moisture.

CORGARD – nadolol

RX

Class: Nonselective beta blocker

Hypersensitivity to catecholamines observed upon withdrawal; exacerbation of angina and, in some cases, myocardial infarction reported after abrupt discontinuation. When discontinuing chronically administered nadolol, particularly in patients with ischemic heart disease, reduce dose gradually over a period of 1-2 weeks and monitor carefully. If angina markedly worsens or acute coronary insufficiency develops, administration of therapy should be reinstituted promptly, at least temporarily, and other measures appropriate for the management of unstable angina should be taken. Warn against interruption or discontinuation of therapy without the physician's advice. Coronary artery disease (CAD) is common and may be unrecognized; it may be prudent not to d/c therapy abruptly even in patients treated only for HTN.

ADULT DOSAGE

Angina Pectoris

Initial: 40mg qd
Titrate: May gradually increase in 40-80mg increments at 3- to 7-day intervals until optimum response is obtained or there is pronounced slowing of the HR
Usual Maint: 40 or 80mg qd; doses up to 160 or 240mg qd may be needed
Max: 240mg/day

Reduce gradually over a period of 1-2 weeks if treatment is to d/c

Hypertension

Initial: 40mg qd
Titrate: May gradually increase in 40-80mg increments until optimum BP reduction is achieved
Usual Maint: 40 or 80mg qd; doses up to 240 or 320mg qd may be needed

PEDIATRIC DOSAGE

Pediatric use may not have been established

C

DOSING CONSIDERATIONS

__Renal Impairment__

CrCl >50mL/min: Dose q24h
CrCl 31-50mL/min: Dose q24-36h
CrCl 10-30mL/min: Dose q24-48h
CrCl <10mL/min: Dose q40-60h

ADMINISTRATION

Oral route

May be administered without regard to meals.

HOW SUPPLIED

Tab: 20mg*, 40mg*, 80mg* *scored

CONTRAINDICATIONS

Bronchial asthma, sinus bradycardia and >1st degree conduction block, cardiogenic shock, overt cardiac failure.

WARNINGS/PRECAUTIONS

May precipitate more severe heart failure (HF) in patients with congestive heart failure (CHF); caution with history of well-compensated HF. May lead to cardiac failure in patients without a history of HF; digitalize and/or treat with diuretics at the first sign or symptom of HF and observe response closely or d/c. Avoid in patients with bronchospastic diseases. Chronically administered therapy should not be routinely withdrawn prior to major surgery. May prevent premonitory signs and symptoms of acute hypoglycemia (eg, tachycardia, BP changes). May mask certain clinical signs (eg, tachycardia) of hyperthyroidism. May precipitate thyroid storm with abrupt withdrawal. Caution in patients with renal impairment. Patients with a history of severe anaphylactic reaction to variety of allergens may be more reactive to repeated challenge and may be unresponsive to usual doses of epinephrine.

ADVERSE REACTIONS

Bradycardia, dizziness, fatigue, nausea, diarrhea, anorexia, abdominal discomfort, rash, pruritus, weight gain, blurred vision, peripheral vascular insufficiency, cardiac failure, hypotension, rhythm/conduction disturbances.

DRUG INTERACTIONS

Additive hypotension and/or bradycardia with catecholamine-depleting drugs (eg, reserpine); monitor closely. Increased risk of bradycardia with digitalis glycosides. Hyperglycemia or hypoglycemia may occur with antidiabetic drugs (oral agents and insulin); adjust dose of antidiabetic agents accordingly. May exaggerate hypotension induced by general anesthetics.

PATIENT CONSIDERATIONS

Assessment: Assess for bronchial asthma, sinus bradycardia, AV heart block, cardiogenic shock, CHF, bronchospastic diseases, CAD, hyperthyroidism, diabetes, renal impairment, hypersensitivity to drug, pregnancy/nursing status, and possible drug interactions.

Monitoring: Monitor for signs/symptoms of CHF, hypoglycemia, thyrotoxicosis, withdrawal symptoms, renal dysfunction, hypersensitivity reactions, and other adverse reactions

Counseling: Warn against interruption or discontinuation of therapy without consulting physician. Advise to consult physician at 1st sign/symptom of impending cardiac failure. Advise of proper course in the event of an inadvertently missed dose.

STORAGE: Room temperature; avoid excessive heat. Protect from light.

CORLANOR – ivabradine RX

Class: Hyperpolarization-activated cyclic nucleotide-gated channel blocker

ADULT DOSAGE

Heart Failure

To reduce the risk of hospitalization for worsening heart failure (HF) in patients w/ stable, symptomatic chronic HF w/ left ventricular ejection fraction ≤35%, who are in sinus rhythm w/ resting HR ≥70 bpm and either are on maximally tolerated doses of β-blockers or have a contraindication to β-blocker use

Initial: 5mg bid

Titrate: After 2 weeks, assess patient and adjust dose to achieve a resting HR of 50-60 bpm

PEDIATRIC DOSAGE

Pediatric use may not have been established

C

Max: 7.5mg bid

HR <50 bpm or Signs/Symptoms of Bradycardia: Decrease dose by 2.5mg (given bid); if current dose is 2.5mg bid, d/c therapy

HR 50-60 bpm: Maintain dose

HR >60 bpm: Increase dose by 2.5mg (given bid) up to a max dose of 7.5mg bid

Thereafter, adjust dose prn based on resting HR and tolerability

DOSING CONSIDERATIONS

Hepatic Impairment

Severe (Child-Pugh C): Contraindicated

Other Important Considerations

History of Conduction Defects or Bradycardia Leading to Hemodynamic Compromise:

Initial: 2.5mg bid

Titrate: Increase dose based on HR

ADMINISTRATION

Oral route

Take w/ meals.

HOW SUPPLIED

Tab: 5mg*, 7.5mg, *scored

CONTRAINDICATIONS

Acute decompensated HF; BP <90/50mmHg; sick sinus syndrome, sinoatrial block, or 3rd degree atrioventricular (AV) block, unless a functioning demand pacemaker is present; resting HR <60 bpm prior to treatment; severe hepatic impairment; pacemaker dependence (HR maintained exclusively by the pacemaker). Concomitant use of strong CYP3A4 inhibitors.

WARNINGS/PRECAUTIONS

May cause fetal toxicity. Increases the risk of A-fib; d/c if this develops. Bradycardia, sinus arrest, and heart block reported. Risk factors for bradycardia include sinus node dysfunction, conduction defects (eg, 1st/2nd degree AV block, bundle branch block), and ventricular dyssynchrony; avoid use in patients w/ 2nd degree AV block, unless a functioning demand pacemaker is present. Not recommended in patients w/ demand pacemakers set to rates ≥60 bpm.

ADVERSE REACTIONS

Bradycardia, HTN, A-fib.

DRUG INTERACTIONS

See Contraindications. CYP3A4 inhibitors/inducers increase/decrease levels respectively; increased levels may exacerbate bradycardia and conduction disturbances; avoid concomitant use of moderate CYP3A4 inhibitors (eg, diltiazem, verapamil, grapefruit juice) and CYP3A4 inducers (eg, St. John's wort, rifampicin, barbiturates, phenytoin). Increased risk of bradycardia w/ other drugs that slow HR (eg, digoxin, diltiazem, verapamil, amiodarone, β-blockers); monitor HR.

PATIENT CONSIDERATIONS

Assessment: Assess for acute decompensated HF, BP <90/50mmHg, sick sinus syndrome, sinoatrial block, 2nd or 3rd degree AV block, presence of a functioning demand pacemaker, resting HR <60 bpm prior to treatment, severe hepatic impairment, pacemaker dependence, risk factors for bradycardia, history of conduction defects, pregnancy/nursing status, and possible drug interactions.

Monitoring: Monitor for A-fib, bradycardia, sinus arrest, heart block, and other adverse reactions. Monitor cardiac rhythm regularly.

Counseling: Advise pregnant women of the potential risks to a fetus. Advise females of reproductive potential to use effective contraception and to notify their healthcare provider w/ a known/suspected pregnancy. Advise to report significant decreases in HR or symptoms such as dizziness, fatigue, or hypotension. Advise to report symptoms of A-fib (eg, heart palpitations or racing, chest pressure, worsened SOB). Advise about the possible occurrence of luminous phenomena (phosphenes) and that phosphenes may subside spontaneously during continued treatment. Advise to use caution if driving or using machines in situations where sudden changes in light intensity may occur, especially when driving at night. Advise to avoid ingestion of grapefruit juice and St. John's wort.

STORAGE: 25°C (77°F); excursions permitted to 15-30°C (59-86°F).

CORTEF – hydrocortisone

RX

Class: Glucocorticoid

C

ADULT DOSAGE

Steroid-Responsive Disorders

Initial: 20-240mg/day depending on disease

Adjust/maintain initial dose until a satisfactory response observed. If no satisfactory clinical response after a reasonable period, D/C and transfer to appropriate therapy

Maint: Decrease dose by small amounts to lowest effective dose

Multiple Sclerosis

Acute Exacerbations:

Usual: 200mg/day of prednisolone for 1 week followed by 80mg qod for 1 month (20mg hydrocortisone=5mg prednisolone)

PEDIATRIC DOSAGE

Steroid-Responsive Disorders

Initial: 20-240mg/day depending on disease

Adjust/maintain initial dose until a satisfactory response observed. If no satisfactory clinical response after a reasonable period, D/C and transfer to appropriate therapy

Maint: Decrease dose by small amounts to lowest effective dose

Multiple Sclerosis

Acute Exacerbations:

Usual: 200mg/day of prednisolone for 1 week followed by 80mg qod for 1 month (20mg hydrocortisone=5mg prednisolone)

DOSING CONSIDERATIONS

Discontinuation

Withdraw gradually after long-term therapy

ADMINISTRATION

Oral route

HOW SUPPLIED

Tab: 5mg, 10mg, 20mg

CONTRAINDICATIONS

Systemic fungal infections, known hypersensitivity to components.

WARNINGS/PRECAUTIONS

May need to increase dose before, during, and after stressful situations. May mask signs of infection or cause new infections. Prolonged use may produce posterior subcapsular cataract, glaucoma with possible optic nerve damage, may enhance secondary ocular infections. Weigh benefit versus risk in use during pregnancy; may cause hypoadrenalism in infants. May cause elevation of BP, salt/water retention, and increased excretion of K^+ and calcium. Dietary salt restriction and K^+ supplementation may be necessary. More serious/fatal course of chickenpox and measles reported. Drug-induced secondary adrenocortical insufficiency may be minimized by gradual reduction of dosage. Enhanced effects with hypothyroidism and cirrhosis. Avoid abrupt withdrawal. Psychic derangements may appear and existing emotional instability or psychotic tendencies may be aggravated. Caution with active or latent tuberculosis (TB), *Strongyloides* infestation, ocular herpes simplex, nonspecific ulcerative colitis, diverticulitis, fresh intestinal anastomosis, active or latent peptic ulcer, renal insufficiency, HTN, osteoporosis, and myasthenia gravis. Growth and development of children on prolonged therapy should be monitored. Kaposi's sarcoma reported.

ADVERSE REACTIONS

Fluid and electrolyte disturbances, HTN, osteoporosis, muscle weakness, cushingoid state, menstrual irregularities, impaired wound healing, ulcerative esophagitis, increased sweating, increased intracranial pressure, carbohydrate intolerance, glaucoma, cataracts.

DRUG INTERACTIONS

Live or live, attenuated vaccines are contraindicated with immunosuppressive doses. May diminish response to killed or inactivated vaccines. Hepatic enzyme inducers (eg, phenobarbital, phenytoin, and rifampin) may decrease levels; may need to increase dose. Troleandomycin and ketoconazole may increase levels. May decrease levels of chronic high dose aspirin; caution with hypoprothrombinemia. Variable effects on oral anticoagulants; monitor coagulation indices. May increase insulin or oral hypoglycemic agents requirements in diabetics.

PATIENT CONSIDERATIONS

Assessment: Assess for systemic fungal infections, history/active TB, vaccination history, hypersensitivity to the drug, stress level, *Strongyloides* infestation, ocular herpes simplex, psychotic tendencies, cirrhosis, ulcerative colitis, diverticulitis, intestinal anastomosis, peptic ulcer, renal insufficiency, HTN, osteoporosis, myasthenia gravis, thyroid status, pregnancy/nursing status, and possible drug interactions. Obtain baseline of K^+ and calcium levels, blood sugar, and BP.

Monitoring: Monitor for occurrence of infections, cataracts, glaucoma, ocular infection, reactivation of TB, *Strongyloides* hyperinfection, adrenocortical insufficiency, psychic derangement, psychotic tendencies, myopathy, edema and Kaposi's sarcoma. Monitor for growth and development of children on prolonged therapy. Monitor BP, blood glucose levels, and serum electrolytes.

Counseling: Advise of benefits/risks of therapy. Inform that susceptibility to infections may increase. Advise to avoid exposure to chickenpox and measles; report immediately to physician if exposed. Advise that dietary salt restriction and supplementation of K^+ and calcium may be necessary. Instruct not to d/c therapy abruptly or without medical supervision.

STORAGE: 20-25°C (68-77°F).

C

CORTIFOAM – hydrocortisone acetate

RX

Class: Corticosteroid

ADULT DOSAGE

Ulcerative Proctitis

Adjunctive treatment of ulcerative proctitis of the distal portion of the rectum in patients who cannot retain hydrocortisone or other corticosteroid enemas

Usual: 1 applicatorful rectally qd or bid for 2 or 3 weeks, and every 2nd day thereafter

Maint: After a favorable response is noted, decrease initial dose in small decrements at appropriate time intervals until lowest effective dose is reached

PEDIATRIC DOSAGE

Pediatric use may not have been established

DOSING CONSIDERATIONS

Discontinuation

If drug is to be stopped after long-term therapy, withdraw gradually rather than abruptly

ADMINISTRATION

Rectal route

Directions for Use

1. Shake foam container vigorously for 5-10 sec before each use; do not remove container cap during use of product
2. Hold container upright on a level surface and gently place the tip of the applicator onto the nose of the container cap
3. Pull plunger past the fill line on the applicator barrel
4. To fill applicator barrel, press down firmly on cap flanges, hold for 1-2 sec and release; pause 5-10 sec to allow foam to expand in applicator barrel and repeat until foam reaches fill line
5. Remove applicator from container cap; allow some foam to remain on the applicator tip. A burst of air may come out of container w/ 1st pump
6. Hold applicator firmly by barrel, making sure thumb and middle finger are positioned securely underneath and resting against barrel wings; place index finger over the plunger
7. Gently insert tip into anus; once in place, push plunger to expel foam, then withdraw applicator
8. Do not insert any part of the aerosol container directly into the anus; apply to anus only w/ enclosed applicator

HOW SUPPLIED

Foam: 10% [15g]

CONTRAINDICATIONS

Hypersensitivity to any components of the medication. Obstruction, abscess, perforation, peritonitis, fresh intestinal anastomoses, extensive fistulas and sinus tracts.

WARNINGS/PRECAUTIONS

Do not insert any part of the aerosol container directly into the anus. Systemic absorption may be greater than from other corticosteroid enema formulations. D/C if no improvement in 2 or 3 weeks, or if condition worsens. Anaphylactoid reactions reported rarely. May cause BP elevation, salt and water retention, increase K^+ and Ca^{2+} excretion. May produce reversible hypothalamic-pituitary-adrenal (HPA) axis suppression w/ the potential for glucocorticosteroid insufficiency after d/c. Decreased metabolic clearance in hypothyroidism and increased in hyperthyroidism; may necessitate dosage adjustment. May mask signs of current infection or increase susceptibility to infections. May exacerbate systemic fungal infections; avoid use in the presence of such infections unless needed to control drug reactions. Latent disease may be activated or intercurrent infections may be exacerbated. Rule out latent or active amebiasis prior to initiation in any patient who spent time in the tropics or w/ unexplained diarrhea. May cause a more serious/fatal course of chickenpox and measles; avoid exposure. May produce posterior subcapsular cataracts, glaucoma w/ possible optic nerve damage, and enhance the establishment of secondary ocular infections. Kaposi's sarcoma reported most often w/ chronic conditions. Drug-induced secondary adrenocortical insufficiency may be minimized by gradual dose reduction. Signs of peritoneal irritation following

GI perforation may be minimal or absent. Enhanced effect w/ cirrhosis. May decrease bone formation and increase bone resorption, and may lead to inhibition of bone growth in pediatrics and development of osteoporosis at any age. Acute myopathy observed w/ high doses, especially in patients w/ neuromuscular transmission disorders (eg, myasthenia gravis). Creatinine kinase elevation, psychic derangements, and emotional instability or aggravation of psychotic tendencies may occur. May elevate IOP; monitor IOP if used for >6 weeks. Caution w/ recent MI, *Strongyloides* (threadworm) infestation, active/latent tuberculosis (TB) or tuberculin reactivity, CHF, HTN, renal insufficiency, active or latent peptic ulcers, diverticulitis, fresh intestinal anastomoses, nonspecific ulcerative colitis, and risk of osteoporosis. Avoid w/ cerebral malaria, active ocular herpes simplex, and immediate or early postoperative period following ileorectostomy. May suppress reactions to skin tests.

ADVERSE REACTIONS

Bradycardia, acne, abdominal distention, convulsions, depression, abnormal fat deposits, fluid retention, muscle weakness, pancreatitis, headache, exophthalmos.

DRUG INTERACTIONS

Live or live, attenuated vaccines are contraindicated w/ immunosuppressive doses. May diminish response to toxoids and live or inactivated vaccines. May potentiate replication of some organisms contained in live attenuated vaccines. Aminoglutethimide may lead to a loss of corticosteroid-induced adrenal suppression. K^+-depleting agents (eg, amphotericin B, diuretics) may cause hypokalemia; observe closely. Concomitant amphotericin B may cause cardiac enlargement and CHF. Macrolide antibiotics may decrease clearance. Withdraw anticholinesterase agents at least 24 hrs prior to initiation of therapy. Monitor coagulation indices w/ warfarin. Dosage adjustments of antidiabetic agents may be required. May decrease levels of isoniazid. Convulsions and increased activity of both drugs reported w/ cyclosporine. Cholestyramine may increase clearance. May increase risk of arrhythmias w/ digitalis glycosides. Estrogens and ketoconazole may decrease metabolism. Hepatic enzyme inducers (eg, barbiturates, phenytoin, carbamazepine, rifampin) may enhance metabolism; may need to increase corticosteroid dose. Aspirin (ASA) (or other NSAIDs) may increase risk of GI side effects; use ASA cautiously in hypoprothrombinemia. May increase clearance of salicylates. Acute myopathy reported w/ neuromuscular-blocking drugs (eg, pancuronium).

PATIENT CONSIDERATIONS

Assessment: Assess for hypersensitivity to any components of the drug, obstruction, abscess, perforation, peritonitis, fresh intestinal anastomoses, extensive fistulas and sinus tracts, recent MI, thyroid status changes, infections, amebiasis, *Strongyloides* infestation, cerebral malaria, TB, active ocular herpes simplex, CHF, HTN, renal insufficiency, peptic ulcer, diverticulitis, nonspecific ulcerative colitis, recent ileorectostomy, cirrhosis, risk of osteoporosis, emotional instability, psychotic tendencies, pregnancy/nursing status, and possible drug interactions.

Monitoring: Monitor for signs/symptoms of HTN, salt and water retention, increased excretion of K^+, left ventricular free wall rupture (in patients w/ recent MI), glucocorticosteroid insufficiency (upon d/c), infections, reactivation of TB, posterior subcapsular cataracts, glaucoma, Kaposi's sarcoma, acute myopathy, improvement or worsening of condition, and other adverse reactions.

Counseling: Counsel not to d/c abruptly or w/o medical supervision. Advise to inform medical attendants that corticosteroids are being taken. Advise that contents of container are under pressure; do not burn or puncture. Instruct to seek medical advice if fever or other signs of infection develop. Advise to avoid exposure to chickenpox or measles; if exposed, advise to seek medical advice w/o delay.

STORAGE: 20-25°C (68-77°F). Do not refrigerate.

CORTISPORIN TOPICAL – bacitracin zinc/hydrocortisone/neomycin sulfate/polymyxin B sulfate; hydrocortisone acetate/neomycin sulfate/polymyxin B sulfate

RX

Class: Antibacterial/corticosteroid combination

ADULT DOSAGE

Dermatoses

Corticosteroid Responsive w/ Secondary Infection:

Apply thin film bid-qid to the affected area(s)

Max: 7 days

PEDIATRIC DOSAGE

Pediatric use may not have been established

C

ADMINISTRATION
Topical route

HOW SUPPLIED
Cre: (Hydrocortisone acetate/Neomycin sulfate/Polymyxin sulfate) (5mg/3.5mg/10,000 U)/g [7.5g]; **Oint:** (Bacitracin zinc/Hydrocortisone/Neomycin sulfate/Polymyxin sulfate) (400 U/10mg/3.5mg/5000 U)/g

CONTRAINDICATIONS
Use in eyes or external ear canal if eardrum is perforated. Tuberculous, fungal, or viral (eg, herpes simplex or varicella zoster) skin lesions. Hypersensitivity to any of the components.

WARNINGS/PRECAUTIONS
Avoid prolonged use; may result in superinfection, nephrotoxicity and ototoxicity. Limit treatment to 7 days. Exogenous hyperadrenocorticism may occur. Application over extensive body surface areas or use of occlusive dressings will increase systemic absorption. Percutaneous absorption may cause growth cessation in pediatrics. D/C if redness, irritation, swelling, or pain persists. May cause cutaneous sensitization; d/c if occurs. Caution in elderly.

ADVERSE REACTIONS
Allergic sensitization, burning, itching, irritation, dryness, folliculitis, hypertrichosis, acneiform eruptions, secondary infection, skin maceration, striae.

PATIENT CONSIDERATIONS

Assessment: Assess for proper diagnosis (eg, cultures, susceptibility tests), perforated eardrum, TB, fungal or viral lesions of skin, pregnancy/nursing status.

Monitoring: Monitor for signs/symptoms of ototoxicity, nephrotoxicity, cutaneous sensitization (eg, swelling, dry scaling, itching, failure to heal), overgrowth of nonsusceptible organisms (eg, fungi), allergic cross reactions, spread of infection, and adrenal suppression. Monitor for clinical response; if infection is not improved after 1 week, repeat diagnostic tests (eg, cultures, susceptibility tests).

Counseling: Instruct to d/c use and contact physician if redness, irritation, swelling, or increased pain occur. Use medication topically and avoid contact with eyes. Advise that medication should not be used for longer than 7 days due to risk of adverse events (eg, ototoxicity, nephrotoxicity).

STORAGE: 15-25°C (59-77°F).

CORVERT – ibutilide fumarate

RX

Class: Class III antiarrhythmic

May cause potentially fatal arrhythmias, particularly sustained polymorphic ventricular tachycardia, usually in association w/ QT prolongation (torsades de pointes), but sometimes w/o documented QT prolongation. Administer in a setting of continuous ECG monitoring and by personnel trained in identification and treatment of acute ventricular arrhythmias. Patients w/ A-fib of >2-3 days' duration must be adequately anticoagulated, generally for ≥2 weeks. Patients should be carefully selected such that the expected benefits of maintaining sinus rhythm outweigh the immediate and maintenance therapy risks.

ADULT DOSAGE

Atrial Fibrillation/Flutter

Rapid Conversion to Sinus Rhythm in Recent Onset A-Fib/A-Flutter:

Initial:

<60kg: 0.01mg/kg over 10 min

≥60kg: 1mg over 10 min

If arrhythmia still present w/in 10 min after the end of the initial infusion, repeat infusion 10 min after completion of 1st infusion

PEDIATRIC DOSAGE

Pediatric use may not have been established

DOSING CONSIDERATIONS

Elderly
Start at lower end of dosing range

ADMINISTRATION
IV route

Dilution
May be administered undiluted or diluted in 50mL of diluent
May be added to 0.9% NaCl or D5 inj before infusion
The contents of one 10mL vial (0.1mg/mL) may be added to a 50mL infusion bag to form an admixture of approx 0.017mg/mL ibutilide

Compatibility

The following diluents are compatible w/ ibutilide inj (0.1mg/mL):
D5 inj; 0.9% NaCl inj
The following IV sol containers are compatible w/ admixtures of ibutilide inj (0.1mg/mL):
polyvinyl chloride plastic bags, polyolefin bags

HOW SUPPLIED

Inj: 0.1mg/mL [10mL]

CONTRAINDICATIONS

Previously demonstrated hypersensitivity to ibutilide fumarate or any other components of the medication.

WARNINGS/PRECAUTIONS

May induce/worsen ventricular arrhythmias. Not recommended in patients who have previously demonstrated polymorphic ventricular tachycardia (eg, torsades de pointes). Anticipate proarrhythmic events. Correct hypokalemia and hypomagnesemia before therapy. Reversible heart block reported. Caution in elderly.

ADVERSE REACTIONS

Sustained/nonsustained polymorphic ventricular tachycardia, nonsustained monomorphic ventricular tachycardia, ventricular extrasystoles, headache.

DRUG INTERACTIONS

Avoid Class IA (eg, disopyramide, quinidine, procainamide) and other Class III (eg, amiodarone, sotalol) antiarrhythmics w/ or w/in 4 hrs postinfusion. Increased proarrhythmia potential w/ drugs that prolong the QT interval (eg, phenothiazines, TCAs, tetracyclic antidepressants, antihistamine drugs [H_1-receptor antagonists]). Caution in patients w/ elevated or above the usual therapeutic range of plasma digoxin levels.

PATIENT CONSIDERATIONS

Assessment: Assess for arrhythmia, bradycardia, polymorphic ventricular tachycardia, electrolyte imbalance, CHF, low ejection fraction, renal/hepatic function, pregnancy/nursing status, and for possible drug interactions. Perform ECG. Obtain baseline QTc.

Monitoring: Monitor for worsening of induction of new ventricular arrhythmia, torsades de pointes (polymorphic ventricular tachycardia), and any arrhythmic activity. Monitor ECG continuously for ≥4 hrs following infusion.

Counseling: Inform about benefits/risks of therapy. Instruct to report any adverse reactions to physician.

STORAGE: Vial: 20-25°C (68-77°F). Admixture: 0.9% NaCl or D5 Inj: Stable at 15-30°C (59-86°F) for 24 hrs and 2-8°C (36-46°F) for 48 hrs in polyvinyl chloride plastic bags or polyolefin bags.

COSENTYX – secukinumab

RX

Class: Monoclonal antibody/IL-17A antagonist

ADULT DOSAGE

Plaque Psoriasis

In Patients Who Are Candidates for Systemic/Phototherapy:

Moderate to Severe:
300mg at Weeks 0, 1, 2, 3, and 4, followed by 300mg every 4 weeks; a dose of 150mg may be acceptable for some patients

Each 300mg dose is given as two 150mg inj

Psoriatic Arthritis

W/ Coexistent Moderate to Severe Plaque Psoriasis:
Use the dosing recommendations for plaque psoriasis

Other Psoriatic Arthritis:
Administer w/ or w/o a LD
W/ a LD: 150mg at Weeks 0, 1, 2, 3, and 4 and every 4 weeks thereafter
W/O a LD: 150mg every 4 weeks
If active psoriatic arthritis continues, consider a dosage of 300mg

May administer w/ or w/o methotrexate

PEDIATRIC DOSAGE

Pediatric use may not have been established

Ankylosing Spondylitis
Administer w/ or w/o a LD
W/ a LD: 150mg at Weeks 0, 1, 2, 3, and 4 and every 4 weeks thereafter
W/O a LD: 150mg every 4 weeks

ADMINISTRATION

SQ route

Administer each inj at a different anatomic location (eg, upper arms, thighs, any quadrant of abdomen) than previous inj.
Do not inject into areas where the skin is tender, bruised, erythematous, indurated, or affected by psoriasis.

Preparation

Pen and Prefilled Syringe:
Before inj, remove from refrigerator and allow to reach room temperature (15-30 min) w/o removing needle cap.
Administer w/in 1 hr after removal from refrigerator and discard any unused product remaining in the pen/prefilled syringe.

Single-Use Vial:
Preparation time from piercing the stopper until end of reconstitution should not exceed 90 min.
1. Remove vial from refrigerator and allow to stand for 15-30 min to reach room temperature; ensure sterile water for inj (SWFI) is at room temperature.
2. Slowly inject 1mL of SWFI into vial.
3. Tilt vial at a 45° angle and gently rotate between fingertips for 1 min; do not shake/invert vial.
4. Allow vial to stand for 10 min at room temperature, then tilt vial at a 45° angle and gently rotate between fingertips for 1 min; do not shake/invert vial.
5. Allow vial to stand undisturbed at room temperature for approx 5 min.
6. Prepare the required number for vials and use immediately or store in refrigerator at 2-8°C (36-46°F) for up to 24 hrs. Do not freeze. After refrigeration, allow reconstituted sol to reach room temperature (15-30 min) before administration; administer w/in 1 hr after removal from 2-8°C (36-46°F) storage.

HOW SUPPLIED

Inj: 150mg/mL [prefilled syringe, Sensoready pen], 150mg [vial]

CONTRAINDICATIONS

Previous serious hypersensitivity reaction to secukinumab or any components of the medication.

WARNINGS/PRECAUTIONS

May increase risk of infections; exercise caution when considering use in patients w/ a chronic infection or a history of recurrent infection. If serious infection develops, closely monitor and d/c until infection resolves. Evaluate for tuberculosis (TB) infection prior to initiating treatment; do not administer to patients w/ active TB infection. Initiate treatment of latent TB prior to administering therapy; consider anti-TB therapy prior to initiation in patients w/ a past history of latent or active TB in whom an adequate course of treatment cannot be confirmed. Caution w/ inflammatory bowel disease; exacerbations and new onset reported. Trend towards greater disease activity and increased adverse events seen w/ active Crohn's disease. Anaphylaxis and urticaria reported; d/c immediately and initiate appropriate therapy if an anaphylactic or other serious allergic reaction occurs. Removable cap of the Sensoready pen and prefilled syringe contains natural rubber latex, which may cause an allergic reaction in latex-sensitive individuals. Prior to initiating therapy, consider completion of all age appropriate immunizations according to current immunization guidelines.

ADVERSE REACTIONS

Ankylosing Spondylitis: Nasopharyngitis, nausea, URTI, infections.
Plaque Psoriasis: Nasopharyngitis, diarrhea, URTI, infections.
Psoriatic Arthritis: Nasopharyngitis, URTI, headache, nausea, hypercholesterolemia, infections.

DRUG INTERACTIONS

Avoid w/ live vaccines. Non-live vaccinations received during a course of therapy may not elicit an immune response sufficient to prevent disease. May normalize formation of CYP450 enzymes; upon initiation or discontinuation of therapy in patients who are receiving concomitant CYP450 substrates, particularly those w/ a narrow therapeutic index, consider monitoring for therapeutic effect (eg, warfarin) or drug concentration (eg, cyclosporine) and consider dosage modification of the CYP450 substrate.

PATIENT CONSIDERATIONS

Assessment: Assess for previous hypersensitivity to the drug, chronic infection or history of recurrent infection, TB infection, inflammatory bowel disease, latex sensitivity, immunization status, pregnancy/nursing status, and possible drug interactions.

Monitoring: Monitor for signs/symptoms of infection, inflammatory bowel disease, anaphylactic/allergic reactions, and other adverse reactions. Monitor for signs/symptoms of active TB during and after treatment.

Counseling: Advise of the potential benefits and risks of therapy. Inform that drug may lower the ability of immune system to fight infections; instruct to contact physician if any symptoms of infection develop. Advise to seek immediate medical attention if any symptoms of a serious hypersensitivity reaction occur. Instruct in inj techniques, as well as proper syringe and needle disposal, and caution against reuse of needles and syringes.

STORAGE: 2-8°C (36-46°F). Protect from light. Do not freeze. To avoid foaming, do not shake.

Cosopt – dorzolamide hydrochloride/timolol maleate RX

Class: Carbonic anhydrase inhibitor/nonselective beta blocker

OTHER BRAND NAMES

Cosopt PF

ADULT DOSAGE

Elevated Intraocular Pressure

Reduction of elevated IOP in patients w/ open-angle glaucoma or ocular HTN who are insufficiently responsive to β-blockers

1 drop in the affected eye(s) bid

PEDIATRIC DOSAGE

Elevated Intraocular Pressure

Reduction of elevated IOP in patients w/ open-angle glaucoma or ocular HTN who are insufficiently responsive to β-blockers

≥2 Years:

1 drop in the affected eye(s) bid

DOSING CONSIDERATIONS

Concomitant Medications

If >1 topical ophthalmic drug is being used, administer at least 5 min apart

ADMINISTRATION

Ocular route

Cosopt PF

Use the sol from 1 individual unit immediately after opening, and discard the remaining contents immediately after administration.

HOW SUPPLIED

Ophthalmic Sol: (Dorzolamide/Timolol) (Cosopt) 2%/0.5% [10mL]; (Cosopt PF) 2%/0.5% [0.2mL, 60[s] 180[s]]

CONTRAINDICATIONS

Bronchial asthma or history thereof, severe COPD, sinus bradycardia, 2nd- or 3rd-degree atrioventricular (AV) block, overt cardiac failure, cardiogenic shock, hypersensitivity to any component of the medication.

WARNINGS/PRECAUTIONS

Bacterial keratitis associated w/ the use of multiple-dose containers of topical ophthalmic products. **Dorzolamide:** Absorbed systemically. Fatalities reported (rare) due to severe reactions to sulfonamides; sensitization may recur when readministered irrespective of the route of administration. D/C if signs of serious reactions or hypersensitivity occur. Not recommended w/ severe renal impairment (CrCl <30mL/min). Caution w/ hepatic impairment. Increased potential for developing corneal edema in patients w/ low endothelial cell counts. **Timolol:** Absorbed systemically; severe respiratory reactions and rarely death in association w/ cardiac failure reported. Inhibition of sympathetic stimulation may precipitate more severe failure in patients w/ diminished myocardial contractility; d/c at the first sign/symptom of cardiac failure. Avoid w/ mild or moderate COPD (eg, chronic bronchitis, emphysema), bronchospastic disease, or history of bronchospastic disease. Patients w/ a history of atopy or a history of severe anaphylactic reactions to a variety of allergens may be more reactive to repeated challenge w/ such allergens, and may be unresponsive to usual doses of epinephrine used to treat anaphylactic reactions. May potentiate muscle weakness. May mask signs/symptoms of acute hypoglycemia; caution in patients subject to spontaneous hypoglycemia and in diabetic patients receiving insulin or oral hypoglycemic agents. May mask certain clinical signs of hyperthyroidism (eg, tachycardia); carefully manage patients suspected of developing thyrotoxicosis to avoid abrupt withdrawal that may precipitate a thyroid storm. Withdrawal of therapy prior to major surgery is controversial. β-adrenergic receptor blockade may impair the ability of the heart to respond to β-adrenergically mediated reflex stimuli; gradual withdrawal of β-blocking agents may be recommended in patients undergoing elective surgery.

ADVERSE REACTIONS

Taste perversion, ocular burning and/or stinging, conjunctival hyperemia, blurred vision, superficial punctate keratitis, or eye itching.

DRUG INTERACTIONS

Dorzolamide: Not recommended w/ oral carbonic anhydrase inhibitors. Acid-base and electrolyte disturbances reported w/ oral carbonic anhydrase inhibitors and have, in some instances, resulted in drug interactions; consider potential for such interactions in patients receiving therapy.
Timolol: Monitor for potential additive effects, both systemic and on IOP, w/ concomitant oral β-blockers; concomitant use of 2 topical β-blocking agents is not recommended. Caution w/ oral or IV calcium antagonists because of possible AV conduction disturbances, left ventricular failure, and hypotension; avoid coadministration in patients w/ impaired cardiac function. Closely observe patients receiving catecholamine-depleting drugs (eg, reserpine) because of possible additive effects and the production of hypotension and/or marked bradycardia. Concomitant use w/ digitalis or calcium antagonists may have additive effects in prolonging AV-conduction time. Potentiated systemic β-blockade (eg, decreased HR, depression) reported w/ concomitant CYP2D6 inhibitors (eg, quinidine, SSRIs). Oral β-blockers may exacerbate the rebound HTN that can follow the withdrawal of clonidine.

PATIENT CONSIDERATIONS

Assessment: Assess for hypersensitivity to any component of product or to sulfonamides, bronchial asthma or history thereof, COPD, sinus bradycardia, 2nd- or 3rd-degree AV block, cardiac failure, cardiogenic shock, patients subject to spontaneous hypoglycemia, diabetes, renal/hepatic impairment, any other conditions where the treatment is contraindicated or cautioned, pregnancy/nursing status, and possible drug interactions.

Monitoring: Monitor for respiratory reactions, signs/symptoms of cardiac failure, hypersensitivity reactions, increased reactivity to allergens, muscle weakness, corneal edema, bacterial keratitis, and other adverse reactions.

Counseling: Advise patients w/ bronchial asthma or history thereof, severe COPD, sinus bradycardia, 2nd- or 3rd-degree AV block, or cardiac failure not to take this product. Inform that medication contains dorzolamide (a sulfonamide) and is absorbed systemically; instruct to d/c use and seek physician's advice if serious/unusual reactions or signs of hypersensitivity develop. Advise to immediately contact physician concerning the continued use of the product if undergoing ocular surgery or if an intercurrent ocular condition (eg, trauma, infection) develops. Explain that if >1 topical ophthalmic drug is being used, the drugs should be administered at least 5 min apart.
Cosopt: Inform that if handled improperly or if the tip of the dispensing container contacts the eye or surrounding structures, the sol can become contaminated. Inform that serious damage to the eye and subsequent loss of vision may result from using contaminated sol. Inform that medication contains benzalkonium chloride, which may be absorbed by soft contact lenses. Instruct to remove contact lenses prior to administration; lenses may be reinserted 15 min following administration.
Cosopt PF: Inform that drug does not contain a preservative; instruct to use immediately after opening and to discard remaining contents immediately after administration.

STORAGE: **Cosopt:** 15-30°C (59-86°F). Protect from light. **Cosopt PF:** 20-25°C (68-77°F). Do not freeze. Store in original pouch; after pouch is opened, store remaining containers in foil pouch to protect from light. Discard any unused containers 15 days after 1st opening the pouch.

COTELLIC — cobimetinib

RX

Class: Kinase inhibitor

ADULT DOSAGE

Unresectable or Metastatic Melanoma with BRAF V600E or V600K Mutations

60mg qd for 21 days of each 28-day cycle in combination w/ vemurafenib

Take until disease progression or unacceptable toxicity

PEDIATRIC DOSAGE

Pediatric use may not have been established

DOSING CONSIDERATIONS

Concomitant Medications

Do not take strong or moderate CYP3A inhibitors; use an alternative to a strong or moderate CYP3A inhibitor in patients who are taking a reduced dose of cobimetinib (40 or 20mg daily)
If short term (≤14 days) use of moderate CYP3A inhibitors is unavoidable, reduce cobimetinib dose to 20mg; after discontinuation of a moderate CYP3A inhibitor, resume previous dose of cobimetinib 60mg

Adverse Reactions

Recommended Dose Reductions:
1st Dose Reduction: 40mg qd

2nd Dose Reduction: 20mg qd
Subsequent Modification: Permanently d/c if unable to tolerate 20mg qd
Hemorrhage:
Grade 3: Withhold for ≤4 weeks; if improved to Grade 0 or 1, resume at the next lower dose level. If not improved w/in 4 weeks, permanently d/c
Grade 4: Permanently d/c
Cardiomyopathy:
Asymptomatic, Absolute Decrease in LVEF from Baseline of >10% and <Lower Limit of Normal (LLN):
Withhold for 2 weeks; repeat LVEF
Resume at next lower dose if LVEF is ≥LLN and absolute decrease from baseline LVEF is ≤10%
Permanently d/c if LVEF is <LLN or absolute decrease from baseline LVEF is >10%
Symptomatic LVEF Decrease from Baseline:
Withhold for ≤4 weeks, repeat LVEF
Resume at next lower dose if symptoms resolve, LVEF is ≥LLN, and absolute decrease from baseline LVEF is ≤10%
Permanently d/c if symptoms persist, LVEF is <LLN, or absolute decrease from baseline LVEF is >10%
Dermatologic Reactions:
Grade 2 (Intolerable), Grade 3 or 4: Withhold or reduce dose
Serous Retinopathy:
Withhold for ≤4 weeks; if signs and symptoms improve, resume at the next lower dose level. If not improved or symptoms recur at the lower dose w/in 4 weeks, permanently d/c
Retinal Vein Occlusion: Permanently d/c
Liver Lab Abnormalities and Hepatotoxicity:
1st Occurrence Grade 4: Withhold for ≤4 weeks; if improved to Grade 0 or 1, then resume at the next lower dose level. If not improved to Grade 0 or 1 w/in 4 weeks, permanently d/c
Recurrent Grade 4: Permanently d/c
Rhabdomyolysis and Creatine Phosphokinase (CPK) Elevations:
Grade 4 CPK Elevation/Any CPK Elevation and Myalgia: Withhold for ≤4 weeks; if improved to Grade 3 or lower, resume at the next lower dose level. If not improved w/in 4 weeks, permanently d/c
Photosensitivity:
Grade 2 (Intolerable), Grade 3 or Grade 4: Withhold for ≤4 weeks; if improved to Grade 0 or 1, resume at the next lower dose level. If not improved w/in 4 weeks, permanently d/c
Other:
Grade 2 (Intolerable)/Any Grade 3 Adverse Reactions: Withhold for ≤4 weeks; if improved to Grade 0 or 1, resume at the next lower dose level. If not improved w/in 4 weeks, permanently d/c
1st Occurrence of Any Grade 4 Adverse Reaction: Withhold until adverse reaction improves to Grade 0 or 1, then resume at the next lower dose level, or permanently d/c
Recurrent Grade 4 Adverse Reaction: Permanently d/c

ADMINISTRATION
Oral route

Take w/ or w/o food.

HOW SUPPLIED
Tab: 20mg

WARNINGS/PRECAUTIONS
See Dosing Considerations. Not indicated for patients w/ wild-type BRAF melanoma. New primary malignancies, cutaneous and non-cutaneous, may occur; monitor patients for signs or symptoms of non-cutaneous malignancies. Cardiomyopathy may occur; evaluate LVEF prior to initiation, 1 month after initiation, and every 3 months thereafter until discontinuation. If restarting treatment after a dose reduction/ interruption, evaluate LVEF at approx 2 weeks, 4 weeks, 10 weeks, and 16 weeks, and then as clinically indicated. Photosensitivity (including severe cases), severe rash and other skin reactions, and hemorrhage (including major hemorrhages) may occur. Ocular toxicities, including serous retinopathy, may occur; perform an ophthalmological evaluation at regular intervals and any time a patient reports new or worsening visual disturbances. Hepatotoxicity may occur; monitor liver lab tests before initiation and monthly during treatment, or more frequently as clinically indicated. Rhabdomyolysis may occur; obtain baseline serum CPK and creatinine levels prior to initiation, periodically during treatment, and as clinically indicated. May cause fetal harm.

ADVERSE REACTIONS
Diarrhea, photosensitivity reaction, N/V, pyrexia.

DRUG INTERACTIONS
See Dosing Considerations. Strong CYP3A4 inhibitors (itraconazole) may increase systemic exposure. Strong CYP3A inducers may decrease systemic exposure and reduce efficacy; avoid concurrent use w/ strong or moderate CYP3A inducers (eg, carbamazepine, efavirenz, phenytoin).

PATIENT CONSIDERATIONS

Assessment: Confirm the presence of BRAF V600E or V600K mutation in tumor specimens and evaluate LVEF, liver lab tests, and baseline serum CPK and creatinine levels prior to initiation. Perform dermatologic evaluations. Assess pregnancy/nursing status.

Monitoring: Monitor for signs or symptoms of non-cutaneous malignancies, hemorrhage, photosensitivity, pregnancy, and other adverse reactions. Perform dermatologic evaluations every 2 months during therapy and monitor for 6 months following discontinuation when administered w/ vemurafenib. Monitor LVEF 1 month after initiation, and every 3 months thereafter until discontinuation; if restarting treatment after a dose reduction/interruption, evaluate LVEF at approx 2 weeks, 4 weeks, 10 weeks, and 16 weeks, and then as clinically indicated. Perform ophthalmological evaluations at regular intervals and any time a patient reports new or worsening visual disturbances. Monitor liver lab tests monthly during treatment or as indicated. Obtain serum CPK and creatinine levels periodically.

Counseling: Advise to contact healthcare provider immediately for change in or development of new skin lesions, severe skin changes, any changes in vision, muscle pain or weakness, and any signs/symptoms of unusual severe bleeding/hemorrhage, left ventricular dysfunction, or liver dysfunction. Advise to report any history of cardiac disease and of the requirement for cardiac monitoring prior to and during treatment. Advise that treatment requires monitoring of their liver function. Advise to avoid sun exposure, wear protective clothing, and use broad-spectrum UVA/UVB sunscreen and lip balm (SPF ≥30) when outdoors. Advise females of reproductive potential of the potential risk to a fetus and to use effective contraception during treatment and for at least 2 weeks after the final dose; advise to contact healthcare provider if they become pregnant, or if pregnancy is suspected, during treatment. Advise not to breastfeed during treatment and for 2 weeks after the final dose.

STORAGE: <30°C (86°F).

COUMADIN — warfarin sodium

RX

Class: Vitamin K-dependent coagulation factor inhibitor

May cause major or fatal bleeding; monitor INR regularly. Drugs, dietary changes, and other factors affect INR levels achieved w/ therapy. Instruct patients about prevention measures to minimize risk of bleeding and to report signs/symptoms of bleeding.

OTHER BRAND NAMES

Jantoven

ADULT DOSAGE

Venous Thromboembolism

Including Deep Vein Thrombosis (DVT) and Pulmonary Embolism (PE):
Target INR: 2.5 (INR Range, 2-3) for all treatment durations

Duration of Therapy:
DVT/PE Secondary to Transient Risk Factor: 3 months
Unprovoked DVT/PE: At least 3 months; evaluate risk-benefit ratio of long-term treatment after 3 months of therapy
2 Episodes of Unprovoked DVT/PE: Long-term treatment recommended

Nonvalvular Atrial Fibrillation

Target INR: 2.5 (INR Range, 2-3)

Duration of Therapy:
Persistent/Paroxysmal A-Fib and High Risk of Stroke: Long-term treatment recommended
Persistent/Paroxysmal A-Fib and Intermediate Risk of Ischemic Stroke: Long-term treatment recommended
A-Fib and Mitral Stenosis: Long-term treatment recommended
A-Fib and Prosthetic Heart Valves: Long-term treatment recommended; target INR may be increased and aspirin (ASA) added depending on valve type and position, and on patient factors

PEDIATRIC DOSAGE

General Dosing

Adequate and well-controlled studies have not been conducted in any pediatric population; optimum dosing and safety/efficacy unknown. Pediatric use is based on adult data and recommendations, and available limited pediatric data

C

Mechanical/Bioprosthetic Heart Valves

Bileaflet Mechanical Valve/Medtronic Hall Tilting Disk Valve in the Aortic Position in Sinus Rhythm and w/o Left Atrial Enlargement:
Target INR: 2.5 (INR Range, 2-3)

Tilting Disk Valves and Bileaflet Mechanical Valves in the Mitral Position:
Target INR: 3 (INR Range, 2.5-3.5)

Caged Ball or Caged Disk Valves:
Target INR: 3 (INR Range, 2.5-3.5)

Bioprosthetic Valve in the Mitral Position:
Target INR: 2.5 (INR Range, 2-3) for the first 3 months after valve insertion. If additional risk factors for thromboembolism present, target INR 2.5 (INR Range, 2-3)

Post-Myocardial Infarction

High Risk Patients w/ MI:
Treat w/ combined moderate-intensity (INR, 2-3) warfarin plus low-dose ASA (≤100 mg/day) for at least 3 months after MI

Recurrent Systemic Embolism

Unknown Etiology:
Use a moderate dose regimen (INR, 2-3)

Dosing Based on Genotype Consideration

Expected Maint Daily Doses Based on CYP2C9 and VKORC1 Genotypes:

VKORC1-GG:
CYP2C9 *1/*1: 5-7mg
CYP2C9 *1/*2: 5-7mg
CYP2C9 *1/*3: 3-4mg
CYP2C9 *2/*2: 3-4mg
CYP2C9 *2/*3: 3-4mg
CYP2C9 *3/*3: 0.5-2mg

VKORC1-AG:
CYP2C9 *1/*1: 5-7mg
CYP2C9 *1/*2: 3-4mg
CYP2C9 *1/*3: 3-4mg
CYP2C9 *2/*2: 3-4mg
CYP2C9 *2/*3: 0.5-2mg
CYP2C9 *3/*3: 0.5-2mg

VKORC1-AA:
CYP2C9 *1/*1: 3-4mg
CYP2C9 *1/*2: 3-4mg
CYP2C9 *1/*3: 0.5-2mg
CYP2C9 *2/*2: 0.5-2mg
CYP2C9 *2/*3: 0.5-2mg
CYP2C9 *3/*3: 0.5-2mg

CYP2C9 *1/*3, *2/*2, *2/*3, and *3/*3:
May require more prolonged time (>2-4 weeks) to achieve max INR effect

If CYP2C9 and VKORC1 Genotypes Are Unknown:
Initial: 2-5mg qd
Maint: 2-10mg qd

Other Indications

Mitral Stenosis/Valvular Disease Associated w/ A-Fib:
Use a moderate dose regimen (INR, 2-3)

Conversions

From Heparin:
Conversion may begin concomitantly w/ heparin therapy or may be delayed 3-6 days. Continue full dose heparin therapy and overlap

warfarin therapy w/ heparin for 4-5 days; may d/c heparin once warfarin has produced the desired therapeutic response as determined by INR.

Patients receiving both heparin and warfarin should have INR monitoring at least:
- Five hrs after the last IV bolus heparin dose, or
- Four hrs after cessation of continuous IV heparin infusion, or
- Twenty-four hrs after the last SQ heparin inj

Warfarin may increase the aPTT test, even in the absence of heparin; severe elevation (>50 sec) in aPTT w/ INR in desired range has been identified as an indication of increased risk of postoperative hemorrhage

From Other Anticoagulants:
Consult the labeling of other anticoagulants for conversion instructions

DOSING CONSIDERATIONS

Elderly

Elderly/Debilitated: Consider lower initial and maint doses

Other Important Considerations

Asian Patients: Consider lower initial and maint doses

Treatment During Dentistry or Surgery: Some dental or surgical procedures may necessitate an interruption or change in dose. Determine the INR immediately prior to any procedure

ADMINISTRATION

Oral route (Coumadin, Jantoven) or IV route (Coumadin)

Coumadin

IV dose is the same as oral dose.

IV:
Reconstitute vial w/ 2.7mL of sterile water for inj; resulting yield is 2.5mL of a 2mg/mL sol.
After reconstitution, administer as a slow bolus inj into a peripheral vein over 1-2 min.
Reconstituted sol is stable for 4 hrs at room temperature; discard any unused sol.

HOW SUPPLIED

Inj: (Coumadin) 5mg; **Tab:** (Coumadin, Jantoven) 1mg*, 2mg*, 2.5mg*, 3mg*, 4mg*, 5mg*, 6mg*, 7.5mg*, 10mg* *scored

CONTRAINDICATIONS

Pregnancy, except in pregnant women w/ mechanical heart valves, who are at high risk of thromboembolism. Hemorrhagic tendencies or blood dyscrasias. Recent or contemplated surgery of the CNS, eye, or traumatic surgery resulting in large open surfaces. Bleeding tendencies associated w/ active ulceration or overt bleeding of GI/genitourinary/respiratory tract, CNS hemorrhage, cerebral aneurysms, dissecting aorta, pericarditis and pericardial effusions, or bacterial endocarditis. Threatened abortion, eclampsia, and preeclampsia. Unsupervised patients w/ conditions associated w/ potential high level of noncompliance. Spinal puncture and other diagnostic/therapeutic procedures w/ potential for uncontrollable bleeding. Hypersensitivity to warfarin or to any other components of the medication (eg, anaphylaxis). Major regional, lumbar block anesthesia. Malignant HTN.

WARNINGS/PRECAUTIONS

Has no direct effect on established thrombus, nor does it reverse ischemic tissue damage; once a thrombus has occurred, the goals of anticoagulant treatment are to prevent further extension of the formed clot and to prevent secondary thromboembolic complications that may result in serious and possibly fatal sequelae. INR >4 provides no additional therapeutic benefit in most patients and is associated w/ higher risk of bleeding. Bleeding is more likely to occur w/in the 1st month; patients at high risk of bleeding may benefit from more frequent INR monitoring, careful dose adjustment to desired INR, and a shortest duration of therapy. Has a narrow therapeutic range (index) and its action may be affected by endogenous factors, other drugs, and dietary vitamin K. Determine the INR daily after initial dose administration until INR results stabilize in the therapeutic range; after stabilization, perform INR monitoring based on the clinical situation (acceptable interval 1-4 weeks). Risk of necrosis and/or gangrene of skin and other tissues; d/c if necrosis occurs and consider alternative therapy. May enhance the release of atheromatous plaque emboli, and systemic atheroemboli and cholesterol microemboli may occur. D/C if distinct syndrome resulting from microemboli to the feet ("purple toes syndrome") occurs and consider alternative therapy. Do not use as initial therapy w/ heparin-induced thrombocytopenia (HIT) and w/ heparin-induced thrombocytopenia w/ thrombosis syndrome (HITTS); limb ischemia, necrosis, and gangrene reported when heparin was discontinued and warfarin started or continued. Can cause fetal harm in pregnant women. Increased risks of therapy in patients w/ moderate-severe hepatic impairment, infectious diseases/disturbances of intestinal flora, indwelling catheter, severe/moderate HTN, deficiency in protein C-mediated anticoagulant response, polycythemia vera, vasculitis, or diabetes mellitus, or who are undergoing eye surgery. Caution in elderly. Caution w/ hepatic impairment; can potentiate the response to warfarin.

ADVERSE REACTIONS

Hemorrhage, necrosis of the skin and other tissues, systemic atheroemboli, cholesterol microemboli, hypersensitivity/allergic reactions, vasculitis, hepatitis, elevated liver enzymes, N/V, diarrhea, rash, dermatitis, tracheal/tracheobronchial calcifications, chills.

DRUG INTERACTIONS

Inhibitors of CYP2C9, 1A2, and/or 3A4 may increase effect (increase INR) by increasing exposure of warfarin. Inducers of CYP2C9, 1A2, and/or 3A4 may decrease effect (decrease INR) by decreasing exposure of warfarin. Increased risk of bleeding w/ anticoagulants (argatroban, bivalirudin, heparin), antiplatelet agents (ASA, cilostazol, clopidogrel), NSAIDs (celecoxib, diclofenac, diflunisal), and serotonin reuptake inhibitors (eg, citalopram, desvenlafaxine, duloxetine). Changes in INR reported w/ antibiotics or antifungals; closely monitor INR when starting or stopping any antibiotics or antifungals. Perform more frequent INR monitoring when starting or stopping botanicals; some botanicals (eg, garlic, *Ginkgo biloba*) may cause additive anticoagulant effects, while some botanicals (eg, coenzyme Q10, St. John's wort, ginseng) may decrease effects. Some botanicals and foods can interact w/ warfarin through CYP450 interactions (eg, *echinacea*, grapefruit juice, ginkgo, goldenseal, St. John's wort). Cholestatic hepatitis has been associated w/ coadministration of warfarin and ticlopidine. Perform more frequent INR monitoring when starting or stopping other drugs, including botanicals, or when changing dosages of other drugs, including drugs intended for short-term use (eg, antibiotics, antifungals, corticosteroids).

PATIENT CONSIDERATIONS

Assessment: Assess for risk factors for bleeding (eg, INR>4, age ≥65 yrs, history of highly variable INR, history of GI bleeding, HTN, cerebrovascular disease, malignancy, anemia, trauma, renal impairment, certain genetic factors, long duration of warfarin therapy), factors affecting INR (eg, diarrhea, hepatic disorders, poor nutritional state, steatorrhea, vitamin K deficiency, increased vitamin K intake, hereditary warfarin resistance), pregnancy/nursing status, other conditions where treatment is contraindicated or cautioned, and possible drug interactions. Assess INR. Obtain platelet counts in patients w/ HIT or HITTS.

Monitoring: Monitor for signs/symptoms of bleeding, necrosis/gangrene of skin and other tissues, systemic atheroemboli, cholesterol microemboli, "purple toes syndrome," and other adverse reactions. For patients receiving long-term anticoagulant treatment, periodically reassess risk-benefit ratio of continuing such treatment. Perform regular INR monitoring.

Counseling: Instruct to inform physician if patient falls often as this may increase risk for complications. Counsel to maintain strict adherence to dosing regimen. Advise not to start or stop other medications, including salicylates (eg, ASA, topical analgesics), OTC drugs, or herbal medications, except on advice of physician. Instruct to inform physician if pregnancy is suspected (to discuss pregnancy planning) or if considering breastfeeding. Counsel to avoid any activity or sport that may result in traumatic injury. Instruct that regular PT tests and visits to physician are required during therapy. Advise patient to carry ID card stating drug is being taken. Instruct to eat a normal, balanced diet to maintain consistent intake of vitamin K and to avoid drastic changes in diet, such as eating large amounts of leafy, green vegetables. Advise to take ud. Advise to immediately report unusual bleeding or symptoms or any serious illness, such as severe diarrhea, infection, or fever. Inform that anticoagulant effects may persist for about 2-5 days after discontinuation.

STORAGE: Tab: (Coumadin) 15-30°C (59-86°F). Protect from light and moisture. (Jantoven) 20-25°C (68-77°F); excursions permitted at 15-30°C (59-86°F). Protect from light and moisture. **Inj:** (Coumadin) 15-30°C (59-86°F). Protect from light. Use reconstituted sol w/in 4 hrs; do not refrigerate. Discard any unused sol.

COZAAR – losartan potassium

RX

Class: Angiotensin II receptor blocker (ARB)

D/C when pregnancy is detected. Drugs that act directly on the renin-angiotensin system (RAS) can cause injury/death to the developing fetus.

ADULT DOSAGE

Hypertension

Initial: 50mg qd
Max: 100mg qd

Hypertension with Left Ventricular Hypertrophy

Reduction in Risk of Stroke:
Initial: 50mg qd
Titrate: Add hydrochlorothiazide (HCTZ) 12.5mg qd and/or increase losartan to 100mg qd, followed by an increase in HCTZ to 25mg qd based on BP response

This may not apply to black patients

Diabetic Nephropathy

Elevated SrCr/Proteinuria (Urinary Albumin to Creatinine Ratio ≥300mg/g) in Patients w/ Type 2 Diabetes and a History of HTN:
Initial: 50mg qd
Titrate: Increase to 100mg qd based on BP response

PEDIATRIC DOSAGE

Hypertension

≥6 Years:
Initial: 0.7mg/kg qd (up to 50mg total) administered as a tab or sus
Titrate: Adjust dose according to BP response
Max: 1.4mg/kg/day (or 100mg/day)

DOSING CONSIDERATIONS

Renal Impairment
Pediatric HTN:
GFR <30mL/min/1.73m²: Not recommended

Hepatic Impairment
Mild-to-Moderate:
Initial: 25mg qd

Other Important Considerations
Adult HTN: Starting dose of 25mg is recommended for patients w/ possible intravascular depletion

ADMINISTRATION

Oral route

Preparation of Sus (for 200mL of a 2.5mg/mL Sus)

1. Add 10mL of purified water to an 8 oz (240mL) amber polyethylene terephthalate (PET) bottle containing ten 50mg Cozaar tabs.
2. Immediately shake for at least 2 min.
3. Let the concentrate stand for 1 hr and then shake for 1 min to disperse the tab contents.
4. Separately prepare a 50/50 volumetric mixture of Ora-Plus and Ora-Sweet SF.
5. Add 190mL of the 50/50 Ora-Plus/Ora-Sweet SF mixture to the tab and water slurry in the PET bottle and shake for 1 min to disperse the ingredients.
6. The sus should be refrigerated at 2-8°C (36-46°F) and can be stored for up to 4 weeks.
7. Shake the sus prior to each use and return promptly to the refrigerator.

HOW SUPPLIED

Tab: 25mg, 50mg*, 100mg *scored

CONTRAINDICATIONS

Hypersensitivity to any component of the medication, coadministration w/ aliskiren in patients w/ diabetes.

WARNINGS/PRECAUTIONS

Symptomatic hypotension may occur in patients w/ an activated RAS (eg, volume- or salt-depleted patients); correct volume or salt depletion prior to administration of therapy. Patients whose renal function may depend in part on the activity of the RAS may be at risk of developing acute renal failure; monitor renal function periodically. Consider withholding or discontinuing therapy in patients who develop a clinically significant decrease in renal function on losartan. Monitor serum K^+ periodically and treat appropriately; dosage reduction or discontinuation of losartan may be required.

ADVERSE REACTIONS

Dizziness, URI, nasal congestion, back pain.

DRUG INTERACTIONS

See Contraindications. Use w/ other drugs that raise serum K^+ may result in hyperkalemia; monitor serum K^+. Increases in serum lithium concentrations and lithium toxicity reported; monitor serum lithium levels during concomitant use. In patients who are elderly, volume-depleted (including those on diuretic therapy), or w/ compromised renal function, coadministration w/ NSAIDs, including selective COX-2 inhibitors, may result in deterioration in renal function, including possible acute renal failure. Antihypertensive effect may be attenuated by NSAIDs, including selective COX-2 inhibitors. Dual blockade of the RAS is associated w/ increased risks of hypotension, syncope, hyperkalemia, and changes in renal function (including acute renal failure); avoid combined use of RAS inhibitors. Closely monitor BP, renal function, and electrolytes w/ concomitant agents that affect the RAS. Avoid w/ aliskiren in patients w/ renal impairment (GFR <60mL/min).

PATIENT CONSIDERATIONS

Assessment: Assess for history of hypersensitivity, volume/salt depletion, CHF, diabetes mellitus, renal artery stenosis, hepatic/renal impairment, pregnancy/nursing status, and possible drug interactions.

Monitoring: Monitor for signs/symptoms of hypotension, changes in renal function, and other adverse reactions. Monitor BP, serum K^+ levels, and renal function periodically.

Counseling: Inform of pregnancy risks and discuss treatment options w/ women planning to become pregnant; instruct to report pregnancy to physician as soon as possible. Instruct not to use K^+ supplements or salt substitutes containing K^+ w/o consulting physician.

STORAGE: (Tab) 25°C (77°F); excursions permitted to 15-30°C (59-86°F). Protect from light. (Sus) 2-8°C (36-46°F) for up to 4 weeks.

Creon – pancrelipase

RX

Class: Pancreatic enzyme supplement

ADULT DOSAGE

Exocrine Pancreatic Insufficiency

Due to Cystic Fibrosis, Chronic Pancreatitis, Pancreatectomy, or Other Conditions:
Start at the lowest recommended dose and increase gradually
Initial: 500 lipase U/kg/meal
Max: 2500 lipase U/kg/meal (or ≤10,000 lipase U/kg/day) or <4000 lipase U/g fat ingested/day
Half of the dose used for meals should be given w/ each snack

Refer to PI for dosing limitations

PEDIATRIC DOSAGE

Exocrine Pancreatic Insufficiency

Due to Cystic Fibrosis, Chronic Pancreatitis, Pancreatectomy, or Other Conditions:
Start at the lowest recommended dose and increase gradually

≤12 Months:
3000 lipase U/120mL of formula or per breastfeeding; administer immediately prior to each feeding

>12 Months-<4 Years:
Initial: 1000 lipase U/kg/meal
Max: 2500 lipase U/kg/meal (or ≤10,000 lipase U/kg/day) or <4000 lipase U/g fat ingested/day

≥4 Years:
Initial: 500 lipase U/kg/meal
Max: 2500 lipase U/kg/meal (or ≤10,000 lipase U/kg/day) or <4000 lipase U/g fat ingested/day
Half of the dose used for meals should be given w/ each snack

Refer to PI for dosing limitations

DOSING CONSIDERATIONS

Elderly
Reduce dose

ADMINISTRATION

Oral route

Take during meals or snacks, w/ sufficient fluid
Swallow whole; do not crush or chew caps/cap contents
Do not retain in mouth
Do not mix directly into formula or breast milk
For patients who are unable to swallow intact capsules, open the contents and add to a small amount of acidic soft food w/ a pH of 4.5 or less, such as applesauce. The mixture should be swallowed immediately and followed w/ water or juice to ensure complete ingestion

HOW SUPPLIED

Cap, Delayed-Release: (Lipase/Protease/Amylase) 3000 U/9500 U/15,000 U; 6000 U/19,000 U/30,000 U; 12,000 U/38,000 U/60,000 U; 24,000 U/76,000 U/120,000 U; 36,000 U/114,000 U/180,000 U

WARNINGS/PRECAUTIONS

Not interchangeable with other pancrelipase products. Fibrosing colonopathy reported; monitor closely for progression to stricture formation. Caution with doses >2500 lipase U/kg/meal (or

>10,000 lipase U/kg/day); use only if these doses are documented to be effective by 3-day fecal fat measures indicating significant improvement. Examine patients receiving >6000 lipase U/kg/meal; immediately decrease or titrate dose downward to a lower range. Ensure that no drug is retained in the mouth. Should not be crushed or chewed, or mixed in foods with pH >4.5; may disrupt enteric coating of cap, resulting in early release of enzymes, irritation of oral mucosa, and/or loss of enzyme activity. Caution in patients with gout, renal impairment, or hyperuricemia; may increase blood uric acid levels. Risk for transmission of viral diseases. Caution with known allergy to proteins of porcine origin; severe allergic reactions reported.

ADVERSE REACTIONS

Vomiting, flatulence, abdominal pain, headache, cough, dizziness, frequent bowel movements, abnormal feces, hyperglycemia, hypoglycemia, nasopharyngitis, decreased appetite, irritability.

PATIENT CONSIDERATIONS

Assessment: Assess for known allergy to porcine proteins, gout, renal impairment, hyperuricemia, and pregnancy/nursing status.

Monitoring: Monitor for fibrosing colonopathy, stricture formation, oral mucosa irritation, viral diseases, and allergic reactions. Monitor serum uric acid levels.

Counseling: Instruct to take ud and with food and fluids. Inform that if a dose is missed, take the next dose with the next meal/snack ud; instruct not to double doses. Inform that cap contents can also be sprinkled on soft acidic foods (eg, applesauce), if necessary. Instruct to notify physician if pregnant/breastfeeding or planning to become pregnant/breastfeed during treatment. Advise to contact physician immediately if allergic reactions develop.

STORAGE: Room temperature up to 25°C (77°F); excursions permitted between 25-40°C (77-104°F) for up to 30 days. Discard if exposed to higher temperature and moisture conditions >70%. Protect from moisture. Store in original container.

CRESEMBA – isavuconazonium sulfate RX

Class: Azole antifungal

ADULT DOSAGE

Aspergillosis

Treatment of invasive aspergillosis

Cap/IV:
LD: 372mg q8h for 6 doses (48 hrs)
Maint: 372mg qd

Start maint doses 12-24 hrs after the last LD

Switching between the IV and oral formulations is acceptable as bioequivalence has been demonstrated; LD is not required when switching between formulations

Mucormycosis

Treatment of invasive mucormycosis

Cap/IV:
LD: 372mg q8h for 6 doses (48 hrs)
Maint: 372mg qd

Start maint doses 12-24 hrs after the last LD

Switching between the IV and oral formulations is acceptable as bioequivalence has been demonstrated; LD is not required when switching between formulations

PEDIATRIC DOSAGE

Pediatric use may not have been established

ADMINISTRATION

Oral/IV route

Cap

Swallow whole; do not chew, crush, dissolve, or open the cap.
Take w/ or w/o food.

IV

Administer via an infusion set w/ an in-line filter (pore size 0.2-1.2 micron).
Infuse over a minimum of 1 hr in 250mL of a compatible diluent; do not administer as an IV bolus inj.
Do not infuse w/ other IV medications.
Flush IV lines w/ 0.9% NaCl inj or D5 inj prior to and after infusion.

After dilution, avoid unnecessary vibration or vigorous shaking of the sol; do not use a pneumatic transport system.

Reconstitution:
Reconstitute 1 vial by adding 5mL water for inj to the vial.
Gently shake to dissolve the powder completely.
May store at <25°C (77°F) for max 1 hr prior to preparation of infusion sol.

Dilution and Preparation:
Add 5mL of the reconstituted sol to an infusion bag containing 250mL of a compatible diluent.
Use gentle mixing or roll bag to minimize the formation of particulates.
Apply in-line filter w/ a microporous membrane pore size of 0.2-1.2 micron and in-line filter reminder sticker to the infusion bag.
Complete administration w/in 6 hrs of dilution at room temperature; if not possible, immediately refrigerate (2-8°C [36-46°F]) the infusion sol after dilution and complete the infusion w/in 24 hrs. Do not freeze.

Compatible Diluents:
0.9% NaCl inj and D5 inj

HOW SUPPLIED

Cap: 186mg; **Inj:** 372mg

CONTRAINDICATIONS

Known hypersensitivity to isavuconazole. Coadministration of strong CYP3A4 inhibitors (eg, ketoconazole, high-dose ritonavir (RTV) [400mg q12h]) and strong CYP3A4 inducers (eg, rifampin, carbamazepine, St. John's wort, long-acting barbiturates). Familial short QT syndrome.

WARNINGS/PRECAUTIONS

Hepatic adverse drug reactions (eg, elevations in ALT, AST, alkaline phosphate, total bilirubin) reported. Cases of more severe hepatic adverse drug reactions including hepatitis, cholestasis or hepatic failure including death reported in patients w/ serious underlying medical conditions (eg, hematologic malignancy); d/c if clinical signs and symptoms consistent w/ liver disease develop. Infusion-related reactions reported during IV administration; d/c infusion if these reactions occur. Serious hypersensitivity and severe skin reactions such as anaphylaxis or Stevens Johnson syndrome reported during treatment w/ other azole antifungal agents; d/c if a severe cutaneous adverse reaction develops. Caution when prescribing to patients w/ hypersensitivity to other azoles. May cause fetal harm when administered to pregnant woman; use only if the potential benefit to the patient outweighs the risk to the fetus.

ADVERSE REACTIONS

N/V, diarrhea, hypokalemia, elevated LFTs, dyspnea, abdominal pain, headache, peripheral edema, constipation, fatigue, insomnia, back pain, renal failure, chest pain, decreased appetite.

DRUG INTERACTIONS

See Contraindications. CYP3A4 inhibitors/inducers may alter the plasma concentrations of isavuconazole. Ketoconazole may increase isavuconazole exposure. Rifampin may decrease isavuconazole exposure. Caution w/ lopinavir/RTV; coadministration may increase isavuconazole exposure and decrease lopinavir/RTV exposure. May increase atorvastatin exposure; use w/ caution and monitor for adverse reactions that are typical of atorvastatin. May increase cyclosporine, sirolimus, and tacrolimus exposures; use w/ caution and monitor drug concentrations of cyclosporine, sirolimus, and tacrolimus and adjust dose prn. May increase midazolam exposure; use w/ caution and consider dose reduction of midazolam. May decrease bupropion exposure, therefore use w/ caution; may be necessary to increase bupropion dose (do not exceed max recommended dose). May increase mycophenolate mofetil exposure; use w/ caution and monitor for mycophenolic acid-related toxicities. May increase digoxin exposure; use w/ caution and monitor serum digoxin concentrations.

PATIENT CONSIDERATIONS

Assessment: Assess for hypersensitivity to the drug or to other azole antifungal agents, familial short QT syndrome, serious underlying medical conditions, pregnancy/nursing status, and for possible drug interactions. Evaluate liver-related laboratory tests prior to therapy. Obtain specimens for fungal culture and other relevant laboratory studies in order to identify causative organism(s).

Monitoring: Monitor for hepatic adverse reactions, infusion-related reactions, serious hypersensitivity and severe skin reactions, and other adverse reactions. Monitor liver-related laboratory tests.

Counseling: Inform of benefits/risks of therapy. Advise to inform physician if taking other drugs or before beginning to take other drugs. Advise to inform physician if pregnant, planning to become pregnant, or nursing.

STORAGE: Cap: 20-25°C (68-77°F); excursions permitted between 15-30°C (59-86°F). Store in original container to protect from moisture. **Inj:** Unreconstituted: 2-8°C (36-46°F). Prepared infusion sol should be kept for ≤6 hrs at 20-25°C (68-77°F) or 24 hrs at 2-8°C (36-46°F) prior to use.

CRESTOR – rosuvastatin calcium

RX

Class: HMG-CoA reductase inhibitor (statin)

ADULT DOSAGE

Hypercholesterolemia

Hyperlipidemia and Mixed Dyslipidemia/ Hypertriglyceridemia/Primary Dysbetalipoproteinemia (Type III Hyperlipoproteinemia)/Slowing of the Progression of Atherosclerosis:

General Dose:
Initial: 10-20mg qd
Range: 5-40mg qd

When initiating treatment or switching from another HMG-CoA reductase inhibitor, use the appropriate starting dose 1st, then titrate according to patient's response and individualized goal of therapy

Analyze lipid levels w/in 2-4 weeks and adjust dose accordingly

Use 40mg dose only if LDL goal is not achieved w/ 20mg dose

Homozygous Familial Hypercholesterolemia

Initial: 20mg qd

Prevention of Cardiovascular Disease

Reduce the risk of stroke, MI, and arterial revascularization procedures in patients w/o clinically evident coronary heart disease but w/ an increased risk of cardiovascular disease (CVD) based on age (men ≥50 yrs of age and women ≥60 yrs of age), hsCRP ≥2mg/L, and the presence of at least 1 additional CVD risk factor

PEDIATRIC DOSAGE

Heterozygous Familial Hypercholesterolemia

Individualize dose

8-<10 Years:
Usual: 5-10mg qd
Titrate: Adjust dose at intervals of ≥4 weeks
Max: 10mg qd

10-17 Years:
Usual: 5-20mg qd
Titrate: Adjust dose at intervals of ≥4 weeks
Max: 20mg qd

DOSING CONSIDERATIONS

Concomitant Medications

Cyclosporine:
Max: 5mg qd

Atazanavir/Ritonavir, Lopinavir/Ritonavir, Simeprevir, or Gemfibrozil:
Initial: 5mg qd
Max: 10mg qd

Renal Impairment

Severe (CrCl <30mL/min) Not on Hemodialysis:
Initial: 5mg qd
Max: 10mg qd

Hepatic Impairment

Chronic Alcohol Liver Disease: Use w/ caution

Other Important Considerations

Asian Patients:
Initial: 5mg qd

ADMINISTRATION

Oral route

Take at any time of day, w/ or w/o food.
Swallow tab whole.
Do not take 2 doses w/in 12 hrs of each other.

HOW SUPPLIED

Tab: 5mg, 10mg, 20mg, 40mg

CONTRAINDICATIONS

Known hypersensitivity to any component of the medication, active liver disease including unexplained persistent elevations of hepatic transaminase levels, women who are pregnant or may become pregnant, nursing mothers.

C

WARNINGS/PRECAUTIONS

Myopathy (including immune-mediated necrotizing myopathy [IMNM]) and rhabdomyolysis reported, w/ increased risk at 40mg; caution in patients w/ predisposing factors for myopathy (eg, age ≥65 yrs, inadequately treated hypothyroidism, renal impairment). D/C if markedly elevated creatine phosphokinase (CPK) levels occur or myopathy is diagnosed or suspected. Temporarily withhold in any patient w/ an acute, serious condition suggestive of myopathy or predisposing to the development of renal failure secondary to rhabdomyolysis. Increases in serum transaminases reported. Fatal and nonfatal hepatic failure reported (rare); promptly interrupt therapy if serious liver injury w/ clinical symptoms and/or hyperbilirubinemia or jaundice occurs, and do not restart if no alternate etiology is found. Caution in patients who consume substantial quantities of alcohol and/or have a history of chronic liver disease, or who are elderly. Dipstick-positive proteinuria and microscopic hematuria reported; consider dose reduction for patients w/ unexplained persistent proteinuria and/or hematuria. Increases in HbA1c and FPG levels reported.

ADVERSE REACTIONS

Headache, myalgia, nausea, asthenia, abdominal pain.

DRUG INTERACTIONS

See Dosing Considerations. Cyclosporine, gemfibrozil, lopinavir/ritonavir, atazanavir/ritonavir, and simeprevir may increase levels. Increased risk of myopathy w/ some other lipid-lowering therapies (fibrates or niacin), gemfibrozil, cyclosporine, lopinavir/ritonavir, or atazanavir/ritonavir. Avoid w/ gemfibrozil. Caution w/ coumarin anticoagulants. May enhance the risk of skeletal muscle effects w/ ≥1g/day of niacin. Caution w/ drugs that may decrease levels or activity of endogenous steroid hormones (eg, ketoconazole, spironolactone, cimetidine), fenofibrates, or protease inhibitors. Caution w/ colchicine; cases of myopathy, including rhabdomyolysis, reported.

PATIENT CONSIDERATIONS

Assessment: Assess for active liver disease (including chronic alcohol liver disease), unexplained persistent elevations in serum transaminases, risk factors for developing myopathy or rhabdomyolysis, pregnancy/nursing status, and possible drug interactions. Obtain baseline lipid profile, LFTs, and evaluate renal function. Check INR w/ coumarin anticoagulants.

Monitoring: Monitor for signs/symptoms of myopathy (including IMNM), rhabdomyolysis, endocrine dysfunction, proteinuria, hematuria, and other adverse reactions. Monitor lipid levels, CPK, and LFTs. Monitor INR w/ coumarin anticoagulants frequently during early therapy.

Counseling: Advise to report promptly any unexplained muscle pain, tenderness, or weakness, particularly if accompanied by malaise or fever or if muscle signs/symptoms persist after discontinuing therapy. Advise to wait at least 2 hrs if taking an antacid containing a combination of aluminum and magnesium hydroxide. Inform of potential hazard to fetus if patient becomes pregnant while on therapy. Advise to promptly report any symptoms that may indicate liver injury (eg, fatigue, anorexia, right upper abdominal discomfort, dark urine, jaundice).

STORAGE: 20-25°C (68-77°F). Protect from moisture.

CUBICIN — daptomycin

RX

Class: Cyclic lipopeptide

ADULT DOSAGE

Skin and Skin Structure Infections

Complicated:

4mg/kg IV once q24h for 7-14 days

Bacteremia

Staphylococcus aureus bloodstream infections, including those w/ right-sided infective endocarditis, caused by methicillin-susceptible and methicillin-resistant isolates

6mg/kg IV once q24h for 2-6 weeks

PEDIATRIC DOSAGE

Pediatric use may not have been established

DOSING CONSIDERATIONS

Renal Impairment

CrCl <30mL/min, Including Hemodialysis and Continuous Ambulatory Peritoneal Dialysis:

Complicated Skin and Skin Structure Infections: 4mg/kg IV once q48h

***Staphylococcus aureus* Bacteremia:** 6mg/kg IV once q48h

When possible, administer following completion of hemodialysis on hemodialysis days

ADMINISTRATION

IV route

Administer either by IV inj over 2 min or by IV infusion over 30 min.

RX

C

C

Preparation for Administration
Reconstitute 500mg vial to 50mg/mL as follows:
1. Slowly transfer 10mL of 0.9% NaCl inj into daptomycin vial, pointing the transfer needle toward the wall of the vial.
2. Gently rotate vial to ensure that all of the powder is wetted; allow the wetted product to stand undisturbed for 10 min.
3. Gently rotate or swirl vial contents for a few min, prn, to obtain a completely reconstituted sol. Avoid vigorous agitation or shaking of the vial during or after reconstitution, to minimize foaming.

IV Inj: For IV inj over 2 min, administer appropriate volume of the reconstituted sol (concentration of 50mg/mL).

IV Infusion: For IV infusion over 30 min, further dilute appropriate volume of the reconstituted sol into a 50mL IV infusion bag containing 0.9% NaCl inj.

Stability:
Reconstituted sol is stable in the vial for 12 hrs at room temperature and up to 48 hrs if stored under refrigeration at 2-8°C (36-46°F).
Diluted sol is stable in the infusion bag for 12 hrs at room temperature and 48 hrs if stored under refrigeration.
The combined storage time (reconstituted sol in vial and diluted sol in infusion bag) should not exceed 12 hrs at room temperature or 48 hrs under refrigeration.

Compatible IV Sol
0.9% NaCl inj.
Lactated Ringer's inj.

Incompatibilities
Not compatible w/ dextrose-containing diluents.
Do not use in conjunction w/ ReadyMED elastomeric infusion pumps.
Additives and other medications should not be added to daptomycin vials or infusion bags, or infused simultaneously through the same IV line; if the same IV line is used for sequential infusion of different drugs, flush line w/ a compatible IV sol before and after infusion w/ daptomycin.

HOW SUPPLIED
Inj: 500mg

CONTRAINDICATIONS
Known hypersensitivity to daptomycin.

WARNINGS/PRECAUTIONS
Not for treatment of pneumonia or of left-sided infective endocarditis due to *S. aureus*. Anaphylaxis/hypersensitivity reactions reported; d/c and institute appropriate therapy if an allergic reaction occurs. Myopathy, CPK elevation, and rhabdomyolysis (w/ or w/o acute renal failure) reported; do not dose more frequently than qd. Monitor CPK levels weekly, and more frequently in patients who received recent prior or concomitant therapy w/ HMG-CoA reductase inhibitor or in whom CPK elevations occur during treatment. D/C in patients w/ unexplained signs/symptoms of myopathy in conjunction w/ CPK elevations to levels >1000 U/L (~5X ULN), and in patients w/o reported symptoms who have marked CPK elevations, w/ levels >2000 U/L (≥10X ULN). Eosinophilic pneumonia reported; d/c therapy immediately and treat w/ systemic steroids if signs and symptoms develop. Peripheral neuropathy reported. Avoid use in pediatric patients <12 months of age due to potential nervous system and/or muscular system effects. *Clostridium difficile*-associated diarrhea (CDAD) reported; may need to d/c if CDAD is suspected or confirmed. Patients w/ persisting or relapsing *S. aureus* bacteremia/endocarditis or poor clinical response should have repeat blood cultures. If a blood culture is positive for *S. aureus*, perform MIC susceptibility testing of the isolate and diagnostic evaluation of the patient to rule out sequestered foci of infection; appropriate surgical intervention and/or change in antibacterial regimen may be required. Decreased efficacy in patients w/ moderate baseline renal impairment. Clinically relevant plasma concentrations of daptomycin observed to cause a significant concentration-dependent false prolongation of PT and elevation of INR when certain recombinant thromboplastin reagents are utilized for the assay. May result in bacterial resistance if used in the absence of a proven or suspected bacterial infection; take appropriate measures if superinfection develops.

ADVERSE REACTIONS
Headache, diarrhea, insomnia, CPK increased, chest pain, abdominal pain, pharyngolaryngeal pain, rash, abnormal LFTs, sepsis, bacteremia, edema, pruritus, sweating increased, HTN.

DRUG INTERACTIONS
Elevated CPK reported in patients who received prior or concomitant treatment w/ HMG-CoA reductase inhibitor; consider suspending use of HMG-CoA reductase inhibitors temporarily in patients receiving daptomycin.

PATIENT CONSIDERATIONS
Assessment: Assess for hypersensitivity to the drug, renal impairment, pregnancy/nursing status, and possible drug interactions.

Monitoring: Monitor for allergic reactions, myopathy, rhabdomyolysis, eosinophilic pneumonia, peripheral neuropathy, CDAD, superinfection, persisting or relapsing *S. aureus* bacteremia/

endocarditis or poor clinical response, and other adverse reactions. Monitor CPK levels weekly, and more frequently in patients who received recent prior or concomitant therapy w/ HMG-CoA reductase inhibitor or in whom CPK elevations occur during treatment. Monitor both renal function and CPK more frequently than once weekly in patients w/ renal impairment. Monitor for muscle pain or weakness, particularly of the distal extremities.

C

Counseling: Advise that allergic reactions, including serious allergic reactions, could occur and that serious reactions require immediate treatment; instruct to report any previous allergic reactions to the drug. Instruct to report muscle pain/weakness, especially in the forearms and lower legs, as well as tingling/numbness. Advise to report any symptoms of cough, breathlessness, or fever. Advise to contact physician immediately if watery and bloody stools (w/ or w/o stomach cramps and fever) develop, even as late as ≥2 months after the last dose. Inform that therapy should be used to treat bacterial, not viral, infections. Instruct to take exactly ud even if the patient feels better early in the course of therapy; inform that skipping doses or not completing the full course of therapy may decrease effectiveness and increase resistance.

STORAGE: 2-8°C (36-46°F). Avoid excessive heat.

CYMBALTA – duloxetine

RX

Class: Serotonin and norepinephrine reuptake inhibitor (SNRI)

Antidepressants increased the risk of suicidal thoughts and behavior in children, adolescents, and young adults in short-term studies. Monitor and observe closely for worsening, and for emergence of suicidal thoughts and behaviors in all patients started on antidepressant therapy.

ADULT DOSAGE

Musculoskeletal Pain

Chronic:
Initial: 30mg qd for 1 week before increasing to 60mg qd
Maint: 60mg qd
Max: 60mg/day

Major Depressive Disorder

Initial: 40mg/day (given as 20mg bid) to 60mg/day (given qd or as 30mg bid); may start at 30mg qd for 1 week before increasing to 60mg qd in some patients
Maint: 60mg qd
Max: 120mg/day

Generalized Anxiety Disorder

Initial: 60mg qd; may start at 30mg qd for 1 week before increasing to 60mg qd in some patients
Maint: 60mg qd
Titrate: Dose increases beyond 60mg qd should be in increments of 30mg qd
Max: 120mg/day

Diabetic Peripheral Neuropathy

Initial: 60mg qd. May lower starting dose if tolerability is a concern
Max: 60mg qd

Fibromyalgia

Initial: 30mg qd for 1 week before increasing to 60mg qd; some patients may respond to the starting dose
Maint: 60mg qd
Max: 60mg/day

PEDIATRIC DOSAGE

Generalized Anxiety Disorder

7-17 Years:
Initial: 30mg qd for 2 weeks before considering an increase to 60mg
Maint: 30-60mg qd
Titrate: Dose increases beyond 60mg qd should be in increments of 30mg qd
Max: 120mg/day

DOSING CONSIDERATIONS

Concomitant Medications

Other MAOIs (eg, Linezolid, IV Methylene Blue):
Do not start duloxetine in patients being treated with linezolid or IV methylene blue. Consider other interventions (eg, hospitalization) in patients who require more urgent treatment of a psychiatric condition

If acceptable alternatives are not available, d/c duloxetine and administer linezolid or IV methylene blue. Monitor for serotonin syndrome for 5 days or until 24 hrs after the last dose of linezolid or IV methylene blue, whichever comes first. May resume duloxetine therapy 24 hrs after last dose of linezolid or IV methylene blue

Renal Impairment
Avoid in patients with severe renal impairment (GFR <30mL/min)

Diabetic Peripheral Neuropathy:
Consider lower starting dose and gradual increase

Hepatic Impairment
Avoid in patients with chronic liver disease or cirrhosis

Elderly
Generalized Anxiety Disorder:
Initial: 30mg qd for 2 weeks before considering increasing to target dose of 60mg
Maint: 60mg qd
Titrate: Dose increases beyond 60mg qd should be in increments of 30mg qd
Max: 120mg/day

Discontinuation
Gradually reduce dose

Other Important Considerations
Switching to/from an MAOI for Psychiatric Disorders:
Allow at least 14 days between discontinuation of an MAOI and initiation of treatment, and allow at least 5 days between discontinuation of treatment and initiation of an MAOI

ADMINISTRATION

Oral route

Swallow cap whole; do not chew, crush, or open to sprinkle on food or mix with liquids
Take without regard to meals

HOW SUPPLIED

Cap, Delayed-Release: 20mg, 30mg, 60mg

CONTRAINDICATIONS

Use of an MAOI for psychiatric disorders either concomitantly or within 5 days of stopping treatment. Treatment within 14 days of stopping an MAOI for psychiatric disorders. Starting treatment in patients being treated with other MAOIs (eg, linezolid, IV methylene blue).

WARNINGS/PRECAUTIONS

Not approved for the treatment of bipolar depression; may precipitate mixed/manic episode for those at risk for bipolar disorder. Hepatic failure (sometimes fatal) and cholestatic jaundice with minimal elevation of serum transaminases reported; d/c if jaundice or other evidence of clinically significant hepatic dysfunction occurs. Avoid with substantial alcohol use or evidence of chronic liver disease or cirrhosis. Orthostatic hypotension, falls, and syncope reported; increased risk with doses >60mg/day. Consider dose reduction or discontinuation in patients who experience symptomatic orthostatic hypotension, falls, and/or syncope during therapy. Serotonin syndrome reported; d/c immediately if symptoms occur and initiate supportive symptomatic treatment. May increase risk of bleeding events. Severe skin reactions (eg, erythema multiforme, Stevens-Johnson syndrome [SJS]) may occur; d/c at the 1st appearance of blisters, peeling rash, mucosal erosions, or any other signs of hypersensitivity if no other etiology can be identified. Adverse events reported upon discontinuation. Activation of mania or hypomania reported in patients with MDD; caution with history of mania. Seizures/convulsions reported; caution with history of seizure disorder. Pupillary dilation that occurs following use may trigger an angle-closure attack in a patient with anatomically narrow angles who does not have a patent iridectomy. May increase BP. Hyponatremia may occur; caution in elderly and volume-depleted patients. Consider discontinuation and institute appropriate medical intervention in patients with symptomatic hyponatremia. Urinary hesitation and retention reported. Caution with conditions that may slow gastric emptying and with diabetes; worsening glycemic control observed in some patients with diabetes. Avoid in severe renal impairment (GFR <30mL/min).

ADVERSE REACTIONS

Nausea, dry mouth, somnolence, constipation, decreased appetite, hyperhidrosis, diarrhea, fatigue, dizziness, headache, insomnia, abdominal pain.

DRUG INTERACTIONS

See Contraindications. Greater risk of hypotension with concomitant use of medications that induce orthostatic hypotension (eg, antihypertensives) and potent CYP1A2 inhibitors. May cause serotonin syndrome with other serotonergic drugs (eg, triptans, TCAs, fentanyl) and with drugs that impair metabolism of serotonin; d/c immediately if this occurs. Caution with NSAIDs, aspirin (ASA), warfarin, or other drugs that affect coagulation due to potential increased risk of bleeding. Avoid use with thioridazine, potent CYP1A2 inhibitors (eg, fluvoxamine, cimetidine, some quinolone antibiotics), and substantial alcohol use. CYP2D6 inhibitors (eg, paroxetine, fluoxetine, quinidine) may increase levels. Caution with drugs metabolized by CYP2D6 having a narrow therapeutic index (eg, TCAs, phenothiazines, type 1C antiarrhythmics); may need to monitor levels/reduce dose of TCA. Caution with CNS-acting drugs, including those with a similar mechanism of action. Increased risk of hyponatremia with diuretics. Potential for interaction with drugs that affect gastric acidity. May increase theophylline and desipramine exposure. May increase free concentrations of highly protein-bound drugs.

PATIENT CONSIDERATIONS

C

Assessment: Assess for bipolar disorder risk, history of mania, history of seizures, substantial alcohol use, diseases/conditions that slow gastric emptying (eg, diabetes mellitus), risk factors for hyponatremia, susceptibility to angle-closure glaucoma/urinary retention, hepatic/renal impairment, pregnancy/nursing status, and possible drug interactions. Assess BP.

Monitoring: Monitor for signs/symptoms of clinical worsening (eg, suicidality, unusual changes in behavior), activation of mania/hypomania, serotonin syndrome, hepatotoxicity, bleeding events, skin reactions (eg, erythema multiforme, SJS), hyponatremia, seizures, orthostatic hypotension, falls, worsened glycemic control, urinary hesitation/retention, angle-closure glaucoma, and other adverse reactions. Periodically monitor BP. Carefully monitor patients receiving concomitant warfarin therapy when duloxetine is initiated or discontinued. Periodically reassess need for maintenance treatment and appropriate dose.

Counseling: Inform about benefits, risks, and appropriate use of therapy. Advise to avoid substantial alcohol use. Instruct to seek medical attention for clinical worsening, signs/symptoms of manic episodes, and symptoms of serotonin syndrome. Inform that abnormal bleeding (especially with the use of NSAIDs, ASA, warfarin), orthostatic hypotension, falls, syncope, hepatotoxicity, urinary hesitation/retention, seizures, BP increase, or discontinuation symptoms may occur. Caution about risk of angle-closure glaucoma. Advise of the signs/symptoms of hyponatremia. Counsel to immediately contact physician if skin blisters, peeling rash, mouth sores, hives, or any other allergic reactions occur. Advise to inform physician if taking/planning to take any prescription or OTC medications, if pregnant, intending to become pregnant, or if breastfeeding. Inform that therapy may impair judgment, thinking, or motor skills; instruct to use caution when operating hazardous machinery, including automobiles. Inform that improvement may be noticed within 1-4 weeks; instruct to continue therapy ud. Advise not to alter dosing regimen or d/c treatment without consulting physician.

STORAGE: 25°C (77°F); excursions permitted to 15-30°C (59-86°F).

CYRAMZA — ramucirumab

RX

Class: Monoclonal antibody/VEGFR2 blocker

Increased risk of hemorrhage and GI hemorrhage, including severe and sometimes fatal hemorrhagic events; permanently d/c if severe bleeding occurs. May increase risk of GI perforation; permanently d/c if this occurs. Impaired wound healing may occur; d/c therapy in patients w/ impaired wound healing. Withhold therapy prior to surgery and d/c therapy if wound healing complications develop.

ADULT DOSAGE

Advanced or Metastatic, Gastric or Gastroesophageal Junction Adenocarcinoma

W/ Disease Progression on or After Prior Fluoropyrimidine- or Platinum-Containing Chemotherapy:

As a Single Agent, or in Combination w/ Paclitaxel:

Usual: 8mg/kg every 2 weeks administered as an IV infusion over 60 min. Continue until disease progression or unacceptable toxicity

When given in combination, administer prior to administration of paclitaxel

Metastatic Non-Small Cell Lung Cancer

W/ Disease Progression:

On or After Platinum-Based Chemotherapy:

Usual: 10mg/kg IV over 60 min on Day 1 of a 21-day cycle prior to docetaxel infusion. Continue until disease progression or unacceptable toxicity

Metastatic Colorectal Cancer

W/ Disease Progression:

On or After Prior Therapy w/ Bevacizumab, Oxaliplatin, and a Fluoropyrimidine:

Usual: 8mg/kg IV over 60 min every 2 weeks prior to FOLFIRI (irinotecan, folinic acid, and 5-fluorouracil) administration. Continue until disease progression or unacceptable toxicity

PEDIATRIC DOSAGE

Pediatric use may not have been established

Premedication

Prior to each infusion, premedicate all patients w/ an IV histamine H_1 antagonist (eg, diphenhydramine)
For patients who have experienced a Grade 1 or 2 infusion-related reaction, also premedicate w/ dexamethasone (or equivalent) and acetaminophen prior to each infusion

DOSING CONSIDERATIONS

Adverse Reactions

Infusion Related Reactions (IRRs):
- Reduce infusion rate by 50% for Grade 1 or 2 IRRs
- Permanently d/c for Grade 3 or 4 IRRs

HTN:
- Interrupt for severe HTN until controlled w/ medical management
- Permanently d/c for severe HTN that cannot be controlled w/ antihypertensive therapy

Proteinuria:
- Interrupt for urine protein levels ≥2g/24 hrs
- Reinitiate at a reduced dose (6mg/kg, if initial dose was 8mg/kg; or 8mg/kg, if initial dose was 10mg/kg) once the urine protein level returns to <2g/24 hrs. If protein level ≥2g/24 hrs reoccurs, interrupt and reduce dose (5mg/kg, if initial dose was 8mg/kg; or 6mg/kg, if initial dose was 10mg/kg) once the urine protein level returns to <2g/24 hrs
- Permanently d/c for urine protein level >3g/24 hrs or in the setting of nephrotic syndrome

Wound Healing Complications:
Interrupt prior to scheduled surgery until the wound is fully healed

Arterial Thromboembolic Events, GI Perforation, or Grade 3 or 4 Bleeding:
Permanently d/c

ADMINISTRATION

IV route

Calculate dose and required volume of ramucirumab needed to prepare the infusion sol.
Withdraw required volume of ramucirumab and further dilute w/ only 0.9% NaCl Inj in an IV infusion container to a final volume of 250mL.
Do not use dextrose containing sol.
Gently invert container to ensure adequate mixing.
Do not dilute w/ other sol or coinfuse w/ other electrolytes or medications.
Administer diluted ramucirumab infusion via infusion pump over 60 min through a separate infusion line. Use of a protein sparing 0.22-micron filter is recommended. Flush line w/ sterile NaCl 0.9% sol for inj at the end of infusion.
Do not administer as an IV push or bolus.

Refer to PI for further administration and preparation instructions

HOW SUPPLIED

Inj: 10mg/mL [10mL, 50mL]

WARNINGS/PRECAUTIONS

Serious, sometimes fatal, arterial thromboembolic events (ATEs) (eg, MI, cardiac arrest, cerebrovascular accident) reported. Increased incidence of severe HTN reported; control HTN prior to initiation of treatment. Permanently d/c treatment in patients w/ hypertensive crisis or hypertensive encephalopathy. IRRs reported; monitor during infusion for signs and symptoms of IRRs in a setting w/ available resuscitation equipment. Clinical deterioration, manifested by new onset or worsening encephalopathy, ascites, or hepatorenal syndrome, reported in patients w/ Child-Pugh B or C cirrhosis. Use in patients w/ Child-Pugh B or C cirrhosis only if potential benefits of treatment are judged to outweigh risks of clinical deterioration. Reversible posterior leukoencephalopathy syndrome (RPLS) reported; confirm diagnosis of RPLS w/ MRI and d/c if RPLS develops. Severe proteinuria and hypothyroidism reported. May cause fetal harm.

ADVERSE REACTIONS

Hemorrhage, GI hemorrhage/perforation, impaired wound healing, HTN, diarrhea, hyponatremia, headache, neutropenia, epistaxis, proteinuria, fatigue/asthenia, stomatitis/mucosal inflammation.

PATIENT CONSIDERATIONS

Assessment: Assess for HTN, presence of wound, upcoming surgery, Child-Pugh B or C cirrhosis, and pregnancy/nursing status.

Monitoring: Monitor for hemorrhage, ATEs, IRRs, GI perforation, wound healing complications, clinical deterioration in patients w/ Child-Pugh B or C cirrhosis patients, RPLS, and other adverse reactions. Monitor BP (every 2 weeks or more frequently as indicated). Monitor proteinuria by urine dipstick and/or urinary protein creatinine ratio for the development of worsening of proteinuria. Monitor thyroid function.

Counseling: Inform of the risks and benefits of therapy. Instruct to contact physician for bleeding or symptoms of bleeding, BP elevation or symptoms of HTN, severe diarrhea, vomiting, or severe abdominal pain. Advise to undergo routine BP monitoring. Inform that drug has the potential to impair wound healing; instruct not to undergo surgery w/o first discussing this potential risk w/ physician. Advise females of reproductive potential regarding potential infertility effects of therapy, and to use effective contraception during treatment and for at least 3 months after the last dose of treatment. Counsel not to breastfeed during treatment.

STORAGE: 2-8°C (36-46°F). Protect from light. Do not freeze or shake. Diluted Sol: 2-8°C (36-46°F) for no >24 hrs or <25°C (77°F) for 4 hrs. Do not freeze or shake.

CYTOTEC – misoprostol

RX

Class: Prostaglandin E_1 analogue

Can cause birth defects, abortion, or premature birth. Uterine rupture reported when used to induce labor or induce abortion beyond 8th week of pregnancy. Not for use by pregnant women to reduce risk of NSAID-induced ulcers. Patients must be advised of the abortifacient property and warned not to give the drug to others. Use only in women of childbearing potential if the patient has had a negative serum pregnancy test within 2 weeks of starting therapy, is capable of complying with effective contraceptive measures, has received both oral and written warnings of the hazards of drug use, the risk of contraception failure, and the danger to other women of childbearing potential should the drug be taken by mistake, and will begin therapy only on 2nd or 3rd day of next normal menstrual period.

ADULT DOSAGE

NSAID-Associated Gastric Ulcer

Risk reduction in patients at high risk of complications from gastric ulcer, as well as patients at high risk of developing gastric ulceration

200mcg qid (last dose of the day should be hs); take for the duration of NSAID therapy. May use 100mcg qid if dose not tolerated

PEDIATRIC DOSAGE

Pediatric use may not have been established

DOSING CONSIDERATIONS

Renal Impairment

May reduce dose if the 200mcg dose is not tolerated

ADMINISTRATION

Oral route

Take w/ a meal

HOW SUPPLIED

Tab: 100mcg, 200mcg

CONTRAINDICATIONS

Pregnant women, history of allergy to prostaglandins.

WARNINGS/PRECAUTIONS

Has not been shown to reduce the risk of duodenal ulcers in patients taking NSAIDs. Caution with preexisting cardiovascular disease (CVD).

ADVERSE REACTIONS

Diarrhea, abdominal pain, nausea.

DRUG INTERACTIONS

May augment the activity of oxytocic agents, especially when given <4 hrs prior to initiating oxytocin treatment; concomitant use is not recommended. Avoid coadministration with Mg^{2+}-containing antacids to decrease incidence of diarrhea. Reduced total availability with antacids.

PATIENT CONSIDERATIONS

Assessment: In women of childbearing potential, assess pregnancy status (negative test within 2 weeks of starting therapy), the ability to comply with effective contraceptive measures, and menstrual cycle. Assess for CVD, risks for gastric ulcer, underlying condition (eg, inflammatory bowel disease), nursing status, previous hypersensitivity to the drug, and possible drug interactions.

Monitoring: Monitor patients with an underlying condition, or those in whom dehydration, were it to occur, would be dangerous.

Counseling: Inform women of childbearing potential that they must not take medication if pregnant and they must use an effective contraception method during therapy. Inform that drug is intended for administration along with NSAIDs, including aspirin, to reduce risk of developing NSAID-induced gastric ulcer. Instruct to take drug only according to directions of physician and contact physician if patient has questions about or problems with the drug. Instruct not to give medication to anyone else.

STORAGE: ≤25°C (77°F), in a dry area.

DAKLINZA – daclatasvir

RX

Class: HCV NS5A inhibitor

D

ADULT DOSAGE

Chronic Hepatitis C

Indicated for use w/ sofosbuvir, w/ or w/o ribavirin, for the treatment of patients w/ chronic hepatitis C virus (HCV) genotype 1 or genotype 3 infection

Recommended Daclatasvir Dose:
60mg qd

Recommended Treatment Regimen and Duration:

Genotype 1:

W/O Cirrhosis or w/ Compensated (Child-Pugh A) Cirrhosis: daclatasvir + sofosbuvir for 12 weeks

Decompensated (Child-Pugh B or C) Cirrhosis or Post-Transplant: daclatasvir + sofosbuvir + ribavirin for 12 weeks

Genotype 3:

W/O Cirrhosis: daclatasvir + sofosbuvir for 12 weeks

Compensated (Child-Pugh A) or Decompensated (Child-Pugh B or C) Cirrhosis, or Post-Transplant: daclatasvir + sofosbuvir + ribavirin for 12 weeks

The recommended treatment durations are also applicable to patients w/ HCV/HIV-1 coinfection

For specific sofosbuvir and ribavirin dosage recommendations, refer to the individual PIs

PEDIATRIC DOSAGE

Pediatric use may not have been established

DOSING CONSIDERATIONS

Concomitant Medications

Strong CYP3A Inhibitors and Certain HIV Antiviral Agents:
Reduce daclatasvir dose to 30mg qd

Moderate CYP3A Inducers and Nevirapine:
Increase daclatasvir dose to 90mg qd

Discontinuation

D/C daclatasvir if sofosbuvir is permanently discontinued

ADMINISTRATION

Oral route

Take w/ or w/o food.

HOW SUPPLIED

Tab: 30mg, 60mg

CONTRAINDICATIONS

In combination w/ strong CYP3A inducers (eg, phenytoin, carbamazepine, rifampin, St. John's wort). When used w/ sofosbuvir and ribavirin, refer to the individual monographs.

WARNINGS/PRECAUTIONS

Consider screening for the presence of NS5A polymorphisms at amino acid positions M28, Q30, L31, and Y93 in patients w/ cirrhosis who are infected w/ HCV genotype 1a prior to treatment initiation. Symptomatic bradycardia and cases requiring pacemaker intervention have been reported when amiodarone is coadministered w/ sofosbuvir in combination w/ another chronic HCV direct-acting antiviral, including daclatasvir. Patients also taking β-blockers or those w/ underlying cardiac comorbidities and/or advanced liver disease may be at increased risk for symptomatic bradycardia w/ coadministration of amiodarone. Coadministration of amiodarone w/ daclatasvir in combination w/ sofosbuvir is not recommended; if coadministration is required, cardiac monitoring in an inpatient setting for the first 48 hrs of coadministration is recommended, after which outpatient or self-monitoring of HR should occur on a daily basis through at least the first 2 weeks of treatment. Patients discontinuing amiodarone just prior to starting sofosbuvir in combination w/ daclatasvir should also undergo similar cardiac monitoring. Immediately evaluate patients who develop signs/

symptoms of bradycardia. If administered w/ ribavirin, refer to the ribavirin PI for a full list of the warnings and precautions for ribavirin.

ADVERSE REACTIONS

Daclatasvir in Combination w/ Sofosbuvir: Headache, fatigue.

Daclatasvir in Combination w/ Sofosbuvir and Ribavirin: Headache, anemia, fatigue, nausea.

DRUG INTERACTIONS

See Dosing Considerations, Contraindications, and Warnings/Precautions. Strong CYP3A inducers or moderate CYP3A inducers (eg, bosentan, dexamethasone, nafcillin) may decrease levels and therapeutic effect. Strong CYP3A inhibitors (eg, clarithromycin, itraconazole, nefazodone) may increase levels. May increase systemic exposure to medicinal products that are substrates of P-gp, OATP 1B1 or 1B3, or breast cancer resistance protein, which could increase or prolong their therapeutic effect or adverse reactions. HIV protease inhibitors (eg, atazanavir w/ ritonavir, indinavir, nelfinavir, saquinavir) may increase levels; decrease daclatasvir dose to 30mg qd. Cobicistat-containing antiretroviral regimens (eg, atazanavir/cobicistat, elvitegravir/cobicistat/emtricitabine/tenofovir disoproxil fumarate) may increase levels; decrease daclatasvir dose to 30mg qd except w/ darunavir combined w/ cobicistat. Non-nucleoside reverse transcriptase inhibitors (eg, efavirenz, etravirine, nevirapine) may decrease levels; increase daclatasvir dose to 90mg qd. May increase levels of dabigatran. Use w/ dabigatran is not recommended in specific renal impairment groups, depending on the indication; refer to dabigatran PI for specific recommendations. May increase digoxin levels; monitor digoxin levels. May increase levels of HMG-CoA reductase inhibitors (eg, atorvastatin, rosuvastatin, simvastatin); monitor for HMG-CoA reductase inhibitor-associated adverse events (eg, myopathy). May increase levels of buprenorphine and norbuprenorphine; monitor for buprenorphine-associated adverse events. Refer to PI for further information on drug interactions.

PATIENT CONSIDERATIONS

Assessment: Assess for hypersensitivity to drug, pregnancy/nursing status, and possible drug interactions. Perform cardiac monitoring in patients discontinuing amiodarone just prior to starting daclatasvir. Consider screening for the presence of NS5A polymorphisms at amino acid positions M28, Q30, L31, and Y93 in patients w/ cirrhosis who are infected w/ HCV genotype 1a prior to treatment initiation.

Monitoring: Monitor for bradycardia if coadministering daclatasvir w/ sofosbuvir and amiodarone. Monitor for other adverse reactions.

Counseling: Inform that therapy may interact w/ other drugs; advise to report to physician the use of any other medication or herbal products. Advise to seek medical evaluation immediately for symptoms of bradycardia (eg, fainting, dizziness, lightheadedness, weakness). Inform that therapy should not be used alone and that it should be used in combination w/ sofosbuvir w/ or w/o ribavirin. Advise to avoid pregnancy during combination treatment w/ daclatasvir and sofosbuvir w/ ribavirin for 6 months after completion of treatment; instruct to notify physician immediately in the event of a pregnancy.

STORAGE: 25°C (77°F); excursions permitted between 15-30°C (59-86°F).

DALIRESP — roflumilast

RX

Class: Selective phosphodiesterase-4 (PDE-4) inhibitor

ADULT DOSAGE

Chronic Obstructive Pulmonary Disease

Reduce risk of exacerbations in patients w/ severe COPD associated w/ chronic bronchitis and a history of exacerbations

500mcg qd

PEDIATRIC DOSAGE

Pediatric use may not have been established

ADMINISTRATION

Oral route

Take w/ or w/o food.

HOW SUPPLIED

Tab: 500mcg

CONTRAINDICATIONS

Moderate to severe liver impairment (Child-Pugh B or C).

WARNINGS/PRECAUTIONS

Not a bronchodilator; not indicated for the relief of acute bronchospasm. Psychiatric adverse reactions, including suicidality, reported; carefully evaluate the risks and benefits of treatment in patients w/ history of depression and/or suicidal thoughts or behavior, and of continuing treatment if such reactions occur. Weight loss reported; evaluate and consider discontinuation if unexplained or clinically significant weight loss occurs. Caution w/ mild liver impairment (Child-Pugh A).

ADVERSE REACTIONS

Diarrhea, weight decreased, nausea, headache, back pain.

DRUG INTERACTIONS

Strong CYP450 inducers (eg, rifampicin, phenobarbital, carbamazepine, phenytoin) decrease exposure and may reduce therapeutic effectiveness; concomitant use is not recommended. CYP3A4 inhibitors or dual inhibitors that inhibit both CYP3A4 and CYP1A2 simultaneously (eg, erythromycin, ketoconazole, fluvoxamine, enoxacin, cimetidine) and oral contraceptives containing gestodene and ethinyl estradiol may increase exposure and may result in increased adverse reactions; use w/ caution.

PATIENT CONSIDERATIONS

Assessment: Assess for liver impairment, history of depression and/or suicidal thoughts or behavior, pregnancy/nursing status, and possible drug interactions.

Monitoring: Monitor for psychiatric events (including suicidality) and other adverse reactions. Monitor weight regularly.

Counseling: Inform that drug is not a bronchodilator and should not be used for the relief of acute bronchospasm. Advise of the need to be alert for the emergence or worsening of insomnia, anxiety, depression, suicidal thoughts, or other mood changes; instruct to contact physician if such changes occur. Instruct to monitor weight regularly and to consult physician if unexplained or clinically significant weight loss occurs. Instruct to notify physician of all medications being taken.

STORAGE: 20-25°C (68-77°F); excursions permitted to 15-30°C (59-86°F).

DALVANCE – dalbavancin RX

Class: Lipoglycopeptide

ADULT DOSAGE

Skin and Skin Structure Infections

Acute Bacterial Infections:
Single Dose Regimen: 1500mg
2-Dose Regimen: 1000mg, followed 1 week later by 500mg

Administer over 30 min by IV infusion

PEDIATRIC DOSAGE

Pediatric use may not have been established

DOSING CONSIDERATIONS

Renal Impairment

CrCl <30mL/min and Not Receiving Regularly Scheduled Hemodialysis:
Single Dose Regimen: 1125mg
2-Dose Regimen: 750mg, followed 1 week later by 375mg

Patients Receiving Regularly Scheduled Hemodialysis:
No dosage adjustment is recommended and may administer w/o regard to timing of hemodialysis

ADMINISTRATION

IV route

Do not co-infuse w/ other medications or electrolytes.
Do not use saline-based infusion sol.
If a common IV line is being used to administer other drugs in addition to dalbavancin, flush the line before and after each infusion w/ D5 inj.

Reconstitution

1. Reconstitute using 25mL of either sterile water for inj or D5 inj for each 500mg vial.
2. Alternate between gentle swirling and inversion of vial to avoid foaming; do not shake.
3. The reconstituted vial contains 20mg/mL dalbavancin.
4. Store reconstituted vials either at 2-8°C (36-46°F), or at 20-25°C (68-77°F); do not freeze.

Dilution

1. Aseptically transfer the required dose of reconstituted dalbavancin sol from the vial(s) to an IV bag or bottle containing D5 inj.
2. The diluted sol must have a final concentration of 1-5mg/mL.
3. Once diluted into an IV bag or bottle, may store either at 2-8°C (36-46°F), or at 20-25°C (68-77°F); do not freeze.

The total time from reconstitution to dilution to administration should not exceed 48 hrs.

HOW SUPPLIED

Inj: 500mg

CONTRAINDICATIONS

Known hypersensitivity to dalbavancin.

WARNINGS/PRECAUTIONS

Serious hypersensitivity (anaphylactic) and skin reactions reported; d/c if an allergic reaction occurs. Caution w/ history of glycopeptide allergy. Rapid IV infusion of therapy can cause reactions that resemble "Red-Man syndrome" (eg, flushing of the upper body, urticaria, pruritus, rash); stopping or slowing infusion may result in cessation of these reactions. ALT elevations reported. *Clostridium difficile*-associated diarrhea (CDAD) reported; may need to d/c if CDAD is suspected or confirmed. May result in bacterial resistance if used in the absence of proven or suspected bacterial infection. Caution w/ moderate or severe hepatic impairment (Child-Pugh Class B or C) and in elderly.

ADVERSE REACTIONS

Nausea, headache, diarrhea.

PATIENT CONSIDERATIONS

Assessment: Assess for hypersensitivity to drug or other glycopeptides, renal/hepatic impairment, and pregnancy/nursing status. Perform culture and susceptibility testing.

Monitoring: Monitor for hypersensitivity reactions, infusion-related reactions, hepatic effects, CDAD, development of drug-resistant bacteria, and other adverse reactions.

Counseling: Advise that allergic reactions may occur and that serious allergic reactions require immediate treatment. Instruct to inform physician about any previous hypersensitivity reactions to dalbavancin, or other glycopeptides. Counsel that therapy should only be used to treat bacterial, not viral, infections. Instruct to take exactly ud, even if the patient feels better early in the course of therapy; inform that skipping doses or not completing full course of therapy may decrease effectiveness of treatment and increase bacterial resistance. Inform that diarrhea is a common problem caused by therapy and usually resolves when therapy is discontinued; instruct to contact physician if severe watery or bloody diarrhea develops.

STORAGE: Unreconstituted: 25°C (77°F); excursions permitted to 15-30°C (59-86°F).

DARZALEX – daratumumab

RX

Class: Monoclonal antibody/CD38 blocker

ADULT DOSAGE

Multiple Myeloma

Patients w/ multiple myeloma who have received at least 3 prior lines of therapy including a proteasome inhibitor (PI) and an immunomodulatory agent or who are double-refractory to a PI and an immunomodulatory agent

Recommended Dose: 16mg/kg IV
Weeks 1-8: Administer weekly
Weeks 9-24: Administer every 2 weeks
Week 25 Onwards Until Disease Progression: Administer every 4 weeks

Infusion Rates:
1st Infusion:
Dilution Volume: 1000mL
Initial Rate (1st hr): 50mL/hr
Rate Increment: 50mL/hr every hr
Max Rate: 200mL/hr

2nd Infusion:
Dilution Volume: 500mL
Initial Rate (1st hr): 50mL/hr
Rate Increment: 50mL/hr every hr
Max Rate: 200mL/hr

Escalate infusion rate only if there were no Grade 1 or greater infusion reactions during the first 3 hrs of the 1st infusion

PEDIATRIC DOSAGE

Pediatric use may not have been established

Subsequent Infusions:
Dilution Volume: 500mL
Initial Rate (1st hr): 100mL/hr
Rate Increment: 50mL/hr every hr
Max Rate: 200mL/hr

Escalate infusion rate only if there were no Grade 1 or greater infusion reactions during a final infusion rate of ≥100 mL/hr in the first 2 infusions

Premedication

IV corticosteroid (methylprednisolone 100mg, or equivalent dose of an intermediate-acting or long-acting corticosteroid) + oral antipyretics (acetaminophen 650-1000mg) + oral or IV antihistamine (diphenhydramine 25-50mg or equivalent)

Administer to all patients 1 hr prior to every infusion; following 2nd infusion, may reduce the corticosteroid dose (methylprednisolone 60mg IV)

Post-Infusion Medication

Administer to all patients oral corticosteroid (20mg methylprednisolone or equivalent dose of a corticosteroid in accordance w/ local standards) on the 1st and 2nd day after all infusions

For patients w/ a history of obstructive pulmonary disorder, consider prescribing post-infusion medications (eg, short and long-acting bronchodilators, inhaled corticosteroids). Following the first 4 infusions, if patient experiences no major infusion reactions, may d/c additional inhaled post-infusion medications

Missed Dose

If a planned dose is missed, administer the dose as soon as possible and adjust dosing schedule accordingly, maintaining the treatment interval

DOSING CONSIDERATIONS

Adverse Reactions

Infusion Reactions:
Immediately interrupt infusion and manage symptoms if an infusion reaction of any grade/severity develops
Grade 1-2: Once reaction symptoms resolve, resume the infusion at no more than 1/2 the rate at which the reaction occurred; may resume infusion rate escalation at increments and intervals as appropriate if patient does not experience any further reaction symptoms
Grade 3: Consider restarting infusion at no more than 1/2 the rate at which the reaction occurred if the intensity of the reaction decreases to Grade 2 or lower. Resume infusion rate escalation if the patient does not experience additional symptoms. Repeat these steps in the event of recurrence of Grade 3 symptoms; permanently d/c upon the 3rd occurrence of a Grade 3 or greater infusion reaction
Grade 4: Permanently d/c treatment

Other Important Considerations

Prophylaxis for Herpes Zoster Reactivation:
Initiate antiviral prophylaxis to prevent herpes zoster reactivation w/in 1 week of starting daratumumab and continue for 3 months following treatment

ADMINISTRATION

IV route

Administer only as an IV infusion after dilution.
Administer diluted sol using an infusion set fitted w/ a flow regulator and w/ an in-line, sterile, non-pyrogenic, low protein-binding polyethersulfone filter (pore size 0.22 or 0.2µm).
Must use polyurethane, polybutadiene, polyvinyl chloride (PVC), polypropylene (PP), or polyethylene (PE) administration sets.

Infusion should be completed w/in 15 hrs.
Do not store any unused portion of the infusion sol for reuse.
Do not infuse concomitantly in the same IV line w/ other agents.

Preparation

1. Calculate the dose (mg), total volume (mL) of daratumumab sol required, and the number of daratumumab vials needed based on patient actual body weight.
2. Aseptically, remove a volume of 0.9% NaCl inj from the infusion bag/container that is equal to the required volume of daratumumab sol.
3. Withdraw the necessary amount of daratumumab sol and dilute to the appropriate volume by adding to the infusion bag/container containing 0.9% NaCl inj; infusion bags/containers must be made of PVC, PP, PE, or polyolefin blend (PE+PP).
4. Gently invert the bag/container to mix the sol; do not shake.

Following dilution, may store the infusion bag/container for up to 24 hrs in a refrigerator at 2-8°C (36-46°F), protected from light; do not freeze.
Use immediately after allowing the bag/container to come to room temperature.
Diluted sol may develop very small, translucent to white proteinaceous particles; do not use if visibly opaque particles, discoloration, or foreign particles are observed.

HOW SUPPLIED

Inj: 20mg/mL [5mL, 20mL]

WARNINGS/PRECAUTIONS

See Dosing Considerations. Should be administered by a healthcare professional, w/ immediate access to emergency equipment and appropriate medical support. Severe infusion reactions (eg, bronchospasm, hypoxia, dyspnea, HTN) reported; interrupt infusion for reactions of any severity and institute medical management as needed. Binds to CD38 on RBCs and results in a positive Indirect Antiglobulin Test (Coombs test); may persist for up to 6 months after the last infusion. Daratumumab bound to RBCs masks detection of antibodies to minor antigens in the patient's serum; determination of a patient's ABO and Rh blood type are not impacted. Notify blood transfusion centers of this interference w/ serological testing and inform blood banks that a patient has received daratumumab. Type and screen patients prior to starting therapy. If an emergency transfusion is required, non-cross-matched ABO/RhD-compatible RBCs can be given per local blood bank practices. Daratumumab may be detected on both, the serum protein electrophoresis and immunofixation assays used for the clinical monitoring of endogenous M-protein; this interference may impact the determination of complete response and of disease progression in some patients w/ IgG kappa myeloma protein; consider other methods to evaluate the depth of response in patients w/ persistent very good partial response.

ADVERSE REACTIONS

Infusion reaction, fatigue, N/V, pyrexia, back pain, cough, URTI, arthralgia, nasal congestion, diarrhea, dyspnea, pain in extremity, nasopharyngitis, decreased appetite, constipation.

PATIENT CONSIDERATIONS

Assessment: Assess for hypersensitivity to drug, history of an obstructive pulmonary disorder, history of herpes zoster, and pregnancy/nursing status. Type and screen patient's blood.

Monitoring: Monitor for infusion reactions, lab test interactions, and for other adverse reactions.

Counseling: Advise to seek immediate medical attention if any signs/symptoms of an infusion reaction develop. Advise patients to inform healthcare providers including blood transfusion centers/personnel that they are taking daratumumab, in the event of a planned transfusion.

STORAGE: 2-8°C (36-46°F). Do not freeze or shake. Protect from light.

DAYTRANA – methylphenidate

CII

Class: CNS stimulant

Caution w/ history of drug dependence or alcoholism. Chronic abusive use may lead to marked tolerance and psychological dependence w/ varying degrees of abnormal behavior. Frank psychotic episodes may occur, especially w/ parenteral abuse. Careful supervision is required during withdrawal from abusive use, since severe depression may occur. Withdrawal following chronic use may unmask symptoms of underlying disorder that may require follow-up.

PEDIATRIC DOSAGE

Attention-Deficit Hyperactivity Disorder

≥6 Years:
Apply to hip area 2 hrs before effect is needed and remove 9 hrs after application

Titration Schedule:
Week 1: 10mg/9 hrs

Week 2: 15mg/9 hrs
Week 3: 20mg/9 hrs
Week 4: 30mg/9 hrs
Dose/Wear Time Reduction and Discontinuation:
May remove patch earlier than 9 hrs if a shorter duration of effect is desired or late day side effects appear

DOSING CONSIDERATIONS

Adverse Reactions

Reduce dose/wear time or, if necessary, d/c drug if aggravation of symptoms or other adverse events occur

ADMINISTRATION

Transdermal route

Apply patch immediately upon removal from the individual protective pouch; press firmly for approx 30 sec.
Apply to clean, dry area of the hip; area should not be oily, damaged, or irritated.
Avoid application to waistline.
Alternate sides when applying the next am.
Do not cut patches.
Do not use w/ dressings, tape, or other adhesives.
Refer to PI for further application, removal, and disposal instructions.

HOW SUPPLIED

Patch: 10mg/9 hrs, 15mg/9 hrs, 20mg/9 hrs, 30mg/9 hrs [30^{s}]

CONTRAINDICATIONS

Known hypersensitivity to methylphenidate or other components of the medication (polyester/ethylene vinyl acetate laminate film backing, acrylic adhesive, silicone adhesive, fluoropolymer-coated polyester); marked anxiety, tension, and agitation; glaucoma; motor tics or family history or diagnosis of Tourette's syndrome. Treatment w/ MAOIs or w/in a minimum of 14 days following discontinuation of an MAOI.

WARNINGS/PRECAUTIONS

Avoid w/ known serious structural cardiac abnormalities, cardiomyopathy, serious heart rhythm abnormalities, coronary artery disease, or other serious cardiac problems. Sudden death reported in children and adolescents w/ structural cardiac abnormalities or other serious heart problems. Sudden deaths, stroke, and MI reported in adults. May increase BP and HR; caution w/ conditions that might be compromised by increases in BP/HR (eg, preexisting HTN, heart failure, recent MI, ventricular arrhythmia). Prior to treatment, obtain medical history (including assessment for family history of sudden death or ventricular arrhythmia) and perform a physical exam to assess for the presence of cardiac disease. Promptly perform cardiac evaluation if symptoms of cardiac disease develop. May exacerbate symptoms of behavior disturbance and thought disorder in patients w/ preexisting psychotic disorder. Caution in patients w/ comorbid bipolar disorder; may induce mixed/manic episode. May cause treatment-emergent psychotic or manic symptoms (eg, hallucinations, delusional thinking, mania) in children and adolescents w/o prior history of psychotic illness or mania; consider discontinuation if such symptoms occur. Aggressive behavior or hostility reported in children and adolescents. May lower convulsive threshold; d/c if seizures occur. Priapism, sometimes requiring surgical intervention, reported. Associated w/ peripheral vasculopathy, including Raynaud's phenomenon; carefully observe for digital changes. May cause long-term suppression of growth in children; monitor growth, and may need to interrupt treatment in patients not growing or gaining height or weight as expected. May result in a persistent loss of skin pigmentation at and around the application site; d/c in patients w/ chemical leukoderma. May lead to contact sensitization; d/c if suspected. Patients who develop contact sensitization to therapy and require oral treatment w/ methylphenidate should be initiated on oral medication under close medical supervision. Difficulties w/ accommodation and blurring of vision reported. Avoid exposing application site to direct external heat sources while wearing the patch; may increase absorption.

ADVERSE REACTIONS

Decreased appetite, headache, insomnia, N/V, decreased weight, irritability, tic, affect lability, anorexia, abdominal pain, dizziness.

DRUG INTERACTIONS

See Contraindications. Caution w/ pressor agents. May decrease effectiveness of drugs used to treat HTN. May inhibit metabolism of coumarin anticoagulants, anticonvulsants (eg, phenobarbital, phenytoin, primidone), and some TCAs (eg, imipramine, clomipramine, desipramine) and SSRIs; downward dose adjustments and monitoring of plasma drug concentrations (or coagulation times for coumarin) of these drugs may be necessary when initiating or discontinuing methylphenidate.

PATIENT CONSIDERATIONS

Assessment: Assess for hypersensitivity to the drug, marked anxiety, tension, agitation, glaucoma, motor tics, family history or diagnosis of Tourette's syndrome, cardiovascular conditions, history of drug dependence or alcoholism, psychotic disorder, comorbid bipolar disorder, any other conditions where treatment is contraindicated or cautioned, pregnancy/nursing status, and possible drug interactions.

Monitoring: Monitor for changes in HR and BP, signs/symptoms of cardiac disease, exacerbation of behavior disturbance and thought disorder, psychosis, mania, appearance of or worsening of aggressive behavior or hostility, seizures, priapism, peripheral vasculopathy (including Raynaud's phenomenon), skin depigmentation, contact sensitization, visual disturbances, and other adverse reactions. In pediatric patients, monitor growth. Perform periodic monitoring of CBC, differential, and platelet counts during prolonged therapy. Periodically reevaluate long-term usefulness of drug.

Counseling: Inform about the benefits and risks of therapy. Counsel on the appropriate use of the medication. Instruct to seek immediate medical attention in the event of priapism. Inform of the risk of peripheral vasculopathy, including Reynaud's syndrome and instruct to contact physician immediately if symptoms occur or w/ any signs of unexplained wounds appearing on fingers or toes while taking the drug. Advise of the possibility of a persistent loss of skin pigmentation at, around, and distant from the application site and to contact physician if this occurs. Advise to avoid exposing application site to direct external heat sources (eg, hair dryers, heating pads, electric blankets, heated water beds) while wearing the patch. Instruct to avoid touching the adhesive side of the patch during application, and to immediately wash hands after application if adhesive side is touched. Advise to take patch off earlier if there is an unacceptable duration of appetite loss or insomnia in the pm. Counsel to not wear the patch and to consult physician if any swelling or blistering occurs. Instruct not to apply hydrocortisone or other sol, cre, oint, or emollients immediately prior to patch application. Caution against operating potentially hazardous machinery or vehicles until accustomed to effects of medication.

STORAGE: 25°C (77°F); excursions permitted to 15-30°C (59-86°F). Do not store patches unpouched. Do not refrigerate or freeze patches. Once the sealed tray or outer pouch is opened, use contents w/in 2 months.

DDAVP NASAL — desmopressin acetate

RX

Class: Synthetic vasopressin analogue

OTHER BRAND NAMES

DDAVP Rhinal Tube

ADULT DOSAGE

Central Cranial Diabetes Insipidus

Usual: 0.1-0.4mL/day, as single dose or divided into 2 or 3 doses; separately adjust am and pm dose for an adequate diurnal rhythm of water turnover

PEDIATRIC DOSAGE

Central Cranial Diabetes Insipidus

3 Months-12 Years:

Usual: 0.05-0.3mL/day, as single dose or divided into 2 doses; separately adjust am and pm dose for an adequate diurnal rhythm of water turnover

DOSING CONSIDERATIONS

Elderly

Start at lower end of dosing range

ADMINISTRATION

Intranasal route

Nasal Spray

Pump must be primed prior to 1st use.

To Prime Pump:

1. Press down 4 times.
2. The bottle will now deliver 10mcg/spray.

Discard after 50 sprays.

HOW SUPPLIED

Sol: 10mcg/0.1mL [2.5mL (Rhinal Tube), 5mL (Nasal Spray)]

CONTRAINDICATIONS

Known hypersensitivity to desmopressin acetate or any components of the medication, moderate to severe renal impairment (CrCl <50mL/min), hyponatremia, or history of hyponatremia.

WARNINGS/PRECAUTIONS

For intranasal use only. Use only when oral formulations are not feasible. May use inj if intranasal route is compromised. May cause water intoxication and/or hyponatremia; fluid restriction is recommended. May decrease plasma osmolality, resulting in seizures or coma. Caution w/ habitual or psychogenic polydipsia, conditions associated w/ fluid and electrolyte imbalance (eg, cystic fibrosis, heart failure, renal disorders), coronary artery insufficiency, and/or hypertensive cardiovascular disease (CVD). Severe allergic reactions reported (rare). Estimate response by adequate duration of sleep and adequate, not excessive, water turnover. Caution in elderly.

ADVERSE REACTIONS

Headache, rhinitis, epistaxis, dizziness.

DRUG INTERACTIONS

Carefully monitor w/ other pressor agents. Caution w/ drugs that may increase the risk of water intoxication w/ hyponatremia (eg, TCAs, SSRIs, chlorpromazine, opiate analgesics, NSAIDs, lamotrigine, carbamazepine).

PATIENT CONSIDERATIONS

Assessment: Assess for renal function, hyponatremia, history of hyponatremia, compromised intranasal route, habitual or psychogenic polydipsia, coronary artery insufficiency, hypertensive CVD, fluid/electrolyte imbalance disorders, hypersensitivity to drug, pregnancy/nursing status, and possible drug interactions.

Monitoring: Monitor for signs/symptoms of hyponatremia, water intoxication, compromised intranasal route, and allergic reactions. Monitor BP, fluid and electrolyte levels, renal function, urine volume and osmolality periodically, and plasma osmolality.

Counseling: Inform that administration in children should be under adult supervision. Instruct to seek medical attention if symptoms of hyponatremia or allergic reactions occur. Instruct to inform physician if symptoms of nasal blockage, discharge, congestion, or other adverse events occur.

STORAGE: **Nasal Spray:** 20-25°C (68-77°F). Store bottle in upright position. **Rhinal Tube:** 2-8°C (36-46°F). When traveling, closed bottles stable for 3 weeks at 20-25°C (68-77°F).

DEMEROL INJECTION – meperidine hydrochloride CII

Class: Opioid analgesic

ADULT DOSAGE

Moderate to Severe Pain

Usual: 50-150mg IM/SQ q3-4h prn
Adjust dose according to severity of pain and patient's response

Preoperative Medication

Usual: 50-100mg IM/SQ 30-90 min before beginning of anesthesia

Support of Anesthesia

Use repeated slow IV inj of fractional doses (eg, 10mg/mL) or continuous IV infusion of a more dilute sol (eg, 1mg/mL)
Titrate: Dependent on the premedication and type of anesthesia being employed, patient characteristics, and nature/duration of operative procedure

Obstetrical Anesthesia

Usual: 50-100mg IM/SQ when pain is regular; may repeat at 1- to 3-hr intervals

PEDIATRIC DOSAGE

Moderate to Severe Pain

Usual: 0.5-0.8mg/lb IM/SQ, up to the adult dose, q3-4h prn
Adjust dose according to severity of pain and patient's response

Preoperative Medication

Usual: 0.5-1mg/lb IM/SQ, up to the adult dose, 30-90 min before beginning of anesthesia

DOSING CONSIDERATIONS

Concomitant Medications

Phenothiazines/Other Tranquilizers: Reduce dose by 25-50%

Renal Impairment

Caution; initial dose should be reduced in patients w/ severe renal impairment

Hepatic Impairment

Caution; initial dose should be reduced in patients w/ severe hepatic impairment

Elderly

Start at lower end of dosage range and observe closely

D

Other Important Modifications
Debilitated/Sickle Cell Anemia/Hypothyroidism/Addison's Disease/Pheochromocytoma/ Prostatic Hypertrophy/Urethral Stricture:
Use w/ caution; initial dose should be reduced

ADMINISTRATION
IM, IV, SQ route

SQ
Suitable for occasional use.

IM
Preferred if repeated doses are required.
Inj should be injected well into the body of a large muscle.

IV
Dosage should be decreased and inj should be made very slowly, preferably utilizing a diluted sol.

HOW SUPPLIED
Inj: 25mg/0.5mL [0.5mL, Uni-Amp], 25mg/mL [1mL, Carpuject], 50mg/mL [1mL, 1.5mL, 2mL, Uni-Amp; 30mL, multiple-dose vial; 1mL Carpuject]; 75mg/mL [1mL, Carpuject], 100mg/mL [1mL, Carpuject; 1mL, Uni-Amp; 20mL, multiple-dose vial]

CONTRAINDICATIONS
Hypersensitivity to meperidine, during or w/in 14 days of MAOI use, severe respiratory insufficiency. Sol of meperidine and barbiturates are chemically incompatible.

WARNINGS/PRECAUTIONS
Prolonged use may increase the risk of toxicity (eg, seizures) from the accumulation of the meperidine metabolite, normeperidine. May produce drug dependence and tolerance and has potential for abuse; prescribe and administer w/ caution. Respiratory depressant effects and capacity to elevate CSF pressure may be markedly exaggerated in the presence of head injury, other intracranial lesions, or a preexisting increase in intracranial pressure. May obscure the clinical course of patients w/ head injuries; use w/ extreme caution and only if deemed essential. Rapid IV inj increases the incidence of adverse reactions; do not administer IV unless a narcotic antagonist and the facilities for assisted/controlled respiration are immediately available. Extreme caution w/ acute asthmatic attack, COPD or cor pulmonale, substantially decreased respiratory reserve, preexisting respiratory depression, hypoxia, or hypercapnia. May cause severe hypotension in postoperative patients or any individual whose ability to maintain BP has been compromised by a depleted blood volume. May impair mental/physical abilities. May produce orthostatic hypotension in ambulatory patients. Not for use in pregnant women prior to labor. Not recommended during labor; may produce depression of respiration and psychophysiologic functions in the newborn when used as an obstetrical analgesic. Caution w/ sickle cell anemia; pheochromocytoma; acute alcoholism; adrenocortical insufficiency (eg, Addison's disease); CNS depression or coma; delirium tremens; debilitated patients; kyphoscoliosis associated w/ respiratory depression; myxedema or hypothyroidism; prostatic hypertrophy or urethral stricture; severe impairment of hepatic, pulmonary, or renal function; and toxic psychosis. Caution w/ A-flutter and other supraventricular tachycardias; may produce a significant increase in the ventricular response rate. May obscure the diagnosis or clinical course in patients w/ acute abdominal conditions. May aggravate convulsions w/ convulsive disorders. Avoid discontinuing abruptly.

ADVERSE REACTIONS
Lightheadedness, dizziness, sedation, N/V, sweating.

DRUG INTERACTIONS
See Contraindications and Dosing Considerations. Respiratory depression, hypotension, and profound sedation, coma, or death may occur w/ concurrent use w/ other CNS depressants (eg, sedatives/hypnotics, general anesthetics, phenothiazines, tranquilizers, alcohol); use meperidine w/ caution and consider starting at a reduced dosage in patients who are concurrently receiving other CNS depressants. Mixed agonist/antagonist opioid analgesics (eg, pentazocine, nalbuphine, butorphanol, buprenorphine) may reduce analgesic effect and/or may precipitate withdrawal symptoms; use w/ caution. Acyclovir may increase levels of meperidine and its metabolite, normeperidine; use w/ caution. Cimetidine may reduce clearance and V_d and also the formation of normeperidine; use w/ caution. Phenytoin may enhance hepatic metabolism and may increase levels of normeperidine; use w/ caution. Ritonavir may increase levels of normeperidine; avoid coadministration. May enhance neuromuscular-blocking action of skeletal muscle relaxants and increase respiratory depression.

PATIENT CONSIDERATIONS
Assessment: Assess for level of pain intensity, patient's general condition and medical status, hypersensitivity to the drug, renal/hepatic impairment, respiratory depression, pregnancy/nursing status, any other conditions where treatment is contraindicated or cautioned, and possible drug interactions.

Monitoring: Monitor for respiratory depression, elevations in CSF pressure, hypotension, convulsions/seizures, drug abuse/tolerance/dependence, and other adverse reactions.

Counseling: Inform of the risks/benefits of therapy. Inform that medication may impair mental/physical abilities required to perform hazardous tasks (eg, driving, operating machinery). Advise about potential for dependence upon repeated administration. Advise to consult physician if pregnant, planning to become pregnant, or breastfeeding.

STORAGE: 20-25°C (68-77°F).

DEPAKENE – valproic acid

RX

Class: Carboxylic acid derivative

Fatal hepatic failure reported, usually during first 6 months of treatment. Serious/fatal hepatotoxicity may be preceded by nonspecific symptoms (eg, malaise, weakness, lethargy, facial edema, anorexia, vomiting) or a loss of seizure control in patients w/ epilepsy; monitor closely. Increased risk of developing fatal hepatotoxicity in children <2 yrs of age, especially if on multiple anticonvulsants, w/ congenital metabolic disorders, severe seizure disorders w/ mental retardation, and organic brain disease; use w/ extreme caution and as a sole agent. Increased risk of drug-induced acute liver failure and resultant deaths in patients w/ hereditary neurometabolic syndromes caused by DNA mutations of the mitochondrial DNA polymerase gamma (POLG) gene (eg, Alpers-Huttenlocher syndrome). Contraindicated in patients known to have mitochondrial disorders caused by POLG mutations and children <2 yrs of age who are clinically suspected of having a mitochondrial disorder. In patients >2 yrs of age who are clinically suspected of having a hereditary mitochondrial disease, drug should only be used after other anticonvulsants have failed; closely monitor for the development of acute liver injury. May cause major congenital malformations, particularly neural tube defects (eg, spina bifida). May cause decreased IQ scores following in utero exposure. Should only be used to treat pregnant women w/ epilepsy if other medications have failed to control their symptoms or are otherwise unacceptable. Do not administer to a woman of childbearing potential unless the drug is essential to the management of her medical condition; use effective contraception. Life-threatening pancreatitis reported; d/c if pancreatitis is diagnosed and initiate appropriate treatment.

ADULT DOSAGE

Epilepsy

Complex Partial Seizures:
Monotherapy/Conversion to Monotherapy/Adjunctive Therapy:
Initial: 10-15mg/kg/day
Titrate: Increase by 5-10mg/kg/week until optimal response is achieved
Usual Therapeutic Range: 50-100mcg/mL
For adjunctive therapy, if total dose exceeds 250mg/day, give in divided doses
No recommendation regarding safety at doses >60mg/kg/day

Simple/Complex Absence Seizures:
Initial: 15mg/kg/day
Titrate: Increase weekly by 5-10mg/kg/day until seizures are controlled or side effects preclude further increases
Max: 60mg/kg/day
Usual Therapeutic Range: 50-100mcg/mL
If total dose exceeds 250mg/day, give in divided doses
Refer to PI for initial daily dose guide

Adjunctive therapy for multiple seizure types that include absence seizures

PEDIATRIC DOSAGE

Epilepsy

Complex Partial Seizures:
Monotherapy/Conversion to Monotherapy/Adjunctive Therapy:
≥10 Years:
Initial: 10-15mg/kg/day
Titrate: Increase by 5-10mg/kg/week until optimal response is achieved
Usual Therapeutic Range: 50-100mcg/mL
For adjunctive therapy, if total dose exceeds 250mg/day, give in divided doses
No recommendation regarding safety at doses >60mg/kg/day

Simple/Complex Absence Seizures:
Initial: 15mg/kg/day
Titrate: Increase weekly by 5-10mg/kg/day until seizures are controlled or side effects preclude further increases
Max: 60mg/kg/day
Usual Therapeutic Range: 50-100mcg/mL
If total dose exceeds 250mg/day, give in divided doses
Refer to PI for initial daily dose guide

Adjunctive therapy for multiple seizure types that include absence seizures

DOSING CONSIDERATIONS

Concomitant Medications

Conversion to Monotherapy from Concomitant Antiepilepsy Drug: Reduce concomitant antiepilepsy drug by approx 25% every 2 weeks (starting at initiation or 1-2 weeks after start of therapy)

Elderly

Reduce initial dose and titrate slowly
Consider dose reduction or discontinuation in patients w/ decreased food or fluid intake or excessive somnolence

Discontinuation

Do not abruptly d/c

ADMINISTRATION

Oral route

Swallow caps whole; do not chew.
Take w/ food or slowly build up the dose from an initial low level if experiencing GI irritation.

HOW SUPPLIED

Cap: 250mg; **Sol:** 250mg/5mL

CONTRAINDICATIONS

Hepatic disease, significant hepatic dysfunction, mitochondrial disorders caused by mutations in mitochondrial POLG (eg, Alpers-Huttenlocher syndrome) and children <2 yrs of age who are suspected of having a POLG-related disorder, known hypersensitivity to the medication, known urea cycle disorders (UCDs).

WARNINGS/PRECAUTIONS

Caution w/ prior history of hepatic disease. D/C immediately if significant hepatic dysfunction (suspected or apparent) occurs. Hyperammonemic encephalopathy reported in patients w/ UCDs; d/c and initiate treatment if symptoms develop. Increased risk of suicidal thoughts or behavior reported. Dose-related thrombocytopenia, and decreases in other cell lines and myelodysplasia reported; reduce dose or d/c if hemorrhage, bruising, or a disorder of hemostasis/coagulation occurs. Hyperammonemia reported and may be present despite normal LFTs; consider discontinuation if elevation persists. Measure ammonia levels if unexplained lethargy, vomiting, or mental status changes occur; hyperammonemic encephalopathy should be considered. Hypothermia reported w/ and in the absence of hyperammonemia; consider discontinuation. Drug reaction w/ eosinophilia and systemic symptoms (DRESS), also known as multiorgan hypersensitivity, reported; evaluate immediately if signs/symptoms (eg, fever, lymphadenopathy) are present, and d/c and do not resume if an alternative etiology cannot be established. Altered thyroid function tests and urine ketone tests reported. May stimulate replication of HIV and CMV.

ADVERSE REACTIONS

N/V, somnolence, dizziness, abdominal pain, anorexia, blurred vision, diarrhea, tremor, asthenia, diplopia, headache, flu syndrome, infection.

DRUG INTERACTIONS

Drugs that affect the level of expression of hepatic enzymes (eg, phenytoin, carbamazepine, phenobarbital) may increase clearance; monitor valproate and concomitant drug concentrations whenever enzyme-inducing drugs are introduced or withdrawn. Concomitant use w/ aspirin decreases protein binding and inhibits metabolism; use w/ caution. Carbapenem antibiotics (eg, ertapenem, imipenem, meropenem) may reduce serum concentrations to subtherapeutic levels, resulting in loss of seizure control. Concomitant use w/ felbamate may increase C_{max}; may require decrease in valproate dosage. Rifampin increases oral clearance; may require valproate dosage adjustment. Reduces the clearance of amitriptyline and nortriptyline; consider lowering the dose of amitriptyline/nortriptyline. Decreases serum levels of carbamazepine while increasing carbamazepine-10,11-epoxide serum levels. Use w/ clonazepam may induce absence status in patients w/ absence seizures. Inhibits metabolism of diazepam, ethosuximide, phenobarbital, and phenytoin; monitor drug serum concentrations and adjust dose appropriately. Increased $T_{1/2}$ of lamotrigine, and serious skin reactions reported; reduce lamotrigine dose. Breakthrough seizures reported w/ concomitant phenytoin. Monitor for neurological toxicity w/ concomitant barbiturate therapy. May displace protein-bound drugs (eg, diazepam, phenytoin, carbamazepine, tolbutamide, warfarin); monitor coagulation tests when coadministered w/ warfarin. May decrease zidovudine clearance in HIV-seropositive patients. May decrease plasma clearance of lorazepam. Concomitant use w/ topiramate has been associated w/ hypothermia and hyperammonemia, w/ or w/o encephalopathy.

PATIENT CONSIDERATIONS

Assessment: Assess for hepatic dysfunction, history of hepatic disease, UCDs (especially in high-risk patients [eg, history of unexplained encephalopathy, coma]), pancreatitis, history of hypersensitivity to the drug, mitochondrial disorders caused by mutations in mitochondrial POLG and children <2 yrs of age who are suspected of having a POLG-related disorder, other conditions where treatment is contraindicated or cautioned, pregnancy/nursing status, and possible drug interactions. Assess LFTs, CBCs, and coagulation parameters.

Monitoring: Monitor for hypersensitivity reactions, pancreatitis, hepatotoxicity, hyperammonemia, hypothermia, DRESS, drug-induced acute liver failure, acute liver injury, emergence/worsening of depression, suicidality or unusual changes in behavior, and other adverse reactions. Monitor LFTs frequently, especially during first 6 months. Monitor fluid/nutritional intake, ammonia levels, CBCs, and coagulation parameters. Perform periodic plasma concentration determinations of valproate and concomitant drugs during the early course of therapy.

Counseling: Instruct to take ud. Inform pregnant women and women of childbearing potential about the risk in pregnancy (eg, birth defects, decreased IQ); advise to use effective contraception while on therapy and counsel about alternative therapeutic options. Instruct to notify physician if pregnant/intending to become pregnant. Encourage patients to enroll in NAAED Pregnancy

Registry. Advise to notify physician if depression, suicidal thoughts/behavior, or thoughts about self-harm emerge; instruct to report behaviors of concern. Counsel about signs/symptoms of pancreatitis, hepatotoxicity, hyperammonemia, or hyperammonemic encephalopathy; advise to notify physician if any symptoms or adverse effects occur. Advise not to engage in hazardous activities (eg, driving, operating machinery) until the effects of the drug are known. Inform that a fever associated w/ other organ system involvement (eg, rash, lymphadenopathy) may be drug-related; instruct to report to physician.

STORAGE: Cap: 15-25°C (59-77°F). **Sol:** <30°C (86°F).

D

DEPAKOTE – divalproex sodium

RX

Class: Valproate compound

Fatal hepatic failure reported, usually during first 6 months of treatment. Serious/fatal hepatotoxicity may be preceded by nonspecific symptoms (eg, malaise, weakness, lethargy, facial edema, anorexia, vomiting) or a loss of seizure control in patients w/ epilepsy; monitor closely. Monitor LFTs prior to therapy and at frequent intervals thereafter, especially during first 6 months of treatment. Increased risk of developing fatal hepatotoxicity in children <2 yrs of age, especially if on multiple anticonvulsants, w/ congenital metabolic disorders, w/ severe seizure disorders accompanied by mental retardation, and w/ organic brain disease; use w/ extreme caution and as a sole agent. Increased risk of drug-induced acute liver failure and resultant death in patients w/ hereditary neurometabolic syndromes caused by DNA mutations of the mitochondrial DNA polymerase gamma (POLG) gene (eg, Alpers-Huttenlocher syndrome). Contraindicated in patients known to have mitochondrial disorders caused by POLG mutations and in children <2 yrs of age who are clinically suspected of having a mitochondrial disorder. In patients >2 yrs of age who are clinically suspected of having a hereditary mitochondrial disease, drug should only be used after other anticonvulsants have failed; closely monitor for the development of acute liver injury. May cause major congenital malformations, particularly neural tube defects (eg, spina bifida). May cause decreased IQ scores following in utero exposure. Should only be used to treat pregnant women w/ epilepsy or bipolar disorder if other medications have failed to control their symptoms or are otherwise unacceptable. Do not administer to a woman of childbearing potential unless the drug is essential to the management of her medical condition; use effective contraception. Life-threatening pancreatitis reported; d/c if pancreatitis is diagnosed and initiate alternative treatment. Tab: Contraindicated in pregnant women treated for migraine prophylaxis.

OTHER BRAND NAMES

Depakote Sprinkle

ADULT DOSAGE

Epilepsy

Monotherapy and Adjunctive Therapy for Complex Partial Seizures and Simple and Complex Absence Seizures; Adjunctive Therapy w/ Multiple Seizure Types (eg, Absence Seizures):

Cap/Tab:

Complex Partial Seizures:
Initial: 10-15mg/kg/day
Titrate: Increase by 5-10mg/kg/week
Usual Therapeutic Range: 50-100mcg/mL
No recommendation regarding safety at doses >60mg/kg/day

Simple and Complex Absence Seizures:
Initial: 15mg/kg/day
Titrate: Increase weekly by 5-10mg/kg/day
Max: 60mg/kg/day

If daily dose >250mg/day, give in divided doses

Mania

Associated w/ Bipolar Disorder:
Tab:
Initial: 750mg/day in divided doses
Titrate: Increase dose as rapidly as possible to achieve lowest therapeutic dose
Max: 60mg/kg/day

Migraine

Prophylaxis:
Tab:
Initial: 250mg bid
Max: 1000mg/day

PEDIATRIC DOSAGE

Epilepsy

Monotherapy and Adjunctive Therapy for Complex Partial Seizures and Simple and Complex Absence Seizures; Adjunctive Therapy w/ Multiple Seizure Types (eg, Absence Seizures):

Cap/Tab:

Simple and Complex Absence Seizure:
Initial: 15mg/kg/day
Titrate: Increase weekly by 5-10mg/kg/day
Max: 60mg/kg/day

Complex Partial Seizures:
≥10 Years:
Initial: 10-15mg/kg/day
Titrate: Increase by 5-10mg/kg/week
Usual Therapeutic Range: 50-100mcg/mL
No recommendation regarding safety at doses >60mg/kg/day

If daily dose >250mg/day, give in divided doses

DOSING CONSIDERATIONS

Concomitant Medications

Complex Partial Seizures:

Conversion to Monotherapy: Reduce concomitant antiepilepsy drug dosage by approx 25% every 2 weeks; reduction may be started at initiation of divalproex therapy, or delayed by 1-2 weeks if seizures are likely to occur w/ a reduction

D

Elderly

Reduce initial dose and titrate slowly; consider dose reductions or discontinuation in patients w/ decreased food/fluid intake or excessive somnolence

Adverse Reactions

Thrombocytopenia: Probability appears to increase significantly at total valproate concentrations of ≥110mcg/mL (females) or ≥135mcg/mL (males)

Discontinuation

Do not abruptly d/c

Other Important Considerations

In epileptic patients previously receiving valproic acid, initiate at the same daily dose and frequency; once the patient is stabilized, the frequency of divalproex may be adjusted to bid-tid

ADMINISTRATION

Oral route

Give w/ food or slowly titrate from initial dose in patients w/ GI irritation.

Cap

May be swallowed whole or the contents may be sprinkled on small amount of soft food.

To Administer w/ Food:

1. Hold the cap so that the end marked "THIS END UP" is straight up and the arrow on the cap is up.
2. To open the cap, gently twist it apart to separate the top from the bottom. It may be helpful to hold the cap over the food to which you will add the sprinkles. If you spill any of the cap contents, start over w/ a new cap and a new portion of food.
3. Place all the sprinkles onto a small amount (about a tsp) of soft food such as applesauce or pudding.
4. Make sure that all of the sprinkle/food mixture is swallowed right away. Do not chew the sprinkle/food mixture.
5. Drinking water right after taking the sprinkle/food mixture will help make sure all sprinkles are swallowed.
6. Throw away any unused sprinkle/food mixture; do not store any for future use.

Tab

Swallow whole; do not crush or chew.

HOW SUPPLIED

Cap, Delayed-Release: (Sprinkle) 125mg; **Tab, Delayed-Release:** 125mg, 250mg, 500mg

CONTRAINDICATIONS

Hepatic disease, significant hepatic dysfunction, mitochondrial disorders caused by mutations in mitochondrial DNA POLG (eg, Alpers-Huttenlocher syndrome) and children <2 yrs of age who are suspected of having a POLG-related disorder, known hypersensitivity to the medication, known urea cycle disorders (UCDs). **Tab:** Prophylaxis of migraine headaches in pregnant women.

WARNINGS/PRECAUTIONS

Caution w/ prior history of hepatic disease. D/C immediately if significant hepatic dysfunction (suspected or apparent) occurs. Hyperammonemic encephalopathy reported in patients w/ UCDs; d/c and initiate treatment if symptoms develop. Increased risk of suicidal thoughts or behavior reported. Dose-related thrombocytopenia and decreases in other cell lines and myelodysplasia reported; reduce dose or d/c if hemorrhage, bruising, or a disorder of hemostasis/coagulation occurs. Hyperammonemia reported and may be present despite normal LFTs. Measure ammonia levels if unexplained lethargy, vomiting, or mental status changes occur; hyperammonemic encephalopathy should be considered. Hypothermia w/ and in absence of hyperammonemia reported; consider discontinuation. Drug reaction w/ eosinophilia and systemic symptoms (DRESS), also known as multiorgan hypersensitivity, reported; evaluate immediately if signs/symptoms (eg, fever, lymphadenopathy) are present, and d/c and do not resume if an alternative etiology cannot be established. Altered thyroid function tests and urine ketone tests reported. May stimulate replication of HIV and CMV. Medication residue in stool reported; check valproate levels and monitor clinical condition, and consider alternative treatment if clinically indicated.

ADVERSE REACTIONS

Diarrhea, N/V, somnolence, dizziness, dyspepsia, thrombocytopenia, asthenia, abdominal pain, tremor, headache, anorexia, diplopia, blurred vision, flu syndrome, infection.

DRUG INTERACTIONS

Drugs that affect the level of expression of hepatic enzymes (eg, phenytoin, carbamazepine, phenobarbital) may increase valproate clearance; monitor valproate and concomitant drug concentrations whenever enzyme-inducing drugs are introduced or withdrawn. Concomitant use w/

aspirin decreases protein binding and inhibits metabolism of valproate; use w/ caution. Carbapenem antibiotics may reduce serum concentrations to subtherapeutic levels, resulting in loss of seizure control. Concomitant use w/ felbamate increases valproate C_{max}; may require decrease in valproate dosage. Rifampin increases oral clearance; may require valproate dosage adjustment. Reduces the clearance of amitriptyline and nortriptyline; consider lowering the dose of amitriptyline/nortriptyline. May decrease levels of carbamazepine while increasing carbamazepine-10,11-epoxide serum levels. Inhibits metabolism of diazepam, ethosuximide, phenobarbital, and phenytoin; monitor drug serum concentrations and adjust dose appropriately. Monitor for neurological toxicity w/ concomitant barbiturate therapy. Breakthrough seizures reported w/ concomitant use w/ phenytoin. Use w/ clonazepam may induce absence status in patients w/ history of absence seizures. Increased $T_{1/2}$ of lamotrigine, and serious skin reactions reported; reduce lamotrigine dose. Monitor coagulation tests when coadministered w/ anticoagulants. May decrease zidovudine clearance in HIV-seropositive patients. Concomitant use w/ topiramate has been associated w/ hypothermia and hyperammonemia, w/ or w/o encephalopathy.

D

PATIENT CONSIDERATIONS

Assessment: Assess for hepatic dysfunction, history of hepatic disease, pancreatitis, history of hypersensitivity to the drug, mitochondrial disorders caused by mutations in mitochondrial POLG, children <2 yrs of age who are suspected of having a POLG-related disorder, other conditions where treatment is contraindicated or cautioned, pregnancy/nursing status, and possible drug interactions. Assess LFTs, CBCs, and coagulation parameters. Evaluate for UCDs, especially in high-risk patients (eg, history of unexplained encephalopathy or coma).

Monitoring: Monitor for hypersensitivity reactions, pancreatitis, hepatotoxicity, hyperammonemia, hypothermia, DRESS, drug-induced acute liver failure, acute liver injury, emergence/worsening of depression, suicidality or unusual changes in behavior, medication residue in stool, and other adverse reactions. Monitor LFTs frequently, especially during first 6 months. Monitor fluid/nutritional intake, ammonia levels, CBCs, and coagulation parameters. Perform periodic plasma concentration determinations of valproate and concomitant drugs during the early course of therapy.

Counseling: Instruct to take ud. Inform pregnant women and women of childbearing potential about the risk in pregnancy (eg, birth defects, decreased IQ); advise to use effective contraception while on therapy and counsel about alternative therapeutic options. Instruct to notify physician if pregnant/intending to become pregnant. Encourage patients to enroll in the NAAED Pregnancy Registry. Advise to notify physician if depression, suicidal thoughts/behavior, or thoughts about self-harm emerge; instruct to report behaviors of concern. Counsel about signs/symptoms of pancreatitis, hepatotoxicity, hyperammonemia, or hyperammonemic encephalopathy; advise to notify physician if any symptoms or adverse effects occur. Advise not to engage in hazardous activities (eg, driving/operating machinery) until the effects of the drug are known. Inform that a fever associated w/ other organ system involvement (eg, rash, lymphadenopathy) may be drug-related; instruct to report to physician. Instruct patients to notify their healthcare provider if they notice medication residue in the stool.

STORAGE: **Cap:** <25°C (77°F). **Tab:** <30°C (86°F).

DEPAKOTE ER – divalproex sodium

RX

Class: Valproate compound

Fatal hepatic failure may occur, usually during first 6 months of treatment. Serious/fatal hepatotoxicity may be preceded by nonspecific symptoms (eg, malaise, weakness, lethargy, facial edema, anorexia, vomiting) or loss of seizure control in patients w/ epilepsy; monitor closely. Monitor LFTs prior to therapy and at frequent intervals thereafter, especially during first 6 months of treatment. Increased risk of developing fatal hepatotoxicity in children <2 yrs of age, especially if on multiple anticonvulsants, w/ congenital metabolic disorders, severe seizure disorders w/ mental retardation, and organic brain disease; use w/ extreme caution and as a sole agent. Increased risk of drug-induced acute liver failure and resultant death in patients w/ hereditary neurometabolic syndromes caused by DNA mutations of the mitochondrial DNA polymerase gamma (POLG) gene (eg, Alpers-Huttenlocher syndrome). Contraindicated in patients known to have mitochondrial disorders caused by POLG mutations and children <2 yrs of age who are clinically suspected of having a mitochondrial disorder. In patients >2 yrs of age who are clinically suspected of having a hereditary mitochondrial disease, drug should only be used after other anticonvulsants have failed; closely monitor for the development of acute liver injury. May cause major congenital malformations, particularly neural tube defects (eg, spina bifida). May cause decreased IQ scores following in utero exposure. Contraindicated in pregnant women treated for prophylaxis of migraine; should only be used to treat pregnant women w/ epilepsy or bipolar disorder if other medications have failed to control their symptoms or are otherwise unacceptable. Do not administer to a woman of childbearing potential unless the drug is essential to the management of her medical condition; use effective contraception. Life-threatening pancreatitis reported; d/c if pancreatitis is diagnosed and initiate appropriate treatment.

D

ADULT DOSAGE

Mania

Acute Mania/Mixed Episodes:
Initial: 25mg/kg qd
Titrate: May increase as rapidly as possible to achieve clinical effect
Max: 60mg/kg/day

Epilepsy

Complex Partial Seizures:
Initial: 10-15mg/kg/day
Titrate: Increase by 5-10mg/kg/week
Max: 60mg/kg/day

Simple/Complex Absence Seizures:
Initial: 15mg/kg/day
Titrate: Increase weekly by 5-10mg/kg/day
Max: 60mg/kg/day

Migraine

Prophylaxis:
Initial: 500mg qd for 1 week
Titrate: Increase to 1000mg qd

Use Depakote instead if a patient requires smaller dosage adjustments than that available w/ Depakote ER

Conversions

Conversion from Depakote to Depakote ER in Patients w/ Epilepsy:
Depakote 500-625mg/day: 750mg Depakote ER
Depakote 750-875mg/day: 1000mg Depakote ER
Depakote 1000-1125mg/day: 1250mg Depakote ER
Depakote 1250-1375mg/day: 1500mg Depakote ER
Depakote 1500-1625mg/day: 1750mg Depakote ER
Depakote 1750mg/day: 2000mg Depakote ER
Depakote 1875-2000mg/day: 2250mg Depakote ER
Depakote 2125-2250mg/day: 2500mg Depakote ER
Depakote 2375mg/day: 2750mg Depakote ER
Depakote 2500-2750mg/day: 3000mg Depakote ER
Depakote 2875mg/day: 3250mg Depakote ER
Depakote 3000-3125mg/day: 3500mg Depakote ER

PEDIATRIC DOSAGE

Epilepsy

≥10 Years:
Complex Partial Seizures:
Initial: 10-15mg/kg/day
Titrate: Increase by 5-10mg/kg/week
Max: 60mg/kg/day

Simple/Complex Absence Seizures:
Initial: 15mg/kg/day
Titrate: Increase weekly by 5-10mg/kg/day
Max: 60mg/kg/day

Conversions

≥10 Years:
Conversion from Depakote to Depakote ER:
Depakote 500-625mg/day: 750mg Depakote ER
Depakote 750-875mg/day: 1000mg Depakote ER
Depakote 1000-1125mg/day: 1250mg Depakote ER
Depakote 1250-1375mg/day: 1500mg Depakote ER
Depakote 1500-1625mg/day: 1750mg Depakote ER
Depakote 1750mg/day: 2000mg Depakote ER
Depakote 1875-2000mg/day: 2250mg Depakote ER
Depakote 2125-2250mg/day: 2500mg Depakote ER
Depakote 2375mg/day: 2750mg Depakote ER
Depakote 2500-2750mg/day: 3000mg Depakote ER
Depakote 2875mg/day: 3250mg Depakote ER
Depakote 3000-3125mg/day: 3500mg Depakote ER

DOSING CONSIDERATIONS

Concomitant Medications

Complex Partial Seizures:
Conversion to Monotherapy: Reduce concomitant antiepilepsy drugs by 25% every 2 weeks; begin reduction at the initiation of Depakote ER, or delay by 1-2 weeks if seizures are likely to occur w/ a reduction

Elderly

Reduce initial dose and titrate more slowly; consider dose reductions/discontinuation in patients w/ decreased food/fluid intake and w/ excessive somnolence

Adverse Reactions

Thrombocytopenia: Probability increases significantly at total valproate concentrations of ≥110mcg/mL (females) or ≥135mcg/mL (males)

GI Irritation: Administer w/ food or slowly build up the dose from an initial low level

ADMINISTRATION

Oral route

Swallow tab whole; do not crush or chew.

HOW SUPPLIED

Tab, Extended-Release: 250mg, 500mg

CONTRAINDICATIONS

Hepatic disease, significant hepatic dysfunction, mitochondrial disorders caused by mutations in mitochondrial POLG (eg, Alpers-Huttenlocher syndrome) and children <2 yrs of age who are suspected of having a POLG-related disorder, known hypersensitivity to the medication, known urea cycle disorders (UCDs), prophylaxis of migraine headaches in pregnant women.

WARNINGS/PRECAUTIONS

Caution w/ prior history of hepatic disease. D/C immediately if significant hepatic dysfunction (suspected or apparent) occurs. Increased risk of suicidal thoughts or behavior reported. Dose-related thrombocytopenia, inhibition of secondary phase of platelet aggregation, and abnormal coagulation parameters reported; associated w/ decreases in other cell lines and myelodysplasia. Hyperammonemic encephalopathy reported in UCD patients; d/c and initiate treatment if symptoms develop. Hyperammonemia reported and may be present despite normal LFTs. Measure ammonia levels if unexplained lethargy, vomiting, or mental status changes occur; consider discontinuation if ammonia elevation persists. Somnolence in elderly reported; monitor fluid/nutritional intake, and for dehydration, somnolence, and other adverse reactions. Altered thyroid function tests and urine ketone tests reported. Avoid abrupt discontinuation. May stimulate replication of HIV and cytomegalovirus. Hypothermia reported. Drug reaction w/ eosinophilia and systemic symptoms (DRESS) reported; d/c if signs/symptoms are present. Medication residue in stool reported; check valproate levels, monitor clinical condition, and consider alternative treatment if clinically indicated.

ADVERSE REACTIONS

Hepatotoxicity, pancreatitis, N/V, somnolence, dizziness, abdominal pain, dyspepsia, amblyopia/blurred vision, diarrhea, tremor, weight gain, asthenia, thrombocytopenia, headache.

DRUG INTERACTIONS

Drugs that affect the level of expression of hepatic enzymes (eg, phenytoin, carbamazepine, phenobarbital, primidone) may increase valproate clearance; monitor valproate and concomitant drug concentrations whenever enzyme-inducing drugs are introduced or withdrawn. Aspirin may decrease protein binding and inhibit metabolism of valproate; use w/ caution. Carbapenem antibiotics may reduce serum concentrations to subtherapeutic levels, resulting in loss of seizure control; monitor serum valproic acid concentrations frequently after initiating carbapenem therapy. Rifampin increases oral clearance; may require valproate dosage adjustment. Felbamate may lead to an increase in valproate C_{max}; may require decrease in valproate dosage. Reduces the clearance of amitriptyline and nortriptyline. Induces metabolism of carbamazepine. Inhibits metabolism of diazepam, ethosuximide, phenobarbital, and phenytoin; monitor drug serum concentrations and adjust dose appropriately. Breakthrough seizures reported w/ phenytoin. Use w/ clonazepam may induce absence status in patients w/ absence seizures. Increases $T_{1/2}$ of lamotrigine; serious skin reactions reported. May increase $T_{1/2}$ and decrease clearance of phenobarbital; monitor for neurological toxicity w/ barbiturate therapy. Concomitant use w/ topiramate has been associated w/ hyperammonemia w/ or w/o encephalopathy, and hypothermia. May displace protein-bound drugs (eg, phenytoin, tolbutamide, warfarin); monitor coagulation tests when coadministered w/ warfarin. May decrease clearance of zidovudine in HIV-seropositive patients.

PATIENT CONSIDERATIONS

Assessment: Assess for hepatic dysfunction, history of hepatic disease, pancreatitis, history of hypersensitivity to the drug, mitochondrial disorders caused by mutations in mitochondrial POLG, children <2 yrs of age who are suspected of having a POLG-related disorder, other conditions where treatment is cautioned, pregnancy/nursing status, and possible drug interactions. Evaluate for UCD in high-risk patients (eg, history of unexplained encephalopathy, coma). Assess LFTs, CBC w/ platelet counts, and coagulation parameters.

Monitoring: Monitor for hypersensitivity reactions, DRESS, pancreatitis, hepatotoxicity, hyperammonemia, hypothermia, drug-induced acute liver failure, acute liver injury, emergence/worsening of depression, suicidality or unusual changes in behavior, medication residue in stool, and other adverse reactions. Monitor LFTs frequently, especially during first 6 months. Monitor fluid/nutritional intake, ammonia levels, CBC w/ platelets, and coagulation parameters.

Counseling: Instruct to take ud. Inform pregnant women and women of childbearing potential about the risk in pregnancy; advise to use effective contraception while on therapy and counsel about alternative therapeutic options. Advise to read the medication guide. Instruct to notify physician if pregnant or intending to become pregnant. Encourage pregnant patients to enroll in North American Antiepileptic Drug Pregnancy Registry. Advise to notify physician if depression, suicidal thoughts, behavior, or thoughts about self-harm emerge; instruct to report behaviors of concern. Counsel about signs/symptoms of pancreatitis, hepatotoxicity, hyperammonemia, or hyperammonemic encephalopathy; advise to notify physician if any symptoms or adverse effects occur. Advise not to engage in hazardous activities (eg, driving/operating machinery) until the effects of the drug are known. Inform that a fever associated w/ other organ system involvement (eg, rash, lymphadenopathy) may be drug related; instruct to report to physician. Instruct patients to notify their physician if they notice medication residue in the stool.

STORAGE: 25°C (77°F); excursions permitted to 15-30°C (59-86°F).

DEPO-PROVERA – medroxyprogesterone acetate

RX

Class: Progestogen

ADULT DOSAGE

Inoperable, Recurrent, and Metastatic Endometrial or Renal Carcinoma

Adjunctive Therapy and Palliative Treatment:

Initial: 400-1000mg/week

If improvement is noted w/in a few weeks or months and the disease appears stabilized, may be possible to maintain improvement w/ as little as 400mg/month

PEDIATRIC DOSAGE

Pediatric use may not have been established

ADMINISTRATION

IM route

Cleanse the vial top prior to aspiration of contents of multidose vial.

HOW SUPPLIED

Inj: 400mg/mL [2.5mL]

CONTRAINDICATIONS

Active thrombophlebitis, or current or past history of thromboembolic disorders, or cerebral vascular disease. Known sensitivity to medroxyprogesterone acetate or to any of the other ingredients.

WARNINGS/PRECAUTIONS

D/C if early manifestations of thrombotic disorder (thrombophlebitis, cerebrovascular disorder, pulmonary embolism, retinal thrombosis) occur or are suspected. D/C, pending examination, if there is a sudden partial or complete loss of vision, or a sudden onset of proptosis, diplopia, or migraine. If examination reveals papilledema or retinal vascular lesions, withdraw therapy. Avoid contamination of multidose vials. In cases of undiagnosed, persistent, or recurrent vaginal bleeding, perform adequate diagnostic measures to rule out malignancies. Advise women who have or have had a history of breast cancer against the use of medroxyprogesterone. Perform annual history and physical examination; physical examination should include special reference to BP, breasts, abdomen and pelvic organs, including cervical cytology and relevant lab tests. Carefully monitor women who have a strong family history of breast cancer. May cause fluid retention. Caution w/ history of psychic depression; d/c if depression recurs to a serious degree. May mask the onset of the climacteric. Use w/ estrogen may produce adverse effects on carbohydrate and lipid metabolism. Decrease in glucose tolerance reported in patients on estrogen-progestin combination treatment; caution in diabetic patients. Should not be used by women w/ significant liver disease. Periodically monitor for hepatic dysfunction and temporarily interrupt therapy if hepatic dysfunction develops; do not resume therapy until markers of liver function return to normal. Medroxyprogesterone given as 150mg IM every 3 months reduces serum estrogen levels and is associated w/ loss of bone mineral density (BMD). Some patients may exhibit suppressed adrenal function; medroxyprogesterone may have cortisol-like glucocorticoid activity and provide (-) feedback to the hypothalamus or pituitary; this may result in decreased plasma cortisol levels, decreased cortisol secretion, and low plasma ACTH levels. May produce cushingoid symptoms (eg, weight gain, edema/fluid retention, facial swelling). May change the results of some lab tests (eg, coagulation factors, lipids, glucose tolerance, binding proteins).

ADVERSE REACTIONS

Breakthrough bleeding, change in menstrual flow, changes in cervical erosion and cervical secretions, breast tenderness, headache, dizziness, somnolence, nervousness, euphoria, edema, pyrexia, change in weight, cholestatic jaundice, anaphylactoid reactions.

DRUG INTERACTIONS

Aminoglutethimide may decrease levels. Avoid w/ strong CYP3A inhibitors (eg, ketoconazole, clarithromycin, atazanavir) or strong CYP3A inducers (eg, phenytoin, carbamazepine, St. John's wort).

PATIENT CONSIDERATIONS

Assessment: Assess for drug hypersensitivity; presence, history, or family history of breast cancer; active thrombophlebitis; current or past history of thromboembolic disorders; and for any other conditions where treatment is contraindicated or cautioned. Assess pregnancy/nursing status and for possible drug interactions.

Monitoring: Monitor for thromboembolic disorders, ocular disorders, breakthrough bleeding, recurrence of depression, fluid retention, hepatic dysfunction, suppressed adrenal function, and other adverse reactions. Perform annual history and physical examination. If undiagnosed, persistent or recurrent abnormal vaginal bleeding occurs, take appropriate measures to rule out malignancy. Monitor BMD. Monitor for adverse effects on carbohydrate and lipid metabolism if used w/ estrogen therapy.

Counseling: Inform of risks/benefits of treatment. Instruct to notify physician if any adverse reactions occur while on therapy.

STORAGE: 20-25°C (68-77°F) in upright position.

DEPO-TESTOSTERONE — testosterone cypionate

CIII

Class: Androgen

ADULT DOSAGE

Testosterone Replacement Therapy

Congenital/Acquired Primary Hypogonadism or Hypogonadotropic Hypogonadism in Males:

Individualize dose based on age, sex, and diagnosis
50-400mg every 2-4 weeks

PEDIATRIC DOSAGE

Testosterone Replacement Therapy

Congenital/Acquired Primary Hypogonadism or Hypogonadotropic Hypogonadism in Males:

≥12 Years:
Individualize dose based on age, sex, and diagnosis
50-400mg every 2-4 weeks

ADMINISTRATION

IM route

Administer deep into gluteal muscle
Warm and shake the vial to redissolve any crystals that may have formed during storage at temperatures lower than recommended.

HOW SUPPLIED

Inj: 100mg/mL [10mL], 200mg/mL [1mL, 10mL]

CONTRAINDICATIONS

Known hypersensitivity to the medication. Males w/ carcinoma of the breast or known/suspected carcinoma of the prostate gland. Women who are or may become pregnant. Serious cardiac, hepatic, or renal disease.

WARNINGS/PRECAUTIONS

May cause hypercalcemia in immobilized patients; d/c if this occurs. Peliosis hepatis, hepatocellular carcinoma, and hepatic adenomas reported w/ prolonged use of high doses. May increase risk of prostatic hypertrophy and prostatic carcinoma in elderly. Venous thromboembolic events reported; evaluate patients who report symptoms of pain, edema, warmth, and erythema in the lower extremity for deep vein thrombosis and those who present w/ acute SOB for pulmonary embolism. D/C treatment and initiate appropriate workup and management if venous thromboembolic event is suspected. Increased risk of major adverse cardiovascular events (MACE) reported. Edema w/ or w/o CHF may be a serious complication in patients w/ preexisting cardiac, renal, or hepatic disease. Gynecomastia may develop and persist. Contains benzyl alcohol; has been associated w/ serious adverse events, including gasping syndrome and death, in pediatric patients. Caution in healthy males w/ delayed puberty; monitor bone maturation by assessing bone age of wrist and hand every 6 months. May accelerate bone maturation w/o producing compensatory gain in linear growth in children; compromised adult stature may result. Acute urethral obstruction in patients w/ benign prostatic hypertrophy (BPH), priapism or excessive sexual stimulation, and oligospermia after prolonged use or excessive dosage may develop; if these effects appear d/c therapy and if restarted, use a lower dose. Do not use interchangeably w/ testosterone propionate and for enhancement of athletic performance. May increase serum cholesterol. May decrease levels of thyroxin-binding globulins, resulting in decreased total T4 serum concentrations and increased resin uptake of T3 and T4.

ADVERSE REACTIONS

Gynecomastia, excessive frequency/duration of penile erections, oligospermia (if at high doses), male pattern baldness, increased/decreased libido, hirsutism, acne, MI, stroke, nausea, clotting factor suppression, polycythemia, altered LFTs, headache, anxiety.

DRUG INTERACTIONS

May increase sensitivity to oral anticoagulants; may require dose reduction in anticoagulants. May increase levels of oxyphenbutazone. May decrease blood glucose and insulin requirements in diabetic patients.

PATIENT CONSIDERATIONS

Assessment: Assess for breast carcinoma in males, prostate carcinoma, cardiac/hepatic/renal disease, delayed puberty, BPH, drug hypersensitivity, any other conditions where treatment is contraindicated/cautioned, and possible drug interactions. Confirm diagnosis of hypogonadism by measuring testosterone levels on at least 2 separate days prior to initiation.

Monitoring: Monitor for signs/symptoms of hypercalcemia, edema w/ or w/o CHF, prostatic hypertrophy/carcinoma in elderly, venous thromboembolic events, MACE and other adverse reactions. Monitor bone maturation by assessing bone age of wrist and hand every 6 months. Periodically check Hgb and Hct in patients receiving long-term androgen therapy. Monitor serum cholesterol levels and LFTs.

Counseling: Instruct to report to physician if N/V, changes in skin color, ankle swelling, or too frequent or persistent penile erections occurs. Inform of the possible risk of MACE when deciding whether to use or continue to use drug.

STORAGE: 20-25°C (68-77°F). Protect from light.

DERMA-SMOOTHE/FS – fluocinolone acetonide

RX

Class: Corticosteroid

ADULT DOSAGE

Atopic Dermatitis

Body Oil:

Apply as a thin film to the affected area(s) tid

D/C when control is achieved

Reassess if no improvement seen w/in 2 weeks

Scalp Psoriasis

Scalp Oil:

Apply a thin film on the scalp; wet hair and scalp thoroughly

Massage well and cover scalp w/ supplied shower cap

PEDIATRIC DOSAGE

Atopic Dermatitis

Moderate to Severe:

≥3 Months of Age:

Body Oil:

Moisten skin and apply as a thin film to the affected area(s) bid for up to 4 weeks

D/C when control is achieved

ADMINISTRATION

Topical route

Do not apply to diaper area

Body Oil

Apply the least amount needed to cover the affected areas

Scalp Oil

Leave on overnight or for a minimum of 4 hours before washing off

Wash hair w/ regular shampoo and rinse thoroughly

HOW SUPPLIED

Oil: 0.01% [4 fl. oz.]

CONTRAINDICATIONS

Scalp Oil: History of hypersensitivity to any components of the medication.

WARNINGS/PRECAUTIONS

May produce reversible hypothalamic-pituitary-adrenal (HPA) axis suppression with potential for glucocorticosteroid insufficiency; when noted, gradually withdraw the drug, reduce frequency of application, or substitute with a less potent steroid. Use over large areas, over prolonged periods, and use with occlusive dressings may increase systemic absorption. May produce Cushing's syndrome, hyperglycemia, and glucosuria. Children may be more susceptible to systemic toxicity due to larger skin surface to body mass ratio. Allergic contact dermatitis may occur; confirm via patch testing. Use appropriate antifungal or antibacterial agent with skin infections; d/c until infection has been adequately treated. Local reactions reported (eg, telangiectasias, burning, itching, dryness, folliculitis, acneiform eruption); may occur with occlusive dressing, prolonged use, or use of higher potency corticosteroids. Not for use on the face, groin, axillae, or eyes. Caution in peanut-sensitive individuals; hypersensitivity or disease exacerbation may occur. Do not apply to the diaper area.

ADVERSE REACTIONS

Telangiectasias, erythema, itching, irritation, hypopigmentation, burning, cough, rhinorrhea, pyrexia, nasopharyngitis, upper respiratory infection, eczema, molluscum, abscess, rash.

PATIENT CONSIDERATIONS

Assessment: Assess for peanut-sensitive individuals, hypersensitivity to corticosteroids, conditions that increase systemic absorption of corticosteroids, concomitant skin infections, and pregnancy/nursing status.

Monitoring: Monitor for HPA-axis suppression, manifestation of Cushing's syndrome, hyperglycemia, glucosuria, skin irritation, allergic contact dermatitis (eg, failure to heal), local adverse reactions, systemic toxicity in children, and skin infections.

Counseling: Instruct to use ud; for external use only. Inform to avoid contact with eyes; instruct to wash eyes liberally with water in case of contact. Instruct not to use for any disorder other than that for which it was prescribed. Instruct to notify physician if any worsening of skin condition occurs. Instruct not to apply on the face, axillae, groin, or under occlusion, unless directed by physician. Instruct to consult a physician first before using other corticosteroid-containing products. Instruct to d/c when control disease is achieved; contact physician if no improvement is seen within 2 weeks. Instruct not to apply to the diaper area, unless directed by physician.

STORAGE: 25°C (68°-77°F); excursion permitted to 15-30°C (59-86°F).

DESLORATADINE – desloratadine

RX

Class: H_1 antagonist

OTHER BRAND NAMES

Clarinex

ADULT DOSAGE

Seasonal Allergic Rhinitis

Relief of Nasal and Non-Nasal Symptoms:
Usual: 5mg or 10mL qd

Perennial Allergic Rhinitis

Relief of Nasal and Non-Nasal Symptoms:
Usual: 5mg or 10mL qd

Chronic Idiopathic Urticaria

Clarinex Tab/Sol:
Relief of pruritus and reduction in number/size of hives

Usual: 5mg or 10mL qd

PEDIATRIC DOSAGE

Seasonal Allergic Rhinitis

Relief of Nasal and Non-Nasal Symptoms:
2-5 Years:
2.5mL qd

6-11 Years:
2.5mg or 5mL qd

≥12 Years:
5mg or 10mL qd

Perennial Allergic Rhinitis

Relief of Nasal And Non-Nasal Symptoms:
6-11 Months of Age:
2mL qd

12 Months-5 Years:
2.5mL qd

6-11 Years:
2.5mg or 5mL qd

≥12 Years:
5mg or 10mL qd

Chronic Idiopathic Urticaria

Clarinex Tab/Sol:
Relief of pruritus and reduction in number/size of hives

6-11 Months of Age:
2mL qd

12 Months-5 Years:
2.5mL qd

6-11 Years:
2.5mg or 5mL qd

≥12 Years:
5mg or 10mL qd

DOSING CONSIDERATIONS

Renal Impairment

Adults:
Initial: 5mg qod

Hepatic Impairment

Adults:
Initial: 5mg qod

ADMINISTRATION

Oral route

May take w/o regard to meals

Sol

Administer w/ a measuring dropper or syringe calibrated to deliver 2mL and 2.5mL

Tab, Disintegrating

Place on tongue and allow to disintegrate before swallowing

Take immediately after opening the blister

Administer w/ or w/o water

HOW SUPPLIED

Tab, Disintegrating: 2.5mg, 5mg; (Clarinex) **Sol:** 0.5mg/mL [4 oz, 16 oz]; **Tab:** 5mg

CONTRAINDICATIONS

Hypersensitivity to this medication or to any of its ingredients or to loratadine.

WARNINGS/PRECAUTIONS

Hypersensitivity reactions reported; d/c therapy if any occur and consider alternative treatment. Caution in elderly.

ADVERSE REACTIONS

Pharyngitis, dry mouth, headache, N/V, fatigue, myalgia, fever, diarrhea, cough, URTI, irritability, somnolence, bronchitis, otitis media, dizziness.

DRUG INTERACTIONS

CYP450 3A4 inhibitors (eg, ketoconazole, erythromycin, azithromycin), fluoxetine, and cimetidine may increase levels.

PATIENT CONSIDERATIONS

Assessment: Assess for hypersensitivity to drug, renal/hepatic impairment, pregnancy/nursing status, and possible drug interactions.

Monitoring: Monitor for hypersensitivity reactions and other adverse reactions.

Counseling: Instruct to take ud; advise not to increase dose or dosing frequency. Inform that disintegrating tabs contain phenylalanine.

STORAGE: (Tab/Sol) 25°C (77°F); excursions permitted to 15-30°C (59-86°F). (Tab) Avoid exposure ≥30°C (86°F). (Sol) Protect from light. (Tab, Disintegrating) 20-25°C (68-77°F); excursions permitted to 15-30°C (59-86°F).

DESONATE – desonide

RX

Class: Corticosteroid

ADULT DOSAGE

Atopic Dermatitis

Mild to Moderate:

Apply thin layer bid to affected area(s)

D/C when control is achieved

If no improvement seen within 4 weeks, reassessment of diagnosis may be necessary

Max Duration: 4 consecutive weeks

PEDIATRIC DOSAGE

Atopic Dermatitis

Mild to Moderate:

≥3 Months of Age:

Apply thin layer bid to affected area(s)

D/C when control is achieved

If no improvement seen within 4 weeks, reassessment of diagnosis may be necessary

Max Duration: 4 consecutive weeks

ADMINISTRATION

Topical route

Rub in gently

Do not use with occlusive dressings

Avoid contact with eyes or other mucous membranes

HOW SUPPLIED

Gel: 0.05% [60g]

CONTRAINDICATIONS

History of hypersensitivity to any of the components of the preparation.

WARNINGS/PRECAUTIONS

May produce reversible hypothalamic-pituitary-adrenal (HPA) axis suppression, Cushing's syndrome, hyperglycemia, and may unmask latent diabetes mellitus (DM). Predisposing factors in patients using topical corticosteroids to HPA axis suppression include use of more potent steroids, over large surface areas, over prolonged periods, under occlusion, on an altered skin barrier, and use in patients with liver failure. Periodic evaluation for HPA axis suppression maybe required due to potential absorption. Pediatric patients may be more susceptible to systemic toxicity. Striae, linear growth retardation, delayed weight gain and intracranial hypertension reported in infants and children. Local adverse reactions may be more likely to occur with occlusive dressings, prolonged use or use of higher potency corticosteroids. If concomitant skin infections are present or develop during treatment, appropriate antifungal or antibacterial agent should be used; if favorable response does not occur promptly, d/c until infection is adequately controlled. D/C if skin irritation develops. Not for oral, ophthalmic, or intravaginal use.

ADVERSE REACTIONS

Application-site reactions, adrenal suppression.

DRUG INTERACTIONS

Use of desonide with other corticosteroid-containing products may increase the total systemic exposure.

PATIENT CONSIDERATIONS

Assessment: Assess for use with other potent steroids, altered skin barrier, liver failure, DM, infections, hypersensitivity and pregnancy/nursing status.

Monitoring: Monitor for signs/symptoms of HPA-axis suppression, Cushing's syndrome, hyperglycemia, and unmasked latent DM. Perform periodic monitoring for HPA-axis suppression through the cosyntropin or ACTH stimulation test. Monitor for local irritation and allergic dermatitis. In pediatric patients, monitor for systemic toxicity, HPA-axis suppression, Cushing's syndrome, linear growth retardation, delayed weight gain, and intracranial HTN.

Counseling: Advise to use exactly as directed. Inform that medication is for external use only; avoid contact with eyes and other mucous membranes. Instruct not to bandage or cover treated skin area unless directed by a physician. Advise that medication should not be used on underarm or in groin areas unless directed by a physician. Advise not to use in treatment of diaper dermatitis; should not be applied in the diaper area, or with diapers or plastic pants. Instruct to notify physician before using any other corticosteroids, if local adverse effects develop, or if no clinical improvement is seen after 4 weeks of therapy.

STORAGE: 25°C (77°F), excursions permitted to 15-30°C (59-86°F).

DETROL LA – tolterodine tartrate

RX

Class: Muscarinic antagonist

OTHER BRAND NAMES

Detrol

ADULT DOSAGE

Overactive Bladder

Cap, Extended-Release:

Usual: 4mg qd; may be lowered to 2mg qd based on response and tolerability

Tab:

Usual: 2mg bid; may be lowered to 1mg bid based on response and tolerability

PEDIATRIC DOSAGE

Pediatric use may not have been established

DOSING CONSIDERATIONS

Concomitant Medications

Potent CYP3A4 Inhibitors:

Cap, ER:

Usual: 2mg qd

Tab:

Usual: 1mg bid

Renal Impairment

Cap, ER:

CrCl 10-30mL/min:

Usual: 2mg qd

CrCl <10mL/min: Not recommended

Tab:

Significantly Reduced Renal Function:

Usual: 1mg bid

Hepatic Impairment
Cap, ER:
Mild to Moderate (Child-Pugh Class A or B):
Usual: 2mg qd
Severe (Child-Pugh Class C): Not recommended
Tab:
Significantly Reduced Hepatic Function:
Usual: 1mg bid

ADMINISTRATION
Oral route

Cap, ER
Take w/ water and swallow whole

HOW SUPPLIED
Cap, ER: (Detrol LA) 2mg, 4mg; **Tab:** (Detrol) 1mg, 2mg

CONTRAINDICATIONS
Urinary/gastric retention, uncontrolled narrow-angle glaucoma, known hypersensitivity to the drug or its ingredients, or to fesoterodine fumarate extended-release tablets.

WARNINGS/PRECAUTIONS
Anaphylaxis/angioedema requiring hospitalization and emergency treatment occurred with 1st or subsequent doses; d/c and provide appropriate therapy if difficulty in breathing, upper airway obstruction, or fall in BP occurs. Risk of urinary retention; caution in patients with clinically significant bladder outflow obstruction. Risk of gastric retention; caution in patients with GI obstructive disorders (eg, pyloric stenosis). Caution with decreased GI motility (eg, intestinal atony), myasthenia gravis, known history of QT prolongation, hepatic/renal impairment, and in patients being treated for narrow-angle glaucoma. CNS anticholinergic effects (eg, dizziness, somnolence) reported; may impair physical/mental abilities. Monitor for signs of anticholinergic CNS effects (particularly after beginning treatment and increasing the dose); consider dose reduction or d/c if such effects occur.

ADVERSE REACTIONS
Dry mouth, dizziness, headache, abdominal pain, constipation.

DRUG INTERACTIONS
Caution with Class IA (eg, quinidine, procainamide) or Class III (eg, amiodarone, sotalol) antiarrhythmics. May aggravate dementia symptoms when initiating therapy in patients taking cholinesterase inhibitors. Increased concentrations with ketoconazole or other potent CYP3A4 inhibitors (eg, itraconazole, miconazole, clarithromycin). Increased levels with fluoxetine reported with IR tolterodine. May increase the frequency and/or severity of anticholinergic effects with other anticholinergic (antimuscarinic) agents.

PATIENT CONSIDERATIONS

Assessment: Assess for hypersensitivity to the drug or fesoterodine fumarate, urinary/gastric retention, bladder outflow obstruction, GI obstructive disorders, decreased GI motility, narrow-angle glaucoma, myasthenia gravis, history of QT prolongation, hepatic/renal impairment, pregnancy/nursing status, and possible drug interactions.

Monitoring: Monitor for anaphylaxis, angioedema, difficulty breathing, upper airway obstruction, fall in BP, urinary retention, gastric retention, CNS anticholinergic effects, QT prolongation, hypersensitivity reactions, and other adverse reactions.

Counseling: Inform patients that drug may produce blurred vision, dizziness, or drowsiness. Advise to exercise caution against potentially dangerous activities until drug's effects have been determined.

STORAGE: (Tab): 25°C (77°F); excursions permitted to 15-30°C (59-86°F). (Cap, ER): 20-25°C (68-77°F); excursions permitted to 15-30°C (59-86°F). Protect from light.

DEXAMETHASONE ORAL – dexamethasone

RX

Class: Glucocorticoid

ADULT DOSAGE
Steroid-Responsive Disorders
Initial: 0.75-9mg/day depending on disease
Maint: Decrease in small amounts at appropriate time intervals to lowest effective dose; may need to increase dose for a period of time in stressful situations

PEDIATRIC DOSAGE
Steroid-Responsive Disorders
Sol/Tab:
Initial: 0.02-0.3mg/kg/day in 3 or 4 divided doses (0.6-9mg/m²BSA/day) depending on the disease
Maint: Decrease in small amounts at

Upon discontinuation after long-term therapy, withdraw gradually

Cushing's Syndrome Test:
1mg at 11pm; draw blood at 8 am next morning
Alternatively, may give 0.5mg q6h for 48 hrs for greater accuracy
Obtain 24-hr urine collections

Test to Distinguish Cushing's Syndrome Due to Pituitary ACTH Excess from Cushing's Syndrome Due to Other Causes:
2mg q6h for 48 hrs; obtain 24-hr urine collections

Elixir:
Less Severe Diseases: <0.75mg may suffice
Severe Diseases: >9mg may be required

D/C and transfer to other therapy, if satisfactory clinical response does not occur

Sol/Tab:
Acute Exacerbations of Multiple Sclerosis:
30mg/day for 1 week, then 4-12mg qod for 1 month

Acute, Self-Limited Allergic Disorders/ Acute Exacerbations of Chronic Allergic Disorders:
Day 1: 1 or 2mL IM of 4mg/mL dexamethasone sodium phosphate inj
Day 2-3: Four 0.75mg tabs in 2 divided doses
Day 4: Two 0.75mg tabs in 2 divided doses
Day 5-6: One 0.75mg tab/day
Day 7: No treatment
Day 8: Follow-up visit

Palliative Management of Recurrent or Inoperable Brain Tumors:
Maint: 2mg bid or tid

appropriate time intervals to lowest effective dose; may need to increase dose for a period of time in stressful situations

Upon discontinuation after long-term therapy, withdraw gradually

Cushing's Syndrome Test:
1mg at 11 pm; draw blood at 8 am next morning
Alternatively, may give 0.5mg q6h for 48 hrs for greater accuracy
Obtain 24-hr urine collections

Test to Distinguish Cushing's Syndrome Due to Pituitary ACTH Excess from Cushing's Syndrome Due to Other Causes:
2mg q6h for 48 hrs; obtain 24-hr urine collections

DOSING CONSIDERATIONS

Elderly
Start at lower end of dosing range

ADMINISTRATION

Oral route

Intensol
Mixed w/ liquid or semi-solid food (eg, water, juices, soda or soda-like beverages, applesauce, pudding); stir liquid or food gently for a few seconds
Consume immediately; do not store for future use
Use only calibrated dropper provided

Elixir
When large doses are given, may take w/ meals and antacids in between meals to help prevent peptic ulcer

HOW SUPPLIED

Elixir: 0.5mg/5mL [237mL]; **Sol:** 0.5mg/5mL [240mL, 500mL], (Intensol) 1mg/mL [30mL]; **Tab:** 0.5mg*, 0.75mg*, 1mg*, 1.5mg*, 2mg*, 4mg*, 6mg* *scored

CONTRAINDICATIONS

Known systemic fungal infections, known hypersensitivity to the medication.

WARNINGS/PRECAUTIONS

May cause BP elevation, Na^+/water retention, and increased K^+ and Ca^{2+} excretion. May cause left ventricular free-wall rupture after a recent MI; use w/ caution. May mask signs of current infection. May increase susceptibility to infections. Rule out latent or active amebiasis before initiating therapy. Use lowest possible dose to control treatment condition; reduce gradually if dosage reduction is possible. Caution w/ active/latent tuberculosis or tuberculin reactivity, active/latent peptic ulcers, diverticulitis, fresh intestinal anastomoses, nonspecific ulcerative colitis, HTN, and renal insufficiency. May have negative effects on pediatric growth; monitor growth and development of pediatric patients on prolonged use. May increase or decrease motility and number of spermatozoa in some patients. Enhanced effect in patients w/ cirrhosis. More serious/

fatal course of chickenpox and measles reported; avoid exposure in patients who have not had these diseases. May produce posterior subcapsular cataracts, glaucoma w/ possible optic nerve damage, and enhance establishment of secondary ocular infections. Drug-induced secondary adrenocortical insufficiency may be minimized by gradual dose reduction. Psychic derangements, and aggravation of emotional instability or psychotic tendencies may occur. Fat embolism reported. May suppress reactions to skin tests. False (-) dexamethasone suppression test results in patients being treated w/ indomethacin reported. (Elixir) Prolongation of coma and high incidence of pneumonia and GI bleeding in patients w/ cerebral malaria reported. Enhanced effect in patients w/ hypothyroidism. Caution w/ ocular herpes simplex, osteoporosis, myasthenia gravis. Withdrawal syndrome reported following prolonged use. May affect the nitroblue-tetrazolium test for bacterial infection and produce false-negative results. (Sol/Tab) Anaphylactoid reactions may occur. Caution w/ CHF. May produce reversible hypothalamic-pituitary-adrenal axis suppression w/ the potential for corticosteroid insufficiency after withdrawal. Changes in thyroid status may necessitate dose adjustment. May activate latent disease or exacerbate intercurrent infections. May exacerbate systemic fungal infections; avoid use unless needed to control life-threatening drug reactions. May increase risk of GI perforation w/ certain GI disorders. Caution w/ known or suspected *Strongyloides* infestation. Not for use in cerebral malaria and active ocular herpes simplex. Not recommended in optic neuritis treatment. Kaposi's sarcoma reported. Acute myopathy reported w/ use of high doses. Creatinine kinase elevation may occur. May elevate IOP; monitor IOP if used for >6 weeks.

ADVERSE REACTIONS

Fluid retention, Na^+ retention, muscle weakness, osteoporosis, peptic ulcer, pancreatitis, ulcerative esophagitis, impaired wound healing, headache, psychic disturbances, growth suppression (pediatrics), glaucoma, weight gain, nausea, malaise.

DRUG INTERACTIONS

Live or live, attenuated vaccines are contraindicated w/ immunosuppressive doses. May diminish response to toxoids and live or inactivated vaccines. Observe closely for hypokalemia w/ K^+-depleting agents (eg, amphotericin B, diuretics). Dose adjustment of antidiabetic agents may be required. Barbiturates, phenytoin, and rifampin may enhance metabolism; may need to increase corticosteroid dose. Caution w/ aspirin (ASA) in patients w/ hypoprothrombinemia. Ephedrine may enhance metabolic clearance; may require an increase in corticosteroid dose. (Elixir) Phenobarbital may enhance the metabolic clearance; may require adjustment of corticosteroid dose. Monitor PT frequently w/ coumarin anticoagulants. (Sol/Tab) May potentiate replication of some organisms contained in live, attenuated vaccines. D/C anticholinesterase agents at least 24 hrs before start of therapy. Monitor coagulation indices w/ warfarin. Hepatic enzyme inducers (eg, carbamazepine) may enhance metabolism; may need to increase corticosteroid dose. CYP3A4 inhibitors may increase plasma concentrations. May decrease plasma concentrations of CYP3A4 substrates (eg, indinavir). Convulsions and increased activity of both drugs reported w/ cyclosporine. May increase risk of arrhythmias due to hypokalemia w/ digitalis glycosides. Estrogens and ketoconazole may decrease metabolism. ASA or other NSAIDs may increase risk of GI side effects. May increase clearance of salicylates. Acute myopathy reported w/ neuromuscular-blocking drugs (eg, pancuronium). May decrease concentrations of isoniazid. Cholestyramine may increase clearance. Cardiac enlargement and CHF reported when hydrocortisone is used w/ amphotericin B. Aminoglutethimide may diminish adrenal suppression. Macrolide antibiotics may decrease clearance. May increase and decrease levels of phenytoin, leading to alterations in seizure control. Caution w/ thalidomide; toxic epidermal necrolysis reported.

PATIENT CONSIDERATIONS

Assessment: Assess for current infections, systemic fungal infections, latent/active amebiasis, cerebral malaria, ocular herpes simplex, cirrhosis, emotional instability or psychotic tendencies, any condition where treatment is cautioned, pregnancy/nursing status, and possible drug interactions. Assess thyroid status and vaccination history.

Monitoring: Monitor for Na^+/water retention, infections/secondary ocular infections, changes in thyroid status, posterior subcapsular cataracts, glaucoma, optic nerve damage, Kaposi's sarcoma, development of osteoporosis, acute myopathy, creatinine kinase elevation, psychic derangements, emotional instability or psychotic tendencies aggravation, and other adverse effects. Monitor IOP, BP, and serum K^+ and Ca^{2+} levels. Monitor bone growth and development in pediatric patients.

Counseling: Instruct not to d/c therapy abruptly or w/o medical supervision. Advise to inform any medical attendants about current corticosteroid therapies. Instruct to seek medical advice if an acute illness including fever or other signs of infection develop. Advise to avoid exposure to chickenpox or measles; if exposed, instruct to seek medical advice w/o delay.

STORAGE: 20-25°C (68-77°F). (Tab) Protect from moisture. (Intensol/Elixir) Do not freeze. (Intensol) Discard opened bottle after 90 days.

DEXEDRINE SPANSULE – dextroamphetamine sulfate CII

Class: CNS stimulant

High potential for abuse. Prolonged use may lead to drug dependence and must be avoided. Misuse may cause sudden death and serious cardiovascular (CV) adverse events.

D

ADULT DOSAGE

Narcolepsy

Individualize dose and administer at the lowest effective dose

Initial: 10mg/day

Titrate: May increase daily dose in increments of 10mg at weekly intervals until optimal response is obtained

Usual: 5-60mg/day in divided doses

PEDIATRIC DOSAGE

Narcolepsy

Individualize dose and administer at the lowest effective dose

Usual: 5-60mg/day in divided doses

6-12 Years:

Initial: 5mg/day

Titrate: May increase daily dose in increments of 5mg at weekly intervals until optimal response is obtained

≥12 Years:

Initial: 10mg/day

Titrate: May increase daily dose in increments of 10mg at weekly intervals until optimal response is obtained

Attention-Deficit Hyperactivity Disorder

Individualize dose and administer at the lowest effective dose

≥6 Years:

Initial: 5mg qd or bid

Titrate: May increase daily dose in increments of 5mg at weekly intervals until optimal response is obtained

Only rarely will it be necessary to exceed 40mg/day

DOSING CONSIDERATIONS

Adverse Reactions

Narcolepsy:

Reduce dose if bothersome adverse reactions appear (eg, insomnia or anorexia)

ADMINISTRATION

Oral route

Avoid late pm doses

May be used for once-a-day dosage wherever appropriate

HOW SUPPLIED

Cap, Sustained-Release: 5mg, 10mg, 15mg

CONTRAINDICATIONS

Advanced arteriosclerosis, symptomatic CV disease (CVD), moderate to severe HTN, hyperthyroidism, known hypersensitivity or idiosyncrasy to sympathomimetic amines, glaucoma, agitated states, and history of drug abuse. During or w/in 14 days following MAOI use.

WARNINGS/PRECAUTIONS

Avoid w/ known serious structural cardiac abnormalities, cardiomyopathy, serious heart rhythm abnormalities, coronary artery disease, or other serious cardiac problems. Sudden death reported in children and adolescents w/ structural cardiac abnormalities or other serious heart problems. Sudden death, stroke, and MI reported in adults. May cause a modest increase in average BP and HR. Promptly perform cardiac evaluation if symptoms suggestive of cardiac disease develop during treatment. May exacerbate symptoms of behavior disturbance and thought disorder in patients w/ preexisting psychotic disorder. Caution w/ comorbid bipolar disorder; may induce mixed/manic episode. May cause treatment-emergent psychotic or manic symptoms in children and adolescents w/o a prior history of psychotic illness or mania; consider discontinuation if such symptoms occur. Aggressive behavior or hostility reported in children and adolescents w/ ADHD. May cause long-term suppression of growth in children. May lower convulsive threshold; d/c if seizures occur. Associated w/ peripheral vasculopathy, including Raynaud's phenomenon. Difficulties w/ accommodation and blurring of vision reported. May exacerbate motor and phonic tics, and Tourette's syndrome. May significantly elevate plasma corticosteroid levels and interfere w/ urinary steroid determinations. In patients w/ ADHD, where possible, interrupt administration occasionally to determine if there is a recurrence of behavioral symptoms sufficient to require continued therapy.

ADVERSE REACTIONS
Palpitations, tachycardia, BP elevation, dizziness, insomnia, euphoria, dyskinesia, headache, dryness of mouth, diarrhea, constipation, urticaria, impotence, changes in libido, rhabdomyolysis.

DRUG INTERACTIONS
See Contraindications. GI acidifying agents (eg, guanethidine, reserpine, glutamic acid HCl) and urinary acidifying agents (eg, ammonium chloride, sodium acid phosphate) lower blood levels and efficacy. Inhibits adrenergic blockers. GI alkalinizing agents (eg, sodium bicarbonate) and urinary alkalinizing agents (eg, acetazolamide, some thiazides) increase blood levels and therefore potentiate actions. May enhance activity of TCAs or sympathomimetic agents. Desipramine or protriptyline and possibly other TCAs cause striking and sustained increases in the concentration of *d*-amphetamine in the brain; CV effects can be potentiated. May counteract sedative effect of antihistamines. May antagonize hypotensive effects of antihypertensives. Chlorpromazine and haloperidol inhibit central stimulant effects. May delay intestinal absorption of ethosuximide, phenobarbital, and phenytoin; coadministration w/ phenobarbital or phenytoin may produce a synergistic anticonvulsant action. Lithium carbonate may inhibit stimulatory effects. Potentiates analgesic effect of meperidine. Acidifying agents used in methenamine therapy increase urinary excretion and reduce efficacy. Enhances adrenergic effect of norepinephrine. In cases of propoxyphene overdosage, CNS stimulation is potentiated and fatal convulsions can occur. Inhibits hypotensive effect of veratrum alkaloids.

PATIENT CONSIDERATIONS

Assessment: Assess for hypersensitivity/idiosyncrasy to sympathomimetic amines, advanced arteriosclerosis, symptomatic CVD, moderate to severe HTN, hyperthyroidism, glaucoma, agitated states, history of drug abuse, tics, Tourette's syndrome, preexisting psychotic disorder, risk for/comorbid bipolar disorder, cardiac disease, medical conditions that might be compromised by increases in BP or HR, family history of sudden death or ventricular arrhythmia, any other conditions where treatment is cautioned, pregnancy/nursing status, and possible drug interactions.

Monitoring: Monitor for changes in HR and BP, signs/symptoms of cardiac disease, exacerbation of behavioral disturbance and thought disorder, psychosis, mania, appearance of or worsening of aggressive behavior or hostility, seizures, peripheral vasculopathy, visual disturbances, exacerbation of motor and phonic tics or Tourette's syndrome, and other adverse reactions. In pediatric patients, monitor growth.

Counseling: Inform about benefits and risks of treatment and counsel about appropriate use. Counsel that drug has high potential for abuse. Caution against engaging in potentially hazardous activities (eg, operating machinery/vehicles). Instruct to report to physician any new numbness, pain, skin color change, or sensitivity to temperature in fingers or toes, and to contact physician immediately w/ any signs of unexplained wounds appearing on fingers or toes while taking the drug.

STORAGE: 20-25°C (68-77°F).

DEXILANT – dexlansoprazole RX

Class: Proton pump inhibitor (PPI)

OTHER BRAND NAMES
Dexilant SoluTab

ADULT DOSAGE

Erosive Esophagitis

Healing:
Cap:
60mg qd for up to 8 weeks

Maint of Healed Erosive Esophagitis (EE) and Relief of Heartburn:
Cap/Tab, Disintegrating:
30mg qd for up to 6 months

Symptomatic Nonerosive Gastroesophageal Reflux Disease

Cap/Tab, Disintegrating:
30mg qd for 4 weeks

PEDIATRIC DOSAGE
Pediatric use may not have been established

DOSING CONSIDERATIONS

Hepatic Impairment
Healing of EE:
Moderate (Child-Pugh Class B): 30mg qd for up to 8 weeks
Severe (Child-Pugh Class C): Not recommended

ADMINISTRATION

Oral route

Two 30mg orally disintegrating tabs are not interchangeable w/ one 60mg cap.

Cap

Take w/o regard to food.
Swallow cap whole; do not chew.

Administration w/ Applesauce:

1. Open cap and sprinkle intact granules on 1 tbsp of applesauce.
2. Swallow immediately; do not chew granules.
3. Do not save applesauce and granules for later use.

Administration w/ Water in an Oral Syringe:

1. Open the cap and empty granules into 20mL of water.
2. Withdraw entire mixture into a syringe and gently swirl syringe.
3. Administer immediately.
4. Refill syringe 2 more times w/ 10mL of water, swirl gently, and administer.

Administration w/ Water via NG Tube (≥16 French):

1. Open the cap and empty the granules into 20mL of water.
2. Withdraw entire mixture into a catheter-tip syringe.
3. Swirl catheter-tip syringe gently and immediately inject the mixture through the NG tube into the stomach. Do not save water and granule mixture for later use.
4. Refill catheter-tip syringe w/ 10mL of water, swirl gently, and flush the tube.
5. Refill catheter-tip syringe again w/ 10mL of water, swirl gently, and administer.

Tab, Disintegrating

Take at least 30 min before a meal.
Do not break or cut.
Place tab on tongue, allow it to disintegrate, and swallow w/o water; do not chew.
May also be swallowed whole w/ water.

Administration w/ Water in an Oral Syringe:

1. Place 1 tab in an oral syringe and draw up 20mL of water.
2. Swirl gently.
3. After tab has dispersed, immediately administer contents into the mouth; do not save water and microgranule mixture for later use.
4. Refill syringe w/ approx 10mL of water, swirl gently, and administer any remaining contents.
5. Refill syringe again w/ approx 10mL of water, swirl gently, and administer any remaining contents.

Administration w/ Water via NG Tube (≥8 French):

1. Place tab in a catheter-tip syringe and draw up 20mL of water.
2. Shake gently.
3. After tab has dispersed, swirl catheter-tip syringe gently, and immediately inject the mixture through the NG tube into the stomach; do not save the water and microgranule mixture for later use.
4. Refill catheter-tip syringe w/ approx 10mL of water, shake gently, and flush the tube.
5. Refill the catheter-tip syringe again w/ 10mL of water, swirl gently, and administer.

HOW SUPPLIED

Cap, Delayed-Release: 30mg, 60mg; **Tab, Disintegrating:** 30mg

CONTRAINDICATIONS

Hypersensitivity to any component of the formulation. Concomitant use w/ rilpivirine-containing products.

WARNINGS/PRECAUTIONS

Symptomatic response does not preclude the presence of gastric malignancy. Acute interstitial nephritis reported; d/c if this develops. Cyanocobalamin (vitamin B12) deficiency may occur due to malabsorption w/ daily long-term treatment (eg, >3 yrs) w/ any acid-suppressing medications. May increase risk of *Clostridium difficile*-associated diarrhea (CDAD), especially in hospitalized patients. May increase risk for osteoporosis-related fractures of the hip, wrist, or spine, especially w/ high-dose and long-term therapy (≥1 yr). Use lowest dose and shortest duration appropriate to the conditions being treated. Hypomagnesemia reported and may require Mg^{2+} replacement and discontinuation of therapy; consider monitoring Mg^{2+} levels prior to and periodically during therapy w/ prolonged treatment. Serum chromogranin A (CgA) levels increase secondary to drug-induced decreases in gastric acidity. Increased CgA level may cause false positive results in diagnostic investigations for neuroendocrine tumors; temporarily stop therapy at least 14 days before assessing CgA levels and consider repeating test if initial CgA levels are high. The same commercial laboratory should be used for testing if serial tests are performed (eg, for monitoring). May interact w/ secretin stimulation test; temporarily stop dexlansoprazole treatment at least 30 days before assessing to allow gastrin levels to return to baseline. False positive urine screening tests for tetrahydrocannabinol reported; consider an alternative confirmatory method to verify positive results.

ADVERSE REACTIONS
Diarrhea, abdominal pain, N/V, URTI, flatulence.

DRUG INTERACTIONS
See Contraindications. May decrease exposure of some antiretroviral drugs (eg, rilpivirine, atazanavir, nelfinavir) and may reduce antiviral effect and promote the development of drug resistance; avoid use w/ nelfinavir. May increase exposure of some antiretroviral drugs (eg, saquinavir) and may increase toxicity of the antiretroviral drugs; monitor for potential saquinavir toxicities. Concomitant use w/ warfarin may increase INR and PT; monitor INR and PT. Dose adjustment of warfarin may be needed. May elevate and prolong levels of methotrexate (MTX) and/or its metabolite, possibly leading to toxicities; consider temporary withdrawal of dexlansoprazole in some patients receiving high-dose MTX. May increase digoxin exposure; monitor digoxin concentrations. A dose adjustment of digoxin may be needed to maintain therapeutic drug concentrations. May reduce absorption of drugs dependent on gastric pH for absorption (eg, iron salts, erlotinib, dasatinib, nilotinib, mycophenolate mofetil [MMF], ketoconazole, itraconazole). Caution in transplant patients receiving MMF. May increase exposure of tacrolimus, especially in transplant patients who are intermediate or poor metabolizers of CYP2C19; monitor tacrolimus whole blood trough concentrations. A dose adjustment of tacrolimus may be needed. Strong CYP2C19 or CYP3A4 inducers (St. John's wort, rifampin, ritonavir-containing products) may decrease exposure; avoid concomitant use w/ St. John's wort or rifampin. Strong CYP2C19 or CYP3A4 inhibitors (eg, voriconazole) may increase exposure. Alcohol may modify the release rate of dexlansoprazole from the orally disintegrating tab (ODT) and may lead to decreased efficacy; avoid alcoholic beverages when taking the ODT. Refer to the prescribing information of the concomitant medication used w/ dexlansoprazole for further information.

PATIENT CONSIDERATIONS

Assessment: Assess for hypersensitivity to the drug, risk for osteoporosis-related fractures, hepatic impairment, pregnancy/nursing status, possible lab test interactions, and for possible drug interactions. Obtain baseline Mg^{2+} levels.

Monitoring: Monitor for signs/symptoms of acute interstitial nephritis, cyanocobalamin deficiency, CDAD, bone fractures, hypersensitivity reactions, and other adverse reactions. Monitor Mg^{2+} levels periodically. Monitor INR and PT when given w/ warfarin.

Counseling: Advise to notify physician if any signs/symptoms consistent w/ a hypersensitivity reaction, acute interstitial nephritis, cyanocobalamin deficiency, CDAD, bone fracture, and/or hypomagnesemia occur. Instruct to notify physician if taking any concomitant medication (eg, high-dose MTX). Instruct how to take cap and ODT.

STORAGE: 20-25°C (68-77°F); excursions permitted to 15-30°C (59-86°F).

DiaBeta — glyburide RX

Class: Sulfonylurea (2nd generation)

ADULT DOSAGE

Type 2 Diabetes Mellitus

Initial: 2.5-5mg qd; 1.25mg qd if more sensitive to hypoglycemic drugs
Titrate: Increase by ≤2.5mg at weekly intervals
Maint: 1.25-20mg/day as single dose or in divided doses
Max: 20mg/day

Transferring from Other Oral Antidiabetic Agents:
Initial: 2.5-5mg qd
No transition period or initial priming dose necessary

Monitor carefully during 1st two weeks when transitioning from chlorpropamide, due to overlapping drug effects

Transferring from Insulin:
Insulin Dose <20 U/Day:
2.5-5mg qd

Insulin Dose 20-40 U/Day:
5mg qd

PEDIATRIC DOSAGE

Pediatric use may not have been established

Insulin Dose >40 U/Day:
Decrease insulin dose by 50% and start w/ 5mg qd
Progressively withdraw insulin and increase dose in increments of 1.25-2.5mg every 2-10 days

DOSING CONSIDERATIONS

Renal Impairment
Initial/Maint: Dose conservatively

Hepatic Impairment
Initial/Maint: Dose conservatively

Concomitant Medications
Colesevelam: Administer at least 4 hrs prior to colesevelam

Elderly
Elderly/Debilitated/Malnourished:
Initial/Maint: Dose conservatively

ADMINISTRATION

Oral route

Take w/ breakfast or 1st main meal

HOW SUPPLIED

Tab: 1.25mg*, 2.5mg*, 5mg* *scored

CONTRAINDICATIONS

Known hypersensitivity or allergy to the drug or any of its excipients. Type 1 DM or diabetic ketoacidosis, with or without coma. Coadministration with bosentan.

WARNINGS/PRECAUTIONS

Caution during the first 2 weeks of therapy if transferring from chlorpropamide. May be associated with increased cardiovascular (CV) mortality. May produce severe hypoglycemia; increased risk when caloric intake is deficient, after severe/prolonged exercise, with severe renal/hepatic insufficiency, with adrenal/pituitary insufficiency, or in elderly, debilitated, or malnourished patients. Loss of glycemic control may occur when exposed to stress (eg, fever, trauma, infection, surgery); may be necessary to d/c therapy and administer insulin. Secondary failure may occur over a period of time. May cause hemolytic anemia; caution with G6PD deficiency and consider a non-sulfonylurea alternative. Caution in elderly. Not bioequivalent to Glynase PresTab and therefore not substitutable.

ADVERSE REACTIONS

Hypoglycemia, nausea, epigastric fullness, heartburn, hyponatremia, LFT abnormalities, photosensitivity reactions, leukopenia, agranulocytosis, thrombocytopenia, porphyria cutanea tarda, blurred vision, changes in accommodation, angioedema, arthralgia.

DRUG INTERACTIONS

See Contraindications and Dosage. Hypoglycemic effects may be potentiated by NSAIDs, ACE-inhibitors, disopyramide, fluoxetine, clarithromycin, fluoroquinolones, other highly protein-bound drugs, salicylates, sulfonamides, chloramphenicol, probenecid, MAOIs, and β-adrenergic blocking drugs; monitor closely for hypoglycemia during coadministration and for loss of glycemic control when such drugs are withdrawn. Increased risk of hypoglycemia with alcohol or use of >1 glucose-lowering drug. May be difficult to recognize hypoglycemia with β-adrenergic blocking drugs or other sympatholytics. Potential interaction leading to severe hypoglycemia reported with oral miconazole. Potentiates or weakens effects of coumarin derivatives. Rifampin may worsen glucose control. Thiazides and other diuretics, corticosteroids, phenothiazines, thyroid products, estrogens, oral contraceptives, phenytoin, nicotinic acid, sympathomimetics, calcium channel blockers, and isoniazid may produce hyperglycemia and may lead to loss of glycemic control; monitor closely for loss of control during coadministration and for hypoglycemia when such drugs are withdrawn. May increase cyclosporine plasma levels and toxicity; monitor and adjust dosage of cyclosporine. Colesevelam may decrease levels. Caution with inducers/inhibitors of CYP2C9.

PATIENT CONSIDERATIONS

Assessment: Assess for previous hypersensitivity to drug or other sulfonamide derivatives, type of DM, risk factors of hypoglycemia, renal/hepatic impairment, G6PD deficiency, pregnancy/nursing status, and possible drug interactions. Obtain baseline FPG and HbA1c levels.

Monitoring: Monitor for CV effects, hypoglycemia, loss of glycemic control when exposed to stress, hypersensitivity reactions, secondary failure, hemolytic anemia, and other adverse reactions. Monitor FPG and HbA1c levels periodically.

Counseling: Inform of the potential risks, benefits, and alternative modes of therapy. Counsel about importance of adherence to dietary instructions, regular exercise program, and regular testing of blood glucose. Inform about the symptoms, treatment, and predisposing conditions of hypoglycemia, as well as primary and secondary failure. During the insulin withdrawal period, instruct patients to test blood glucose and acetone in urine at least tid and report results to physician.

STORAGE: 25°C (77°F); excursions permitted to 15-30°C (59-86°F).

DICLEGIS — doxylamine succinate/pyridoxine hydrochloride RX

Class: Antihistamine/vitamin B6 analogue

ADULT DOSAGE

Nausea/Vomiting

Treatment of N/V of Pregnancy in Women Who Do Not Respond to Conservative Management:

Initial: 2 tabs hs (Day 1)

Titrate: If this dose adequately controls symptoms the next day, continue taking 2 tabs/day hs; if symptoms persist into the afternoon of Day 2, take the usual dose of 2 tabs hs that night then take 3 tabs starting on Day 3 (1 tab in the am and 2 tabs hs)

If dose adequately controls symptoms on Day 4, continue taking 3 tabs/day; otherwise take 4 tabs starting on Day 4 (1 tab in the am, 1 tab mid-afternoon, and 2 tabs hs)

Max: 4 tabs/day (1 tab in the am, 1 tab mid-afternoon, and 2 tabs hs)

Reassess for continued need as pregnancy progresses

PEDIATRIC DOSAGE

Pediatric use may not have been established

ADMINISTRATION

Oral route

Take on an empty stomach w/ a glass of water

Swallow tab whole; do not crush, chew, or split

Take as a daily prescription and not prn

HOW SUPPLIED

Tab, Delayed Release: (Doxylamine/Pyridoxine) 10mg/10mg

CONTRAINDICATIONS

Known hypersensitivity to doxylamine succinate, other ethanolamine derivative antihistamines, pyridoxine HCl, or any inactive ingredient in the formulation. Concomitant MAOIs.

WARNINGS/PRECAUTIONS

Not studied in women with hyperemesis gravidarum. May cause somnolence and impair physical/mental abilities. Caution with asthma, increased intraocular pressure (IOP), narrow-angle glaucoma, stenosing peptic ulcer, pyloroduodenal obstruction, and urinary bladder-neck obstruction.

ADVERSE REACTIONS

Somnolence, dyspnea, vertigo, visual disturbances, abdominal pain, fatigue, dizziness, anxiety, dysuria, pruritus, palpitation, constipation, malaise, paresthesia, rash.

DRUG INTERACTIONS

See Contraindications. Not recommended with alcohol and other CNS depressants (eg, hypnotic sedatives, tranquilizers).

PATIENT CONSIDERATIONS

Assessment: Assess for hypersensitivity reaction to the drug or to its components, hyperemesis gravidarum, asthma, IOP, narrow-angle glaucoma, stenosing peptic ulcer, pyloroduodenal obstruction, urinary bladder-neck obstruction, nursing status, and possible drug interactions.

Monitoring: Monitor for somnolence and other adverse reactions. Reassess for continued need as pregnancy progresses.

Counseling: Instruct to avoid engaging in activities requiring complete mental alertness (eg, driving, operating heavy machinery), until cleared to do so. Inform of the importance of not taking the medication with alcohol or sedating medications including other antihistamines, opiates, and sleep aids.

STORAGE: 20-25°C (68-77°F); excursions permitted between 15-30°C (59-86°F). Protect from moisture.

DICYCLOMINE HCL – dicyclomine hydrochloride

RX

Class: Anticholinergic

OTHER BRAND NAMES

Bentyl

ADULT DOSAGE

Functional Bowel/Irritable Bowel Syndrome

PO:

Initial: 20mg qid

Titrate: May increase to 40mg qid after 1 week of initial dose, unless side effects limit dose escalation. D/C if efficacy not achieved w/in 2 weeks or side effects require doses below 80mg/day

Inj:

Initial: 10-20mg IM qid for 1-2 days if unable to take oral medication

PEDIATRIC DOSAGE

Pediatric use may not have been established

D

DOSING CONSIDERATIONS

Elderly

Start at lower end of dosing range

ADMINISTRATION

Oral, IM route

Aspirate the syringe before injecting to avoid intravascular inj

HOW SUPPLIED

Oral Sol: 10mg/5mL [473mL]; (Bentyl) **Cap:** 10mg; **Inj:** 10mg/mL; **Tab:** 20mg

CONTRAINDICATIONS

Infants <6 months of age, nursing mothers, unstable cardiovascular status in acute hemorrhage, myasthenia gravis, glaucoma, obstructive uropathy, GI tract obstructive disease, severe ulcerative colitis, reflux esophagitis. **Oral Sol:** Prior hypersensitivity to dicyclomine HCl or other ingredients in the formulation.

WARNINGS/PRECAUTIONS

Caution in conditions characterized by tachyarrhythmia (eg, thyrotoxicosis, CHF, in cardiac surgery). Caution with coronary heart disease; ischemia and infarction may worsen. Peripheral effects (eg, dryness of mouth with difficulty in swallowing/talking) and CNS signs/symptoms (eg, confusional state, disorientation, amnesia) reported. Psychosis and delirium reported in sensitive individuals (eg, elderly patients and/or in patients with mental illness) given anticholinergic drugs. Heat prostration may occur in high environmental temperatures; d/c if symptoms occur and institute supportive measures. May impair mental abilities. Diarrhea may be the early symptom of incomplete intestinal obstruction, especially with ileostomy/colostomy patients; treatment would be inappropriate and possibly harmful. Caution with ulcerative colitis; large doses may suppress intestinal motility and produce paralytic ileus, and use of this drug may precipitate or aggravate the serious complication of toxic megacolon. Caution in patients with HTN, fever, autonomic neuropathy, prostatic enlargement, hepatic/renal impairment, and in the elderly. (Cap/Tab/Inj) Avoid with myasthenia gravis except to reduce adverse muscarinic effects of an anticholinesterase. Ogilvie's syndrome (colonic pseudo-obstruction) rarely reported. Caution with Salmonella dysentery; toxic dilation of intestine and intestinal perforation may occur. (Inj) For IM use only; inadvertent IV use may result in thrombosis, thrombophlebitis, and inj-site reactions. (Sol) Caution with hyperthyroidism and hiatal hernia.

ADVERSE REACTIONS

Dry mouth, dizziness, blurred vision, nausea, somnolence, asthenia, nervousness.

DRUG INTERACTIONS

May antagonize the effect of antiglaucoma agents and drugs that alter GI motility (eg, metoclopramide). Avoid concomitant use with corticosteroids in glaucoma patients. Potentiated by amantadine, Class I antiarrhythmics (eg, quinidine), antihistamines, antipsychotics (eg, phenothiazines), benzodiazepines, MAOIs, narcotic analgesics (eg, meperidine), nitrates/nitrites, sympathomimetics, TCAs, and other drugs with anticholinergic activity. Antacids may interfere with absorption; avoid simultaneous use. May affect GI absorption of various drugs by affecting GI motility; increased serum digoxin concentration may result with slowly dissolving forms of digoxin. Inhibiting effects on gastric hydrochloric acid secretion are antagonized by drugs used to treat achlorhydria and those used to test gastric secretion.

PATIENT CONSIDERATIONS

Assessment: Assess for cardiovascular conditions, myasthenia gravis, glaucoma, intestinal obstruction, psychosis, ulcerative colitis, tachycardia, or any other conditions where treatment is contraindicated or cautioned. Assess for history of hypersensitivity, pregnancy/nursing status, renal/hepatic dysfunction, and for possible drug interactions.

Monitoring: Monitor for increased HR, worsening of ischemia/infarction, heat prostration, drowsiness, blurred vision, confusion, disorientation, hallucinations, paralytic ileus with large doses, urinary retention, hypersensitivity reactions, and for other adverse reactions. Monitor renal function.

Counseling: Counsel on proper administration. Advise not to breastfeed while on therapy and not to administer to infants <6 months of age. Advise not to engage in activities requiring mental alertness (eg, operating motor vehicle or other machinery) or to perform hazardous work while taking the drug. Inform of risk of heat prostration in high environmental temperature; instruct to d/c if symptoms occur and to consult a physician.

STORAGE: (Cap/Tab/Inj) Room temperature <30°C (86°F). Sol: 20-25°C (68-77°F). Inj: Protect from freezing. Tab: Avoid exposure to direct sunlight.

DIFFERIN – adapalene

RX

Class: Naphthoic acid derivative (retinoid-like)

ADULT DOSAGE

Acne Vulgaris

Cre:
Apply a thin film qpm

0.1% Gel:
Apply a thin film qpm after washing

0.3% Gel:
Apply a thin film qpm after washing

Reevaluate if therapeutic results are not noticed after 12 weeks of treatment

Lot:
Apply a thin film (3-4 actuations of the pump) qd after washing

PEDIATRIC DOSAGE

Acne Vulgaris

≥12 Years:

Cre:
Apply a thin film qpm

0.1% Gel:
Apply a thin film qpm after washing

0.3% Gel:
Apply a thin film qpm after washing

Reevaluate if therapeutic results are not noticed after 12 weeks of treatment

Lot:
Apply a thin film (3-4 actuations of the pump) qd after washing

ADMINISTRATION

Topical route

Apply enough to cover the entire face or other affected areas completely and lightly

HOW SUPPLIED

Cre: 0.1% [45g]; **Gel:** 0.1% [45g], 0.3% [15g, 45g tube; 45g pump]; **Lot:** 0.1% [2 oz]

CONTRAINDICATIONS

Hypersensitivity to adapalene or any components in the vehicle.

WARNINGS/PRECAUTIONS

Not for ophthalmic, oral, or intravaginal use. Avoid exposure to sunlight, including sunlamps; caution in patients with high levels of sun exposure and those with inherent sensitivity to sun. Extreme weather (eg, wind, cold) may cause irritation. Local skin irritation may be experienced; depending on severity, may use moisturizer, reduce frequency of application, or d/c use. (Cre/Gel) Apparent exacerbation of acne may occur. (Cre/0.1% Gel) D/C if reaction suggesting sensitivity or chemical irritation occurs. (Cre/0.3% Gel) A mild transitory sensation of warmth or slight stinging may occur shortly after application. (0.1% Gel) Avoid in patients with sunburn until fully recovered. (0.3% Gel) Reactions characterized by pruritus, face edema, eyelid edema, and lip swelling, requiring medical treatment reported; d/c use if experiencing allergic or anaphylactoid/anaphylactic reactions during therapy.

ADVERSE REACTIONS

Local cutaneous irritation. (0.3% Gel) Skin discomfort.

DRUG INTERACTIONS

Caution with preparations containing sulfur, resorcinol, or salicylic acid. (Cre/Gel) Do not start therapy until effects of such preparations in the skin have subsided. Caution with other potentially irritating topical products (medicated/abrasive soaps and cleansers, soaps and cosmetics that have a strong drying effect, and products with high concentrations of alcohol, astringents, spices, or lime). (Lot) Caution with concomitant topical acne therapy, especially with peeling, desquamating, or abrasive agents. Avoid with other potentially irritating topical products.

PATIENT CONSIDERATIONS

Assessment: Assess for excessive sun exposure, sun sensitivity, hypersensitivity to any of the components of the drug, pregnancy/nursing status, and for possible drug interactions. Assess for presence of cuts, abrasions, eczematous, or sunburned skin at the treatment site.

Monitoring: Monitor for sensitivity or chemical irritation, cutaneous signs/symptoms, and other adverse reactions.

Counseling: Advise to cleanse area with mild or soapless cleanser before applying the medication. Instruct to avoid or minimize exposure to sunlight and sunlamps. Instruct to use sunscreen products and protective clothing when exposure cannot be avoided. Instruct not to use more than the recommended amount. Instruct to avoid contact with eyes, lips, angles of the nose, and mucous membranes. Advise not to apply medication to cuts, abrasions, eczematous, or sunburned skin. Counsel to avoid use of waxing as depilatory method. Advise to use moisturizers if necessary and to avoid products containing α-hydroxyl or glycolic acids. Instruct to use externally and ud. Inform that an apparent exacerbation of acne may occur during the early weeks of therapy and that it should not be considered a reason for discontinuation. Instruct to contact the physician if signs of allergy or hypersensitivity develop. (Cre/0.3% Gel/Lot) Avoid waxing as a depilatory method.

STORAGE: 20-25°C (68-77°F); excursions permitted to 15-30°C (59-86°F). Protect from freezing. (Lot) Do not refrigerate. Protect from light. Keep away from heat.

D

DIFICID – fidaxomicin

RX

Class: Macrolide

ADULT DOSAGE

***Clostridium difficile*-Associated Diarrhea**

200mg bid for 10 days

PEDIATRIC DOSAGE

Pediatric use may not have been established

ADMINISTRATION

Oral route

Take w/ or w/o food

HOW SUPPLIED

Tab: 200mg

CONTRAINDICATIONS

Hypersensitivity to fidaxomicin.

WARNINGS/PRECAUTIONS

Not effective for treatment of systemic infections. Acute hypersensitivity reactions (eg, dyspnea, rash, pruritus) reported; d/c therapy if severe hypersensitivity reaction occurs. May increase the risk of the development of drug resistant bacteria when prescribed in the absence of a proven or strongly suspected *C. difficile* infection.

ADVERSE REACTIONS

N/V, abdominal pain, GI hemorrhage.

PATIENT CONSIDERATIONS

Assessment: Assess for hypersensitivity to the drug, macrolide allergy, and pregnancy/nursing status.

Monitoring: Monitor for development of drug resistant bacteria, hypersensitivity reactions, and other adverse reactions.

Counseling: Inform that drug only treats CDAD infections, not other bacterial or viral infections. Instruct to take exactly ud; inform that skipping doses or not completing full course may decrease effectiveness and increase antibiotic resistance.

STORAGE: 20-25°C (68-77°F); excursions permitted 15-30°C (59-86°F).

DIFLUCAN ORAL – fluconazole

RX

Class: Azole antifungal

ADULT DOSAGE

Prophylaxis in Bone Marrow Transplant

Decrease Incidence of Candidiasis:
400mg qd

Start prophylaxis several days before the anticipated onset of neutropenia in

PEDIATRIC DOSAGE

Cryptococcal Meningitis

12mg/kg on 1st day, followed by 6mg/kg qd for 10-12 weeks after the CSF becomes culture (-); a dose of 12mg/kg qd may be used (not to exceed 600mg/day)

patients who are anticipated to have severe granulocytopenia (<500 neutrophils/mm^3); continue for 7 days after the neutrophil count rises >1000 cells/mm^3

Cryptococcal Meningitis

400mg on 1st day, followed by 200mg qd for 10-12 weeks after the CSF becomes culture (-); a dose of 400mg qd may be used

Suppression of Cryptococcal Meningitis Relapse in AIDS:
200mg qd

Vaginal Candidiasis

PO Single Dose:
150mg

Oropharyngeal Candidiasis

200mg on 1st day, followed by 100mg qd for ≥2 weeks

Esophageal Candidiasis

200mg on 1st day, followed by 100mg qd for a minimum of 3 weeks and for ≥2 weeks following resolution of symptoms
Doses up to 400mg/day may be used

***Candida* Infections**

Systemic Infections:
Max: 400mg qd

UTIs/Peritonitis:
50-200mg/day

Suppression of Cryptococcal Meningitis Relapse in AIDS:
6mg/kg qd

***Candida* Infections**

Systemic:
6-12mg/kg/day (not to exceed 600mg/day)

Esophageal Candidiasis

6mg/kg on 1st day, followed by 3mg/kg qd for a minimum of 3 weeks and for ≥2 weeks following resolution of symptoms; doses up to 12mg/kg/day may be used (not to exceed 600mg/day)

Oropharyngeal Candidiasis

6mg/kg on 1st day, followed by 3mg/kg qd for ≥2 weeks

DOSING CONSIDERATIONS

Renal Impairment
Multiple Doses:
Initial LD: 50-400mg
Maint:
CrCl ≤50mL/min (No Dialysis): Give 50% of recommended dose
Regular Dialysis: Give 100% of recommended dose after each dialysis; on non-dialysis days, administer a reduced dose based on CrCl

ADMINISTRATION

Oral route
Take w/ or w/o food
Shake sus well before using

Sus
To reconstitute, add 24mL of distilled or purified water to bottle

HOW SUPPLIED

Sus: 10mg/mL, 40mg/mL [35mL]; **Tab:** 50mg, 100mg, 150mg, 200mg

CONTRAINDICATIONS

Hypersensitivity to fluconazole or to any excipients. Coadministration with terfenadine (with multiple doses ≥400mg of fluconazole), other drugs known to prolong the QT interval and that are metabolized via the enzyme CYP3A4 (eg, cisapride, astemizole, erythromycin, pimozide, quinidine).

WARNINGS/PRECAUTIONS

Associated with rare cases of serious hepatic toxicity; monitor for more severe hepatic injury if abnormal LFTs develop. D/C if clinical signs and symptoms consistent with liver disease develop. Anaphylaxis reported (rare). Exfoliative skin disorders reported; closely monitor patients with deep seated fungal infections who develop rashes during treatment and d/c if lesions progress. D/C therapy if rash develops in patients treated for superficial fungal infection. QT prolongation and torsades de pointes reported (rare); caution with potentially proarrhythmic conditions. Caution in elderly or with renal/hepatic dysfunction. May impair mental/physical abilities. (Sus) Contains sucrose; do not use in patients with hereditary fructose, glucose/galactose malabsorption, and sucrase-isomaltase deficiency. (Tab) Consider risk versus benefits of single dose oral tab versus intravaginal agent therapy for the treatment of vaginal yeast infections.

ADVERSE REACTIONS

Headache, N/V, abdominal pain, diarrhea.

DRUG INTERACTIONS

See Contraindications. Carefully monitor coadministration of fluconazole at doses <400mg/day with terfenadine. Avoid with voriconazole. Risk of increased plasma concentration of compounds metabolized by CYP2C9 and CYP3A4; caution when coadministered and monitor patients carefully. May precipitate clinically significant hypoglycemia with oral hypoglycemics; monitor blood glucose and adjust dose of sulfonylurea as necessary. May increase PT with coumarin-type anticoagulants; monitor PT and, if necessary, adjust warfarin dose. May increase levels of phenytoin, cyclosporine, theophylline, rifabutin, oral tacrolimus, triazolam, celecoxib, halofantrine, flurbiprofen, racemic ibuprofen, methadone, saquinavir, sirolimus, and vinca alkaloids (eg, vincristine, vinblastine). May increase exposure of ethinyl estradiol and levonorgestrel. May reduce the metabolism and increase levels of tolbutamide, glyburide, and glipizide. Monitor SrCr with cyclosporine. Rifampin may enhance metabolism. May increase levels and psychomotor effects of oral midazolam; consider dose reduction of short-acting benzodiazepines metabolized by CYP450, and monitor appropriately. May increase systemic exposure to tofacitinib; reduce tofacitinib dose when given concomitantly. HCTZ may increase levels. May reduce clearance/distribution volume and prolong $T_{1/2}$ of alfentanil. May increase effect of amitriptyline and nortriptyline. May increase levels of zidovudine; consider dose reduction. May potentially increase systemic exposure of other NSAIDs that are metabolized by CYP2C9 (eg, naproxen, lornoxicam, meloxicam, diclofenac), and calcium channel antagonists. Risk of carbamazepine toxicity. May increase serum bilirubin and SrCr with cyclophosphamide. May significantly delay elimination of fentanyl, leading to respiratory depression. May increase risk of myopathy and rhabdomyolysis with HMG-CoA reductase inhibitors metabolized through CYP3A4 (eg, atorvastatin, simvastatin) or through CYP2C9 (eg, fluvastatin); monitor for symptoms and d/c statin if a marked increase in creatinine kinase is observed or myopathy/rhabdomyolysis is diagnosed or suspected. May inhibit the metabolism of losartan; monitor BP continuously. Acute adrenal cortex insufficiency reported after discontinuation of a 3-month therapy with fluconazole in a liver-transplanted patient treated with prednisone. CNS-related undesirable effects reported with all-trans-retinoid acid (an acid form of vitamin A).

PATIENT CONSIDERATIONS

Assessment: Assess for hypersensitivity to the drug, renal/hepatic impairment, AIDS, malignancies, risk factors for QT prolongation, any other conditions where treatment is contraindicated or cautioned, pregnancy/nursing status, and possible drug interactions. Obtain specimens for fungal culture and other relevant lab studies (serology, histopathology) to isolate and identify causative organisms. (Sus) Assess for hereditary fructose, glucose/galactose malabsorption, and sucrase-isomaltase deficiency.

Monitoring: Monitor for signs/symptoms of liver disease, rash, and other adverse reactions. Monitor LFTs and renal function. Monitor PT when used with coumarin-type anticoagulants.

Counseling: Inform about risks/benefits of therapy. Advise to notify physician if pregnant/nursing and counsel about potential hazard to the fetus if pregnant or pregnancy occurs. Instruct to inform physician of all medications currently being taken.

STORAGE: Tab: <30°C (86°F). Sus: Dry Powder: <30°C (86°F). Reconstituted: 5-30°C (41-86°F); discard unused portion after 2 weeks. Protect from freezing.

DIGOXIN ORAL – digoxin

RX

Class: Cardiac glycoside

OTHER BRAND NAMES

Lanoxin

ADULT DOSAGE

Atrial Fibrillation

Control of Ventricular Response Rate in Chronic A-Fib:

Dosing can be either initiated w/ a LD followed by maint dosing if rapid titration is desired or initiated w/ maint dosing w/o a LD

Sol:

LD: 10-15mcg/kg

Maint: 3.0-4.5mcg/kg/dose qd

Tab:

LD: 10-15mcg/kg; administer 1/2 the total LD initially, then 1/4 the LD q6-8h twice

Maint:

Initial: 3.4-5.1mcg/kg qd

PEDIATRIC DOSAGE

Heart Failure

Increase Myocardial Contractility:

Dosing can be either initiated w/ a LD followed by maint dosing if rapid titration is desired or initiated w/ maint dosing w/o a LD

Sol:

If a LD is needed, administer w/ roughly 1/2 the total given as the 1st dose; additional fractions of the total dose may be given at 4- to 8-hr intervals, w/ careful assessment of clinical response before each additional dose. If the clinical response necessitates a change from the calculated LD, then calculation of the maint dose should be based on the amount actually given as the LD

Titrate: May increase dose every 2 weeks according to clinical response, serum drug levels, and toxicity

Heart Failure

Mild to Moderate:

Dosing can be either initiated w/ a LD followed by maint dosing if rapid titration is desired or initiated w/ maint dosing w/o a LD

Sol:

LD: 10-15mcg/kg

Maint: 3.0-4.5mcg/kg/dose qd

Tab:

LD: 10-15mcg/kg; administer 1/2 the total LD initially, then 1/4 the LD q6-8h twice

Maint:

Initial: 3.4-5.1mcg/kg qd

Titrate: May increase dose every 2 weeks according to clinical response, serum drug levels, and toxicity

Where possible, use in combination w/ a diuretic and an ACE inhibitor

Conversions

IV to Oral Conversion:

50mcg inj = 62.5mcg tab

100mcg inj = 125mcg tab

200mcg inj = 250mcg tab

400mcg inj = 500mcg tab

LD:

Premature Infants: 20-30mcg/kg

Full-Term Infants: 25-35mcg/kg

1-24 Months: 35-60mcg/kg

2-5 Years: 30-45mcg/kg

5-10 Years: 20-35mcg/kg

>10 Years: 10-15mcg/kg

Maint:

Premature Infants: 2.3-3.9mcg/kg/dose bid

Full-Term Infants: 3.8-5.6mcg/kg/dose bid

1-24 Months: 5.6-9.4mcg/kg/dose bid

2-5 Years: 4.7-6.6mcg/kg/dose bid

5-10 Years: 2.8-5.6mcg/kg/dose bid

>10 Years: 3-4.5mcg/kg/dose qd

Tab:

LD:

Administer 1/2 the total LD initially, then 1/4 the LD q6-8h twice

5-10 Years: 20-45mcg/kg

>10 Years: 10-15mcg/kg

Maint:

Initial:

5-10 Years: 3.2-6.4mcg/kg/dose bid

>10 Years: 3.4-5.1mcg/kg qd

Titrate: May increase dose every 2 weeks according to clinical response, serum drug levels, and toxicity

Conversions

IV to Oral Conversion:

50mcg inj = 62.5mcg tab

100mcg inj = 125mcg tab

200mcg inj = 250mcg tab

400mcg inj = 500mcg tab

DOSING CONSIDERATIONS

Renal Impairment

Refer to PI for recommended maint doses based on lean body weight and renal function

ADMINISTRATION

Oral route

Sol

The provided calibrated dropper is not appropriate to measure doses <0.2mL.

HOW SUPPLIED

Sol: 0.05mg/mL [60mL]; (Lanoxin) **Tab:** 62.5mcg, 125mcg*, 187.5mcg, 250mcg* *scored

CONTRAINDICATIONS

Ventricular fibrillation. Known hypersensitivity to digoxin (reactions seen include unexplained rash, swelling of the mouth, lips, or throat or a difficulty in breathing) or to other digitalis preparations.

WARNINGS/PRECAUTIONS

Increased risk of ventricular fibrillation in patients w/ Wolff-Parkinson-White syndrome who develop A-fib. May cause severe sinus bradycardia or sinoatrial block particularly in patients w/ preexisting sinus node disease and may cause advanced or complete heart block in patients w/ preexisting incomplete atrioventricular (AV) block; consider insertion of a pacemaker before treatment. Signs/symptoms of digoxin toxicity may be mistaken for worsening symptoms of heart failure (HF). May be desirable to reduce dose or d/c therapy 1-2 days prior to electrical cardioversion of A-fib. If digitalis toxicity is suspected, delay elective cardioversion, and if it is not prudent to delay cardioversion, select the lowest possible energy level to avoid provoking ventricular arrhythmias. May increase myocardial oxygen demand and lead to ischemia in patients w/ acute MI (AMI). May precipitate vasoconstriction and promote production of pro-inflammatory cytokines in patients w/ myocarditis; avoid use in these patients. Patients w/ certain disorders involving HF associated w/ preserved left ventricular ejection fraction (eg, restrictive cardiomyopathy, constrictive pericarditis, amyloid heart disease, idiopathic hypertrophic subaortic stenosis) may not benefit from treatment and may be particularly susceptible to adverse reactions. Hypercalcemia increased the risk of toxicity, while hypocalcemia may nullify the effects of treatment. Hypothyroidism may reduce the requirements for therapy. HF and/or atrial arrhythmias resulting from hypermetabolic or hyperdynamic states (eg, hyperthyroidism, hypoxia, arteriovenous shunt) are best treated by addressing the underlying condition. Endogenous substances of unknown composition (digoxin-like immunoreactive substances) may interfere w/ standard radioimmunoassays for digoxin. Caution in the elderly. **Sol:** Toxicity may occur at concentrations w/in therapeutic range in patients w/ hypokalemia or hypomagnesemia; maintain normal K^+ levels and Mg^+ levels while on therapy. May result in potentially detrimental increases in coronary vascular resistance. May prolong the PR interval and depress the ST segment on the ECG. May produce false positive ST-T changes on the ECG during exercise testing that may be indistinguishable from those of ischemia. **Tab:** Patients w/ low body weight, advanced age or impaired renal function, hypokalemia, or hypomagnesemia may be predisposed to digoxin toxicity. Not recommended in patients w/ AMI. Avoid in patients w/ restrictive cardiomyopathy, constrictive pericarditis, amyloid heart disease, acute cor pulmonale, and idiopathic hypertrophic subaortic stenosis. Patients w/ beri beri heart disease may fail to respond adequately to therapy if the underlying thiamine deficiency is not treated concomitantly.

ADVERSE REACTIONS

Cardiac arrhythmias, N/V, abdominal pain, intestinal ischemia, hemorrhagic necrosis of the intestines, headache, weakness, dizziness, apathy, mental disturbances.

DRUG INTERACTIONS

Drugs that induce/inhibit P-gp may alter digoxin pharmacokinetics. Increased levels or exposure w/ amiodarone, captopril, clarithromycin, erythromycin, dronedarone, gentamicin, erythromycin, itraconazole, nitrendipine, propafenone, quinidine, ranolazine, ritonavir, telaprevir, tetracycline, verapamil, atorvastatin, carvedilol, conivaptan, diltiazem, indomethacin, nifedipine, nefazodone, propantheline, quinine, saquinavir, spironolactone, telmisartan, ticagrelor, tolvaptan, trimethoprim, alprazolam, azithromycin, cyclosporine, diclofenac, diphenoxylate, epoprostenol, esomeprazole, ketoconazole, lansoprazole, metformin, omeprazole, and rabeprazole. Decreased levels w/ acarbose, activated charcoal, albuterol, antacids, certain cancer chemotherapy or radiation therapy, cholestyramine, colestipol, exenatide, kaolin-pectin, meals high in bran, metoclopramide, miglitol, neomycin, rifampin, St. John's wort, sucralfate, and sulfasalazine. Proarrhythmic events reported to be more common in patients receiving concomitant therapy w/ sotalol. May increase risk of arrhythmias w/ rapid IV Ca^{2+} administration, sympathomimetics (eg, epinephrine, norepinephrine, dopamine), and succinylcholine. Increased digoxin dose requirement w/ thyroid supplements. Calcium channel blockers and β-adrenergic blockers produce additive effects on AV node conduction, which can result in bradycardia and advanced or complete heart block. Higher rate of torsades de pointes w/ dofetilide. Teriparatide transiently increases serum Ca^{2+}. Refer to PI for dose adjustment information when used w/ certain concomitant therapies. **Sol:** Increased PR interval and QRS duration reported w/ moricizine. **Tab:** Decreased levels w/ penicillamine, and phenytoin. ACE inhibitors, ARBs, NSAIDs, and COX-2 inhibitors may impair digoxin excretion. Sudden death reported to be more common in patients receiving concomitant therapy w/ dronedarone.

PATIENT CONSIDERATIONS

Assessment: Assess for known hypersensitivity to the drug or other digitalis preparations, ventricular fibrillation, myocarditis, hypermetabolic or hyperdynamic states, sinus node disease, AV block, pregnancy/nursing status, possible drug interactions, and any other conditions where treatment is cautioned. Assess serum electrolytes and renal function. Obtain a baseline digoxin level.

Monitoring: Monitor for signs/symptoms of severe sinus bradycardia, sinoatrial block, advanced or complete heart block, digoxin toxicity, vasoconstriction, and other adverse reactions. Monitor serum electrolytes and renal function periodically. Obtain serum digoxin concentrations just before the next dose or at least 6 hrs after the last dose. Monitor for clinical response.

Counseling: Advise that digoxin is used to treat HF and heart arrhythmias. Advise to inform physician if taking any OTC medications, including herbal medication, or if started on a new prescription. Inform that blood tests will be necessary to ensure the appropriate digoxin dose. Instruct to contact physician if N/V, persistent diarrhea, confusion, weakness, or visual disturbances occur. Advise parents or caregivers that symptoms of having too high doses may be difficult to recognize in infants and pediatric patients; symptoms such as weight loss, failure to thrive in infants, abdominal pain, and behavioral disturbances may be indications of digoxin toxicity. Suggest to monitor and record HR and BP daily. Instruct women of childbearing potential who become or are planning to become pregnant to consult physician prior to initiation or continuing therapy. **Sol:** Instruct to use calibrated dropper to measure the dose and to avoid less precise measuring tools (eg, tsp).

STORAGE: 25°C (77°F); excursions permitted to 15-30°C (59-86°F). Protect from light. **Tab:** Store in dry place.

D

DILANTIN CAPSULES – phenytoin sodium RX

Class: Hydantoin

ADULT DOSAGE

Seizures

Tonic-Clonic (Grand Mal) and Psychomotor (Temporal Lobe) Seizures and Prevention/ Treatment of Neurosurgery-Associated Seizures:

Divided Daily Dosing:
Initial: (Treatment naive) 100mg tid
Maint: 100mg tid-qid
Titrate: May increase up to 200mg tid, if necessary

QD Dosing:
May consider 300mg qd if seizure is controlled w/ divided doses of three 100mg caps daily

LD (Clinic/Hospital):
Rapid steady-state serum levels required and where IV administration is not desirable
Initial: 1g in 3 divided doses (400mg, 300mg, 300mg) at 2-hr intervals
Maint: Start maint dose 24 hrs after LD

Clinically effective serum level is usually 10-20mcg/mL; do not change dose at intervals <7-10 days

Conversions

May require dose adjustment when switching from product formulated w/ free acid to product formulated w/ Na^+ salt and vice versa

PEDIATRIC DOSAGE

Seizures

Tonic-Clonic (Grand Mal) and Psychomotor (Temporal Lobe) Seizures and Prevention/ Treatment of Neurosurgery-Associated Seizures:
Initial: 5mg/kg/day in 2 or 3 equally divided doses
Maint: 4-8mg/kg/day
Max: 300mg/day

>6 Years: May require the minimum adult dose (300mg/day)

Clinically effective serum level is usually 10-20mcg/mL; do not change dose at intervals <7-10 days

Conversions

May require dose adjustment when switching from product formulated w/ free acid to product formulated w/ Na^+ salt and vice versa

DOSING CONSIDERATIONS

Renal Impairment

Caution when interpreting total phenytoin plasma concentrations; unbound phenytoin concentrations may be more useful.
Do not use LD regimen w/ history of renal disease.

Hepatic Impairment

Caution when interpreting total phenytoin plasma concentrations; unbound phenytoin concentrations may be more useful.
Do not use LD regimen w/ history of liver disease.

Elderly

May require lower or less frequent dosing

Other Important Considerations

Hypoalbuminemia:
Caution when interpreting total phenytoin plasma concentrations; unbound phenytoin concentrations may be more useful

ADMINISTRATION

Oral route

HOW SUPPLIED

Cap, Extended-Release: 30mg, 100mg

CONTRAINDICATIONS

History of hypersensitivity to phenytoin or its inactive ingredients, or other hydantoins. Coadministration w/ delavirdine.

WARNINGS/PRECAUTIONS

Avoid abrupt withdrawal; may precipitate status epilepticus. May increase risk of suicidal thoughts/ behavior; monitor for emergence/worsening of depression, suicidal thoughts/behavior, and/or any unusual changes in mood/behavior. Serious and sometimes fatal dermatologic reactions, including toxic epidermal necrolysis (TEN) and Stevens-Johnson syndrome (SJS), reported; d/c at 1st sign of rash, unless the rash is clearly not drug-related. Do not resume therapy, and consider alternative therapy if signs/symptoms suggest SJS/TEN. Avoid use as an alternative for carbamazepine in patients positive for HLA-B*1502. Drug reaction w/ eosinophilia and systemic symptoms (DRESS)/ multiorgan hypersensitivity reported; evaluate immediately if signs and symptoms (eg, rash, fever, lymphadenopathy) are present and d/c if an alternative etiology cannot be established.

Caution w/ history of hypersensitivity to structurally similar drugs (eg, carboxamides, barbiturates, succinimides, oxazolidinediones); consider alternatives to therapy. Acute hepatotoxicity (eg, acute hepatic failure) reported; d/c immediately and do not readminister. Hematopoietic complications and lymphadenopathy reported; extended follow-up observation is indicated and every effort should be made to achieve seizure control using alternative antiepileptic drugs in all cases of lymphadenopathy. Decreased bone mineral density and bone fractures reported during chronic use; consider screening and initiating treatment plans as appropriate. Caution w/ porphyria, hepatic impairment, and in elderly or gravely ill patients. An increase in seizure frequency may occur during pregnancy due to altered phenytoin pharmacokinetics. May cause fetal harm. Bleeding disorder in newborns may occur; give vitamin K to mother before delivery and to neonate after birth. Check plasma levels immediately if early signs of dose-related CNS toxicity develop. Hyperglycemia reported; may increase serum glucose levels in diabetics. Not indicated for seizures due to hypoglycemia or other metabolic causes. Not effective for absence (petit mal) seizures; if tonic-clonic (grand mal) and absence (petit mal) seizures are present, combined drug therapy is needed. Serum levels of phenytoin sustained above the optimal range may produce confusional states or rarely irreversible cerebellar dysfunction and/or cerebellar atrophy; reduce dose if plasma levels are excessive, or d/c if symptoms persist. Lab test interactions may occur. Do not use if discolored.

ADVERSE REACTIONS

Rash, nystagmus, ataxia, slurred speech, decreased coordination, somnolence, mental confusion, dizziness, insomnia, transient nervousness, motor twitching, acute hepatic failure, thrombocytopenia, altered taste sensation, Peyronie's disease.

DRUG INTERACTIONS

See Contraindications. Acute alcohol intake, amiodarone, antiepileptic agents (eg, ethosuximide, felbamate, oxcarbazepine), azoles (eg, fluconazole, ketoconazole, itraconazole), capecitabine, chloramphenicol, chlordiazepoxide, disulfiram, estrogens, fluorouracil, fluoxetine, fluvastatin, fluvoxamine, H_2-antagonists (eg, cimetidine), halothane, isoniazid, methylphenidate, omeprazole, phenothiazines, salicylates, sertraline, succinimides, sulfonamides (eg, sulfamethizole, sulfadiazine, sulfamethoxazole-trimethoprim), ticlopidine, tolbutamide, trazodone, and warfarin may increase levels. Anticancer drugs usually in combination (eg, bleomycin, carboplatin, cisplatin), carbamazepine, chronic alcohol abuse, diazepam, diazoxide, folic acid, fosamprenavir, nelfinavir, reserpine, rifampin, ritonavir (RTV), St. John's wort, sucralfate, vigabatrin, and theophylline may decrease levels. Administration w/ preparations that increase gastric pH (eg, supplements or antacids containing calcium carbonate, aluminum hydroxide, and magnesium hydroxide) may affect absorption; do not take at the same time of day. Phenobarbital, sodium valproate, and valproic acid may increase or decrease levels. May impair efficacy of azoles (eg, fluconazole, ketoconazole, itraconazole), corticosteroids, doxycycline, estrogens, furosemide, irinotecan, oral contraceptives, paclitaxel, paroxetine, quinidine, rifampin, sertraline, teniposide, theophylline, and vitamin D. Increased and decreased PT/INR responses reported w/ warfarin. May decrease levels of active metabolites of albendazole, certain HIV antivirals (eg, efavirenz, lopinavir/RTV, indinavir), antiepileptic agents (eg, carbamazepine, felbamate, lamotrigine), atorvastatin, chlorpropamide, clozapine, cyclosporine, digoxin, fluvastatin, folic acid, methadone, mexiletine, nifedipine, nimodipine, nisoldipine, praziquantel, simvastatin, and verapamil. May decrease levels of amprenavir (active metabolite) when given w/ fosamprenavir alone. May increase levels of amprenavir when given w/ the combination of fosamprenavir and RTV. Resistance to the neuromuscular blocking action of pancuronium, vecuronium, rocuronium, and cisatracurium reported in patients chronically administered phenytoin; monitor closely for more rapid recovery from neuromuscular blockade than expected and for higher infusion rate requirements. Enteral feeding preparations and/or related nutritional supplements may decrease levels; avoid w/ enteral feeding preparations.

PATIENT CONSIDERATIONS

Assessment: Assess for hypersensitivity to the drug or other hydantoins, alcohol use, hepatic/renal impairment, porphyria, grave illness, seizures due to hypoglycemia or other metabolic causes, absence seizures, any other conditions where treatment is contraindicated or cautioned, pregnancy/nursing status, and possible drug interactions.

Monitoring: Monitor for hypersensitivity reactions, dermatologic reactions, DRESS/multiorgan hypersensitivity, hepatotoxicity, hematopoietic complications, lymphadenopathy, decreased bone mineral density, bone fractures, exacerbation of porphyria, hyperglycemia, and other adverse reactions. Monitor for emergence/worsening of depression, suicidal thoughts/behavior, and/or any unusual changes in mood/behavior. Monitor serum levels when switching from Na^+ salt to free acid form and vice versa.

Counseling: Instruct to read medication guide and to take ud. Advise of the importance of adhering strictly to the prescribed dosage regimen, and of informing the physician of any clinical condition in which it is not possible to take the drug orally as prescribed (eg, surgery). Inform about the early toxic signs and symptoms of potential hematologic, dermatologic, hypersensitivity, or hepatic reactions; instruct to immediately contact physician if these develop. Caution on the use of other drugs or alcoholic beverages w/o first seeking physician's advice. Stress the importance of good dental hygiene to minimize the development of gingival hyperplasia and its complications. Advise to notify physician immediately if depression, suicidal thoughts/behavior, or thoughts about self-harm emerge. Encourage patients to enroll in the NAAED Pregnancy Registry if they become pregnant.

STORAGE: 20-25°C (68-77°F). Protect from moisture. Preserve in tight, light-resistant containers.

DILANTIN INFATABS – phenytoin

RX

Class: Hydantoin

ADULT DOSAGE

Seizures

Generalized Tonic-Clonic (Grand Mal) and Complex Partial (Psychomotor/Temporal Lobe) Seizures and Prevention/Treatment of Neurosurgery-Associated Seizures:

Initial: (treatment naive) 100mg (2 tabs) tid

Maint: 300-400mg (6-8 tabs) daily

Titrate: May increase to 600mg (12 tabs) daily, if necessary

Clinically effective serum level usually 10-20mcg/mL; do not change dose at intervals <7-10 days

Conversions

May require dose adjustment when switching from product formulated w/ free acid to product formulated w/ Na^+ salt and vice versa

PEDIATRIC DOSAGE

Seizures

Generalized Tonic-Clonic (Grand Mal) and Complex Partial (Psychomotor/Temporal Lobe) Seizures and Prevention/Treatment of Neurosurgery-Associated Seizures:

Initial: 5mg/kg/day in 2 or 3 equally divided doses

Maint: 4-8mg/kg/day

Max: 300mg/day

>6 Years: May require the minimum adult dose (300mg/day)

If daily dose cannot be divided equally, give larger dose hs

Clinically effective serum level usually 10-20mcg/mL; do not change dose at intervals <7-10 days

Conversions

May require dose adjustment when switching from product formulated w/ free acid to product formulated w/ Na^+ salt and vice versa

DOSING CONSIDERATIONS

Renal Impairment

Caution when interpreting total phenytoin plasma concentrations; unbound phenytoin concentrations may be more useful

Hepatic Impairment

Caution when interpreting total phenytoin plasma concentrations; unbound phenytoin concentrations may be more useful

Elderly

May require lower or less frequent dosing

Other Important Considerations

Hypoalbuminemia:

Caution when interpreting total phenytoin plasma concentrations; unbound phenytoin concentrations may be more useful

ADMINISTRATION

Oral route

May chew or swallow tab whole.

Not for once-a-day dosing.

HOW SUPPLIED

Tab, Chewable: 50mg* *scored

CONTRAINDICATIONS

History of hypersensitivity to phenytoin or its inactive ingredients, or other hydantoins. Coadministration w/ delavirdine.

WARNINGS/PRECAUTIONS

Avoid abrupt withdrawal; may precipitate status epilepticus. May increase risk of suicidal thoughts/behavior; monitor for emergence/worsening of depression, suicidal thoughts/behavior, and/or any unusual changes in mood/behavior. Serious and sometimes fatal dermatologic reactions, including toxic epidermal necrolysis (TEN) and Stevens-Johnson syndrome (SJS), reported; d/c at 1st sign of rash, unless the rash is clearly not drug-related. Do not resume therapy, and consider alternative therapy if signs/symptoms suggest SJS/TEN. Avoid use as an alternative for carbamazepine in patients positive for HLA-B*1502. Drug reaction w/ eosinophilia and systemic symptoms (DRESS)/multiorgan hypersensitivity reported; evaluate immediately if signs and symptoms (eg, rash, fever, lymphadenopathy) are present and d/c if an alternative etiology cannot be established. Caution w/ history of hypersensitivity to structurally similar drugs (eg, carboxamides, barbiturates, succinimides, oxazolidinediones); consider alternatives to therapy. Acute hepatotoxicity (eg, acute hepatic failure) reported; d/c immediately and do not readminister. Hematopoietic complications and lymphadenopathy reported; extended follow-up observation is indicated and every effort should be made to achieve seizure control using alternative antiepileptic drugs in all cases of lymphadenopathy. Decreased bone mineral density and bone fractures reported during chronic use; consider screening and initiating treatment plans as appropriate. Caution w/ porphyria, hepatic impairment, and in elderly or gravely ill patients. An increase in seizure frequency may occur during pregnancy due to altered phenytoin pharmacokinetics. May cause fetal harm. Bleeding disorder in newborns may occur; give vitamin K to mother before delivery and to neonate after birth. Check plasma levels immediately if early signs of dose-related CNS toxicity develop. Hyperglycemia reported; may increase serum glucose levels in diabetics. Not indicated for seizures due to hypoglycemia or other metabolic causes. Not effective for absence (petit mal) seizures; if tonic-clonic (grand mal) and absence (petit mal) seizures are present, combined drug therapy is needed. Serum levels of phenytoin sustained above the optimal range may produce confusional states or rarely irreversible cerebellar dysfunction and/or cerebellar atrophy; reduce dose if plasma levels are excessive, or d/c if symptoms persist. Lab test interactions may occur.

ADVERSE REACTIONS

Rash, nystagmus, ataxia, slurred speech, decreased coordination, somnolence, mental confusion, dizziness, insomnia, transient nervousness, motor twitching, acute hepatic failure, thrombocytopenia, altered taste sensation, Peyronie's disease.

DRUG INTERACTIONS

See Contraindications. Acute alcohol intake, amiodarone, antiepileptic agents (eg, ethosuximide, felbamate, oxcarbazepine), azoles (eg, fluconazole, ketoconazole, itraconazole), capecitabine, chloramphenicol, chlordiazepoxide, disulfiram, estrogens, fluorouracil, fluoxetine, fluvastatin, fluvoxamine, H_2-antagonists (eg, cimetidine), halothane, isoniazid, methylphenidate, omeprazole, phenothiazines, salicylates, sertraline, succinimides, sulfonamides (eg, sulfamethizole, sulfadiazine, sulfamethoxazole-trimethoprim), ticlopidine, tolbutamide, trazodone, and warfarin may increase levels. Anticancer drugs usually in combination (eg, bleomycin, carboplatin, cisplatin), carbamazepine, chronic alcohol abuse, diazepam, diazoxide, folic acid, fosamprenavir, nelfinavir, reserpine, rifampin, ritonavir (RTV), St. John's wort, sucralfate, vigabatrin, and theophylline may decrease levels. Administration w/ preparations that increase gastric pH (eg, supplements or antacids containing calcium carbonate, aluminum hydroxide, and magnesium hydroxide) may affect absorption; do not take at the same time of day. Phenobarbital, sodium valproate, and valproic acid may increase or decrease levels. May impair efficacy of azoles (eg, fluconazole, ketoconazole, itraconazole), corticosteroids, doxycycline, estrogens, furosemide, irinotecan, oral contraceptives, paclitaxel, paroxetine, quinidine, rifampin, sertraline, teniposide, theophylline, and vitamin D. Increased and decreased PT/INR responses reported w/ warfarin. May decrease levels of active metabolites of albendazole, certain HIV antivirals (eg, efavirenz, lopinavir/RTV, indinavir), antiepileptic agents (eg, carbamazepine, felbamate, lamotrigine), atorvastatin, chlorpropamide, clozapine, cyclosporine, digoxin, fluvastatin, folic acid, methadone, mexiletine, nifedipine, nimodipine, nisoldipine, praziquantel, simvastatin, and verapamil. May decrease levels of amprenavir (active metabolite) when given w/ fosamprenavir alone. May increase levels of amprenavir when given w/ the combination of fosamprenavir and RTV. Resistance to the neuromuscular blocking action of pancuronium, vecuronium, rocuronium, and cisatracurium reported in patients chronically administered phenytoin; monitor closely for more rapid recovery from neuromuscular blockade than expected and for higher infusion rate requirements. Enteral feeding preparations and/or related nutritional supplements may decrease levels; avoid w/ enteral feeding preparations.

PATIENT CONSIDERATIONS

Assessment: Assess for hypersensitivity to the drug or other hydantoins, alcohol use, hepatic/renal impairment, porphyria, grave illness, seizures due to hypoglycemia or other metabolic causes, absence seizures, any other conditions where treatment is contraindicated or cautioned, pregnancy/nursing status, and possible drug interactions.

Monitoring: Monitor for hypersensitivity reactions, dermatologic reactions, DRESS/multiorgan hypersensitivity, hepatotoxicity, hematopoietic complications, lymphadenopathy, decreased bone mineral density, bone fractures, exacerbation of porphyria, hyperglycemia, and other adverse reactions. Monitor for emergence/worsening of depression, suicidal thoughts/behavior, and/or any unusual changes in mood/behavior. Monitor serum levels when switching from Na^+ salt to free acid form and vice versa.

Counseling: Instruct to read medication guide and to take ud. Advise of the importance of adhering strictly to the prescribed dosage regimen, and of informing the physician of any clinical condition in which it is not possible to take the drug orally as prescribed (eg, surgery). Inform about the early toxic signs and symptoms of potential hematologic, dermatologic, hypersensitivity, or hepatic reactions; instruct to immediately contact physician if these develop. Caution on the use of other drugs or alcoholic beverages w/o first seeking physician's advice. Stress the importance of good dental hygiene to minimize the development of gingival hyperplasia and its complications. Advise to notify physician immediately if depression, suicidal thoughts/behavior, or thoughts about self-harm emerge. Encourage patients to enroll in the NAAED Pregnancy Registry if they become pregnant.

STORAGE: 20-25°C (68-77°F). Protect from moisture.

D

DILANTIN-125 – phenytoin RX

Class: Hydantoin

ADULT DOSAGE

Seizures

Tonic-Clonic (Grand Mal) and Psychomotor (Temporal Lobe) Seizures:

Initial: (Treatment naive) 125mg (1 tsp) tid

Titrate: May increase to 625mg (5 tsp) daily, if necessary

Clinically effective serum level is usually 10-20mcg/mL; do not change dose at intervals <7-10 days

Conversions

May require dose adjustment when switching from product formulated w/ free acid to product formulated w/ Na+ salt and vice versa

PEDIATRIC DOSAGE

Seizures

Tonic-Clonic (Grand Mal) and Psychomotor (Temporal Lobe) Seizures:

Initial: 5mg/kg/day in 2 or 3 equally divided doses

Maint: 4-8mg/kg/day

Max: 300mg/day

>6 Years: May require the minimum adult dose (300mg/day)

Clinically effective serum level is usually 10-20mcg/mL; do not change dose at intervals <7-10 days

Conversions

May require dose adjustment when switching from product formulated w/ free acid to product formulated w/ Na+ salt and vice versa

DOSING CONSIDERATIONS

Renal Impairment

Caution when interpreting total phenytoin plasma concentrations; unbound phenytoin concentrations may be more useful

Hepatic Impairment

Caution when interpreting total phenytoin plasma concentrations; unbound phenytoin concentrations may be more useful

Elderly

May require lower or less frequent dosing

Other Important Considerations

Hypoalbuminemia:

Caution when interpreting total phenytoin plasma concentrations; unbound phenytoin concentrations may be more useful

ADMINISTRATION

Oral route

Use an accurately calibrated measuring device to ensure accurate dosing.

HOW SUPPLIED

Oral Sus: 125mg/5mL [237mL]

CONTRAINDICATIONS

History of hypersensitivity to phenytoin or its inactive ingredients, or other hydantoins. Coadministration w/ delavirdine.

WARNINGS/PRECAUTIONS

Avoid abrupt withdrawal; may precipitate status epilepticus. May increase risk of suicidal thoughts/behavior; monitor for emergence/worsening of depression, suicidal thoughts/behavior, and/or any unusual changes in mood/behavior. Serious and sometimes fatal dermatologic reactions, including toxic epidermal necrolysis (TEN) and Stevens-Johnson syndrome (SJS), reported; d/c at 1st sign of rash, unless the rash is clearly not drug-related. Do not resume therapy, and consider alternative therapy if signs/symptoms suggest SJS/TEN. Avoid use as an alternative for carbamazepine in patients positive for HLA-B*1502. Drug reaction w/ eosinophilia and systemic symptoms (DRESS)/multiorgan hypersensitivity reported; evaluate immediately if signs and symptoms (eg, rash, fever, lymphadenopathy) are present and d/c if an alternative etiology cannot be established. Caution w/ history of hypersensitivity to structurally similar drugs (eg, carboxamides, barbiturates, succinimides, oxazolidinediones); consider alternatives to therapy. Acute hepatotoxicity (eg, acute hepatic failure) reported; d/c immediately and do not readminister. Hematopoietic complications and lymphadenopathy reported; extended follow-up observation is indicated and every effort should be made to achieve seizure control using alternative antiepileptic drugs in all cases of lymphadenopathy. Decreased bone mineral density and bone fractures reported during chronic use; consider screening and initiating treatment plans as appropriate. Caution w/ porphyria, hepatic impairment, and in elderly or gravely ill patients. An increase in seizure frequency may occur during pregnancy due to altered phenytoin pharmacokinetics. May cause fetal harm. Bleeding disorder in newborns may occur; give vitamin K to mother before delivery and to neonate after birth. Check plasma levels immediately if early signs of dose-related CNS toxicity develop. Hyperglycemia reported; may increase serum glucose levels in diabetics. Not indicated for seizures due to hypoglycemia or other metabolic causes. Not effective for absence (petit mal) seizures; if tonic-clonic (grand mal) and absence (petit mal) seizures are present, combined drug therapy is needed. Serum levels of phenytoin sustained above the optimal range may produce confusional states or rarely irreversible cerebellar dysfunction and/or cerebellar atrophy; reduce dose if plasma levels are excessive, or d/c if symptoms persist. Lab test interactions may occur.

D

ADVERSE REACTIONS

Rash, nystagmus, ataxia, slurred speech, decreased coordination, somnolence, mental confusion, dizziness, insomnia, transient nervousness, motor twitching, acute hepatic failure, thrombocytopenia, altered taste sensation, Peyronie's disease.

DRUG INTERACTIONS

See Contraindications. Acute alcohol intake, amiodarone, antiepileptic agents (eg, ethosuximide, felbamate, oxcarbazepine), azoles (eg, fluconazole, ketoconazole, itraconazole), capecitabine, chloramphenicol, chlordiazepoxide, disulfiram, estrogens, fluorouracil, fluoxetine, fluvastatin, fluvoxamine, H_2-antagonists (eg, cimetidine), halothane, isoniazid, methylphenidate, omeprazole, phenothiazines, salicylates, sertraline, succinimides, sulfonamides (eg, sulfamethizole, sulfadiazine, sulfamethoxazole-trimethoprim), ticlopidine, tolbutamide, trazodone, and warfarin may increase levels. Anticancer drugs usually in combination (eg, bleomycin, carboplatin, cisplatin), carbamazepine, chronic alcohol abuse, diazepam, diazoxide, folic acid, fosamprenavir, nelfinavir, reserpine, rifampin, ritonavir (RTV), St. John's wort, sucralfate, vigabatrin, and theophylline may decrease levels. Administration w/ preparations that increase gastric pH (eg, supplements or antacids containing calcium carbonate, aluminum hydroxide, and magnesium hydroxide) may affect absorption; do not take at the same time of day. Phenobarbital, sodium valproate, and valproic acid may increase or decrease levels. May impair efficacy of azoles (eg, fluconazole, ketoconazole, itraconazole), corticosteroids, doxycycline, estrogens, furosemide, irinotecan, oral contraceptives, paclitaxel, paroxetine, quinidine, rifampin, sertraline, teniposide, theophylline, and vitamin D. Increased and decreased PT/INR responses reported w/ warfarin. May decrease levels of active metabolites of albendazole, certain HIV antivirals (eg, efavirenz, lopinavir/RTV, indinavir), antiepileptic agents (eg, carbamazepine, felbamate, lamotrigine), atorvastatin, chlorpropamide, clozapine, cyclosporine, digoxin, fluvastatin, folic acid, methadone, mexiletine, nifedipine, nimodipine, nisoldipine, praziquantel, simvastatin, and verapamil. May decrease levels of amprenavir (active metabolite) when given w/ fosamprenavir alone. May increase levels of amprenavir when given w/ the combination of fosamprenavir and RTV. Resistance to the neuromuscular blocking action of pancuronium, vecuronium, rocuronium, and cisatracurium reported in patients chronically administered phenytoin; monitor closely for more rapid recovery from neuromuscular blockade than expected and for higher infusion rate requirements. Enteral feeding preparations and/or related nutritional supplements may decrease levels; avoid w/ enteral feeding preparations.

PATIENT CONSIDERATIONS

Assessment: Assess for hypersensitivity to the drug or other hydantoins, alcohol use, hepatic/renal impairment, porphyria, grave illness, seizures due to hypoglycemia or other metabolic causes, absence seizures, any other conditions where treatment is contraindicated or cautioned, pregnancy/nursing status, and possible drug interactions.

Monitoring: Monitor for hypersensitivity reactions, dermatologic reactions, DRESS/multiorgan hypersensitivity, hepatotoxicity, hematopoietic complications, lymphadenopathy, decreased bone mineral density, bone fractures, exacerbation of porphyria, hyperglycemia, and other adverse reactions. Monitor for emergence/worsening of depression, suicidal thoughts/behavior, and/or any unusual changes in mood/behavior. Monitor serum levels when switching from Na^+ salt to free acid form and vice versa.

Counseling: Instruct to read medication guide and to take ud. Advise of the importance of adhering strictly to the prescribed dosage regimen, and of informing the physician of any clinical condition in which it is not possible to take the drug orally as prescribed (eg, surgery). Inform about the early toxic signs and symptoms of potential hematologic, dermatologic, hypersensitivity, or hepatic reactions; instruct to immediately contact physician if these develop. Caution on the use of other drugs or alcoholic beverages w/o first seeking physician's advice. Stress the importance of good dental hygiene to minimize the development of gingival hyperplasia and its complications. Advise to notify physician immediately if depression, suicidal thoughts/behavior, or thoughts about self-harm emerge. Encourage patients to enroll in the NAAED Pregnancy Registry if they become pregnant.

STORAGE: 20-25°C (68-77°F). Protect from freezing and light.

DILAUDID ORAL – hydromorphone hydrochloride

CII

Class: Opioid analgesic

Contains hydromorphone, a Schedule II controlled opioid agonist with the highest potential for abuse and risk of respiratory depression. Alcohol, other opioids, and CNS depressants (eg, sedative-hypnotics) potentiate respiratory depressant effects, increasing the risk of respiratory depression that may result in death.

ADULT DOSAGE

Pain

Periodically reassess after the initial dosing

Sol:
Usual: 2.5-10mg q3-6h ud by clinical situation

Tab:
Initial: 2-4mg q4-6h
Titrate: May increase gradually if analgesia is inadequate, as tolerance develops, or if pain severity increases

Sol/Tab:
Nonopioid-Tolerant:
Initial: 2-4mg q4h

Taking Opioids:
Base starting dose on prior opioid usage
Give only 1/2 to 2/3 of the estimated dose for the 1st few doses, then increase prn according to response

Chronic Pain:
Administer dose around-the-clock
May give a supplemental dose of 5-15% of the total daily usage q2h prn

Conversions

From Morphine Sulfate: 10mg parenteral or 40-60mg oral
From Hydromorphone HCl: 1.3-2mg parenteral or 6.5-7.5mg oral
From Oxymorphone HCl: 1-1.1mg parenteral or 6.6mg oral
From Levorphanol Tartrate: 2-2.3mg parenteral or 4mg oral
From Meperidine HCl: 75-100mg parenteral or 300-400mg oral
From Methadone HCl: 10mg parenteral or 10-20mg oral

PEDIATRIC DOSAGE

Pediatric use may not have been established

DOSING CONSIDERATIONS

Renal Impairment

Moderate-Severe:
Start on a lower dose and closely monitor during titration
Use oral liquid to adjust the dose

Hepatic Impairment

Moderate:
Start on a lower dose and closely monitor during titration
Use oral liquid to adjust the dose

Elderly

Start at lower end of dosing range

ADMINISTRATION

Oral route

HOW SUPPLIED

Sol: 1mg/mL [473mL]; **Tab:** 2mg, 4mg, 8mg* *scored

CONTRAINDICATIONS

Known hypersensitivity to hydromorphone, respiratory depression in the absence of resuscitative equipment, status asthmaticus, obstetrical analgesia.

WARNINGS/PRECAUTIONS

Respiratory depression is more likely to occur in elderly, debilitated, and those suffering from conditions accompanied by hypoxia or hypercapnia; extreme caution with chronic obstructive pulmonary disease (COPD) or cor pulmonale, substantially decreased respiratory reserve, hypoxia, hypercapnia, or preexisting respiratory depression. May cause neonatal withdrawal syndrome. Respiratory depressant effects with carbon dioxide retention and secondary elevation of CSF pressure may be markedly exaggerated in the presence of head injury, other intracranial lesions, or preexisting increase in intracranial pressure (ICP). May produce effects on pupillary response and consciousness, which can obscure the clinical course and neurologic signs of further increase in ICP in patients with head injuries. May cause severe hypotension; caution with circulatory shock. Contains sodium metabisulfite; may cause allergic-type reactions, including anaphylactic symptoms and life-threatening or less severe asthmatic episodes in certain susceptible people. Caution in elderly/debilitated and those with severe pulmonary/hepatic/renal impairment, myxedema/hypothyroidism, adrenocortical insufficiency (eg, Addison's disease), CNS depression or coma, toxic psychoses, prostatic hypertrophy, urethral stricture, gallbladder disease, acute alcoholism, delirium tremens, kyphoscoliosis, or following GI surgery; reduce initial dose. May obscure the diagnosis or clinical course in patients with acute abdominal conditions. May aggravate preexisting convulsions in patients with convulsive disorders. Mild to severe seizures and myoclonus reported in severely compromised patients administered high doses of parenteral hydromorphone. Caution with alcoholism and other drug dependencies. May impair mental/physical abilities. May produce orthostatic hypotension in ambulatory patients. May cause spasm of the sphincter of Oddi; caution in patients about to undergo biliary tract surgery. Physical dependence and tolerance may occur. Do not abruptly d/c.

ADVERSE REACTIONS

Respiratory depression, apnea, lightheadedness, dizziness, sedation, N/V, sweating, flushing, dysphoria, euphoria, dry mouth, pruritus.

DRUG INTERACTIONS

See Boxed Warning. Concomitant use with other CNS depressants (eg, general anesthetics, phenothiazines, tranquilizers) may produce additive depressant effects; use with caution and in reduced dosages. Do not give with alcohol. May enhance action of neuromuscular blocking agents and produce an excessive degree of respiratory depression. May cause severe hypotension with phenothiazines or general anesthetics. Mixed agonist/antagonist analgesics (pentazocine, nalbuphine, butorphanol, buprenorphine) may reduce the analgesic effect and/or may precipitate withdrawal symptoms; use with caution.

PATIENT CONSIDERATIONS

Assessment: Assess for risk factors for drug abuse or addiction, pain type/severity, prior opioid therapy, opioid tolerance, respiratory depression, COPD, cor pulmonale, decreased respiratory reserve, hypoxia, hypercapnia, asthma, renal/hepatic impairment, pregnancy/nursing status, possible drug interactions, or any other conditions where treatment is contraindicated or cautioned.

Monitoring: Monitor for respiratory depression, sedation, CNS depression, aggravation/induction of seizures/convulsions, increase in ICP, hypotension, tolerance, physical dependence, and other adverse reactions. Routinely monitor for signs of misuse, abuse, and addiction.

Counseling: Inform that medication may cause severe adverse effects (eg, respiratory depression) if not taken ud. Instruct to report pain and adverse experiences occurring during therapy. Advise not to adjust dose or combine with alcohol or other CNS depressants without prescriber's consent. Inform that drug may impair mental/physical abilities; instruct to use caution when performing hazardous tasks (eg, operating machinery/driving). Advise to consult physician if pregnant or planning to become pregnant. Inform that drug has potential for abuse; instruct to protect it from theft and never to share with others. Advise to avoid abrupt withdrawal if taking medication for more than a few weeks and cessation of therapy is indicated. Instruct to keep drug in a secure place, and to destroy unused tabs by flushing down toilet.

STORAGE: 25°C (77°F); excursions permitted to 15-30°C (59-86°F). Protect from light.

DIOVAN – valsartan

RX

Class: Angiotensin II receptor blocker (ARB)

D/C when pregnancy is detected. Drugs that act directly on the renin-angiotensin system (RAS) can cause injury/death to the developing fetus.

ADULT DOSAGE

Hypertension

Initial: 80mg or 160mg qd
Titrate: May increase to a max of 320mg qd
May add diuretic if BP not controlled

PEDIATRIC DOSAGE

Hypertension

6-16 Years:
Initial: 1.3mg/kg qd (up to 40mg total)
Titrate: Adjust dose according to BP response
Max: 2.7mg/kg (up to 160mg) qd

Heart Failure

NYHA Class II-IV
Initial: 40mg bid
Titrate: May increase to 80mg and 160mg bid (use highest dose tolerated)
Max: 320mg/day in divided doses

Post-Myocardial Infarction

Initial: 20mg bid as early as 12 hrs after MI
Titrate: May increase to 40mg bid w/in 7 days, w/ subsequent titrations to 160mg bid as tolerated
Maint: 160mg bid
Consider reducing dose if symptomatic hypotension or renal dysfunction occurs

DOSING CONSIDERATIONS

Concomitant Medications

Consider reducing concomitant diuretic dose in patients w/ heart failure (HF)

ADMINISTRATION

Oral route

Take w/ or w/o food.
Use of sus is recommended for children who cannot swallow tabs, or if calculated dosage does not correspond to available tab strength.
Adjust dose accordingly when switching dosage forms; exposure w/ sus is 1.6X greater than w/ tab.

Preparation of Sus (for 160mL of a 4mg/mL Sus)

1. Add 80mL of Ora-Plus oral suspending vehicle to an amber glass bottle containing 8 Diovan 80mg tabs, and shake for a minimum of 2 min
2. Allow the sus to stand for a minimum of 1 hr
3. After the standing time, shake the sus for a minimum of 1 additional min
4. Add 80mL of Ora-Sweet SF oral sweetening vehicle to the bottle and shake the sus for at least 10 sec to disperse the ingredients
5. The sus is homogenous and can be stored for either up to 30 days at room temperature (below 30°C/86°F) or up to 75 days at refrigerated conditions (2-8°C/35-46°F) in the glass bottle
6. Shake the bottle well (at least 10 sec) prior to dispensing the sus

HOW SUPPLIED

Tab: 40mg*, 80mg, 160mg, 320mg *scored

CONTRAINDICATIONS

Known hypersensitivity to any component of this medication. Coadministration w/ aliskiren in patients w/ diabetes.

WARNINGS/PRECAUTIONS

Symptomatic hypotension may occur in patients w/ an activated RAS (eg, volume- and/or salt-depleted patients receiving high doses of diuretics); correct this condition prior to therapy. Caution when initiating therapy in patients w/ HF or post-MI. Renal function changes may occur; caution in patients whose renal function depend in part on the activity of the RAS (eg, renal artery stenosis, chronic kidney disease, severe CHF, volume depletion). Consider withholding or discontinuing therapy if clinically significant decrease in renal function develops. Increased K^+ in some patients w/ HF reported, and more likely to occur in patients w/ preexisting renal impairment; dose reduction and/or discontinuation of therapy may be required. Do not readminister to patients who have had angioedema. Caution w/ dosing in patients w/ hepatic or severe renal impairment.

ADVERSE REACTIONS

Headache, abdominal pain, cough, increased BUN, hyperkalemia, dizziness, hypotension, SrCr elevation, viral infection, fatigue, diarrhea, arthralgia, back pain.

DRUG INTERACTIONS

See Contraindications. Dual blockade of the RAS is associated w/ increased risk of hypotension, hyperkalemia, and changes in renal function (including acute renal failure); avoid combined use of RAS inhibitors, or closely monitor BP, renal function, and electrolytes w/ concomitant agents that also affect the RAS. Avoid w/ aliskiren in patients w/ renal impairment (GFR <60mL/min). Inhibitors of the hepatic uptake transporter OATP1B1 (rifampin, cyclosporine) and the hepatic efflux transporter MRP2 (ritonavir) may increase exposure. Other agents that block the RAS, K^+-sparing diuretics, K^+ supplements, salt substitutes containing K^+, or other drugs that may increase K^+ levels (heparin), may increase serum K^+ levels, and in HF patients may increase SrCr; monitor serum K^+ levels. Greater antihypertensive effect w/ atenolol. NSAIDs, including selective COX-2 inhibitors, may result in deterioration of renal function, including possible acute renal failure, and may attenuate antihypertensive effect. Increased lithium levels and lithium toxicity reported; monitor serum lithium levels during concomitant use.

PATIENT CONSIDERATIONS

Assessment: Assess for hypersensitivity to the drug and its components, hepatic/renal impairment, volume/salt depletion, renal artery stenosis, HF, pregnancy/nursing status, and possible drug interactions.

Monitoring: Monitor for signs/symptoms of hypotension and other adverse reactions. Monitor electrolytes, BP, and renal function.

Counseling: Counsel about the risk/benefits of therapy and possible adverse effects. Inform of consequences of exposure during pregnancy and discuss treatment options w/ women planning to become pregnant. Instruct to report pregnancies to physician as soon as possible.

STORAGE: (Tab) 25°C (77°F); excursions permitted to 15-30°C (59-86°F). Protect from moisture. (Sus) <30°C (86°F) for up to 30 days or at 2-8°C (35-46°F) for up to 75 days.

DIOVAN HCT – hydrochlorothiazide/valsartan

RX

Class: Angiotensin II receptor blocker (ARB)/thiazide diuretic

D/C when pregnancy is detected. Drugs that act directly on the renin-angiotensin system (RAS) can cause injury/death to the developing fetus.

ADULT DOSAGE

Hypertension

Initial: 160mg/12.5mg qd
Titrate: May increase after 1-2 weeks of therapy
Max: 320mg/25mg qd

Add-On Therapy:

Use if not adequately controlled w/ valsartan (or another ARB) alone or HCTZ alone
W/ dose-limiting adverse reactions to either component alone, may switch to therapy containing a lower dose of that component
Titrate: May increase after 3-4 weeks of therapy if BP uncontrolled
Max: 320mg/25mg

Replacement Therapy:

May substitute for titrated components

PEDIATRIC DOSAGE

Pediatric use may not have been established

ADMINISTRATION

Oral route

Take w/ or w/o food.

HOW SUPPLIED

Tab: (Valsartan/HCTZ) 80mg/12.5mg, 160mg/12.5mg, 160mg/25mg, 320mg/12.5mg, 320mg/25mg

CONTRAINDICATIONS

Anuria, sulfonamide-derived drug hypersensitivity, hypersensitivity to any component of this product. Coadministration w/ aliskiren in patients w/ diabetes.

WARNINGS/PRECAUTIONS

Not for initial therapy w/ intravascular volume depletion. Symptomatic hypotension may occur in patients w/ activated RAS (eg, volume- and/or salt-depleted patients receiving high doses of diuretics); correct this condition prior to therapy. Renal function changes may occur including acute renal failure; caution in patients whose renal function depends in part on the activity of the RAS (eg, renal artery stenosis, chronic kidney disease, severe CHF, volume depletion). Consider withholding or discontinuing therapy if clinically significant decrease in renal function develops. May cause serum electrolyte abnormalities (eg, hyperkalemia, hypokalemia, hyponatremia, hypomagnesemia); correct hypokalemia and any coexisting hypomagnesemia prior to initiation of therapy and monitor periodically. D/C if hypokalemia is accompanied by clinical signs (eg, muscular weakness, paresis, ECG alterations). Increased K^+ in patients w/ heart failure (HF) reported; dose reduction or discontinuation of therapy may be required. Do not readminister to patients w/ angioedema. **HCTZ:** May cause hypersensitivity reactions and exacerbation or activation of systemic lupus erythematosus (SLE). May precipitate hepatic coma w/ hepatic impairment or progressive liver disease. May cause idiosyncratic reaction, resulting in acute transient myopia and acute angle-closure glaucoma; d/c as rapidly as possible. May alter glucose tolerance and increase serum cholesterol and TG levels. May cause or exacerbate hyperuricemia and precipitate gout in susceptible patients. May cause hypercalcemia.

ADVERSE REACTIONS

Dizziness, BUN elevations, hypokalemia, angioedema, dry cough, nasopharyngitis.

D

DRUG INTERACTIONS

See Contraindications. Increased lithium levels and lithium toxicity reported; monitor lithium levels during concomitant use. **Valsartan:** Dual blockade of the RAS is associated w/ increased risk of hypotension, hyperkalemia, and changes in renal function (including acute renal failure); avoid combined use of RAS inhibitors, or closely monitor BP, renal function, and electrolytes w/ concomitant agents that also affect the RAS. Avoid w/ aliskiren in patients w/ renal impairment (GFR <60mL/min). Greater antihypertensive effect w/ atenolol. Inhibitors of the hepatic uptake transporter OATP1B1 (rifampin, cyclosporine) or the hepatic efflux transporter MRP2 (ritonavir) may increase exposure. NSAIDs, including selective COX-2 inhibitors, may result in deterioration of renal function, including possible acute renal failure, and may attenuate antihypertensive effect. Other agents that block the RAS, K^+-sparing diuretics, K^+ supplements, salt substitutes containing K^+, or other drugs that may increase K^+ levels (heparin), may increase serum K^+ levels, and in HF patients may increase SrCr; monitor serum K^+ levels. **HCTZ:** Dosage adjustment of antidiabetic drugs (eg, oral agents, insulin) may be required. May lead to symptomatic hyponatremia w/ carbamazepine. Ion exchange resins (eg, cholestyramine, colestipol) may reduce exposure; space dosing at least 4 hrs before or 4-6 hrs after the administration of ion exchange resins. Cyclosporine may increase risk of hyperuricemia and gout-type complications.

PATIENT CONSIDERATIONS

Assessment: Assess for hypersensitivity to the drug and its components, anuria, history of sulfonamide-derived hypersensitivity or penicillin allergy, renal/hepatic impairment, volume/salt depletion, risk for acute renal failure, SLE, electrolyte imbalances, pregnancy/nursing status, and possible drug interactions.

Monitoring: Monitor for signs/symptoms of hypotension, hypersensitivity/idiosyncratic reactions, exacerbation or activation of SLE, myopia, angle-closure glaucoma, precipitation of gout or hyperuricemia, and other adverse reactions. Monitor BP, serum electrolytes, cholesterol, TG levels, and renal function periodically.

Counseling: Inform about the consequences of exposure during pregnancy and discuss treatment options in women planning to become pregnant. Instruct to report pregnancies to physician as soon as possible. Caution about lightheadedness, especially during the 1st days of therapy; instruct to d/c and consult physician if syncope occurs. Caution that inadequate fluid intake, excessive perspiration, diarrhea, and vomiting may lead to an excessive fall in BP, w/ the same consequences of lightheadedness and possible syncope. Instruct to avoid use of K^+ supplements or salt substitutes containing K^+ w/o consulting a physician.

STORAGE: 25°C (77°F); excursions permitted to 15-30°C (59-86°F). Protect from moisture.

DIPROLENE – betamethasone dipropionate

RX

Class: Corticosteroid

OTHER BRAND NAMES

Diprolene AF

ADULT DOSAGE

Inflammatory and Pruritic Manifestations of Corticosteroid-Responsive Dermatoses

Lot:
Usual: Apply a few drops to affected skin qd or bid and massage lightly until it disappears
Max: 50mL/week; limit treatment to 2 weeks
D/C when control is achieved; reassess diagnosis if no improvement seen w/in 2 weeks

Oint:
Usual: Apply a thin film to affected skin qd or bid
Max: 50g/week
D/C when control is achieved; reassess diagnosis if no improvement seen w/in 2 weeks

Cre:
Usual: Apply a thin film to affected skin qd or bid
Max: 50g/week
D/C when control is achieved

PEDIATRIC DOSAGE

Inflammatory and Pruritic Manifestations of Corticosteroid-Responsive Dermatoses

≥13 Years:

Lot:
Usual: Apply a few drops to affected skin qd or bid and massage lightly until it disappears
Max: 50mL/week; limit treatment to 2 weeks
D/C when control is achieved; reassess diagnosis if no improvement seen w/in 2 weeks

Oint:
Usual: Apply a thin film to affected skin qd or bid
Max: 50g/week
D/C when control is achieved; reassess diagnosis if no improvement seen w/in 2 weeks

Cre:
Usual: Apply a thin film to affected skin qd or bid
Max: 50g/week
D/C when control is achieved

ADMINISTRATION
Topical route

Avoid use w/ occlusive dressings unless directed

HOW SUPPLIED
Cre (AF)/Oint: 0.05% [15g, 50g]; **Lot:** 0.05% [30mL, 60mL]

CONTRAINDICATIONS
Hypersensitivity to betamethasone dipropionate, to other corticosteroids, or to any ingredient in this preparation.

WARNINGS/PRECAUTIONS
Avoid use with occlusive dressings. Avoid use on the face, groin, or axillae or if skin atrophy is present at the treatment site. May produce reversible hypothalamic-pituitary-adrenal (HPA) axis suppression with the potential for glucocorticosteroid insufficiency; may occur during or after withdrawal of treatment. Periodically evaluate for HPA axis suppression and, if noted, gradually withdraw drug, reduce frequency of application, or substitute a less potent corticosteroid. Infrequently, signs/symptoms of steroid withdrawal may occur, requiring supplemental systemic corticosteroids. Cushing's syndrome and hyperglycemia may occur. Pediatric patients may be more susceptible to systemic toxicity. Allergic contact dermatitis reported; confirm by patch testing. D/C and institute appropriate therapy if irritation develops. Not for treatment of diaper dermatitis.

ADVERSE REACTIONS
(Cre) Skin atrophy (telangiectasia, bruising, shininess). (Oint/Lot) Erythema, folliculitis, pruritus, vesiculation.

PATIENT CONSIDERATIONS

Assessment: Assess for hypersensitivity to corticosteroids, factors that predispose to HPA axis suppression, pregnancy/nursing status, and possible drug interactions. Evaluate for HPA axis suppression using the adrenocorticotropic hormone (ACTH) stimulation test.

Monitoring: Monitor for signs/symptoms of HPA axis suppression, Cushing's syndrome, hyperglycemia, irritation, and other adverse reactions. Perform periodic monitoring of HPA axis suppression using ACTH stimulation test. Monitor for systemic toxicity in pediatric patients. Monitor response to therapy.

Counseling: Inform to d/c therapy when control is achieved, unless directed otherwise by physician. Counsel to avoid contact with eyes. Instruct not to use on face, underarms, or groin areas unless directed by physician. Instruct not to occlude the treatment area with bandage or other covering, unless directed by the physician. Inform that local reactions and skin atrophy are more likely to occur with occlusive use, prolonged use or use of higher potency corticosteroids. (Lot/Oint) Instruct to use no longer than 2 consecutive weeks.

STORAGE: 25°C (77°F); excursions permitted to 15-30°C (59-86°F).

DITROPAN XL – oxybutynin chloride

RX

Class: Anticholinergic

ADULT DOSAGE
Overactive Bladder
Initial: 5 or 10mg qd at the same time each day
Titrate: May adjust dose in 5mg increments weekly
Max: 30mg/day

PEDIATRIC DOSAGE
Detrusor Overactivity
Associated w/ a Neurological Condition (eg, Spina Bifida):
≥6 Years:
Initial: 5mg qd at the same time each day
Titrate: May adjust dose in 5mg increments
Max: 20mg/day

ADMINISTRATION
Oral route

May be taken w/ or w/o food
Swallow tab whole w/ aid of liquids; do not chew, divide, or crush

HOW SUPPLIED
Tab, Extended-Release: 5mg, 10mg, 15mg

CONTRAINDICATIONS
Urinary retention, gastric retention and other severe decreased GI motility conditions, uncontrolled narrow-angle glaucoma. Hypersensitivity to the drug substance or other components of the product.

WARNINGS/PRECAUTIONS
Angioedema of the face, lips, tongue, and/or larynx reported; d/c promptly and provide appropriate therapy if angioedema occurs. Associated w/ anticholinergic CNS effects; consider dose reduction or discontinuation if any occur. Caution w/ preexisting dementia treated w/ cholinesterase inhibitors, Parkinson's disease, myasthenia gravis, autonomic neuropathy, clinically significant bladder outflow obstruction, GI obstructive disorders, ulcerative colitis, intestinal atony, GERD, and preexisting severe GI narrowing (pathologic or iatrogenic). May decrease GI motility. May impair mental/physical abilities. Not recommended in pediatric patients who cannot swallow tab whole w/o chewing, dividing, or crushing.

ADVERSE REACTIONS
Dry mouth, constipation, diarrhea, headache, somnolence, dizziness, dyspepsia, nausea, blurred vision, dry eyes, insomnia.

DRUG INTERACTIONS
Concomitant use w/ other anticholinergic drugs may increase the frequency and/or severity of anticholinergic-like effects. May alter GI absorption of other drugs due to GI motility effects; caution w/ drugs w/ narrow therapeutic index. May antagonize effects of prokinetic agents (eg, metoclopramide). Increased levels w/ ketoconazole. Caution w/ CYP3A4 inhibitors (eg, antimycotics, macrolides); may alter mean pharmacokinetic parameters. Caution w/ drugs that may cause/exacerbate esophagitis (eg, bisphosphonates).

PATIENT CONSIDERATIONS

Assessment: Assess for urinary/gastric retention, bladder outflow obstruction, GI narrowing/obstructive disorder, GERD, ulcerative colitis, uncontrolled narrow-angle glaucoma, Parkinson's disease, myasthenia gravis, autonomic neuropathy, dementia, hypersensitivity to the drug substance or other components of the product, any other conditions where treatment is contraindicated or cautioned, pregnancy/nursing status, and possible drug interactions.

Monitoring: Monitor for aggravation of myasthenia gravis or autonomic neuropathy, angioedema, hypersensitivity reactions, anticholinergic CNS effects, GI adverse reactions (eg, urinary retention, esophagitis, gastric retention), and other adverse reactions.

Counseling: Inform that angioedema may occur and could result in life-threatening airway obstruction; advise to promptly d/c therapy and seek medical attention if experiencing swelling of the tongue, edema of the laryngopharynx, or difficulty breathing. Inform that heat prostration may occur when administered in high environmental temperature. Inform that drug may produce drowsiness, dizziness, or blurred vision; advise to exercise caution. Inform that alcohol may enhance drowsiness. Advise not to drive or operate heavy machinery until effects have been determined.

STORAGE: 25°C (77°F); excursions permitted to 15-30°C (59-86°F). Protect from moisture and humidity.

DIVIGEL – estradiol

RX

Class: Estrogen

Estrogens increase the risk of endometrial cancer in women w/ uterus. Perform adequate diagnostic measures (eg, endometrial sampling) to rule out malignancy w/ undiagnosed persistent or recurring abnormal genital bleeding. Should not be used for the prevention of cardiovascular disease (CVD) or dementia. Increased risk of MI, stroke, pulmonary embolism (PE), and deep vein thrombosis (DVT) in postmenopausal women (50-79 yrs of age) reported. May increase risk of invasive breast cancer. Increased risk of developing probable dementia in postmenopausal women ≥65 yrs of age reported. Should be prescribed at the lowest effective dose and for the shortest duration consistent w/ treatment goals and risks.

ADULT DOSAGE

Menopausal Vasomotor Symptoms

Moderate to Severe:
Initial: 0.25g qd applied on skin of right or left upper thigh

Reevaluate periodically to determine need for treatment

PEDIATRIC DOSAGE

Pediatric use may not have been established

ADMINISTRATION
Topical route
Application surface area should be about 5 by 7 inches (approx the size of 2 palm prints)
Entire contents of a unit dose pkt should be applied each day
Apply to right or left upper thigh on alternating days to avoid skin irritation

Do not apply on face, breasts, irritated skin, or in or around vagina
Allow gel to dry before dressing
Do not wash the application site w/in 1 hr after application
Contact of gel w/ eyes should be avoided
Wash hands after application

HOW SUPPLIED

Gel: 0.1% [0.25g, 0.5g, 1g pkts]

CONTRAINDICATIONS

Undiagnosed abnormal genital bleeding, known/suspected/history of breast cancer, known/suspected estrogen-dependent neoplasia, active/history of DVT, PE, or arterial thromboembolic disease (eg, stroke, MI), liver impairment/disease, protein C/protein S/antithrombin deficiency, or other known thrombophilic disorders, known/suspected pregnancy.

WARNINGS/PRECAUTIONS

D/C immediately if PE, DVT, stroke, or MI occurs or is suspected. Caution in patients w/ risk factors for arterial vascular disease and/or venous thromboembolism (VTE). If feasible, d/c at least 4-6 weeks before surgery of the type associated w/ increased risk of thromboembolism, or during periods of prolonged immobilization. May increase risk of gallbladder disease requiring surgery and ovarian cancer. Consider addition of progestin for women w/ a uterus or w/ residual endometriosis posthysterectomy. May lead to severe hypercalcemia in patients w/ breast cancer and bone metastases; d/c and take appropriate measures if this occurs. Retinal vascular thrombosis reported; d/c pending examination if sudden partial/complete loss of vision, sudden onset of proptosis, diplopia, or migraine occurs. D/C permanently if examination reveals papilledema or retinal vascular lesions. May elevate BP and thyroid-binding globulin levels. May elevate plasma TG levels (w/ preexisting hypertriglyceridemia); consider discontinuation if pancreatitis occurs. Caution w/ history of cholestatic jaundice; d/c in case of recurrence. May cause fluid retention; caution w/ cardiac or renal impairment. Caution w/ hypoparathyroidism; hypocalcemia may occur. May exacerbate symptoms of angioedema in women w/ hereditary angioedema. May exacerbate endometriosis, asthma, diabetes mellitus (DM), epilepsy, migraine, porphyria, systemic lupus erythematosus, and hepatic hemangiomas; use w/ caution. May affect certain endocrine, and blood components in lab tests. Alcohol-based gels are flammable; avoid fire, flame, or smoking until applied dose has dried. Potential for drug transfer following physical contact; cover application site after drying.

ADVERSE REACTIONS

Nasopharyngitis, URTI(s), vaginal mycosis, breast tenderness, metrorrhagia.

DRUG INTERACTIONS

CYP3A4 inducers (eg, St. John's wort, phenobarbital, carbamazepine, rifampin) may decrease levels; may decrease therapeutic effects and/or change uterine bleeding profile. CYP3A4 inhibitors (eg, erythromycin, clarithromycin, ketoconazole) may increase levels; may result in side effects. Patients concomitantly receiving thyroid replacement therapy and estrogens may require increased doses of thyroid replacement therapy. May change systemic exposure w/ sunscreens.

PATIENT CONSIDERATIONS

Assessment: Assess for undiagnosed abnormal genital bleeding, liver impairment/disease, presence/history of breast cancer, estrogen-dependent neoplasia, DVT, PE, or arterial thromboembolic disease, pregnancy/nursing status, any other conditions where treatment is contraindicated or cautioned, need for progestin therapy, and possible drug interactions. Assess for protein C, protein S, or antithrombin deficiency, or other known thrombophilic disorders.

Monitoring: Monitor for signs/symptoms of CVD, arterial vascular disease, VTE, malignant neoplasms, dementia, gallbladder disease, hypercalcemia, BP and plasma TG elevations, visual abnormalities, pancreatitis, cholestatic jaundice, hypothyroidism, fluid retention, exacerbation of endometriosis and other adverse reactions. Perform annual breast exam; schedule mammography based on age, risk factors, and prior mammogram results. Monitor thyroid function in patients on thyroid replacement therapy. Perform adequate diagnostic measures (eg, endometrial sampling) in patients w/ undiagnosed persistent or recurrent genital bleeding. Perform periodic evaluation to determine treatment need.

Counseling: Inform postmenopausal women of the importance of reporting vaginal bleeding as soon as possible and of possible serious adverse reactions of therapy and possible less serious but common adverse reactions. Advise to have yearly breast exams by a physician and to perform monthly self-breast exams. Instruct on the proper application and use. Inform that gel contains alcohol that is flammable; instruct to avoid fire, flame, or smoking until the gel has dried. Inform of potential for drug transfer from one individual to the other following physical contact; advise to avoid skin contact w/ other subjects until the gel is completely dried.

STORAGE: 20-25°C (68-77°F); excursions permitted to 15-30°C (59-86°F).

DOCETAXEL – docetaxel

RX

Class: Antimicrotubule agent

Increased incidence of treatment-related mortality reported in patients w/ hepatic dysfunction, in patients receiving higher-doses, and in patients w/ non-small cell lung cancer (NSCLC) and a history of prior treatment w/ platinum-based chemotherapy who receive docetaxel as a single agent at a dose of 100mg/m². Avoid if bilirubin >ULN, or AST/ALT >1.5X ULN concomitant w/ alkaline phosphatase >2.5X ULN; may increase risk for the development of Grade 4 neutropenia, febrile neutropenia, infections, severe thrombocytopenia, severe stomatitis, severe skin toxicity, and toxic death. Patients w/ isolated elevations of transaminase >1.5X ULN reported to have a higher rate of febrile neutropenia Grade 4 but did not have an increased incidence of toxic death. Obtain bilirubin, AST or ALT, and alkaline phosphatase values prior to each cycle. Avoid therapy if neutrophils <1500 cells/mm³. Monitor for the occurrence of neutropenia; perform frequent blood cell counts on all patients. Severe hypersensitivity reactions reported w/ dexamethasone premedication; d/c immediately if symptoms occur. Contraindicated w/ history of severe hypersensitivity reactions to docetaxel or other drugs formulated w/ polysorbate 80. Severe fluid retention may occur despite dexamethasone premedication.

OTHER BRAND NAMES

Taxotere

ADULT DOSAGE

Breast Cancer

Locally advanced or metastatic breast cancer after failure of prior chemotherapy

60-100mg/m² IV over 1 hr every 3 weeks

Combination w/ Doxorubicin and Cyclophosphamide:

Adjuvant treatment of operable node-positive breast cancer

75mg/m² 1 hr after doxorubicin 50mg/m² and cyclophosphamide 500mg/m² every 3 weeks for 6 courses

Prophylactic G-CSF may be used to mitigate risk of hematological toxicities

Non-Small Cell Lung Cancer

Single Agent:

Locally advanced or metastatic NSCLC after failure of prior platinum-based chemotherapy

75mg/m² IV over 1 hr every 3 weeks

Combination w/ Cisplatin:

Unresectable, locally advanced or metastatic NSCLC in chemotherapy-naive patients

75mg/m² IV over 1 hr immediately followed by cisplatin 75mg/m² over 30-60 min every 3 weeks

Metastatic Prostate Cancer

Combination w/ prednisone for androgen-independent (hormone refractory) metastatic prostate cancer

75mg/m² IV over 1 hr every 3 weeks + prednisone 5mg PO bid

Gastric Adenocarcinoma

Combination w/ cisplatin and fluorouracil for advanced gastric adenocarcinoma, including adenocarcinoma of the gastroesophageal junction, in chemotherapy-naive patients

75mg/m² IV over 1 hr, followed by cisplatin 75mg/m² IV over 1-3 hrs (both on Day 1 only), followed by fluorouracil 750mg/m²/day IV over 24 hrs x 5 days, starting at end of cisplatin infusion

Repeat treatment every 3 weeks

Squamous Cell Carcinoma of the Head and Neck

Combination w/ cisplatin and fluorouracil for induction treatment of locally advanced

PEDIATRIC DOSAGE

Pediatric use may not have been established

squamous cell carcinoma of the head and neck (SCCHN)

Administer prophylaxis for neutropenic infections

Induction Followed by Radiotherapy:
Locally advanced inoperable SCCHN

75mg/m^2 IV over 1 hr, followed by cisplatin 75mg/m^2 IV over 1 hr, on Day 1, followed by fluorouracil as a continuous IV infusion at 750mg/m^2/day x 5 days

Administer every 3 weeks for 4 cycles; following chemotherapy, patients should receive radiotherapy

Induction Followed by Chemoradiotherapy:
Locally advanced (unresectable, low surgical cure, or organ preservation) SCCHN

75mg/m^2 IV over 1 hr on Day 1, followed by cisplatin 100mg/m^2 IV over 30 min to 3 hrs, followed by fluorouracil 1000mg/m^2/day as a continuous IV infusion from Day 1 to Day 4

Administer every 3 weeks for 3 cycles; following chemotherapy, patients should receive chemoradiotherapy

Premedication

All Patients:
Oral corticosteroids (see below for prostate cancer) such as dexamethasone 16mg/day (8mg bid) for 3 days starting 1 day prior to docetaxel administration

Prostate Cancer:
Given the concurrent use of prednisone, the recommended regimen is dexamethasone 8mg PO, at 12 hrs, 3 hrs, and 1 hr before docetaxel infusion

Gastric Adenocarcinoma/Head and Neck Cancer:
Patients must receive antiemetics and appropriate hydration for cisplatin administration

DOSING CONSIDERATIONS

Concomitant Medications

Strong CYP3A4 Inhibitors: Avoid use; consider a 50% docetaxel dose reduction if patients require coadministration of a strong CYP3A4 inhibitor

Hepatic Impairment

AST/ALT >2.5 to ≤5X ULN and Alkaline Phosphatase ≤2.5X ULN, or AST/ALT >1.5 to ≤5X ULN and Alkaline Phosphatase >2.5 to ≤5X ULN: Reduce docetaxel dose by 20%
AST/ALT >5X ULN and/or Alkaline Phosphatase >5X ULN: D/C treatment

Adverse Reactions

Breast Cancer:
Initial Dose 100mg/m^2:
Experience Febrile Neutropenia, Neutrophils <500 cells/mm^3 for >1 Week, or Severe/Cumulative Cutaneous Reactions: Reduce dose to 75mg/m^2; if reactions continue, either reduce dose to 55mg/m^2 or d/c treatment
Initial Dose 60mg/m^2:
Do Not Experience Febrile Neutropenia, Neutrophils <500 cells/mm^3 for >1 Week, Severe/Cumulative Cutaneous Reactions, or Severe Peripheral Neuropathy: May tolerate higher doses
≥Grade 3 Peripheral Neuropathy: D/C treatment

Combination Therapy in Adjuvant Treatment of Breast Cancer:
Febrile Neutropenia: Administer G-CSF in all subsequent cycles; if reaction continues, continue G-CSF and reduce docetaxel dose to 60mg/m^2
Grade 3 or 4 Stomatitis: Reduce docetaxel dose to 60mg/m^2
Severe/Cumulative Cutaneous Reactions or Moderate Neurosensory Signs and/or Symptoms: Reduce docetaxel dose to 60mg/m^2; if reactions continue at 60mg/m^2, d/c treatment

NSCLC:
Monotherapy:
Experience Febrile Neutropenia, Neutrophils <500 cells/mm³ for >1 Week, or Severe/Cumulative Cutaneous Reactions, or Other Grade 3-4 Nonhematological Toxicities: Withhold treatment until toxicity resolves, then resume at 55mg/m²
≥Grade 3 Peripheral Neuropathy: D/C treatment

Combination Therapy:
Nadir of Platelet Count During Previous Course of Therapy is <25,000 cells/mm³ w/ Febrile Neutropenia/Serious Nonhematologic Toxicities: Reduce docetaxel dose in subsequent cycles to 65mg/m²; if further dose reduction is required, 50mg/m² is recommended

Prostate Cancer:
Experience Febrile Neutropenia, Neutrophils <500 cells/mm³ for >1 Week, Severe/Cumulative Cutaneous Reactions, or Moderate Neurosensory Signs and/or Symptoms: Reduce docetaxel dose to 60mg/m²; if reactions continue at 60mg/m², d/c treatment

Gastric Adenocarcinoma/Head and Neck Cancer:
Experience Episode of Febrile Neutropenia or Prolonged Neutropenia/Neutropenic Infection Occurs Despite G-CSF Use: Reduce docetaxel dose to 60mg/m²; if subsequent episodes of complicated neutropenia occur, reduce docetaxel dose to 45mg/m². D/C if toxicities persist
Grade 4 Thrombocytopenia: Reduce docetaxel dose to 60mg/m²; do not retreat w/ subsequent cycles until neutrophils recover to >1500 cells/mm³ and platelets recover to >100,000 cells/mm³. D/C if toxicities persist

Toxicities w/ Docetaxel in Combination w/ Cisplatin and Fluorouracil:
Grade 3 Diarrhea:
1st Episode: Reduce fluorouracil dose by 20%
2nd Episode: Reduce docetaxel dose by 20%

Grade 4 Diarrhea:
1st Episode: Reduce docetaxel and fluorouracil doses by 20%
2nd Episode: D/C treatment

Grade 3 Stomatitis/Mucositis:
1st Episode: Reduce fluorouracil dose by 20%
2nd Episode: Stop fluorouracil only, at all subsequent cycles
3rd Episode: Reduce docetaxel dose by 20%

Grade 4 Stomatitis/Mucositis:
1st Episode: Stop fluorouracil only, at all subsequent cycles
2nd Episode: Reduce docetaxel dose by 20%

Refer to PI for cisplatin and fluorouracil dose modifications

ADMINISTRATION

IV route

Administration Precautions

Contact of the docetaxel inj w/ plasticized PVC equipment or devices used to prepare sol for infusion is not recommended; store the final docetaxel dilution for infusion in bottles (glass, polypropylene) or plastic bags (polypropylene, polyolefin) and administer through polyethylene-lined administration sets.

Preparation

Requires no prior dilution w/ a diluent and is ready to add to the infusion sol.

Docetaxel Inj Concentrate (20mg/mL):
Do not use the two-vial formulation (inj concentrate and diluent) w/ the one-vial formulation.

Refer to PI for further administration instructions.

HOW SUPPLIED

Inj: 10mg/mL [2mL, 8mL, 16mL], (Taxotere) 20mg/mL [1mL, 4mL]

CONTRAINDICATIONS

History of severe hypersensitivity reactions to docetaxel or to other drugs formulated w/ polysorbate 80. Neutrophils <1500 cells/mm³.

WARNINGS/PRECAUTIONS

Avoid subsequent cycles until neutrophils recover to level >1500 cells/mm³ and platelets to >100,000 cells/mm³. Severe fluid retention reported; monitor from the 1st dose for possible exacerbation of preexisting effusions. Acute myeloid leukemia or myelodysplasia may occur in adjuvant therapy (eg, adjuvant therapy in breast cancer). Localized erythema of the extremities w/ edema followed by desquamation reported; adjust dose if severe skin toxicity occurs. Severe neurosensory symptoms (eg, paresthesia, dysesthesia, pain) may develop; adjust dose if symptoms occur and d/c treatment if symptoms persist. Cystoid macular edema (CME) reported; d/c and initiate appropriate treatment if CME is diagnosed, and/or consider alternative non-taxane cancer treatment. Severe asthenia reported. May cause fetal harm. Caution in elderly. Intoxication reported due to alcohol content. Alcohol content of the drug may affect CNS; caution in whom alcohol intake should be avoided or minimized. Alcohol content of the drug may impair physical/mental abilities.

ADVERSE REACTIONS

Infections, neutropenia, anemia, febrile neutropenia, hypersensitivity, thrombocytopenia, neuropathy, dysgeusia, dyspnea, constipation, anorexia, nail disorders, fluid retention, asthenia, pain.

DRUG INTERACTIONS

See Dosing Considerations. Avoid w/ CYP3A4 inhibitors (eg, ketoconazole, clarithromycin, atazanavir); may increase docetaxel exposure. CYP3A4 inducers and substrates may alter metabolism. Protease inhibitors (eg, ritonavir) may increase exposure. Renal insufficiency and renal failure reported w/ concomitant nephrotoxic drugs. Radiation pneumonitis may occur in patients receiving concomitant radiotherapy (rare).

PATIENT CONSIDERATIONS

Assessment: Assess for history of severe hypersensitivity reactions to the drug or other drugs w/ polysorbate 80, preexisting effusion, hepatic impairment, pregnancy/nursing status, and possible drug interactions. Obtain baseline weight, CBC w/ platelets, and differential count. Obtain bilirubin, AST or ALT, and alkaline phosphatase values prior to each cycle of therapy.

Monitoring: Monitor for fluid retention, acute myeloid leukemia, hematologic effects, skin toxicities, exacerbation of effusions, neurosensory symptoms, hepatic impairment, hypersensitivity reactions, asthenia, CME, and other adverse reactions. Monitor weight, CBC w/ platelets, and differential count. Perform a comprehensive ophthalmologic examination in patients w/ impaired vision.

Counseling: Inform about risks and benefits of therapy. Inform that drug may cause fetal harm; advise to avoid pregnancy and to use effective contraceptives. Explain the significance of oral corticosteroid administration to help facilitate compliance; instruct to report if not compliant. Instruct to report signs of hypersensitivity reactions, fluid retention, myalgia, or cutaneous/neurologic reactions. Counsel about side effects that are associated w/ the drug. Explain the significance of routine blood cell counts. Instruct to monitor temperature frequently and to immediately report any occurrence of fever. Explain about the possible side effects of the alcohol content in the drug, including possible side effects on the CNS. Advise patients in whom alcohol should be avoided or minimized to consider the alcohol content of the drug; inform that alcohol could impair their ability to drive or use machines immediately after infusion.

STORAGE: 20-25°C (68-77°F), (Taxotere) 2-25°C (36-77°F). Multi-use vials are stable for up to 28 days when stored at 2-8°C (36-46°F) after use. Protect from light. **Reconstituted Sol:** 0.9% NaCl or D5: Stable at 2-25°C (36-77°F) for 4 hrs or (Taxotere) 6 hrs. (Taxotere) Infusion sol is stable in non-PVC bags up to 48 hrs at 2-8°C (36-46°F).

DOLOPHINE – methadone hydrochloride

CII

Class: Opioid analgesic

Exposes patients and other users to the risk of opioid addiction, abuse, and misuse, leading to overdose and death; assess each patient's risk prior to prescribing, and monitor regularly for development of these behaviors/conditions. Serious, life-threatening, or fatal respiratory depression may occur; monitor for respiratory depression, especially during initiation or following a dose increase. Accidental ingestion, especially in children, can result in fatal overdose. QT interval prolongation and serious arrhythmia (torsades de pointes) occurred; closely monitor for changes in cardiac rhythm during initiation and titration. Prolonged use during pregnancy can result in neonatal opioid withdrawal syndrome; advise pregnant women of the risk and ensure availability of appropriate treatment. For detoxification and maintenance of opioid dependence, methadone should be administered in accordance w/ treatment standards, including limitations on unsupervised administration.

ADULT DOSAGE

Severe Pain (Daily, Around-the-Clock Management)

Management of pain severe enough to require daily, around-the-clock, long-term opioid treatment and for which alternative treatment options are inadequate

1st Opioid Analgesic: 2.5mg q8-12h
Titration/Maint:
Individually titrate to a dose that provides adequate analgesia and minimizes adverse reactions
Titrate slowly, w/ dose increases no more frequent than every 3-5 days; some patients may require longer intervals of up to 12 days

PEDIATRIC DOSAGE

Pediatric use may not have been established

If breakthrough pain is experienced, patient may require a dose increase or need rescue medication w/ an appropriate dose of an immediate-release medication

Detoxification/Maintenance Treatment of Opioid Addiction

Induction/Initial:
Initial: 20-30mg single dose; use lower initial doses for patients whose tolerance is expected to be low at treatment entry
Max Initial: 30mg
May administer an additional 5-10mg if withdrawal symptoms are not suppressed or if symptoms reappear
Max Total Day 1 Dose: 40mg
Adjust dose over the 1st week of treatment based on control of withdrawal symptoms at the time of expected peak activity (eg, 2-4 hrs after dosing)

Short-Term Detoxification:
Titrate to a total daily dose of 40mg in divided doses to achieve an adequate stabilizing level
Gradually decrease methadone dose on a daily basis or at 2-day intervals, 2-3 days after stabilization
Hospitalized patients may tolerate a daily reduction of 20% of the total daily dose; ambulatory patients may need a slower schedule

Titration and Maint:
Usual: 80-120mg/day

Medically Supervised Withdrawal After a Period of Maint Treatment:
Dose reductions should be <10% of the established tolerance or maint dose w/ 10- to 14-day intervals

Management of Acute Pain During Methadone Maint Treatment:
May require somewhat higher and/or more frequent doses than in nontolerant patients

Conversions

D/C all other around-the-clock opioid drugs when therapy is initiated
From Parenteral Methadone: Use conversion ratio of 1:2mg for parenteral to oral methadone (eg, 5mg parenteral to 10mg oral)

Conversion Factors to Dolophine:
Total daily baseline oral morphine equivalent dose: Calculate the estimated daily oral methadone requirement as a percent of morphine equivalent dose:
<100mg: 20-30%
100-300mg: 10-20%
300-600mg: 8-12%
600-1000mg: 5-10%
>1000mg: <5%

Calculation for Estimated Daily Dose for Dolophine:
Always round down, if necessary, to the appropriate Dolophine strength(s) available
On a Single Opioid: Sum the total daily dose of opioid, convert to morphine equivalent dose, then multiply the morphine equivalent dose by the corresponding percentage to calculate approximate daily oral methadone dose

On >1 Opioid: Calculate approximate oral methadone dose for each opioid and sum the totals to obtain approximate daily total methadone dose
On Fixed-Ratio Opioid/Nonopioid Analgesics: Only use the opioid component of these products in the conversion

DOSING CONSIDERATIONS

Renal Impairment

Start on lower dose and w/ longer dosing intervals and titrate slowly

Hepatic Impairment

Start on lower dose and titrate slowly

Pregnancy

May need to increase dose or decrease dosing interval

Elderly

Start at lower end of dosing range

Discontinuation

Avoid abrupt discontinuation; use a gradual downward titration every 2-4 days

ADMINISTRATION

Oral route

HOW SUPPLIED

Tab: 5mg*, 10mg* *scored

CONTRAINDICATIONS

Significant respiratory depression, acute or severe bronchial asthma in an unmonitored setting or in the absence of resuscitative equipment, known or suspected paralytic ileus, hypersensitivity to methadone.

WARNINGS/PRECAUTIONS

Reserve for use in patients for whom alternative analgesic treatment options (eg, nonopioid or immediate-release opioid analgesics) are ineffective, not tolerated, or would be otherwise inadequate to provide sufficient management of pain. Not indicated as a prn analgesic. Deaths reported during conversion from chronic, high-dose treatment w/ other opioid agonists and during initiation of treatment of addiction in subjects previously abusing high doses of other agonists. Retained in the liver and then slowly released, prolonging the duration of potential toxicity, w/ repeated dosing. Life-threatening respiratory depression is more likely to occur in elderly, cachectic, or debilitated patients; monitor closely when initiating and titrating, and when given w/ drugs that depress respiration. Consider alternative nonopioid analgesics in patients w/ significant COPD or cor pulmonale, and in patients having a substantially decreased respiratory reserve, hypoxia, hypercapnia, or preexisting respiratory depression. May cause severe hypotension including orthostatic hypotension and syncope in ambulatory patients; increased risk in patients w/ compromised ability to maintain BP. Monitor for signs of sedation and respiratory depression in patients susceptible to the intracranial effects of carbon dioxide retention (eg, those w/ increased intracranial pressure or brain tumors). May obscure the clinical course in patients w/ head injury. Avoid w/ GI obstruction and impaired consciousness or coma. May cause spasm of sphincter of Oddi or increase serum amylase. May aggravate convulsions in patients w/ convulsive disorders and may induce or aggravate seizures. May impair mental/physical abilities. Abrupt discontinuation may lead to opioid withdrawal symptoms. Infants born to opioid-dependent mothers may be physically dependent and may exhibit respiratory difficulties and withdrawal symptoms.

ADVERSE REACTIONS

Respiratory depression, QT prolongation, arrhythmia, systemic hypotension, lightheadedness, dizziness, sedation, sweating, N/V.

DRUG INTERACTIONS

Concomitant use w/ other CNS depressants (eg, sedatives, tranquilizers, phenothiazines) may result in hypotension, profound sedation, coma, respiratory depression, and death; reduce dose of one or both drugs when combined therapy is considered. Deaths reported when therapy has been abused in conjunction w/ benzodiazepines. CYP3A4 inhibitors may cause decreased clearance leading to an increase in plasma levels and increased or prolonged opioid effects; these effects could be more pronounced w/ concomitant use of CYP2C9 and 3A4 inhibitors. CYP3A4 inducers may induce metabolism and, therefore, may increase clearance, leading to a decrease in plasma concentrations, lack of efficacy, or (possibly) development of a withdrawal syndrome in a patient who had developed physical dependence to therapy. Antiretroviral agents w/ CYP3A4 inhibitory activity (eg, abacavir, darunavir + ritonavir [RTV], efavirenz, lopinavir + RTV) may increase clearance or decrease plasma levels. May decrease levels of didanosine and stavudine. May increase AUC of zidovudine. Monitor for cardiac conduction changes w/ drugs known to have potential to prolong QT interval. Pharmacodynamic interactions may occur w/ potentially arrhythmogenic agents (eg, Class I and III antiarrhythmics, neuroleptics, TCAs, calcium channel blockers). Monitor closely w/ drugs capable of inducing electrolyte disturbances that may prolong QT interval, including diuretics, laxatives, and mineralocorticoid hormones. Mixed agonist/antagonist (eg, pentazocine, nalbuphine, butorphanol), and partial agonist (buprenorphine) analgesics may reduce the analgesic effect or precipitate withdrawal symptoms; avoid use. Severe reactions may occur w/ concurrent use or w/in 14 days of MAOI use. May increase levels of desipramine. Anticholinergics may increase risk of urinary retention and/or severe constipation, which may lead to paralytic ileus.

PATIENT CONSIDERATIONS

Assessment: Assess for personal/family history or risk factors for drug abuse or addiction, general condition and medical status, opioid experience/tolerance, pain type/severity, previous opioid daily dose, type of prior analgesics used, respiratory depression, cardiac conduction abnormalities, COPD or other respiratory complications, GI obstruction, paralytic ileus, hepatic/renal impairment, previous hypersensitivity to drug, pregnancy/nursing status, possible drug interactions, and any other conditions where treatment is contraindicated or cautioned.

Monitoring: Monitor for signs/symptoms of respiratory depression, QT prolongation and arrhythmias, orthostatic hypotension, syncope, symptoms of worsening biliary tract disease, aggravation/induction of seizures, tolerance, physical dependence, mental/physical impairment, withdrawal syndrome, hypersensitivity reactions, and other adverse reactions. Monitor for signs of increased intracranial pressure w/ head injuries. Routinely monitor for signs of misuse, abuse, and addiction.

Counseling: Inform that use of medication, even when taken as recommended, may result in addiction, abuse, and misuse. Instruct not to share w/ others and to take steps to protect from theft or misuse. Inform of the risks of life-threatening respiratory depression; advise how to recognize respiratory depression and to seek medical attention if breathing difficulties develop. Inform that accidental ingestion, especially in children, may result in respiratory depression or death. Instruct to dispose of unused tab by flushing down the toilet. Instruct to seek medical attention immediately if patient experiences symptoms suggestive of an arrhythmia. Inform female patients of reproductive potential that prolonged use of drug during pregnancy may result in neonatal opioid withdrawal syndrome, which may be life threatening if not recognized and treated. Inform that potentially serious additive effects may occur if drug is used w/ alcohol or other CNS depressants, and instruct not to use such drugs unless supervised by a healthcare provider. Advise to use drug exactly ud and not to d/c w/o 1st discussing the need for tapering regimen w/ prescriber. Inform that drug may impair ability to perform potentially hazardous activities (eg, driving a car, operating heavy machinery). Advise about potential for severe constipation, including management instructions and when to seek medical attention. Inform that anaphylaxis may occur; advise how to recognize such a reaction and when to seek medical attention. Instruct nursing mothers to watch for signs of methadone toxicity in their infants (eg, increased sleepiness [more than usual], difficulty breastfeeding, breathing difficulties, limpness); instruct to inform physician immediately if these signs occur.

STORAGE: 20-25°C (68-77°F).

DONNATAL — atropine sulfate/hyoscyamine sulfate/phenobarbital/scopolamine hydrobromide

RX

Class: Anticholinergic/barbiturate

ADULT DOSAGE

Irritable Bowel Syndrome

Adjunctive Therapy:

Elixir:

1 or 2 tsp tid or qid

Tab:

1 or 2 tabs tid or qid

Extentabs:

1 tab q12h. May give 1 tab q8h if indicated

Acute Enterocolitis

Adjunctive Therapy:

Elixir:

1 or 2 tsp tid or qid

Tab:

1 or 2 tabs tid or qid

PEDIATRIC DOSAGE

Irritable Bowel Syndrome

Adjunctive Therapy:

Elixir:

Initial:

4.5kg: 0.5mL q4h or 0.75mL q6h

9.1kg: 1mL q4h or 1.5mL q6h

13.6kg: 1.5mL q4h or 2mL q6h

22.7kg: 2.5mL q4h or 3.75mL q6h

34kg: 3.75mL q4h or 5mL q6h

45.4kg: 5mL q4h or 7.5mL q6h

Acute Enterocolitis

Adjunctive Therapy:

Elixir:

Initial:

Extentabs:
1 tab q12h. May give 1 tab q8h if indicated

Duodenal Ulcers

Adjunctive Therapy:
Elixir:
1 or 2 tsp tid or qid

Tab:
1 or 2 tabs tid or qid

Extentabs:
1 tab q12h. May give 1 tab q8h if indicated

4.5kg: 0.5mL q4h or 0.75mL q6h
9.1kg: 1mL q4h or 1.5mL q6h
13.6kg: 1.5mL q4h or 2mL q6h
22.7kg: 2.5mL q4h or 3.75mL q6h
34kg: 3.75mL q4h or 5mL q6h
45.4kg: 5mL q4h or 7.5mL q6h

Duodenal Ulcers

Adjunctive Therapy:
Elixir:
Initial:
4.5kg: 0.5mL q4h or 0.75mL q6h
9.1kg: 1mL q4h or 1.5mL q6h
13.6kg: 1.5mL q4h or 2mL q6h
22.7kg: 2.5mL q4h or 3.75mL q6h
34kg: 3.75mL q4h or 5mL q6h
45.4kg: 5mL q4h or 7.5mL q6h

DOSING CONSIDERATIONS

Hepatic Impairment
Use small initial doses

ADMINISTRATION

Oral route

Elixir
Use pediatric dosing device or oral syringe to measure the dose

HOW SUPPLIED

(Atropine/Hyoscyamine/Phenobarbital/Scopolamine) **Elixir:** (0.0194mg/0.1037mg/16.2mg/0.0065mg)/5mL [10mL, 4 fl. oz., 1 pint]; **Tab:** 0.0194mg/0.1037mg/16.2mg/0.0065mg; **Tab, Extended-Release:** (Extentabs) 0.0582mg/0.3111mg/48.6mg/0.0195mg

CONTRAINDICATIONS

Glaucoma; obstructive uropathy (eg, bladder-neck obstruction due to prostatic hypertrophy); obstructive GI disease (achalasia, pyloroduodenal stenosis, etc.); paralytic ileus, intestinal atony in elderly/debilitated; unstable cardiovascular status in acute hemorrhage; severe ulcerative colitis (especially if complicated by toxic megacolon); myasthenia gravis; hiatal hernia associated w/ reflux esophagitis; known hypersensitivity to any of the ingredients; acute intermittent porphyria; patients in whom phenobarbital produces restlessness and/or excitement.

WARNINGS/PRECAUTIONS

Heat prostration can occur in high environmental temperatures. Diarrhea may be an early symptom of incomplete intestinal obstruction, especially w/ ileostomy or colostomy; treatment would be inappropriate and possibly harmful. May impair physical/mental abilities. Phenobarbital may be habit forming; avoid in patients prone to addiction or w/ history of physical and/or psychological drug dependence. Caution w/ autonomic neuropathy, renal disease, hyperthyroidism, coronary heart disease, CHF, arrhythmias, tachycardia, and HTN. May delay gastric emptying. Curare-like action may occur w/ overdosage. Abrupt withdrawal may produce delirium or convulsions in patients habituated to barbiturates. Elderly patients may react w/ symptoms of excitement, agitation, drowsiness, and other untoward manifestations to even small doses of the drug. (Elixir/Tab) May cause fetal harm when administered to pregnant women. Do not rely on the use of the drug in the presence of biliary tract disease complications. (Elixir [Mint]) Contains tartrazine, which may cause allergic-type reactions (including bronchial asthma) in certain susceptible persons; frequently seen in patients who also have aspirin sensitivity.

ADVERSE REACTIONS

Xerostomia, urinary hesitancy/retention, blurred vision, tachycardia, mydriasis, cycloplegia, increased ocular tension, loss of taste, headache, nervousness, drowsiness, weakness, dizziness, insomnia.

DRUG INTERACTIONS

Phenobarbital may decrease the effect of anticoagulants; may need larger doses of anticoagulant for optimal effect.

PATIENT CONSIDERATIONS

Assessment: Assess for previous hypersensitivity to the drug or any of its components, diarrhea, ileostomy, colostomy, history of physical and/or psychological drug dependence, biliary tract disease, hepatic dysfunction, pregnancy/nursing status, possible drug interactions, and any other conditions where treatment is contraindicated or cautioned.

Monitoring: Monitor for signs/symptoms of heat prostration, drowsiness, blurred vision, constipation, diarrhea, urinary hesitancy/retention, hypersensitivity reactions, and other adverse reactions.

Counseling: Counsel about possible side effects and advise to notify physician if any occur. Inform that the drug may be habit forming. If drowsiness or blurring of vision occurs, warn patients not to engage in activities requiring mental alertness (eg, operating a motor vehicle or other machinery) and not to perform hazardous work. Inform that treatment may decrease sweating, resulting in heat prostration, fever, or heat strokes. (Elixir/Tab) Advise to notify physician if pregnant or intending to become pregnant during therapy; apprise of the potential hazard to the fetus.

STORAGE: 20-25°C (68-77°F). Protect from light and moisture. (Elixir) Avoid freezing.

DORYX — doxycycline hyclate RX

Class: Tetracyclines

ADULT DOSAGE

General Dosing

Initial: 100mg q12h on 1st day
Maint: 100mg qd or 50mg q12h

More Severe Infections (eg, Chronic UTIs):
100mg q12h

Streptococcal Infections: Continue therapy for 10 days

Acute Epididymo-Orchitis

Caused by *Chlamydia trachomatis*:
100mg bid for at least 10 days

Malaria

Prophylaxis:
100mg qd beginning 1 or 2 days before travel and continuing daily during travel and for 4 weeks after departure from malarious area

Inhalational Anthrax (Postexposure)

100mg bid for 60 days

Chlamydia trachomatis Infections

Uncomplicated Urethral/Endocervical/Rectal Infections:
100mg bid for 7 days

Alternate Dosing for Uncomplicated Urethral/Endocervical Infections:
200mg qd for 7 days (Doryx)

Gonococcal Infections

Uncomplicated Infections (Except Anorectal Infections in Men):
100mg bid for 7 days

Alternate Dosing:
Single visit dose of 300mg stat followed in 1 hr by a second 300mg dose

Nongonococcal Urethritis

Caused by *Ureaplasma urealyticum*:
100mg bid for 7 days

Syphilis

Patients Allergic to Penicillin (PCN):
Early:
100mg bid for 2 weeks

>1-Year Duration:
100mg bid for 4 weeks

Other Indications

Rickettsial infections (eg, Rocky Mountain spotted fever, typhus fever and the typhus group, Q fever, rickettsialpox, tick fevers)

PEDIATRIC DOSAGE

General Dosing

>8 Years:
≤45kg:
4.4mg/kg divided into 2 doses on 1st day, followed by 2.2mg/kg qd or as 2 divided doses, on subsequent days
More Severe Infections: May use up to 4.4mg/kg

>45kg:
Initial: 100mg q12h on 1st day
Maint: 100mg qd or 50mg q12h
More Severe Infections (eg, Chronic UTIs):
100mg q12h

Streptococcal Infections: Continue therapy for 10 days

Malaria

Prophylaxis:
>8 Years:
2mg/kg qd up to 100mg qd beginning 1 or 2 days before travel and continuing daily during travel and for 4 weeks after departure from malarious area

Inhalational Anthrax (Postexposure)

<45kg:
2.2mg/kg bid for 60 days
≥45kg:
100mg bid for 60 days

Lymphogranuloma venereum
Granuloma inguinale
Chancroid
Respiratory tract infections
Psittacosis (ornithosis)
Relapsing fever
Plague
Tularemia
Cholera
Campylobacter fetus infections
Brucellosis (in conjunction w/ streptomycin)
Bartonellosis
UTIs
Trachoma
Inclusion conjunctivitis
Escherichia coli infections
Enterobacter aerogenes infections
Shigella species infections
Acinetobacter species infections

When PCN is contraindicated, treatment of the following infections: yaws, Vincent's infection, actinomycosis, and infections caused by *Clostridium* species

Adjunctive therapy in acute intestinal amebiasis and severe acne

ADMINISTRATION

Oral route

Administer w/ adequate amounts of fluid.
May be given w/ food or milk if gastric irritation occurs.

Administering w/ Applesauce

May break up tab and sprinkle contents (delayed-release pellets) over a spoonful of applesauce.
Do not crush or damage the pellets when breaking up the tab.
Swallow applesauce/pellet mixture immediately w/o chewing; may follow w/ a glass of water.

HOW SUPPLIED

Tab, Delayed-Release: 50mg, 200mg*; (Generic) 75mg*, 100mg*, 150mg* *scored

CONTRAINDICATIONS

Hypersensitivity to any of the tetracyclines.

WARNINGS/PRECAUTIONS

May cause permanent discoloration of the teeth (yellow-gray-brown) if used during tooth development (last 1/2 of pregnancy, infancy, and childhood to 8 yrs of age); do not use in this age group, except for anthrax. Enamel hypoplasia reported. *Clostridium difficile*-associated diarrhea (CDAD) reported; may need to d/c if CDAD is suspected or confirmed. Photosensitivity reported; d/c at the 1st evidence of skin erythema. May result in bacterial resistance if used in the absence of proven or suspected bacterial infection or a prophylactic indication. May result in overgrowth of non-susceptible organisms (including fungi); d/c and institute appropriate therapy if superinfection occurs. Associated w/ intracranial HTN (pseudotumor cerebri); increased risk in women of childbearing age who are overweight or have a history of intracranial HTN. If visual disturbance occurs, prompt ophthalmologic evaluation is warranted. Intracranial pressure can remain elevated for weeks after drug cessation; monitor patients until they stabilize. May decrease fibula growth rate in prematures. May cause an increase in BUN. When used for malaria prophylaxis, patient may still transmit the infection to mosquitoes outside endemic areas. False elevations of urinary catecholamines may occur due to interference w/ the fluorescence test.

ADVERSE REACTIONS

N/V, diarrhea, bacterial vaginitis.

DRUG INTERACTIONS

Avoid concomitant use w/ isotretinoin; may also cause pseudotumor cerebri. Depresses plasma prothrombin activity; may require downward adjustment of anticoagulant dose. May interfere w/ bactericidal action of PCN; avoid concurrent use. Impaired absorption w/ bismuth subsalicylate, antacids containing aluminum, Ca^{2+}, or Mg^{2+}, and iron-containing preparations. May render oral contraceptives less effective. Decreased $T_{1/2}$ w/ barbiturates, carbamazepine, and phenytoin. Fatal renal toxicity reported w/ methoxyflurane.

PATIENT CONSIDERATIONS

Assessment: Assess for hypersensitivity to drug or any tetracyclines, pregnancy/nursing status, and possible drug interactions. Perform culture and susceptibility testing.

Monitoring: Monitor for CDAD, photosensitivity, skin erythema, superinfection, intracranial HTN, visual disturbance, and other adverse reactions. In long-term therapy, perform periodic lab evaluation of organ systems, including hematopoietic, renal, and hepatic studies.

Counseling: Apprise of the potential hazard to fetus if used during pregnancy. Inform that therapy does not guarantee protection against malaria; advise to use measures that help avoid contact w/ mosquitoes. Advise to avoid excessive sunlight or artificial UV light and to d/c therapy if phototoxicity (eg, skin eruptions) occurs; advise to consider use of sunscreen or sunblock. Inform that absorption of drug is reduced when taken w/ bismuth subsalicylate, antacids containing aluminum, Ca^{2+}, or Mg^{2+}, iron-containing preparations, and w/ foods, especially those that contain Ca^{2+}. Advise to drink fluids liberally. Inform that drug may increase the incidence of vaginal candidiasis. Inform that diarrhea may be experienced and instruct to immediately contact physician if watery and bloody stools (w/ or w/o stomach cramps and fever) occur, even as late as ≥2 months after the last dose. Inform that therapy should only be used to treat bacterial, not viral, infections. Instruct to take exactly ud even if the patient feels better early in the course of therapy. Inform that skipping doses or not completing the full course of therapy may decrease effectiveness of treatment and increase bacterial resistance.

STORAGE: 25°C (77°F); excursions permitted to 15-30°C (59-86°F). **Generic:** Protect from light.

DOVONEX – calcipotriene

RX

Class: Vitamin D3 derivative

ADULT DOSAGE

Plaque Psoriasis

Usual: Apply a thin layer to the affected skin bid and rub in gently and completely

Safety and efficacy demonstrated in patients treated for 8 weeks

PEDIATRIC DOSAGE

Pediatric use may not have been established

ADMINISTRATION

Topical route

Wash hands thoroughly after use

HOW SUPPLIED

Cre: 0.005% [60g, 120g]

CONTRAINDICATIONS

History of hypersensitivity to any components of the preparation, hypercalcemia, evidence of vitamin D toxicity. Do not use on the face.

WARNINGS/PRECAUTIONS

Contact dermatitis, including allergic contact dermatitis, reported. Transient irritation of both lesions and surrounding uninvolved skin may occur; d/c if irritation develops. Reversible elevation of serum Ca^{2+} reported; d/c until normal Ca^{2+} levels are restored. For external use only; not for ophthalmic, oral, or intravaginal use.

ADVERSE REACTIONS

Skin irritation, rash, pruritus, dermatitis, worsening of psoriasis.

PATIENT CONSIDERATIONS

Assessment: Assess for history of hypersensitivity to any of the components of the preparation, hypercalcemia, evidence of vitamin D toxicity, and pregnancy/nursing status.

Monitoring: Monitor for serum Ca^{2+} elevation, irritation, contact dermatitis, and other adverse reactions.

Counseling: Advise to use drug only ud by the physician. Inform that the medication is for external use only; instruct to avoid contact w/ face or eyes. Advise to wash hands after application. Counsel that the drug should not be used for any disorder other than for which it was prescribed. Instruct to report any signs of adverse reactions to the physician. Instruct patients who apply medication to the exposed portions of the body to avoid excessive exposure to either natural or artificial sunlight (eg, tanning booths, sun lamps).

STORAGE: 15-25°C (59-77°F). Do not freeze.

Doxil — doxorubicin hydrochloride liposome

RX

Class: Anthracycline

D

May cause myocardial damage, including CHF, as the total cumulative dose approaches 550mg/m²; include prior use of other anthracyclines or anthracenediones in total cumulative dose calculations. Risk of cardiomyopathy may be increased at lower cumulative doses w/ prior mediastinal irradiation. Acute infusion-related reactions occurred in patients w/ solid tumors. Serious, life-threatening, and fatal infusion reactions reported.

ADULT DOSAGE

Ovarian Carcinoma

Progressed/Recurred After Platinum-Based Therapy:
50mg/m² IV over 60 min every 28 days until disease progression or unacceptable toxicity

AIDS-Related Kaposi's Sarcoma

After Failure of Prior Systemic Chemotherapy or Intolerance to Such Therapy:
20mg/m² IV over 60 min every 21 days until disease progression or unacceptable toxicity

Multiple Myeloma

In combination w/ bortezomib in patients who have not previously received bortezomib and have received at least 1 prior therapy

30mg/m² IV over 60 min on Day 4 of each 21-day cycle for 8 cycles or until disease progression or unacceptable toxicity

Administer therapy after bortezomib on Day 4 of each cycle

PEDIATRIC DOSAGE

Pediatric use may not have been established

DOSING CONSIDERATIONS

Hepatic Impairment

Serum Bilirubin ≥1.2mg/dL: Reduce dose

Adverse Reactions

Hand-Foot Syndrome (HFS):

Grade 1:
If previous Grade 3 or 4 HFS, delay dose up to 2 weeks, then decrease dose by 25%

Grade 2:
Delay dosing up to 2 weeks or until resolved to Grade 0-1
If resolved to Grade 0-1 w/in 2 weeks, continue treatment at previous dose if no previous Grade 3 or 4 HFS, or decrease dose by 25% if previous Grade 3 or 4 toxicity
D/C if no resolution after 2 weeks

Grade 3 or 4:
Delay dosing up to 2 weeks or until resolved to Grade 0-1, then decrease dose by 25%
D/C if no resolution after 2 weeks

Stomatitis:

Grade 1:
If previous Grade 3 or 4 toxicity, delay dose up to 2 weeks, then decrease by 25%

Grade 2:
Delay dosing up to 2 weeks or until resolved to Grade 0-1
If resolved to Grade 0-1 w/in 2 weeks, resume treatment at previous dose if no previous Grade 3 or 4 stomatitis, or decrease dose by 25% if previous Grade 3 or 4 toxicity
D/C if no resolution after 2 weeks

Grade 3 or 4:
Delay dosing up to 2 weeks or until resolved to Grade 0-1; decrease dose by 25% and return to original dose interval
D/C if no resolution after 2 weeks

Neutropenia/Thrombocytopenia:

Grade 2 or 3:
Delay until ANC ≥1500 and platelet count ≥75,000; resume treatment at previous dose

Grade 4:
Delay until ANC ≥1500 and platelet count ≥75,000; resume at 25% dose reduction or continue previous dose w/ prophylactic granulocyte growth factor

Toxicities When Administered in Combination w/ Bortezomib:
Fever ≥38°C and ANC <1000/mm³: Withhold dose for this cycle if before Day 4; decrease dose by 25% if after Day 4 of previous cycle
On any Day of Administration After Day 1 of Each Cycle:
Platelet Count <25,000/mm³ or Hgb <8g/dL or ANC <500/mm³: Withhold dose for this cycle if before Day 4; decrease dose by 25% if after Day 4 of previous cycle and if bortezomib is reduced for hematologic toxicity
Grade 3 or 4 Nonhematologic Toxicity: Do not dose until recovered to Grade <2, then reduce dose by 25%

Suspected Extravasation:
D/C for burning or stinging sensation or other evidence indicating perivenous infiltration or extravasation
Manage confirmed or suspected extravasation as follows:
1. Do not remove the needle until attempts are made to aspirate extravasated fluid
2. Do not flush the line; avoid applying pressure to the site
3. Apply ice to the site intermittently for 15 min qid for 3 days
4. Elevate extremity if extravasation is in an extremity

ADMINISTRATION

IV route

Do not substitute for doxorubicin HCl inj.
Administer 1st dose at an initial rate of 1mg/min; if no infusion-related adverse reactions are observed, increase infusion rate to complete the administration of the drug over 1 hr.
Do not administer as an undiluted sus or as an IV bolus.
Do not use w/ in-line filters.
Do not rapidly flush the IV line.
Do not mix w/ other drugs.

Preparation
Dilute doses up to 90mg in 250mL of D5 inj prior to administration.
Dilute doses >90mg in 500mL of D5 inj prior to administration.
Refrigerate diluted Doxil at 2-8°C (36-46°F) and administer w/in 24 hrs.

HOW SUPPLIED

Inj: 20mg/10mL, 50mg/25mL

CONTRAINDICATIONS

History of severe hypersensitivity reactions, including anaphylaxis, to doxorubicin HCl.

WARNINGS/PRECAUTIONS

Do not substitute for doxorubicin HCl inj. Administer only when potential benefits outweigh the risk in patients w/ a history of cardiovascular disease (CVD). Temporarily stop therapy in the event of an infusion-related reaction until resolution, then resume at a reduced infusion rate; d/c infusion for serious or life-threatening infusion-related reactions. HFS reported; d/c if HFS is severe and debilitating. Secondary oral cancers, primarily squamous cell carcinoma, reported w/ long-term (>1 yr) exposure; malignancies were diagnosed both during treatment and up to 6 yrs after last dose. Examine patients at regular intervals for the presence of oral ulceration or w/ any oral discomfort that may be indicative of secondary oral cancer. May cause fetal harm.

ADVERSE REACTIONS

Asthenia, fatigue, fever, N/V, stomatitis, diarrhea, constipation, anorexia, HFS, rash, neutropenia, thrombocytopenia, anemia.

PATIENT CONSIDERATIONS

Assessment: Assess for drug hypersensitivity, history of CVD, hepatic dysfunction, pregnancy/nursing status. Assess left ventricular cardiac function (eg, multigated acquisition, echocardiogram) prior to initiation of therapy.

Monitoring: Monitor for signs/symptoms of myocardial damage, infusion-related reactions, HFS, secondary oral cancers, and other adverse reactions. Monitor cardiac function.

Counseling: Instruct to contact physician if a new onset of fever, symptoms of an infection, or symptoms of HF develop. Advise about the symptoms of infusion-related reactions and instruct to seek immediate medical attention if any of these symptoms develop. Instruct to notify physician if symptoms of HFS or stomatitis develop. Advise females of reproductive potential of the potential risk to a fetus and to inform physician w/ a known or suspected pregnancy. Advise females and males of reproductive potential to use effective contraception during and for 6 months following treatment, and inform that therapy may cause temporary or permanent infertility. Instruct females not to breastfeed during treatment. Inform that a reddish-orange color may appear in urine and other body fluids.

STORAGE: **Unopened Vials:** 2-8°C (36-46°F). Do not freeze.

DRISDOL – ergocalciferol

RX

Class: Vitamin D analogue

D

ADULT DOSAGE

Hypoparathyroidism

50,000-200,000 IU daily given concomitantly w/ calcium lactate 4g, 6X/day

Vitamin D Resistant Rickets

12,000-500,000 IU daily

Other Indications

Familial Hypophosphatemia

PEDIATRIC DOSAGE

Hypoparathyroidism

50,000-200,000 IU daily given concomitantly w/ calcium lactate 4g, 6X/day

Vitamin D Resistant Rickets

12,000-500,000 IU daily

Other Indications

Familial Hypophosphatemia

DOSING CONSIDERATIONS

Elderly

Start at lower end of dosing range

ADMINISTRATION

Oral route

HOW SUPPLIED

Cap: 1.25mg (50,000 IU vitamin D)

CONTRAINDICATIONS

Hypercalcemia, malabsorption syndrome, abnormal sensitivity to the toxic effects of vitamin D, hypervitaminosis D.

WARNINGS/PRECAUTIONS

Avoid in infants w/ idiopathic hypercalcemia. Readjust the therapeutic dosage as soon as there is clinical improvement. Exercise great care in dose adjustment to prevent serious toxic effects; the range between therapeutic and toxic doses is narrow in vitamin D resistant rickets. IV Ca^{2+}, parathyroid hormone, and/or dihydrotachysterol may be required when treating hypoparathyroidism. Maintain normal serum phosphorus (P) levels (eg, dietary phosphate restriction and/or administration of aluminum gels) when treating hyperphosphatemia to prevent metastatic calcification. Adequate dietary Ca^{2+} is necessary for clinical response to vitamin D therapy. Contains FD&C Yellow No. 5 (tartrazine), which may cause allergic reactions (including bronchial asthma) in susceptible individuals. Avoid excess use of vitamin D during normal pregnancy, unless unique case outweighs the significant hazards.

ADVERSE REACTIONS

Anemia, anorexia, constipation, nausea, stiffness, weakness, calcification of soft tissues, impaired renal function, weight loss.

DRUG INTERACTIONS

Impaired absorption w/ mineral oil. Thiazide diuretics may cause hypercalcemia in hypoparathyroid patients.

PATIENT CONSIDERATIONS

Assessment: Assess for hypercalcemia, malabsorption syndrome, hypervitaminosis D, sensitivity to tartrazine, hypersensitivity to vitamin D in infants w/ idiopathic hypercalcemia, pregnancy/nursing status, and possible drug interactions. Evaluate vitamin D administration from fortified foods, dietary supplements, self-administered and prescription drug sources.

Monitoring: Monitor for clinical response to therapy and for adverse reactions. Monitor serum Ca^{2+} levels frequently in high doses. Perform monthly bone x-rays until condition is corrected and stabilized. In patients treated for hypoparathyroidism, monitor need for IV Ca^{2+}, parathyroid hormone, and/or dihydrotachysterol, have blood Ca^{2+} and P levels checked every 2 weeks or more frequently if necessary. Monitor serum Ca^{2+} in infants if a nursing mother is given large doses of vitamin D.

Counseling: Inform about risks/benefits of therapy and instruct to take ud. Counsel about signs/symptoms of hypervitaminosis D (eg, hypercalcemia, impaired renal function, calcification of soft tissues).

STORAGE: 25°C (77°F); excursions permitted to 15-30°C (59-86°F). Protect from light.

DUAVEE – bazedoxifene/conjugated estrogens

RX

Class: Estrogen/estrogen agonist and antagonist

D

Do not take additional estrogens. Increased risk of endometrial cancer in a woman w/ a uterus who uses unopposed estrogens. Perform adequate diagnostic measures to rule out malignancy in postmenopausal women w/ undiagnosed persistent or recurring abnormal genital bleeding. Should not be used for the prevention of cardiovascular disease (CVD) or dementia. Increased risk of stroke and deep vein thrombosis (DVT) reported in postmenopausal women (50-79 yrs of age) treated w/ daily oral conjugated estrogens (CEs) alone. Increased risk of probable dementia reported in postmenopausal women ≥65 yrs of age treated w/ daily conjugated estrogens alone. Estrogens should be prescribed at the lowest effective dose and for the shortest duration consistent w/ treatment goals and risks.

ADULT DOSAGE

Menopausal Vasomotor Symptoms

Moderate to Severe:
1 tab daily

Postmenopausal Osteoporosis

Prevention:
1 tab daily
Add supplemental Ca^{2+}/vitamin D if patient has inadequate dietary intake

PEDIATRIC DOSAGE

Pediatric use may not have been established

DOSING CONSIDERATIONS

Renal Impairment
Use not recommended

Elderly
Not recommended in women >75 years of age

ADMINISTRATION

Oral route
Swallow tab whole; take w/o regard to meals.

HOW SUPPLIED

Tab: (CEs/Bazedoxifene) 0.45mg/20mg

CONTRAINDICATIONS

Undiagnosed abnormal uterine bleeding; known/suspected/history of breast cancer; known/suspected estrogen-dependent neoplasia; active/history of DVT/pulmonary embolism (PE); active/history of arterial thromboembolic disease (eg, stroke, MI); hypersensitivity (eg, anaphylaxis, angioedema) to estrogens, bazedoxifene, or any ingredients; known hepatic impairment or disease; known protein C/protein S/antithrombin deficiency or other known thrombophilic disorders; pregnancy, women who may become pregnant, and nursing mothers.

WARNINGS/PRECAUTIONS

D/C immediately if stroke or DVT occurs or is suspected. If feasible, d/c at least 4-6 weeks before surgery of the type associated w/ an increased risk of thromboembolism, or during periods of prolonged immobilization. Not recommended for use in patients >75 yrs of age or in patients w/ renal impairment. May affect certain endocrine and blood components in lab tests. **CEs:** May increase risk of ovarian cancer and gallbladder disease requiring surgery. Retinal vascular thrombosis reported; d/c pending exam if sudden partial/complete loss of vision, or sudden onset of proptosis, diplopia, or migraine occurs. D/C permanently if exam reveals papilledema or retinal vascular lesions. May elevate BP and thyroid-binding globulin levels. May elevate plasma TGs, leading to pancreatitis in patients w/ preexisting hypertriglyceridemia; consider discontinuation of therapy if pancreatitis occurs. Caution w/ history of cholestatic jaundice associated w/ past estrogen use or w/ pregnancy; d/c in case of recurrence. May cause fluid retention. Caution w/ hypoparathyroidism; hypocalcemia may occur. May exacerbate symptoms of angioedema in women w/ hereditary angioedema. May exacerbate asthma, diabetes mellitus (DM), epilepsy, migraine, porphyria, systemic lupus erythematosus (SLE), and hepatic hemangiomas; caution in women w/ these conditions.

ADVERSE REACTIONS

Muscle spasms, nausea, diarrhea, dyspepsia, upper abdominal pain, oropharyngeal pain, dizziness, neck pain.

DRUG INTERACTIONS

Do not take progestins, additional estrogens, or additional estrogen agonist/antagonists. Itraconazole, a strong CYP3A4 inhibitor, reported to increase bazedoxifene and CE exposure. **CEs:** CYP3A4 inducers (eg, St. John's wort preparations, phenobarbital, carbamazepine) may decrease levels and may decrease therapeutic effects and/or result in changes in the uterine bleeding profile. Women dependent on thyroid hormone replacement therapy who are also receiving estrogens may require increased doses of their thyroid replacement therapy; monitor thyroid function.

Bazedoxifene: Substances known to induce uridine diphosphate glucuronosyltransferase (eg, rifampin, phenobarbital, carbamazepine) may increase metabolism, decrease exposure, and may be associated w/ an increase in risk of endometrial hyperplasia.

PATIENT CONSIDERATIONS

Assessment: Assess for undiagnosed abnormal uterine bleeding, presence/history of breast cancer, estrogen-dependent neoplasia, active/history of DVT/PE/arterial thromboembolic disease, hepatic impairment/disease, history of cholestatic jaundice, drug hypersensitivity, renal impairment, pregnancy/nursing status, any other conditions where treatment may be contraindicated or cautioned, and possible drug interactions.

Monitoring: Monitor for signs/symptoms of CVD; malignant neoplasms; gallbladder disease; dementia; visual abnormalities; BP and plasma TG elevations; pancreatitis; hypothyroidism; fluid retention; exacerbation of asthma, DM, epilepsy, migraine, porphyria, SLE, and hepatic hemangiomas; and other adverse reactions. Perform annual breast exam; schedule mammography based on age, risk factors, and prior mammogram results. Perform adequate diagnostic measures in patients w/ undiagnosed persistent or recurring genital bleeding. Perform periodic evaluation to determine treatment need.

Counseling: Advise to immediately report to physician any signs/symptoms related to venous thrombosis and thromboembolic events. Inform postmenopausal women of the importance of reporting vaginal bleeding to physician as soon as possible. Inform postmenopausal women of possible serious reactions of therapy (eg, cardiovascular disorders, malignant neoplasms, probable dementia), and possible less serious but common adverse reactions (eg, muscle spasms, nausea, diarrhea). Advise to add supplemental Ca^{2+} and/or vitamin D to the diet if daily intake is inadequate. Instruct to remove only 1 tab from the blister package at the time of use.

STORAGE: 20-25°C (68-77°F); excursions permitted to 15-30°C (59-86°F). Protect from moisture; do not place in pill boxes or pill organizers. After opening foil pouch, use w/in 60 days.

DUEXIS – famotidine/ibuprofen

RX

Class: H_2 blocker/NSAID

NSAIDs may increase risk of serious cardiovascular (CV) thrombotic events, myocardial infarction (MI), and stroke; increased risk with duration of use and with CV disease (CVD) or risk factors for CVD. Increased risk of serious GI adverse reactions (eg, bleeding, ulceration, and perforation of stomach/intestines) that can be fatal and occur anytime during use and without warning symptoms; elderly patients are at greater risk. Contraindicated for the treatment of perioperative pain in the setting of coronary artery bypass graft (CABG) surgery.

ADULT DOSAGE

Rheumatoid Arthritis

Relief of signs/symptoms of rheumatoid arthritis and to decrease the risk of developing upper GI ulcers in patients taking ibuprofen for this indication

1 tab tid

Osteoarthritis

Relief of signs/symptoms of osteoarthritis and to decrease the risk of developing upper GI ulcers in patients taking ibuprofen for this indication

1 tab tid

PEDIATRIC DOSAGE

Pediatric use may not have been established

ADMINISTRATION

Oral route

Swallow whole; do not cut, chew, divide, or crush

HOW SUPPLIED

Tab: (Ibuprofen/Famotidine) 800mg/26.6mg

CONTRAINDICATIONS

Patients who have experienced asthma, urticaria, or allergic reactions after taking aspirin (ASA) or other NSAIDs. Treatment of perioperative pain in the setting of CABG surgery. Patients in the late stages of pregnancy. History of hypersensitivity to other H_2-receptor antagonists.

WARNINGS/PRECAUTIONS

Use for the shortest possible duration. Symptomatic response does not preclude the presence of gastric malignancy. D/C with active and clinically significant bleeding. Periodically monitor Hgb if initial Hgb ≤10g and long-term therapy is going to be received. D/C if visual disturbances occur and perform ophthalmologic exam. May mask signs of inflammation and fever. Ibuprofen: May cause HTN or worsen preexisting HTN; caution with HTN, and monitor BP closely. Fluid retention and edema reported; caution with fluid retention or heart failure (HF). Caution with history of ulcer disease or GI bleeding, or risk factors for GI bleeding (eg, prolonged NSAID therapy, older age, poor general health status); monitor for GI ulceration/bleeding, and d/c if serious GI adverse reaction occurs. May exacerbate inflammatory bowel disease (IBD). Renal injury reported with long-term use; increased risk with renal/hepatic impairment, HF, and in elderly. D/C if clinical signs and symptoms consistent with renal disease develop. Anaphylaxis may occur; avoid with ASA triad. May cause serious skin adverse reactions; d/c at 1st appearance of skin rash or any sign of hypersensitivity. May cause elevated LFTs or severe hepatic reactions; d/c if liver disease or systemic manifestations occur. Anemia may occur; monitor Hgb/Hct if signs/symptoms of anemia develop with long-term use. May inhibit platelet aggregation and prolong bleeding time; monitor patients with coagulation disorders. Caution with preexisting asthma and avoid with ASA-sensitive asthma. Aseptic meningitis with fever and coma observed on rare occasions. Not a substitute for corticosteroids or for the treatment of corticosteroid insufficiency. Caution in elderly and debilitated. Famotidine: CNS adverse effects reported with moderate (CrCl <50mL/min) and severe renal insufficiency (CrCl <10mL/min); not recommended with CrCl <50mL/min.

ADVERSE REACTIONS

CV thrombotic events, MI, stroke, GI bleeding/ulceration/perforation, nausea, diarrhea, constipation, upper abdominal pain, headache, dyspepsia, upper respiratory tract infection, HTN.

DRUG INTERACTIONS

Increased risk of GI bleeding with oral corticosteroids, anticoagulants (eg, warfarin), antiplatelet drugs (including low-dose ASA), smoking, alcohol, and SSRIs. Risk of renal toxicity when coadministered with diuretics and ACE inhibitors. Avoid with other ibuprofen-containing products. Bleeding reported with coumarin-type anticoagulants. Increased risk of adverse events with ASA. May diminish effects of ACE inhibitors, thiazides, and loop (eg, furosemide) diuretics. May increase lithium levels; monitor for lithium toxicity. May enhance methotrexate toxicity; use with caution. Delayed absorption with cholestyramine.

PATIENT CONSIDERATIONS

Assessment: Assess for CABG surgery, CVD, a history of hypersensitivity to ASA or other NSAIDs, or any other conditions where treatment is contraindicated or cautioned. Assess for pregnancy/nursing status and for possible drug interactions. Obtain baseline BP, LFTs, CBC, and renal function.

Monitoring: Monitor for CV thrombotic events, GI events, active bleeding, anemia, anaphylaxis, skin reactions, visual disturbances, and other adverse reactions. Monitor BP, LFTs, renal function, CBC, and chemistry profiles.

Counseling: Inform of possible serious CV and GI side effects. Advise to d/c drug immediately and contact physician if any type of rash develops. Instruct to d/c therapy and seek immediate medical therapy if nephrotoxicity, hepatotoxicity, or anaphylaxis occurs. Advise to report signs/symptoms of unexplained weight gain or edema to physician. Inform that medication should be avoided in late pregnancy. Instruct on what to do if a dose is missed.

STORAGE: 25°C (77°F); excursions permitted to 15-30°C (59-86°F).

DULERA — formoterol fumarate dihydrate/mometasone furoate RX

Class: $Beta_2$ agonist/corticosteroid

Long-acting β_2-adrenergic agonists (LABAs), such as formoterol, increase the risk of asthma-related death. LABAs may increase the risk of asthma-related hospitalization in pediatric patients and adolescents. Use only for patients not adequately controlled on a long-term asthma control medication (eg, inhaled corticosteroid) or whose disease severity clearly warrants initiation of treatment with both an inhaled corticosteroid and LABA. Do not use if asthma is adequately controlled on low- or medium-dose inhaled corticosteroids.

ADULT DOSAGE

Asthma

Previously on Inhaled Medium Dose Corticosteroids:
2 inh of 100mcg-5mcg bid (am and pm)
Max: 400mcg-20mcg daily

Previously on Inhaled High Dose Corticosteroids:
2 inh of 200mcg-5mcg bid (am and pm)

PEDIATRIC DOSAGE

Asthma

≥12 Years:

Previously on Inhaled Medium Dose Corticosteroids:
2 inh of 100mcg-5mcg bid (am and pm)
Max: 400mcg-20mcg daily

Previously on Inhaled High Dose Corticosteroids:
2 inh of 200mcg-5mcg bid (am and pm)

Max: 800mcg-20mcg daily Do not use >2 inh bid of the prescribed strength. If inadequate response after 2 weeks of therapy, higher strength may provide additional asthma control	**Max:** 800mcg-20mcg daily Do not use >2 inh bid of the prescribed strength. If inadequate response after 2 weeks of therapy, higher strength may provide additional asthma control

ADMINISTRATION

Oral inh route

After inh, rinse mouth w/ water w/o swallowing

Shake well before use

Refer to PI for proper administration

Priming

Hold in the upright position and release 4 actuations (puffs) into the air, away from your face

After priming 4 times, the dose counter should read either "60" or "120"

If Dulera is not used for more than 5 days, prime again before use

HOW SUPPLIED

MDI: (Mometasone-Formoterol) 100mcg-5mcg/inh, 200mcg-5mcg/inh [60, 120 inh]

CONTRAINDICATIONS

Primary treatment of status asthmaticus or other acute episodes of asthma where intensive measures are required. Known hypersensitivity to mometasone furoate, formoterol fumarate, or any ingredients in the medication.

WARNINGS/PRECAUTIONS

Not indicated for the relief of acute bronchospasm. Do not initiate during rapidly deteriorating/potentially life-threatening episodes of asthma. D/C regular use of oral/inhaled short-acting β_2-agonists (SABAs) prior to treatment. Cardiovascular (CV) effects and fatalities reported with excessive use; do not use an additional LABA. *Candida albicans* infections of mouth and pharynx reported; treat and, if needed, interrupt therapy. Increased susceptibility to infections. May lead to serious/fatal course of chickenpox or measles; avoid exposure and, if exposed, consider prophylaxis/treatment. Caution with active/quiescent tuberculosis (TB), untreated systemic fungal, bacterial, viral, or parasitic infections, or ocular herpes simplex. Deaths due to adrenal insufficiency reported with transfer from systemic to inhaled corticosteroids; wean slowly from systemic corticosteroid use after transferring to therapy. Resume oral corticosteroids during periods of stress or a severe asthma attack if patient previously withdrawn from systemic corticosteroid. Transferring from systemic to inhalation therapy may unmask previously suppressed allergic conditions (eg, rhinitis, conjunctivitis, eczema). Observe for systemic corticosteroid withdrawal effects. Reduce dose slowly if hypercorticism and adrenal suppression appear. Inhalation induced bronchospasm with immediate increase in wheezing may occur; d/c immediately and institute alternative therapy. Immediate hypersensitivity reactions, and CV and CNS effects may occur. Decreases in bone mineral density (BMD) reported; caution with major risk factors for decreased bone mineral content, including chronic use of drugs that can reduce bone mass (eg, anticonvulsants, corticosteroids). May reduce growth velocity in pediatric patients. Glaucoma, increased intraocular pressure (IOP), and cataracts reported. Caution in elderly and patients with CV disorders, aneurysm, pheochromocytoma, convulsive disorders, thyrotoxicosis, and in patients unusually responsive to sympathomimetic amines. May cause changes in blood glucose and serum K^+ levels.

ADVERSE REACTIONS

Nasopharyngitis, sinusitis, headache, dysphonia.

DRUG INTERACTIONS

Do not use with other medications containing LABA; increased risk of CV effects. Caution with ketoconazole, other known strong CYP3A4 inhibitors (eg, ritonavir, clarithromycin, itraconazole), and non-K^+-sparing diuretics (eg, loop or thiazide diuretics). Elevated risk of arrhythmias with concomitant anesthesia with halogenated hydrocarbons. Mometasone: Increased plasma concentration with oral ketoconazole and increased systemic exposure with CYP3A4 inhibitors. Formoterol: Potentiation of sympathetic effects with additional adrenergic drugs; use with caution. Potentiation of hypokalemic effect with xanthine derivatives and diuretics. Caution with MAOIs, TCAs, macrolides, drugs known to prolong QTc interval or within 2 weeks of discontinuing such agents; effect on CV system may be potentiated. Use with β-blockers may block effects and produce severe bronchospasm in asthma patients; if needed, consider cardioselective β-blocker with caution.

PATIENT CONSIDERATIONS

Assessment: Assess for status asthmaticus, acute asthma episodes, rapidly deteriorating asthma, known hypersensitivity to any drug component, risk factors for decreased bone mineral content, CV or convulsive disorders, thyrotoxicosis, other conditions where treatment is contraindicated or cautioned, pregnancy/nursing status, and possible drug interactions. Obtain baseline BMD and lung function.

Monitoring: Monitor for localized oral *C. albicans* infections, glaucoma, increased IOP, cataracts, CV/CNS effects, hypercorticism, adrenal suppression, inhalation induced bronchospasm, hypokalemia, hyperglycemia, hypersensitivity reactions, signs of increased drug exposure with hepatic impairment, and other adverse reactions. Monitor BMD and lung function. Perform regular eye examinations. Monitor growth in pediatric patients routinely.

Counseling: Inform about increased risk of asthma-related hospitalization in pediatric patients/adolescents and asthma-related death. Instruct not to use to relieve acute asthma symptoms, if symptoms arise between doses, use an inhaled SABA for immediate relief. Instruct to seek medical attention if symptoms worsen, if lung function decreases, or if more inhalations than usual of a SABA are needed. If a dose is missed, instruct to take next dose at the same time patients normally do. Instruct not to d/c or reduce therapy without physician's guidance. Instruct not to use with other LABAs. Advise to avoid exposure to chickenpox or measles and, if exposed, consult physician without delay. Inform of potential worsening of existing TB, fungal, bacterial, viral, or parasitic infections, or ocular herpes simplex. Inform about risks of hypercorticism and adrenal suppression, decreased BMD, cataracts or glaucoma, oropharyngeal candidiasis, and reduced growth velocity in pediatric patients. Inform of adverse events associated with β_2-agonists. Instruct regarding use of therapy.

STORAGE: 20-25°C (68-77°F); excursions permitted to 15-30°C (59-86°F). Do not puncture. Do not use or store near heat or open flame. 60-inhalation inhaler: Store with the mouthpiece down or in a horizontal position after priming.

DUONEB – albuterol sulfate/ipratropium bromide — RX

Class: Anticholinergic/beta$_2$ agonist

ADULT DOSAGE

Bronchospasm

Associated w/ COPD:
3mL qid via nebulizer
May give up to 2 additional 3mL doses/day, prn

PEDIATRIC DOSAGE

Pediatric use may not have been established

ADMINISTRATION

Inh route

Administer via jet nebulizer connected to an air compressor w/ an adequate air flow, equipped w/ a mouthpiece or suitable face mask

HOW SUPPLIED

Sol, Inhalation: (Ipratropium Bromide-Albuterol Sulfate) 0.5mg-3mg/3mL

CONTRAINDICATIONS

History of hypersensitivity to any components in the medication, or to atropine and its derivatives.

WARNINGS/PRECAUTIONS

Paradoxical bronchospasm may occur; d/c immediately and institute alternative therapy if occurs. Fatalities reported with excessive use of inhaled products containing sympathomimetic amines and with home use of nebulizers. May produce significant cardiovascular (CV) effects (eg, ECG changes). Immediate hypersensitivity reactions reported. Caution with CV disorders (eg, coronary insufficiency, cardiac arrhythmias, HTN), convulsive disorders, hyperthyroidism, diabetes mellitus (DM), narrow-angle glaucoma, prostatic hypertrophy, bladder neck obstruction, hepatic/renal insufficiency, and in patients unusually responsive to sympathomimetic amines. Aggravation of preexisting DM and ketoacidosis reported with large doses of IV albuterol. May decrease serum K^+.

ADVERSE REACTIONS

Lung disease, pharyngitis, pain, chest pain, diarrhea, dyspepsia, nausea, leg cramps, bronchitis, pneumonia, UTI, constipation, voice alterations.

DRUG INTERACTIONS

Additive effects with other anticholinergic drugs; use with caution. Other sympathomimetic agents may increase risk of adverse CV effects; use with caution. β-blockers and albuterol inhibit the effect of each other; use β-blockers with caution in patients with hyperreactive airways. ECG changes and/or hypokalemia that may result from non-K^+-sparing diuretics (eg, loop or thiazide diuretics) may be worsened by β-agonists; use with caution. Administration with MAOIs or TCAs, or within 2 weeks of discontinuation of such agents may potentiate the action of albuterol on CV system; use with extreme caution.

PATIENT CONSIDERATIONS

Assessment: Assess for history of hypersensitivity to atropine and its derivatives, CV disorders, convulsive disorders, hyperthyroidism, DM, narrow-angle glaucoma, prostatic hypertrophy, bladder neck obstruction, hepatic/renal insufficiency, pregnancy/nursing status, and possible drug interactions. Assess use in patients unusually responsive to sympathomimetic amines.

Monitoring: Monitor for signs/symptoms of hypersensitivity reactions, paradoxical bronchospasm, CV effects, and other adverse reactions. Monitor pulse rate and BP. Reassess therapy if signs of worsening COPD occur.

Counseling: Advise not to exceed recommended dose or frequency without consulting physician. Instruct to contact physician if symptoms worsen. Instruct to avoid exposing eyes to this product as temporary pupillary dilation, blurred vision, eye pain, or precipitation/worsening of narrow-angle glaucoma may occur. Inform that proper nebulizer technique should be assured, particularly if a mask is used. Instruct to contact physician if pregnancy occurs or nursing is started while on therapy.

STORAGE: 2-25°C (36-77°F). Store in pouch until time of use. Protect from light.

DUOPA – carbidopa/levodopa

RX

Class: Dopa-decarboxylase inhibitor/dopamine precursor

ADULT DOSAGE

Parkinson's Disease

Prior to initiation of therapy, convert patient from all other forms of levodopa to oral immediate-release (IR) carbidopa-levodopa (1:4 ratio)

Initial:

Step 1: Calculate/Administer Morning Dose for Day 1:

a. Determine total amount of levodopa (in mg) in the 1st dose of oral IR carbidopa-levodopa that was taken on the previous day

b. Convert the levodopa dose from mg to mL by multiplying the oral dose by 0.8 and dividing by 20mg/mL (Morning Dose)

c. Add 3mL to the Morning Dose to prime the intestinal tube (Total Morning Dose)

d. Administer Total Morning Dose over 10-30 min

Step 2: Calculate/Administer Continuous Dose for Day 1:

a. Determine amount of oral IR levodopa the patient received from the oral IR carbidopa-levodopa doses throughout the previous day (16 waking hrs) in mg; do not include doses taken at night when calculating the levodopa amount

b. Subtract 1st oral levodopa dose taken by the patient on the previous day (determined in Step 1 (a)) from total oral levodopa dose (determined in Step 2 (a)) and divide the result by 20mg/mL to get the Continuous Dose (in mL) over 16 hrs

c. The hourly infusion rate (mL/hr) is obtained by dividing the Continuous Dose by 16 (hrs)

d. If persistent/numerous "Off" periods occur during the 16-hr infusion, consider increasing the Continuous Dose or using the Extra Dose function. If dyskinesia/levodopa-related adverse reactions occur, consider decreasing the Continuous Dose or stopping infusion until adverse reactions subside

Titrate:

Morning Dose:

Inadequate Response w/in 1 hr of Morning Dose on Preceding Day:

Morning Dose on Preceding Day ≤6mL:

Increase Morning Dose by 1 mL

PEDIATRIC DOSAGE

Pediatric use may not have been established

Morning Dose on Preceding Day >6mL:
Increase Morning Dose by 2mL
Exclude the 3mL to prime tube
Continuous Dose Adjustment:
Consider increasing dose based on clinical response and on the number/volume of Extra Doses that was needed for the previous day
Max: 2g of levodopa component (eg, 1 cassette/day) over 16 hrs
Extra Doses:
Initial: 1mL (20mg of levodopa)
Titrate: Increase in 0.2mL increments
Limit frequency to 1 extra dose q2h

D

DOSING CONSIDERATIONS

Adverse Reactions

Dyskinesia/Therapy-Related Adverse Reactions on Preceding Day:
Morning Dose: If patient experienced dyskinesias or therapy-related adverse reactions w/in 1 hr of Morning Dose on preceding day, then decrease morning dose by 1mL
Continuous Dose:
Troublesome Adverse Reactions Lasting for a Period of ≥1 hr: Decrease dose by 0.3mL/hr
Troublesome Adverse Reactions Lasting for 2 or More Periods of ≥1 hr: Decrease dose by 0.6mL/hr

Discontinuation

Avoid sudden discontinuation/rapid dose reduction; if patients need to d/c therapy, taper dose or switch to oral IR carbidopa-levodopa tabs
When using a PEG-J tube, may d/c by withdrawing tube and letting the stoma heal

ADMINISTRATION

Naso-jejunal/PEG-J route

Bring to room temperature before administration; 20 min prior to use, take 1 cassette out of the refrigerator/carton
Deliver as 16-hr infusion through either a naso-jejunal tube (short-term administration) or through a PEG-J tube (long-term administration)
Do not use cassettes for longer than 16 hrs; do not reuse an opened cassette
At the end of daily infusion, disconnect PEG-J tube from the pump, flush w/ room temperature potable water using a syringe, and take night-time dose of oral IR carbidopa-levodopa
Cassettes are specifically designed to be connected to the CADD-Legacy 1400 pump

Morning of PEG-J Procedure

Ensure patients take their oral Parkinson's disease medications

Refer to PI for tubing sets recommendations for long-term and short-term administration

HOW SUPPLIED

Sus: (Carbidopa/Levodopa) (4.63mg/20mg)/mL [100mL]

CONTRAINDICATIONS

Patients who are currently taking a nonselective MAOI (eg, phenelzine, tranylcypromine) or have recently (w/in 2 weeks) taken a nonselective MAOI.

WARNINGS/PRECAUTIONS

GI complications may occur and may result in serious outcomes (eg, need for surgery, death). Orthostatic hypotension reported; monitor especially after starting or increasing dose. Hallucinations, psychosis, and confusion reported; hallucinations may be responsive to a dose reduction of levodopa. Do not use in patients w/ a major psychotic disorder. Intense urges to gamble, increased sexual urges, intense urges to spend money, binge or compulsive eating, and/or other intense urges, and the inability to control these urges may occur; consider dose reduction or discontinuation if such urges develop. Depression reported. A symptom complex resembling neuroleptic malignant syndrome (hyperpyrexia and confusion) reported in association w/ rapid dose reduction, withdrawal of, or changes in dopaminergic therapy; avoid sudden discontinuation/rapid dose reduction and taper dose if discontinuing therapy. May cause or exacerbate dyskinesias; may require dose reduction of therapy or other medications used to treat PD. Polyneuropathy reported; monitor periodically for signs of neuropathy after starting therapy, especially in patients w/ preexisting neuropathy and in patients taking medications or those who have medical conditions associated w/ neuropathy. MI and arrhythmia reported; monitor for symptoms, especially those w/ a history of MI or cardiac arrhythmias. Perform periodic skin examinations to monitor for melanoma. May increase risk for elevated BUN and CPK. May increase levels of catecholamines and metabolites in plasma and urine, giving false-positive results suggesting the diagnosis of pheochromocytoma. May cause increased IOP in patients w/ glaucoma. Levodopa: Falling asleep during activities of daily living and somnolence reported; consider discontinuation if significant daytime sleepiness or episodes of falling asleep during activities that require active participation occur.

ADVERSE REACTIONS
Complication of device insertion, nausea, depression, peripheral edema, HTN, URTI, oropharyngeal pain, incision-site erythema, constipation, dyskinesia, atelectasis, confusional state, anxiety, dizziness, hiatal hernia.

DRUG INTERACTIONS
See Contraindications. Selective MAO-B inhibitors (eg, rasagiline, selegiline) may be associated w/ orthostatic hypotension; monitor patients. Antihypertensive medications may cause symptomatic postural hypotension; may need a dose reduction of antihypertensive medication after starting or increasing the dose of Duopa. Iron salts or multivitamins containing iron salts may form chelates and may reduce bioavailability; monitor for worsening Parkinson's symptoms. Levodopa: Caution w/ concomitant use of sedating medications; may increase the risk for somnolence. Dopamine D2 receptor antagonists (eg, phenothiazines, butyrophenones, risperidone, metoclopramide, papaverine) and isoniazid may reduce the effectiveness of levodopa; monitor for worsening Parkinson's symptoms. Absorption may be decreased in patients on a high-protein diet.

PATIENT CONSIDERATIONS

Assessment: Assess for major psychotic disorder, risk factors that may increase risk for somnolence (eg, presence of sleep disorders), peripheral neuropathy, history of MI or cardiac arrhythmias, glaucoma, pregnancy/nursing status, and possible drug interactions.

Monitoring: Monitor for GI complications, drowsiness or falling asleep during activities of daily living, orthostatic hypotension, hallucinations/psychosis/confusion, impulse control/compulsive behaviors, depression w/ suicidal tendencies, dyskinesias, neuropathy, ischemic heart disease, arrhythmia, and other adverse reactions. Monitor for hyperpyrexia and confusion if sudden discontinuation or rapid dose reduction occurs. Perform periodic skin examinations to monitor for melanoma. Monitor IOP in patients w/ glaucoma after starting therapy.

Counseling: Inform of risks and benefits of therapy. Instruct to inform physician of any previous surgery in the upper part of the abdomen. Advise that foods that are high in protein may reduce the effectiveness of therapy. Instruct to contact physician if experiencing symptoms of GI complications, depression or worsening of depression, suicidal thoughts, hallucinations, abnormal thinking, psychotic behavior, confusion, new/increased gambling urges, sexual urges, uncontrolled spending, binge/compulsive eating or other urges, or if any symptoms or features suggesting neuropathy develop. Inform of the potential sedating effects caused by therapy. Advise not to drive a car, operate machinery, or engage in other potentially dangerous activities until patient effects of therapy are known. Advise of possible additive effects when taking other sedating medications, alcohol, or other CNS depressants in combination w/ therapy. Inform that syncope and hypotension w/ or w/o symptoms may develop; caution against standing rapidly after sitting or lying down, especially if patient has been doing so for prolonged periods and especially at the initiation of treatment. Advise to contact physician before stopping therapy and to notify physician if withdrawal symptoms develop. Inform that therapy may cause or exacerbate preexisting dyskinesia. Advise to have a regular skin examination by a qualified healthcare provider.

STORAGE: -20°C (-4°F). Thaw at 2-8°C (36-46°F) prior to dispensing; refer to PI for thawing instructions. Protect from light.

DURAGESIC – fentanyl

CII

Class: Opioid analgesic

Exposes patients and other users to the risk of opioid addiction/abuse/misuse, which may lead to overdose and death; assess risk prior to therapy and monitor all patients regularly for development of these behaviors or conditions. Serious, life-threatening, or fatal respiratory depression may occur; monitor especially during initiation or following a dose increase. Contraindicated for use as a prn analgesic, in nonopioid tolerant patients, in acute pain, and in postoperative pain. Deaths due to fatal overdose have occurred from accidental exposure; strict adherence to handling/disposal instructions is of utmost importance to prevent accidental exposure. Prolonged use during pregnancy may result in neonatal opioid withdrawal syndrome. Concomitant use with all CYP3A4 inhibitors and discontinuation of a concomitantly administered CYP3A4 inducer may increase plasma concentrations and potentially cause fatal respiratory depression; monitor patients during concomitant therapy. Exposure of application site and surrounding area to direct external heat sources may increase absorption and result in fatal overdose and death; patients who develop fever or increased core body temperature due to strenuous exertion are at increased risk and may require dose adjustment.

ADULT DOSAGE

Severe Pain (Daily, Around-the-Clock Management)

Opioid-Tolerant Patients:
D/C or taper all other ER and around-the-clock opioids when beginning therapy

PEDIATRIC DOSAGE

Severe Pain (Daily, Around-the-Clock Management)

Opioid-Tolerant Patients:
≥2 Years:
D/C or taper all other ER and around-the-clock opioids when beginning therapy

D

25-300mcg/hr reapplied q72hr; initiate dosing regimen for each patient individually, taking into account the patient's prior analgesic treatment (refer to PI for dose conversions)

Titrate dose based on daily dose of supplemental opioid analgesics required on the 2nd or 3rd day of initial application; use the ratio of 45mg/24 hrs of oral morphine to a 12mcg/hr increase in fentanyl dose

Evaluate for further titration after no less than two 3-day applications before any further increase in dose

A small portion of patients may require systems to be applied q48h; an increase in dose should be evaluated before changing dosing interval

25-300mcg/hr reapplied q72hr; initiate dosing regimen for each patient individually, taking into account the patient's prior analgesic treatment (refer to PI for dose conversions)

Titrate dose based on daily dose of supplemental opioid analgesics required on the 2nd or 3rd day of initial application; use the ratio of 45mg/24 hrs of oral morphine to a 12mcg/hr increase in fentanyl dose

Evaluate for further titration after no less than two 3-day applications before any further increase in dose

A small portion of patients may require systems to be applied q48h; an increase in dose should be evaluated before changing dosing interval

DOSING CONSIDERATIONS

Renal Impairment

Mild to Moderate: Start w/ one half of the usual dosage

Severe: Avoid use

Hepatic Impairment

Mild to Moderate: Start w/ one half of the usual dosage

Severe: Avoid use

Discontinuation

Significant amounts of fentanyl continue to be absorbed from the skin for ≥24 hrs after the patch is removed

Converting to Another Opioid:

1. Remove patch and titrate the dose of the new analgesic based upon the patient's report of pain until adequate analgesia has been attained
2. Upon system removal, ≥17 hrs are required for a 50% decrease in serum fentanyl concentrations

Not Converting to Another Opioid:

Use a gradual downward titration (eg, having the dose every 6 days), in order to reduce the possibility of withdrawal symptoms; it is not known at what dose level fentanyl may be discontinued w/o producing the signs and symptoms of opioid withdrawal

Elderly

Start at lower end of the dosing range

ADMINISTRATION

Transdermal route

Application and Handling Instructions

1. Apply to intact, non-irritated, and non-irradiated skin on a flat surface such as the chest, back, flank, or upper arm; in young children and persons w/ cognitive impairment, adhesion should be monitored and the upper back is the preferred location to minimize the potential of inappropriate patch removal
2. Hair at the application site may be clipped (not shaved) prior to system application
3. If the application site must be cleansed prior to application of the patch, do so w/ clear water; do not use soaps, oils, lotions, alcohol, or any other agents that might irritate the skin or alter its characteristics. Allow the skin to dry completely prior to patch application
4. Apply immediately upon removal from the sealed package; the patch must not be altered (eg, cut) in any way prior to application. Do not use if the pouch seal is broken or if the patch is cut or damaged
5. Press the transdermal system firmly in place w/ the palm of the hand for 30 sec, making sure the contact is complete, especially around the edges
6. Each patch may be worn continuously for 72 hrs; the next patch is applied to a different skin site after removal of the previous transdermal system
7. If problems w/ adhesion of the patch occur, the edges of the patch may be taped w/ first aid tape; if adhesion problems persist, the patch may be overlaid w/ a transparent adhesive film dressing
8. If the patch falls off before 72 hrs, dispose of it by folding in 1/2 and flushing down the toilet; a new patch may be applied to a different skin site
9. Patients (or caregivers) should wash their hands immediately w/ soap and water after applying patch
10. Contact w/ unwashed or unclothed application sites can result in secondary exposure and should be avoided

Disposal Instructions
1. Patients should dispose of used patches immediately upon removal by folding the adhesive side of the patch to itself, then flushing down the toilet
2. Unused patches should be removed from their pouches, the protective liners removed, the patches folded so that the adhesive side of the patch adheres to itself, and immediately flushed down the toilet
3. Patients should dispose of any patches remaining from a prescription as soon as they are no longer needed

HOW SUPPLIED

Patch: 12mcg/hr, 25mcg/hr, 50mcg/hr, 75mcg/hr, 100mcg/hr [5[s]]

CONTRAINDICATIONS

Opioid-intolerant patients; management of acute/intermittent pain, or in patients who require opioid analgesia for a short period; management of postoperative pain, including use after outpatient/day surgeries (eg, tonsillectomies); management of mild pain; significant respiratory compromise, especially if adequate monitoring and resuscitative equipment are not readily available; acute or severe bronchial asthma; diagnosis or suspicion of paralytic ileus; known hypersensitivity to fentanyl or any components of the transdermal system.

WARNINGS/PRECAUTIONS

Should be prescribed only by healthcare professionals knowledgeable in the use of potent opioids for the management of chronic pain. Reserve for use in patients for whom alternative treatment options (eg, nonopioid analgesics, immediate-release opioids) are ineffective, not tolerated, or would be otherwise inadequate to provide sufficient management of pain. Do not use as the 1st opioid. Risk of addiction is increased with personal/family history of substance abuse or mental illness. Prescribe smallest appropriate quantity. Closely monitor elderly, cachectic, or debilitated patients for respiratory depression. May decrease respiratory drive to the point of apnea in patients with chronic pulmonary disease; consider use of other nonopioid analgesic alternatives if possible. Avoid in patients who may be susceptible to the intracranial effects of CO_2 retention. May obscure clinical course of head injury and may increase intracranial pressure (ICP); monitor patients with brain tumors. May cause severe hypotension, including orthostatic hypotension and syncope, in ambulatory patients; increased risk with reduced blood volume. May produce bradycardia. Avoid use with severe hepatic/renal impairment. May cause spasm of the sphincter of Oddi; monitor patients with biliary tract disease (eg, acute pancreatitis). May cause increases in serum amylase concentration. Tolerance and physical dependence may develop during chronic therapy. May impair mental/physical abilities. Significant absorption from the skin continues for ≥24 hrs after patch removal. Avoid abrupt discontinuation; use a gradual downward dose titration. Not for use in women during and immediately prior to labor.

ADVERSE REACTIONS

Respiratory depression, N/V, constipation, diarrhea, headache, muscle spasms, malaise, palpitations, dizziness, insomnia, somnolence, fatigue, feeling cold, hyperhidrosis, anorexia.

DRUG INTERACTIONS

See Boxed Warning. Monitor respiratory depression when given with other drugs that depress respiration. Concomitant use with CNS depressants (eg, other opioids, sedatives, alcohol) may cause respiratory depression, hypotension, profound sedation, coma, or death; closely monitor and reduce dose of 1 or both agents. Coadministration with CYP3A4 inducers may lead to lack of efficacy of fentanyl or development of withdrawal; monitor for signs of opioid withdrawal and consider dose adjustments until stable drug effects are achieved. Avoid concomitant use with MAOIs or within 14 days of stopping such treatment. Mixed agonist/antagonist (eg, pentazocine, nalbuphine, butorphanol) or partial agonist (buprenorphine) analgesics may reduce analgesic effect or may precipitate withdrawal symptoms; avoid concomitant use. Monitor for signs of urinary retention or reduced GI motility with anticholinergics or other medications with anticholinergic activity.

PATIENT CONSIDERATIONS

Assessment: Assess for degree of opioid tolerance, type and severity of pain, risks for opioid abuse, addiction, or misuse, paralytic ileus, acute/severe bronchial asthma, history of hypersensitivity to drug or any component of patch, debilitation, seizures, biliary tract disease, any other conditions where treatment is contraindicated or cautioned, pregnancy/nursing status, and possible drug interactions.

Monitoring: Monitor for signs/symptoms of respiratory depression, bradycardia, worsening of biliary tract disease, increased ICP, increased serum amylase levels, increased body temperature/fever, abuse, misuse, addiction, tolerance/physical dependence, opioid withdrawal syndrome in neonates born to mothers on prolonged therapy during pregnancy, and other adverse reactions.

Counseling: Inform that use of patch may result in addiction, abuse, and misuse, which may lead to overdose or death; instruct not to share with others and protect from theft, misuse, and from children. Inform of the risk of life-threatening respiratory depression; advise on how to recognize respiratory depression and to seek medical attention. Instruct to avoid accidental contact when holding or caring for children. Instruct to immediately take patch off if it dislodges and accidentally sticks to the skin of another person, wash exposed area with water, and seek medical attention. Advise to never change the dose/number of patches unless instructed. Advise how to safely taper medication and not to stop abruptly. Warn of the potential for temperature-dependent increases in drug release from patch; instruct to avoid strenuous exertion that may increase body temperature and avoid exposing application site and surrounding area to direct external heat sources. Counsel that medication may impair mental and/or physical ability; instruct patients to refrain from potentially hazardous tasks until therapy is established that they have not been adversely affected. Inform of pregnancy risks and advise women of childbearing potential who become/are planning to become pregnant to consult physician prior to initiating or continuing therapy. Advise to notify physician of all medications currently being taken and avoid using other CNS depressants and alcohol. Inform that severe constipation may develop. Instruct to refer to the instructions for use for proper disposal of patch.

STORAGE: Up to 25°C (77°F); excursions permitted to 15-30°C (59-86°F). Store in original unopened pouch.

DYANAVEL XR – amphetamine

CII

Class: CNS stimulant

High potential for abuse and dependence; assess risk of abuse prior to prescribing and monitor for signs of abuse/dependence while on therapy.

PEDIATRIC DOSAGE

Attention-Deficit Hyperactivity Disorder

≥6 Years:

Initial: 2.5mg or 5mg qam

Titrate: May increase in increments of 2.5-10mg/day every 4-7 days

Max: 20mg/day

Conversions

If switching from other amphetamine products, d/c that treatment, and titrate w/ Dyanavel XR using above titration schedule.

Do not substitute for other amphetamine products on a mg-per-mg basis.

DOSING CONSIDERATIONS

Concomitant Medications

Agents that alter urinary pH can impact urinary excretion and alter blood levels of amphetamine. Acidifying agents (eg, ascorbic acid) decrease blood levels, while alkalinizing agents (eg, sodium bicarbonate) increase blood levels; adjust dose accordingly.

ADMINISTRATION

Oral route

Administer w/ or w/o food.

Shake bottle before use.

HOW SUPPLIED

Oral Sus, Extended-Release: 2.5mg/mL [464mL]

CONTRAINDICATIONS

Known hypersensitivity to amphetamine or other components of this medication. During treatment w/ MAOIs and w/in 14 days following discontinuation of an MAOI.

WARNINGS/PRECAUTIONS

Prior to treatment, assess for the presence of cardiac disease. Sudden death, stroke, and MI reported in adults. Sudden death reported in children and adolescents w/ structural cardiac abnormalities and other serious heart problems. Avoid use in patients w/ known structural cardiac abnormalities, cardiomyopathy, serious heart arrhythmia, coronary artery disease, and other serious heart problems. Further evaluate patients who develop exertional chest pain, unexplained syncope, or arrhythmias during treatment. May increase BP and HR; monitor for tachycardia and HTN. May exacerbate symptoms of behavior disturbance and thought disorder in patients w/ preexisting psychotic disorder. May induce a mixed or manic episode in patients w/ bipolar disorder. Prior to initiation, screen patients for risk factors for developing a manic episode (eg, comorbid/history of depressive symptoms, family history of suicide, bipolar disorder, depression). May cause psychotic or manic symptoms in patients w/o prior history of psychotic illness or mania; consider discontinuing if such symptoms occur. May cause weight loss and slowing of growth rate in children; closely monitor growth (weight and height). Associated w/ peripheral vasculopathy, including Raynaud's phenomenon; signs/symptoms are usually intermittent and mild. Observe carefully for digital changes.

ADVERSE REACTIONS

Epistaxis, allergic rhinitis, upper abdominal pain.

DRUG INTERACTIONS

See Dosing Considerations and Contraindications. GI alkalinizing agents (eg, sodium bicarbonate) and urinary alkalinizing agents (eg, acetazolamide, some thiazides) increase blood levels and potentiate effects; avoid coadministration w/ GI alkalinizing agents. GI acidifying agents (eg, guanethidine, reserpine, glutamic acid HCl) and urinary acidifying agents (eg, ammonium chloride, sodium acid phosphate, methenamine salts) lower blood levels and efficacy. May enhance activity of TCAs (eg, desipramine, protriptyline) or sympathomimetic agents causing increases of d-amphetamine levels in the brain and possibly potentiating cardiovascular (CV) effects; monitor frequently, adjust dose, or use alternative therapy. Proton pump inhibitors (eg, omeprazole) increase T_{max} of amphetamine; monitor for changes in clinical effect and adjust therapy based on clinical response. May cause significant elevations in plasma corticosteroid levels; increase is greatest in evening. May interfere w/ urinary steroid determinations.

PATIENT CONSIDERATIONS

Assessment: Assess for presence of cardiac disease, risk of abuse, preexisting psychotic disorder, risk factors for developing a manic episode, pregnancy/nursing status, and possible drug interactions.

Monitoring: Monitor for CV reactions, tachycardia, HTN, psychiatric adverse reactions, peripheral vasculopathy including Raynaud's phenomenon, and other adverse reactions. Monitor growth (weight and height) in children. Periodically reevaluate long-term use of therapy. Monitor for signs of abuse and dependence while on therapy. Monitor infants born to mothers taking amphetamines for symptoms of withdrawal.

Counseling: Inform about benefits and risks of treatment, appropriate administration instructions, and about the potential for abuse/dependence. Advise of serious CV risk and elevations in BP/pulse rate; instruct to contact physician immediately if symptoms such as exertional chest pain, unexplained syncope, or other symptoms suggestive of cardiac disease develop. Advise that at recommended doses, treatment may cause psychotic or manic symptoms, even w/o a prior history of psychotic symptoms or mania. Inform that treatment may cause slowing of growth and weight loss. Inform about the risk of peripheral vasculopathy, including Raynaud's phenomenon; instruct to report to physician any new numbness, pain, skin color change, or sensitivity to temperature in fingers or toes, and to call physician immediately if any signs of unexplained wounds appear on fingers or toes while on therapy. Advise patients of the potential fetal effects from the use of therapy during pregnancy; instruct to notify physician if pregnant/planning to become pregnant during treatment. Advise to avoid breastfeeding. Advise patients to avoid alcohol while taking drug.

STORAGE: 20-25°C (68-77°F); excursions permitted from 15-30°C (59-86°F).

DYAZIDE – hydrochlorothiazide/triamterene

RX

Class: Potassium-sparing diuretic/thiazide diuretic

Abnormal elevation of serum K^+ levels (≥5.5mEq/L) may occur w/ all K^+-sparing diuretic combinations. Hyperkalemia is more likely to occur w/ renal impairment and diabetes (even w/o evidence of renal impairment), and in elderly or severely ill; monitor serum K^+ levels at frequent intervals.

ADULT DOSAGE

Edema

1-2 caps PO qd

Hypertension

1-2 caps PO qd

PEDIATRIC DOSAGE

Pediatric use may not have been established

ADMINISTRATION

Oral route

HOW SUPPLIED

Cap: (HCTZ-Triamterene) 25mg-37.5mg

CONTRAINDICATIONS

Anuria, acute and chronic renal insufficiency or significant renal impairment, hypersensitivity to the drug or to other sulfonamide-derived drugs, preexisting elevated serum K^+ (hyperkalemia), K^+-sparing agents (eg, spironolactone, amiloride, or other formulations containing triamterene), K^+ salt substitutes, K^+ supplements (except w/ severe hypokalemia).

WARNINGS/PRECAUTIONS

Avoid in severely ill in whom respiratory or metabolic acidosis may occur; if used, frequent evaluations of acid/base balance and serum electrolytes are necessary. May cause idiosyncratic reaction, resulting in acute transient myopia and acute angle-closure glaucoma; d/c as rapidly as possible. Caution w/ diabetes; may cause hyperglycemia and glycosuria. Diabetes mellitus (DM) may become manifest. Caution w/ hepatic impairment; may precipitate hepatic coma w/ severe liver disease. Corrective measures must be taken if hypokalemia develops; d/c and initiate potassium chloride (KCl) supplementation if serious hypokalemia develops (serum K^+ <3.0mEq/L). May potentiate electrolyte imbalance w/ heart failure, renal disease, or cirrhosis of the liver. May cause hypochloremia. Dilutional hyponatremia may occur in edematous patients in hot weather. Caution w/ history of renal stones. May increase BUN and SrCr. May decrease serum PBI levels. Decreased Ca^{2+} excretion reported. Changes in parathyroid glands w/ hypercalcemia and hypophosphatemia reported during prolonged therapy. May interfere w/ the fluorescent measurement of quinidine.

ADVERSE REACTIONS

Muscle cramps, N/V, pancreatitis, weakness, arrhythmia, impotence, dry mouth, jaundice, paresthesia, renal stones, anaphylaxis, acute renal failure, hyperkalemia, hyponatremia.

DRUG INTERACTIONS

See Contraindications. Increased risk of hyperkalemia w/ ACE inhibitors, blood from blood bank, and low-salt milk. Increased risk of severe hyponatremia w/ chlorpropamide. Possible interaction resulting in acute renal failure w/ indomethacin; caution w/ NSAIDs. Avoid w/ lithium due to risk of lithium toxicity. Decreased arterial responsiveness to norepinephrine. Amphotericin B, corticosteroids, and corticotropin may intensify electrolyte imbalance, particularly hypokalemia. Adjust dose of antigout drugs to control hyperuricemia and gout. May decrease effect of oral anticoagulants. May alter insulin requirements. Increased paralyzing effects of nondepolarizing muscle relaxants (eg, tubocurarine). Reduced K^+ levels w/ chronic or overuse of laxatives or use of exchange resins (eg, sodium polystyrene sulfonate). May reduce effectiveness of methenamine. May potentiate action of other antihypertensive drugs (eg, β-blockers).

PATIENT CONSIDERATIONS

Assessment: Assess for anuria, renal/hepatic impairment, sulfonamide hypersensitivity, hyperkalemia, diabetes, history of renal stones, pregnancy/nursing status, and for possible drug interactions. Obtain baseline BUN, SrCr, and serum electrolytes.

Monitoring: Monitor for signs/symptoms of hype/hypokalemia, hyperglycemia, hypochloremia, renal stones, and for electrolyte imbalance. Monitor for hepatic coma in patients w/ severe liver disease. Monitor serum K^+ levels, BUN, SrCr, and serum electrolytes.

Counseling: Inform about risks/benefits of therapy. Advise to seek medical attention if symptoms of hyperkalemia (eg, paresthesias, muscular weakness, fatigue), hypokalemia, hyperglycemia, renal stones, electrolyte imbalance (eg, dry mouth, thirst, weakness), or hypersensitivity reactions occur.

STORAGE: 20-25°C (68-77°F); excursions permitted to 15-30°C (59-86°F). Protect from light. Dispense in a tight, light-resistant container.

DYMISTA – azelastine hydrochloride/fluticasone propionate RX

Class: Corticosteroid/H_1 antagonist

ADULT DOSAGE

Seasonal Allergic Rhinitis

1 spray in each nostril bid

PEDIATRIC DOSAGE

Seasonal Allergic Rhinitis

≥6 Years:
1 spray in each nostril bid

DOSING CONSIDERATIONS

Elderly

Dose cautiously; start at lower end of dosing range

ADMINISTRATION

Intranasal route

Shake the bottle gently before each use

Priming

Prime pump before initial use by releasing 6 sprays or until a fine mist appears
Reprime w/ 1 spray or until a fine mist appears if not used for ≥14 days

HOW SUPPLIED

Spray: (Azelastine/Fluticasone) (137mcg/50mcg)/spray [23g]

WARNINGS/PRECAUTIONS

Somnolence reported; may impair mental/physical abilities. Epistaxis reported. Nasal ulceration and septal perforation reported; avoid w/ recent nasal ulcers, nasal surgery, or nasal trauma. Development of localized infections of the nose and pharynx w/ *Candida albicans* may occur; may require discontinuation and treatment w/ appropriate local therapy if infection develops. Examine periodically for evidence of *Candida* infection or other signs of adverse effects on nasal mucosa if used over several months or longer. D/C slowly if hypercorticism and adrenal suppression occur. Fluticasone: May result in development of glaucoma and/or cataracts; closely monitor patients w/ change in vision or w/ history of increased IOP, glaucoma, and/or cataracts. May increase susceptibility to infections; caution w/ active or quiescent tuberculosis (TB) of the respiratory tract; untreated local or systemic fungal or bacterial infections; systemic viral or parasitic infections; or ocular herpes simplex. Avoid exposure to chickenpox and measles. Risk of adrenal insufficiency and withdrawal symptoms when replacing systemic corticosteroids w/ topical corticosteroids. May cause growth velocity reduction in pediatric patients.

ADVERSE REACTIONS

Dysgeusia, headache, epistaxis, pyrexia, cough, nasal congestion, rhinitis, viral infection, URTI, pharyngitis, pain, diarrhea, N/V, otitis media/externa.

DRUG INTERACTIONS

Avoid w/ alcohol or other CNS depressants. Fluticasone: Ritonavir and other strong CYP3A4 inhibitors may increase exposure; not recommended w/ ritonavir and caution w/ other potent CYP3A4 inhibitors (eg, ketoconazole). Concomitant use of intranasal corticosteroids w/ other inhaled corticosteroids could increase the risk of signs/symptoms of hypercorticism and/or hypothalamic-pituitary-adrenal axis suppression.

PATIENT CONSIDERATIONS

Assessment: Assess for recent nasal ulcers/surgery/trauma, active or quiescent TB, systemic viral/parasitic infections, ocular herpes simplex, untreated fungal/bacterial infections, history of IOP, glaucoma, cataracts, pregnancy/nursing status, and possible drug interactions.

Monitoring: Monitor for somnolence, epistaxis, nasal ulceration, nasal septal perforation, changes in vision, glaucoma, cataracts, hypercorticism, adrenal suppression, and for the development/exacerbation of infections. Routinely monitor growth of pediatric patients.

Counseling: Caution against engaging in hazardous occupations requiring complete mental alertness and motor coordination (eg, driving, operating machinery). Advise to avoid w/ alcohol and other CNS depressants. Instruct to inform physician if a change in vision is noted. Instruct to avoid exposure to chickenpox or measles and, if exposed, to consult physician w/o delay. Inform of potential worsening of existing TB, fungal, bacterial, viral or parasitic infections, or ocular herpes simplex. Counsel that corticosteroids may cause reduction in growth velocity in pediatric patients. Instruct to avoid spraying into eyes; if sprayed in the eyes, instruct to flush eyes w/ water for at least 10 min. Discard the bottle after 120 medicated sprays have been used. Instruct to notify physician of all medications currently taking.

STORAGE: 20-25°C (68-77°F). Store upright w/ dust cap in place. Protect from light. Do not store in the freezer or refrigerator.

ECONAZOLE CREAM — econazole nitrate

RX

Class: Azole antifungal

OTHER BRAND NAMES

Spectazole (Discontinued)

ADULT DOSAGE

Fungal Infections

Cutaneous Candidiasis:
Apply bid (am/pm) for 2 weeks

Tinea Versicolor:
Apply qd for 2 weeks

Tinea Corporis, Tinea Cruris, and Tinea Pedis caused by *Trichophyton rubrum*, *T. mentagrophytes*, *T. tonsurans*, *Microsporum canis*, *M. audouini*, *M. gypseum*, and *Epidermophyton floccosum*:
Apply qd

Tinea Corporis and Tinea Cruris:
Treat for 2 weeks

Tinea Pedis:
Treat for 4 weeks

Reevaluate if no improvement after treatment period

PEDIATRIC DOSAGE

Pediatric use may not have been established

ADMINISTRATION
Topical route

HOW SUPPLIED
Cre: 1% [15g, 30g, 85g]

CONTRAINDICATIONS
Hypersensitivity to any of the ingredients.

WARNINGS/PRECAUTIONS
D/C if sensitivity or chemical irritation occurs.

ADVERSE REACTIONS
Burning, itching, stinging, erythema.

DRUG INTERACTIONS
Coadministration with warfarin resulted in enhancement of anticoagulation effect; monitoring of INR/PT may be indicated especially in patients who apply the medication to large BSAs, in the genital area, or under occlusion.

PATIENT CONSIDERATIONS

Assessment: Assess for hypersensitivity to drug, pregnancy/nursing status, and possible drug interactions.

Monitoring: Monitor for signs/symptoms of sensitivity reaction or chemical irritation, and other adverse reactions. Monitor clinical improvement. May need to monitor INR/PT with warfarin, especially in patients who apply the medication to large BSA, in the genital area, or under occlusion.

Counseling: Counsel that medication is for external use only and to avoid contact with eyes. Instruct to notify physician if any signs of a sensitivity reaction or chemical irritation develop or if signs/symptoms do not improve by end of treatment period.

STORAGE: <30°C (86°F).

EDARBI – azilsartan medoxomil RX

Class: Angiotensin II receptor blocker (ARB)

D/C when pregnancy is detected. Drugs that act directly on the renin-angiotensin system (RAS) can cause injury/death to the developing fetus.

ADULT DOSAGE

Hypertension

Usual: 80mg qd

W/ High Dose Diuretics:
Initial: 40mg qd

PEDIATRIC DOSAGE
Pediatric use may not have been established

ADMINISTRATION
Oral route

Take w/ or w/o food

HOW SUPPLIED
Tab: 40mg, 80mg

CONTRAINDICATIONS
Coadministration with aliskiren in patients with diabetes.

WARNINGS/PRECAUTIONS
Symptomatic hypotension may occur in patients with an activated RAS (eg, volume- and/or salt-depleted patients receiving high doses of diuretics); correct this condition prior to therapy or start treatment at 40mg. Changes in renal function may occur. Oliguria and/or progressive azotemia and (rarely) acute renal failure and/or death may occur in patients whose renal function is dependent on the RAS (eg, severe CHF, renal artery stenosis, volume depletion). Increases in SrCr or BUN in patients with renal artery stenosis reported.

ADVERSE REACTIONS
Dizziness, postural dizziness, nausea, asthenia, fatigue, muscle spasm, cough, diarrhea.

DRUG INTERACTIONS
See Contraindications. NSAIDs, including selective COX-2 inhibitors, may deteriorate renal function and attenuate the antihypertensive effect. Dual blockade of the RAS is associated with increased risks of hypotension, hyperkalemia, and changes in renal function (including acute renal failure); avoid combined use of RAS inhibitors. Closely monitor BP, renal function, and electrolytes with concomitant agents that also affect the RAS. Avoid with aliskiren in patients with renal impairment

(GFR <60mL/min). Increases in lithium levels and lithium toxicity reported; monitor lithium levels. Increases in SrCr may be larger with chlorthalidone or HCTZ.

PATIENT CONSIDERATIONS

Assessment: Assess for volume/salt depletion, renal impairment, CHF, renal artery stenosis, diabetes, pregnancy/nursing status, and possible drug interactions.

Monitoring: Monitor for signs/symptoms of hypotension and other adverse reactions. Monitor BP and renal function.

Counseling: Inform of pregnancy risks; instruct to notify physician as soon as possible if pregnant/planning to become pregnant. Advise to seek medical attention if symptoms of hypotension or other adverse events occur.

STORAGE: 25°C (77°F); excursions permitted to 15-30°C (59-86°F). Protect from moisture and light.

EDARBYCLOR – azilsartan medoxomil/chlorthalidone

RX

Class: Angiotensin II receptor blocker (ARB)/monosulfamyl diuretic

D/C when pregnancy is detected. Drugs that act directly on the renin-angiotensin system (RAS) can cause injury/death to the developing fetus.

ADULT DOSAGE

Hypertension

Initial: 40mg/12.5mg qd
Titrate: May increase to 40mg/25mg after 2-4 weeks prn to achieve BP goals
Max: 40mg/25mg

Add-On Therapy:
Use if not adequately controlled on ARBs or diuretic monotherapy

Replacement Therapy:
May receive the corresponding dose of the titrated individual components

May be administered w/ other antihypertensive agents

PEDIATRIC DOSAGE

Pediatric use may not have been established

DOSING CONSIDERATIONS

Adverse Reactions

Dose-Limiting Adverse Reaction on Chlorthalidone: Initially give w/ a lower dose of chlorthalidone

ADMINISTRATION

Oral route

Take w/ or w/o food

HOW SUPPLIED

Tab: (Azilsartan/Chlorthalidone) 40mg/12.5mg, 40mg/25mg

CONTRAINDICATIONS

Anuria. Coadministration w/ aliskiren in patients w/ diabetes.

WARNINGS/PRECAUTIONS

Symptomatic hypotension may occur in patients w/ activated RAS (eg, volume- and/or salt-depleted patients receiving high doses of diuretics); correct this condition prior to therapy. Consider withholding or discontinuing therapy if progressive renal impairment becomes evident. Azilsartan: Changes in renal function may occur. Oliguria and/or progressive azotemia and (rarely) acute renal failure and/or death may occur in patients whose renal function is dependent on the RAS (eg, severe CHF). Increases in BUN or SrCr in patients w/ renal artery stenosis reported. May cause hyperkalemia. Chlorthalidone: May cause fetal/neonatal jaundice and thrombocytopenia. May precipitate azotemia w/ renal disease. May cause hyponatremia and hypokalemia. Hyperuricemia may occur or frank gout may be precipitated. May precipitate hepatic coma in patients w/ hepatic dysfunction or progressive liver disease.

ADVERSE REACTIONS

Dizziness, syncope, hypotension, diarrhea, nausea, asthenia, fatigue, muscle spasm, cough, rash, headache, GI upset, elevation of uric acid and cholesterol.

DRUG INTERACTIONS

See Contraindications. May increase risk of symptomatic hypotension w/ high-dose diuretics. May increase risk of lithium toxicity; monitor lithium levels. Azilsartan: NSAIDs, including selective COX-2 inhibitors, may deteriorate renal function and attenuate the antihypertensive effect. Dual blockade of the RAS is associated w/ increased risks of hypotension, hyperkalemia, and changes in renal function, including acute renal failure; avoid combined use of RAS inhibitors. Closely monitor BP, renal function, and electrolytes w/ concomitant agents that affect the RAS. Avoid w/ aliskiren in patients w/ renal impairment (GFR <60mL/min). Chlorthalidone: Coadministration w/ digitalis may exacerbate the adverse effect of hypokalemia.

PATIENT CONSIDERATIONS

Assessment: Assess for anuria, volume/salt depletion, CHF, renal/hepatic function, renal artery stenosis, pregnancy/nursing status, and possible drug interactions. Obtain baseline BP.

Monitoring: Monitor for signs/symptoms of hypotension, hyperuricemia, precipitation of frank gout, and other adverse reactions. Monitor BP and hepatic/renal function. Monitor serum electrolytes periodically.

Counseling: Inform about the consequences of exposure during pregnancy and discuss treatment options in women planning to become pregnant. Instruct to report pregnancy to the physician as soon as possible. If a dose is missed, instruct to take it later in the same day; advise not to double the dose on the following day. Instruct to report gout symptoms and lightheadedness; advise to d/c and consult physician if syncope occurs. Inform that dehydration from excessive perspiration, vomiting, and diarrhea may lead to an excessive fall in BP; advise to consult physician if these occur. Advise patients w/ renal impairment to receive periodic blood tests while on therapy.

STORAGE: 25°C (77°F); excursions permitted to 15-30°C (59-86°F). Protect from moisture and light.

EDURANT – rilpivirine

RX

Class: Non-nucleoside reverse transcriptase inhibitor (NNRTI)

ADULT DOSAGE

HIV-1 Infection

In combination w/ other antiretrovirals, in antiretroviral treatment-naive patients w/ HIV-1 RNA ≤100,000 copies/mL at the start of therapy

25mg qd

PEDIATRIC DOSAGE

HIV-1 Infection

In combination w/ other antiretrovirals, in antiretroviral treatment-naive patients w/ HIV-1 RNA ≤100,000 copies/mL at the start of therapy

≥12 Years:
≥35kg:
25mg qd

DOSING CONSIDERATIONS

Concomitant Medications

W/ Rifabutin: Increase Edurant dose to 50mg qd; when coadministration is stopped, decrease dose to 25mg qd

ADMINISTRATION

Oral route

Take w/ a meal.

HOW SUPPLIED

Tab: 25mg

CONTRAINDICATIONS

Concomitant use w/ carbamazepine, oxcarbazepine, phenobarbital, phenytoin, rifampin, rifapentine, proton pump inhibitors (eg, esomeprazole, lansoprazole, omeprazole, pantoprazole, rabeprazole), systemic dexamethasone (more than a single dose), and St. John's wort.

WARNINGS/PRECAUTIONS

Severe skin and hypersensitivity reactions reported, including cases of drug reaction w/ eosinophilia and systemic symptoms; d/c immediately and initiate appropriate therapy if signs/symptoms develop. Depressive disorders reported; immediate medical evaluation is recommended if severe depressive symptoms occur. Hepatotoxicity reported; underlying hepatitis B or C, or marked elevation in transaminases prior to treatment may increase risk for worsening or development of transaminase elevations. Consider liver enzyme monitoring in patients w/o preexisting hepatic dysfunction or other risk factors. Immune reconstitution syndrome, redistribution/accumulation of body fat, and autoimmune disorders (eg, Graves' disease, polymyositis, Guillain-Barre syndrome) in the setting of immune reconstitution reported. Caution w/ severe renal impairment or ESRD; monitor for adverse effects. Caution in elderly.

ADVERSE REACTIONS

Lab abnormalities (increased SrCr, AST/ALT, total bilirubin, total cholesterol, LDL), depressive disorders, insomnia, headache, rash, somnolence, N/V, dizziness, abdominal pain.

DRUG INTERACTIONS

See Dosing Considerations and Contraindications. Caution w/ drugs that may reduce exposure. Coadministration w/ CYP3A inducers or drugs that increase gastric pH may result in decreased levels, loss of virologic response, and possible resistance to rilpivirine or to the class of non-nucleoside reverse transcriptase inhibitors (NNRTIs). CYP3A inhibitors may increase levels. Not recommended w/ delavirdine and other NNRTIs (eg, efavirenz, etravirine, nevirapine). Concomitant didanosine should be given on an empty stomach and at least 2 hrs before or at least 4 hrs after therapy. Darunavir/ritonavir (RTV), lopinavir/RTV, unboosted protease inhibitors (PIs) or other boosted PIs (w/ RTV), may increase levels. Azole antifungals may increase levels; monitor for breakthrough fungal infections w/ azole antifungals. May decrease ketoconazole levels. Clarithromycin, erythromycin, or telithromycin may increase levels; consider alternatives (eg, azithromycin) when possible. Rifabutin may decrease levels. Antacids and H_2-receptor antagonists may significantly decrease levels. Administer antacids either at least 2 hrs before or at least 4 hrs after therapy. Administer H_2-receptor antagonists at least 12 hrs before or at least 4 hrs after therapy. Clinical monitoring is recommended w/ methadone as methadone maintenance therapy may need to be adjusted in some patients. Caution w/ drugs that have a known risk of torsades de pointes.

PATIENT CONSIDERATIONS

Assessment: Assess for severe renal impairment or ESRD, underlying hepatic disease, marked transaminase elevations, pregnancy/nursing status, and possible drug interactions. Perform appropriate lab testing in patients w/ underlying hepatic disease or w/ marked transaminase elevations.

Monitoring: Monitor for severe skin and hypersensitivity reactions, depressive disorders, immune reconstitution syndrome, autoimmune disorders, fat redistribution/accumulation, hepatotoxicity, and other adverse reactions.

Counseling: Inform that product is not a cure for HIV infection; advise that continuous therapy is necessary to control HIV infection and decrease HIV-related illnesses. Advise to continue to practice safer sex and to use latex or polyurethane condoms. Instruct never to reuse or share needles. Inform mothers to avoid nursing to reduce risk of transmission of HIV to their baby. Advise to take medication ud. Advise not to alter the dose or d/c therapy w/o consulting physician. If a dose is missed w/in 12 hrs of the time it is usually taken, instruct to take as soon as possible w/ a meal and then to take the next dose at the regular scheduled time. If dose is missed by >12 hrs of the time it is usually taken, instruct not to take the missed dose, but resume the usual dosing schedule. Advise to report to physician the use of any other prescription/nonprescription or herbal products (eg, St. John's wort). Inform of the signs/symptoms of severe skin and hypersensitivity reactions and instruct to immediately stop taking therapy and seek medical attention if a rash develops associated w/ such symptoms. Inform patients that lab tests will be performed and appropriate therapy will be initiated if severe rash occurs. Instruct to seek medical evaluation if depressive symptoms are experienced. Inform that hepatotoxicity has been reported and redistribution/accumulation of body fat may occur.

STORAGE: 25°C (77°F); excursions permitted to 15-30°C (59-86°F). Protect from light.

EFFEXOR XR – venlafaxine

RX

Class: Serotonin and norepinephrine reuptake inhibitor (SNRI)

Antidepressants increased the risk of suicidal thoughts and behavior in children, adolescents, and young adults in short-term studies. Monitor closely for clinical worsening and emergence of suicidal thoughts and behaviors.

ADULT DOSAGE

Major Depressive Disorder

Initial: 75mg/day as a single dose, or 37.5mg/day for 4-7 days and then increase to 75mg/day

Titrate: May increase by increments of up to 75mg/day at ≥4-day intervals

Max: 225mg/day

Anxiety Disorders

Generalized Anxiety Disorder:

Initial: 75mg/day as a single dose, or 37.5mg/day for 4-7 days and then increase to 75mg/day

PEDIATRIC DOSAGE

Pediatric use may not have been established

Titrate: May increase by increments of up to 75mg/day at ≥4-day intervals
Max: 225mg/day

Social Anxiety Disorder:
75mg/day as a single dose

Panic Disorder

W/ or w/o Agoraphobia:
Initial: 37.5mg/day for 7 days
Titrate: May increase by increments of up to 75mg/day at ≥7-day intervals
Max: 225mg/day

Conversions

Switching from Effexor Immediate-Release (IR) Tabs:
Depressed patients currently being treated at a therapeutic dose w/ Effexor IR tabs may be switched to Effexor XR at the nearest equivalent dose (mg/day); individual dose adjustments may be necessary

Dosing Considerations with MAOIs

Switching to/from an MAOI for Psychiatric Disorders:
Allow at least 14 days between discontinuation of an MAOI and initiation of treatment, and allow at least 7 days between discontinuation of treatment and initiation of an MAOI

W/ Other MAOIs (eg, Linezolid, IV Methylene Blue):
Do not start venlafaxine in patients being treated w/ linezolid or IV methylene blue. Consider other interventions (eg, hospitalization) in patients who require more urgent treatment of a psychiatric condition

If acceptable alternatives are not available, d/c venlafaxine and administer linezolid or IV methylene blue. Monitor for serotonin syndrome for 7 days or until 24 hrs after the last dose of linezolid or IV methylene blue, whichever comes 1st. May resume venlafaxine therapy 24 hrs after last dose of linezolid or IV methylene blue

DOSING CONSIDERATIONS

Renal Impairment
Mild (CrCl 60-89mL/min) or Moderate (CrCl 30-59mL/min): Reduce total daily dose by 25-50%
Severe (CrCl <30mL/min) or Hemodialysis: Reduce total daily dose by ≥50%

Hepatic Impairment
Mild (Child-Pugh 5-6) to Moderate (Child-Pugh 7-9): Reduce total daily dose by 50%
Severe (Child-Pugh 10-15) or Hepatic Cirrhosis: May need to reduce by ≥50%

Discontinuation
Gradually reduce dose (eg, reducing daily dose by 75mg at 1-week intervals)

ADMINISTRATION

Oral route

Take w/ food at same time each day, either in am or pm.
Swallow whole w/ fluid and do not divide, crush, chew, or place in water.
May take by carefully opening the cap and sprinkling the entire contents on a spoonful of applesauce; swallow immediately w/o chewing and follow w/ glass of water.

HOW SUPPLIED

Cap, Extended-Release: 37.5mg, 75mg, 150mg

CONTRAINDICATIONS

Hypersensitivity to venlafaxine HCl, desvenlafaxine succinate, or to any excipients in the formulation. Use of an MAOI for psychiatric disorders either concomitantly or w/in 7 days of discontinuing treatment. Treatment w/in 14 days of discontinuing an MAOI for psychiatric disorders. Starting treatment in patients being treated w/ other MAOIs (eg, linezolid, IV methylene blue).

WARNINGS/PRECAUTIONS

Not approved for the treatment of bipolar depression. Serotonin syndrome reported; d/c immediately and initiate supportive symptomatic treatment. Dose-related increases in systolic and diastolic BP, as well as sustained HTN, reported; control preexisting HTN before initiating treatment and consider dose reduction or discontinuation for patients who experience a sustained increase in BP. May increase the risk of bleeding events. Pupillary dilation that occurs following use may trigger an angle-closure attack in a patient w/ anatomically narrow angles who does not have a patent iridectomy. Mania/hypomania reported. Avoid abrupt discontinuation; gradually reduce dose. Seizures reported; d/c if seizures develop. Hyponatremia may occur; consider discontinuation in patients w/ symptomatic hyponatremia. Interstitial lung disease (ILD) and eosinophilic pneumonia rarely reported; consider discontinuation if symptoms occur. Caution w/ preexisting HTN or cardiovascular (CV) or cerebrovascular conditions that might be compromised by increases in BP, history of mania/hypomania, history of seizures, and in the elderly. False (+) urine immunoassay screening tests for phencyclidine and amphetamines reported.

ADVERSE REACTIONS

Asthenia, sweating, N/V, constipation, anorexia, dry mouth, dizziness, insomnia, nervousness, somnolence, abnormal ejaculation/orgasm, impotence, decreased libido.

DRUG INTERACTIONS

See Contraindications. May cause serotonin syndrome w/ other serotonergic drugs (eg, triptans, TCAs, fentanyl) and w/ drugs that impair metabolism of serotonin; d/c therapy and any concomitant serotonergic agents immediately if this occurs. Not recommended w/ weight-loss agents or tryptophan supplements. Increased risk of hyponatremia w/ diuretics. Increased risk of bleeding w/ aspirin (ASA), NSAIDs, warfarin, and other anticoagulants or other drugs known to affect platelet function. Avoid w/ ethanol. Increased levels w/ cimetidine; use w/ caution in patients w/ HTN, hepatic dysfunction, or in the elderly. Increased levels w/ ketoconazole; use w/ caution. May increase metoprolol levels; use w/ caution and monitor BP. Caution w/ other CNS-active drugs.

PATIENT CONSIDERATIONS

Assessment: Assess for history of mania/hypomania, seizures, HTN, susceptibility to angle-closure glaucoma, CV/cerebrovascular conditions, volume depletion, hepatic/renal impairment, hypersensitivity to the drug, pregnancy/nursing status, and possible drug interactions. Perform adequate screening to determine if patient is at risk for bipolar disorder; such screening should include a detailed psychiatric history, including a family history of suicide, bipolar disorder, and depression. Monitor BP before initiating treatment.

Monitoring: Monitor for signs/symptoms of clinical worsening, suicidality, unusual behavior, serotonin syndrome, sustained HTN, abnormal bleeding, angle-closure glaucoma, activation of mania/hypomania, hyponatremia, seizures, ILD, eosinophilic pneumonia, and other adverse reactions. Monitor BP regularly during treatment. If discontinued abruptly, monitor for discontinuation symptoms (eg, dysphoric mood, confusion, agitation). Carefully monitor patients receiving concomitant warfarin therapy when treatment is initiated or discontinued. Periodically reassess to determine the need for maintenance or continued treatment.

Counseling: Inform about the risks and benefits of therapy. Advise to look for emergence of suicidality, worsening of depression, and unusual changes in behavior, especially early during treatment and when the dose is adjusted up or down. Advise not to use concomitantly w/ other venlafaxine- or desvenlafaxine-containing products. Instruct not to take w/ an MAOI or w/in 14 days of stopping an MAOI and to allow 7 days after stopping treatment before starting an MAOI. Caution about the risk of serotonin syndrome. Advise to have regular BP monitoring during therapy. Caution that concomitant use w/ ASA, NSAIDs, warfarin, or other drugs that affect coagulation may increase the risk of bleeding. Inform about the risk of angle-closure glaucoma in susceptible individuals. Advise patients, families, and caregivers to observe for signs of activation of mania/hypomania. Advise that elevations in total cholesterol, LDL, and TGs may occur and that measurement of serum lipids may be considered. Advise not to stop taking medication w/o first talking w/ a healthcare professional; inform that discontinuation effects may occur when stopping treatment. Caution against operating hazardous machinery (including automobiles) until reasonably certain that therapy does not adversely affect ability to engage in such activities. Advise to avoid alcohol while on therapy. Advise to notify physician if allergic phenomena develops, or if pregnant, intending to become pregnant, or if breastfeeding. Inform that spheroids may be passed in the stool or via colostomy.

STORAGE: 20-25°C (68-77°F).

EFFIENT – prasugrel

RX

Class: Antiplatelet agent

May cause significant, sometimes fatal, bleeding; risk factors include <60kg body weight, propensity to bleed, and concomitant use of medications that increase risk of bleeding (eg, warfarin, heparin, fibrinolytic therapy, chronic use of NSAIDs). Do not use in patients w/ active pathological bleeding or a history of transient ischemic attack (TIA) or stroke. Not recommended in patients ≥75 yrs of age, due to increased risk of fatal and intracranial bleeding and uncertain benefit, except in high-risk situations (diabetes or history of prior MI) where the effect appears to be greater and use may be considered. Do not start in patients likely to undergo urgent CABG; d/c at least 7 days prior to any surgery, when possible. Suspect bleeding in any patient who is hypotensive and has recently undergone coronary angiography, percutaneous coronary intervention (PCI), CABG, or other surgical procedures. If possible, manage bleeding w/o discontinuing the drug. Discontinuing therapy, particularly in the 1st few weeks after acute coronary syndrome (ACS), increases the risk of subsequent cardiovascular (CV) events.

E

ADULT DOSAGE

Acute Coronary Syndrome

To reduce the rate of thrombotic CV events (including stent thrombosis) in patients who are to be managed w/ PCI as follows: patients w/ unstable angina or non-ST-elevation MI or patients w/ ST-elevation MI when managed w/ primary or delayed PCI

LD: 60mg as a single dose

Maint: 10mg qd

Take w/ aspirin (75-325mg/day)

PEDIATRIC DOSAGE

Pediatric use may not have been established

DOSING CONSIDERATIONS

Other Important Considerations

Low Body Weight:

<60kg: Consider lowering the maint dose to 5mg qd

ADMINISTRATION

Oral route

Take w/ or w/o food

Do not break the tab

HOW SUPPLIED

Tab: 5mg, 10mg

CONTRAINDICATIONS

Active pathological bleeding (eg, peptic ulcer, intracranial hemorrhage), history of prior TIA or stroke, hypersensitivity (eg, anaphylaxis) to prasugrel or any component of the product.

WARNINGS/PRECAUTIONS

Withholding a dose will not be useful in managing a bleeding event or the risk of bleeding associated w/ an invasive procedure. D/C for active bleeding, elective surgery, stroke, or TIA. Avoid therapy lapses; if temporary discontinuation is needed because of an adverse event(s), restart as soon as possible. Thrombotic thrombocytopenic purpura (TTP) reported; may occur after a brief exposure (<2 weeks) and requires urgent treatment (eg, plasmapheresis). Hypersensitivity including angioedema reported. Increased risk for bleeding w/ severe hepatic impairment or moderate to severe renal impairment.

ADVERSE REACTIONS

Bleeding, HTN, hypercholesterolemia/hyperlipidemia, headache, back pain, dyspnea, nausea, dizziness, cough, hypotension, fatigue, noncardiac chest pain.

DRUG INTERACTIONS

See Boxed Warning.

PATIENT CONSIDERATIONS

Assessment: Assess for active pathological bleeding, history of prior TIA or stroke, other risk factors for bleeding, hypersensitivity, pregnancy/nursing status, and possible drug interactions. Assess likelihood of undergoing urgent CABG.

Monitoring: Monitor for signs/symptoms of bleeding, TTP, hypersensitivity, stroke, TIA, and other adverse reactions.

Counseling: Inform about the benefits and risks of treatment. Instruct to take exactly as prescribed and not to d/c w/o consulting the prescribing physician. Inform that patient may bruise and bleed more easily and that bleeding will take longer than usual to stop. Advise to report to physician any unanticipated, prolonged, or excessive bleeding, or blood in stool/urine. Inform that TTP, a rare but serious condition, has been reported; instruct to seek prompt medical attention if experiencing unexplained fever, weakness, extreme skin paleness, purple skin patches, yellowing of skin/eyes, or neurological changes. Inform that hypersensitivity reactions may occur. Instruct to notify physicians and dentists about therapy before scheduling any invasive procedure.

STORAGE: 25°C (77°F); excursions permitted to 15-30°C (59-86°F).

EFUDEX – fluorouracil

RX

Class: Antimetabolite

ADULT DOSAGE

Multiple Actinic or Solar Keratoses

Apply sufficient amount to cover the lesions bid. Continue use until inflammatory response reaches the erosion stage

Usual Duration: 2-4 weeks

Superficial Basal Cell Carcinomas

5%:

Apply sufficient amount to cover the lesions bid. Continue use for at least 3-6 weeks

May be required for as long as 10-12 weeks before lesions are obliterated

Use when conventional methods are impractical (eg, w/ multiple lesions or difficult treatment sites)

PEDIATRIC DOSAGE

Pediatric use may not have been established

ADMINISTRATION

Topical route

Apply preferably w/ a nonmetal applicator or suitable glove

If applied w/ the fingers, wash the hands immediately afterward

HOW SUPPLIED

Cre: 5% [40g]; **Sol:** 2%, 5% [10mL, 25mL]

CONTRAINDICATIONS

Women who are or may become pregnant, dihydropyrimidine dehydrogenase (DPD) enzyme deficiency, known hypersensitivity to any of the components.

WARNINGS/PRECAUTIONS

Avoid application to mucous membranes; local inflammation and ulceration may occur. If any occlusive dressing is used in treatment of basal cell carcinoma, there may be an increase in the severity of inflammatory reactions in the adjacent normal skin; a porous gauze dressing may be applied for cosmetic reasons without increase in reaction. Minimize exposure to UV rays during and immediately following treatment; intensity of the reaction may be increased. D/C if symptoms of DPD enzyme deficiency develop. Increased absorption through ulcerated or inflamed skin may occur. Not for ophthalmic, oral, or intravaginal use.

ADVERSE REACTIONS

Burning, crusting, allergic contact dermatitis, pruritus, scarring, rash, soreness, ulceration, leukocytosis.

PATIENT CONSIDERATIONS

Assessment: Assess for drug hypersensitivity, DPD enzyme deficiency, skin ulceration/inflammation, and pregnancy/nursing status.

Monitoring: Monitor for local reactions, and other adverse effects. Biopsy solar keratoses that do not respond to confirm the diagnosis. Perform follow-up biopsies as indicated in the management of superficial basal cell carcinoma.

Counseling: Inform that the reaction in the treated areas may be unsightly during therapy and, usually, for several weeks following cessation of therapy. Instruct to avoid exposure to UV rays during and immediately following treatment. Advise not to apply on the eyelids or directly into the eyes, nose, or mouth.

STORAGE: 25°C (77°F); excursions permitted to 15-30°C (59-86°F).

Elepsia XR – levetiracetam

RX

Class: Pyrrolidine derivative

ADULT DOSAGE

Partial Onset Seizures

Adjunctive Therapy in Patients w/ Epilepsy:
Initial: 1000mg qd
Titrate: May adjust dose in increments of 1000mg every 2 weeks
Max: 3000mg qd

PEDIATRIC DOSAGE

Partial Onset Seizures

Adjunctive Therapy in Patients w/ Epilepsy:
≥12 Years:
Initial: 1000mg qd
Titrate: May adjust dose in increments of 1000mg every 2 weeks
Max: 3000mg qd

E

DOSING CONSIDERATIONS

Renal Impairment

Mild (CrCl 50-80mL/min): 1000-2000mg q24h
Moderate/Severe: Not recommended

ADMINISTRATION

Oral route

Swallow whole; do not split or cut tab

HOW SUPPLIED

Tab, Extended-Release: 1000mg, 1500mg

WARNINGS/PRECAUTIONS

Increased risk of suicidal thoughts/behavior. May cause behavioral abnormalities, somnolence, fatigue, and coordination difficulties. May impair mental/physical abilities. Serious dermatological reactions (eg, Stevens-Johnson syndrome [SJS], toxic epidermal necrolysis [TEN]) reported. Recurrence of serious skin reactions following rechallenge reported; d/c at 1st sign of rash, unless rash is clearly not drug-related. If signs/symptoms suggest SJS/TEN, do not resume therapy; consider alternative therapy. Withdraw gradually to minimize potential of increased seizure frequency. Hematologic abnormalities may occur. Physiological changes may gradually decrease plasma levels throughout pregnancy; decrease is more pronounced during 3rd trimester. Caution in elderly.

ADVERSE REACTIONS

Nausea, influenza, nasopharyngitis, somnolence, dizziness, irritability.

PATIENT CONSIDERATIONS

Assessment: Assess for renal impairment, depression, suicidal thoughts/behavior, and pregnancy/nursing status.

Monitoring: Monitor for emergence or worsening of depression, suicidal thoughts/behavior, and/or any unusual changes in mood or behavior; somnolence/fatigue; coordination difficulties; serious dermatological reactions; hematologic abnormalities; and other adverse reactions. Monitor patients carefully during pregnancy and continue close monitoring through the postpartum period, especially if the dose was changed during pregnancy.

Counseling: Counsel patients, their caregivers, and/or families that drug may increase risk of suicidal thoughts/behavior; instruct to immediately report emergence or worsening of symptoms of depression, any unusual changes in mood/behavior, or suicidal thoughts, behavior, or thoughts about self-harm to physician. Counsel that medication may cause changes in behavior (eg, irritability, aggression). Inform that dizziness and somnolence may occur; advise not to drive or operate heavy machinery or engage in other hazardous activities until patient has gained sufficient experience to gauge whether drug adversely affects patient's performance of these activities. Advise that serious dermatological adverse reactions may occur; instruct to notify physician immediately if rash develops. Inform that each coated bilayer tab consists of a distinctly visible blue layer and a white to off-white layer; advise not to consume tab if 1 layer is absent and to report this to the pharmacist. Advise to notify physician if pregnancy occurs or is intended while on drug; encourage to enroll in the North American Antiepileptic Drug pregnancy registry if pregnant.

STORAGE: 20-25°C (68-77°F); excursions permitted between 15-30°C (59-86°F).

ELIDEL – pimecrolimus

RX

Class: Calcineurin-inhibitor immunosuppressant

Rare cases of malignancy (eg, skin and lymphoma) reported with topical calcineurin inhibitors, including pimecrolimus, although causal relationship is not established. Avoid long-term use, and application should be limited to areas of involvement with atopic dermatitis. Not indicated for children <2 yrs or age.

ADULT DOSAGE

Atopic Dermatitis

Short-term/noncontinuous chronic treatment (2nd line) of mild to moderate atopic dermatitis in patients who have failed to respond adequately to other topical treatments, or when those treatments are not advisable

Apply thin layer to the affected skin bid until signs and symptoms resolve

Reexamine if signs and symptoms persist beyond 6 weeks

PEDIATRIC DOSAGE

Atopic Dermatitis

Short-term/noncontinuous chronic treatment (2nd line) of mild to moderate atopic dermatitis in patients who have failed to respond adequately to other topical treatments, or when those treatments are not advisable

≥2 Years:

Apply thin layer to the affected skin bid until signs and symptoms resolve

Reexamine if signs and symptoms persist beyond 6 weeks

ADMINISTRATION

Topical route

HOW SUPPLIED

Cre: 1% [30g, 60g, 100g]

CONTRAINDICATIONS

History of hypersensitivity to pimecrolimus or any components of the medication.

WARNINGS/PRECAUTIONS

Avoid with malignant or premalignant skin conditions, Netherton's syndrome, or other skin diseases that may increase the potential for systemic absorption. Avoid in immunocompromised patients. May cause local symptoms, such as skin burning or pruritus, and may improve as the lesions of atopic dermatitis resolve. Resolve bacterial or viral infections at treatment sites before starting treatment. Increased risk of varicella zoster and herpes simplex virus infection, or eczema herpeticum. Skin papilloma/warts reported; consider discontinuation until complete resolution is achieved if skin papillomas worsen or do not respond to conventional therapy. Lymphadenopathy reported; d/c if lymphadenopathy of uncertain etiology or in the presence of acute infectious mononucleosis. Minimize or avoid natural or artificial sunlight exposure during treatment.

ADVERSE REACTIONS

Application-site burning, application-site reaction, influenza, nasopharyngitis, headache, URTI, sore throat, hypersensitivity, cough, pyrexia, N/V, skin infection, abdominal pain.

DRUG INTERACTIONS

Caution with CYP3A4 inhibitors (eg, erythromycin, ketoconazole, calcium channel blockers) in patients with widespread and/or erythrodermic disease.

PATIENT CONSIDERATIONS

Assessment: Assess for malignant or premalignant skin conditions, Netherton's syndrome, or other skin diseases that may increase the potential for systemic absorption, immunocompromised state, viral/bacterial skin infections, pregnancy/nursing status, and possible drug interactions.

Monitoring: Monitor for varicella virus infection, herpes simplex virus infection, eczema herpeticum, skin papilloma/warts, lymphomas, lymphadenopathy, skin malignancies, local symptoms, and other adverse reactions.

Counseling: Instruct to use ud. Inform not to use continuously for a long time and to use only on areas of skin with eczema. Instruct not to use sun lamps, tanning beds, or get treatment with UV light therapy. Advise to limit sun exposure, wear loose fitting clothing that protects the treated area from the sun, and not to cover treated skin area with bandages, dressings, or wraps. Inform that the medication is for use on the skin only; instruct to avoid contact with eyes, nose, mouth, vagina, or rectum (mucous membranes). Instruct to wash hands and dry skin before applying cre and not to bathe, shower, or swim after application.

STORAGE: 25°C (77°F); excursions permitted to 15-30°C (59-86°F). Do not freeze.

ELIQUIS – apixaban

RX

Class: Selective factor Xa inhibitor

Premature discontinuation increases the risk of thrombotic events. If therapy is discontinued for a reason other than pathological bleeding or completion of a course of therapy, consider coverage w/ another anticoagulant. Epidural or spinal hematomas may occur in patients treated w/ apixaban who are receiving neuraxial anesthesia or undergoing spinal puncture; long-term or permanent paralysis may result. Increased risk of developing epidural/spinal hematomas w/ the use of indwelling epidural catheters, concomitant use of other drugs that affect hemostasis, (eg, NSAIDs, platelet inhibitors, other anticoagulants), history of traumatic or repeated epidural or spinal punctures, history of spinal deformity or spinal surgery, and when optimal timing between the administration of apixaban and neuraxial procedure is not known. Monitor frequently for signs/symptoms of neurologic impairment; urgent treatment is necessary if neurologic compromise is noted. Consider benefits and risks before neuraxial intervention in patients anticoagulated or to be anticoagulated.

E

ADULT DOSAGE

Reduce Risk of Stroke and Systemic Embolism in Nonvalvular Atrial Fibrillation

5mg bid

Patients w/ at Least 2 of the Following Characteristics:
≥80 Years, ≤60kg, or SrCr ≥1.5mg/dL:
2.5mg bid

Deep Vein Thrombosis/Pulmonary Embolism

Deep Vein Thrombosis (DVT) Prophylaxis Following Hip/Knee Replacement Surgery:
2.5mg bid; give initial dose 12-24 hrs after surgery

Duration:
Hip Replacement Surgery: 35 days
Knee Replacement Surgery: 12 days

DVT/Pulmonary Embolism (PE) Treatment:
10mg bid for the first 7 days, followed by 5mg bid

Risk Reduction of Recurrent DVT/PE:
2.5mg bid after at least 6 months of treatment for DVT/PE

Conversions

Switching from Warfarin:
D/C warfarin and start apixaban when INR <2.0

Switching to Warfarin:
D/C apixaban and begin both a parenteral anticoagulant and warfarin at the time the next dose of apixaban would have been taken; d/c parenteral anticoagulant when INR reaches an acceptable range

Switching from Anticoagulants Other Than Warfarin (Oral or Parenteral):
D/C the anticoagulant and begin apixaban at the usual time of the next dose of the anticoagulant

Switching to Anticoagulants Other Than Warfarin (Oral or Parenteral):
D/C apixaban and begin the new anticoagulant at the usual time of the next dose of apixaban

PEDIATRIC DOSAGE

Pediatric use may not have been established

DOSING CONSIDERATIONS

Concomitant Medications

Strong Dual CYP3A4 and P-gp Inhibitors (eg, Ketoconazole, Itraconazole, Ritonavir):
For patients receiving apixaban doses of 5mg or 10mg bid, reduce apixaban dose by 50%; if already taking 2.5mg bid, avoid coadministration w/ strong dual inhibitors of CYP3A4 and P-gp

Hepatic Impairment

Severe (Child-Pugh Class C): Not recommended

Other Important Considerations

Temporary Interruption for Surgery and Other Interventions:
D/C at least 48 hrs prior to elective surgery or invasive procedures w/ a moderate/high risk of unacceptable/clinically significant bleeding, or at least 24 hrs prior w/ a low risk of bleeding or where

bleeding would be noncritical in location and easily controlled. Bridging anticoagulation during the 24-48 hrs after discontinuing therapy and prior to the intervention is not generally required. Restart therapy after the surgical or other procedures as soon as adequate hemostasis has been established

ADMINISTRATION

Oral route

Patients Unable to Swallow Tabs Whole

Tabs may be crushed and suspended in 60mL D5W and immediately delivered through a NG tube.

HOW SUPPLIED

Tab: 2.5mg, 5mg

CONTRAINDICATIONS

Active pathological bleeding, severe hypersensitivity reaction to apixaban (eg, anaphylactic reactions).

WARNINGS/PRECAUTIONS

Not recommended in patients w/ prosthetic heart valves. Increases the risk of bleeding and may cause serious, potentially fatal, bleeding; d/c in patients w/ active pathological hemorrhage. Specific antidote for apixaban is not available; activated oral charcoal reduces apixaban absorption. In patients who receive both apixaban and neuraxial anesthesia, removal of indwelling epidural or intrathecal catheters should not be earlier than 24 hrs after the last administration of apixaban; next dose of apixaban should not be administered earlier than 5 hrs after the removal of the catheter. If traumatic spinal/epidural puncture occurs, delay administration of apixaban for 48 hrs. Initiation of apixaban is not recommended as an alternative to unfractionated heparin for the initial treatment of patients w/ PE who present w/ hemodynamic instability or who may receive thrombolysis or pulmonary embolectomy.

ADVERSE REACTIONS

Bleeding.

DRUG INTERACTIONS

See Boxed Warning and Dosing Considerations. CYP3A4 and P-gp inhibitors increase exposure and increase the risk of bleeding. CYP3A4 and P-gp inducers decrease exposure and increase the risk of stroke and other thromboembolic events. Avoid w/ strong dual inducers of CYP3A4 and P-gp (eg, rifampin, carbamazepine, phenytoin, St. John's wort). Increased risk of bleeding w/ drugs affecting hemostasis, including aspirin (ASA) and other antiplatelet agents, other anticoagulants, heparin, thrombolytics, SSRIs, SNRIs, NSAIDs, and fibrinolytics.

PATIENT CONSIDERATIONS

Assessment: Assess for drug hypersensitivity, active pathological bleeding, prosthetic heart valves, PE w/ hemodynamic instability or in patients who may receive thrombolysis or pulmonary embolectomy, hepatic/renal impairment, pregnancy/nursing status, and possible drug interactions.

Monitoring: Monitor for active pathological hemorrhage and other adverse reactions. Monitor for thrombotic events in patients discontinuing therapy. In patients undergoing neuraxial anesthesia or spinal puncture, monitor for epidural or spinal hematomas and neurological impairment.

Counseling: Instruct not to d/c w/o consulting physician. Inform that it may take longer than usual for bleeding to stop, and that bruising/bleeding may occur more easily. Advise on how to recognize bleeding/symptoms of hypovolemia and of the urgent need to report any unusual bleeding to physician. Instruct to inform physicians and dentists of apixaban use, and/or any other product known to affect bleeding (eg, ASA or NSAIDs), before any surgery/medical/dental procedure is scheduled and before any new drug is taken. Advise patients having neuraxial anesthesia or spinal puncture to watch for signs/symptoms of spinal/epidural hematomas (eg, numbness, weakness of legs, bowel/bladder dysfunction); instruct to contact physician immediately if symptoms occur. Advise to inform physician if pregnant/planning to become pregnant, or if breastfeeding/intending to breastfeed during treatment. If a dose is missed, instruct to take it as soon as possible on the same day and that bid administration should be resumed; instruct not to double the dose to make up for a missed dose.

STORAGE: 20-25°C (68-77°F); excursions permitted to 15-30°C (59-86°F).

ELLA — ulipristal acetate

RX

Class: Emergency contraceptive kit

ADULT DOSAGE

Emergency Contraception

1 tab as soon as possible w/in 120 hrs (5 days) after unprotected intercourse or a known or suspected contraceptive failure

Consider repeating the dose if vomiting occurs w/in 3 hrs of intake

PEDIATRIC DOSAGE

Emergency Contraception

Postpubertal:

1 tab as soon as possible w/in 120 hrs (5 days) after unprotected intercourse or a known or suspected contraceptive failure

Consider repeating the dose if vomiting occurs w/in 3 hrs of intake

ADMINISTRATION

Oral route

Can be taken at any time during the menstrual cycle, w/ or w/o food

HOW SUPPLIED

Tab: 30mg

CONTRAINDICATIONS

Known or suspected pregnancy.

WARNINGS/PRECAUTIONS

Not for routine use as a contraceptive. Not indicated for termination of existing pregnancy. Exclude pregnancy prior to prescribing; perform pregnancy test if pregnancy cannot be excluded based on history and/or physical examination. Consider possibility of ectopic pregnancy if lower abdominal pain or pregnancy occurs following use. Repeated use within the same menstrual cycle is not recommended. Rapid return of fertility may occur following treatment; continue or initiate routine contraception as soon as possible following use. After intake, menses sometimes occur earlier or later than expected by a few days; rule out pregnancy if there is a delay in the onset of expected menses beyond 1 week. Intermenstrual bleeding reported. Does not protect against HIV infection (AIDS) or other sexually transmitted infections.

ADVERSE REACTIONS

Headache, abdominal/upper abdominal pain, nausea, dysmenorrhea, fatigue, dizziness.

DRUG INTERACTIONS

Drugs or herbal products that induce CYP3A4 (eg, barbiturates, carbamazepine, St. John's wort) decrease plasma concentrations and may decrease effectiveness; avoid coadministration. CYP3A4 inhibitors (eg, itraconazole, ketoconazole) may increase plasma concentrations. May reduce contraceptive action of regular hormonal contraceptive methods. May increase the concentration of P-glycoprotein (P-gp) substrates (eg, dabigatran etexilate, digoxin) due to inhibition of P-gp at clinically relevant concentrations.

PATIENT CONSIDERATIONS

Assessment: Assess pregnancy/nursing status and for possible drug interactions.

Monitoring: Monitor for ectopic pregnancy and effect on menstrual cycle. Perform follow-up physical/pelvic examination if in doubt concerning general health or pregnancy status.

Counseling: Instruct to take as soon as possible and not >120 hrs after unprotected intercourse or a known or suspected contraceptive failure. Advise not to take if pregnancy is known or suspected and that drug is not indicated for termination of an existing pregnancy. Advise to contact physician immediately if vomiting occurs within 3 hrs of intake, if period is delayed after taking the drug by >1 week beyond expected date, or if experiencing severe lower abdominal pain 3-5 weeks after use. Advise not to use as routine contraception or repeatedly in the same menstrual cycle. Inform that therapy may reduce contraceptive action of regular hormonal contraceptive methods and to use a reliable barrier method of contraception after using medication, for any subsequent acts of intercourse that occur in that same menstrual cycle. Inform that drug does not protect against HIV infection (AIDS) and other sexually transmitted diseases/infections. Instruct not to use if breastfeeding.

STORAGE: 20-25°C (68-77°F). Keep blister in the outer carton to protect from light.

ELMIRON — pentosan polysulfate sodium

RX

Class: Urinary tract analgesic

ADULT DOSAGE

Interstitial Cystitis

Bladder Pain/Discomfort:

100mg tid

Reassess patient after 3 months; may continue for another 3 months if no improvement and no limiting adverse events

PEDIATRIC DOSAGE

Interstitial Cystitis

Bladder Pain/Discomfort:

≥16 Years:

100mg tid

Reassess patient after 3 months; may continue for another 3 months if no improvement and no limiting adverse events

ADMINISTRATION

Oral route

Take with water ≥1 hr ac or 2 hrs pc

HOW SUPPLIED

Cap: 100mg

CONTRAINDICATIONS

Known hypersensitivity to the drug, structurally related compounds, or excipients.

WARNINGS/PRECAUTIONS

Rectal hemorrhage, bleeding complications of ecchymosis, epistaxis, gum hemorrhage, and alopecia reported. Evaluate patients undergoing invasive procedures or having signs/symptoms of underlying coagulopathy for hemorrhage. Evaluate patients with aneurysms, thrombocytopenia, hemophilia, GI ulcers, polyps, or diverticula prior to therapy. Caution with history of heparin-induced thrombocytopenia and hepatic impairment. Mildly elevated transaminase, alkaline phosphatase, GGT, and lactic dehydrogenase, and increases in PTT and PT, or thrombocytopenia reported.

ADVERSE REACTIONS

Nausea, diarrhea, alopecia, headache, rash, rectal hemorrhage.

DRUG INTERACTIONS

Coumarin anticoagulants, heparin, tissue plasminogen activator, streptokinase, high-dose aspirin, or NSAIDs may increase risk of bleeding; evaluate for hemorrhage.

PATIENT CONSIDERATIONS

Assessment: Assess for increased risk of bleeding, aneurysms, thrombocytopenia, hemophilia, GI ulcers, polyps, diverticula, history of heparin-induced thrombocytopenia, hepatic impairment, hypersensitivity to drug, pregnancy/nursing status, and possible drug interactions.

Monitoring: Monitor for improvement, bleeding complications, and other adverse reactions.

Counseling: Instruct to take drug as prescribed and no more frequently than prescribed. Inform that drug has a weak anticoagulant effect which may increase bleeding time.

STORAGE: 15-30°C (59-86°F).

ELOXATIN – oxaliplatin

RX

Class: Platinum analogue

Anaphylactic reactions reported, and may occur w/in min of administration. Epinephrine, corticosteroids, and antihistamines have been employed to alleviate symptoms of anaphylaxis.

ADULT DOSAGE

Colon Cancer

Stage III:

In combination w/ 5-fluorouracil (5-FU)/leucovorin (LV) for adjuvant treatment in patients who have undergone complete resection of the primary tumor

Day 1: Oxaliplatin 85mg/m^2 IV infusion + LV 200mg/m^2 IV infusion; both given over 120 min at the same time in separate bags using a Y-line, followed by 5-FU 400mg/m^2 IV bolus given over 2-4 min, followed by 5-FU 600mg/m^2 IV infusion as a 22-hr continuous infusion

Day 2: LV 200 mg/m^2 IV infusion over 120 min, followed by 5-FU 400mg/m^2 IV bolus given over 2-4 min, followed by 5-FU 600 mg/m^2 IV infusion as a 22-hr continuous infusion

Administer every 2 weeks; treatment is recommended for a total of 6 months (12 cycles)

Advanced Colorectal Cancer

Combination w/ 5-FU/LV:

Day 1: Oxaliplatin 85mg/m^2 IV infusion + LV 200mg/m^2 IV infusion; both given over 120 min at the same time in separate bags using a Y-line, followed by 5-FU 400mg/m^2 IV bolus given over 2-4 min, followed by 5-FU 600mg/m^2 IV infusion as a 22-hr continuous infusion

Day 2: LV 200 mg/m^2 IV infusion over 120 min, followed by 5-FU 400mg/m^2 IV bolus given over 2-4 min, followed by 5-FU 600 mg/m^2 IV infusion as a 22-hr continuous infusion

PEDIATRIC DOSAGE

Pediatric use may not have been established

Administer every 2 weeks. Continue treatment until disease progression or unacceptable toxicity

Premedication

Antiemetics, including 5-HT_3 blockers w/ or w/o dexamethasone, are recommended

DOSING CONSIDERATIONS

Renal Impairment

Severe:
Initial: 65mg/m^2

Adverse Reactions

Adjuvant Therapy in Stage III Colon Cancer:
Persistent Grade 2 Neurosensory Events That Do Not Resolve:
Consider reducing dose to 75mg/m^2; 5-FU/LV regimen need not be altered
Persistent Grade 3 Neurosensory Events:
Consider discontinuing; 5-FU/LV regimen need not be altered
After Recovery from Grade 3/4 GI (Despite Prophylactic Treatment), or Grade 4 Neutropenia, or Febrile Neutropenia, or Grade 3/4 Thrombocytopenia:
Reduce oxaliplatin dose to 75mg/m^2 and 5-FU to 300mg/m^2 bolus and 500mg/m^2 22-hr infusion; delay next dose until neutrophils $\geq$1.5 x 10^9/L and platelets $\geq$75 x 10^9/L

Advanced Colorectal Cancer (Previously Treated/Untreated):
Persistent Grade 2 Neurosensory Events That Do Not Resolve:
Consider reducing dose to 65mg/m^2; 5-FU/LV regimen need not be altered
Persistent Grade 3 Neurosensory Events:
Consider discontinuing therapy; 5-FU/LV regimen need not be altered
After Recovery from Grade 3/4 GI (Despite Prophylactic Treatment), or Grade 4 Neutropenia, or Febrile Neutropenia, or Grade 3/4 Thrombocytopenia:
Reduce oxaliplatin dose to 65mg/m^2 and 5-FU by 20% (300mg/m^2 bolus and 500mg/m^2 22-hr infusion); delay next dose until neutrophils $\geq$1.5 x 10^9/L and platelets $\geq$75 x 10^9/L

ADMINISTRATION

IV route

Incompatible in sol w/ alkaline medications or media (eg, basic sol of 5-FU); do not mix w/ these or administer simultaneously through the same infusion line.
Flush the infusion line w/ D5 inj prior to administration of any concomitant medication.
Do not use needles or IV administration sets containing aluminum parts to prepare or mix the drug; aluminum has been reported to cause degradation of platinum compounds.
Prolongation of infusion time for oxaliplatin from 2 hrs to 6 hrs may mitigate acute toxicities; infusion times for 5-FU and LV do not need to be changed.

Preparation of Infusion Sol

The sol must be further diluted in an infusion sol of 250-500mL of D5 inj; never perform a final dilution w/ a NaCl sol or other Cl^- containing sol.
After dilution, the shelf life is 6 hrs at 20-25°C (68-77°F) or up to 24 hrs at 2-8°C (36-46°F).
After final dilution, protection from light is not required.

HOW SUPPLIED

Inj: 5mg/mL [50mg, 100mg]

CONTRAINDICATIONS

History of known allergy to oxaliplatin or other platinum compounds.

WARNINGS/PRECAUTIONS

Should be administered under the supervision of a physician experienced in the use of cancer chemotherapeutic agents. An early onset, acute, reversible, primarily peripheral, sensory neuropathy and a persistent (>14 days), primarily peripheral, sensory neuropathy, reported. Cold temperature/objects may precipitate or exacerbate acute neurological symptoms; avoid ice for mucositis prophylaxis during infusion. Reversible posterior leukoencephalopathy syndrome (RPLS), also known as posterior reversible encephalopathy syndrome (PRES), reported. Grade 3 or 4 neutropenia reported in patients w/ colorectal cancer treated w/ oxaliplatin in combination w/ 5-FU and LV. Sepsis, neutropenic sepsis, and septic shock reported; withhold oxaliplatin for sepsis or septic shock. Potentially fatal pulmonary fibrosis reported. If unexplained respiratory symptoms develop, d/c until further pulmonary investigation excludes interstitial lung disease or pulmonary fibrosis. Hepatotoxicity observed; consider hepatic vascular disorders, and if appropriate, investigate in case of abnormal LFT results or portal HTN, which cannot be explained by liver metastases. QT prolongation and ventricular arrhythmias including fatal torsades de pointes reported; correct hypokalemia or hypomagnesemia prior to initiating therapy and monitor these electrolytes periodically during therapy. Avoid in patients w/ congenital long QT syndrome. ECG monitoring is recommended if therapy is initiated in patients w/ CHF, bradyarrhythmias, drugs known to prolong the QT interval (eg, Class Ia and III antiarrhythmics), and electrolyte abnormalities. Rhabdomyolysis, including fatal cases reported; d/c if any signs/symptoms of rhabdomyolysis occur. May cause fetal harm. Caution w/ renal impairment.

ADVERSE REACTIONS

Peripheral sensory neuropathy, neutropenia, thrombocytopenia, anemia, N/V, increased transaminases/alkaline phosphatase, diarrhea, fatigue, stomatitis, abdominal pain, fever, skin disorder, anorexia, dyspnea.

DRUG INTERACTIONS

Increased 5-FU plasma levels reported w/ doses of 130mg/m^2 oxaliplatin dosed every 3 weeks. Potentially nephrotoxic agents may decrease clearance. Prolonged PT and INR occasionally associated w/ hemorrhage reported in patients who concomitantly received oxaliplatin plus 5-FU/LV and anticoagulants; monitor patients requiring oral anticoagulants closely.

PATIENT CONSIDERATIONS

Assessment: Assess for history of known allergy to the drug or other platinum compounds, renal impairment, congenital long QT syndrome, hypokalemia, hypomagnesemia, pregnancy/nursing status, and possible drug interactions. Assess LFTs, WBC count w/ differential, Hgb, platelet count, and blood chemistries before each cycle.

Monitoring: Monitor for signs/symptoms of anaphylactic reactions, neurosensory toxicity, pulmonary toxicity, hepatotoxicity, RPLS, neutropenia, sepsis, septic shock, QT prolongation, ventricular arrhythmias, rhabdomyolysis, and other adverse reactions. Monitor patients w/ renal impairment closely and monitor patients requiring oral anticoagulants closely. Monitor Mg^{2+} and K^+ levels periodically. Perform ECG monitoring in patients w/ CHF, bradyarrhythmias, patients taking drugs known to prolong the QT interval, and in patients w/ electrolyte abnormalities.

Counseling: Inform of pregnancy risks. Advise to expect side effects, particularly neurologic effects, both the acute, reversible effects and the persistent neurosensory toxicity. Inform that acute neurosensory toxicity may be precipitated or exacerbated by exposure to cold or cold objects. Instruct to avoid cold drinks and ice, and to cover exposed skin prior to exposure to cold temperature or cold objects. Inform of the risk of low blood cell counts and to contact physician immediately if fever, particularly if associated w/ persistent diarrhea, or evidence of infection develops. Advise to contact physician if persistent vomiting, diarrhea, fever, signs of dehydration, cough or breathing difficulties, or signs of an allergic reaction occur. Advise of the potential effects of vision abnormalities; instruct to use caution when driving and using machines.

STORAGE: 25°C (77°F); excursions permitted to 15-30°C (59-86°F). Do not freeze and protect from light (keep in original outer carton).

EMEND CAPSULES AND ORAL SUSPENSION – aprepitant RX

Class: Substance P/neurokinin-1 (NK1) receptor antagonist

ADULT DOSAGE

Chemotherapy-Induced Nausea/Vomiting

Prevention of N/V associated w/ initial and repeat courses of highly emetogenic chemotherapy (HEC) or moderately emetogenic chemotherapy (MEC)

Caps:

Day 1: 125mg, 1 hr prior to chemotherapy

Days 2 and 3: 80mg, 1 hr prior to chemotherapy; administer in the am if no chemotherapy is given on Days 2 and 3

Oral Sus:

Patients Unable to Swallow Caps:

Day 1: 3mg/kg (max dose of 125mg), 1 hr prior to chemotherapy

Days 2 and 3: 2mg/kg (max dose of 80mg), 1 hr prior to chemotherapy; administer in the am if no chemotherapy is given on Days 2 and 3

Administer as part of a regimen that includes a corticosteroid and a 5-HT_3 antagonist; refer to PI

Postoperative Nausea/Vomiting

Prevention:

Caps:

40mg w/in 3 hrs prior to induction of anesthesia

PEDIATRIC DOSAGE

Chemotherapy-Induced Nausea/Vomiting

Prevention of N/V associated w/ initial and repeat courses of HEC or MEC

Oral Sus:

6 Months to <12 Years of Age or Pediatric Patients Unable to Swallow Caps:

Day 1: 3mg/kg (max dose of 125mg), 1 hr prior to chemotherapy

Days 2 and 3: 2mg/kg (max dose of 80mg), 1 hr prior to chemotherapy; administer in the am if no chemotherapy is given on Days 2 and 3

Caps:

≥12 Years:

Day 1: 125mg, 1 hr prior to chemotherapy

Days 2 and 3: 80mg, 1 hr prior to chemotherapy; administer in the am if no chemotherapy is given on Days 2 and 3

Administer as part of a regimen that includes a corticosteroid and a 5-HT_3 antagonist; refer to PI

DOSING CONSIDERATIONS

Other Important Considerations

Pediatric Patients <6kg: Not recommended

ADMINISTRATION

Oral route

Take w/ or w/o food.
Swallow caps whole.

Oral Sus

Should be prepared by a healthcare provider.
When ready to use, take the cap off the dispenser, place the dispenser in the patient's mouth along the inner cheek on either the right or left side; slowly dispense.
Discard any doses remaining after 72 hrs.

Preparation:

1. Fill the mixing cup w/ room temperature drinking water.
2. Fill the 5mL oral dosing dispenser w/ 4.6mL of water from the mixing cup; make sure no air is in the dispenser.
3. Discard all the unused water remaining in the mixing cup, and then add the 4.6mL of water from the dispenser back into the mixing cup.
4. Shake the pouch and pour the entire contents of the pouch into the 4.6mL of water in the mixing cup and snap the lid shut.
5. Gently swirl 20X; then gently invert the mixing cup 5X.
6. Check for any clumps or foaming and if there are clumps present, repeat step 5 until there are no clumps; if there is foam, wait until it disappears.
7. The final concentration is 25mg/mL; fill the appropriate dispenser w/ the prescribed dose.
8. Place the cap on the dispenser until it clicks.
9. Discard the mixing cup along w/ any remaining sus.

Storage:

Store the pouch at room temperature between 20-25°C (68-77°F).
Store filled dosing dispenser(s) in the refrigerator (2-8°C [36-46°F]) for up to 72 hrs prior to use if the dose is not administered immediately after measuring.
When ready to use, mixture may be kept at room temperature (20-25°C [68-77°F]) for up to 3 hours.

HOW SUPPLIED

Cap: 40mg, 80mg, 125mg; **Oral Sus:** 125mg

CONTRAINDICATIONS

Hypersensitivity to any component of the product, concomitant use w/ pimozide.

WARNINGS/PRECAUTIONS

Not recommended for chronic continuous use. Additional monitoring for adverse reactions in patients w/ severe hepatic impairment (Child-Pugh score >9) may be warranted. Caution in elderly.

ADVERSE REACTIONS

Prevention of Chemotherapy Induced N/V (CINV): (Adults) Fatigue, diarrhea, asthenia, dyspepsia, abdominal pain, hiccups, decreased WBC count, dehydration, increased alanine aminotransferase. (Pediatrics) Neutropenia, headache, diarrhea, decreased appetite, cough, fatigue, decreased Hgb, dizziness, hiccups.
Prevention of Postoperative N/V (PONV): (Adults) Constipation, hypotension.

DRUG INTERACTIONS

See Contraindications. Use w/ other drugs that are CYP3A4 substrates may result in increased concentration of the concomitant drug. Use w/ strong or moderate CYP3A4 inhibitors (eg, ketoconazole, diltiazem) may increase concentrations and result in increased risk of adverse reactions; avoid concomitant use. Use w/ strong CYP3A4 inducers (eg, rifampin) may reduce concentrations and decrease efficacy; avoid concomitant use. Coadministration w/ warfarin may decrease PT/INR; monitor INR for chronic warfarin therapy in the 2-week period, particularly at 7-10 days, following initiation of aprepitant w/ each chemotherapy cycle, or following single administration for the prevention of PONV. Efficacy of hormonal contraceptives may be reduced; alternative or backup methods of contraception should be used during therapy and for 1 month following the last dose. Increased exposure to midazolam or other benzodiazepines metabolized via CYP3A4 (eg, alprazolam, triazolam); monitor for benzodiazepine-related adverse reactions during use for prevention of CINV and may consider reducing the dose of IV midazolam. Increased dexamethasone exposure; reduce dose of oral dexamethasone by approx 50% during use for prevention of CINV. Increased methylprednisolone exposure; reduce dose of IV methylprednisolone by approx 25% and oral methylprednisolone by approx 50% during use for prevention of CINV. May increase exposure of chemotherapeutic agents metabolized by CYP3A4 (eg, vinblastine, vincristine, ifosfamide); monitor for adverse events.

PATIENT CONSIDERATIONS

Assessment: Assess for hypersensitivity to drug, severe hepatic impairment, ability to swallow caps, pregnancy/nursing status, and possible drug interactions.

Monitoring: Monitor for hypersensitivity reactions and other adverse reactions. Monitor INR closely w/ warfarin.

Counseling: Advise that hypersensitivity reactions, including anaphylaxis, have been reported; instruct to d/c medication and contact physician immediately if an allergic reaction occurs. Advise to inform physician if using any other prescription, nonprescription medication, or herbal products. Inform that drug may reduce efficacy of hormonal contraceptives; advise to use alternative or backup methods of contraception (eg, condoms, spermicides) during therapy and for 1 month after the last dose. Instruct patients on chronic warfarin therapy to follow instructions from physician regarding blood draws to monitor INR.

STORAGE: Caps: 20-25°C (68-77°F). **Oral Sus:** (Unopened pouch) 20-25°C (68-77°F); excursions permitted at 15-30°C (59-86°F). Do not open until ready for use. (Prepared sus) If not used immediately, refrigerate at 2-8°C (36-46°F) for up to 72 hrs prior to use; when ready to use, mixture can be kept at 20-25°C (68-77°F) for up to 3 hrs.

EMLA – lidocaine/prilocaine

RX

Class: Acetamide local anesthetic

ADULT DOSAGE

Topical Anesthetic

Apply thick layer of cre to intact skin and cover w/ occlusive dressing

Minor Dermal Procedure:
Apply 2.5g over 20-25cm^2 of skin surface for at least 1 hr

Major Dermal Procedure:
Apply 2g/10cm^2 of skin for 2 hrs

As an Adjunct Prior to Local Anesthetic Infiltration on Adult Male Genital Skin:
Apply 1g/10cm^2 of skin surface for 15 min

Minor Procedures on the Female External Genitalia (eg, Removal of Condylomata Acuminata) and Pretreatment for Anesthetic Infiltration:
Apply 5-10g for 5-10 min

PEDIATRIC DOSAGE

Topical Anesthetic

Intact Skin:

0-3 Months of Age:
<5kg:
Max: 1g/10cm^2 for up to 1 hr

3-12 Months of Age:
>5kg:
Max: 2g/20cm^2 for up to 4 hrs

1-6 Years:
>10kg:
Max: 10g/100cm^2 for up to 4 hrs

7-12 Years:
>20kg:
Max: 20g/200cm^2 for up to 4 hrs

If >3 months and does not meet minimum weight requirement, max dose restricted to corresponding weight

ADMINISTRATION

Topical route

Not for ophthalmic use

HOW SUPPLIED

Cre: (Lidocaine-Prilocaine) 2.5%-2.5%

CONTRAINDICATIONS

Known history of sensitivity to local anesthetics of the amide type or to any other component of the product.

WARNINGS/PRECAUTIONS

Application to larger areas or for longer than recommended times may result in serious adverse effects. Should not be used where penetration or migration beyond the tympanic membrane into the middle ear is possible. Avoid w/ congenital or idiopathic methemoglobinemia and in infants <12 months of age receiving treatment w/ methemoglobin-inducing agents. Very young or patients w/ G6PD deficiency are more susceptible to methemoglobinemia. Reports of methemoglobinemia in infants and children following excessive applications. Monitor neonates and infants up to 3 months of age for Met-Hb levels before, during, and after application. Repeated doses may increase blood levels; caution in patients who may be more susceptible to systemic effects (eg, acutely ill, debilitated, elderly). Avoid eye contact and application to open wounds. Has been shown to inhibit viral and bacterial growth. Caution w/ severe hepatic disease and in patients w/ drug sensitivities.

ADVERSE REACTIONS

Erythema, edema, abnormal sensations, paleness (pallor or blanching), altered temperature sensations, burning sensation, itching, rash.

E

DRUG INTERACTIONS

Additive and potentially synergistic toxic effects w/ Class I antiarrhythmic drugs (eg, tocainide, mexiletine). May have additive cardiac effects w/ Class III antiarrhythmic drugs (eg, amiodarone, bretylium, sotalol, dofetilide). Avoid drugs associated w/ drug-induced methemoglobinemia (eg, sulfonamides, acetaminophen, acetanilid, aniline dyes, benzocaine, chloroquine, dapsone, naphthalene, nitrates/nitrites, nitrofurantoin, nitroglycerin, nitroprusside, phenobarbital, phenytoin, primaquine, pamaquine, para-aminosalicylic acid, phenacetin, quinine). Caution w/ other products containing lidocaine/prilocaine; consider the amount absorbed from all formulations.

PATIENT CONSIDERATIONS

Assessment: Assess for congenital or idiopathic methemoglobinemia, G6PD deficiency, hepatic disease, open wounds, presence of acute illness, presence of debilitation, history of drug sensitivities, pregnancy/nursing status, and for possible drug interactions. In neonates and infants ≤3 months of age, obtain Met-Hb levels prior to application.

Monitoring: Monitor for signs/symptoms of methemoglobinemia, ototoxicity, local skin reactions and for allergic/anaphylactoid reactions. Monitor Met-Hb levels in neonates and infants ≤3 months of age during and after application.

Counseling: Inform about potential risks/benefits of drug. Advise to avoid inadvertent trauma to treated area. Instruct not to apply near eyes or on open wounds. Apply ud by physician. Advise to notify physician if pregnant/nursing or planning to become pregnant. Instruct to remove cre and consult physician if child becomes very dizzy, excessively sleepy, or develops duskiness on the face or lips after application.

STORAGE: 20-25°C (68-77°F). Keep tightly closed.

EMPLICITI — elotuzumab RX

Class: Monoclonal antibody/SLAMF7-directed

ADULT DOSAGE

Multiple Myeloma

Use in combination w/ lenalidomide and dexamethasone for the treatment of patients w/ multiple myeloma who have received 1-3 prior therapies; continue treatment until disease progression or unacceptable toxicity

Recommended Dose: 10mg/kg IV every week for the first 2 cycles and every 2 weeks thereafter; each cycle consists of 28 days

Dexamethasone:
Administer 28mg PO 3-24 hrs before elotuzumab plus 8mg IV 45-90 min before elotuzumab, on days that elotuzumab is administered.
Administer 40mg PO on days that elotuzumab is not administered but a dose of dexamethasone is scheduled (Days 8 and 22 of cycle 3 and all subsequent cycles).

Lenalidomide:
25mg PO qd on Days 1-21 of a 28-day treatment cycle

Infusion Rate:
Cycle 1, Dose 1:
0-30 min: 0.5mL/min
30-60 min: 1mL/min
≥60 min: 2mL/min

Cycle 1, Dose 2:
0-30 min: 1mL/min
≥30 min: 2mL/min

Cycle 1, Dose 3 and 4 and All Subsequent Cycles:
2 mL/min

Max: 2mL/min; 5mL/min in patients who have received 4 cycles of treatment

PEDIATRIC DOSAGE

Pediatric use may not have been established

Premedication

Premedicate w/ the Following 45-90 min Prior to Each Elotuzumab Infusion:
8mg IV dexamethasone;
25-50mg PO or IV diphenhydramine or equivalent H1 blocker;
50mg IV or 150mg oral ranitidine or equivalent H2 blocker;
650-1000mg oral acetaminophen

DOSING CONSIDERATIONS

Adverse Reactions

Infusion Reactions:

≥Grade 2: Interrupt elotuzumab infusion and institute appropriate medical/supportive measures. Upon resolution to ≤Grade 1, restart at 0.5mL/min and gradually increase at a rate of 0.5mL/min every 30 min as tolerated to the rate at which the infusion reaction occurred; resume escalation regimen if there is no recurrence of the infusion reaction. Monitor vital signs every 30 min for 2 hrs after end of infusion, in patients who experience an infusion reaction; if infusion reaction recurs, d/c elotuzumab infusion and do not restart on that day

Severe: May require permanent discontinuation and emergency treatment

Other Important Modifications

If the dose of 1 drug in the regimen is delayed, interrupted, or discontinued, treatment w/ the other drugs may continue as scheduled. If dexamethasone is delayed or discontinued, base decision whether to administer elotuzumab on clinical judgment (risk of hypersensitivity)

ADMINISTRATION

IV route

Administer w/ an infusion set and sterile, nonpyrogenic, low-protein-binding filter (w/ a pore size of 0.2-1.2μm) using an automated infusion pump.
Do not mix w/, or administer as an infusion w/, other medicinal products.

Reconstitution

1. Reconstitute 300mg vial w/ 13mL sterile water for injection (SWFI) and 400mg vial w/ 17mL SWFI; post-reconstitution concentration is 25mg/mL.
2. Use a syringe of adequate size and ≤18-gauge needle.
3. Dissolve by swirling/inverting vial; avoid vigorous agitation/shaking. The lyophilized powder should dissolve in <10 min.
4. Allow reconstituted sol to stand for 5-10 min.

Dilution

1. Once the reconstitution is completed, withdraw necessary volume for calculated dose from each vial, up to a max of 16mL from 400mg vial and 12mL from 300 mg vial.
2. Further dilute w/ 230mL of either 0.9% NaCl inj or D5 inj into an infusion bag made of polyvinyl chloride or polyolefin.
3. Volume of 0.9% NaCl inj or D5 inj can be adjusted so as not to exceed 5mL/kg of patient weight at any given dose.

Complete infusion w/in 24 hrs of reconstitution. If not used immediately, may store at 2-8°C (36-46°F) and protect from light for up to 24 hrs (max of 8 hrs of the total 24 hrs can be at 20-25°C [68-77°F] and room light).

HOW SUPPLIED

Inj: 300mg, 400mg

CONTRAINDICATIONS

Refer to the individual monographs for lenalidomide and dexamethasone.

WARNINGS/PRECAUTIONS

See Dosing Considerations. May cause infusion reactions. Infections reported; monitor and treat promptly. Invasive second primary malignancies (SPMs) reported; monitor for development of SPMs. Elevations in liver enzymes consistent w/ hepatotoxicity reported; monitor liver enzymes periodically. D/C treatment upon ≥Grade 3 elevation of liver enzymes; may consider treatment continuation after return to baseline values. Can be detected on both serum protein electrophoresis and immunofixation assays; may impact determination of complete response and possibly relapse from complete response in patients w/ IgG kappa myeloma protein.

ADVERSE REACTIONS

Fatigue, diarrhea, pyrexia, constipation, cough, peripheral neuropathy, nasopharyngitis, URTI, decreased appetite, pneumonia, pain in extremities, headache, vomiting, decreased weight, lymphopenia.

PATIENT CONSIDERATIONS

Assessment: Assess baseline liver enzyme values.

Monitoring: Monitor for infusion reactions, infections, SPMs, hepatotoxicity, and other adverse reactions. Monitor liver enzymes periodically.

Counseling: Inform of risks/benefits of therapy. Advise to contact physician if experiencing signs/symptoms of infusion reactions w/in 24 hrs of infusion. Inform that oral premedication is necessary prior to infusion to reduce the risk of infusion reaction. Advise that lenalidomide has the potential to cause fetal harm and has specific requirements regarding contraception, pregnancy testing, blood and sperm donation, and transmission in sperm. Inform of the risk of developing infections and SPMs during treatment; instruct to report any symptoms of infection. Inform of the risk of hepatotoxicity and instruct to report any signs/symptoms associated w/ this event.

STORAGE: 2-8°C (36-46°F). Protect from light. Do not freeze or shake.

ENALAPRIL/HCTZ – enalapril maleate/hydrochlorothiazide RX

Class: ACE inhibitor/thiazide diuretic

D/C when pregnancy is detected. Drugs that act directly on the renin-angiotensin system (RAS) can cause injury/death to the developing fetus.

OTHER BRAND NAMES
Vaseretic

ADULT DOSAGE
Hypertension

Uncontrolled BP w/ Either Enalapril or HCTZ Monotherapy:
5mg/12.5mg or 10mg/25mg qd. Further increases of enalapril, HCTZ or both depend on clinical response; may increase HCTZ dose after 2-3 weeks
Max: 20mg/50mg qd

Replacement Therapy: Combination may be substituted for titrated components

PEDIATRIC DOSAGE
Pediatric use may not have been established

DOSING CONSIDERATIONS
Elderly
Start at lower end of dosing range

Renal Impairment
Severe: Not recommended; loop diuretics preferred

ADMINISTRATION
Oral route

HOW SUPPLIED
Tab: (Enalapril/HCTZ) 5mg/12.5mg; (Vaseretic) 10mg/25mg* *scored

CONTRAINDICATIONS
Hypersensitivity to any component of this product, hereditary/idiopathic angioedema, anuria, hypersensitivity to other sulfonamide-derived drugs, history of ACE inhibitor-associated angioedema. Coadministration w/ aliskiren in patients w/ diabetes.

WARNINGS/PRECAUTIONS
Not for initial therapy. Syncope reported. **Enalapril:** Excessive hypotension may occur in salt/volume-depleted patients (eg, patients treated vigorously w/ diuretics or on dialysis). Excessive hypotension reported and may be associated w/ oliguria and/or progressive azotemia, and rarely, w/ acute renal failure and/or death in patients w/ severe CHF; monitor closely during first 2 weeks of therapy and when dose is increased. Caution w/ ischemic heart or cerebrovascular disease in whom an excessive fall in BP could result in a MI or cerebrovascular accident. Head/neck angioedema reported; d/c and administer appropriate therapy. Intestinal angioedema reported. Higher incidence of angioedema in blacks than nonblacks. Patients w/ a history of angioedema unrelated to ACE inhibitor therapy may be at increased risk of angioedema during therapy. Anaphylactoid reactions reported during desensitization w/ hymenoptera venom, dialysis w/ high-flux membranes, and LDL apheresis w/ dextran sulfate absorption. Neutropenia/agranulocytosis may occur; consider monitoring WBCs in patients w/ collagen vascular disease and renal disease. Associated w/ syndrome that starts w/ cholestatic jaundice and progresses to fulminant hepatic necrosis and sometimes death (rare); d/c if jaundice or marked elevations of hepatic enzymes occur. Caution w/ left ventricular outflow obstruction. May cause changes in renal function; may be associated w/ oliguria and/or progressive azotemia and rarely w/ acute renal failure or death in severe CHF patients whose renal function depends on the renin-angiotensin-aldosterone system. May increase BUN/SrCr in patients

w/ renal artery stenosis or w/ no preexisting renal vascular disease; may need to reduce dose or d/c therapy. Monitor renal function during the 1st few weeks of therapy in patients w/ renal artery stenosis. Hyperkalemia and persistent nonproductive cough reported. Hypotension may occur w/ major surgery or during anesthesia. **HCTZ:** May precipitate azotemia in patients w/ renal disease. Consider withholding or discontinuing therapy if progressive renal impairment occurs. Caution w/ hepatic impairment or progressive liver disease; may precipitate hepatic coma. Sensitivity reactions may occur. May exacerbate/activate systemic lupus erythematosus (SLE). May cause idiosyncratic reaction, resulting in acute transient myopia and acute angle-closure glaucoma; d/c as rapidly as possible. Observe for signs of fluid or electrolyte imbalance (eg, hyponatremia, hypochloremic alkalosis, hypokalemia). Hyperuricemia, gout precipitation, hyperglycemia and manifestations of latent diabetes mellitus (DM), hypomagnesemia, hypercalcemia, and increased cholesterol and TG levels may occur. D/C before testing for parathyroid function. Enhanced effects in postsympathectomy patients. Hypokalemia may sensitize or exaggerate the response of the heart to toxic effects of digitalis.

E

ADVERSE REACTIONS

Dizziness, cough, fatigue, headache.

DRUG INTERACTIONS

See Contraindications. Increased risk of lithium toxicity; avoid w/ lithium. **Enalapril:** Dual blockade of the RAS is associated w/ increased risks of hypotension, hyperkalemia, and changes in renal function (including acute renal failure); in general, avoid combined use of RAS inhibitors, or closely monitor BP, renal function, and electrolytes w/ concomitant agents that affect the RAS. Avoid w/ aliskiren in patients w/ renal impairment (GFR <60mL/min). Hypotension risk and increased BUN and SrCr w/ diuretics. Antihypertensive agents that cause renin release (eg, diuretics) may augment effect. NSAIDs, including selective COX-2 inhibitors, may diminish antihypertensive effect and may cause deterioration of renal function, including possible acute renal failure. Increased risk of hyperkalemia w/ K^+-sparing diuretics, K^+ supplements, or K^+-containing salt substitutes; use w/ caution and monitor serum K^+. Nitritoid reactions reported w/ injectable gold. Coadministration w/ mTOR inhibitors (e.g., temsirolimus, sirolimus, everolimus) may increase risk for angioedema. **HCTZ:** Potentiation of orthostatic hypotension may occur w/ alcohol, barbiturates, or narcotics. Dose adjustment of the antidiabetic drug (oral agents and insulin) may be required. Additive effect or potentiation may occur w/ other antihypertensives. Cholestyramine and colestipol resins impair absorption. Corticosteroids and ACTH may intensify electrolyte depletion, particularly hypokalemia. May decrease response to pressor amines (eg, norepinephrine). May increase responsiveness to nondepolarizing skeletal muscle relaxants (eg, tubocurarine). NSAIDs may reduce diuretic effect.

PATIENT CONSIDERATIONS

Assessment: Assess for hereditary/idiopathic or history of ACE inhibitor-associated angioedema, anuria, DM, volume/salt depletion, hypersensitivity to the drug or sulfonamide-derived drugs, CHF, left ventricular outflow obstruction, collagen vascular disease, SLE, risk factors for hyperkalemia, renal/hepatic impairment, pregnancy/nursing status, and possible drug interactions.

Monitoring: Monitor for signs/symptoms of angioedema, exacerbation/activation of SLE, idiosyncratic reaction, latent DM, fluid/electrolyte imbalance, hypercalcemia, hypomagnesemia, hyperuricemia or precipitation of gout, sensitivity reactions, and other adverse reactions. Periodically monitor WBCs in patients w/ collagen vascular disease and renal disease. Monitor BP, serum electrolytes, renal/hepatic function, and cholesterol/TG levels.

Counseling: Inform about fetal risks if taken during pregnancy and discuss treatment options in women planning to become pregnant; instruct to report pregnancy to physician as soon as possible. Instruct to d/c therapy and immediately report any signs/symptoms of angioedema. Instruct to report lightheadedness and to d/c therapy if actual syncope occurs. Inform that excessive perspiration, dehydration, and other causes of volume depletion may lead to an excessive fall in BP. Instruct not to use salt substitutes containing K^+ w/o consulting physician, and to report promptly any signs/symptoms of infection.

STORAGE: Protect from moisture. **Enalapril/HCTZ:** 20-25°C (68-77°F). **Vaseretic:** 25°C (77°F); excursions permitted to 15-30°C (59-86°F).

ENBREL – etanercept

RX

Class: Tumor necrosis factor (TNF) blocker

Increased risk for developing serious infections (eg, active tuberculosis [TB], latent TB reactivation, invasive fungal infections, bacterial/viral infections, opportunistic infections) leading to hospitalization or death, mostly w/ concomitant use w/ immunosuppressants (eg, methotrexate [MTX], corticosteroids). D/C if serious infection or sepsis develops. Active/latent reactivation of TB may present w/ disseminated or extrapulmonary disease; test for latent TB before and during therapy and initiate treatment for latent TB prior to therapy. Consider empiric antifungal therapy in patients at risk for invasive fungal infections who develop severe systemic illness. Monitor for development of infection during and after treatment, including development of TB in patients who tested (-) for latent TB infection prior to therapy. Lymphoma and other malignancies, some fatal, reported in children and adolescents.

E

ADULT DOSAGE

Plaque Psoriasis

Initial: 50mg twice weekly for 3 months; initial doses of 25mg or 50mg/week were also shown to be efficacious
Maint: 50mg once weekly

Rheumatoid Arthritis

50mg weekly
Max: 50mg/week

May continue MTX, glucocorticoids, salicylates, NSAIDs, or analgesics during treatment

Psoriatic Arthritis

50mg weekly
Max: 50mg/week

May continue MTX, glucocorticoids, salicylates, NSAIDs, or analgesics during treatment

Ankylosing Spondylitis

50mg weekly
Max: 50mg/week

May continue MTX, glucocorticoids, salicylates, NSAIDs, or analgesics during treatment

PEDIATRIC DOSAGE

Juvenile Idiopathic Arthritis

Moderately to Severely Active:
≥2 Years:
<63kg: 0.8mg/kg weekly
≥63kg: 50mg weekly

May continue glucocorticoids, NSAIDs, or analgesics during treatment

ADMINISTRATION

SQ route

Do not mix contents of 1 vial of Enbrel sol w/ the contents of another vial of Enbrel
Do not add any other medications to sol containing Enbrel
Do not reconstitute Enbrel w/ other diluents
Do not filter reconstituted sol during preparation or administration

Preparation Using the Single-Use Prefilled Syringe

Leave at room temperature for about 15-30 min before injecting
Check to see if the amount of liquid in the prefilled syringe falls between the 2 purple fill level indicator lines; do not use if the syringe does not have the right amount of liquid

Preparation Using the SureClick Autoinjector

Leave at room temperature for at least 30 min before injecting

Preparation Using the Multiple-Use Vial

Reconstitute w/ 1mL of sterile bacteriostatic water for inj (0.9% benzyl alcohol)
Do not use vial adaptor if multiple doses are to be withdrawn from the vial; use a 25-gauge needle if the vial will be used for multiple doses
Reconstituted sol must be refrigerated at 36-46°F (2-8°C) and used w/in 14 days; discard reconstituted sol after 14 days
Leave at room temperature for about 15-30 min before injecting

If Using Vial Adapter:

1. Twist adapter onto the diluents syringe
2. Place vial adapter over Enbrel vial and insert vial adapter into vial stopper
3. Push down on plunger to inject diluent into Enbrel vial; inject the diluent very slowly into the Enbrel vial if using a 25-gauge needle
4. Keeping the diluent syringe in place, gently swirl the contents of the Enbrel vial during dissolution
5. Withdraw the correct dose of reconstituted sol into the syringe
6. Remove the syringe from the vial adapter or remove the 25-gauge needle from the syringe
7. Attach a 27-gauge needle to inject Enbrel

HOW SUPPLIED

Inj: 25mg [multiple-use vial, single-use prefilled syringe], 50mg [single-use prefilled syringe, single-use prefilled SureClick autoinjector]

CONTRAINDICATIONS

Sepsis.

WARNINGS/PRECAUTIONS

Do not initiate in patients w/ an active infection. Increased risk of infection in patients >65 yrs of age and in patients w/ comorbid conditions. New onset or exacerbation of CNS and peripheral nervous system demyelinating disorders, acute and chronic leukemia, new onset and worsening of CHF, melanoma and non-melanoma skin cancer, and Merkel cell carcinoma reported; consider periodic skin examinations for all patients at increased risk for skin cancer. Pancytopenia, including aplastic anemia, reported; consider discontinuation of therapy in patients w/ confirmed significant hematologic abnormalities. Reactivation of hepatitis B in patients who were previously infected w/ hepatitis B virus (HBV) reported; closely monitor for signs of active HBV infection during and for several months after therapy. Consider discontinuing therapy and initiating antiviral therapy w/ appropriate supportive treatment if HBV reactivation develops. Allergic reactions reported; d/c immediately and initiate appropriate therapy if an anaphylactic or other serious allergic reaction occurs. Needle cover of prefilled syringe and needle cover w/in the needle cap of autoinjector contain dry natural rubber; may cause allergic reactions in latex-sensitive individuals. If possible, pediatric patients should be brought up-to-date w/ all immunizations in agreement w/ current immunization guidelines prior to initiating therapy. May result in the formation of autoantibodies and in the development of a lupus-like syndrome or autoimmune hepatitis; d/c and evaluate patient if a lupus-like syndrome or autoimmune hepatitis develops. Caution w/ moderate to severe alcoholic hepatitis and in the elderly. Patients w/ a significant exposure to varicella virus should temporarily d/c therapy and be considered for prophylactic treatment w/ varicella zoster immune globulin.

ADVERSE REACTIONS

Infections, sepsis, malignancies, inj-site reactions, diarrhea, rash, pyrexia, pruritus.

DRUG INTERACTIONS

See Boxed Warning. Avoid w/ live vaccines. Not recommended w/ anakinra or abatacept; may increase risk of serious infections. Not recommended in patients w/ Wegener's granulomatosis receiving immunosuppressive agents; increased incidence of noncutaneous solid malignancies when added to standard therapy (eg, cyclophosphamide). Not recommended w/ cyclophosphamide. Mild decrease in mean neutrophil counts reported w/ sulfasalazine. Hypoglycemia reported following initiation of therapy in patients receiving antidiabetic medication; reduction in antidiabetic medication may be necessary.

PATIENT CONSIDERATIONS

Assessment: Assess for sepsis, active/chronic/recurrent infection, history of an opportunistic infection, recent travel in areas of endemic TB or endemic mycoses, underlying conditions that may predispose to infection, central or peripheral nervous system demyelinating disorders, CHF, history of significant hematologic abnormalities, latex sensitivity, alcoholic hepatitis, risk for skin cancer, pregnancy/nursing status, and possible drug interactions. Test for latent TB infection and for HBV infection. Assess immunization history in pediatric patients.

Monitoring: Monitor for development of infection during and after treatment. Monitor for sepsis, central or peripheral nervous system demyelinating disorders, malignancies, new or worsening CHF, hematologic abnormalities, allergic reactions, lupus-like syndrome, autoimmune hepatitis, and other adverse reactions. Monitor for active TB and periodically test for latent TB. Monitor for HBV reactivation during therapy and for several months following termination of therapy. Consider periodic skin examinations for all patients at increased risk for skin cancer.

Counseling: Advise of the potential risks and benefits of therapy. Inform that therapy may lower the ability of immune system to fight infections; instruct to contact physician if any symptoms of infection, TB, or HBV develop. Advise to report any signs of new/worsening medical conditions (eg, CNS demyelinating disorders, CHF, autoimmune disorders) or any symptoms suggestive of pancytopenia. Counsel about the risk of lymphoma and other malignancies. Instruct to seek immediate medical attention if any symptoms of a severe allergic reaction develop. Advise that the needle cover of prefilled syringe and the needle cover w/in the needle cap of the autoinjector contain dry natural rubber (a derivative of latex), which may cause allergic reactions in individuals sensitive to latex. Instruct in inj technique, as well as proper syringe and needle disposal, and caution against reuse of needles and syringes. Advise to inform physician if pregnant/breastfeeding.

STORAGE: 2-8°C (36-46°F). Do not shake. Protect from light or physical damage. Storage at room temperature at 20-25°C (68-77°F) for a max single period of 14 days is permissible, w/ protection from light, sources of heat, and (vial) humidity; once the product has been stored at room temperature, do not place back into the refrigerator. Discard if not used w/in 14 days at room temperature. Do not store in extreme heat or cold. Do not freeze. (Vial) Reconstituted Sol: Use immediately or may refrigerate for up to 14 days.

ENDOMETRIN – progesterone

RX

Class: Progesterone

ADULT DOSAGE

Assisted Reproductive Technology

To support embryo implantation and early pregnancy by supplementation of corpus luteal function in infertile women

General Dosing: 100mg vaginally bid or tid starting the day after oocyte retrieval and continuing for up to 10 weeks

PEDIATRIC DOSAGE

Pediatric use may not have been established

ADMINISTRATION
Intravaginal route

HOW SUPPLIED
Vaginal Insert: 100mg [21[s]]

CONTRAINDICATIONS
Previous allergic reactions to progesterone or any of the ingredients of the medication; known missed abortion or ectopic pregnancy; liver disease; known/suspected breast cancer; active arterial/venous thromboembolism or severe thrombophlebitis, or a history of these events.

WARNINGS/PRECAUTIONS
D/C if signs/symptoms of myocardial infarction (MI), cerebrovascular disorders, arterial or venous thromboembolism (venous thromboembolism or pulmonary embolism), thrombophlebitis, or retinal thrombosis suspected. Caution with history of depression; d/c if symptoms of depression worsen.

ADVERSE REACTIONS
Post-oocyte retrieval pain, abdominal pain, N/V, ovarian hyperstimulation syndrome, abdominal distention, headache, uterine spasm, vaginal bleeding.

DRUG INTERACTIONS
Not recommended for use with other vaginal products (eg, antifungals); progesterone release and absorption from vaginal insert may be altered. CYP450 3A4 inducers (eg, rifampin, carbamazepine) may increase elimination.

PATIENT CONSIDERATIONS

Assessment: Assess for known sensitivity to product, known missed or ectopic abortion, liver disease, breast cancer, active/history of arterial/venous thromboembolism, thrombophlebitis, MI, cerebrovascular disorders, depression, use of other vaginal products, pregnancy/nursing status, and possible drug interactions.

Monitoring: Monitor for signs/symptoms of MI, cerebrovascular disorder, arterial/venous thromboembolism, ovarian hyperstimulation syndrome, vaginal bleeding, worsening of depression, and other adverse reactions.

Counseling: Inform of the importance of reporting irregular vaginal bleeding to physician as soon as possible. Counsel about possible side effects (eg, headaches, breast tenderness, bloating, mood swings, irritability, and drowsiness); advise to seek prompt medical attention if any occur. Inform that product is not recommended for use with other vaginal products.

STORAGE: 25°C (77°F); excursions permitted to 15-30°C (59-86°F).

Engerix-B – hepatitis B vaccine (recombinant) RX

Class: Vaccine

ADULT DOSAGE

Hepatitis B Vaccine

Immunization Against Infection Caused by All Known Subtypes:

≥20 Years:

Primary Immunization: 1mL IM dose as a 3-dose series given on a 0, 1, and 6-month schedule

Booster: 1mL IM

Alternate Schedule:
1mL IM at 0, 1, 2, and 12 months

Known or Presumed Exposure to Hepatitis B Virus (HBV):
Hepatitis B immune globulin should be given in addition to vaccine w/ known or presumed exposure to the hepatitis B virus

PEDIATRIC DOSAGE

Hepatitis B Vaccine

Immunization Against Infection Caused by All Known Subtypes:

≤19 Years:

Primary Immunization: 0.5mL IM dose as a 3-dose series given on a 0, 1, and 6-month schedule

Booster:
≤10 Years: 0.5mL IM
11-19 Years: 1mL IM

Alternate Schedule:
≤10 Years/Infants Born of HBsAg-Positive Mothers: 0.5mL IM at 0, 1, 2, 12 months
5-16 Years: 0.5mL IM at 0, 12, and 24 months
11-19 Years: 1mL IM at 0, 1, 6 months or at 0, 1, 2, and 12 months

Known or Presumed Exposure to HBV:
Hepatitis B immune globulin should be given in addition to vaccine w/ known or presumed exposure to the HBV

DOSING CONSIDERATIONS

Renal Impairment

Hemodialysis:

Adults:

Primary Immunization: 2mL IM dose as a 4-dose series (given as a single 2mL dose or two 1mL doses) on a 0, 1, 2, and 6-month schedule

Booster: 2mL IM dose when antibody levels decline <10 mIU/mL

Alternate Schedule: 1mL IM at 0, 1, 2, and 12 months

ADMINISTRATION

IM route

Preferred site of administration is the anterolateral aspect of the thigh (<1 yr of age) and deltoid muscle (older children [whose deltoid is large enough for IM inj] and adults); do not administer in the gluteal region.
May give SQ if at risk of hemorrhage (eg, hemophiliacs).
Shake well before use.
Do not dilute to administer.
Do not mix w/ any other vaccine or product in the same syringe or vial.

HOW SUPPLIED

Inj: 10mcg/0.5mL, 20mcg/mL [vial, prefilled syringe]

CONTRAINDICATIONS

Severe allergic reaction (eg, anaphylaxis) after a previous dose of any hepatitis B-containing vaccine, or to any component of Engerix-B, including yeast.

WARNINGS/PRECAUTIONS

Tip caps of prefilled syringes may contain natural rubber latex; allergic reactions may occur in latex-sensitive individuals. Syncope may occur and can be accompanied by transient neurological signs (eg, visual disturbance, paresthesia, tonic-clonic limb movements). Defer vaccine for infants w/ a birth weight <2000g if mother is documented to be HBsAg negative at the time of infant's birth; vaccination can commence at chronological age 1 month or hospital discharge. Infants born weighing <2000g to HBsAg-positive mothers should receive vaccine and hepatitis B immune globulin (HBIG) w/in 12 hrs after birth. Infants born weighing <2000 g to mothers of unknown HBsAg status should receive vaccine and HBIG w/in 12 hrs after birth if the mother's HBsAg status cannot be determined w/in the first 12 hrs of life. The birth dose in infants born weighing <2000g should not be counted as the 1st dose in the vaccine series and it should be followed w/ a full 3-dose standard regimen (total of 4 doses). Apnea in premature infants following IM administration observed; decisions about when to administer vaccine should be based on consideration of medical status, and the potential benefits and possible risks of vaccination. Review immunization history for possible vaccine sensitivity and previous vaccination-related adverse reactions; appropriate treatment must be available for possible anaphylactic reactions. Postpone vaccination w/ moderate or severe acute febrile illness unless at immediate risk of hepatitis B infection (eg, infants born of HBsAg-positive mothers). Immunocompromised persons may have a diminished immune response to vaccine. May not prevent hepatitis B infection in individuals who had an unrecognized hepatitis B infection at the time of vaccination. May not prevent infection in individuals who do not achieve protective antibody titers.

ADVERSE REACTIONS

Inj-site reactions (soreness, erythema, swelling, induration), fatigue, fever, headache, dizziness.

DRUG INTERACTIONS

May diminish immune response w/ immunosuppressant therapy.

PATIENT CONSIDERATIONS

Assessment: Assess for hypersensitivity to yeast or latex, moderate or severe acute febrile illness, immunosuppression, unrecognized hepatitis B infection, pregnancy/nursing status, and for possible drug interactions. Review immunization history for possible vaccine sensitivity and previous vaccination-related adverse reactions. If an infant is receiving the vaccine, assess the birth weight.

Monitoring: Monitor for allergic and inj-site reactions, syncope, and other adverse reactions. Monitor immune response. Perform annual antibody testing in hemodialysis patients to assess the need for booster doses.

Counseling: Inform of potential benefits/risks of immunization. Educate about potential side effects and instruct to notify physician if any side effects develop. Inform that vaccine contains noninfectious purified HBsAg and cannot cause hepatitis B infection.

STORAGE: 2-8°C (36-46°F). Do not freeze; discard if has been frozen.

Entocort EC – budesonide

RX

Class: Corticosteroid

ADULT DOSAGE

Crohn's Disease

Mild to Moderate Active Crohn's Disease of the Ileum and/or Ascending Colon:
9mg qd, in the am for up to 8 weeks; repeated 8-week courses may be given for recurring episodes of active disease

PEDIATRIC DOSAGE

Pediatric use may not have been established

Maint of Clinical Remission:
6mg qd for up to 3 months; if symptom control is still maintained at 3 months, attempt to taper to complete cessation

DOSING CONSIDERATIONS

Concomitant Medications

CYP3A4 Inhibitors: Monitor for increased signs and/or symptoms of hypercorticism if concomitant administration w/ ketoconazole or any other CYP3A4 inhibitor is indicated; consider reducing dose

Hepatic Impairment

Moderate to Severe: Monitor for increased signs and/or symptoms of hypercorticism; consider reducing dose

Elderly

Start at lower end of dosing range

ADMINISTRATION

Oral route

Swallow caps whole; do not chew or break

HOW SUPPLIED

Cap: 3mg

CONTRAINDICATIONS

Known hypersensitivity to budesonide.

WARNINGS/PRECAUTIONS

May reduce response of hypothalamic-pituitary-adrenal axis to stress. Supplement with systemic glucocorticosteroids if undergoing surgery or other stressful situations. Increased risk of infection; avoid exposure to varicella/varicella zoster and measles. Caution with tuberculosis (TB), HTN, diabetes mellitus (DM), osteoporosis, peptic ulcer, glaucoma, cirrhosis, cataracts, or family history of DM or glaucoma. Replacement of systemic glucocorticosteroids may unmask allergies. Chronic use may cause hypercorticism and adrenal suppression.

ADVERSE REACTIONS

Headache, respiratory infection, N/V, back pain, dyspepsia, dizziness, abdominal pain, diarrhea, flatulence, sinusitis, viral infection, arthralgia, benign intracranial HTN, signs/symptoms of hypercorticism.

DRUG INTERACTIONS

Ketoconazole caused an eight-fold increase of systemic exposure to oral budesonide. Increased levels with CYP3A4 inhibitors (eg, ketoconazole, saquinavir, erythromycin, grapefruit); monitor for increased signs and symptoms of hypercorticism and reduce budesonide dose if coadministered.

PATIENT CONSIDERATIONS

Assessment: Assess for liver disease, history of chickenpox or measles, TB, HTN, osteoporosis, peptic ulcers, cataracts, history and/or family history of DM or glaucoma, and possible drug interactions. Obtain baseline LFTs.

Monitoring: Monitor LFTs periodically and for signs/symptoms of hypercorticism and hypersensitivity reactions.

Counseling: Advise to swallow whole; do not chew or break. Instruct to avoid consumption of grapefruit and grapefruit juice during therapy. Caution to take particular care to avoid exposure to chickenpox or measles.

STORAGE: 25° (77°F); excursions permitted to 15-30°C (59-86°F). Keep container tightly closed.

ENTRESTO — sacubitril/valsartan RX

Class: Angiotensin II receptor blocker (ARB)/neprilysin inhibitor

D/C when pregnancy is detected. Drugs that act directly on the renin-angiotensin system (RAS) can cause injury/death to the developing fetus.

ADULT DOSAGE

Heart Failure

Risk reduction of cardiovascular death and hospitalization for heart failure (HF) in patients w/ chronic HF (NYHA Class II-IV) and reduced ejection fraction

Initial: 49mg/51mg bid
Titrate: Double the dose after 2-4 weeks to the target maint dose of 97mg/103mg bid, as tolerated

Patients Not Taking an ACE Inhibitor/ARB or Previously Taking Low Doses of These Agents:
Initial: 24mg/26mg bid
Titrate: Double the dose every 2-4 weeks to the target maint dose of 97mg/103mg bid, as tolerated

Conversions

Switching from an ACE Inhibitor:
Allow a washout period of 36 hrs between administration of the two drugs

PEDIATRIC DOSAGE

Pediatric use may not have been established

DOSING CONSIDERATIONS

Renal Impairment
Severe (eGFR <30mL/min/1.73m²):
Initial: 24mg/26mg bid
Titrate: Double the dose every 2-4 weeks to the target maint dose of 97mg/103mg bid, as tolerated

Hepatic Impairment
Moderate (Child-Pugh B):
Initial: 24mg/26mg bid
Titrate: Double the dose every 2-4 weeks to the target maint dose of 97mg/103mg bid, as tolerated

Severe: Not recommended

ADMINISTRATION

Oral route

Usually administered in conjunction w/ other heart failure therapies, in place of an ACE inhibitor or other ARB

Take w/ or w/o food

HOW SUPPLIED

Tab: (Sacubitril/Valsartan) 24mg/26mg, 49mg/51mg, 97mg/103mg

CONTRAINDICATIONS

Hypersensitivity to any component, history of angioedema related to previous ACE inhibitor or ARB therapy, concomitant use of ACE inhibitors or use w/in 36 hrs of switching from or to an ACE inhibitor, coadministration w/ aliskiren in patients w/ diabetes.

WARNINGS/PRECAUTIONS

May cause angioedema; d/c immediately and do not readminister if angioedema occurs. Associated w/ a higher rate of angioedema in black than in non-black patients. May cause symptomatic hypotension; patients w/ an activated RAS (eg, volume- and/or salt-depleted patients [including those on high doses of diuretics]) are at greater risk. Correct volume or salt depletion prior to therapy or start at a lower dose. If hypotension occurs, consider dose adjustment of diuretics, concomitant antihypertensive drugs, and treatment of other causes of hypotension. If hypotension persists despite such measures, reduce the dosage or temporarily d/c therapy. Decreased renal function may occur; caution w/ patients whose renal function depends upon the activity of the RAS (eg, severe CHF). Closely monitor SrCr, and down-titrate or interrupt therapy in patients who develop a clinically significant decrease in renal function. May increase blood urea and SrCr levels in patients w/ bilateral or unilateral renal artery stenosis. Hyperkalemia may occur; dosage reduction or interruption may be required.

ADVERSE REACTIONS

Hypotension, hyperkalemia, cough, dizziness, renal failure.

DRUG INTERACTIONS

See Contraindications. Avoid use w/ an ARB. Avoid use w/ aliskiren in patients w/ renal impairment (eGFR <60mL/min/1.73m²). Concomitant use of K^+-sparing diuretics, K^+ supplements, or salt substitutes containing K^+ may increase serum K^+ levels. Concomitant use of NSAIDs, including COX-2 inhibitors, may result in worsening of renal function, including possible acute renal failure, in patients who are elderly, volume-depleted, or w/ compromised renal function; monitor renal function periodically. Increases in lithium levels and lithium toxicity reported during concomitant administration w/ ARBs; monitor serum lithium levels during concomitant use.

PATIENT CONSIDERATIONS

Assessment: Assess for hypersensitivity to any component of the drug, history of angioedema related to previous ACE inhibitor/ARB therapy, diabetes, activated RAS, renal artery stenosis, risk factors for hyperkalemia, renal/hepatic impairment, pregnancy/nursing status, and possible drug interactions.

Monitoring: Monitor for signs/symptoms of angioedema and hypotension. Closely monitor SrCr in patients who develop a clinically significant decrease in renal function. Monitor renal function. Monitor serum K^+ periodically, especially in patients w/ risk factors for hyperkalemia.

Counseling: Advise females of childbearing age about the consequences of exposure to drug during pregnancy. Discuss treatment options w/ women planning to become pregnant. Advise to report pregnancies to physicians as soon as possible. Advise to d/c use of previous ACE inhibitor or ARB and to allow a 36-hr washout period if switching from or to an ACE inhibitor.

STORAGE: 25°C (77°F); excursions permitted to 15-30°C (59-86°F). Protect from moisture.

ENTYVIO – vedolizumab RX

Class: Monoclonal antibody/integrin receptor antagonist

ADULT DOSAGE

Ulcerative Colitis

Moderately to Severely Active:

For inducing/maintaining clinical response and remission, improving endoscopic appearance of the mucosa, and achieving corticosteroid-free remission in patients who have had an inadequate response w/, lost response to, or were intolerant to a TNF blocker or immunomodulator; or had an inadequate response w/, were intolerant to, or demonstrated dependence on corticosteroids

300mg IV infusion over 30 min at 0, 2, and 6 weeks and then every 8 weeks thereafter

D/C if no evidence of therapeutic benefit seen by Week 14

Crohn's Disease

Moderately to Severely Active:

For achieving clinical response and remission, and achieving corticosteroid-free remission in patients who have had an inadequate response w/, lost response to, or were intolerant to a TNF blocker or immunomodulator; or had an inadequate response w/, were intolerant to, or demonstrated dependence on corticosteroids

300mg IV infusion over 30 min at 0, 2, and 6 weeks and then every 8 weeks thereafter

D/C if no evidence of therapeutic benefit seen by Week 14

PEDIATRIC DOSAGE

Pediatric use may not have been established

ADMINISTRATION

IV route

Do not administer as an IV push or bolus

Lyophilized powder must be reconstituted w/ sterile water for inj (SWFI) and diluted in 250mL of sterile 0.9% NaCl inj prior to administration

After infusion is complete, flush w/ 30mL of sterile 0.9% NaCl inj

Reconstitution

1. Reconstitute vial containing lyophilized powder w/ 4.8mL of SWFI using a syringe w/ a 21- to 25-gauge needle
2. Insert the syringe needle into the vial through the center of the stopper and direct the stream of SWFI to the glass wall of the vial to avoid excessive foaming

3. Gently swirl vial for at least 15 sec; do not vigorously shake or invert
4. Allow sol to sit for up to 20 min at room temperature to allow for reconstitution and for any foam to settle; may swirl and inspect for dissolution during this time. If not fully dissolved after 20 min, allow another 10 min for dissolution; do not use vial if the drug product is not dissolved w/in 30 min
5. Prior to withdrawing the reconstituted sol from vial, gently invert vial 3X
6. Withdraw 5mL (300mg) of reconstituted sol using a syringe w/ a 21- to 25- gauge needle

Dilution

Add the 5mL (300mg) of reconstituted sol to 250mL of 0.9% NaCl and gently mix infusion bag; once reconstituted and diluted, use infusion sol as soon as possible

Do not add other medicinal products to the prepared infusion sol or IV infusion set

May store infusion sol for up to 4 hrs at 2°-8°C (36°-46°F), if necessary; do not freeze

E

HOW SUPPLIED

Inj: 300mg

CONTRAINDICATIONS

Known serious or severe hypersensitivity reaction to vedolizumab or any of the excipients (eg, dyspnea, bronchospasm, urticaria, flushing, rash, increased HR).

WARNINGS/PRECAUTIONS

Hypersensitivity reactions reported; d/c immediately and initiate appropriate treatment if anaphylaxis or other serious allergic reactions occur. Increased risk for developing infections; not recommended in patients with active, severe infections until the infections are controlled. Consider withholding treatment if a severe infection develops. Consider screening for tuberculosis according to the local practice. Progressive multifocal leukoencephalopathy (PML) may occur; monitor for any new onset, or worsening, of neurological signs and symptoms. If PML is suspected, withhold dosing and refer to a neurologist; if confirmed, d/c dosing permanently. Elevations of transaminase and/or bilirubin reported; d/c if jaundice or other evidence of significant liver injury develops. Prior to initiating treatment, all patients should be brought up to date with all immunizations according to current immunization guidelines.

ADVERSE REACTIONS

Nasopharyngitis, headache, arthralgia, nausea, pyrexia, upper respiratory tract infection, fatigue, cough, bronchitis, influenza, back pain, rash, pruritus, sinusitis, oropharyngeal pain, pain in extremities.

DRUG INTERACTIONS

Avoid with natalizumab; potential for increased risk of PML and other infections. Avoid with TNF blockers; potential for increased risk of infections. Live vaccines may be administered concurrently with therapy only if the benefits outweigh the risks.

PATIENT CONSIDERATIONS

Assessment: Assess for hypersensitivity to drug, infections, history of recurring severe infections, pregnancy/nursing status, and possible drug interactions. Assess immunization history.

Monitoring: Monitor for infusion/hypersensitivity reactions, infections, PML, liver injury, and other adverse reactions.

Counseling: Instruct to report immediately if symptoms consistent with a hypersensitivity reaction occur during or following infusion. Advise to notify physician if any signs/symptoms of infection develop. Instruct to report immediately any symptoms that may indicate PML (new onset or worsening of neurological signs/symptoms) and/or liver injury (eg, fatigue, anorexia, right upper abdominal discomfort, dark urine, jaundice).

STORAGE: 2-8°C (36-46°F). Protect from light. Infusion Sol: 2-8°C (36-46°F) for up to 4 hrs. Do not freeze.

ENULOSE – lactulose

RX

Class: Ammonium detoxicant/osmotic laxative

OTHER BRAND NAMES

Generlac

ADULT DOSAGE

Portal-Systemic Encephalopathy

Including Stages of Hepatic Pre-Coma and Coma:

Oral Route:

Usual: 30-45mL (containing 20-30g of lactulose) tid or qid

Titrate: Adjust dose every day or two, to produce 2 or 3 soft stools daily

PEDIATRIC DOSAGE

Portal-Systemic Encephalopathy

Including Stages of Hepatic Pre-Coma and Coma:

Oral Route:

Infants:

Initial: 2.5-10mL/day in divided doses, to produce 2-3 soft stools daily

Hourly doses of 30-45mL may be used to induce the rapid laxation indicated in the initial phase of the therapy; when the laxative effect has been achieved, the dose may then be reduced to the recommended daily dose

Rectal Route:
When the patient is in the impending coma or coma stage and the danger of aspiration exists, or when the necessary endoscopic or intubation procedures physically interfere w/ the administration of the recommended oral doses, lactulose sol may be given as a retention enema via a rectal balloon catheter

Mix 300mL of lactulose sol w/ 700mL of water or physiologic saline and retain for 30-60 min; may repeat q4-6h

If the enema is inadvertently evacuated too promptly, it may be repeated immediately

Start oral therapy before the enema is stopped entirely

Older Children and Adolescents:
40-90mL/day, to produce 2-3 soft stools daily

If initial dose causes diarrhea, reduce dose immediately; if diarrhea persists, d/c lactulose

E

ADMINISTRATION
Oral/Rectal route

HOW SUPPLIED
Sol: 10g/15mL [473mL], Generlac [1892mL]

CONTRAINDICATIONS
Patients who require a low-galactose diet.

WARNINGS/PRECAUTIONS
Potential explosive reaction with electrocautery procedures during proctoscopy or colonoscopy; patients on therapy undergoing such procedures should have a thorough bowel cleansing with a non-fermentable solution. Contains galactose and lactose; caution with diabetes. May develop hyponatremia and dehydration in infants.

ADVERSE REACTIONS
Flatulence/belching, abdominal discomfort, diarrhea, N/V.

DRUG INTERACTIONS
May interfere the desired degradation and prevent the acidification of colonic contents with neomycin; closely monitor the status of the treated patients. Nonabsorbable antacids may decrease effects. Avoid use with other laxatives, especially during the initial phase of therapy.

PATIENT CONSIDERATIONS

Assessment: Assess for diabetes, patients requiring a low-galactose diet, pregnancy/nursing status, and possible drug interactions. Assess use in electrocautery procedures during proctoscopy or colonoscopy.

Monitoring: Monitor for hyponatremia and dehydration in infants, diarrhea, vomiting, and other adverse reactions.

Counseling: Inform about the risks and benefits of therapy. Instruct to take exactly ud. Advise to report any potential adverse effects.

STORAGE: Do not freeze. Prolonged exposure >30°C (86°F) or to direct light may cause extreme darkening and turbidity; do not use if this condition develops. Prolonged exposure to freezing temperature may cause change to a semi-solid, too viscous to pour; viscosity will return to normal upon warming to room temperature. (Enulose) 2-30°C (36-86°F). (Generlac) 20-25°C (68-77°F).

EPANOVA — omega-3-carboxylic acids

RX

Class: Lipid-regulating agent

ADULT DOSAGE
Hypertriglyceridemia

Adjunct to Diet in Patients w/ Severe (≥500mg/dL) Hypertriglyceridemia:
2g/day (2 caps qd) or 4g/day (4 caps qd)

PEDIATRIC DOSAGE
Pediatric use may not have been established

E

DOSING CONSIDERATIONS

Elderly

Start at lower end of dosing range

ADMINISTRATION

Oral route

Take w/o regard to meals

Swallow caps whole; do not break open, crush, dissolve, or chew

HOW SUPPLIED

Cap: 1g

CONTRAINDICATIONS

Known hypersensitivity (eg, anaphylactic reaction) to Epanova or any of its components.

WARNINGS/PRECAUTIONS

Attempt to control serum lipids w/ appropriate diet, exercise, weight loss in obese patients, and control of any medical problems that are contributing to the lipid abnormalities (eg, diabetes mellitus, hypothyroidism). D/C or change medications known to exacerbate hypertriglyceridemia (eg, β-blockers, thiazides, estrogens) if possible prior to consideration of TG-lowering drug therapy. May increase LDL levels. Monitor ALT and AST levels periodically during therapy in patients w/ hepatic impairment. Use w/ caution in patients w/ known hypersensitivity to fish and/or shellfish.

ADVERSE REACTIONS

Diarrhea, nausea, abdominal pain/discomfort, eructation.

DRUG INTERACTIONS

Periodically monitor patients receiving concomitant treatment w/ drugs affecting coagulation (eg, antiplatelet agents).

PATIENT CONSIDERATIONS

Assessment: Assess for hypersensitivity to drug, fish, and/or shellfish. Assess for hepatic impairment, pregnancy/nursing status, and possible drug interactions. Attempt to control serum lipids w/ appropriate diet, exercise, weight loss in obese patients, and control of any medical problems (eg, diabetes mellitus, hypothyroidism) that may contribute to lipid abnormalities prior to therapy. Assess lipid levels.

Monitoring: Monitor for allergic reactions and other adverse reactions. Monitor lipid levels. Periodically monitor ALT/AST levels in patients w/ hepatic impairment.

Counseling: Instruct to notify physician if allergic to fish and/or shellfish. Inform that use of lipid-regulating agents does not reduce the importance of adhering to diet. Instruct to take ud. Advise not to alter caps in any way and to ingest intact caps only.

STORAGE: 25°C (77°F); excursions permitted to 15-30°C (59-86°F). Do not freeze.

EPIDUO – adapalene/benzoyl peroxide

RX

Class: Antibacterial/keratolytic

ADULT DOSAGE

Acne Vulgaris

Apply a thin film to affected areas of the face and/or trunk qd after washing. Use a pea-sized amount for each area of the face (eg, forehead, chin, each cheek)

PEDIATRIC DOSAGE

Acne Vulgaris

≥9 Years:

Apply a thin film to affected areas of the face and/or trunk qd after washing. Use a pea-sized amount for each area of the face (eg, forehead, chin, each cheek)

ADMINISTRATION

Topical route

Apply after washing.

Not for oral, ophthalmic, or intravaginal use.

HOW SUPPLIED

Gel: (Adapalene/Benzoyl Peroxide) 0.1%/2.5% [45g]

WARNINGS/PRECAUTIONS

Minimize exposure to sunlight and sunlamps; use sunscreen and protective apparel if exposure cannot be avoided. Exercise caution in patients w/ high levels of sun exposure and those w/ inherent sensitivity to sun. Extreme weather may cause irritation. Avoid contact w/ the eyes, lips, and mucous membranes. Avoid application to cuts, abrasions, or eczematous or sunburned skin. Erythema, scaling, dryness, stinging/burning, and irritant and allergic contact dermatitis may occur; depending on severity, may apply moisturizer, reduce frequency of application, or d/c use. Avoid waxing as a depilatory method on the treated skin.

ADVERSE REACTIONS
Dry skin, contact dermatitis, application-site burning, application-site irritation, skin irritation.

DRUG INTERACTIONS
Caution w/ concomitant topical acne therapy, especially w/ peeling, desquamating, or abrasive agents. Avoid w/ other potentially irritating topical products (medicated or abrasive soaps and cleansers, soaps and cosmetics that have strong skin-drying effect, and products w/ high concentrations of alcohol, astringents, spices, or limes).

PATIENT CONSIDERATIONS

E

Assessment: Assess for presence of cuts, abrasions, or eczematous or sunburned skin at the treatment site. Assess for pregnancy/nursing status and possible drug interactions. Assess if patient has high levels of sun exposure or inherent sensitivity to the sun.

Monitoring: Monitor for irritation, erythema, scaling, dryness, stinging/burning, and other adverse reactions.

Counseling: Advise to cleanse area w/ mild or soapless cleanser and to pat dry. Advise to avoid contact w/ the eyes, lips, and mucous membranes. Instruct not to use more than the recommended amount. Inform that drug may cause irritation and may bleach hair and colored fabric. Instruct to minimize exposure to sunlight and sunlamps. Recommend to use sunscreen products and protective apparel when exposure to sunlight cannot be avoided.

STORAGE: 25°C (77°F); excursions permitted to 15-30°C (59-86°F). Keep tube tightly closed. Protect from light. Keep away from heat.

EpiPen – epinephrine

RX

Class: Sympathomimetic catecholamine

OTHER BRAND NAMES
EpiPen Jr.

ADULT DOSAGE
Emergency Treatment of Type I Allergic Reactions

Including anaphylaxis to stinging and biting insects, allergen immunotherapy, foods, drugs, diagnostic testing substances, and other allergens, as well as idiopathic or exercise-induced anaphylaxis

15-30kg:
EpiPen Jr: 0.15mg

≥30kg:
EpiPen: 0.3mg

Severe Persistent Anaphylaxis:
Repeat inj may be necessary

PEDIATRIC DOSAGE
Emergency Treatment of Type I Allergic Reactions

Including anaphylaxis to stinging and biting insects, allergen immunotherapy, foods, drugs, diagnostic testing substances, and other allergens, as well as idiopathic or exercise-induced anaphylaxis

15-30kg:
EpiPen Jr: 0.15mg

≥30kg:
EpiPen: 0.3mg

Severe Persistent Anaphylaxis:
Repeat inj may be necessary

ADMINISTRATION
IM/SQ route

Inject into the anterolateral aspect of the thigh, through clothing if necessary

Consider using other forms of injectable epinephrine if doses <0.15mg are deemed necessary

HOW SUPPLIED
Inj: (EpiPen Jr) 0.15mg/0.3mL; (EpiPen) 0.3mg/0.3mL

WARNINGS/PRECAUTIONS
Intended for immediate administration in patients who are determined to be at increased risk for anaphylaxis, including those with a history of anaphylactic reactions. Intended for immediate administration as emergency supportive therapy only and is not a substitute for immediate medical care. More than 2 sequential doses should only be administered under direct medical supervision. Do not inject IV. Large doses or accidental IV inj use may result in cerebral hemorrhage due to sharp rise in BP; rapidly acting vasodilators can counteract the marked pressor effects of epinephrine. Do not inject into buttock; may not provide effective treatment of anaphylaxis. Do not inject into digits, hands, or feet; may result in loss of blood flow to the affected area. Contains sodium metabisulfite; may cause allergic-type reactions, including anaphylactic symptoms or life-threatening or less severe asthmatic episodes in certain susceptible persons. Caution in patients with heart disease, hyperthyroidism, diabetes mellitus (DM), elderly, pregnant women. May temporarily worsen symptoms of Parkinson's disease.

ADVERSE REACTIONS
Anxiety, apprehensiveness, restlessness, tremor, weakness, dizziness, sweating, palpitations, pallor, N/V, headache, respiratory difficulties.

DRUG INTERACTIONS
May precipitate/aggravate angina pectoris as well as produce ventricular arrhythmias with drugs that may sensitize the heart to arrhythmias; use with caution. Monitor for cardiac arrhythmias with antiarrhythmics, cardiac glycosides, and diuretics. Effects may be potentiated by TCAs, MAOIs, levothyroxine sodium, and certain antihistamines (notably, chlorpheniramine, tripelennamine, diphenhydramine). Cardiostimulating and bronchodilating effects are antagonized by β-adrenergic blockers (eg, propranolol). Vasoconstricting and hypertensive effects are antagonized by α-adrenergic blockers (eg, phentolamine). Ergot alkaloids may reverse pressor effects.

E

PATIENT CONSIDERATIONS

Assessment: Assess for risk of anaphylaxis, heart disease, hyperthyroidism, DM, Parkinson's disease, pregnancy/nursing status, and for possible drug interactions.

Monitoring: Monitor for allergic-type reactions, angina pectoris, ventricular arrhythmias, cerebral hemorrhage, and other adverse reactions. Monitor HR and BP.

Counseling: Advise that therapy may produce signs and symptoms that include increased HR, sensation of more forceful heartbeat, palpitations, sweating, N/V, difficulty breathing, pallor, dizziness, weakness or shakiness, headache, apprehension, nervousness, or anxiety; advise that these signs and symptoms usually subside rapidly, especially with rest, quiet, and recumbency. Inform that patients may develop more severe or persistent effects if they have HTN or hyperthyroidism. Inform that patients may experience angina if they have coronary artery disease. Advise that patients may develop increased blood glucose levels following administration if they have DM. Advise that a temporary worsening of symptoms may be noticed if patient has Parkinson's disease. Instruct to seek immediate medical care in case of accidental inj.

STORAGE: 20-25°C (68-77°F); excursions permitted to 15-30°C (59-86°F). Store in the carrier tube provided. Protect from light. Do not refrigerate.

EPIVIR — lamivudine

RX

Class: Nucleoside reverse transcriptase inhibitor (NRTI)

Lactic acidosis and severe hepatomegaly w/ steatosis, including fatal cases, reported w/ nucleoside analogues; d/c treatment if lactic acidosis or pronounced hepatotoxicity occurs. Severe acute exacerbations of hepatitis B reported in patients coinfected w/ hepatitis B virus (HBV) upon discontinuation of therapy; closely monitor hepatic function for at least several months. If appropriate, initiation of antihepatitis B therapy may be warranted. Epivir tabs and sol (used to treat HIV-1 infection) contain a higher dose of lamivudine than Epivir-HBV tabs and sol (used to treat chronic HBV infection); patients w/ HIV-1 infection should only receive dosage forms appropriate for HIV-1 treatment.

ADULT DOSAGE

HIV-1 Infection

In Combination w/ Other Antiretrovirals:
150mg bid or 300mg qd

If lamivudine is administered to a patient infected w/ HIV-1 and HBV, the dosage indicated for HIV-1 therapy should be used as part of an appropriate combination regimen

PEDIATRIC DOSAGE

HIV-1 Infection

In Combination w/ Other Antiretrovirals:
≥3 Months:
Sol:
4mg/kg bid or 8mg/kg qd
Max: 300mg/day

Tab:
QD Dosing Regimen:
14 to <20kg: 150mg
≥20 to <25kg: 225mg
≥25kg: 300mg

BID Dosing Regimen (Using Scored 150mg Tab):
14 to <20kg:
AM Dose: 75mg
PM Dose: 75mg
Total Daily Dose: 150mg

≥20 to <25kg:
AM Dose: 75mg
PM Dose: 150mg
Total Daily Dose: 225mg

≥25kg:
AM Dose: 150mg
PM Dose: 150mg
Total Daily Dose: 300mg

DOSING CONSIDERATIONS

Renal Impairment

Adults and Adolescents ≥25kg:

CrCl 30-49mL/min: 150mg qd

CrCl 15-29mL/min: 150mg 1st dose, then 100mg qd

CrCl 5-14mL/min: 150mg 1st dose, then 50mg qd

CrCl <5mL/min: 50mg 1st dose, then 25mg qd

No additional dosing is required after routine (4-hr) hemodialysis or peritoneal dialysis

Pediatric Patients:

Consider dose reduction and/or increase in dosing interval

ADMINISTRATION

Oral route

Take w/ or w/o food.

HOW SUPPLIED

Oral Sol: 10mg/mL [240mL]; **Tab:** 150mg*, 300mg *scored

CONTRAINDICATIONS

Previous hypersensitivity reaction to lamivudine.

WARNINGS/PRECAUTIONS

Obesity and prolonged nucleoside exposure may be risk factors for lactic acidosis and severe hepatomegaly w/ steatosis. Caution w/ known risk factors for liver disease. Emergence of lamivudine-resistant HBV reported. Caution in pediatric patients w/ a history of prior antiretroviral nucleoside exposure, history of pancreatitis, or other significant risk factors for development of pancreatitis; d/c if pancreatitis develops. Immune reconstitution syndrome reported. Autoimmune disorders (eg, Graves' disease, polymyositis, Guillain-Barre syndrome) reported to occur in the setting of immune reconstitution and can occur many months after initiation of treatment. Redistribution/accumulation of body fat may occur. Caution in elderly.

ADVERSE REACTIONS

Headache, malaise, fatigue, N/V, diarrhea, nasal signs/symptoms, neuropathy, insomnia, musculoskeletal pain, cough, fever, dizziness.

DRUG INTERACTIONS

Not recommended w/ other lamivudine- and emtricitabine-containing products. Hepatic decompensation reported in HIV-1/hepatitis C virus coinfected patients receiving antiretroviral therapy for HIV-1 and interferon-alfa w/ or w/o ribavirin; closely monitor for treatment-associated toxicities during coadministration. Possible interaction w/ drugs whose main route of elimination is active renal secretion via the organic cationic transport system (eg, trimethoprim).

PATIENT CONSIDERATIONS

Assessment: Assess for renal impairment, risk factors for lactic acidosis and liver disease, HIV-1 and HBV coinfection, previous hypersensitivity, pregnancy/nursing status, and possible drug interactions. In pediatric patients, assess for a history of prior antiretroviral nucleoside exposure, a history of pancreatitis, or risk factors for pancreatitis. Consider HIV-1 viral load and CD4+ cell count/percentage when selecting the dosing interval for patients initiating treatment w/ oral sol.

Monitoring: Monitor for signs/symptoms of pancreatitis, immune reconstitution syndrome, autoimmune disorders, fat redistribution/accumulation, lactic acidosis, hepatomegaly w/ steatosis, hepatitis B exacerbation, renal dysfunction, and hypersensitivity reactions. Monitor hepatic function closely for several months in patients w/ HIV/HBV coinfection who d/c therapy. Monitor CBC.

Counseling: Inform that drug may cause a rare, but serious condition called lactic acidosis w/ liver enlargement. Instruct to discuss any changes in regimen w/ physician. Instruct not to take concomitantly w/ emtricitabine- or other lamivudine-containing products. Advise parents/guardians of pediatric patients to monitor for signs and symptoms of pancreatitis. Advise that drug is not a cure for HIV-1 infection and continuous therapy is necessary to control HIV-1 infection and decrease HIV-related illness. Inform that redistribution/accumulation of body fat may occur. Advise diabetic patients that each 15mL dose of sol contains 3g of sucrose. Advise to avoid doing things that can spread HIV-1 to others. Inform to take all HIV medications exactly as prescribed.

STORAGE: **Tab:** 25°C (77°F); excursions permitted to 15-30°C (59-86°F). **Sol:** 25°C (77°F).

Epivir-HBV – lamivudine

RX

Class: Nucleoside reverse transcriptase inhibitor (NRTI)

Lactic acidosis and severe hepatomegaly with steatosis, including fatal cases, reported with nucleoside analogues. Suspend treatment if lactic acidosis or pronounced hepatotoxicity occurs. Severe acute exacerbations of hepatitis B reported upon discontinuation of therapy; closely monitor hepatic function for at least several months. If appropriate, initiation of antihepatitis B therapy may be warranted. Not approved for treatment of HIV infection. Lamivudine dosage in Epivir-HBV is subtherapeutic and monotherapy is inappropriate for treatment of HIV infection. HIV-1 resistance may emerge in chronic hepatitis B-infected patients with unrecognized/untreated HIV infection. Offer HIV counseling and testing to all patients prior to therapy and periodically thereafter.

ADULT DOSAGE

Chronic Hepatitis B

100mg qd

PEDIATRIC DOSAGE

Chronic Hepatitis B

2-17 Years:

3mg/kg qd

Max: 100mg/day

DOSING CONSIDERATIONS

Renal Impairment

CrCl 30-49mL/min: 100mg 1st dose, then 50mg qd

CrCl 15-29mL/min: 100mg 1st dose, then 25mg qd

CrCl 5-14mL/min: 35mg 1st dose, then 15mg qd

CrCl <5mL/min: 35mg 1st dose, then 10mg qd

ADMINISTRATION

Oral route

Take w/ or w/o food

Tabs and oral sol are interchangeable

Use oral sol for doses <100mg

Do not use w/ other medications that contain lamivudine or emtricitabine

Refer to PI for assessing patients during treatment

HOW SUPPLIED

Sol: 5mg/mL [240mL]; **Tab:** 100mg

CONTRAINDICATIONS

Previous hypersensitivity reaction (eg, anaphylaxis) to lamivudine or to any component of the tabs or oral sol.

WARNINGS/PRECAUTIONS

Consider initiation of treatment only when use of an alternative antiviral agent with a higher genetic barrier to resistance is not available/appropriate. Obesity and prolonged nucleoside exposure may be risk factors for lactic acidosis and severe hepatomegaly with steatosis. Caution with known risk factors for liver disease. Emergence of resistance-associated HBV substitutions reported; monitor ALT and HBV DNA levels if suspected. Not approved for patients dually infected with HBV and HIV. Epivir HBV contains a lower lamivudine dose than Epivir, Combivir, Epzicom, and Trizivir. If a decision is made to administer lamivudine to such coinfected patients, use the higher dosage indicated for HIV therapy as part of an appropriate combination regimen and refer to PI of such drugs. Caution in elderly patients.

ADVERSE REACTIONS

Lactic acidosis, severe hepatomegaly with steatosis, exacerbations of hepatitis B, ear/nose/throat infections, sore throat, diarrhea, serum lipase increase, CPK increase, ALT increase, thrombocytopenia.

DRUG INTERACTIONS

Avoid with other lamivudine- and emtricitabine-containing products. Possible interaction with other drugs whose main route of elimination is active renal secretion via the organic cationic transport system (eg, trimethoprim).

PATIENT CONSIDERATIONS

Assessment: Assess for hepatic/renal impairment, previous nucleoside exposure, risk factors for liver disease, HIV infection, hypersensitivity to drug, pregnancy/nursing status, and possible drug interactions. Perform HIV counseling and testing. Obtain baseline ALT and HBV DNA levels.

Monitoring: Monitor for renal/hepatic dysfunction, loss of therapeutic response (eg, persistent ALT elevation, increasing HBV DNA levels after an initial decline below assay limit, progression of clinical signs/symptoms of hepatic disease, worsening of hepatic necroinflammatory findings), signs/symptoms of lactic acidosis, hepatomegaly with steatosis, emergence of resistant HIV, hepatitis B exacerbation, and hypersensitivity reactions. Monitor hepatic function closely for several months in patients who d/c therapy.

Counseling: Advise to remain under the care of a physician during therapy and to report any new symptoms or concurrent medications. Inform that drug is not a cure for hepatitis B and that long-term benefits and relationship of initial treatment response to outcomes (eg, hepatocellular carcinoma, decompensated cirrhosis) are unknown. Inform that liver disease deterioration may occur upon discontinuation. Instruct to discuss any changes in regimen with physician. Inform that emergence of resistant HBV and worsening of disease can occur; advise to report any new symptoms to physician. Counsel on importance of HIV testing to avoid inappropriate therapy and development of resistant HIV. Inform that drug contains a lower dose of lamivudine than Epivir, Combivir, Epzicom, and Trizivir; instruct not to take concurrently with these products. Instruct not to take concurrently with emtricitabine-containing products (eg, Atripla, Complera, Emtriva, Stribild, Truvada). Inform that therapy has not been shown to reduce the risk of HBV transmission through sexual contact/blood contamination. Instruct to avoid doing things that can spread HBV infection to others. Inform diabetics that each 20mL dose of oral sol contains 4g of sucrose.

STORAGE: Tab: 25°C (77°F); excursions permitted to 15-30°C (59-86°F). Sol: 20-25°C (68-77°F); store in tightly closed bottles.

EPOGEN — epoetin alfa

RX

Class: Erythropoiesis stimulator

Increased risk of death, MI, stroke, venous thromboembolism (VTE), thrombosis of vascular access, and tumor progression or recurrence. Use the lowest dose sufficient to reduce/avoid the need for RBC transfusions. Chronic Kidney Disease (CKD): Greater risks for death, serious adverse cardiovascular (CV) reactions, and stroke when administered to target Hgb level >11g/dL. Cancer: Shortened overall survival and/or increased risk of tumor progression or recurrence in patients with breast, non-small cell lung, head and neck, lymphoid, and cervical cancers. Must enroll in and comply with the ESA APPRISE Oncology Program to prescribe and/or dispense drug to patients. Use only for anemia from myelosuppressive chemotherapy. Not indicated for patients receiving myelosuppressive chemotherapy when anticipated outcome is cure. D/C following completion of a chemotherapy course. Perisurgery: Due to increased risk of deep venous thrombosis (DVT), DVT prophylaxis is recommended.

ADULT DOSAGE

Anemia

Chronic Kidney Disease Associated Anemia:
Initiate When:
On Dialysis: Hgb <10g/dL
Not On Dialysis: Hgb <10g/dL, the rate of Hgb decline indicates likelihood of requiring a RBC transfusion, and reducing the risk of alloimmunization and/or other RBC transfusion-related risks is a goal

Initial: 50-100 U/kg IV/SQ 3X/week
Titrate:
On Dialysis: When Hgb approaches/exceeds 11g/dL, reduce or interrupt dose
Not On Dialysis: When Hgb approaches/exceeds 10g/dL, reduce or interrupt dose

All Chronic Kidney Disease Patients:
Do not increase dose more frequently than once every 4 weeks; decreases in dose may occur more frequently
If Hgb rises rapidly (eg, >1g/dL in any 2-week period), decrease dose by 25% or more prn to reduce rapid responses
If Hgb has not increased by >1g/dL after 4 weeks, increase dose by 25%
If no response after 12-week escalation period, use lowest dose to maintain sufficient Hgb level to reduce need for RBC transfusions and evaluate other causes of anemia

Zidovudine (≤4200mg) Associated Anemia in HIV-Infected Patients w/ Endogenous Serum Erythropoietin Levels of ≤500 mU/mL:
Initial: 100 U/kg IV/SQ 3X/week
Titrate:
Hgb Does Not Increase After 8 Weeks of Therapy: Increase by 50-100 U/kg at 4- to 8- week intervals until Hgb reaches a level needed to avoid RBC transfusions or 300 U/kg

PEDIATRIC DOSAGE

Anemia

Chronic Kidney Disease Associated Anemia:
1 Month-16 Years:
On Dialysis:
Initial: 50 U/kg IV/SQ 3X weekly
Titrate: When Hgb approaches/exceeds 11g/dL, reduce or interrupt dose
Do not increase dose more frequently than once every 4 weeks; decreases in dose may occur more frequently
If Hgb rises rapidly (eg, >1g/dL in any 2-week period), decrease dose by 25% or more prn to reduce rapid responses
If Hgb has not increased by >1g/dL after 4 weeks, increase dose by 25%
If no response after 12-week escalation period, use lowest dose to maintain sufficient Hgb level to reduce need for RBC transfusions and evaluate other causes of anemia

Chemotherapy Associated Anemia:
5-18 Years:
Initial: 600 U/kg IV weekly until completion of a chemotherapy course
Titrate:
Dose Reduction: Reduce by 25% if Hgb increases >1g/dL in any 2-week period or Hgb reaches a level needed to avoid RBC transfusions. Withhold if Hgb exceeds level needed to avoid RBC transfusions; reinitiate at 25% below previous dose when Hgb approaches a level where RBC transfusions may be required
Dose Increase: If Hgb increases by <1g/dL and remains below 10g/dL after initial 4 weeks, increase dose to 900 U/kg weekly
D/C therapy if there is no response in Hgb levels or if RBC transfusions are still required after 8 weeks
Max: 60,000 U/week

Hgb >12g/dL: Withhold dose. When Hgb <11g/dL, resume at 25% below the previous dose

D/C if increase in Hgb is not achieved at a dose of 300 U/kg for 8 weeks

Chemotherapy Associated Anemia:
Initiate when Hgb <10g/dL and if there is a minimum of 2 additional months of planned chemotherapy
Initial: 150 U/kg SQ 3X/week or 40,000 U SQ weekly until completion of a chemotherapy course
Titrate:
Dose Reduction: Reduce by 25% if Hgb increases >1g/dL in any 2-week period or reaches a level needed to avoid RBC transfusions. Withhold if Hgb exceeds level needed to avoid RBC transfusions; reinitiate at 25% below previous dose when Hgb approaches a level where RBC transfusions may be required
Dose Increase: If Hgb increases by <1g/dL and remains below 10g/dL after initial 4 weeks, increase dose to 300 U/kg 3X/week or 60,000 U/week
D/C therapy if there is no response in Hgb levels or if RBC transfusions are still required after 8 weeks
Surgery Patients:
Used to reduce the need for allogeneic RBC transfusions among patients w/ perioperative Hgb >10-≤13g/dL who are at high risk for perioperative blood loss from elective, noncardiac, nonvascular surgery
Usual: 300 U/kg/day SQ qd for 10 days before, on the day of, and for 4 days after surgery; or 600 U/kg SQ in 4 doses administered 21, 14, and 7 days before surgery and on the day of surgery. Deep vein thrombosis prophylaxis is recommended

DOSING CONSIDERATIONS

Elderly
Individualize dose selection and adjustment to achieve and maintain target Hgb

ADMINISTRATION

IV/SQ route

IV route is recommended for chronic kidney disease patients on hemodialysis

Preparation/Administration
Do not shake; do not use if shaken or frozen
Preservative-free single-use vials may be admixed in a syringe w/ bacteriostatic 0.9% NaCl inj, w/ benzyl alcohol 0.9% in a 1:1 ratio
Do not dilute or mix w/ other drug sol
Do not re-enter preservative-free vials; discard unused portions
Store unused portions of multidose vials at 36-46°F (2-8°C); discard after 21 days after initial entry

HOW SUPPLIED

Inj: 2000 U/mL, 3000 U/mL, 4000 U/mL, 10,000 U/mL [single-dose vial]; 10,000 U/mL [2mL], 20,000 U/mL [1mL] [multidose vial]

CONTRAINDICATIONS

Uncontrolled HTN, pure red cell aplasia (PRCA) that begins after treatment with epoetin alfa or other erythropoietin protein drugs, serious allergic reactions to epoetin alfa. **Multidose Vials:** Neonates, infants, pregnant women, and nursing mothers.

WARNINGS/PRECAUTIONS

Not indicated for use in patients with cancer receiving hormonal agents, biologic products, or radiotherapy, unless also receiving concomitant myelosuppressive chemotherapy; in patients scheduled for surgery who are willing to donate autologous blood; in patients undergoing cardiac/

vascular surgery; or as a substitute for RBC transfusions in patients requiring immediate correction of anemia. Evaluate transferrin saturation and serum ferritin prior to and during treatment; administer supplemental iron when serum ferritin is <100mcg/L or serum transferrin saturation is <20%. Correct/exclude other causes of anemia (eg, vitamin deficiency, metabolic/chronic inflammatory conditions, bleeding) before initiating therapy. Hypertensive encephalopathy and seizures reported in patients with CKD; increases risk of seizures in CKD patients. Appropriately control HTN prior to initiation of and during treatment; reduce/withhold therapy if BP becomes difficult to control. PRCA and severe anemia, with or without other cytopenias that arise following the development of neutralizing antibodies to erythropoietin, reported. Withhold and evaluate for neutralizing antibodies to erythropoietin if severe anemia and low reticulocyte count develop; d/c permanently if PRCA develops, and do not switch to other erythropoiesis-stimulating agents. Serious allergic reactions may occur; immediately and permanently d/c therapy. Contains albumin; may carry an extremely remote risk for transmission of viral diseases or Creutzfeldt-Jakob disease. Patients may require adjustments in their dialysis prescriptions after initiation of therapy, or require increased anticoagulation with heparin to prevent clotting of extracorporeal circuit during hemodialysis. Multidose vial contains benzyl alcohol; benzyl alcohol is associated with serious adverse events and death, particularly in pediatric patients.

ADVERSE REACTIONS

MI, stroke, VTE, thrombosis of vascular access, tumor progression/recurrence, pyrexia, N/V, HTN, cough, arthralgia, dizziness, pruritus, rash, headache.

PATIENT CONSIDERATIONS

Assessment: Assess for uncontrolled HTN, previous hypersensitivity to the drug, causes of anemia, pregnancy/nursing status, and other conditions where treatment is contraindicated or cautioned. Obtain baseline Hgb levels, transferrin saturation, and serum ferritin.

Monitoring: Monitor for signs/symptoms of an allergic reaction, CV/thromboembolic events, stroke, premonitory neurologic symptoms, PRCA, severe anemia, progression/recurrence of tumor, and other adverse reactions. Monitor BP, transferrin saturation, and serum ferritin. Following initiation of therapy and after each dose adjustment, monitor Hgb weekly until Hgb is stable, then at least monthly, and to maintain Hgb sufficient to minimize need for RBC transfusions.

Counseling: Inform of the risks and benefits of therapy, and of the increased risks of mortality, serious CV reactions, thromboembolic reactions, stroke, and tumor progression. Advise of the need to have regular lab tests for Hgb. Inform cancer patients that they must sign the patient-physician acknowledgment form prior to therapy. Instruct to undergo regular BP monitoring, adhere to prescribed antihypertensive regimen, and follow recommended dietary restrictions. Advise to contact physician for new-onset neurologic symptoms or change in seizure frequency. Instruct regarding proper disposal and caution against reuse of needles, syringes, or unused portions of single-dose vials.

STORAGE: 2-8°C (36-46°F). Do not freeze; do not use if it has been frozen. Protect from light. Discard unused portions of multidose vials 21 days after initial entry.

EPZICOM — abacavir sulfate/lamivudine

RX

Class: Nucleoside reverse transcriptase inhibitor (NRTI)

Lactic acidosis and severe hepatomegaly w/ steatosis, including fatal cases, reported w/ nucleoside analogues. Abacavir: Serious and sometimes fatal hypersensitivity reactions (multiorgan clinical syndrome) reported; d/c as soon as suspected and never restart therapy w/ any abacavir-containing product. Patients w/ HLA-B*5701 allele are at high risk for hypersensitivity; screen for HLA-B*5701 allele prior to therapy. Lamivudine: Severe acute exacerbations of hepatitis B reported in patients coinfected w/ hepatitis B virus (HBV) upon discontinuation of therapy; closely monitor hepatic function for at least several months. If appropriate, initiation of antihepatitis B therapy may be warranted.

ADULT DOSAGE

HIV-1 Infection

Combination w/ Other Antiretrovirals:
1 tab qd

PEDIATRIC DOSAGE

HIV-1 Infection

Combination w/ Other Antiretrovirals:
≥25kg: 1 tab qd

DOSING CONSIDERATIONS

Renal Impairment

CrCl <50mL/min: Not recommended

Hepatic Impairment

Contraindicated

ADMINISTRATION

Oral route

Take w/ or w/o food.

HOW SUPPLIED

Tab: (Abacavir/Lamivudine) 600mg/300mg

CONTRAINDICATIONS

Previous demonstrated hypersensitivity to abacavir or any components of the medication, hepatic impairment.

WARNINGS/PRECAUTIONS

Obesity and prolonged nucleoside exposure may be risk factors for lactic acidosis and severe hepatomegaly w/ steatosis. Caution w/ known risk factors for liver disease; suspend therapy if clinical or lab findings suggestive of lactic acidosis or pronounced hepatotoxicity develop. Immune reconstitution syndrome reported. Autoimmune disorders (eg, Graves' disease, polymyositis, Guillain-Barre syndrome) reported to occur in the setting of immune reconstitution and can occur many months after initiation of treatment. Redistribution/accumulation of body fat reported. Cross-resistance potential w/ nucleoside reverse transcriptase inhibitors reported. Caution in elderly. **Abacavir:** Consider the underlying risk of coronary heart disease when prescribing therapy. **Lamivudine:** Emergence of lamivudine-resistant HBV reported.

ADVERSE REACTIONS

Hypersensitivity, insomnia, depression/depressed mood, headache/migraine, fatigue/malaise, dizziness/vertigo, nausea, diarrhea, rash, pyrexia, abdominal pain/gastritis, abnormal dreams, anxiety.

DRUG INTERACTIONS

Avoid w/ other abacavir-, lamivudine-, and/or emtricitabine-containing products. **Abacavir:** Ethanol may decrease elimination causing an increase in overall exposure. May increase oral methadone clearance. **Lamivudine:** Hepatic decompensation reported in HIV-1/hepatitis C virus (HCV) coinfected patients receiving combination antiretroviral therapy for HIV-1 and interferon-alfa w/ or w/o ribavirin; closely monitor for treatment-associated toxicities, and consider discontinuation of Epzicom and dose reduction/discontinuation of interferon-alfa, ribavirin, or both.

PATIENT CONSIDERATIONS

Assessment: Assess medical history for prior exposure to any abacavir-containing product. Assess for HBV infection, history of hypersensitivity reactions, HLA-B*5701 status (including patients of unknown HLA-B*5701 status who have previously tolerated abacavir), hepatic/renal impairment, risk factors for coronary heart disease and lactic acidosis, pregnancy/nursing status, and possible drug interactions.

Monitoring: Monitor for signs/symptoms of hypersensitivity reactions, lactic acidosis, hepatomegaly w/ steatosis, immune reconstitution syndrome (eg, opportunistic infections), autoimmune disorders, fat redistribution/accumulation, and other adverse reactions. Monitor hepatic/renal function. Closely monitor hepatic function for several months after discontinuing therapy in patients coinfected w/ HIV-1 and HBV.

Counseling: Inform patients regarding hypersensitivity reactions w/ abacavir; instruct to contact physician immediately if symptoms develop and not to restart or replace w/ any other abacavir-containing products w/o medical consultation. Inform that the drug may cause lactic acidosis w/ hepatomegaly. Inform patients coinfected w/ HIV-1 and HBV that deterioration of liver disease has occurred in some cases when treatment w/ lamivudine was discontinued; instruct to discuss any changes in regimen w/ the physician. Inform that hepatic decompensation has occurred in HIV-1/HCV coinfected patients receiving combination antiretroviral therapy for HIV-1 and interferon alfa w/ or w/o ribavirin. Inform that redistribution/accumulation of body fat may occur. Advise that drug is not a cure for HIV-1 infection and continuous therapy is necessary to control HIV-1 infection and decrease HIV-related illness. Inform patients to take all HIV medications exactly as prescribed. Advise not to re-use or share needles/other inj equipment and not to share personal items (eg, toothbrush, razor blades), to continue to practice safer sex by using latex or polyurethane condoms, and not to breastfeed.

STORAGE: 25°C (77°F); excursions permitted to 15-30°C (59-86°F).

ERBITUX – cetuximab

RX

Class: Monoclonal antibody/EGFR blocker

Serious infusion reactions, some fatal, reported; immediately interrupt and permanently d/c infusion if these reactions occur. Cardiopulmonary arrest and/or sudden death occurred in patients w/ squamous cell carcinoma of the head and neck (SCCHN) treated w/ cetuximab in combination w/ radiation therapy or w/ European Union-approved cetuximab in combination w/ platinum-based therapy w/ 5-fluorouracil (5-FU); closely monitor serum electrolytes during and after therapy.

E

ADULT DOSAGE

Squamous Cell Carcinoma of the Head and Neck

W/ Radiation Therapy for the Initial Treatment of Locally or Regionally Advanced Squamous Cell Carcinoma of the Head and Neck (SCCHN):
Initial: 400mg/m^2 administered 1 week prior to initiation of a course of radiation therapy as a 120 min IV infusion
Maint: 250mg/m^2 infused over 60 min weekly for the duration of radiation therapy (6-7 weeks)
Max Infusion Rate: 10mg/min

Complete administration 60 min prior to radiation therapy

W/ Platinum-Based Therapy w/ 5-fluorouracil (5-FU) for the 1st-Line Treatment of Patients w/ Recurrent Locoregional Disease or Metastatic SCCHN:
Initial: 400mg/m^2 administered on the day of initiation of platinum-based therapy w/ 5-FU as a 120 min IV infusion
Maint: 250mg/m^2 infused over 60 min weekly until disease progression or unacceptable toxicity
Max Infusion Rate: 10mg/min

Complete administration 60 min prior to platinum-based therapy w/ 5-FU

As Monotherapy in Patients w/ Recurrent/Metastatic SCCHN for Whom Prior Platinum-Based Therapy Failed:
Initial: 400mg/m^2 administered as a 120 min IV infusion
Maint: 250mg/m^2 infused over 60 min weekly until disease progression or unacceptable toxicity
Max Infusion Rate: 10mg/min

Metastatic Colorectal Cancer

Treatment of *K-Ras* wild-type, epidermal growth factor receptor-expressing, metastatic colorectal cancer in combination w/ FOLFIRI (irinotecan, 5-fluorouracil, leucovorin) for 1st-line treatment, in combination w/ irinotecan in patients who are refractory to irinotecan-based chemotherapy, and as monotherapy in patients who have failed oxaliplatin- and irinotecan-based chemotherapy or are intolerant to irinotecan
Initial: 400mg/m^2 administered as a 120-min IV infusion; complete administration 60 min prior to FOLFIRI
Maint: 250mg/m^2 infused over 60 min weekly until disease progression or unacceptable toxicity; complete administration 60 min prior to FOLFIRI
Max Infusion Rate: 10mg/min

Premedication

H_1-antagonist (eg, 50mg diphenhydramine) IV 30-60 min prior to 1st dose; premedication for subsequent doses should be based on clinical judgment and presence/severity of prior infusion reactions

PEDIATRIC DOSAGE

Pediatric use may not have been established

E

DOSING CONSIDERATIONS

Adverse Reactions

NCI CTC Grade 1 or 2 and Non-Serious NCI CTC Grade 3 Infusion Reaction:
Reduce infusion rate by 50%; immediately and permanently d/c for serious infusion reactions, requiring medical intervention and/or hospitalization

Severe Acneiform Rash (NCI CTC Grade 3 or 4):
1st Occurrence: Delay infusion 1-2 weeks
W/ Improvement: Continue at 250mg/m^2
No Improvement: D/C treatment

2nd Occurrence: Delay infusion 1-2 weeks
W/ Improvement: Reduce to 200mg/m^2
No Improvement: D/C treatment

3rd Occurrence: Delay infusion 1-2 weeks
W/ Improvement: Reduce to 150mg/m^2
No Improvement: D/C treatment

4th Occurrence: D/C treatment

ADMINISTRATION

IV route

Do not administer as IV push or bolus
Administer via infusion pump or syringe pump
Administer through low protein binding 0.22μm in-line filter
Do not shake or dilute

HOW SUPPLIED

Inj: 2mg/mL [50mL, 100mL]

WARNINGS/PRECAUTIONS

Caution when used in combination w/ radiation therapy or platinum-based therapy w/ 5-FU in head and neck cancer patients w/ history of coronary artery disease (CAD), CHF, or arrhythmias. Interstitial lung disease (ILD) reported; interrupt for acute onset or worsening of pulmonary symptoms and permanently d/c if ILD is confirmed. Dermatologic toxicities (eg, acneiform rash, skin drying/fissuring, paronychial inflammation, infectious sequelae, hypertrichosis) reported. Life-threatening and fatal bullous mucocutaneous disease w/ blisters, erosions, and skin sloughing has also been observed; limit sun exposure during therapy. Addition of cetuximab to radiation and cisplatin in patients reported to increase incidence of Grade 3-4 mucositis, radiation recall syndrome, acneiform rash, cardiac events, and electrolyte disturbances compared to radiation and cisplatin alone; addition of cetuximab did not improve progression-free survival. Hypomagnesemia and electrolyte abnormalities reported; replete electrolytes as necessary. Do not resume nursing earlier than 60 days following the last dose of therapy if nursing is interrupted. Not indicated for the treatment of *Ras* mutant colorectal cancer or when *Ras* mutation test results are unknown, or for the treatment of patients w/ colorectal cancer that harbor somatic mutations in exon 2 (codons 12 and 13), exon 3 (codons 59 and 61), and exon 4 (codons 117 and 146) of either *K-ras* or *N-ras*.

ADVERSE REACTIONS

Cardiopulmonary arrest, infusion reactions, cutaneous reactions (eg, rash, pruritus, nail changes), headache, diarrhea, infection, sepsis, asthenia, nausea, emesis, fatigue, fever, pain, dyspnea, cough.

PATIENT CONSIDERATIONS

Assessment: Assess for history of CAD, CHF, arrhythmias, pulmonary disorders, pregnancy/nursing status, and possible drug interactions. Obtain serum electrolyte levels (including Mg^{2+}, K^{+}, Ca^{2+}). Determine EGFR-expression status and confirm the absence of a *Ras* mutation in colorectal tumors using FDA-approved tests.

Monitoring: Monitor for signs/symptoms of infusion reactions, cardiopulmonary arrest, acute onset or worsening of pulmonary symptoms, dermatologic toxicities and infectious sequelae, and for other adverse reactions. Monitor patients for 1 hr after infusion in a setting w/ resuscitation equipment and other agents necessary to treat anaphylaxis; monitor longer to confirm resolution of the event in patients requiring treatment for infusion reactions. Periodically monitor for hypomagnesemia, hypocalcemia, and hypokalemia during and for at least 8 weeks after therapy.

Counseling: Advise to report to physician signs/symptoms of infusion reactions. Inform of pregnancy/nursing risks; advise to use adequate contraception during and for 6 months after last dose for both males and females. Inform that nursing is not recommended during and for 2 months following last dose of therapy. Instruct to limit sun exposure (eg, use of sunscreen, wear hats) during and for 2 months after last dose of therapy.

STORAGE: Vials: 2-8°C (36-46°F). Do not freeze. Infusion Containers: Stable for up to 12 hrs at 2-8°C (36-46°F) and up to 8 hrs at 20-25°C (68-77°F).

E

ERTACZO – sertaconazole nitrate

RX

Class: Azole antifungal

ADULT DOSAGE

Fungal Infections

Interdigital Tinea Pedis Caused by *Trichophyton rubrum*, *Trichophyton mentagrophytes*, and *Epidermophyton floccosum*:

Apply sufficient amount to cover both the affected areas between the toes and the immediately surrounding healthy skin bid for 4 weeks

PEDIATRIC DOSAGE

Fungal Infections

Interdigital Tinea Pedis Caused by *Trichophyton rubrum*, *Trichophyton mentagrophytes*, and *Epidermophyton floccosum*:

≥12 Years:

Apply sufficient amount to cover both the affected areas between the toes and the immediately surrounding healthy skin bid for 4 weeks

ADMINISTRATION

Topical route

Wash hands after applying medication

Dry affected area(s) thoroughly before application if used after bathing

HOW SUPPLIED

Cre: 2% [60g]

WARNINGS/PRECAUTIONS

D/C and institute appropriate therapy if irritation occurs. Caution in patients sensitive to imidazole antifungals; cross-reactivity may occur.

ADVERSE REACTIONS

Contact dermatitis, dry skin, burning skin, application site skin tenderness.

PATIENT CONSIDERATIONS

Assessment: Assess for hypersensitivity to imidazole antifungals and pregnancy/nursing status.

Monitoring: Monitor for irritation and other adverse reactions.

Counseling: Instruct to use externally and ud. Instruct to use medication for the full treatment time, even though symptoms may have improved. Instruct to inform physician if area of application shows signs of increased irritation, redness, itching, burning, blistering, swelling, or oozing. Instruct to avoid the use of occlusive dressings unless directed by physician. Advise not to use for any disorder other than that for which it was prescribed.

STORAGE: 20-25°C (68-77°F); excursions permitted to 15-30°C (59-86°F).

ERY-TAB – erythromycin

RX

Class: Macrolide

ADULT DOSAGE

General Dosing

Mild to moderate upper/lower respiratory tract and skin and skin structure infections, listeriosis, diphtheria infections, and erythrasma, caused by susceptible strains of microorganisms

250mg qid in equally spaced doses, 333mg q8h, or 500mg q12h; may increase to 4g/day according to severity of infection

When dose is >1g/day, bid dosing is not recommended

Streptococcal Infections of the Upper Respiratory Tract:

Treat for at least 10 days

Rheumatic Fever

Prevention of Initial Attacks of Rheumatic Fever in Penicillin (PCN)-Allergic Patients:

Administer therapeutic dose for 10 days

PEDIATRIC DOSAGE

General Dosing

30-50mg/kg/day in equally divided doses; may double dose for more severe infections

Max: 4g/day

Streptococcal Infections of the Upper Respiratory Tract:

Treat for at least 10 days

Bacterial Conjunctivitis

Sus:

Conjunctivitis of the Newborn Caused by *Chlamydia trachomatis*:

50mg/kg/day in 4 divided doses for at least 2 weeks

Pneumonia

Sus:

Pneumonia of Infancy Caused by *Chlamydia trachomatis*:

50mg/kg/day in 4 divided doses for at least 3 weeks

Long-Term Prophylaxis of Streptococcal URTIs to Prevent Recurrent Attacks of Rheumatic Fever in Patients Allergic to PCN and Sulfonamides:
250mg bid

Urogenital Infections

During Pregnancy Due to *Chlamydia trachomatis*:
500mg qid or two 333mg tab q8h on an empty stomach for at least 7 days; if not tolerated, reduce to 500mg q12h, 333mg q8h, or 250mg qid for at least 14 days

Chlamydia trachomatis Infections

Uncomplicated Urethral, Endocervical, or Rectal Infections When Tetracycline is Contraindicated/Not Tolerated:
500mg qid, or two 333mg tabs q8h for at least 7 days

Nongonococcal Urethritis

Caused by *Ureaplasma urealyticum* When Tetracycline is Contraindicated/Not Tolerated:
500mg qid, or two 333mg tabs q8h for at least 7 days

Syphilis

30-40g given in divided doses for 10-15 days

Acute Pelvic Inflammatory Disease

Caused by *Neisseria gonorrhoeae*:
500mg (erythromycin lactobionate) IV q6h for 3 days, followed by 500mg PO q12h or 333mg PO q8h for 7 days

Amebiasis

Intestinal:
500mg q12h, 333mg q8h, or 250mg q6h for 10-14 days

Pertussis

40-50mg/kg/day in divided doses for 5-14 days

Legionnaires' Disease

1-4g/day in divided doses

Prophylaxis of Postoperative Infections

For Elective Colorectal Surgery:
(If proposed surgery time is 8:00 am)

Preop Day 1: Two 500mg tabs, three 333mg tabs, or four 250mg tabs PO at 1:00 pm, 2:00 pm, and 11:00 pm

Refer to PI for additional recommendations

Amebiasis

Intestinal:
30-50mg/kg/day in divided doses for 10-14 days

Pertussis

40-50mg/kg/day in divided doses for 5-14 days

E

ADMINISTRATION

Oral route

May dose w/o regard to meals; optimal levels are obtained when administered in the fasting state, at least 1/2 hr and preferably 2 hrs ac

HOW SUPPLIED

Tab, Delayed-Release: 250mg, 333mg, 500mg

CONTRAINDICATIONS

Known hypersensitivity to this antibiotic. Concomitant use of terfenadine, astemizole, cisapride, pimozide, ergotamine, or dihydroergotamine.

WARNINGS/PRECAUTIONS

Hepatic dysfunction, including increased LFTs, and hepatocellular and/or cholestatic hepatitis, with or without jaundice, reported; caution with impaired hepatic function. Associated with QT interval prolongation and arrhythmia (infrequent); cases of torsades de pointes reported. Avoid with known QT interval prolongation and with ongoing proarrhythmic conditions. Cardiovascular malformations reported when used during early pregnancy. Infants born to women treated during pregnancy for early syphilis should be treated with an appropriate PCN regimen. *Clostridium difficile*-associated diarrhea (CDAD) reported; d/c if CDAD is suspected or confirmed. Use in the absence of a proven or strongly suspected bacterial infection or prophylactic indication is unlikely to provide benefit and increases the risk of development of drug-resistant bacteria. Exacerbation of symptoms of myasthenia gravis, new onset of symptoms of myasthenic syndrome, and infantile hypertrophic pyloric stenosis (IHPS) reported. Prolonged and repeated use may result in an overgrowth of nonsusceptible bacteria or fungi; d/c and take appropriate measures if superinfection develops. Lab test interactions may occur. Caution in elderly.

ADVERSE REACTIONS

N/V, abdominal pain, diarrhea, anorexia.

DRUG INTERACTIONS

See Contraindications. Avoid with Class IA (quinidine, procainamide) or Class III (dofetilide, amiodarone, sotalol) antiarrhythmic agents. Serious adverse reactions reported with CYP3A4 substrates such as hypotension with calcium channel blockers (eg, verapamil, amlodipine, diltiazem). Monitor for colchicine toxicity with coadministration; starting dose of colchicine may need to be reduced, and max colchicine dose should be lowered. May increase theophylline levels and potential toxicity with high doses of theophylline; reduce theophylline dose in these cases. Decreased levels with theophylline. Hypotension, bradyarrhythmias, and lactic acidosis observed with verapamil. May elevate digoxin levels. May elevate concentrations that could increase or prolong both therapeutic and adverse effects of drugs primarily metabolized by CYP3A; closely monitor concentrations and consider dose adjustment. May increase the pharmacological effect of triazolam and midazolam. Increased systemic exposure of sildenafil; consider dose reduction of sildenafil. Increased anticoagulant effects of oral anticoagulants; may be more pronounced in elderly. Increased levels of HMG-CoA reductase inhibitors (eg, lovastatin, simvastatin); rhabdomyolysis (rare) reported. Carefully monitor for creatine kinase and serum transaminase levels with lovastatin. Interactions with drugs metabolized by CYP3A (eg, cyclosporine, carbamazepine, tacrolimus, alfentanil, disopyramide, rifabutin, quinidine, methylprednisolone, cilostazol, vinblastine, bromocriptine), hexobarbital, phenytoin, and valproate reported.

PATIENT CONSIDERATIONS

Assessment: Assess for hypersensitivity to drug, hepatic impairment, QT interval prolongation, ongoing proarrhythmic conditions, myasthenia gravis, pregnancy/nursing status, and possible drug interactions. Perform culture and susceptibility tests to confirm diagnosis of causative organism. Perform serologic test for syphilis (if treating gonorrhea) and spinal fluid exam (primary syphilis).

Monitoring: Monitor for hepatic dysfunction, CDAD, QT interval prolongation, arrhythmia, exacerbation of myasthenia gravis symptoms, new onset of symptoms of myasthenic syndrome, IHPS, superinfection, and other adverse reactions. Perform follow-up serologic test for syphilis (after 3 months) and spinal fluid exam (primary syphilis).

Counseling: Inform that therapy should only be used to treat bacterial, not viral, infections. Instruct to take exactly ud. Inform that skipping doses or not completing full course may decrease effectiveness and increase bacterial resistance. Inform that diarrhea is a common problem caused by therapy and will usually end upon discontinuation of therapy. Instruct to immediately contact physician if watery and bloody stools (with or without stomach cramps and fever) occur, even as late as ≥2 months after discontinuation of therapy. Inform caregivers of infant patients to contact physician if vomiting or irritability with feeding occurs.

STORAGE: <30°C (86°F).

ESBRIET – pirfenidone

RX

Class: Pyridone

ADULT DOSAGE

Idiopathic Pulmonary Fibrosis

Days 1-7: 1 cap tid
Days 8-14: 2 caps tid
Day 15 Onward: 3 caps tid
Maint/Max: 2403mg/day (9 caps/day)

PEDIATRIC DOSAGE

Pediatric use may not have been established

DOSING CONSIDERATIONS

Concomitant Medications

Strong CYP1A2 Inhibitors (eg, Fluvoxamine, Enoxacin):
Reduce to 1 cap tid

Moderate CYP1A2 Inhibitors (eg, Ciprofloxacin 750mg bid):
Reduce to 2 caps tid

Adverse Reactions

Significant (eg, GI, Photosensitivity, Rash):
Consider temporary dosage reductions or interruptions to allow for resolution of symptoms

Elevated Liver Enzymes:

ALT and/or AST >3 but ≤5X ULN w/o Symptoms or Hyperbilirubinemia:
1. D/C confounding medications, exclude other causes, and monitor patient closely
2. Repeat LFTs as clinically indicated
3. Full daily dosage may be maintained, if clinically appropriate, or reduced or interrupted (eg, until LFTs are w/in normal limits) w/ subsequent retitration to full dosage as tolerated

ALT and/or AST >3 but ≤5X ULN w/ Symptoms or Hyperbilirubinemia:
D/C permanently and do not rechallenge

ALT and/or AST >5X ULN:
D/C permanently and do not rechallenge

Other Important Considerations

Treatment Interruption ≥14 Days:
Reinitiate by undergoing the initial 2-week titration regimen up to full maint dose

Treatment Interruption <14 Days:
Resume w/ dosage prior to the interruption

ADMINISTRATION

Oral route

Take at the same time each day w/ food.

HOW SUPPLIED

Cap: 267mg

WARNINGS/PRECAUTIONS

Increases in ALT and AST >3X ULN reported; rarely associated w/ concomitant bilirubin elevations. Photosensitivity reactions reported. GI events (eg, N/V, diarrhea, dyspepsia, GERD, abdominal pain) reported. Caution w/ mild (Child-Pugh Class A) to moderate (Child-Pugh Class B) hepatic impairment, or mild (CrCl 50-80mL/min)/moderate (CrCl 30-50mL/min)/severe (CrCl <30mL/min) renal impairment. Not recommended w/ severe (Child-Pugh Class C) hepatic impairment or ESRD requiring dialysis.

ADVERSE REACTIONS

N/V, rash, abdominal pain, URTI, diarrhea, fatigue, headache, dyspepsia, dizziness, anorexia, GERD, sinusitis, insomnia, weight decreased, arthralgia.

DRUG INTERACTIONS

See Dosing Considerations. Fluvoxamine or other strong CYP1A2 inhibitors (eg, enoxacin) significantly increase exposure; d/c use of such agents prior to treatment, and avoid during treatment. If such agents are the only drug of choice, dosage reductions are recommended; monitor for adverse reactions and consider discontinuation of pirfenidone prn. Ciprofloxacin (moderate CYP1A2 inhibitor) moderately increases exposure; if ciprofloxacin at the dosage of 750mg bid cannot be avoided, dosage reductions are recommended. Monitor closely when ciprofloxacin is used at a dosage of 250mg or 500mg qd. Agents or combinations of agents that are moderate or strong inhibitors of both CYP1A2 and ≥1 other CYP isoenzymes involved in the metabolism of pirfenidone (CYP2C9, 2C19, 2D6, 2E1) should be discontinued prior to and avoided during treatment. CYP1A2 inducers may decrease exposure, which may lead to loss of efficacy; d/c use of strong CYP1A2 inducers prior to treatment and avoid concomitant use. Avoid concomitant medications known to cause photosensitivity. Smoking causes decreased exposure, which may alter the efficacy profile; stop smoking prior to treatment and avoid smoking during treatment.

PATIENT CONSIDERATIONS

Assessment: Assess for renal/hepatic impairment, smoking, pregnancy/nursing status, and possible drug interactions. Conduct LFTs.

Monitoring: Monitor for photosensitivity reaction, rash, GI events, and other adverse reactions. Conduct LFTs monthly for the first 6 months and every 3 months thereafter.

Counseling: Inform that periodic monitoring of LFTs may be required. Instruct to immediately report any symptoms of a liver problem, photosensitivity reaction, rash, or persistent GI effects to physician. Advise to avoid or minimize exposure to sunlight (eg, sunlamps) during therapy; instruct to use a sunblock (SPF ≥50) and to wear clothing that protects against sun exposure. Encourage to stop smoking prior to treatment and to avoid smoking while on therapy.

STORAGE: 25°C (77°F); excursions permitted to 15-30°C (59-86°F).

ESTERIFIED ESTROGENS AND METHYLTESTOSTERONE — CIII

esterified estrogens/methyltestosterone

Class: Androgen/estrogen

E

Estrogens increase the risk of endometrial cancer. Perform adequate diagnostic measures, including endometrial sampling when indicated, to rule out malignancy in all cases of undiagnosed persistent or recurring abnormal vaginal bleeding. Estrogens with or without progestins should not be used for the prevention of cardiovascular disease (CVD). Increased risk of myocardial infarction (MI), stroke, invasive breast cancer, pulmonary embolism (PE), and deep vein thrombosis (DVT) reported in postmenopausal women (50-79 yrs of age) treated with oral conjugated estrogens combined with medroxyprogesterone acetate. Increased risk of developing probable dementia reported in postmenopausal women ≥65 yrs of age treated with oral conjugated estrogens combined with medroxyprogesterone acetate. Estrogens with or without progestins should be prescribed at the lowest effective dose and for the shortest duration consistent with treatment goals and risks.

ADULT DOSAGE

Menopausal Vasomotor Symptoms

Moderate to Severe Symptoms Not Improved by Estrogens Alone:

Usual: 1 tab or 1-2 half-strength tabs qd given cyclically (eg, 3 weeks on and 1 week off)

Short-term use only; attempt to d/c or taper medication at 3- to 6-month intervals

PEDIATRIC DOSAGE

Pediatric use may not have been established

DOSING CONSIDERATIONS

Elderly

Start at lower end of dosing range

ADMINISTRATION

Oral route

HOW SUPPLIED

Tab: (Esterified Estrogens-Methyltestosterone) 0.625mg-1.25mg (Half Strength), 1.25mg-2.5mg

CONTRAINDICATIONS

Undiagnosed abnormal genital bleeding, known/suspected/history of breast cancer, known/suspected estrogen-dependent neoplasia, active/history of DVT/PE, active/recent (eg, within the past year) arterial thromboembolic disease (eg, stroke, MI), liver dysfunction or disease, known hypersensitivity to the ingredients, known or suspected pregnancy. **Methyltestosterone:** Severe liver damage, breastfeeding mothers.

WARNINGS/PRECAUTIONS

Esterified Estrogens: D/C immediately if an MI, stroke, DVT, or PE occurs or is suspected. If feasible, d/c at least 4-6 weeks before surgery associated with an increased risk of thromboembolism, or during periods of prolonged immobilization. May increase risk of ovarian cancer. Consider addition of a progestin in women with a uterus or in patients with residual endometriosis post-hysterectomy. May increase risk of gallbladder disease requiring surgery. Worsening of glucose tolerance reported; carefully observe diabetic patients during therapy. May lead to severe hypercalcemia in patients with breast cancer and bone metastases; d/c and take appropriate measures if hypercalcemia occurs. Retinal vascular thrombosis reported; d/c pending examination if sudden partial/complete loss of vision, or sudden onset of proptosis, diplopia, or migraine occurs. If examination reveals papilledema or retinal vascular lesions, d/c therapy permanently. May increase BP, thyroid-binding globulin levels, and plasma TG, leading to pancreatitis or other complications. Caution with history of cholestatic jaundice associated with past estrogen use or with pregnancy; d/c in the case of recurrence. May cause fluid retention. Caution with severe hypocalcemia. May exacerbate endometriosis, asthma, DM, epilepsy, migraine or porphyria, systemic lupus erythematosus, and hepatic hemangiomas; use with caution. May affect certain endocrine and blood components in lab tests. **Methyltestosterone:** May cause hypercalcemia in patients with breast cancer; d/c if this occurs. Peliosis hepatis and hepatic neoplasms, including hepatocellular carcinoma, reported with prolonged use of high doses. D/C if cholestatic hepatitis with jaundice appears or if abnormal LFTs occur. Edema with or without heart failure may be a serious complication in patients with preexisting cardiac, renal, or hepatic disease; may require diuretic therapy in addition to discontinuation of therapy. Monitor for signs of virilization; d/c at the time of evidence of mild virilism. Prolonged use may result in sodium and fluid retention; caution with compromised cardiac reserve or renal disease. May decrease protein-bound iodine.

ADVERSE REACTIONS

Amenorrhea, menstrual irregularities, voice deepening, clitoral enlargement, thromboembolism, N/V, chloasma, headache, urticaria, hirsutism, cholestatic jaundice, depression, anxiety, breast tenderness, pruritus.

DRUG INTERACTIONS

Esterified Estrogens: CYP3A4 inducers (eg, St. John's wort preparations, phenobarbital, carbamazepine) may decrease therapeutic effects and/or result in changes in uterine bleeding profile. CYP3A4 inhibitors (eg, erythromycin, ketoconazole, ritonavir) may result in side effects. Patients concomitantly receiving thyroid hormone replacement therapy and estrogens may require increased doses of their thyroid replacement therapy. **Methyltestosterone:** May decrease oral anticoagulant requirement; close monitoring is required, especially when androgens are started or stopped. May increase oxyphenbutazone levels. May decrease blood glucose and insulin requirements in diabetics.

PATIENT CONSIDERATIONS

Assessment: Assess for undiagnosed abnormal genital bleeding, presence or history of breast cancer, estrogen-dependent neoplasia, active/history deep vein thrombosis, active or recent (within past yr) arterial thromboembolic disease, liver dysfunction, pregnancy/nursing status, any other conditions where treatment is contraindicated or cautioned, need for progestin therapy, and for possible drug interactions.

Monitoring: Monitor for signs/symptoms of hypercalcemia and fluid retention, CVD, malignant neoplasms, gallbladder disease, visual abnormalities, cholestatic jaundice, hypertriglyceridemia, exacerbation of endometriosis, virilization, and for other adverse reactions. In cases of undiagnosed persistent or recurrent vaginal bleeding in women with a uterus, perform adequate diagnostic measures to rule out malignancies. Perform annual breast exam; schedule mammography based on age, risk factors, and prior mammogram results. Periodically monitor BP, thyroid function if on thyroid hormone replacement therapy, and reassess need for therapy every 3-6 months. Monitor LFTs periodically. Frequently monitor urine and serum Ca^{2+} in women with disseminated breast carcinoma. Periodically check Hgb and Hct for polycythemia in patients receiving high doses of androgens.

Counseling: Inform of the risks/benefits of therapy. Inform of the possible adverse reactions of therapy and instruct to contact physician if any adverse reactions occur.

STORAGE: 20-25°C (68-77°F); excursions permitted to 15-30°C (59-86°F).

ESTRACE – estradiol

RX

Class: Estrogen

Estrogens increase the risk of endometrial cancer. Perform adequate diagnostic measures, including endometrial sampling, to rule out malignancy w/ undiagnosed persistent or recurrent abnormal vaginal bleeding. Should not be used for the prevention of cardiovascular disease. Increased risk of MI, stroke, invasive breast cancer, pulmonary embolism (PE), and DVT in postmenopausal women (50-79 yrs of age) reported. Increased risk of developing probable dementia in postmenopausal women ≥65 yrs of age reported. Should be prescribed at the lowest effective dose and for the shortest duration consistent w/ treatment goals and risks.

ADULT DOSAGE

Menopausal Vasomotor Symptoms

Moderate to Severe:
Tab:
Initial: 1-2mg/day
Maint: Minimal effective dose should be determined by titration; Administer cyclically (eg, 3 weeks on and 1 week off)

Use the lowest effective dose for the shortest duration; reevaluate at 3- to 6-month intervals

Menopausal Vulvar/Vaginal Atrophy

Cre:
Usual: 2-4g/day for 1-2 weeks; then gradually reduce to 1/2 initial dose for a similar period
Maint: 1g 1-3X/week

Tab:
Moderate to Severe:
Initial: 1-2mg/day
Maint: Minimal effective dose should be determined by titration; Administer cyclically (eg, 3 weeks on and 1 week off)

Use the lowest effective dose for the shortest duration; reevaluate at 3- to 6-month intervals

PEDIATRIC DOSAGE

Pediatric use may not have been established

Hypoestrogenism

Due to Hypogonadism, Castration, or Primary Ovarian Failure:
Tab:
Initial: 1-2mg/day
Titrate: Adjust as necessary to control presenting symptoms
Maint: Minimal effective dose should be determined by titration

Breast Cancer

Palliative Treatment in Appropriately Selected Women and Men w/ Metastatic Disease:
Tab:
10mg tid for at least 3 months

Prostate Carcinoma

Palliative Treatment of Advanced Androgen-Dependent Carcinoma:
Tab:
1-2mg tid

Osteoporosis

Prevention:
Tab:
Consider therapy for women at risk of osteoporosis and for whom non-estrogen medications are not appropriate, when used solely for prevention of postmenopausal osteoporosis

ADMINISTRATION

Cre
Intravaginal route

Tab
Oral route

HOW SUPPLIED

Cre: 0.01% [42.5g]; **Tab:** 0.5mg*, 1mg*, 2mg* *scored

CONTRAINDICATIONS

Undiagnosed abnormal genital bleeding, known/suspected/history of breast cancer, known/suspected estrogen-dependent neoplasia, active/history of DVT/PE, active or recent arterial thromboembolic disease (eg, stroke, MI), liver dysfunction or disease, known hypersensitivity to the ingredients, known/suspected pregnancy.

WARNINGS/PRECAUTIONS

D/C immediately if stroke, DVT, PE, or MI occur or is suspected. Caution in patients w/ risk factors for arterial vascular disease and/or venous thromboembolism. If feasible, d/c at least 4-6 weeks before surgery of the type associated w/ an increased risk of thromboembolism, or during periods of prolonged immobilization. May increase the risk of gallbladder disease and ovarian cancer. May lead to severe hypercalcemia in patients w/ breast cancer and bone metastases; d/c and take appropriate measures if hypercalcemia occurs. Retinal vascular thrombosis reported; d/c pending exam if sudden partial/complete loss of vision, or sudden onset of proptosis, diplopia, or migraine occurs. D/C permanently if exam reveals papilledema or retinal vascular lesions. Consider addition of progestin for women w/ a uterus or w/ residual endometriosis post-hysterectomy. May elevate BP and thyroid-binding globulin levels. May elevate plasma TGs leading to pancreatitis in patients w/ preexisting hypertriglyceridemia. Caution w/ impaired liver function, and history of cholestatic jaundice associated w/ past estrogen use or w/ pregnancy; d/c in case of recurrence. May cause fluid retention; caution w/ cardiac/renal impairment. Caution w/ severe hypocalcemia. May exacerbate endometriosis, asthma, diabetes mellitus, epilepsy, migraine, porphyria, systemic lupus erythematosus, and hepatic hemangiomas; use w/ caution. May affect certain endocrine and blood components in lab tests. (Tab) 2mg tab contains tartrazine, which may cause allergic-type reactions (eg, bronchial asthma) in certain susceptible individuals.

ADVERSE REACTIONS

Vaginal bleeding pattern changes, vaginitis, breast tenderness, galactorrhea, N/V, thrombophlebitis, melasma, abdominal cramps, headache, mental depression, weight changes, edema, libido changes, MI, PE.

DRUG INTERACTIONS

CYP3A4 inducers (eg, St. John's wort preparations, phenobarbital, carbamazepine, rifampin) may decrease levels, which may decrease therapeutic effects and/or change uterine bleeding profile. CYP3A4 inhibitors (eg, erythromycin, ketoconazole, ritonavir, grapefruit juice) may increase levels, which may result in side effects. Patients concomitantly receiving thyroid replacement therapy and estrogens may require increased doses of thyroid replacement therapy; monitor thyroid function.

PATIENT CONSIDERATIONS

Assessment: Assess for undiagnosed abnormal genital bleeding, presence/history of breast cancer, estrogen-dependent neoplasia, active/history of DVT/PE/arterial thromboembolic disease, liver impairment/disease, history of cholestatic jaundice, drug hypersensitivity, pregnancy/nursing status, any other conditions where treatment is contraindicated or cautioned, need for progestin therapy, and possible drug interactions.

Monitoring: Monitor for signs/symptoms of CV events, malignant neoplasms, dementia, gallbladder disease, hypercalcemia, visual abnormalities, BP and serum TG elevations, pancreatitis, fluid retention, cholestatic jaundice, exacerbation of endometriosis and other conditions, and other adverse reactions. Perform annual breast exam; schedule mammography based on age, risk factors, and prior mammogram results. Monitor thyroid function in patients on thyroid hormone replacement therapy. Periodically evaluate (every 3-6 months) to determine need for therapy. In cases of undiagnosed, persistent, or recurrent abnormal vaginal bleeding, perform adequate diagnostic measures (eg, endometrial sampling) to rule out malignancy.

Counseling: Inform of the risks/benefits of therapy. Inform that medication increases risk for breast/uterine cancer. Advise to contact physician if breast lumps, unusual vaginal bleeding, dizziness or faintness, changes in speech, severe headaches, chest pain, SOB, leg pain, visual changes, or vomiting occur. Advise to have yearly breast exams by a physician and perform monthly breast self-exams. Advise to notify physician if pregnant/nursing.

STORAGE: (Cre) Room temperature. Protect from temperatures in excess of 40°C (104°F). (Tab) 20-25°C (68-77°F).

ESTRING — estradiol

RX

Class: Estrogen

Increased risk of endometrial cancer in a woman w/ a uterus who uses unopposed estrogens. Adding a progestin to estrogen therapy reduces the risk of endometrial hyperplasia. Adequate diagnostic measures should be undertaken to rule out malignancy in all cases of undiagnosed, persistent or recurring abnormal genital bleeding. Should not be used for the prevention of cardiovascular (CV) disease or dementia. Increased risk of stroke and DVT reported in postmenopausal women (50-79 yrs of age) treated w/ daily oral conjugated estrogens (CE) alone and when combined w/ medroxyprogesterone acetate (MPA). Increased risk of developing probable dementia reported in postmenopausal women ≥65 yrs of age treated w/ daily CE alone and when combined w/ MPA. Increased risks of pulmonary embolism (PE), MI, and invasive breast cancer reported in postmenopausal women (50-79 yrs of age) treated w/ daily oral CE combined w/ MPA. Should be prescribed at the lowest effective dose and for the shortest duration consistent w/ treatment goals and risks.

ADULT DOSAGE

Menopausal Vulvar/Vaginal Atrophy

Moderate to Severe Symptoms:

Insert 1 ring as deeply as possible into the upper 1/3 of the vaginal vault; the ring is to remain in place continuously for 3 months, after which it is to be removed and, if appropriate, replaced by a new ring

Reassess need to continue treatment at 3- or 6-month intervals

PEDIATRIC DOSAGE

Pediatric use may not have been established

ADMINISTRATION

Intravaginal route

Retention of the ring for >90 days does not represent overdosage, but will result in progressively greater underdosage w/ the risk of loss of efficacy and increasing risk of vaginal infections and/or erosions

Insertion

1. Press ring into an oval and insert into upper 3rd of the vaginal vault; exact position is not critical
2. If patient feels discomfort, the ring is probably not far enough inside
3. Gently push ring further into the vagina

Use

The patient should not feel Estring when it is in place and it should not interfere w/ sexual intercourse. Straining at defecation may make Estring move down in the lower part of the vagina; if so, it may be pushed up again w/ a finger. Should the ring be removed or fall out at any time during the 90-day treatment period, it should be rinsed in lukewarm water and re-inserted by the patient (or by a physician/nurse if necessary)

Removal

Remove by hooking a finger through the ring and pulling it out

HOW SUPPLIED

Vaginal Ring: 2mg

CONTRAINDICATIONS

Undiagnosed abnormal genital bleeding, known/suspected/history of breast cancer, known/suspected estrogen-dependent neoplasia, active/history of DVT/PE/arterial thromboembolic disease (eg, stroke, MI), known anaphylactic reaction or angioedema or hypersensitivity to the medication, known liver impairment/disease, known protein C/protein S/antithrombin deficiency or other known thrombophilic disorders, known/suspected pregnancy.

WARNINGS/PRECAUTIONS

D/C immediately if stroke, DVT, PE, or MI occurs or is suspected. If feasible, d/c at least 4-6 weeks before surgery of the type associated w/ an increased risk of thromboembolism, or during periods of prolonged immobilization. May increase risk of gallbladder disease requiring surgery and risk of ovarian cancer. May lead to severe hypercalcemia in patients w/ breast cancer and bone metastases; d/c and take appropriate measures if hypercalcemia occurs. Retinal vascular thrombosis reported; d/c therapy pending exam if sudden partial/complete loss of vision, or sudden onset of proptosis, diplopia, or migraine occurs. D/C if exam reveals papilledema or retinal vascular lesions. May exacerbate symptoms of angioedema in women w/ hereditary angioedema. May increase BP and thyroid-binding globulin levels. May be associated w/ elevations of plasma TGs, leading to pancreatitis in patients w/ preexisting hypertriglyceridemia; consider discontinuation if pancreatitis occurs. Caution w/ history of cholestatic jaundice associated w/ past estrogen use or w/ pregnancy; d/c in case of recurrence. Caution w/ hypoparathyroidism; hypocalcemia may occur. May cause fluid retention. Cases of malignant transformation of residual endometrial implants reported in women treated posthysterectomy w/ estrogen therapy alone; consider addition of progestin for these patients. May exacerbate asthma, diabetes mellitus, epilepsy, migraine, porphyria, systemic lupus erythematosus, and hepatic hemangiomas. A narrow vagina, vaginal stenosis, prolapse, or a vaginal infection may make the vagina more susceptible to irritation/ulceration. If a vaginal infection develops, remove and reinsert only after the infection is appropriately treated. May affect certain endocrine and blood components in lab tests.

ADVERSE REACTIONS

Headache, leukorrhea, back pain, genital moniliasis, sinusitis, vaginitis, vaginal discomfort/pain, vaginal hemorrhage, arthritis, insomnia, abdominal pain, upper respiratory tract infection, asymptomatic genital bacterial growth, arthralgia.

DRUG INTERACTIONS

CYP3A4 inducers (eg, St. John's wort preparations, phenobarbital, carbamazepine) may decrease levels, possibly resulting in a decrease in systemic effects and/or changes in the uterine bleeding profile. CYP3A4 inhibitors (eg, erythromycin, ketoconazole, grapefruit juice) may increase levels, and may result in side effects. Patients concomitantly receiving thyroid hormone replacement therapy and estrogens may require increased doses of thyroid replacement therapy; monitor thyroid function.

PATIENT CONSIDERATIONS

Assessment: Assess for abnormal genital bleeding, presence/history of breast cancer, estrogen-dependent neoplasia, active/history of DVT/PE/arterial thromboembolic disease, liver impairment/disease, thrombophilic disorders, known anaphylactic reaction or angioedema/hypersensitivity to the drug, pregnancy/nursing status, and any other conditions where treatment is contraindicated or cautioned, need for progestin therapy, and possible drug interactions.

Monitoring: Monitor for signs/symptoms of CV disorders, malignant neoplasms, dementia, gallbladder disease, hypercalcemia, visual abnormalities, BP and plasma TG elevations, pancreatitis, cholestatic jaundice, hypothyroidism, fluid retention, exacerbation of endometriosis or other conditions, vaginal irritation/infection, and other adverse reactions. Perform adequate diagnostic measures (eg, endometrial sampling) in patients w/ undiagnosed, persistent or recurring abnormal genital bleeding. Perform annual breast exam; schedule mammography based on age, risk factors, and prior mammogram results. Monitor thyroid function if on thyroid hormone replacement therapy. Reassess need to continue treatment at 3- or 6-month intervals.

Counseling: Inform of risks and benefits of therapy. Instruct to use ud. Advise of possible serious adverse reactions of therapy (eg, CV disorders, malignant neoplasms, probable dementia). Instruct to notify physician if signs/symptoms of vaginal irritation, abnormal vaginal bleeding, or any adverse reactions occur. Advise to have yearly breast exams by a physician and to perform monthly breast self-exams. Inform that the ring may be expelled from the vagina during bowel movement, straining or w/ constipation; if this occurs, rinse in lukewarm water and reinsert.

STORAGE: 15-30°C (59-86°F).

ETODOLAC – etodolac

RX

Class: NSAID

NSAIDs cause an increased risk of serious cardiovascular (CV) thrombotic events, including MI and stroke, which can be fatal; risk may occur early in treatment and may increase w/ duration of use. Contraindicated in the setting of CABG surgery. NSAIDs cause an increased risk of serious GI adverse events (eg, bleeding, ulceration, perforation of the stomach/intestines), which can be fatal and may occur at any time during use w/o warning symptoms; elderly patients are at greater risk.

OTHER BRAND NAMES

Lodine (Discontinued)

ADULT DOSAGE

Acute Pain

200-400mg q6-8h, up to 1000mg

Doses >1000mg/day have not been adequately evaluated

Osteoarthritis

Acute and Long-Term Management of Signs/ Symptoms:

Initial: 300mg bid-tid, or 400mg bid, or 500mg bid

May give a lower dose of 600mg/day for long-term use

Doses >1000mg/day have not been adequately evaluated

Rheumatoid Arthritis

Acute and Long-Term Management of Signs/ Symptoms:

Initial: 300mg bid-tid, or 400mg bid, or 500mg bid

May give a lower dose of 600mg/day for long-term use

Doses >1000mg/day have not been adequately evaluated

PEDIATRIC DOSAGE

Pediatric use may not have been established

ADMINISTRATION

Oral route

HOW SUPPLIED

Cap: 200mg, 300mg; **Tab:** 400mg, 500mg

CONTRAINDICATIONS

Known hypersensitivity to etodolac or other ingredients in the medication; asthma, urticaria, or other allergic-type reactions after taking aspirin (ASA) or other NSAIDs; in the setting of CABG surgery.

WARNINGS/PRECAUTIONS

Use lowest effective dose for the shortest duration possible. Increased CV thrombotic risk w/ higher doses reported. Avoid in patients w/ a recent MI unless benefits outweigh the risks; if used, monitor for signs of cardiac ischemia. May cause HTN or worsen preexisting HTN. Fluid retention and edema reported. Avoid use in patients w/ severe heart failure (HF) unless benefits outweigh risk of worsening HF; if used, monitor for signs of worsening HF. Use w/ extreme caution in patients w/ prior history of ulcer disease, GI bleeding, or risk factors for GI bleeding (eg, longer duration of NSAID therapy, older age, poor general health status). D/C if a serious GI adverse event is suspected, until event is ruled out; for high-risk patients, consider alternate therapies that do not involve NSAIDs. Renal papillary necrosis and other renal injury reported after long-term use. Renal toxicity also reported in patients in whom renal prostaglandins have a compensatory role in the maintenance of renal perfusion; increased risk w/ renal/hepatic impairment, HF, and in elderly. Not recommended w/ advanced renal disease; if therapy must be initiated, closely monitor renal function. D/C if renal disease develops. Anaphylactoid reactions may occur; avoid w/ ASA triad.

May cause serious skin reactions (eg, exfoliative dermatitis, Stevens-Johnson syndrome, toxic epidermal necrolysis); d/c at 1st appearance of skin rash or any other sign of hypersensitivity. Avoid in late pregnancy; may cause premature closure of ductus arteriosus. Not a substitute for corticosteroids or for the treatment of corticosteroid insufficiency; may mask signs of inflammation and fever. May cause elevations of LFTs or severe hepatic reactions (eg, jaundice, fulminant hepatitis, liver necrosis, hepatic failure); d/c if liver disease develops, systemic manifestations occur, or if abnormal LFTs persist/worsen. Anemia may occur; monitor Hgb/Hct if any signs/symptoms of anemia develop in patients on long-term therapy. May inhibit platelet aggregation and prolong bleeding time; monitor patients w/ coagulation disorders. Caution in debilitated and elderly. Lab test interactions may occur. Caution w/ preexisting asthma.

ADVERSE REACTIONS

Abdominal pain, constipation, diarrhea, dyspepsia, flatulence, heartburn, N/V, GI ulcers, abnormal renal function, anemia, dizziness, headaches, increased bleeding time, pruritus, rashes.

DRUG INTERACTIONS

May diminish the antihypertensive effect of ACE inhibitors. Increased risk of renal toxicity w/ diuretics and ACE inhibitors. May decrease peak concentration w/ antacids. Not recommended w/ ASA due to potential for increased adverse effects. May reduce the natriuretic effect of thiazide and loop diuretics. May increase lithium levels; monitor for lithium toxicity. May increase levels of cyclosporine, digoxin, and methotrexate (MTX), leading to increased toxicity. May enhance nephrotoxicity associated w/ cyclosporine. Avoid use prior to or concomitantly w/ high doses of MTX. May enhance MTX toxicity; caution w/ concomitant use. Increased free fraction of etodolac w/ phenylbutazone; coadministration not recommended. Synergistic effect on GI bleeding w/ warfarin; closely monitor. Increased risk of GI bleeding w/ oral corticosteroids, anticoagulants, smoking, and alcohol use. May blunt the CV effects of several therapeutic agents used to treat fluid retention and edema (eg, diuretics, ACE inhibitors, ARBs).

PATIENT CONSIDERATIONS

Assessment: Assess for history of asthma, urticaria, or allergic-type reactions w/ ASA or other NSAIDs, ASA triad, HTN, recent MI, severe HF, history of ulcer disease or GI bleeding, coagulation disorders, renal/hepatic impairment, pregnancy/nursing status, any other conditions where treatment is contraindicated or cautioned, and possible drug interactions. Obtain baseline BP.

Monitoring: Monitor for GI bleeding/ulceration/perforation, CV thrombotic events, HTN, fluid retention, edema, serious skin reactions, anaphylactoid reactions, and other adverse reactions. Monitor BP, CBC, bleeding time, LFTs, renal function, and chemistry profile periodically.

Counseling: Instruct to seek medical advice if symptoms of CV events, GI ulceration/bleeding, skin/hypersensitivity reactions, congestive HF, hepatotoxicity, or anaphylactoid reactions occur. Inform that medication should be avoided in late pregnancy.

STORAGE: 20-25°C (68-77°F). **Cap:** Protect from moisture.

Evekeo – amphetamine sulfate

CII

Class: CNS stimulant

High potential for abuse; prolonged use may lead to drug dependence and must be avoided. Misuse may cause sudden death and serious cardiovascular (CV) adverse events.

ADULT DOSAGE

Narcolepsy

Initial: 10mg/day

Titrate: May increase in increments of 10mg at weekly intervals until optimal response is obtained

Usual: 5-60mg/day in divided doses

Give 1st dose on awakening; additional doses (5 or 10mg) at intervals of 4-6 hrs

Obesity

Management of exogenous obesity as a short-term (few weeks) adjunct in a regimen of weight reduction based on caloric restriction, for patients refractory to alternative therapy

Usual: Up to 30mg/day in divided doses of 5-10mg, 30-60 min ac

PEDIATRIC DOSAGE

Narcolepsy

Usual: 5-60mg/day in divided doses

Give 1st dose on awakening; additional doses (5 or 10mg) at intervals of 4-6 hrs

6-12 Years:

Initial: 5mg/day

Titrate: May increase in increments of 5mg at weekly intervals until optimal response is obtained

≥12 Years:

Initial: 10mg/day

Titrate: May increase in increments of 10mg at weekly intervals until optimal response is obtained

Attention-Deficit Hyperactivity Disorder

3-5 Years:
Initial: 2.5mg/day
Titrate: May increase in increments of 2.5mg at weekly intervals until optimal response is obtained

≥6 Years:
Initial: 5mg qd or bid
Titrate: May increase in increments of 5mg at weekly intervals until optimal response is obtained
Only in rare cases will it be necessary to exceed a total of 40mg/day

Give 1st dose on awakening; additional doses (1-2 tabs) at intervals of 4-6 hrs
Where possible, interrupt therapy occasionally to determine if there is a recurrence of behavioral symptoms sufficient to require continued therapy

Obesity

Management of exogenous obesity as a short-term (few weeks) adjunct in a regimen of weight reduction based on caloric restriction, for patients refractory to alternative therapy

≥12 Years:
Usual: Up to 30mg/day in divided doses of 5-10mg, 30-60 min ac

DOSING CONSIDERATIONS

Adverse Reactions

Narcolepsy:
Reduce dose if bothersome adverse reactions (eg, insomnia, anorexia) appear

ADMINISTRATION

Oral route

Avoid late pm dosing.

HOW SUPPLIED

Tab: 5mg*, 10mg* *scored

CONTRAINDICATIONS

Advanced arteriosclerosis, symptomatic cardiovascular disease (CVD), moderate to severe HTN, hyperthyroidism, agitated states, history of drug abuse, during or w/in 14 days following MAOI use, known hypersensitivity or idiosyncrasy to the sympathomimetic amines.

WARNINGS/PRECAUTIONS

Sudden death reported in children and adolescents w/ structural cardiac abnormalities or other serious heart problems. Sudden deaths, stroke, and MI reported in adults. Avoid w/ serious structural cardiac abnormalities, cardiomyopathy, serious heart rhythm abnormalities, coronary artery disease, or other serious cardiac problems. May cause modest increase in average BP and HR; caution w/ underlying medical conditions that may be compromised (eg, preexisting HTN, heart failure, recent MI). Perform prompt cardiac evaluation when symptoms suggestive of cardiac disease develop. May exacerbate symptoms of behavior disturbance and thought disorder in patients w/ preexisting psychotic disorder. Caution in patients w/ comorbid bipolar disorder; may induce mixed/manic episodes. May cause treatment-emergent psychotic/manic symptoms (eg, hallucinations, delusional thinking, mania) in children and adolescents w/o prior history of psychotic illness or mania; consider discontinuation if such symptoms occur. Aggressive behavior or hostility reported in children and adolescents w/ ADHD. May cause suppression of growth in children; may need to interrupt treatment in patients not growing or gaining weight as expected. May lower convulsive threshold; d/c if seizures develop. Associated w/ peripheral vasculopathy, including Raynaud's phenomenon. Difficulties w/ accommodation and blurring of vision reported. Caution w/ even mild HTN. May exacerbate motor and phonic tics and Tourette's syndrome. May cause a significant elevation in plasma corticosteroid levels and interfere w/ urinary steroid determinations.

ADVERSE REACTIONS

Palpitations, tachycardia, elevation of BP, overstimulation, restlessness, dizziness, insomnia, euphoria, dryness of the mouth, unpleasant taste, diarrhea, urticaria, impotence, changes in libido, rhabdomyolysis.

DRUG INTERACTIONS

See Contraindications. GI acidifying agents (eg, guanethidine, reserpine, glutamic acid HCl) and urinary acidifying agents (eg, ammonium chloride, sodium acid phosphate) lower blood levels and efficacy. Inhibits adrenergic blockers. GI alkalinizing agents (eg, sodium bicarbonate) and urinary alkalinizing agents (eg, acetazolamide, some thiazides) increase blood levels and potentiate action of amphetamines. May enhance activity of TCAs or sympathomimetic agents. Desipramine or protriptyline and possibly other TCAs cause striking and sustained increases in the concentration of d-amphetamine in the brain; CV effects can be potentiated. May counteract sedative effect of antihistamines. May antagonize the hypotensive effects of antihypertensives. Chlorpromazine and haloperidol block dopamine and norepinephrine reuptake, thus inhibiting the central stimulant effects. Lithium carbonate may inhibit the antiobesity and stimulatory effects. Potentiates the analgesic effect of meperidine. Acidifying agents used in methenamine therapy increase urinary excretion and reduce efficacy. Enhances adrenergic effect of norepinephrine. May delay intestinal absorption of ethosuximide, phenobarbital, and phenytoin; may produce a synergistic anticonvulsant action if coadministered w/ phenobarbital or phenytoin. In cases of propoxyphene overdosage, CNS stimulation and fatal convulsions may occur. Inhibits the hypotensive effect of veratrum alkaloids.

PATIENT CONSIDERATIONS

Assessment: Assess for hypersensitivity/idiosyncrasy to sympathomimetic amines, structural cardiac abnormalities, advanced arteriosclerosis, symptomatic CVD, HTN, hyperthyroidism, history of drug abuse, tics, Tourette's syndrome, psychotic disorder, any other conditions where treatment is contraindicated or cautioned, pregnancy/nursing status, and possible drug interactions. Adequately screen patients w/ comorbid depressive symptoms to determine if they are at risk for bipolar disorder.

Monitoring: Monitor for changes in HR and BP, signs/symptoms of cardiac disease, exacerbation of symptoms of behavior disturbance and thought disorder, psychosis, mania, appearance of or worsening of aggressive behavior or hostility, seizures, peripheral vasculopathy (eg, digital changes), visual disturbances, exacerbation of motor and phone tics or Tourette's syndrome, and other adverse reactions. In pediatric patients, monitor growth.

Counseling: Inform about benefits and risks of treatment. Advise that drug has high potential for abuse. Caution that therapy may impair the ability to engage in potentially hazardous activities (eg, operating machinery or vehicles). Inform about the risk of peripheral vasculopathy (eg, Raynaud's phenomenon); instruct to report to physician any numbness, pain, skin color change, or sensitivity to temperature in fingers or toes and to call physician immediately if any signs of unexplained wounds appearing on fingers or toes while on therapy. Advise to avoid breastfeeding and to notify physician if pregnant/planning to become pregnant.

STORAGE: 20-25°C (68-77°F).

EVISTA – raloxifene hydrochloride

RX

Class: Selective estrogen receptor modulator

Increased risk of deep vein thrombosis (DVT) and pulmonary embolism (PE) reported. Avoid use in women with active or past history of venous thromboembolism (VTE). Increased risk of death due to stroke in postmenopausal women with documented coronary heart disease or at increased risk for major coronary events; consider risk-benefit balance in women at risk for stroke.

ADULT DOSAGE

Osteoporosis

Treatment and Prevention in Postmenopausal Women:
60mg qd

Reduction in Risk of Invasive Breast Cancer

Postmenopausal Women w/ Osteoporosis/ Postmenopausal Women at High Risk for Invasive Breast Cancer:
60mg qd

PEDIATRIC DOSAGE

Pediatric use may not have been established

DOSING CONSIDERATIONS

Other Important Considerations

Ca^{2+} and Vitamin D Supplementation:
Total Daily Ca^{2+} Requirement: 1500mg/day
Total Daily Vitamin D: 400-800 IU/day

ADMINISTRATION

Oral route

May be given at any time of day w/o regard to meals

HOW SUPPLIED

Tab: 60mg

CONTRAINDICATIONS

Active/past history of VTE (eg, DVT, PE, retinal vein thrombosis), pregnancy, women who may become pregnant, nursing mothers.

WARNINGS/PRECAUTIONS

VTE events, including superficial venous thrombophlebitis, reported. D/C at least 72 hrs prior to and during prolonged immobilization (eg, postsurgical recovery, prolonged bed rest); resume therapy only after patient is fully ambulatory. Caution in women at risk of thromboembolic disease for other reasons (eg, CHF, superficial thrombophlebitis, active malignancy). Should not be used for primary or secondary prevention of cardiovascular disease (CVD). Avoid use in premenopausal women. Monitor serum TG levels in women with history of hypertriglyceridemia in response to treatment with estrogen or estrogen plus progestin. Use in women with history of breast cancer has not been adequately studied. Caution with hepatic impairment or with moderate or severe renal impairment. Not recommended for use in men. Monitor for unexplained uterine bleeding and breast abnormalities.

ADVERSE REACTIONS

DVT, PE, hot flashes, leg cramps, infection, flu syndrome, headache, N/V, diarrhea, peripheral edema, arthralgia, vaginal bleeding, pharyngitis, sinusitis, cough increased.

DRUG INTERACTIONS

Avoid concomitant administration with cholestyramine, other anion exchange resins, and systemic estrogens. Monitor PT with warfarin and other warfarin derivatives. Caution with certain other highly protein-bound drugs (eg, diazepam, diazoxide, lidocaine).

PATIENT CONSIDERATIONS

Assessment: Assess for active or history of VTE (eg, DVT, PE, retinal vein thrombosis), CVD, risk factors for stroke, history of breast cancer, history of hypertriglyceridemia, prolonged immobilization, renal/hepatic impairment, pregnancy/nursing status, and for possible drug interactions. Perform breast exams and mammograms prior to treatment.

Monitoring: Monitor for VTE (eg, DVT, PE, retinal vein thrombosis), stroke, unexplained uterine bleeding, breast abnormalities, and other adverse reactions. Monitor serum TG levels with history of hypertriglyceridemia. Monitor PT with warfarin and other warfarin derivatives. Perform regular breast exams and mammograms after initial treatment.

Counseling: For osteoporosis treatment/prevention, instruct to take supplemental Ca^{2+} and/or vitamin D if intake is inadequate. Counsel on weight-bearing exercise and modification of certain behavioral factors (eg, smoking, excessive alcohol consumption) for osteoporosis treatment/prevention. Advise to d/c therapy at least 72 hrs prior to and during prolonged immobilization. Instruct to avoid prolonged restrictions of movement during travel. Counsel that therapy may increase incidence of hot flashes or hot flashes may occur upon initiation of therapy. Inform that regular breast exams and mammography should be done before initiation of therapy and should continue during therapy.

STORAGE: 20-25°C (68-77°F); excursions permitted to 15-30°C (59-86°F).

EVOTAZ – atazanavir/cobicistat

RX

Class: CYP3A inhibitor/protease inhibitor

ADULT DOSAGE

HIV-1 Infection

In Combination w/ Other Antiretroviral Agents in Treatment Naive/Experienced Patients:

1 tab qd

PEDIATRIC DOSAGE

Pediatric use may not have been established

DOSING CONSIDERATIONS

Concomitant Medications

Dose separation may be required when coadministered w/ H_2-receptor antagonists (H_2RAs) or proton-pump inhibitors (PPIs)

Renal Impairment
CrCl <70mL/min: Coadministration w/ tenofovir disoproxil fumarate (TDF) is not recommended
ESRD on Hemodialysis (Treatment-Experienced Patients): Not recommended

Hepatic Impairment
Not recommended

ADMINISTRATION

Oral route

Take w/ food.

HOW SUPPLIED

E

Tab: (Atazanavir [ATV]/Cobicistat) 300mg/150mg

CONTRAINDICATIONS

Hypersensitivity to Evotaz. Coadministration w/ drugs that are highly dependent on CYP3A or UGT1A1 for clearance, and for which elevated plasma concentrations of the interacting drugs are associated w/ serious and/or life-threatening events, and w/ strong CYP3A inducers that may lead to lower exposure and loss of efficacy of therapy (alfuzosin, ranolazine, dronedarone, carbamazepine, phenobarbital, phenytoin, colchicine, rifampin, irinotecan, lurasidone, triazolam, oral midazolam, dihydroergotamine, ergotamine, methylergonovine, cisapride, St. John's wort, lovastatin, simvastatin, pimozide, nevirapine, sildenafil [when used for the treatment of pulmonary HTN], indinavir).

WARNINGS/PRECAUTIONS

Use in treatment-experienced patients should be guided by the number of baseline primary protease inhibitor resistance substitutions. Patients w/ underlying hepatitis B or C infections or marked elevations in transaminases may be at increased risk for developing further transaminase elevations or hepatic decompensation. Redistribution/accumulation of body fat reported. Caution in elderly. **ATV:** May prolong the PR interval. 2nd-degree atrioventricular block and other conduction abnormalities reported; consider ECG monitoring in patients w/ preexisting conduction system disease. Cases of Stevens-Johnson syndrome, erythema multiforme, mild-to-moderate maculopapular skin eruptions, and toxic skin eruptions, including drug rash eosinophilia and systemic symptoms (DRESS) syndrome, reported; d/c if severe rash develops. Cases of nephrolithiasis and/or cholelithiasis reported; consider temporary interruption or discontinuation of therapy if signs/symptoms occur. Asymptomatic elevations in indirect (unconjugated) bilirubin may occur. Hepatic transaminase elevations that occur w/ hyperbilirubinemia should be evaluated for alternative etiologies. Consider alternative therapy if jaundice or scleral icterus associated w/ bilirubin elevations presents cosmetic concerns for patients. Immune reconstitution syndrome and autoimmune disorders (eg, Graves' disease, polymyositis, Guillain-Barre syndrome) in the setting of immune reconstitution reported. New-onset or exacerbation of diabetes mellitus (DM), hyperglycemia, and diabetic ketoacidosis reported; may require either initiation or dose adjustments of insulin or oral hypoglycemic agents. Increased bleeding in patients w/ hemophilia A and B reported. **Cobicistat:** Decreases estimated CrCl w/o affecting actual renal glomerular function; consider effect when interpreting changes in estimated CrCl in patients initiating therapy, particularly w/ medical conditions or receiving drugs needing monitoring w/ estimated CrCl. Closely monitor patients w/ confirmed increase in SrCr >0.4mg/dL from baseline for renal safety. Consider alternative medications that do not require dosage adjustments in patients w/ renal impairment.

ADVERSE REACTIONS

Jaundice, ocular icterus, nausea.

DRUG INTERACTIONS

See Dosing Considerations and Contraindications. Coadministration of therapy w/ TDF in combination w/ concomitant or recent use of a nephrotoxic agent is not recommended. Not recommended w/ products containing the individual components of Evotaz, ritonavir (RTV) or products containing RTV, other antiretroviral drugs that require CYP3A inhibition to achieve adequate exposures (eg, other HIV protease inhibitors, elvitegravir), efavirenz, etravirine, boceprevir, telaprevir, simeprevir, voriconazole, apixaban, rivaroxaban, dabigatran etexilate (in specific renal impairment groups), salmeterol, inhaled/nasal corticosteroids that are metabolized by CYP3A, or avanafil. Not recommended w/ drugs highly dependent on CYP2C8 for clearance w/ narrow therapeutic indices (eg, paclitaxel, repaglinide). Coadministration w/ TDF and H_2RA in treatment-experienced patients is not recommended; administer either at the same time or at a minimum of 10 hrs after H_2RA dose. Coadministration w/ PPIs in treatment-experienced patients is not recommended; give therapy a minimum of 12 hrs after PPI administration in treatment-naive patients. CYP3A4 inhibitors may increase levels. Clarithromycin, erythromycin, telithromycin, ketoconazole, and itraconazole may increase levels; consider alternative antibiotics. Bosentan may decrease levels. CYP3A4 inducers may decrease levels and reduce the therapeutic effect leading to development of resistance to ATV. Anticonvulsants that induce CYP3A (eg, oxcarbazepine) may decrease levels; consider alternative anticonvulsant or antiretroviral therapy, if coadministration is necessary, monitor for lack/loss of virologic response and clinical monitoring of anticonvulsants is recommended. May increase levels of maraviroc, antiarrhythmics, digoxin, clarithromycin, erythromycin, telithromycin, dasatinib, nilotinib, vinblastine, vincristine, anticonvulsants metabolized by CYP3A (eg, clonazepam), TCAs, trazodone, ketoconazole, itraconazole, colchicine, rifabutin, quetiapine, β-blockers, calcium channel blockers, corticosteroids, bosentan, atorvastatin, fluvastatin, pravastatin, rosuvastatin, immunosuppressants (eg, cyclosporine, everolimus, sirolimus, tacrolimus), fentanyl, tramadol, neuroleptics, PDE-5 inhibitors, and sedatives/hypnotics (eg, buspirone, diazepam, zolpidem). May increase levels of drugs that are primarily metabolized by CYP3A, UGT1A1 and/or CYP2D6 or substrates of P-gp, BCRP, OATP1B1, and/or OATP1B3, increasing/prolonging their therapeutic effects and adverse reactions, and requiring dose adjustments and/or additional monitoring of these drugs. Monitor for tenofovir-associated adverse reactions w/ TDF. Monitor INR w/ warfarin. Caution w/ antidepressants (eg, SSRIs, TCAs) and w/ narcotics used for treatment of opioid dependence (buprenorphine, naloxone, methadone). Coadministration w/ corticosteroids that are metabolized by CYP3A, particularly long-term use, may increase the risk for development of systemic corticosteroid effects. Coadministration w/ dexamethasone or other corticosteroids that induce CYP3A may result in loss of therapeutic effect and development of resistance to ATV. Consider alternative nonhormonal forms of contraception if taking hormonal contraceptives. Coadministration w/ parenteral midazolam should be done in a setting that ensures close clinical monitoring and appropriate medical management in case of respiratory depression and/or prolonged sedation. **ATV:** Reduced levels w/ PPIs, antacids, buffered medications, or H_2RAs. Administer a minimum of 2 hrs apart w/ concomitant use of antacids. Coadministration w/ didanosine buffered tabs may decrease atazanavir exposure. Simultaneous coadministration w/ didanosine enteric coated caps and atazanavir w/ food, may decrease didanosine exposure. **Cobicistat:** Renal impairment, including cases of acute renal failure and Fanconi syndrome, reported when used in an antiretroviral regimen containing TDF. Refer to PI for further detailed information on drug interactions, including dosing modifications required when used w/ certain concomitant therapies.

PATIENT CONSIDERATIONS

Assessment: Assess for previous hypersensitivity to the drug, preexisting conduction system disease, hemophilia, preexisting DM, renal/hepatic impairment, pregnancy/nursing status, and possible drug interactions. Assess estimated CrCl. Assess for primary protease inhibitor resistance substitutions in treatment-experienced patients. When coadministering w/ TDF, assess estimated CrCl, urine glucose, and urine protein at baseline. Perform baseline hepatic laboratory testing in patients w/ underlying hepatitis B or C infections or marked transaminase elevations.

Monitoring: Monitor for fat redistribution/accumulation, cardiac conduction abnormalities, rash, Stevens-Johnson syndrome, DRESS syndrome, nephrolithiasis, cholelithiasis, hyperbilirubinemia, new onset or exacerbation of DM, hyperglycemia, diabetic ketoacidosis, immune reconstitution syndrome, autoimmune disorders, and other adverse reactions. Monitor for bleeding in patients w/ hemophilia. Perform routine monitoring of estimated CrCl, urine glucose, and urine protein when used w/ TDF. Monitor serum phosphorus levels in patients at risk for renal impairment when used w/ TDF. Perform hepatic laboratory testing in patients w/ underlying hepatitis B or C infections or marked transaminase elevations.

Counseling: Inform that therapy is not a cure for HIV and that illnesses associated w/ HIV may continue. Advise to remain under the care of a physician during therapy. Advise to avoid activities that can spread HIV infection to others. Instruct to take ud and not to d/c therapy w/o consulting physician. Advise not to miss a dose, but if a dose is missed by ≤12 hrs, instruct to take the missed dose right away and take next dose at the usual time, or if missed by >12 hrs, instruct to wait and take next dose at the usual time and not to double next dose. Inform of the potential for serious drug interactions, and explain that some drugs should not be taken concomitantly, or some drugs may need a change in dose. Advise to report use of any prescription/nonprescription medication or herbal products, particularly St. John's wort. Instruct patients receiving hormonal contraceptives to use additional or alternative nonhormonal contraceptive measures during therapy. Inform that therapy may produce ECG changes; advise to consult physician if symptoms (eg, dizziness, lightheadedness) are experienced. Inform that mild rashes w/o other symptoms and severe skin reactions have been reported; advise to immediately contact physician if signs/symptoms of severe skin/hypersensitivity reactions develop. Inform that kidney stones and/or gallstones, and fat redistribution/accumulation have been reported. Inform that asymptomatic elevations in indirect bilirubin accompanied by yellowing of the skin or whites of the eyes have occurred and that alternative antiretroviral therapy may be considered if patients have cosmetic concerns.

STORAGE: 25°C (77°F); excursions permitted to 15-30°C (59-86°F).

EXELON — rivastigmine

RX

Class: Acetylcholinesterase (AChE) inhibitor

ADULT DOSAGE

Alzheimer's Disease

Cap/Sol:

Mild to Moderate Dementia:

Initial: 1.5mg bid

PEDIATRIC DOSAGE

Pediatric use may not have been established

Titrate: May increase to 3mg bid after at least 2 weeks; subsequent increases to 4.5mg bid and 6mg bid should be attempted after a minimum of 2 weeks at the previous dose
Usual: 6-12mg/day (3-6mg bid)
Max: 12mg/day (6mg bid)

Patch:
Mild to Moderate Dementia:
Initial: Apply one 4.6mg/24 hrs patch qd
Titrate: Increase dose only after a minimum of 4 weeks at the previous dose
Maint: 9.5mg/24 hrs qd or 13.3mg/24 hrs qd
Max: 13.3mg/24 hrs

Severe Dementia:
Initial: Apply one 4.6mg/24 hrs patch qd
Titrate: Increase dose only after a minimum of 4 weeks at the previous dose
Maint: 13.3mg/24 hrs qd
Max: 13.3mg/24 hrs

Parkinson's Disease

Mild to Moderate Dementia:
Cap/Sol:
Initial: 1.5mg bid
Titrate: May increase to 3mg bid after at least 4 weeks; subsequent increases to 4.5mg bid and 6mg bid should be attempted after a minimum of 4 weeks at the previous dose
Max: 12mg/day (6mg bid)

Patch:
Initial: Apply one 4.6mg/24 hrs patch qd
Titrate: Increase dose only after a minimum of 4 weeks at the previous dose
Maint: 9.5mg/24 hrs qd or 13.3mg/24 hrs qd
Max: 13.3mg/24 hrs

Conversions

Switching to Patch from Cap/Sol:
Total Daily PO Dose <6mg: 4.6mg/24 hrs patch
Total Daily PO Dose 6-12mg: 9.5mg/24 hrs patch

Apply first patch on the day following the last oral dose

DOSING CONSIDERATIONS

Renal Impairment
Moderate to Severe:
Cap/Sol: May only be able to tolerate lower doses

Hepatic Impairment
Mild to Moderate (Child-Pugh 5-9):
Cap/Sol: May only be able to tolerate lower doses
Patch: Consider using the 4.6mg/24 hrs patch as both initial and maint dose

Adverse Reactions
Treatment Interruption w/ Adverse Reactions:
Cap/Sol:
≤3-Day Interruption: Restart treatment w/ same or lower dose
>3-Day Interruption: Restart treatment w/ 1.5mg bid and titrate
Patch:
≤3-Day Interruption: Restart w/ same or lower strength patch
>3-Day Interruption: Restart w/ 4.6mg/24 hrs patch and titrate

Other Important Considerations
Low Body Weight (<50kg):
Cap/Sol: Consider reducing dose if toxicities develop
Patch: Consider reducing maint dose to the 4.6mg/24 hrs patch if toxicities develop

E

ADMINISTRATION

Oral/Transdermal route

Oral

Take w/ meals in divided doses in am and pm
Cap and sol may be interchanged at equal doses

Sol Administration Instructions:

Remove the oral dosing syringe provided in its protective case, and using the provided syringe, withdraw the prescribed amount of sol from container
Each dose of sol may be swallowed directly from the syringe or 1st mixed w/ a small glass of water, cold fruit juice, or soda

Patch

Do not use the patch if the pouch seal is broken or the patch is cut, damaged, or changed in any way
Apply once a day; press down firmly for 30 sec until the edges stick well when applying to clean, dry, hairless, intact, healthy skin in a place that will not be rubbed against by tight clothing
Use the upper or lower back as the site of application. If sites on the back are not accessible, apply the patch to the upper arm or chest; do not apply to a skin area where cre, lotion, or powder has recently been applied
Do not apply to skin that is red, irritated, or cut
Replace w/ a new patch every 24 hrs. Instruct patients to only wear 1 patch at a time. If a patch falls off or if a dose is missed, apply a new patch immediately and then replace this patch the following day at the usual application time
Change the site of patch application daily, although a new patch can be applied to the same general area (eg, another spot on the upper back) on consecutive days. Do not apply a new patch to the same location for at least 14 days
Patch may be worn during bathing and in hot weather; avoid long exposure to external heat sources (excessive sunlight, saunas, solariums)
Place used patches in the previously saved pouch and discard in the trash, away from pets or children

HOW SUPPLIED

Cap: 1.5mg, 3mg, 4.5mg, 6mg; **Sol:** 2mg/mL [120mL]; **Patch:** 4.6mg/24 hrs, 9.5mg/24 hrs, 13.3mg/24 hrs [30[s]]

CONTRAINDICATIONS

Known hypersensitivity to rivastigmine, other carbamate derivatives, or other components of the formulation. Previous history of application-site reactions w/ rivastigmine transdermal patch suggestive of allergic contact dermatitis, (Oral) in the absence of negative allergy testing.

WARNINGS/PRECAUTIONS

May cause dose-related GI adverse reactions (eg, significant N/V, diarrhea, anorexia/decreased appetite, and weight loss). Disseminated allergic dermatitis irrespective of route of administration reported; d/c if these occur. In patients who develop application-site reactions to patch suggestive of allergic contact dermatitis and who still require therapy, switch to oral therapy only after negative allergy testing and under close medical supervision. May increase gastric acid secretion; monitor for symptoms of active/occult bleeding. Caution in those at increased risk of developing ulcers. May have vagotonic effects on HR (eg, bradycardia), which may be particularly important in sick sinus syndrome or supraventricular cardiac conduction conditions. May cause urinary obstruction and seizures. Caution in patients w/ asthma and obstructive pulmonary disease. May exacerbate or induce extrapyramidal symptoms and impair mental/physical abilities. Caution in patients w/ low or high body weights. (Oral) Syncopal episodes reported. Worsening of parkinsonian symptoms, particularly tremor, observed in patients treated w/ cap. (Patch) Skin application-site reactions may occur. Allergic contact dermatitis should be suspected if application-site reactions spread beyond the patch size; d/c treatment if there is evidence of more intense local reaction (eg, increasing erythema, edema, papules), and if symptoms do not significantly improve w/in 48 hrs after patch removal.

ADVERSE REACTIONS

N/V, anxiety, decreased weight, anorexia, headache, dizziness, fatigue, diarrhea, depression, asthenia, tremor, dyspepsia. (Oral) Abdominal pain.

DRUG INTERACTIONS

Increased risk of additive extrapyramidal adverse reactions w/ metoclopramide; avoid concomitant use. May increase cholinergic effects of other cholinomimetics and may interfere w/ the activity of anticholinergics (eg, oxybutynin, tolterodine); avoid concomitant use unless clinically necessary. Additive bradycardic effects resulting in syncope may occur w/ β-blockers, especially cardioselective β-blockers (eg, atenolol); avoid concomitant use. May exaggerate succinylcholine-type muscle relaxation during anesthesia. Caution w/ NSAIDs; monitor for symptoms of active/occult bleeding.

PATIENT CONSIDERATIONS

Assessment: Assess for hypersensitivity to drug, history of GI ulcer disease, sick sinus syndrome, supraventricular cardiac conduction conditions, asthma or obstructive pulmonary disease, pregnancy/nursing status, and possible drug interactions. Assess body weight, for history of application-site reactions w/ rivastigmine patch suggestive of allergic contact dermatitis, and hepatic impairment. (Oral) Assess for renal impairment.

Monitoring: Monitor for signs/symptoms of active or occult GI bleeding, hypersensitivity reactions, extrapyramidal symptoms, urinary obstruction, seizures, GI adverse events, cardiac conduction effects, and other adverse reactions. Closely monitor patients w/ high or low body weight. Monitor for toxicities (eg, excessive N/V) in patients w/ low body weight. (Patch) Monitor for skin reactions (allergic contact dermatitis).

Counseling: Instruct caregivers to monitor for GI adverse reactions and to inform physician if these occur. Inform that allergic skin reactions have been reported regardless of formulation; instruct to consult physician immediately in case of skin reaction while on therapy. Instruct to d/c if disseminated skin hypersensitivity reaction occurs. Advise that therapy may exacerbate or induce extrapyramidal symptoms. (Patch) Instruct to rotate application site, not to use the same site w/in 14 days, to replace patch q24h at consistent time of day, and to wear only 1 patch at a time. Instruct to avoid exposure to external heat for long periods. Instruct on proper usage and discarding of patch. In case of accidental contact w/ eyes or if eyes become red after handling the patch, instruct to rinse immediately w/ plenty of water and seek medical advice if symptoms do not resolve. Advise not to take rivastigmine cap or oral sol, or other drugs w/ cholinergic effects while wearing patch. Instruct to inform physician if application-site reactions spread beyond the patch size, if there is evidence of more intense local reaction, and if symptoms do not significantly improve w/in 48 hrs after patch removal.

STORAGE: 25°C (77°F); excursions permitted to 15-30°C (59-86°F). (Sol) Store in upright position and protect from freezing. Stable for up to 4 hrs at room temperature if combined w/ cold fruit juice or soda. (Patch) Keep in sealed pouch until use.

EXFORGE — amlodipine/valsartan

RX

Class: Angiotensin II receptor blocker (ARB)/calcium channel blocker (CCB) (dihydropyridine)

D/C therapy as soon as possible when pregnancy is detected. Drugs that act directly on the renin-angiotensin system (RAS) can cause injury/death to the developing fetus.

ADULT DOSAGE

Hypertension

Initial Therapy:
Initial: 5mg/160mg qd in patients who are not volume-depleted
Titrate: May increase after 1-2 weeks
Max: 10mg/320mg qd

Add-On Therapy:
May be used if BP is not adequately controlled w/ amlodipine (or another dihydropyridine calcium channel blocker) or valsartan (or another ARB) alone. Patients w/ dose-limiting adverse reactions to either component alone may be switched to therapy containing a lower dose of that component in combination w/ the other to achieve similar BP reductions
Titrate: May increase dose if BP remains uncontrolled after 3-4 weeks
Max: 10mg/320mg qd

Replacement Therapy:
May substitute for individually titrated components

May be administered w/ other antihypertensive agents

PEDIATRIC DOSAGE

Pediatric use may not have been established

E

DOSING CONSIDERATIONS

Hepatic Impairment

Initial: 2.5mg of amlodipine

Elderly

Initial: 2.5mg of amlodipine

ADMINISTRATION

Oral route

Take w/ or w/o food.

HOW SUPPLIED

Tab: (Amlodipine/Valsartan) 5mg/160mg, 10mg/160mg, 5mg/320mg, 10mg/320mg

CONTRAINDICATIONS

Known hypersensitivity to any component, coadministration w/ aliskiren in patients w/ diabetes.

WARNINGS/PRECAUTIONS

Excessive hypotension reported. Symptomatic hypotension may occur in patients w/ an activated RAS (eg, volume- and/or salt-depleted patients receiving high doses of diuretics); correct volume depletion prior to therapy. Initiate therapy cautiously in patients w/ heart failure (HF) or recent MI, and in patients undergoing surgery/dialysis. Changes in renal function may occur; consider withholding or discontinuing therapy if clinically significant decrease in renal function develops. Patients whose renal function may depend in part on the activity of the RAS (eg, patients w/ renal artery stenosis, chronic kidney disease, severe CHF, volume depletion) may be at particular risk of developing acute renal failure; periodically monitor renal function in these patients. Hyperkalemia may occur; dose reduction and/or discontinuation of therapy may be required. **Amlodipine:** Acute hypotension reported (rare); caution w/ severe aortic stenosis. Worsening angina and acute MI may develop after starting or increasing dose, particularly w/ severe obstructive coronary artery disease (CAD). **Valsartan:** Increases in K^+ reported in some patients w/ HF; more likely to occur in patients w/ preexisting renal impairment.

ADVERSE REACTIONS

Peripheral edema, nasopharyngitis, URTI, dizziness.

DRUG INTERACTIONS

See Contraindications. **Amlodipine:** CYP3A inhibitors (moderate and strong) increased systemic exposure and may require dose reduction; monitor for symptoms of hypotension and edema to determine the need for dose adjustment. Monitor BP closely when coadministered w/ CYP3A inducers. Monitor for hypotension when coadministered w/ sildenafil. Increases systemic exposure of simvastatin; limit simvastatin dose to 20mg/day. May increase systemic exposure of cyclosporine or tacrolimus; frequently monitor trough levels of cyclosporine and tacrolimus and adjust dose when appropriate. **Valsartan:** NSAIDs, including selective COX-2 inhibitors, may attenuate antihypertensive effect and result in deterioration of renal function, including possible acute renal failure; monitor renal function periodically. Concomitant use w/ other agents that block the RAS, K^+-sparing diuretics (eg, spironolactone, triamterene, amiloride), K^+ supplements, salt substitutes containing K^+, or other drugs that may increase K^+ levels (eg, heparin) may lead to increases in serum K^+, and in HF patients to increases in SrCr; monitor serum K^+ if comedication is necessary. Inhibitors of the hepatic uptake transporter OATP1B1 (rifampin, cyclosporine) or the hepatic efflux transporter MRP2 (ritonavir) may increase systemic exposure. Dual blockade of the RAS is associated w/ increased risks of hypotension, hyperkalemia, and changes in renal function (including acute renal failure); in general, avoid combined use of RAS inhibitors, or closely monitor BP, renal function, and electrolytes w/ concomitant agents that affect the RAS. Avoid w/ aliskiren in patients w/ renal impairment (GFR <60mL/min). Increases in lithium levels and lithium toxicity reported; monitor serum lithium levels during concomitant use.

PATIENT CONSIDERATIONS

Assessment: Assess for hypersensitivity to any component of the drug, volume/salt depletion, HF, recent MI, renal artery stenosis, severe aortic stenosis, severe obstructive CAD, renal/hepatic impairment, pregnancy/nursing status, and possible drug interactions.

Monitoring: Monitor for signs/symptoms of hypotension, hyperkalemia, hypersensitivity reactions, and other adverse reactions. Monitor for symptoms of angina or MI, particularly in patients w/ severe obstructive CAD, after initiation of therapy or dose increase. Monitor BP, serum electrolytes, and renal function.

Counseling: Counsel about risks/benefits of therapy. Inform females of childbearing age about the consequences of exposure to therapy during pregnancy; discuss treatment options w/ women planning to become pregnant. Instruct to report pregnancies to physician as soon as possible.

STORAGE: 25°C (77°F); excursions permitted to 15-30°C (59-86°F). Protect from moisture.

EXFORGE HCT – amlodipine/hydrochlorothiazide/valsartan RX

Class: Angiotensin II receptor blocker (ARB)/calcium channel blocker (CCB) (dihydropyridine)/thiazide diuretic

D/C therapy as soon as possible when pregnancy is detected. Drugs that act directly on the renin-angiotensin system (RAS) can cause injury/death to the developing fetus.

E

ADULT DOSAGE

Hypertension

Usual: Dose qd
Titrate: May increase dose after 2 weeks
Max: 10mg/320mg/25mg qd

Add-On/Switch Therapy:
May use for patients not adequately controlled on any 2 of the following classes: CCBs, ARBs, and diuretics. Patients w/ dose-limiting adverse reactions to an individual component while on any dual combination of the components of therapy may be switched to therapy containing a lower dose of that component

Replacement Therapy:
May substitute for individually titrated components

May be administered w/ other antihypertensive agents

PEDIATRIC DOSAGE

Pediatric use may not have been established

DOSING CONSIDERATIONS

Hepatic Impairment
Initial: 2.5mg of amlodipine

Elderly
Initial: 2.5mg of amlodipine

ADMINISTRATION

Oral route

Take w/ or w/o food.

HOW SUPPLIED

Tab: (Amlodipine/Valsartan/Hydrochlorothiazide [HCTZ]) 5mg/160mg/12.5mg, 5mg/160mg/25mg, 10mg/160mg/12.5mg, 10mg/160mg/25mg, 10mg/320mg/25mg

CONTRAINDICATIONS

Anuria, sulfonamide-derived drug hypersensitivity, hypersensitivity to any component of the product, coadministration w/ aliskiren in patients w/ diabetes.

WARNINGS/PRECAUTIONS

This fixed combination drug is not indicated for initial therapy of HTN. Excessive hypotension, including orthostatic hypotension, reported. Symptomatic hypotension may occur in patients w/ an activated RAS (eg, volume- and/or salt-depleted patients receiving high doses of diuretics); correct this condition prior to therapy. Avoid w/ aortic or mitral stenosis or obstructive hypertrophic cardiomyopathy. Changes in renal function, including acute renal failure, may occur; consider withholding or discontinuing therapy if clinically significant decrease in renal function develops. Patients whose renal function may depend in part on the activity of the RAS (eg, patients w/ renal artery stenosis, chronic kidney disease, severe CHF, volume depletion) may be at particular risk of developing acute renal failure; periodically monitor renal function in these patients. Hyperkalemia may occur. HCTZ may cause hypokalemia, hyponatremia, and hypomagnesemia. D/C therapy if hypokalemia is accompanied by clinical signs (eg, muscular weakness, paresis, ECG alterations); correct hypokalemia and any coexisting hypomagnesemia prior to the initiation of thiazides. **Amlodipine:** Worsening angina and acute MI may develop after starting or increasing dose, particularly in patients w/ severe obstructive coronary artery disease (CAD). **Valsartan:** Increases in K^+ reported in some patients w/ heart failure (HF), and are more likely to occur in patients w/ preexisting renal impairment; dose reduction and/or discontinuation of diuretic and/or valsartan may be required. **HCTZ:** May cause hypersensitivity reactions and exacerbation/activation of systemic lupus erythematosus (SLE). May alter glucose tolerance and increase serum cholesterol and TG levels. May cause or exacerbate hyperuricemia and precipitate gout in susceptible patients. Decreases urinary Ca^{2+} excretion and may cause elevations of serum Ca^{2+}; monitor Ca^{2+} levels in patients w/ hypercalcemia. May cause idiosyncratic reaction, resulting in acute transient myopia and acute angle-closure glaucoma; d/c as rapidly as possible. Minor alterations of fluid and electrolyte balance may precipitate hepatic coma in patients w/ impaired hepatic function or progressive liver disease.

ADVERSE REACTIONS

Dizziness, edema, headache, dyspepsia, fatigue, muscle spasms, back pain, nausea, nasopharyngitis.

DRUG INTERACTIONS

See Contraindications. **Amlodipine:** CYP3A inhibitors (moderate and strong) increased systemic exposure and may require dose reduction; monitor for symptoms of hypotension and edema to determine the need for dose adjustment. Monitor BP closely when coadministered w/ CYP3A inducers. Monitor for hypotension when coadministered w/ sildenafil. Increases systemic exposure of simvastatin; limit simvastatin dose to 20mg/day. May increase systemic exposure of cyclosporine or tacrolimus; frequently monitor trough levels of cyclosporine and tacrolimus and adjust dose when appropriate. **Valsartan:** Concomitant use w/ other agents that block the RAS, K^+-sparing diuretics (eg, spironolactone, triamterene, amiloride), K^+ supplements, salt substitutes containing K^+, or other drugs that may increase K^+ levels (eg, heparin) may lead to increases in serum K^+, and in HF patients to increases in SrCr; monitor serum K^+ levels if comedication is necessary. NSAIDs, including selective COX-2 inhibitors, may attenuate antihypertensive effect and result in deterioration of renal function, including possible acute renal failure; monitor renal function periodically. Dual blockade of the RAS is associated w/ increased risks of hypotension, hyperkalemia, and changes in renal function (including acute renal failure); in general, avoid combined use of RAS inhibitors, or closely monitor BP, renal function, and electrolytes w/ concomitant agents that affect the RAS. Avoid w/ aliskiren in patients w/ renal impairment (GFR <60mL/min). **HCTZ:** Dosage adjustment of antidiabetic drugs (eg, oral agents, insulin) may be required. When used concomitantly w/ NSAIDs, monitor closely to determine if the desired effect of diuretic is obtained. May lead to symptomatic hyponatremia w/ carbamazepine. Staggering the dose of HCTZ and ion exchange resins (eg, cholestyramine, colestipol) such that HCTZ is administered at least 4 hrs before or 4-6 hrs after the administration of resins would potentially minimize the interaction. Cyclosporine may increase risk of hyperuricemia and gout-type complications. **Valsartan and HCTZ:** Increases in lithium levels and lithium toxicity reported; monitor serum lithium levels during concomitant use.

PATIENT CONSIDERATIONS

Assessment: Assess for hypersensitivity to the drug and its components, anuria, sulfonamide-derived drug or penicillin hypersensitivity, renal/hepatic impairment, HF, aortic or mitral stenosis, renal artery stenosis, obstructive hypertrophic cardiomyopathy, SLE, volume/salt depletion, electrolyte imbalances, CAD, pregnancy/nursing status, and possible drug interactions.

Monitoring: Monitor for signs/symptoms of hypotension, hypersensitivity/idiosyncratic reactions, metabolic disturbances, myopia and angle-closure glaucoma, worsening angina or acute MI, fluid imbalance, exacerbation or activation of SLE, hyperglycemia, hyperuricemia or precipitation of gout, increases in cholesterol and TG levels, and other adverse reactions. Monitor BP, serum electrolytes, and renal function.

Counseling: Counsel about risks/benefits of therapy. Inform females of childbearing age about the consequences of exposure to therapy during pregnancy; discuss treatment options w/ women planning to become pregnant. Instruct to report pregnancies to physician as soon as possible. Caution that lightheadedness may occur, especially during the 1st days of therapy, and that it should be reported to physician. Instruct to d/c therapy until the physician has been consulted if syncope occurs. Caution that inadequate fluid intake, excessive perspiration, diarrhea, or vomiting may lead to an excessive fall in BP, w/ the same consequences of lightheadedness and possible syncope. Instruct patients not to use K^+ supplements or salt substitutes containing K^+ w/o consulting prescribing physician.

STORAGE: 25°C (77°F); excursions permitted to 15-30°C (59-86°F). Protect from moisture.

FAMVIR – famciclovir

RX

Class: Nucleoside analogue

ADULT DOSAGE

Herpes Zoster

500mg q8h for 7 days
Initiate as soon as diagnosed

Herpes

Orolabial/Genital:
Recurrent in HIV-Infected Patients:
500mg bid for 7 days
Initiate at 1st sign/symptom

PEDIATRIC DOSAGE

Pediatric use may not have been established

Herpes Labialis (Cold Sores)

Recurrent:
1500mg single dose
Initiate at 1st sign/symptom

Genital Herpes

Recurrent Episodes:
1000mg bid for 1 day
Initiate at 1st sign/symptom

Suppressive Therapy:
250mg bid

DOSING CONSIDERATIONS

Renal Impairment

Recurrent Herpes Labialis:
CrCl 40-59mL/min: 750mg single dose
CrCl 20-39mL/min: 500mg single dose
CrCl <20mL/min: 250mg single dose
Hemodialysis: 250mg single dose following dialysis

Recurrent Genital Herpes:
CrCl 40-59mL/min: 500mg q12h for 1 day
CrCl 20-39mL/min: 500mg single dose
CrCl <20mL/min: 250mg single dose
Hemodialysis: 250mg single dose following dialysis

Suppression of Recurrent Genital Herpes:
CrCl 20-39mL/min: 125mg q12h
CrCl <20mL/min: 125mg q24h
Hemodialysis: 125mg following each dialysis

Herpes Zoster:
CrCl 40-59mL/min: 500mg q12h
CrCl 20-39mL/min: 500mg q24h
CrCl <20mL/min: 250mg q24h
Hemodialysis: 250mg following each dialysis

Recurrent Orolabial/Genital Herpes in HIV-Infected Patients:
CrCl 20-39mL/min: 500mg q24h
CrCl <20mL/min: 250mg q24h
Hemodialysis: 250mg following each dialysis

ADMINISTRATION

Oral route
Take w/ or w/o food

HOW SUPPLIED

Tab: 125mg, 250mg, 500mg

CONTRAINDICATIONS

Known hypersensitivity to the product, its components, or penciclovir.

WARNINGS/PRECAUTIONS

Acute renal failure reported in patients with underlying renal disease who have received inappropriately high doses. Caution in elderly and with renal impairment.

ADVERSE REACTIONS

Headache, N/V, diarrhea, elevated lipase, ALT elevation, fatigue, flatulence, pruritus, rash, neutropenia, abdominal pain, dysmenorrhea, migraine.

DRUG INTERACTIONS

Probenecid or other drugs significantly eliminated by active renal tubular secretion may increase levels of penciclovir. Potential interaction with drugs metabolized by and/or inhibiting aldehyde oxidase. Raloxifene may decrease formation of penciclovir.

PATIENT CONSIDERATIONS

Assessment: Assess for hypersensitivity to the drug, renal impairment, pregnancy/nursing status, and possible drug interactions.

Monitoring: Monitor renal function and for adverse reactions.

Counseling: Inform to take exactly ud. Advise to initiate treatment at earliest signs/symptoms of recurrence of cold sores, at the 1st sign/symptom of recurrent genital herpes if episodic therapy is indicated, and as soon as possible after a diagnosis of herpes zoster. Inform that drug is not a cure for cold sores or genital herpes. Advise to avoid contact with lesions or intercourse when lesions and/or symptoms are present to avoid infecting partners. Counsel to use safer sex practices.

Instruct to refrain from driving or operating machinery if dizziness, somnolence, confusion, or other CNS disturbances occur. Inform that drug contains lactose; instruct to notify physician if with rare hereditary problems of galactose intolerance, a severe lactase deficiency, or glucose-galactose malabsorption.

STORAGE: 25°C (77°F); excursions permitted to 15-30°C (59-86°F).

FANAPT – iloperidone

RX

Class: Atypical antipsychotic

Elderly patients with dementia-related psychosis treated with antipsychotic drugs are at an increased risk of death; most deaths appeared to be cardiovascular (CV) (eg, heart failure, sudden death) or infectious (eg, pneumonia) in nature. Not approved for the treatment of patients with dementia-related psychosis.

ADULT DOSAGE

Schizophrenia

Initial: 1mg bid
Titrate: Dose increases may be made w/ daily dosage adjustments not to exceed 2mg bid (4mg/day) to reach the target range of 6-12mg bid (12-24mg/day)
Max: 12mg bid (24mg/day)
Responding patients may continue beyond acute response; periodically reassess need for maint treatment

Reinitiation of Treatment:
Follow initiation titration schedule if patients have had an interval off therapy for >3 days

Conversions

Switching from Other Antipsychotics:
Minimize overlapping period of antipsychotics

PEDIATRIC DOSAGE

Pediatric use may not have been established

DOSING CONSIDERATIONS

Concomitant Medications

Strong CYP2D6 Inhibitors or Strong CYP3A4 Inhibitors:
Reduce dose by 50%; increase to previous iloperidone dose upon withdrawal of strong CYP2D6/CYP3A4 inhibitors

Hepatic Impairment

Severe: Not recommended

Other Important Considerations

Poor CYP2D6 Metabolizers:
Reduce dose by 50%

ADMINISTRATION

Oral route

Take w/o regard to meals

HOW SUPPLIED

Tab: 1mg, 2mg, 4mg, 6mg, 8mg, 10mg, 12mg

CONTRAINDICATIONS

Known hypersensitivity reaction to the product.

WARNINGS/PRECAUTIONS

Not recommended in patients with severe hepatic impairment and caution with moderate hepatic impairment. QT prolongation reported; avoid with congenital long QT syndrome, history of cardiac arrhythmias, or history of significant CV illnesses. D/C if persistent QTc measurements are >500 msec. Obtain baseline measurements and periodically monitor K^+ and Mg^{2+} levels in patients at risk of electrolyte disturbances. Risk of tardive dyskinesia (TD), especially in the elderly; consider discontinuation if signs/symptoms develop. Neuroleptic malignant syndrome (NMS) reported; immediately d/c and treat. May cause metabolic changes (eg, hyperglycemia, dyslipidemia, weight gain) that may increase CV and cerebrovascular risk. Hyperglycemia, in some cases extreme and associated with ketoacidosis or hyperosmolar coma or death, reported; monitor for worsening of glucose control, and perform FPG testing at the beginning of therapy and periodically in patients at risk for diabetes mellitus (DM). Caution with a history of seizures, conditions that lower the seizure threshold, or in patients with reduced CYP2D6 activity. May induce orthostatic hypotension; caution with CV disease (CVD), cerebrovascular disease, or conditions that predispose to hypotension. Leukopenia, neutropenia, and agranulocytosis reported; d/c in cases of severe neutropenia (absolute neutrophil count <1000/mm^3). Monitor CBC and d/c at 1st sign of decline in WBC count if with preexisting low WBC count or history of drug-induced leukopenia/neutropenia and in the absence of other causative factors. May elevate prolactin levels. May disrupt body's ability to reduce core body temperature. Esophageal dysmotility and aspiration reported; caution in patients at risk of aspiration pneumonia. Closely supervise high-risk patients for suicide attempt. Priapism reported. May impair mental/physical abilities. Evaluate for history of drug abuse; monitor for drug misuse/abuse in these patients.

ADVERSE REACTIONS

Dizziness, somnolence, tachycardia, nausea, dry mouth, weight gain, nasal congestion, diarrhea, fatigue, extrapyramidal disorder, orthostatic hypotension, nasopharyngitis, arthralgia, tremor, upper respiratory tract infection.

F

DRUG INTERACTIONS

See Dosage. Caution with CYP3A4 (eg, ketoconazole, clarithromycin) or CYP2D6 (eg, fluoxetine, paroxetine) inhibitors; may increase levels and may augment effect on the QTc interval. May increase total exposure of dextromethorphan with concomitant use. Avoid with Class IA (eg, quinidine, procainamide) or Class III (eg, amiodarone, sotalol) antiarrhythmics, antipsychotics (eg, chlorpromazine, thioridazine), antibiotics (eg, gatifloxacin, moxifloxacin), or other drugs known to prolong the QTc interval (eg, pentamidine, levomethadyl acetate, methadone). Caution with other centrally acting drugs and alcohol. May enhance hypotensive effects of antihypertensive agents. Concomitant use with medications with anticholinergic activity may contribute to an elevation in core body temperature. May increase levels of drugs that are predominantly eliminated by CYP3A4.

PATIENT CONSIDERATIONS

Assessment: Assess for known hypersensitivity to the drug, dementia-related psychosis, hepatic impairment, DM, risk factors for DM, CVD, cerebrovascular disease, congenital long QT syndrome, history of cardiac arrhythmias, conditions that predispose to hypotension, conditions that may contribute to an elevation in core body temperature, history of low WBCs or drug-induced leukopenia/neutropenia, history of seizures, conditions that lower the seizure threshold, history of drug abuse, poor metabolizers of CYP2D6, risk for aspiration pneumonia, risk for suicide, pregnancy/nursing status, and possible drug interactions. Obtain baseline FPG in patients with DM or with risk factors for DM. Perform baseline CBC, orthostatic vital signs, serum K^+ and Mg^{2+} levels.

Monitoring: Monitor for TD, NMS, hyperprolactinemia, priapism, extrapyramidal symptoms, esophageal dysmotility, aspiration, orthostatic hypotension, body temperature lability, seizures, weight gain, dyslipidemia, QT prolongation, cognitive/motor impairment, and other adverse effects. Monitor for signs of hyperglycemia; monitor FPG levels in patients with DM or at risk for DM. Monitor for suicide attempts, and drug misuse/abuse in patients with a history of drug misuse/abuse. Monitor for signs/symptoms of leukopenia, neutropenia, and agranulocytosis; frequently monitor CBC in patients with risk factors for leukopenia/neutropenia. Monitor serum K^+ and Mg^{2+} levels, and orthostatic vital signs.

Counseling: Advise to inform physician immediately if feeling faint, or if loss of consciousness or heart palpitations occur. Counsel to avoid drugs that cause QT interval prolongation and instruct to inform physician of all medications currently being taken or plan to take (prescription or OTC drugs). Inform about the signs/symptoms of NMS, hyperglycemia, and DM. Counsel that weight gain may occur during treatment. Advise of risk of orthostatic hypotension, particularly during initiation/reinitiation/dose increases. Inform that the drug may impair judgment, thinking, or motor skills; advise to use caution against driving or operating hazardous machinery. Instruct to notify physician if pregnant/intending to become pregnant. Advise not to breastfeed. Advise to avoid alcohol during treatment. Counsel about appropriate care to avoid overheating and dehydration.

STORAGE: 25°C (77°F); excursions permitted to 15-30°C (59-86°F). Protect from light and moisture.

FARXIGA – dapagliflozin

RX

Class: Sodium-glucose cotransporter 2 (SGLT2) inhibitor

ADULT DOSAGE

Type 2 Diabetes Mellitus

Initial: 5mg qam

Titrate: May increase to 10mg qd in patients tolerating 5mg qd who require additional glycemic control

PEDIATRIC DOSAGE

Pediatric use may not have been established

DOSING CONSIDERATIONS

Renal Impairment

eGFR <60mL/min/1.73m²: Do not initiate treatment

D/C therapy when eGFR is persistently <60mL/min/1.73m²

Other Important Considerations

Patients w/ Volume-Depletion:

Correct this condition before initiating treatment

ADMINISTRATION

Oral route

Take w/ or w/o food.

HOW SUPPLIED

Tab: 5mg, 10mg

CONTRAINDICATIONS

Severe renal impairment, ESRD, patients on dialysis. History of a serious hypersensitivity reaction to dapagliflozin.

WARNINGS/PRECAUTIONS

Not recommended for type 1 diabetes mellitus (DM) or for treatment of diabetic ketoacidosis. Causes intravascular volume contraction. Symptomatic hypotension may occur after initiating therapy, particularly in patients w/ renal impairment (eGFR <60mL/min/1.73m²), elderly patients, or patients on loop diuretics; assess and correct volume status before initiating treatment in patients w/ ≥1 of these characteristics. Ketoacidosis reported; if suspected, d/c and institute prompt treatment. Assess for ketoacidosis in patients presenting w/ signs/symptoms consistent w/ severe metabolic acidosis regardless of presenting blood glucose levels. Consider temporarily discontinuing therapy in clinical situations known to predispose to ketoacidosis (eg, prolonged fasting due to acute illness or surgery). Increases SrCr and decreases eGFR; caution in elderly patients and patients w/ renal impairment. Adverse reactions related to renal function may occur. Serious UTIs (eg, urosepsis, pyelonephritis), requiring hospitalization, reported; evaluate for signs/symptoms of UTIs and treat promptly, if indicated. Increases risk of genital mycotic infections; monitor and treat appropriately. Increases in LDL levels reported. Newly diagnosed cases of bladder cancer reported; do not use in patients w/ active bladder cancer and caution in patients w/ prior history of bladder cancer. Caution in patients w/ severe hepatic impairment. Monitoring glycemic control w/ urine glucose tests or 1,5-anhydroglucitol assay is not recommended.

ADVERSE REACTIONS

Genital mycotic infections, nasopharyngitis, UTIs, back pain, increased urination.

DRUG INTERACTIONS

May increase risk of hypoglycemia when combined w/ insulin or an insulin secretagogue; a lower dose of insulin or insulin secretagogue may be required.

PATIENT CONSIDERATIONS

Assessment: Assess for diabetic ketoacidosis, type of DM, volume depletion, history of genital mycotic infections, active/history of bladder cancer, drug hypersensitivity, predisposition to ketoacidosis, pregnancy/nursing status, and possible drug interactions. Assess baseline renal/hepatic function, LDL levels, and BP.

Monitoring: Monitor for signs/symptoms of hypotension, ketoacidosis, UTIs, genital mycotic infections, and other adverse reactions. Monitor renal function and LDL levels.

Counseling: Inform of the risks, benefits, and alternative modes of therapy. Advise about the importance of adherence to dietary instructions, regular physical activity, periodic blood glucose monitoring and HbA1c testing, recognition and management of hypo/hyperglycemia, and assessment of diabetes complications. Instruct to seek medical advice promptly during periods of stress (eg, fever, trauma, infection, surgery) as medication requirements may change. Instruct to immediately inform physician if pregnant, breastfeeding, planning to become pregnant or to breastfeed, or if experiencing signs/symptoms of hypotension or bladder cancer. Inform of the most common adverse reactions associated w/ therapy. Instruct to have adequate fluid intake. Instruct to d/c and seek medical advice immediately if symptoms of ketoacidosis occur. Counsel on the signs/symptoms of vaginal yeast infections, UTIs, balanitis, and balanoposthitis; inform of treatment options and when to seek medical advice. Instruct to d/c therapy and consult physician if any signs/symptoms suggesting an allergic reaction or angioedema develop.

STORAGE: 20-25°C (68-77°F); excursions permitted between 15-30°C (59-86°F).

FARYDAK – panobinostat

RX

Class: Histone deacetylase (HDAC) inhibitor

Severe diarrhea reported; monitor for symptoms, institute antidiarrheal treatment, interrupt panobinostat, and then reduce dose or d/c panobinostat. Severe and fatal cardiac ischemic events, severe arrhythmias, and ECG changes reported. Arrhythmias may be exacerbated by electrolyte abnormalities. Obtain ECG and electrolytes at baseline and periodically during treatment as clinically indicated.

F

ADULT DOSAGE

Multiple Myeloma

In combination w/ bortezomib (BTZ) and dexamethasone for the treatment of patients w/ multiple myeloma who have received at least 2 prior regimens, including BTZ and an immunomodulatory agent

Initial: 20mg once qod for 3 doses/week in Weeks 1 and 2 of each 21-day cycle for up to 8 cycles

Consider continuing treatment for an additional 8 cycles for patients w/ clinical benefit who do not experience unresolved severe or medically significant toxicity; total duration of treatment may be up to 16 cycles (48 weeks)

Recommended Dosing Schedule w/ BTZ and Dexamethasone:

Cycles 1-8:

- Panobinostat on Days 1, 3, 5, 8, 10, 12, and then rest for 1 week
- BTZ (1.3mg/m^2 IV) on Days 1, 4, 8, 11, and then rest for 1 week
- Dexamethasone (20mg PO) on Days 1, 2, 4, 5, 8, 9, 11, 12, and then rest for 1 week

Cycles 9-16:

- Panobinostat on Days 1, 3, 5, 8, 10, 12, and then rest for 1 week
- BTZ (1.3mg/m^2 IV) on Days 1, 8, and then rest for 1 week
- Dexamethasone (20mg PO) on Days 1, 2, 8, 9, and then rest for 1 week

Missed Dose

If a dose is missed it can be taken up to 12 hrs after the specified time

If vomiting occurs, patient should not repeat the dose but should take the next usual scheduled dose

PEDIATRIC DOSAGE

Pediatric use may not have been established

DOSING CONSIDERATIONS

Hepatic Impairment

Mild: Reduce starting dose to 15mg

Moderate: Reduce starting dose to 10mg

Severe: Avoid use

Concomitant Medications

Strong CYP3A Inhibitors:

Reduce starting dose to 10mg

Adverse Reactions

Management of adverse reactions may require treatment interruption and/or dose reductions.

If dose reduction is required, the dose of panobinostat should be reduced in increments of 5mg.

If the dosing of panobinostat is reduced <10mg given 3X per week, d/c panobinostat.

Keep the same treatment schedule (3-week treatment cycle) when reducing dose.

Thrombocytopenia:

Platelets <50 x 10^9/L (CTCAE Grade 3): Maintain panobinostat dose; monitor platelet counts at least weekly.

Maintain BTZ dose.

Platelets <50 x 10^9/L w/ Bleeding (CTCAE Grade 3) or Platelets <25 x 10^9/L (CTCAE Grade 4): Interrupt panobinostat; monitor platelet counts at least weekly until ≥50 x 10^9/L, then restart at reduced dose.
Interrupt BTZ until thrombocytopenia resolves to ≥75 x 10^9/L.
If only 1 dose was omitted prior to correction to these levels, restart BTZ at same dose.
If ≥2 doses were omitted consecutively, or w/in the same cycle, BTZ should be restarted at a reduced dose.

Neutropenia:
ANC 0.75 to 1.0 x 10^9/L (CTCAE Grade 3): Maintain panobinostat dose.
Maintain BTZ dose.
ANC 0.5 to 0.75 x 10^9/L (CTCAE Grade 3) (2 or More Occurrences): Interrupt panobinostat until ANC ≥1.0 x 10^9/L, then restart at same dose.
Maintain BTZ dose.
ANC <1.0 x 10^9/L (CTCAE Grade 3) w/ Febrile Neutropenia (Any Grade): Interrupt panobinostat until febrile neutropenia resolves and ANC ≥1.0 x 10^9/L, then restart at reduced dose.
Interrupt BTZ until febrile neutropenia resolves and ANC ≥1.0 x 10^9/L.
If only 1 dose was omitted prior to correction to these levels, restart BTZ at same dose.
If ≥2 doses were omitted consecutively, or w/in the same cycle, BTZ should be restarted at a reduced dose.
ANC <0.5 x 10^9/L (CTCAE Grade 4): Interrupt panobinostat until ANC ≥1.0 x 10^9/L, then restart at reduced dose.
Interrupt BTZ until febrile neutropenia resolves and ANC ≥1.0 x 10^9/L.
If only 1 dose was omitted prior to correction to these levels, restart BTZ at same dose.
If ≥2 doses were omitted consecutively, or w/in the same cycle, BTZ should be restarted at a reduced dose.

Anemia:
Hgb <8g/dL (CTCAE Grade 3): Interrupt panobinostat until Hgb ≥10g/dL.
Restart at reduced dose.

Diarrhea:
Moderate Diarrhea, 4-6 Stools/Day (CTCAE Grade 2): Interrupt panobinostat until resolved, then restart at same dose.
Consider interruption of BTZ until resolved; restart at same dose.
Severe Diarrhea (≥7 Stools/Day) IV Fluids or Hospitalization Required (CTCAE Grade 3): Interrupt panobinostat until resolved, then restart at reduced dose.
Interrupt BTZ until resolved, then restart at reduced dose.
Life-Threatening Diarrhea (CTCAE Grade 4): Permanently d/c panobinostat.
Permanently d/c BTZ.

N/V:
Severe Nausea (CTCAE Grade 3/4) or Severe/Life-Threatening Vomiting (CTCAE Grade 3/4): Interrupt panobinostat until resolved, then restart at reduced dose

Myelosuppression:
Interrupt or reduce dose of panobinostat in patients who have thrombocytopenia, neutropenia, or anemia according to instructions listed above.
Consider platelet transfusions in patients w/ severe thrombocytopenia.
D/C panobinostat treatment if thrombocytopenia does not improve despite the recommended treatment modifications or if repeated platelet transfusions are required.
Consider dose reduction and/or use of growth factors (eg, granulocyte colony-stimulating factor) in the event of Grade 3 or 4 neutropenia.
D/C panobinostat if neutropenia does not improve despite dose modifications, colony-stimulating factors, or in case of severe infection.

GI Toxicity:
May require treatment interruption or dose reduction if diarrhea, nausea, or vomiting occurs.
Treat w/ antidiarrheal medication (eg, loperamide) at 1st sign of abdominal cramping, loose stools, or onset of diarrhea.
Consider and administer prophylactic antiemetics as clinically indicated.

Other Adverse Drug Reactions:
Patients Experiencing Grade 3/4 Adverse Drug Reactions Other Than Thrombocytopenia, Neutropenia, or GI Toxicity:
CTC Grade 2 Toxicity Recurrence and CTC Grade 3 and 4: Omit dose until recovery to CTC ≤Grade 1 and restart treatment at a reduced dose
CTC Grade 3 or 4 Toxicity Recurrence: May consider further dose reduction once the adverse events have resolved to CTC ≤Grade 1

ADMINISTRATION

Oral route

Take on each scheduled day at about the same time, either w/ or w/o food.
Swallow cap whole w/ a cup of water; do not open, crush, or chew.

Direct contact of the powder in cap w/ skin or mucous membranes should be avoided; wash thoroughly if such contact occurs.

HOW SUPPLIED

Cap: 10mg, 15mg, 20mg

WARNINGS/PRECAUTIONS

Do not initiate in patients w/ history of recent MI or unstable angina. May prolong cardiac ventricular repolarization (QT interval); do not initiate in patients w/ a QTcF >450 msec or clinically significant baseline ST-segment or T-wave abnormalities. If during therapy the QTcF increases to ≥480 msec, interrupt therapy. If QT prolongation does not resolve, d/c therapy permanently. Fatal and serious hemorrhage reported. Myelosuppression (eg, severe thrombocytopenia, neutropenia, anemia) may occur. Localized and systemic infections (eg, pneumonia, bacterial infections, invasive fungal infections, viral infections) reported; if diagnosis of infection is made, institute appropriate anti-infective treatment promptly and consider interruption or discontinuation of therapy. Should not be initiated in patients w/ active infections. Hepatic dysfunction reported; if abnormal LFTs are observed, may consider dose adjustment until values return to normal or pretreatment levels.

ADVERSE REACTIONS

Diarrhea, fatigue, nausea, peripheral edema, decreased appetite, pyrexia, vomiting, hypophosphatemia, hypokalemia, hyponatremia, increased creatinine, thrombocytopenia, lymphopenia, leukopenia, neutropenia, anemia.

DRUG INTERACTIONS

See Dosing Considerations. Avoid w/ strong CYP3A inducers. Increased levels w/ strong CYP3A inhibitors; avoid star fruit, pomegranate or pomegranate juice, and grapefruit or grapefruit juice. Avoid coadministration w/ sensitive CYP2D6 substrates (eg, atomoxetine, metoprolol, venlafaxine) or CYP2D6 substrates that have a narrow therapeutic index (eg, thioridazine, pimozide); if concomitant use of CYP2D6 substrates is unavoidable, monitor patients frequently for adverse reactions. Not recommended w/ antiarrhythmics (eg, amiodarone, disopyramide, procainamide) and other drugs known to prolong the QT interval (eg, chloroquine, halofantrine, clarithromycin). Antiemetic drugs w/ known QT prolonging risk (eg, dolasetron, ondansetron, tropisetron) can be used w/ frequent ECG monitoring.

PATIENT CONSIDERATIONS

Assessment: Assess for history of recent MI or unstable angina, active infection, pregnancy/nursing status, and possible drug interactions. Obtain baseline CBC, LFTs, ECG, and electrolyte levels (including K^+, Mg^{2+}, and phosphate). Assess hydration status.

Monitoring: Monitor for signs/symptoms of diarrhea, cardiac ischemic events, arrhythmias, hemorrhage, infection, and other adverse reactions. Monitor ECG periodically as clinically indicated. Monitor CBC, hydration status, and electrolyte blood levels weekly (or more frequently if clinically indicated). Monitor LFTs regularly. Monitor for toxicity more frequently in patients >65 yrs of age, especially for GI toxicity, myelosuppression, and cardiac toxicity.

Counseling: Instruct to take exactly ud. If a dose is missed, advise to take dose as soon as possible and up to 12 hrs after the specified dose time. If vomiting occurs, advise not to repeat dose, but to take the next usual prescribed dose on schedule. Instruct to avoid star fruit, pomegranate/pomegranate juice, and grapefruit/grapefruit juice while on therapy. Advise to report to physician if any signs/symptoms of a heart problem develop while on therapy (eg, chest pain/discomfort, changes in heartbeat, palpitations). Inform about risk of thrombocytopenia; advise to contact physician right away if any signs of bleeding occur. Explain the need to perform laboratory tests prior to start of therapy and while on therapy. Inform about the risk of neutropenia and severe, life-threatening infections; instruct to contact physician immediately if fever and/or any sign of infection develops. Inform that drug may cause severe N/V and diarrhea that may require medication for treatment; advise to contact physician at the start of diarrhea, if persistent vomiting develops, or if any signs of dehydration develop. Instruct to consult w/ physician prior to using medications w/ laxative properties. Inform that drug may cause fetal harm. Advise women of reproductive potential to use effective contraception while taking therapy and for at least 1 month after the last dose of the drug. Counsel sexually active men to use condoms while receiving therapy and for at least 3 months following the last dose of the drug. Instruct not to breastfeed during therapy.

STORAGE: 20-25°C (68-77°F); excursions permitted between 15-30°C (59-86°F). Protect from light.

FELODIPINE ER – felodipine

RX

Class: Calcium channel blocker (CCB) (dihydropyridine)

OTHER BRAND NAMES

Plendil (Discontinued)

ADULT DOSAGE

Hypertension

Initial: 5mg qd
Titrate: May decrease to 2.5mg qd or increase to 10mg qd at intervals of not <2 weeks, depending on the patient's response
Range: 2.5-10mg qd

PEDIATRIC DOSAGE

Pediatric use may not have been established

DOSING CONSIDERATIONS

Hepatic Impairment
Initial: 2.5mg qd

Elderly
Initial: 2.5mg qd

ADMINISTRATION

Oral route

Take regularly either w/o food or w/ a light meal
Swallow whole; do not crush or chew

HOW SUPPLIED

Tab, Extended-Release: 2.5mg, 5mg, 10mg

CONTRAINDICATIONS

Hypersensitivity to this product.

WARNINGS/PRECAUTIONS

May occasionally precipitate significant hypotension and, rarely, syncope. May lead to reflex tachycardia, which may precipitate angina pectoris. Caution with heart failure (HF) or compromised ventricular function, particularly in combination with a β-blocker. Closely monitor BP during dose adjustment in patients with hepatic impairment and in elderly. Peripheral edema reported. Caution in elderly.

ADVERSE REACTIONS

Peripheral edema, headache, asthenia, dyspepsia, dizziness, upper respiratory infection, flushing.

DRUG INTERACTIONS

CYP3A4 inhibitors (eg, ketoconazole, erythromycin, grapefruit juice, cimetidine) may increase plasma levels by several-fold. Decreased levels with long-term anticonvulsant therapy (eg, phenytoin, carbamazepine, phenobarbital); consider alternative antihypertensive therapy. May increase metoprolol and tacrolimus levels; monitor tacrolimus blood concentration and adjust tacrolimus dose if needed.

PATIENT CONSIDERATIONS

Assessment: Assess for hypersensitivity to the drug, HF, compromised ventricular function, hepatic impairment, pregnancy/nursing status, and possible drug interactions.

Monitoring: Monitor for syncope, angina pectoris, peripheral edema, and other adverse reactions. Monitor BP.

Counseling: Inform that mild gingival hyperplasia (gum swelling) has been reported and that good dental hygiene decreases its incidence and severity.

STORAGE: 20-25°C (68-77°F). Protect from light.

FEMARA – letrozole

RX

Class: Nonsteroidal aromatase inhibitor

ADULT DOSAGE

Breast Cancer

Adjuvant Treatment of Postmenopausal Women w/ Hormone Receptor Positive Early Breast Cancer:
2.5mg qd; d/c at relapse

Extended Adjuvant Treatment of Early Breast Cancer in Postmenopausal Women,

PEDIATRIC DOSAGE

Pediatric use may not have been established

Who Have Received 5 Years of Adjuvant Tamoxifen Therapy:
2.5mg qd; d/c at tumor relapse

1st-Line Treatment of Postmenopausal Women w/ Hormone Receptor Positive or Unknown, Locally Advanced or Metastatic Breast Cancer; Treatment of Advanced Breast Cancer in Postmenopausal Women w/ Disease Progression Following Antiestrogen Therapy:
2.5mg qd; continue until tumor progression is evident

DOSING CONSIDERATIONS

Hepatic Impairment

Cirrhosis/Severe Hepatic Dysfunction: 2.5mg qod

ADMINISTRATION

Oral route

Take w/o regard to meals

HOW SUPPLIED

Tab: 2.5mg

CONTRAINDICATIONS

Women who are or may become pregnant.

WARNINGS/PRECAUTIONS

May decrease bone mineral density (BMD); consider monitoring BMD. Bone fractures and osteoporosis reported. Hypercholesterolemia reported; consider monitoring serum cholesterol levels. Reduce dose by 50% with cirrhosis and severe hepatic impairment. May impair physical/mental abilities. Moderate decreases in lymphocyte counts and thrombocytopenia reported.

ADVERSE REACTIONS

Hypercholesterolemia, hot flushes, fatigue, edema, arthralgia/arthritis, myalgia, headache, dizziness, night sweats, nausea, back pain, bone fractures, weight increase, depression, osteopenia.

DRUG INTERACTIONS

Reduced plasma levels with coadministered tamoxifen.

PATIENT CONSIDERATIONS

Assessment: Assess for premenopausal endocrine status, cirrhosis or hepatic impairment, pregnancy/nursing status, and possible drug interactions.

Monitoring: Monitor for bone fractures, osteoporosis, fatigue, dizziness, somnolence, and other adverse reactions. Monitor BMD and serum cholesterol levels.

Counseling: Inform that the drug is contraindicated in pregnant women and women of premenopausal endocrine status. Counsel perimenopausal and recently postmenopausal women to use contraception until postmenopausal status is fully established. Advise about possible fatigue, dizziness, and somnolence; caution against operating machinery/driving. Advise that BMD may be monitored while on therapy.

STORAGE: 25°C (77°F); excursions permitted to 15-30°C (59-86°F).

FERRALET 90 – docusate sodium/iron (carbonyl iron, ferrous gluconate)/vitamin B9 (folic acid)/vitamin B12 (cyanocobalamin)/vitamin C (ascorbic acid)

RX

Class: Iron/mineral/vitamin

Accidental overdose of iron-containing products is a leading cause of fatal poisoning in children <6 yrs; keep out of reach of children. In case of accidental overdose, call a physician or poison control center immediately.

ADULT DOSAGE

Anemia

Anemias responsive to oral iron therapy (eg, hypochromic anemia associated w/ pregnancy, chronic and/or acute blood loss, metabolic disease, postsurgical convalescence, dietary needs)

1 tab qd or ud

PEDIATRIC DOSAGE

Pediatric use may not have been established

DOSING CONSIDERATIONS

Elderly

Start at lower end of dosing range

ADMINISTRATION

Oral route

Do not chew tab
Take 2 hrs pc

HOW SUPPLIED

Tab: Iron 90mg-Folic Acid 1mg-Vitamin B12 12mcg-Vitamin C 120mg-Docusate 50mg

CONTRAINDICATIONS

Hypersensitivity to any of the ingredients; hemolytic anemia, hemochromatosis, and hemosiderosis.

WARNINGS/PRECAUTIONS

Folic acid alone is improper therapy in the treatment of pernicious anemia and other megaloblastic anemias where vitamin B12 is deficient. D/C use if symptoms of intolerance appear. Determine type of anemia and underlying causes before starting therapy. Determine Hgb, Hct, and reticulocyte counts before starting therapy and periodically thereafter during prolonged treatment. Periodically review therapy to determine if it needs to be continued without change or if a dose change is indicated. Contains FD&C Yellow No. 5 (tartrazine), which may cause allergic-type reactions (including bronchial asthma). Folic acid in doses >0.1mg/day may obscure pernicious anemia; hematologic remission may occur while neurological manifestations remain progressive. Exclude pernicious anemia before use. Caution in elderly.

ADVERSE REACTIONS

GI irritation, constipation, diarrhea, N/V, dark stools, allergic sensitization.

DRUG INTERACTIONS

Iron may interact with antacids, tetracyclines, or fluoroquinolones.

PATIENT CONSIDERATIONS

Assessment: Assess for hemolytic anemia, hemochromatosis, hemosiderosis, type of anemia, underlying causes of anemia, hypersensitivity to drug, nursing status, and possible drug interactions. Determine Hgb, Hct, and reticulocyte counts.

Monitoring: Monitor for symptoms of intolerance, allergic-type reactions, and masking of pernicious anemia. Determine Hgb, Hct, and reticulocyte counts periodically during prolonged therapy. Periodically review therapy to determine if it needs to be continued without change or if a dose change is indicated.

Counseling: Instruct to use qd or ud, and to d/c use and consult physician if symptoms of intolerance appear. Advise to keep drug out of reach of children, and to immediately call a doctor or poison control center in case of accidental overdose.

STORAGE: 25°C (77°F); excursions permitted to 15-30°C (59-86°F). Avoid moisture.

FETZIMA – levomilnacipran

RX

Class: Serotonin and norepinephrine reuptake inhibitor (SNRI)

Antidepressants increased the risk of suicidal thoughts and behavior in children, adolescents, and young adults in short-term studies. Monitor and observe closely for worsening, and for emergence of suicidal thoughts and behaviors. Not approved for use in pediatric patients.

ADULT DOSAGE

Major Depressive Disorder

Initial: 20mg qd for 2 days
Titrate: Increase to 40mg qd. Based on efficacy and tolerability, may then be increased in increments of 40mg at intervals of ≥2 days
Range: 40-120mg qd
Max: 120mg qd

Periodically reassess need for maint treatment and the appropriate dose

Dosing Considerations with MAOIs

Switching to/from an MAOI for Psychiatric Disorders:
Allow at least 14 days between discontinuation of an MAOI and initiation of treatment, and allow at least 7 days between discontinuation of treatment and initiation of an MAOI

PEDIATRIC DOSAGE

Pediatric use may not have been established

W/ Other MAOIs (eg, Linezolid, IV Methylene Blue):
Do not start levomilnacipran in patients being treated w/ linezolid or IV methylene blue
In patients already receiving levomilnacipran, if acceptable alternatives are not available and benefits outweigh risks, d/c levomilnacipran and administer linezolid or IV methylene blue; monitor for serotonin syndrome for 2 weeks or until 24 hrs after the last dose of linezolid or IV methylene blue, whichever comes 1st. May resume levomilnacipran therapy 24 hrs after the last dose of linezolid or IV methylene blue

F

DOSING CONSIDERATIONS

Concomitant Medications

Use w/ Strong CYP3A4 Inhibitors:
Max: 80mg qd

Renal Impairment

Moderate (CrCl 30-59mL/min):
Max Maint: 80mg qd

Severe (CrCl 15-29mL/min):
Max Maint: 40mg qd

ESRD: Not recommended

Discontinuation

Gradually reduce dose, whenever possible; if intolerable symptoms occur following a dose decrease or upon discontinuation of treatment, consider resuming previously prescribed dose and decreasing the dose at a more gradual rate

ADMINISTRATION

Oral route

Take at the same time each day, w/ or w/o food.
Swallow cap whole; do not open, chew, or crush.

HOW SUPPLIED

Cap, Extended-Release: 20mg, 40mg, 80mg, 120mg; (Titration Pack) 20mg [2^{s}], 40mg [26^{s}]

CONTRAINDICATIONS

Hypersensitivity to levomilnacipran, milnacipran HCl, or to any excipient in the formulation. Use of MAOIs intended to treat psychiatric disorders w/ levomilnacipran or w/in 7 days of stopping treatment w/ levomilnacipran. Use of levomilnacipran w/in 14 days of stopping an MAOI intended to treat psychiatric disorders. Starting levomilnacipran in a patient who is being treated w/ MAOIs (eg, linezolid or IV methylene blue).

WARNINGS/PRECAUTIONS

Not recommended for patients with end-stage renal disease. Not approved for the treatment of bipolar depression. Serotonin syndrome reported; d/c immediately if symptoms occur and initiate supportive symptomatic treatment. Associated with increases in BP and HR; control preexisting HTN or treat preexisting tachyarrhythmias and other cardiac disease before initiating treatment. Caution with preexisting HTN, cardiovascular (CV) or cerebrovascular conditions that might be compromised by increases in BP. Consider discontinuation or other appropriate medical intervention if sustained increase in BP or HR occurs. May increase risk of bleeding events. Pupillary dilation that occurs following therapy may trigger an angle-closure attack in a patient with anatomically narrow angles who does not have a patent iridectomy. May affect urethral resistance; caution in patients prone to obstructive urinary disorders. If symptoms of urinary hesitation, urinary retention, or dysuria develop, consider discontinuation or other appropriate medical intervention. Activation of mania/hypomania reported; caution with history or family history of bipolar disorder, mania, or hypomania. Seizures reported; caution in patients with a seizure disorder. Discontinuation symptoms may occur. Avoid abrupt discontinuation; reduce dose gradually whenever possible. Hyponatremia may occur; elderly and volume-depleted patients may be at greater risk. D/C in patients with symptomatic hyponatremia and institute appropriate medical intervention.

ADVERSE REACTIONS

N/V, constipation, hyperhidrosis, HR/BP increased, erectile dysfunction, tachycardia, palpitations, testicular pain, ejaculation disorder, urinary hesitation, hot flush, hypotension, HTN, decreased appetite.

DRUG INTERACTIONS

See Contraindications and Dosage. May cause serotonin syndrome with other serotonergic drugs (eg, triptans, TCAs, fentanyl, lithium, St. John's wort) and with drugs that impair metabolism of serotonin; d/c immediately if serotonin syndrome occurs. Caution with NSAIDs, aspirin (ASA), warfarin, and other drugs that affect coagulation or bleeding due to potential increased risk of bleeding. Increased exposure with CYP3A4 inhibitor ketoconazole. Caution with other CNS-active drugs, including those with a similar mechanism of action. Do not give with alcohol; pronounced accelerated drug release may occur. Caution with drugs that increase BP and HR. Increased risk of hyponatremia with diuretics.

PATIENT CONSIDERATIONS

Assessment: Assess for risk for bipolar disorder, HTN, CV/cerebrovascular conditions, tachyarrhythmias, susceptibility to angle-closure glaucoma/obstructive urinary disorders, history of mania/hypomania, seizure disorder, volume depletion, hypersensitivity to the drug, renal impairment, pregnancy/nursing status, and possible drug interactions.

Monitoring: Monitor for signs/symptoms of clinical worsening, suicidality, unusual changes in behavior, serotonin syndrome, bleeding events, angle-closure glaucoma, urinary hesitation/ retention, dysuria, activation of mania/hypomania, seizures, discontinuation symptoms, hyponatremia, and other adverse reactions. Monitor BP and HR periodically. Periodically reassess the need for maintenance treatment and the appropriate dose.

Counseling: Advise about the benefits and risks of therapy and counsel on its appropriate use. Counsel to look for the emergence of suicidality, especially early during treatment and when the dose is adjusted up or down. Caution about the risk of serotonin syndrome, particularly with the concomitant use with other serotonergic agents. Inform that concomitant use with ASA, NSAIDs, warfarin, or other drugs that affect coagulation may increase the risk of abnormal bleeding. Inform that drug can cause mild pupillary dilation, which in susceptible individuals, can lead to an episode of angle-closure glaucoma. Advise to have BP and HR monitored regularly, to observe for signs of activation of mania/hypomania, to avoid alcohol consumption, and not to d/c therapy without notifying physician. Caution against operating hazardous machinery until reasonably certain that therapy does not adversely affect ability to engage in such activities. Advise to notify physician if allergic reactions develop, if pregnant/intending to become pregnant, or if breastfeeding.

STORAGE: 25°C (77°F); excursions permitted between 15-30°C (59-86°F).

FINACEA FOAM – azelaic acid

RX

Class: Dicarboxylic acid antimicrobial

ADULT DOSAGE

Rosacea

Inflammatory Papules/Pustules of Mild to Moderate Rosacea:

Apply a thin layer to the entire facial area (cheeks, chin, forehead, and nose) bid (am and pm)

Use continuously over 12 weeks; reassess if no improvement is observed upon completing 12 weeks of therapy

PEDIATRIC DOSAGE

Pediatric use may not have been established

ADMINISTRATION

Topical route

Shake well before use.

Cosmetics may be applied after the application of foam has dried.

Avoid the use of occlusive dressings or wrappings.

HOW SUPPLIED

Foam: 15% [50g]

WARNINGS/PRECAUTIONS

Hypopigmentation reported; monitor patients w/ dark complexion for early signs of hypopigmentation. Irritation of the eyes reported; avoid contact w/ the eyes, mouth, and other mucous membranes. Propellant in foam is flammable; avoid fire, flame, and smoking during and immediately following application. Caution in elderly.

ADVERSE REACTIONS

Application-site pain.

PATIENT CONSIDERATIONS

Assessment: Assess hypersensitivity to drug and pregnancy/nursing status.

Monitoring: Monitor for skin reactions; eyes, mouth, and other mucous membranes irritation; and for other adverse reactions. Monitor for early signs of hypopigmentation in patients w/ dark complexion. Monitor response to therapy; reassess if no improvement is observed upon completing 12 weeks of therapy.

Counseling: Advise to cleanse affected area(s) w/ a very mild soap or a soapless cleansing lotion and pat dry w/ a soft towel. Instruct to avoid use of alcoholic cleansers, tinctures and astringents, abrasives, and peeling agents. Instruct to avoid contact w/ the eyes, mouth, and other mucous membranes explaining that if contact w/ the eyes occurs, patient should wash eyes w/ large amounts of water and consult physician if eye irritation persists. Instruct to d/c use and consult physician if an allergic reaction occurs. Advise to wash hands immediately following application of the foam. Inform that cosmetics may be applied after the application of foam has dried. Advise to avoid the use of occlusive dressings and wrappings. Instruct to avoid any triggers that may provoke erythema, flushing, and blushing (eg, spicy and thermally hot food and drinks, alcoholic beverages). Inform that the propellant in the foam is flammable; instruct to avoid fire, flame, or smoking during and immediately following application. Instruct to discard the product 8 weeks after opening.

STORAGE: 25°C (77°F); excursions permitted between 15-30°C (59-86°F). Product is flammable; avoid fire, flame, or smoking during and immediately following application. Do not puncture or incinerate drug container, expose to heat, or store at temperatures >49°C (120°F).

FIORINAL – aspirin/butalbital/caffeine CIII

Class: Analgesic/barbiturate

ADULT DOSAGE

Tension Headache

1-2 caps q4h

Max: 6 caps/day

PEDIATRIC DOSAGE

Pediatric use may not have been established

ADMINISTRATION

Oral route

HOW SUPPLIED

Cap: (Butalbital/Aspirin [ASA]/Caffeine) 50mg/325mg/40mg

CONTRAINDICATIONS

Hypersensitivity or intolerance to ASA, caffeine, or butalbital; hemorrhagic diathesis (eg, hemophilia, hypoprothrombinemia, von Willebrand's disease, the thrombocytopenias, thrombasthenia and other ill-defined hereditary platelet dysfunctions, severe vitamin K deficiency and severe liver damage); syndrome of nasal polyps, angioedema, and bronchospastic reactivity to ASA or other NSAIDs; peptic ulcer or other serious GI lesions; porphyria.

WARNINGS/PRECAUTIONS

Not for extended and repeated use. May be habit-forming. Caution in elderly, debilitated, with severe renal/hepatic impairment, hypothyroidism, urethral stricture, head injuries, elevated intracranial pressure, acute abdominal conditions, Addison's disease, prostatic hypertrophy, presence of peptic ulcer, and coagulation disorders. Therapeutic doses of ASA can lead to anaphylactic shock and severe allergic reactions. Significant bleeding possible with peptic ulcers, GI lesions, or bleeding disorders. Caution in children, including teenagers, with chickenpox or flu. Preoperative ASA may prolong bleeding time.

ADVERSE REACTIONS

Drowsiness, lightheadedness, dizziness, N/V, flatulence.

DRUG INTERACTIONS

Caution with anticoagulant therapy; may enhance bleeding. CNS effects enhanced by MAOIs. Additive CNS depression with alcohol, other narcotic analgesics, general anesthetics, tranquilizers (eg, chlordiazepoxide), sedatives/hypnotics, other CNS depressants. May cause hypoglycemia with oral antidiabetic agents and insulin. May cause bone marrow toxicity and blood dyscrasias with 6-mercaptopurine and methotrexate. Increased risk of peptic ulceration and bleeding with NSAIDs. Decreased effects of uricosuric agents (eg, probenecid, sulfinpyrazone). Withdrawal of corticosteroids may cause salicylism with chronic ASA use.

PATIENT CONSIDERATIONS

Assessment: Assess for previous hypersensitivity to drug, renal/hepatic function, porphyria, peptic ulcer, other serious GI lesions, bleeding disorders, or any other conditions where treatment is cautioned or contraindicated. Assess for pregnancy/nursing status and possible drug interactions.

Monitoring: Serial monitoring of LFTs and/or renal function with severe hepatic/renal disease. Monitor for anaphylactoid/hypersensitivity reactions, drug abuse/dependence and bleeding.

Counseling: Advise not to take if patient has ASA allergy. Instruct to take exactly as prescribed; instruct to avoid coadministration with alcohol or other CNS depressants. Advise to avoid hazardous tasks (eg, operating machinery/driving) while on therapy. Counsel that drug may be habit-forming.

STORAGE: Below 25°C (77°F); tight container. Protect from moisture.

FLAGYL — metronidazole

RX

Class: Nitroimidazole

Shown to be carcinogenic in mice and rats. Avoid unnecessary use. Should be reserved for the conditions for which it is indicated.

F

ADULT DOSAGE

Anaerobic Bacterial Infections

IV metronidazole is usually administered initially in the treatment of most serious infections

Cap/Tab:

Usual: 7.5mg/kg q6h

Max: 4g/24 hrs

Duration: 7-10 days; bone and joint, lower respiratory tract, and endocardium infections may require longer treatment

Trichomoniasis

Female:

7-Day Course of Treatment:

Cap: 375mg bid for 7 consecutive days

Tab: 250mg tid for 7 consecutive days

1-Day Treatment:

Tab: 2g given as a single dose or in 2 divided doses of 1g each, given in the same day

When repeat courses are required, allow an interval of 4-6 weeks between courses, and reconfirm presence of the trichomonad

Male:

Individualize treatment as it is for the female

Amebiasis

Acute Intestinal Amebiasis (Acute Amebic Dysentery):

Cap/Tab:

750mg tid for 5-10 days

Amebic Liver Abscess:

Cap:

750mg tid for 5-10 days

Tab:

500mg or 750mg tid for 5-10 days

PEDIATRIC DOSAGE

Amebiasis

Cap/Tab:

35-50mg/kg/24 hrs, divided into 3 doses, for 10 days

DOSING CONSIDERATIONS

Renal Impairment

Hemodialysis: If administration cannot be separated from hemodialysis session, consider supplementation of metronidazole dosage following hemodialysis session

Hepatic Impairment

Severe (Child-Pugh C):

Cap:

Amebiasis: 375mg q8h for 5-10 days

Trichomoniasis: 375mg q24h for 7 days

Tab:

Reduce dosage by 50%

ADMINISTRATION

Oral route

HOW SUPPLIED

Cap: 375mg; **Tab:** 250mg, 500mg

CONTRAINDICATIONS

Prior history of hypersensitivity to metronidazole or other nitroimidazole derivatives. Disulfiram use w/in the last 2 weeks. Consumption of alcohol or products containing propylene glycol during and for at least 3 days after therapy w/ metronidazole. Use during the 1st trimester of pregnancy in trichomoniasis patients.

WARNINGS/PRECAUTIONS

Cases of encephalopathy and peripheral neuropathy (including optic neuropathy), convulsive seizures, and aseptic meningitis reported; promptly evaluate benefit/risk ratio of the continuation of therapy if abnormal neurologic signs/symptoms appear. Known or previously unrecognized candidiasis may present more prominent symptoms during therapy and requires treatment w/ a candidacidal agent. Caution w/ hepatic/renal impairment, evidence of or history of blood dyscrasia, and in the elderly. Mild leukopenia reported; monitor total and differential leukocyte counts before and after therapy. May result in bacterial/parasitic resistance if used in the absence of proven or suspected bacterial/parasitic infection, or a prophylactic indication. Lab test interactions may occur. **Tab:** In pregnant patients for whom alternative treatment has been inadequate, the 1-day course of therapy should not be used for trichomoniasis.

ADVERSE REACTIONS

Headache, syncope, dizziness, vertigo, incoordination, nausea, diarrhea, epigastric distress, abdominal cramping, constipation, unpleasant metallic taste, erythematous rash, pruritus, urticaria, dysuria.

DRUG INTERACTIONS

See Contraindications. May potentiate anticoagulant effect of warfarin and other oral coumarin anticoagulants, resulting in PT prolongation; carefully monitor PT and INR. May increase serum lithium, and may cause lithium toxicity; obtain serum lithium and serum creatinine levels several days after beginning metronidazole. May increase busulfan levels, which may increase risk for serious busulfan toxicity; avoid concomitant use, or, if coadministration is medically needed, frequently monitor busulfan concentration and adjust busulfan dose accordingly. Simultaneous administration of drugs that decrease microsomal liver enzyme activity (eg, cimetidine) may prolong $T_{1/2}$ and decrease clearance. Simultaneous administration of drugs that induce microsomal liver enzymes (eg, phenytoin, phenobarbital) may accelerate elimination, resulting in reduced levels. Impaired clearance of phenytoin reported.

PATIENT CONSIDERATIONS

Assessment: Assess for candidiasis, alcohol use, hepatic/renal impairment, evidence/history of blood dyscrasia, hypersensitivity to drug or other nitroimidazole derivatives, pregnancy/nursing status, and possible drug interactions. Obtain total and differential leukocyte counts.

Monitoring: Monitor for abnormal neurologic signs/symptoms, candidiasis, and other adverse reactions. Monitor total and differential leukocyte counts after therapy. Monitor PT and INR w/ oral coumarin anticoagulants (eg, warfarin).

Counseling: Instruct to d/c consumption of alcoholic beverages or products containing propylene glycol while taking the drug and for at least 3 days afterward. Inform that therapy should only be used to treat bacterial and parasitic, not viral, infections. Instruct to take exactly ud. Inform that skipping doses or not completing the full course of therapy may decrease effectiveness of treatment and increase bacterial resistance.

STORAGE: Cap: 15-25°C (59-77°F). **Tab:** <25°C (77°F). Protect from light.

FLECAINIDE – flecainide acetate

RX

Class: Class IC antiarrhythmic

Excessive mortality or nonfatal cardiac arrest rate reported in patients with asymptomatic non-life-threatening ventricular arrhythmias who had MI >6 days but <2 yrs previously. It is prudent to consider the risks of Class IC agents, coupled with the lack of any evidence of improved survival, generally unacceptable in patients without life-threatening ventricular arrhythmias, even if patients are experiencing unpleasant, but not life-threatening, symptoms or signs. Ventricular tachycardia (VT) reported in patients treated for paroxysmal atrial fibrillation/flutter (PAF). Use not recommended in patients with chronic A-fib. Case reports of ventricular proarrhythmic effects in patients treated for A-fib/atrial flutter (A-flutter) have included increased premature ventricular contractions (PVCs), VT, ventricular fibrillation (VF), and death. Patients treated for A-flutter have been reported with 1:1 atrioventricular (AV) conduction due to slowing the atrial rate. A paradoxical increase in ventricular rate also may occur in patients with A-fib. Concomitant negative chronotropic therapy (eg, digoxin, β-blockers) may lower the risk of this complication.

F

OTHER BRAND NAMES

Tambocor (Discontinued)

ADULT DOSAGE

Paroxysmal Supraventricular Tachycardia

Prevention of paroxysmal supraventricular tachycardias, including atrioventricular nodal reentrant tachycardia, atrioventricular reentrant tachycardia, and other supraventricular tachycardias of unspecified mechanism associated w/ disabling symptoms in patients w/o structural heart disease
Initial: 50mg q12h
Titrate: May increase in increments of 50mg bid every 4 days until efficacy is achieved
Max: 300mg/day
Inadequately Controlled: May dose at 8h intervals

Paroxysmal Atrial Fibrillation/Flutter

Prevention of paroxysmal atrial fibrillation/ flutter associated w/ disabling symptoms in patients w/o structural heart disease
Initial: 50mg q12h
Titrate: May increase in increments of 50mg bid every 4 days until efficacy is achieved
Inadequately Controlled: May dose at 8h intervals

May achieve substantial increase in efficacy w/o a substantial increase in discontinuations for adverse experiences by increasing the dose from 50-100mg bid

Ventricular Arrhythmias

Prevention of documented ventricular arrhythmias (life-threatening)
Sustained Ventricular Tachycardia:
Initial: 100mg q12h
Titrate: May increase in increments of 50mg bid every 4 days until efficacy is achieved
Max: 400mg/day

PEDIATRIC DOSAGE

Arrhythmias

<6 Months of Age:
Initial: 50mg/m^2/day divided into 2 or 3 equally spaced doses
>6 Months of Age:
Initial: 100mg/m^2/day divided into 2 or 3 equally spaced doses
Max: 200mg/m^2/day

DOSING CONSIDERATIONS

Concomitant Medications
Amiodarone: Reduce dose by 50%

Renal Impairment
Less Severe Renal Disease:
Initial: 100mg q12h
Severe (CrCl ≤35mL/min):
Initial: 100mg qd or 50mg bid

Other Important Considerations
Transferring from Another Antiarrhythmic: Allow at least 2-4 plasma half-lives to elapse for the drug being discontinued before starting therapy

Inadequately Controlled Patients: May dose at 8h intervals. Once adequate control is achieved, may be possible to reduce the dose as necessary in some patients. Evaluate efficacy at lower dose in these patients

ADMINISTRATION

Oral route

Initiate therapy in-hospital w/ rhythm monitoring for patients w/ sustained ventricular tachycardia

HOW SUPPLIED

Tab: 50mg, 100mg*, 150mg* *scored

CONTRAINDICATIONS

Pre-existing 2nd- or 3rd-degree AV block, or right bundle branch block when associated w/ a left hemiblock (bifascicular block), unless a pacemaker is present to sustain the cardiac rhythm should complete heart block occur; presence of cardiogenic shock; known hypersensitivity to the drug.

WARNINGS/PRECAUTIONS

May cause new or worsened supraventricular or ventricular arrhythmias. May cause or worsen CHF; caution with history of CHF or myocardial dysfunction. Close attention must be given to maintenance of cardiac function. Slows cardiac conduction, producing dose-related increases in PR, QRS, and QT intervals; may consider dose reduction. Rare cases of torsades de pointes-type arrhythmia reported. Conduction changes (eg, sinus pause, sinus arrest, symptomatic bradycardia, 2nd- or 3rd-degree AV block) reported; manage on the lowest effective dose. D/C therapy if 2nd- or 3rd-degree AV block, or right bundle branch block associated with a left hemiblock occurs, unless a temporary or implanted ventricular pacemaker is in place to ensure an adequate ventricular rate. Extreme caution with sick sinus syndrome. May increase endocardial pacing thresholds and suppress ventricular escape rhythms; caution in patients with permanent pacemakers or temporary pacing electrodes. Should not be administered with existing poor thresholds or nonprogrammable pacemakers unless suitable pacing rescue is available. Hypokalemia/hyperkalemia may alter effects. Should not be used in hepatic impairment unless benefits clearly outweigh the risks; if used, caution in dosage increases. Start therapy of patients with sustained VT and pediatric patients in the hospital with rhythm monitoring.

F

ADVERSE REACTIONS

Cardiac arrest, increased PVCs, VT, VF, arrhythmias, CHF, dizziness, visual disturbances, headache, fatigue, nausea, palpitation, dyspnea, chest pain, asthenia.

DRUG INTERACTIONS

Coadministration may increase digoxin levels. Additive negative inotropic effects with β-blockers (eg, propranolol). Concomitant enzyme inducers (phenytoin, phenobarbital, carbamazepine) may increase the rate of elimination. Cimetidine may increase levels and $T_{1/2}$. CYP2D6 inhibitors (eg, quinidine) may increase levels in patients that are on chronic flecainide therapy, especially if they are extensive metabolizers. Amiodarone may increase levels, if flecainide dosage is not reduced. Avoid with disopyramide, verapamil, nifedipine, or diltiazem. Milk may inhibit absorption in infants; consider a reduction in flecainide dosage when milk is removed from diet of infants.

PATIENT CONSIDERATIONS

Assessment: Assess for preexisting 2nd- or 3rd-degree AV block, right bundle branch block associated with a left hemiblock, implanted pacemaker, asymptomatic non-life-threatening ventricular arrhythmia, A-fib/A-flutter, cardiogenic shock, MI, cardiomyopathy, preexisting CHF or low ejection fractions (<30%), sick sinus syndrome, hypersensitivity, pregnancy/nursing status, renal/hepatic impairment, and possible drug interactions. Correct preexisting hypokalemia or hyperkalemia prior to therapy. Determine pacing threshold in patients with pacemaker.

Monitoring: Monitor for paradoxical increase in ventricular rate, new or worsened supraventricular/ventricular arrhythmias, worsening of CHF, effects on cardiac conduction, bradycardia, hypersensitivity reactions, and other adverse reactions. Monitor for plasma trough levels and ECGs either after initiation or change in dose, whether the dose was increased for lack of effectiveness, or increased growth of pediatric patient. Periodically monitor plasma levels with renal/hepatic impairment, CHF, and/or if on concurrent amiodarone therapy. Determine pacing threshold in patients with pacemakers after 1 week and at regular intervals thereafter.

Counseling: Inform about risks/benefits of therapy and instruct to report any adverse reactions to physician.

STORAGE: 20-25°C (68-77°F).

FLECTOR – diclofenac epolamine

RX

Class: NSAID

NSAIDs may cause an increased risk of serious cardiovascular (CV) thrombotic events, MI, stroke, and serious GI adverse events including bleeding, ulceration, and perforation of the stomach or intestines that can be fatal. Patients with CV disease (CVD) or risk factors for CVD may be at greater risk. Elderly patients are at a greater risk for GI events. Contraindicated in the perioperative setting of coronary artery bypass graft (CABG) surgery.

ADULT DOSAGE

Acute Pain

Due to Minor Strains, Sprains, and Contusions:
Apply 1 patch to most painful area bid

PEDIATRIC DOSAGE

Pediatric use may not have been established

ADMINISTRATION

Transdermal route

HOW SUPPLIED

Patch: 180mg (1.3%) [5[s]]

CONTRAINDICATIONS
History of asthma, urticaria, or allergic-type reactions after taking aspirin (ASA) or other NSAIDs. Treatment of perioperative pain in the setting of CABG surgery. Use on non-intact or damaged skin. Known hypersensitivity to diclofenac.

WARNINGS/PRECAUTIONS
Use lowest effective dose for shortest duration possible. Extreme caution with history of ulcer disease/GI bleeding. Cases of severe hepatic reactions reported. May cause elevations of LFTs; d/c if abnormal LFTs persist or worsen, liver disease develops, or systemic manifestations occur. May lead to new onset or worsening of preexisting HTN; monitor BP closely. Fluid retention and edema reported; caution with fluid retention/heart failure (HF). Caution when initiating treatment in patients with considerable dehydration. Renal papillary necrosis and other renal injury reported after long-term use; increased risk with renal/hepatic impairment, HF, and elderly. Not recommended for use with advanced renal disease; if therapy must be initiated, monitor renal function. Anaphylactic reactions may occur; avoid in patients with aspirin (ASA) triad. May cause serious skin adverse events (eg, exfoliative dermatitis, Stevens-Johnson syndrome [SJS], toxic epidermal necrolysis [TEN]); d/c at 1st appearance of skin rash or any other signs of hypersensitivity. Avoid starting at 30 weeks gestation; may cause premature closure of ductus arteriosus. Cannot replace corticosteroids or treat corticosteroid insufficiency. May diminish the utility of diagnostic signs in detecting complications of presumed noninfectious, painful conditions. Anemia may occur; monitor Hgb/Hct if signs/symptoms of anemia develop with long-term use. May inhibit platelet aggregation and prolong bleeding time; monitor patients with coagulation disorders. Caution with preexisting asthma and avoid with ASA-sensitive asthma. Avoid contact with eyes and mucosa. D/C if abnormal renal tests persist or worsen. Caution in elderly and debilitated patients.

ADVERSE REACTIONS
CV thrombotic events, MI, stroke, GI adverse events, application-site reactions (eg, pruritus, dermatitis), headache, paresthesia, somnolence.

DRUG INTERACTIONS
Increased adverse effects with ASA; avoid use. May result in higher rate of hemorrhage, more frequent abnormal creatinine, urea, and Hgb with oral NSAIDs; avoid combination unless benefit outweighs risk. May diminish antihypertensive effect of ACE inhibitors. Patients taking thiazides or loop diuretics may have impaired response to these therapies. Increased risk of renal toxicity with diuretics and ACE inhibitors. May reduce natriuretic effect of furosemide and thiazides; monitor for signs of renal failure and diuretic efficacy. May increase lithium levels; monitor for toxicity. May enhance methotrexate toxicity and cyclosporine nephrotoxicity; caution with coadministration. Increased risk of GI bleeding with oral corticosteroids, anticoagulants (eg, warfarin), smoking, and alcohol. Synergistic effects on GI bleeding with anticoagulants (eg, warfarin). Caution with drugs known to be potentially hepatotoxic (eg, acetaminophen [APAP], certain antibiotics, antiepileptics).

PATIENT CONSIDERATIONS

Assessment: Assess for history of asthma, urticaria, or allergic-type reactions with ASA or other NSAIDs, ASA triad, CVD, risk factors for CVD, HTN, fluid retention, HF, history of ulcer disease, history of/risk factors for GI bleeding, general health status, history of renal/hepatic impairment, coagulation disorders, dehydration, tobacco/alcohol use, pregnancy/nursing status, and for possible drug interactions. Assess that skin at application site is intact and not damaged. Obtain baseline CBC and BP.

Monitoring: Monitor BP, CBC, LFTs, renal function, and chemistry profile periodically. Monitor for GI bleeding/ulceration/perforation, CV thrombotic events, MI, stroke, HTN, fluid retention, edema, skin/allergic reactions, and other adverse reactions.

Counseling: Instruct only to use on intact skin. Advise to wash hands after applying, handling, or removing the patch. Instruct not to wear patch during bathing or showering. Instruct to avoid contact with eyes and mucosa; advise that if eye contact occurs, to wash out the eye with water or saline immediately and consult physician if irritation persists for >1 hr. Counsel to seek medical attention if symptoms of hepatotoxicity, anaphylactic reactions, skin and hypersensitivity reactions, CV events, GI ulceration and bleeding, bronchospasm, weight gain, or edema occurs. Inform of pregnancy risks. Instruct to tape down edges of patch if it begins to peel-off; if problems with adhesion persist, recommend to overlay the patch with a mesh netting sleeve. Advise to avoid coadministration with unprescribed APAP.

STORAGE: 25°C (77°F); excursions permitted to 15-30°C (59-86°F). Keep sealed at all times when not in use.

FLO-PRED – prednisolone acetate

RX

Class: Glucocorticoid

ADULT DOSAGE

Steroid-Responsive Disorders

Initial: 5-60mg/day depending on disease and response

Maintain or adjust dose until response is satisfactory. If no satisfactory clinical response after a reasonable period, D/C and transfer to appropriate therapy

Maint: Decrease dose by small amounts to lowest effective dose at appropriate time intervals

May need to increase dose for a period of time in stressful situations

D/C if period of spontaneous remission occurs in a chronic condition

Multiple Sclerosis

Acute Exacerbations:

Usual: 200mg qd for 1 week, followed by 80mg qod for 1 month

PEDIATRIC DOSAGE

Steroid-Responsive Disorders

Initial: 0.14-2mg/kg/day in 3 or 4 divided doses (4-60mg/m^2/day) depending on disease and response

Nephrotic Syndrome

>2 Years:

Usual: 60mg/m^2/day in 3 divided doses for 4 weeks, followed by 4 weeks of single-dose alternate-day therapy at 40mg/m^2/day

Asthma

Uncontrolled by Inhaled Corticosteroids and Long-Acting Bronchodilators:

Usual: 1-2mg/kg/day in single or divided doses; continue short course ("burst" therapy) until peak expiratory flow rate of 80% of personal best is achieved or symptoms resolve (usually 3-10 days)

DOSING CONSIDERATIONS

Elderly

Start at low end of dosing range

Discontinuation

Withdraw gradually after long-term therapy

ADMINISTRATION

Oral route

May take w/ food to avoid GI irritation

HOW SUPPLIED

Sus: 15mg/5mL [37mL, 52mL, 65mL]

CONTRAINDICATIONS

Hypersensitivity to corticosteroids (eg, prednisolone), or any components of this product.

WARNINGS/PRECAUTIONS

May cause hypothalamic-pituitary-adrenal (HPA) axis suppression, Cushing's syndrome, and hyperglycemia; monitor patients and taper doses gradually. May cause reversible HPA axis suppression with potential for glucocorticosteroid insufficiency after withdrawal. May impair mineralocorticoid secretion; administer salt and/or mineralocorticoid concurrently. Changes in thyroid status may necessitate dose adjustment; clearance may be decreased in hypothyroidism and increased in hyperthyroidism. May mask/exacerbate infections, reduce resistance to new infections, increase risk of disseminated infection, increase risk of reactivation/exacerbation of latent infection. Avoid exposure to chickenpox and measles. Caution in patients with known or suspected *Strongyloides* infestation, active/latent tuberculosis or tuberculin reactivity, active/latent peptic ulcers, diverticulitis, and fresh intestinal anastomoses. Avoid with systemic fungal infections unless needed to control drug reactions. Rule out latent/active amebiasis before initiating therapy. Not for use in cerebral malaria and active ocular herpes simplex. May cause BP elevation, salt/water retention, and increase excretion of K^+ and calcium; caution with HTN, congestive heart failure (CHF), or renal insufficiency. May cause left ventricular free wall rupture after recent myocardial infarction; use caution. May increase risk of GI perforation with certain GI disorders. May be associated with CNS effects (eg, euphoria, insomnia, mood swings, personality changes, severe depression, frank psychotic manifestations). Emotional instability or psychotic tendency aggravation may occur. May inhibit bone growth in pediatrics and adolescents and cause osteoporosis at any age. Caution in patients at risk for osteoporosis. May produce posterior subcapsular cataracts, glaucoma with possible optic nerve damage, and enhance establishment of secondary ocular infections. Not recommended in optic neuritis treatment. May elevate intraocular pressure (IOP); monitor IOP if used for >6 weeks. May have negative effect on growth and development in children; monitor growth and development with prolonged therapy. May cause fetal harm. Acute myopathy reported with use of high doses. Creatine kinase elevation may occur. Kaposi's sarcoma reported. May suppress reaction to skin tests.

ADVERSE REACTIONS

Fluid retention, alteration in glucose tolerance, elevation in BP, behavioral and mood changes, increased appetite, weight gain.

DRUG INTERACTIONS

May lead to a loss of corticosteroid-induced adrenal suppression with aminoglutethimide. May develop hypokalemia with K^+-depleting agents (eg, amphotericin B, diuretics). Cases of cardiac enlargement and CHF with amphotericin B reported. Anticholinesterase agents may produce severe weakness in patients with myasthenia gravis; d/c anticholinesterase agents at least 24 hours before start of therapy. May inhibit response to warfarin; frequently monitor coagulation indices. May require dose adjustments of antidiabetic agents. May decrease isoniazid levels. Cholestyramine may increase clearance. Convulsions and increased activity of both drugs reported with cyclosporine. May increase risk of arrhythmias with digitalis glycosides. Estrogens, including oral contraceptives, may decrease hepatic metabolism and enhance effect. May enhance metabolism and require dosage increase with CYP3A4 inducers (eg, barbiturates, phenytoin, carbamazepine, rifampin). May decrease metabolism and increase risk of corticosteroid side effects with CYP3A4 inhibitors (eg, ketoconazole). May increase risk of GI side effects with aspirin (ASA) or other NSAIDs. Caution with ASA in patients with hypoprothrombinemia. May increase clearance of salicylates. Live or live, attenuated vaccines is contraindicated in patients receiving immunosuppressive doses. Killed or inactivated vaccines may be administered, although response is unpredictable. May diminish response to toxoids and live or inactivated vaccines. May potentiate replication of some organisms contained in live attenuated vaccines. Acute myopathy reported with neuromuscular blocking drugs (eg, pancuronium).

PATIENT CONSIDERATIONS

Assessment: Assess for vaccination history, current infections, systemic fungal infections, thyroid status, latent/active amebiasis, cerebral malaria, active ocular herpes simplex, emotional instability or psychotic tendencies, any condition where treatment is cautioned, pregnancy/nursing status, and possible drug interactions.

Monitoring: Monitor for salt/water retention, infections/secondary ocular infections, changes in thyroid status, posterior subcapsular cataracts, glaucoma, optic nerve damage, Kaposi's sarcoma, development of osteoporosis, acute myopathy, creatine kinase elevation, and emotional instability or psychotic tendencies aggravation. Monitor IOP, BP, body weight, routine laboratory studies, including two-hour postprandial blood glucose and serum K^+, chest x-ray, bone density, and bone growth and development in pediatrics. Obtain upper GI x-rays with known/suspected peptic ulcer disease.

Counseling: Advise not to d/c abruptly or without medical supervision, to inform any medical attendants about therapy, and to seek medical advice at once if fever or other signs of infection develop. Instruct to notify physician if had recent or ongoing infection or have recently received a vaccine. Counsel to avoid exposure to chickenpox or measles; instruct to immediately report if exposed. Inform of possibility of developing fluid retention, alteration in glucose tolerance, elevation in BP, behavioral and mood changes, increased appetite and weight gain. Advise that if a dose is missed, to take it as soon as remember, if it is almost time for next dose, skip the missed dose and take it at the next regular scheduled time, and not to take an extra dose to make up for the missed dose. Advise to take with food. Instruct to notify physician if using other Rx/OTC medications, dietary supplements, or herbal products.

STORAGE: 20-25°C (68-77°F). Do not refrigerate.

FLOMAX – tamsulosin hydrochloride

RX

Class: $Alpha_1$ antagonist

ADULT DOSAGE

Benign Prostatic Hyperplasia

0.4mg qd 30 min after the same meal each day

Titrate: May increase to 0.8mg qd after 2-4 weeks if response is inadequate

If therapy is discontinued or interrupted for several days at either the 0.4mg or 0.8mg dose, restart w/ 0.4mg qd

PEDIATRIC DOSAGE

Pediatric use may not have been established

DOSING CONSIDERATIONS

Concomitant Medications

Do not combine w/ strong CYP3A4 (eg, ketoconazole)

ADMINISTRATION
Oral route

Do not crush, chew, or open cap.

HOW SUPPLIED
Cap: 0.4mg

CONTRAINDICATIONS
Hypersensitivity to tamsulosin HCl or any component of this product.

WARNINGS/PRECAUTIONS
Orthostasis/syncope may occur; caution to avoid situations in which injury could result should syncope occur. May cause priapism. Prostate cancer and BPH frequently coexist; screen patients for the presence of prostate cancer prior to treatment and at regular intervals afterwards. Intraoperative floppy iris syndrome (IFIS) observed during cataract and glaucoma surgery; initiation of therapy in patients who are scheduled for cataract or glaucoma surgery is not recommended. Allergic reaction reported (rare) in patients w/ sulfa allergy. Caution in patients known to be CYP2D6 poor metabolizers particularly at a dose >0.4mg.

ADVERSE REACTIONS
Headache, dizziness, rhinitis, infection, abnormal ejaculation, asthenia, back pain, diarrhea, pharyngitis, chest pain, cough increased, somnolence, insomnia, sinusitis, nausea.

DRUG INTERACTIONS
See Dosing Considerations. Ketoconazole (a strong CYP3A4 inhibitor) and paroxetine (a strong CYP2D6 inhibitor) increased levels. Potential for significant increase in exposure when tamsulosin 0.4mg is coadministered w/ a combination of both CYP3A4 and CYP2D6 inhibitors. Caution w/ moderate CYP3A4 inhibitors (eg, erythromycin), and w/ strong (eg, paroxetine) or moderate (eg, terbinafine) CYP2D6 inhibitors. Cimetidine increased exposure; caution w/ cimetidine, particularly at a tamsulosin dose >0.4mg. Avoid w/ other α-adrenergic blockers. Caution w/ PDE-5 inhibitors; concomitant use may cause symptomatic hypotension. Caution w/ warfarin.

PATIENT CONSIDERATIONS

Assessment: Assess for known hypersensitivity to the drug, sulfa allergy, and possible drug interactions. Assess if patient is planning to undergo cataract/glaucoma surgery. Screen for the presence of prostate cancer.

Monitoring: Monitor for signs/symptoms of orthostasis, syncope, priapism, IFIS, allergic reactions, and other adverse reactions. Monitor for the presence of prostate cancer at regular intervals.

Counseling: Advise patient about the possible occurrence of symptoms related to orthostatic hypotension; caution about driving, operating machinery, or performing hazardous tasks. Advise that therapy should not be used in combination w/ strong inhibitors of CYP3A4. Advise about the possibility of priapism as a result of treatment and instruct to seek immediate medical attention if it occurs. Inform of the importance of screening for prostate cancer prior to therapy and at regular intervals afterwards. Advise to inform ophthalmologist of drug use if considering cataract or glaucoma surgery.

STORAGE: 25°C (77°F); excursions permitted to 15-30°C (59-86°F).

FLOVENT DISKUS – fluticasone propionate RX

Class: Corticosteroid

ADULT DOSAGE
Asthma

Maintenance Treatment

Previous Therapy:

Bronchodilators Alone:
Initial: 100mcg bid
Max: 500mcg bid

Inhaled Corticosteroids:
Initial: 100-250mcg bid
Max: 500mcg bid
May consider starting doses >100mcg bid with poorer asthma control or previous high-dose inhaled corticosteroid requirement

Oral Corticosteroids:
Initial: 500-1000mcg bid

PEDIATRIC DOSAGE
Asthma

Maintenance Treatment

4-11 Years:
Previous Therapy:
Oral Corticosteroids:
Initial: 50mcg bid
May consider starting doses >50mcg bid with poorer asthma control or previous high-dose inhaled corticosteroid requirement
Max: 100mcg bid

≥12 Years:
Previous Therapy:
Bronchodilators Alone:
Initial: 100mcg bid
Max: 500mcg bid

Max: 1000mcg bid
Reduce oral prednisone no faster than 2.5-5mg/day on a weekly basis beginning after at least 1 week of fluticasone therapy

Titrate: Reduce to lowest effective dose once asthma stability is achieved. Higher dosages may provide additional asthma control if response to initial dose is inadequate after 2 weeks

Inhaled Corticosteroids:
Initial: 100-250mcg bid
May consider starting doses >100mcg bid with poorer asthma control or previous high-dose inhaled corticosteroid requirement
Max: 500mcg bid

Oral Corticosteroids:
Initial: 500-1000mcg bid
Max: 1000mcg bid
Reduce oral prednisone no faster than 2.5-5mg/day on a weekly basis beginning after at least 1 week of fluticasone therapy

Titrate: Reduce to lowest effective dose once asthma stability is achieved. Higher dosages may provide additional asthma control if response to initial dose is inadequate after 2 weeks

ADMINISTRATION
Orally inhaled powder

Rinse mouth after inhalation

HOW SUPPLIED
Disk: 50mcg/inh [60 blisters]; 100mcg/inh, 250mcg/inh [28, 60 blisters]

CONTRAINDICATIONS
Primary treatment of status asthmaticus or other acute episodes of asthma where intensive measures are required. Milk protein hypersensitivity.

WARNINGS/PRECAUTIONS
Not indicated for acute bronchospasm relief. *Candida albicans* infections of mouth and pharynx reported; treat and/or interrupt therapy if needed. Increased susceptibility to infections. May lead to serious/fatal course of chickenpox or measles; avoid exposure and, if exposed, consider prophylaxis/treatment. Caution with active/quiescent tuberculosis (TB), systemic fungal/bacterial/viral/parasitic infections, or ocular herpes simplex. Deaths due to adrenal insufficiency reported during and after transfer from systemic to inhaled corticosteroids; wean slowly from systemic corticosteroid use after transferring to therapy. Resume oral corticosteroids during periods of stress or a severe asthma attack in patients previously withdrawn from systemic corticosteroids. Transfer from systemic to inhaled corticosteroids may unmask allergic conditions previously suppressed by systemic therapy (eg, rhinitis, conjunctivitis, eczema). Monitor for systemic corticosteroid effects. Reduce dose slowly if hypercorticism and adrenal suppression/crisis occur. Immediate hypersensitivity reactions may occur. Decreases in bone mineral density (BMD) reported with long-term use; caution with major risk factors for decreased bone mineral content, including chronic use of drugs that can reduce bone mass (eg, anticonvulsants, oral corticosteroids). May cause reduction in growth velocity in pediatric patients; routinely monitor growth. Glaucoma, increased intraocular pressure (IOP), and cataracts reported with long-term use. Systemic eosinophilic conditions and vasculitis consistent with Churg-Strauss syndrome may occur. Paradoxical bronchospasm with immediate increase in wheezing may occur; treat immediately with an inhaled, short-acting bronchodilator; d/c and institute alternative therapy. Closely monitor patients with hepatic disease.

ADVERSE REACTIONS
Upper respiratory tract infection, throat irritation, headache, sinusitis, N/V, rhinitis, cough, muscle pain, oral candidiasis, arthralgia, fatigue, fever, nasal congestion, bronchitis, GI discomfort.

DRUG INTERACTIONS
Not recommended with strong CYP3A4 inhibitors (eg, ritonavir, clarithromycin, itraconazole); increased systemic corticosteroid adverse effects may occur. Ritonavir and ketoconazole may increase levels and reduce cortisol levels.

PATIENT CONSIDERATIONS

Assessment: Assess for hypersensitivity to drug or to milk proteins, status asthmaticus, acute bronchospasm, risk factors for decreased bone mineral content, history of increased IOP, glaucoma, cataracts, active/quiescent TB, ocular herpes simplex, systemic infections, hepatic impairment, pregnancy/nursing status, and possible drug interactions.

Monitoring: Monitor for signs of infections, systemic corticosteroid effects (eg, hypercorticism, adrenal suppression), hypersensitivity reactions, decreased BMD, glaucoma, increased IOP, cataracts, paradoxical bronchospasm, eosinophilic conditions, asthma instability, and other adverse reactions. Monitor growth of pediatric patients routinely. Closely monitor patients with hepatic disease.

Counseling: Advise to contact physician if oropharyngeal candidiasis develops. Inform that product is not a bronchodilator and not intended for use as rescue medication for acute asthma exacerbations; instruct to contact physician immediately if deterioration of asthma occurs. Instruct to avoid exposure to chickenpox or measles and to consult physician without delay if exposed. Inform about risks of immunosuppression, hypercorticism, adrenal suppression, reduction in BMD, reduced growth velocity in pediatric patients, and ocular effects. Instruct to d/c therapy if immediate hypersensitivity reaction occurs. Instruct to use at regular intervals ud and not to stop use abruptly; advise to contact physician immediately if use is discontinued.

STORAGE: 20-25°C (68-77°F); excursions permitted from 15-30°C (59-86°F). Store in a dry place away from direct heat or sunlight. Store inside unopened moisture-protective pouch and only remove immediately before initial use. Discard 6 weeks (50-mcg strength) or 2 months (100-mcg and 250-mcg strengths) after opening the foil pouch or when counter reads "0," whichever comes 1st.

Flovent HFA – fluticasone propionate RX

Class: Corticosteroid

ADULT DOSAGE

Asthma

Prophylactic Maint Treatment:

Previous Therapy:

Bronchodilators Alone:
Initial: 88mcg bid
Max: 440mcg bid

Inhaled Corticosteroids:
Initial: 88-220mcg bid
Max: 440mcg bid

Oral Corticosteroids:
Initial: 440mcg bid
Max: 880mcg bid

Reduce oral prednisone no faster than 2.5-5mg/day on a weekly basis beginning after at least 1 week of fluticasone therapy

Titrate:
Reduce to lowest effective dose once asthma stability is achieved. Higher dosages may provide additional asthma control if response to initial dose is inadequate after 2 weeks

PEDIATRIC DOSAGE

Asthma

Prophylactic Maint Treatment:

4-11 Years:
Initial/Max: 88mcg bid

≥12 Years:

Previous Therapy:

Bronchodilators Alone:
Initial: 88mcg bid
Max: 440mcg bid

Inhaled Corticosteroids:
Initial: 88-220mcg bid
Max: 440mcg bid

Oral Corticosteroids:
Initial: 440mcg bid
Max: 880mcg bid

Reduce oral prednisone no faster than 2.5-5mg/day on a weekly basis beginning after at least 1 week of fluticasone therapy

Titrate:
Reduce to lowest effective dose once asthma stability is achieved. Higher dosages may provide additional asthma control if response to initial dose is inadequate after 2 weeks

ADMINISTRATION

Oral inh route

Rinse mouth after inh
Shake well for 5 sec before each spray

Priming
Prime the inhaler before using for the first time by releasing 4 test sprays into the air, shaking well for 5 sec before each spray
If the inhaler has not been used for more than 7 days or has been dropped, prime inhaler by shaking well for 5 sec and releasing 1 spray into the air

HOW SUPPLIED

MDI: 44mcg/inh, 110mcg/inh, 220mcg/inh [120 inhalations]

CONTRAINDICATIONS

Primary treatment of status asthmaticus or other acute episodes of asthma where intensive measures are required, hypersensitivity to any of the ingredients.

WARNINGS/PRECAUTIONS

Not indicated for acute bronchospasm relief. *Candida albicans* infections of mouth and pharynx reported; treat and/or interrupt therapy if needed. Increased susceptibility to infections. May lead to serious/fatal course of chickenpox or measles in children; avoid exposure, and if exposed, consider prophylaxis/treatment. Caution with active/quiescent tuberculosis (TB), systemic fungal/bacterial/viral/parasitic infections, or ocular herpes simplex. Deaths due to adrenal insufficiency reported during and after transfer from systemic to inhaled corticosteroids; wean slowly from systemic corticosteroid use after transferring to therapy. Resume oral corticosteroids during periods of stress or a severe asthma attack in patients previously withdrawn from systemic corticosteroids. Transfer from systemic to inhaled corticosteroids may unmask allergic conditions previously suppressed by systemic therapy (eg, rhinitis, conjunctivitis, eczema). Monitor for systemic corticosteroid effects. Reduce dose slowly and consider other treatments if hypercorticism and adrenal suppression/crisis occur. Immediate hypersensitivity reactions may occur. Decreases in bone mineral density (BMD) reported with long-term use; caution with major risk factors for decreased bone mineral content, including chronic use of drugs that can reduce bone mass (eg, anticonvulsants, oral corticosteroids). May cause reduction in growth velocity in pediatric patients; routinely monitor growth. Glaucoma, increased intraocular pressure (IOP), and cataracts reported with long-term use. Systemic eosinophilic conditions, and vasculitis consistent with Churg-Strauss syndrome may occur. Paradoxical bronchospasm with immediate increase in wheezing may occur; treat immediately with an inhaled short-acting bronchodilator; d/c and institute alternative therapy. Closely monitor patients with hepatic disease.

F

ADVERSE REACTIONS

Upper respiratory tract infection/inflammation, throat irritation, sinusitis/sinus infection, hoarseness/dysphonia, candidiasis, cough, bronchitis, headache.

DRUG INTERACTIONS

Not recommended with strong CYP3A4 inhibitors (eg, ritonavir [RTV], atazanavir, clarithromycin, indinavir, itraconazole, nefazodone, nelfinavir, saquinavir, ketoconazole, telithromycin); increased systemic corticosteroid adverse effects may occur. RTV and ketoconazole may increase exposure and reduce cortisol levels.

PATIENT CONSIDERATIONS

Assessment: Assess for hypersensitivity to drug, status asthmaticus, acute bronchospasm, active/quiescent TB, ocular herpes simplex, systemic infections, risk factors for decreased bone mineral content, history of increased IOP, glaucoma, cataracts, hepatic impairment, pregnancy/nursing status, and possible drug interactions.

Monitoring: Monitor for signs of infection, systemic corticosteroid effects (eg, hypercorticism, adrenal suppression), hypersensitivity reactions, decreased BMD, glaucoma, increased IOP, cataracts, paradoxical bronchospasm, eosinophilic conditions, asthma instability, hypoadrenalism (in infants born to a mother who received corticosteroids during pregnancy), and other adverse reactions. Monitor growth in pediatric patients routinely. Closely monitor patients with hepatic disease.

Counseling: Advise to contact physician if oropharyngeal candidiasis develops. Advise to rinse the mouth with water without swallowing after inh to help reduce the risk of thrush. Inform that product is not a bronchodilator and not intended for use as rescue medicine for acute asthma exacerbations; instruct to contact physician immediately if deterioration of asthma occurs. Instruct to avoid exposure to chickenpox or measles and to consult physician without delay if exposed. Inform about risks of immunosuppression, hypercorticism, adrenal suppression, reduction in BMD, reduced growth velocity in pediatric patients, and ocular effects. Instruct to d/c therapy if immediate hypersensitivity reactions occur. Instruct to use at regular intervals ud and not to stop use abruptly; advise to contact physician immediately if use is discontinued. Instruct to avoid spraying in eyes. Advise women to contact physician if they become pregnant while on therapy.

STORAGE: 20-25°C (68-77°F); excursions permitted to 15-30°C (59-86°F). Store with mouthpiece down. Do not puncture, use/store near heat or open flame, or throw canister into fire/incinerator. Exposure to temperatures >49°C (120°F) may cause bursting. Discard when counter reads 000.

FLUDROCORTISONE – fludrocortisone acetate

RX

Class: Corticosteroid

OTHER BRAND NAMES

Florinef (Discontinued)

ADULT DOSAGE

Addison's Disease

Primary and Secondary Adrenocortical Insufficiency:
Usual: 0.1mg/day
Range: 0.1mg 3X weekly to 0.2mg/day

Preferably administered w/ cortisone (10-37.5mg/day in divided doses) or hydrocortisone (10-30mg/day in divided doses)

Salt-Losing Adrenogenital Syndrome

0.1-0.2mg/day

PEDIATRIC DOSAGE

Pediatric use may not have been established

DOSING CONSIDERATIONS

Adverse Reactions

Addison's Disease:

Transient HTN: Reduce dose to 0.05mg/day

ADMINISTRATION

Oral route

HOW SUPPLIED

Tab: 0.1mg* *scored

CONTRAINDICATIONS

Systemic fungal infections, history of possible or known hypersensitivity to these agents.

WARNINGS/PRECAUTIONS

May mask signs of infection, and new infections may appear during therapy. There may be decreased resistance and inability to localize infection; promptly control infection with suitable antimicrobial therapy. Prolonged use may produce posterior subcapsular cataracts, glaucoma with possible damage to optic nerves, and secondary ocular infections due to fungi or viruses. May cause elevation of BP, salt and water retention, and increased K^+ excretion; carefully monitor dosage and salt intake to avoid HTN, edema, or weight gain. Periodic serum electrolyte monitoring is advisable during prolonged therapy; dietary salt restriction and K^+ supplementation may be necessary. May increase Ca^{2+} excretion. Use in patients with active tuberculosis (TB) should be restricted to fulminating or disseminated cases in conjunction with an appropriate antituberculous regimen. Reactivation of TB may occur; caution in patients with latent TB or tuberculin reactivity; patients on prolonged therapy should receive chemoprophylaxis. Avoid exposure to chickenpox or measles. Adverse effects may occur by too rapid withdrawal or by continued use of large doses. Enhanced effects with hypothyroidism and cirrhosis. To avoid drug-induced adrenal insufficiency, supportive dosage may be required in times of stress (eg, trauma, surgery, severe illness) both during treatment and for a yr afterwards. Use lowest possible dose; gradually reduce dosage when possible. Caution with ocular herpes simplex, nonspecific ulcerative colitis, HTN, diverticulitis, fresh intestinal anastomoses, active/latent peptic ulcer, renal insufficiency, osteoporosis, and myasthenia gravis. Psychic derangements may appear and existing emotional instability or psychotic tendencies may be aggravated. Lab test interactions may occur.

ADVERSE REACTIONS

HTN, CHF, edema, cardiac enlargement, K^+ loss, hypokalemic alkalosis.

DRUG INTERACTIONS

Decreased pharmacologic effect and increased ulcerogenic effect of aspirin (ASA); monitor salicylate levels or therapeutic effect of ASA and adjust salicylate dosage accordingly if effect is altered. Caution with ASA in patients with hypoprothrombinemia. Enhanced hypokalemia with amphotericin B or K^+-depleting diuretics (eg, benzothiadiazines, furosemide, ethacrynic acid) and enhanced possibility of arrhythmias or digitalis toxicity associated with hypokalemia with digitalis glycosides; monitor serum K^+ levels and use K^+ supplements if necessary. Rifampin, barbiturates, or phenytoin may diminish steroid effect; increase steroid dosage accordingly. Decreased PT response with oral anticoagulants; monitor prothrombin levels and adjust anticoagulant dosage accordingly. Diminished effect of oral hypoglycemics and insulin; monitor for symptoms of hyperglycemia and adjust dosage of antidiabetic drug upward if necessary. Enhanced tendency toward edema with anabolic steroids (particularly C-17 alkylated androgens [eg, oxymetholone, methandrostenolone, norethandrolone]); use with caution especially in patients with hepatic/cardiac disease. May require a reduction of corticosteroid dose when estrogen therapy is initiated, and may require increased amounts when estrogen is terminated. Avoid smallpox vaccination and other immunizations; possible hazards of neurologic complications and a lack of antibody response.

PATIENT CONSIDERATIONS

Assessment: Assess for hypersensitivity to drug, systemic fungal infections, active/latent TB, HTN, renal insufficiency, psychotic tendencies, hypothyroidism, osteoporosis, myasthenia gravis, peptic ulcer, fresh intestinal anastomoses, ocular herpes simplex, diverticulitis, ulcerative colitis, other conditions where treatment is cautioned, pregnancy/nursing status, and possible drug interactions.

Monitoring: Monitor for infections, edema, weight gain, psychic derangement, cataracts, latent TB reactivation, and other adverse reactions. Monitor dosage, salt intake, serum electrolytes, and BP. Monitor for remission or exacerbations of disease and stress (surgery, infection, trauma). Monitor prothrombin levels if used with oral anticoagulants.

Counseling: Advise to report any medical history of heart disease, high BP, and kidney/liver disease, and to report current use of any medicines. Instruct to avoid exposure to chickenpox or measles and, if exposed, to obtain medical advice. Inform of steroid-dependent status and of increased dosage requirement with stress; advise to carry medical identification indicating this dependence and, if necessary, instruct to carry an adequate supply of medication for emergency use. Inform of the importance of regular follow-up visits and the need to promptly notify physician of dizziness, severe or continuing headaches, swelling of feet or lower legs, or unusual weight gain. Instruct to take only ud, to take a missed dose as soon as possible, unless it is almost time for next dose, and not to double next dose.

STORAGE: 15-30°C (59-86°F). Avoid excessive heat.

FLUMIST QUADRIVALENT – influenza vaccine live, intranasal RX

Class: Vaccine

ADULT DOSAGE

Influenza

Active Immunization Against Influenza A Subtype Viruses and Type B Viruses:

≤49 Years:

One 0.2mL dose (0.1mL/nostril)

PEDIATRIC DOSAGE

Influenza

Active Immunization Against Influenza A Subtype Viruses and Type B Viruses:

2-8 Years:

One or two 0.2mL doses (0.1mL/nostril), depending on vaccination history. If 2 doses, administer at least 1 month apart

≥9 Years:

One 0.2mL dose (0.1mL/nostril)

ADMINISTRATION

Intranasal route

For administration by a healthcare provider.

Each sprayer contains a single dose (0.2mL); administer approx 1/2 of the contents of the single-dose intranasal sprayer into each nostril.

HOW SUPPLIED

Intranasal Spray: 0.2mL [10s]

CONTRAINDICATIONS

Severe allergic reaction (eg, anaphylaxis) to egg protein, or after a previous dose of any influenza vaccine. Children and adolescents through 17 yrs of age who are receiving aspirin (ASA) or ASA-containing therapy.

WARNINGS/PRECAUTIONS

Increased risk of hospitalization and wheezing in children <2 yrs of age. Children <5 yrs of age w/ recurrent wheezing and persons of any age w/ asthma may be at increased risk of wheezing following administration of vaccine. Caution if Guillain-Barre syndrome (GBS) has occurred w/in 6 weeks of any prior influenza vaccination. Appropriate treatment and supervision must be available to manage possible anaphylactic reactions. May not protect all individuals receiving the vaccine.

ADVERSE REACTIONS

Runny nose/nasal congestion, headache, lethargy, sore throat, decreased appetite, muscle aches, fever, cough.

DRUG INTERACTIONS

See Contraindications. Avoid ASA-containing therapy in children and adolescents (through 17 yrs of age) during the first 4 weeks after vaccination unless clearly needed. Antiviral drugs that are active against influenza A and/or B viruses may reduce the effectiveness of vaccine if administered w/in 48 hrs before, or w/in 2 weeks after vaccination; consider revaccination when appropriate if administered concomitantly w/ antiviral agents.

PATIENT CONSIDERATIONS

Assessment: Assess for history of severe allergic reaction to any component of the vaccine (eg, egg protein) or after a previous dose of any influenza vaccination, history of asthma, recurrent wheezing in children <5 yrs of age, development of GBS following a prior dose of influenza vaccine, pregnancy/nursing status, and possible drug interactions. Review current health/medical status and immunization history.

Monitoring: Monitor for signs/symptoms of GBS, acute allergic reactions, and other adverse reactions.

Counseling: Inform vaccinee/caregivers of benefits/risks and the need for 2 doses at least 1 month apart in children 2-8 yrs of age, depending on vaccination history. Inform that the vaccine is an attenuated live virus vaccine and has the potential for transmission to immunocompromised household contacts. Inform vaccinee/caregiver that there may be an increased risk of wheezing associated w/ vaccine in persons <5 yrs of age w/ recurrent wheezing and persons of any age w/ asthma. Instruct to inform physician if adverse reactions occur.

STORAGE: 2-8°C (35-46°F). Do not freeze. Keep sprayer in outer carton in order to protect from light. A single temperature excursion up to 25°C (77°F) for 12 hrs permitted. After a temperature excursion, the vaccine should be returned immediately to the recommended storage condition and used as soon as feasible. Subsequent excursions are not permitted.

FLUPHENAZINE DECANOATE – fluphenazine decanoate

RX

Class: Piperazine phenothiazine

F

OTHER BRAND NAMES

Prolixin Decanoate (Discontinued)

ADULT DOSAGE

Psychotic Disorders

Management of Patients Requiring Prolonged Parenteral Neuroleptic Therapy (eg, Chronic Schizophrenics):
Initial: 12.5-25mg IM/SQ
Titrate: Determine subsequent inj and dose interval based on response; single inj given as maint therapy may be effective for up to 4-6 weeks. If doses >50mg are necessary, cautiously increase next and succeeding doses in increments of 12.5mg
Max: 100mg/dose

Phenothiazine-Naive:
Treat initially w/ shorter-acting form of fluphenazine before administering decanoate to determine response and establish appropriate dose

Severely Agitated Patients:
May treat initially w/ rapid-acting phenothiazine (eg, fluphenazine HCl), then give 25mg of fluphenazine decanoate when acute symptoms subside; adjust subsequent doses as necessary

"Poor Risk" Patients:
May initiate therapy cautiously w/ PO or parenteral fluphenazine HCl, then administer equivalent dose of fluphenazine decanoate when pharmacologic effects and appropriate dose are apparent; adjust subsequent dose according to response

Stabilized on a Fixed Daily Dosage of Fluphenazine HCl Tab/Elixir:
Conversion from these short-acting oral forms to the long-acting fluphenazine decanoate inj may be indicated; approximate conversion ratio of 12.5mg of decanoate every 3 weeks for every 10mg/day of fluphenazine HCl
Carefully monitor and adjust dose appropriately at the time of each inj

PEDIATRIC DOSAGE

Pediatric use may not have been established

ADMINISTRATION

IM/SQ route

Use a dry syringe and needle of at least 21 gauge

HOW SUPPLIED

Inj: 25mg/mL [5mL]

CONTRAINDICATIONS

Suspected or established subcortical brain damage, patients receiving large doses of hypnotics, comatose or severely depressed states, presence of blood dyscrasia or liver damage, children <12 yrs of age, hypersensitivity to fluphenazine.

WARNINGS/PRECAUTIONS

May develop tardive dyskinesia (TD); consider discontinuation if signs/symptoms develop. Neuroleptic malignant syndrome (NMS) reported; d/c therapy immediately and institute symptomatic treatment. May impair mental/physical abilities. Leukopenia, neutropenia, and agranulocytosis reported; d/c with severe neutropenia (absolute neutrophil count <1000/mm^3). D/C at 1st sign of WBC decline in absence of other causative factors in patients with preexisting low WBC or history of drug induced leukopenia/neutropenia. Monitor for fever or other signs/symptoms of infections in patients with neutropenia; treat promptly if such signs/symptoms occur.

Caution in patients who developed cholestatic jaundice, dermatoses, or other allergic reactions to phenothiazine derivatives. May cause hypotension phenomena in patients on large doses undergoing surgery. Caution in patients exposed to extreme heat, with mitral insufficiency or other cardiovascular disease (CVD), and pheochromocytoma. Caution with history of convulsive disorders; grand mal convulsions reported. May develop liver damage, pigmentary retinopathy, lenticular and corneal deposits, and irreversible dyskinesia with prolonged therapy. Monitor renal function with long-term therapy; d/c if BUN becomes abnormal. May develop "silent pneumonias". May elevate prolactin levels; galactorrhea, amenorrhea, gynecomastia, and impotence reported.

ADVERSE REACTIONS

Extrapyramidal symptoms, TD, HTN, hypotension, allergic reactions, nausea, loss of appetite, dry mouth, constipation, perspiration, salivation, liver damage, fever, muscle rigidity, blood dyscrasias.

DRUG INTERACTIONS

See Contraindications. May potentiate the effects of CNS depressants (eg, opiates, analgesics, antihistamines, barbiturates, alcohol) and atropine. Avoid epinephrine in treating severe hypotension caused by phenothiazine derivatives; reversal of action, resulting in further lowering of BP, may occur. Dose of anesthetics or CNS depressants may need to be reduced. Caution with phosphorus insecticides.

PATIENT CONSIDERATIONS

Assessment: Assess for previous hypersensitivity to the drug or cross-sensitivity to phenothiazine derivatives, subcortical brain damage, comatose or severely depressed states, current use of hypnotics, blood dyscrasias, liver damage, history of convulsive disorders, mitral insufficiency or other CVD, pheochromocytoma, renal/hepatic impairment, any conditions where treatment is contraindicated or cautioned, pregnancy/nursing status, and possible drug interactions.

Monitoring: Monitor for signs/symptoms of TD, NMS, grand mal convulsions, liver damage, pigmentary retinopathy, lenticular and corneal deposits, irreversible dyskinesia, elevated prolactin levels, infection, and other adverse reactions. Monitor for hypotensive phenomena in patients undergoing surgery. Monitor CBC, hepatic and renal function periodically. Frequently monitor CBC during 1st few months of therapy in patients with preexisting low WBC or history of drug induced leukopenia/neutropenia. Periodically reassess the need for continued treatment.

Counseling: Inform about the risks and benefits of therapy. Inform that therapy may impair mental and physical abilities.

STORAGE: 20-25°C (68-77°F). Protect from light.

FOCALIN – dexmethylphenidate hydrochloride   CII

Class: CNS stimulant

Caution with history of drug dependence or alcoholism. Chronic, abusive use may lead to marked tolerance and psychological dependence with varying degrees of abnormal behavior may occur with chronic abusive use. Frank psychotic episodes may occur, especially with parenteral abuse. Careful supervision is required during withdrawal from abusive use, since severe depression may occur. Withdrawal following chronic use may unmask symptoms of underlying disorder that may require follow-up.

ADULT DOSAGE

Attention-Deficit Hyperactivity Disorder

Refer to pediatric dosing

PEDIATRIC DOSAGE

Attention-Deficit Hyperactivity Disorder

≥6 Years:

Methylphenidate-Naive:

Initial: 5mg/day (2.5mg bid)

Titrate: May adjust weekly in 2.5-5mg increments

Max: 20mg/day (10mg bid)

Currently on Methylphenidate:

Initial: 1/2 the dose of racemic methylphenidate

Max: 20mg/day (10mg bid)

DOSING CONSIDERATIONS

Adverse Reactions

Reduce dose or d/c if paradoxical aggravation of symptoms or other adverse events occur

D/C if no improvement seen after appropriate dosage adjustment over 1 month

ADMINISTRATION

Oral route

Take w/ or w/o food.

Administer bid, at least 4 hrs apart.

HOW SUPPLIED

Tab: 2.5mg, 5mg, 10mg

CONTRAINDICATIONS

Marked anxiety, tension, and agitation; hypersensitivity to methylphenidate or other components of the product; glaucoma; motor tics or family history or diagnosis of Tourette's syndrome; during treatment w/ MAOIs, and w/in a minimum of 14 days following discontinuation of an MAOI.

WARNINGS/PRECAUTIONS

Avoid in patients with known serious structural cardiac abnormalities, cardiomyopathy, serious heart rhythm abnormalities, coronary artery disease, or other serious cardiac problems. Sudden death reported in children and adolescents with structural cardiac abnormalities or other serious heart problems. Sudden death, stroke, and myocardial infarction (MI) reported in adults. May cause modest increase in average BP and HR; caution in patients whose underlying medical conditions might be compromised by increases in BP or HR. Prior to treatment, perform medical history (including assessment for family history of sudden death or ventricular arrhythmia) and physical exam to assess for presence of cardiac disease. Promptly perform cardiac evaluation if symptoms of cardiac disease develop during treatment. May exacerbate symptoms of behavior disturbance and thought disorder in patients with a preexisting psychotic disorder. May induce mixed/manic episode in patients with comorbid bipolar disorder. May cause treatment-emergent psychotic or manic symptoms at usual doses in children and adolescents without a prior history of psychotic illness or mania; discontinuation may be appropriate if such symptoms occur. Aggressive behavior or hostility reported in children and adolescents. May cause long-term suppression of growth in children; may need to interrupt treatment in patients not growing or gaining height or weight as expected. May lower convulsive threshold; d/c in the presence of seizures. Priapism reported; immediate medical attention should be sought if abnormally sustained or frequent and painful erections develop. Associated with peripheral vasculopathy, including Raynaud's phenomenon; monitor for digital changes. Difficulties with accommodation and blurring of vision reported. Periodically monitor CBC, differential, and platelet counts during prolonged therapy.

ADVERSE REACTIONS

Abdominal pain, fever, anorexia, nausea.

DRUG INTERACTIONS

See Contraindications. May decrease the effectiveness of drugs used to treat HTN. Caution with pressor agents. May inhibit metabolism of coumarin anticoagulants, anticonvulsants (eg, phenobarbital, phenytoin, primidone) and some antidepressants (eg, TCAs, SSRIs); downward dose adjustments and monitoring of plasma drug concentration (or coagulation times for coumarin) of these drugs may be necessary when initiating or discontinuing dexmethylphenidate.

PATIENT CONSIDERATIONS

Assessment: Assess for previous hypersensitivity to the drug, history of drug dependence or alcoholism, marked anxiety, agitation, tension, glaucoma, motor tics, family history or diagnosis of Tourette's syndrome, preexisting psychotic disorder, comorbid bipolar disorder, history of seizures, medical conditions that might be compromised by increases in BP or HR, any other conditions where treatment is contraindicated or cautioned, pregnancy/nursing status, and possible drug interactions. Perform a careful history (including assessment for a family history of sudden death or ventricular arrhythmia) and physical exam to assess for the presence of cardiac disease, and perform further cardiac evaluation if findings suggest such disease (eg, ECG, echocardiogram). Adequately screen patients with comorbid depressive symptoms to determine if they are at risk for bipolar disorder (eg, detailed psychiatric history, including a family history of suicide, bipolar disorder, and depression).

Monitoring: Monitor for signs/symptoms of cardiac disease, exacerbation of behavioral disturbance and thought disorder, psychosis, mania, appearance of or worsening of aggressive behavior or hostility, seizures, priapism, digital changes, visual disturbances, and other adverse reactions. Monitor BP and HR. During prolonged use, periodically evaluate usefulness of therapy and monitor CBC, differential, and platelet counts. In pediatric patients, monitor growth.

Counseling: Inform about risks and benefits of treatment. Counsel on the appropriate use of the medication. Advise of the possibility of priapism; instruct to seek immediate medical attention in the event of priapism. Instruct to report to physician any new numbness, pain, skin color change, sensitivity to temperature in fingers or toes, or any signs of unexplained wounds appearing on the fingers or toes.

STORAGE: 25°C (77°F); excursions permitted to 15-30°C (59-86°F). Protect from light and moisture.

FOCALIN XR – dexmethylphenidate hydrochloride CII

Class: CNS stimulant

Caution w/ history of drug dependence or alcoholism. Marked tolerance and psychological dependence w/ varying degrees of abnormal behavior may occur w/ chronic abusive use. Frank psychotic episodes may occur, especially w/ parenteral abuse. Careful supervision is required during withdrawal from abusive use, since severe depression may occur. Withdrawal following chronic therapeutic use may unmask symptoms of underlying disorder that may require follow-up.

ADULT DOSAGE

Attention-Deficit Hyperactivity Disorder

New to Methylphenidate:
Initial: 10mg qam
Titrate: May adjust weekly in 10mg increments
Max: 40mg/day

Currently on Methylphenidate:
Initial: 1/2 of methylphenidate total daily dose

Currently on Dexmethylphenidate Immediate-Release:
May switch to the same daily dose of the extended-release

D/C if no improvement seen after appropriate dosage adjustment over 1 month

PEDIATRIC DOSAGE

Attention-Deficit Hyperactivity Disorder

≥6 Years:
New to Methylphenidate:
Initial: 5mg qam
Titrate: May adjust weekly in 5mg increments
Max: 30mg/day

Currently on Methylphenidate:
Initial: 1/2 of methylphenidate total daily dose

Currently on Dexmethylphenidate Immediate-Release:
May switch to the same daily dose of the extended-release

D/C if no improvement seen after appropriate dosage adjustment over 1 month

DOSING CONSIDERATIONS

Adverse Reactions

Reduce dose or d/c if paradoxical aggravation of symptoms or other adverse events occur

ADMINISTRATION

Oral route

Swallow caps whole or sprinkle contents on a spoonful of applesauce.

Do not crush, chew, or divide.

Consume drug and applesauce mixture immediately; do not store for future use.

HOW SUPPLIED

Cap, Extended-Release: 5mg, 10mg, 15mg, 20mg, 25mg, 30mg, 35mg, 40mg

CONTRAINDICATIONS

Marked anxiety, tension, and agitation; hypersensitivity to methylphenidate or other components of the product; glaucoma; motor tics or family history or diagnosis of Tourette's syndrome; during treatment w/ MAOIs, and w/in a minimum of 14 days following discontinuation of an MAOI.

WARNINGS/PRECAUTIONS

Avoid in patients w/ known serious structural cardiac abnormalities, cardiomyopathy, serious heart rhythm abnormalities, coronary artery disease, or other serious cardiac problems. Sudden death reported in children and adolescents w/ structural cardiac abnormalities or other serious heart problems. Sudden death, stroke, MI reported in adults. May cause modest increase in average BP and HR; caution w/ HTN, heart failure, recent MI, or ventricular arrhythmia. Promptly perform cardiac evaluation if symptoms of cardiac disease develop during treatment. May exacerbate symptoms of behavior disturbance and thought disorder in patients w/ preexisting psychotic disorder. Caution in patients w/ comorbid bipolar disorder; may induce mixed/manic episodes. May cause treatment-emergent psychotic or manic symptoms (eg, hallucinations, delusional thinking, mania) in children and adolescents w/o prior history of psychotic illness or mania; discontinuation may be appropriate if such symptoms occur. Aggressive behavior or hostility reported in children and adolescents. May cause long-term suppression of growth in children; monitor growth, and may need to interrupt treatment in patients not growing or gaining height or weight as expected. May lower convulsive threshold; d/c in the presence of seizures. Priapism reported; seek immediate medical attention if abnormally sustained or frequent and painful erections develop. Associated w/ peripheral vasculopathy, including Raynaud's phenomenon; monitor for digital changes. Difficulties w/ accommodation and blurring of vision reported.

ADVERSE REACTIONS

Dyspepsia, headache, anxiety, insomnia, anorexia, dry mouth, pharyngolaryngeal pain, feeling jittery, dizziness, decreased appetite, vomiting.

DRUG INTERACTIONS

See Contraindications. Caution w/ pressor agents. May decrease the effectiveness of drugs used to treat HTN. May inhibit metabolism of coumarin anticoagulants, anticonvulsants (eg, phenobarbital, phenytoin, primidone), and tricyclic drugs (eg, imipramine, clomipramine, desipramine); downward dose adjustments and monitoring of plasma drug concentration (or coagulation times for coumarin) of these drugs may be necessary when initiating or discontinuing therapy. Antacids or acid suppressants could alter drug release.

PATIENT CONSIDERATIONS

Assessment: Assess for previous hypersensitivity to the drug, history of drug dependence or alcoholism, marked anxiety, tension, agitation, glaucoma, motor tics, family history or diagnosis of Tourette's syndrome, preexisting psychotic disorder, comorbid bipolar disorder, cardiac disease, medical conditions that might be compromised by increases in BP and HR, any other conditions where treatment is cautioned, pregnancy/nursing status, and possible drug interactions.

Monitoring: Monitor BP, HR, and for signs/symptoms of cardiac disease (eg, exertional chest pain, unexplained syncope), exacerbation of behavioral disturbance and thought disorder, psychosis, mania, appearance of or worsening of aggressive behavior or hostility, seizures, priapism, digital changes, visual disturbances, and other adverse reactions. During prolonged use, periodically reevaluate usefulness of therapy and monitor CBC, differential, and platelet counts. In pediatric patients, monitor growth.

Counseling: Inform about benefits and risks of treatment. Counsel on the appropriate use of the medication. Advise of the possibility of priapism; instruct to seek immediate medical attention in the event of priapism. Instruct to report to physician any new numbness, pain, skin color change, sensitivity to temperature in fingers or toes, or any signs of unexplained wounds appearing on fingers or toes.

STORAGE: 25°C (77°F); excursions permitted to 15-30°C (59-86°F).

FORTAMET – metformin hydrochloride

RX

Class: Biguanide

Lactic acidosis reported (rare). May occur in association w/ other conditions such as diabetes mellitus (DM) w/ significant renal insufficiency, CHF, and conditions w/ risk of hypoperfusion and hypoxemia. Risk increases w/ the degree of renal dysfunction and age. Avoid in patients ≥80 yrs unless renal function is normal. Avoid w/ clinical/lab evidence of hepatic disease. Temporarily d/c prior to IV radiocontrast studies or surgical procedures. Caution against excessive alcohol intake; may potentiate effects of metformin on lactate metabolism. Withhold in the presence of any condition associated w/ hypoxemia, dehydration, or sepsis. Regularly monitor renal function and use minimum effective dose to decrease risk. If lactic acidosis is suspected, immediately d/c and institute general supportive measures.

ADULT DOSAGE

Type 2 Diabetes Mellitus

≥17 Years:
Initial: 500-1000mg qd
Titrate: May increase in increments of 500mg weekly
Max: 2500mg/day

Transfer from Other Antidiabetic Therapy:
From Standard Oral Hypoglycemic Agents Other Than Chlorpropamide: No transition period necessary
From Chlorpropamide: Exercise care during first 2 weeks for overlapping drug effects and possible hypoglycemia

PEDIATRIC DOSAGE

Pediatric use may not have been established

DOSING CONSIDERATIONS

Concomitant Medications

Oral Sulfonylurea Therapy:
If unresponsive to 4 weeks of max dose of metformin HCl extended-release (ER) monotherapy, consider gradual addition of an oral sulfonylurea while continuing metformin HCl ER at max dose
If patients have not satisfactorily responded to 1-3 months of concomitant therapy (max dose of metformin HCl ER and max dose of an oral sulfonylurea), consider therapeutic alternatives (eg, switching to insulin w/ or w/o metformin HCl ER)

Insulin Therapy:
Initial: 500mg qd while continuing current insulin dose
Titrate: May increase by 500mg after approx 1 week and by 500mg every week thereafter
Max: 2500mg/day
Decrease insulin dose by 10-25% if FPG <120mg/dL

Elderly
Initial/Maint: Use conservative dosing
Do not titrate to max dose

Other Important Considerations
Debilitated/Malnourished Patients:
Do not titrate to max dose

ADMINISTRATION

Oral route

Take w/ a full glass of water w/ pm meal

HOW SUPPLIED

Tab, ER: 500mg, 1000mg

CONTRAINDICATIONS

Renal disease/dysfunction (eg, SrCr ≥1.5mg/dL [males], ≥1.4mg/dL [females], or abnormal CrCl); known hypersensitivity to metformin; acute or chronic metabolic acidosis, including diabetic ketoacidosis, w/ or w/o coma.

WARNINGS/PRECAUTIONS

Lactic acidosis may be suspected in diabetic patients w/ metabolic acidosis lacking evidence of ketoacidosis (ketonuria and ketonemia). Caution w/ concomitant medications that may affect renal function, result in significant hemodynamic change, or interfere w/ the disposition of metformin. Temporarily d/c prior to surgical procedures associated w/ restricted oral intake. Temporarily withhold drug before, during, and 48 hrs after radiologic studies w/ IV iodinated contrast materials; reinstitute only when renal function is normal. D/C in hypoxic states (eg, shock, CHF, acute myocardial infarction [MI]), dehydration, and sepsis. Avoid w/ clinical or lab evidence of hepatic disease. May decrease vitamin B12 levels. Increased risk of hypoglycemia in elderly, debilitated/malnourished, adrenal or pituitary insufficiency, or alcohol intoxication. Temporarily withhold metformin and administer insulin if loss of glycemic control occurs due to stress; reinstitute metformin after acute episode is resolved.

ADVERSE REACTIONS

Lactic acidosis, infection, diarrhea, nausea, headache, dyspepsia, rhinitis, flatulence, abdominal pain.

DRUG INTERACTIONS

Furosemide, nifedipine, cimetidine, and cationic drugs (eg, amiloride, digoxin, morphine) may increase metformin levels. Thiazides, other diuretics, corticosteroids, phenothiazines, thyroid products, estrogens, oral contraceptives, phenytoin, nicotinic acid, sympathomimetics, calcium channel blockers, and isoniazid may cause hyperglycemia and loss of glycemic control. May decrease furosemide levels.

PATIENT CONSIDERATIONS

Assessment: Assess for hypoxic states (eg, acute CHF, acute MI, cardiovascular collapse), septicemia, acute/chronic metabolic acidosis, adrenal/pituitary insufficiency, alcoholism, pregnancy/nursing status, and possible drug interactions. Evaluate for other medical conditions, and for any IV radiocontrast study or surgical procedure. Assess FPG, HbA1c, renal function, LFTs, and hematologic parameters (eg, Hgb/Hct, RBC indices).

Monitoring: Monitor for lactic acidosis, hypoglycemia, prerenal azotemia, hypoxic states, hypersensitivity reactions, and other adverse reactions. Monitor FPG, HbA1c, renal function (eg, SrCr), LFTs, and hematologic parameters (eg, Hgb/Hct, RBC indices).

Counseling: Inform of the potential risks, benefits, and alternative modes of therapy. Inform about the importance of adherence to dietary instructions, regular exercise programs, and regular testing of blood glucose, HbA1c, renal function, and hematologic parameters. Inform of the risk of lactic acidosis w/ therapy and to contact physician if unexplained hyperventilation, myalgia, malaise, unusual somnolence, or other nonspecific symptoms occur. Counsel against excessive alcohol intake. Explain risks, symptoms, and conditions that predispose to the development of hypoglycemia when initiating combination therapy. Instruct that drug must be taken w/ food, swallowed whole w/ a full glass of water and should not be chewed, cut, or crushed, and that inactive ingredients may be eliminated in the feces as a soft mass.

STORAGE: 20-25°C (68-77°F); excursions permitted to 15-30°C (59-86°F). Keep tightly closed. Protect from light and moisture. Avoid excessive heat and humidity.

FORTEO — teriparatide (rDNA origin)

RX

Class: Recombinant human parathyroid hormone

Increased incidence of osteosarcoma seen in animal studies; prescribe only when benefits outweigh risks. Do not prescribe for patients who are at increased baseline risk for osteosarcoma (including those w/ Paget's disease of bone or unexplained alkaline phosphatase elevations, pediatric and young adult patients w/ open epiphyses, or prior external beam or implant radiation therapy involving the skeleton).

ADULT DOSAGE

Osteoporosis

High Risk for Fracture:

Postmenopausal Women w/ Osteoporosis:
20mcg qd

Primary or Hypogonadal Osteoporosis in Men:
20mcg qd

Glucocorticoid-Induced Osteoporosis in Men and Women:
20mcg qd

Use for >2 yrs during a patient's lifetime is not recommended

PEDIATRIC DOSAGE

Pediatric use may not have been established

ADMINISTRATION

SQ route

Inject into the thigh or abdominal wall

Administer initially under circumstances where the patient can sit or lie down if symptoms of orthostatic hypotension occur

HOW SUPPLIED

Inj: 20mcg/dose [28 doses]

CONTRAINDICATIONS

Hypersensitivity to teriparatide or to any of its excipients.

WARNINGS/PRECAUTIONS

Use for >2 yrs during a patient's lifetime is not recommended. Do not give in patients w/ bone metastases or history of skeletal malignancies, metabolic bone diseases other than osteoporosis, preexisting hypercalcemia, or underlying hypercalcemic disorder (eg, primary hyperparathyroidism). Transiently increases serum Ca^{2+}. Consider measurement of urinary Ca^{2+} excretion if active urolithiasis or preexisting hypercalciuria are suspected; caution w/ active or recent urolithiasis. Transient episodes of symptomatic orthostatic hypotension reported w/ administration of initial doses; administer initially under circumstances where the patient can sit or lie down if symptoms of orthostatic hypotension occur.

ADVERSE REACTIONS

Pain, arthralgia, rhinitis, asthenia, N/V, dizziness, headache, HTN, increased cough, pharyngitis, constipation, dyspepsia, diarrhea, rash, insomnia.

DRUG INTERACTIONS

Hypercalcemia may predispose to digitalis toxicity; caution if taking digoxin concomitantly.

PATIENT CONSIDERATIONS

Assessment: Assess for increased baseline risk for osteosarcoma, bone metastases or history of skeletal malignancies, metabolic bone disease other than osteoporosis, hypercalcemia, hypercalcemic disorder, hypercalciuria, active or recent urolithiasis, hypersensitivity to drug, pregnancy/nursing status, and possible drug interactions. Consider measurement of urinary Ca^{2+} excretion if active urolithiasis or preexisting hypercalciuria are suspected.

Monitoring: Monitor for signs/symptoms of osteosarcoma, orthostatic hypotension, and other adverse reactions.

Counseling: Inform of potential risk of osteosarcoma and encourage to enroll in the voluntary Forteo Patient Registry. Instruct to sit or lie down if lightheadedness or palpitations following inj develop; if symptoms persist or worsen, advise to consult physician before continuing treatment. Instruct to contact physician if persistent symptoms of hypercalcemia (eg, N/V, constipation, lethargy, muscle weakness) develop. Counsel on roles of supplemental Ca^{2+} and/or vitamin D, weight-bearing exercise, and modification of certain behavioral factors (eg, smoking, alcohol consumption). Instruct on proper use of delivery device (pen) and proper disposal of needles; advise not to share pen w/ other patients and not to transfer contents to a syringe.

STORAGE: 2-8°C (36-46°F). Recap pen when not in use. Minimize time out of the refrigerator during the use period; may deliver dose immediately following removal from the refrigerator. Do not freeze; do not use if it has been frozen. Discard after the 28-day use period.

FORTICAL – calcitonin-salmon (rDNA origin) RX

Class: Hormonal bone resorption inhibitor

ADULT DOSAGE

Postmenopausal Osteoporosis

In Women >5 Years Postmenopause:
1 spray qd intranasally, alternating nostrils daily

Calcium and Vitamin D Supplementation:
Patients should receive adequate Ca^{2+} (≥1000mg elemental Ca^{2+}/day) and vitamin D (≥400 IU/day)

Periodically reevaluate the need for continued therapy

PEDIATRIC DOSAGE

Pediatric use may not have been established

F

ADMINISTRATION

Intranasal route

Wait until the bottle has reached room temperature before using the 1st dose

To prime the pump before it is used for the 1st time, hold the bottle upright and depress the 2 white side arms of the pump toward the bottle at least 5 times until a full spray is produced; the pump is primed once the 1st full spray is emitted

To administer, carefully place the nozzle into the nostril w/ the patient's head in the upright position, then firmly depress the pump toward the bottle

Do not prime the pump before each daily use

HOW SUPPLIED

Spray: 200 IU/spray [3.7mL]

CONTRAINDICATIONS

Hypersensitivity to calcitonin-salmon or any of the excipients.

WARNINGS/PRECAUTIONS

Reserve for patients for whom alternative treatments are not suitable. Serious hypersensitivity reactions reported; usual provisions should be made for emergency treatment if such a reaction occurs. Consider skin testing prior to treatment for patients with suspected hypersensitivity to drug. Hypocalcemia associated with tetany and seizure activity reported. Correct hypocalcemia and treat other disorders affecting mineral metabolism (eg, vitamin D deficiency) before initiating therapy. Adequate intake of Ca^{2+} and vitamin D is recommended. Nasal adverse reactions (eg, rhinitis, epistaxis) reported, and development of mucosal alterations may occur; perform periodic nasal exams prior to start of treatment and during therapy, and at any time nasal symptoms occur. D/C if severe ulceration of the nasal mucosa occurs; d/c temporarily until healing occurs in patients with smaller ulcers. Increased risk of malignancies; carefully consider benefits against possible risks. Consider possibility of antibody formation in any patient with an initial response to therapy who later stops responding to treatment. Urine sediment abnormalities may occur; consider periodic exam of urine sediment.

ADVERSE REACTIONS

Rhinitis, nasal symptoms, back pain, arthralgia, epistaxis, headache.

DRUG INTERACTIONS

May reduce lithium concentrations; dose of lithium may require adjustment.

PATIENT CONSIDERATIONS

Assessment: Assess for hypersensitivity to drug, hypocalcemia or other disorders affecting mineral metabolism, pregnancy/nursing status, and possible drug interactions. Consider skin testing for patients with suspected hypersensitivity to drug. Perform baseline nasal exam.

Monitoring: Monitor for signs/symptoms of hypersensitivity reactions, hypocalcemia, nasal adverse reactions, malignancy, antibody formation, and other adverse reactions. Perform nasal exams periodically during therapy and at any time nasal symptoms occur. Perform periodic exams of urine sediment. Periodically reevaluate the need for continued therapy.

Counseling: Instruct on pump assembly, priming of the pump, and nasal introduction of medication. Advise to notify physician if significant nasal irritation develops. Inform of the potential increase in risk of malignancy. Advise to maintain an adequate Ca^{2+} and vitamin D intake. Instruct to seek emergency medical help if any signs/symptoms of a serious allergic reaction develop.

STORAGE: Unopened: 2-8°C (36-46°F). Protect from freezing. Opened: 20-25°C (68-77°F); excursions permitted to 15-30°C (59-86°F). Discard after 30 doses have been used.

FOSAMAX PLUS D – alendronate sodium/cholecalciferol

RX

Class: Bisphosphonate/vitamin D analogue

ADULT DOSAGE

Osteoporosis

Treatment of Osteoporosis in Postmenopausal Women/Treatment to Increase Bone Mass in Men w/ Osteoporosis:

1 tab (70mg/2800 IU or 70mg/5600 IU) once weekly

For most osteoporotic women/men, appropriate dose is 70mg/5600 IU once weekly

Missed Dose

If once-weekly dose is missed, administer 1 tab on am after patient remembers; do not take 2 tabs on same day, but return to taking 1 tab once a week, as originally scheduled on chosen day

PEDIATRIC DOSAGE

Pediatric use may not have been established

DOSING CONSIDERATIONS

Renal Impairment

CrCl <35mL/min: Not recommended

ADMINISTRATION

Oral route

Take upon arising for the day

Swallow tabs w/ full glass of water (6-8 oz); do not chew or suck on the tab

Take at least 1/2 hr before the 1st food, beverage, or medication of the day w/ plain water only

Do not lie down for at least 30 min and until after 1st food of the day

HOW SUPPLIED

Tab: (Alendronate/Cholecalciferol) 70mg/2800 IU, 70mg/5600 IU

CONTRAINDICATIONS

Esophageal abnormalities that delay esophageal emptying (eg, stricture, achalasia), inability to stand or sit upright for at least 30 min, hypocalcemia. Hypersensitivity to any component of this product.

WARNINGS/PRECAUTIONS

Do not use alone to treat vitamin D deficiency. Consider discontinuation after 3-5 yrs of use in patients at low-risk for fracture; periodically reevaluate risk for fracture in patients who d/c therapy. May cause local irritation of the upper GI mucosa; caution w/ active upper GI problems (eg, Barrett's esophagus, dysphagia, other esophageal diseases, gastritis, duodenitis, ulcers). Esophageal reactions (eg, esophagitis, esophageal ulcers/erosions) reported; d/c and seek medical attention if dysphagia, odynophagia, retrosternal pain, or new/worsening heartburn develops. Use under appropriate supervision in patients who cannot comply w/ dosing instructions due to mental disability. Gastric and duodenal ulcers reported. Treat hypocalcemia or other disorders affecting mineral metabolism (eg, vitamin D deficiency) prior to therapy. Asymptomatic decreases in serum Ca^{2+} and phosphate may occur. Severe and occasionally incapacitating bone, joint, and/or muscle pain reported; d/c if severe symptoms develop. Osteonecrosis of the jaw (ONJ) reported; risk may increase w/ duration of exposure to drug. If invasive dental procedures are required, discontinuation of treatment may reduce risk for ONJ. Consider discontinuation if ONJ develops. Atypical, low-energy, or low trauma fractures of the femoral shaft reported; evaluate any patient w/ a history of bisphosphonate exposure who presents w/ thigh/groin pain to rule out incomplete femur fracture, and consider interruption of therapy. Vitamin D3 supplementation may worsen hypercalcemia and/or hypercalciuria in patients w/ diseases associated w/ unregulated overproduction of 1,25-dihydroxyvitamin D (eg, leukemia, lymphoma, sarcoidosis).

ADVERSE REACTIONS

Abdominal pain, musculoskeletal pain, nausea, dyspepsia, constipation, diarrhea.

DRUG INTERACTIONS

Ca^{2+} supplements, antacids, or oral medications containing multivalent cations will interfere w/ absorption of alendronate; wait at least 1/2 hr after dosing before taking any other oral medications. NSAID use is associated w/ GI irritation; use w/ caution. Alendronate: Increased incidence of upper GI adverse events in patients receiving concomitant therapy w/ daily doses of alendronate >10mg and aspirin-containing products. Cholecalciferol: Olestra, mineral oils, orlistat, and bile acid sequestrants (eg, cholestyramine, colestipol) may impair absorption; consider additional supplementation. Anticonvulsants, cimetidine, and thiazides may increase catabolism; consider additional supplementation.

PATIENT CONSIDERATIONS

Assessment: Assess for esophageal abnormalities, ability to stand or sit upright for at least 30 min, hypocalcemia, risk for ONJ, active upper GI problems, mental disability, renal impairment, drug hypersensitivity, any other conditions where treatment is contraindicated or cautioned, pregnancy/nursing status, and possible drug interactions.

Monitoring: Monitor for signs/symptoms of ONJ, atypical fractures, esophageal reactions, musculoskeletal pain, hypocalcemia, and other adverse events. Monitor urine and serum Ca^{2+} in patients w/ diseases associated w/ unregulated overproduction of 1,25-dihydroxyvitamin D. Periodically reevaluate the need for continued therapy.

Counseling: Instruct to take supplemental Ca^{2+} and vitamin D if dietary intake is inadequate. Counsel to consider weight-bearing exercise along w/ the modification of certain behavioral factors (eg, cigarette smoking, excessive alcohol consumption), if these factors exist. Instruct to take upon arising for the day and at least 1/2 hr before the 1st food, beverage, or other medication of the day w/ plain water only; advise to swallow tab w/ 6-8 oz of water. Advise to avoid lying down for at least 30 min after taking the drug and until after 1st food of the day. Instruct to follow all dosing instructions and inform that failure to follow them may increase risk of esophageal problems. Advise to d/c and consult physician if symptoms of esophageal disease develop. Instruct that if a once-weekly dose is missed, to take 1 dose on the am after patient remembers and to return to taking 1 dose once a week, as originally scheduled on patient's chosen day; instruct not to take 2 doses on the same day.

STORAGE: 20-25°C (68-77°F); excursions permitted to 15-30°C (59-86°F). Protect from moisture and light.

FOSINOPRIL – fosinopril sodium

RX

Class: ACE inhibitor

May cause injury and even death to the developing fetus during the 2nd and 3rd trimesters of pregnancy. D/C when pregnancy is detected.

OTHER BRAND NAMES

Monopril (Discontinued)

ADULT DOSAGE

Hypertension

Initial: 10mg qd
Titrate: May adjust dosage based on BP response
Usual: 20-40mg qd

Divide daily dose if trough response is inadequate
Diuretic may be added if BP is not adequately controlled with therapy alone

Currently Treated w/ Diuretic:
D/C diuretic 2-3 days prior to initiating therapy, if possible. May resume diuretic therapy if BP is not controlled w/ therapy alone
Initial: 10mg qd w/ careful monitoring until BP is stabilized

Heart Failure

Adjunct to Diuretics w/ or w/o Digitalis:
Initial: 10mg qd
Titrate: Increase over several weeks as tolerated
Usual: 20-40mg qd
Max: 40mg qd

PEDIATRIC DOSAGE

Hypertension

≥6 Years:
>50kg: 5-10mg qd

DOSING CONSIDERATIONS

Renal Impairment

HF:

Moderate to Severe Renal Failure/Vigorous Diuresis:

Initial: 5mg

Elderly

Start at lower end of dosing range

ADMINISTRATION

Oral route

HOW SUPPLIED

Tab: 10mg*, 20mg, 40mg *scored

CONTRAINDICATIONS

F

Hypersensitivity to this product or to any other ACE inhibitor (eg, angioedema).

WARNINGS/PRECAUTIONS

Head and neck angioedema reported; d/c and administer appropriate therapy if laryngeal stridor or angioedema of the face, lips, tongue, mucous membranes, glottis, or extremities occurs. More reports of angioedema in blacks than nonblacks. Intestinal angioedema reported; monitor for abdominal pain. Anaphylactoid reactions reported during desensitization with hymenoptera venom, dialysis with high-flux membranes, and LDL apheresis with dextran sulfate absorption. Symptomatic hypotension may occur, most likely in patients with volume and/or salt depletion; correct depletion prior to therapy. Excessive hypotension associated with oliguria, azotemia, and rarely acute renal failure and death may occur in patients with HF, with or without associated renal insufficiency; monitor closely during the first 2 weeks of treatment and whenever dose of therapy or diuretic is increased. May cause agranulocytosis and bone marrow depression; consider monitoring of WBC in patients with collagen-vascular disease, especially with renal impairment. Rarely, associated with syndrome that starts with cholestatic jaundice and progresses to fulminant hepatic necrosis and sometimes death; d/c if jaundice or marked elevation of hepatic enzymes occur. May cause renal function changes. May increase BUN and SrCr levels with renal artery stenosis or with no preexisting renal vascular disease; may need to reduce dose of therapy and/or d/c diuretic. Hyperkalemia reported; risk factors include diabetes mellitus (DM) and renal insufficiency. Hypotension may occur with surgery or during anesthesia. Persistent nonproductive cough reported. Caution in elderly.

ADVERSE REACTIONS

Dizziness, cough, hypotension, musculoskeletal pain.

DRUG INTERACTIONS

May increase lithium levels and symptoms of lithium toxicity; frequently monitor serum lithium levels. Hypotension risk with diuretics. Increased risk of hyperkalemia with K^+-sparing diuretics (eg, spironolactone, amiloride, triamterene), K^+-containing salt substitutes, or K^+ supplements; use with caution. Antacids may impair absorption; separate doses by 2 hrs. Nitritoid reactions reported rarely with injectable gold (sodium aurothiomalate).

PATIENT CONSIDERATIONS

Assessment: Assess for history of angioedema, hypersensitivity to drug, volume/salt depletion, collagen vascular disease, DM, renal artery stenosis, HF, renal impairment, pregnancy/nursing status, and possible drug interactions.

Monitoring: Monitor for signs/symptoms of hypotension, anaphylactoid or hypersensitivity reactions, head/neck/intestinal angioedema, agranulocytosis, neutropenia, bone marrow depression, hyperkalemia, and other adverse reactions. Monitor BP and renal/hepatic function. Consider monitoring WBCs in patients with collagen vascular disease, especially if with renal impairment.

Counseling: Instruct to d/c therapy and immediately report signs/symptoms of angioedema. Caution about lightheadedness, especially during the 1st few days of therapy; advise to d/c therapy and consult physician if syncope occurs. Caution that inadequate fluid intake or excessive perspiration, diarrhea, or vomiting may lead to an excessive fall in BP resulting in lightheadedness or syncope. Instruct to avoid using K^+ supplements or salt substitutes-containing K^+ without consulting physician. Advise to report any symptoms of infection. Inform of pregnancy risks during the 2nd or 3rd trimesters and instruct to report to physician as soon as possible if pregnant.

STORAGE: 20-25°C (68-77°F). Protect from moisture.

FOSINOPRIL/HCTZ – fosinopril sodium/hydrochlorothiazide

RX

Class: ACE inhibitor/thiazide diuretic

D/C when pregnancy is detected. Drugs that act directly on the renin-angiotensin system (RAS) can cause injury/death to developing fetus.

OTHER BRAND NAMES
Monopril-HCT (Discontinued)

ADULT DOSAGE

Hypertension

Not Controlled w/ Fosinopril/HCTZ Monotherapy:
10mg/12.5mg tab or 20mg/12.5mg tab qd
Titrate: Dosage must be guided by clinical response

PEDIATRIC DOSAGE
Pediatric use may not have been established

DOSING CONSIDERATIONS

Elderly
Start at lower end of dosing range

ADMINISTRATION
Oral route

HOW SUPPLIED
Tab: (Fosinopril/HCTZ) 10mg/12.5mg, 20mg/12.5mg* *scored

CONTRAINDICATIONS
Anuria; hypersensitivity to fosinopril, to any other ACE inhibitor, to hydrochlorothiazide, or other sulfonamide-derived drugs, or any other ingredient or component in the formulation.

WARNINGS/PRECAUTIONS
Not indicated for initial therapy. Caution in elderly and with severe renal disease. Avoid if CrCl <30mL/min. Caution with impaired hepatic function or progressive liver disease; may precipitate hepatic coma. Fosinopril: Angioedema reported; d/c and administer appropriate therapy if laryngeal stridor or angioedema of the face, tongue, or glottis occurs. Higher rate of angioedema in blacks than nonblacks. Intestinal angioedema reported; monitor for abdominal pain. Anaphylactoid reactions reported during desensitization with hymenoptera venom, dialysis with high-flux membranes, and LDL apheresis with dextran sulfate absorption. Symptomatic hypotension may occur, most likely in patients with volume and/or salt depletion; correct volume and/or salt depletion prior to therapy. Excessive hypotension associated with oliguria, azotemia, and rarely acute renal failure and/or death may occur in patients with CHF; monitor closely during the first 2 weeks of treatment and when dose is increased. May cause changes in renal function. May increase BUN and SrCr levels with renal artery stenosis and with no preexisting renal vascular disease; monitor renal function during 1st few weeks of therapy in patients with renal artery stenosis. May cause agranulocytosis and bone marrow depression; consider monitoring of WBCs in patients with collagen vascular disease and renal disease. Rarely, associated with syndrome that starts with cholestatic jaundice and progresses to fulminant necrosis and sometimes death; d/c if jaundice or marked hepatic enzyme elevations occur. Hyperkalemia and persistent nonproductive cough reported. Hypotension may occur with surgery or during anesthesia. HCTZ: May precipitate azotemia with severe renal disease. May exacerbate or activate systemic lupus erythematosus (SLE). Dilutional hyponatremia may occur in edematous patients; institute appropriate therapy of water restriction rather than salt administration, except for life-threatening hyponatremia. May increase cholesterol, TGs, uric acid levels, and decrease glucose tolerance. Hyponatremia, hypokalemia, and hypochloremic alkalosis reported. Hypokalemia may sensitize or exaggerate the response of the heart to toxic effects of digitalis. Pathological changes in the parathyroid glands, with hypercalcemia and hypophosphatemia observed with prolonged therapy. May enhance effects in postsympathectomy patients. Neutropenia/agranulocytosis reported. Lab test interactions may occur.

ADVERSE REACTIONS
Headache, cough, fatigue, dizziness.

DRUG INTERACTIONS
Dual blockade of the RAS is associated with increased risks of hypotension, hyperkalemia, and changes in renal function (including acute renal failure); closely monitor BP, renal function, and electrolytes with concomitant agents that also affect the RAS. Avoid concomitant use of aliskiren in patients with diabetes and with renal impairment (GFR <60mL/min). Increased risk of hyperkalemia with K^+-sparing diuretics, K^+ supplements, or K^+-containing salt substitutes; use with caution and monitor serum K+ frequently. Caution with other antihypertensives. May alter insulin requirements in diabetic patients. May increase lithium levels and risk of toxicity; use with caution and monitor serum lithium levels frequently. Nitritoid reactions reported rarely with injectable gold (eg, sodium aurothiomalate). Fosinopril: Antacids (aluminum hydroxide, magnesium hydroxide, simethicone) may impair absorption; separate doses by 2 hrs. HCTZ: May potentiate action of other antihypertensives, especially ganglionic or peripheral adrenergic-blocking drugs. May decrease effectiveness of methenamine. May increase responsiveness to tubocurarine. May decrease arterial responsiveness to norepinephrine. NSAIDs may decrease diuretic, natriuretic, and antihypertensive effects. Cholestyramine or colestipol resins reduce absorption. Increased risk of hypokalemia with corticosteroids and adrenocorticotropic hormone.

PATIENT CONSIDERATIONS

Assessment: Assess for anuria, history of allergy or bronchial asthma, hypersensitivity to drug or to sulfonamides, volume/salt depletion, CHF, SLE, renal/hepatic function, collagen vascular disease, risk factors for hyperkalemia, pregnancy/nursing status, and possible drug interactions.

Monitoring: Monitor for signs/symptoms of angioedema, agranulocytosis, anaphylactoid/hypersensitivity reactions, hypotension, exacerbation/activation of SLE, and other adverse reactions. Monitor BP, serum electrolytes, serum uric acid levels, hepatic/renal function, cholesterol/TG levels, and glucose tolerance. Monitor WBCs in patients with collagen vascular disease and renal impairment.

Counseling: Inform females of childbearing age of the consequences of exposure during pregnancy and of the treatment options for women planning to become pregnant; report pregnancy to physician as soon as possible. Instruct to d/c therapy and immediately report signs/symptoms of angioedema (eg, swelling of face, eyes, lips, tongue, difficulty breathing). Caution that lightheadedness can occur, especially during the 1st days of therapy and advise to report to physician; instruct to d/c therapy and consult physician if syncope occurs. Caution that inadequate fluid intake, excessive perspiration, diarrhea, or vomiting can lead to excessive fall in BP, resulting in lightheadedness or syncope. Instruct not to use salt substitutes containing K^+ or K^+ supplements without consulting physician. Instruct to promptly report any indication of infection (eg, sore throat, fever).

STORAGE: 20-25°C (68-77°F). Protect from moisture.

FROVA – frovatriptan succinate

RX

Class: 5-$HT_{1B/1D}$ agonist (triptans)

ADULT DOSAGE

Migraine

W/ or w/o Aura:
2.5mg w/ fluids
May administer 2nd dose 2 hrs after 1st dose if migraine recurs after initial relief
Max: 7.5mg/day
Safety of treating >4 migraines/30 days not known

PEDIATRIC DOSAGE

Pediatric use may not have been established

ADMINISTRATION

Oral route

HOW SUPPLIED

Tab: 2.5mg

CONTRAINDICATIONS

Ischemic coronary artery disease (CAD) (eg, angina pectoris, history of MI, or documented silent ischemia), or coronary artery vasospasm, including Prinzmetal's angina; Wolff-Parkinson-White syndrome or arrhythmias associated w/ other cardiac accessory conduction pathway disorders; history of stroke, transient ischemic attack, or history of hemiplegic or basilar migraine; peripheral vascular disease; ischemic bowel disease; uncontrolled HTN; recent use (w/in 24 hours) of another 5-HT1 agonist or an ergotamine containing or ergot-type medication (eg, dihydroergotamine or methysergide); hypersensitivity to frovatriptan succinate.

WARNINGS/PRECAUTIONS

Use only if a clear diagnosis of migraine has been established. If no treatment response for the 1st migraine attack, reconsider diagnosis before treating any subsequent attacks. Not indicated for prevention of migraine attacks. Serious cardiac adverse reactions, including acute MI, reported. May cause coronary artery vasospasm (Prinzmetal's angina). Perform cardiovascular (CV) evaluation in triptan-naive patients who have multiple CV risk factors prior to therapy; consider administering 1st dose in a medically supervised setting and perform ECG immediately following administration in patients with a negative CV evaluation. Consider periodic CV evaluation in intermittent long-term users who have CV risk factors. Life-threatening cardiac rhythm disturbances (eg, ventricular tachycardia/fibrillation leading to death) reported; d/c if these occur. Sensations of pain, tightness, pressure, and heaviness reported in the chest, throat, neck, and jaw after treatment and are usually noncardiac in origin; perform a cardiac evaluation if at high cardiac risk. Cerebral/subarachnoid hemorrhage, stroke, and other cerebrovascular events reported. Care should be taken to exclude other potentially serious neurological conditions before treatment. May cause noncoronary vasospastic reactions (eg, peripheral vascular ischemia, GI vascular ischemia and infarction [presenting with abdominal pain and bloody diarrhea], splenic infarction, Raynaud's syndrome); rule out vasospastic reaction before using if experiencing signs/symptoms suggestive of noncoronary vasospasm reaction. Transient and permanent blindness and significant partial vision loss reported. Overuse of acute migraine drugs may lead to exacerbation of headache (medication overuse headache); detoxification, including withdrawal of the overused drugs, and treatment of withdrawal symptoms may be necessary. Serotonin syndrome may occur; d/c if serotonin syndrome is suspected. Significant elevation in BP, including hypertensive crisis with acute impairment of organ systems, reported; monitor BP. Anaphylaxis, anaphylactoid, and hypersensitivity reactions including angioedema reported; more likely to occur in patients with history of sensitivity to multiple allergens. Caution with severe hepatic impairment.

ADVERSE REACTIONS

Dizziness, fatigue, headache, paresthesia, flushing, dry mouth, hot or cold sensation, skeletal pain.

DRUG INTERACTIONS

See Contraindications. Serotonin syndrome reported with SSRIs, SNRIs, TCAs, and MAOIs.

PATIENT CONSIDERATIONS

Assessment: Assess for ischemic CAD, coronary artery vasospasm, uncontrolled HTN, neurological conditions, hepatic impairment, history of sensitivity to multiple allergens, drug hypersensitivity, any conditions where treatment is cautioned or contraindicated, pregnancy/nursing status, and possible drug interactions. Perform CV evaluation in triptan-naive patients prior to therapy who have multiple CV risk factors.

Monitoring: Monitor for cardiac adverse reactions, coronary artery vasospasm, cardiac rhythm disturbances, cerebrovascular events, noncoronary vasospastic reactions, serotonin syndrome, BP elevation, exacerbation of headache, anaphylactic/hypersensitivity reactions, ophthalmic changes, and other adverse events. Consider periodic CV evaluation in intermittent long-term users who have CV risk factors. Perform ECG immediately following administration in patients with a negative CV evaluation.

Counseling: Inform that drug may cause serious CV side effects, to be alert for the signs/symptoms of chest pain, SOB, weakness, and slurring of speech, and to ask for medical advice when observing any indicative signs/symptoms. Inform that anaphylactic/anaphylactoid reactions have occurred and that they are more likely to occur in patients with history of sensitivity to multiple allergens. Inform that overuse (≥10 days/month) may lead to exacerbation of headache; encourage to record headache frequency and drug use. Caution about the risk of serotonin syndrome. Advise to notify physician if pregnant/nursing or planning to become pregnant.

STORAGE: 25°C (77°F); excursions permitted to 15-30°C (59-86°F). Protect from moisture.

FULYZAQ – crofelemer

RX

Class: Antidiarrheal

ADULT DOSAGE

Noninfectious Diarrhea

Symptomatic Relief in Patients w/ HIV/AIDS on Antiretroviral Therapy

125mg bid

PEDIATRIC DOSAGE

Pediatric use may not have been established

ADMINISTRATION

Oral route

Take w/ or w/o food

Swallow whole; do not crush or chew

HOW SUPPLIED

Tab, Delayed-Release: 125mg

WARNINGS/PRECAUTIONS

Not indicated for the treatment of infectious diarrhea; rule out infectious etiologies of diarrhea before initiating therapy.

ADVERSE REACTIONS

URTI, bronchitis, cough, flatulence, increased bilirubin.

PATIENT CONSIDERATIONS

Assessment: Assess etiology of diarrhea and pregnancy/nursing status.

Monitoring: Monitor for adverse reactions.

Counseling: Instruct to take ud.

STORAGE: 20-25°C (68-77°F); excursions permitted between 15-30°C (59-86°F).

FUROSEMIDE — furosemide

RX

Class: Loop diuretic

OTHER BRAND NAMES

Lasix

ADULT DOSAGE

Edema

Associated w/ CHF, Liver Cirrhosis, and Renal Disease (Nephrotic Syndrome):

Oral:

Initial: 20-80mg as a single dose

Titrate: May repeat the same dose if needed or increase dose by 20mg or 40mg. Give dose no sooner than 6-8 hrs after the previous dose until desired diuretic effect has been obtained; give individually determined single dose qd or bid

Severe Edematous States: May carefully titrate dose up to 600mg/day

Consider giving on 2-4 consecutive days each week

Closely monitor when exceeding 80mg/day for prolonged periods

Inj:

Initial: 20-40mg as a single dose IV/IM; give IV dose slowly (1-2 min)

Titrate: May repeat the same dose if needed or increase by 20mg no sooner than 2 hrs after the previous dose; give individually determined single dose qd or bid

Closely monitor when given for prolonged periods

Hypertension

Oral:

Initial: 40mg bid

Titrate: Adjust dose according to response

Add other antihypertensive agents if response is not satisfactory

Acute Pulmonary Edema

Inj:

Initial: 40mg IV slowly (over 1-2 min)

Titrate: May increase to 80mg IV slowly (over 1-2 min), if satisfactory response does not occur w/in 1 hr

Additional therapy (eg, digitalis, oxygen) may be administered concomitantly if necessary

PEDIATRIC DOSAGE

Edema

Associated w/ CHF, Liver Cirrhosis, and Renal Disease (Nephrotic Syndrome):

Oral:

Initial: 2mg/kg as a single dose

Titrate: May increase by 1 or 2mg/kg no sooner than 6-8 hrs after the previous dose, if diuretic response is not satisfactory after the initial dose

Maint: Adjust to the minimum effective level

Max: 6mg/kg

Inj:

Initial: 1mg/kg IV/IM

Titrate: If response is not satisfactory, may increase by 1mg/kg no sooner than 2 hrs after the previous dose, until the desired diuretic effect has been obtained

Max: 6mg/kg

Premature Infants: Max: 1mg/kg/day

DOSING CONSIDERATIONS

Elderly

Oral/Inj:

Start at lower end of dosing range

Concomitant Medications

Antihypertensives:

Oral:

Reduce dose of other agents by at least 50%

May further reduce dose or d/c therapy of other antihypertensive drugs as BP falls

ADMINISTRATION

Oral/IV/IM route

IV

Add furosemide inj to NaCl inj, D5, or lactated Ringer's inj after pH has been adjusted to above 5.5. Administer as a controlled IV infusion at a rate no greater than 4mg/min.

Care must be taken to ensure that the pH of the prepared infusion sol is in the weakly alkaline to neutral range.

Acid sol, including other parenteral medications (eg, labetalol, ciprofloxacin, amrinone, milrinone), must not be administered concurrently in the same infusion because they may cause precipitation of the furosemide; furosemide inj should not be added to a running IV line containing any of these acidic products.

HOW SUPPLIED

Inj: 10mg/mL [2mL, 4mL, 10mL]; **Sol:** 10mg/mL [60mL, 120mL], 40mg/5mL [500mL]; **Tab:** (Lasix) 20mg, 40mg*, 80mg *scored

CONTRAINDICATIONS

Anuria. History of hypersensitivity to furosemide.

WARNINGS/PRECAUTIONS

May lead to profound diuresis w/ water and electrolyte depletion if given in excessive amounts; careful medical supervision required and dose and dose schedule must be adjusted to individual patient's needs. Initiate therapy in hospital w/ hepatic cirrhosis and ascites. Do not institute therapy until basic condition is improved in patients w/ hepatic coma and in states of electrolyte depletion. D/C if increasing azotemia and oliguria occur during treatment of severe progressive renal disease. Tinnitus, reversible or irreversible hearing impairment, and deafness reported. Ototoxicity is associated w/ rapid inj, severe renal impairment, use of higher than recommended doses, hypoproteinemia, or concomitant use w/ aminoglycoside antibiotics, ethacrynic acid, or other ototoxic drugs; control IV infusion rate if using high-dose parenteral therapy. Excessive diuresis may cause dehydration, blood volume reduction w/ circulatory collapse, vascular thrombosis, and embolism, particularly in elderly. Monitor for fluid/electrolyte imbalance (hyponatremia, hypochloremic alkalosis, hypokalemia, hypomagnesemia, or hypocalcemia), liver/kidney damage, blood dyscrasias, or other idiosyncratic reactions. Increases in blood glucose and alterations in glucose tolerance tests, and rarely, precipitation of diabetes mellitus (DM) reported. May cause acute urinary retention in patients w/ severe symptoms of urinary retention; monitor carefully, especially during the initial stages of treatment. May lead to a higher incidence of deterioration in renal function after receiving radiocontrast in patients at high risk for radiocontrast nephropathy. May potentiate ototoxicity and effect of therapy may be weakened in patients w/ hypoproteinemia. Asymptomatic hyperuricemia may occur and gout may rarely be precipitated. Caution in patients w/ sulfonamide allergy. May activate/exacerbate systemic lupus erythematosus (SLE). May precipitate nephrocalcinosis/nephrolithiasis in premature infants and children <4 yrs of age w/ no history of prematurity; monitor renal function and consider renal ultrasonography. May increase risk of persistence of patent ductus arteriosus if administered to premature infants during the 1st weeks of life. Caution in elderly. (Inj) Use only in patients unable to take oral medication or in emergency situations; replace w/ oral therapy as soon as practical. Premature infants w/ post conceptual age (gestational plus postnatal) <31 weeks receiving doses >1mg/kg/24 hrs may develop plasma levels which could be associated w/ potential toxic effects. May cause hearing loss in neonates.

ADVERSE REACTIONS

Pancreatitis, jaundice, increased liver enzymes, anorexia, severe anaphylactic/anaphylactoid reactions, systemic vasculitis, tinnitus/hearing loss, paresthesias, aplastic anemia, thrombocytopenia, toxic epidermal necrolysis, orthostatic hypotension, hyperglycemia.

DRUG INTERACTIONS

See Dosing Considerations. May increase ototoxic potential of aminoglycoside antibiotics, especially in the presence of impaired renal function; avoid this combination, except in life-threatening situations. Avoid w/ ethacrynic acid and lithium. Patients receiving high doses of salicylates concomitantly w/ furosemide may experience salicylate toxicity at lower doses because of competitive renal excretory sites. Risk of ototoxic effects if given concomitantly w/ cisplatin. Nephrotoxicity of nephrotoxic drugs such as cisplatin may be enhanced if furosemide is not given in lower doses and w/ positive fluid balance when used to achieve forced diuresis during cisplatin treatment. May antagonize skeletal muscle relaxing effect of tubocurarine. May potentiate action of succinylcholine. Concomitant use w/ ACE inhibitors or ARBs may lead to severe hypotension and deterioration in renal function, including renal failure; an interruption or reduction in the dosage of furosemide, ACE inhibitors, or ARBs may be necessary. Potentiation occurs w/ ganglionic or peripheral adrenergic blockers. May decrease arterial responsiveness to norepinephrine. Reduced CrCl in patients w/ chronic renal insufficiency w/ acetylsalicylic acid. Increased BUN, SrCr, and K^+ levels, and weight gain reported w/ NSAIDs. Hypokalemia may develop w/ adrenocorticotropic hormone and corticosteroids. Reduced natriuretic and antihypertensive effects w/ indomethacin. Indomethacin may affect plasma renin levels, aldosterone excretion, and renin profile evaluation. Digitalis may exaggerate metabolic effects of hypokalemia. Avoid w/ chloral hydrate. Phenytoin interferes w/ renal action of furosemide. Methotrexate and other drugs that undergo significant renal tubular secretion may reduce the effect of furosemide. May decrease renal elimination of other drugs that undergo tubular secretion; high-dose treatment of both furosemide and these other drugs may result in elevated serum levels of these drugs and may potentiate their toxicity as well as the toxicity of furosemide. May increase the risk of cephalosporin-induced nephrotoxicity. Increased risk of gouty arthritis w/ cyclosporine. (Inj/Tab) Hypokalemia may develop w/ licorice in large amounts or w/ prolonged use of laxatives. (Tab/Sol) Reduced natriuretic and antihypertensive effects w/ sucralfate; separate intake by at least 2 hrs. Phenytoin may decrease levels. (Inj) May add to or potentiate the therapeutic effect of other antihypertensive drugs.

PATIENT CONSIDERATIONS

Assessment: Assess for anuria, sulfonamide/drug hypersensitivity, SLE, hepatic/renal impairment, hypoproteinemia, pregnancy/nursing status, and possible drug interactions.

Monitoring: Monitor for signs/symptoms of fluid/electrolyte imbalance, blood dyscrasias, hyperglycemia, hyperuricemia, precipitation of gout or DM, ototoxicity, dehydration, activation or exacerbation of SLE, blood volume reduction w/ circulatory collapse, vascular thrombosis and embolism, liver or kidney damage, and other adverse reactions. Monitor serum electrolytes, carbon dioxide, creatinine, and BUN frequently during 1st few months of therapy, then periodically thereafter. Monitor urine and blood glucose periodically in diabetics. Periodically monitor Mg^{2+} and Ca^{2+} levels. Monitor renal function and perform renal ultrasonography in pediatric patients. Carefully monitor patients w/ severe symptoms of urinary retention, especially during the initial stages of treatment.

G

Counseling: Advise that patient may experience symptoms from excessive fluid and/or electrolyte losses. Advise that postural hypotension can be managed by getting up slowly. Inform patients w/ DM that drug may increase blood glucose levels and affect urine glucose tests. Advise that skin may be more sensitive to sunlight during therapy. Advise hypertensive patients to avoid medications that may increase BP, including OTC products for appetite suppression and cold symptoms.

STORAGE: Protect from light. (Inj/Sol) 20-25°C (68-77°F). (Lasix) 25°C (77°F); excursions permitted to 15-30°C (59-86°F).

GARDASIL — human papillomavirus quadrivalent (types 6, 11, 16, and 18) vaccine, recombinant

RX

Class: Vaccine

ADULT DOSAGE

Human Papillomavirus

Vaccination of girls and women 9-26 yrs of age for the prevention of cervical, vulvar, vaginal, and anal cancer caused by human papillomavirus (HPV) types 16 and 18; genital warts (condyloma acuminata) caused by HPV types 6 and 11; and cervical intraepithelial neoplasia (CIN) grade 2/3 and cervical adenocarcinoma in situ, CIN grade 1, vulvar intraepithelial neoplasia grades 2 and 3, vaginal intraepithelial neoplasia grades 2 and 3, and anal intraepithelial neoplasia (AIN) grades 1, 2, and 3 caused by HPV types 6, 11, 16, and 18. Vaccination of boys and men 9-26 yrs of age for the prevention of anal cancer caused by HPV types 16 and 18; genital warts (condyloma acuminata) caused by HPV types 6 and 11; and AIN grades 1, 2, and 3 caused by HPV types 6, 11, 16, and 18

9-26 Years:

0.5mL dose at the following schedule: 0, 2, and 6 months

PEDIATRIC DOSAGE

Human Papillomavirus

Vaccination of girls and women 9-26 yrs of age for the prevention of cervical, vulvar, vaginal, and anal cancer caused by human papillomavirus (HPV) types 16 and 18; genital warts (condyloma acuminata) caused by HPV types 6 and 11; and cervical intraepithelial neoplasia (CIN) grade 2/3 and cervical adenocarcinoma in situ, CIN grade 1, vulvar intraepithelial neoplasia grades 2 and 3, vaginal intraepithelial neoplasia grades 2 and 3, and anal intraepithelial neoplasia (AIN) grades 1, 2, and 3 caused by HPV types 6, 11, 16, and 18. Vaccination of boys and men 9-26 yrs of age for the prevention of anal cancer caused by HPV types 16 and 18; genital warts (condyloma acuminata) caused by HPV types 6 and 11; and AIN grades 1, 2, and 3 caused by HPV types 6, 11, 16, and 18

9-26 Years:

0.5mL dose at the following schedule: 0, 2, and 6 months

ADMINISTRATION

IM route

Shake well before use

Administer in the deltoid region of the upper arm or in the higher anterolateral area of the thigh

Do not dilute or mix w/ other vaccines

Administer as soon as possible after being removed from refrigeration; can be out of refrigeration (≤25°C [77°F]) for a total time of not more than 72 hrs

Single-Dose Vial

Withdraw the 0.5mL dose of vaccine using a sterile needle and syringe and use promptly

Prefilled Syringe

Attach needle by twisting in clockwise direction until needle fits securely on syringe; administer entire dose as per standard protocol

HOW SUPPLIED

Inj: 0.5mL [prefilled syringe, vial]

CONTRAINDICATIONS

Hypersensitivity to Gardasil or any of its components (eg, severe allergic reactions to yeast), or after a previous dose of Gardasil.

WARNINGS/PRECAUTIONS

Syncope may occur; observe for 15 min after administration. Appropriate medical treatment and supervision must be readily available in case of anaphylactic reactions. Women should continue to undergo cervical cancer screening. Recipients should not d/c anal cancer screening if it has been recommended by healthcare provider. Does not protect against disease from vaccine and non-vaccine HPV types to which a person has previously been exposed through sexual activity. Not intended for treatment of active external genital lesions; cervical, vulvar, vaginal, and anal cancers; CIN; VIN; VaIN; or AIN. Vaccination may not result in protection in all vaccine recipients. Response to vaccine may be diminished in immunocompromised individuals.

ADVERSE REACTIONS

Inj-site pain/swelling/erythema/pruritus, pyrexia, nausea, dizziness, diarrhea, headache.

DRUG INTERACTIONS

Immunosuppressive therapies, including irradiation, antimetabolites, alkylating agents, cytotoxic drugs, and corticosteroids (used in greater than physiologic doses), may reduce the immune responses to vaccines.

PATIENT CONSIDERATIONS

Assessment: Assess for hypersensitivity to yeast or the vaccine, immunocompromised conditions, pregnancy/nursing status, and possible drug interactions.

Monitoring: Monitor for syncope, anaphylactic reactions, and other adverse reactions.

Counseling: Inform about benefits and risks associated w/ vaccine. Instruct women to continue to undergo cervical cancer screening per standard of care. Advise not to d/c anal cancer screening if recommended by physician. Inform that vaccine does not provide protection against disease from vaccine and non-vaccine HPV types to which a person has previously been exposed through sexual activity. Inform that syncope may occur following vaccination. Advise that vaccine is not recommended during pregnancy. Counsel about the importance of completing the immunization series unless contraindicated. Instruct to report any adverse reactions to physician.

STORAGE: 2-8°C (36-46°F). Do not freeze. Protect from light.

GARDASIL 9 – human papillomavirus 9-valent vaccine, recombinant RX

Class: Vaccine

ADULT DOSAGE

Human Papillomavirus

Vaccination of females 9-26 yrs of age for the prevention of cervical, vulvar, vaginal, and anal cancer caused by human papillomavirus (HPV) types 16, 18, 31, 33, 45, 52, and 58; genital warts (condyloma acuminata) caused by HPV types 6 and 11; and cervical intraepithelial neoplasia (CIN) grade 2/3 and cervical adenocarcinoma in situ, CIN grade 1, vulvar intraepithelial neoplasia (VIN) grades 2 and 3, vaginal intraepithelial neoplasia (VaIN) grades 2 and 3, and anal intraepithelial neoplasia (AIN) grades 1, 2, and 3 caused by HPV types 6, 11, 16, 18, 31, 33, 45, 52, and 58

Vaccination of males 9-26 yrs of age for the prevention of anal cancer caused by HPV types 16, 18, 31, 33, 45, 52, and 58; genital warts (condyloma acuminata) caused by HPV types 6 and 11; and AIN grades 1, 2, and 3 caused by HPV types 6, 11, 16, 18, 31, 33, 45, 52, and 58

9-26 Years:

0.5mL dose at the following schedule: 0, 2, and 6 months

PEDIATRIC DOSAGE

Human Papillomavirus

Vaccination of females 9-26 yrs of age for the prevention of cervical, vulvar, vaginal, and anal cancer caused by HPV types 16, 18, 31, 33, 45, 52, and 58; genital warts (condyloma acuminata) caused by HPV types 6 and 11; and CIN grade 2/3 and cervical adenocarcinoma in situ, CIN grade 1, VIN grades 2 and 3, VaIN grades 2 and 3, and AIN grades 1, 2, and 3 caused by HPV types 6, 11, 16, 18, 31, 33, 45, 52, and 58

Vaccination of males 9-26 yrs of age for the prevention of anal cancer caused by HPV types 16, 18, 31, 33, 45, 52, and 58; genital warts (condyloma acuminata) caused by HPV types 6 and 11; and AIN grades 1, 2, and 3 caused by HPV types 6, 11, 16, 18, 31, 33, 45, 52, and 58

9-26 Years:

0.5mL dose at the following schedule: 0, 2, and 6 months

ADMINISTRATION

IM route

Shake well before use.
Administer in the deltoid region of the upper arm or in the higher anterolateral area of the thigh.
Do not dilute or mix w/ other vaccines.
Administer as soon as possible after being removed from refrigeration; cumulative multiple excursions out of refrigeration (8-25°C [46-77°F]) or between 0-2°C (32-36°F) are permitted for a total time of not more than 72 hrs.

HOW SUPPLIED

Inj: 0.5mL [prefilled syringe, single-dose vial]

CONTRAINDICATIONS

Hypersensitivity, including severe allergic reactions to yeast (a vaccine component), or after a previous dose of this vaccine or to Gardasil.

WARNINGS/PRECAUTIONS

Women should continue to undergo cervical cancer screening per standard of care. Recipients should not d/c anal cancer screening if it has been recommended by healthcare provider. Has not been demonstrated to provide protection against disease from vaccine HPV types to which a person has previously been exposed through sexual activity. Not a treatment for external genital lesions; cervical, vulvar, vaginal, and anal cancers; CIN; VIN; VaIN; or AIN. Vaccination may not result in protection in all vaccine recipients. Syncope may occur; observe for 15 min after administration. Appropriate medical treatment and supervision must be readily available in case of anaphylactic reactions following administration. Response to vaccine may be diminished in immunocompromised individuals.

ADVERSE REACTIONS

Females 9-15 Years: Inj-site pain/swelling/erythema, headache, pyrexia, nausea.
Females 16-26 Years: Inj-site pain/swelling/erythema, headache, pyrexia, nausea, dizziness.
Males 9-15 Years: Inj-site pain/swelling/erythema, headache, pyrexia.
Males 16-26 Years: Inj-site pain/swelling/erythema, headache.

DRUG INTERACTIONS

Immunosuppressive therapies, including irradiation, antimetabolites, alkylating agents, cytotoxic drugs, and corticosteroids (used in greater than physiologic doses), may reduce the immune responses to vaccines.

PATIENT CONSIDERATIONS

Assessment: Assess for hypersensitivity to yeast or the vaccine, immunocompromised conditions, pregnancy/nursing status, and possible drug interactions.

Monitoring: Monitor for syncope, anaphylactic reactions, and other adverse reactions.

Counseling: Inform about benefits and risks associated w/ vaccine. Instruct women to continue to undergo cervical cancer screening per standard of care. Advise not to d/c anal cancer screening if recommended by healthcare provider. Inform that vaccine has not been demonstrated to provide protection against disease from vaccine and non-vaccine HPV types to which a person has previously been exposed through sexual activity. Inform that syncope may occur following vaccination. Instruct female patients to notify physician if pregnant or nursing; encourage women exposed to vaccine around time of conception or during pregnancy to register. Counsel about the importance of completing the immunization series unless contraindicated. Instruct to report any adverse reactions to physician.

STORAGE: 2-8°C (36-46°F). Do not freeze. Protect from light.

GENGRAF – cyclosporine

RX

Class: Calcineurin-inhibitor immunosuppressant

Should only be prescribed by physicians experienced in the management of systemic immunosuppressive therapy for indicated diseases. Manage patients in facilities equipped and staffed w/ adequate lab and supportive medical resources. Increased susceptibility to infection and development of neoplasia (eg, lymphoma) may result from immunosuppression. May be coadministered w/ other immunosuppressive agents in kidney, liver, and heart transplant patients. Not bioequivalent to Sandimmune and cannot be used interchangeably w/o physician supervision. Caution in switching from Sandimmune. Monitor cyclosporine blood levels in transplant and rheumatoid arthritis (RA) patients to avoid toxicity due to high levels. Dose adjustments should be made in transplant patients to minimize possible organ rejection due to low levels. (Psoriasis) Increased risk of developing skin malignancies in psoriasis patients previously treated w/ PUVA, methotrexate (MTX) or other immunosuppressive agents, UVB, coal tar, or radiation therapy. May cause systemic HTN and nephrotoxicity; risk increases w/ increasing dose and duration. Monitor for renal dysfunction, including structural kidney damage, during therapy.

ADULT DOSAGE

Organ Rejection Prophylaxis

Kidney, Liver, and Heart Allogeneic Transplants:

Newly Transplanted Patients:

Initial dose may be given 4-12 hrs prior to transplant or postoperatively; dose varies depending on transplanted organ and other immunosuppressive agents included in protocol

Suggested Initial Doses:

Renal Transplant: 9mg/kg/day ± 3mg/kg/day
Liver Transplant: 8mg/kg/day ± 4mg/kg/day
Heart Transplant: 7mg/kg/day ± 3mg/kg/day

Always administer daily dose in 2 divided doses (bid) and adjust subsequent dose to achieve a predefined cyclosporine blood concentration

Adjunct therapy w/ adrenal corticosteroids is recommended initially

Conversion from Sandimmune:

Start w/ the same daily dose as was previously used w/ Sandimmune (1:1 dose conversion); dose should subsequently be adjusted to attain the pre-conversion blood trough concentration

It is strongly recommended that the blood trough concentration be monitored every 4-7 days after conversion to Gengraf, until the blood trough concentration attains the pre-conversion value

Patients w/ Poor Absorption of Sandimmune:

Due to the increase in bioavailability of cyclosporine following conversion to Gengraf, the blood trough concentration may exceed the target range; caution when converting patients at doses >10mg/kg/day

Titrate dose individually based on trough levels, tolerability, and clinical response; measure blood trough concentrations more frequently, at least 2X a week (daily, if initial dose >10mg/kg/day) until the concentration stabilizes w/in the desired range

Has been used in combination w/ azathioprine and corticosteroids

Rheumatoid Arthritis

Severe active rheumatoid arthritis where the disease has not adequately responded to methotrexate (MTX)

Initial: 2.5mg/kg/day, taken in 2 divided doses

Titrate: May increase by 0.5-0.75mg/kg/day after 8 weeks and again after 12 weeks

Max: 4mg/kg/day

Salicylates, NSAIDs, and oral corticosteroids may be continued

D/C if no benefit is seen by 16 weeks of therapy

Combination w/ MTX:

Use same initial dose and dosage range; most patients can be treated w/ Gengraf doses of ≤3mg/kg/day when combined w/ MTX doses of up to 15mg/week

PEDIATRIC DOSAGE

Organ Rejection Prophylaxis

Kidney, Liver, and Heart Allogeneic Transplants:

Transplant recipients as young as 1 year of age have received cyclosporine (MODIFIED) w/ no unusual adverse effects

Plaque Psoriasis

In immunocompetent patients w/ severe, recalcitrant, plaque psoriasis who failed to respond to at least 1 systemic therapy (eg, PUVA, retinoids, methotrexate) or in patients for whom other systemic therapies are contraindicated, or cannot be tolerated

Initial: 2.5mg/kg/day, taken in 2 divided doses for at least 4 weeks
Titrate: If significant clinical improvement does not occur, increase the dose at 2-week intervals by approx 0.5mg/kg/day
Max: 4mg/kg/day

D/C if satisfactory response cannot be achieved after 6 weeks at 4mg/kg/day or the patient's max tolerated dose

Once a patient is adequately controlled and appears stable, the dose should be lowered, and the patient treated w/ the lowest dose that maintains an adequate response

DOSING CONSIDERATIONS

Renal Impairment
In Kidney, Liver, and Heart Transplant: Reduce dose if indicated
In Rheumatoid Arthritis/Psoriasis: Not recommended for use

Hepatic Impairment
Severe: Dose reduction may be necessary

Elderly
Start at lower end of dosing range

Adverse Reactions
Rheumatoid Arthritis/Psoriasis: Decrease dose by 25-50% at any time to control adverse events or clinically significant lab abnormalities; d/c if dose reduction is not effective in controlling abnormalities or if the adverse event or abnormality is severe

Other Important Considerations
Avoid consumption of grapefruit or grapefruit juice during therapy

ADMINISTRATION

Oral route

Always administer daily dose in 2 divided doses (bid).
Administer on a consistent schedule w/ regard to time of day and relation to meals.

Sol
To make the sol more palatable, dilute w/ room temperature orange or apple juice; avoid switching diluents frequently.

Instructions:
1. Take the prescribed amount of sol from the container using the dosing syringe supplied, and transfer the sol to a glass of orange or apple juice; use a glass container, not plastic.
2. Stir well and drink at once; do not allow diluted sol to stand before drinking.
3. Rinse the glass w/ more diluent to ensure that the total dose is consumed.
4. After use, dry the outside of the dosing syringe w/ a clean towel and store in a clean, dry place; do not rinse the dosing syringe w/ water or other cleaning agents.
5. If the syringe requires cleaning, it must be completely dry before resuming use.

HOW SUPPLIED

Cap: 25mg, 100mg, (Generic) 50mg; **Sol:** 100mg/mL [50mL]

CONTRAINDICATIONS

RA/Psoriasis: Abnormal renal function, uncontrolled HTN, malignancies. Psoriasis: Concomitant PUVA or UVB therapy, MTX or other immunosuppressants, coal tar or radiation therapy. Hypersensitivity to cyclosporine or to any components of the medication.

WARNINGS/PRECAUTIONS

Elevations in SrCr and BUN may occur and reflect a reduction in GFR; impaired renal function at any time requires close monitoring, and frequent dose adjustment may be indicated. Elevations in SrCr and BUN levels in renal transplant patients do not necessarily indicate rejection; evaluate patient before initiating dose adjustment. Thrombocytopenia and microangiopathic hemolytic anemia, resulting in graft failure reported. Significant hyperkalemia (sometimes associated w/ hyperchloremic metabolic acidosis) and hyperuricemia reported. May cause hepatotoxicity and liver injury (eg, cholestasis, jaundice, hepatitis, liver failure). Avoid excessive ultraviolet light exposure.

Oversuppression of the immune system may result in an increased risk of infection/malignancy; caution when using a treatment regimen containing multiple immunosuppressants. Increased risk of developing bacterial, viral, fungal, protozoal, and opportunistic infections (eg, polyoma virus infections). JC virus-associated progressive multifocal leukoencephalopathy and polyomavirus-associated nephropathy, especially due to BK virus infection, reported; consider reduction in immunosuppression if either develops. Convulsions and encephalopathy including posterior reversible encephalopathy syndrome, and rarely, optic disc edema, reported. HTN may occur and persist, and may require antihypertensive therapy. (Cap) Consider the alcohol content of the drug when given to patients in whom alcohol intake should be avoided or minimized (eg, pregnant or breastfeeding women, patients presenting w/ liver disease or epilepsy, alcoholic patients, pediatric patients).

ADVERSE REACTIONS

Increased susceptibility to infection, lymphoma, renal dysfunction, HTN, hirsutism, hypertrichosis, tremor, headache, gum hyperplasia, diarrhea, hypertriglyceridemia, paresthesia, hyperesthesia, influenza-like symptoms, N/V.

DRUG INTERACTIONS

See Boxed Warning, Dosing Considerations, and Contraindications. Avoid w/ K^+-sparing diuretics, aliskiren, bosentan, dabigatran, and compounds that decrease drug absorption (eg, orlistat). Vaccination may be less effective; avoid live vaccines during therapy. Caution w/ rifabutin, nephrotoxic drugs, HIV protease inhibitors, K^+-sparing drugs (eg, ACE inhibitors, ARBs), K^+-containing drugs, and K^+-rich diet. Ciprofloxacin, gentamicin, tobramycin, vancomycin, trimethoprim w/ sulfamethoxazole, melphalan, amphotericin B, ketoconazole, azapropazone, colchicine, diclofenac, naproxen, sulindac, cimetidine, ranitidine, tacrolimus, fibric acid derivatives (eg, bezafibrate, fenofibrate), MTX, and NSAIDs may potentiate renal dysfunction; closely monitor renal function and reduce dose of coadministered drug or consider alternative treatment. CYP3A4 and/or P-gp inducers/inhibitors may alter levels; adjust cyclosporine dose appropriately. Diltiazem, nicardipine, verapamil, fluconazole, itraconazole, ketoconazole, voriconazole, azithromycin, clarithromycin, erythromycin, quinupristin/dalfopristin, methylprednisolone, allopurinol, amiodarone, bromocriptine, colchicine, danazol, imatinib, metoclopramide, nefazodone, oral contraceptives, HIV protease inhibitors, grapefruit, grapefruit juice, boceprevir, and telaprevir may increase levels. St. John's wort, nafcillin, rifampin, carbamazepine, oxcarbazepine, phenobarbital, phenytoin, bosentan, octreotide, sulfinpyrazone, terbinafine, and ticlopidine may decrease levels. May increase plasma levels of bosentan, dabigatran, and substrates of CYP3A4, P-gp, or organic anion transporter proteins. May increase levels of ambrisentan; do not titrate ambrisentan dose to the recommended max daily dose when coadministering w/ cyclosporine. May reduce clearance of digoxin, colchicine, prednisolone, HMG-CoA reductase inhibitors (statins), aliskiren, bosentan, dabigatran, repaglinide, NSAIDs, sirolimus, and etoposide. Digitalis toxicity reported; monitor digoxin levels. May increase levels and enhance toxic effects of colchicine; reduce colchicine dose. Myotoxicity cases seen w/ statins; temporarily withhold or d/c statin therapy if signs of myopathy develop or w/ risk factors predisposing to severe renal injury. May increase levels of repaglinide and thereby increase the risk of hypoglycemia; closely monitor blood glucose levels. High doses of cyclosporine may increase the exposure to anthracycline antibiotics in cancer patients. May double diclofenac blood levels; dose of diclofenac should be in the lower end of the therapeutic range. May increase MTX levels and decrease levels of MTX metabolite. Increases levels of sirolimus w/ elevations of SrCr; give 4 hrs after cyclosporine. Frequent gingival hyperplasia reported w/ nifedipine; avoid concomitant use w/ nifedipine in patients in whom gingival hyperplasia develops as a side effect of cyclosporine. Convulsions reported w/ high-dose methylprednisolone. Calcium antagonists may interfere w/ cyclosporine metabolism.

PATIENT CONSIDERATIONS

Assessment: Assess for hypersensitivity to the drug, renal dysfunction, uncontrolled HTN, presence of malignancies, pregnancy/nursing status, and for possible drug interactions. RA: Before initiating treatment, assess BP (on at least 2 occasions) and obtain 2 SrCr levels. Psoriasis: Prior to treatment, perform a dermatological and physical examination, including measuring BP (on at least 2 occasions). Assess for presence of occult infection and for the presence of tumors. Assess for atypical skin lesions and biopsy them. Obtain baseline SrCr (on 2 occasions), BUN, CBC, Mg^{2+}, K^+, uric acid, and lipid levels.

Monitoring: Monitor for signs/symptoms of hepatotoxicity, liver injury, nephrotoxicity, thrombocytopenia, microangiopathic hemolytic anemia, HTN, hyperkalemia, lymphomas and other malignancies, serious/opportunistic/polyomavirus infections, convulsions and other neurotoxicities, and other adverse reactions. Monitor cyclosporine blood levels routinely in transplant patients and periodically in RA patients. RA: Monitor BP and SrCr every 2 weeks during the initial 3 months of therapy and then monthly if patient is stable. Monitor SrCr and BP after an increase of the dose of NSAIDs and after initiation of new NSAID therapy. If coadministered w/ MTX, monitor CBC and LFTs monthly. Psoriasis: Monitor for occult infection and for the presence of tumors. Monitor SrCr, BUN, BP, CBC, uric acid, K^+, lipids, and Mg^{2+} every 2 weeks during first 3 months of treatment, then monthly if stable, or more frequently during dose adjustments.

Counseling: Instruct to contact physician before changing formulations of cyclosporine, which may require dose changes. Inform that repeated lab tests are required while on therapy. Advise of the potential risks if used during pregnancy and inform of the increased risk of neoplasia, HTN, and renal dysfunction. Inform that vaccinations may be less effective and instruct to avoid live vaccines during therapy. Advise to avoid grapefruit/grapefruit juice and excessive sun exposure.

STORAGE: 20-25°C (68-77°F). (Sol) Do not refrigerate. Use w/in 2 months once opened. May form gel at <20°C (68°F); light flocculation, or formation of light sediment may occur. Allow to warm to 25°C (77°F) to reverse these changes.

GENTAMICIN INJECTION – gentamicin sulfate RX

Class: Aminoglycoside

G

Potential for nephrotoxicity, neurotoxicity, and ototoxicity; adjust dose or d/c on evidence of ototoxicity/nephrotoxicity. Risk of nephrotoxicity is greater w/ impaired renal function and in those who receive high dosage or prolonged therapy. Neurotoxicity (eg, vestibular and auditory ototoxicity) can occur w/ preexisting renal damage or w/ normal renal function treated at higher doses and/or longer treatment periods than recommended. Closely monitor renal and 8th cranial nerve function, especially in patients w/ known or suspected reduced renal function at onset of therapy and also in those whose renal function is initially normal but who develop signs of renal dysfunction during therapy. Examine urine for decreased specific gravity, increased protein excretion, and presence of cells/casts. Monitor BUN, SrCr, or CrCl periodically. Obtain serial audiograms in patients old enough to be tested, particularly high-risk patients, when feasible. Periodically monitor peak and trough serum concentrations to assure adequate levels and to avoid toxicity. Dose should be adjusted when monitoring peak and trough concentrations; avoid prolonged peak levels >12mcg/mL and trough levels >2mcg/mL. Hemodialysis may aid in the removal of gentamicin from the blood, especially if renal function is or becomes compromised. Consider exchange transfusions in the newborn infant. Avoid concurrent and/or sequential systemic or topical use of other potentially neurotoxic and/or nephrotoxic drugs (eg, cisplatin, cephaloridine, kanamycin, amikacin, neomycin, polymyxin B, colistin, paromomycin, streptomycin, tobramycin, vancomycin, viomycin). Advanced age and dehydration may increase risk of toxicity. Avoid w/ potent diuretics (eg, ethacrynic acid, furosemide). May cause fetal harm.

OTHER BRAND NAMES

Gentamicin in 0.9% Sodium Chloride

ADULT DOSAGE

General Dosing

Treatment of bacterial neonatal sepsis, bacterial septicemia, and infections of the CNS (meningitis), urinary tract, respiratory tract, GI tract (including peritonitis), skin, bone, and soft tissue (including burns) caused by susceptible strains of microorganisms; for initial therapy in suspected/confirmed gram-negative infections or as initial therapy in conjunction w/ a penicillin (PCN)-type or cephalosporin-type drug in serious infections when the causative organisms are unknown; for treatment of life-threatening infections caused by *Pseudomonas aeruginosa* in combination w/ carbenicillin, and endocarditis caused by group D streptococci in combination w/ a PCN-type drug; in treatment of serious staphylococcal infections; and for treatment of mixed infections caused by susceptible strains of staphylococci and gram-negative infections

Serious Infections: 3mg/kg/day given in 3 equal doses q8h

Life-Threatening Infections: 5mg/kg/day in 3 or 4 equal doses; reduce to 3mg/kg/day as soon as clinically indicated

Treat for 7-10 days; may need longer course in difficult and complicated infections. Reduce dose if clinically indicated.

PEDIATRIC DOSAGE

General Dosing

Use concomitantly w/ PCN-type drug in neonates w/ suspected bacterial sepsis or staphylococcal pneumonia

Premature or Full-Term Neonates ≤1 Week of Age:

5mg/kg/day (2.5mg/kg q12h)

Infants and Neonates:

7.5mg/kg/day (2.5mg/kg q8h)

Children:

6-7.5mg/kg/day (2-2.5mg/kg q8h)

Treat for 7-10 days; may need longer course in difficult and complicated infections. Reduce dose if clinically indicated.

DOSING CONSIDERATIONS

Renal Impairment

Increasing Intervals:

Multiply SrCr level (mg/100mL) by 8 (eg, SrCr of 2mg/100mL x 8 = q16h)

Reducing Dosage at 8-Hour Intervals After Initial Dose:

CrCl 70-100mL/min: 80% of usual dose
CrCl 55-70mL/min: 65% of usual dose
CrCl 45-55mL/min: 55% of usual dose
CrCl 40-45mL/min: 50% of usual dose
CrCl 35-40mL/min: 40% of usual dose
CrCl 30-35mL/min: 35% of usual dose
CrCl 25-30mL/min: 30% of usual dose
CrCl 20-25mL/min: 25% of usual dose
CrCl 15-20mL/min: 20% of usual dose
CrCl 10-15mL/min: 15% of usual dose
CrCl <10mL/min: 10% of usual dose

Hemodialysis:

Adults: 1-1.7mg/kg at the end of each dialysis period, depending on the severity of infection
Pediatrics: May administer 2mg/kg

Other Important Considerations

Obese Patients:

Base dose on estimate of lean body mass

Extensive Burns:

Adjust dose based on serum concentrations

ADMINISTRATION

IM/IV route

Do not physically premix w/ other drugs; administer separately.
IV route may be preferred w/ bacterial septicemia, CHF, hematologic disorders, severe burns, reduced muscle mass, or those in shock.
Infuse over a period of 1/2 to 2 hrs.

0.9% NaCl

No dilution or buffering required.
If administration is controlled by a pumping device, use caution when discontinuing pumping action before container runs dry.
Intended for use only as an IV secondary medication unit.
Do not use in plastic containers in series connection.

Intermittent IV Administration

10mg/mL: May dilute a single-dose in 0.9% NaCl or in D5 inj.
40mg/mL: May dilute in 50-200mL of sterile isotonic saline sol or in a sterile sol of D5W; in infants and children, the volume of diluent should be less.
0.9% NaCl: Single dose of gentamicin sulfate may be administered according to individual requirements from appropriate premixed container.

HOW SUPPLIED

Inj: 10mg/mL [2mL], 40mg/mL [2mL, 20mL]; (0.9% NaCl) 60mg [50mL], 80mg, 100mg [50mL, 100mL], 120mg [100mL]

CONTRAINDICATIONS

Hypersensitivity to gentamicin, history of hypersensitivity or serious toxic reactions to aminoglycosides.

WARNINGS/PRECAUTIONS

Neuromuscular blockade, respiratory paralysis, ototoxicity, and nephrotoxicity may occur after local irrigation or topical application of neurotoxic and nephrotoxic antibiotics during surgical procedures. Caution w/ neuromuscular disorders (eg, myasthenia gravis, parkinsonism); may aggravate muscle weakness. During or following therapy, paresthesia, tetany, mental confusion, and positive Chvostek and Trousseau signs have been described in patients w/ hypomagnesemia, hypocalcemia, and hypokalemia; appropriate corrective electrolyte therapy is required. Fanconi-like syndrome w/ aminoaciduria and metabolic acidosis reported. Cross-allergenicity among aminoglycosides demonstrated. Maintain adequate hydration. May result in overgrowth of nonsusceptible organisms; take appropriate measures if this occurs. Not for uncomplicated initial episodes of UTI unless the causative organisms are susceptible and are not susceptible to antibiotics having less potential for toxicity. (40mg/mL, 0.9% NaCl) Caution in elderly. (40mg/mL) Contains sodium metabisulfite; allergic-type reactions may occur more frequently in asthmatics. (0.9% NaCl) Contains Na^+; caution w/ CHF, severe renal insufficiency, and edema w/ Na^+ retention.

ADVERSE REACTIONS

Peripheral neuropathy, encephalopathy, respiratory depression, lethargy, confusion, depression, visual disturbances, decreased appetite, weight loss, hypo/hypertension, rash, N/V, fever, headache.

DRUG INTERACTIONS

See Boxed Warning. Increased nephrotoxicity w/ cephalosporins. Neuromuscular blockade and respiratory paralysis may occur in anesthetized patients, those receiving neuromuscular blockers (eg, succinylcholine, tubocurarine, decamethonium), or those receiving massive transfusions of citrate-anticoagulated blood. May increase risk of toxicity w/ previous exposure to ototoxic drugs. Rapid and significant inactivation of gentamicin w/ carbenicillin in vitro; concomitant use w/ carbenicillin in patients w/ severe renal impairment reported a reduction in gentamicin serum $T_{1/2}$.

PATIENT CONSIDERATIONS

Assessment: Obtain pretreatment body weight for calculation of correct dosage. Assess and document bacterial infection using culture and susceptibility techniques. Assess for history of hypersensitivity to drug, other aminoglycosides, or to sulfites. Assess for CHF, hypomagnesemia, hypocalcemia, hypokalemia, neuromuscular disorders, pregnancy/nursing status, and for possible drug interactions. Assess renal function.

Monitoring: Monitor for signs/symptoms of ototoxicity, neurotoxicity, nephrotoxicity, hypersensitivity reactions, Fanconi-like syndrome w/ aminoaciduria and metabolic acidosis, and other adverse reactions. Monitor hydration status, LFTs, BUN, SrCr, CrCl, CBC, and serum electrolytes. Monitor peak and trough serum levels of gentamicin periodically. Repeat culture and susceptibility test.

Counseling: Inform that drug only treats bacterial, not viral, infections. Instruct to take ud; inform that skipping doses or not completing full course may decrease effectiveness and may increase likelihood of bacterial resistance. Advise to keep well hydrated during treatment. Instruct to inform physician if pregnant/breastfeeding.

STORAGE: (10mg/mL, 40mg/mL) 20-25°C (68-77°F). (0.9% NaCl) 25°C (77°F); brief exposure up to 40°C (104°F) does not adversely affect the product. Avoid excessive heat.

GENVOYA – cobicistat/elvitegravir/emtricitabine/tenofovir alafenamide RX

Class: CYP3A inhibitor/HIV integrase strand transfer inhibitor/nucleoside analogue combination

Lactic acidosis and severe hepatomegaly w/ steatosis, including fatal cases, reported w/ the use of nucleoside analogues in combination w/ other antiretrovirals. Not approved for the treatment of chronic hepatitis B virus (HBV) infection. Severe acute exacerbations of hepatitis B reported in patients who are coinfected w/ HBV and HIV-1 and have discontinued products containing emtricitabine and/or tenofovir disoproxil fumarate (TDF); closely monitor hepatic function w/ both clinical and lab follow-up for at least several months in patients who are coinfected w/ HIV-1 and HBV and d/c therapy. If appropriate, initiation of anti-hepatitis B therapy may be warranted.

ADULT DOSAGE

HIV-1 Infection

For use as a complete regimen in adults who have no antiretroviral treatment history or to replace the current antiretroviral regimen in those who are virologically-suppressed (HIV-1 RNA <50 copies/mL) on a stable antiretroviral regimen for at least 6 months w/ no history of treatment failure and no known substitutions associated w/ resistance to the individual components of the drug

≥35kg:
1 tab qd

PEDIATRIC DOSAGE

HIV-1 Infection

For use as a complete regimen in pediatrics who have no antiretroviral treatment history or to replace the current antiretroviral regimen in those who are virologically-suppressed (HIV-1 RNA <50 copies/mL) on a stable antiretroviral regimen for at least 6 months w/ no history of treatment failure and no known substitutions associated w/ resistance to the individual components of the drug

≥12 Years and ≥35kg:
1 tab qd

DOSING CONSIDERATIONS

Renal Impairment

CrCl <30mL/min: Not recommended for use

Hepatic Impairment

Severe (Child-Pugh Class C): Not recommended for use

ADMINISTRATION

Oral route

Take w/ food.

HOW SUPPLIED

Tab: (Cobicistat/Elvitegravir/Emtricitabine/Tenofovir Alafenamide [TAF]) 150mg/150mg/200mg/10mg

CONTRAINDICATIONS

Concomitant use w/ drugs that are highly dependent on CYP3A for clearance and for which elevated plasma concentrations are associated w/ serious and/or life-threatening events (eg, alfuzosin, carbamazepine, phenobarbital, phenytoin, rifampin, dihydroergotamine, ergotamine, methylergonovine, cisapride, St. John's wort, lovastatin, simvastatin, pimozide, sildenafil [when dosed as Revatio for the treatment of pulmonary arterial HTN], triazolam, oral midazolam).

WARNINGS/PRECAUTIONS

Test for HBV infection prior to initiation of therapy. Redistribution/accumulation of body fat reported. Not recommended in patients w/ estimated CrCl <30mL/min. **Emtricitabine and TAF:** Obesity and prolonged nucleoside exposure may be risk factors for lactic acidosis and severe hepatomegaly. Caution in any patient w/ known risk factors for liver disease. **Emtricitabine:** Immune reconstitution syndrome and autoimmune disorders (eg, Graves' disease, polymyositis, Guillain-Barre syndrome) in the setting of immune reconstitution reported. **TAF:** Renal impairment, including cases of acute renal failure and Fanconi syndrome reported. Decreased bone mineral density (BMD) and increased biochemical markers of bone metabolism reported. Osteomalacia associated w/ proximal renal tubulopathy reported in association w/ the use of TDF-containing products. Hypophosphatemia and osteomalacia secondary to proximal renal tubulopathy have occurred in patients at risk of renal dysfunction who present w/ persistent or worsening bone or muscle symptoms while receiving products containing TDF. **Cobicistat:** May produce elevations of SrCr.

ADVERSE REACTIONS

Nausea.

DRUG INTERACTIONS

See Contraindications. Avoid w/ elvitegravir, cobicistat, emtricitabine, TDF, lamivudine, adefovir dipivoxil, ritonavir, other antiretrovirals, rifabutin, rifapentine, or salmeterol. CYP3A inducers may decrease plasma concentration of cobicistat, elvitegravir, and TAF and may lead to loss of therapeutic effect and development of resistance. Coadministration w/ drugs that reduce renal function or compete for active tubular secretion (eg, acyclovir, cidofovir, ganciclovir, valacyclovir, valganciclovir, aminoglycosides [eg, gentamicin]) may increase concentrations of emtricitabine, tenofovir, and other renally eliminated drugs and this may increase the risk of adverse reactions. May increase levels of antiarrhythmics (eg, digoxin), itraconazole, ketoconazole, voriconazole, colchicine, ethosuximide, β-blockers, calcium channel blockers, inhaled or nasal fluticasone, bosentan, atorvastatin, immunosuppressants, salmeterol, neuroleptics, PDE-5 inhibitors, and sedatives/hypnotics. May increase levels of clarithromycin and telithromycin; reduce clarithromycin dose by 50% in patients w/ CrCl 50-60mL/min. Monitor INR upon coadministration w/ warfarin. Ethosuximide and oxcarbazepine may decrease elvitegravir, cobicistat, and TAF levels; consider alternative anticonvulsants w/ oxcarbazepine and monitor upon coadministration w/ ethosuximide. May increase levels of antidepressants (eg, SSRIs [except sertraline], TCAs, trazodone); carefully titrate antidepressant dose and monitor response. Ketoconazole, itraconazole, and voriconazole may increase levels of elvitegravir and cobicistat. Avoid w/ colchicine in patients w/ renal or hepatic impairment. Rifabutin and rifapentine may decrease elvitegravir, cobicistat, and TAF levels. Dexamethasone may decrease elvitegravir and cobicistat levels; consider an alternative corticosteroid. May increase levels of diazepam and parenterally administered midazolam; consider dose reduction for midazolam. May increase norgestimate and decrease ethinyl estradiol levels; consider alternative (nonhormonal) methods of contraception. Cyclosporine may increase elvitegravir and cobicistat levels. May increase levels of buprenorphine and norbuprenorphine and may decrease levels of naloxone. **TAF:** Patients taking nephrotoxic agents (eg, NSAIDs) are at increased risk of developing renal-related adverse reactions. P-gp inducers may decrease levels. **Cobicistat:** May increase levels of CYP3A substrates or CYP2D6 substrates, and substrates of P-gp, BCRP, OATP1B1, or OATP1B3. CYP3A inhibitors may increase levels. Clarithromycin and telithromycin may increase levels. **Elvitegravir:** May decrease plasma levels of CYP2C9 substrates. Antacids (eg, aluminum and magnesium hydroxide) may decrease levels; separate administration by at least 2 hrs. Refer to PI for dosing modifications when used w/ certain concomitant therapies.

PATIENT CONSIDERATIONS

Assessment: Assess for obesity, prolonged nucleoside exposure, risk factors for liver disease, renal/hepatic impairment, pregnancy/nursing status, and possible drug interactions. Assess BMD in patients who have a history of pathological bone fracture or w/ other risk factors for osteoporosis or bone loss. Obtain baseline estimated CrCl, urine glucose, urine protein, and SrCr. Perform test for HBV infection prior to therapy.

Monitoring: Monitor for signs/symptoms of lactic acidosis, severe hepatomegaly w/ steatosis, new onset/worsening renal impairment, immune reconstitution syndrome, autoimmune disorders, fat redistribution/accumulation, decreased BMD, increased biochemical markers for bone metabolism, osteomalacia, and other adverse reactions. Monitor for exacerbations of hepatitis B in patients w/ coinfection for at least several months upon discontinuation of therapy. Monitor BMD, estimated CrCl, urine glucose, urine protein, and SrCr. Monitor serum phosphorus levels in patients w/ chronic kidney disease. Monitor INR upon coadministration w/ warfarin.

Counseling: Instruct to take on a regular dosing schedule w/ food and to avoid missing doses. Advise to report use of any prescription or nonprescription medication or herbal products, including St. John's wort. Instruct to contact physician if symptoms of lactic acidosis/pronounced hepatotoxicity or any symptoms of infection occur. Inform that hepatitis B testing is recommended prior to initiating therapy. Advise that fat redistribution/accumulation, renal impairment, and decreases in BMD may occur. Inform that there is an antiretroviral pregnancy registry to monitor fetal outcomes of pregnant women exposed to the drug. Instruct mothers not to breastfeed.

STORAGE: <30°C (86°F).

GEODON – ziprasidone hydrochloride; ziprasidone mesylate RX

Class: Atypical antipsychotic

Elderly patients w/ dementia-related psychosis treated w/ antipsychotic drugs are at an increased risk of death; most deaths appeared to be cardiovascular (CV) (eg, heart failure [HF], sudden death) or infectious (eg, pneumonia) in nature. Not approved for treatment of dementia-related psychosis.

G

ADULT DOSAGE

Schizophrenia

Cap:
Initial: 20mg bid
Titrate: May adjust up to 80mg bid at intervals of not <2 days
Max: 80mg bid

Maint Treatment: No additional benefit demonstrated for doses >20mg bid

Acute Agitation in Schizophrenia:
IM:
10mg (may give q2h) to 20mg (may give q4h)
Max: 40mg/day

IM administration for >3 consecutive days has not been studied; if long-term therapy is indicated, replace w/ oral formulation as soon as possible

Bipolar I Disorder

Mixed or Manic Episodes:
Cap:
Acute (Monotherapy):
Initial: 40mg bid
Titrate: May increase to 60mg or 80mg bid on 2nd day of treatment, and subsequently adjust based on tolerance and efficacy w/in the range 40-80mg bid

Maint (Adjunct to Lithium or Valproate):
Continue treatment at the same dose on which the patient was initially stabilized, w/in the range of 40-80mg bid

PEDIATRIC DOSAGE

Pediatric use may not have been established

DOSING CONSIDERATIONS

Elderly
Start at lower end of dosing range

ADMINISTRATION

Oral/IM route

Cap
Take w/ food.

IM
Add 1.2mL of sterile water for inj (SWFI) to vial and shake vigorously until all the drug is dissolved. Draw up 0.5mL of reconstituted sol to administer a 10mg dose; draw up 1mL of reconstituted sol to administer a 20mg dose.
Do not mix w/ other medicinal products or solvents other than SWFI.

HOW SUPPLIED

Cap: 20mg, 40mg, 60mg, 80mg; **Inj:** 20mg/mL

CONTRAINDICATIONS

Known history of QT prolongation (including congenital long QT syndrome); recent acute MI; uncompensated HF; concomitant use w/ dofetilide, sotalol, quinidine, other Class Ia and III antiarrhythmics, mesoridazine, thioridazine, chlorpromazine, droperidol, pimozide, sparfloxacin, gatifloxacin, moxifloxacin, halofantrine, mefloquine, pentamidine, arsenic trioxide, levomethadyl acetate, dolasetron mesylate, probucol or tacrolimus, or other drugs that have demonstrated QT prolongation; known hypersensitivity to the product.

WARNINGS/PRECAUTIONS

Avoid in patients w/ history of cardiac arrhythmias. D/C in patients w/ persistent QTc measurements >500 msec. Hypokalemia and/or hypomagnesemia may increase risk of QT prolongation and arrhythmia; replete those electrolytes before treatment. Initiate further evaluation if symptoms of torsades de pointes occur. Neuroleptic malignant syndrome (NMS) reported; d/c therapy and institute symptomatic treatment. Drug reaction w/ eosinophilia and systemic symptoms (DRESS) and other severe cutaneous reactions reported; d/c if suspected. May cause tardive dyskinesia (TD), especially in the elderly; consider discontinuation if this occurs. Associated w/ metabolic changes (eg, hyperglycemia, dyslipidemia, weight gain) that may increase CV/cerebrovascular risk. Rash and/or urticaria reported; d/c upon appearance of rash. May induce orthostatic hypotension and syncope; caution w/ CV disease, cerebrovascular disease, or conditions that predispose to hypotension. Leukopenia, neutropenia, and agranulocytosis reported; d/c in patients w/ severe neutropenia (ANC <1000/mm^3) or at 1st sign of decline in WBCs in patients w/ preexisting low WBC count or history of drug-induced leukopenia/ neutropenia. Seizures reported. May cause esophageal dysmotility and aspiration; caution in patients at risk for aspiration pneumonia. May elevate prolactin levels. May impair physical/ mental abilities. Somnolence and priapism reported. May disrupt the body's ability to reduce core body temperature. Caution in cardiac patients and in those at risk for suicide. Caution w/ renal impairment when administered IM. Concomitant use of IM and oral preparations in schizophrenic patients is not recommended.

ADVERSE REACTIONS

Schizophrenia: Somnolence, respiratory tract infection.
Bipolar I Disorder: Somnolence, extrapyramidal symptoms, dizziness, akathisia, abnormal vision, asthenia, vomiting.
IM: Headache, nausea, somnolence.

DRUG INTERACTIONS

See Contraindications. Caution w/ centrally acting drugs and medications w/ anticholinergic activity. May enhance effects of certain antihypertensives. May antagonize effects of levodopa and dopamine agonists. Decreased exposure w/ carbamazepine. Increased levels w/ CYP3A4 inhibitors (eg, ketoconazole). Periodically monitor serum electrolytes w/ diuretics.

PATIENT CONSIDERATIONS

Assessment: Assess for drug hypersensitivity, history of QT prolongation, recent acute MI, uncompensated HF, dementia-related psychosis, history of seizures/conditions that lower seizure threshold, other conditions where treatment is contraindicated or cautioned, pregnancy/ nursing status, and possible drug interactions. Obtain baseline serum electrolytes (K^+, Mg^{2+}) in patients at risk for significant electrolyte disturbances. Obtain baseline FPG in patients w/ diabetes mellitus (DM) or at risk for DM. Obtain baseline CBC if at risk for leukopenia/ neutropenia.

Monitoring: Monitor for QT prolongation, torsades de pointes, NMS, DRESS and other severe cutaneous reactions, TD, metabolic changes, rash, orthostatic hypotension, seizures, esophageal dysmotility, aspiration, suicidal ideation, hypokalemia, hypomagnesemia, and other adverse reactions. Monitor CBC frequently during the 1st few months of therapy in patients w/ preexisting low WBCs or history of drug-induced leukopenia/neutropenia. Monitor for fever or other signs/ symptoms of infection in patients w/ neutropenia. Monitor for worsening of glucose control in patients w/ DM and monitor FPG in patients at risk for DM. Reassess periodically to determine need for maintenance treatment.

Counseling: Inform of the risks and benefits of therapy. Advise to inform physician of any history of QT prolongation, recent acute MI, uncompensated HF, risk for electrolyte abnormalities, history of cardiac arrhythmia, or if taking other QT-prolonging drugs. Instruct to report conditions that increase risk for electrolyte disturbances (eg, hypokalemia, taking diuretics, prolonged diarrhea) and if dizziness, palpitations, or syncope occurs. Instruct to report to physician at the earliest onset any signs/symptoms that may be associated w/ DRESS or w/ severe cutaneous reactions (eg, Stevens-Johnson syndrome).

STORAGE: 25°C (77°F); excursions permitted to 15-30°C (59-86°F). **Inj:** Protect from light. **Reconstituted Sol:** 15-30°C (59-86°F) for up to 24 hrs when protected from light, or at 2-8°C (36-46°F) for up to 7 days.

GIAZO – balsalazide disodium

RX

Class: 5-aminosalicylic acid derivative

ADULT DOSAGE

Ulcerative Colitis

Mildly to Moderately Active:

Males: 3 tabs bid (6.6g/day) for up to 8 weeks

PEDIATRIC DOSAGE

Pediatric use may not have been established

ADMINISTRATION

Oral route

Take w/ or w/o food.

HOW SUPPLIED

Tab: 1.1g

CONTRAINDICATIONS

Hypersensitivity to salicylates, aminosalicylates, or their metabolites, or to any of the components of this medication.

WARNINGS/PRECAUTIONS

Associated w/ acute intolerance syndrome (eg, cramping, acute abdominal pain and bloody diarrhea, fever, headache, and rash) that may be difficult to distinguish from exacerbation of ulcerative colitis; observe closely for worsening of symptoms and d/c therapy if acute intolerance syndrome is suspected. Renal impairment, including minimal change nephropathy, acute/chronic interstitial nephritis, and renal failure, reported; evaluate renal function prior to initiation and periodically while on therapy. Caution w/ known renal dysfunction or history of renal disease. Hepatic failure reported in patients w/ preexisting liver disease; use caution and consider LFTs in patients w/ liver disease. Caution in elderly; closely monitor blood cell counts during therapy.

ADVERSE REACTIONS

Headache, nasopharyngitis, anemia, diarrhea, fatigue, pharyngolaryngeal pain, urinary tract infection, GI disorders.

PATIENT CONSIDERATIONS

Assessment: Assess for hypersensitivity to salicylates, aminosalicylates, or their metabolites, and renal/hepatic function.

Monitoring: Monitor for signs/symptoms of acute intolerance syndrome, renal/hepatic impairment, and other adverse reactions. Monitor blood cell counts in elderly.

Counseling: Instruct not to take drug if hypersensitive to salicylates (eg, aspirin). Advise patients who need to control Na^+ intake that the recommended dosing of 6.6g/day provides about 756mg of Na^+/day. Instruct to contact physician if worsening of ulcerative colitis symptoms is experienced. Instruct to inform physician if they have or are later diagnosed w/ renal dysfunction and/or liver disease.

STORAGE: 20-25°C (68-77°F); excursions permitted between 15-30°C (59-86°F).

GILENYA – fingolimod

RX

Class: Sphingosine 1-phosphate receptor modulator

ADULT DOSAGE

Multiple Sclerosis

Treatment of relapsing forms of multiple sclerosis (MS) to reduce the frequency of clinical exacerbations and to delay the accumulation of physical disability

0.5mg qd

PEDIATRIC DOSAGE

Pediatric use may not have been established

ADMINISTRATION

Oral route

Take w/ or w/o food.

First Dose Monitoring

Administer the 1st dose in a setting in which resources to appropriately manage symptomatic bradycardia are available. Observe all patients for 6 hrs for signs/symptoms of bradycardia w/ hourly pulse and BP measurement. Obtain an ECG prior to dosing and at the end of the observation period.

Additional observation should be instituted until the finding has resolved in the following situations:
1. HR 6 hrs post-dose is <45 bpm.
2. HR 6 hrs post-dose is at the lowest value post-dose (suggesting that the max pharmacodynamics effect on the heart may not have occurred).
3. ECG 6 hrs post-dose shows onset 2nd degree or higher atrioventricular (AV) block.

Should post-dose symptomatic bradycardia occur, initiate appropriate management, begin continuous ECG monitoring, and continue observation until the symptoms have resolved.

Should a patient require pharmacologic intervention for symptomatic bradycardia, continuous overnight ECG monitoring in a medical facility should be instituted, and the 1st dose monitoring strategy should be repeated after the 2nd dose.

Reinitiation of Therapy Following Discontinuation

If therapy is discontinued for >14 days, after the 1st month of treatment, the same precautions (1st dose monitoring) as for initial dosing should apply. W/in the first 2 weeks of treatment, 1st dose procedures are recommended after interruption of ≥1 day; during weeks 3 and 4 of treatment, 1st dose procedures are recommended after treatment interruption of >7 days.

HOW SUPPLIED

Cap: 0.5mg

CONTRAINDICATIONS

Patients who in the last 6 months experienced MI, unstable angina, stroke, transient ischemic attack (TIA), decompensated heart failure (HF) requiring hospitalization, or Class III/IV HF. History/presence of Mobitz Type II 2nd- or 3rd-degree AV block or sick sinus syndrome (unless w/ functioning pacemaker), baseline QTc interval ≥500 msec, and treatment w/ Class IA/III anti-arrhythmic drugs.

WARNINGS/PRECAUTIONS

Bradyarrhythmia and AV blocks may occur; monitor during treatment initiation. Cases of syncope reported after 1st dose. May increase risk of infections; consider suspending treatment if a serious infection develops. Do not start treatment in patients w/ active acute/chronic infections until the infection(s) is resolved. Include disseminated herpetic infections in the differential diagnosis of patients receiving therapy and present w/ an atypical MS relapse or multiorgan failure. Cryptococcal infections reported; initiate prompt diagnostic evaluation and treatment if signs/symptoms occur. Caution when switching to fingolimod from immune-modulating or immunosuppressive medications to avoid unintended additive effects. Test for antibodies to varicella zoster virus (VZV) prior to commencing treatment in patients w/o a healthcare professional confirmed history of chickenpox or w/o a documentation of a full course of vaccination against VZV. Give VZV vaccination to antibody-negative patients; initiate therapy 1 month after vaccination. Progressive multifocal leukoencephalopathy (PML) and probable PML reported; withhold therapy and perform appropriate diagnostic evaluation at the 1st sign/symptom suggestive of PML. May increase risk of macular edema; patients w/ history of uveitis or w/ diabetes mellitus (DM) are at increased risk. Posterior reversible encephalopathy syndrome (PRES) reported rarely; d/c if suspected. Dose-dependent reductions in forced expiratory volume over 1 sec and diffusion lung capacity for carbon monoxide (DLCO) reported. Liver transaminase elevations reported; d/c if significant liver injury confirmed. May cause fetal harm; women of childbearing potential should use effective contraception during and for 2 months after stopping therapy. May cause HTN and decreased lymphocyte counts. Caution w/ severe hepatic impairment and in elderly.

ADVERSE REACTIONS

Headache, liver transaminase elevations, influenza, abdominal/back pain, diarrhea, cough, sinusitis, pain in extremity, bronchitis, dyspnea, HTN.

DRUG INTERACTIONS

See Contraindications. Monitor patients on QT prolonging drugs w/ known risk of torsades de pointes (eg, citalopram, methadone, erythromycin) overnight w/ continuous ECG in a medical facility. Severe bradycardia or heart block may occur w/ drugs that slow the HR or AV conduction (eg, β-blockers, digoxin, HR-slowing calcium channel blockers). Increased blood levels w/ ketoconazole. May reduce the immune response to vaccination. Vaccination may be less effective during and for up to 2 months after discontinuation of treatment; avoid live attenuated vaccines during and for 2 months after treatment. Prior or concurrent use w/ antineoplastic, immune-modulating, or immunosuppressive therapies (eg, corticosteroids) may increase the risk of immunosuppression; consider the risk of additive immune system effects if these therapies are coadministered w/ fingolimod. Consider the duration and mode of action when switching from drugs w/ prolonged immune effects (eg, natalizumab, teriflunomide, mitoxantrone) to avoid unintended additive immunosuppressive effects.

PATIENT CONSIDERATIONS

Assessment: Assess if MI, unstable angina, stroke, TIA, decompensated HF requiring hospitalization, or Class III/IV HF was experienced in the last 6 months. Assess for history or presence of Mobitz Type II 2nd- or 3rd-degree AV block or sick sinus syndrome, pregnancy/nursing status, any other conditions where treatment is cautioned or contraindicated, and for drug interactions. Assess ECG, CBC, and LFTs. Perform an examination of the fundus including the macula.

Monitoring: Monitor for signs/symptoms of bradyarrhythmia, AV blocks, hepatic dysfunction, infection, PML, macular edema, PRES, and other adverse reactions. Monitor BP and lymphocyte counts. Perform spirometric evaluation of respiratory function and evaluation of DLCO if clinically indicated. Perform an examination of the fundus including the macula 3-4 months after starting therapy, at any time after a patient reports visual disturbances while on therapy, and regularly in patients w/ DM or history of uveitis.

Counseling: Instruct not to d/c w/o 1st consulting the prescribing physician. Advise to contact physician if patient accidently takes more drug than prescribed. Advise that decreased HR may occur upon initiation of treatment and that observation in the clinic or other facility for at least 6 hrs after the 1st dose will be required. Instruct to contact physician if symptoms of infection, new onset/worsening of dyspnea, unexplained N/V, abdominal pain, fatigue, anorexia, jaundice, dark urine, and/or any changes in vision develop. Instruct to delay treatment w/ fingolimod until after VZV vaccination if patient has not had chickenpox or a previous VZV vaccination. Counsel on the importance of contacting the physician if symptoms suggestive of PML develop; inform that typical symptoms are diverse, progress over days to weeks, and include progressive weakness on one side of the body or clumsiness of limbs, disturbance of vision, and changes in thinking, memory, and orientation leading to confusion and personality changes. Advise women of childbearing age to use effective contraception during and for 2 months after stopping treatment. Inform that drug remains in the blood and continues to have effects for up to 2 months following the last dose.

G

STORAGE: 25°C (77°F); excursions permitted to 15-30°C (59-86°F). Protect from moisture.

GLEEVEC – imatinib mesylate

RX

Class: Kinase inhibitor

ADULT DOSAGE

Hypereosinophilic Syndrome/Chronic Eosinophilic Leukemia

FIP1L1-PDGFRα Fusion Kinase-Negative/Unknown:
400mg qd

Demonstrated FIP1L1-PDGFRα Fusion Kinase:
Initial: 100mg qd
Titrate: May increase to 400mg qd

Dermatofibrosarcoma Protuberans

Unresectable, Recurrent, and/or Metastatic:
800mg/day (as 400mg bid)

Kit (CD117)-Positive Gastrointestinal Stromal Tumors

Unresectable and/or Metastatic Malignant:
400mg qd
Titrate: May increase up to 800mg/day (as 400mg bid)

Adjuvant Treatment Following Complete Gross Resection:
400mg qd; optimal treatment duration unknown

Ph+ Chronic Myeloid Leukemia

Chronic Phase:
400mg qd
Titrate: May increase to 600mg qd

Accelerated Phase/Blast Crisis:
600mg qd
Titrate: May increase to 800mg/day (as 400mg bid)

Ph+ Acute Lymphoblastic Leukemia

Relapsed/Refractory:
600mg qd

Myelodysplastic/Myeloproliferative Diseases

Associated w/ PDGFR Gene Re-Arrangements:
400mg qd

PEDIATRIC DOSAGE

Ph+ Chronic Myeloid Leukemia

Newly Diagnosed Patients in Chronic Phase:
≥1 Year:
340mg/m^2/day
Max: 600mg/day
Dose can be given qd or split in 2 (am and pm)

Ph+ Acute Lymphoblastic Leukemia

In Combination w/ Chemotherapy for Newly Diagnosed Patients:
≥1 Year:
340mg/m^2 qd
Max: 600mg qd

Aggressive Systemic Mastocytosis

W/O D816V c-Kit Mutation:
400mg qd

c-Kit Mutational Status Unknown/Unavailable:
400mg qd may be considered for patients not responding satisfactorily to other therapies

Associated w/ Eosinophilia:
Initial: 100mg qd
Titrate: May increase to 400mg qd

DOSING CONSIDERATIONS

Concomitant Medications

Strong CYP3A4 Inducers: Avoid use; if necessary, increase imatinib dose by at least 50%

Renal Impairment

Mild (CrCl 40-59mL/min):
Max: 600mg

Moderate (CrCl 20-39mL/min):
Initial: Reduce dose by 50%
Max: 400mg

Hepatic Impairment

Severe: Reduce dose by 25%

Adverse Reactions

Bilirubin >3X Institutional ULN (IULN)/Liver Transaminases >5X IULN:
1. Withhold therapy until bilirubin levels return to <1.5X IULN and transaminase levels to <2.5X IULN
2. Continue treatment at a reduced daily dose:

Adults: 400mg to 300mg, 600mg to 400mg, or 800mg to 600mg
Pediatrics: 340mg/m²/day to 260mg/m²/day

Severe Nonhematologic (eg, Severe Hepatotoxicity, Severe Fluid Retention):
Withhold therapy until the event has resolved; resume treatment as appropriate depending on initial severity of event

Neutropenia/Thrombocytopenia:

ANC <1.0 x 10⁹/L and/or Platelets <50 x 10⁹/L:

Adults:

Initial Dose 100mg:
1. Withhold treatment until ANC ≥1.5 x 10⁹/L and platelets ≥75 x 10⁹/L
2. Resume treatment at previous dose (dose before severe adverse reaction)

Initial Dose 400mg:
1. Withhold treatment until ANC ≥1.5 x 10⁹/L and platelets ≥75 x 10⁹/L
2. Resume treatment at the original starting dose of 400mg
3. If recurrence of ANC <1.0 x 10⁹/L and/or platelets <50 x 10⁹/L, repeat step 1 and resume at a reduced dose of 300mg

Initial Dose 800mg:
1. Withhold treatment until ANC ≥1.5 x 10⁹/L and platelets ≥75 x 10⁹/L
2. Resume treatment at 600mg
3. In the event of recurrence of ANC <1.0 x 10⁹/L and/or platelets <50 x 10⁹/L, repeat step 1 and resume at reduced dose of 400mg

Pediatrics:

Initial Dose 340mg/m²:
1. Withhold treatment until ANC ≥1.5 x 10⁹/L and platelets ≥75 x 10⁹/L
2. Resume treatment at previous dose (dose before severe adverse reaction)
3. In the event of recurrence of ANC <1.0 x 10⁹/L and/or platelets <50 x 10⁹/L, repeat step 1 and resume at reduced dose of 260mg/m²

ANC <0.5 x 10⁹/L and/or Platelets <10 x 10⁹/L:

Adults:

Initial Dose 600mg:
1. Check if cytopenia is related to leukemia (marrow aspirate or biopsy)
2. If cytopenia is unrelated to leukemia, reduce dose to 400mg
3. If cytopenia persists 2 weeks, reduce further to 300mg
4. If cytopenia persists 4 weeks and is still unrelated to leukemia, withhold treatment until ANC ≥1 x 10⁹/L and platelets ≥20 x 10⁹/L and then resume treatment at 300mg

ADMINISTRATION

Oral route

Take w/ a meal and a large glass of water
Do not crush tab

G

Patients Unable to Swallow Tabs

1. Disperse tabs in a glass of water or apple juice
2. Required number of tabs should be placed in the appropriate volume of beverage (approx 50mL for a 100mg tab and 200mL for a 400mg tab)
3. Stir w/ a spoon and administer immediately after complete disintegration of tab

HOW SUPPLIED

Tab: 100mg*, 400mg* *scored

WARNINGS/PRECAUTIONS

Edema and serious fluid retention reported. Hematologic toxicity (eg, anemia/neutropenia/thrombocytopenia) reported. CHF and left ventricular dysfunction reported; carefully monitor patients w/ cardiac disease or risk factors for cardiac failure or history of renal failure, and evaluate/treat any patient w/ cardiac or renal failure. Hepatotoxicity may occur. Grade 3/4 hemorrhages in clinical studies in patients w/ newly diagnosed CML and w/ GIST reported. GI tumor sites may be the source of GI hemorrhages; GI hemorrhage in patients w/ newly diagnosed Ph+ CML, and gastric antral vascular ectasia reported. GI irritation/perforation reported. In patients w/ HES w/ occult infiltration of HES cells w/in the myocardium, cases of cardiogenic shock/left ventricular dysfunction have been associated w/ HES cell degranulation upon initiation of therapy; reversible w/ administration of systemic steroids, circulatory support measures, and temporarily withholding treatment. Consider echocardiogram and determination of serum troponin in patients w/ HES/CEL, MDS/MPD, or ASM associated w/ high eosinophil levels; if either is abnormal, consider prophylactic use of systemic steroids (1-2mg/kg) for 1-2 weeks concomitantly at initiation of therapy. Bullous dermatologic reactions, including erythema multiforme and Stevens-Johnson syndrome, reported. May cause fetal harm; sexually active female patients of reproductive potential should use highly effective contraception. Growth retardation reported in children and preadolescents; closely monitor growth. Tumor lysis syndrome (TLS) reported in patients w/ CML, GIST, ALL, and eosinophilic leukemia; caution in patients at risk of TLS (those w/ tumors w/ high proliferative rate or high tumor burden prior to treatment), and correct dehydration and treat high uric acid levels prior to initiation of treatment. May impair mental/physical abilities.

ADVERSE REACTIONS

N/V, edema, muscle cramps, musculoskeletal pain, diarrhea, rash, fatigue, headache, asthenia, abdominal pain, hemorrhage, malaise, neutropenia, anemia, anorexia.

DRUG INTERACTIONS

See Dosing Considerations. Increased levels w/ CYP3A4 inhibitors; caution w/ strong CYP3A4 inhibitors (eg, ketoconazole, nefazodone, clarithromycin); avoid w/ grapefruit juice. Decreased levels w/ CYP3A4 inducers (eg, rifampin, St. John's wort, enzyme-inducing antiepileptic drugs); consider alternative therapeutic agents w/ less enzyme induction potential when CYP3A4 inducers are indicated. Increases levels of simvastatin, metoprolol, and CYP3A4 metabolized drugs (eg, dihydropyridine calcium channel blockers, triazolo-benzodiazepines, certain HMG-CoA reductase inhibitors); caution w/ CYP3A4/CYP2D6 substrates that have a narrow therapeutic window (eg, alfentanil, cyclosporine, ergotamine). Switch from warfarin to low molecular weight or standard heparin if anticoagulation is required during therapy. When concomitantly used w/ chemotherapy, liver toxicity reported; monitor hepatic function. Hypothyroidism reported in thyroidectomy patients undergoing levothyroxine replacement; closely monitor TSH levels.

PATIENT CONSIDERATIONS

Assessment: Assess for cardiac disease, renal impairment, dehydration, high uric acid levels, pregnancy/nursing status, and possible drug interactions. Perform echocardiogram and determine troponin levels in patients w/ HES/CEL and w/ MDS/MPD or ASM associated w/ high eosinophil levels. Obtain baseline CBC and LFTs.

Monitoring: Monitor for signs and symptoms of fluid retention, CHF, left ventricular dysfunction, hemorrhage, GI disorders, TLS, bullous dermatologic reactions, and other adverse events. Perform CBCs weekly for the 1st month, biweekly for the 2nd month, and periodically thereafter. Monitor LFTs monthly or as clinically indicated. Monitor growth in children, and TSH levels in thyroidectomy patients undergoing levothyroxine replacement.

Counseling: Instruct to take drug exactly as prescribed and not to change the dose or to stop taking the medication unless told to do so by physician. Advise women of reproductive potential to avoid becoming pregnant and instruct to notify physician if pregnant. Instruct sexually active females to use highly effective contraception. Instruct to avoid breastfeeding while on therapy. Advise to contact physician if patient is experiencing any side effects during therapy or has a history of cardiac disease or risk factors for cardiac failure. Inform that the drug and certain other medicines can interact w/ each other; advise to inform physician if taking/planning to take iron supplements. Inform to avoid grapefruit juice and other foods known to inhibit CYP3A4 while on therapy. Advise that growth retardation has been reported in children and preadolescents, and that growth should be monitored. Caution about driving a car or operating machinery.

STORAGE: 25°C (77°F); excursions permitted to 15-30°C (59-86°F). Protect from moisture.

GLIMEPIRIDE – glimepiride

RX

Class: Sulfonylurea (2nd generation)

OTHER BRAND NAMES

Amaryl

ADULT DOSAGE

Type 2 Diabetes Mellitus

Initial: 1mg or 2mg qd
Titrate: After reaching 2mg/day, may further increase dose in increments of 1mg or 2mg based on glycemic response, not more frequently than every 1-2 weeks
Max: 8mg qd

PEDIATRIC DOSAGE

Pediatric use may not have been established

DOSING CONSIDERATIONS

Concomitant Medications

Colesevelam: Administer at least 4 hrs prior to colesevelam

Renal Impairment

Initial: 1mg qd
Titrate: Adjust conservatively
Max: 8mg qd

Elderly

Initial: 1mg qd
Titrate: Adjust conservatively
Max: 8mg qd

ADMINISTRATION

Oral route

Administer w/ breakfast or the 1st main meal of the day

HOW SUPPLIED

Tab: 3mg*, 6mg*, 8mg*; (Amaryl) 1mg*, 2mg*, 4mg* *scored

CONTRAINDICATIONS

History of a hypersensitivity reaction to glimepiride or any of the product's ingredients, history of an allergic reaction to sulfonamide derivatives.

WARNINGS/PRECAUTIONS

Not for treatment of type 1 DM or diabetic ketoacidosis. Patients being transferred from longer $T_{1/2}$ sulfonylureas (eg, chlorpropamide) may have overlapping drug effect for 1-2 weeks; monitor for hypoglycemia. May cause severe hypoglycemia, which may impair mental/physical abilities; caution in patients predisposed to hypoglycemia. Early warning symptoms of hypoglycemia may be different/less pronounced in patients with autonomic neuropathy and in the elderly. Hypersensitivity reactions (eg, anaphylaxis, angioedema, Stevens-Johnson syndrome) reported; if suspected, promptly d/c therapy, assess for other potential causes for the reaction, and institute alternative treatment. May cause hemolytic anemia; caution with G6PD deficiency and consider the use of a non-sulfonylurea alternative. Increased risk of cardiovascular mortality. Caution in elderly.

ADVERSE REACTIONS

Dizziness, nausea, asthenia, headache, hypoglycemia, flu syndrome.

DRUG INTERACTIONS

See Dosage. Oral antidiabetic medications, pramlintide acetate, insulin, ACE inhibitors, H_2-receptor antagonists, fibrates, propoxyphene, pentoxifylline, somatostatin analogues, anabolic steroids and androgens, cyclophosphamide, phenyramidol, guanethidine, fluconazole, sulfinpyrazone, tetracyclines, clarithromycin, disopyramide, quinolones, and drugs that are highly protein-bound (eg, fluoxetine, NSAIDs, salicylates, sulfonamides, chloramphenicol, coumarins, probenecid, MAOIs) may increase glucose-lowering effect; monitor for hypoglycemia during coadministration and for worsening glycemic control during withdrawal of these drugs. Danazol, glucagon, somatropin, protease inhibitors, atypical antipsychotics (eg, olanzapine, clozapine), barbiturates, diazoxide, laxatives, rifampin, thiazides and other diuretics, corticosteroids, phenothiazines, thyroid hormones, estrogens, oral contraceptives, phenytoin, nicotinic acid, sympathomimetics (eg, epinephrine, albuterol, terbutaline), and isoniazid may reduce glucose-lowering effect; monitor for worsening glycemic control during coadministration and for hypoglycemia during withdrawal of these drugs. β-blockers, clonidine, reserpine, and alcohol intake may potentiate or weaken glucose-lowering effect. Signs of hypoglycemia may be reduced or absent with sympatholytic drugs (eg, β-blockers, clonidine, guanethidine, reserpine). Potential interaction leading to severe hypoglycemia reported with oral miconazole. May interact with inhibitors (eg, fluconazole) and inducers (eg, rifampin) of CYP2C9. Colesevelam may reduce levels.

PATIENT CONSIDERATIONS

Assessment: Assess for hypersensitivity to drug or sulfonamide derivatives, predisposition to hypoglycemia, autonomic neuropathy, G6PD deficiency, pregnancy/nursing status, and possible drug interactions.

Monitoring: Monitor for hypoglycemia, hypersensitivity reactions, hemolytic anemia, and other adverse reactions.

Counseling: Inform about importance of adherence to dietary instructions, a regular exercise program, and regular testing of blood glucose. Advise about potential side effects (eg, hypoglycemia, weight gain). Inform about the symptoms and treatment of hypoglycemia, and the conditions that predispose to it. Inform that ability to concentrate and react may be impaired as a result of hypoglycemia; caution when driving/operating machinery. Advise to inform physician if pregnant/breastfeeding or contemplating pregnancy/breastfeeding.

STORAGE: 20-25°C (68-77°F). (Amaryl) 25°C (77°F); excursions permitted to 20-25°C (68-77°F).

G

GLIPIZIDE/METFORMIN – glipizide/metformin hydrochloride RX

Class: Biguanide/sulfonylurea

Lactic acidosis may occur due to metformin accumulation; risk increases with CHF, degree of renal dysfunction, and patient's age. Regularly monitor renal function and use the minimum effective dose of metformin. Do not initiate in patients ≥80 yrs of age unless measurement of CrCl demonstrates that renal function is not reduced. Promptly withhold therapy in the presence of any condition associated with hypoxemia, dehydration, or sepsis. Avoid with clinical or lab evidence of hepatic disease. Caution against excessive alcohol intake; alcohol potentiates the effects of metformin on lactate metabolism. Temporarily d/c therapy prior to any intravascular radiocontrast study or for any surgical procedure. D/C use immediately and promptly institute general supportive measures if lactic acidosis occurs. Prompt hemodialysis is recommended to correct the acidosis and remove the accumulated metformin.

OTHER BRAND NAMES

Metaglip (Discontinued)

ADULT DOSAGE

Type 2 Diabetes Mellitus

Initial: 2.5mg/250mg qd w/ a meal; may consider an initial dose of 2.5mg/500mg bid if FPG is 280-320mg/dL
Titrate: Increase by 1 tab/day every 2 weeks
Max: (10mg/2000mg)/day in divided doses

Inadequately Controlled on a Sulfonylurea and/or Metformin:
Initial: 2.5mg/500mg or 5mg/500mg bid w/ am and pm meals; starting dose should not exceed the daily doses of the individual components
Titrate: Increase by no more than (5mg/500mg)/day
Max: (20mg/2000mg)/day

PEDIATRIC DOSAGE

Pediatric use may not have been established

DOSING CONSIDERATIONS

Concomitant Medications
Colesevelam: Administer at least 4 hrs prior to colesevelam

Elderly
Elderly/Debilitated/Malnourished:
Initial/Maint: Dose conservatively; do not titrate to max dose

ADMINISTRATION

Oral route

Take w/ meals.

HOW SUPPLIED

Tab: (Glipizide/Metformin) 2.5mg/250mg, 2.5mg/500mg, 5mg/500mg

CONTRAINDICATIONS

Renal disease or dysfunction (eg, SrCr ≥1.5mg/dL [males], ≥1.4mg/dL [females], or abnormal CrCl); known hypersensitivity to glipizide or metformin HCl; acute or chronic metabolic acidosis, including diabetic ketoacidosis, w/ or w/o coma.

WARNINGS/PRECAUTIONS

May be associated with increased cardiovascular (CV) mortality. May cause hypoglycemia; increased risk when caloric intake is deficient, when strenuous exercise is not compensated by caloric supplementation, with renal/hepatic insufficiency, adrenal/pituitary insufficiency, alcohol intoxication, and in elderly, debilitated, or malnourished patients. Use not recommended during pregnancy. Caution in elderly. **Glipizide:** May cause hemolytic anemia; caution with G6PD deficiency. **Metformin:** Assess renal function before initiation of therapy and at least annually thereafter; d/c with evidence of renal impairment. Temporarily d/c at the time of or prior to radiologic studies involving the use of intravascular iodinated contrast materials, withhold for 48 hrs subsequent to the procedure, and reinstitute only if renal function is normal. D/C promptly if CV collapse (shock), acute CHF, acute myocardial infarction, and other conditions characterized by hypoxemia occur. Temporarily suspend for any surgical procedure (except minor procedures not associated with restricted intake of food and fluids); should not be restarted until oral intake has resumed and renal function is normal. May decrease serum vitamin B12 levels; monitor hematologic parameters annually. Evaluate patients previously well controlled on therapy who develop lab abnormalities or clinical illness for evidence of ketoacidosis or lactic acidosis; d/c if acidosis occurs.

ADVERSE REACTIONS

Lactic acidosis, upper respiratory infection, HTN, headache, diarrhea, dizziness, musculoskeletal pain, N/V, abdominal pain.

DRUG INTERACTIONS

See Boxed Warning and Dosage. Increased risk of hypoglycemia with other glucose-lowering agents or ethanol. May be difficult to recognize hypoglycemia with β-blockers. Thiazides and other diuretics, corticosteroids, phenothiazines, thyroid products, estrogens, oral contraceptives, phenytoin, nicotinic acid, sympathomimetics, calcium channel blockers, and isoniazid may produce hyperglycemia and may lead to loss of blood glucose control; monitor closely for loss of control during coadministration and for hypoglycemia during withdrawal of these drugs. **Glipizide:** Hypoglycemic action may be potentiated by NSAIDs, some azoles, and other highly protein-bound drugs, salicylates, sulfonamides, chloramphenicol, probenecid, coumarins, MAOIs, and β-blockers; monitor closely for hypoglycemia during coadministration and for loss of blood glucose control during withdrawal of these drugs. Potential interaction leading to severe hypoglycemia reported with oral miconazole. Fluconazole may increase exposure. Colesevelam may reduce levels. **Metformin:** Furosemide, nifedipine, and cimetidine may increase levels. May decrease furosemide levels and may decrease furosemide $T_{1/2}$. Caution with drugs that may affect renal function or result in significant hemodynamic change or may interfere with the disposition of metformin, such as cationic drugs eliminated by renal tubular secretion (eg, cimetidine, amiloride, digoxin, morphine, procainamide); monitor and adjust dose of glipizide and metformin and/or the interfering drug.

PATIENT CONSIDERATIONS

Assessment: Assess for metabolic acidosis, diabetic ketoacidosis, risk factors for lactic acidosis, renal/hepatic impairment, presence of malnourishment or debilitation, adrenal/pituitary insufficiency, alcoholism, G6PD deficiency, hypoxemia, inadequate vitamin B12 or Ca^{2+} intake/absorption, previous hypersensitivity to the drug, any other conditions where treatment is cautioned, pregnancy/nursing status, and possible drug interactions. Assess if patient is planning to undergo any surgical procedure, or radiologic studies involving the use of intravascular iodinated contrast materials. Obtain baseline FPG and HbA1c levels, and hematologic parameters.

Monitoring: Monitor for signs/symptoms of lactic acidosis, CV effects, hypoglycemia, hemolytic anemia, and other adverse reactions. Monitor for changes in clinical status. Monitor renal function, especially in elderly, at least annually. Monitor hematologic parameters annually. Perform routine serum vitamin B12 measurements at 2- to 3-yr intervals in patients predisposed to developing subnormal vitamin B12 levels. Monitor FPG and HbA1c levels periodically.

Counseling: Inform of the potential risks, benefits, and alternative modes of therapy. Advise on the importance of adherence to dietary instructions, regular exercise program, and regular testing of blood glucose, HbA1c, renal function, and hematologic parameters. Inform of the risk of lactic acidosis; instruct to d/c therapy immediately and notify physician if unexplained hyperventilation, myalgia, malaise, unusual somnolence, or other nonspecific symptoms occur. Inform of the risk of hypoglycemia. Counsel against excessive alcohol intake.

STORAGE: 20-25°C (68-77°F).

GLUCOPHAGE XR – metformin hydrochloride

RX

Class: Biguanide

Lactic acidosis reported (rare); increased risk w/ increased age, renal dysfunction, or CHF. Risk of lactic acidosis may be significantly decreased by regular monitoring of renal function and by use of the minimum effective dose of metformin. Avoid use in patients ≥80 yrs of age unless renal function is normal. Withhold therapy in the presence of any condition associated w/ hypoxemia, dehydration, or sepsis. Avoid w/ clinical or lab evidence of hepatic disease. Caution against excessive alcohol intake; may potentiate the effects of metformin on lactate metabolism. Temporarily d/c prior to any IV radiocontrast study and for any surgical procedure. Lactic acidosis should be suspected in any diabetic patient w/ metabolic acidosis lacking evidence of ketoacidosis (ketonuria and ketonemia). D/C use and institute appropriate therapy if lactic acidosis occurs.

OTHER BRAND NAMES
Glucophage

ADULT DOSAGE
Type 2 Diabetes Mellitus

Tab:
Initial: 500mg bid or 850mg qd w/ meals
Titrate: Increase by 500mg/week or 850mg every 2 weeks, up to a total of 2000mg/day, given in divided doses; may also titrate from 500mg bid to 850mg bid after 2 weeks
Max: 2550mg/day; doses >2000mg/day may be better tolerated given tid

Tab, Extended-Release (ER):
Initial: 500mg qd w/ pm meal
Titrate: Increase by 500mg/week
Max: 2000mg/day; consider 1000mg bid if unable to achieve glycemic control on 2000mg qd

PEDIATRIC DOSAGE
Type 2 Diabetes Mellitus

10-16 Years:
Tab:
Initial: 500mg bid w/ meals
Titrate: Increase by 500mg/week
Max: 2000mg/day

G

DOSING CONSIDERATIONS
Concomitant Medications
Insulin Therapy in Adults:
Initial: 500mg qd while continuing current insulin dose
Titrate: Increase by 500mg/week; decrease insulin dose by 10-25% when FPG <120mg/dL
Max: 2500mg/day (tab) and 2000mg/day (tab, extended-release [ER])
Oral Sulfonylurea Therapy in Adults:
Consider gradual addition of an oral sulfonylurea if unresponsive to 4 weeks of max dose of Glucophage or Glucophage XR monotherapy; if patient has not satisfactorily responded to 1-3 months of concomitant therapy w/ the max dose of Glucophage or Glucophage XR and the max dose of an oral sulfonylurea, consider therapeutic alternatives (eg, switching to insulin w/ or w/o Glucophage or Glucophage XR)

Elderly
Dose conservatively; do not titrate to max dose

Other Important Considerations
Transferring Patients from Chlorpropamide: Exercise care during the first 2 weeks because of the prolonged retention of chlorpropamide in the body
Debilitated/Malnourished: Do not titrate to max dose

ADMINISTRATION
Oral route

Tab
Give in divided doses w/ meals.

Tab, ER
Give qd w/ the pm meal.
Must be swallowed whole; do not crush or chew.

HOW SUPPLIED
Tab: (Glucophage) 500mg, 850mg, 1000mg; **Tab, ER:** (Glucophage XR) 500mg, 750mg

CONTRAINDICATIONS
Renal disease or dysfunction (eg, SrCr ≥1.5mg/dL [males], ≥1.4mg/dL [females] or abnormal CrCl); known hypersensitivity to metformin HCl; acute or chronic metabolic acidosis, including diabetic ketoacidosis, w/ or w/o coma.

WARNINGS/PRECAUTIONS
D/C therapy if conditions associated w/ lactic acidosis and characterized by hypoxemia states (eg, acute CHF, cardiovascular [CV] collapse, acute MI), or prerenal azotemia develop. Temporary loss of glycemic control may occur when a patient stabilized on a diabetic regimen is exposed to stress (eg, fever, trauma, infection, surgery); may be necessary to withhold metformin and temporarily administer insulin; may reinstitute metformin after acute episode is resolved. May decrease serum vitamin B12 levels. Increased risk of hypoglycemia in elderly, debilitated/malnourished or w/ adrenal or pituitary insufficiency or alcohol intoxication. Consider therapeutic alternatives, including initiation of insulin, if secondary failure w/ combined metformin/sulfonylurea therapy occurs. Hypoglycemia may be difficult to recognize in the elderly; caution in elderly.

ADVERSE REACTIONS
Diarrhea, N/V, flatulence, asthenia, indigestion, abdominal discomfort, headache.

DRUG INTERACTIONS

See Boxed Warning and Contraindications. Furosemide, nifedipine, cimetidine, and cationic drugs that are eliminated by renal tubular secretion (eg, digoxin, amiloride, procainamide, quinidine, quinine, ranitidine, trimethoprim, vancomycin, triamterene, morphine) may increase levels. Observe for loss of glycemic control w/ thiazides, other diuretics, corticosteroids, phenothiazines, thyroid products, estrogens, oral contraceptives, phenytoin, nicotinic acid, sympathomimetics, calcium channel blockers, and isoniazid. May interact w/ highly protein-bound drugs (eg, salicylates, sulfonamides, chloramphenicol, probenecid). May decrease furosemide or glyburide levels. Caution w/ drugs that may affect renal function or result in significant hemodynamic change or may interfere w/ the disposition of metformin (eg, cationic drugs that are eliminated by renal tubular secretion). Hypoglycemia may occur w/ concomitant use of other glucose-lowering agents (eg, sulfonylureas, insulin) or ethanol. Hypoglycemia may be difficult to recognize w/ β-adrenergic blocking drugs.

PATIENT CONSIDERATIONS

Assessment: Assess for renal disease or renal dysfunction, hepatic impairment, acute/chronic metabolic acidosis, presence of a hypoxic state (eg, acute CHF, acute MI, CV collapse), dehydration, sepsis, alcoholism, nutritional status, adrenal/pituitary insufficiency, pregnancy/nursing status, or any other conditions where treatment is contraindicated or cautioned. Assess for possible drug interactions. Assess baseline renal function, FPG, HbA1c, and hematological parameters (eg, Hct, Hgb, RBC indices).

Monitoring: Monitor for lactic acidosis, hypoglycemia, hypoxemia (eg, CV collapse, acute CHF, acute MI), prerenal azotemia, decreases in vitamin B12 levels, and for any other adverse reactions. Monitor FPG, HbA1c, renal function, and hematological parameters (eg, Hgb, Hct, RBC indices).

Counseling: Inform of the potential risks/benefits of therapy. Inform about the importance of adherence to dietary instructions, a regular exercise program, and of regular testing of blood glucose, HbA1c, renal function, and hematologic parameters. Inform of the risk of developing lactic acidosis during therapy; advise to d/c therapy immediately and contact physician if unexplained hyperventilation, myalgia, malaise, unusual somnolence, or other nonspecific symptoms occur. Instruct to avoid excessive alcohol intake. Counsel to take tab w/ meals and ER tab w/ pm meal. Instruct that ER tab must be swallowed whole and not crushed or chewed.

STORAGE: 20-25°C (68-77°F); excursions permitted to 15-30°C (59-86°F).

GLUCOTROL – glipizide

RX

Class: Sulfonylurea (2nd generation)

ADULT DOSAGE

Type 2 Diabetes Mellitus

Initial: 5mg qd

Titrate: Increase by 2.5-5mg every several days; may divide dose if response to single dose is not satisfactory

Max qd Dose: 15mg

Max Total Daily Dose: 40mg

Doses >15mg/day should be divided

Switching from Insulin:

Daily Insulin Requirement:

≤20 U/day: D/C insulin and begin glipizide at usual dose

>20 U/day: Reduce insulin dose by 50% and begin glipizide at usual dose; subsequent insulin reductions should depend on individual patient response

Switching from Longer Half-Life Sulfonylureas (eg, Chlorpropamide):

Observe patient carefully for 1-2 weeks

PEDIATRIC DOSAGE

Pediatric use may not have been established

DOSING CONSIDERATIONS

Concomitant Medications

Colesevelam: Administer glipizide at least 4 hrs prior to colesevelam

Renal Impairment

Initial/Maint: Dose conservatively

Hepatic Impairment
Initial: 2.5mg qd
Maint: Dose conservatively

Elderly
Initial: 2.5mg qd
Maint: Dose conservatively

Other Important Considerations
Debilitated/Malnourished Patients:
Initial/Maint: Dose conservatively

ADMINISTRATION
Oral route

Administer approx 30 min ac.

HOW SUPPLIED
Tab: 5mg*, 10mg* *scored

CONTRAINDICATIONS
Known hypersensitivity to the drug; type 1 diabetes mellitus; diabetic ketoacidosis, w/ or w/o coma.

WARNINGS/PRECAUTIONS
Caution during first 1-2 weeks of therapy if transferring from longer $T_{1/2}$ sulfonylureas (eg, chlorpropamide). Consider hospitalization during the insulin withdrawal period if patient has been receiving >40 U/day of insulin. May be associated with increased risk of cardiovascular mortality. May produce severe hypoglycemia; increased risk in elderly, debilitated, or malnourished patients; with renal/hepatic impairment, or adrenal/pituitary insufficiency; when caloric intake is deficient; or after severe/prolonged exercise. Loss of glycemic control may occur when exposed to stress (eg, fever, trauma, infection, surgery); may be necessary to d/c therapy and administer insulin. Secondary failure may occur over time. May cause hemolytic anemia; caution with G6PD deficiency and consider a non-sulfonylurea alternative. Caution in elderly.

ADVERSE REACTIONS
Hypoglycemia, GI disturbances, dizziness, drowsiness, headache, porphyria cutanea tarda, photosensitivity reactions, leukopenia, agranulocytosis, thrombocytopenia, hemolytic anemia.

DRUG INTERACTIONS
See Dosage. Hypoglycemic effects may be potentiated by NSAIDs, some azoles, other highly protein-bound drugs, salicylates, sulfonamides, chloramphenicol, probenecid, coumarins, MAOIs, and β-blockers; monitor closely for hypoglycemia during coadministration and for loss of glycemic control when such drugs are withdrawn. Potential interaction leading to severe hypoglycemia reported with oral miconazole. Fluconazole may increase levels. Thiazides and other diuretics, corticosteroids, phenothiazines, thyroid products, estrogens, oral contraceptives, phenytoin, nicotinic acid, sympathomimetics, calcium channel blockers, and isoniazid may produce hyperglycemia and may lead to loss of glycemic control; monitor closely for loss of control during coadministration and for hypoglycemia when such drugs are withdrawn. Increased likelihood of hypoglycemia with alcohol and use of >1 glucose-lowering drug. May be difficult to recognize hypoglycemia with β-blockers. Caution with salicylate or dicumarol. Colesevelam may reduce levels.

PATIENT CONSIDERATIONS

Assessment: Assess for previous hypersensitivity to drug, renal/hepatic impairment, type of DM, diabetic ketoacidosis, risk factors for hypoglycemia, G6PD deficiency, pregnancy/nursing status, and possible drug interactions. Obtain baseline FPG and HbA1c levels.

Monitoring: Monitor for hypoglycemia, loss of glycemic control when exposed to stress, hypersensitivity reactions, secondary failure, hemolytic anemia, and other adverse reactions. Monitor blood/urine glucose and HbA1c levels periodically.

Counseling: Inform of the risks, benefits, and alternative modes of therapy. Counsel about the importance of adherence to dietary instructions, regular exercise program, and regular testing of urine and/or blood glucose. Inform about the symptoms, treatment, and predisposing conditions of hypoglycemia, as well as primary and secondary failure. During the insulin withdrawal period, instruct to test for sugar and ketone bodies in urine at least tid and to contact physician immediately if these tests are abnormal.

STORAGE: <30°C (86°F).

GLUCOTROL XL – glipizide

RX

Class: Sulfonylurea (2nd generation)

ADULT DOSAGE

Type 2 Diabetes Mellitus

Initial: 5mg qd; start at 2.5mg qd if at increased risk of hypoglycemia
Titrate: Adjust dose based on patient's glycemic control
Max: 20mg qd

Switching from Immediate-Release Glipizide:
May give qd dose at the nearest equivalent total daily dose

PEDIATRIC DOSAGE

Pediatric use may not have been established

DOSING CONSIDERATIONS

Concomitant Medications

Other Blood-Glucose-Lowering Agents: Initiate Glucotrol XL at 5mg qd; start at lower dose if at increased risk for hypoglycemia
Colesevelam: Administer at least 4 hrs prior to colesevelam

Renal Impairment

Initial: 2.5mg qd

Hepatic Impairment

Initial: 2.5mg qd
Dose conservatively

Elderly

Initial: 2.5mg qd
Dose conservatively

Other Important Considerations

Debilitated/Malnourished/Adrenal Impairment/Pituitary Impairment:
Initial: 2.5mg qd

ADMINISTRATION

Oral route

Administer w/ breakfast or the first main meal of the day.
Swallow tab whole; do not chew, divide, or crush.

HOW SUPPLIED

Tab, Extended-Release (ER): 2.5mg, 5mg, 10mg

CONTRAINDICATIONS

Known hypersensitivity to glipizide or any components of the medication, hypersensitivity to sulfonamide derivatives.

WARNINGS/PRECAUTIONS

Not recommended for the treatment of type 1 diabetes mellitus (DM) or diabetic ketoacidosis. May produce severe hypoglycemia. There is an increased risk for hypoglycemia w/ debilitated or malnourished patients; adrenal, pituitary, or hepatic impairment; deficient caloric intake; or after severe/prolonged exercise. May cause hemolytic anemia; avoid in patients w/ G6PD deficiency. May be associated w/ increased risk of cardiovascular mortality. Obstructive symptoms reported in patients w/ known strictures in association w/ ingestion of another drug w/ non-dissolvable ER formulation; avoid in patients w/ preexisting severe GI narrowing (pathologic or iatrogenic).

ADVERSE REACTIONS

Hypoglycemia, dizziness, diarrhea, nervousness, tremor, flatulence.

DRUG INTERACTIONS

See Dosing Considerations. Ingestion of alcohol may increase likelihood of hypoglycemia. Potential interaction leading to severe hypoglycemia reported w/ oral miconazole; monitor for hypoglycemia. Fluconazole may increase levels which may lead to hypoglycemia; monitor for hypoglycemia. Colesevelam may reduce max plasma concentration and total exposure of glipizide. Concomitant use w/ other anti-diabetic medications may increase the risk of hypoglycemia; a lower dose of glipizide may be required. Early warning symptoms of hypoglycemia may be different or less pronounced in patients who are taking β-adrenergic blocking medications or other sympatholytic agents.

PATIENT CONSIDERATIONS

Assessment: Assess for hypersensitivity to glipizide or any components of the medication, hypersensitivity to sulfonamide derivatives, renal/hepatic impairment, type of DM, diabetic ketoacidosis, risk factors for hypoglycemia, G6PD deficiency, severe GI narrowing (pathologic or iatrogenic), pregnancy/nursing status, and for possible drug interactions. Obtain baseline FPG and HbA1c levels.

Monitoring: Monitor for hypoglycemia, hypersensitivity reactions, secondary failure, hemolytic anemia, and other adverse reactions. Periodically monitor blood glucose levels and HbA1c levels.

Counseling: Advise of the risks and benefits of therapy. Inform about the risk of hypoglycemia, its symptoms and treatment, and conditions that predispose to its development. Counsel about the importance of adherence to dietary instructions, of a regular exercise program, and of regular testing of glycemic control. Advise patients that they may occasionally notice something that looks like a tablet in their stool. Advise to inform healthcare provider if pregnant, contemplating pregnancy, breastfeeding, or contemplating breastfeeding.

STORAGE: 20-25°C (68-77°F); excursions permitted between 15-30°C (59-86°F). Protect from moisture and humidity.

GLUCOVANCE – glyburide/metformin hydrochloride RX

Class: Biguanide/sulfonylurea

Lactic acidosis may occur due to metformin accumulation; risk increases w/ CHF, degree of renal dysfunction, and patient's age. Regularly monitor renal function and use the minimum effective dose of metformin. Do not initiate in patients ≥80 yrs of age unless measurement of CrCl demonstrates that renal function is not reduced. Promptly withhold therapy in the presence of any condition associated w/ hypoxemia, dehydration, or sepsis. Avoid w/ clinical or lab evidence of hepatic disease. Caution against excessive alcohol intake; alcohol potentiates the effects of metformin on lactate metabolism. Temporarily d/c therapy prior to any intravascular radiocontrast study and for any surgical procedure. D/C use immediately and promptly institute general supportive measures if lactic acidosis occurs. Prompt hemodialysis is recommended to correct the acidosis and remove the accumulated metformin.

ADULT DOSAGE

Type 2 Diabetes Mellitus

Currently on Diet and Exercise:
Initial: 1.25mg/250mg qd w/ a meal; may use 1.25mg/250mg bid w/ the am and pm meals if baseline HbA1c >9% or FPG >200mg/dL
Titrate: Increase by 1.25mg/250mg/day every 2 weeks
Max: 20mg/2000mg/day

Currently on a Sulfonylurea and/or Metformin:
Initial: 2.5mg/500mg or 5mg/500mg bid w/ the am and pm meals; starting dose should not exceed daily doses of the sulfonylurea or metformin already being taken
Titrate: Increase by no more than 5mg/500mg/day
Max: 20mg/2000mg/day

Addition of Thiazolidinediones:
Continue current dose of Glucovance and initiate thiazolidinedione at its recommended starting dose

PEDIATRIC DOSAGE

Pediatric use may not have been established

DOSING CONSIDERATIONS

Concomitant Medications

Colesevelam: Administer Glucovance at least 4 hrs prior to colesevelam

Elderly

Initial/Maint: Dose conservatively; do not titrate to max dose

Adverse Reactions

Hypoglycemia w/ Glucovance/Thiazolidinedione Combination: Consider reducing the dose of the glyburide component; consider adjusting the dosages of the other components of the regimen as clinically warranted

Other Important Considerations

Debilitated/Malnourished Patients: Do not titrate to max dose

ADMINISTRATION

Oral route

HOW SUPPLIED

Tab: (Glyburide/Metformin) 1.25mg/250mg, 2.5mg/500mg, 5mg/500mg

CONTRAINDICATIONS

Renal disease or dysfunction (eg, SrCr ≥1.5mg/dL [males], ≥1.4mg/dL [females], or abnormal CrCl); known hypersensitivity to metformin HCl or glyburide; acute or chronic metabolic acidosis, including diabetic ketoacidosis, w/ or w/o coma; concomitant administration of bosentan.

WARNINGS/PRECAUTIONS

May be associated w/ increased cardiovascular (CV) mortality. May cause hypoglycemia; increased risk when caloric intake is deficient; when strenuous exercise is not compensated by caloric supplementation; w/ renal/hepatic insufficiency, adrenal/pituitary insufficiency, alcohol intoxication; or in elderly, debilitated, or malnourished patients. Not recommended during pregnancy. Caution in elderly. Glyburide: May cause hemolytic anemia; caution w/ G6PD deficiency. Metformin: Assess renal function before initiation of therapy and at least annually thereafter; d/c w/ evidence of renal impairment. Temporarily d/c at the time of or prior to radiologic studies involving the use of intravascular iodinated contrast materials, withhold for 48 hrs subsequent to the procedure, and reinstitute only if renal function is normal. D/C promptly if CV collapse (shock), acute CHF, acute MI and other conditions characterized by hypoxemia occur. Temporarily suspend for any surgical procedure (except minor procedures not associated w/ restricted intake of food and fluids); restart when oral intake is resumed and renal function is normal. May decrease serum vitamin B12 levels; monitor hematologic parameters annually. Caution in patients predisposed to developing subnormal vitamin B12 levels (eg, those w/ inadequate vitamin B12 or Ca^{2+} intake or absorption). Evaluate patients previously well controlled on therapy who develop lab abnormalities or clinical illness for evidence of ketoacidosis or lactic acidosis; d/c if acidosis occurs.

G

ADVERSE REACTIONS

Lactic acidosis, upper respiratory infection, N/V, abdominal pain, headache, dizziness, diarrhea.

DRUG INTERACTIONS

See Boxed Warning, Dosage, Dosing Considerations, and Contraindications. Increased risk of hypoglycemia w/ other glucose-lowering agents or ethanol. May be difficult to recognize hypoglycemia w/ β-blockers. Thiazides and other diuretics, corticosteroids, phenothiazines, thyroid products, estrogens, oral contraceptives, phenytoin, nicotinic acid, sympathomimetics, calcium channel blockers, and isoniazid may produce hyperglycemia and may lead to loss of glycemic control; monitor closely for loss of control during coadministration and for hypoglycemia during withdrawal of these drugs. Weight gain observed w/ the addition of rosiglitazone to therapy. Monitor LFTs during coadministration w/ a thiazolidinedione. Metformin: Caution w/ drugs that may affect renal function or result in significant hemodynamic change or may interfere w/ the disposition of metformin (eg, cationic drugs eliminated by renal tubular secretion). Furosemide, nifedipine, and cimetidine may increase levels. May decrease furosemide levels. Cationic drugs that are eliminated by renal tubular secretion (eg, cimetidine, amiloride, digoxin, morphine, quinidine, vancomycin) may potentially produce an interaction; monitor and adjust dose of therapy and/or the interfering drug. Glyburide: Hypoglycemic effects may be potentiated by NSAIDs and other highly protein-bound drugs, salicylates, sulfonamides, chloramphenicol, probenecid, coumarins, MAOIs, and β-blockers; monitor closely for hypoglycemia during coadministration and for loss of glycemic control during withdrawal of these drugs. Possible interaction w/ ciprofloxacin (a fluoroquinolone antibiotic), resulting in potentiation of hypoglycemic action. Potential interaction leading to severe hypoglycemia reported w/ oral miconazole. Colesevelam may reduce levels.

PATIENT CONSIDERATIONS

Assessment: Assess for metabolic acidosis, diabetic ketoacidosis, risk factors for lactic acidosis, renal/hepatic impairment, presence of malnourishment or debilitation, adrenal/pituitary insufficiency, alcoholism, G6PD deficiency, hypoxemia, inadequate vitamin B12 or Ca^{2+} intake/absorption, previous hypersensitivity to the drug, pregnancy/nursing status, and possible drug interactions. Assess if patient is planning to undergo any surgical procedure, or radiologic studies involving the use of intravascular iodinated contrast materials. Obtain baseline FPG and HbA1c levels, and hematologic parameters.

Monitoring: Monitor for signs/symptoms of lactic acidosis, CV effects, hypoglycemia, hemolytic anemia, and other adverse reactions. Monitor for changes in clinical status. Monitor renal function, especially in elderly, at least annually. Monitor hematologic parameters annually. Perform routine serum vitamin B12 measurements at 2- to 3-yr intervals in patients predisposed to developing subnormal vitamin B12 levels. Monitor FPG and HbA1c levels periodically.

Counseling: Inform of the risks, benefits, and alternative modes of therapy. Advise on the importance of adherence to dietary instructions, regular exercise program, and regular testing of blood glucose, HbA1c, renal function, and hematologic parameters. Inform of the risk of lactic acidosis; instruct to d/c therapy immediately and notify physician if unexplained hyperventilation, myalgia, malaise, unusual somnolence, or other nonspecific symptoms occur. Inform of the risk of hypoglycemia. Counsel against excessive alcohol intake.

STORAGE: Up to 25°C (77°F).

GLYXAMBI – empagliflozin/linagliptin RX

Class: Dipeptidyl peptidase-4 (DPP-4) inhibitor/sodium-glucose cotransporter 2 (SGLT2) inhibitor

ADULT DOSAGE

Type 2 Diabetes Mellitus

Recommended Dose: 10mg/5mg qam

Titrate: May increase to 25mg/5mg qd in patients tolerating therapy

PEDIATRIC DOSAGE

Pediatric use may not have been established

DOSING CONSIDERATIONS

Renal Impairment

eGFR <45mL/min/1.73m^2: Do not initiate treatment

eGFR is Persistently <45mL/min/1.73m^2: D/C therapy

Other Important Considerations

Patients w/ Volume Depletion:

Correct this condition prior to initiating therapy

ADMINISTRATION

Oral route

Take w/ or w/o food.

HOW SUPPLIED

Tab: (Empagliflozin/Linagliptin) 10mg/5mg, 25mg/5mg

CONTRAINDICATIONS

History of hypersensitivity reaction (eg, anaphylaxis, angioedema, exfoliative skin conditions, urticaria, bronchial hyperreactivity) to linagliptin; history of serious hypersensitivity reaction to empagliflozin. Severe renal impairment, ESRD, dialysis.

WARNINGS/PRECAUTIONS

Not recommended w/ type 1 diabetes mellitus (DM) or for treatment of diabetic ketoacidosis. **Empagliflozin:** May cause intravascular volume contraction. Symptomatic hypotension may occur, particularly w/ renal impairment, the elderly, patients w/ low systolic BP, and in patients on diuretics. Ketoacidosis reported; if suspected, d/c and institute prompt treatment. Assess for ketoacidosis in patients presenting w/ signs/symptoms consistent w/ severe metabolic acidosis regardless of presenting blood glucose levels. Consider temporarily discontinuing therapy in clinical situations known to predispose to ketoacidosis (eg, prolonged fasting due to acute illness or surgery). May increase SrCr and decrease eGFR; risk of impaired renal function is increased in elderly and in patients w/ moderate renal impairment. Serious UTIs (eg, urosepsis, pyelonephritis), requiring hospitalization, reported; evaluate for signs/symptoms of UTIs and treat promptly, if indicated. Increases risk for genital mycotic infections and UTIs; monitor and treat as appropriate. Increases in LDL may occur; monitor and treat as appropriate. Monitoring glycemic control w/ urine glucose tests or 1,5-anhydroglucitol assay is not recommended. **Linagliptin:** Acute pancreatitis, including fatal pancreatitis, reported; d/c therapy and initiate appropriate management if pancreatitis is suspected. Serious hypersensitivity reactions reported; if suspected, d/c therapy, assess for other potential causes, and institute alternative treatment for DM. Caution in patients w/ history of angioedema to another DPP-4 inhibitor. Severe and disabling arthralgia may occur; consider as a possible cause for severe joint pain and d/c therapy if appropriate.

ADVERSE REACTIONS

UTI, URTI, nasopharyngitis, hypoglycemia.

DRUG INTERACTIONS

Use in combination w/ an insulin secretagogue (eg, sulfonylurea) or insulin may be associated w/ a higher rate of hypoglycemia; may require a lower dose of insulin secretagogue or insulin. **Empagliflozin:** Coadministration w/ diuretics resulted in increased urine volume and frequency of voids; may enhance potential for volume depletion. **Linagliptin:** Rifampin decreased exposure. Strong P-gp or CYP3A4 inducers may reduce linagliptin efficacy; use of alternative treatments is strongly recommended.

PATIENT CONSIDERATIONS

Assessment: Assess for history of hypersensitivity to either drug, type of DM, diabetic ketoacidosis, renal impairment, history of chronic or recurrent genital mycotic infections, history of angioedema w/ another DPP-4 inhibitor, pregnancy/nursing status, and possible drug interactions. Obtain baseline FPG and HbA1c levels. Assess for volume contraction and correct volume status if indicated.

Monitoring: Monitor for signs/symptoms of pancreatitis, hypotension, ketoacidosis, genital mycotic infections, UTIs, hypersensitivity reactions, LDL increase, severe joint pain, and other adverse reactions. Monitor FPG, HbA1c levels, and renal function periodically.

Counseling: Inform of the potential risks and benefits of therapy, alternative modes of therapy, importance of adherence to dietary instructions, regular physical activity, periodic blood glucose monitoring and HbA1c testing, recognition/management of hypo/hyperglycemia, and assessment of diabetes complications. Advise to seek medical advice promptly during periods of stress (eg, fever, trauma, infection), as medication requirements may change. Instruct to immediately report to physician if pregnant/nursing, if experiencing symptoms of hypotension, if any unusual symptom develops, or if any known symptom persists or worsens. Instruct to d/c use and notify physician if signs/symptoms of pancreatitis (eg, severe abdominal pain) or allergic reactions (eg, rash) occur. Instruct to d/c and seek medical advice immediately if symptoms of ketoacidosis occur. Inform that dehydration may increase the risk for hypotension, and to have adequate fluid intake. Advise on the signs/symptoms of UTIs, vaginal yeast infections, balanitis, and balanoposthitis; explain of treatment options and when to seek medical advice. Inform that severe and disabling joint pain may occur and to seek medical advice if this occurs.

STORAGE: 25°C (77°F); excursions permitted to 15-30°C (59-86°F).

G

GoLYTELY – polyethylene glycol 3350/potassium chloride/sodium bicarbonate/sodium chloride/sodium sulfate

RX

Class: Bowel cleanser

ADULT DOSAGE

Bowel Cleansing

Prior to Colonoscopy and Barium Enema X-Ray Examination:

PO:

240mL (8 oz) every 10 min until 4L consumed or rectal effluent is clear

NG Tube:

20-30mL/min (1.2-1.8L/hr).

PEDIATRIC DOSAGE

Pediatric use may not have been established

ADMINISTRATION

Oral/NG tube route

Must be reconstituted w/ water before use; not for direct ingestion

May consume water or clear liquids during bowel preparation and after completion of bowel preparation up until 2 hrs before the time of colonoscopy; sol is more palatable if chilled prior to administration

Rapid drinking of each portion is preferred to drinking small amounts continuously

First bowel movements should occur approx 1 hr after the start of administration

Administration Instructions Prior to Dosage

On the day prior to the colonoscopy, instruct patients to:

1. Take only clear liquids; avoid red and purple liquids. Patients may consume a light breakfast
2. Early in the pm prior to colonoscopy, fill the supplied container containing powder w/ lukewarm water to the 4L fill line; sol is clear and colorless when reconstituted
3. Shake vigorously several times to ensure that the ingredients are dissolved; use w/in 48 hrs when reconstituted

HOW SUPPLIED

Sol (Powder): (Polyethylene Glycol (PEG) 3350/Sodium Sulfate/Sodium Bicarbonate/Sodium Chloride/Potassium Chloride) 236g/22.74g/6.74g/5.86g/2.97g [4L], 227.1g/21.5g/6.36g/5.53g/2.82g [1 gallon]

CONTRAINDICATIONS

GI obstruction, ileus, or gastric retention; bowel perforation; toxic colitis or toxic megacolon; known allergy or hypersensitivity to any component of this product.

WARNINGS/PRECAUTIONS

Adequately hydrate before, during, and after use; caution with congestive heart failure when replacing fluids. Consider performing postcolonoscopy lab tests (electrolytes, SrCr, BUN) and treat accordingly if significant vomiting or signs of dehydration develop. Correct fluid and electrolyte abnormalities before treatment. Caution with conditions that increase risk for fluid and electrolyte disturbances or may increase risk of adverse events (eg, seizures, arrhythmias, and renal impairment). Serious arrhythmias reported rarely; caution in patients at increased risk of arrhythmias and consider predose and postcolonoscopy ECGs. Generalized tonic-clonic seizures and/or loss of consciousness reported; caution in patients with a history of or at increased risk of seizures (eg, with known/suspected hyponatremia). Caution with impaired renal function; consider performing baseline and postcolonoscopy lab tests. May produce colonic mucosal aphthous ulcerations; consider this when interpreting colonoscopy findings in patients with known/suspected inflammatory bowel disease. Serious cases of ischemic colitis reported. Slow administration or temporarily d/c if severe bloating, distention, or abdominal pain develops; caution with severe ulcerative colitis. Caution in patients with impaired gag reflex, unconscious or semiconscious patients, and patients prone to regurgitation or aspiration; observe during administration especially if administered via NG tube. Not for direct ingestion; direct ingestion of undissolved powder may increase risk of N/V, dehydration, and electrolyte disturbances.

ADVERSE REACTIONS

Nausea, abdominal fullness/bloating.

DRUG INTERACTIONS

Caution with medications that increase risk for fluid and electrolyte disturbances or may increase risk of adverse events (eg, seizures, arrhythmias, prolonged QT, renal impairment). Caution with drugs that lower seizure threshold (eg, TCAs) and in patients withdrawing from alcohol or benzodiazepines. Caution with drugs that may affect renal function (eg, diuretics, ACE inhibitors, ARBs, NSAIDs). Oral medication administered within 1 hr of start of administration may be flushed from GI tract and may not be absorbed properly. Avoid with stimulant laxatives (eg, bisacodyl, sodium picosulfate); may increase the risk of mucosal ulceration or ischemic colitis.

PATIENT CONSIDERATIONS

Assessment: Assess for drug hypersensitivity, GI obstruction, gastric retention, bowel perforation, ileus, toxic colitis, toxic megacolon, fluid and electrolyte abnormalities, renal impairment, any other conditions where treatment is cautioned, pregnancy/nursing status, and possible drug interactions. Consider predose ECG in patients at increased risk of serious cardiac arrhythmias.

Monitoring: Monitor for arrhythmias, generalized tonic-clonic seizures, loss of consciousness, colonic mucosal aphthous ulceration, ischemic colitis, and other adverse reactions. Monitor patients with impaired gag reflex, unconscious or semiconscious patients, and patients prone to regurgitation or aspiration, especially if administered via NG tube. Consider performing postcolonoscopy lab tests (electrolytes, SrCr, BUN) in patients with dehydration or renal impairment.

Counseling: Inform that sol is more palatable if chilled. Instruct to inform physician if have trouble swallowing or are prone to regurgitation or aspiration. Instruct not to take other laxatives. Instruct to consume water or clear liquids during the bowel preparation and after completion of the bowel preparation up until 2 hrs before the time of the colonoscopy. If severe bloating, distention, or abdominal pain occur, instruct to slow or temporarily d/c administration until symptoms abate; advise to report these events to physician. Instruct to d/c and contact physician if hives, rashes, or any allergic reaction develop. Instruct to notify physician if signs/symptoms of dehydration develop. Inform that oral medication administered within 1 hr of the start of administration may be flushed from the GI tract and the medication may not be absorbed completely. Counsel that rapid drinking of each portion is preferred rather than drinking small amounts continuously. Inform that the 1st bowel movement should occur approximately 1 hr after start of administration and to continue drinking until the watery stool is clear and free of solid matter.

STORAGE: 15-30°C (59-86°F). Reconstituted Sol: Keep refrigerated. Use within 48 hrs.

GRANIX – tbo-filgrastim

RX

Class: Granulocyte colony-stimulating factor (G-CSF)

ADULT DOSAGE

Chemotherapy-Associated Neutropenia

Reducing the Duration of Severe Neutropenia in Patients with Non-Myeloid Malignancies Receiving Myelosuppressive Anticancer Drugs:

5mcg/kg/day SQ

Continue daily dosing until the expected neutrophil nadir is passed and the neutrophil count has recovered to the normal range

PEDIATRIC DOSAGE

Pediatric use may not have been established

ADMINISTRATION

SQ route

Administer the 1st dose no earlier than 24 hrs following myelosuppressive chemotherapy; do not administer w/in 24 hrs prior to chemotherapy

Prefilled syringes are for single use only; discard unused portions

Recommended sites of administration include abdomen (except for the 2-inch area around the navel), the front of the middle thighs, the upper outer areas of the buttocks, or the upper back portion of the upper arms
Vary inj site daily
Do not inject into an area that is tender, red, bruised, hard, or that has scars or stretch marks
Avoid shaking syringe

HOW SUPPLIED

Inj: 300mcg/0.5mL, 480mcg/0.8mL

WARNINGS/PRECAUTIONS

May be administered by either a healthcare professional or by a patient/caregiver; before a decision is made to allow therapy to be administered by a patient/caregiver, ensure that the patient is an appropriate candidate for self-administration or administration by a caregiver. Splenic rupture, including fatal cases, may occur; d/c therapy and evaluate for an enlarged spleen or splenic rupture if upper abdominal or shoulder pain occurs. Acute respiratory distress syndrome (ARDS) may occur; evaluate for ARDS if fever and lung infiltrates or respiratory distress develops, and d/c if ARDS occurs. Serious allergic reactions may occur; permanently d/c if such reactions occur. Severe and sometimes fatal sickle cell crises may occur in patients with sickle cell disease; d/c in patients undergoing a sickle cell crisis. Capillary leak syndrome (CLS) may occur; closely monitor and give standard symptomatic treatment if symptoms develop. May act as a growth factor for any tumor type. Increased hematopoietic activity of the bone marrow in response to therapy has been associated with transient positive bone imaging changes; consider this when interpreting bone-imaging results.

H

ADVERSE REACTIONS

Bone pain.

DRUG INTERACTIONS

Caution with drugs that may potentiate the release of neutrophils (eg, lithium).

PATIENT CONSIDERATIONS

Assessment: Assess for history of hypersensitivity to the drug, history of serious allergic reactions to filgrastim or pegfilgrastim, sickle cell disease, pregnancy/nursing status, and possible drug interactions. Assess CBC prior to chemotherapy.

Monitoring: Monitor for enlarged spleen/splenic rupture, ARDS, serious allergic reactions, sickle cell crisis (in patients with sickle cell disease), CLS, and other adverse reactions. Monitor CBC twice per week until recovery.

Counseling: Instruct patient or caregivers on the proper storage, preparation, and administration technique once it is determined that a patient is an appropriate candidate for self-administration or administration by a caregiver. Instruct to report any symptoms of adverse reactions to physician. Inform that bone pain is common and analgesics may be necessary. Counsel to be alert for signs of infection and to report these findings to physician immediately. Inform not to become pregnant while on therapy; advise of the possibility of fetal harm if pregnancy occurs.

STORAGE: 2-8°C (36-46°F). Protect from light. May be removed from 2-8°C (36-46°F) storage for a single period of up to 5 days between 23-27°C (73-81°F); if not used within 5 days, may be returned to 2-8°C (36-46°F).

HALCION – triazolam

CIV

Class: Benzodiazepine

ADULT DOSAGE

Insomnia

Short-Term Treatment (Generally 7-10 Days):
0.25mg qhs; 0.125mg may be sufficient for some patients (eg, low body weight)
Max: 0.5mg

PEDIATRIC DOSAGE

Pediatric use may not have been established

DOSING CONSIDERATIONS

Elderly

Elderly/Debilitated:
Initial: 0.125mg
Max: 0.25mg

ADMINISTRATION

Oral route

HOW SUPPLIED

Tab: 0.25mg* *scored

CONTRAINDICATIONS
Known hypersensitivity to this drug or other benzodiazepines; pregnancy; concomitant use w/ medications that significantly impair the oxidative metabolism mediated by CYP3A (eg, ketoconazole, itraconazole, nefazodone, HIV protease inhibitors).

WARNINGS/PRECAUTIONS
Initiate only after careful evaluation; failure of insomnia to remit after 7-10 days of treatment may indicate presence of a primary psychiatric and/or medical illness. Use lowest effective dose, especially in elderly. Complex behaviors (eg, sleep-driving, preparing/eating food, making phone calls, having sex) reported; consider discontinuation if sleep-driving occurs. Severe anaphylactic and anaphylactoid reactions reported; do not rechallenge if angioedema develops. Increased daytime anxiety reported; may d/c if observed. Abnormal thinking, behavior changes, anterograde amnesia, paradoxical reactions, traveler's amnesia, and dose-related side effects (eg, drowsiness, dizziness, lightheadedness, amnesia) reported. Worsening of depression, including suicidal thinking, reported in primarily depressed patients. May impair mental/physical abilities. Respiratory depression and apnea reported in patients with compromised respiratory function. Caution in patients with signs or symptoms of depression that could be intensified by hypnotic drugs, renal/hepatic impairment, chronic pulmonary insufficiency, and sleep apnea. Dependence and tolerance to drug may develop; caution with history of alcoholism, drug abuse, or with marked personality disorders, due to increased risk of dependence. Withdrawal symptoms reported following abrupt discontinuation; avoid abrupt discontinuation, and taper dose gradually in any patient taking more than the lowest dose for more than a few weeks or with history of seizure.

ADVERSE REACTIONS
Drowsiness, dizziness, lightheadedness, headache, nervousness, coordination disorders/ataxia, N/V.

DRUG INTERACTIONS
See Contraindications. Avoid with very potent CYP3A inhibitors (eg, azole-type antifungals). Caution and consider triazolam dose reduction with drugs inhibiting CYP3A to a lesser but significant degree. Macrolide antibiotics (eg, erythromycin, clarithromycin) and cimetidine may increase levels; use with caution and consider triazolam dose reduction. Isoniazid, oral contraceptives, grapefruit juice, and ranitidine may increase levels; use with caution. Additive CNS depressant effects with psychotropic medications, anticonvulsants, antihistamines, ethanol, and other CNS depressants. Increased risk of complex behaviors with alcohol and other CNS depressants. Caution with fluvoxamine, diltiazem, verapamil, sertraline, paroxetine, ergotamine, cyclosporine, amiodarone, nicardipine, and nifedipine.

PATIENT CONSIDERATIONS

Assessment: Assess for physical and/or psychiatric disorder, depression, compromised respiratory function, renal/hepatic impairment, chronic pulmonary insufficiency, sleep apnea, history of seizures, alcoholism or drug abuse, marked personality disorders, hypersensitivity to the drug, pregnancy/nursing status, and possible drug interactions.

Monitoring: Monitor for complex behaviors, anaphylactic/anaphylactoid reactions, increased daytime anxiety, emergence of any new behavioral signs/symptoms of concern, tolerance, dependence, withdrawal symptoms, and other adverse reactions.

Counseling: Inform of the risks and benefits of therapy. Caution against engaging in hazardous activities requiring complete mental alertness (eg, operating machinery, driving). Instruct to immediately report to physician if any adverse reactions (eg, sleep-driving, other complex behaviors) develop. Caution about the concomitant ingestion of alcohol and other CNS depressant drugs during treatment. Instruct to notify physician if pregnant, planning to become pregnant, or if nursing.

STORAGE: 20-25°C (68-77°F).

HALOPERIDOL – haloperidol

RX

Class: Butyrophenone

Elderly patients w/ dementia-related psychosis treated w/ antipsychotic drugs are at an increased risk of death; most deaths appeared to be cardiovascular (CV) (eg, heart failure, sudden death) or infectious (eg, pneumonia) in nature. Not approved for the treatment of patients w/ dementia-related psychosis.

OTHER BRAND NAMES
Haldol

ADULT DOSAGE

Psychosis

Sol/Tab:
Initial:
Moderate Symptoms:
0.5-2mg bid or tid

PEDIATRIC DOSAGE

Psychosis

Sol/Tab:
3-12 Years (15-40kg):
Initial: 0.5mg/day

Severe Symptoms/Chronic or Resistant Patients:
3-5mg bid or tid
Remain Severely Disturbed/Inadequately Controlled:
May need up to 100mg/day; >100mg/day has been used for severely resistant patients but safety of prolonged use not demonstrated

Maint:
Gradually reduce to lowest effective dose

Schizophrenia

Inj:
Acutely Agitated:
Moderately Severe to Very Severe Symptoms:
2-5mg
Subsequent Doses: May give as often as every hr; 4- to 8-hr intervals may be satisfactory
Max: 20mg/day

Tourette's Disorder

Sol/Tab:
Initial:
Moderate Symptoms:
0.5-2mg bid or tid
Severe Symptoms/Chronic or Resistant Patients:
3-5mg bid or tid
Remain Severely Disturbed/Inadequately Controlled:
May need up to 100mg/day; >100mg/day has been used for severely resistant patients but safety of prolonged use not demonstrated

Maint:
Gradually reduce to lowest effective dose

Conversions

From IM to Oral Formulations:
For the initial approximation of the total daily dose required, the parenteral dose administered in the preceding 24 hrs should be used w/in 12-24 hrs following the last parenteral dose

Monitor clinical signs and symptoms periodically for the 1st several days

Titrate: Increase by 0.5mg increments at 5- to 7-day intervals
Maint: Gradually reduce to lowest effective dose; 0.05-0.15mg/kg/day
Severely disturbed psychotic children may require higher doses

Total dose may be given bid or tid

Behavioral Problems

Failed Response to Psychotherapy/Non-Antipsychotic Medications:
Sol/Tab:
3-12 Years (15-40kg):
Initial: 0.5mg/day
Titrate: Increase by 0.5mg increments at 5- to 7-day intervals
Maint: Gradually reduce to lowest effective dose; 0.05-0.075mg/kg/day

Short-term treatment may suffice for severely disturbed, nonpsychotic/hyperactive children w/ conduct disorders

There is no evidence establishing a max effective dose; little evidence exists that behavior improvement is further enhanced in dosages beyond 6mg/day

Total dose may be given bid or tid

Tourette's Disorder

Sol/Tab:
3-12 Years (15-40kg):
Initial: 0.5mg/day
Titrate: Increase by 0.5mg increments at 5- to 7-day intervals
Maint: Gradually reduce to lowest effective dose; 0.05-0.075mg/kg/day

Total dose may be given bid or tid

DOSING CONSIDERATIONS

Elderly
Inj:
Initial: May require lower dose

Sol/Tab:
Initial: 0.5-2mg bid or tid

Other Important Considerations
Debilitated Patients:
Inj:
Initial: May require lower dose

Sol/Tab:
Initial: 0.5-2mg bid or tid

History of Adverse Reactions to Antipsychotic Drugs:
Inj:
Initial: May require lower dose

ADMINISTRATION

Oral/IM route

HOW SUPPLIED

Inj: (Haldol) 5mg/mL; **Sol:** 2mg/mL [15mL, 120mL]; **Tab:** 0.5mg*, 1mg*, 2mg*, 5mg*, 10mg*, 20mg*
*scored

H

CONTRAINDICATIONS

Severe toxic CNS depression or comatose states, Parkinson's disease, hypersensitivity to haloperidol.

WARNINGS/PRECAUTIONS

Risk of tardive dyskinesia (TD), especially in the elderly; consider discontinuation if signs/symptoms develop. Neuroleptic malignant syndrome (NMS) reported; d/c immediately, institute symptomatic treatment, and monitor. Hyperpyrexia, heat stroke, and bronchopneumonia reported. Dehydration, hemoconcentration, and reduced pulmonary ventilation may develop; institute prompt remedial therapy if signs/symptoms appear. Decreased serum cholesterol and/or cutaneous and ocular changes reported in patients receiving chemically related drugs. Leukopenia, neutropenia, and agranulocytosis reported; d/c if severe neutropenia (ANC <1000/mm^3) develops. Monitor CBC frequently during the 1st few months of therapy and consider discontinuation at 1st sign of clinically significant decline in WBCs in the absence of other causative factors if history of clinically significant preexisting low WBCs or drug-induced leukopenia/neutropenia exists. Caution w/ severe CV disease (CVD), in the elderly, and in patients w/ known/history of allergic reactions to drugs. May cause transient hypotension and/or precipitation of anginal pain in patients w/ severe CV disorders. If hypotension occurs and a vasopressor is required, treat w/ metaraminol, phenylephrine, or norepinephrine. There may be a rapid mood swing to depression when haloperidol is used to control mania in cyclic disorders. Severe neurotoxicity may occur in patients w/ thyrotoxicosis. May increase prolactin levels. May impair mental/physical abilities. May lower convulsive threshold; caution w/ history of seizures or EEG abnormalities. **Inj/Tab:** Sudden death, QT prolongation, and torsades de pointes reported. Caution w/ other QT-prolonging conditions (eg, electrolyte imbalance, underlying cardiac abnormalities, hypothyroidism, familial long QT syndrome).

ADVERSE REACTIONS

Extrapyramidal symptoms, TD, dystonia, ECG changes, insomnia, restlessness, tachycardia, hypotension, HTN, N/V, constipation, diarrhea, dry mouth, blurred vision, urinary retention.

DRUG INTERACTIONS

Encephalopathic syndrome followed by irreversible brain damage may occur w/ lithium; monitor closely for early evidence of neurological toxicity and promptly d/c treatment if such signs appear. Caution w/ anticonvulsants and anticoagulants (eg, phenindione). Anticholinergics, including antiparkinson agents, may increase IOP. If an antiparkinson medication is discontinued simultaneously w/ haloperidol, extrapyramidal symptoms may occur. May potentiate CNS depressants (eg, alcohol, anesthetics, opiates); avoid w/ alcohol. Avoid w/ epinephrine for hypotension treatment; vasopressor activity may be blocked and paradoxical further lowering of BP may occur. **Inj/Tab:** Caution w/ drugs known to prolong the QT interval or cause electrolyte imbalance. Rifampin may decrease levels. **Inj:** Ketoconazole (400mg/day) and paroxetine (20mg/day) may increase QTc. Potential increased levels and risk of certain adverse events w/ inhibitors of CYP450 or glucuronidation. CYP3A4 or CYP2D6 substrates/inhibitors (eg, itraconazole, nefazodone, buspirone, venlafaxine) may increase levels. A significant reduction of haloperidol plasma levels may occur when prolonged treatment (1-2 weeks) w/ enzyme-inducing drugs (eg, carbamazepine) is added to haloperidol; carefully monitor clinical status when enzyme inducing drugs are administered or discontinued; haloperidol dose may need to be adjusted during concomitant use; may be necessary to reduce the haloperidol dose after discontinuation of such drugs.

PATIENT CONSIDERATIONS

Assessment: Assess for severe toxic CNS depression or comatose states, Parkinson's disease, CVD, history of seizures, EEG abnormalities, hypersensitivity to drug, pregnancy/nursing status, and for any other conditions where treatment is contraindicated or cautioned. Assess for possible drug interactions.

Monitoring: Monitor for signs/symptoms of NMS, TD, bronchopneumonia, hyperpyrexia, heat stroke, QT prolongation, torsades de pointes, leukopenia, neutropenia, agranulocytosis, and for other adverse reactions. Monitor for neurotoxicity in patients w/ thyrotoxicosis. Monitor CBC frequently during the first few months of therapy in patients w/ a preexisting low WBC count or a history of drug-induced leukopenia/neutropenia. Carefully monitor for fever or other symptoms or signs of infection in patients w/ neutropenia. Monitor vital signs, ECG, EEG, serum electrolytes, and cholesterol levels.

Counseling: Inform about risks/benefits of therapy. Instruct to use caution when performing hazardous tasks (eg, operating machinery/driving). Instruct to avoid alcohol due to possible additive effects and hypotension. Advise to inform physician if nursing, pregnant, or planning to get pregnant.

STORAGE: Protect from light. **Tab/Sol:** 20-25°C (68-77°F). **Inj:** 15-30°C (59-86°F). **Inj/Sol:** Do not freeze.

HARVONI – ledipasvir/sofosbuvir

RX

Class: HCV NS5A inhibitor/HCV nucleotide analogue NS5B polymerase inhibitor

ADULT DOSAGE

Chronic Hepatitis C

Chronic Hepatitis C Virus (HCV) Genotype 1, 4, 5, or 6 Infection:
1 tab qd w/ or w/o ribavirin

Treatment Duration:

Genotype 1:

Treatment-Naive w/o Cirrhosis or w/ Compensated Cirrhosis (Child-Pugh A): 12 weeks; may consider treatment duration of 8 weeks in patients w/o cirrhosis who have pre-treatment HCV RNA <6 million IU/mL

Treatment-Experienced w/o Cirrhosis: 12 weeks

Treatment-Experienced w/ Compensated Cirrhosis: 24 weeks; may consider Harvoni + ribavirin for 12 weeks in patients w/ cirrhosis who are eligible for ribavirin

Treatment-Naive and Treatment-Experienced w/ Decompensated Cirrhosis (Child-Pugh B or C): Harvoni + ribavirin for 12 weeks

Genotype 1 or 4:

Treatment-Naive and Treatment-Experienced Liver Transplant Recipients w/o Cirrhosis, or w/ Compensated Cirrhosis: Harvoni + ribavirin for 12 weeks

Genotype 4, 5, or 6:

Treatment-Naive and Treatment-Experienced w/o Cirrhosis or w/ Compensated Cirrhosis: 12 weeks

The recommended treatment durations are also applicable to patients w/ HCV/HIV-1 coinfection

For further information on ribavirin dosing and dosing modifications, refer to the ribavirin PI

PEDIATRIC DOSAGE

Pediatric use may not have been established

H

DOSING CONSIDERATIONS

Renal Impairment

Severe/ESRD: No dosage recommendation can be given due to higher exposures of the predominant sofosbuvir metabolite

ADMINISTRATION

Oral route

Take w/ or w/o food.

HOW SUPPLIED

Tab: (Ledipasvir/Sofosbuvir) 90mg/400mg

CONTRAINDICATIONS

If administered w/ ribavirin, refer to the ribavirin prescribing information for a list of contraindications for ribavirin.

WARNINGS/PRECAUTIONS

Symptomatic bradycardia, as well as fatal cardiac arrest and cases requiring pacemaker intervention, reported when coadministered w/ amiodarone. Patients also taking β-blockers, or those w/ underlying cardiac comorbidities and/or advanced liver disease, may be at increased risk for symptomatic bradycardia w/ coadministration of amiodarone. Not recommended w/ amiodarone. If coadministration is required, cardiac monitoring in an in-patient setting for the first 48 hrs of coadministration is recommended, after which outpatient or self-monitoring of HR should occur on a daily basis through at least the first 2 weeks of therapy. Patients discontinuing amiodarone just prior to starting therapy should also undergo similar cardiac monitoring.
P-gp inducers (eg, rifampin, St. John's wort) may decrease levels and may lead to a reduced therapeutic effect; not recommended w/ P-gp inducers. Not recommended w/ other products containing sofosbuvir. If administered w/ ribavirin, refer to the ribavirin prescribing information

for the warnings and precautions for ribavirin. Safety and efficacy not established w/ severe renal impairment or ESRD requiring hemodialysis.

ADVERSE REACTIONS

Fatigue, headache, asthenia.

DRUG INTERACTIONS

See Warnings/Precautions. Not recommended w/ carbamazepine, phenytoin, phenobarbital, oxcarbazepine, rifabutin, rifapentine, or tipranavir/ritonavir (RTV); may decrease levels. Not recommended w/ rosuvastatin; may increase rosuvastatin levels and consequently increase risk of myopathy, including rhabdomyolysis. May increase digoxin levels; monitor digoxin levels. Monitor for tenofovir-associated adverse reactions in patients receiving concomitant therapy w/ a regimen containing tenofovir disoproxil fumarate (TDF) w/o a HIV protease inhibitor/RTV or cobicistat. Coadministration w/ regimens containing TDF and an HIV protease inhibitor/RTV or cobicistat may increase tenofovir levels; consider alternative HCV or antiretroviral therapy to avoid increases in tenofovir exposures; if coadministration is necessary, monitor for tenofovir-associated adverse reactions. Coadministration w/ combination of elvitegravir, cobicistat, emtricitabine, and TDF is not recommended; may increase tenofovir levels. **Ledipasvir:** May increase intestinal absorption of coadministered substrates of P-gp or breast cancer resistance protein. Drugs that increase gastric pH may decrease levels. Separate administration w/ antacids by 4 hrs. May administer H_2-receptor antagonists (eg, famotidine) simultaneously or 12 hrs apart from Harvoni at a dose that does not exceed doses comparable to famotidine 40mg bid. Proton-pump inhibitor doses comparable to omeprazole ≤20mg can be administered simultaneously under fasted conditions. Not recommended w/ simeprevir; may increase levels. Refer to PI for further information on drug interactions.

PATIENT CONSIDERATIONS

Assessment: Assess for hypersensitivity to drug, pregnancy/nursing status, and possible drug interactions.

Monitoring: Monitor for bradycardia if coadministering w/ amiodarone or if discontinuing amiodarone just prior to starting therapy; perform cardiac monitoring in an in-patient setting for the first 48 hrs of coadministration, after which outpatient or self-monitoring of the HR should occur on a daily basis through at least the first 2 weeks of treatment. Perform clinical and hepatic lab monitoring for patients w/ decompensated cirrhosis receiving concomitant treatment w/ ribavirin. Monitor for other adverse reactions.

Counseling: Advise to seek medical evaluation immediately for symptoms of bradycardia. Inform that therapy may interact w/ other drugs; advise to report to physician the use of any other medication or herbal products. Advise to avoid pregnancy during combination treatment w/ ribavirin and for 6 months after completion of treatment; instruct to notify physician immediately in the event of a pregnancy. Advise to take therapy at the regularly schedule time w/ or w/o food.

STORAGE: Room temperature <30°C (86°F).

HAVRIX – hepatitis A vaccine

RX

Class: Vaccine

ADULT DOSAGE

Hepatitis A Vaccine

Active Immunization:

Single 1mL dose, then 1mL booster dose anytime between 6-12 months later

PEDIATRIC DOSAGE

Hepatitis A Vaccine

Active Immunization:

≥12 Months of Age:

Single 0.5mL dose, then 0.5mL booster dose anytime between 6-12 months later

ADMINISTRATION

IM route

Administer primary immunization at least 2 weeks prior to expected exposure to hepatitis A virus

Preparation

1. Shake well before use
2. For the prefilled syringes, attach a sterile needle and administer IM
3. For the vials, use a sterile needle and sterile syringe to withdraw the vaccine dose and administer IM
4. Changing needles between drawing vaccine from a vial and injecting it into a recipient is not necessary unless the needle has been damaged or contaminated
5. Use a separate sterile needle and syringe for each individual
6. Do not dilute to administer

Administration
1. Administer in the anterolateral aspect of the thigh in young children or in deltoid muscle of the upper arm in older children and adults; do not administer in the gluteal region
2. When concomitant administration of other vaccines or immune globulin is required, administer w/ different syringes and at different inj sites
3. Do not mix w/ any other vaccine or product in the same syringe or vial

HOW SUPPLIED
Inj: 720 EL.U./0.5mL, 1440 EL.U./mL [vial, prefilled syringe]

CONTRAINDICATIONS
Severe allergic reaction (eg, anaphylaxis) after a previous dose of any hepatitis A-containing vaccine, or to any component of Havrix, including neomycin.

WARNINGS/PRECAUTIONS
Tip caps of prefilled syringes may contain natural rubber latex; may cause allergic reactions in latex-sensitive individuals. Syncope may occur and can be accompanied by transient neurological signs (eg, visual disturbance, paresthesia, tonic-clonic limb movements); procedures should be in place to avoid falling injury and to restore cerebral perfusion following syncope. Appropriate treatment and supervision must be available for possible anaphylactic reactions. Immunocompromised persons may have a diminished immune response to vaccine. May not prevent hepatitis A infection in individuals who have an unrecognized hepatitis A infection at the time of vaccination. May not protect all individuals. Lower antibody response reported in patients with chronic liver disease.

ADVERSE REACTIONS
Inj-site reactions (eg, soreness, pain, redness, swelling, induration), headache, irritability, drowsiness, loss of appetite, fever, fatigue, malaise, anorexia, nausea.

DRUG INTERACTIONS
Immunosuppressive therapies, including irradiation, antimetabolites, alkylating agents, cytotoxic drugs, and corticosteroids (used in greater than physiologic doses), may reduce the immune response to vaccine.

PATIENT CONSIDERATIONS
Assessment: Assess for history of severe allergic reaction to hepatitis A vaccine or neomycin. Assess for latex sensitivity, immunosuppression, chronic liver disease, unrecognized hepatitis A infection, immunization status/vaccination history, pregnancy/nursing status, and possible drug interactions.

Monitoring: Monitor for allergic reactions, syncope, neurological signs, and other adverse reactions. Monitor immune response to vaccine.

Counseling: Inform of the potential benefits and risks of immunization. Counsel about potential side effects and emphasize that the vaccine contains noninfectious killed viruses and cannot cause hepatitis A infection. Instruct to report any adverse events to physician.

STORAGE: 2-8°C (36-46°F). Do not freeze; discard if vaccine has been frozen.

HERCEPTIN – trastuzumab
RX

Class: Monoclonal antibody/HER2 blocker

May result in cardiac failure; incidence and severity were highest w/ anthracycline-containing chemotherapy regimens. Evaluate left ventricular function prior to and during treatment; d/c in patients receiving adjuvant therapy and withhold in patients w/ metastatic disease for clinically significant decrease in left ventricular function. May result in serious and fatal infusion reactions and pulmonary toxicity; interrupt infusion for dyspnea or clinically significant hypotension, and monitor until symptoms completely resolve. D/C for anaphylaxis, angioedema, interstitial pneumonitis, or acute respiratory distress syndrome. Exposure during pregnancy may result in oligohydramnios and oligohydramnios sequence manifesting as pulmonary hypoplasia, skeletal abnormalities, and neonatal death.

ADULT DOSAGE
HER2 Overexpressing Node Positive or Node Negative Breast Cancer

Adjuvant Treatment:
During and Following Paclitaxel, Docetaxel, or Docetaxel/Carboplatin:
Initial: 4mg/kg IV infusion over 90 min, then at 2mg/kg IV infusion over 30 min weekly during chemotherapy for the first 12 weeks (paclitaxel or docetaxel) or 18 weeks (docetaxel/carboplatin)
Subsequent Doses: 1 week following the last weekly dose, give 6mg/kg IV infusion over 30-90 min every 3 weeks

PEDIATRIC DOSAGE
Pediatric use may not have been established

Single Agent w/in 3 Weeks Following Completion of Multimodality Anthracycline-Based Chemotherapy Regimens:
Initial: 8mg/kg IV infusion over 90 min
Subsequent Doses: 6mg/kg IV infusion over 30-90 min every 3 weeks

Administer for a total of 52 weeks; extending adjuvant treatment >1 yr is not recommended

HER2 Overexpressing Metastatic Breast Cancer

Alone or in Combination w/ Paclitaxel:
Initial: 4mg/kg IV infusion over 90 min
Subsequent Doses: 2mg/kg IV infusion over 30 min once a week until disease progression

HER2 Overexpressing Metastatic Gastric or Gastroesophageal Junction Adenocarcinoma

Patients Who Have Not Received Prior Treatment for Metastatic Disease:
Combination w/ Cisplatin and Capecitabine or 5-Fluorouracil:
Initial: 8mg/kg IV infusion over 90 min
Subsequent Doses: 6mg/kg IV infusion over 30-90 min every 3 weeks until disease progression

Missed Dose

Dose Missed by ≤1 Week:
Administer the usual maint dose (weekly schedule: 2mg/kg; 3-weekly schedule: 6mg/kg) as soon as possible; do not wait until the next planned cycle
Administer subsequent maint doses 7 days or 21 days later according to the weekly or 3-weekly schedules, respectively

Dose Missed by >1 Week:
Administer a reloading dose over approx 90 min (weekly schedule: 4mg/kg; 3-weekly schedule: 8mg/kg) as soon as possible
Administer subsequent maint doses (weekly schedule: 2mg/kg; 3-weekly schedule: 6mg/kg) 7 days or 21 days later according to the weekly or 3-weekly schedules, respectively

DOSING CONSIDERATIONS

Adverse Reactions
Infusion Reactions:
Mild or Moderate: Decrease rate of infusion
Dyspnea/Clinically Significant Hypotension: Interrupt infusion
Severe/Life-threatening: D/C therapy

Cardiomyopathy:
Withhold Therapy for at Least 4 Weeks for Either of the Following:
1. ≥16% absolute decrease in left ventricular ejection fraction (LVEF) from pretreatment values
2. LVEF below institutional limits of normal and ≥10% absolute decrease in LVEF from pretreatment values
May Resume Therapy if:
LVEF returns to normal limits and absolute decrease from baseline is ≤15% w/in 4-8 weeks
Permanently D/C Therapy for:
Persistent (>8 weeks) LVEF decline or for suspension of dosing on more than 3 occasions for cardiomyopathy

ADMINISTRATION

IV route
Do not administer as IV push or bolus
Do not mix w/ other drugs
Do not substitute for or w/ ado-trastuzumab emtansine

Reconstitution
Reconstitute each 440mg vial w/ 20mL of bacteriostatic water for inj, containing 1.1% benzyl alcohol as a preservative to yield a multidose sol containing 21mg/mL

In patients w/ known hypersensitivity to benzyl alcohol, reconstitute w/ 20mL of sterile water for inj (SWFI) w/o preservative to yield a single use sol
Swirl vial gently; do not shake
Allow vial to stand undisturbed for approx 5 min after reconstitution
If reconstituted w/ SWFI w/o preservative, use immediately

Dilution

1. Determine the dose (mg) and calculate the volume of the 21mg/mL reconstituted sol needed
2. Withdraw this amount from the vial and add it to an infusion bag containing 250mL of 0.9% NaCl inj
3. Gently invert the bag to mix the sol

HOW SUPPLIED

Inj: 440mg

WARNINGS/PRECAUTIONS

Patients w/ symptomatic intrinsic lung disease or extensive tumor involvement of the lungs, resulting in dyspnea at rest, may have more severe pulmonary toxicity. Detection of HER2 protein overexpression is necessary for appropriate patient selection; use FDA-approved tests for the specific tumor type to assess HER2 protein overexpression and HER2 gene amplification. Avoid pregnancy during treatment; if contraceptive methods are being considered, use effective contraception during treatment and for at least 7 months following the last dose of therapy.

ADVERSE REACTIONS

Cardiac failure, infusion reactions, pulmonary toxicity, fever, N/V, headache, nasopharyngitis, diarrhea, infections, fatigue, anemia, neutropenia, rash, weight loss, increased cough.

DRUG INTERACTIONS

See Boxed Warning. Higher incidence of neutropenia w/ myelosuppressive chemotherapy. Increased risk of cardiac dysfunction in patients who receive anthracycline after stopping trastuzumab; if possible, avoid anthracycline-based therapy for up to 7 months after stopping trastuzumab, but if anthracyclines are used, carefully monitor cardiac function.

PATIENT CONSIDERATIONS

Assessment: Assess cardiac function, including baseline left ventricular ejection fraction (LVEF). Assess HER2 protein overexpression and HER2 gene amplification. Assess for symptomatic intrinsic lung disease or extensive tumor involvement of lungs, pregnancy/nursing status, and possible drug interactions.

Monitoring: Monitor for infusion reactions, pulmonary toxicity, neutropenia, and other adverse reactions. Monitor LVEF every 3 months during and upon completion of therapy, and every 6 months for at least 2 yrs following completion of therapy as a component of adjuvant therapy. Repeat LVEF measurement at 4-week intervals if therapy is withheld for significant left ventricular cardiac dysfunction.

Counseling: Advise to contact physician immediately for new onset or worsening SOB, cough, swelling of ankles/legs/face, palpitations, weight gain of >5 lbs in 24 hrs, dizziness, or loss of consciousness. Inform that drug may cause fetal harm. Advise women who are exposed to drug during pregnancy or become pregnant w/in 7 months following the last dose of therapy, to immediately report exposure to Genentech Adverse Event Line. Encourage women who may be exposed to therapy during pregnancy or w/in 7 months of conception, to enroll in the MotHER Pregnancy Registry. Advise females of reproductive potential to avoid becoming pregnant during therapy; if contraceptive methods are being considered, instruct to use effective contraception during treatment and for at least 7 months following the last dose of therapy. Instruct not to breastfeed during treatment.

STORAGE: 2-8°C (36-46°F). Reconstituted w/ Bacteriostatic Water for Inj: 2-8°C (36-46°F) for 28 days. Diluted in Polyvinylchloride or Polyethylene Bags Containing 0.9% NaCl Inj: 2-8°C (36-46°F) for no more than 24 hrs prior to use. Do not freeze following reconstitution/dilution.

HETLIOZ – tasimelteon

RX

Class: Melatonin receptor agonist

ADULT DOSAGE

Non-24-Hour Sleep-Wake Disorder

20mg/day before hs, at the same time every night

PEDIATRIC DOSAGE

Pediatric use may not have been established

DOSING CONSIDERATIONS

Hepatic Impairment

Severe (Child-Pugh Class C): Not recommended

ADMINISTRATION
Oral route

Take w/o food
Swallow cap whole

HOW SUPPLIED
Cap: 20mg

WARNINGS/PRECAUTIONS
Effects of therapy may not occur for weeks or months because of individual differences in circadian rhythms. May cause somnolence; limit activity before going to bed. May impair mental/physical abilities. Not recommended with severe hepatic impairment.

ADVERSE REACTIONS
Headache, increased ALT, nightmare/abnormal dreams, URTI, UTI.

DRUG INTERACTIONS
Large increase in exposure with fluvoxamine or other strong CYP1A2 inhibitors; avoid concomitant use. Decreased exposure with reduced efficacy with rifampin or other CYP3A4 inducers; avoid concomitant use. Efficacy may be reduced in smokers due to induction of CYP1A2 levels.

PATIENT CONSIDERATIONS

Assessment: Assess for severe hepatic impairment, smoking, pregnancy/nursing status, and possible drug interactions.

Monitoring: Monitor for somnolence, impairment of mental/physical abilities, and other adverse reactions.

Counseling: Inform about the potential risks and benefits of therapy. Advise to take therapy before hs at the same time every night; advise to skip dose if unable to take at scheduled time. Instruct to limit activity before going to bed after taking drug. Inform that daily use for several weeks or months may be necessary before benefit from therapy is observed.

STORAGE: 25°C (77°F); excursions permitted to 15-30°C (59-86°F). Protect from exposure to light and moisture.

HIBERIX — haemophilus b conjugate vaccine (tetanus toxoid conjugate) RX

Class: Vaccine

PEDIATRIC DOSAGE
***Haemophilus influenza* Type B**

Active Immunization for Prevention of Invasive Disease:
6 Weeks-4 Years (Prior to 5th Birthday):
0.5mL IM single dose

Administer as a 4-dose series; series consists of a primary immunization course of 3 doses administered at 2, 4, and 6 months of age, followed by a booster dose administered at 15-18 months of age. May give first dose as early as 6 weeks of age

ADMINISTRATION
IM route

Administer into anterolateral aspect of thigh or deltoid.
Do not mix w/ any other vaccine in the same syringe or vial.
Administer other vaccines at different inj sites.

Reconstitution
1. Withdraw 0.6mL of saline diluent from accompanying vial; reconstitute only w/ accompanying saline diluent.
2. Transfer 0.6mL saline diluent into lyophilized vaccine vial; shake the vial well.
3. Withdraw 0.5mL of reconstituted vaccine and administer.

Administer immediately after reconstitution or store refrigerated between 2-8°C (35- 46°F) and administer w/in 24 hrs; if not administered immediately, shake sol well again before administration.

HOW SUPPLIED
Inj: 0.5mL

CONTRAINDICATIONS
Severe allergic reaction (eg, anaphylaxis) after a previous dose of any *Haemophilus influenzae* type b- or tetanus toxoid-containing vaccine or any component of the vaccine.

WARNINGS/PRECAUTIONS

Evaluate potential benefits and risks if Guillain-Barre syndrome has occurred w/in 6 weeks of receipt of a prior tetanus toxoid-containing vaccine. Syncope may occur and can be accompanied by transient neurological signs. Apnea following IM vaccination reported in some infants born prematurely; decision on when to administer to premature infants should be based on the individual infant's medical status, and the potential benefits and possible risks of vaccination. Review immunization history for possible vaccine hypersensitivity; epinephrine and other appropriate agents must be immediately available if an anaphylactic reaction occurs. Expected immune response may not be obtained in immunosuppressed children. Urine antigen detection may not have a diagnostic value in suspected disease due to *H. influenzae* type b w/in 1-2 weeks after receipt of vaccine. Not a substitute for routine tetanus immunization.

ADVERSE REACTIONS

Pain and redness at inj site, irritability, drowsiness, fever, loss of appetite, fussiness, restlessness.

DRUG INTERACTIONS

Immunosuppressive therapies, including irradiation, antimetabolites, alkylating agents, cytotoxic drugs, and corticosteroids (used in greater than physiologic doses) may reduce immune response to vaccine.

PATIENT CONSIDERATIONS

Assessment: Assess for history of a severe allergic reaction to previous dose of any *H. influenzae* type b vaccination, tetanus toxoid-containing vaccine, or any component of the vaccine; history of Guillain-Barre syndrome w/in 6 weeks of receipt of a prior vaccine containing tetanus toxoid; immunosuppression; and for possible drug interactions. Review immunization history.

Monitoring: Monitor for allergic reactions, signs/symptoms of Guillain-Barre syndrome, inj-site reactions (eg, pain, redness, swelling), syncope, apnea in premature infants, and for any other possible adverse events. Monitor immune response.

Counseling: Inform patient's parents/guardians about benefits/risks of immunization. Counsel about the potential for adverse reactions; instruct to notify physician if any adverse reactions occur.

STORAGE: 2-8°C (36-46°F). Protect from light. **Diluent:** 2-25°C (36-77°F). Do not freeze. **After Reconstitution:** 2-8°C (36-46°F). Do not freeze. Discard if not used w/in 24 hrs or if has been frozen.

HORIZANT – gabapentin enacarbil

RX

Class: GABA analogue

ADULT DOSAGE

Restless Legs Syndrome

Moderate-Severe Primary Restless Legs Syndrome:
Usual: 600mg qd at about 5 pm

If dose is not taken at the recommended time, the next dose should be taken the following day as prescribed

Postherpetic Neuralgia

Initial: 600mg qam for 3 days
Titrate: Increase to 600mg bid (1200mg/day) on Day 4
Usual: 600mg bid

PEDIATRIC DOSAGE

Pediatric use may not have been established

DOSING CONSIDERATIONS

Renal Impairment

Restless Leg Syndrome:
CrCl ≥60mL/min:
600mg/day
CrCl 30-59mL/min:
Initial: 300mg/day
Titrate: Increase to 600mg prn
CrCl 15-29mL/min:
300mg/day
CrCl <15mL/min:
300mg qod
CrCl <15mL/min on Hemodialysis:
Not recommended

Postherpetic Neuralgia:
CrCl ≥60mL/min:
Titration: 600mg qam for 3 days
Maint: 600mg bid
Tapering: 600mg qam for 1 week

CrCl 30-59mL/min:
Titration: 300mg qam for 3 days
Maint: 300mg bid; increase to 600mg bid if needed based on tolerability and efficacy
Tapering: Reduce current maint dose to qd in am for 1 week

CrCl 15-29mL/min:
Titration: 300mg qam on Day 1 and Day 3
Maint: 300mg qam; increase to 300mg bid if needed based on tolerability and efficacy
Tapering: If taking 300mg bid, reduce to 300mg qd in am for 1 week. If taking 300mg qd, no taper needed

CrCl <15mL/min:
Maint: 300mg qod in am; increase to 300mg qd in am if needed based on tolerability and efficacy

CrCl <15mL/min on Hemodialysis:
Maint: 300mg following every dialysis; increase to 600mg following every dialysis if needed based on tolerability and efficacy

H

ADMINISTRATION
Oral route

Take w/ food
Swallow tab whole; do not cut, crush, or chew

HOW SUPPLIED
Tab, Extended-Release: 300mg, 600mg

WARNINGS/PRECAUTIONS
Not recommended for patients who are required to sleep during the day and remain awake at night or in restless legs syndrome patients with CrCl <15mL/min on hemodialysis. May cause significant driving impairment, somnolence/sedation, and dizziness. Not interchangeable with other gabapentin products. Increases the risk of suicidal thoughts or behavior; monitor for the emergence or worsening of depression, suicidal thoughts/behavior, and/or any unusual changes in mood or behavior. Drug reaction with eosinophilia and systemic symptoms (DRESS)/multiorgan hypersensitivity reported; evaluate immediately if signs/symptoms (eg, hypersensitivity, fever, lymphadenopathy) are present and d/c if alternative etiology cannot be established. For RLS patients, if recommended daily dose is exceeded, reduce dose to 600mg daily for 1 week prior to discontinuation to minimize potential for withdrawal seizure. For postherpetic neuralgia patients receiving bid dose, reduce dose to qd for 1 week prior to discontinuation to minimize potential for withdrawal seizure. May have tumorigenic potential. Caution in elderly and with renal impairment.

ADVERSE REACTIONS
Somnolence/sedation, dizziness, headache, nausea, dry mouth, flatulence, fatigue, insomnia, irritability, feeling drunk/abnormal, peripheral edema, weight increase, vertigo.

DRUG INTERACTIONS
Drug is released faster from extended-release tab in the presence of alcohol; avoid alcohol consumption. Increased somnolence/sedation, dizziness, and nausea when taken in conjunction with morphine.

PATIENT CONSIDERATIONS

Assessment: Assess for preexisting tumors, history of depression, pregnancy/nursing status, renal function (CrCl), and possible drug interactions.

Monitoring: Monitor for withdrawal seizures with discontinuation, somnolence/sedation, dizziness, emergence or worsening of depression, suicidal thoughts/behavior, and/or any unusual changes in mood/behavior, DRESS, development or worsening of tumors, renal function, and hypersensitivity reactions.

Counseling: Inform that therapy may cause significant driving impairment, somnolence, and dizziness; advise not to drive or operate dangerous machinery until sufficient experience on therapy is gained. Counsel that treatment may increase the risk of suicidal thoughts and behavior; advise to report to physician any behaviors of concern. Advise that multiorgan hypersensitivity reactions may occur; instruct to contact physician if experiencing any signs or symptoms of this condition. Advise not to interchange with other gabapentin products. If the dose is missed, instruct to take the next dose at the time of the next scheduled dose. Instruct about how to d/c therapy. Advise to avoid alcohol when taking the drug.

STORAGE: 25°C (77°F); excursions permitted to 15-30°C (59-86°F). Protect from moisture.

HUMALOG – insulin lispro

RX

Class: Insulin (rapid-acting)

ADULT DOSAGE

Diabetes Mellitus

IV/SQ:

Individualize and adjust dose based on route of administration, metabolic needs, blood glucose monitoring results, and glycemic control goal

PEDIATRIC DOSAGE

Type 1 Diabetes Mellitus

≥3 Years:

SQ (Humalog U-100):

Individualize and adjust dose based on metabolic needs, blood glucose monitoring results, and glycemic control goal

DOSING CONSIDERATIONS

Renal Impairment

May require more frequent dose adjustment

Hepatic Impairment

May require more frequent dose adjustment

Other Important Considerations

May require dose adjustments w/ changes in physical activity/meal patterns, or during acute illness

ADMINISTRATION

IV/SQ route

Do not transfer Humalog U-200 from the KwikPen to a syringe for administration.
Do not perform dose conversion when using either Humalog U-100 or Humalog U-200 KwikPens.
Do not mix Humalog U-200 w/ any other insulins.

SQ (Humalog U-100 or U-200)

Administer w/in 15 min ac or immediately pc by inj into the SQ tissue of the abdominal wall, thigh, upper arm, or buttocks; rotate inj sites w/in the same region
Generally used w/ an intermediate- or long-acting insulin

Continuous SQ Infusion (Insulin Pump); Humalog U-100 Only

Administer into the SQ tissue of the abdominal wall; rotate infusion sites w/in the same region
Do not dilute or mix w/ other insulins
Change Humalog U-100 in the pump reservoir at least every 7 days; change infusion sets and infusion set insertion site at least every 3 days
Do not expose Humalog U-100 in the pump reservoir to temperatures >37°C (98.6°F)
Use Humalog U-100 in pump systems suitable for insulin infusion

IV (Humalog U-100 Only)

Dilute to concentrations from 0.1 U/mL to 1.0 U/mL using 0.9% NaCl

Instructions for Mixing Humalog U-100 w/ Other Insulins

SQ:

May be mixed w/ NPH insulin preparations only; draw insulin lispro into syringe 1st and inject immediately after mixing

HOW SUPPLIED

Inj: 100 U/mL [3mL, cartridge, KwikPen, vial; 10mL, vial], 200 U/mL [3mL, KwikPen]

CONTRAINDICATIONS

During episodes of hypoglycemia. Hypersensitivity to Humalog or to any of its excipients.

WARNINGS/PRECAUTIONS

KwikPen, cartridges, reusable pens, and syringes must never be shared between patients, even if needle is changed; may carry a risk for transmission of blood-borne pathogens. Changes in strength, manufacturer, type, or method of administration may affect glycemic control and predispose to hypo/hyperglycemia; these changes should be made cautiously and under close medical supervision and the frequency of blood glucose monitoring should be increased. Hypoglycemia may occur; increase frequency of blood glucose monitoring in patients at higher risk for hypoglycemia and patients who have reduced symptomatic awareness of hypoglycemia. Hypoglycemia may impair concentration ability and reaction time. Accidental mix-ups between insulin products and other insulins, particularly rapid-acting insulins, reported. Severe, life-threatening, generalized allergy, including anaphylaxis, may occur; if hypersensitivity reactions occur, d/c therapy, treat per standard of care, and monitor until symptoms and signs resolve. Hypokalemia may occur. Malfunction of the insulin pump or infusion set or insulin degradation can rapidly lead to hyperglycemia and ketoacidosis; prompt identification and correction of the cause is necessary. Train patients using continuous SQ infusion pump therapy to administer by inj and have alternate insulin therapy available in case of pump failure. IV administration should be under medical supervision w/ close monitoring of blood glucose and K^+ levels. More frequent glucose monitoring may be necessary w/ renal/hepatic impairment.

ADVERSE REACTIONS

Flu syndrome, pharyngitis, rhinitis, headache, pain, cough increased, infection, diarrhea, nausea, fever, abdominal pain, asthenia, bronchitis, myalgia, UTI.

DRUG INTERACTIONS

Dose adjustment and increased frequency of glucose monitoring may be required w/ drugs that may increase the risk of hypoglycemia (eg, salicylates, sulfonamide antibiotics, MAOIs, ACE inhibitors, somatostatin analogues [eg, octreotide]), drugs that may decrease blood glucose-lowering effect (eg, corticosteroids, oral contraceptives, sympathomimetic agents [eg, epinephrine, albuterol, terbutaline], atypical antipsychotics, protease inhibitors), or drugs that may increase or decrease blood glucose-lowering effect (eg, β-blockers, clonidine, lithium salts, alcohol). Pentamidine may cause hypoglycemia, sometimes followed by hyperglycemia. Signs and symptoms of hypoglycemia may be blunted w/ β-blockers, clonidine, guanethidine, and reserpine. Monitor K^+ levels w/ K^+-lowering medications or medications sensitive to serum K^+ concentrations. Observe for signs/symptoms of heart failure (HF) if treated concomitantly w/ a peroxisome proliferator-activated receptor (PPAR)-gamma agonist (eg, thiazolidinedione); consider discontinuation or dose reduction of the PPAR-gamma agonist if HF develops.

H

PATIENT CONSIDERATIONS

Assessment: Assess for predisposition to hypoglycemia, risk for hypokalemia, hypersensitivity, renal/hepatic impairment, pregnancy/nursing status, and possible drug interactions. Obtain baseline blood glucose and HbA1c levels.

Monitoring: Monitor for signs/symptoms of hypoglycemia, hypokalemia, hypersensitivity reactions, and other adverse effects. Monitor blood glucose, HbA1c, K^+ levels, and renal/hepatic function.

Counseling: Advise to never share KwikPen, cartridge, reusable pen, or syringe w/ another person, even if needle is changed. Instruct on self-management procedures (eg, glucose monitoring, proper inj technique, management of hypo/hyperglycemia), especially at initiation of therapy. Advise on handling of special situations, such as intercurrent conditions (eg, illness, stress, emotional disturbances), inadequate or skipped doses, inadvertent administration of an increased dose, inadequate food intake, and skipped meals. Inform that the ability to concentrate and react may be impaired as a result of hypoglycemia; advise patients who have frequent hypoglycemia or reduced/absent warning signs of hypoglycemia to use caution when driving/operating machinery. Advise that hypersensitivity reactions may occur; inform about the symptoms of hypersensitivity reactions. Instruct to always check the label before each inj to avoid mix-ups between insulin products. Advise females of reproductive potential w/ diabetes to inform physician if pregnant or contemplating pregnancy. Instruct on how to use external infusion pump, and to follow healthcare provider recommendations when setting basal and meal time infusion rate.

STORAGE: Unused: 2-8°C (36-46°F) until expiration date. Do not freeze; do not use if it has been frozen. **Opened:** <30°C (86°F) for up to 28 days. Protect from direct heat and light. (Vials) May refrigerate. (Cartridge/KwikPen) Do not refrigerate. Discard cartridge used in the D-Tron pumps after 7 days, even if it still contains the drug. **Diluted Humalog U-100 for SQ Inj:** 5°C (41°F) for 28 days or 30°C (86°F) for 14 days. Do not dilute drug contained in a cartridge or drug used in an external insulin pump. **IV Admixture:** 2-8°C (36-46°F) for 48 hrs; may be used at room temperature for up to an additional 48 hrs.

HUMALOG MIX 50/50 – insulin lispro protamine (rDNA origin)/ insulin lispro (rDNA origin) RX

Class: Insulin (combination)

ADULT DOSAGE

Diabetes Mellitus

Individualize dose

PEDIATRIC DOSAGE

Pediatric use may not have been established

DOSING CONSIDERATIONS

Renal Impairment

Dose adjustments may be necessary

Hepatic Impairment

Dose adjustments may be necessary

ADMINISTRATION

SQ route

Inject w/in 15 min ac.

HOW SUPPLIED

Inj: (Insulin Lispro Protamine/Insulin Lispro) (50 U/50 U)/mL [3mL, KwikPen; 10mL, vial]

CONTRAINDICATIONS

During episodes of hypoglycemia. Sensitivity to insulin lispro or any of the excipients contained in the formulation.

WARNINGS/PRECAUTIONS

KwikPens and syringes must never be shared between patients, even if needle is changed; may carry a risk for transmission of blood-borne pathogens. Any change of insulin should be made cautiously and only under medical supervision. Changes in strength, manufacturer, type, species, or method of manufacture may result in the need for a change in dosage. Hypoglycemia and hypokalemia may occur; caution in patients in whom such potential side effects may be clinically relevant (eg, patients w/ autonomic neuropathy). Lipodystrophy and hypersensitivity may occur. Dosage adjustment may be necessary if patient changes physical activity or usual meal plan. Illness, emotional disturbances, or other stress may alter insulin requirements. Careful glucose monitoring and insulin dose adjustment may be necessary w/ hepatic/renal impairment. Inj-site redness/swelling/itching and severe, life-threatening, generalized allergy may occur. Contains cresol as excipient; localized reactions and generalized myalgias reported. Antibody production reported. Caution in elderly.

ADVERSE REACTIONS

Hypoglycemia, allergic reactions, inj-site reactions, lipodystrophy, pruritus, rash.

DRUG INTERACTIONS

Drugs w/ hyperglycemic activity (eg, corticosteroids, certain lipid-lowering drugs [eg, niacin], oral contraceptives, phenothiazines, thyroid replacement therapy) may increase insulin requirements. Drugs that increase insulin sensitivity or have hypoglycemic activity (eg, salicylates, sulfa antibiotics, MAOIs, ACE inhibitors, inhibitors of pancreatic function [eg, octreotide]) may decrease insulin requirements. β-blockers may mask symptoms of hypoglycemia. Caution w/ K^+-lowering drugs or drugs sensitive to serum K^+ levels. Observe for signs/symptoms of heart failure (HF) if treated concomitantly w/ a peroxisome proliferator-activated receptor (PPAR)-gamma agonist (eg, thiazolidinedione); consider discontinuation or dose reduction of the PPAR-gamma agonist if HF develops.

PATIENT CONSIDERATIONS

Assessment: Assess for presence of hypoglycemia or hypokalemia and for conditions where such potential side effects might be clinically relevant. Assess for hypersensitivity, renal/hepatic impairment, pregnancy/nursing status, and possible drug interactions. Obtain baseline blood glucose and HbA1c levels.

Monitoring: Monitor for signs/symptoms of hypoglycemia, hypokalemia, lipodystrophy, allergic reactions, antibody production, and other adverse effects. Monitor blood glucose, HbA1c, K^+ levels, and renal/hepatic function.

Counseling: Inform of the potential risks and advantages of therapy and alternative therapies. Instruct not to mix drug w/ any other insulin. Inform of the importance of proper insulin storage, inj technique, timing of dosage, adherence to meal planning, regular physical activity, regular blood glucose monitoring, periodic HbA1c testing, recognition and management of hypo/hyperglycemia, and periodic assessment for diabetes complications. Advise to inform physician if pregnant or planning to become pregnant. Instruct patients using insulin pen delivery device on how to properly use the delivery device, prime the pen to a stream of insulin, and properly dispose of needles. Advise not to share insulin pen w/ others.

STORAGE: Unopened: 2-8°C (36-46°F) until expiration date, or at room temperature (<30°C [86°F]) for 28 days (vial) or 10 days (KwikPen). Do not freeze; do not use if it has been frozen. Opened: <30°C (86°F) for 28 days (vial) or 10 days (KwikPen). Do not refrigerate KwikPen. Protect from direct heat and light.

HUMALOG MIX 75/25 – insulin lispro protamine (rDNA origin)/insulin lispro (rDNA origin) RX

Class: Insulin (combination)

ADULT DOSAGE

Diabetes Mellitus

Individualize dose

PEDIATRIC DOSAGE

Pediatric use may not have been established

DOSING CONSIDERATIONS

Renal Impairment

Dose adjustments may be necessary

Hepatic Impairment

Dose adjustments may be necessary

ADMINISTRATION

SQ route

Inject w/in 15 min ac.

HOW SUPPLIED

Inj: (Insulin Lispro Protamine/Insulin Lispro) (75 U/25 U)/mL [3mL, KwikPen; 10mL, vial]

CONTRAINDICATIONS

During episodes of hypoglycemia. Sensitivity to insulin lispro or any of the excipients contained in the formulation.

WARNINGS/PRECAUTIONS

KwikPens and syringes must never be shared between patients, even if needle is changed; may carry a risk for transmission of blood-borne pathogens. Any change of insulin should be made cautiously and only under medical supervision. Changes in strength, manufacturer, type, species, or method of manufacture may result in the need for a change in dosage. Hypoglycemia and hypokalemia may occur; caution in patients in whom such potential side effects might be clinically relevant (eg, patients w/ autonomic neuropathy). Lipodystrophy and hypersensitivity may occur. Dosage adjustment may be necessary if patient changes physical activity or usual meal plan. Illness, emotional disturbances, or other stress may alter insulin requirements. Careful glucose monitoring and insulin dose adjustment may be necessary w/ hepatic/renal impairment. Inj-site redness/swelling/itching, and severe, life-threatening, generalized allergy may occur. Contains cresol as excipient; localized reactions and generalized myalgias reported. Antibody production reported. Caution in elderly.

H

ADVERSE REACTIONS

Hypoglycemia, allergic reactions, inj-site reactions, lipodystrophy, pruritus, rash.

DRUG INTERACTIONS

Drugs w/ hyperglycemic activity (eg, corticosteroids, certain lipid-lowering drugs [eg, niacin], oral contraceptives, phenothiazines, thyroid replacement therapy) may increase insulin requirements. Drugs that increase insulin sensitivity or have hypoglycemic activity (eg, salicylates, sulfa antibiotics, MAOIs, ACE inhibitors, inhibitors of pancreatic function [eg, octreotide]) may decrease insulin requirements. β-blockers may mask symptoms of hypoglycemia. Caution w/ K^+-lowering drugs or drugs sensitive to serum K^+ levels. Observe for signs/symptoms of heart failure (HF) if treated concomitantly w/ a peroxisome proliferator-activated receptor (PPAR)-gamma agonist (eg, thiazolidinedione); consider discontinuation or dose reduction of the PPAR-gamma agonist if HF develops.

PATIENT CONSIDERATIONS

Assessment: Assess for presence of hypoglycemia or hypokalemia and for conditions where such potential side effects might be clinically relevant. Assess for hypersensitivity, renal/hepatic impairment, pregnancy/nursing status, and possible drug interactions. Obtain baseline blood glucose and HbA1c levels.

Monitoring: Monitor for signs/symptoms of hypoglycemia, hypokalemia, lipodystrophy, allergic reactions, antibody production, and other adverse effects. Monitor blood glucose, HbA1c, K^+ levels, and renal/hepatic function.

Counseling: Inform of the potential risks and advantages of therapy and alternative therapies. Instruct not to mix drug w/ any other insulin. Inform of the importance of proper insulin storage, inj technique, timing of dosage, adherence to meal planning, regular physical activity, regular blood glucose monitoring, periodic HbA1c testing, recognition and management of hypo/hyperglycemia, and periodic assessment for diabetes complications. Advise to inform physician if pregnant/planning to become pregnant. Instruct patients using insulin pen delivery device on how to properly use delivery device, prime the pen to a stream of insulin, and properly dispose of needles. Advise not to share insulin pen w/ others.

STORAGE: Unopened: 2-8°C (36-46°F) until expiration date, or room temperature (<30°C [86°F]) for 28 days (vial) or 10 days (KwikPen). Do not freeze; do not use if it has been frozen. **Opened:** <30°C (86°F) for 28 days (vial) or 10 days (KwikPen). Do not refrigerate KwikPen. Protect from direct heat and light.

HUMIRA – adalimumab

RX

Class: Monoclonal antibody/TNF blocker

Increased risk of serious infections (eg, active tuberculosis [TB], including latent TB reactivation; invasive fungal infections; bacterial, viral, and other infections due to opportunistic pathogens) that may lead to hospitalization or death, mostly w/ concomitant use of immunosuppressants (eg, methotrexate [MTX], corticosteroids). D/C if serious infection or sepsis develops. TB patients have frequently presented w/ disseminated or extrapulmonary disease; test for latent TB before and during therapy and initiate treatment for latent TB prior to adalimumab use. Consider empiric antifungal therapy in patients at risk for invasive fungal infections who develop severe systemic illness. Monitor patients closely for development of infection during and after treatment, including development of TB in patients who tested negative for latent TB infection prior to therapy. Lymphoma and other malignancies, some fatal, reported in children and adolescents. Postmarketing cases of aggressive and fatal hepatosplenic T-cell lymphoma reported; the majority of cases occurred in patients w/ Crohn's disease (CD) or ulcerative colitis (UC) and the majority were in adolescent and young adult males. Almost all of these patients were treated concomitantly w/ azathioprine or 6-mercaptopurine.

ADULT DOSAGE

Rheumatoid Arthritis

Reduce signs/symptoms, induce major clinical response, inhibit progression of structural damage, and improve physical function in patients w/ moderately to severely active rheumatoid arthritis

40mg every other week; may increase to 40mg every week in patients not taking concomitant methotrexate (MTX)

May be used alone or in combination w/ MTX or other nonbiologic disease-modifying anti-rheumatic drugs

Psoriatic Arthritis

Reduce signs/symptoms, inhibit progression of structural damage, and improve physical function in patients w/ active psoriatic arthritis

40mg every other week

May be used alone or in combination w/ nonbiologic disease-modifying anti-rheumatic drugs

Ankylosing Spondylitis

Reduce signs/symptoms in patients w/ active ankylosing spondylitis

40mg every other week

Crohn's Disease

Reduce signs/symptoms and induce/maintain clinical remission in patients w/ moderately to severely active Crohn's disease who have had an inadequate response to conventional therapy and/or lost response to or are intolerant to infliximab

Day 1: 160mg (given as four 40mg inj in 1 day or as two 40mg inj/day for 2 consecutive days)
Day 15: 80mg
Day 29 and Onward: 40mg every other week

Use beyond 1 year has not been evaluated

Plaque Psoriasis

Treatment of moderate to severe chronic plaque psoriasis in candidates for systemic therapy or phototherapy when other systemic therapies are medically less appropriate

Initial: 80mg
Maint: 40mg every other week starting 1 week after initial dose

PEDIATRIC DOSAGE

Juvenile Idiopathic Arthritis

Reduce signs/symptoms of moderately to severely active polyarticular juvenile idiopathic arthritis

≥2 Years:
10-<15kg: 10mg every other week
15-<30kg: 20mg every other week
≥30kg: 40mg every other week

May be used alone or in combination w/ methotrexate

Crohn's Disease

Reduce signs/symptoms and induce/maintain clinical remission in patients w/ moderately to severely active Crohn's disease who have had an inadequate response to corticosteroids or immunomodulators

≥6 Years:
17-<40kg:
Day 1: 80mg (given as two 40mg inj in 1 day)
Day 15: 40mg
Day 29 and Onward: 20mg every other week

≥40kg:
Day 1: 160mg (given as four 40mg inj in 1 day or as two 40mg inj/day for 2 consecutive days)
Day 15: 80mg (given as two 40mg inj in 1 day)
Day 29 and Onward: 40mg every other week

H

Ulcerative Colitis

Induce and sustain clinical remission in patients w/ moderately to severely active ulcerative colitis who have had an inadequate response to immunosuppressants

Day 1: 160mg (given as four 40mg inj in 1 day or as two 40mg inj/day for 2 consecutive days)
Day 15: 80mg
Day 29 and Onward: 40mg every other week

Only continue if clinical remission is evident by 8 weeks (Day 57) of therapy

ADMINISTRATION

SQ route

May be left at room temperature for about 15-30 min before injecting; do not remove the cap or cover while allowing it to reach room temperature

Inject at separate sites in the thigh or abdomen. Rotate inj sites; avoid areas where skin is tender, bruised, red, or hard

H

HOW SUPPLIED

Inj: 10mg/0.2mL [prefilled syringe], 20mg/0.4mL [prefilled syringe], 40mg/0.8mL [prefilled syringe, prefilled pen, vial]

WARNINGS/PRECAUTIONS

Do not initiate in patients w/ an active infection. Increased risk of infection in patients >65 yrs of age and in patients w/ comorbid conditions. Malignancies, including acute and chronic leukemia, lymphoma, and nonmelanoma skin cancer (NMSC), reported in adults. Anaphylaxis and angioneurotic edema reported; d/c immediately and institute appropriate therapy if an anaphylactic or other serious allergic reaction occurs. May increase risk of hepatitis B virus (HBV) reactivation in chronic carriers; closely monitor for signs of active HBV infection during and for several months after therapy termination. D/C if HBV reactivation develops and start effective antiviral therapy w/ appropriate supportive treatment. New onset or exacerbation of CNS and peripheral demyelinating diseases, new or worsening congestive heart failure (CHF), and hematologic system adverse reactions, including significant cytopenia (eg, thrombocytopenia, leukopenia) reported. May result in the formation of autoantibodies and development of a lupus-like syndrome; d/c if symptoms suggestive of a lupus-like syndrome develop. If possible, pediatric patients should be brought up to date w/ all immunizations in agreement w/ current immunization guidelines prior to initiating therapy. Avoid having latex-sensitive patients handle the needle cover of the prefilled syringe; it contains dry rubber (latex). Caution in elderly.

ADVERSE REACTIONS

URTI, sinusitis, inj-site reactions, headache, rash, nausea, flu syndrome, abdominal pain, hyperlipidemia, hypercholesterolemia, back pain, hematuria, increased alkaline phosphatase, UTI, HTN.

DRUG INTERACTIONS

See Boxed Warning. Reduced clearance w/ MTX. Concomitant administration w/ other biologic DMARDs (eg, anakinra, abatacept) or other TNF blockers is not recommended due to possible increased risk for infections and other potential pharmacological interactions. Avoid w/ live vaccines. Upon initiation or discontinuation of adalimumab in patients being treated w/ CYP450 substrates w/ a narrow therapeutic index, monitor therapeutic effect (eg, warfarin) or drug concentration (eg, cyclosporine, theophylline) and adjust individual dose of the drug product prn.

PATIENT CONSIDERATIONS

Assessment: Assess for active/chronic/recurrent infection, history of an opportunistic infection, recent travel in areas of endemic TB or endemic mycoses, underlying conditions that may predispose to infection, central or peripheral nervous system demyelinating disorders, CHF, latex sensitivity, drug hypersensitivity, pregnancy/nursing status, and for possible drug interactions. Test for latent TB infection and for HBV infection. Assess immunization history in pediatric patients. Perform a skin examination, particularly in patients w/ a medical history of prior prolonged immunosuppressant therapy or psoriasis patients w/ a history of psoralen plus ultraviolet light (PUVA) treatment for the presence of NMSC.

Monitoring: Monitor for development of infection during and after treatment. Monitor for malignancies, hypersensitivity reactions, neurological reactions, hematological reactions, worsening/new-onset CHF, lupus-like syndrome, and other adverse reactions. Monitor for active TB and periodically test for latent TB. Monitor for HBV reactivation during therapy and for several months following termination of therapy. Perform periodic skin examinations, particularly in patients w/ a medical history of prior prolonged immunosuppressant therapy or psoriasis patients w/ a history of PUVA treatment for the presence of NMSC.

Counseling: Inform about the potential benefits/risks of therapy. Inform that therapy may lower the ability of the immune system to fight infections; instruct to contact physician if any symptoms of infection, including TB, invasive fungal infections, or reactivation of HBV infections, develop. Counsel about the risk of malignancies. Advise to seek immediate medical attention if any symptoms of a severe allergic reaction develop. Advise latex-sensitive patients that the needle cap of the prefilled syringe contains latex. Advise to report to physician any signs of new/worsening medical conditions (eg, CHF, neurological disease, autoimmune disorders) or any symptoms suggestive of a cytopenia (eg, bleeding, bruising, persistent fever). Instruct on proper inj technique, as well as proper syringe and needle disposal.

STORAGE: 2-8°C (36-46°F). Do not freeze; do not use if frozen even if it has been thawed. Store in original carton until time of administration to protect from light. May be stored up to a max of 25°C (77°F) for up to 14 days, if needed. Do not store in extreme heat or cold.

HUMULIN 70/30 – NPH, human insulin isophane (rDNA origin)/ regular, human insulin (rDNA origin) — OTC

Class: Insulin (combination)

ADULT DOSAGE

Diabetes Mellitus

Individualize dose

May need to adjust dosage based on metabolic needs, blood glucose monitoring results, and glycemic control goal

Administer SQ approx 30-45 min ac

PEDIATRIC DOSAGE

Pediatric use may not have been established

DOSING CONSIDERATIONS

Renal Impairment

May require more frequent dose adjustment

Hepatic Impairment

May require more frequent dose adjustment

Other Important Considerations

May require dose adjustments w/ changes in physical activity/meal patterns, or during acute illness

ADMINISTRATION

SQ route

Should appear uniformly cloudy after mixing; do not use if particulate matter is seen.
Do not mix w/ any other insulins/diluents.
Administer in the abdominal wall, thigh, upper arm, or buttocks; rotate the inj site w/in the same region from 1 inj to the next.
Do not use in an insulin infusion pump.

HOW SUPPLIED

Inj: (Insulin Isophane/Regular) (70 U/30 U)/mL [3mL, vial, pen, KwikPen; 10mL, vial]

CONTRAINDICATIONS

During episodes of hypoglycemia. Hypersensitivity reactions to Humulin 70/30 or any of its excipients.

WARNINGS/PRECAUTIONS

Pens and KwikPens must never be shared between patients, even if the needle is changed; may carry a risk for transmission of blood-borne pathogens. Changes in strength, manufacturer, type, or method of administration may affect glycemic control and predispose to hypo/hyperglycemia; these changes should be made cautiously and under close medical supervision and the frequency of blood glucose monitoring should be increased. Hypoglycemia may occur; increase frequency of blood glucose monitoring in patients at higher risk for hypoglycemia and patients who have reduced symptomatic awareness of hypoglycemia. Hypoglycemia may impair concentration ability and reaction time. Severe, life-threatening, generalized allergy, including anaphylaxis, may occur; if hypersensitivity reactions occur, d/c therapy, treat per standard of care, and monitor until symptoms and signs resolve. May cause hypokalemia.

ADVERSE REACTIONS

Hypoglycemia, allergic reactions, peripheral edema, lipodystrophy, weight gain, immunogenicity.

DRUG INTERACTIONS

May require dose adjustment and increased frequency of glucose monitoring w/ drugs that may increase the risk of hypoglycemia (eg, antidiabetic agents, salicylates, sulfonamide antibiotics), drugs that may decrease the glucose-lowering effect (eg, corticosteroids, isoniazid, niacin), or drugs that may increase or decrease glucose-lowering effect (eg, β-blockers, clonidine, lithium salts, alcohol). Pentamidine may cause hypoglycemia, sometimes followed by hyperglycemia. Signs and symptoms of hypoglycemia may be blunted w/ β-blockers, clonidine, guanethidine, and reserpine. Monitor K^+ levels w/ K^+-lowering medications or medications sensitive to serum K^+ concentrations. Observe for signs/symptoms of heart failure (HF) if treated concomitantly w/ a peroxisome proliferator-activated receptor (PPAR)-gamma agonist (eg, thiazolidinedione); consider discontinuation or dose reduction of the PPAR-gamma agonist if HF develops.

PATIENT CONSIDERATIONS

Assessment: Assess for risk of hypoglycemia or hypokalemia, hypersensitivity, renal/hepatic impairment, pregnancy/nursing status, and possible drug interactions. Obtain baseline FPG and HbA1c.

Monitoring: Monitor for signs and symptoms of hypoglycemia, hypokalemia, hypersensitivity reactions, and other adverse reactions. Monitor FPG, HbA1c, and renal/hepatic function.

Counseling: Advise never to share a pen or KwikPen w/ another person, even if the needle is changed. Instruct on self-management procedures, including glucose monitoring, proper inj technique, and management of hypo/hyperglycemia, and on handling of special situations, such as intercurrent conditions, inadequate or skipped insulin dose, inadvertent administration of an increased insulin dose, inadequate food intake, and skipped meals. Inform that hypoglycemia may impair ability to concentrate and react; advise to use caution when driving or operating machinery. Instruct to always check the label before each inj to avoid medication errors/accidental mix-ups. Inform on the symptoms of hypersensitivity reactions. Advise to inform physician if pregnant/contemplating pregnancy. Advise to use only if product contains no particulate matter and appears uniformly cloudy after mixing.

STORAGE: Protect from heat and light. Do not freeze; do not use if it has been frozen. **Vial: Unopened:** 2-8°C (36-46°F) until expiration date, or room temperature <30°C (86°F) for 31 days. **Opened:** 2-8°C (36-46°F) or room temperature <30°C (86°F) for 31 days. **Pen/KwikPen: Unopened:** 2-8°C (36-46°F) until expiration date, or room temperature <30°C (86°F) for 10 days. **Opened:** Room temperature <30°C (86°F) for 10 days. Do not refrigerate.

HUMULIN N – NPH, human insulin isophane (rDNA origin) OTC

Class: Insulin (intermediate-acting)

ADULT DOSAGE

Diabetes Mellitus

Individualize dose

May need to adjust dosage based on metabolic needs, blood glucose monitoring results, and glycemic control goal

PEDIATRIC DOSAGE

Diabetes Mellitus

Individualize dose

May need to adjust dosage based on metabolic needs, blood glucose monitoring results, and glycemic control goal

DOSING CONSIDERATIONS

Renal Impairment

May require more frequent dose adjustment

Hepatic Impairment

May require more frequent dose adjustment

Other Important Considerations

May require dose adjustments w/ changes in physical activity/meal patterns, or during acute illness

ADMINISTRATION

SQ route

Should appear uniformly cloudy after mixing; do not use if particulate matter is seen.
Administer in the abdominal wall, thigh, upper arm, or buttocks; rotate the inj site w/in the same region from 1 inj to the next.
Do not administer IV/IM and do not use in an insulin infusion pump.

Mixing w/ Other Insulins

If Humulin N is mixed w/ Humulin R or Humalog, draw Humulin R or Humalog into syringe 1st; inject immediately after mixing.

HOW SUPPLIED

Inj: 100 U/mL [3mL, vial, pen, KwikPen; 10mL, vial]

CONTRAINDICATIONS

During episodes of hypoglycemia. Hypersensitivity reactions to Humulin N or any of its excipients.

WARNINGS/PRECAUTIONS

Pens and KwikPens must never be shared between patients, even if needle is changed; may carry a risk for transmission of blood-borne pathogens. Changes in strength, manufacturer, type, or method of administration may affect glycemic control and predispose to hypo/hyperglycemia; these changes should be made cautiously and under close medical supervision and the frequency of blood glucose monitoring should be increased. Hypoglycemia may occur; increase frequency of blood glucose monitoring in patients at higher risk for hypoglycemia and in patients who have reduced symptomatic awareness of hypoglycemia. Hypoglycemia may impair concentration ability and reaction time. Severe, life-threatening, generalized allergy, including anaphylaxis, may occur; if hypersensitivity reactions occur, d/c therapy, treat per standard of care, and monitor until symptoms and signs resolve. May cause hypokalemia. May require more frequent glucose monitoring w/ hepatic/renal impairment.

ADVERSE REACTIONS

Hypoglycemia, allergic reactions, peripheral edema, lipodystrophy, weight gain, immunogenicity.

DRUG INTERACTIONS

May require dose adjustment and increased frequency of glucose monitoring w/ drugs that may increase the risk of hypoglycemia (eg, antidiabetic agents, salicylates, sulfonamide antibiotics), drugs that may decrease the glucose-lowering effect (eg, corticosteroids, isoniazid, niacin), or drugs that may increase or decrease glucose-lowering effect (eg, β-blockers, clonidine, lithium salts, alcohol). Pentamidine may cause hypoglycemia, sometimes followed by hyperglycemia. Signs and symptoms of hypoglycemia may be blunted w/ β-blockers, clonidine, guanethidine, and reserpine. Monitor K^+ levels w/ K^+-lowering medications or medications sensitive to serum K^+ concentrations. Observe for signs/symptoms of heart failure (HF) if treated concomitantly w/ a peroxisome proliferator-activated receptor (PPAR)-gamma agonist (eg, thiazolidinedione); consider discontinuation or dose reduction of the PPAR-gamma agonist if HF develops.

H

PATIENT CONSIDERATIONS

Assessment: Assess for risk of hypoglycemia or hypokalemia, hypersensitivity, renal/hepatic impairment, pregnancy/nursing status, and possible drug interactions. Obtain baseline FPG and HbA1c.

Monitoring: Monitor for signs and symptoms of hypoglycemia, hypokalemia, hypersensitivity reactions, and other adverse reactions. Monitor FPG, HbA1c, and renal/hepatic function.

Counseling: Advise never to share a pen or KwikPen w/ another person even if needle is changed. Instruct on self-management procedures, including glucose monitoring, proper inj technique, management of hypo/hyperglycemia, and on handling of special situations such as intercurrent conditions, inadequate or skipped insulin dose, inadvertent administration of an increased insulin dose, inadequate food intake, and skipped meals. Inform that hypoglycemia may impair ability to concentrate and react; advise to use caution when driving or operating machinery. Instruct to always check the label before each inj to avoid medication errors/accidental mix-ups. Educate on the symptoms of hypersensitivity reactions. Advise to inform physician if pregnant/contemplating pregnancy. Advise to use only if product contains no particulate matter and appears uniformly cloudy after mixing.

STORAGE: Protect from heat and light. Do not freeze; do not use if it has been frozen. **Vial:** (Unopened) 2-8°C (36-46°F) until expiration date, or room temperature <30°C (86°F) for 31 days. (Opened) 2-8°C (36-46°F) or room temperature <30°C (86°F) for 31 days. **Pen/KwikPen:** (Unopened) 2-8°C (36-46°F) until expiration date, or room temperature <30°C (86°F) for 14 days. (Opened) Room temperature <30°C (86°F) for 14 days. Do not refrigerate.

HUMULIN R – regular, human insulin (rDNA origin) OTC

Class: Insulin (short-acting)

ADULT DOSAGE

Diabetes Mellitus

Initial: 0.2-0.4 U/kg/day

Maint:

Total Daily Insulin Requirement: 0.5-1 U/kg/day; requirement may be substantially higher in insulin-resistant patients

PEDIATRIC DOSAGE

Diabetes Mellitus

Initial: 0.2-0.4 U/kg/day

Maint:

Total Daily Insulin Requirement: 0.5-1 U/kg/day; requirement may be substantially higher in insulin-resistant patients

Prepubertal Children: Average total daily insulin requirement varies from 0.7-1 U/kg/day, but may be much lower during the period of partial remission

DOSING CONSIDERATIONS

Renal Impairment

May require frequent dose reduction

Hepatic Impairment

May require frequent dose reduction

ADMINISTRATION

SQ/IV route

May be used in combination w/ oral antihyperglycemics or longer-acting insulin products.

SQ

Usually given ≥3X daily ac.

Inj should be followed by a meal w/in approx 30 min.

Inject in the abdominal wall, thigh, gluteal region, or upper arm; rotate inj sites w/in the same region.

IV

Use at concentrations from 0.1-1 U/mL in infusion systems w/ the infusion fluids 0.9% NaCl using polyvinyl chloride infusion bags.

Mixing of Insulins

Humulin R is often used in combination w/ intermediate- or long-acting insulins; when mixed w/ an intermediate-acting insulin (eg, NPH insulin isophane sus), draw Humulin R into the syringe first. A U-100 insulin syringe should always be used.

HOW SUPPLIED

Inj: 100 U/mL [3mL, 10mL]

CONTRAINDICATIONS

During episodes of hypoglycemia. Hypersensitivity to Humulin R U-100 or any of its excipients.

WARNINGS/PRECAUTIONS

Needles or syringes must never be reused or shared between patients; may carry a risk for transmission of blood-borne pathogens. Any change in insulin should be made cautiously and only under medical supervision. Changes in strength, manufacturer, type, species, or method of administration may result in the need for a change in dosage. May require dosage adjustments w/ change in physical activity or usual meal plan. Stress, illness, or emotional disturbances may alter insulin requirements. Hypoglycemia may occur and may impair ability to concentrate and react; caution in patients w/ hypoglycemia unawareness and those predisposed to hypoglycemia (eg, pediatric population, those who fast or have erratic food intake). Hyperglycemia, diabetic ketoacidosis, or hyperosmolar coma may develop if taken less than needed. Hypokalemia may occur. Severe, life-threatening, generalized allergy, including anaphylaxis, may occur. Contains metacresol as excipient; localized reactions and generalized myalgias reported. Frequent glucose monitoring and dose reduction may be required w/ hepatic/renal impairment. May be administered IV under medical supervision; close monitoring of blood glucose and K^+ is required.

ADVERSE REACTIONS

Hypoglycemia, lipodystrophy, weight gain, peripheral edema.

DRUG INTERACTIONS

May require dose adjustment and close monitoring w/ drugs that may increase blood-glucose-lowering effect and susceptibility to hypoglycemia (eg, oral antihyperglycemics, salicylates, sulfa antibiotics), drugs that may reduce blood-glucose-lowering effect (eg, corticosteroids, isoniazid, certain lipid-lowering drugs [eg, niacin]), or drugs that may increase or decrease blood-glucose-lowering effect (eg, β-blockers, clonidine, lithium salts, alcohol). Pentamidine may cause hypoglycemia, which may sometimes be followed by hyperglycemia. β-blockers, clonidine, guanethidine, and reserpine may mask the signs of hypoglycemia. Caution w/ K^+-lowering medications or medications sensitive to serum K^+ concentrations. Observe for signs/symptoms of heart failure (HF) if treated concomitantly w/ a peroxisome proliferator-activated receptor (PPAR)-gamma agonist (eg, thiazolidinedione); consider discontinuation or dose reduction of the PPAR-gamma agonist if HF develops.

PATIENT CONSIDERATIONS

Assessment: Assess for risk of hypoglycemia or hypokalemia, hypersensitivity, renal/hepatic impairment, pregnancy/nursing status, and possible drug interactions. Obtain baseline FPG and HbA1c.

Monitoring: Monitor for signs and symptoms of hypoglycemia, hypokalemia, allergic reactions, and other adverse reactions. Monitor FPG, HbA1c, and renal/hepatic function.

Counseling: Instruct not to share syringes w/ other people, even if the needle has been changed. Instruct to always carry a quick source of sugar (eg, hard candy or glucose tabs). Counsel about proper dose preparation, administration technique, signs/symptoms of hypoglycemia, importance of frequent monitoring of blood glucose levels, and need for a balanced diet and regular exercise. Advise to always keep an extra supply of insulin as well as a spare syringe and needle on hand, and to always wear diabetic identification. Instruct to exercise caution when driving or operating machinery. Instruct to notify physician if pregnant/nursing, planning to become pregnant, or taking any other medications.

STORAGE: Do not use if it has been frozen. **Unopened:** 2-8°C (36-46°F). Do not freeze. **Opened:** <30°C (86°F). Protect from heat and light. Use w/in 31 days. **Admixture:** 2-8°C (36-46°F) for 48 hrs, then may use at room temperature for up to an additional 48 hrs.

HUMULIN R U-500 – insulin human

RX

Class: Insulin (short-acting)

ADULT DOSAGE

Diabetes Mellitus

To improve glycemic control in patients w/ diabetes mellitus (DM) requiring >200 U of insulin per day

Individualize and titrate dose based on the patient's metabolic needs, blood glucose monitoring results, and glycemic control goal

Give bid-tid approx 30 min ac

PEDIATRIC DOSAGE

Diabetes Mellitus

To improve glycemic control in patients w/ DM requiring >200 U of insulin per day

Individualize and titrate dose based on the patient's metabolic needs, blood glucose monitoring results, and glycemic control goal

Give bid-tid approx 30 min ac

DOSING CONSIDERATIONS

Renal Impairment

May require frequent glucose monitoring and insulin dose reduction

Hepatic Impairment

May require frequent glucose monitoring and insulin dose reduction

Other Important Considerations

May require dose adjustments w/ changes in physical activity/meal patterns/medications, or during acute illness

ADMINISTRATION

SQ route

Inject into the thigh, upper arm, abdomen, or buttocks; rotate inj sites w/in the same region.
Do not dilute or mix w/ any other insulin products or sol.
Do not administer IV or IM.

Delivery of Humulin R U-500 Using the Humulin R U-500 Disposable Prefilled KwikPen Device

Do not perform dose conversion when using the Humulin R U-500 KwikPen; dose window of the Humulin R U-500 KwikPen shows the number of units of Humulin R U-500 to be injected.
Do not transfer Humulin R U-500 from the Humulin R U-500 KwikPen into a syringe for administration as overdose and severe hypoglycemia can occur.
Humulin R U-500 KwikPen is for single patient use only.

Refer to PI for dose conversion information when using U-100 insulin syringe or a tuberculin syringe.

HOW SUPPLIED

Inj: 500 U/mL [3mL, KwikPen; 20mL, vial]

CONTRAINDICATIONS

Episodes of hypoglycemia. Hypersensitivity to Humulin R U-500 or any of its components.

WARNINGS/PRECAUTIONS

Medication errors in dispensing, prescribing, and administration have occurred and resulted in patients experiencing hyperglycemia, hypoglycemia, or death. Never share a KwikPen or syringe between patients; may carry a risk for transmission of blood-borne pathogens. Changes in insulin, manufacturer, type, or method of administration may affect glycemic control and predispose to hypoglycemia or hyperglycemia; changes should be made cautiously and only under medical supervision w/ increased frequency of blood glucose monitoring. Patients w/ type 2 DM who have a change in their insulin regimen may require adjustments in concomitant oral anti-diabetic treatment. Hypoglycemia may occur and may impair concentration ability and reaction time. Severe hypoglycemia may develop as long as 18-24 hrs after the original inj and may cause seizures, be life threatening, or cause death. Symptomatic awareness of hypoglycemia may be less pronounced in patients w/ longstanding diabetes, in patients w/ diabetic nerve disease, in patients using medications that block the sympathetic nervous system, or in patients who experience recurrent hypoglycemia. Monitor blood glucose levels more frequently in patients at higher risk for hypoglycemia, and in patients who have reduced symptomatic awareness of hypoglycemia. Severe, life-threatening, generalized allergy, including anaphylaxis, may occur; d/c and treat appropriately if a hypersensitivity reaction occurs. Hypokalemia may occur.

ADVERSE REACTIONS

Hypoglycemia, allergic reactions, lipodystrophy, inj-site reactions, weight gain, peripheral edema.

DRUG INTERACTIONS

May require dose adjustment and increased frequency of glucose monitoring w/ drugs that may increase the risk of hypoglycemia (eg, antidiabetic agents, salicylates, sulfonamide antibiotics), drugs that may decrease the glucose-lowering effect (eg, corticosteroids, isoniazid, niacin), or drugs that may increase or decrease glucose-lowering effect (eg, alcohol, β-blockers, clonidine, lithium salts). Signs/symptoms of hypoglycemia may be blunted w/ alcohol, β-blockers, clonidine, guanethidine, and reserpine. Caution w/ K^+-lowering medications or medications sensitive to serum K^+ concentrations. Observe for signs/symptoms of heart failure (HF) if treated concomitantly w/ a peroxisome proliferator-activated receptor (PPAR)-gamma agonist (eg, thiazolidinedione); consider discontinuation or dose reduction of the PPAR-gamma agonist if HF develops.

PATIENT CONSIDERATIONS

Assessment: Assess for risk of hypoglycemia or hypokalemia, hypersensitivity, renal/hepatic impairment, pregnancy/nursing status, and possible drug interactions. Obtain baseline FPG and HbA1c.

Monitoring: Monitor for signs and symptoms of hypoglycemia, hypokalemia, hypersensitivity reactions, and other adverse reactions. Monitor FPG, HbA1c, and renal/hepatic function.

H

Counseling: Inform that this formulation is concentrated and that extreme caution must be observed in the measurement of dosage because inadvertent overdose may result in serious adverse reaction or life-threatening hypoglycemia. Instruct to always check the label before each inj to avoid medication errors/accidental mix-ups. If using the KwikPen, counsel to dial and dose the prescribed number of units of insulin. When using the insulin from a vial, counsel to calculate the conversion and measure the amount of delivered insulin using the unit of measurement that corresponds to the type of syringe being used. Instruct on self-management procedures, including glucose monitoring, proper inj technique, management of hypo/hyperglycemia, and handling of special situations (eg, intercurrent conditions, inadequate or skipped insulin dose, inadvertent administration of an increased insulin dose, inadequate food intake, skipped meals). Advise to inform physician if pregnant/contemplating pregnancy.

STORAGE: Protect from heat and light. Do not freeze; do not use if it has been frozen. **KwikPen:** (Unopened) 2-8°C (36-46°F); or <30°C (86°F) for 28 days. (Opened) <30°C (86°F) for 28 days. Do not refrigerate. **Vial:** (Unopened) 2-8°C (36-46°F); or <30°C (86°F) for 40 days. (Opened) 2-8°C (36-46°F) for 40 days; or <30°C (86°F) for 40 days.

HYDROCHLOROTHIAZIDE TABLETS – hydrochlorothiazide

RX

Class: Thiazide diuretic

ADULT DOSAGE

Edema

For edema due to renal dysfunction (eg, nephrotic syndrome, acute glomerulonephritis, chronic renal failure), edema in pregnancy due to pathologic causes and adjunctive therapy for edema associated w/ congestive heart failure, hepatic cirrhosis, and corticosteroid and estrogen therapy

Usual: 25-100mg/day as a single or divided dose. May give qod or 3-5 days/week

Hypertension

Initial: 25mg qd

Titrate: May increase to 50mg/day as a single or 2 divided doses

PEDIATRIC DOSAGE

Diuresis

Usual: 1-2mg/kg/day in single or 2 divided doses

Max:

<6 Months: 3mg/kg/day in 2 divided doses

Infants up to 2 Years: 37.5mg/day

2-12 Years: 100mg/day

Hypertension

Usual: 1-2mg/kg/day in single or 2 divided doses

Max:

<6 Months: 3mg/kg/day in 2 divided doses

Infants up to 2 Years: 37.5mg/day

2-12 Years: 100mg/day

ADMINISTRATION

Oral route

HOW SUPPLIED

Tab: 12.5mg, 25mg*, 50mg* *scored

CONTRAINDICATIONS

Anuria, hypersensitivity to this product or to other sulfonamide-derived drugs.

WARNINGS/PRECAUTIONS

Caution with severe renal disease; may precipitate azotemia. Caution with hepatic impairment or progressive liver disease; may precipitate hepatic coma. Sensitivity reactions may occur in patients with or without a history of allergy or bronchial asthma. Possibility of exacerbation/activation of systemic lupus erythematosus (SLE) reported. May cause idiosyncratic reaction, resulting in acute transient myopia and acute angle-closure glaucoma; d/c as rapidly as possible. Observe for evidence of fluid/electrolyte imbalance (eg, hyponatremia, hypochloremic alkalosis, hypokalemia). Hypokalemia may sensitize or exaggerate the response of the heart to toxic effects of digitalis. Hyperuricemia or precipitation of acute gout, hyperglycemia, manifestations of latent diabetes mellitus (DM), hypomagnesemia, hypercalcemia, and increases in cholesterol and TG levels may occur. Enhanced antihypertensive effects in postsympathectomy patients. Consider withholding or discontinuing therapy if progressive renal impairment becomes evident. D/C before testing for parathyroid function.

ADVERSE REACTIONS

Weakness, hypotension, pancreatitis, jaundice, diarrhea, aplastic anemia, agranulocytosis, anaphylactic reactions, muscle spasm, vertigo, paresthesia, renal failure, erythema multiforme, transient blurred vision, impotence.

DRUG INTERACTIONS

Potentiation of orthostatic hypotension may occur with alcohol, barbiturates, or narcotics. Dosage adjustment of antidiabetic drugs (oral agents and insulin) may be required. Additive effect or potentiation with other antihypertensives. Anionic exchange resins (eg, cholestyramine, colestipol) may impair absorption. Corticosteroids and adrenocorticotropic hormone may intensify electrolyte depletion, particularly hypokalemia. May decrease response to pressor amines (eg, norepinephrine). May increase responsiveness to nondepolarizing skeletal muscle relaxants (eg, tubocurarine). May increase risk of lithium toxicity; avoid concomitant use. NSAIDs may reduce diuretic, natriuretic, and antihypertensive effects.

PATIENT CONSIDERATIONS

Assessment: Assess for anuria, hypersensitivity to drug or sulfonamide-derived drugs, renal/hepatic impairment, history of allergy or bronchial asthma, SLE, DM, postsympathectomy status, pregnancy/nursing status, and possible drug interactions.

Monitoring: Monitor for signs/symptoms of fluid/electrolyte imbalance, sensitivity reactions, exacerbation/activation of SLE, idiosyncratic reaction, hyperuricemia or precipitation of acute gout, hyperglycemia, latent DM, increases in cholesterol and TG levels, and other adverse reactions. Monitor serum electrolytes.

Counseling: Inform of the risks and benefits of therapy. Advise to report to physician any adverse reactions.

STORAGE: 20-25°C (68-77°F).

HYDROCORTISONE – hydrocortisone RX

Class: Corticosteroid

OTHER BRAND NAMES

Anusol-HC Cream, Proctozone-HC

ADULT DOSAGE

Inflammatory and Pruritic Manifestations of Corticosteroid-Responsive Dermatoses

Apply a thin film to the affected area bid-qid depending on the severity of the condition

PEDIATRIC DOSAGE

Inflammatory and Pruritic Manifestations of Corticosteroid-Responsive Dermatoses

Apply a thin film to the affected area bid-qid depending on the severity of the condition

Use least effective amount

ADMINISTRATION

Topical route

May use occlusive dressings for the management of psoriasis or recalcitrant conditions; d/c use of occlusive dressings and institute appropriate antimicrobial therapy if an infection develops.

Lot

Shake well before use.

HOW SUPPLIED

Cre: (Proctozone/Anusol) 2.5% [30g]; **Lot:** 2.5% [59mL]; **Oint:** 2.5% [28.35g, 453.6g]

CONTRAINDICATIONS

History of hypersensitivity to any of the components of the preparation.

WARNINGS/PRECAUTIONS

Systemic absorption may produce reversible hypothalamic-pituitary-adrenal (HPA) axis suppression, manifestations of Cushing's syndrome, hyperglycemia, and glucosuria. Application of more potent steroids, use over large surface areas, prolonged use, and the addition of occlusive dressings may augment systemic absorption. Periodically evaluate for evidence of HPA axis suppression when a large dose of a potent topical steroid is applied to a large surface area and under an occlusive dressing; if noted, withdraw treatment, reduce frequency of application, or substitute w/ a less potent steroid. Infrequently, signs/symptoms of steroid withdrawal may occur requiring supplemental systemic corticosteroids. D/C and institute appropriate therapy if irritation occurs. Use appropriate antifungal or antibacterial agent in the presence of dermatological infections; if favorable response does not occur promptly, d/c until infection is controlled. Children may be more susceptible to systemic toxicity. Chronic therapy may interfere w/ growth and development of children.

ADVERSE REACTIONS

Burning, itching, irritation, dryness, folliculitis, hypertrichosis, acneiform eruptions, hypopigmentation, perioral dermatitis, allergic contact dermatitis, maceration of the skin, secondary infection, skin atrophy, striae, miliaria.

PATIENT CONSIDERATIONS

Assessment: Assess for previous hypersensitivity to any of the components of the drug, dermatological infections, conditions that augment systemic absorption, and pregnancy/nursing status.

Monitoring: Monitor for signs/symptoms of reversible HPA axis suppression, Cushing's syndrome, hyperglycemia, glucosuria, skin irritation, systemic toxicity in children, hypersensitivity reactions, steroid withdrawal, and other adverse reactions. When a large dose is applied to a large surface area or under occlusive dressings, monitor for HPA axis suppression by using urinary free cortisol and adrenocorticotropic hormone stimulation tests.

Counseling: Instruct to use externally ud and to avoid contact w/ eyes. Advise not to use for any disorder other than for which it was prescribed. Instruct not to bandage, cover, or wrap treated skin area, unless directed by physician. Advise to report any signs of local adverse reactions, especially under occlusive dressing. Instruct not to use tight-fitting diapers or plastic pants on a child being treated in the diaper area, as these garments may constitute occlusive dressings.

STORAGE: Lot/Oint: 15-30°C (59-86°F). **Cre:** (Anusol) 20-25°C (68-77°F). Store away from heat. Protect from freezing. (Proctozone) 20-25°C (68-77°F); excursion permitted to 15-30°C (59-86°F).

HYDROMET — homatropine methylbromide/hydrocodone bitartrate CII

Class: Opioid antitussive

OTHER BRAND NAMES

Tussigon

ADULT DOSAGE

Cough

Hydromet:
1 tsp (5mL) q4-6h prn
Max: 6 tsp (30mL)/24 hrs

Tussigon:
1 tab q4-6h prn
Max: 6 tabs/24 hrs

PEDIATRIC DOSAGE

Cough

6-12 Years:
Hydromet:
1/2 tsp (2.5mL) q4-6h prn
Max: 3 tsp (15mL)/24 hrs

Tussigon:
1/2 tab q4-6h prn
Max: 3 tabs/24 hrs

ADMINISTRATION

Oral route

HOW SUPPLIED

(Hydrocodone-Homatropine) **Syrup:** (Hydromet) 5mg-1.5mg/5mL [473mL]; **Tab:** (Tussigon) 5mg-1.5mg* *scored

CONTRAINDICATIONS

Hypersensitivity to hydrocodone or homatropine methylbromide.

WARNINGS/PRECAUTIONS

May be habit forming and has potential for abuse. Psychic/physical dependence and tolerance may develop upon repeated administration; use with caution. May produce dose-related respiratory depression; may be antagonized by the use of naloxone HCl and other supportive measures when indicated. Respiratory depression effects and the capacity to elevate CSF pressure may be markedly exaggerated in the presence of head injury, other intracranial lesions, or preexisting increased intracranial pressure (ICP). May obscure clinical course of head injuries and acute abdominal conditions. Carefully consider benefit to risk ratio, especially in pediatric patients with respiratory embarrassment (eg, croup). Before prescribing medication to suppress or modify cough, it is important to ascertain the underlying cause of cough, that the modification of cough does not increase the risk of clinical or physiological complications, and that appropriate therapy for the primary disease is provided. Caution in elderly, debilitated, severe hepatic/renal impairment, hypothyroidism, Addison's disease, prostatic hypertrophy or urethral stricture, asthma, and narrow-angle glaucoma.

ADVERSE REACTIONS

Sedation, drowsiness, lethargy, mental/physical impairment, anxiety, fear, dizziness, psychic dependence, N/V, ureteral spasm, urinary retention, respiratory depression, skin rash, pruritus.

DRUG INTERACTIONS

Additive CNS depression with other narcotics, antihistamines, antipsychotics, antianxiety agents, or other CNS depressants (including alcohol); reduce dose of 1 or both agents. May increase effects of either antidepressants or hydrocodone with MAOIs or TCAs.

PATIENT CONSIDERATIONS

Assessment: Assess for drug hypersensitivity, cough cause, head injury, intracranial lesions, preexisting increased ICP, acute abdominal conditions, respiratory embarrassment in pediatric patients, presence of debilitation, hepatic/renal impairment, hypothyroidism, Addison's disease, prostatic hypertrophy or urethral stricture, asthma, narrow-angle glaucoma, pregnancy/nursing status, and possible drug interactions.

Monitoring: Monitor for drug abuse/dependence, respiratory depression, and other adverse reactions.

Counseling: Inform about risks and benefits of therapy. Advise to take caution with hazardous activities (eg, operating machinery/driving); inform that medication may impair mental and physical abilities.

STORAGE: 15-30°C (59-86°F).

HYDROMET – homatropine methylbromide/hydrocodone bitartrate CII

Class: Opioid antitussive

OTHER BRAND NAMES

Tussigon

ADULT DOSAGE

Cough

Hydromet:
1 tsp (5mL) q4-6h prn
Max: 6 tsp (30mL)/24 hrs

Tussigon:
1 tab q4-6h prn
Max: 6 tabs/24 hrs

PEDIATRIC DOSAGE

Cough

6-12 Years:
Hydromet:
1/2 tsp (2.5mL) q4-6h prn
Max: 3 tsp (15mL)/24 hrs

Tussigon:
1/2 tab q4-6h prn
Max: 3 tabs/24 hrs

ADMINISTRATION

Oral route

HOW SUPPLIED

(Hydrocodone-Homatropine) **Syrup:** (Hydromet) 5mg-1.5mg/5mL [473mL]; **Tab:** (Tussigon) 5mg-1.5mg* *scored

CONTRAINDICATIONS

Hypersensitivity to hydrocodone or homatropine methylbromide.

WARNINGS/PRECAUTIONS

May be habit forming and has potential for abuse. Psychic/physical dependence and tolerance may develop upon repeated administration; use with caution. May produce dose-related respiratory depression; may be antagonized by the use of naloxone HCl and other supportive measures when indicated. Respiratory depression effects and the capacity to elevate CSF pressure may be markedly exaggerated in the presence of head injury, other intracranial lesions, or preexisting increased intracranial pressure (ICP). May obscure clinical course of head injuries and acute abdominal conditions. Carefully consider benefit to risk ratio, especially in pediatric patients with respiratory embarrassment (eg, croup). Before prescribing medication to suppress or modify cough, it is important to ascertain the underlying cause of cough, that the modification of cough does not increase the risk of clinical or physiological complications, and that appropriate therapy for the primary disease is provided. Caution in elderly, debilitated, severe hepatic/renal impairment, hypothyroidism, Addison's disease, prostatic hypertrophy or urethral stricture, asthma, and narrow-angle glaucoma.

ADVERSE REACTIONS

Sedation, drowsiness, lethargy, mental/physical impairment, anxiety, fear, dizziness, psychic dependence, N/V, ureteral spasm, urinary retention, respiratory depression, skin rash, pruritus.

DRUG INTERACTIONS

Additive CNS depression with other narcotics, antihistamines, antipsychotics, antianxiety agents, or other CNS depressants (including alcohol); reduce dose of 1 or both agents. May increase effects of either antidepressants or hydrocodone with MAOIs or TCAs.

PATIENT CONSIDERATIONS

Assessment: Assess for drug hypersensitivity, cough cause, head injury, intracranial lesions, preexisting increased ICP, acute abdominal conditions, respiratory embarrassment in pediatric patients, presence of debilitation, hepatic/renal impairment, hypothyroidism, Addison's disease, prostatic hypertrophy or urethral stricture, asthma, narrow-angle glaucoma, pregnancy/nursing status, and possible drug interactions.

Monitoring: Monitor for drug abuse/dependence, respiratory depression, and other adverse reactions.

Counseling: Inform about risks and benefits of therapy. Advise to take caution with hazardous activities (eg, operating machinery/driving); inform that medication may impair mental and physical abilities.

STORAGE: 15-30°C (59-86°F).

H

HYDROXYZINE HCL — hydroxyzine hydrochloride

RX

Class: Piperazine antihistamine

OTHER BRAND NAMES

Vistaril Injection (Discontinued)

ADULT DOSAGE

Pruritus

Management of pruritus due to allergic conditions (eg, chronic urticaria, atopic/contact dermatoses) and histamine-mediated pruritus

Syrup/Tab:
25mg tid or qid

Sedation

As premedication and following general anesthesia

Syrup/Tab:
50-100mg

Nausea/Vomiting

IM:
25-100mg; not for use in N/V of pregnancy

Surgery

As pre- and postoperative adjunctive medication to permit reduction in narcotic dosage, allay anxiety, and control emesis

IM:
25-100mg

Anxiety

Syrup/Tab:
Symptomatic relief of anxiety and tension associated w/ psychoneurosis and as an adjunct in organic disease states

50-100mg qid

IM:
Management of anxiety, tension, and psychomotor agitation in conditions of emotional stress. Useful in alleviating manifestations of anxiety/tension as in the preparation for dental procedures and in

PEDIATRIC DOSAGE

Pruritus

Management of pruritus due to allergic conditions (eg, chronic urticaria, atopic/contact dermatoses) and histamine-mediated pruritus

Syrup/Tab:
<6 Years:
50mg/day in divided doses
>6 Years:
50-100mg/day in divided doses

Sedation

As premedication and following general anesthesia

Syrup/Tab:
0.6mg/kg

Nausea/Vomiting

Excluding N/V of pregnancy

IM:
0.5mg/lb

Surgery

As pre- and postoperative adjunctive medication to permit reduction in narcotic dosage, allay anxiety, and control emesis

IM:
0.5mg/lb

Anxiety

Symptomatic relief of anxiety and tension associated w/ psychoneurosis and as an adjunct in organic disease states

Syrup/Tab:
<6 Years:
50mg/day in divided doses
>6 Years:
50-100mg/day in divided doses

acute emotional problems. Management of anxiety associated w/ organic disturbances and as adjunctive therapy in alcoholism and allergic conditions w/ strong emotional overlay (eg, asthma, chronic urticaria, pruritus). Treatment of acutely disturbed or hysterical patient and acute/chronic alcoholic w/ anxiety withdrawal symptoms or delirium tremens

50-100mg immediately, and q4-6h prn

Pregnancy

As pre- and postpartum adjunctive medication to permit reduction in narcotic dosage, allay anxiety, and control emesis

IM:
25-100mg

DOSING CONSIDERATIONS

Elderly

Start at lower end of dosing range

ADMINISTRATION

Oral/IM route

Adjust dose according to response.

When treatment is initiated by IM route, subsequent doses may be administered orally.

IM

May be administered w/o further dilution.

Inject well w/in the body of a relatively large muscle; preferred site in adults is the upper outer quadrant of the buttock or midlateral thigh and in children is the midlateral thigh.

HOW SUPPLIED

Inj: 25mg/mL [1mL], 50mg/mL [1mL, 2mL, 10mL]; **Syrup:** 10mg/5mL [118mL, 473mL]; **Tab:** 10mg, 25mg, 50mg

CONTRAINDICATIONS

Prolonged QT interval, known hypersensitivity to hydroxyzine HCl, early pregnancy. **Inj:** SQ, intra-arterial, or IV administration. **Syrup/Tab:** Known hypersensitivity to cetirizine or levocetirizine.

WARNINGS/PRECAUTIONS

Patients may be started on IM therapy when indicated and should be maintained on oral therapy whenever this route is practicable. QT prolongation and torsades de pointes reported; caution in patients w/ risk factors for QT prolongation, congenital long QT syndrome, a family history of long QT syndrome, other conditions that predispose to QT prolongation, ventricular arrhythmia, recent MI, uncompensated heart failure, and bradyarrhythmias. Drowsiness may occur. May impair mental/physical abilities. Caution in elderly. **Inj:** Should not be used as sole treatment of psychosis or for clearly demonstrated cases of depression. Inadvertent SQ inj may result in significant tissue damage. IM inj may result in severe inj-site reactions requiring surgical intervention. Inj into the deltoid area should be used only if well developed (eg, certain adults and older children), and then only w/ caution to avoid radial nerve injury. In infants and small children, inj into the periphery of the upper outer quadrant of the gluteal region should be used only when necessary, in order to minimize the possibility of damage to the sciatic nerve. IM inj in children should not be made into the lower and mid-third of the upper arm.

ADVERSE REACTIONS

Dry mouth, drowsiness, involuntary motor activity.

DRUG INTERACTIONS

May potentiate CNS depressants (eg, narcotics, non-narcotic analgesics and barbiturates, alcohol); reduce dose of CNS depressants when administered concomitantly. Modify use of meperidine and barbiturates, on an individual basis, when used in preanesthetic adjunctive therapy. Caution during the concomitant use of drugs known to prolong the QT interval (eg, quinidine, amiodarone, sotalol, ziprasidone, clozapine, quetiapine, chlorpromazine, fluoxetine, azithromycin, erythromycin, moxifloxacin, pentamidine, methadone, ondansetron, droperidol). **Inj:** Cardiac arrests and death reported when combined w/ other CNS depressants. Administration of meperidine may result in severe hypotension in the postoperative patient or any individual whose ability to maintain BP has been compromised by a depleted blood volume. Use meperidine w/ great caution and in reduced dosage in patients who are receiving other pre- and/or postoperative medications and in whom there is a risk of respiratory depression, hypotension, and profound sedation or coma occurring.

PATIENT CONSIDERATIONS

Assessment: Assess for hypersensitivity to drug, QT prolongation, risk factors for QT prolongation, pregnancy/nursing status, and for possible drug interactions. **Syrup/Tab:** Assess for hypersensitivity to cetirizine or levocetirizine.

Monitoring: Monitor for hypersensitivity reactions, QT prolongation, torsades de pointes, drowsiness, and other adverse reactions. Periodically reassess the usefulness of therapy.

Counseling: Inform about risks/benefits of therapy. Inform that drowsiness may occur; instruct to use caution when driving or operating heavy machinery. Instruct to notify physician if pregnant, nursing, or taking any other concomitant therapy.

STORAGE: 20-25°C (68-77°F). **Inj:** Excursions permitted to 15-30°C (59-86°F). **Syrup:** Protect from freezing. **Inj/Syrup:** Protect from light.

HYSINGLA ER – hydrocodone bitartrate CII

Class: Opioid analgesic

H

Exposes users to risks of addiction, abuse, and misuse, which can lead to overdose and death; assess each patient's risk prior to prescribing, and monitor regularly for development of these behaviors/conditions. Serious, life-threatening, or fatal respiratory depression may occur; monitor for respiratory depression, especially during initiation or following a dose increase. Swallow tab whole; crushing, chewing, or dissolving tab can cause rapid release and absorption of a potentially fatal dose. Accidental ingestion of even 1 dose, especially by children, can result in a fatal overdose. Prolonged use during pregnancy can result in neonatal opioid withdrawal syndrome, which may be life threatening if not recognized and treated, and requires management according to protocols developed by neonatology experts; advise pregnant women of the risk and ensure availability of appropriate treatment. Concomitant use w/ all CYP3A4 inhibitors may result in an increase in plasma concentrations, which could increase or prolong adverse drug effects and may cause potentially fatal respiratory depression. Discontinuation of a concomitantly used CYP3A4 inducer may result in an increase in plasma concentrations. Monitor patients receiving concomitant therapy w/ any CYP3A4 inhibitor or inducer.

ADULT DOSAGE

Chronic Pain

Management of Pain Severe Enough to Require Daily, Around-the-Clock, Long-Term Opioid Treatment and for Which Alternative Treatment Options are Inadequate:

Initial Dosing:
1st Opioid Analgesic/Opioid Intolerant: 20mg q24h

Titration and Maint of Therapy:
Adjust in increments of 10-20mg every 3-5 days prn
Patients who experience breakthrough pain may require a dose increase, or may need rescue medication w/ an appropriate dose of an immediate-release analgesic. If level of pain increases after dose stabilization, attempt to identify source of increased pain before increasing dose

If unacceptable opioid-related adverse reactions are observed, next daily dose may be reduced

Daily doses ≥80mg are only for use in opioid-tolerant patients

Conversions

Initial Dosing:
From Oral Hydrocodone Formulations:
Administer patient's total daily oral hydrocodone dose as extended-release hydrocodone qd
From Other Oral Opioids:
D/C all other around-the-clock opioids when extended-release hydrocodone is initiated

Conversion Factors from Other Oral Opioids (Previous Oral Opioid: Approximate Oral Conversion Factor):
Codeine 133mg: 0.15

PEDIATRIC DOSAGE

Pediatric use may not have been established

Hydromorphone 5mg: 4
Methadone 13.3mg: 1.5
Morphine 40mg: 0.5
Oxycodone 20mg: 1
Oxymorphone 10mg: 2
Tramadol 200mg: 0.1

Calculation of Estimated Total Hydrocodone Daily Dose:
On Single Opioid: Sum current total daily dose of opioid, then multiply the total daily dose by the approximate oral conversion factor
On >1 Opioid: Calculate approximate oral hydrocodone dose for each opioid and sum the totals to obtain the approximate oral hydrocodone daily dose
On Fixed-Ratio Opioid/Nonopioid Analgesic Products: Use only the opioid component of these products in the conversion
Reduce calculated daily oral hydrocodone dose by 25%

From Methadone:
Close monitoring is of particular importance. Ratio between methadone and other opioid agonists may vary widely as a function of previous dose exposure. Methadone has a long $T_{1/2}$ and can accumulate in the plasma

From Transdermal Fentanyl:
May initiate 18 hrs following removal of patch; for each 25mcg/hr fentanyl transdermal patch, a dose of 20mg q24h represents a conservative initial dose

From Transdermal Buprenorphine:
All patients receiving transdermal buprenorphine (≤20mcg/hr) should initiate w/ 20mg q24h

Refer to PI for further conversion information

DOSING CONSIDERATIONS

Elderly

Start on low doses and monitor closely for adverse events (eg, respiratory depression, sedation, confusion)

Renal Impairment

Moderate to Severe Impairment and ESRD:
Initial: 1/2 initial dose and monitor closely for respiratory depression and sedation

Hepatic Impairment

Severe Impairment:
Initial: 1/2 initial dose and monitor closely for respiratory depression and sedation

Discontinuation

Gradually reduce dose every 2-4 days; next dose should be at least 50% of the prior dose
After reaching 20mg dose for 2-4 days, may d/c

ADMINISTRATION

Oral route

Take whole, w/ enough water to ensure complete swallowing immediately after placing in the mouth
Do not crush, chew, or dissolve
Do not pre-soak, lick or otherwise wet tab prior to placing in mouth

HOW SUPPLIED

Tab, Extended-Release: 20mg, 30mg, 40mg, 60mg, 80mg, 100mg, 120mg

CONTRAINDICATIONS

Significant respiratory depression, acute or severe bronchial asthma in an unmonitored setting or in the absence of resuscitative equipment, known/suspected paralytic ileus and GI obstruction, hypersensitivity to any component of this medication or the active ingredient, hydrocodone bitartrate.

WARNINGS/PRECAUTIONS

Reserve for use in patients for whom alternative treatment options are ineffective, not tolerated, or would be otherwise inadequate to provide sufficient management of pain. Should be prescribed only by healthcare professionals knowledgeable in the use of potent opioids for the management of chronic pain. Overestimating the dose when converting from another opioid product may result in fatal overdose w/ the 1st dose. Life-threatening respiratory depression is more likely to occur in elderly, cachectic, or debilitated patients. Consider alternative nonopioid analgesics in patients w/ significant COPD or cor pulmonale, and in patients having a substantially decreased respiratory reserve, hypoxia, hypercapnia, or preexisting respiratory depression. Respiratory depressant effects and elevation of CSF pressure (resulting from vasodilation following carbon dioxide retention) may be markedly exaggerated in the presence of head injury, intracranial lesions, or preexisting increase in intracranial pressure (ICP). May produce effects on pupillary response and consciousness, which can obscure neurologic signs of further increases in ICP in patients w/ head injuries. Monitor patients closely who may be susceptible to intracranial effects of carbon dioxide retention. May obscure clinical course of a patient w/ a head injury. Avoid w/ impaired consciousness, coma, or circulatory shock. May cause severe hypotension, including orthostatic hypotension and syncope in ambulatory patients; increased risk in patients whose ability to maintain BP has been compromised by depleted blood volume, or after concurrent administration w/ drugs such as phenothiazines or other agents that compromise vasomotor tone. Esophageal obstruction, dysphagia, and choking reported; consider use of an alternative analgesic in patients who have difficulty swallowing and patients at risk for underlying GI disorders resulting in a small GI lumen. Diminishes propulsive peristaltic waves in the GI tract and decreases bowel motility. May obscure diagnosis or clinical course in patients w/ acute abdominal conditions. May cause spasm of the sphincter of Oddi; monitor patients w/ biliary tract disease, including acute pancreatitis. May impair mental/physical abilities. QTc prolongation reported following daily doses of 160mg; consider this in making clinical decisions regarding patient monitoring when prescribing in patients w/ CHF, bradyarrhythmias, electrolyte abnormalities, or who are taking medications that are known to prolong the QTc interval. Avoid in patients w/ congenital long QT syndrome; consider reducing dose by 33-50% or changing to an alternate analgesic in patients who develop QTc prolongation. Caution w/ severe hepatic impairment, moderate or severe renal impairment or ESRD, and in elderly.

ADVERSE REACTIONS

Respiratory depression, constipation, N/V, fatigue, URTI, dizziness, headache, somnolence, pruritus, insomnia, influenza.

DRUG INTERACTIONS

See Boxed Warning. Caution when initiating treatment in patients currently taking, or discontinuing, CYP3A4 inhibitors or inducers; evaluate at frequent intervals and consider dose adjustments until stable drug effects are achieved. Concomitant use w/ alcohol or other CNS depressants (eg, sedatives, hypnotics, tranquilizers, general anesthetics, phenothiazines, other opioids) may increase the risk of respiratory depression, profound sedation, coma, and death; if coadministration is considered, reduce dose of 1 or both agents. Monitor use in elderly, cachectic, and debilitated patients when given concomitantly w/ other drugs that depress respiration. Mixed agonist/antagonist (eg, pentazocine, nalbuphine, butorphanol) and partial agonist (buprenorphine) analgesics may reduce analgesic effect or precipitate withdrawal symptoms; avoid use. Severe and unpredictable potentiation by MAOIs reported; not recommended for use in patients who have received MAOIs w/in 14 days. Anticholinergics or other drugs w/ anticholinergic activity may increase the risk of urinary retention or severe constipation, which may lead to paralytic ileus; monitor for signs of urinary retention and constipation in addition to respiratory and CNS depression when used concurrently. Strong laxatives (eg, lactulose) that rapidly increase GI motility may decrease hydrocodone absorption and result in decreased plasma levels; closely monitor for development of adverse events and changing analgesic requirements.

PATIENT CONSIDERATIONS

Assessment: Assess for abuse/addiction risk, pain type/severity, prior opioid therapy, opioid tolerance, respiratory depression, COPD or other respiratory complications, head injury, paralytic ileus, drug hypersensitivity, pregnancy/nursing status, possible drug interactions, and any other conditions where treatment is contraindicated or cautioned.

Monitoring: Monitor for respiratory depression (especially w/in the first 24-72 hrs of initiating therapy), hypotension, decreased bowel motility in postoperative patients, QTc prolongation, and other adverse reactions. Monitor for development of addiction, abuse, or misuse. Periodically reassess the continued need for therapy.

Counseling: Inform that use of drug can result in addiction, abuse, and misuse; instruct not to share w/ others and to take steps to protect from theft or misuse. Inform of the risk of life-threatening respiratory depression; advise how to recognize respiratory depression and to seek medical attention if experiencing breathing difficulties. Inform that accidental exposure, especially in children, may result in respiratory depression or death. Advise to store securely and to dispose of unused tabs in accordance w/ local state guidelines and/or regulations. Inform female patients of reproductive potential that use during pregnancy may cause fetal harm; instruct to notify physician if pregnant/planning to become pregnant. Inform that potentially serious additive effects may occur if used w/ alcohol or other CNS depressants, and not to use such drugs unless supervised by a healthcare provider. Instruct how to properly take the drug. Inform that drug may cause orthostatic hypotension and syncope; instruct how to recognize symptoms of low BP and how to reduce risk of serious consequences should hypotension occur. Inform that drug may impair the ability to perform potentially hazardous activities; advise not to perform such tasks until patients know how they will react to the medication. Advise of potential for severe constipation, including management instructions and when to seek medical attention; instruct to monitor analgesic response following the use of strong laxatives and to contact the prescriber if changes are noted. Instruct patients w/ a history of CHF or bradyarrhythmias, and patients at risk for electrolyte abnormalities or who are taking other medications known to prolong QT interval that periodic monitoring of ECGs and electrolytes may be necessary during therapy. Advise how to recognize anaphylaxis and when to seek medical attention.

STORAGE: 25°C (77°F); excursions permitted between 15-30°C (59-86°F).

HYZAAR – hydrochlorothiazide/losartan potassium RX

Class: Angiotensin II receptor blocker (ARB)/thiazide diuretic

D/C when pregnancy is detected. Drugs that act directly on the renin-angiotensin system (RAS) can cause injury/death to the developing fetus.

H

ADULT DOSAGE

Hypertension

Initial: 50mg/12.5mg qd
Titrate: May increase after 3 weeks
Max: 100mg/25mg qd

BP Not Adequately Controlled w/ Losartan 50mg Monotherapy:
Initial: 50mg/12.5mg qd
Titrate: May increase after 3 weeks to 100mg/25mg qd

BP Not Adequately Controlled w/ Losartan 100mg Monotherapy:
Initial: 100mg/12.5mg qd
Titrate: May increase after 3 weeks to 100mg/25mg qd

BP Not Adequately Controlled w/ Hydrochlorothiazide (HCTZ) 25mg QD/ Hypokalemia Develops w/ HCTZ 25mg QD:
Initial: 50mg/12.5mg qd
Titrate: May increase after 3 weeks to 100mg/25mg qd

Hypertension with Left Ventricular Hypertrophy

Reduction in Risk of Stroke:
Initial (BP Uncontrolled on Losartan 50mg QD): 50mg/12.5mg
Titrate: Increase to 100mg/12.5mg, followed by 100mg/25mg; add other antihypertensives for further reduction

This benefit may not apply to black patients

PEDIATRIC DOSAGE

Pediatric use may not have been established

DOSING CONSIDERATIONS

Renal Impairment

Consider withholding or discontinuing therapy in patients who develop a clinically significant decrease in renal function

ADMINISTRATION

Oral route

HOW SUPPLIED

Tab: (Losartan/HCTZ) 50mg/12.5mg, 100mg/12.5mg, 100mg/25mg

CONTRAINDICATIONS

Hypersensitivity to any component, anuria, coadministration w/ aliskiren in patients w/ diabetes.

WARNINGS/PRECAUTIONS

Not indicated for initial therapy of HTN except when HTN is severe enough that the value of achieving prompt BP control exceeds the risk of initiating combination therapy. Symptomatic hypotension may occur in patients w/ an activated RAS (eg, volume- or salt-depleted patients); do not use as initial therapy in patients w/ intravascular volume depletion. Correct volume or salt depletion prior to administration of therapy. Patients whose renal function may depend in part on the activity of the RAS may be at risk of developing acute renal failure; monitor renal function periodically. Can cause hypokalemia, hyponatremia, and hypomagnesemia; monitor serum electrolytes periodically. The antihypertensive effects of the drug may be enhanced in the postsympathectomy patient. Initiation not recommended for patients w/ hepatic impairment. **HCTZ:** Hypersensitivity reactions may occur; more likely to occur in patients w/ history of allergy or bronchial asthma. May alter glucose tolerance and raise serum levels of cholesterol and TGs. Decreases urinary calcium excretion and may cause elevations of serum calcium; monitor calcium levels. May cause idiosyncratic reaction, resulting in acute transient myopia and acute angle-closure glaucoma; d/c as rapidly as possible. May cause exacerbation or activation of systemic lupus erythematosus (SLE). May cause hyperuricemia or frank gout may be precipitated.

ADVERSE REACTIONS

Dizziness, URI, cough, back pain.

DRUG INTERACTIONS

See Contraindications. Increases in serum lithium concentrations and lithium toxicity reported; monitor serum lithium levels during concomitant use. NSAIDs, including selective COX-2 inhibitors, may decrease effects of diuretics and ARBs and may deteriorate renal function (possible acute renal failure). Avoid w/ aliskiren in patients w/ renal impairment (GFR <60mL/min). **Losartan:** Use w/ other drugs that raise serum K^+ may result in hyperkalemia; monitor serum K^+. Dual blockade of the RAS is associated w/ increased risks of hypotension, syncope, hyperkalemia, and changes in renal function (including acute renal failure); closely monitor BP, renal function, and electrolytes w/ concomitant agents that affect the RAS. **HCTZ:** Dose adjustment of antidiabetic drugs (oral agents, insulin) may be required. Anionic exchange resins (eg, cholestyramine, colestipol) may impair absorption; stagger the dose of HCTZ and the resin such that HCTZ is administered at least 4 hrs before or 4-6 hrs after the administration of the resin.

PATIENT CONSIDERATIONS

Assessment: Assess for hypersensitivity to drugs and their components, anuria, history of sulfonamide or penicillin allergy, volume/salt depletion, SLE, diabetes, hepatic/renal impairment, postsympathectomy status, pregnancy/nursing status, and possible drug interactions. Obtain baseline BP.

Monitoring: Monitor for signs/symptoms of fluid/electrolyte imbalance, exacerbation/activation of SLE, idiosyncratic reaction, precipitation of gout, hypersensitivity reactions, and other adverse reactions. Monitor BP, serum electrolytes, renal/hepatic function, Ca^{2+} levels, cholesterol, and TG levels periodically.

Counseling: Inform females of childbearing potential of the consequences of exposure during pregnancy and of the treatment options for women planning to become pregnant. Instruct to report pregnancy to the physician as soon as possible. Counsel that lightheadedness may occur, especially during the 1st days of therapy; instruct to report to physician. Instruct to consult physician if syncope occurs. Inform that dehydration from inadequate fluid intake, excessive perspiration, vomiting, or diarrhea may lead to an excessive fall in blood pressure. Instruct not to use K^+ supplements or salt substitutes containing K^+ w/o consulting physician. Advise to d/c and seek immediate medical attention if experiencing symptoms of acute myopia or secondary angle closure glaucoma.

STORAGE: 25°C (77°F); excursions permitted to 15-30°C (59-86°F). Protect from light.

IBRANCE – palbociclib

RX

Class: Kinase inhibitor

ADULT DOSAGE

HR Positive, HER2 Negative Advanced or Metastatic Breast Cancer

Initial Endocrine-Based Therapy in Postmenopausal Women:
125mg qd for 21 consecutive days followed by 7 days off treatment + 2.5mg letrozole qd continuously throughout the 28-day cycle

Women w/ Disease Progression Following Endocrine Therapy:
125mg qd for 21 consecutive days followed by 7 days off treatment + 500mg fulvestrant on Days 1, 15, 29, and once monthly thereafter

PEDIATRIC DOSAGE

Pediatric use may not have been established

Pre/perimenopausal should be treated w/ luteinizing hormone-releasing hormone agonists according to current clinical practice standards

Missed Dose

If patient vomits/misses dose, patient should not take an additional dose that day; patient should take next prescribed dose at usual time

DOSING CONSIDERATIONS

Concomitant Medications

Strong CYP3A Inhibitors:

Avoid concomitant use and consider alternative concomitant medication w/ no/minimal CYP3A inhibition

If Concomitant Use Cannot Be Avoided: Reduce palbociclib dose to 75mg qd. If strong inhibitor is discontinued, increase dose (after 3-5 half lives of the inhibitor) to the dose used prior to initiating the strong inhibitor

Adverse Reactions

Recommended Starting Dose: 125mg/day

1st Dose Reduction: 100mg/day

2nd Dose Reduction: 75mg/day

If further dose reduction below 75mg/day is required, d/c treatment

Hematologic Toxicities (Except Lymphopenia Unless Associated w/ Clinical Events):

Monitor CBC prior to start of therapy, at the beginning of each cycle, as well as on Day 14 of the first 2 cycles, and as clinically indicated

Grade 1 or 2: No dose adjustment required

Grade 3:

Day 1 of Cycle:

Withhold, repeat CBC monitoring w/in 1 week. When recovered to Grade ≤2, start the next cycle at the same dose

Day 14 of First 2 Cycles:

Continue at current dose to complete cycle. Repeat CBC on Day 21

Consider dose reduction in cases of prolonged (>1 week) recovery from Grade 3 neutropenia or recurrent Grade 3 neutropenia in subsequent cycles

Grade 3 Neutropenia w/ Fever ≥38.5°C and/or Infection:

Withhold until recovery to Grade ≤2; resume at the next lower dose

Grade 4:

Withhold until recovery to Grade ≤2; resume at the next lower dose

Nonhematologic Toxicities:

Grade 1 or 2: No dose adjustment required

Grade ≥3: If persisting despite medical treatment, withhold until symptoms resolve to Grade ≤1 or Grade ≤2 (if not considered a safety risk for patient). Resume at next lower dose

ADMINISTRATION

Oral route

Take w/ food at the same time each day.

Swallow whole; do not chew, crush, or open prior to swallowing.

HOW SUPPLIED

Cap: 75mg, 100mg, 125mg

WARNINGS/PRECAUTIONS

Decreased neutrophil counts and febrile neutropenia reported; dose interruption, reduction, or delay in starting treatment cycles is recommended for patients who develop Grade 3 or 4 neutropenia. Pulmonary embolism (PE) reported; monitor and treat as medically appropriate. May cause fetal harm.

ADVERSE REACTIONS

Neutropenia, leukopenia, infections, fatigue, nausea, anemia, stomatitis, headache, diarrhea, thrombocytopenia, constipation, alopecia, vomiting, rash, decreased appetite.

DRUG INTERACTIONS

See Dosing Considerations. Increased plasma exposure w/ strong CYP3A inhibitors (itraconazole). Avoid grapefruit or grapefruit juice. Decreased plasma exposure w/ strong CYP3A inducers (eg, rifampin); avoid concomitant use w/ strong CYP3A inducers (eg, phenytoin, carbamazepine, St John's wort). Multiple doses increased midazolam plasma exposure. May need to reduce dose of sensitive CYP3A substrate w/ a narrow therapeutic index (eg, alfentanil, cyclosporine, ergotamine) as therapy may increase their exposure.

PATIENT CONSIDERATIONS

Assessment: Assess for pregnancy/nursing status and possible drug interactions. Obtain baseline CBC.

Monitoring: Monitor for signs/symptoms of PE, and other adverse reactions. Monitor CBC at the beginning of each cycle, as well as on Day 14 of the first 2 cycles, and as clinically indicated.

Counseling: Advise to immediately report any signs/symptoms of myelosuppression/infection, or PE. Instruct not to consume grapefruit products while on therapy. Inform patients to avoid strong CYP3A inhibitors/inducers. Advise to inform physician of all concomitant medications, including prescription medicines, OTC drugs, vitamins, and herbal products. Instruct not to take additional dose if the patient vomits or misses a dose and to take the next dose at the usual time. Advise females of reproductive potential to use effective contraception during therapy and for at least 3 weeks after the last dose. Advise women not to breastfeed during treatment and for 3 weeks after the last dose. Advise to contact physician if patient becomes pregnant, or if pregnancy is suspected, during treatment.

STORAGE: 20-25°C (68-77°F); excursions permitted between 15-30°C (59-86°F).

ILARIS – canakinumab

RX

Class: Monoclonal antibody/interleukin-1 (IL-1) beta

I

ADULT DOSAGE

Cryopyrin-Associated Periodic Syndromes

Including familial cold autoinflammatory syndrome and Muckle-Wells syndrome

15-40kg:
Usual: 2mg/kg

>40kg:
Usual: 150mg

Administer every 8 weeks as a single dose via SQ inj

PEDIATRIC DOSAGE

Cryopyrin-Associated Periodic Syndromes

Including familial cold autoinflammatory syndrome and Muckle-Wells syndrome

≥4 Years:
15-40kg:
Usual: 2mg/kg
Titrate: May increase to 3mg/kg if response is inadequate

>40kg:
Usual: 150mg

Administer every 8 weeks as a single dose via SQ inj

Systemic Juvenile Idiopathic Arthritis

≥2 Years:
≥7.5kg:
Usual: 4mg/kg SQ every 4 weeks
Max: 300mg/dose

ADMINISTRATION

SQ route

Supplied in a single-use vial; discard any unused product or waste material
Avoid inj into scar tissue as this may result in insufficient exposure

Preparation and Administration

1. Reconstitute each vial by slowly injecting 1mL of preservative-free sterile water for inj w/ a 1mL syringe and an 18-gauge x 2- inches needle
2. Swirl the vial slowly at an angle of about 45° for approx 1 min and allow to stand for 5 min; do not shake. Then gently turn the vial upside down and back again 10X
3. Allow to stand for about 15 min at room temperature to obtain a clear sol
4. The reconstituted sol has a final concentration of 150mg/mL
5. Tap the side of the vial to remove any residual liquid from the stopper; the reconstituted sol should be essentially free from particulates, and clear to opalescent
6. The sol should be colorless or may have a slight brownish-yellow tint; if the sol has a distinctly brown discoloration it should not be used
7. Slight foaming of the product upon reconstitution is not unusual
8. Using a sterile syringe and needle carefully withdraw the required volume depending on the dose to be administered (0.2-1mL) and subcutaneously inject using a 27-gauge x 0.5-inches needle

HOW SUPPLIED

Inj: 180mg

CONTRAINDICATIONS

Confirmed hypersensitivity to the active substance or to any of the excipients.

WARNINGS/PRECAUTIONS

Associated with an increased risk of serious infections; caution in patients with infections, history of recurring infections or underlying conditions that may predispose to infections, and do not administer during an active infection requiring medical intervention. D/C if serious infection develops. May increase risk of tuberculosis (TB) reactivation or of opportunistic infections (eg, aspergillosis, atypical mycobacterial infections, cytomegalovirus). Evaluate for active and latent TB infection prior to treatment initiation; perform appropriate screening tests in all patients, and treat those testing positive according to standard medical practice prior to therapy. May increase risk of malignancies. Hypersensitivity reactions reported. Prior to initiation of therapy, patients should receive all recommended vaccinations, as appropriate, including pneumococcal and inactivated influenza vaccine. Macrophage activation syndrome (MAS) reported in SJIA patients.

ADVERSE REACTIONS

Nasopharyngitis, diarrhea, influenza, headache, nausea, rhinitis, bronchitis, gastroenteritis, pharyngitis, weight increase, musculoskeletal pain, vertigo, inj-site reactions, infections, abdominal pain.

DRUG INTERACTIONS

Increased risk of serious infections with TNF inhibitors; coadministration is not recommended. Not recommended with other agents that block interleukin-1 (IL-1) or its receptors. Do not give with live vaccines. May alter effect or concentration of drugs metabolized by CYP450 enzymes; monitor effect or concentration and may need to adjust dose of CYP450 substrates with a narrow therapeutic index (eg, warfarin).

PATIENT CONSIDERATIONS

Assessment: Assess for drug hypersensitivity, infections, history of recurring infections or underlying conditions that may predispose to infections, active/latent TB, vaccination history, pregnancy/nursing status, and possible drug interactions.

Monitoring: Monitor for serious infections, signs/symptoms of TB, malignancies, hypersensitivity reactions, MAS or triggers for MAS, and other adverse reactions.

Counseling: Advise of the potential benefits and risks of therapy. Inform that healthcare providers should perform administration of drug. Instruct to immediately contact physician if an infection, signs of an allergic reaction, persistent inj-site reaction, or signs/symptoms or high risk exposure suggestive of TB (eg, persistent cough, weight loss, subfebrile temperature) develop.

STORAGE: 2-8°C (36-46°F). Do not freeze. Protect from light. Reconstituted Sol: Room temperature if used within 60 min of reconstitution, or 2-8°C (36-46°F) if used within 4 hrs of reconstitution. Protect from light.

ILEVRO — nepafenac

RX

Class: NSAID

ADULT DOSAGE

Ocular Pain and Inflammation

1 drop to the affected eye qd, beginning 1 day prior to cataract surgery, continued on the day of surgery, and through the first 2 weeks of postoperative period

Administer additional drop 30-120 min prior to surgery

PEDIATRIC DOSAGE

Ocular Pain and Inflammation

≥10 Years:

1 drop to the affected eye qd, beginning 1 day prior to cataract surgery, continued on the day of surgery, and through the first 2 weeks of postoperative period

Administer additional drop 30-120 min prior to surgery

DOSING CONSIDERATIONS

Concomitant Medications

Space dosing ≥5 min apart w/ other topical ophthalmic medications

ADMINISTRATION

Ocular route

Shake well before use.

HOW SUPPLIED

Sus: 0.3% [1.7mL, 3mL]

CONTRAINDICATIONS

Previously demonstrated hypersensitivity to any of the ingredients in the formula or to other NSAIDs.

WARNINGS/PRECAUTIONS

Potential for increased bleeding time due to interference w/ thrombocyte aggregation. Increased bleeding of ocular tissues (eg, hyphemas) reported in conjunction w/ ocular surgery; caution w/ known bleeding tendencies. May slow or delay healing, or result in keratitis. Continued use may result in sight threatening epithelial breakdown, corneal thinning/erosion/ulceration/perforation; d/c if evidence of corneal epithelial breakdown occurs and monitor for corneal health. Caution w/ complicated ocular surgeries, corneal denervation, corneal epithelial defects, diabetes mellitus (DM), ocular surface diseases (eg, dry eye syndrome), rheumatoid arthritis (RA), or repeat ocular surgeries w/in a short period of time. Use >1 day prior to surgery or beyond 14 days post-surgery may increase risk and severity of corneal adverse events. Avoid use w/ contact lenses and during late pregnancy.

ADVERSE REACTIONS

Capsular opacity, decreased visual acuity, foreign body sensation, IOP, sticky sensation, conjunctival edema, corneal edema, dry eye, lid margin crusting, ocular discomfort, ocular hyperemia/pain/pruritus, photophobia, tearing, vitreous detachment.

DRUG INTERACTIONS

May increase potential for healing problems w/ topical steroids. Caution w/ agents that may prolong bleeding time.

PATIENT CONSIDERATIONS

I

Assessment: Assess for previous hypersensitivity to the drug, bleeding tendencies, complicated or repeated ocular surgeries, corneal denervation, corneal epithelial defects, DM, ocular surface diseases, RA, contact lens use, pregnancy/nursing status, and possible drug interactions.

Monitoring: Monitor for hypersensitivity reactions, wound healing problems, keratitis, increased bleeding time, bleeding of ocular tissues in conjunction w/ ocular surgery, epithelial breakdown, corneal thinning/erosion/ulceration/perforation, and other adverse reactions.

Counseling: Inform of possibility that slow or delayed healing may occur. Instruct to avoid allowing the tip of the container to contact the eye or surrounding structures. Advise that use of the same bottle for both eyes is not recommended. Instruct not to use while wearing contact lens. Advise to notify physician if an intercurrent ocular condition (eg, trauma or infection) develops or if undergoing ocular surgery.

STORAGE: 2-25°C (36-77°F). Protect from light.

IMDUR – isosorbide mononitrate

RX

Class: Nitrate vasodilator

ADULT DOSAGE

Angina Pectoris

Prevention:

Initial: 30mg or 60mg qam

Titrate: Increase to 120mg qam after several days; rarely, 240mg qam may be required

PEDIATRIC DOSAGE

Pediatric use may not have been established

DOSING CONSIDERATIONS

Elderly

Start at lower end of dosing range

ADMINISTRATION

Oral route

Take qam on arising

Swallow tab whole w/ a half-glassful of fluid; do not crush or chew

Do not break 30mg tab

HOW SUPPLIED

Tab, Extended-Release: 30mg*, 60mg*, 120mg *scored

CONTRAINDICATIONS

Hypersensitivity or idiosyncratic reactions to other nitrates or nitrites.

WARNINGS/PRECAUTIONS

Not useful in aborting acute anginal episode. Not recommended for use in patients w/ acute MI or congestive heart failure; perform careful clinical or hemodynamic monitoring if used in these conditions. Severe hypotension, particularly w/ upright posture, may occur; caution in volume depleted, hypotensive, or elderly patients. Nitrate-induced hypotension may be accompanied by paradoxical bradycardia and increased angina pectoris. May aggravate angina caused by hypertrophic cardiomyopathy. May develop tolerance. Chest pain, acute MI, and sudden death reported during temporary withdrawal.

ADVERSE REACTIONS
Headache, dizziness, dry mouth, asthenia, cardiac failure, abdominal pain, earache, arrhythmia, hyperuricemia, arthralgia, purpura, anxiety, hypochromic anemia, atrophic vaginitis, bacterial infection.

DRUG INTERACTIONS
Sildenafil amplifies vasodilatory effects that can result in severe hypotension. Additive vasodilating effects w/ other vasodilators (eg, alcohol). Marked symptomatic orthostatic hypotension reported w/ calcium channel blockers; dose adjustments of either class of agents may be necessary.

PATIENT CONSIDERATIONS

Assessment: Assess for drug hypersensitivity, hypotension, volume depletion, angina caused by hypertrophic cardiomyopathy, pregnancy/nursing status, possible drug interactions, and any other conditions where treatment is cautioned or contraindicated.

Monitoring: Monitor for hypotension w/ paradoxical bradycardia and increased angina pectoris, tachycardia, aggravation of angina caused by hypertrophic cardiomyopathy, tolerance, manifestations of true physical dependence (eg, chest pain, acute MI), and other adverse reactions.

Counseling: Inform about the risks and benefits of therapy. Counsel to carefully follow the prescribed schedule of dosing. Advise that daily headaches may accompany treatment and instruct to avoid altering schedule of treatment as the headaches are a marker of the activity of the medication and loss of headache may be associated w/ loss of antianginal efficacy. Inform that treatment may be associated w/ lightheadedness on standing, especially just after rising from a recumbent/seated position and may be more frequent w/ alcohol consumption.

STORAGE: 20-25°C (68-77°F).

I

IMITREX – sumatriptan

RX

Class: 5-$HT_{1B/1D}$ agonist (triptans)

ADULT DOSAGE

Cluster Headache

Inj:
Max Single Dose: 6mg SQ
Max Dose/24 Hrs: Two 6mg inj separated by at least 1 hr; consider a 2nd dose only if some response to 1st inj was observed

Migraine

W/ or w/o Aura:
May use lower doses (1-5mg) if side effects are dose limiting

Inj:
Max Single Dose: 6mg SQ
Max Dose/24 hrs: Two 6mg inj separated by at least 1 hr; consider a 2nd dose only if some response to 1st inj was observed

Spray:
5mg, 10mg, or 20mg
Additional Dose: May administer 1 additional dose at least 2 hrs after 1st dose if migraine has not resolved or returns after transient improvement
Max: 40mg/24 hrs
The 5mg and 20mg doses are given as a single spray in 1 nostril; 10mg dose may be achieved by administering a single 5mg dose in each nostril

Tab:
25mg, 50mg, or 100mg
Additional Dose: May administer a 2nd dose at least 2 hrs after 1st dose if migraine has not resolved or returns after transient improvement
Use After Inj: If migraine returns after initial treatment w/ inj, may give additional single tab (up to 100mg/day), w/ an interval of at least 2 hrs between tab doses
Max: 200mg/24 hrs

PEDIATRIC DOSAGE
Pediatric use may not have been established

DOSING CONSIDERATIONS

Hepatic Impairment

Mild to Moderate:

Max Tab Single Dose: 50mg

Elderly

Start at lower end of dosing range

ADMINISTRATION

Oral/SQ/Nasal route

SQ

Use the 6mg single dose vial for patients receiving doses other than 4mg or 6mg; do not use autoinjector.

Avoid IM or intravascular delivery.

HOW SUPPLIED

Inj: 4mg, 6mg [prefilled syringe], 6mg/0.5mL [vial]; **Spray:** 5mg, 20mg [6^s]; **Tab:** 25mg, 50mg, 100mg

CONTRAINDICATIONS

Ischemic coronary artery disease (CAD) (eg, angina pectoris, history of MI, documented silent ischemia), coronary artery vasospasm (eg, Prinzmetal's angina), Wolff-Parkinson-White syndrome or arrhythmias associated w/ other cardiac accessory conduction pathway disorders, history of stroke or transient ischemic attack, history of hemiplegic/basilar migraine, peripheral vascular disease, ischemic bowel disease, uncontrolled HTN, hypersensitivity to sumatriptan, and severe hepatic impairment. Recent use (w/in 24 hrs) of another $5\text{-}HT_1$ agonist, or of an ergotamine-containing or ergot-type medication (eg, dihydroergotamine, methysergide). Concurrent administration or recent use (w/in 2 weeks) of an MAO-A inhibitor.

WARNINGS/PRECAUTIONS

Use only where a clear diagnosis of migraine headache or (Inj) cluster headache has been established. Reconsider diagnosis of migraine or (Inj) cluster headache before treating any subsequent attacks if patient does not respond to the 1st dose of therapy. Serious cardiac adverse reactions (eg, acute MI) reported. May cause coronary artery vasospasm. Perform cardiovascular (CV) evaluation in triptan-naive patients w/ multiple CV risk factors (eg, increased age, diabetes, HTN, smoking, obesity, strong family history of CAD) prior to therapy; if negative, consider administering 1st dose under medical supervision and perform an ECG immediately following administration. Consider periodic CV evaluation in intermittent long-term users w/ multiple CV risk factors. Sensations of tightness, pain, pressure, and heaviness in the precordium, throat, neck, and jaw, usually noncardiac in origin, reported; perform cardiac evaluation if at high cardiac risk. Life-threatening cardiac rhythm disturbances (eg, ventricular tachycardia, ventricular fibrillation leading to death) reported; d/c if these occur. Cerebral/subarachnoid hemorrhage and stroke reported; d/c therapy if a cerebrovascular event occurs. Patients w/ migraine may be at increased risk of certain cerebrovascular events. Exclude other potentially serious neurological conditions prior to therapy in patients not previously diagnosed w/ migraine or (Inj) cluster headache or in patients who present w/ atypical symptoms. May cause noncoronary vasospastic reactions (eg, peripheral vascular ischemia, GI vascular ischemia/infarction, splenic infarction, Raynaud's syndrome); rule out therapy-related vasospastic reactions before additional therapy is given. May cause transient/permanent blindness and significant partial vision loss. Overuse of acute migraine drugs may lead to exacerbation of headache; detoxification, including drug withdrawal, and treatment of withdrawal symptoms may be necessary. Serotonin syndrome may occur; d/c if suspected. Significant elevation in BP, including hypertensive crisis w/ acute impairment of organ systems, reported. Anaphylactic/anaphylactoid reactions may occur. Seizures reported; caution w/ history of epilepsy or conditions associated w/ a lowered seizure threshold. **Spray/Tab:** Safety of treating >4 headaches/30 days not known. **Spray:** Local irritative symptoms reported.

ADVERSE REACTIONS

Inj: Tingling, warm/hot/burning/pressure sensation, feeling of heaviness, tightness, numbness, flushing, chest/throat discomfort, inj-site reaction, weakness, neck pain/stiffness, dizziness/vertigo, drowsiness/sedation.

Spray: Disorder/discomfort of nasal cavity/sinuses, N/V, bad/unusual taste.

Tab: Paresthesia, warm/cold sensation, chest/neck/throat/jaw pain and other pressure sensations, malaise/fatigue.

DRUG INTERACTIONS

See Contraindications. Serotonin syndrome reported w/ SSRIs, SNRIs, TCAs, or MAOIs.

PATIENT CONSIDERATIONS

Assessment: Confirm diagnosis of migraine or (Inj) cluster headache and exclude other potentially serious neurologic conditions and noncoronary vasospastic reactions prior to therapy. Assess for CV disease, HTN, hemiplegic/basilar migraine, hypersensitivity to drug, and any other conditions where treatment is cautioned or contraindicated. Assess hepatic function, pregnancy/nursing status, and for possible drug interactions. Perform CV evaluation in triptan-naive patients w/ multiple CV risk factors.

Monitoring: Monitor for signs/symptoms of cardiac events, cerebrovascular events, peripheral vascular ischemia, GI vascular ischemia/infarction, serotonin syndrome, hypersensitivity reactions, BP, and other adverse reactions. Perform periodic CV evaluation in intermittent long-term users w/ risk factors for CAD.

Counseling: Inform that therapy may cause CV side effects and anaphylactic/anaphylactoid reactions. Instruct to seek medical attention if such signs/symptoms occur. Inform that use of acute migraine drugs for ≥10 days/month may lead to an exacerbation of headache; encourage to record headache frequency and drug use (eg, by keeping a headache diary). Inform about the risk of serotonin syndrome. Inform that drug may cause somnolence and dizziness; instruct to evaluate ability to perform complex tasks after administration of drug. Inform that medication should not be used during pregnancy unless the potential benefit justifies the potential risk to the fetus; instruct to notify physician if breastfeeding or planning to breastfeed. **Inj:** Instruct to read instructions prior to use and advise on proper use, storage, and disposal of inj. Advise to avoid IM or intravascular delivery, and to use inj sites w/ adequate skin and SQ thickness to accommodate length of needle. **Spray:** Inform that local irritation of the nose and throat may occur and that symptoms will generally resolve in <2 hrs. Instruct on proper use of spray and caution to avoid spraying in eyes.

STORAGE: 2-30°C (36-86°F). **Spray/Inj:** Protect from light.

IMLYGIC – talimogene laherparepvec

RX

Class: Oncolytic viral therapy

ADULT DOSAGE

Melanoma

Local treatment of unresectable cutaneous, subcutaneous, and nodal lesions in patients w/ melanoma recurrent after initial surgery

The total inj volume for each treatment visit should not exceed 4mL for all injected lesions combined

Initial Treatment:
Up to 4mL at a concentration of 10^6 (1 million) plaque-forming units (PFU)/mL

Second Treatment (3 Weeks After Initial Treatment):
Up to 4mL at a concentration of 10^8 (100 million) PFU/mL

All Subsequent Treatments Including Reinitiation (2 Weeks After Previous Treatment):
Up to 4mL at a concentration of 10^8 (100 million) PFU/mL

Continue treatment for at least 6 months unless other treatment is required or until there are no injectable lesions to treat

Reinitiate treatment if new unresectable cutaneous, subcutaneous, or nodal lesions appear after a complete response

PEDIATRIC DOSAGE

Pediatric use may not have been established

ADMINISTRATION

Intralesional route

Administer by inj into cutaneous, subcutaneous, and/or nodal lesions that are visible, palpable, or detectable by ultrasound guidance.

Prioritization of Lesions to be Injected

Initial Treatment:
-Inject largest lesion(s) first.
-Prioritize inj of remaining lesion(s) based on lesion size until max inj volume is reached or until all injectable lesion(s) have been treated.

Second and All Subsequent Treatments:
-Inject any new lesion(s) (lesions that have developed since initial or previous treatment) first.
-Prioritize inj of remaining lesion(s) based on lesion size until max inj volume is reached or until all injectable lesion(s) have been treated.

Inj Volume Determination (Per Lesion)
>5cm Lesion: Up to 4mL inj
>2.5-5cm Lesion: Up to 2mL inj
>1.5-2.5cm Lesion: Up to 1mL inj
>0.5-1.5cm Lesion: Up to 0.5mL inj
≤0.5cm Lesion: Up to 0.1mL inj
When lesions are clustered together, inject them as a single lesion according to above.

Preparation and Handling
Healthcare providers who are immunocompromised or pregnant should not prepare or administer talimogene laherparepvec and should not come into direct contact w/ the inj sites, dressings, or body fluids of treated patients.
Avoid accidental exposure and follow universal biohazard precautions for preparation, administration, and handling.

1. Determine the total volume required for inj, up to 4mL.
2. Thaw frozen vials at room temperature (20-25°C [68-77°F]) until talimogene laherparepvec is liquid (approx 30 min). Do not expose the vial to higher temperatures. Keep the vial in original carton during thawing.
3. Swirl gently. Do not shake.
4. After thawing, administer immediately or store in original vial and carton, protected from light in a refrigerator (2-8°C [36-46°F]) for no longer than the following:

10^6 (1 million) PFU/mL: 12 hrs
10^8 (100 million) PFU/mL: 48 hrs
NOTE: Do not refreeze after thawing. Discard any vial left in the refrigerator longer than the specified times.

5. Prepare sterile syringes and needles. A detachable needle of 18-26G may be used for withdrawal and a detachable needle of 22-26G may be used for inj. Small unit syringes (eg, 0.5mL insulin syringes) are recommended for better inj control.
6. Using aseptic technique, remove the vial cap and withdraw the product from the vial into the syringe(s), noting the total volume. Avoid generating aerosols when loading syringes w/ product, and use a biologic safety cabinet if available.

Administration
1. Treat the inj site w/ a topical or local anesthetic agent, if necessary. Do not inject anesthetic agent directly into the lesion. Inject anesthetic agent around the periphery of the lesion.
2. Using a single insertion point, inject talimogene laherparepvec along multiple tracks as far as the radial reach of the needle allows w/in the lesion to achieve even and complete dispersion. Multiple insertion points may be used if a lesion is larger than the radial reach of the needle.
3. Inject talimogene laherparepvec evenly and completely w/in the lesion by pulling the needle back w/o exiting the lesion. Redirect the needle as many times as necessary while injecting the remainder of the dose. Continue until the full dose is evenly and completely dispersed.
4. When removing the needle, withdraw it from the lesion slowly to avoid leakage of talimogene laherparepvec at the insertion point.
5. Repeat steps 1-4 for other lesions to be injected.
6. Use a new needle any time the needle is completely removed from a lesion and each time a different lesion is injected.

Post-Inj
1. Apply pressure to the inj site(s) w/ sterile gauze for at least 30 sec.
2. Swab the inj site(s) and surrounding area w/ alcohol.
3. Change gloves and cover the injected lesion(s) w/ an absorbent pad and dry occlusive dressing.
4. Wipe the exterior of occlusive dressing w/ alcohol.
5. Advise patients to:

-Keep the inj site(s) covered for at least the 1st week after each treatment visit or longer if the inj site is weeping or oozing.
-Replace the dressing if it falls off.

HOW SUPPLIED
Inj: 10^6 (1 million) PFU/mL, 10^8 (100 million) PFU/mL [1mL]

CONTRAINDICATIONS
Immunocompromised patients, including those w/ a history of primary or acquired immunodeficient states, leukemia, lymphoma, AIDS or other clinical manifestations of infection w/ HIV, and those on immunosuppressive therapy. Pregnant patients.

WARNINGS/PRECAUTIONS
Accidental exposure may lead to transmission of talimogene laherparepvec and herpetic infection. Healthcare providers, close contacts (household members, caregivers, sex partners, or persons sharing the same bed), pregnant women, and newborns should avoid direct contact w/ injected lesions, dressings, or body fluids of treated patients. Caregivers should wear protective gloves when assisting patients in applying or changing occlusive dressings and observe safety precautions for disposal of used dressings, gloves, and cleaning materials. In the event of an accidental exposure, exposed individuals should clean the affected area thoroughly w/ soap and water and/

or a disinfectant. If signs or symptoms of herpetic infection develop, the exposed individuals should contact their healthcare provider for appropriate treatment. Patients should avoid touching or scratching inj sites or their occlusive dressings. Patients who develop suspicious herpes-like lesions should follow standard hygienic practices to prevent viral transmission. Patients or close contacts w/ suspected herpetic infections should also contact their healthcare provider to evaluate the lesions. Necrosis or ulceration of tumor tissue may occur; careful wound care and infection precautions are recommended, particularly if tissue necrosis results in open wounds. Impaired healing at the inj site reported. May increase the risk of impaired healing in patients w/ underlying risk factors (eg, previous radiation at the inj site or lesions in poorly vascularized areas); consider risks and benefits of continuing treatment if there is persistent infection or delayed healing of the inj site(s). Immune-mediated events, including glomerulonephritis, vasculitis, pneumonitis, worsening psoriasis, and vitiligo, reported; consider risks and benefits before initiating treatment in patients who have underlying autoimmune disease or before continuing treatment in patients who develop immune-mediated events. Plasmacytoma reported in proximity to the inj site after administration in a patient w/ smoldering multiple myeloma. Consider risks and benefits of treatment in patients w/ multiple myeloma or in whom plasmacytoma develops during treatment.

ADVERSE REACTIONS

Fatigue, chills, pyrexia, nausea, influenza-like illness, inj-site pain.

DRUG INTERACTIONS

Acyclovir or other antiherpetic viral agents may interfere w/ effectiveness; consider the risks and benefits before administering antiviral agents to manage herpetic infection.

PATIENT CONSIDERATIONS

Assessment: Assess for history of primary or acquired immunodeficient states, leukemia, lymphoma, AIDS or other clinical manifestations of infection w/ HIV, immunosuppressive therapy, underlying autoimmune disease, multiple myeloma, pregnancy/nursing status, and possible drug interactions.

Monitoring: Monitor for accidental exposure, herpetic infection, inj-site complications, immune-mediated events, and plasmacytoma at the inj site.

Counseling: Advise to avoid direct contact w/ inj sites, dressings, or body fluids; wear gloves when changing dressing; and avoid touching or scratching inj sites. Advise to keep inj sites covered for at least the first week after each treatment visit or longer if the inj site is weeping or oozing. Advise to dispose of used dressings and cleaning materials in household waste in a sealed plastic bag. Instruct females of childbearing potential to use an effective method of contraception during treatment. Advise that close contacts who are pregnant or immunocompromised should not change dressings or clean inj sites. In case of accidental exposure, instruct to clean the exposed area w/ soap and water and/or a disinfectant.

STORAGE: Store at -90 to -70°C (-130 to -94°F). Protect from light and store in the carton until use.

IMPAVIDO – miltefosine

RX

Class: Antileishmanial agent

May cause fetal harm; do not administer to pregnant women. Obtain a serum or urine pregnancy test in females of reproductive potential prior to prescribing therapy; advise to use effective contraception during therapy and for 5 months after therapy.

ADULT DOSAGE

Leishmaniasis

Treatment of visceral, cutaneous, and mucosal leishmaniasis caused by susceptible *Leishmania* species

30-44kg:
50mg bid w/ food (breakfast and dinner)
≥45kg:
50mg tid w/ food (breakfast, lunch, and dinner)

Treat for 28 consecutive days

PEDIATRIC DOSAGE

Leishmaniasis

Treatment of visceral, cutaneous, and mucosal leishmaniasis caused by susceptible *Leishmania* species

≥12 Years:
30-44kg:
50mg bid w/ food (breakfast and dinner)
≥45kg:
50mg tid w/ food (breakfast, lunch, and dinner)

Treat for 28 consecutive days

ADMINISTRATION

Oral route

Take w/ food to ameliorate GI adverse reactions.
Swallow caps whole; do not chew or break.

HOW SUPPLIED

Cap: 50mg

CONTRAINDICATIONS
Pregnancy, Sjogren-Larsson syndrome, hypersensitivity to miltefosine or any of its excipients.

WARNINGS/PRECAUTIONS
Leishmania species studied in clinical trials were based on epidemiologic data. There may be geographic variation in clinical response of the same *Leishmania* species to therapy. May cause reproductive effects (eg, impaired fertility). Scrotal pain and decreased/absent ejaculation during therapy reported. Elevations of SrCr reported. Elevations in liver transaminases (ALT, AST) and bilirubin reported in the treatment of visceral leishmaniasis. Vomiting and/or diarrhea commonly occur during administration and may result in volume depletion; encourage fluid intake. Vomiting and/or diarrhea occurring during therapy may affect absorption of oral contraceptives, and therefore compromise their efficacy; additional nonhormonal or alternative method(s) of effective contraception should be used if vomiting and/or diarrhea occur. Thrombocytopenia reported in patients treated for visceral leishmaniasis. Stevens-Johnson syndrome (SJS) reported; d/c if an exfoliative or bullous rash is noted. Avoid breastfeeding for 5 months after therapy.

ADVERSE REACTIONS
N/V, decreased appetite, diarrhea, asthenia, motion sickness, headache, dizziness, abdominal pain, lymphangitis, pruritus, malaise, pyrexia, somnolence.

PATIENT CONSIDERATIONS

Assessment: Assess for drug hypersensitivity, Sjogren-Larsson syndrome, pregnancy/nursing status, and possible drug interactions. Obtain a serum or urine pregnancy test in females of reproductive potential.

Monitoring: Monitor for reproductive effects, vomiting/diarrhea, volume depletion, SJS, and other adverse reactions. Monitor renal function weekly during therapy and for 4 weeks after end of therapy. Monitor liver transaminases and bilirubin. Monitor platelet count during therapy for visceral leishmaniasis.

Counseling: Instruct to complete the full course of therapy. Inform that abdominal pain, N/V, and diarrhea are common side effects of therapy and instruct to inform physician if these GI side effects are severe or persistent. Instruct to consume sufficient fluids to avoid dehydration and, consequently, the risk of kidney injury. Advise women of reproductive potential to use effective contraception during therapy and for 5 months after therapy ends. Advise women who use oral contraceptives to use additional nonhormonal or alternative method(s) of effective contraception during therapy if vomiting and/or diarrhea occurs. Advise nursing mothers not to breastfeed during therapy and for 5 months after therapy is completed. Inform that drug may cause reproductive effects (eg, impaired fertility).

STORAGE: 20-25°C (68-77°F); excursions permitted to 15-30°C (59-86°F). Protect from light.

IMURAN – azathioprine

RX

Class: Purine antagonist antimetabolite

Increased risk of malignancy w/ chronic immunosuppression. Malignancy (eg, post-transplant lymphoma, hepatosplenic T-cell lymphoma) reported in patients w/ inflammatory bowel disease. Physician should be familiar w/ this risk as well as mutagenic potential to both men and women and possible hematologic toxicities.

OTHER BRAND NAMES
Azasan

ADULT DOSAGE

Renal Transplant

Adjunct Therapy for Prevention of Rejection in Renal Homotransplantation:
Initial: 3-5mg/kg/day, beginning at the time of transplant
Usually given as a single daily dose on the day of, and in a minority of cases 1-3 days before, transplantation
Maint: 1-3mg/kg/day
Discontinuation may be necessary for severe hematologic or other toxicity, even if rejection of the homograft may be a consequence of drug withdrawal

Rheumatoid Arthritis

Treatment of Active Rheumatoid Arthritis (RA) to Reduce Signs/Symptoms:
Initial: 1mg/kg/day (50-100mg) given qd or bid

PEDIATRIC DOSAGE
Pediatric use may not have been established

Titrate: May increase dose by 0.5mg/kg/day increments beginning at 6-8 weeks and thereafter by steps at 4-week intervals
Max: 2.5mg/kg/day

May be considered refractory if no improvement after 12 weeks

Maint Therapy:
Use lowest effective dose; decrease by 0.5mg/kg/day or 25mg/day every 4 weeks to lowest effective dose while other therapy is kept constant

During treatment, may continue aspirin, NSAIDs, and/or low dose glucocorticoids

DOSING CONSIDERATIONS

Renal Impairment

Oliguric patients may have delayed clearance; give lower doses

ADMINISTRATION

Oral route

HOW SUPPLIED

Tab: 50mg*, (Azasan) 75mg*, 100mg* *scored

CONTRAINDICATIONS

Hypersensitivity to the drug. **RA:** Pregnancy, patients previously treated w/ alkylating agents (eg, cyclophosphamide, chlorambucil, melphalan).

WARNINGS/PRECAUTIONS

Renal transplant patients are known to have an increased risk of malignancy, predominantly skin cancer and reticulum cell or lymphomatous tumors. Risk of post-transplant lymphomas may be increased w/ aggressive immunosuppressive treatment; maintain therapy at the lowest effective levels. Acute myelogenous leukemia as well as solid tumors reported in patients w/ RA. Severe leukopenia, thrombocytopenia, anemias (eg, macrocytic anemia, pancytopenia), and severe bone marrow suppression may occur. Hematologic toxicities are dose-related and may be more severe in renal transplant patients whose homograft is undergoing rejection. Monitor CBCs, including platelet counts, weekly during the 1st month, twice monthly for the 2nd and 3rd months of therapy, then monthly or more frequently if dose/therapy changes are necessary. Delayed hematologic suppression may occur. Prompt dose reduction or temporary drug withdrawal may be necessary if there is a rapid fall in or persistently low leukocyte count, or other evidence of bone marrow depression. Increased risk for bacterial, viral, fungal, protozoal, and opportunistic infections, including reactivation of latent infections that may lead to serious, including fatal, outcomes. JC virus-associated infection resulting in progressive multifocal leukoencephalopathy (PML) reported; consider reducing the amount of immunosuppression in patients who develop PML. May cause fetal harm. GI hypersensitivity reaction characterized by severe N/V reported. Myelotoxicity risk may be increased in patients w/ intermediate thiopurine S-methyl transferase (TPMT) activity. Increased risk of severe, life-threatening myelotoxicity in patients w/ low or absent TPMT activity; consider alternative therapies. Caution in patients having one non-functional allele who are at risk for reduced TPMT activity; dose reduction is recommended in patients w/ reduced TPMT activity. TPMT testing cannot be a substitute for CBC monitoring. Consider early drug discontinuation in patients w/ abnormal CBC results that do not respond to dose reduction.

ADVERSE REACTIONS

Hematologic toxicities, infections, N/V.

DRUG INTERACTIONS

See Contraindications. Combined use w/ disease-modifying antirheumatic drugs cannot be recommended. Caution w/ concomitant aminosalicylate derivatives (eg, sulfasalazine, mesalazine, olsalazine); may inhibit TPMT enzyme. Allopurinol inhibits one of the inactivation pathways; reduce azathioprine dose to approx 1/3-1/4 of the usual dose and consider further dose reduction or alternative therapies for patients w/ low or absent TPMT activity. Drugs that may affect leukocyte production (eg, co-trimoxazole) may lead to exaggerated leukopenia, especially in renal transplant recipients. ACE inhibitors may induce anemia and severe leukopenia. May inhibit anticoagulant effect of warfarin. Use of ribavirin for hepatitis C has been reported to induce severe pancytopenia and may increase the risk of azathioprine-related myelotoxicity.

PATIENT CONSIDERATIONS

Assessment: Assess for drug hypersensitivity, renal/hepatic dysfunction, previous treatment of RA w/ alkylating agents, pregnancy/nursing status, and for possible drug interactions. Conduct TPMT genotyping/phenotyping to identify absent or reduced TPMT activity.

Monitoring: Monitor for signs/symptoms of cytopenias, malignancies, infections, GI hypersensitivity reactions, and other adverse reactions. Monitor CBCs, including platelet counts, weekly during the 1st month, twice monthly for the 2nd and 3rd months of therapy, then monthly or more frequently if dose/therapy changes are necessary. Periodically monitor serum transaminases, alkaline phosphatase, and bilirubin levels. Consider TPMT testing in patients w/ abnormal CBC results unresponsive to dose reduction.

Counseling: Inform about necessity of periodic blood counts while on therapy and risks of malignancy and infection. Instruct to report to physician any unusual bleeding/bruising or signs/symptoms of infections. Educate about proper dosage instructions, especially w/ impaired renal function or concomitant use w/ allopurinol. Inform of the potential risks during pregnancy and nursing; advise to notify physician if pregnant or nursing. Instruct patients w/ increased risk for skin cancer to limit exposure to sunlight and UV light (eg, wearing protective clothing, using a sunscreen).

STORAGE: 20-25°C (68-77°F). Store in a dry place and protect from light.

INCRUSE ELLIPTA – umeclidinium RX

Class: Anticholinergic

ADULT DOSAGE

Chronic Obstructive Pulmonary Disease

Long-Term Maint Treatment of Airflow Obstruction:
1 inh qd at the same time every day; do not use >1 time q24h

PEDIATRIC DOSAGE

Pediatric use may not have been established

DOSING CONSIDERATIONS

Hepatic Impairment

Severe: Not studied

ADMINISTRATION

Oral inh route

HOW SUPPLIED

Powder, Inh: 62.5mcg/blister [7, 30 blisters]

CONTRAINDICATIONS

Severe hypersensitivity to milk proteins, hypersensitivity to umeclidinium or any of the excipients.

WARNINGS/PRECAUTIONS

Do not initiate during rapidly deteriorating or potentially life-threatening episodes of COPD. Not for relief of acute symptoms. May produce paradoxical bronchospasm; treat immediately w/ an inhaled, short-acting bronchodilator; d/c umeclidinium and institute alternative therapy. Hypersensitivity reactions may occur. Caution w/ narrow-angle glaucoma and urinary retention. Monitor for signs and symptoms of acute narrow-angle glaucoma and urinary retention (especially in those w/ prostatic hyperplasia or bladder neck obstruction).

ADVERSE REACTIONS

Nasopharyngitis, URTI, cough.

DRUG INTERACTIONS

Avoid w/ other anticholinergic-containing drugs; may increase anticholinergic adverse effects.

PATIENT CONSIDERATIONS

Assessment: Assess for hypersensitivity to drug or to milk proteins, COPD status, narrow-angle glaucoma, urinary retention, prostatic hyperplasia, bladder neck obstruction, pregnancy/nursing status, and possible drug interactions.

Monitoring: Monitor for deteriorating disease, paradoxical bronchospasm, hypersensitivity reactions, narrow-angle glaucoma, urinary retention, and other adverse reactions.

Counseling: Inform that drug is not meant to relieve acute symptoms of COPD. Advise that acute symptoms should be treated w/ a rescue inhaler (eg, albuterol). Instruct to seek medical attention immediately if experiencing worsening of symptoms, decreased effectiveness of the rescue inhaler, or a need for more inhalations than usual of the rescue inhaler. Advise not to d/c therapy w/o physician guidance. Instruct to d/c therapy if paradoxical bronchospasm occurs. Inform about risk of worsening narrow-angle glaucoma and urinary retention; instruct to consult physician immediately if any signs/symptoms develop. Advise to contact physician if pregnancy occurs while on therapy. Inform that the inhaler is not reusable and advise not to take the inhaler apart.

STORAGE: 20-25°C (68-77°F); excursions permitted from 15-30°C (59-86°F). Store in a dry place away from direct heat or sunlight. Store inside the unopened moisture-protective foil tray and only remove from the tray immediately before initial use. Discard 6 weeks after opening the foil tray or when the counter reads "0" (after all blisters have been used), whichever comes 1st.

INDERAL LA – propranolol hydrochloride

RX

Class: Nonselective beta blocker

ADULT DOSAGE

Hypertension

Initial: 80mg qd
Titrate: May increase to 120mg qd or higher until adequate BP control is achieved
Maint: 120-160mg qd; 640mg/day may be required

Angina Pectoris

To decrease angina frequency and increase exercise tolerance

Initial: 80mg qd
Titrate: Increase gradually at 3- to 7-day intervals until optimal response is obtained
Maint: 160mg qd
Max: 320mg qd

Reduce dose gradually over a period of a few weeks if therapy is to be discontinued

Migraine

For Prophylaxis:
Initial: 80mg qd; may increase gradually to achieve optimal response
Usual: 160-240mg qd

D/C gradually over a period of several weeks if a satisfactory response is not obtained w/in 4-6 weeks after reaching maximal dose

Hypertrophic Subaortic Stenosis

Usual: 80-160mg qd

PEDIATRIC DOSAGE

Pediatric use may not have been established

DOSING CONSIDERATIONS

Elderly

Start at lower end of dosing range

ADMINISTRATION

Oral route

HOW SUPPLIED

Cap, Extended-Release: 60mg, 80mg, 120mg, 160mg

CONTRAINDICATIONS

Cardiogenic shock, sinus bradycardia and greater than 1st-degree block, bronchial asthma, known hypersensitivity to propranolol HCl.

WARNINGS/PRECAUTIONS

Exacerbation of angina and MI following abrupt discontinuation reported; when discontinuation is planned, reduce dose gradually over at least a few weeks. Reinstitute therapy if exacerbation of angina occurs upon interruption and take other measures for management of angina pectoris; follow same procedure in patients at risk of occult atherosclerotic heart disease who are given propranolol for other indications since coronary artery disease may be unrecognized. Hypersensitivity reactions (eg, anaphylactic/anaphylactoid reactions) and cutaneous reactions (eg, Stevens-Johnson syndrome, toxic epidermal necrolysis, exfoliative dermatitis) reported. May precipitate more severe failure in patients w/ CHF; avoid w/ overt CHF and caution in patients w/ history of heart failure (HF) who are well compensated and are receiving diuretics prn. Continued use in patients w/o history of HF may cause cardiac failure. Caution w/ bronchospastic lung disease; may provoke a bronchial asthmatic attack. Chronically administered therapy should not be routinely withdrawn prior to major surgery; however, may augment risks of general anesthesia and surgical procedures. May prevent the appearance of signs/symptoms of acute hypoglycemia, especially w/ labile insulin-dependent diabetics; may be more difficult to adjust insulin dose. Hypoglycemia reported. May mask certain clinical signs of hyperthyroidism; abrupt withdrawal may be followed by an exacerbation of symptoms of hyperthyroidism, including thyroid storm. Associated w/ severe bradycardia requiring treatment w/ a pacemaker in patients w/ Wolff-Parkinson-White (WPW) syndrome and tachycardia. Caution w/ hepatic/renal impairment. May reduce IOP. Patients w/ history of severe anaphylactic reaction to a variety of allergens may be more reactive to repeated accidental/diagnostic/therapeutic challenge; may be unresponsive to usual doses of epinephrine. Lab test interactions may occur (eg, changes to thyroid function tests). Not for treatment of hypertensive emergencies. Inderal LA should not be considered a simple mg-for-mg substitute for Inderal.

ADVERSE REACTIONS

Bradycardia, CHF, hypotension, lightheadedness, mental depression, N/V, agranulocytosis, bronchospasm, urticaria, alopecia.

DRUG INTERACTIONS

Caution w/ drugs that have an effect on CYP2D6, 1A2, or 2C19 metabolic pathways; may lead to clinically relevant drug interactions and changes on its efficacy and/or toxicity. Alcohol may increase levels. Propafenone and amiodarone may cause additive effects. Quinidine may increase levels and may cause postural hypotension. Reduced clearance of lidocaine and lidocaine toxicity reported following coadministration. Caution w/ drugs that slow atrioventricular (AV) nodal conduction (eg, digitalis, lidocaine, calcium channel blocker); increased risk of bradycardia w/ digitalis. Bradycardia, HF, and cardiovascular collapse reported w/ verapamil. Bradycardia, hypotension, high-degree heart block, and HF reported w/ diltiazem. ACE inhibitors may cause hypotension, particularly in the setting of acute MI. May antagonize effects of clonidine; administer cautiously to patients withdrawing from clonidine. May prolong 1st dose hypotension w/ prazosin. Postural hypotension reported w/ terazosin or doxazosin. May cause excessive reduction of resting sympathetic nervous activity w/ catecholamine-depleting drugs (eg, reserpine). May experience uncontrolled HTN w/ epinephrine. Effects can be reversed by β-receptor agonists (eg, dobutamine, isoproterenol). May reduce sensitivity to dobutamine stress echocardiography in patients undergoing evaluation for myocardial ischemia. Indomethacin may reduce efficacy and NSAIDs may blunt antihypertensive effects. May exacerbate hypotensive effects of MAOIs or TCAs. May depress myocardial contractility w/ methoxyflurane and trichloroethylene. May increase levels of warfarin; monitor PT. Hypotension and cardiac arrest reported w/ haloperidol. May lower T3 concentration w/ thyroxine.

PATIENT CONSIDERATIONS

Assessment: Assess for cardiogenic shock, sinus bradycardia, AV heart block, bronchial asthma, CHF, bronchospastic lung disease, hyperthyroidism, diabetes, WPW syndrome, tachycardia, hepatic/renal impairment, history of HF, risk for occult atherosclerotic heart disease, hypersensitivity to drug, pregnancy/nursing status, and possible drug interactions.

Monitoring: Monitor for signs/symptoms of cardiac failure, hypoglycemia, decreased IOP, hyperthyroidism, withdrawal symptoms, hypersensitivity reactions, and other adverse reactions. Monitor PT w/ warfarin.

Counseling: Inform of the risks/benefits of therapy. Instruct not to interrupt or d/c therapy w/o consulting physician. Inform that therapy may interfere w/ glaucoma screening test.

STORAGE: 20-25°C (68-77°F); excursions permitted to 15-30°C (59-86°F). Protect from light, moisture, freezing, and excessive heat.

INDOMETHACIN – indomethacin

RX

Class: NSAID

NSAIDs may cause an increased risk of serious cardiovascular (CV) thrombotic events, including MI and stroke; increased risk w/ duration of use. NSAIDs may cause an increased risk of serious GI adverse events, including bleeding, ulceration, and perforation of the stomach or intestines. Contraindicated in the setting of CABG surgery.

OTHER BRAND NAMES

Indocin

ADULT DOSAGE

Ankylosing Spondylitis

Moderate to Severe Active Stages:

Initial: 25mg (5mL) bid-tid

Titrate: May increase by 25mg (5mL) or 50mg (10mL) at weekly intervals

Max: 150-200mg (30-40mL)/day

May give a large portion (up to a max of

PEDIATRIC DOSAGE

General Dosing

Safety and effectiveness in patients ≤14 yrs of age has not been established and should not be prescribed unless toxicity or lack of efficacy associated w/ other drugs warrants the risk

100mg [20mL]) of the total daily dose hs in patients who have persistent night pain and/or morning stiffness

Rheumatoid Arthritis

Moderate to Severe Active Stages (Including Acute Flares of Chronic Disease):
Initial: 25mg (5mL) bid-tid
Titrate: May increase by 25mg (5mL) or 50mg (10mL) at weekly intervals
Max: 150-200mg (30-40mL)/day

May give a large portion (up to a max of 100mg [20mL]) of the total daily dose hs in patients who have persistent night pain and/or morning stiffness

Osteoarthritis

Moderate to Severe Active Stages:
Initial: 25mg (5mL) bid-tid
Titrate: May increase by 25mg (5mL) or 50mg (10mL) at weekly intervals
Max: 150-200mg (30-40mL)/day

May give a large portion (up to a max of 100mg [20mL]) of the total daily dose hs in patients who have persistent night pain and/or morning stiffness

Bursitis/Tendinitis

Acute Painful Shoulder:
Active Stages:
75-150mg (15-30mL)/day given in 3 or 4 divided doses; d/c after signs/symptoms of inflammation have been controlled for several days
Usual Duration: 7-14 days

Acute Gouty Arthritis

Active Stages:
50mg (10mL) tid until pain is tolerable, then reduce dose to complete cessation of therapy

≥2 Years:
Initial: 1-2mg/kg/day given in divided doses
Max: 3mg/kg/day or 150-200mg/day, whichever is less

DOSING CONSIDERATIONS

Adverse Reactions
Rheumatoid Arthritis:
Minor: Reduce dose rapidly to a tolerated dose and observe closely
Severe: D/C therapy; after acute phase of the disease is under control, reduce daily dose repeatedly until smallest effective dose or therapy is discontinued

ADMINISTRATION

Oral route

HOW SUPPLIED

Cap: 50mg; **Sus:** (Indocin) 25mg/5mL [237mL]

CONTRAINDICATIONS

Known hypersensitivity to indomethacin or the excipients; asthma, urticaria, or allergic-type reactions after taking aspirin or other NSAIDs; in the setting of CABG surgery.

WARNINGS/PRECAUTIONS

Use the lowest effective dose for the shortest duration possible. Increased CV thrombotic risk at higher doses reported. Avoid use in patients w/ a recent MI unless benefits outweigh the risks; if used, monitor for signs of cardiac ischemia. May lead to onset of new HTN or worsening of preexisting HTN. Avoid use in patients w/ severe heart failure (HF) unless benefits outweigh the risks; if used, monitor for signs of worsening HF. Fluid retention and edema reported. Intestinal ulceration associated w/ stenosis and obstruction; GI bleeding w/o obvious ulcer formation and perforation of preexisting sigmoid lesions; and increased abdominal pain in ulcerative colitis or development of ulcerative colitis and regional ileitis reported. Use extreme caution w/ prior history of ulcer disease/GI bleeding; increased risk of a GI bleed w/ prolonged NSAID therapy, older age, and poor general health status. D/C if serious GI adverse event occurs. Renal papillary necrosis and other renal injury reported after long-term use. Renal toxicity reported; increased risk w/ renal/hepatic impairment, HF, volume depletion, and elderly. Increases in serum K^+ levels, including hyperkalemia reported. Not recommended for use w/ advanced renal disease; if therapy must be initiated, monitor renal function. Anaphylactoid reactions may occur; avoid in patient w/ ASA triad. May cause serious skin adverse events (eg, exfoliative dermatitis, Stevens-Johnson syndrome, toxic epidermal necrolysis); d/c at the 1st appearance of skin rash or any other signs of hypersensitivity. Avoid in late pregnancy; may cause premature closure of ductus arteriosus. Corneal deposits and retinal disturbances reported w/ prolonged therapy; d/c if such changes are observed. Blurred vision may occur; perform eye exams at periodic intervals during prolonged therapy. May aggravate depression or other psychiatric disturbances, epilepsy, and parkinsonism; use w/ caution. D/C if severe CNS adverse reactions develop. May impair mental/physical abilities. Not a substitute for corticosteroids or to treat corticosteroid insufficiency. May cause elevations of LFTs; d/c if liver disease develops or systemic manifestations occur. Anemia may occur; w/ long-term use, monitor Hgb/Hct if signs or symptoms of anemia develop. May inhibit platelet aggregation and prolong bleeding time; monitor w/ coagulation disorders. Caution w/ preexisting asthma and avoid w/ ASA-sensitive asthma. Caution in elderly. Lab interactions may occur.

ADVERSE REACTIONS

Headache, dizziness, N/V, dyspepsia.

DRUG INTERACTIONS

May diminish antihypertensive effect of ACE inhibitors and angiotensin II antagonists; concomitant use may further deteriorate renal function. Avoid w/ ASA, salicylates, diflunisal, triamterene, and other NSAIDs. Blunting of the antihypertensive effects of β-blockers reported. May increase cyclosporine toxicity; use w/ caution and monitor renal function. May increase digoxin levels and prolong $T_{1/2}$ of digoxin; monitor serum digoxin levels. May reduce the diuretic, natriuretic, and antihypertensive effects of loop, K^+-sparing, and thiazide diuretics. Reduced basal plasma renin activity (PRA), as well as those elevations of PRA induced by furosemide reported. May decrease lithium clearance; monitor for toxicity. Caution w/ methotrexate (MTX); may enhance MTX toxicity. Caution w/ anticoagulants; increased risk of serious GI bleeding w/ warfarin. Probenecid increases levels. May increase risk of serious GI bleeding when used concomitantly w/ oral corticosteroids or anticoagulants, alcohol, or smoking.

PATIENT CONSIDERATIONS

Assessment: Confirm that use is not in the setting of CABG surgery. Assess for CV disorders, HTN, history of hypersensitivity reactions to ASA or other NSAIDs, history of ulcer disease or GI bleeding, coagulation disorders, renal/hepatic impairment, hypersensitivity to the drug, pregnancy/nursing status, possible drug interactions, or any other conditions where treatment is contraindicated or cautioned. Obtain baseline BP.

Monitoring: Monitor for signs/symptoms of CV thrombotic events, GI events, anaphylactoid/hypersensitivity/skin reactions, corneal deposits/retinal disturbances, CNS effects, aggravation of depression or other psychiatric disturbances, hematological effects, and other adverse reactions. Monitor BP, LFTs, renal function, CBC, and chemistry profiles.

Counseling: Inform of the benefits/risks of therapy. Instruct to seek medical advice if symptoms of CV events, GI ulceration/bleeding, skin/hypersensitivity reactions, CHF, hepatotoxicity, or anaphylactoid reactions occur. Advise to d/c drug immediately if any type of rash or signs/symptoms of hepatotoxicity occur. Instruct to avoid therapy in late pregnancy.

STORAGE: Cap: 20-25°C (68-77°F). Protect from light. **Sus:** <30°C (86°F); avoid >50°C (122°F). Protect from freezing.

INSPRA — eplerenone

RX

Class: Aldosterone blocker

ADULT DOSAGE

Congestive Heart Failure Post-Myocardial Infarction

Initial: 25mg qd
Titrate: Increase to 50mg qd, preferably w/in 4 weeks as tolerated
Dose Adjustment in CHF Post-MI Once Treatment Has Begun:
Serum K^+ <5.0mEq/L:
Increase from 25mg qod to 25mg qd
Increase from 25mg qd to 50mg qd
Serum K^+ 5.0-5.4mEq/L:
No adjustment
Serum K^+ 5.5-5.9mEq/L:
Decrease from 50mg qd to 25mg qd
Decrease from 25mg qd to 25mg qod
Decrease from 25mg qod to withhold

PEDIATRIC DOSAGE

Pediatric use may not have been established

Serum K$^+$ ≥6mEq/L:
Withhold and restart at 25mg qod when serum K$^+$ <5.5mEq/L

Hypertension

Initial: 50mg qd
Titrate: Increase to 50mg bid if BP response is inadequate
Max: 100mg/day

DOSING CONSIDERATIONS

Concomitant Medications

Hypertensive Patients Receiving Moderate CYP3A4 Inhibitors:
Initial: 25mg qd

ADMINISTRATION

Oral route

May be administered w/ or w/o food

HOW SUPPLIED

Tab: 25mg, 50mg

CONTRAINDICATIONS

All Patients: Serum K$^+$ >5.5mEq/L at initiation, CrCl ≤30mL/min, concomitant administration of strong CYP3A4 inhibitors (eg, ketoconazole, itraconazole, nefazodone, troleandomycin, clarithromycin, ritonavir, nelfinavir). Patients Treated for HTN: Type 2 diabetes w/ microalbuminuria, SrCr >2mg/dL (males) or >1.8mg/dL (females), CrCl <50mL/min, concomitant administration of K$^+$ supplements or K$^+$-sparing diuretics (eg, amiloride, spironolactone, triamterene).

WARNINGS/PRECAUTIONS

Minimize the risk of hyperkalemia w/ proper patient selection and monitoring. Caution in patients w/ CHF post-MI who have SrCr >2mg/dL (males) or >1.8mg/dL (females), or CrCl ≤50mL/min, or who are diabetic (especially those w/ proteinuria). Increased risk of hyperkalemia in patients w/ decreased renal function.

ADVERSE REACTIONS

Hyperkalemia, dizziness, increased SrCr/TGs.

DRUG INTERACTIONS

See Contraindications and Dosing Considerations. Monitor serum K$^+$ and SrCr in 3-7 days in patients who start taking a moderate CYP3A4 inhibitor. Increased risk of hyperkalemia w/ an ACE inhibitor and/or an ARB; closely monitor serum K$^+$ and renal function, especially in patients at risk for impaired renal function (eg, elderly). Monitor serum lithium levels frequently if coadministered w/ lithium. When used w/ NSAIDs, observe to determine whether the desired effect on BP is obtained and monitor for changes in serum K$^+$ levels.

PATIENT CONSIDERATIONS

Assessment: Assess for type 2 diabetes w/ microalbuminuria/proteinuria, pregnancy/nursing status, and possible drug interactions. Assess serum K$^+$ levels and renal function (eg, CrCl, SrCr).

Monitoring: Monitor for signs/symptoms of hyperkalemia and other adverse reactions. Monitor serum K$^+$ w/in the 1st week, at 1 month after start of treatment or dose adjustment, and periodically thereafter. Monitor BP and renal function.

Counseling: Advise not to use K$^+$ supplements or salt substitutes containing K$^+$ w/o consulting the prescribing physician. Instruct to contact physician if dizziness, diarrhea, vomiting, rapid or irregular heartbeat, lower extremity edema, or difficulty breathing occurs. Inform that periodic monitoring of BP and serum K$^+$ is important.

STORAGE: 25°C (77°F); excursions permitted to 15-30°C (59-86°F).

INTELENCE – etravirine

RX

Class: Non-nucleoside reverse transcriptase inhibitor (NNRTI)

ADULT DOSAGE

HIV-1 Infection

Combination w/ Other Antiretrovirals
Treatment-Experienced:
Evidence of Viral Replication and HIV-1 Strains Resistant to an NNRTI and Other Antiretrovirals:
200mg bid

PEDIATRIC DOSAGE

HIV-1 Infection

Combination w/ Other Antiretrovirals
Treatment-Experienced:
Evidence of Viral Replication and HIV-1 Strains Resistant to an NNRTI and Other Antiretrovirals:
6-<18 Years:

≥16-<20kg: 100mg bid
≥20-<25kg: 125mg bid
≥25-<30kg: 150mg bid
≥30kg: 200mg bid

ADMINISTRATION

Oral route

Take after a meal.
Swallow whole w/ liquid
May be dispersed in a glass of water if unable to swallow whole

Dispersion Instructions

- Place the tablet(s) in 5mL (1 tsp) of water, or at least enough liquid to cover the medication, stir well until the water looks milky
- If desired, add more water or alternatively orange juice or milk (Do not place the tablets in orange juice or milk w/out first adding water). The use of grapefruit juice or warm (>40°C) or carbonated beverages should be avoided
- Drink it immediately, rinse the glass several times w/ water, orange juice, or milk and completely swallow the rinse each time to takes the entire dose

HOW SUPPLIED

Tab: 25mg*, 100mg, 200mg *scored

WARNINGS/PRECAUTIONS

Severe, potentially life-threatening, and fatal skin reactions (eg, erythema multiforme, toxic epidermal necrolysis, Stevens-Johnson syndrome), and hypersensitivity reactions including drug rash with eosinophilia and systemic symptoms reported; d/c immediately if these occur and initiate appropriate therapy. Immune reconstitution syndrome, autoimmune disorders (eg, Graves' disease, polymyositis, Guillain-Barre syndrome) in the setting of immune reconstitution, and redistribution/accumulation of body fat reported. Caution in elderly.

ADVERSE REACTIONS

Rash, peripheral neuropathy.

DRUG INTERACTIONS

May alter therapeutic effect and adverse reaction profile with drugs that induce, inhibit, or are substrates of CYP3A, CYP2C9, and CYP2C19, or are transported by P-glycoprotein. Avoid with other NNRTIs, delavirdine, rilpivirine, atazanavir (ATV) without low-dose ritonavir (RTV), fosamprenavir (FPV) without low-dose RTV, FPV/RTV, tipranavir/RTV, indinavir without low-dose RTV, nelfinavir without low-dose RTV, RTV (600mg bid), carbamazepine, phenobarbital, phenytoin, rifampin, rifapentine, and St. John's wort. Coadministration with boceprevir is not recommended in the presence of other drugs which may further decrease etravirine exposure (eg, darunavir/RTV, lopinavir/RTV, saquinavir/RTV, tenofovir disoproxil fumarate, or rifabutin). Caution with digoxin; use lowest dose initially. May increase levels of nelfinavir without RTV, digoxin, warfarin (monitor INR), anticoagulants, 14-OH-clarithromycin, voriconazole, diazepam, boceprevir, fluvastatin, and pitavastatin. May increase maraviroc levels in the presence of a potent CYP3A inhibitor (eg, RTV boosted protease inhibitor). May decrease levels of maraviroc, antiarrhythmics, itraconazole, ketoconazole, rifabutin, telaprevir, atorvastatin, lovastatin, simvastatin, immunosuppressant, and clopidogrel (active) metabolite. May decrease dolutegravir levels; should only be used with dolutegravir when coadministered with ATV/RTV, darunavir/RTV, or lopinavir/RTV. Fluconazole and voriconazole may increase exposure. Posaconazole, itraconazole, or ketoconazole may increase levels. May decrease clarithromycin exposure. Caution with artemether/lumefantrine. Efavirenz, nevirapine, rifabutin, systemic dexamethasone, and boceprevir may decrease levels. Darunavir/RTV, lopinavir/RTV, and saquinavir/RTV may decrease exposure. Consider alternatives to clarithromycin, such as azithromycin, for treatment of *Mycobacterium avium* complex. Monitor for withdrawal symptoms when coadministered with methadone, buprenorphine, buprenorphine/naloxone. May need to alter sildenafil dose. Refer to PI for additional drug interaction information.

PATIENT CONSIDERATIONS

Assessment: Assess treatment history, pregnancy/nursing status, and for possible drug interactions. Perform resistance testing where possible.

Monitoring: Monitor for signs/symptoms of severe skin/hypersensitivity reactions, body fat redistribution/accumulation, immune reconstitution syndrome (eg, opportunistic infections), autoimmune disorders, and other adverse reactions. Monitor clinical status, including liver transaminases. Monitor INR when combined with warfarin.

Counseling: Inform that product is not a cure for HIV infection and patients may continue to develop opportunistic infections and other complications associated with HIV disease. Advise to avoid doing things that can spread HIV-1 infection to others. Advise to take medication ud. Instruct to always use in combination with other antiretrovirals. Advise not to alter dose or d/c therapy without consulting physician. If a dose is missed within 6 hrs of time usually taken, instruct to take as soon as possible following a meal. If scheduled time exceeds 6 hrs, instruct not to take the missed dose and resume the usual dosing schedule. Advise to report to physician the use of any other prescription/nonprescription or herbal products (eg, St. John's wort). Counsel to d/c and notify physician if severe rash develops. Advise that redistribution or accumulation of body fat may occur.

STORAGE: 25°C (77°F); excursions permitted to 15-30°C (59-86°F). Store in the original bottle. Protect from moisture.

INTUNIV – guanfacine

RX

Class: $Alpha_{2A}$ agonist

PEDIATRIC DOSAGE

Attention-Deficit Hyperactivity Disorder

Monotherapy/Adjunctive Therapy to Stimulant Medications:

6-17 Years:
Initial: 1mg/day
Titrate: Adjust in increments of no more than 1mg/week
Target Dose Range: 0.05-0.12mg/kg/day (total daily dose 1-7mg), depending on clinical response and tolerability
Max: Doses above 4mg/day in children 6-12 yrs of age and doses above 7mg/day in adolescents 13-17 yrs of age have not been evaluated
Weight-Based Target Dose Range:
25-33.9kg: 2-3mg/day
34-41.4kg: 2-4mg/day
41.5-49.4kg: 3-5mg/day
49.5-58.4kg: 3-6mg/day
58.5-91kg: 4-7mg/day
>91kg: 5-7mg/day
Maint Treatment:
Periodically reevaluate the long-term use of the drug and adjust weight-based dose prn

Missed Dose

When reinitiating to the previous maint dose after ≥2 missed consecutive doses, consider titration based on tolerability

Conversions

Switching from Immediate-Release (IR):
D/C IR, and titrate w/ extended-release following the recommended schedule
Do not substitute for IR tabs on a mg-per-mg basis

DOSING CONSIDERATIONS

Concomitant Medications

Strong CYP3A4 Inhibitors:
(Based on Weight-Based Target Dose Range)
Continue CYP3A4 Inhibitor/Initiate Guanfacine: Decrease guanfacine dose by 1/2
Continue Guanfacine/Initiate CYP3A4 Inhibitor: Decrease guanfacine dose by 1/2
Stop CYP3A4 Inhibitor/Continue Guanfacine: Increase guanfacine to recommended level

Strong CYP3A4 Inducers:
(Based on Weight-Based Target Dose Range)
Continue CYP3A4 Inducer/Initiate Guanfacine: Consider increasing guanfacine up to twice the recommended dose
Continue Guanfacine/Initiate CYP3A4 Inducer: Consider increasing guanfacine up to twice the recommended dose over 1-2 weeks
Stop CYP3A4 Inducer/Continue Guanfacine: Decrease guanfacine dose to recommended level over 1-2 weeks

Renal Impairment
Significant Impairment: May need to reduce dose

Hepatic Impairment
Significant Impairment: May need to reduce dose

Discontinuation
Taper dose in decrements of no more than 1mg every 3-7 days

ADMINISTRATION

Oral route

Take either in am or pm, at approx same time each day.
Swallow tabs whole w/ water, milk, or other liquid; do not crush, chew, or break.
Do not administer w/ high-fat meals.

HOW SUPPLIED

Tab, Extended-Release: 1mg, 2mg, 3mg, 4mg

CONTRAINDICATIONS

History of a hypersensitivity reaction to Intuniv or its inactive ingredients, or other products containing guanfacine.

WARNINGS/PRECAUTIONS

May experience increase in BP and HR following discontinuation of therapy. May cause dose-dependent decreases in BP and HR. Orthostatic hypotension and syncope reported. Titrate slowly in patients w/ a history of hypotension, and those w/ underlying conditions that may be worsened by hypotension and bradycardia (eg, heart block, cardiovascular disease, vascular disease). In patients who have a history of syncope or may have a condition that predisposes to syncope (eg, hypotension, orthostatic hypotension, bradycardia), avoid dehydration or overheating. Somnolence and sedation commonly reported. May impair mental/physical abilities. May worsen sinus node dysfunction and atrioventricular (AV) block; titrate slowly and monitor vital signs frequently in patients w/ cardiac conduction abnormalities.

ADVERSE REACTIONS

Somnolence, fatigue, abdominal pain, hypotension, N/V, lethargy, dizziness, irritability, decreased appetite, dry mouth, insomnia, enuresis, bradycardia.

DRUG INTERACTIONS

See Dosing Considerations. CYP3A4 inhibitors (eg, ketoconazole) may increase exposure. CYP3A4 inducers (eg, rifampin) may decrease exposure. Monitor BP and HR, and adjust dosages accordingly w/ antihypertensives or other drugs that can reduce BP/HR or increase the risk of syncope. Consider the potential for additive sedative effects before using w/ other centrally active depressants. Avoid w/ alcohol. May worsen sinus node dysfunction and AV block, especially w/ other sympatholytic drugs; titrate slowly and monitor vital signs frequently w/ other sympatholytic drugs.

PATIENT CONSIDERATIONS

Assessment: Assess for history of hypotension, underlying conditions that may be worsened by hypotension and bradycardia, history of syncope, condition that predisposes to syncope, cardiac conduction abnormalities, hypersensitivity to drug, renal/hepatic impairment, pregnancy/nursing status, and possible drug interactions. Assess HR and BP.

Monitoring: Monitor for hypotension, bradycardia, syncope, somnolence, sedation, cardiac conduction abnormalities, and other adverse reactions. Monitor HR and BP following dose increases, and periodically while on therapy. Monitor BP and pulse when reducing the dose or discontinuing the drug. Observe human milk-fed infants for sedation and somnolence. Monitor vital signs frequently in patients w/ cardiac conduction abnormalities. Periodically reevaluate the long term use of the drug.

Counseling: Instruct caregiver to supervise the child or adolescent taking the drug. Counsel on how to properly taper the medication, if the physician decides to d/c treatment. Instruct patients not to d/c therapy w/o consulting their physician. Inform of the adverse reactions (eg, sedation, headache, abdominal pain) that may occur; advise to consult physician if any of these symptoms persist or other symptoms occur. Caution patients against operating heavy equipment or driving until accustomed to effects of medication. Advise to avoid becoming dehydrated or overheated, and to avoid use w/ alcohol.

STORAGE: 20-25°C (68-77°F); excursions permitted to 15-30°C (59-86°F).

INVEGA – paliperidone

RX

Class: Atypical antipsychotic

Elderly patients with dementia-related psychosis treated with antipsychotic drugs are at an increased risk of death; most deaths appeared to be cardiovascular (CV) (eg, heart failure, sudden death) or infectious (eg, pneumonia) in nature. Not approved for the treatment of patients with dementia-related psychosis.

ADULT DOSAGE

Schizophrenia

6mg qd; a lower dose of 3mg qd may be sufficient
Titrate: If indicated, may increase by 3mg/day; dose increases >6mg/day should be made at intervals >5 days
Max: 12mg/day

Schizoaffective Disorder

Monotherapy or Adjunct to Mood Stabilizers and/or Antidepressants:
6mg qd
Range: 3-12mg/day
Titrate: If indicated, may increase by 3mg/day at intervals of >4 days
Max: 12mg/day

PEDIATRIC DOSAGE

Schizophrenia

12-17 Years:
Initial: 3mg qd
Titrate: If indicated, may increase by 3mg/day at intervals of >5 days

DOSING CONSIDERATIONS

Renal Impairment

Mild (CrCl ≥50-<80mL/min):
Initial: 3mg qd
Max: 6mg qd

Moderate to Severe (CrCl ≥10-<50mL/min):
Initial: 1.5mg qd
Max: 3mg qd

Elderly

Adjust dose according to renal function

ADMINISTRATION

Oral route

Take w/ or w/o food
Swallow whole with liquids; do not crush, divide, or chew

HOW SUPPLIED

Tab, Extended-Release: 1.5mg, 3mg, 6mg, 9mg

CONTRAINDICATIONS

Known hypersensitivity to either paliperidone or risperidone, or to any of the excipients in this medication.

WARNINGS/PRECAUTIONS

Neuroleptic malignant syndrome (NMS) reported; d/c if this occurs. May increase QTc interval; avoid with congenital long QT syndrome and history of cardiac arrhythmias. Tardive dyskinesia (TD) may develop; consider discontinuation if signs/symptoms of TD appear. Hyperglycemia and diabetes mellitus (DM), in some cases extreme and associated with ketoacidosis or hyperosmolar coma or death, reported. Undesirable alterations in lipids and weight gain reported. May elevate prolactin levels. Avoid with preexisting severe GI narrowing. May induce orthostatic hypotension and syncope; caution with known CV disease, cerebrovascular disease, or conditions that predispose to hypotension. Leukopenia, neutropenia, and agranulocytosis reported; d/c in cases of severe neutropenia (absolute neutrophil count <1000/mm^3). Somnolence reported. May impair mental/physical abilities. Seizures reported; caution with history of seizures or conditions that lower the seizure threshold. May cause esophageal dysmotility and aspiration; caution with risk of aspiration pneumonia. May induce priapism; severe cases may require surgical intervention. May disrupt body's ability to reduce core body temperature; caution with conditions that may contribute to an elevated core body temperature. May have an antiemetic effect that may mask signs/symptoms of overdosage with certain drugs or of conditions (eg, intestinal obstruction, Reye's syndrome, brain tumor). Patients with Parkinson's disease or dementia with Lewy bodies may have increased sensitivity to therapy. Caution with suicidal tendencies, renal impairment, and in elderly. Not recommended with CrCl <10mL/min.

ADVERSE REACTIONS

Extrapyramidal symptoms, tachycardia, somnolence, akathisia, dyskinesia, dyspepsia, dizziness, nasopharyngitis, headache, nausea, hyperkinesia, constipation, weight gain, parkinsonism, tremors.

DRUG INTERACTIONS

Consider additive exposure with risperidone. Avoid with other drugs known to prolong QTc interval, including Class 1A (eg, quinidine, procainamide) or Class III (eg, amiodarone, sotalol) antiarrhythmics, antipsychotics (eg, chlorpromazine, thioridazine), and antibiotics (eg, gatifloxacin, moxifloxacin). Caution with other centrally acting drugs, alcohol, and drugs with anticholinergic activity. May antagonize the effect of levodopa and other dopamine agonists. Additive effect may be observed with other agents that cause orthostatic hypotension. Carbamazepine may decrease levels. Paroxetine (a potent CYP2D6 inhibitor) may increase exposure in CYP2D6 extensive metabolizers. Divalproex sodium may increase levels; consider dose reduction with valproate.

PATIENT CONSIDERATIONS

Assessment: Assess for dementia-related psychosis, congenital long QT syndrome, history of cardiac arrhythmias, DM, risk factors for DM, severe GI narrowing, history of clinically significant low WBCs or drug-induced leukopenia/neutropenia, Parkinson's disease, dementia with Lewy bodies, renal impairment, any other conditions where treatment is contraindicated or cautioned, pregnancy/nursing status, and possible drug interactions. Obtain baseline FPG in patients at risk for DM.

I

Monitoring: Monitor for NMS, TD, QT prolongation, hyperprolactinemia, orthostatic hypotension, syncope, cognitive and motor impairment, seizures, esophageal dysmotility, aspiration, priapism, disruption of body temperature, and other adverse reactions. Monitor for signs of hyperglycemia; perform periodic monitoring of FPG levels in patients with DM or at risk for DM. Monitor for signs/symptoms of leukopenia/neutropenia; frequently monitor CBC in patients with a history of clinically significant low WBC or drug-induced leukopenia/neutropenia. Monitor weight and renal function.

Counseling: Inform of the risk of orthostatic hypotension during initiation/reinitiation or dose increases. Inform that therapy has the potential to impair judgment, thinking, or motor skills; advise to use caution when operating hazardous machinery (eg, automobiles). Advise to avoid alcohol during therapy. Instruct to notify physician of all prescription and nonprescription drugs currently taking, and if pregnant, intending to become pregnant, or breastfeeding. Counsel on appropriate care in avoiding overheating and dehydration. Advise that the tab shell, along with insoluble core components, may be found in stool.

STORAGE: Up to 25°C (77°F); excursions permitted to 15-30°C (59-86°F). Protect from moisture.

INVEGA SUSTENNA – paliperidone palmitate

RX

Class: Atypical antipsychotic

Elderly patients w/ dementia-related psychosis treated w/ antipsychotic drugs are at an increased risk of death. Not approved for use in patients w/ dementia-related psychosis.

ADULT DOSAGE

Schizophrenia

Initial: 234mg on Day 1, then 156mg on Day 8 (both in deltoid muscle)
Maint: 117mg/month (in deltoid/gluteal muscle), administer 5 weeks after 1st inj; some may benefit from lower or higher dose w/in the available strengths (39-234mg)
Max: 234mg/month

Establish tolerability w/ oral paliperidone/risperidone prior to initiating therapy in oral paliperidone- or oral/injectable risperidone-naive patients

Schizoaffective Disorder

Monotherapy and Adjunctive Therapy to Mood Stabilizers/Antidepressants:
Initial: 234mg on Day 1, then 156mg on Day 8 (both in deltoid muscle)
Maint: 78-234mg/month (in deltoid/gluteal muscle), administer 5 weeks after 1st inj; adjust maint dose monthly based on tolerability and/or efficacy using available strengths

PEDIATRIC DOSAGE

Pediatric use may not have been established

Max: 234mg/month

Establish tolerability w/ oral paliperidone/risperidone prior to initiating therapy in oral paliperidone- or oral/injectable risperidone-naive patients

Conversions

Switching from Oral Antipsychotics:
Gradually d/c oral antipsychotics at the time of initiation of therapy

Tab, Extended-Release to Inj Maint Dose Conversion:
3mg PO qd: 39-78mg IM every 4 weeks
6mg PO qd: 117mg IM every 4 weeks
12mg PO qd: 234mg IM every 4 weeks

Switching from Long-Acting Injectable Antipsychotics:
Initiate therapy in place of the next scheduled inj and continue w/ monthly maint dose; the 1-week initiation dosing regimen is not required

Missed Dose

Avoiding Missed Doses:
May give 2nd initiation dose 4 days before/after the 1-week time point
May give 3rd and subsequent monthly inj up to 7 days before/after the monthly time point

Management of a Missed 2nd Initiation Dose:
<4 Weeks Since 1st Inj:
Administer 2nd inj (156mg) as soon as possible. A 3rd inj (117mg) is recommended 5 weeks after 1st inj (regardless of timing of 2nd inj), followed thereafter by normal monthly inj
4-7 Weeks Since 1st Inj:
Resume dosing w/ 2 inj of 156mg, administered in the deltoid 1 week apart, then resume usual monthly inj cycle
>7 Weeks Since 1st Inj:
Restart therapy

Management of a Missed Maint Dose:
4-6 Weeks Since Last Inj:
Resume regular monthly dosing as soon as possible at previously stabilized dose, followed by inj at monthly intervals
>6 Weeks to 6 Months Since Last Inj:
Resume the same previously stabilized dose as soon as possible into the deltoid, followed by another deltoid inj at the same dose 1 week later. Resume monthly dosing thereafter. If previous stabilized dose was 234mg, then 1st two inj should be 156mg each
>6 Months Since Last Inj:
Restart therapy

DOSING CONSIDERATIONS

Concomitant Medications

Strong CYP3A4/P-gp Inducers:
May need to increase dose; may need to decrease the dose when the strong inducer is discontinued
Risperidone/Oral Paliperidone:
Caution when coadministered for extended periods of time

Renal Impairment

Mild (CrCl 50 to <80mL/min):
Initial: 156mg on Day 1, then 117mg 1 week later (both in the deltoid muscle)
Maint: 78mg/month (in deltoid or gluteal muscle)
Moderate or Severe (CrCl <50mL/min): Not recommended

ADMINISTRATION

IM route

Inject slowly, deep into muscle
Administer as a single inj; do not administer dose in divided inj
Avoid inadvertent inj into a blood vessel

Deltoid Muscle Inj
Alternate deltoid inj between the 2 deltoid muscles
Needle Size Recommendations:
<90kg: 1-inch, 23-gauge needle
≥90kg: 1.5-inch, 22-gauge needle

Gluteal Muscle Inj
Administer into the upper outer quadrant of gluteal muscle; alternate gluteal inj between the 2 gluteal muscles
Needle Size Recommendations:
1.5-inch, 22-gauge needle size regardless of weight

HOW SUPPLIED
Inj, Extended-Release: 39mg, 78mg, 117mg, 156mg, 234mg

CONTRAINDICATIONS
Known hypersensitivity to either paliperidone or risperidone, or to any of the excipients in this formulation.

WARNINGS/PRECAUTIONS
Neuroleptic malignant syndrome (NMS) reported; d/c immediately if this occurs. May increase QTc interval; avoid w/ congenital long QT syndrome and history of cardiac arrhythmias. May develop tardive dyskinesia (TD); consider discontinuing if this occurs. Hyperglycemia and diabetes mellitus (DM), in some cases extreme and associated w/ ketoacidosis or hyperosmolar coma or death, reported. Dyslipidemia, weight gain, and hyperprolactinemia reported. May induce orthostatic hypotension and syncope; caution w/ known cardiovascular/cerebrovascular disease or conditions that predispose the patient to hypotension. Leukopenia, neutropenia, and agranulocytosis reported; d/c in cases of severe neutropenia (ANC <1000/mm^3). Somnolence, sedation, and dizziness reported. May impair mental/physical abilities. Seizures reported; caution w/ history of seizures or conditions that potentially lower the seizure threshold. May cause esophageal dysmotility and aspiration; use w/ caution in patients w/ a risk of aspiration pneumonia. May induce priapism; severe cases may require surgical intervention. May disrupt body's ability to reduce core body temperature; caution w/ conditions that may contribute to an elevated core body temperature. Patients w/ Parkinson's disease or dementia w/ Lewy bodies may have increased sensitivity to therapy. Caution in elderly.

ADVERSE REACTIONS
N/V, inj-site reactions, nasopharyngitis, weight gain, dizziness, akathisia, extrapyramidal disorder, headache, somnolence/sedation, agitation, anxiety, pyrexia, hyperprolactinemia.

DRUG INTERACTIONS
See Dosing Considerations. May antagonize the effect of levodopa and other dopamine agonists. An additive effect may occur w/ other agents that also cause orthostatic hypotension. Avoid w/ other drugs known to prolong QTc interval, including Class 1A (eg, quinidine, procainamide) or Class III (eg, amiodarone, sotalol) antiarrhythmics, antipsychotics (eg, chlorpromazine, thioridazine), or antibiotics (eg, gatifloxacin, moxifloxacin). Caution w/ anticholinergics; may contribute to an elevated body temperature.

PATIENT CONSIDERATIONS

Assessment: Assess for known hypersensitivity to drug/risperidone/any of the excipients, dementia-related psychosis, congenital long QT syndrome, history of cardiac arrhythmias, DM, risk factors for DM, history of clinically significant low WBC counts or drug-induced leukopenia/neutropenia, Parkinson's disease, dementia w/ Lewy bodies, renal impairment, any other conditions where treatment is contraindicated or cautioned, pregnancy/nursing status, and possible drug interactions. Obtain baseline FPG in patients at risk for DM.

Monitoring: Monitor for hypersensitivity reactions, NMS, QT prolongation, TD, hyperprolactinemia, orthostatic hypotension, syncope, seizures, aspiration, priapism, disruption of body temperature, and other adverse reactions. Monitor for signs of hyperglycemia; perform periodic monitoring of FPG levels in patients w/ DM or at risk for DM. Monitor for signs/symptoms of leukopenia/neutropenia; frequently monitor CBC in patients w/ a history of clinically significant low WBC counts or drug-induced leukopenia/neutropenia. Monitor weight and renal function. Reassess periodically to determine need for continued treatment.

Counseling: Advise patients on risk of orthostatic hypotension. Caution about operating machinery/driving until certain that therapy does not affect the patient adversely. Advise to avoid overheating and becoming dehydrated. Instruct to inform physician about any concomitant prescription or OTC medications. Advise to notify physician if pregnancy occurs or is intended. Instruct not to breastfeed.

STORAGE: 25°C (77°F); excursions permitted to 15-30°C (59-86°F).

INVEGA TRINZA – paliperidone palmitate

RX

Class: Atypical antipsychotic

Elderly patients w/ dementia-related psychosis treated w/ antipsychotic drugs are at an increased risk of death. Not approved for use in patients w/ dementia-related psychosis.

ADULT DOSAGE

Schizophrenia

3-month inj for the treatment of schizophrenia in patients after they have been adequately treated w/ Invega Sustenna (1-month paliperidone palmitate ER injectable sus) for at least 4 months

Initiate when the next 1-month paliperidone dose is scheduled w/ an Invega Trinza dose based on the previous 1-month inj dose, using the equivalent 3.5-fold higher dose; refer to initial Invega Trinza dose listed below

Administer up to 7 days before or after the monthly time point of the next scheduled paliperidone 1-month dose

Initial Invega Trinza Dose Based on Last Dose of Invega Sustenna:

Invega Sustenna 78mg: 273mg Invega Trinza every 3 months

Invega Sustenna 117mg: 410mg Invega Trinza every 3 months

Invega Sustenna 156mg: 546mg Invega Trinza every 3 months

Invega Sustenna 234mg: 819mg Invega Trinza every 3 months

If needed, dose adjustment can be made every 3 months in increments w/in the range of 273-819mg based on individual patient tolerability and/or efficacy

In order to establish a consistent maint dose, it is recommended that the last 2 doses of Invega Sustenna be the same dosage strength before starting Invega Trinza

Missed Dose

Dosing Window:

Avoid missing doses; may give the inj up to 2 weeks before or after the 3-month time point if necessary

Missed Dose 3.5-4 Months Since Last Inj:

Administer the previously administered dose as soon as possible, then continue w/ the 3-month inj following this dose

Missed Dose 4-9 Months Since Last Inj:

Do not administer the next dose; refer to PI for reinitiation regimen

Missed Dose Longer Than 9 Months Since Last Inj:

Reinitiate treatment w/ the 1-month paliperidone ER injectable sus; may resume Invega Trinza after the patient has been adequately treated w/ the 1-month paliperidone ER injectable sus for at least 4 months

Conversions

Switching from Invega Trinza (Last Dose) to Invega Sustenna (1-Month Paliperidone ER Injectable Sus):

Invega Trinza 273mg: Initiate 78mg Invega

PEDIATRIC DOSAGE

Pediatric use may not have been established

Sustenna 3 months later
Invega Trinza 410mg: Initiate 117mg Invega Sustenna 3 months later
Invega Trinza 546mg: Initiate 156mg Invega Sustenna 3 months later
Invega Trinza 819mg: Initiate 234mg Invega Sustenna 3 months later

The 1-month paliperidone ER injectable sus should then continue, dosed at monthly intervals

Switching from Invega Trinza to Oral Paliperidone ER Tabs:
Daily dosing of the paliperidone ER tabs should start 3 months after the last Invega Trinza dose and be transitioned over the next several months following the last Invega Trinza dose; refer to PI for Invega Trinza doses and once daily paliperidone ER conversion regimens needed to attain similar paliperidone exposures

DOSING CONSIDERATIONS

Concomitant Medications
Use w/ Risperidone or w/ Oral Paliperidone: Use w/ caution when coadministered for extended periods of time

Renal Impairment
Mild (CrCl ≥50 to <80mL/min): Adjust dose and stabilize the patient using the 1-month paliperidone ER injectable sus, then transition to Invega Trinza
Moderate/Severe (CrCl <50mL/min): Not recommended

ADMINISTRATION

IM route

Administer once every 3 months
Each inj must be administered only by a healthcare professional
Shake syringe vigorously for at least 15 sec; inject w/in 5 min of shaking vigorously to ensure a homogeneous sus and ensure needle does not get clogged during inj
Avoid inadvertent inj into a blood vessel
Administer as a single inj; do not administer dose in divided inj
Inject slowly, deep into the deltoid or gluteal muscle
Administer using only the thin wall needles that are provided in the pack; do not use needles from the 1-month paliperidone ER injectable sus pack or other commercially-available needles
Do not re-inject dose remaining in the syringe and do not administer another dose in the event of an incompletely administered dose

Needle Size Recommendations
Deltoid Muscle:
<90kg: 1-inch, 22-gauge needle
≥90kg: 1.5-inch, 22-gauge needle
Gluteal Muscle:
1.5-inch, 22-gauge needle size, regardless of weight

HOW SUPPLIED

Inj, ER: 273mg, 410mg, 546mg, 819mg

WARNINGS/PRECAUTIONS

Neuroleptic malignant syndrome (NMS) reported; d/c therapy and institute symptomatic treatment. May increase QTc interval; avoid in patients w/ congenital long QT syndrome and in patients w/ history of cardiac arrhythmias. May cause tardive dyskinesia (TD), especially in the elderly; consider discontinuation if this occurs. Hyperglycemia and diabetes mellitus (DM), in some cases extreme and associated w/ ketoacidosis or hyperosmolar coma or death, reported. Dyslipidemia, weight gain, and hyperprolactinemia reported. May induce orthostatic hypotension and syncope; caution w/ known cardiovascular/cerebrovascular disease or conditions that predispose to hypotension. Leukopenia, neutropenia, and agranulocytosis reported; consider discontinuation at 1st sign of a clinically significant decline in WBC count in the absence of other causative factors in patients w/ a history of a clinically significant low WBC count/ANC or a drug-induced leukopenia/neutropenia. D/C therapy and follow WBC count until recovery in patients w/ severe neutropenia (ANC <1000/ mm^3). Somnolence, sedation, and dizziness reported. May impair mental/physical abilities. Caution w/ history of seizures or other conditions that potentially lower the seizure threshold. May cause esophageal dysmotility and aspiration; caution in patients at risk for aspiration pneumonia. May induce priapism; severe cases may require surgical intervention. May disrupt body's ability to reduce core body temperature; caution w/ conditions that may contribute to an elevated core body temperature. Patients w/ Parkinson's disease or dementia w/ Lewy bodies may experience increased sensitivity to therapy.

ADVERSE REACTIONS

Inj-site reaction, URTI, weight increase, akathisia, headache, parkinsonism, UTI.

DRUG INTERACTIONS

Avoid in combination w/ other drugs that are known to prolong QTc interval including Class 1A (eg, quinidine, procainamide) or Class III (eg, amiodarone, sotalol) antiarrhythmics, antipsychotics (eg, chlorpromazine, thioridazine), antibiotics (eg, gatifloxacin, moxifloxacin), and any other class of medications known to prolong the QTc interval. An additive effect may occur w/ drugs that have potential for inducing orthostatic hypotension; monitor orthostatic vital signs in patients who are vulnerable to hypotension. Strong inducers of CYP3A4 and P-gp (eg, carbamazepine, rifampin, St. John's wort) may decrease exposure; avoid using CYP3A4 and/or P-gp inducers during the 3-month dosing interval, if possible, and consider managing the patient using paliperidone ER tabs if administering a strong inducer is necessary. Caution if receiving a concomitant medication w/ anticholinergic activity. May antagonize the effect of levodopa and other dopamine agonists; monitor and manage patients as clinically appropriate.

PATIENT CONSIDERATIONS

Assessment: Assess for known hypersensitivity to the drug, dementia-related psychosis, congenital long QT syndrome, history of cardiac arrhythmias, DM, history of clinically significant low WBCs or drug-induced leukopenia/neutropenia, renal impairment, any other conditions where treatment is contraindicated or cautioned, pregnancy/nursing status, and possible drug interactions. Obtain baseline FPG in patients at risk for DM.

Monitoring: Monitor for hypersensitivity reactions, NMS, QT prolongation, TD, hyperglycemia, weight gain, dyslipidemia, orthostatic hypotension, syncope, seizures, esophageal dysmotility, aspiration, priapism, cognitive and motor impairment, disruption of body temperature, and other adverse reactions. Monitor CBC frequently in patients w/ a history of a clinically significant low WBC count/ANC or drug-induced leukopenia/neutropenia. Monitor for fever or other signs/symptoms of infection in patients w/ neutropenia. Monitor for worsening of glucose control in patients w/ DM. Monitor FPG levels in patients at risk for DM periodically during therapy. Reassess periodically to determine need for continued treatment.

Counseling: Inform of the risks/benefits of therapy. Inform about risk of developing NMS and explain its signs and symptoms. Counsel on the signs and symptoms of TD and advise to contact physician if these abnormal movements occur. Counsel about the risk of metabolic changes, how to recognize symptoms of hyperglycemia and DM, and the need for specific monitoring. Inform about risk of orthostatic hypotension, particularly at the time of initiating treatment, reinitiating treatment, or increasing the dose. Advise patients w/ preexisting low WBC counts or history of drug-induced leukopenia/neutropenia to have their CBC monitored. Counsel on signs and symptoms of hyperprolactinemia that may be associated w/ chronic use; advise to seek medical attention if a female patient experiences amenorrhea or galactorrhea or if a male patient experiences erectile dysfunction or gynecomastia. Caution about operating hazardous machinery, including automobiles. Advise of the possibility of painful or prolonged penile erections; instruct to seek immediate medical attention in the event of priapism. Counsel on the importance of avoiding overheating and dehydration. Advise to inform physician if taking/planning to take any prescription or OTC drugs. Advise female patients to notify physician if pregnancy occurs or is intended during treatment. Advise that there is a pregnancy registry that monitors pregnancy outcomes in women exposed to paliperidone during pregnancy.

STORAGE: 20-25°C (68-77°F); excursions permitted between 15-30°C (59-86°F).

INVOKANA — canagliflozin

RX

Class: Sodium-glucose cotransporter 2 (SGLT2) inhibitor

ADULT DOSAGE

Type 2 Diabetes Mellitus

Initial: 100mg qd before the 1st meal of the day

Titrate: May increase to 300mg qd in patients tolerating therapy who have an eGFR ≥60mL/min/1.73m^2 and require additional glycemic control

PEDIATRIC DOSAGE

Pediatric use may not have been established

DOSING CONSIDERATIONS

Concomitant Medications

UDP-Glucuronosyl Transferase Enzyme Inducers (eg, Rifampin, Phenytoin, Phenobarbital, Ritonavir):

eGFR ≥60mL/min/1.73m²: Consider increasing canagliflozin dose to 300mg qd in patients tolerating 100mg qd and requiring additional glycemic control

eGFR 45 to <60mL/min/1.73m²: Consider another antihyperglycemic agent

Renal Impairment

Moderate (eGFR 45 to <60mL/min/1.73m²): Limit dose to 100mg qd

eGFR <45mL/min/1.73m²: Do not initiate treatment

D/C therapy when eGFR is persistently <45mL/min/1.73m²

Other Important Considerations

Patients w/ Volume-Depletion:

Correct this condition before initiating treatment

ADMINISTRATION

Oral route

Take w/ or w/o food.

HOW SUPPLIED

Tab: 100mg, 300mg

CONTRAINDICATIONS

History of a serious hypersensitivity reaction to canagliflozin. Severe renal impairment (eGFR <30mL/min/1.73m²), ESRD, patients on dialysis.

WARNINGS/PRECAUTIONS

Not recommended w/ type 1 diabetes mellitus (DM) or severe hepatic impairment, or for treatment of diabetic ketoacidosis. Ketoacidosis reported; if suspected, d/c and institute prompt treatment. Assess for ketoacidosis in patients presenting w/ signs/symptoms consistent w/ severe metabolic acidosis regardless of presenting blood glucose levels. Consider temporarily discontinuing therapy in clinical situations known to predispose to ketoacidosis (eg, prolonged fasting due to acute illness or surgery). Causes intravascular volume contraction. Symptomatic hypotension may occur, particularly in patients w/ renal impairment (eGFR <60mL/min/1.73m²), elderly patients, patients on either diuretics or medications that interfere w/ the renin-angiotensin-aldosterone system (RAAS), or patients w/ low systolic BP; assess and correct volume status before initiating treatment in patients w/ ≥1 of these characteristics. Increases SrCr and decreases eGFR; caution in patients w/ hypovolemia. Renal function abnormalities may occur; monitor renal function more frequently in patients w/ an eGFR <60mL/min/1.73m². May lead to hyperkalemia; increased risk in patients w/ moderate renal impairment who are taking medications that interfere w/ K^+ excretion or medications that interfere w/ the RAAS. Serious UTIs (eg, urosepsis, pyelonephritis), requiring hospitalization, reported; evaluate for signs/symptoms of UTIs and treat promptly, if indicated. Increases risk of genital mycotic infections; increased risk w/ a history of genital mycotic infections and uncircumcised males. Hypersensitivity reactions, some serious, reported; d/c and treat if this occurs and monitor until signs/symptoms resolve. Increased risk on bone fractures observed; consider factors that contribute to fracture risk prior to initiation. Dose-related increases in LDL levels reported. Monitoring glycemic control w/ urine glucose tests or 1,5-anhydroglucitol assay is not recommended.

ADVERSE REACTIONS

Genital mycotic infections, UTIs, increased urination, vulvovaginal pruritus, hypersensitivity reactions, hypoglycemia, increases in serum K^+ levels.

DRUG INTERACTIONS

See Dosing Considerations. May increase risk of hypoglycemia when combined w/ insulin or an insulin secretagogue; lower dose of insulin or insulin secretagogue may be required. Rifampin decreases exposure. Increases levels of digoxin; monitor appropriately.

PATIENT CONSIDERATIONS

Assessment: Assess for diabetic ketoacidosis, type of DM, volume status, predisposition to hyperkalemia, risk for genital mycotic infections, drug hypersensitivity, risk factors for fractures, predisposition to ketoacidosis, pregnancy/nursing status, and possible drug interactions. Assess baseline renal/hepatic function, LDL levels, and BP.

Monitoring: Monitor for signs/symptoms of hypotension, ketoacidosis, urosepsis, pyelonephritis, genital mycotic infections, hypersensitivity reactions, bone fractures, and other adverse reactions. Monitor renal function, serum K^+ levels, and LDL levels.

Counseling: Inform of the risks, benefits, and alternative modes of therapy. Advise about the importance of adherence to dietary instructions, regular physical activity, periodic blood glucose monitoring and HbA1C testing, recognition and management of hypo/hyperglycemia, and assessment for diabetes complications. Instruct to seek medical advice promptly during periods of stress (eg, fever, trauma, infection, surgery) as medication requirements may change. Instruct to report to physician if pregnant, nursing, or experiencing symptoms of hypotension. Instruct to have adequate fluid intake. Instruct to d/c and seek medical advice immediately if symptoms of ketoacidosis occur. Counsel on the signs/symptoms of UTI, vaginal yeast infection, balanitis, and balanoposthitis; inform of treatment options and when to seek medical advice. Instruct to d/c therapy and consult physician if any signs/symptoms suggesting an allergic reaction or angioedema develop. Inform that bone fractures have been reported and provide information on factors that may contribute to fracture risk.

STORAGE: 25°C (77°F); excursions permitted to 15-30°C (59-86°F).

ISENTRESS – raltegravir

RX

Class: HIV-integrase strand transfer inhibitor

ADULT DOSAGE

HIV-1 Infection

Combination w/ Other Antiretrovirals:

Tab:
400mg bid

In Combination w/ Rifampin:
800mg bid

PEDIATRIC DOSAGE

HIV-1 Infection

Combination w/ Other Antiretrovirals:

≥4 Weeks of Age:
Tab:
≥25kg: 400mg bid

Tab, Chewable:
11-<14kg: 75mg bid
14-<20kg: 100mg bid
20-<28kg: 150mg bid
28-<40kg: 200mg bid
≥40kg: 300mg bid
Max: 300mg bid

Sus:
3-<4kg: 1mL (20mg) bid
4-<6kg: 1.5mL (30mg) bid
6-<8kg: 2mL (40mg) bid
8-<11kg: 3mL (60mg) bid
11-<14kg: 4mL (80mg) bid
14-<20kg: 5mL (100mg) bid
Max: 100mg bid

ADMINISTRATION

Oral route

Take w/ or w/o food

Tab
Swallow whole

Tab, Chewable
Chew or swallow whole

Sus
1. Pour sus pack contents into mixing cup, add 5mL of water, and mix
2. To mix, swirl mixing cup w/ a gentle circular motion for 30-60 sec; do not turn mixing cup upside down
3. Measure the recommended dose w/ provided syringe and administer w/in 30 min of mixing
4. Discard any remaining sus

HOW SUPPLIED

Sus (Powder): 100mg/pkt; **Tab:** 400mg; **Tab, Chewable:** 25mg, 100mg* *scored

WARNINGS/PRECAUTIONS

Do not substitute chewable tabs or oral sus for the 400mg film-coated tab; not bioequivalent. Severe, potentially life-threatening, and fatal skin reactions (eg, Stevens-Johnson syndrome, toxic epidermal necrolysis), and hypersensitivity reactions reported; d/c therapy and other suspect agents immediately if signs/symptoms develop. Immune reconstitution syndrome reported. Autoimmune disorders (eg, Graves' disease, polymyositis, Guillain-Barre syndrome) reported in the setting of immune reconstitution and can occur many months after initiation of treatment. Caution in patients at increased risk of myopathy or rhabdomyolysis and in elderly. Avoid dosing before a dialysis session. (Tab, Chewable) Contains phenylalanine.

ADVERSE REACTIONS

Insomnia, headache, nausea, hyperglycemia, ALT/AST elevation, hyperbilirubinemia, low ANC, serum lipase/creatine kinase/pancreatic amylase increase, thrombocytopenia.

DRUG INTERACTIONS

See Dosage. UGT1A1 inhibitors may increase levels. UGT1A1 inducers (eg, rifampin) may decrease levels. Coadministration or staggered administration w/ aluminum- and/or magnesium hydroxide-containing antacids is not recommended.

PATIENT CONSIDERATIONS

Assessment: Assess for risk of myopathy or rhabdomyolysis, previous hypersensitivity to the drug, pregnancy/nursing status, and possible drug interactions. Assess if patient is undergoing dialysis session. (Tab, Chewable) Assess for phenylketonuria.

Monitoring: Monitor for signs/symptoms of severe skin/hypersensitivity reactions, immune reconstitution syndrome, autoimmune disorders, and other adverse reactions. If a severe skin reaction or hypersensitivity reaction develops, monitor clinical status, including liver aminotransferases.

Counseling: Instruct to inform physician if any unusual symptom develops, or if any known symptom persists or worsens. Inform that drug is not a cure for HIV-1 infection and that illnesses associated w/ HIV-1 may still be experienced. Advise to avoid doing things that can spread HIV-1 to others. Instruct to always practice safe sex by using a latex or polyurethane condom. Instruct to immediately d/c therapy and seek medical attention if rash develops w/ signs/symptoms of a more serious skin reaction. Instruct to immediately report to physician if any unexplained muscle pain, tenderness, or weakness occurs. Instruct to avoid taking aluminum- and/or magnesium hydroxide-containing antacids. (Tab, Chewable) Inform patients w/ phenylketonuria that product contains phenylalanine. (Sus) Instruct to administer w/in 30 min of mixing.

STORAGE: 20-25°C (68-77°F); excursions permitted to 15-30°C (59-86°F). (Tab, Chewable) Protect from moisture. (Sus) Do not open foil pkt until ready for use.

ISONIAZID — isoniazid

RX

Class: Isonicotinic acid hydrazide

Severe and sometimes fatal hepatitis associated w/ isoniazid (INH) therapy reported and may develop even after many months of treatment. The risk of developing hepatitis is age related and is increased w/ daily alcohol consumption. Carefully monitor and interview at monthly intervals. Measure hepatic enzymes prior to starting therapy and periodically throughout treatment in addition to monthly symptom reviews in patients ≥35 years old. Strongly consider discontinuation if abnormalities of liver function exceed 3-5X ULN. D/C drug promptly if signs and symptoms of hepatic damage occur. Patients w/ tuberculosis (TB) who have INH-induced hepatitis should be given appropriate treatment w/ alternative drugs. If INH must be reinstituted, do so only after symptoms and lab abnormalities have cleared. Restart in very small and gradually increasing doses and withdraw immediately if there is any indication of recurrent liver involvement. Defer preventive treatment in persons w/ acute hepatic disease.

ADULT DOSAGE

Tuberculosis

In conjunction w/ other effective antituberculous agents

Treatment:

Usual: 5mg/kg (up to 300mg/day) in a single dose; or 15mg/kg (up to 900mg/day) 2 or 3X/week

Patients w/ Pulmonary TB w/o HIV Infection:

Option 1: Daily INH + rifampin + pyrazinamide for 8 weeks followed by 16 weeks of INH + rifampin daily or 2-3X/week; ethambutol or streptomycin should be added to the initial regimen until sensitivity to INH and rifampin is demonstrated

Option 2: Daily INH + rifampin + pyrazinamide + streptomycin or ethambutol for 2 weeks followed by 2X/week administration of the same drugs for 6 weeks, subsequently 2X/week INH + rifampin for 16 weeks

PEDIATRIC DOSAGE

Tuberculosis

In conjunction w/ other effective antituberculous agents

Treatment:

Usual: 10-15mg/kg (up to 300mg/day) as a single dose; or 20-40mg/kg (up to 900mg/day), 2 or 3X/week

Patients w/ Pulmonary TB w/o HIV Infection:

Option 1: Daily INH + rifampin + pyrazinamide for 8 weeks followed by 16 weeks of INH + rifampin, daily or 2-3X/week; ethambutol or streptomycin should be added to the initial regimen until sensitivity to INH and rifampin is demonstrated

Option 2: Daily INH + rifampin + pyrazinamide + streptomycin or ethambutol for 2 weeks followed by 2X/week administration of the same drugs for 6 weeks, subsequently 2X/week INH + rifampin for 16 weeks

Option 3: INH + rifampin + pyrazinamide + ethambutol or streptomycin 3X/week for 6 months All regimens given 2 or 3X/week should be administered by directly observed therapy **Prevention:** **>30kg:** 300mg/day as a single dose **Concomitant Administration of Pyridoxine (B6):** Recommended in malnourished patients and in those predisposed to neuropathy (eg, alcoholics and diabetics) Refer to PI for additional information (eg, treatment of patients w/ pulmonary TB and HIV infection, extrapulmonary TB, pregnant women w/ TB, multi-drug resistant TB)	**Option 3:** INH + rifampin + pyrazinamide + ethambutol or streptomycin 3X/week for 6 months All regimens given 2 or 3X/week should be administered by directly observed therapy **Prevention:** 10mg/kg (up to 300mg/day) as a single dose or 20-30mg/kg (not to exceed 900mg/day) 2X/week, under the direct observation of a healthcare worker at the time of administration **Concomitant Administration of Pyridoxine (B6):** Recommended in malnourished patients and in those predisposed to neuropathy (eg, alcoholics and diabetics) Refer to PI for additional information (eg, treatment of patients w/ pulmonary TB and HIV infection, extrapulmonary TB, multi-drug resistant TB)

ADMINISTRATION
Oral and IM routes

Do not administer w/ food.
IM administration is intended for use whenever oral administration is not possible.

HOW SUPPLIED
Inj: 100mg/mL [10mL]; **Syrup:** 50mg/5mL [473mL]; **Tab:** 100mg*, 300mg* *scored

CONTRAINDICATIONS
Severe hypersensitivity reactions, including drug-induced hepatitis, previous INH-associated hepatic injury, severe adverse effects to INH (eg, drug fever, chills, arthritis), acute liver disease of any etiology.

WARNINGS/PRECAUTIONS
D/C all drugs and evaluate patient at 1st sign of a hypersensitivity reaction. Carefully monitor w/ daily alcohol use, active chronic liver disease, severe renal dysfunction, age >35, concurrent use of any chronically administered medication, history of previous discontinuation of INH, peripheral neuropathy or conditions predisposing to neuropathy, pregnancy, inj drug use, women belonging to minority groups (particularly in the postpartum period), and HIV-seropositive patients. **Inj:** Periodic ophthalmologic examinations during therapy are recommended when visual symptoms occur.

ADVERSE REACTIONS
Peripheral neuropathy, elevated serum transaminases, bilirubinemia, jaundice, hepatitis.

DRUG INTERACTIONS
Severe acetaminophen toxicity reported. Known to increase levels of carbamazepine; determine carbamazepine levels prior to concurrent INH administration, monitor for signs/symptoms of carbamazepine toxicity, and appropriately adjust dose of the anticonvulsant. Decreased ketoconazole exposure when given in combination w/ INH and rifampin. May increase levels of phenytoin; appropriately adjust dose of the anticonvulsant. May increase levels of theophylline and valproate; monitor levels and appropriately adjust dose of theophylline/valproate. **Inj/Tab:** Avoid tyramine- and histamine-containing foods.

PATIENT CONSIDERATIONS

Assessment: Assess for severe hypersensitivity reactions, previous INH-associated hepatic injury, severe adverse reactions to INH, acute/active chronic liver disease, daily alcohol use, severe renal dysfunction, peripheral neuropathy or conditions predisposing to neuropathy, any other conditions where treatment is contraindicated or cautioned, and possible drug interactions. Assess age, pregnancy/nursing status, and HIV status. Measure hepatic enzymes prior to therapy.

Monitoring: Monitor for hepatitis, hypersensitivity reactions, and other adverse reactions. Periodically measure hepatic enzymes.

Counseling: Instruct to immediately report signs/symptoms consistent w/ liver damage or other adverse events (unexplained anorexia, N/V, dark urine). Instruct to take drug w/o food.

STORAGE: **Tab:** 20-25°C (68-77°F). Protect from light and moisture. **Syrup:** 15-30°C (59-86°F). Protect from light and moisture. **Inj:** 20-25°C (68-77°F). Protect from light. If vial contents crystallize, warm vial to room temperature to redissolve crystals before use.

ISOSORBIDE DINITRATE – isosorbide dinitrate

RX

Class: Nitrate vasodilator

OTHER BRAND NAMES

Isordil Titradose

ADULT DOSAGE

Angina Pectoris

Due to Coronary Artery Disease:

Prevention:
Tab/Isordil Titradose:
Initial: 5-20mg bid-tid
Maint: 10-40mg bid-tid
Allow a dose-free interval of ≥14 hrs

Tab, Extended Release:
Refer to PI for dosing based on clinical trials

Tab, SL:
Prevention: 1 tab (2.5mg-5mg) 15 min before activity
Treatment: Use to abort acute angina episode recommended only in patients who fail to respond to SL nitroglycerin
Must provide a daily dose-free interval; 1 of the daily dose-free intervals must be somewhat >14 hrs

PEDIATRIC DOSAGE

Pediatric use may not have been established

DOSING CONSIDERATIONS

Elderly
Start at lower end of dosing range

ADMINISTRATION

Oral/SL route

HOW SUPPLIED

Tab, Extended Release (ER): 40mg*; **Tab, SL:** 2.5mg, 5mg; **Tab:** 10mg*, 20mg*, 30mg*, (Isordil Titradose) 5mg*, 40mg* *scored

CONTRAINDICATIONS

Allergic to isosorbide dinitrate or any of its other ingredients. **Tab:** Coadministration w/ certain drugs for erectile dysfunction (PDE inhibitors) (eg, sildenafil, tadalafil, or vardenafil); concomitant use w/ the soluble guanylate cyclase stimulator riociguat.

WARNINGS/PRECAUTIONS

Severe hypotension, particularly w/ upright posture, may occur. Perform careful clinical or hemodynamic monitoring if used in patients w/ acute MI or CHF to avoid the hazards of hypotension and tachycardia. Hypotension may be accompanied by paradoxical bradycardia and increased angina pectoris. May aggravate angina caused by hypertrophic cardiomyopathy. Caution w/ volume depletion and hypotension. May develop tolerance. Chest pain, acute MI, and sudden death reported during temporary withdrawal in patients w/ long term exposure to therapy. (Tab, SL) Not the 1st drug of choice for abortion of acute anginal episode.

ADVERSE REACTIONS

Headache, lightheadedness, hypotension, syncope, crescendo angina, rebound HTN.

DRUG INTERACTIONS

See Contraindications. Additive vasodilation w/ other vasodilators (eg, alcohol).

PATIENT CONSIDERATIONS

Assessment: Assess for drug hypersensitivity, hypotension, acute MI, CHF, volume depletion, hypertrophic cardiomyopathy, alcohol intake, pregnancy/nursing status, and possible drug interactions.

Monitoring: Monitor for paradoxical bradycardia, increased angina pectoris, hypotension, hemodynamic rebound, decreased exercise tolerance, chest pain, acute MI, and other adverse reactions. In patients w/ MI or CHF, perform careful clinical or hemodynamic monitoring.

Counseling: Counsel to carefully follow prescribed dosing regimen. Inform that headaches sometimes accompany therapy and are markers of drug activity; instruct not to alter schedule of therapy since loss of headache may be associated w/ simultaneous loss of antianginal efficacy.

Inform that lightheadedness on standing may occur, which may be more frequent w/ alcohol consumption.

STORAGE: (Tab) 25°C (77°F); (Isordil Titradose) excursions permitted to 15-30°C (59-86°F). Protect from light. (Tab, SL/Tab, ER) 20-25°C (68-77°F). (Tab, SL) Protect from light and moisture.

JADENU – deferasirox

RX

Class: Iron-chelating agent

May cause acute renal failure and death, particularly in patients w/ comorbidities and those in the advanced stages of their hematologic disorders. Measure SrCr and determine CrCl in duplicate prior to initiation of therapy and monitor renal function at least monthly thereafter. Monitor creatinine weekly for the 1st month, then at least monthly for patients w/ baseline renal impairment or increased risk of acute renal failure. Consider dose reduction, interruption, or discontinuation based on increases in SrCr. May cause hepatic injury, including hepatic failure and death. Measure serum transaminases and bilirubin prior to initiating treatment, every 2 weeks during the 1st month, and at least monthly thereafter. Avoid in patients w/ severe (Child-Pugh C) hepatic impairment and reduce dose w/ moderate (Child-Pugh B) hepatic impairment. May cause GI hemorrhages, which may be fatal, especially in elderly who have advanced hematologic malignancies and/or low platelet counts. Monitor patients and d/c therapy if GI ulceration or hemorrhage is suspected.

ADULT DOSAGE

Chronic Iron Overload

Transfusional Iron Overload:
Only consider when a patient has evidence of chronic transfusional iron overload. Evidence should include the transfusion of ≥100mL/kg of packed RBCs (eg, ≥20 U of packed RBCs for a 40kg person or more in individuals weighing >40kg), and a serum ferritin consistently >1000mcg/L

Initial: 14mg/kg qd; calculate doses (mg/kg/day) to the nearest whole tab
Titrate: May adjust dose every 3-6 months based on serum ferritin trends. Make dose adjustments in steps of 3.5 or 7mg/kg and tailor adjustments to individual response and therapeutic goals. If patient is inadequately controlled w/ doses of 21mg/kg (eg, serum ferritin levels persistently >2500mcg/L and not showing a decreasing trend over time), doses of up to 28mg/kg may be considered
Max: 28mg/kg

Consider temporarily interrupting therapy if serum ferritin falls consistently <500mcg/L

Iron Overload in Non-Transfusion-Dependent Thalassemia (NTDT) Syndromes:
Only consider in a patient w/ a liver iron concentration (LIC) of ≥5mg of iron per gram of liver dry weight (mg Fe/g dw) and a serum ferritin >300mcg/L

Initial: 7mg/kg qd; calculate doses (mg/kg/day) to the nearest whole tab
Titrate: Consider increasing dose to 14mg/kg/day after 4 weeks if baseline LIC is >15mg Fe/g dw
Max: 14mg/kg/day

Interrupt treatment when serum ferritin is <300mcg/L and obtain an LIC to determine whether LIC has fallen to <3mg Fe/g dw. After 6 months of therapy, if LIC remains >7mg Fe/g dw, increase dose to a max of 14mg/kg/day. If after 6 months of therapy, LIC is 3-7mg Fe/g dw, continue treatment at no more than 7mg/kg/day. When LIC is <3mg Fe/g dw, interrupt treatment and

PEDIATRIC DOSAGE

Chronic Iron Overload

Transfusional Iron Overload:
Only consider when a patient has evidence of chronic transfusional iron overload. Evidence should include the transfusion of ≥100mL/kg of packed red blood cells (eg, ≥20 U of packed RBCs for a 40kg person or more in individuals weighing >40kg), and a serum ferritin consistently >1000mcg/L

≥2 Years:
Initial: 14mg/kg qd; calculate doses (mg/kg/day) to the nearest whole tab
Titrate: May adjust dose every 3-6 months based on serum ferritin trends. Make dose adjustments in steps of 3.5 or 7mg/kg and tailor adjustments to individual response and therapeutic goals. If patient is inadequately controlled w/ doses of 21mg/kg (eg, serum ferritin levels persistently >2500mcg/L and not showing a decreasing trend over time), doses of up to 28mg/kg may be considered
Max: 28mg/kg

Consider temporarily interrupting therapy if serum ferritin falls consistently <500mcg/L

Iron Overload in NTDT Syndromes:
Only consider in a patient w/ a LIC of ≥5mg of iron per gram of liver dry weight (mg Fe/g dw) and a serum ferritin >300mcg/L

≥10 Years:
Initial: 7mg/kg qd; calculate doses (mg/kg/day) to the nearest whole tab
Titrate: Consider increasing dose to 14mg/kg/day after 4 weeks if baseline LIC is >15mg Fe/g dw
Max: 14mg/kg/day

Interrupt treatment when serum ferritin is <300mcg/L and obtain an LIC to determine whether LIC has fallen to <3mg Fe/g dw. After 6 months of therapy, if LIC remains >7mg Fe/g dw, increase dose to a max of 14mg/kg/day. If after 6 months of therapy, LIC is 3-7mg Fe/g dw, continue treatment at no more than 7mg/

continue to monitor LIC. Restart treatment when LIC rises again to >5mg Fe/g dw

Conversions

Converting from Exjade to Jadenu: Jadenu dose should be about 30% lower, rounded to nearest whole tab

Transfusion-Dependent Iron Overload:
Initial: 14mg/kg/day (for 20mg/kg/day Exjade)
Titration Increments: 3.5-7mg/kg (for 5-10mg/kg Exjade)
Max: 28mg/kg/day (for 40mg/kg/day Exjade)
NTDT Syndromes:
Initial: 7mg/kg/day (for 10mg/kg/day Exjade)
Titration Increments: 3.5-7mg/kg (for 5-10mg/kg Exjade)
Max: 14mg/kg/day (for 20mg/kg/day Exjade)

kg/day. When LIC is <3mg Fe/g dw, interrupt treatment and continue to monitor LIC. Restart treatment when LIC rises again to >5mg Fe/g dw

Conversions

Converting from Exjade to Jadenu: Jadenu dose should be about 30% lower, rounded to nearest whole tab

Transfusion-Dependent Iron Overload:
Initial: 14mg/kg/day (for 20mg/kg/day Exjade)
Titration Increments: 3.5-7mg/kg (for 5-10mg/kg Exjade)
Max: 28mg/kg/day (for 40mg/kg/day Exjade)
NTDT Syndromes:
Initial: 7mg/kg/day (for 10mg/kg/day Exjade)
Titration Increments: 3.5-7mg/kg (for 5-10mg/kg Exjade)
Max: 14mg/kg/day (for 20mg/kg/day Exjade)

DOSING CONSIDERATIONS

Concomitant Medications

Bile Acid Sequestrants/Potent UDP-Glucuronosyltransferase (UGT) Inducers: Avoid concomitant use of bile acid sequestrants (eg, cholestyramine, colesevelam, colestipol) or potent UGT inducers (eg, rifampicin, phenytoin, phenobarbital, ritonavir) w/ Jadenu. If coadministration cannot be avoided, consider increasing initial deferasirox dose by 50%, and monitor serum ferritin levels and clinical responses for further dose modification

Renal Impairment

Baseline Renal Impairment:
CrCl 40-60mL/min: Reduce initial dose by 50%

Increases in SrCr During Therapy:
Transfusional Iron Overload:
Adults and Adolescents (≥16 Years): If SrCr increases by ≥33% above the average baseline measurement, repeat SrCr w/in 1 week, and if still elevated by ≥33%, reduce dose by 7mg/kg
Pediatric Patients (2-15 Years): Reduce dose by 7mg/kg if SrCr increases to >33% above the average baseline measurement and greater than the age-appropriate ULN
All Patients (Regardless of Age): D/C therapy for SrCr >2X the age-appropriate ULN or for CrCl <40mL/min

Non-Transfusion-Dependent Thalassemia Syndromes:
Adults and Adolescents (≥16 Years): If SrCr increases by ≥33% above the average baseline measurement, repeat SrCr w/in 1 week, and if still elevated by ≥33%, interrupt therapy if the dose is 3.5mg/kg, or reduce by 50% if the dose is 7 or 14mg/kg
Pediatric Patients (10-15 Years): Reduce dose by 3.5mg/kg if SrCr increases to >33% above the average baseline measurement and greater than the age-appropriate ULN
All Patients (Regardless of Age): D/C therapy for SrCr >2X the age-appropriate ULN or for CrCl <40mL/min

Hepatic Impairment

Baseline Hepatic Impairment:
Moderate (Child-Pugh B): Reduce initial dose by 50%
Severe (Child-Pugh C): Avoid therapy

Elderly

Start at lower end of dosing range

ADMINISTRATION

Oral route

Swallow tab w/ water or other liquids, preferably at the same time each day.
May be taken on an empty stomach or w/ a light meal (containing <7% fat content and approx 250 calories).
Do not take w/ aluminum-containing antacid products.

For patients who have difficulty swallowing whole tabs, may crush tabs and mix w/ soft foods (eg, yogurt, apple sauce) immediately prior to use; dose should be immediately and completely consumed and not stored for future use. Avoid commercial crushers w/ serrated surfaces for crushing a single 90mg tab.

HOW SUPPLIED

Tab: 90mg, 180mg, 360mg

CONTRAINDICATIONS

SrCr >2X the age-appropriate ULN or CrCl <40mL/min, poor performance status, high-risk myelodysplastic syndrome (MDS), advanced malignancies, platelet counts <50 x 10^9/L, known hypersensitivity to deferasirox or any component of this medication.

WARNINGS/PRECAUTIONS

Renal tubular damage, including Fanconi's syndrome, reported, most commonly in children and adolescents w/ β-thalassemia and serum ferritin levels <1500mcg/L. Intermittent proteinuria reported. Hepatic failure reported more commonly in patients w/ significant comorbidities, including liver cirrhosis and multiorgan failure. Consider dose modifications or interruption of treatment for severe or persistent elevations in serum transaminases and bilirubin. Patients w/ mild (Child-Pugh A) or moderate (Child-Pugh B) hepatic impairment may be at higher risk for hepatic toxicity. Nonfatal upper GI irritation, ulceration, and hemorrhage reported. Neutropenia, agranulocytosis, worsening anemia, and thrombocytopenia, including fatal events, reported; risk may increase w/ preexisting hematologic disorders. Interrupt treatment in patients who develop cytopenias until the cause has been determined. Increased risk of toxicity in elderly. May cause serious hypersensitivity reactions (eg, anaphylaxis, angioedema); d/c and institute appropriate medical intervention if reactions are severe. Severe skin reactions (including Stevens-Johnson syndrome [SJS] and erythema multiforme) reported; d/c immediately and do not reintroduce therapy if SJS or erythema multiforme is suspected. Therapy may be continued w/o dose adjustment for rashes of mild to moderate severity; interrupt therapy in severe cases. Reintroduction at a lower dose w/ escalation may be considered after resolution of the rash. Auditory and ocular disturbances reported; consider dose reduction or interruption if disturbances are noted. Measure serum ferritin monthly for possible overchelation of iron for patients w/ transfusional iron overload. For patients w/ NTDT, measure LIC by liver biopsy or by using an FDA-cleared/approved method for monitoring patients receiving therapy every 6 months on treatment.

ADVERSE REACTIONS

Transfusional Iron Overload: Abdominal pain, N/V, diarrhea, skin rash, increased SrCr.
Non-Transfusion-Dependent Thalassemia Syndromes: Nausea, rash, diarrhea.

DRUG INTERACTIONS

See Dosing Considerations. Avoid w/ aluminum-containing antacid preparations. Avoid w/ theophylline or other CYP1A2 substrates w/ a narrow therapeutic index (eg, tizanidine); monitor theophylline concentrations and consider theophylline dose modification if coadministration is necessary. Bile acid sequestrants may decrease deferasirox concentrations. Potent UGT inducers may decrease deferasirox efficacy due to possible decrease in deferasirox concentrations. Increased risk of GI hemorrhage w/ drugs that have ulcerogenic or hemorrhagic potential (eg, NSAIDs, corticosteroids, oral bisphosphonates, anticoagulants). May induce CYP3A4, resulting in a decrease in CYP3A4 substrate concentration; monitor closely for signs of reduced effectiveness when given w/ drugs metabolized by CYP3A4 (eg, alfentanil, aprepitant, budesonide). Inhibits CYP2C8 and CYP1A2, resulting in an increase in CYP2C8 (eg, repaglinide, paclitaxel) and CYP1A2 (eg, alosetron, caffeine, duloxetine) substrate concentration; closely monitor for signs of exposure-related toxicity. Consider decreasing the dose of repaglinide and monitor blood glucose levels carefully.

PATIENT CONSIDERATIONS

Assessment: Assess for high-risk MDS, performance status, renal/hepatic impairment, advanced malignancies, hematological disorders, comorbidities, hypersensitivity to the drug, any other conditions where treatment is contraindicated or cautioned, pregnancy/nursing status, and possible drug interactions. Perform baseline auditory and ophthalmic examinations. Determine CrCl (Cockcroft-Gault method). Obtain baseline SrCr in duplicate, serum transaminases, bilirubin, and blood counts. In patients w/ transfusional iron overload, obtain baseline serum ferritin level. In patients w/ iron overload in NTDT syndromes, obtain LIC by liver biopsy or by an FDA cleared or approved method for identifying patients for treatment w/ deferasirox therapy, and obtain baseline serum ferritin level on at least 2 measurements 1 month apart.

Monitoring: Monitor for acute renal failure, hepatic failure, GI ulceration/hemorrhage, neutropenia, agranulocytosis, worsening anemia, thrombocytopenia, hypersensitivity reactions, rashes, SJS, erythema multiforme, and other adverse reactions. Monitor blood counts. Perform auditory and ophthalmic tests every 12 months. Monitor closely for efficacy and adverse reactions that may require dose titration in patients w/ mild or moderate hepatic impairment. Monitor serum transaminases and bilirubin every 2 weeks during the 1st month of therapy and at least monthly thereafter. Monitor SrCr weekly during the 1st month after initiation or modification of therapy and at least monthly thereafter. Monitor SrCr and/or CrCl more frequently if creatinine levels are increasing. Monitor serum ferritin and for proteinuria monthly.

In patients w/ iron overload in NTDT syndromes, monitor LIC every 6 months. Monitor elderly more frequently for toxicity.

Counseling: Instruct to take ud. Instruct not to take the medication simultaneously w/ aluminum-containing antacids. Inform of the importance of auditory and ophthalmic testing before starting treatment and thereafter at regular intervals. Caution patients experiencing dizziness to avoid driving or operating machinery. Advise to notify physician of all prescription and nonprescription medications currently being taken. Explain that blood tests will be performed every month or more frequently if at increased risk of complications. Inform that skin rashes/serious allergic reactions have been reported; advise to d/c therapy and contact physician immediately if a severe allergic reaction/rash occurs.

STORAGE: 25°C (77°F); excursions permitted to 15-30°C (59-86°F). Protect from moisture.

JALYN – dutasteride/tamsulosin hydrochloride RX

Class: 5-alpha-reductase inhibitor (5-ARI)/alpha antagonist

ADULT DOSAGE	PEDIATRIC DOSAGE
Benign Prostatic Hyperplasia 1 cap qd, 30 min after the same meal each day	Pediatric use may not have been established

J

ADMINISTRATION

Oral route

Swallow cap whole; do not chew, crush, or open

HOW SUPPLIED

Cap: (Dutasteride/Tamsulosin) 0.5mg/0.4mg

CONTRAINDICATIONS

Pregnancy, women of childbearing potential, pediatric patients. Previously demonstrated, clinically significant hypersensitivity (eg, serious skin reactions, angioedema, urticaria, pruritus, respiratory symptoms) to dutasteride, other 5-alpha-reductase inhibitors, tamsulosin, or any other component of Jalyn.

WARNINGS/PRECAUTIONS

Not approved for the prevention of prostate cancer. Orthostatic hypotension/syncope may occur; avoid situations where syncope may result in an injury. May reduce serum prostate specific antigen (PSA) concentration during therapy; establish a new baseline PSA at least 3 months after starting therapy and monitor PSA periodically thereafter. Any confirmed increase from the lowest PSA value during treatment may signal the presence of prostate cancer and should be evaluated. May increase the risk of high-grade prostate cancer. Prior to initiating treatment, consideration should be given to other urological conditions that may cause similar symptoms; BPH and prostate cancer may coexist. Risk to male fetus; cap should not be handled by pregnant women or women who may become pregnant. May cause priapism; may lead to permanent impotence if not properly treated. Avoid blood donation until at least 6 months following the last dose. Intraoperative floppy iris syndrome (IFIS) reported during cataract surgery; initiation of therapy is not recommended in patients for whom cataract surgery is scheduled. Caution w/ sulfa allergy; allergic reaction rarely reported. Reduced total sperm count, semen volume, and sperm motility reported.

ADVERSE REACTIONS

Ejaculation disorders, impotence, decreased libido, breast disorders, dizziness.

DRUG INTERACTIONS

Avoid w/ strong CYP3A4 inhibitors (eg, ketoconazole); may increase tamsulosin exposure. Caution w/ potent, chronic CYP3A4 inhibitors (eg, ritonavir), moderate CYP3A4 inhibitors (eg, erythromycin), strong (eg, paroxetine) or moderate (eg, terbinafine) CYP2D6 inhibitors; potential for significant increase in tamsulosin exposure. Potential for significant increase in tamsulosin exposure when coadministered w/ a combination of both CYP3A4 and CYP2D6 inhibitors. Caution w/ cimetidine and warfarin. Avoid w/ other α-adrenergic antagonists; may increase the risk of symptomatic hypotension. Caution w/ PDE-5 inhibitors; may cause symptomatic hypotension.

PATIENT CONSIDERATIONS

Assessment: Assess for urological conditions that may cause similar symptoms, previous hypersensitivity to the drug, sulfa allergy, and possible drug interactions. Assess if patient is planning to undergo cataract surgery.

Monitoring: Monitor for signs/symptoms of prostate cancer, other urological diseases, orthostatic hypotension, syncope, priapism, IFIS, and allergic reactions. Obtain new baseline PSA at least 3 months after starting treatment and monitor PSA periodically thereafter.

Counseling: Inform about the possible occurrence of symptoms related to orthostatic hypotension and the potential risk of syncope; instruct to avoid situations where injury may result if syncope occurs. Inform that an increase in high-grade prostate cancer was reported. Inform females who are pregnant or who may become pregnant not to handle the drug due to potential risk to the fetus. Instruct that if a pregnant woman or woman of childbearing potential comes in contact w/ a leaking cap to wash the area immediately w/ soap and water. Inform that cap may become deformed and/or discolored if kept at high temperatures; instruct to avoid use if this occurs. Advise about the possibility of priapism (rare) that may lead to permanent erectile dysfunction if not brought to immediate medical attention. Advise not to donate blood for at least 6 months following the last dose. Instruct to inform ophthalmologist of drug if considering cataract surgery.

STORAGE: 25°C (77°F); excursions permitted to 15-30°C (59-86°F).

JANUMET – metformin hydrochloride/sitagliptin RX

Class: Biguanide/dipeptidyl peptidase-4 (DPP-4) inhibitor

Lactic acidosis may occur due to metformin accumulation; risk increases w/ conditions such as sepsis, dehydration, excess alcohol intake, hepatic/renal impairment, and acute CHF. If acidosis is suspected, d/c therapy and hospitalize patient immediately.

ADULT DOSAGE

Type 2 Diabetes Mellitus

Adjunct to diet and exercise to improve glycemic control when treatment w/ both sitagliptin and metformin is appropriate

Initial:

Not Currently on Metformin: 50mg/500mg bid

Currently on Metformin: 50mg bid of sitagliptin + current metformin dose

Currently on Metformin 850mg bid: 50mg/1000mg bid

Titrate: Gradually escalate dose to reduce GI side effects

Max: (100mg/2000mg)/day

PEDIATRIC DOSAGE

Pediatric use may not have been established

DOSING CONSIDERATIONS

Concomitant Medications

Insulin Secretagogue (eg, Sulfonylurea)/Insulin: May require lower doses of insulin secretagogue or insulin

ADMINISTRATION

Oral route

Take bid w/ meals.

Do not split or divide tab before swallowing.

HOW SUPPLIED

Tab: (Sitagliptin/Metformin) 50mg/500mg, 50mg/1000mg

CONTRAINDICATIONS

Renal impairment (eg, SrCr ≥1.5mg/dL [men], ≥1.4mg/dL [women], or abnormal CrCl), acute or chronic metabolic acidosis, including diabetic ketoacidosis. Hypersensitivity to metformin HCl, history of a serious hypersensitivity reaction to Janumet or sitagliptin (eg, anaphylaxis or angioedema).

WARNINGS/PRECAUTIONS

Not for use in type 1 diabetes mellitus (DM) or for treatment of diabetic ketoacidosis. Acute pancreatitis, including fatal and nonfatal hemorrhagic or necrotizing pancreatitis, reported; d/c if pancreatitis is suspected and initiate appropriate management. Avoid in patients w/ clinical or lab evidence of hepatic disease. Worsening renal function, including acute renal failure, reported. Assess renal function before initiation of therapy and at least annually thereafter; d/c w/ evidence of renal impairment. Temporarily d/c for any surgical procedure (except minor procedures not associated w/ restricted food and fluid intake); restart when oral intake is resumed and renal function is evaluated as normal. Evaluate patients previously well controlled on therapy who develop lab abnormalities or clinical illness for evidence of ketoacidosis or lactic acidosis; d/c if acidosis of either form occurs. Promptly d/c in the event of cardiovascular collapse (shock) from whatever cause, acute CHF, acute MI, and other conditions characterized by hypoxemia. Temporary loss of glycemic control may occur when a patient is exposed to stress (eg, fever, trauma, infection, surgery); may be necessary to withhold therapy and temporarily administer insulin. Caution in elderly. **Sitagliptin:** Serious hypersensitivity reactions reported; d/c if suspected, assess for other potential causes, and institute alternative treatment for DM. Caution in patients w/ history of angioedema to another DPP-4 inhibitor. Severe and disabling arthralgia reported in patients taking DPP-4 inhibitors; d/c if appropriate. **Metformin:** May decrease serum vitamin B12 levels; monitor hematologic parameters annually. Elderly, debilitated, or malnourished patients, and those w/ adrenal/pituitary insufficiency or alcohol intoxication are particularly susceptible to hypoglycemic effects. Temporarily d/c at the time of or prior to radiologic studies involving the use of intravascular iodinated contrast materials, withhold for 48 hrs subsequent to the procedure, and reinstitute only after renal function is confirmed to be normal.

ADVERSE REACTIONS

Diarrhea, URTI, headache, nausea, abdominal pain.

DRUG INTERACTIONS

See Dosing Considerations. Hypoglycemia may occur w/ other glucose-lowering agents (eg, sulfonylureas, insulin) or ethanol. Topiramate or other carbonic anhydrase inhibitors (eg, zonisamide, acetazolamide, dichlorphenamide) may induce metabolic acidosis; use w/ caution. Thiazides and other diuretics, corticosteroids, phenothiazines, thyroid products, estrogens, oral contraceptives, phenytoin, nicotinic acid, sympathomimetics, calcium channel blockers, and isoniazid tend to produce hyperglycemia and may lead to loss of glycemic control; observe closely when such drugs are administered. **Metformin:** Hypoglycemia may be difficult to recognize w/ β-adrenergic blocking drugs. Alcohol potentiates the effect of metformin on lactate metabolism; avoid excessive alcohol intake. Caution w/ drugs that may affect renal function or result in significant hemodynamic change or interfere w/ the disposition of metformin. Cationic drugs (eg, cimetidine, amiloride, digoxin) that are eliminated by renal tubular secretion may interact w/ metformin; monitor and adjust dose of Janumet and/or the interfering drug.

PATIENT CONSIDERATIONS

Assessment: Assess for previous hypersensitivity to the drug, metabolic acidosis including diabetic ketoacidosis, risk factors for lactic acidosis, renal/hepatic impairment, history of pancreatitis, inadequate vitamin B12 or Ca^{2+} absorption, type of DM, alcoholism, hypoxemia, presence of malnourishment or debilitation, adrenal/pituitary insufficiency, history of angioedema w/ another DPP-4 inhibitor, pregnancy/nursing status, and possible drug interactions. Assess if patient is planning to undergo any surgical procedure, radiologic studies involving the use of intravascular iodinated contrast materials, or is under any form of stress. Obtain baseline FPG and HbA1c levels, and hematologic parameters.

Monitoring: Monitor for signs/symptoms of lactic acidosis, pancreatitis, hypoxic states, hypersensitivity reactions, severe and disabling arthralgia, and other adverse reactions. Monitor for changes in clinical status. Monitor renal function, especially in elderly, at least annually. Monitor hematologic parameters annually. Perform routine serum vitamin B12 measurements at 2- to 3-yr intervals in patients predisposed to developing subnormal vitamin B12 levels. Monitor FPG and HbA1c levels, and hepatic function periodically.

Counseling: Inform of the risks, benefits, and alternative modes of therapy. Advise on the importance of adherence to dietary instructions, regular physical activity, periodic blood glucose monitoring and HbA1c testing, recognition/management of hypo/hyperglycemia, and assessment of diabetic complications. Instruct to seek medical advice during periods of stress (eg, fever, trauma, infection, surgery) as medication needs may change. Inform of the risk of lactic acidosis; instruct to d/c therapy immediately and contact physician if unexplained hyperventilation, myalgia, malaise, unusual somnolence, dizziness, slow or irregular heartbeat, sensation of feeling cold (especially in the extremities), or other nonspecific symptoms occur. Counsel against excessive alcohol intake. Inform that GI symptoms and acute pancreatitis may occur; instruct to d/c therapy promptly and contact physician if persistent severe abdominal pain occurs. Inform that allergic reactions may occur; instruct to d/c therapy and seek medical advice promptly if symptoms occur. Inform that severe and disabling joint pain may occur. Instruct not to split or divide the tabs before swallowing. Instruct to inform physician if any bothersome or unusual symptoms develop, or if any symptoms persist or worsen.

STORAGE: 20-25°C (68-77°F); excursions permitted to 15-30°C (59-86°F).

Janumet XR – metformin hydrochloride/sitagliptin

RX

Class: Biguanide/dipeptidyl peptidase-4 (DPP-4) inhibitor

Lactic acidosis may occur due to metformin accumulation; risk increases w/ conditions such as sepsis, dehydration, excess alcohol intake, hepatic/renal impairment, and acute CHF. If acidosis is suspected, d/c therapy and hospitalize patient immediately.

ADULT DOSAGE

Type 2 Diabetes Mellitus

Adjunct to diet and exercise to improve glycemic control when treatment w/ both sitagliptin and metformin extended-release (ER) is appropriate

Initial:

Not Currently on Metformin: (100mg/1000mg)/day

Currently on Metformin: 100mg/day of sitagliptin + current metformin dose

Currently on Metformin Immediate-Release 850mg bid or 1000mg bid: Two 50mg/1000mg tabs qd

Changing Between Janumet and Janumet XR: Maintain the same total daily dose of sitagliptin and metformin

Titrate: If metformin dose is inadequate to achieve glycemic control, gradually titrate dose to reduce GI side effects

Max: (100mg/2000mg)/day

PEDIATRIC DOSAGE

Pediatric use may not have been established

J

DOSING CONSIDERATIONS

Concomitant Medications

Insulin Secretagogue (eg, Sulfonylurea)/Insulin: May require lower doses of insulin secretagogue or insulin

ADMINISTRATION

Oral route

Take qd w/ a meal, preferably in pm.
Swallow tab whole; do not split, crush, or chew.
Patients taking 2 tabs should take the 2 tabs together qd.
Reports of incompletely dissolved tabs being eliminated in the feces; assess adequacy of glycemic control if patient reports repeatedly seeing tabs in feces.

HOW SUPPLIED

Tab, ER: (Sitagliptin/Metformin ER) 50mg/500mg, 50mg/1000mg, 100mg/1000mg

CONTRAINDICATIONS

Renal impairment (eg, SrCr ≥1.5 mg/dL [men], ≥1.4mg/dL [women] or abnormal CrCl); hypersensitivity to metformin HCl; acute or chronic metabolic acidosis, including diabetic ketoacidosis; history of a serious hypersensitivity reaction to Janumet XR or sitagliptin (eg, anaphylaxis or angioedema).

WARNINGS/PRECAUTIONS

Not for use in type 1 diabetes mellitus or for treatment of diabetic ketoacidosis. Acute pancreatitis, including fatal and nonfatal hemorrhagic or necrotizing pancreatitis, reported; d/c if pancreatitis is suspected and initiate appropriate management. Avoid in patients w/ clinical or lab evidence of hepatic disease. Worsening renal function, including acute renal failure, reported. Assess renal function before initiation of therapy and at least annually thereafter; d/c w/ evidence of renal impairment. Temporarily suspend for any surgical procedure (except minor procedures not associated w/ restricted food and fluid intake); restart when oral intake is resumed and renal function is normal. Evaluate patients previously well controlled on therapy who develop lab abnormalities or clinical illness for evidence of ketoacidosis or lactic acidosis; d/c if acidosis occurs. Promptly d/c in the event of cardiovascular collapse (shock) from whatever cause, acute CHF, acute MI, and other conditions characterized by hypoxemia. Temporary loss of glycemic control may occur when exposed to stress (eg, fever, trauma, infection, surgery); may be necessary to withhold therapy and temporarily administer insulin. Caution in elderly. **Sitagliptin:** Serious hypersensitivity reactions reported; if suspected, d/c therapy, assess for other potential causes, and institute alternative treatment for DM. Caution in patients w/ history of angioedema w/ another DPP-4 inhibitor. Severe and disabling arthralgia reported w/ DPP-4 inhibitors; d/c if appropriate. **Metformin:** May decrease vitamin B12 levels; monitor hematologic parameters annually. Elderly or debilitated/malnourished patients, and those w/ adrenal/pituitary insufficiency or alcohol intoxication are particularly susceptible to hypoglycemic effects. Temporarily d/c at the time of or prior to radiologic studies involving the use of intravascular iodinated contrast materials, withhold for 48 hrs subsequent to the procedure, and reinstitute only if renal function is normal.

ADVERSE REACTIONS

Diarrhea, URTI, headache, nausea, abdominal pain.

DRUG INTERACTIONS

See Dosing Considerations. Hypoglycemia may occur w/ other glucose-lowering agents (eg, sulfonylureas, insulin) or ethanol. Topiramate or other carbonic anhydrase inhibitors (eg, zonisamide, acetazolamide, dichlorphenamide) may induce metabolic acidosis; use w/ caution as risk of lactic acidosis may increase. Thiazides and other diuretics, corticosteroids, phenothiazines, thyroid products, estrogens, oral contraceptives, phenytoin, nicotinic acid, sympathomimetics, calcium channel blockers, and isoniazid may produce hyperglycemia and lead to loss of glycemic control; observe closely when such drugs are administered. **Metformin:** May be difficult to recognize hypoglycemia w/ β-adrenergic blocking drugs. Alcohol potentiates the effects of metformin on lactate metabolism; avoid excessive alcohol intake. Caution w/ drugs that may affect renal function or result in significant hemodynamic change. Cationic drugs (eg, cimetidine, amiloride, digoxin) that are eliminated by renal tubular secretion may potentially produce an interaction; monitor and adjust dose of Janumet XR and/or the interfering drug.

J

PATIENT CONSIDERATIONS

Assessment: Assess for metabolic acidosis including diabetic ketoacidosis, risk factors for lactic acidosis, renal/hepatic impairment, previous hypersensitivity to the drug, history of pancreatitis, inadequate vitamin B12 or Ca^{2+} intake/absorption, type of DM, alcoholism, hypoxemia, presence of malnourishment or debilitation, adrenal/pituitary insufficiency, history of angioedema w/ another DPP-4 inhibitor, pregnancy/nursing status, and possible drug interactions. Assess if patient is planning to undergo any surgical procedure, radiologic studies involving the use of intravascular iodinated contrast materials, or is under any form of stress. Obtain baseline FPG and HbA1c levels, and hematologic parameters.

Monitoring: Monitor for signs/symptoms of lactic acidosis, pancreatitis, hypoxic states, hypersensitivity reactions, and other adverse reactions. Monitor for changes in clinical status. Monitor renal function, especially in elderly, at least annually. Monitor hematologic parameters annually. Perform routine serum vitamin B12 measurements at 2- to 3-yr intervals in patients predisposed to developing subnormal vitamin B12 levels. Monitor FPG and HbA1c levels, and hepatic function periodically.

Counseling: Inform of the risks, benefits, and alternative modes of therapy. Advise on the importance of adherence to dietary instructions, regular physical activity, periodic blood glucose monitoring and HbA1c testing, regular testing of renal function and hematologic parameters, recognition/management of hypo/hyperglycemia, and assessment of diabetes complications. Instruct to seek medical advice during periods of stress (eg, fever, trauma, infection, surgery) as medication needs may change. Inform of the risk of lactic acidosis; instruct to d/c therapy immediately and notify physician if unexplained hyperventilation, myalgia, malaise, unusual somnolence, dizziness, slow or irregular heartbeat, sensation of feeling cold (especially in the extremities), or other nonspecific symptoms occur. Counsel against excessive alcohol intake. Inform that GI symptoms may occur. Inform that acute pancreatitis may occur; instruct to d/c therapy promptly and contact physician if persistent severe abdominal pain occurs. Inform that allergic reactions may occur; instruct to d/c therapy and seek medical advice promptly if symptoms occur. Inform that severe and disabling joint pain may occur. Inform that incompletely dissolved tabs may be eliminated in the feces; advise to report to physician if patient repeatedly sees tabs in feces. Instruct to inform physician if any bothersome or unusual symptom develops, or if any known symptom persists or worsens.

STORAGE: 20-25°C (68-77°F); excursions permitted to 15-30°C (59-86°F). Store in a dry place.

JANUVIA – sitagliptin

RX

Class: Dipeptidyl peptidase-4 (DPP-4) inhibitor

ADULT DOSAGE

Type 2 Diabetes Mellitus

100mg qd

PEDIATRIC DOSAGE

Pediatric use may not have been established

DOSING CONSIDERATIONS

Concomitant Medications

Insulin Secretagogue (eg, Sulfonylurea)/Insulin: May require lower dose of insulin secretagogue or insulin

Renal Impairment

Moderate (CrCl ≥30 to <50mL/min): 50mg qd
Severe (CrCl <30mL/min): 25mg qd
ESRD Requiring Hemodialysis/Peritoneal Dialysis: 25mg qd; administer w/o regard to timing of dialysis

ADMINISTRATION

Oral route

May be taken w/ or w/o food.

HOW SUPPLIED

Tab: 25mg, 50mg, 100mg

CONTRAINDICATIONS

History of a serious hypersensitivity reaction to sitagliptin (eg, anaphylaxis or angioedema).

WARNINGS/PRECAUTIONS

Not for use w/ type 1 diabetes mellitus (DM) or for treatment of diabetic ketoacidosis. Acute pancreatitis reported; d/c if pancreatitis is suspected. Worsening renal function, including acute renal failure, reported. Severe and disabling arthralgia reported in patients taking DPP-4 inhibitors. Serious hypersensitivity reactions reported; if suspected, d/c therapy, assess for other potential causes, and institute alternative treatment. Caution in patients w/ a history of angioedema w/ another DPP-4 inhibitor and in the elderly.

ADVERSE REACTIONS

Nasopharyngitis, URTI, headache.

DRUG INTERACTIONS

See Dosing Considerations. May slightly increase digoxin levels; monitor appropriately.

PATIENT CONSIDERATIONS

Assessment: Assess for previous hypersensitivity to the drug, type of DM, diabetic ketoacidosis, history of pancreatitis, history of angioedema w/ another DPP-4 inhibitor, pregnancy/nursing status, and possible drug interactions. Obtain baseline renal function, FPG, and HbA1c levels.

Monitoring: Monitor for pancreatitis, hypersensitivity reactions, and other adverse reactions. Monitor FPG, HbA1c, and renal function periodically.

Counseling: Inform of risks, benefits, and alternative modes of therapy. Advise on the importance of adherence to dietary instructions, regular physical activity, periodic blood glucose monitoring, HbA1c testing, recognition/management of hypo/hyperglycemia, and assessment of diabetic complications. Instruct to seek medical advice during periods of stress as medication requirements may change. Instruct to d/c use and notify physician if signs and symptoms of pancreatitis or allergic reactions occur. Instruct to inform physician if any unusual symptom develops, or if any known symptom persists or worsens. Inform patients that severe and disabling joint pain may occur and to seek medical advice if severe joint pain occurs.

STORAGE: 20-25°C (68-77°F); excursions permitted to 15-30°C (59-86°F).

JARDIANCE – empagliflozin RX

Class: Sodium-glucose cotransporter 2 (SGLT2) inhibitor

ADULT DOSAGE

Type 2 Diabetes Mellitus

Recommended Dose: 10mg qam
Titrate: May increase to 25mg in patients tolerating therapy

PEDIATRIC DOSAGE

Pediatric use may not have been established

DOSING CONSIDERATIONS

Renal Impairment

Baseline eGFR <45mL/min/1.73m²: Do not initiate treatment
eGFR Persistently <45mL/min/1.73m²: D/C treatment

Other Important Considerations

Patients w/ Volume Depletion: Correct this condition prior to initiating therapy

ADMINISTRATION

Oral route

Take w/ or w/o food.

HOW SUPPLIED

Tab: 10mg, 25mg

CONTRAINDICATIONS

History of serious hypersensitivity reaction to empagliflozin, severe renal impairment, ESRD, dialysis.

WARNINGS/PRECAUTIONS

Not recommended w/ type 1 diabetes mellitus (DM) or for treatment of diabetic ketoacidosis. Causes intravascular volume contraction. Symptomatic hypotension may occur, particularly in patients w/ renal impairment, the elderly, in patients w/ low systolic BP, and in patients on diuretics; assess for volume contraction and correct volume status before initiating treatment, if indicated. Monitor for signs/symptoms of hypotension after initiating therapy and increase monitoring in clinical situations where volume contraction is expected. Ketoacidosis reported; if suspected, d/c and institute prompt treatment. Assess for ketoacidosis in patients presenting w/ signs/symptoms consistent w/ severe metabolic acidosis regardless of presenting blood glucose levels. Consider temporarily discontinuing therapy in clinical situations known to predispose to ketoacidosis (eg, prolonged fasting due to acute illness or surgery). Increases SrCr and decreases eGFR; risk of impaired renal function is increased in elderly patients and patients w/ moderate renal impairment. Serious UTIs (eg, urosepsis, pyelonephritis), requiring hospitalization, reported; evaluate for signs/symptoms of UTIs and treat promptly, if indicated. Increases risk for genital mycotic infections; monitor and treat as appropriate. Increases in LDL levels may occur. Monitoring glycemic control w/ urine glucose tests or 1,5-anhydroglucitol assay is not recommended.

ADVERSE REACTIONS

UTIs, genital mycotic infections, dyslipidemia, increased urination, URTI.

J

DRUG INTERACTIONS

Increased risk of hypoglycemia w/ insulin secretagogues (eg, sulfonylurea) or insulin; a lower dose of the insulin secretagogue or insulin may be required. Coadministration w/ diuretics resulted in increased urine volume and frequency of voids, which might enhance the potential for volume depletion.

PATIENT CONSIDERATIONS

Assessment: Assess for diabetic ketoacidosis, type of DM, volume contraction, history of chronic/recurrent genital mycotic infections, drug hypersensitivity, predisposition to ketoacidosis, pregnancy/nursing status, and possible drug interactions. Assess baseline renal function, LDL levels, and BP.

Monitoring: Monitor for signs/symptoms of hypotension, ketoacidosis, genital mycotic infections, UTIs, and other adverse reactions. Monitor renal function and LDL levels.

Counseling: Inform of the risks, benefits, and alternative modes of therapy. Advise about the importance of adherence to dietary instructions, regular physical activity, periodic blood glucose monitoring and HbA1c testing, recognition and management of hypoglycemia and hyperglycemia, and assessment for diabetes complications. Instruct to seek medical advice promptly during periods of stress (eg, fever, trauma, infection), as medication requirements may change. Instruct to inform physician if pregnant/nursing, if experiencing symptoms of hypotension, if any unusual symptom develops, or if any known symptom persists or worsens. Instruct to have adequate fluid intake. Instruct to d/c and seek medical advice immediately if symptoms of ketoacidosis occur. Counsel on the signs/symptoms of UTIs, vaginal yeast infections, balanitis, and balanoposthitis; inform of treatment options and when to seek medical advice.

STORAGE: 25°C (77°F); excursions permitted to 15-30°C (59-86°F).

JENTADUETO — linagliptin/metformin hydrochloride — RX

Class: Biguanide/dipeptidyl peptidase-4 (DPP-4) inhibitor

Lactic acidosis may occur due to metformin accumulation; risk increases w/ conditions such as sepsis, dehydration, excess alcohol intake, hepatic/renal impairment, and acute CHF. If acidosis is suspected, d/c therapy and hospitalize patient immediately.

ADULT DOSAGE

Type 2 Diabetes Mellitus

Initial Dose:

Not Currently on Metformin: 2.5mg/500mg bid

Currently on Metformin: 2.5mg linagliptin + current metformin dose taken at each of the 2 daily meals (eg, a patient on

PEDIATRIC DOSAGE

Pediatric use may not have been established

metformin 1000mg bid would be started on 2.5mg/1000mg bid)

Currently on Linagliptin and Metformin Individually: Switch to Jentadueto containing the same doses of each component

Titrate: Dose escalation should be gradual to reduce the GI side effects associated w/ metformin use

Max: 2.5mg/1000mg bid

DOSING CONSIDERATIONS

Concomitant Medications

Insulin Secretagogue (eg, Sulfonylurea)/Insulin: May require lower dose of insulin secretagogue or insulin

ADMINISTRATION

Oral route

Take w/ meals.

HOW SUPPLIED

Tab: (Linagliptin/Metformin) 2.5mg/500mg, 2.5mg/850mg, 2.5mg/1000mg

CONTRAINDICATIONS

Renal impairment (eg, SrCr ≥1.5mg/dL [men], ≥1.4mg/dL [women], or abnormal CrCl); acute or chronic metabolic acidosis, including diabetic ketoacidosis; history of hypersensitivity reaction to linagliptin (eg, anaphylaxis, angioedema, exfoliative skin conditions, urticaria, or bronchial hyperreactivity); hypersensitivity to metformin.

WARNINGS/PRECAUTIONS

Not for use in type 1 diabetes mellitus (DM) or for treatment of diabetic ketoacidosis. Promptly d/c in the event of cardiovascular collapse (shock) from whatever cause (eg, acute CHF, acute MI, other conditions characterized by hypoxemia). Caution in elderly. **Linagliptin:** Acute pancreatitis, including fatal pancreatitis, reported; d/c if suspected and initiate appropriate management. If therapy is discontinued due to renal impairment, may continue linagliptin as a single entity tab. Serious hypersensitivity reactions reported; d/c if suspected, assess for other potential causes, and institute alternative treatment for DM. Caution in patients w/ history of angioedema to another DPP-4 inhibitor. Severe and disabling arthralgia reported; d/c if therapy is a possible cause for severe joint pain. **Metformin:** D/C if evidence of renal impairment is present. Temporarily d/c at the time of or prior to radiologic studies involving the use of intravascular iodinated contrast materials, withhold for 48 hrs subsequent to the procedure, and reinstitute only after renal function is confirmed to be normal. Temporarily d/c for any surgical procedure (except minor procedures not associated w/ restricted food and fluid intake); restart when oral intake is resumed and renal function is evaluated as normal. Avoid in patients w/ clinical or lab evidence of hepatic disease. Elderly, debilitated, or malnourished patients, and those w/ adrenal/pituitary insufficiency or alcohol intoxication are particularly susceptible to hypoglycemic effects. May decrease serum vitamin B12 to subnormal levels; monitor hematologic parameters annually.

ADVERSE REACTIONS

Nasopharyngitis, diarrhea, hypoglycemia.

DRUG INTERACTIONS

See Dosing Considerations. Thiazides and other diuretics, corticosteroids, phenothiazines, thyroid products, estrogens, oral contraceptives, phenytoin, nicotinic acid, sympathomimetics, calcium channel blockers, and isoniazid tend to produce hyperglycemia and may lead to loss of glycemic control; observe closely for hypoglycemia when such drugs are withdrawn. **Linagliptin:** Increased risk of hypoglycemia w/ insulin or insulin secretagogue (eg, sulfonylurea); may require lower dose of insulin or insulin secretagogue. Rifampin decreased linagliptin exposure, suggesting that strong P-gp or CYP3A4 inducers may reduce efficacy; use alternative treatments (not containing linagliptin) when a strong P-gp or CYP3A4 inducer is necessary. **Metformin:** Caution w/ drugs that may affect renal function, result in significant hemodynamic change, or interfere w/ the disposition of metformin. Hypoglycemia may occur w/ other glucose-lowering agents (eg, sulfonylureas, insulin) or ethanol. Hypoglycemia may be difficult to recognize w/ β-adrenergic blocking drugs. Alcohol potentiates the effect of metformin on lactate metabolism; avoid excessive alcohol intake. Cationic drugs (eg, cimetidine, amiloride, digoxin) that are eliminated by renal tubular secretion may potentially produce an interaction; monitor and adjust dose of Jentadueto and/or the interfering drug. Topiramate or other carbonic anhydrase inhibitors (eg, zonisamide, acetazolamide, dichlorphenamide) may induce metabolic acidosis; use w/ caution.

PATIENT CONSIDERATIONS

Assessment: Assess for metabolic acidosis, risk factors for lactic acidosis, renal/hepatic impairment, previous hypersensitivity to the drug, history of pancreatitis, inadequate vitamin B12 or Ca^{2+} intake/absorption, type of DM, diabetic ketoacidosis, alcoholism, hypoxemia, presence of malnourishment or debilitation, adrenal/pituitary insufficiency, history of angioedema w/ another DPP-4 inhibitor, pregnancy/nursing status, and possible drug interactions. Assess if patient is planning to undergo any surgical procedure, radiologic studies involving the use of intravascular iodinated contrast materials, or is under any form of stress. Obtain baseline FPG and HbA1c levels, and hematologic parameters.

Monitoring: Monitor for signs/symptoms of lactic acidosis, pancreatitis, hypoxic states, hypersensitivity reactions, severe joint pain, and other adverse reactions. Monitor renal function, especially in elderly, at least annually. Monitor hematologic parameters annually. Perform routine serum vitamin B12 measurement at 2- to 3-yr intervals in patients predisposed to developing subnormal vitamin B12 levels. Monitor FPG and HbA1c levels and hepatic function periodically.

Counseling: Inform of the risks and benefits of therapy. Advise on the importance of adherence to dietary instructions, regular physical activity, periodic blood glucose monitoring and HbA1c testing, recognition/management of hypo/hyperglycemia, and assessment for diabetes complications. Instruct to seek medical advice promptly during periods of stress as medication needs may change. Inform of the risk of lactic acidosis; instruct to d/c therapy immediately and contact physician if unexplained hyperventilation, malaise, myalgia, unusual somnolence, slow or irregular heartbeat, sensation of feeling cold (especially in the extremities), or other nonspecific symptoms occur. Inform that GI symptoms and acute pancreatitis may occur; instruct to d/c therapy promptly and contact physician if persistent severe abdominal pain occurs. Instruct to inform of Jentadueto use prior to any surgical or radiological procedure. Inform that allergic reactions may occur; instruct to d/c therapy and seek medical advice promptly if symptoms occur. Advise against excessive alcohol intake. Inform that severe and disabling joint pain may occur; instruct to seek medical advice if this occurs.

STORAGE: 25°C (77°F); excursions permitted to 15-30°C (59-86°F). Protect from exposure to high humidity.

JUBLIA – efinaconazole

RX

Class: Azole antifungal

ADULT DOSAGE

Fungal Infections

Onychomycosis of the Toenail(s) Due to Trichophyton rubrum and Trichophyton mentagrophytes:

Apply to affected toenails qd for 48 weeks

PEDIATRIC DOSAGE

Pediatric use may not have been established

ADMINISTRATION

Topical route

Apply using the integrated flow-through brush applicator.

When applying, ensure toenail, toenail folds, toenail bed, hyponychium, and undersurface of toenail plate are completely covered.

HOW SUPPLIED

Sol: 10% [4mL, 8mL]

WARNINGS/PRECAUTIONS

Not for oral, ophthalmic, or intravaginal use.

ADVERSE REACTIONS

Ingrown toenail, application-site dermatitis/vesicles/pain.

PATIENT CONSIDERATIONS

Assessment: Assess pregnancy/nursing status.

Monitoring: Monitor for adverse reactions.

Counseling: Inform that therapy is for use on toenails and immediately adjacent skin only. Instruct to use ud to clean dry toenails and to wait for at least 10 min after showering, bathing, or washing before applying. Advise to inform physician if the area of application shows signs of persistent irritation (eg, redness, itching, swelling). Inform that the impact of nail polish or other cosmetic nail products on the efficacy of therapy has not been evaluated.

STORAGE: 20-25°C (68-77°F); excursions permitted to 15-30°C (59-86°F). Store in upright position. Flammable; keep away from heat or flame. Protect from freezing.

JUXTAPID — lomitapide

RX

Class: Lipid-regulating agent

May cause elevations in transaminases; measure ALT, AST, alkaline phosphatase, and total bilirubin prior to therapy, and then ALT/AST regularly as recommended. Adjust dose if ALT/AST is ≥3X ULN. D/C for clinically significant liver toxicity. May increase hepatic fat w/ or w/o increases in transaminases. Hepatic steatosis associated w/ lomitapide treatment may be a risk factor for progressive liver disease, including steatohepatitis and cirrhosis. Available only through a restricted program under a Risk Evaluation and Mitigation Strategy (REMS) because of the risk of hepatotoxicity.

ADULT DOSAGE

Homozygous Familial Hypercholesterolemia

Prior to treatment, initiate a low-fat diet supplying <20% of energy from fat

Initial: 5mg qd
Titrate: After ≥2 weeks, may increase dose to 10mg qd; and then at ≥4-week intervals, may increase to 20mg qd, then 40mg qd, and then up to a max of 60mg qd
Max: 60mg qd

PEDIATRIC DOSAGE

Pediatric use may not have been established

DOSING CONSIDERATIONS

Concomitant Medications
Weak CYP3A4 Inhibitors:
Max: 30mg/day

Renal Impairment
ESRD Receiving Dialysis:
Max: 40mg/day

Hepatic Impairment
Mild (Child-Pugh A):
Max: 40mg/day

Adverse Reactions
ALT/AST ≥3X and <5X ULN:
Confirm elevation w/ repeat measurement w/in 1 week
If confirmed, reduce dose and obtain additional liver-related tests if not already measured (eg, alkaline phosphatase, total bilirubin, INR)
Repeat tests weekly and withhold dosing if signs of abnormal liver function (increase in bilirubin/INR) are present, if transaminase levels rise above 5X ULN, or if transaminase levels do not fall below 3X ULN w/in approx 4 weeks; investigate to identify probable cause in these cases of persistent or worsening abnormalities
Consider reducing dose and monitor liver-related tests more frequently if resuming therapy after transaminases resolve to <3X ULN

ALT/AST ≥5X ULN:
Withhold dosing, obtain additional liver-related tests if not already measured (eg, alkaline phosphatase, total bilirubin, INR), and investigate to identify probable cause
Reduce dose and monitor liver-related tests more frequently if resuming therapy after transaminases resolve to <3X ULN

If transaminase elevations are accompanied by clinical symptoms of liver injury, increases in bilirubin ≥2X ULN, or active liver disease, d/c treatment and investigate to identify probable cause

ADMINISTRATION

Oral route

Take qd w/ a glass of water, w/o food, at least 2 hrs after pm meal
Swallow cap whole; do not open, crush, dissolve, or chew
Take daily supplements containing 400 IU vitamin E and at least 200mg linoleic acid, 210mg α-linolenic acid, 110mg eicosapentaenoic acid, and 80mg docosahexaenoic acid

HOW SUPPLIED

Cap: 5mg, 10mg, 20mg, 30mg, 40mg, 60mg

CONTRAINDICATIONS

Pregnancy, moderate or severe hepatic impairment (based on Child-Pugh category B or C), active liver disease including unexplained persistent elevations of serum transaminases, concomitant moderate or strong CYP3A4 inhibitors.

WARNINGS/PRECAUTIONS

If baseline LFTs are abnormal, consider initiating therapy after an appropriate work-up and the baseline abnormalities are explained or resolved. May cause fetal harm; females of reproductive potential should have a negative pregnancy test before initiation of therapy and use effective contraception during therapy. May reduce absorption of fat-soluble nutrients, especially in patients w/ chronic bowel or pancreatic diseases that predispose to malabsorption. GI adverse reactions reported; absorption of concomitant oral medications may be affected in patients who develop diarrhea or vomiting. Avoid in patients w/ rare hereditary problems of galactose intolerance, Lapp lactase deficiency, or glucose-galactose malabsorption; may result in diarrhea and malabsorption. Caution in elderly.

ADVERSE REACTIONS

Hepatic steatosis, increased serum transaminases, diarrhea, N/V, dyspepsia, abdominal pain/discomfort/distention, weight loss, constipation, flatulence, chest pain, influenza, nasopharyngitis, fatigue.

DRUG INTERACTIONS

See Dosing Considerations and Contraindications. Not recommended w/ other LDL-lowering agents that can increase hepatic fat. Avoid grapefruit juice. Alcohol may increase levels of hepatic fat and induce/exacerbate liver injury; avoid consumption of >1 alcoholic drink/day. Caution w/ other medications known to have potential for hepatotoxicity (eg, isotretinoin, amiodarone, acetaminophen [>4g/day for ≥3 days/week]). Increased exposure w/ weak CYP3A4 inhibitors (eg, alprazolam, atorvastatin, cimetidine, oral contraceptives). May increase INR and plasma concentrations of both R(+)-warfarin and S(-)-warfarin; regularly monitor INR (particularly after any changes in lomitapide dosage) and adjust dose of warfarin as clinically indicated. May double the exposure of simvastatin; refer to simvastatin PI for dosing recommendations. May increase the exposure of lovastatin; consider reducing dose of lovastatin when initiating therapy. May increase the absorption of P-gp substrates (eg, aliskiren, colchicine, digoxin, sirolimus); consider dose reduction of the P-gp substrate. Separate dosing by at least 4 hrs w/ bile acid sequestrants.

PATIENT CONSIDERATIONS

Assessment: Assess for active liver disease, including unexplained persistent elevations of serum transaminases, bowel/pancreatic disease, galactose intolerance, renal dysfunction, pregnancy/nursing status, and possible drug interactions. Measure ALT/AST, alkaline phosphatase, and serum bilirubin prior to therapy.

Monitoring: Monitor for hepatic steatosis, hepatotoxicity, and GI and other adverse reactions. Monitor renal/hepatic function. During the 1st yr, perform hepatic-related tests (eg, ALT, AST) prior to each increase in dose or monthly, whichever occurs 1st. After the 1st yr, perform these tests at least every 3 months and before any dose increase. Monitor INR w/ warfarin.

Counseling: Encourage to participate in the registry to monitor/evaluate long-term effects and inform that participation is voluntary. Advise that medication is only available from certified pharmacies enrolled in the REMS program. Discuss the importance of liver-related tests before initiation, prior to each dose escalation, and periodically thereafter. Advise of the potential for increased risk of liver injury if alcohol is consumed and instruct to limit alcohol consumption to not >1 drink/day. Advise to report any symptoms of possible liver injury (eg, fever, jaundice, lethargy, flu-like symptoms). Advise females of reproductive potential to have a negative pregnancy test before starting treatment and to use effective contraception while on therapy. Discuss the importance of taking daily supplements. Inform that GI adverse reactions are common and that strict adherence to a low-fat diet (<20% of total calories from fat) may reduce these reactions. Inform that absorption of oral medications may be affected in patients who develop diarrhea or vomiting; instruct to seek physician's advice if symptoms develop. Instruct to omit grapefruit juice from diet; advise to inform physician about all medications, nutritional supplements, and vitamins taken. If a dose is missed, instruct to take the normal dose at the usual time the next day; if dose is interrupted for more than a week, advise to contact physician before restarting treatment.

STORAGE: 20-25°C (68-77°F); excursions permitted to 15-30°C (59-86°F). May tolerate brief exposure up to 40°C (104°F), provided the mean kinetic temperature does not exceed 25°C (77°F); however, such exposure should be minimized. Protect from moisture.

KALETRA – lopinavir/ritonavir

RX

Class: Protease inhibitor

ADULT DOSAGE

HIV-1 Infection

In Combination w/ Other Antiretrovirals:

<3 Lopinavir Resistance-Associated Substitutions:
400mg/100mg bid or 800mg/200mg qd

≥3 Resistance-Associated Substitutions:
400mg/100mg bid

PEDIATRIC DOSAGE

HIV-1 Infection

In Combination w/ Other Antiretrovirals:

14 Days-6 Months of Age:
Sol:
Weight-Based: 16mg/4mg/kg bid
BSA-Based: 300mg/75mg/m² bid
Therapy is not recommended in combination w/ efavirenz, nevirapine, or nelfinavir in patients <6 months or age

6 Months-18 Years:
W/O Concomitant Efavirenz, Nevirapine, or Nelfinavir:
Sol:
Weight-Based:
<15kg: 12mg/3mg/kg bid
≥15-40kg: 10mg/2.5mg/kg bid
Max: 400mg/100mg bid
BSA-Based: 230mg/57.5mg/m² bid
Max: 400mg/100mg bid
Tab:
Weight-Based:
15-25kg: 200mg/50mg bid
>25-35kg: 300mg/75mg bid
>35kg: 400mg/100mg bid
BSA-Based:
≥0.6 to <0.9m²: 200mg/50mg bid
≥0.9 to <1.4m²: 300mg/75mg bid
≥1.4m²: 400mg/100mg bid

DOSING CONSIDERATIONS

Concomitant Medications

Combination w/ Efavirenz/Nevirapine/Nelfinavir:
6 Months-18 Years:
Sol:
Weight-Based:
<15kg: 13mg/3.25mg/kg bid
>15-45kg: 11mg/2.75mg/kg bid
Max: 533mg/133mg bid
BSA-Based: Increase dose to 300mg/75mg/m² bid
Max: 533mg/133mg bid
Tab:
Weight-Based:
15-20kg: 200mg/50mg bid
>20-30kg: 300mg/75mg bid
>30-45kg: 400mg/100mg bid
>45kg: 500mg/125mg bid
BSA-Based:
≥0.6 to <0.8m²: 200mg/50mg bid
≥0.8 to <1.2m²: 300mg/75mg bid
≥1.2 to <1.7m²: 400mg/100mg bid
≥1.7m²: 500mg/125mg bid
Adults:
Increase dose to 500mg/125mg bid

ADMINISTRATION

Oral route

Tab
Take w/ or w/o food.
Swallow whole; do not crush, break, or chew.

Sol
Take w/ food.

HOW SUPPLIED

(Lopinavir/Ritonavir) **Sol:** (80mg/20mg)/mL [160mL]; **Tab:** 100mg/25mg, 200mg/50mg

CONTRAINDICATIONS

Previously demonstrated clinically significant hypersensitivity (eg, toxic epidermal necrolysis, Stevens-Johnson syndrome, erythema multiforme, urticaria, angioedema) to Kaletra or any of its components. Coadministration w/ CYP3A substrates for which elevated plasma concentrations are associated w/ serious and/or life-threatening reactions and w/ potent CYP3A inducers where significantly reduced lopinavir levels may be associated w/ the potential for loss of virologic response and possible resistance and cross-resistance (eg, alfuzosin, rifampin, dihydroergotamine, ergotamine, methylergonovine, St. John's wort, cisapride, lovastatin, simvastatin, sildenafil [when used to treat pulmonary arterial HTN], pimozide, triazolam, oral midazolam).

WARNINGS/PRECAUTIONS

Avoid sol in preterm neonates in the immediate postnatal period; preterm neonates may be at increased risk of propylene glycol-associated adverse events and other toxicities. Pancreatitis, including marked TG elevations, reported; evaluate and suspend therapy if clinically appropriate. Patients w/ underlying hepatitis B or C or marked serum transaminase elevations prior to treatment may be at increased risk for developing or worsening of transaminase elevations or hepatic decompensation; conduct appropriate lab testing prior to therapy and monitor closely during treatment. New onset or exacerbation of diabetes mellitus (DM), hyperglycemia, diabetic ketoacidosis, immune reconstitution syndrome, autoimmune disorders (eg, Graves' disease, polymyositis, Guillain-Barre syndrome) in the setting of immune reconstitution, redistribution/accumulation of body fat, lipid elevations, and increased bleeding w/ hemophilia A and B reported. PR and QT interval prolongation, torsades de pointes, and cases of 2nd- and 3rd-degree atrioventricular block reported; caution w/ underlying structural heart disease, preexisting conduction system abnormalities, ischemic heart disease, or cardiomyopathies. Avoid use w/ congenital long QT syndrome or hypokalemia and w/ other drugs that prolong QT interval. QD regimen is not recommended for adults w/ ≥3 lopinavir resistance-associated substitutions or in pediatric patients <18 yrs. Caution w/ hepatic impairment and in elderly.

ADVERSE REACTIONS

Diarrhea, N/V, hypertriglyceridemia and hypercholesterolemia, dysgeusia, rash, decreased weight, insomnia.

DRUG INTERACTIONS

See Contraindications and Dosing Considerations. Caution w/ drugs that prolong the PR interval (eg, calcium channel blockers [CCBs], β-adrenergic blockers, digoxin, atazanavir). Avoid w/ colchicine in patients w/ renal/hepatic impairment, tadalafil during initiation, tipranavir/ritonavir combination, and drugs that prolong the QT interval. Not recommended w/ voriconazole, high doses of itraconazole or ketoconazole, boceprevir, telaprevir, avanafil, salmeterol, and simeprevir. Not recommended w/ fluticasone or other glucocorticoids that are metabolized by CYP3A unless benefit outweighs the risk of systemic corticosteroid effects. Cushing's syndrome and adrenal suppression reported w/ budesonide and fluticasone propionate. May increase levels of CYP3A substrates, colchicine, fentanyl, tenofovir, indinavir, nelfinavir, saquinavir, maraviroc, antiarrhythmics, vincristine, vinblastine, dasatinib, nilotinib, trazodone, itraconazole, ketoconazole, rifabutin and rifabutin metabolite, clarithromycin in patients w/ renal impairment, IV midazolam, dihydropyridine CCB, bosentan, atorvastatin, rosuvastatin, immunosuppressants, salmeterol, rivaroxaban, glucocorticoids, sildenafil, tadalafil, vardenafil, rilpivirine, simeprevir, and quetiapine. May decrease levels of methadone, phenytoin, bupropion, atovaquone, ethinyl estradiol, abacavir, zidovudine, lamotrigine, valproate, voriconazole, boceprevir, amprenavir, and etravirine. Delavirdine and CYP3A inhibitors may increase levels. May alter concentrations of warfarin; monitor INR. Efavirenz, nevirapine, nelfinavir, carbamazepine, phenobarbital, and phenytoin may decrease levels; not for qd dosing regimen. Rifampin, fosamprenavir/ritonavir, systemic corticosteroids, and CYP3A inducers may decrease levels. May require initiation or dose adjustments of insulin or oral hypoglycemics for treatment of DM. **Sol:** Contains alcohol; may produce disulfiram-like reactions w/ disulfiram or metronidazole. Didanosine should be given 1 hr before or 2 hrs after sol. Refer to PI for further information and dosing modifications when used w/ certain concomitant therapies.

PATIENT CONSIDERATIONS

Assessment: Assess for history of hypersensitivity reactions, history of pancreatitis, hepatitis B or C, cirrhosis, DM or hyperglycemia, dyslipidemia, hemophilia type A or B, structural heart disease, preexisting conduction system abnormalities, ischemic heart disease or cardiomyopathies, congenital long QT syndrome, hypokalemia, renal/hepatic impairment, pregnancy/nursing status, and for possible drug interactions. Assess children for the ability to swallow intact tab.

Monitoring: Monitor for signs/symptoms of pancreatitis, hyperglycemia, hepatic dysfunction, immune reconstitution syndrome, autoimmune disorders, fat redistribution/accumulation, hypersensitivity reactions, and other adverse reactions. Monitor lipid profile, glucose levels, total bilirubin levels, ECG changes, serum lipase levels, and serum amylase levels. Monitor infants for increase in serum osmolality, SrCr, and other toxicities.

Counseling: Instruct to take prescribed dose ud. Advise to inform physician if weight changes in children occur. Inform that if a dose is missed, a dose should be taken as soon as possible and to return to normal schedule; instruct not to double the next dose. Advise that therapy is not a cure for HIV; opportunistic infections may still occur. Instruct to avoid doing things that can spread HIV-1 infection to others. Instruct not to have any kind of sex w/o protection; advise to always practice safe sex by using a latex or polyurethane condom to lower the chance of sexual contact w/ semen, vaginal secretions, or blood. Instruct to notify physician if using other prescription/OTC or herbal products, particularly St. John's wort. Inform that skin rashes, liver function changes, ECG changes, redistribution/accumulation of body fat, new onset or worsening of preexisting diabetes, and hyperglycemia may occur. Instruct to seek medical attention if symptoms of worsening liver disease (eg, loss of appetite, abdominal pain, jaundice, itchy skin), dizziness, abnormal heart rhythm, loss of consciousness, or any other adverse reactions develop.

STORAGE: **Tab:** 20-25°C (68-77°F); excursions permitted to 15-30°C (59-86°F). **Sol:** 2-8°C (36-46°F). Avoid exposure to excessive heat. If stored at room temperature up to 25°C (77°F), sol should be used w/in 2 months.

KANUMA – sebelipase alfa

Class: Enzyme

RX

ADULT DOSAGE

Lysosomal Acid Lipase Deficiency

1mg/kg IV infusion once every other week

PEDIATRIC DOSAGE

Lysosomal Acid Lipase Deficiency

Rapidly Progressive Lysosomal Acid Lipase (LAL) Deficiency Presenting w/in First 6 Months of Life:

Initial: 1mg/kg IV infusion once weekly

Titrate: Increase to 3mg/kg once weekly if optimal response is not achieved

Pediatric Patients w/ LAL Deficiency:

1mg/kg IV infusion once every other week

ADMINISTRATION

IV route

Vials are for single-use only; discard any unused product.

Use immediately after dilution; if immediate use is not possible, store ≤24 hrs at 2-8°C (36-46°F).

Do not freeze or shake.

Protect from light.

Preparation

1. Determine the number of vials needed based on the patient's weight and the recommended dose of 1mg/kg or 3mg/kg.
2. Round to the next whole vial and remove required number of vials from refrigerator and allow to reach room temperature.
3. Mix gently by inversion; do not shake vials or prepared infusion.

Administration

Administer sol as an IV infusion using a low-protein binding infusion set w/ an in-line, low-protein binding 0.2 micron filter.

Infuse over ≥2 hrs; consider further prolonging the infusion time for patients receiving 3mg/kg dose or those who have experienced hypersensitivity reactions.

A 1-hr infusion may be considered for patients receiving 1mg/kg dose who tolerate the infusion.

HOW SUPPLIED

Inj: 20mg/10mL

WARNINGS/PRECAUTIONS

Hypersensitivity reactions, including anaphylaxis, reported; immediately d/c infusion and initiate appropriate medical treatment if anaphylaxis occurs. Management of hypersensitivity reactions should be based on severity of the reaction and may include temporarily interrupting infusion, lowering infusion rate, and/or treatment w/ antihistamines, antipyretics, and/or corticosteroids. If interrupted, infusion may resume at a slower rate w/ increases as tolerated. Pretreatment w/ antipyretics and/or antihistamines may prevent subsequent reactions. Immediately d/c infusion and initiate appropriate medical treatment if a severe hypersensitivity reaction occurs; consider risks/benefits of readministration following a severe reaction. Observe closely during and after infusion. Produced in the egg whites of genetically engineered chickens; caution w/ known systemic hypersensitivity reactions to eggs or egg products.

ADVERSE REACTIONS

Rapidly Progressive Disease Presenting w/in First 6 Months of Life: Diarrhea, vomiting, fever, rhinitis, anemia, cough, nasopharyngitis, urticaria.

Pediatrics and Adults: Headache, fever, oropharyngeal pain, nasopharyngitis, asthenia, constipation, nausea.

PATIENT CONSIDERATIONS

Assessment: Assess for known systemic hypersensitivity reactions to eggs or egg products.

Monitoring: Monitor for hypersensitivity/anaphylactic reactions.

Counseling: Advise that hypersensitivity/anaphylactic reactions may occur during and after treatment. Inform of the signs/symptoms of anaphylaxis/hypersensitivity reactions, and advise to seek immediate medical care should signs/symptoms occur.

STORAGE: 2-8°C (36-46°F) in original carton to protect from light. Do not shake or freeze vials.

KAPVAY – clonidine hydrochloride

RX

Class: $Alpha_2$ agonist

PEDIATRIC DOSAGE

Attention-Deficit Hyperactivity Disorder

Monotherapy or Adjunctive Therapy to Stimulant Medications:

6-17 Years:

Initial: 0.1mg hs

Titrate: Adjust daily dose in increments of 0.1mg/day at weekly intervals until desired response is achieved; doses should be taken bid, w/ either an equal or higher split dosage being given hs

Max: 0.4mg/day

Dosing Guidance:

Total Daily Dose of 0.1mg: 0.1mg qhs

Total Daily Dose of 0.2mg: 0.1mg qam and 0.1mg qhs

Total Daily Dose of 0.3mg: 0.1mg qam and 0.2mg qhs

Total Daily Dose of 0.4mg: 0.2mg qam and 0.2mg qhs

DOSING CONSIDERATIONS

Concomitant Medications

Concomitant Psychostimulant: Adjust psychostimulant dose depending on response to clonidine

Renal Impairment

Give initial dosage based on degree of impairment; titrate to higher doses cautiously

Discontinuation

Taper total daily dose in decrements of no more than 0.1mg every 3-7 days

ADMINISTRATION

Oral route

Take w/ or w/o food

Swallow tabs whole; do not crush, chew, or break

HOW SUPPLIED

Tab, Extended-Release: 0.1mg, 0.2mg

CONTRAINDICATIONS

History of a hypersensitivity reaction to clonidine.

WARNINGS/PRECAUTIONS

Substitution for other clonidine products on mg-per-mg basis is not recommended. May cause dose-related decreases in BP and HR. Titrate slowly in patients with history of hypotension and those with underlying conditions that may be worsened by hypotension and bradycardia (eg, heart block, bradycardia, cardiovascular/vascular/cerebrovascular disease, chronic renal failure). Caution with a history of syncope or with a condition that predisposes to syncope (eg, hypotension, orthostatic hypotension, bradycardia, dehydration); avoid becoming dehydrated or overheated. Somnolence and sedation reported. May impair mental/physical abilities. Abrupt discontinuation may cause rebound HTN; gradually reduce dose when discontinuing therapy. May elicit allergic reactions (eg, generalized rash, urticaria, angioedema) in patients who develop an allergic reaction from clonidine transdermal system. May worsen sinus node dysfunction and atrioventricular (AV) block; titrate slowly and monitor vital signs frequently in patients with cardiac conduction abnormalities.

ADVERSE REACTIONS

Somnolence, fatigue, nausea, dizziness, nasal congestion, nightmare, insomnia, emotional disorder, headache, upper abdominal pain, irritability, constipation, dry mouth, decreased appetite, tremor.

DRUG INTERACTIONS

TCAs increase BP and may counteract hypotensive effects, while antihypertensives potentiate hypotensive effect; monitor BP and adjust dose PRN. Avoid with CNS depressants; may potentiate sedating effects. Avoid with drugs that affect sinus node function or AV node conduction (eg, digitalis, calcium channel blockers, β-blockers); may potentiate bradycardia and risk of AV block. Monitor BP and HR, and adjust dosages accordingly in patients treated concomitantly with antihypertensives or other drugs that can reduce BP/HR or increase risk of syncope. Consider the potential for additive sedative effects with other centrally active depressants (eg, phenothiazines, barbiturates, benzodiazepines). Titrate slowly and monitor vital signs frequently with other sympatholytics. Avoid use with alcohol.

PATIENT CONSIDERATIONS

Assessment: Assess for drug hypersensitivity, history of hypotension, underlying conditions that may be worsened by hypotension and bradycardia, history of syncope or conditions that predispose to syncope, cardiac conduction abnormalities, renal impairment, pregnancy/nursing status, and for possible drug interactions. Obtain baseline HR and BP.

Monitoring: Monitor for somnolence, sedation, hypotension, bradycardia, allergic reactions, dehydration, overheating, and for other adverse reactions. Monitor BP and HR following dose increases and periodically while on therapy. Monitor vital signs frequently in patients with cardiac conduction abnormalities.

Counseling: Inform about risks/benefits of therapy and instruct to take ud. If a dose is missed, instruct to skip that dose and take the next dose as scheduled; advise not to take more than the prescribed total daily amount in any 24-hr period. Advise patients with a history of syncope or who may have a condition that predisposes them to syncope (eg, hypotension, orthostatic hypotension, bradycardia, dehydration) to avoid becoming dehydrated or overheated. Instruct to use caution when driving or operating hazardous machinery until they know how they will respond to treatment. Advise to avoid use of therapy with other centrally active depressants and with alcohol. Advise not to d/c therapy abruptly. Instruct to d/c therapy and seek immediate medical attention if any signs/symptoms of a hypersensitivity reaction (eg, generalized rash, urticaria, angioedema) occur.

STORAGE: 20-25°C (68-77°F).

KAZANO – alogliptin/metformin hydrochloride

RX

Class: Biguanide/dipeptidyl peptidase-4 (DPP-4) inhibitor

Lactic acidosis may occur due to metformin accumulation; risk increases w/ conditions such as sepsis, dehydration, excess alcohol intake, hepatic/renal impairment, and acute CHF. If acidosis is suspected, d/c therapy and hospitalize patient immediately.

ADULT DOSAGE

Type 2 Diabetes Mellitus

When treatment w/ both alogliptin and metformin is appropriate

Initial: Base on current regimen

May adjust dose based on effectiveness and tolerability; gradually escalate dose to reduce GI side effects of metformin

Max: (25mg/2000mg)/day

PEDIATRIC DOSAGE

Pediatric use may not have been established

ADMINISTRATION

Oral route

Take bid w/ food.

Do not split tab before swallowing.

HOW SUPPLIED

Tab: (Alogliptin/Metformin) 12.5mg/500mg, 12.5mg/1000mg

CONTRAINDICATIONS

Renal impairment (eg, SrCr ≥1.5mg/dL [men], ≥1.4mg/dL [women] or abnormal CrCl); acute or chronic metabolic acidosis, including diabetic ketoacidosis; history of a serious hypersensitivity reaction to alogliptin or metformin (eg, anaphylaxis, angioedema or severe cutaneous adverse reactions).

WARNINGS/PRECAUTIONS

Not for use in type 1 diabetes mellitus (DM) or for treatment of diabetic ketoacidosis. **Alogliptin:** Acute pancreatitis reported; d/c if suspected and initiate appropriate management. Serious hypersensitivity reactions reported; d/c if suspected, assess for other potential causes, and institute alternative treatment for DM. Caution w/ history of angioedema to another DPP-4 inhibitor. Fatal and nonfatal hepatic failure reported; interrupt therapy and investigate probable cause if liver enzymes are significantly elevated or if abnormal LFTs persist/worsen, and do not restart w/o another explanation for the liver test abnormalities. Severe and disabling arthralgia reported; d/c if it is a possible cause for severe join pain. **Metformin:** Avoid in patients w/ clinical or lab evidence of hepatic disease. D/C if evidence of renal impairment is present and do not initiate in patients ≥80 yrs of age unless renal function is normal. Temporarily d/c at time of or prior to radiologic studies involving intravascular iodinated contrast materials, withhold for 48 hrs subsequent to the procedure, and reinstitute only if renal function is normal. Suspend temporarily for any surgical procedure (except minor procedures not associated w/ restricted food and fluid intake); restart when oral intake is resumed and renal function is normal. D/C in hypoxic states (eg, acute CHF, shock, acute MI). May decrease vitamin B12 levels; monitor hematologic parameters annually. Caution in patients susceptible to hypoglycemic effects, such as elderly, debilitated, or malnourished patients, and those w/ adrenal/pituitary insufficiency or alcohol intoxication.

ADVERSE REACTIONS

URTI, nasopharyngitis, diarrhea, HTN, headache, back pain, UTI, hypoglycemia.

DRUG INTERACTIONS

Alogliptin: May require lower doses of insulin or insulin secretagogues. **Metformin:** Topiramate or other carbonic anhydrase inhibitors (eg, zonisamide, acetazolamide, dichlorphenamide) may induce metabolic acidosis; use w/ caution. Cationic drugs (eg, cimetidine, amiloride, digoxin, morphine, procainamide, quinidine, quinine, ranitidine, triamterene, trimethoprim, vancomycin) that are eliminated by renal tubular secretion may potentially produce an interaction; monitor and adjust dose. Observe for loss of glycemic control w/ thiazides and other diuretics, corticosteroids, phenothiazines, thyroid products, estrogens, oral contraceptives, phenytoin, nicotinic acid, sympathomimetics, calcium channel blockers, and isoniazid. Alcohol may potentiate effect of metformin on lactate metabolism; avoid excessive alcohol intake. Caution w/ drugs that may affect renal function or result in significant hemodynamic change or may interfere w/ the disposition of metformin (eg, cationic drugs eliminated by renal tubular secretion). Hypoglycemia may be difficult to recognize w/ β-adrenergic blocking drugs.

PATIENT CONSIDERATIONS

Assessment: Assess for metabolic acidosis, risk factors for lactic acidosis, renal/hepatic impairment, previous hypersensitivity to the drug, history of pancreatitis, inadequate vitamin B12 or calcium absorption, type of DM, diabetic ketoacidosis, history of angioedema w/ another DPP-4 inhibitor, pregnancy/nursing status, and possible drug interactions. Assess if patient is planning to undergo any surgical procedure. Obtain baseline FPG, HbA1c, and hematologic parameters.

Monitoring: Monitor for lactic acidosis, pancreatitis, hypoxic states, decreases in vitamin B12 levels, and hypersensitivity reactions. Monitor renal function, especially in patients in whom development of renal dysfunction is anticipated, at least annually. Monitor FPG, HbA1c, hepatic function, and hematologic parameters periodically.

Counseling: Inform of risks and benefits of therapy. Advise of the risk of lactic acidosis; instruct to d/c therapy immediately and contact physician if unexplained hyperventilation, myalgia, malaise, unusual somnolence, or other nonspecific symptoms occur. Counsel against excessive alcohol intake. Inform that GI symptoms, acute pancreatitis, severe and disabling joint pain, and hypoglycemia may occur. Advise to d/c and seek medical advice if signs/symptoms of allergic reactions, liver injury, severe joint pain, or persistent severe abdominal pain occur. Inform about the importance of regular testing of renal function and hematological parameters during treatment. Instruct to take ud.

STORAGE: 25°C (77°F); excursions permitted to 15-30°C (59-86°F). Keep container tightly closed.

KENALOG-10 – triamcinolone acetonide

RX

Class: Corticosteroid

ADULT DOSAGE

Dermatoses

Intralesional:

For alopecia areata; discoid lupus erythematosus; keloids; localized hypertrophic, infiltrated, inflammatory lesions of granuloma annulare, lichen planus, lichen simplex chronicus (neurodermatitis), and psoriatic plaques;

PEDIATRIC DOSAGE

General Dosing

Initial: 0.11-1.6mg/kg/day (3.2-48mg/m^2/day) in 3 or 4 divided doses depending on disease being treated

Titrate: Adjust to the lowest effective dose

Upon discontinuation after long-term therapy, withdraw gradually necrobiosis lipoidica diabeticorum; and cystic tumors of an aponeurosis or tendon (ganglia)

Initial: Varies depending on the specific disease and lesion being treated; multiple sites separated by 1cm or more may be injected. May be repeated at weekly or less frequent intervals if necessary

Maint: After a favorable response is noted, decrease initial dose in small decrements at appropriate time intervals until lowest dosage achieves adequate clinical response

Arthritic Disorders

Intra-articular/Soft Tissue:
Adjunctive therapy for short-term administration in acute gouty arthritis, acute/subacute bursitis, acute nonspecific tenosynovitis, epicondylitis, rheumatoid arthritis, synovitis, or osteoarthritis

Initial:
Smaller Joints: 2.5-5mg depending on disease being treated
Larger Joints: 5-15mg depending on disease being treated
Single inj into several joints, up to a total of 20mg or more, have been given

Maint: After a favorable response is noted, decrease initial dose in small decrements at appropriate time intervals until lowest dosage achieves adequate clinical response

DOSING CONSIDERATIONS

Other Important Considerations

Localization of Doses:
Lower initial dosage ranges of triamcinolone may produce the desired effect when administered to provide a localized concentration.
Carefully consider the site and volume of the inj when triamcinolone acetonide is administered for this purpose.

ADMINISTRATION

Intra-articular/Soft Tissue/Intralesional route

Inj Technique

Joints: If an excessive amount of synovial fluid is present in the joint, some, but not all, should be aspirated to aid in the relief of pain and to prevent undue dilution of the steroid.
Intra-articular: Carefully inject, particularly in the deltoid region, to avoid injecting sus into the tissues surrounding the site; may lead to tissue atrophy.
Acute Nonspecific Tenosynovitis: Ensure that inj is made into the tendon sheath rather than the tendon substance.
Epicondylitis: Infiltrate the preparation into the area of greatest tenderness.
Intralesional: For accuracy of dosage measurement and ease of administration, it is preferable to employ a tuberculin syringe and a small-bore needle (23-25 gauge). Ethyl chloride spray may be used to alleviate the discomfort of the inj.
Dermal Lesions: Inj directly into the lesion (intradermally or subcutaneously).

HOW SUPPLIED

Inj: 10mg/mL [5mL]

CONTRAINDICATIONS

Hypersensitivity to any components of the medication.

WARNINGS/PRECAUTIONS

Serious neurologic events reported w/ epidural inj; not approved for epidural administration. Not for use in neonates; contains benzyl alcohol, which has been associated w/ gasping syndrome in neonates, and increased incidence of kernicterus in small preterm infants. Anaphylaxis may occur. Not suitable for use in acute stressful situations. High systemic doses should not be used to treat traumatic brain injury. May cause BP elevation, salt/water retention, and increased K^+ and Ca^{2+} excretion; dietary salt restriction and K^+ supplementation may be necessary. Caution w/ a recent MI. May produce reversible hypothalamic-pituitary-adrenal (HPA) axis suppression w/ potential for glucocorticosteroid insufficiency after withdrawal. Drug-induced secondary adrenocortical insufficiency may be minimized by gradual dose reduction. Metabolic clearance is decreased in hypothyroidism and increased in hyperthyroidism; changes in thyroid status may necessitate dose adjustment. May increase susceptibility to infections, mask signs of current infection, activate latent disease, or exacerbate intercurrent infections/systemic fungal infections. Avoid use in the presence of systemic fungal infections unless needed to control drug reactions. Rule out latent or active amebiasis before initiating therapy. Caution w/ *Strongyloides* infestation, active or latent tuberculosis (TB), congestive heart failure (CHF), HTN, and renal insufficiency. Not for use in cerebral malaria or active ocular herpes simplex. May cause more serious/fatal course of chickenpox and measles; avoid exposure. Reports of severe medical events have been associated w/ the intrathecal route of administration; avoid intrathecal administration. May produce posterior subcapsular cataracts, glaucoma w/ possible damage to the optic nerves, and enhance the establishment of secondary ocular infections; not recommended in the treatment of optic neuritis. Endophthalmitis, eye inflammation, increased intraocular pressure (IOP), and visual disturbances including vision loss reported w/ intravitreal administration. Administration intraocularly or into the nasal turbinates is not recommended. Sensitive to heat; should not be autoclaved when it is desirable to sterilize the exterior of the vial. Kaposi's sarcoma reported. Caution w/ active or latent peptic ulcers, diverticulitis, fresh intestinal anastomoses, and nonspecific ulcerative colitis; may increase risk of perforation. Signs of peritoneal irritation following GI perforation may be minimal/absent. Enhanced effect in patients w/ cirrhosis. May decrease bone formation and increase bone resorption and may lead to inhibition of bone growth in pediatric patients and development of osteoporosis at any age; caution w/ increased risk of osteoporosis. Acute myopathy reported w/ high doses, most often in patients w/ neuromuscular transmission disorders (eg, myasthenia gravis). Elevation of creatine kinase (CK) or IOP may occur; monitor IOP if used for >6 weeks. Psychiatric derangements may appear and existing emotional instability or psychotic tendencies may be aggravated. May suppress reactions to skin tests. **Intra-articular/Soft Tissue Administration:** Intra-articularly injected corticosteroids may be systemically absorbed. Appropriate examination of any joint fluid present is necessary to exclude a septic process; institute appropriate antimicrobial therapy if septic arthritis occurs and diagnosis is confirmed. Avoid inj into an infected site/previously infected joint or into unstable joints. Intra-articular inj may result in damage to joint tissues.

ADVERSE REACTIONS

Bradycardia, HTN, edema, allergic dermatitis, impaired wound healing, urticaria, glycosuria, hirsutism, abdominal distention, ulcerative esophagitis, negative nitrogen balance, muscle weakness, osteoporosis, convulsions, depression.

DRUG INTERACTIONS

Administration of live or live, attenuated vaccines is contraindicated in patients receiving immunosuppressive doses. Killed or inactivated vaccines may be administered, although response is unpredictable; if possible, routine vaccine/toxoid administration should be deferred until therapy is discontinued. Aminoglutethimide may lead to loss of corticosteroid-induced adrenal suppression. Closely monitor for hypokalemia w/ K^+-depleting agents (eg, amphotericin B, diuretics). Cardiac enlargement and CHF following concomitant use of amphotericin B and hydrocortisone reported. Macrolide antibiotics may decrease clearance and cholestyramine may increase clearance. Concomitant use w/ anticholinesterase agents may produce severe weakness in patients w/ myasthenia gravis; d/c anticholinesterase agents at least 24 hrs before initiating therapy. May inhibit response to warfarin; frequently monitor coagulation indices. May increase blood glucose levels; dosage adjustments of antidiabetic agents may be required. May decrease concentrations of isoniazid. Increased activity of both drugs may occur w/ cyclosporine; convulsions reported w/ concurrent use. May increase risk of arrhythmias w/ digitalis glycosides. Estrogens, including oral contraceptives, may decrease hepatic metabolism and enhance effect. Hepatic enzyme inducers (eg, barbiturates, phenytoin, carbamazepine, rifampin) may enhance metabolism and require corticosteroid dosage increase. Ketoconazole may increase risk of corticosteroid side effects. Aspirin (ASA) or other NSAIDs may increase the risk of GI side effects; caution w/ ASA in hypoprothrombinemia patients. May increase clearance of salicylates. Acute myopathy reported w/ neuromuscular blocking drugs (eg, pancuronium).

PATIENT CONSIDERATIONS

Assessment: Assess for hypersensitivity to drug, unusual stress, recent MI, systemic fungal infections, other current infections, active/latent TB, cerebral malaria, ocular herpes simplex, CHF, HTN, renal insufficiency, traumatic brain injury, diverticulitis, intestinal anastomoses, ulcerative colitis, psychotic tendencies, cirrhosis, myasthenia gravis, any other conditions where treatment is contraindicated or cautioned, pregnancy/nursing status, and possible drug interactions.

Monitoring: Monitor for anaphylaxis, HPA axis suppression, Kaposi's sarcoma, acute myopathy, infections, psychiatric derangements, intestinal perforation, cataracts, glaucoma, growth/development (in pediatric patients), osteoporosis, and other adverse reactions. Monitor BP, serum electrolytes, CK, and IOP. Frequently monitor coagulation indices w/ warfarin.

Counseling: Instruct not to d/c abruptly or use w/o medical supervision. Instruct to inform any medical attendants of intake of corticosteroids and to seek medical advice at once if fever or signs of infection develop. Advise to avoid exposure to chickenpox or measles; instruct to seek medical advice w/o delay if exposed.

STORAGE: 20-25°C (68-77°F), avoid freezing and protect from light. Do not refrigerate.

KENGREAL – cangrelor

RX

Class: Antiplatelet agent

ADULT DOSAGE

Percutaneous Coronary Intervention

Adjunct to percutaneous coronary intervention (PCI) to reduce the risk of periprocedural MI, repeat coronary revascularization, and stent thrombosis in patients who have not been treated w/ a $P2Y_{12}$ platelet inhibitor and are not being given a glycoprotein IIb/IIIa inhibitor

30mcg/kg IV bolus followed immediately by a 4mcg/kg/min infusion

Initiate the bolus prior to PCI. Maint infusion should be continued for at least 2 hrs or for the duration of PCI, whichever is longer

Conversions

Transitioning to Oral $P2Y_{12}$ Therapy:
Ticagrelor: 180mg at any time during infusion or immediately after discontinuation
Prasugrel: 60mg immediately after discontinuation
Clopidogrel: 600mg immediately after discontinuation

PEDIATRIC DOSAGE

Pediatric use may not have been established

K

ADMINISTRATION

IV route

Administer via a dedicated IV line.
Administer the bolus volume rapidly (<1 min), from the diluted bag via manual IV push or pump. Ensure the bolus is completely administered before the start of PCI. Start the infusion immediately after administration of the bolus.

Preparation

Reconstitute 50mg vial by adding 5mL of sterile water for inj. Swirl gently until all material is dissolved; avoid vigorous mixing and allow any foam to settle. Ensure that reconstituted material is a clear, colorless to pale yellow sol. Reconstitute the vial prior to dilution in a bag.

Do not use w/o dilution. Before administration, each reconstituted vial must be diluted further w/ NaCl 0.9% inj or D5W. Withdraw the contents from 1 reconstituted vial and add to one 250mL saline bag. Mix the bag thoroughly; this dilution will result in a concentration of 200mcg/mL and should be sufficient for at least 2 hrs of dosing. Patients ≥100kg will require a minimum of 2 bags.

Reconstituted vial should be diluted immediately. Diluted sol is stable for up to 12 hrs in D5W and 24 hrs in normal saline at room temperature.

HOW SUPPLIED

Inj: 50mg [10mL]

CONTRAINDICATIONS

Significant active bleeding, known hypersensitivity (eg, anaphylaxis) to cangrelor or any component of the product.

WARNINGS/PRECAUTIONS

Increased risk of bleeding; after discontinuation, there is no antiplatelet effect after an hr. Worsening renal function reported in patients w/ severe renal impairment (CrCl <30mL/min).

ADVERSE REACTIONS

Bleeding.

DRUG INTERACTIONS

If clopidogrel or prasugrel is administered during cangrelor infusion, it will have no antiplatelet effect until the next dose is administered; do not administer until infusion is discontinued.

PATIENT CONSIDERATIONS

Assessment: Assess for hypersensitivity, active bleeding, renal impairment, pregnancy/nursing status, and possible drug interactions.

Monitoring: Monitor for bleeding and other adverse reactions.

Counseling: Inform of the risks and benefits of therapy. Instruct to contact physician if hypersensitivity reactions (eg, anaphylaxis) or unusual bleeding develops.

STORAGE: 20-25°C (68-77°F) w/ excursions between 15-30°C (59-86°F).

KEPPRA – levetiracetam RX

Class: Pyrrolidine derivative

ADULT DOSAGE

Partial Onset Seizures

Adjunctive Therapy for Patients w/ Epilepsy:
≥16 Years:
Initial: 500mg bid
Titrate: May increase by 1000mg/day every 2 weeks
Max: 3000mg/day

Myoclonic Seizures

Adjunctive Therapy for Patients w/ Juvenile Myoclonic Epilepsy:
Initial: 500mg bid
Titrate: Increase by 1000mg/day every 2 weeks to recommended dose of 3000mg/day

Tonic-Clonic Seizures

Adjunctive Therapy in the Treatment of Primary Generalized Tonic-Clonic Seizures w/ Idiopathic Generalized Epilepsy:
≥16 Years:
Initial: 500mg bid
Titrate: Increase by 1000mg/day every 2 weeks to recommended dose of 3000mg/day

Conversions

Switching from Oral Dosing:
Initial total daily IV dose should be equivalent to the total daily dose and frequency of oral formulation
Switching to Oral Dosing:
At the end of IV treatment period, switch at equivalent daily dose and frequency of IV administration

PEDIATRIC DOSAGE

Partial Onset Seizures

Adjunctive Therapy for Patients w/ Epilepsy:
1-<6 Months of Age:
Initial: 7mg/kg bid
Titrate: Increase by 14mg/kg/day every 2 weeks to recommended dose of 21mg/kg bid
6 Months-<4 Years:
Initial: 10mg/kg bid
Titrate: Increase by 20mg/kg/day in 2 weeks to recommended dose of 25mg/kg bid; may reduce dose if 50mg/kg/day cannot be tolerated
4-<16 Years:
Initial: 10mg/kg bid
Titrate: Increase by 20mg/kg/day every 2 weeks to recommended dose of 30mg/kg bid; may reduce dose if 60mg/kg/day cannot be tolerated
Max: 3000mg/day
Tab:
20-40kg:
Initial: 250mg bid
Titrate: Increase by 500mg/day every 2 weeks
Max: 750mg bid
>40kg:
Initial: 500mg bid
Titrate: Increase by 1000mg/day every 2 weeks
Max: 1500mg bid

Myoclonic Seizures

Adjunctive Therapy for Patients w/ Juvenile Myoclonic Epilepsy:
≥12 Years:
Initial: 500mg bid
Titrate: Increase by 1000mg/day every 2 weeks to recommended dose of 3000mg/day

Tonic-Clonic Seizures

Adjunctive Therapy in the Treatment of Primary Generalized Tonic-Clonic Seizures w/ Idiopathic Generalized Epilepsy:
6-<16 Years:
Initial: 10mg/kg bid
Titrate: Increase by 20mg/kg/day every 2 weeks to recommended dose of 30mg/kg bid

Conversions

Switching from Oral Dosing:
Initial total daily IV dose should be equivalent to the total daily dose and frequency of oral formulation
Switching to Oral Dosing:
At the end of IV treatment period, switch at equivalent daily dose and frequency of IV administration

DOSING CONSIDERATIONS

Renal Impairment
Adults:
Mild (CrCl 50-80mL/min): 500-1000mg q12h
Moderate (CrCl 30-50mL/min): 250-750mg q12h

Severe (CrCl <30mL/min): 250-500mg q12h
ESRD Using Dialysis: 500-1000mg q24h
Following dialysis, a supplemental dose of 250-500mg is recommended

ADMINISTRATION

Oral/IV route

Oral

Take w/ or w/o food
Prescribe oral sol for pediatric patients ≤20kg
Prescribe oral sol or tabs for pediatric patients >20kg

Tab:
Swallow whole; do not crush or chew

Sol:
Dosing is weight-based using a calibrated measuring device

IV

Use only as an alternative for patients when oral administration is temporarily not feasible
Administer as a 15-min IV infusion following dilution
Dilute in 100mL of a compatible diluent; if smaller volume is required, amount of diluent should be calculated to not exceed a max levetiracetam concentration of 15mg/mL of diluted sol
Consider total daily fluid intake of patient
Stable for ≥24 hrs when mixed w/ compatible diluents and antiepileptic drugs and stored in polyvinyl chloride bags

Compatible Diluents:
0.9% NaCl inj
Lactated Ringer's inj
D5 inj

Compatible Antiepileptic Drugs:
Lorazepam
Diazepam
Valproate sodium

IV/Sol

Refer to PI for weight-based dosing calculation

HOW SUPPLIED

Inj: 100mg/mL [5mL]; **Sol:** 100mg/mL [16 fl oz]; **Tab:** 250mg*, 500mg*, 750mg*, 1000mg* *scored

WARNINGS/PRECAUTIONS

May cause behavioral abnormalities, psychotic symptoms, somnolence, fatigue, and coordination difficulties. May impair mental/physical abilities. Serious dermatological reactions (eg, Stevens-Johnson syndrome [SJS], toxic epidermal necrolysis [TEN]), and recurrence of serious skin reactions following rechallenge reported; d/c at the 1st sign of rash, unless the rash is clearly not drug-related. Do not resume, and consider alternative therapy if signs/symptoms suggest SJS/TEN. Increased risk of suicidal thoughts or behavior. Withdraw gradually to minimize the potential of increased seizure frequency. Hematologic abnormalities and agranulocytosis reported. Physiological changes may decrease plasma levels throughout pregnancy; monitor patients during pregnancy and through the postpartum period, especially if the dose was changed during pregnancy. Caution in elderly. (Oral) Increased diastolic BP reported.

ADVERSE REACTIONS

Somnolence, asthenia, infection, dizziness, fatigue, aggression, irritability, neck pain, pharyngitis, vertigo, diarrhea, anorexia, pain, depression, nervousness.

PATIENT CONSIDERATIONS

Assessment: Assess for renal impairment, depression, suicidal thoughts/behavior, pregnancy/nursing status, and possible drug interactions.

Monitoring: Monitor for signs/symptoms of psychiatric reactions, behavior abnormalities, somnolence and fatigue, coordination difficulties, suicidal behavior, serious dermatological reactions, hematologic abnormalities, agranulocytosis, and other adverse reactions. Monitor patients during pregnancy and continue close monitoring through the postpartum period, especially if the dose was changed during pregnancy. Monitor for increase in diastolic BP in patients 1 month to <4 yrs of age.

Counseling: Advise patients and their caregivers that the drug may cause behavioral changes and psychotic symptoms. Inform that the drug may increase the risk of suicidal thoughts and behavior; advise to be alert for the emergence or worsening of symptoms of depression, unusual changes in mood/behavior, or the emergence of suicidal thoughts, behavior, or thoughts about self-harm. Instruct to immediately report behaviors of concern to physician. Inform that dizziness and somnolence may occur; advise not to drive, operate heavy machinery, or engage in other hazardous activities until they have gained sufficient experience to gauge whether it adversely affects their performance of these activities. Inform that serious dermatological adverse reactions have been reported; advise to notify physician if a rash develops. Advise to notify physician if patient becomes pregnant or intends to become pregnant; encourage to enroll in the North American Antiepileptic Drug pregnancy registry.

STORAGE: 25°C (77°F); excursions permitted to 15-30°C (59-86°F).

Keppra XR – levetiracetam

RX

Class: Pyrrolidine derivative

ADULT DOSAGE

Partial Onset Seizures

Adjunctive Therapy in Patients w/ Epilepsy:
Initial: 1000mg qd
Titrate: Adjust dose in increments of 1000mg every 2 weeks
Max: 3000mg/day

PEDIATRIC DOSAGE

Partial Onset Seizures

Adjunctive Therapy in Patients w/ Epilepsy:
≥12 Years:
Initial: 1000mg qd
Titrate: Adjust dose in increments of 1000mg every 2 weeks
Max: 3000mg/day

DOSING CONSIDERATIONS

Renal Impairment

Adults:
Mild (CrCl 50-80mL/min): 1000-2000mg q24h
Moderate (CrCl 30-50mL/min): 500-1500mg q24h
Severe (CrCl <30mL/min): 500-1000mg q24h
ESRD on Dialysis: Use immediate-release formulation

K

ADMINISTRATION

Oral route

Swallow tabs whole; do not chew, break, or crush

HOW SUPPLIED

Tab, Extended-Release: 500mg, 750mg

WARNINGS/PRECAUTIONS

Increased risk of suicidal thoughts/behavior. May cause behavioral abnormalities, psychotic symptoms, somnolence, fatigue, and coordination difficulties. May impair mental/physical abilities. Serious dermatological reactions (eg, Stevens-Johnson syndrome [SJS], toxic epidermal necrolysis [TEN]) and recurrence of serious skin reactions following rechallenge reported; d/c at the 1st sign of rash, unless the rash is clearly not drug-related. If signs/symptoms suggest SJS/TEN, do not resume therapy and consider alternative therapy. Withdraw gradually to minimize the potential of increased seizure frequency. Hematologic abnormalities and agranulocytosis reported. Physiological changes may decrease plasma levels throughout pregnancy. Caution in elderly.

ADVERSE REACTIONS

Somnolence, nausea, influenza, nasopharyngitis, dizziness, irritability.

PATIENT CONSIDERATIONS

Assessment: Assess for renal impairment, depression, suicidal thoughts/behavior, and pregnancy/nursing status.

Monitoring: Monitor for emergence or worsening of depression, suicidal thoughts/behavior, and/or any unusual changes in mood or behavior, psychotic symptoms, somnolence, fatigue, coordination difficulties, serious dermatological reactions, hematologic abnormalities, agranulocytosis, and other adverse reactions. Monitor patients during pregnancy and continue close monitoring through the postpartum period, especially if the dose was changed during pregnancy.

Counseling: Inform that the drug may increase the risk of suicidal thoughts/behavior; instruct to immediately report the emergence or worsening of symptoms of depression, any unusual changes in mood/behavior, or suicidal thoughts, behavior, or thoughts about self-harm to physician. Counsel that medication may cause changes in behavior (eg, irritability and aggression). Inform that dizziness and somnolence may occur; advise not to drive or operate heavy machinery or engage in other hazardous activities until patients have gained sufficient experience to gauge whether it adversely affects their performance of these activities. Advise that serious dermatological adverse reactions may occur; instruct to notify physician immediately if rash develops. Instruct to take as directed. Advise to notify physician if patient becomes pregnant or intends to become pregnant; encourage to enroll in the North American Antiepileptic Drug pregnancy registry.

STORAGE: 25°C (77°F); excursions permitted to 15-30°C (59-86°F).

KERYDIN – tavaborole

RX

Class: Antifungal agent

ADULT DOSAGE

Onychomycosis

Onychomycosis of the Toenails Due to *Trichophyton rubrum/Trichophyton mentagrophytes*:

Apply to affected toenails qd for 48 weeks

PEDIATRIC DOSAGE

Pediatric use may not have been established

ADMINISTRATION

Topical route

Apply to the entire toenail surface and under the tip of each toenail being treated

HOW SUPPLIED

Sol: 5% [4mL, 10mL]

ADVERSE REACTIONS

Application-site exfoliation/erythema/dermatitis, ingrown toenail.

PATIENT CONSIDERATIONS

Assessment: Assess pregnancy/nursing status.

Monitoring: Monitor for adverse reactions.

Counseling: Instruct to use ud, and to avoid contact w/ eyes, mouth, or vagina. Advise to avoid contact w/ skin other than skin immediately surrounding the treated nail(s); instruct to wipe away excess sol from surrounding skin. Instruct to clean and dry nails prior to use. Advise to allow sol to dry following application. Inform that the impact of nail polish or other cosmetic nail products on the efficacy of therapy has not been evaluated. Instruct to inform physician if the area of application shows signs of persistent irritation (eg, redness, itching, swelling). Advise not to use for any disorder other than that for which it is prescribed.

STORAGE: 20-25°C (68-77°F); excursions permitted to 15-30°C (59-86°F). Flammable; keep away from heat and flame. Discard w/in 3 months after insertion of the dropper.

KEYTRUDA – pembrolizumab

RX

Class: Monoclonal antibody/programmed death receptor-1 (PD-1) blocker

ADULT DOSAGE

Unresectable or Metastatic Melanoma

2mg/kg every 3 weeks until disease progression or unacceptable toxicity

Metastatic Non-Small Cell Lung Cancer

Treatment of metastatic non-small cell lung cancer (NSCLC) in patients whose tumors express PD-L1 as determined by an FDA-approved test w/ disease progression on or after platinum-containing chemotherapy

Patients w/ EGFR or ALK genomic tumor aberrations should have disease progression on FDA-approved therapy for these aberrations prior to receiving pembrolizumab

2mg/kg every 3 weeks until disease progression or unacceptable toxicity

PEDIATRIC DOSAGE

Pediatric use may not have been established

DOSING CONSIDERATIONS

Adverse Reactions

Withhold for the Following:

- Grade 2 pneumonitis
- Grade 2 or 3 colitis
- Grade 3 or 4 endocrinopathies
- Grade 2 nephritis
- AST/ALT >3 and up to 5X ULN or total bilirubin >1.5 and up to 3X ULN
- Any other severe or Grade 3 treatment-related adverse reaction

Resume Therapy:
In patients whose adverse reactions recover to Grade 0-1

Permanently D/C for the Following:
- Any life-threatening adverse reaction (excluding endocrinopathies controlled w/ hormone replacement therapy)
- Grade 3 or 4 pneumonitis or recurrent pneumonitis of Grade 2 severity
- Grade 3 or 4 nephritis
- AST/ALT >5X ULN or total bilirubin >3X ULN; for patients w/ liver metastasis who begin treatment w/ Grade 2 AST/ALT, if AST/ALT increases by ≥50% relative to baseline and lasts for at least 1 week
- Grade 3 or 4 infusion-related reactions
- Inability to reduce corticosteroid dose to ≤10mg/day of prednisone (or equivalent) w/in 12 weeks
- Persistent Grade 2 or 3 adverse reactions (excluding endocrinopathies controlled w/ hormone replacement therapy) that do not recover to Grade 0-1 w/in 12 weeks after last dose of therapy
- Any severe or Grade 3 treatment-related adverse reaction that recurs

ADMINISTRATION

IV route

Administer infusion sol IV over 30 min through an IV line containing a sterile, non-pyrogenic, low-protein binding 0.2-5 micron in-line/add-on filter.
Do not coadminister other drugs through the same infusion line.

Preparation

Add 2.3mL of sterile water for inj for a resulting concentration of 25mg/mL; inject the water along the walls of the vial, not directly on lyophilized powder.
Slowly swirl vial and allow up to 5 min for bubbles to clear; do not shake.
Dilute inj sol or reconstituted powder prior to IV administration by withdrawing required volume from vial(s) and transferring into an IV bag containing 0.9% NaCl inj or D5 inj.
Mix diluted sol by gentle inversion; final concentration should be 1-10mg/mL.

K

Reconstituted/Diluted Sol from 50mg Vial

Store at room temperature for ≤6 hrs from the time of reconstitution, or at 2-8°C (36-46°F) for ≤24 hrs from the time of reconstitution. If refrigerated, allow the diluted sol to come to room temperature prior to administration. Do not freeze.

Diluted Sol from 25mg/mL Vial

Store at room temperature for ≤6 hrs from the time of dilution, or at 2-8°C (36-46°F) for ≤24 hrs from the time of dilution. If refrigerated, allow the diluted sol to come to room temperature prior to administration. Do not freeze.

HOW SUPPLIED

Inj: (Powder) 50mg; (Sol) 25mg/mL [4mL]

WARNINGS/PRECAUTIONS

Immune-mediated pneumonitis, colitis, hepatitis, hypophysitis, and nephritis reported; administer corticosteroids for ≥Grade 2. Thyroid disorders can occur at any time during treatment. Administer replacement hormones for hypothyroidism and manage hyperthyroidism w/ thionamides and beta-blockers as appropriate. Type 1 diabetes mellitus (DM), including diabetic ketoacidosis, reported; administer insulin for type 1 DM, and withhold therapy and administer antihyperglycemics in patients w/ severe hyperglycemia. Other clinically important immune-mediated reactions may occur; evaluate and administer corticosteroids based on severity of the adverse reaction. Upon improvement to ≤Grade 1, initiate corticosteroid taper and continue to taper over at least 1 month. Severe and life-threatening infusion-related reactions reported. Can cause fetal harm.

ADVERSE REACTIONS

Melanoma: Fatigue, diarrhea, pruritus, rash, constipation, nausea, decreased appetite.
NSCLC: Fatigue, decreased appetite, dyspnea, cough.

PATIENT CONSIDERATIONS

Assessment: Assess pregnancy/nursing status. Obtain baseline liver/renal/thyroid function.

Monitoring: Monitor for signs/symptoms of pneumonitis, colitis, hypophysitis, changes in liver/renal function, hyperglycemia/type 1 DM, infusion-related reactions, and other adverse reactions. Evaluate patients w/ suspected pneumonitis w/ radiographic imaging. Monitor for changes in thyroid function (periodically during treatment, and as indicated based on clinical evaluation) and for signs/symptoms of thyroid disorders. Monitor for immune-mediated adverse reactions; ensure adequate evaluation to confirm etiology or exclude other causes.

Counseling: Inform of the risk of immune-mediated adverse reactions that may require corticosteroid treatment and interruption or discontinuation of therapy (eg, pneumonitis, colitis, hepatitis, hypophysitis, nephritis, hyper/hypothyroidism, type 1 DM); instruct to immediately contact physician if signs/symptoms of an immune-mediated adverse reaction occur. Advise to contact physician immediately for signs/symptoms of infusion-related reactions. Advise of the importance of keeping scheduled appointments for blood work or other lab tests. Advise women that drug may cause fetal harm; instruct women of reproductive potential to use highly effective contraception during and for 4 months after the last dose of therapy. Advise nursing mothers not to breastfeed while taking therapy.

STORAGE: 2-8°C (36-46°F). **Sol:** Protect from light. Do not freeze. Do not shake.

KINRIX – diphtheria and tetanus toxoids and acellular pertussis adsorbed and inactivated poliovirus vaccine

RX

Class: Toxoid/vaccine combination

PEDIATRIC DOSAGE

Active Immunization Against Diphtheria, Tetanus, Pertussis, and Poliomyelitis

For use as the 5th dose in the diphtheria, tetanus, and acellular pertussis (DTaP) vaccine series and 4th dose in the inactivated poliovirus vaccine series in patients whose previous DTaP vaccine doses have been w/ Infanrix and/or Pediarix for the first 3 doses and Infanrix for the 4th dose

4-6 Years:
0.5mL dose IM

ADMINISTRATION

IM route

The preferred site of administration is the deltoid muscle of the upper arm
Do not mix w/ any other vaccine in the same syringe or vial

Preparation

Shake vigorously; do not use if resuspension does not occur w/ vigorous shaking
For prefilled syringes, attach a sterile needle and administer IM
For vials, use a sterile needle and sterile syringe to withdraw dose and administer IM; not necessary to change needles between drawing vaccine from a vial and injecting into recipient, unless needle has been damaged or contaminated

HOW SUPPLIED

Inj: 0.5mL [vial, prefilled syringe]

CONTRAINDICATIONS

Severe allergic reaction (eg, anaphylaxis) after a previous dose of any diphtheria toxoid, tetanus toxoid, pertussis- or poliovirus-containing vaccine, or to any component of Kinrix, including neomycin and polymyxin B; encephalopathy (eg, coma, decreased level of consciousness, prolonged seizures) w/in 7 days of administration of a previous dose of a pertussis-containing vaccine that is not attributable to another identifiable cause; progressive neurologic disorder, including infantile spasms, uncontrolled epilepsy, or progressive encephalopathy.

WARNINGS/PRECAUTIONS

Evaluate potential benefits and risks of vaccine administration if Guillain-Barre syndrome occurs within 6 weeks of receipt of a prior tetanus toxoid-containing vaccine. Tip caps of prefilled syringes may contain natural rubber latex; may cause allergic reactions in latex-sensitive individuals. Syncope may occur and can be accompanied by transient neurological signs. Evaluate the potential benefits and risks of vaccine administration if any of the following events occur in temporal relation to receipt of a pertussis-containing vaccine: temperature ≥40.5°C (105°F) within 48 hrs not due to another identifiable cause; collapse or shock-like state within 48 hrs; persistent, inconsolable crying lasting ≥3 hrs, occurring within 48 hrs; or seizures with or without fever occurring within 3 days. May administer an antipyretic at the time of vaccination and for the ensuing 24 hrs in children at higher risk for seizures. Review immunization history for possible vaccine sensitivity and previous vaccination-related adverse reactions; epinephrine and other appropriate agents must be immediately available should an acute anaphylactic reaction occur.

ADVERSE REACTIONS

Local inj-site reactions (eg, pain, redness, arm circumference increase, swelling), drowsiness, fever, loss of appetite.

DRUG INTERACTIONS

Immunosuppressive therapies, including irradiation, antimetabolites, alkylating agents, cytotoxic drugs, and corticosteroids (used in greater than physiologic doses) may reduce immune response to vaccine.

PATIENT CONSIDERATIONS

Assessment: Assess for history of encephalopathy, development of Guillain-Barre syndrome following a prior tetanus toxoid-containing vaccine, progressive neurologic disorder, immunosuppression, risk for seizures, possible drug interactions, and hypersensitivity to latex, neomycin, or polymyxin B. Review immunization history for possible vaccine sensitivity and previous vaccination-related adverse reactions.

Monitoring: Monitor for signs/symptoms of Guillain-Barre syndrome, allergic reactions, syncope, neurological signs, and other adverse reactions.

Counseling: Inform parents/guardians of the potential benefits and risks of immunization, and about the potential for adverse reactions.

STORAGE: 2-8°C (36-46°F). Do not freeze; discard if vaccine has been frozen.

Kitabis Pak – tobramycin **RX**

Class: Aminoglycoside

ADULT DOSAGE

Cystic Fibrosis

Patients w/ *Pseudomonas aeruginosa*:
1 single-use ampule (300mg/5mL) bid by oral inh in alternating periods of 28 days on drug followed by 28 days off drug

PEDIATRIC DOSAGE

Cystic Fibrosis

Patients w/ *Pseudomonas aeruginosa*:
≥6 Years:
1 single-use ampule (300mg/5mL) bid by oral inh in alternating periods of 28 days on drug followed by 28 days off drug

K

ADMINISTRATION

Oral inh route

Take doses as close to 12 hrs apart as possible; not <6 hrs apart

Administer using only the Pari LC Plus Reusable Nebulizer with a DeVilbiss Pulmo-Aide air compressor

Entire treatment should take approximately 15 min to complete; continue treatment until all inh sol has been delivered and there is no longer any mist being produced

Do not dilute/mix inh sol with other drugs in the nebulizer, including dornase alfa

HOW SUPPLIED

Sol, Inhalation: 300mg/5mL

CONTRAINDICATIONS

Known hypersensitivity to any aminoglycoside.

WARNINGS/PRECAUTIONS

Bronchospasm, ototoxicity (eg, tinnitus), and nephrotoxicity may occur. If ototoxicity is noted, or nephrotoxicity develops, patient should be managed as medically appropriate, including potentially discontinuing tobramycin inh sol. May aggravate muscle weakness because of a potential curare-like effect on neuromuscular function. If neuromuscular blockade occurs, it may be reversed by administration of Ca^{2+} salts but mechanical assistance may be necessary. May cause fetal harm.

ADVERSE REACTIONS

Cough, pharyngitis, increased sputum, dyspnea, hemoptysis, decreased lung function, voice alteration, taste perversion, rash.

DRUG INTERACTIONS

Avoid concurrent and/or sequential use with other drugs with neurotoxic, nephrotoxic, or ototoxic potential. Some diuretics may enhance aminoglycoside toxicity by altering aminoglycoside concentrations in serum and tissue; do not administer with ethacrynic acid, furosemide, urea, or IV mannitol. Monitor for toxicities associated with aminoglycosides if used concomitantly with parenteral aminoglycosides; monitor serum tobramycin levels.

PATIENT CONSIDERATIONS

Assessment: Assess for auditory or vestibular dysfunction, renal dysfunction, neuromuscular disorders, drug hypersensitivity, pregnancy/nursing status, and possible drug interactions.

Monitoring: Monitor for bronchospasm, ototoxicity, nephrotoxicity, neuromuscular effects, and other adverse reactions.

Counseling: Advise to inform physician if SOB or wheezing occurs soon after administration, or if ringing in the ears, dizziness, or any changes in hearing develop. Instruct to notify physician if planning to become pregnant or if nursing. Instruct patients on multiple therapies to take their medications prior to inhaling the tobramycin inh sol, or ud by physician.

STORAGE: 2-8°C (36-46°F). Upon removal from the refrigerator, or if refrigeration is unavailable, may be stored at room temperature (up to 25°C [77°F]) for up to 28 days. Do not expose to intense light.

KLOR-CON M – potassium chloride

RX

Class: Potassium supplement

OTHER BRAND NAMES

Klor-Con

ADULT DOSAGE

Hypokalemia

Prevention:
20mEq/day

Treatment:
≥40-100mEq/day or more; divide dose so that no more than 20mEq is given in a single dose

PEDIATRIC DOSAGE

Pediatric use may not have been established

DOSING CONSIDERATIONS

Elderly

Start at lower end of dosing range

ADMINISTRATION

Oral route

Take w/ meals and w/ a glass of water or other liquid

Klor-Con

Swallow tab whole; do not crush, chew, or suck

Klor-Con M

If Unable to Swallow Whole Tab:

A) Break tab in 1/2 and take each half separately w/ a glass of water, or
B) Prepare an aqueous sus

Aqueous Sus Preparation:

1. Place whole tab in approx 4 fl oz of water
2. Allow 2 min for tab to disintegrate
3. Stir for 30 sec after tab has disintegrated
4. Swirl sus and consume entire contents of the glass immediately by drinking or using a straw
5. Add another 1 fl oz of water, swirl, and consume immediately
6. Then, add an additional 1 fl oz of water, swirl, and consume immediately

HOW SUPPLIED

Tab, Extended-Release (ER): (Klor-Con M) 10mEq, 15mEq, 20mEq; (Klor-Con) 8mEq, 10mEq

CONTRAINDICATIONS

Hyperkalemia. ER formulations should not be used in certain cardiac patients w/ esophageal compression due to an enlarged left atrium; if indicated, give as liquid preparation or aqueous sus. **Solid Dosage Forms:** Structural, pathological (eg, diabetic gastroparesis), or pharmacologic (use of anticholinergic agents or other agents w/ anticholinergic properties) cause for arrest or delay in tab passage through the GI tract.

WARNINGS/PRECAUTIONS

Potentially fatal hyperkalemia and cardiac arrest may occur; monitor serum K^+ levels and adjust dose appropriately. Extreme caution with acidosis and cardiac and renal disease; monitor ECG and electrolytes. Hypokalemia with metabolic acidosis should be treated with an alkalinizing K^+ salt (eg, potassium bicarbonate, potassium citrate, potassium acetate, potassium gluconate). Solid oral dosage forms may produce ulcerative and/or stenotic lesions of the GI tract; d/c use if severe vomiting, abdominal pain, distention, or GI bleeding occurs. Reserve use for those who cannot tolerate, cannot comply, or refuse to take liquid or effervescent preparations. Caution in elderly.

ADVERSE REACTIONS

Hyperkalemia, GI effects (eg, obstruction, bleeding, ulceration), N/V, abdominal pain/discomfort, flatulence, diarrhea.

DRUG INTERACTIONS

See Contraindications. Risk of hyperkalemia with ACE inhibitors (eg, captopril, enalapril). Risk of hyperkalemia with K^+-sparing diuretics (eg, spironolactone, triamterene, amiloride).

PATIENT CONSIDERATIONS

Assessment: Assess for hyperkalemia, chronic renal failure, systemic acidosis, cardiac patients, if patient cannot tolerate, refuses to take, or cannot comply with taking liquid or effervescent K^+ preparations prior to administration of an ER tab formulation. Obtain baseline ECG, serum electrolyte levels, and renal function.

K

Monitoring: Monitor for signs/symptoms of hyperkalemia and other adverse events that may occur. In patients taking solid oral dosage forms, monitor for signs/symptoms of GI lesions. In patients with cardiac disease, acidosis, or renal disease, monitor acid-base balance and perform appropriate monitoring of serum electrolytes, ECG, renal function, and the clinical status of the patient.

Counseling: Inform about benefits and risks of therapy. Instruct to report to physician if patient develops any type of GI symptoms (eg, tarry stools or other evidence of GI bleeding, vomiting, abdominal pain/distention) or if other adverse events occur. Instruct to contact physician if difficulty in swallowing develops or if the tabs are sticking in the throat. (Klor-Con): Instruct to swallow tabs whole and to take with meals and full glass of water or other liquid. Follow the frequency and amount prescribed by the physician, especially if also taking diuretics and/or digitalis preparations. (Klor-Con M): Instruct to take each dose with meals and with full glass of water or other liquid. Inform that patient may break tabs in half or make an oral aqueous sus with tabs and 4 fl oz of water (see PI for proper preparation). Inform that aqueous sus not taken immediately should be discarded and use of other liquids for suspending is not recommended.

STORAGE: Klor-Con: 15-30°C (59-86°F). Klor-Con M: 20-25°C (68-77°F); excursions permitted to 15-30°C (59-86°F).

Kombiglyze XR — metformin hydrochloride/saxagliptin RX

Class: Biguanide/dipeptidyl peptidase-4 (DPP-4) inhibitor

Lactic acidosis may occur due to metformin accumulation; risk increases w/ conditions such as sepsis, dehydration, excess alcohol intake, hepatic impairment, renal impairment, and acute CHF. If acidosis is suspected, d/c and hospitalize patient immediately.

K

ADULT DOSAGE

Type 2 Diabetes Mellitus

Adjunct to diet and exercise to improve glycemic control when treatment w/ both saxagliptin and metformin is appropriate

Patients Requiring 5mg Saxagliptin:
Not Currently Treated w/ Metformin:
Initial: 5mg/500mg qd
Patients Treated w/ Metformin:
Dose should provide metformin at the dose already being taken, or the nearest therapeutically appropriate dose
Patients Requiring 2.5mg Saxagliptin:
Currently on Metformin ER: 2.5mg/1000mg qd
Metformin Naive/Requiring >1000mg Metformin: Use individual components
Max: (5mg/2000mg)/day

PEDIATRIC DOSAGE

Pediatric use may not have been established

DOSING CONSIDERATIONS

Concomitant Medications

Strong CYP3A4/5 Inhibitors:
Max: 2.5mg/1000mg qd
Insulin Secretagogue (eg, Sulfonylurea)/Insulin:
May require lower doses of insulin secretagogue or insulin

ADMINISTRATION

Oral route

Swallow tab whole; do not cut, crush, or chew.
Take qd w/ pm meal.

HOW SUPPLIED

Tab, Extended-Release: (Saxagliptin/Metformin ER) 5mg/500mg, 5mg/1000mg, 2.5mg/1000mg

CONTRAINDICATIONS

Renal impairment (eg, SrCr ≥1.5mg/dL [men], ≥1.4mg/dL [women], or abnormal CrCl); hypersensitivity to metformin HCl; acute or chronic metabolic acidosis, including diabetic ketoacidosis; history of a serious hypersensitivity reaction to Kombiglyze XR or saxagliptin (eg, anaphylaxis, angioedema, or exfoliative skin conditions).

WARNINGS/PRECAUTIONS

Not for use for the treatment of type 1 diabetes mellitus (DM) or diabetic ketoacidosis. Assess renal function before initiation of therapy and at least annually thereafter; d/c w/ evidence of renal impairment. Avoid in patients w/ clinical or lab evidence of hepatic disease. Temporarily suspend for any surgical procedure (except minor procedures not associated w/ restricted intake of foods and fluids); restart when oral intake is resumed and renal function is normal. Evaluate patients previously well controlled on therapy who develop lab abnormalities or clinical illness for evidence of ketoacidosis or lactic acidosis; d/c if acidosis occurs. Elderly or debilitated/malnourished patients and those w/ adrenal/pituitary insufficiency or alcohol intoxication are particularly susceptible to hypoglycemic effects. Promptly d/c in the event of cardiovascular collapse (shock), acute CHF, acute MI, and other conditions characterized by hypoxemia. Caution in elderly. **Metformin:** Do not initiate ≥80 yrs of age unless renal function is not reduced. May decrease vitamin B12 levels; monitor hematological parameters annually. Temporarily d/c at time of or prior to intravascular contrast studies w/ iodinated materials, withhold for 48 hrs subsequent to the procedure, and reinstitute only if renal function is normal. **Saxagliptin:** Acute pancreatitis reported; promptly d/c if pancreatitis is suspected and initiate appropriate management. Serious hypersensitivity reactions reported; d/c if suspected, assess for other potential causes, and institute alternative treatment for DM. Caution in patients w/ history of angioedema to another DPP-4 inhibitor. Severe and disabling arthralgia reported w/ DPP-4 inhibitors; d/c if appropriate.

ADVERSE REACTIONS

Diarrhea, N/V, URTI, UTI, headache, nasopharyngitis.

DRUG INTERACTIONS

See Dosing Considerations. Hypoglycemia may occur w/ other glucose-lowering agents (eg, sulfonylureas, insulin) or ethanol. **Metformin:** Cationic drugs that are eliminated by renal tubular secretion (eg, cimetidine, amiloride, digoxin) may potentially produce an interaction; monitor and adjust dose of Kombiglyze XR and/or the interfering drug. Thiazides and other diuretics, corticosteroids, phenothiazines, thyroid products, estrogens, oral contraceptives, phenytoin, nicotinic acid, sympathomimetics, calcium channel blockers, and isoniazid may predispose to hyperglycemia and may lead to loss of glycemic control; observe closely when such drugs are administered. Alcohol may potentiate the effect of metformin on lactate metabolism; avoid excessive alcohol intake. Caution w/ drugs that may affect renal function or result in significant hemodynamic change. May be difficult to recognize hypoglycemia w/ β-adrenergic blocking drugs. **Saxagliptin:** Ketoconazole and other strong CYP3A4/5 inhibitors (eg, atazanavir, clarithromycin, itraconazole) may significantly increase plasma concentrations.

PATIENT CONSIDERATIONS

Assessment: Assess for metabolic acidosis (including diabetic ketoacidosis), risk factors for lactic acidosis, renal/hepatic impairment, previous hypersensitivity to the drug, history of pancreatitis, inadequate vitamin B12 or Ca^{2+} absorption, type of DM, history of angioedema w/ another DPP-4 inhibitor, pregnancy/nursing status, and possible drug interactions. Assess if patient is planning to undergo any surgical procedure or radiologic studies involving the use of intravascular iodinated contrast materials. Obtain baseline FPG and HbA1c levels, and hematological parameters.

Monitoring: Monitor for signs/symptoms of lactic acidosis, pancreatitis, hypoxic states, hypoglycemia, hypersensitivity reactions, arthralgia, and other adverse reactions. Monitor for changes in clinical status. Monitor renal function, especially in elderly, at least annually. Perform routine serum vitamin B12 measurements at 2- to 3-yr intervals in patients predisposed to develop subnormal vitamin B12 levels. Monitor FPG and HbA1c levels, hepatic function, and hematologic parameters periodically.

Counseling: Inform of the risks, benefits, and alternative modes of therapy. Advise on the importance of adherence to dietary instructions, regular physical activity, periodic blood glucose monitoring and HbA1c testing, recognition/management of hypo/hyperglycemia, and assessment of diabetes complications. Instruct to seek medical advice promptly during periods of stress as medication needs may change. Inform of the risk of lactic acidosis; instruct to d/c therapy immediately and notify physician if unexplained hyperventilation, myalgia, malaise, unusual somnolence, dizziness, slow or irregular heartbeat, sensation of feeling cold (especially in the extremities), or other nonspecific symptoms occur. Inform that GI symptoms may occur. Instruct to inform physician if any unusual symptom develops, or if any known symptom persists or worsens. Counsel against excessive alcohol intake. Inform about the importance of regular testing of renal function and hematological parameters when receiving treatment. Inform that acute pancreatitis may occur; instruct to d/c therapy promptly and contact physician if persistent severe abdominal pain occurs. Inform that allergic reactions may occur; instruct to d/c therapy and seek medical advice promptly if symptoms occur. Inform that severe and disabling joint pain may occur; instruct to seek medical advice if severe joint pain occurs. Inform that inactive ingredients may occasionally be eliminated in the feces as a soft mass that may resemble the original tab.

STORAGE: 20-25°C (68-77°F); excursions permitted to 15-30°C (59-86°F).

KYBELLA – deoxycholic acid

RX

Class: Cytolytic agent

ADULT DOSAGE

Submental Fat

Improvement in appearance of moderate to severe convexity or fullness associated w/ submental fat

Inject using an area-adjusted dose of 2mg/cm^2

Single treatment consists of up to a max of 50 inj, 0.2mL each (up to a total of 10mL), spaced 1cm apart

Up to 6 single treatments may be administered at intervals no <1 month apart

PEDIATRIC DOSAGE

Pediatric use may not have been established

DOSING CONSIDERATIONS

Elderly

Start at the lower end of dosing range

K

ADMINISTRATION

SQ route

Do not dilute

Inject into SQ fat tissue in the submental area

Refer to PI for inj technique

HOW SUPPLIED

Inj: 10mg/mL [2mL]

CONTRAINDICATIONS

Presence of infection at the inj sites.

WARNINGS/PRECAUTIONS

Give careful consideration to the use of drug in patients w/ excessive skin laxity, prominent platysmal bands, or other conditions for which reduction of submental fat may result in an aesthetically undesirable outcome. Caution in patients who have had prior surgical or aesthetic treatment of the submental area. Changes in anatomy/landmarks or the presence of scar tissue may impact the ability to safely administer drug or to obtain the desired aesthetic result. Cases of marginal mandibular nerve injury, manifested as an asymmetric smile or facial muscle weakness (paresis), reported. To avoid potential for nerve injury, do not inject into or in close proximity to the marginal mandibular branch of the facial nerve. Dysphagia may occur; avoid use in patients w/ current or prior history of dysphagia. Inj-site hematoma/bruising reported; caution w/ bleeding abnormalities, as excessive bleeding or bruising in the treatment area may occur. To avoid potential tissue damage, do not inject into or in close proximity (1-1.5cm) to salivary glands, lymph nodes, and muscles.

ADVERSE REACTIONS

Inj-site reactions, headache, oropharyngeal pain, HTN.

DRUG INTERACTIONS

Caution in patients who are currently being treated w/ antiplatelet or anticoagulant therapy.

PATIENT CONSIDERATIONS

Assessment: Assess for presence of infection at the inj site, current or prior history of dysphagia, bleeding abnormalities, any other conditions where treatment is contraindicated or cautioned, pregnancy/nursing status, and for possible drug interactions. Screen for other potential causes of submental convexity/fullness (eg, thyromegaly, cervical lymphadenopathy).

Monitoring: Monitor for marginal mandibular nerve injury, dysphagia, inj-site hematoma/bruising, and other adverse reactions.

Counseling: Advise to inform physician if signs of marginal mandibular nerve paresis (eg, asymmetric smile, facial muscle weakness) or difficulty swallowing develops, or if any existing symptom worsens.

STORAGE: 20-25°C (68-77°F); excursions permitted between 15-30°C (59-86°F).

KYNAMRO – mipomersen sodium

RX

Class: Lipid-regulating agent

May cause elevations in transaminases; measure ALT, AST, alkaline phosphatase, and total bilirubin prior to therapy, and then ALT/AST regularly as recommended. Withhold dose if ALT/AST is ≥3X ULN. D/C for clinically significant liver toxicity. May increase hepatic fat. Hepatic steatosis is a risk factor for advanced liver disease, including steatohepatitis and cirrhosis. Available only through a restricted program under a Risk Evaluation and Mitigation Strategy because of the risk of hepatotoxicity.

ADULT DOSAGE

Homozygous Familial Hypercholesterolemia

200mg SQ once weekly; give on the same day every week, but if dose is missed, give at least 3 days from the next weekly dose

PEDIATRIC DOSAGE

Pediatric use may not have been established

DOSING CONSIDERATIONS

Adverse Reactions

Transaminase Elevations:

ALT/AST ≥3X and <5X ULN:

Confirm elevation w/ repeat measurement w/in 1 week

If confirmed, withhold dosing, and obtain additional liver-related tests if not already measured (eg, total bilirubin, alkaline phosphatase, INR) and investigate to identify probable cause

If resuming therapy after transaminases resolve to <3X ULN, consider monitoring liver-related tests more frequently

ALT/AST ≥5X ULN:

Withhold dosing, obtain additional liver-related tests if not already measured (eg, total bilirubin, alkaline phosphatase, INR) and investigate to identify probable cause

If resuming therapy after transaminases resolve to <3X ULN, monitor liver-related tests more frequently

If transaminase elevations are accompanied by clinical symptoms of liver injury, increases in bilirubin ≥2X ULN, or active liver disease, d/c therapy and investigate to identify probable cause

ADMINISTRATION

SQ route

Remove from refrigerated storage and allow to reach room temperature for at least 30 min prior to administration.

Inject into abdomen, thigh region, or outer area of the upper arm.

Do not inject in areas of active skin disease or injury; avoid areas of tattooed skin and scarring.

HOW SUPPLIED

Inj: 200mg/mL [1mL]

CONTRAINDICATIONS

Moderate or severe hepatic impairment (Child-Pugh B or C); active liver disease, including unexplained persistent elevations of serum transaminases; known hypersensitivity to any component of this product.

WARNINGS/PRECAUTIONS

Not recommended as an adjunct to LDL apheresis. Not recommended in patients w/ severe renal impairment, clinically significant proteinuria, or on renal dialysis. If baseline LFTs are abnormal, consider initiating therapy after an appropriate work-up and the baseline abnormalities are explained or resolved. D/C therapy and identify the probable cause if transaminase elevations are accompanied by clinical symptoms of liver injury (eg, N/V, abdominal pain, fever), increases in bilirubin ≥2X ULN, or active liver disease. Inj-site reactions (eg, erythema, pain, tenderness) reported; follow proper technique for SQ administration. Flu-like symptoms (eg, influenza-like illness, pyrexia, chills) reported. May cause fetal harm; females of reproductive potential should use effective contraception during therapy.

ADVERSE REACTIONS

Hepatic steatosis, increased serum transaminases, N/V, headache, pain in extremity, inj-site reactions, fatigue, influenza-like illness, HTN, pyrexia, chills, angina pectoris, peripheral edema, musculoskeletal pain, insomnia.

DRUG INTERACTIONS

Not recommended w/ other LDL-lowering agents that can increase hepatic fat. Alcohol may increase levels of hepatic fat and induce/exacerbate liver injury; avoid consumption of >1 alcoholic drink/day. Caution w/ other medications known to have potential for hepatotoxicity (eg, isotretinoin, amiodarone, acetaminophen [>4g/day for ≥3 days/week], methotrexate, tetracyclines, tamoxifen); more frequent monitoring of liver-related tests may be warranted.

PATIENT CONSIDERATIONS

Assessment: Assess for hepatic/renal impairment, drug hypersensitivity, pregnancy/nursing status, and possible drug interactions. Obtain baseline lipid levels, ALT/AST, alkaline phosphatase, and total bilirubin.

Monitoring: Monitor for inj-site reactions, flu-like symptoms, and other adverse reactions. Monitor LFTs monthly during 1st yr and at least every 3 months after 1st yr of therapy. Monitor lipid levels at least every 3 months for the 1st yr of therapy. Evaluate LDL level after 6 months to determine if LDL reduction achieved is sufficiently robust to warrant the potential risk of liver toxicity.

Counseling: Inform that transaminase elevations and hepatic steatosis may occur; inform of the importance of monitoring LFTs prior to therapy and periodically thereafter. Advise of the potential for increased risk of liver injury if alcohol is consumed; instruct to limit alcohol consumption to ≤1 drink/day. Advise to report any symptoms of possible liver injury (eg, N/V, fever, anorexia). Inform that inj-site reactions and flu-like symptoms have been reported. Instruct patient or caregiver of the proper technique of administration and safe disposal procedures. Instruct females of reproductive potential to use effective contraception during therapy.

STORAGE: 2-8°C (36-46°F). Protect from light and keep in the original carton until time of use. If refrigeration is unavailable, may store ≤30°C (86°F), away from heat sources, for up to 14 days.

KYPROLIS — carfilzomib

RX

Class: Proteasome inhibitor

K

ADULT DOSAGE

Relapsed or Refractory Multiple Myeloma

In Combination w/ Lenalidomide + Dexamethasone in Patients Who Have Received 1-3 Lines of Therapy:
Each 28-day period is considered 1 treatment cycle; treatment may be continued until disease progression or unacceptable toxicity occurs

Lenalidomide: 25mg PO on Days 1-21 of each cycle
Dexamethasone: 40mg PO or IV on Days 1, 8, 15, and 22 of each cycle

Cycle 1:
Administer 20mg/m^2 carfilzomib on Days 1 and 2. If tolerated, escalate to a target dose of 27mg/m^2 on Day 8; continue w/ tolerated dose on Days 9, 15, and 16

Cycles 2-12:
Administer 27mg/m^2 carfilzomib on Days 1, 2, 8, 9, 15, and 16

Cycles 13 and Thereafter:
Administer 27mg/m^2 carfilzomib on Days 1, 2, 15, and 16
D/C carfilzomib after Cycle 18

In Combination w/ Dexamethasone in Patients Who Have Received 1-3 Lines of Therapy:
Each 28-day period is considered 1 treatment cycle; treatment may be continued until disease progression or unacceptable toxicity occurs

Dexamethasone: 20mg PO or IV on Days 1, 2, 8, 9, 15, 16, 22, and 23 of each cycle

Cycle 1:
Administer 20mg/m^2 carfilzomib on Days 1 and 2. If tolerated, escalate to a target dose of 56mg/m^2 starting on Day 8; continue w/ tolerated dose on Days 9, 15, and 16

Cycles 2 and Thereafter:
Administer 56mg/m^2 carfilzomib on Days 1, 2, 8, 9, 15, and 16

PEDIATRIC DOSAGE

Pediatric use may not have been established

Single Agent in Patients Who Have Received ≥1 Line of Therapy:
Each 28-day period is considered 1 treatment cycle; treatment may be continued until disease progression or unacceptable toxicity occurs

20/27mg/m^2 Regimen:
Cycle 1:
Administer 20mg/m^2 carfilzomib on Days 1 and 2. If tolerated, escalate to a target dose of 27mg/m^2 starting on Day 8; continue w/ tolerated dose on Days 9, 15, and 16

Cycles 2-12:
Administer 27mg/m^2 carfilzomib on Days 1, 2, 8, 9, 15, and 16

Cycles 13 and Thereafter:
Administer 27mg/m^2 carfilzomib on Days 1, 2, 15, and 16

20/56mg/m^2 Regimen:
Cycle 1:
Administer 20mg/m^2 carfilzomib on Days 1 and 2. If tolerated, escalate to a target dose of 56mg/m^2 starting on Day 8; continue w/ tolerated dose on Days 9, 15, and 16

Cycles 2-12:
Administer 56mg/m^2 carfilzomib on Days 1, 2, 8, 9, 15, and 16

Cycles 13 and Thereafter:
Administer 56mg/m^2 carfilzomib on Days 1, 2, 15, and 16

Premedication

Hydration and Fluid Monitoring:
Prior to Each Dose in Cycle 1: Give both oral (30mL/kg at least 48 hrs before Cycle 1, Day 1) and IV fluids (250-500mL of appropriate IV fluid prior to each dose in Cycle 1); if needed, give an additional 250-500mL of IV fluids following administration
Subsequent Cycles: Continue oral and/or IV hydration prn

Dexamethasone:
Administer recommended dexamethasone 30 min to 4 hrs prior to all doses of carfilzomib during Cycle 1 to reduce the incidence and severity of infusion reactions; reinstate dexamethasone premedication if these symptoms occur during subsequent cycles
20/27mg/m^2 Regimen: 4mg PO or IV
20/56mg/m^2 Regimen: 8mg PO or IV

Thromboprophylaxis:
Recommended for patients being treated w/ combination of carfilzomib w/ dexamethasone or w/ lenalidomide + dexamethasone; base regimen on underlying risks

Infection Prophylaxis:
Consider antiviral prophylaxis to decrease the risk of herpes zoster reactivation

DOSING CONSIDERATIONS
Adverse Reactions
Dose Level Reductions:

27mg/m^2 Dose:
First Dose Reduction: 20mg/m^2
Second Dose Reduction: 15mg/m^2; d/c if toxicity persists

56mg/m^2 Dose:
First Dose Reduction: 45mg/m^2

Second Dose Reduction: 36mg/m^2
Third Dose Reduction: 27mg/m^2; d/c if toxicity persists

Hematologic Toxicity:
ANC <0.5 x 10^9/L:
- Withhold dose
- If recovered to ≥0.5 x 10^9/L, continue at same dose level
- For subsequent drop to <0.5 x 10^9/L, follow same recommendations as above and consider 1 dose level reduction when restarting carfilzomib

Febrile Neutropenia (ANC <0.5 x 10^9/L and an Oral Temperature >38.5°C or 2 Consecutive Readings of >38.0°C for 2 Hrs):
- Withhold dose
- If ANC returns to baseline grade and fever resolves, resume at the same dose level

Platelets <10 x 10^9/L or Evidence of Bleeding w/ Thrombocytopenia:
- Withhold dose; if recovered to ≥10 x 10^9/L and/or bleeding is controlled, continue at same dose level
- For subsequent drops <10 x 10^9/L, follow the same recommendations as above and consider 1 dose level reduction when restarting carfilzomib

Renal Toxicity:
SrCr ≥2 x Baseline, or CrCl <15mL/min or CrCl Decreases to ≤50% of Baseline, or Need for Dialysis:
- Withhold dose and continue monitoring renal function (SrCr or CrCl)
- If attributable to carfilzomib, resume when renal function has recovered to w/in 25% of baseline; start at 1 dose level reduction
- If not attributable to carfilzomib, dosing may be resumed at the discretion of the physician
- For patients on dialysis, administer the dose after dialysis

Other Non-Hematologic Toxicity:
All Other Severe or Life-Threatening (CTCAE Grades 3 and 4) Non-Hematological Toxicities:
- Withhold until resolved or returned to baseline
- Consider restarting the next scheduled treatment at 1 dose level reduction

K

ADMINISTRATION

IV route

Calculate dose based on actual BSA at baseline; patients w/ BSA >2.2m^2 should receive a dose based on a BSA of 2.2m^2.

Dose does not need to be adjusted for weight change of ≤20%.

Do not mix w/ or administer as an infusion w/ other medicinal products.

Flush IV line w/ normal saline or D5 inj immediately before and after administration.

Infusion Times

W/ Lenalidomide and Dexamethasone: 10 min
W/ Dexamethasone: 30 min
20/27mg/m^2 Monotherapy Regimen: 10 min
20/56mg/m^2 Monotherapy Regimen: 30 min

Reconstitution/Preparation

1. Slowly inject 29mL of sterile water for inj, directing the sol onto the inside wall of the vial to minimize foaming.
2. Gently swirl and/or invert vial slowly for about 1 min, or until complete dissolution; do not shake. If foaming occurs, allow sol to settle in the vial until foaming subsides (approx 5 min) and the sol is clear.
3. When administering in an IV bag, withdraw calculated dose from vial and dilute into 50mL D5 inj IV bag.
4. Discard any unused portion left in the vial.

Stability of Reconstituted Carfilzomib

Total time from reconstitution to administration should not exceed 24 hrs.
Stable for 24 hrs at 2-8°C (36-46°F).
Stable for 4 hrs at 15-30°C (59-86°F).

HOW SUPPLIED

Inj: 60mg

WARNINGS/PRECAUTIONS

New onset/worsening of preexisting cardiac failure, restrictive cardiomyopathy, myocardial ischemia, and MI including fatalities reported following administration. Death due to cardiac arrest has occurred w/in a day of administration. Renal insufficiency adverse events reported; acute renal failure was reported more frequently in patients w/ advanced relapsed and refractory multiple myeloma who received carfilzomib monotherapy. Cases of tumor lysis syndrome (TLS), including fatal outcomes, reported; monitor for evidence of TLS during treatment and manage promptly, including interruption of therapy until TLS is resolved. Consider uric acid-lowering drugs in patients at risk for TLS. Acute respiratory distress syndrome, acute respiratory failure, and acute diffuse infiltrative pulmonary disease reported; d/c in the event of drug-induced pulmonary toxicity. Pulmonary arterial HTN (PAH) reported; withhold therapy until resolved or returned to baseline and consider whether to restart therapy based on a benefit/risk assessment. Dyspnea reported; evaluate dyspnea to exclude cardiopulmonary conditions. HTN, including hypertensive crisis and hypertensive emergency, reported; withhold carfilzomib and evaluate if HTN cannot be adequately controlled. Venous thromboembolic events (eg, deep venous thrombosis, pulmonary embolism) reported; consider an alternative method of contraception during treatment w/ carfilzomib in combination w/ dexamethasone or lenalidomide + dexamethasone in patients using oral contraceptives or a hormonal method of contraception associated w/ a risk of thrombosis. Infusion reactions may occur immediately following or up to 24 hrs after treatment; administer dexamethasone prior to treatment to reduce the incidence and severity of reactions. Thrombocytopenia reported; reduce or interrupt dose as appropriate. Hepatic failure, including fatal cases, reported; monitor liver enzymes regularly. Thrombotic microangiopathy, including thrombotic thrombocytopenic purpura/hemolytic uremic syndrome (TTP/HUS), reported; if diagnosis is suspected, d/c therapy and evaluate. If diagnosis of TTP/HUS is excluded, therapy can be restarted. Posterior reversible encephalopathy syndrome (PRES) reported; d/c if suspected and evaluate. May cause fetal harm.

ADVERSE REACTIONS

Monotherapy: Anemia, fatigue, thrombocytopenia, nausea, pyrexia, dyspnea, diarrhea, headache, cough, peripheral edema.

Combination Therapy: Anemia, neutropenia, diarrhea, dyspnea, fatigue, thrombocytopenia, pyrexia, insomnia, muscle spasm, cough, URTI, hypokalemia.

PATIENT CONSIDERATIONS

Assessment: Assess for dehydration, hypersensitivity to drug, preexisting cardiac failure, hepatic dysfunction, renal impairment, and pregnancy/nursing status. Obtain baseline CBC, LFTs, SrCr, and weight. Consider antiviral prophylaxis therapy.

Monitoring: Monitor for signs/symptoms of cardiac toxicities, acute renal failure, TLS, dehydration, pulmonary toxicity, PAH, dyspnea, HTN, venous thromboembolic events, infusion reactions, TTP/HUS, PRES, hepatic failure, and other adverse reactions. Monitor CBC, LFTs, and SrCr.

Counseling: Advise to contact physician if SOB, fever, chills, rigors, chest pain, cough, swelling of the feet or legs, bleeding, bruising, weakness, headaches, confusion, seizures, or visual loss develops. Instruct not to drive or operate machinery if fatigue, dizziness, fainting, and/or drop in BP are experienced. Advise regarding appropriate measures to avoid dehydration; instruct to notify physician if symptoms of dizziness, lightheadedness, or fainting spells develop. Advise females of reproductive potential to use effective contraceptive measures to prevent pregnancy during and for at least 30 days after treatment and instruct to inform physician immediately if pregnant. Advise males of reproductive potential to use effective contraceptive measures to prevent pregnancy during and for at least 90 days after treatment. Instruct not to breastfeed while on therapy. Advise to notify physician if using or planning to take other prescription or OTC drugs.

STORAGE: **Unopened Vials:** 2-8°C (36-46°F). Protect from light. **Reconstituted Sol:** 2-8°C (36-46°F) for 24 hrs and 15-30°C (59-86°F) for 4 hrs.

LAMICTAL – lamotrigine

RX

Class: Phenyltriazine

Serious life-threatening rashes, including Stevens-Johnson syndrome, toxic epidermal necrolysis, and/or rash-related death reported. Serious rash occurs more often in pediatric patients than in adults. D/C at 1st sign of rash, unless rash is clearly not drug related. Potential increased risk w/ concomitant valproate (including valproic acid and divalproex sodium) or exceeding the recommended initial dose/dose escalation.

OTHER BRAND NAMES

Lamictal ODT

ADULT DOSAGE

Epilepsy

Adjunctive Therapy for Partial-Onset, Primary Generalized Tonic-Clonic Seizures, or Generalized Seizures of Lennox-Gastaut Syndrome:

Taking Valproate:

Weeks 1 and 2: 25mg qod

Weeks 3 and 4: 25mg qd

Week 5 Onward: Increase every 1-2 weeks by 25-50mg/day

PEDIATRIC DOSAGE

Epilepsy

Adjunctive Therapy for Partial-Onset, Primary Generalized Tonic-Clonic Seizures, or Generalized Seizures of Lennox-Gastaut Syndrome:

2-12 Years:

Round dose down to the nearest whole tab; give in 1-2 divided doses

L

Maint: 100-200mg/day w/ valproate alone or 100-400mg/day w/ valproate and other drugs inducing glucuronidation in 1 or 2 divided doses

Not Taking Carbamazepine, Phenytoin, Phenobarbital, Primidone, or Valproate:
Weeks 1 and 2: 25mg qd
Weeks 3 and 4: 50mg/day
Week 5 Onward: Increase every 1-2 weeks by 50mg/day
Maint: 225-375mg/day in 2 divided doses

Taking Carbamazepine, Phenytoin, Phenobarbital, or Primidone, w/o Valproate:
Weeks 1 and 2: 50mg/day
Weeks 3 and 4: 100mg/day in 2 divided doses
Week 5 Onward: Increase every 1-2 weeks by 100mg/day
Maint: 300-500mg/day in 2 divided doses

Bipolar I Disorder

Maint Treatment to Delay the Time to Occurrence of Mood Episodes in Patients Treated for Acute Mood Episodes w/ Standard Therapy:

Taking Valproate:
Weeks 1 and 2: 25mg qod
Weeks 3 and 4: 25mg/day
Week 5: 50mg/day
Weeks 6 and 7: 100mg/day

Not Taking Carbamazepine, Phenytoin, Phenobarbital, Primidone, or Valproate:
Weeks 1 and 2: 25mg/day
Weeks 3 and 4: 50mg/day
Week 5: 100mg/day
Weeks 6 and 7: 200mg/day

Taking Carbamazepine, Phenytoin, Phenobarbital, or Primidone, w/o Valproate:
Weeks 1 and 2: 50mg/day
Weeks 3 and 4: 100mg/day
Week 5: 200mg/day
Week 6: 300mg/day
Week 7: Up to 400mg/day
Weeks 3-7: Take in divided doses

Conversions

Conversion from Adjunctive Therapy to Monotherapy:
≥16 Years:
Monotherapy Maint: 500mg/day in 2 divided doses

From Adjunctive Therapy w/ Carbamazepine, Phenytoin, Phenobarbital, or Primidone:
After achieving a dose of 500mg/day of lamotrigine, withdraw concomitant antiepileptic drug by 20% decrements each week over a 4-week period

From Adjunctive Therapy w/ Valproate:
1. Maintain lamotrigine at 200mg/day and decrease valproate by decrements no >500mg/day/week to 500mg/day and then maintain for 1 week
2. Increase lamotrigine to 300mg/day and maintain for 1 week; simultaneously decrease valproate to 250mg/day and maintain for 1 week
3. Increase lamotrigine by 100mg/day every week to achieve maint dose of 500mg/day; d/c valproate

Taking Valproate:
Initial Weight-Based Dosing Guide (Weeks 1-4): Refer to PI
Weeks 1 and 2: 0.15mg/kg/day
Weeks 3 and 4: 0.3mg/kg/day
Week 5 Onward: Increase every 1-2 weeks by 0.3mg/kg/day
Maint: 1-5mg/kg/day (max 200mg/day) or 1-3mg/kg/day w/ valproate alone

Not Taking Carbamazepine, Phenytoin, Phenobarbital, Primidone, or Valproate:
Weeks 1 and 2: 0.3mg/kg/day
Weeks 3 and 4: 0.6mg/kg/day
Week 5 Onward: Increase every 1-2 weeks by 0.6mg/kg/day
Maint: 4.5-7.5mg/kg/day
Max: 300mg/day in 2 divided doses

Taking Carbamazepine, Phenytoin, Phenobarbital, or Primidone, w/o Valproate:
Weeks 1 and 2: 0.6mg/kg/day
Weeks 3 and 4: 1.2mg/kg/day
Week 5 Onward: Increase every 1-2 weeks by 1.2mg/kg/day
Maint: 5-15mg/kg/day
Max: 400mg/day in 2 divided doses

>12 Years:
Taking Valproate:
Weeks 1 and 2: 25mg qod
Weeks 3 and 4: 25mg qd
Week 5 Onward: Increase every 1-2 weeks by 25-50mg/day
Maint: 100-200mg/day w/ valproate alone or 100-400mg/day w/ valproate and other drugs inducing glucuronidation in 1 or 2 divided doses

Not Taking Carbamazepine, Phenytoin, Phenobarbital, Primidone, or Valproate:
Weeks 1 and 2: 25mg qd
Weeks 3 and 4: 50mg/day
Week 5 Onward: Increase every 1-2 weeks by 50mg/day
Maint: 225-375mg/day in 2 divided doses

Taking Carbamazepine, Phenytoin, Phenobarbital, or Primidone, w/o Valproate:
Weeks 1 and 2: 50mg/day
Weeks 3 and 4: 100mg/day in 2 divided doses
Week 5 Onward: Increase every 1-2 weeks by 100mg/day
Maint: 300-500mg/day in 2 divided doses

L

DOSING CONSIDERATIONS

Concomitant Medications

Taking Estrogen-Containing Oral Contraceptives w/o Other Drugs Known to Induce Glucuronidation:
May need to increase maint dose of lamotrigine by as much as 2-fold

Starting Estrogen-Containing Oral Contraceptives w/o Other Drugs Known to Induce Glucuronidation:
May need to increase maint dose of lamotrigine by as much as 2-fold
Increase lamotrigine dose at the same time the oral contraceptive is introduced; no more than 50-100mg/day every week
If adverse reactions occur during the pill-free week due to lamotrigine, may need to adjust overall maint dose; dose adjustments limited to pill-free week not recommended

Stopping Estrogen-Containing Oral Contraceptives w/o Other Drugs Known to Induce Glucuronidation:
May need to decrease maint dose of lamotrigine by as much as 50%; decreases should not exceed 25% of total daily dose/week over a 2-week period, unless clinical response or lamotrigine plasma levels indicate otherwise

Taking Atazanavir/Ritonavir But Not Taking Other Glucuronidation Inducers:
Lamotrigine may need to be increased if atazanavir/ritonavir is added or decreased if atazanavir/ritonavir is discontinued

Bipolar Disorder:

Discontinuation of Psychotropic Drugs Excluding Valproate, Carbamazepine, Phenytoin, Phenobarbital, or Primidone:
Maintain current dose of lamotrigine

After Discontinuation of Valproate w/ Current dose of 100mg/day Lamotrigine:
Week 1: 150mg/day
Week 2 Onward: 200mg/day

After Discontinuation of Carbamazepine, Phenytoin, Phenobarbital, or Primidone w/ Current Dose of 400mg/day Lamotrigine:
Week 1: 400mg/day
Week 2: 300mg/day
Week 3 Onward: 200mg/day

Renal Impairment

Significant: Reduce maint doses

Hepatic Impairment

Moderate/Severe w/o Ascites: Reduce initial, escalation, and maint doses by approx 25%
Severe w/ Ascites: Reduce initial, escalation, and maint doses by 50%
Adjust maint and escalation doses based on clinical response

Elderly

Start at lower end of dosing range

Discontinuation

A step-wise reduction over at least 2 weeks (approx 50% per week) is recommended unless safety concerns require a more rapid withdrawal

Other Important Considerations

<30kg: Maint dose may need to be increased by as much as 50%, based on clinical response

ADMINISTRATION

Oral route

Tab, Chewable

May swallow whole, chewed, or dispersed in water or diluted fruit juice
If tabs are chewed, consume a small amount of water or diluted fruit juice to aid in swallowing
To disperse chewable tabs, add tabs to a small amount of liquid (1 tsp, or enough to cover the medication); approx 1 min later when tabs are completely dispersed, swirl sol and consume entire quantity immediately

Tab, Orally Disintegrating

Place onto the tongue and move around in the mouth
Can be swallowed w/ or w/o water and taken w/ or w/ food

HOW SUPPLIED

Tab: 25mg*, 100mg*, 150mg*, 200mg*; **Tab, Chewable:** 2mg, 5mg, 25mg; **Tab, Disintegrating:** (ODT) 25mg, 50mg, 100mg, 200mg *scored

CONTRAINDICATIONS

Hypersensitivity (eg, rash, angioedema, acute urticaria, extensive pruritus, mucosal ulceration) to the drug or its ingredients.

WARNINGS/PRECAUTIONS

Not recommended for treatment of acute manic/mixed episodes. Drug reaction w/ eosinophilia and systemic symptoms (DRESS), also known as multiorgan hypersensitivity reactions, reported.

Fatalities from acute multiorgan failure and various degrees of hepatic failure reported. Isolated liver failure w/o rash or involvement of other organs reported. D/C if alternative etiology for signs/symptoms of early manifestations of hypersensitivity cannot be established. Blood dyscrasias (eg, neutropenia, leukopenia) reported. Increased risk of suicidal thoughts or behavior. Increases risk of developing aseptic meningitis; evaluate for other causes of aseptic meningitis and treat appropriately. Avoid abrupt withdrawal due to risk of withdrawal seizures. Treatment-emergent status epilepticus and sudden unexplained death in epilepsy reported. May cause toxicity in the eyes and other melanin-rich tissues due to melanin binding. Medication errors reported. Do not restart therapy in patients who discontinued due to rash associated w/ prior treatment, unless potential benefits outweigh the risks. If restarting after discontinuation, assess the need to restart w/ initial dosing recommendations. May interfere w/ assay used in some rapid urine screens, which can result in false-positive readings, particularly for phencyclidine; use a more specific analytical method to confirm a positive result.

ADVERSE REACTIONS

Rash, dizziness, diplopia, infection, headache, ataxia, blurred vision, N/V, somnolence, fever, pharyngitis, rhinitis, diarrhea, abdominal pain, tremor.

DRUG INTERACTIONS

See Boxed Warning and Dosing Considerations. Estrogen-containing oral contraceptives, carbamazepine, lopinavir/ritonavir, phenobarbital/primidone, and phenytoin decreased levels. Atazanavir/ritonavir and rifampin decreased exposure. May decrease levels of levonorgestrel. Valproate may increase levels. May increase carbamazepine epoxide levels. Drugs known to induce or inhibit glucuronidation may affect clearance. May increase plasma levels of drugs substantially excreted via organic cationic transporter 2 (OCT2) proteins; avoid w/ OCT2 substrates w/ a narrow therapeutic index (eg, dofetilide).

PATIENT CONSIDERATIONS

Assessment: Assess for history of allergy/rash to other AEDs, renal/hepatic impairment, depression, systemic lupus erythematosus or other autoimmune diseases, hypersensitivity to drug, pregnancy/nursing status, and possible drug interactions.

Monitoring: Monitor for signs/symptoms of rash, DRESS, multiorgan failure, status epilepticus, blood dyscrasias, emergence/worsening of depression, suicidal thoughts or behavior, unusual mood/behavior changes, aseptic meningitis, ophthalmologic effects, and other adverse reactions. Periodically reassess patients w/ bipolar disorder taking lamotrigine for >16 weeks to determine need for maintenance treatment.

Counseling: Inform that a rash or other signs/symptoms of hypersensitivity may herald a serious medical event; instruct to report such symptoms to healthcare providers immediately. Instruct to notify healthcare providers immediately if blood dyscrasias, DRESS, acute multiorgan failure, or aseptic meningitis occur. Inform about increased risk of suicidal thoughts and behavior; instruct to be alert for emergence/worsening of symptoms of depression, any unusual changes in mood/behavior, suicidal thoughts/behavior, or thoughts about self-harm. Instruct to immediately report behaviors of concern to healthcare providers. Instruct to notify healthcare providers if worsening of seizure control occurs. Inform that CNS depression may occur; instruct to avoid operating machinery/driving until effects of the drug are known. Instruct to notify healthcare providers if pregnant, intending to become pregnant, or if breastfeeding. Encourage patients to enroll in the North American Antiepileptic Drug Pregnancy Registry. Instruct women to notify healthcare providers if they plan to start/stop use of oral contraceptives or other hormonal preparations. Instruct to promptly notify healthcare providers of changes in menstrual pattern and adverse reactions. Instruct to notify healthcare providers if medication is discontinued and not to resume therapy w/o consulting healthcare providers. Strongly advise to visually inspect tab to verify if correct drug/formulation was dispensed each time prescription is filled.

STORAGE: (Tab/Tab, Chewable) 25°C (77°F); excursions permitted to 15-30°C (59-86°F) in a dry place. (Tab) Protect from light. (Tab, Disintegrating) 20-25°C (68-77°F); excursions permitted between 15-30°C (59-86°F).

LAMICTAL XR – lamotrigine

RX

Class: Phenyltriazine

Serious life-threatening rashes, including Stevens-Johnson syndrome, toxic epidermal necrolysis, and/or rash-related death reported. Serious rash occurs more often in pediatric patients than in adults. D/C at 1st sign of rash, unless rash is clearly not drug related. Potential increased risk w/ concomitant valproate (including valproic acid and divalproex sodium) or exceeding the recommended initial dose/dose escalation. Not approved for patients <13 yrs of age.

ADULT DOSAGE

Seizures

Adjunctive Therapy for Primary Generalized Tonic-Clonic Seizures and Partial-Onset Seizures w/ or w/o Secondary Generalization:

Taking Valproate:
Weeks 1 and 2: 25mg qod
Weeks 3 and 4: 25mg qd
Week 5: 50mg qd
Week 6: 100mg qd
Week 7: 150mg qd
Week 8 Onward (Maint): 200-250mg qd

Not Taking Carbamazepine, Phenytoin, Phenobarbital, Primidone, or Valproate:
Weeks 1 and 2: 25mg qd
Weeks 3 and 4: 50mg qd
Week 5: 100mg qd
Week 6: 150mg qd
Week 7: 200mg qd
Week 8 Onward (Maint): 300-400mg qd

Taking Carbamazepine, Phenytoin, Phenobarbital, or Primidone, w/o Valproate:
Weeks 1 and 2: 50mg qd
Weeks 3 and 4: 100mg qd
Week 5: 200mg qd
Week 6: 300mg qd
Week 7: 400mg qd
Week 8 Onward (Maint): 400-600mg qd

Dose increases at week 8 or later should not exceed 100mg/day at weekly intervals

Conversions

Conversion from Adjunctive Therapy to Monotherapy:
Monotherapy Maint: 250-300mg qd

From Adjunctive Therapy w/ Carbamazepine, Phenytoin, Phenobarbital, or Primidone:
1. After achieving 500mg/day Lamictal XR, withdraw concomitant antiepileptic drug by 20% decrements/week over a 4-week period
2. Two weeks after withdrawal of the antiepileptic drug, Lamictal XR may be decreased no faster than 100mg/day each week to achieve monotherapy maint dosage range of 250-300mg/day

From Adjunctive Therapy w/ Valproate:
1. Achieve dose of 150mg/day of Lamictal XR; maintain established stable valproate dose
2. Maintain dose of Lamictal XR at 150mg/day; decrease valproate by decrements no >500mg/day/week to 500mg/day and maintain for 1 week
3. Increase Lamictal XR to 200mg/day; simultaneously decrease valproate to 250mg/day and maintain for 1 week
4. Increase Lamictal XR to 250 or 300mg/day; d/c valproate

From Adjunctive Therapy w/ Antiepileptic Drugs Other than Carbamazepine, Phenytoin, Phenobarbital, Primidone, or Valproate:
After achieving 250-300mg/day of Lamictal XR, withdraw concomitant antiepileptic drug by 20% decrements each week over a 4-week period

Conversion from Immediate Release (IR) to Extended Release Tabs:
Initial dose of therapy should match the total daily dose of IR lamotrigine

PEDIATRIC DOSAGE

Seizures

Adjunctive Therapy for Primary Generalized Tonic-Clonic Seizures and Partial-Onset Seizures w/ or w/o Secondary Generalization:
≥13 Years:

Taking Valproate:
Weeks 1 and 2: 25mg qod
Weeks 3 and 4: 25mg qd
Week 5: 50mg qd
Week 6: 100mg qd
Week 7: 150mg qd
Week 8 Onward (Maint): 200-250mg qd

Not Taking Carbamazepine, Phenytoin, Phenobarbital, Primidone, or Valproate:
Weeks 1 and 2: 25mg qd
Weeks 3 and 4: 50mg qd
Week 5: 100mg qd
Week 6: 150mg qd
Week 7: 200mg qd
Week 8 Onward (Maint): 300-400mg qd

Taking Carbamazepine, Phenytoin, Phenobarbital, or Primidone, w/o Valproate:
Weeks 1 and 2: 50mg qd
Weeks 3 and 4: 100mg qd
Week 5: 200mg qd
Week 6: 300mg qd
Week 7: 400mg qd
Week 8 Onward (Maint): 400-600mg qd

Dose increases at week 8 or later should not exceed 100mg/day at weekly intervals

Conversions

≥13 Years:

Conversion from Adjunctive Therapy to Monotherapy:
Monotherapy Maint: 250-300mg qd

From Adjunctive Therapy w/ Carbamazepine, Phenytoin, Phenobarbital, or Primidone:
1. After achieving 500mg/day of Lamictal XR, withdraw concomitant antiepileptic drug by 20% decrements/week over a 4-week period
2. Two weeks after withdrawal of the antiepileptic drug, Lamictal XR may be decreased no faster than 100mg/day each week to monotherapy maint dosage range of 250-300mg/day.

From Adjunctive Therapy w/ Valproate:
1. Achieve dose of 150mg/day of Lamictal XR; maintain established stable valproate dose
2. Maintain dose of Lamictal XR at 150mg/day; decrease valproate by decrements no >500mg/day/week to 500mg/day and maintain for 1 week
3. Increase Lamictal XR to 200mg/day; simultaneously decrease valproate to 250mg/day and maintain for 1 week
4. Increase Lamictal XR to 250 or 300mg/day; d/c valproate

From Adjunctive Therapy w/ Antiepileptic Drugs Other than Carbamazepine, Phenytoin, Phenobarbital, Primidone, or Valproate:
After achieving 250-300mg/day of Lamictal XR, withdraw concomitant antiepileptic drug by 20% decrements each week over a 4-week period

Conversion from Immediate Release (IR) to Extended Release Tabs:
Initial dose of therapy should match the total daily dose of IR lamotrigine

DOSING CONSIDERATIONS

Concomitant Medications

Taking Estrogen-Containing Oral Contraceptives w/o Other Drugs Known to Induce Glucuronidation:
May need to increase maint dose by as much as 2-fold

Starting Estrogen-Containing Oral Contraceptives w/o Other Drugs Known to Induce Glucuronidation:
May need to increase maint dose by as much as 2-fold
Increase at the same time the oral contraceptive is introduced and continue no more rapidly than 50-100mg/day every week
If adverse reactions occur during the pill-free week, may need to adjust overall maint dose; dose adjustments limited to pill-free week are not recommended

Stopping Estrogen-Containing Oral Contraceptives w/o Other Drugs Known to Induce Glucuronidation:
May need to decrease maint dose by as much as 50%; decreases should not exceed 25% of the total daily dose/week over a 2-week period, unless clinical response or lamotrigine plasma levels indicate otherwise

Atazanavir/Ritonavir Not Taking Other Glucuronidation Inducers:
May need to increase dose if atazanavir/ritonavir is added, or decrease if atazanavir/ritonavir is discontinued

Renal Impairment

Significant: Reduce maint doses

Hepatic Impairment

Moderate/Severe w/o Ascites: Reduce initial, escalation, and maint doses by 25%
Severe w/ Ascites: Reduce initial, escalation, and maint doses by 50%
Adjust maint and escalation doses based on clinical response

Elderly

Start at lower end of dosing range

Discontinuation

A step-wise reduction of dose over at least 2 weeks (approx 50% per week) is recommended unless safety concerns require a more rapid withdrawal

ADMINISTRATION

Oral route

May take w/ or w/o food
Swallow whole; do not chew, crush, or divide

HOW SUPPLIED

Tab, Extended Release (ER): 25mg, 50mg, 100mg, 200mg, 250mg, 300mg

CONTRAINDICATIONS

Hypersensitivity (eg, rash, angioedema, acute urticaria, extensive pruritus, mucosal ulceration) to the drug or its ingredients.

WARNINGS/PRECAUTIONS

Drug reaction w/ eosinophilia and systemic symptoms (DRESS), also known as multiorgan hypersensitivity reactions, reported. Fatalities from acute multiorgan failure and various degrees of hepatic failure reported. Isolated liver failure w/o rash or involvement of other organs reported. D/C if alternative etiology for signs/symptoms of early manifestations of hypersensitivity cannot be established. Blood dyscrasias (eg, neutropenia, leukopenia) w/ the IR formulation reported. Increased risk of suicidal thoughts or behavior. Increases risk of developing aseptic meningitis; evaluate for other causes of aseptic meningitis and treat appropriately. Avoid abrupt withdrawal due to risk of withdrawal seizures. Treatment-emergent status epilepticus and sudden unexplained death in epilepsy reported w/ IR formulation. May cause toxicity in the eyes and other melanin-rich tissues due to melanin binding. Medication errors including errors due to product name confusion, reported. Caution w/ significant renal impairment, moderate/severe hepatic impairment, and in the elderly. Do not restart therapy in patients who discontinued due to rash associated w/ prior treatment, unless potential benefits outweigh the risks. If restarting after discontinuation, assess the need to restart w/ initial dosing recommendations. May interfere w/ assay used in some rapid urine screens, which can result in false-positive readings, particularly for phencyclidine; use a more specific analytical method to confirm a positive result. May increase incidence of subnormal values in some hematology analytes (eg, total WBC, monocytes).

ADVERSE REACTIONS

Rash, dizziness, N/V, tremor, asthenia, somnolence, diplopia, diarrhea, vertigo, depression, anxiety, blurred vision, anorexia, pharyngolaryngeal pain, cerebellar coordination and balance disorder.

DRUG INTERACTIONS

See Boxed Warning and Dosing Considerations. Estrogen-containing oral contraceptives, carbamazepine, lopinavir/ritonavir, phenobarbital/primidone, and phenytoin may decrease levels. Atazanavir/ritonavir and rifampin may decrease exposure. May decrease levels of levonorgestrel.

Valproate may increase levels. May increase carbamazepine epoxide levels. Drugs known to induce or inhibit glucuronidation may affect clearance. May increase plasma levels of drugs substantially excreted via organic cationic transporter 2 (OCT2) proteins; avoid w/ OCT2 substrates w/ a narrow therapeutic index (eg, dofetilide).

PATIENT CONSIDERATIONS

Assessment: Assess for history of allergy/rash to other AEDs, renal/hepatic impairment, depression, hypersensitivity to drug, pregnancy/nursing status, and possible drug interactions.

Monitoring: Monitor for signs/symptoms of rash, DRESS, multiorgan failure, status epilepticus, blood dyscrasias, emergence/worsening of depression, suicidal thoughts or behavior, unusual mood/behavior changes, aseptic meningitis, ophthalmologic effects, and other adverse reactions. Monitor for seizure control following conversion to ER, especially those on drugs that induce lamotrigine glucuronidation. If indicated, monitor plasma levels of lamotrigine and concomitant medications, particularly during dosage adjustments.

Counseling: Inform that a rash or other signs/symptoms of hypersensitivity may herald a serious medical event; instruct to report such symptoms to healthcare provider immediately. Instruct to notify healthcare provider immediately if blood dyscrasias, DRESS, acute multiorgan failure, or aseptic meningitis occur. Inform about increased risk of suicidal thoughts and behavior; instruct to be alert for emergence/worsening of signs/symptoms of depression, any unusual changes in mood/behavior, suicidal thoughts/behavior, or thoughts about self-harm. Instruct to immediately report behaviors of concern to healthcare provider. Instruct to notify healthcare provider if worsening of seizure control occurs. Inform that CNS depression may occur; instruct to avoid operating machinery/driving until effects of the drug are known. Advise to notify healthcare provider if pregnant/intending to become pregnant, or breastfeeding. Encourage patients to enroll in the North American Antiepileptic Drug Pregnancy Registry if they become pregnant. Instruct women to notify healthcare provider if they plan to start/stop oral contraceptives or other hormonal preparations. Instruct to promptly notify healthcare provider of changes in menstrual pattern and adverse reactions. Instruct to notify healthcare provider if medication is discontinued and not to resume therapy w/o consulting healthcare provider. Strongly advise to visually inspect tab to verify if correct drug/formulation is dispensed each time prescription is filled.

STORAGE: 25°C (77°F); excursions permitted to 15-30°C (59-86°F).

L

LAMISIL — terbinafine hydrochloride

RX

Class: Allylamine antifungal

ADULT DOSAGE

Tinea Capitis

Granules:
<25kg: 125mg/day qd
25-35kg: 187.5mg/day qd
>35kg: 250mg/day qd

Treatment Duration: 6 weeks

Onychomycosis

Due to Dermatophytes (Tinea Unguium):
Tab:
Fingernail: 250mg qd for 6 weeks
Toenail: 250mg qd for 12 weeks

PEDIATRIC DOSAGE

Tinea Capitis

≥4 Years:
Granules:
<25kg: 125mg/day
25-35kg: 187.5mg/day
>35kg: 250mg/day

Treatment Duration: 6 weeks

DOSING CONSIDERATIONS

Elderly

Tab:
Start at lower end of dosing range

ADMINISTRATION

Oral route

Granules

Take w/ food
Sprinkle contents of 1 pkt on a spoonful of pudding or other soft, nonacidic food (eg, mashed potatoes), and swallow entire spoonful (w/o chewing); do not use applesauce or fruit-based foods
Either the contents of both pkts may be sprinkled on 1 spoonful, or the contents of both pkts may be sprinkled on 2 spoonfuls of nonacidic food if 2 pkts are required/dose

Tab

Take w/ or w/o food

HOW SUPPLIED

Granules: 125mg/pkt, 187.5mg/pkt; **Tab:** 250mg

CONTRAINDICATIONS

History of allergic reaction to oral terbinafine.

WARNINGS/PRECAUTIONS

Cases of liver failure, some leading to liver transplant or death, reported in individuals with and without preexisting liver disease; d/c therapy if evidence of liver injury develops. Hepatotoxicity may occur. Not recommended for patients with chronic or active liver disease; perform LFTs prior to initiating therapy and periodically thereafter. D/C immediately in case of LFTs elevation or if any symptoms of persistent N/V, anorexia, fatigue, right upper abdominal pain, jaundice, dark urine, or pale stools occur. Taste/smell disturbance reported; d/c if symptoms occur. Depressive symptoms reported. Transient decreases in absolute lymphocyte counts and severe neutropenia reported; d/c and start supportive management if neutrophil count is $\leq$1000 cells/mm^3.Consider monitoring CBCs in patients with known or suspected immunodeficiency if treatment continues for >6 weeks. Serious skin/hypersensitivity reactions (eg, Stevens-Johnson syndrome, toxic epidermal necrolysis, erythema multiforme, exfoliative/bullous dermatitis, drug reaction with eosinophilia and systemic symptoms (DRESS) syndrome) reported; d/c if progressive skin rash or signs/symptoms of DRESS occur. Precipitation and exacerbation of cutaneous and systemic lupus erythematosus reported; d/c in patients with clinical signs/symptoms suggestive of lupus erythematosus.

ADVERSE REACTIONS

Headache, diarrhea. (Granules) Nasopharyngitis, pyrexia, cough, vomiting, URTI, upper abdominal pain. (Tab) Dyspepsia, nausea, rash, liver enzyme abnormalities, pruritus, taste disturbances.

DRUG INTERACTIONS

Coadministration with drugs predominantly metabolized by CYP2D6 (eg, TCAs, β-blockers, SSRIs, antiarrhythmics class 1C [eg, flecainide, propafenone], MAOIs type B, dextromethorphan) should be done with careful monitoring; may require dose reduction of the CYP2D6-metabolized drug. Increased dextromethorphan/dextrorphan metabolite ratio in urine in patients who are extensive metabolizers of dextromethorphan; may convert extensive CYP2D6 metabolizers to poor metabolizer status. Increased levels/exposure of desipramine. Increased clearance of cyclosporine. Decreased clearance of caffeine. Fluconazole may increase levels and exposure. May increase systemic exposure with other inhibitors of both CYP2C9 and CYP3A4 (eg, ketoconazole, amiodarone). Clearance increased by rifampin and decreased by cimetidine. Increased or decreased PT with warfarin.

PATIENT CONSIDERATIONS

Assessment: Assess for known hypersensitivity to the drug, active/chronic liver disease, immunodeficiency, lupus erythematosus, pregnancy/nursing status, and possible drug interactions. Confirm diagnosis of onychomycosis (potassium hydroxide preparation, fungal culture, or nail biopsy). Obtain baseline LFTs.

Monitoring: Monitor for signs/symptoms of hepatotoxicity, taste/smell disturbances, progressive skin rash, DRESS, depressive symptoms, lupus erythematosus, and other adverse reactions. Monitor CBC in patients with known or suspected immunodeficiency if therapy continues for >6 weeks, or if signs/symptoms of secondary infection occur. Monitor LFTs periodically.

Counseling: Advise to d/c treatment and report immediately to physician if N/V, right upper abdominal pain, jaundice, dark urine, pale stools, taste/smell disturbance, anorexia, fatigue, depressive symptoms, hives, mouth sores, blistering and peeling of skin, swelling of face, lips, tongue, or throat, difficulty breathing/swallowing, fever, skin eruption, erythema, scaling, loss of pigment, unusual photosensitivity that can result in a rash, and lymph node enlargement occur. Instruct to minimize exposure to natural and artificial sunlight (tanning beds or UVA/B treatment) while on therapy. Advise to call physician if too many doses have been taken. If a dose is missed, advise to take tab as soon as remembered, unless it is <4 hrs before the next dose is due.

STORAGE: (Tab) <25°C (77°F); in a tight container. Protect from light. (Granules) 25°C (77°F); excursions permitted to 15-30°C (59-86°F).

LANOXIN INJECTION — digoxin

RX

Class: Cardiac glycoside

ADULT DOSAGE

Heart Failure

Mild to Moderate:

Dosing can be either initiated w/ a LD followed by maint dosing if rapid titration is desired or initiated w/ maint dosing w/o a LD

PEDIATRIC DOSAGE

Heart Failure

Increase Myocardial Contractility:

Dosing can be either initiated w/ a LD followed by maint dosing if rapid titration is desired or initiated w/ maint dosing w/o a LD

LD: 8-12mcg/kg; administer 1/2 the total LD initially, then 1/4 the LD q6-8h twice

Maint:
Initial: 2.4-3.6mcg/kg qd
Titrate: May increase dose every 2 weeks according to clinical response, serum drug levels, and toxicity
Max: 500mcg in a single site

Atrial Fibrillation

Control of Ventricular Response Rate in Chronic A-Fib:
Dosing can be either initiated w/ a LD followed by maint dosing if rapid titration is desired or initiated w/ maint dosing w/o a LD

LD: 8-12mcg/kg; administer 1/2 the total LD initially, then 1/4 the LD q6-8h twice

Maint:
Initial: 2.4-3.6mcg/kg qd
Titrate: May increase dose every 2 weeks according to clinical response, serum drug levels, and toxicity
Max: 500mcg in a single site

Conversions

IV to Oral Conversion:
50mcg inj = 62.5mcg tab
100mcg inj = 125mcg tab
200mcg inj = 250mcg tab
400mcg inj = 500mcg tab

LD:
Administer 1/2 the total LD initially, then 1/4 the LD q6-8h twice
Premature Infants: 15-25mcg/kg
Full-Term Infants: 20-30mcg/kg
1-24 Months: 30-50mcg/kg
2-5 Years: 25-35mcg/kg
5-10 Years: 15-30mcg/kg
>10 Years: 8-12mcg/kg

Maint:
Initial:
Premature Infants: 1.9-3.1mcg/kg/dose bid
Full-Term: 3.0-4.5mcg/kg/dose bid
1-24 Months: 4.5-7.5mcg/kg/dose bid
2-5 Years: 3.8-5.3mcg/kg/dose bid
5-10 Years: 2.3-4.5mcg/kg/dose bid
>10 Years: 2.4-3.6mcg/kg qd; may be increased every 2 weeks according to clinical response, serum drug levels, and toxicity

Max: 200mcg in a single site

Conversions

IV to Oral Conversion:
50mcg inj = 62.5mcg tab
100mcg inj = 125mcg tab
200mcg inj = 250mcg tab
400mcg inj = 500mcg tab

L

DOSING CONSIDERATIONS

Renal Impairment
Refer to PI for recommended maint doses based on lean body weight and renal function

ADMINISTRATION

IV/IM route

Parenteral administration should be used only when the need for rapid digitalization is urgent or when the drug cannot be taken orally.
IV route is preferred; if IM route is necessary, inject deep into the muscle and follow w/ massage.
Administer over a period of ≥5 min; avoid bolus administration.
May be administered undiluted or diluted w/ a ≥4-fold volume of SWFI, 0.9% NaCl inj, or D5 inj; use of <4-fold volume of diluent could lead to precipitation of digoxin.
Used diluted sol immediately.
Do not mix w/ other drugs in the same container or administer simultaneously in the same IV line.

HOW SUPPLIED

Inj: (Lanoxin) 0.25mg/mL, (Lanoxin Pediatric) 0.1mg/mL

CONTRAINDICATIONS

Ventricular fibrillation. Known hypersensitivity to digoxin (reactions seen include unexplained rash, swelling of the mouth, lips, or throat or a difficulty in breathing) or to other digitalis preparations.

WARNINGS/PRECAUTIONS

Increased risk of ventricular fibrillation in patients w/ Wolff-Parkinson-White syndrome who develop A-fib. May cause severe sinus bradycardia or sinoatrial block particularly in patients w/ preexisting sinus node disease and may cause advanced or complete heart block in patients w/ preexisting incomplete atrioventricular (AV) block; consider insertion of a pacemaker before treatment. Patients w/ low body weight, advanced age or impaired renal function, hypokalemia, hypercalcemia, or hypomagnesemia may be predisposed to digoxin toxicity. Signs/symptoms of digoxin toxicity may be mistaken for worsening symptoms of heart failure (HF). May be desirable to reduce dose or d/c therapy 1-2 days prior to electrical cardioversion of A-fib. If digitalis toxicity is suspected, delay elective cardioversion, and if it is not prudent to delay cardioversion, select the lowest possible energy level to avoid provoking ventricular arrhythmias. May increase myocardial oxygen demand and lead to ischemia in patients w/ acute MI; not recommended in these patients. May precipitate vasoconstriction and promote production of pro-inflammatory cytokines in patients w/ myocarditis; avoid use in these patients. Avoid in patients w/ HF associated w/ preserved left ventricular ejection fraction (eg, restrictive cardiomyopathy, constrictive pericarditis, amyloid heart disease, acute cor pulmonale) and patients w/ idiopathic hypertrophic subaortic stenosis. Hypocalcemia may nullify the effects of treatment. Hypothyroidism may reduce the requirements for therapy. HF and/or atrial arrhythmias resulting from hypermetabolic or hyperdynamic states (eg, hyperthyroidism, hypoxia, arteriovenous shunt) are best treated by addressing the underlying condition. Patients w/ beri beri heart disease may fail to respond adequately to therapy if the underlying thiamine deficiency is not treated concomitantly. Endogenous substances of unknown composition (digoxin-like immunoreactive substances) may interfere w/ standard radioimmunoassays for digoxin. Caution in the elderly.

ADVERSE REACTIONS

Cardiac arrhythmias, N/V, abdominal pain, intestinal ischemia, hemorrhagic necrosis of the intestines, headache, weakness, dizziness, apathy, mental disturbances.

DRUG INTERACTIONS

Drugs that induce/inhibit P-gp may alter digoxin pharmacokinetics. Increased levels w/ quinidine, ritonavir, amiodarone, propafenone, quinine, spironolactone, and verapamil; refer to PI for recommendations to reduce digoxin concentrations. Drugs that affect renal function (eg, ACE inhibitors, ARBs, NSAIDs, COX-2 inhibitors) may impair excretion. Higher rate of torsades de pointes w/ dofetilide. Proarrhythmic events were more common w/ concomitant sotalol. Sudden death was more common w/ concomitant dronedarone. Teriparatide transiently increases serum calcium. Thyroid supplements may increase digoxin dose requirement. Increased risk of arrhythmias w/ epinephrine, norepinephrine, dopamine, and succinylcholine. Rapid IV calcium administration can produce serious arrhythmias in digitalized patients. Additive effects on AV node conduction w/ β-adrenergic blockers and calcium channel blockers.

PATIENT CONSIDERATIONS

Assessment: Assess for known hypersensitivity to the drug or other digitalis preparations, ventricular fibrillation, myocarditis, hypermetabolic or hyperdynamic states, sinus node disease, AV block, pregnancy/nursing status, possible drug interactions, and any other conditions where treatment is cautioned. Assess serum electrolytes and renal function. Obtain a baseline digoxin level; serum digoxin concentrations may be falsely elevated by endogenous digoxin-like substances.

Monitoring: Monitor for signs/symptoms of severe sinus bradycardia, sinoatrial block, advanced or complete heart block, digoxin toxicity, vasoconstriction, and other adverse reactions. Monitor serum electrolytes and renal function periodically. Obtain serum digoxin concentrations just before the next dose or at least 6 hrs after the last dose. Monitor for clinical response.

Counseling: Advise that digoxin is used to treat HF and heart arrhythmias. Advise to inform physician if taking any OTC medications, including herbal medication, or if started on a new prescription. Inform that blood tests will be necessary to ensure the appropriate digoxin dose. Instruct to contact physician if N/V, persistent diarrhea, confusion, weakness, or visual disturbances occur. Advise parents or caregivers that symptoms of having too high doses may be difficult to recognize in infants and pediatric patients; inform that symptoms such as weight loss, failure to thrive in infants, abdominal pain, and behavioral disturbances may be indications of digoxin toxicity. Suggest to monitor and record HR and BP daily. Instruct women of childbearing potential who become or are planning to become pregnant to consult physician prior to initiating or continuing therapy.

STORAGE: 25°C (77°F); excursions permitted to 15-30°C (59-86°F). Protect from light.

LANTUS – insulin glargine

RX

Class: Insulin (long-acting)

ADULT DOSAGE

Type 1 Diabetes Mellitus

Initial: Approx 1/3 of total daily insulin requirements

Titrate: Based on individual's metabolic needs, blood glucose monitoring results, and glycemic control goal

Use short-acting, premeal insulin to satisfy remainder of the daily insulin requirements

Type 2 Diabetes Mellitus

Not Currently Treated w/ Insulin:

Initial: 0.2 U/kg or up to 10 U qd

Titrate: Based on individual's metabolic needs, blood glucose monitoring results, and glycemic control goal

Conversions

From QD Toujeo 300 U/mL:

Initial Lantus dose is 80% of Toujeo that is being discontinued

PEDIATRIC DOSAGE

Type 1 Diabetes Mellitus

≥6 Years:

Initial: Approx 1/3 of total daily insulin requirements

Titrate: Based on individual's metabolic needs, blood glucose monitoring results, and glycemic control goal

Use short-acting, premeal insulin to satisfy remainder of the daily insulin requirements

Conversions

From QD Toujeo 300 U/mL:

Initial Lantus dose is 80% of Toujeo that is being discontinued

From Intermediate- or Long-Acting Insulin:

Change in basal insulin dose may be required and amount and timing of the shorter-acting insulins and doses of any oral antidiabetic drugs may need to be adjusted

From Intermediate- or Long-Acting Insulin:
Change in basal insulin dose may be required and amount and timing of the shorter-acting insulins and doses of any oral antidiabetic drugs may need to be adjusted

From QD NPH Insulin:
Initial Lantus dose is the same as the dose of NPH that is being discontinued

From BID NPH Insulin:
Initial Lantus dose is 80% of total NPH dose that is being discontinued

From QD NPH Insulin:
Initial Lantus dose is the same as the dose of NPH that is being discontinued

From BID NPH Insulin:
Initial Lantus dose is 80% of total NPH dose that is being discontinued

DOSING CONSIDERATIONS

Concomitant Medications
For patients w/ type 2 diabetes, may need to adjust dosage of concomitant oral antidiabetic products

Renal Impairment
Frequent glucose monitoring and dose adjustments may be necessary

Hepatic Impairment
Frequent glucose monitoring and dose adjustments may be necessary

Elderly
Dose conservatively

Other Important Considerations
Dosage adjustments may be needed w/ changes in physical activity, changes in meal patterns (eg, macronutrient content, timing of food intake), changes in hepatic/renal function, or during acute illness

ADMINISTRATION

SQ route

Inject into the abdominal area, thigh, or deltoid, and rotate inj sites w/in the same region from 1 inj to the next.
Inject qd at the same time every day.
Must be used w/ short-acting insulin in patients w/ type 1 diabetes mellitus.
Do not administer IV or via an insulin pump.
Do not dilute or mix w/ any other insulin or sol.
Refrigerate unused (unopened) vials and SoloStar prefilled pens.

SoloStar Prefilled Pen
For single patient use only.

HOW SUPPLIED

Inj: 100 U/mL [3mL SoloStar, 10mL vial]

CONTRAINDICATIONS

During episodes of hypoglycemia; hypersensitivity to Lantus or one of its excipients.

WARNINGS/PRECAUTIONS

Not recommended for the treatment of diabetic ketoacidosis. Insulin pens, syringes, or needles must never be shared between patients, even if the needle is changed; may carry a risk for transmission of blood-borne pathogens. Changes in insulin strength, manufacturer, type, or method of administration may affect glycemic control and predispose to hypo/hyperglycemia. Hypoglycemia may occur and may impair concentration ability and reaction time. Symptomatic awareness of hypoglycemia may be less pronounced in patients w/ longstanding diabetes, diabetic nerve disease, w/ medications that block the sympathetic nervous system (eg, β-blockers), or in patients who experience recurrent hypoglycemia. The long-acting effect of insulin glargine may delay recovery from hypoglycemia. Accidental mix-ups among insulin products reported. Severe, life-threatening, generalized allergy, including anaphylaxis, may occur. If hypersensitivity reactions occur, d/c therapy; treat per standard of care and monitor until signs/symptoms resolve. May cause hypokalemia; monitor K^+ levels in patients at risk for hypokalemia (eg, patients using K^+-lowering medications or medications sensitive to serum K^+ concentrations) if indicated.

ADVERSE REACTIONS

Hypoglycemia, URTI, peripheral edema, HTN, influenza, sinusitis, cataract, bronchitis, arthralgia, infection, pain in extremities, back pain, cough, UTI, diarrhea.

DRUG INTERACTIONS

See Dosing Considerations. Dose adjustments and increased frequency of glucose monitoring may be required w/ drugs that may increase the risk of hypoglycemia (eg, ACE inhibitors, ARBs, disopyramide, fibrates, fluoxetine, MAOIs, pentoxifylline, pramlintide, propoxyphene, salicylates, somatostatin analogues [eg, octreotide], sulfonamide antibiotics), drugs that may decrease blood glucose-lowering effect (eg, atypical antipsychotics [eg, olanzapine, clozapine], corticosteroids, danazol, diuretics, estrogens, glucagon, isoniazid, niacin, oral contraceptives, phenothiazines, progestogens [eg, in oral contraceptives], protease inhibitors, somatropin, sympathomimetic agents [eg, albuterol, epinephrine, terbutaline], thyroid hormones), or drugs that may increase/decrease blood glucose-lowering effect (eg, alcohol, β-blockers, clonidine, lithium salts, pentamidine). Signs/symptoms of hypoglycemia may be blunted w/ β-blockers, clonidine, guanethidine, or reserpine. Observe for signs/symptoms of heart failure (HF) if treated concomitantly w/ a peroxisome proliferator-activated receptor (PPAR)-gamma agonist (eg, thiazolidinediones); consider discontinuation or dose reduction of the PPAR-gamma agonist if HF develops.

PATIENT CONSIDERATIONS

Assessment: Assess for diabetic ketoacidosis, predisposition to hypoglycemia, risk factors for hypokalemia, hypersensitivity, renal/hepatic impairment, pregnancy/nursing status, and possible drug interactions. Obtain baseline blood glucose and HbA1c levels.

Monitoring: Monitor for signs/symptoms of hypoglycemia, allergic reactions, and other adverse reactions. Monitor blood glucose and HbA1c levels, and renal/hepatic function. Monitor K^+ levels in patients at risk for hypokalemia if indicated.

Counseling: Advise to never share SoloStar pen w/ another person, even if needle is changed. Instruct not to reuse or share needles or syringes. Inform of hypoglycemia symptoms, including impairment of the ability to concentrate and react; advise to use caution when driving/operating machinery. Advise that changes in insulin regimen can predispose to hypo/hyperglycemia and that changes should be made under close medical supervision. Instruct to always check the label before each inj to avoid medication errors and to not dilute or mix w/ any other insulin or sol. Instruct on self-management procedures, including glucose monitoring, proper inj technique, management of hypo/hyperglycemia, and on handling of special situations (eg, intercurrent conditions, inadequate or skipped dose, inadvertent administration of increased insulin dose, inadequate food intake, skipped meals). Advise to inform physician if pregnant or contemplating pregnancy.

STORAGE: Do not freeze; discard if drug has been frozen. **Unopened:** 2-8°C (36-46°F) until expiration date or <30°C (86°F) for 28 days. **Open (In-Use):** 2-8°C (36-46°F) or <30°C (86°F) for vials and <30°C (86°F) for SoloStar. Discard after 28 days. Protect from direct heat and light.

LATISSE – bimatoprost

RX

Class: Prostaglandin analogue

ADULT DOSAGE

Hypotrichosis of the Eyelashes

Apply 1 drop qpm

PEDIATRIC DOSAGE

Hypotrichosis of the Eyelashes

≥5 Years:

Apply 1 drop qpm

ADMINISTRATION

Topical route

1. Ensure face is clean, and that makeup and contact lenses are removed
2. Place one drop on disposable sterile applicator and apply evenly along the skin of the upper eyelid margin at the base of eyelashes; do not apply to lower eyelash line
3. Upper lid margin in area of lash growth should feel lightly moist w/o runoff; blot any excess sol runoff outside upper eyelid margin w/ a tissue or other absorbent cloth
4. Dispose of applicator after one use; repeat for the opposite eyelid margin using a new sterile applicator
5. Do not reuse applicators and do not use any other brush/applicator to apply sol

HOW SUPPLIED

Sol: 0.03% [3mL, 5mL]

WARNINGS/PRECAUTIONS

May lower intraocular pressure (IOP) when instilled directly to the eye. Increased iris pigmentation reported; may continue therapy in patients who develop noticeably increased iris pigmentation. May cause pigment changes (darkening) to periorbital pigmented tissues and eyelashes. May cause hair growth to occur in areas where sol comes in repeated contact with skin surface. Caution with active intraocular inflammation (eg, uveitis); inflammation may be exacerbated. Macular edema (eg, cystoid macular edema) reported during treatment of elevated IOP; caution in aphakic patients, pseudophakic patients with a torn posterior lens capsule, or in patients at risk for macular edema. Do not allow the bottle tip to contact any other surface. Use the accompanying sterile applicators on 1 eye and then discard; reuse of applicators increases the potential for contamination and infections. Bacterial keratitis associated with the use of multiple-dose containers reported. Contains benzalkonium chloride, which may be absorbed by and cause discoloration of soft contact lenses; contact lenses should be removed prior to application and may be reinserted 15 min following administration.

ADVERSE REACTIONS

Eye pruritus, conjunctival hyperemia, skin hyperpigmentation, ocular irritation, dry eye symptoms, periorbital erythema.

DRUG INTERACTIONS

May interfere with the desired reduction in IOP when given with other prostaglandin analogues for the treatment of elevated IOP.

PATIENT CONSIDERATIONS

Assessment: Assess for active intraocular inflammation, aphakia, pseudophakia with a torn posterior lens capsule, risk for macular edema, pregnancy/nursing status, and possible drug interactions.

Monitoring: Monitor for IOP changes, increased iris pigmentation, pigment changes (darkening) to periorbital pigmented tissues and eyelashes, macular edema, bacterial keratitis, and other adverse reactions.

Counseling: Instruct to apply medication ud. Counsel that if any sol gets into the eye proper, it will not cause harm, and the eye should not be rinsed. Counsel that the effect is not permanent and can be expected to gradually return to original level upon discontinuation. Instruct that the bottle must be maintained intact and to avoid contaminating the bottle tip or applicator. Advise that serious infections may result from using contaminated sol or applicators. Instruct to consult physician before use if using prostaglandin analogues for IOP reduction. Inform about the possibility of eyelid skin darkening, increased brown iris pigmentation (may be permanent), hair growth outside of the target treatment area, and disparity between eyes in length, thickness, pigmentation, number of eyelashes or vellus hairs, and/or direction of eyelash growth. Advise to consult physician if patient has ocular surgery, develops a new ocular condition (eg, trauma, infection), experiences a sudden decrease in visual acuity, or if any ocular reactions (eg, conjunctivitis, eyelid reactions) develop. Advise that contact lenses should be removed prior to application, and may be reinserted 15 min following administration.

STORAGE: 2-25°C (36-77°F).

L

LATUDA – lurasidone hydrochloride

RX

Class: Atypical antipsychotic

Elderly patients with dementia-related psychosis treated with antipsychotic drugs are at an increased risk of death. Not approved for use in patients with dementia-related psychosis. Antidepressants increased the risk of suicidal thoughts and behavior in children, adolescents, and young adults in short-term studies. Monitor closely for worsening, and for emergence of suicidal thoughts and behaviors in patients who are started on antidepressant therapy.

ADULT DOSAGE

Schizophrenia

Initial: 40mg qd
Range: 40-160mg/day
Max: 160mg/day
Periodically reevaluate long-term usefulness of therapy for individual patient

Bipolar I Disorder

Treatment of major depressive episodes as monotherapy or as adjunctive therapy w/ either lithium or valproate
Initial: 20mg qd
Range: 20-120mg/day
Max: 120mg/day
Periodically reevaluate long-term usefulness of therapy for individual patient

PEDIATRIC DOSAGE

Pediatric use may not have been established

DOSING CONSIDERATIONS

Concomitant Medications

Moderate CYP3A4 Inhibitors (eg, Diltiazem, Atazanavir, Erythromycin, Fluconazole, Verapamil):
Moderate CYP3A4 Inhibitor Added to Current Therapy w/ Lurasidone: Reduce lurasidone dose to 1/2 of the original dose level
Lurasidone Added to Current Therapy w/ a Moderate CYP3A4 Inhibitor:
Initial: 20mg/day
Max: 80mg/day
Moderate CYP3A4 Inducers:
May need to increase lurasidone dose after chronic treatment (≥7 days) w/ the CYP3A4 inducer

Renal Impairment
Moderate (CrCl 30-<50mL/min) and Severe (CrCl <30mL/min):
Initial: 20mg/day
Max: 80mg/day

Hepatic Impairment
Moderate (Child-Pugh Score 7-9):
Initial: 20mg/day
Max: 80mg/day

Severe (Child-Pugh Score 10-15):
Initial: 20mg/day
Max: 40mg/day

ADMINISTRATION

Oral route

Take w/ food (at least 350 calories)

HOW SUPPLIED

Tab: 20mg, 40mg, 60mg, 80mg, 120mg

CONTRAINDICATIONS

Known hypersensitivity to lurasidone HCl or any components in the formulation; concomitant use w/ strong CYP3A4 inhibitors (eg, ketoconazole, clarithromycin, ritonavir, voriconazole, mibefradil) or strong CYP3A4 inducers (eg, rifampin, avasimibe, St. John's wort, phenytoin, carbamazepine).

WARNINGS/PRECAUTIONS

Neuroleptic malignant syndrome (NMS) reported; d/c immediately and institute symptomatic treatment. May cause tardive dyskinesia (TD), especially in the elderly; d/c if this occurs. May cause metabolic changes (eg, hyperglycemia, dyslipidemia, weight gain) that may increase cardiovascular (CV)/cerebrovascular risk. Hyperglycemia, in some cases extreme and associated with ketoacidosis or hyperosmolar coma or death, reported; monitor glucose control regularly in patients with diabetes mellitus (DM) and FPG in patients at risk for DM. May elevate prolactin levels. Leukopenia, neutropenia, and agranulocytosis may occur; monitor CBC frequently during the 1st few months in patients with preexisting low WBCs or history of drug-induced leukopenia/neutropenia, and d/c at 1st sign of decline in WBCs without other causative factors. D/C therapy and follow WBCs until recovery in patients with severe neutropenia (absolute neutrophil count <1000/mm^3). May cause orthostatic hypotension and syncope; consider using a lower starting dose/slower titration and monitor orthostatic vital signs in patients at increased risk of these reactions or at increased risk of developing complications from hypotension (eg, dehydration, hypovolemia, treatment with antihypertensives, history of CV/cerebrovascular disease, antipsychotic-naive patients). Caution with history of seizures or with conditions that lower the seizure threshold. May impair mental/physical abilities. May disrupt body's ability to reduce core body temperature; caution when prescribing for patients who will be experiencing conditions that may contribute to an elevation in core body temperature (eg, concomitant anticholinergics). Closely supervise patients at high risk of suicide. May increase risk of developing a manic or hypomanic episode, particularly in patients with bipolar disorder. May cause esophageal dysmotility and aspiration; caution in patients at risk for aspiration pneumonia. Increased sensitivity reported in patients with Parkinson's disease or dementia with Lewy bodies. Evaluate for history of drug abuse; observe for drug misuse/abuse in these patients.

ADVERSE REACTIONS

Somnolence, akathisia, N/V, extrapyramidal symptoms, agitation, dyspepsia, back pain, dizziness, insomnia, anxiety, restlessness, diarrhea, dry mouth, nasopharyngitis.

DRUG INTERACTIONS

See Contraindications. Grapefruit/grapefruit juice may inhibit CYP3A4 and alter concentrations; avoid concomitant use. Adjust lurasidone dose when used in combination with moderate CYP3A4 inhibitors/inducers.

PATIENT CONSIDERATIONS

Assessment: Assess for dementia-related psychosis, DM, renal/hepatic impairment, drug hypersensitivity, any other conditions where treatment is cautioned, pregnancy/nursing status, and possible drug interactions. Obtain baseline FPG in patients with DM or at risk for DM. Obtain baseline CBC if at risk for leukopenia/neutropenia.

Monitoring: Monitor for signs/symptoms of clinical worsening, suicidality, unusual changes in behavior, NMS, TD, hyperglycemia, hyperprolactinemia, orthostatic hypotension/syncope, cognitive/motor impairment, seizures, disruption of body temperature, manic/hypomanic episodes, esophageal dysmotility, aspiration, and other adverse reactions. Monitor FPG in patients with DM or at risk for DM, lipid profile, and weight. Monitor CBC frequently during the 1st few months in patients with preexisting low WBCs or history of drug-induced leukopenia/neutropenia. Monitor for fever or other signs/symptoms of infection in patients with neutropenia. Periodically reevaluate long-term usefulness for individual patient.

Counseling: Advise to monitor for the emergence of suicidal thoughts and behavior, manic/hypomanic symptoms, irritability, agitation, or unusual changes in behavior and to report such symptoms to physician. Counsel about signs/symptoms of NMS (eg, hyperpyrexia, muscle rigidity, altered mental status, autonomic instability), hyperglycemia, and DM. Advise of the risk of dyslipidemia, weight gain, CV reactions, and orthostatic hypotension. Advise patients with preexisting low WBCs or history of drug-induced leukopenia/neutropenia to have their CBC monitored. Instruct to use caution when performing activities requiring mental alertness (eg, operating hazardous machinery, driving) until patients are reasonably certain that therapy does not affect them adversely. Instruct to notify physician if pregnant/intending to become pregnant, or if taking/planning to take any other medications. Advise to avoid alcohol while on treatment. Counsel regarding appropriate care in avoiding overheating and dehydration.

STORAGE: 25°C (77°F); excursions permitted to 15-30°C (59-86°F).

LAZANDA – fentanyl

CII

Class: Opioid analgesic

Fatal respiratory depression may occur. Contraindicated in the management of acute or postoperative pain (eg, headache/migraine) and in opioid-nontolerant patients. Keep out of reach of children. Concomitant use with CYP3A4 inhibitors may increase plasma levels, and may cause fatal respiratory depression. Do not convert patients on a mcg-per-mcg basis from any other fentanyl products to Lazanda. Do not substitute for any other fentanyl products; may result in fatal overdose. Contains fentanyl with abuse liability similar to other opioid analgesics. Available only through a restricted program called Transmucosal Immediate Release Fentanyl Risk Evaluation Mitigation Strategy (TIRF REMS) Access program, due to risk of misuse, abuse, addiction, and overdose. Outpatients, healthcare professionals who prescribe to outpatients, pharmacies, and distributors must enroll in this program.

ADULT DOSAGE

Pain

Management of Breakthrough Pain in Cancer Patients Already Receiving and Tolerant to Opioid Therapy for Underlying Persistent Cancer Pain:

≥18 Years:

Initial (Including Switching from Another Fentanyl Product):

One 100mcg spray (1 spray in 1 nostril); if adequate analgesia is obtained w/in 30 min, treat subsequent episodes w/ this dose

Titrate:

If adequate analgesia is not achieved w/ the first 100mcg dose, escalate dose in a stepwise manner over consecutive episodes until adequate analgesia w/ tolerable side effects is achieved

100mcg/dose: 1 x 100mcg spray

200mcg/dose: 2 x 100mcg spray (1 in each nostril)

400mcg/dose: 4 x 100mcg spray (2 in each nostril) or 1 x 400mcg spray

800mcg/dose: 2 x 400mcg spray (1 in each nostril)

Confirm dose w/ a 2nd episode of breakthrough pain and review experience if dose is appropriate or further adjustment is warranted

Wait at least 2 hrs before treating another episode of breakthrough cancer pain

Maint:

Use the established dose for each subsequent episode; limit to ≤4 doses/day and wait at least 2 hrs before treating another episode

May use rescue medication if pain relief is inadequate after 30 min following dosing or if a separate episode occurs before the next dose is permitted

Max: 800mcg

PEDIATRIC DOSAGE

Pediatric use may not have been established

DOSING CONSIDERATIONS

Renal Impairment

Severe: Use w/ caution; titrate to clinical effect

Hepatic Impairment

Severe: Use w/ caution; titrate to clinical effect

Discontinuation

No Longer Requires Opioid Therapy: Consider discontinuation along w/ a gradual downward titration of other opioids

Continuing to Take Chronic Opioid Therapy but No Longer Requires Treatment for Breakthrough Pain: Therapy can be discontinued immediately

Other Important Considerations

Dose Readjustment:

Response (Analgesia or Adverse Reactions) to Titrated Dose Markedly Changes: An adjustment may be necessary

>4 Episodes of Breakthrough Pain/Day: Reevaluate the dose of the long-acting opioid used; if the long-acting opioid or dose of long-acting opioid is changed, reevaluate and retitrate the Lazanda dose as necessary

ADMINISTRATION

Intranasal route

Prime device before use by spraying into the pouch (4 sprays total)

If not used for 5 days, reprime by spraying once

Insert nozzle of the bottle a short distance (about 1/2 inch or 1cm) into nose and point towards bridge of nose, tilting bottle slightly

Press down firmly on the finger grips until a click is heard and the number in the counting window advances by 1

Fine mist spray is not always felt; rely on audible click and dose counter to confirm a spray has been administered

Refer to PI for further priming and disposal instructions

L

HOW SUPPLIED

Spray: 100mcg/spray, 400mcg/spray

CONTRAINDICATIONS

Opioid non-tolerant patients; management of acute or postoperative pain, including headache/migraine, or dental pain; known intolerance or hypersensitivity to any of its components or the drug fentanyl.

WARNINGS/PRECAUTIONS

Increased risk of respiratory depression in patients with underlying respiratory disorders and in elderly/debilitated. May impair mental and/or physical abilities. Caution with COPD or preexisting medical conditions predisposing to respiratory depression; may further decrease respiratory drive to the point of respiratory failure. Extreme caution in patients who may be susceptible to intracranial effects of CO_2 retention (eg, with evidence of increased intracranial pressure or impaired consciousness). May obscure the clinical course of head injuries. May produce bradycardia; caution with bradyarrhythmias. Avoid use during labor and delivery. Caution in the elderly.

ADVERSE REACTIONS

Respiratory depression, N/V, somnolence, dizziness, headache, constipation, pyrexia.

DRUG INTERACTIONS

See Boxed Warning. Increase dose conservatively when beginning therapy with or increasing dose of CYP3A4 inhibitors. Not recommended with MAOIs or within 14 days of discontinuation of MAOIs. Increased depressant effects with other CNS depressants (eg, other opioids, sedatives/hypnotics, skeletal muscle relaxants); may require adjustment of Lazanda dose. CYP3A4 inducers (eg, barbiturates, carbamazepine, efavirenz) may decrease levels; adjust dose of Lazanda accordingly. Vasoconstrictive nasal decongestants such as oxymetazoline may decrease efficacy; avoid titration while patient is experiencing an acute episode of rhinitis as it could lead to incorrect dose identification. Respiratory depression reported with other drugs that depress respiration.

PATIENT CONSIDERATIONS

Assessment: Assess for degree of opioid tolerance, previous opioid dose, level of pain intensity, type of pain, patient's general condition and medical status, and any other conditions where treatment is contraindicated or cautioned. Assess for hypersensitivity to the drug, renal/hepatic impairment, pregnancy/nursing status, and possible drug interactions.

Monitoring: Monitor for signs/symptoms of respiratory depression, impairment of mental/physical abilities, drug abuse/addiction, bradycardia, hypersensitivity reactions, and other adverse reactions.

Counseling: Inform outpatients to enroll in the TIRF REMS Access program. Explain that therapy may be fatal in children, in individuals for whom it was not prescribed, and in those who are not opioid tolerant. Counsel on proper administration and disposal. Advise to take drug as prescribed and to avoid sharing it with anyone else. Instruct not to take medication for acute or postoperative pain, pain from injuries, headache, migraine, or any other short-term pain. Instruct to notify physician if breakthrough pain is not alleviated or worsens after taking the drug. Inform that drug may impair mental/physical abilities; caution against performing activities that require high level of attention (eg, driving/using heavy machinery). Advise not to combine with alcohol, sleep aids, or tranquilizers, except if ordered by the physician. Instruct to notify physician if pregnant or planning to become pregnant.

STORAGE: Up to 25°C (77°F). Do not freeze. Protect from light.

LEMTRADA – alemtuzumab

RX

Class: Monoclonal antibody/CD52 blocker

May cause serious, sometimes fatal, autoimmune conditions such as immune thrombocytopenia (ITP) and anti-glomerular basement membrane disease; monitor CBCs with differential, SrCr levels, and urinalysis with urine cell counts at periodic intervals for 48 months after the last dose. May cause serious and life threatening infusion reactions; administer in a setting with appropriate equipment and personnel to manage anaphylaxis or serious infusion reactions. Monitor patients for 2 hrs after each infusion. Serious infusion reactions can also occur after the 2-hr monitoring period. May cause an increased risk of malignancies, including thyroid cancer, melanoma, and lymphoproliferative disorders; perform baseline and yearly skin exams. Available only through a restricted distribution program, Lemtrada Risk Evaluation Mitigation Strategy (REMS).

ADULT DOSAGE

Multiple Sclerosis

Relapsing Forms:

Usual: 12mg/day for 2 treatment courses

First Treatment Course:

12mg/day on 5 consecutive days (60mg total dose)

Second Treatment Course:

12mg/day on 3 consecutive days (36mg total dose) administered 12 months after the first treatment course

Corticosteroids:

Premedicate with high dose corticosteroids (1000mg methylprednisolone or equivalent) immediately prior to infusion and for the first 3 days of each treatment course

Herpes Prophylaxis:

Administer antiviral prophylaxis for herpetic viral infections starting on the first day of each treatment course and continue for at least 2 months following treatment or until CD4+ lymphocyte count is ≥200 cells/µL, whichever occurs later

PEDIATRIC DOSAGE

Pediatric use may not have been established

ADMINISTRATION

IV route

Preparation and Infusion

Withdraw 1.2mL from the vial into a syringe and inject into a 100mL bag of 0.9% NaCl or D5W

Invert the bag to mix the sol

Infuse Lemtrada over 4 hrs starting within 8 hrs after dilution

Do not add or simultaneously infuse other drug substances through the same IV line

Do not give as an IV push or bolus

HOW SUPPLIED

Inj: 10mg/mL

CONTRAINDICATIONS

Human immunodeficiency virus (HIV).

WARNINGS/PRECAUTIONS

Reserve for patients who have had an inadequate response to two or more drugs indicated for the treatment of MS. Determine whether patient has a history of varicella or if has been vaccinated for varicella zoster virus (VZV) prior to treatment; if not, test patient for antibodies to VZV and consider vaccination for those who are antibody-negative. Complete any necessary immunizations at least 6 weeks prior to treatment. Therapy can result in the formation of autoantibodies; autoantibodies may be transferred from the mother to the fetus during pregnancy. Case of transplacental transfer of anti-thyrotropin receptor antibodies resulting in neonatal Graves' disease occurred after alemtuzumab treatment in the mother. May cause cytokinase release syndrome resulting in infusion reactions; consider pretreatment with antihistamines and/or antipyretics prior to therapy. Caution when initiating therapy in patients with preexisting or ongoing malignancies. Immediately obtain CBC if ITP is suspected and promptly initiate appropriate medical intervention if confirmed. Glomerular nephropathies reported. Perform further evaluation for nephropathies if significant changes from baseline in SrCr, unexplained hematuria, or proteinuria are observed. Autoimmune thyroid disorders reported; administer only if potential benefit justifies potential risks in patients with an ongoing thyroid disorder. Autoimmune cytopenias such as neutropenia, hemolytic anemia, and pancytopenia reported; use CBC results to monitor for cytopenias and prompt medical intervention is indicated if a cytopenia is confirmed. Infections (eg, urinary tract infection, appendicitis, gastroenteritis, pneumonia, tooth infection) reported. Consider delaying administration in patients with active infection until the infection is fully controlled. Herpes viral infection, cervical human papilloma virus (HPV) (eg, cervical dysplasia) infection, active/latent tuberculosis (TB), fungal infections (oral and vaginal candidiasis), and Listeria meningitis reported. Avoid or adequately heat foods that are potential sources of *Listeria monocytogenes*. Caution in patients identified as carriers of hepatitis B virus (HBV) and/or hepatitis C virus (HCV) as these patients may be at risk of irreversible liver damage relative to a potential virus reactivation as a consequence of their preexisting status. Hypersensitivity pneumonitis and pneumonitis with fibrosis reported. Contains same active ingredient (alemtuzumab) found in Campath; exercise increased vigilance for additive and long-lasting effects on the immune system if use is considered in a patient who has previously received Campath.

ADVERSE REACTIONS

Autoimmune conditions, infusion reactions, malignancies, rash, headache, pyrexia, nasopharyngitis, N/V, urinary tract infection, fatigue, insomnia, upper respiratory tract infection, herpes viral infection, urticaria, pruritus.

DRUG INTERACTIONS

Do not administer live viral vaccines following a course of therapy; may increase the risk of infection. Concomitant use with antineoplastic or immunosuppressive therapies could increase risk of immunosuppression.

PATIENT CONSIDERATIONS

Assessment: Assess for HIV, history of varicella, thyroid disorder, HBV, HBC, any other conditions where treatment is cautioned, pregnancy/nursing status, and possible drug interactions. Obtain CBC with differential, SrCr levels, and urinalysis with urine cell counts. Perform a test of thyroid function (eg, thyroid-stimulating hormone level). Perform TB screening according to local guidelines. Perform baseline skin examination. Assess vital signs and immunization history.

Monitoring: Monitor for autoimmune conditions (eg, ITP, anti-glomerular basement membrane disease), malignancies (eg, thyroid cancer, melanoma, lymphoproliferative disorders, lymphoma), glomerular nephropathies, infusion reactions, thyroid disorders, autoimmune cytopenias, infections, TB, and other adverse reactions. Monitor CBCs with differential, SrCr levels, and urinalysis with urine cell counts monthly for 48 months after the last dose; perform testing after 48 months based on clinical findings. Monitor vital signs periodically during infusion. Monitor for infusion reactions during and for at least 2 hrs after each infusion. Perform thyroid function test every 3 months until 48 months after the last infusion; continue to test thyroid function after 48 months if clinically indicated. Consider additional monitoring in patients with medical conditions that may predispose to cardiovascular or pulmonary compromise. Perform yearly skin examination. Perform annual HPV screening in female patients.

Counseling: Inform of benefits and risks of therapy. Instruct to contact physician promptly if experience any symptoms of potential autoimmune disease (eg, bleeding, easy bruising, petechiae). Advise of the importance of monthly blood and urine tests for 48 months following the last course of therapy; inform that monitoring may need to continue past 48 months if there are signs/symptoms of autoimmunity. Instruct to contact physician if experience symptoms reflective of a potential thyroid disorder. Inform that infusion reactions can occur after patient leaves the infusion center; instruct to report symptoms that occur during and after each infusion to physician. Inform that must enroll in the Lemtrada REMS Program. Instruct to carry the Lemtrada REMS patient safety information card in case of an emergency. Advise of the risk of malignancies, including thyroid cancer and melanoma; instruct to have yearly skin examinations. Instruct to take prescribed medication for herpes prophylaxis ud. Advise that yearly screening for HPV is recommended. Advise to avoid, or adequately heat foods that are potential sources of *L. monocytogenes* if have had a recent course of therapy. Instruct to notify physician if pregnant, breastfeeding, or if any adverse reactions develop. Instruct patients to inform physician if they have taken Campath.

STORAGE: 2-8°C (36-46°F). Do not freeze or shake. Store in original carton to protect from light. Diluted Sol: Store for as long as 8 hrs either at 15-25°C (59-77°F) or at 2-8°C (36-46°F). Protect from light.

LENVIMA – lenvatinib

RX

Class: Kinase inhibitor

ADULT DOSAGE

Differentiated Thyroid Carcinoma

Locally Recurrent or Metastatic, Progressive, Radioactive Iodine-Refractory:

24mg (two 10mg caps and one 4mg cap) qd

Continue until disease progression or unacceptable toxicity occurs

PEDIATRIC DOSAGE

Pediatric use may not have been established

DOSING CONSIDERATIONS

Renal Impairment

Severe (CrCl <30mL/min): 14mg qd

Hepatic Impairment

Severe (Child-Pugh C): 14mg qd

Adverse Reactions

Hypertension:

- Withhold for Grade 3 HTN that persists despite optimal antihypertensive therapy
- Resume at a reduced dose when HTN is controlled at ≤Grade 2
- D/C for life-threatening HTN

Cardiac Dysfunction or Hemorrhage:

- D/C for a Grade 4 event
- Withhold for development of Grade 3 event until improved to Grade 0 or 1 or baseline
- Either resume at a reduced dose or d/c depending on the severity and persistence of the adverse event

Arterial Thrombotic Event:

- D/C following an arterial thrombotic event

Renal Failure and Impairment or Hepatotoxicity:

- Withhold for development of Grade 3 or 4 renal failure/impairment or hepatotoxicity until resolved to Grade 0 to 1 or baseline
- Either resume at a reduced dose or d/c depending on severity and persistence of renal impairment or hepatotoxicity
- D/C for hepatic failure

Proteinuria:

- Withhold for ≥2g of proteinuria/24 hrs
- Resume at a reduced dose when proteinuria is <2g/24 hrs
- D/C for nephrotic syndrome

GI Perforation or Fistula Formation:

- D/C in patients who develop GI perforation or life-threatening fistula

QT Prolongation:

- Withhold for the development of ≥Grade 3 QT prolongation
- Resume at a reduced dose when QT prolongation resolves to Grade 0 or 1 or baseline

Reversible Posterior Leukoencephalopathy Syndrome (RPLS):

- Withhold until fully resolved
- Upon resolution, resume at a reduced dose or d/c depending on the severity and persistence of neurologic symptoms

Persistent and Intolerable Grade 2 or 3 Adverse Reactions or Grade 4 Lab Abnormalities:

1st Occurrence: Interrupt until resolved to Grade 0-1 or baseline; decrease dose to 20mg (two 10mg caps) qd

2nd Occurrence: Interrupt until resolved to Grade 0-1 or baseline; decrease dose to 14mg (one 10mg cap plus one 4mg cap) qd

3rd Occurrence: Interrupt until resolved to Grade 0-1 or baseline; decrease dose to 10mg (one 10mg cap) qd

- Initiate medical management for N/V or diarrhea prior to interruption or dose reduction
- Reduce dose in succession based on the previous daily dose level (24mg/day, 20mg/day, or 14mg/day)
- 2nd or 3rd occurrence may refer to either the same or a different adverse reaction that requires dose modification

ADMINISTRATION

Oral route

Take w/ or w/o food.

Take at the same time each day.

If a dose is missed and cannot be taken w/in 12 hrs, skip that dose and take the next dose at the usual time of administration.

HOW SUPPLIED

Cap: 4mg, 10mg

WARNINGS/PRECAUTIONS

See Dosing Considerations. HTN, cardiac dysfunction, arterial thromboembolic events, increases in AST/ALT, hepatic failure (including fatal events), acute hepatitis, renal failure/impairment, GI perforation or fistula, and RPLS reported. Proteinuria reported; obtain a 24-hr urine protein if urine dipstick proteinuria ≥2+ is detected. QT interval prolongation reported; monitor ECG in patients w/ congenital long QT syndrome, CHF, bradyarrhythmias, or in patients taking drugs known to prolong the QT interval (eg, Class Ia and III antiarrhythmics). Hypocalcemia reported; monitor blood Ca^{2+} levels at least monthly and replace Ca^{2+} as necessary. Hemorrhagic events including fatal events reported; consider the degree of tumor invasion/infiltration of major blood vessels (eg, carotid artery) prior to initiation of therapy due to the potential risk of severe hemorrhage associated w/ tumor shrinkage/necrosis. May impair exogenous thyroid suppression; monitor TSH levels monthly and adjust thyroid replacement medication prn w/ differentiated thyroid cancer. May cause fetal harm.

ADVERSE REACTIONS

HTN, fatigue, diarrhea, arthralgia/myalgia, decreased appetite, decreased weight, N/V, stomatitis, headache, proteinuria, palmar-plantar erythrodysesthesia syndrome, abdominal pain, dysphonia, pneumonia, dehydration.

PATIENT CONSIDERATIONS

Assessment: Assess for proteinuria, congenital long QT syndrome, CHF, bradyarrhythmias, electrolyte abnormalities, renal/hepatic impairment, pregnancy/nursing status, and if taking drugs known to prolong the QT interval. Assess BP. Consider the degree of tumor invasion/infiltration of major blood vessels (eg, carotid artery).

Monitoring: Monitor for signs/symptoms of cardiac decompensation, arterial thromboembolic events, renal failure/impairment, GI perforation and fistula formation, proteinuria, RPLS, hemorrhagic events, QT interval prolongation, and other adverse reactions. Monitor BP after 1 week, then every 2 weeks for the first 2 months, and then at least monthly thereafter. Monitor LFTs every 2 weeks for the first 2 months, and at least monthly thereafter. Monitor and correct electrolyte abnormalities. Monitor ECG in patients w/ congenital long QT syndrome, CHF, bradyarrhythmias, and in patients taking drugs known to prolong QT interval. Monitor blood Ca^{2+} levels at least monthly. Monitor TSH levels monthly.

Counseling: Advise to undergo regular BP monitoring and to contact physician if BP is elevated. Inform that therapy may cause cardiac dysfunction; instruct to immediately contact physician if any clinical symptoms of cardiac dysfunction is experienced. Advise to seek immediate medical attention for new onset chest pain or acute neurologic symptoms consistent w/ MI or stroke. Inform of the need to undergo lab tests to monitor for kidney function, protein in the urine, and liver function; instruct to report any new symptoms indicating hepatic toxicity or failure. Advise that therapy may increase the risk of GI perforation or fistula; instruct to seek immediate medical attention for severe abdominal pain. Explain that therapy may increase the risk of bleeding; instruct to contact physician for bleeding or symptoms of severe bleeding. Inform females of reproductive potential of the potential risk to a fetus and instruct to inform physician of a known or suspected pregnancy. Instruct females of reproductive potential to use effective contraception during and for at least 2 weeks following completion of therapy. Advise nursing women to d/c breastfeeding during treatment.

STORAGE: 25°C (77°F); excursions permitted to 15-30°C (59-86°F).

LETAIRIS – ambrisentan

RX

Class: Endothelin receptor antagonist

Do not administer to a pregnant female; may cause serious birth defects. Exclude pregnancy before initiation of treatment. Females of reproductive potential must use acceptable methods of contraception during and for 1 month after treatment; obtain monthly pregnancy tests during and 1 month after discontinuation of treatment. Females can only receive the drug through a restricted program called the Letairis Risk Evaluation and Mitigation Strategy (REMS) program.

ADULT DOSAGE

Pulmonary Arterial Hypertension

Treatment of pulmonary arterial HTN (PAH) (WHO Group 1) to improve exercise ability and delay clinical worsening; can be used w/ tadalafil to reduce the risks of disease progression and hospitalization for worsening PAH, and to improve exercise ability

Initial: 5mg qd w/ or w/o tadalafil 20mg qd

PEDIATRIC DOSAGE

Pediatric use may not have been established

Titrate: At 4 wk intervals, either dose of ambrisentan or tadalafil can be increased to ambrisentan 10mg or tadalafil 40mg

DOSING CONSIDERATIONS

Hepatic Impairment

Elevation of Liver Transaminases:

D/C if elevations of ALT/AST >5X ULN or if elevations are accompanied by bilirubin >2X ULN, or by signs/symptoms of liver dysfunction and other causes are excluded

ADMINISTRATION

Oral route

Do not split, crush, or chew tabs.

HOW SUPPLIED

Tab: 5mg, 10mg

CONTRAINDICATIONS

Pregnancy, idiopathic pulmonary fibrosis (IPF), including IPF patients w/ pulmonary HTN (WHO Group 3).

WARNINGS/PRECAUTIONS

May cause peripheral edema; more common w/ concomitant tadalafil and in the elderly. If clinically significant fluid retention develops, evaluate further to determine the cause and the possible need for specific treatment or discontinuation of therapy. If acute pulmonary edema develops during initiation of therapy, consider the possibility of pulmonary veno-occlusive disease (PVOD); d/c if confirmed. May decrease sperm counts. Decreases in Hgb concentration and Hct reported and may result in anemia requiring transfusion. Initiation of therapy is not recommended w/ clinically significant anemia. Consider discontinuation if a clinically significant Hgb decrease is observed and other causes have been excluded. Avoid w/ preexisting moderate/severe hepatic impairment. Fully investigate the cause of liver injury if hepatic impairment develops.

ADVERSE REACTIONS

W/O Tadalafil: peripheral edema, nasal congestion, flushing, sinusitis.

W/ Tadalafil: peripheral edema, headache, nasal congestion, cough, anemia, dyspepsia, bronchitis.

DRUG INTERACTIONS

Cyclosporine may increase exposure; limit dose of ambrisentan to 5mg qd when coadministered w/ cyclosporine.

PATIENT CONSIDERATIONS

Assessment: Assess for IPF, anemia, hepatic impairment, pregnancy/nursing status, and possible drug interactions. Obtain baseline Hgb level.

Monitoring: Monitor for fluid retention, pulmonary edema, PVOD, hepatic impairment, and other adverse reactions. Obtain monthly pregnancy tests in females of reproductive potential during therapy and 1 month after discontinuation of treatment. Measure Hgb at 1 month after initiating therapy and periodically thereafter.

Counseling: Instruct on the risk of fetal harm when used in pregnancy and instruct to immediately contact physician if pregnancy is suspected. Inform female patients that drug is only available through a restricted program called the Letairis REMS program. Inform female patients that they must sign an enrollment form and that female patients of reproductive potential must comply w/ pregnancy testing and contraception requirements. Educate and counsel females of reproductive potential on the use of emergency contraception in the event of unprotected sex or known or suspected contraceptive failure. Advise prepubertal females to immediately report to physician any reproductive status changes. Instruct to contact physician if any symptoms of liver injury occur. Advise of the importance of Hgb testing and of other risks associated w/ therapy (eg, decreases in Hgb, Hct, and sperm count; fluid overload).

STORAGE: 25°C (77°F); excursions permitted to 15-30°C (59-86°F).

Leucovorin Injection – leucovorin calcium RX

Class: Cytoprotective agent

ADULT DOSAGE

Rescue Therapy

After High Dose Methotrexate (MTX) Therapy in Osteosarcoma:

Normal MTX Elimination:

15mg (10mg/m^2) q6h for 10 doses starting 24 hrs after the beginning of MTX infusion

PEDIATRIC DOSAGE

Pediatric use may not have been established

Delayed Late MTX Elimination:
Continue 15mg PO/IM/IV q6h until MTX level is <0.05µm

Delayed Early MTX and/or Evidence of Acute Renal Injury:
150mg IV q3h until MTX level is <1µm, then 15mg IV q3h until MTX level is <0.05µm. Continue therapy, hydration, and urinary alkalization (pH of ≥7) until MTX level is <0.05µm

If significant clinical toxicity w/ less severe abnormalities in MTX elimination/renal function is observed, extend rescue therapy for an additional 24 hrs in subsequent courses of therapy

Methotrexate Toxicity

Used to diminish the toxicity and counteract the effects of impaired MTX elimination and of inadvertent overdosage of folic acid antagonists

Initial: $10mg/m^2$ IV/IM/PO q6h until serum MTX level is $<10^{-8}$ M
Titrate: Increase to $100mg/m^2$ IV q3h until MTX level is $<10^{-8}$ M if 24-hr SrCr has increased 50% over baseline, or if 24-hr MTX level is $>5 \times 10^{-6}$ M, or the 48-hr level is $>9 \times 10^{-7}$ M

Employ concurrent hydration (3L/day) and urinary alkalinization w/ sodium bicarbonate; adjust bicarbonate dose to maintain urine pH at ≥7

Begin rescue therapy as soon as possible after an inadvertent overdosage and w/in 24 hrs of MTX administration when there is delayed excretion

Advanced Colorectal Cancer

Palliative Treatment in Combination w/ 5-Fluorouracil (5-FU):
Usual: $200mg/m^2$ slow IV over a minimum of 3 min, followed by $370mg/m^2$ 5-FU IV, daily for 5 days, or
$20mg/m^2$ IV, followed by $425mg/m^2$ 5-FU IV, daily for 5 days

May repeat at 4-week intervals for 2 courses, then at 4- to 5-week intervals provided that the patient has completely recovered from the toxic effects of the prior treatment course

May increase 5-FU dose by 10% if no toxicity. Reduce 5-FU daily dose by 20% w/ moderate GI/hematologic toxicity and by 30% w/ severe toxicity

Megaloblastic Anemia

Usual: Up to 1mg/day

ADMINISTRATION

IM/IV route
Do not mix in same infusion as 5-FU; may form precipitate
Do not administer intrathecally
Reconstitute 50mg, 100mg, and 200mg vials w/ 5mL, 10mL, and 20mL, respectively, of bacteriostatic water for inj (benzyl alcohol preserved) or sterile water for inj
Reconstitute 350mg vial w/ 17.5mL of bacteriostatic water for inj (benzyl alcohol preserved) or sterile water for inj (SWFI)
Must use sol reconstituted w/ bacteriostatic water for inj w/in 7 days; must use sol reconstituted w/ SWFI immediately and discard any unused portion

When doses >10mg/m² are administered, reconstitute w/ SWFI and use immediately
No more than 160mg/min should be injected IV (16mL/min of 10mg/mL sol, or 8mL/min of 20mg/mL sol)

HOW SUPPLIED

Inj: 10mg/mL [50mL], 50mg, 100mg, 200mg, 350mg

CONTRAINDICATIONS

Pernicious anemia and other megaloblastic anemias secondary to lack of vitamin B12.

WARNINGS/PRECAUTIONS

Do not administer intrathecally; may be harmful or fatal. Monitor serum MTX to determine the optimal dose and duration of treatment. Delayed MTX excretion may be caused by 3rd space fluid accumulation (eg, ascites, pleural effusion), renal insufficiency, or inadequate hydration; higher doses or prolonged administration may be indicated. Bacteriostatic water for inj diluent contains benzyl alcohol; when doses >10mg/m² are administered, reconstitute with sterile water for inj and use immediately. Sol contains Ca^{2+}; no more than 160mg should be injected IV per min (16mL of a 10mg/mL, or 8mL of a 20mg/mL sol per min). Do not initiate or continue therapy with leucovorin and 5-FU in patients with symptoms of GI toxicity until symptoms have completely resolved; caution in elderly and/or debilitated patients. Monitor patients with diarrhea until it has resolved, as rapid clinical deterioration leading to death can occur. Seizures and/or syncope reported rarely in cancer patients, most commonly in those with CNS metastases or other predisposing factors. Leucovorin/5-FU combination therapy for advanced colorectal cancer should be administered under supervision of a physician experienced in the use of antimetabolite cancer chemotherapy. Defer 5-FU/leucovorin treatment until WBCs are 4000/mm³ and platelets 130,000/mm³; d/c if blood counts do not reach these levels within 2 weeks. Follow up with physical exam prior to each treatment course and appropriate radiological exam as needed. D/C when there is clear evidence of tumor progression.

ADVERSE REACTIONS

Allergic sensitization (eg, anaphylactoid reactions, urticaria), stomatitis, N/V, leukopenia, diarrhea, alopecia, dermatitis, thrombocytopenia, infection, lethargy/malaise/fatigue, anorexia, constipation.

DRUG INTERACTIONS

May enhance 5-FU toxicity. Seizures and/or syncope reported with fluoropyrimidine. Use with trimethoprim-sulfamethoxazole for the acute treatment of *Pneumocystis carinii* pneumonia in patients with HIV infection reported to be associated with increased rates of treatment failure and morbidity. Folic acid in large amounts may counteract antiepileptic effect of phenobarbital, phenytoin, and primidone, and increase seizure frequency in susceptible pediatric patients. High doses may reduce efficacy of intrathecally administered MTX.

L

PATIENT CONSIDERATIONS

Assessment: Assess for pernicious anemia and other megaloblastic anemias secondary to lack of vitamin B12, 3rd space fluid accumulation, renal impairment, inadequate hydration, GI toxicity, CNS metastases, pregnancy/nursing status, and possible drug interactions. (Leucovorin/5-FU Combination) Obtain CBC with differential and platelets prior to each treatment. Check electrolytes and LFTs prior to each treatment for the first 3 cycles, then prior to every other cycle.

Monitoring: Monitor for GI toxicity, seizures, syncope, and other adverse reactions. Monitor patients with diarrhea until it has resolved. Monitor fluid and electrolyte status in patients with abnormalities in MTX elimination. Monitor SrCr and MTX levels at least qd. (Leucovorin/5-FU Combination) Monitor CBC with differential and platelets weekly during the first 2 courses, and thereafter once each cycle at the time of anticipated WBC nadir. Perform physical exam prior to each treatment course and appropriate radiological exam as needed.

Counseling: Inform about risks and benefits of therapy. Instruct to notify physician if any adverse reactions occur. Instruct to inform physician if pregnant/nursing.

STORAGE: (Sol) 2-8°C (36-46°F). Protect from light. (Powder) 20-25°C (68-77°F). Protect from light. Reconstitution with Bacteriostatic Water for Inj: Use within 7 days. Reconstitution with Sterile Water for Inj: Use immediately.

LEVAQUIN — levofloxacin

RX

Class: Fluoroquinolone

Fluoroquinolones are associated with an increased risk of tendinitis and tendon rupture in all ages. Risk is further increased in patients >60 yrs of age, patients taking corticosteroids, and with kidney, heart, or lung transplants. May exacerbate muscle weakness with myasthenia gravis; avoid in patients with known history of myasthenia gravis.

ADULT DOSAGE

Pneumonia

Oral/IV:
Nosocomial Pneumonia: 750mg q24h for 7-14 days
Community-Acquired Pneumonia: 750mg q24h for 5 days or 500mg q24h for 7-14 days

Acute Bacterial Sinusitis

750mg q24h for 5 days or 500mg q24h for 10-14 days

Acute Bacterial Exacerbation of Chronic Bronchitis

500mg q24h for 7 days

Skin and Skin Structure Infections

Complicated: 750mg q24h for 7-14 days
Uncomplicated: 500mg q24h for 7-10 days

Chronic Bacterial Prostatitis

500mg q24h for 28 days

Urinary Tract Infections

Complicated/Acute Pyelonephritis: 750mg q24h for 5 days or 250mg q24h for 10 days
Uncomplicated: 250mg q24h for 3 days

Inhalational Anthrax (Postexposure)

>50kg: 500mg q24h for 60 days

Plague

Pneumonic/Septicemic Plague and Prophylaxis:
500mg q24h for 10-14 days

PEDIATRIC DOSAGE

Inhalational Anthrax (Postexposure)

≥6 Months of Age:
<50kg: 8mg/kg q12h for 60 days
Max: 250mg/dose
>50kg: 500mg q24h for 60 days

Plague

Pneumonic/Septicemic Plague and Prophylaxis:
≥6 Months of Age:
<50kg: 8mg/kg q12h for 10-14 days
Max: 250mg/dose
>50kg: 500mg q24h for 10-14 days

DOSING CONSIDERATIONS

Renal Impairment
750mg q24h:
CrCl 20-49mL/min: 750mg q48h
CrCl 10-19mL/min or Hemodialysis/Chronic Ambulatory Peritoneal Dialysis: 750mg initial dose, then 500mg q48h
500mg q24h:
CrCl 20-49mL/min: 500mg initial dose, then 250mg q24h
CrCl 10-19mL/min or Hemodialysis/Chronic Ambulatory Peritoneal Dialysis: 500mg initial dose, then 250mg q48h
250mg q24h:
CrCl 20-49mL/min: No dose adjustment
CrCl 10-19mL/min: 250mg q48h; if treating uncomplicated UTI, no dose adjustment required
Hemodialysis/Chronic Ambulatory Peritoneal Dialysis: No information on dose adjustment available

ADMINISTRATION

IV/Oral route
Drink fluids liberally

Oral
Take antacids, metal cations, and multivitamins at least 2 hrs before or 2 hrs after oral administration
Take at the same time each day
Tab: Take w/ or w/o food
Sol: Take 1 hr before or 2 hrs after eating

IV
Not for rapid or bolus IV infusion
Do not coadminister w/ any sol containing multivalent cations through the same IV line
Infuse over 60 min (250-500mg) or over 90 min (750mg)
Refer to PI for administration, preparation, stability, compatibility, and thawing instructions

HOW SUPPLIED

Inj: 5mg/mL in D5W [50mL, 100mL, 150mL]; **Sol:** 25mg/mL [480mL]; **Tab:** 250mg, 500mg, 750mg

CONTRAINDICATIONS

Known hypersensitivity to levofloxacin, or other quinolone antibacterials.

WARNINGS/PRECAUTIONS

D/C if patient experiences pain, swelling, inflammation, or rupture of a tendon. Serious and occasionally fatal hypersensitivity and/or anaphylactic reactions reported; d/c immediately at the 1st appearance of a skin rash, jaundice, or any other sign of hypersensitivity, and institute supportive measures. Severe hepatotoxicity, including acute hepatitis and fatal events, reported; d/c immediately if signs and symptoms of hepatitis occur. Convulsions, toxic psychoses, and increased intracranial pressure (including pseudotumor cerebri) reported. CNS stimulation may occur; d/c and institute appropriate measures if CNS events occur. Caution with CNS disorders (eg, severe cerebral arteriosclerosis, epilepsy) or risk factors that may predispose to seizures or lower seizure threshold. *Clostridium difficile*-associated diarrhea (CDAD) reported; may need to d/c if CDAD is suspected or confirmed. Cases of sensory or sensorimotor axonal polyneuropathy resulting in paresthesias, hypoesthesias, dysesthesias, and weakness reported; d/c immediately if symptoms of neuropathy occur. May prolong QT interval; avoid with known QT interval prolongation or uncorrected hypokalemia. Increased incidence of musculoskeletal disorders in pediatric patients. Blood glucose disturbances reported in diabetics; d/c and initiate appropriate therapy if hypoglycemic reaction occurs. May cause photosensitivity/phototoxicity reactions; avoid excessive exposure to sun/UV light and d/c if occurs. May increase risk of bacterial resistance if used in the absence of a proven/suspected bacterial infection or a prophylactic indication. Crystalluria and cylindruria reported; maintain adequate hydration. May produce false-positive urine screening results for opiates. Caution in elderly and with renal impairment.

ADVERSE REACTIONS

Tendinitis, tendon rupture, nausea, diarrhea, constipation, headache, insomnia, dizziness.

DRUG INTERACTIONS

See Boxed Warning. Caution with drugs that may lower the seizure threshold. Avoid with Class IA (eg, quinidine, procainamide) and Class III (eg, amiodarone, sotalol) antiarrhythmics. May enhance effects of warfarin; monitor PT and INR. Disturbances of blood glucose in diabetic patients receiving a concomitant antidiabetic agent reported; monitor glucose levels. NSAIDs may increase risk of CNS stimulation and convulsive seizures. May prolong theophylline $T_{1/2}$ and increase theophylline levels/risk of theophylline-related adverse reactions; monitor theophylline levels closely. Probenecid or cimetidine may increase exposure and reduce renal clearance. (PO) Antacids containing Mg^{2+}, aluminum, as well as sucralfate, metal cations such as iron, and multivitamin preparations with zinc or didanosine chewable/buffered tab or pediatric powder for oral sol may substantially interfere with the GI absorption and lower systemic concentrations; take at least 2 hrs before or 2 hrs after oral levofloxacin.

PATIENT CONSIDERATIONS

Assessment: Assess for risk factors for developing tendinitis and tendon rupture, history of myasthenia gravis, drug hypersensitivity, CNS disorders or risk factors that may predispose to seizures or lower seizure threshold, QT interval prolongation, uncorrected hypokalemia, renal/hepatic impairment, pregnancy/nursing status, and possible drug interactions.

Monitoring: Monitor for tendon rupture, tendinitis, exacerbation of myasthenia gravis, hypersensitivity reactions, hepatotoxicity, CNS effects, CDAD, peripheral neuropathy, ECG changes, arrhythmias, musculoskeletal disorders (pediatric patients), photosensitivity/phototoxicity reactions, and other adverse reactions. Monitor hydration status, blood glucose levels, and renal function. Monitor for evidence of bleeding, PT, and INR with warfarin.

Counseling: Inform that drug only treats bacterial, not viral, infections. Advise to take as prescribed; inform that skipping doses or not completing full course of therapy may decrease effectiveness and increase likelihood of drug resistance. Advise to contact physician if pain, swelling, or inflammation of a tendon, or weakness or inability to move joints develops; instruct to d/c therapy and rest/refrain from exercise. Advise to d/c use and notify physician if allergic reaction, skin rash, or signs/symptoms of liver injury occur. Instruct to inform physician if experiencing any symptoms of muscle weakness, including respiratory difficulties. Advise to notify physician of any history of convulsions, QT prolongation, or myasthenia gravis. Inform that peripheral neuropathy has been associated with therapy, and that symptoms may occur soon after initiation of therapy and may be irreversible; instruct to d/c treatment immediately and contact physician if symptoms of peripheral neuropathy develop. Instruct to use caution with activities requiring mental alertness and coordination; advise to notify physician if persistent headache with or without blurred vision occurs. Instruct to contact physician immediately if watery and bloody diarrhea (with or without stomach cramps and fever) develop, even as late as ≥2 months after last dose. Advise to inform physician if child has tendon or joint-related problems prior to, during, or after therapy. Advise to minimize or avoid exposure to natural or artificial sunlight. Instruct diabetic patients being treated with antidiabetic agents to d/c therapy and notify physician if hypoglycemia occurs. Advise to inform physician if taking warfarin.

STORAGE: (Tab) 15-30°C (59-86°F). (Sol) 25°C (77°F); excursions permitted to 15-30°C (59-86°F). (Inj) Single-use Vials: Controlled room temperature. Protect from light. Premixed Sol: ≤25°C (77°F); brief exposure ≤40°C (104°F) does not adversely affect product. Avoid excessive heat and protect from freezing and light. Diluted Sol (5mg/mL): Stable at ≤25°C (77°F) for 72 hrs; 5°C (41°F) for 14 days; -20°C (-4°F) for 6 months.

LEVBID – hyoscyamine sulfate RX

Class: Anticholinergic

ADULT DOSAGE

General Dosing

1-2 tabs q12h

Max: 4 tabs/24 hrs

Other Indications

Adjunctive therapy in the treatment of peptic ulcer, irritable bowel syndrome (irritable colon, spastic colon, mucous colitis), functional GI disorders, neurogenic bladder, neurogenic bowel disturbances (eg, splenic flexure syndrome, neurogenic colon)

May be used to control gastric secretion, visceral spasm and hypermotility in spastic colitis, spastic bladder, cystitis, pylorospasm, and associated abdominal cramps

May be used to reduce symptoms in functional intestinal disorders (eg, mild dysenteries, diverticulitis, acute enterocolitis)

Along w/ morphine or other narcotics in symptomatic relief of biliary and renal colic

As a "drying agent" in the relief of symptoms of acute rhinitis

To reduce rigidity and tremors and to control associated sialorrhea and hyperhidrosis in the therapy of parkinsonism

May be used in the therapy of poisoning by anticholinesterase agents

PEDIATRIC DOSAGE

General Dosing

≥12 Years:

1-2 tabs q12h

Max: 4 tabs/24 hrs

Other Indications

Adjunctive therapy in the treatment of peptic ulcer, irritable bowel syndrome (irritable colon, spastic colon, mucous colitis), functional GI disorders, neurogenic bladder, neurogenic bowel disturbances (eg, splenic flexure syndrome, neurogenic colon)

May be used to control gastric secretion, visceral spasm and hypermotility in spastic colitis, spastic bladder, cystitis, pylorospasm, and associated abdominal cramps

May be used to reduce symptoms in functional intestinal disorders (eg, mild dysenteries, diverticulitis, acute enterocolitis)

Along w/ morphine or other narcotics in symptomatic relief of biliary and renal colic

As a "drying agent" in the relief of symptoms of acute rhinitis

To reduce rigidity and tremors and to control associated sialorrhea and hyperhidrosis in the therapy of parkinsonism

May be used in the therapy of poisoning by anticholinesterase agents

DOSING CONSIDERATIONS

Elderly

Start at lower end of dosing range

ADMINISTRATION

Oral route

Do not crush or chew.

HOW SUPPLIED

Tab, Extended-Release: 0.375mg

CONTRAINDICATIONS

Glaucoma; obstructive uropathy (eg, bladder neck obstruction due to prostatic hypertrophy); obstructive disease of the GI tract (as in achalasia, pyloroduodenal stenosis); paralytic ileus, intestinal atony of elderly/debilitated patients; unstable cardiovascular status in acute hemorrhage; severe ulcerative colitis; toxic megacolon complicating ulcerative colitis; myasthenia gravis.

WARNINGS/PRECAUTIONS

Heat prostration may occur w/ high environmental temperature. Diarrhea may be an early symptom of incomplete intestinal obstruction, especially in patients w/ ileostomy or colostomy; in this instance, treatment would be inappropriate and possibly harmful. May impair physical/mental abilities. Psychosis reported in sensitive individuals. CNS signs/symptoms usually resolve w/in 12-48 hrs after discontinuation of the drug. Caution w/ autonomic neuropathy, hyperthyroidism, coronary heart disease, CHF, cardiac arrhythmias, HTN, renal disease, and hiatal hernia associated w/ reflux esophagitis. May increase HR; investigate any tachycardia prior to therapy.

ADVERSE REACTIONS

Dry mouth, urinary hesitancy/retention, blurred vision, tachycardia, palpitations, mydriasis, increased ocular tension, loss of taste, headache, nervousness, drowsiness, weakness, fatigue, dizziness, N/V.

DRUG INTERACTIONS

Additive adverse effects resulting from cholinergic blockade may occur when administered concomitantly w/ other antimuscarinics, amantadine, haloperidol, phenothiazines, MAOIs, TCAs, or some antihistamines. Antacids may interfere w/ absorption.

PATIENT CONSIDERATIONS

Assessment: Assess for glaucoma, obstructive uropathy, GI obstruction, paralytic ileus, sensitivity towards anticholinergic drugs, tachycardia, any other conditions where treatment is contraindicated or cautioned, pregnancy/nursing status, and possible drug interactions.
Monitoring: Monitor for signs/symptoms of heat prostration, drowsiness, dizziness, blurred vision, psychosis, CNS signs/symptoms, diarrhea, and other adverse reactions.
Counseling: Inform that drug may produce drowsiness, dizziness, or blurred vision; warn not to engage in activities requiring mental alertness (eg, operating a motor vehicle or other machinery) and not to perform hazardous work while taking drug. Advise that treatment may decrease sweating, resulting in heat prostration, fever or heat stroke; instruct to use caution if febrile or exposed to elevated environmental temperatures.
STORAGE: 20-25°C (68-77°F); excursions permitted to 15-30°C (59-86°F).

LEVEMIR – insulin detemir (rDNA origin) RX

Class: Insulin (long-acting)

ADULT DOSAGE

Type 1 Diabetes Mellitus

Initial: Approx 1/3 of total daily insulin requirements
Titrate: Adjust dose based on blood glucose measurements

Use rapid-acting or short-acting, premeal insulin to satisfy the remainder of the daily insulin requirements

Type 2 Diabetes Mellitus

Inadequately Controlled on Oral Antidiabetics:
Initial: 10 U (or 0.1-0.2 U/kg) qpm or divided bid
Titrate: Adjust dose based on blood glucose measurements
Inadequately Controlled on Glucagon-Like Peptide (GLP)-1 Receptor Agonist:
Initial: 10 U qpm
Titrate: Adjust dose based on blood glucose measurements
Administer as separate inj when using w/ a GLP-1 receptor agonist

Conversions

From Insulin Glargine/NPH Insulin:
Convert on a unit-to-unit basis

In converting from NPH insulin, some type 2 diabetes mellitus patients may require more units of therapy than NPH insulin

PEDIATRIC DOSAGE

Type 1 Diabetes Mellitus

≥2 Years:
Initial: Approx 1/3 of total daily insulin requirements
Titrate: Adjust dose based on blood glucose measurements

Use rapid-acting or short-acting, premeal insulin to satisfy the remainder of the daily insulin requirements

Conversions

From Insulin Glargine/NPH Insulin:
Convert on a unit-to-unit basis

In converting from NPH insulin, some type 2 diabetes mellitus patients may require more units of therapy than NPH insulin

L

DOSING CONSIDERATIONS

Elderly
Dose conservatively

ADMINISTRATION

SQ route

Rotate inj sites w/in the same region (abdomen, thigh, or deltoid) from 1 inj to the next
Do not dilute or mix w/ any other insulin or sol

QD Dosing
Administer dose w/ pm meal or hs

BID Dosing
Administer pm dose w/ pm meal, hs, or 12 hrs after am dose

HOW SUPPLIED

Inj: 100 U/mL [3mL, FlexTouch; 10mL, vial]

CONTRAINDICATIONS

Hypersensitivity to Levemir or any of its excipients.

WARNINGS/PRECAUTIONS

Not recommended for treatment of diabetic ketoacidosis. Do not share insulin device between patients, even if the needle is changed; may carry a risk for transmission of blood-borne pathogens. Changes to an insulin regimen should be made cautiously and only under medical supervision. Changes in strength, manufacturer, type, or method of administration may result in the need for a change in dose or an adjustment of concomitant antidiabetic treatment. Not for IV/IM use or use in insulin infusion pumps. Hypoglycemia may occur; caution in patients w/ hypoglycemia unawareness and patients predisposed to hypoglycemia. Hypoglycemia may impair ability to concentrate and react. Severe, life-threatening, generalized allergy, including anaphylaxis, may occur. Caution in renal/hepatic impairment.

ADVERSE REACTIONS

Hypoglycemia, URTI, headache, pharyngitis, influenza-like illness, abdominal pain, back pain, gastroenteritis, bronchitis, pyrexia, cough, viral infection, N/V, rhinitis.

DRUG INTERACTIONS

May require insulin dose adjustment and close monitoring w/ drugs that may increase blood-glucose-lowering effect and susceptibility to hypoglycemia (eg, oral antidiabetic drugs, pramlintide acetate, ACE inhibitors), drugs that may reduce blood-glucose-lowering effect (eg, corticosteroids, niacin, danazol), or drugs that may either increase or decrease blood-glucose-lowering effect (eg, β-blockers, clonidine, lithium salts, alcohol). Pentamidine may cause hypoglycemia, sometimes followed by hyperglycemia. Signs of hypoglycemia may be reduced or absent w/ antiadrenergic drugs (eg, β-blockers, clonidine, guanethidine, reserpine). May need to lower or more conservatively titrate dose when used w/ a GLP-1 receptor agonist to minimize risk of hypoglycemia. Observe for signs/symptoms of heart failure (HF) if treated concomitantly w/ a peroxisome proliferator-activated receptor (PPAR)-gamma agonist (eg, thiazolidinedione); consider discontinuation or dose reduction of the PPAR-gamma agonist if HF develops.

PATIENT CONSIDERATIONS

L

Assessment: Assess for diabetic ketoacidosis, predisposition to hypoglycemia, hypersensitivity, renal/hepatic impairment, pregnancy/nursing status, and possible drug interactions. Obtain baseline blood glucose and HbA1c levels.

Monitoring: Monitor for signs/symptoms of hypoglycemia, allergic reactions, and other adverse reactions. Monitor blood glucose and HbA1c levels, and renal/hepatic function.

Counseling: Inform about the potential side effects, including hypoglycemia, weight gain, lipodystrophy, and allergic reactions. Inform that hypoglycemia may impair ability to concentrate and react; advise to use caution when driving or operating machinery. Instruct to always check the label before each inj to avoid medication errors/accidental mix-ups. Advise to use only if sol is clear and colorless w/ no particles visible. Instruct on self-management procedures, including glucose monitoring, proper inj technique, and management of hypoglycemia and hyperglycemia, and on handling of special situations (eg, intercurrent conditions, inadequate or skipped insulin dose, inadequate food intake). Advise to inform physician if pregnant/contemplating pregnancy. Counsel to never share insulin device w/ another person, even if the needle is changed.

STORAGE: Unopened: 2-8°C (36-46°F) until expiration date. If refrigeration is not possible, may be kept at room temperature <30°C (86°F) for 42 days. Do not freeze. Protect from direct heat and light. Opened: Vial: 2-8°C (36-46°F) or room temperature <30°C (86°F). Discard refrigerated vials 42 days after initial use and discard unrefrigerated vials 42 days after they are 1st kept out of the refrigerator. Do not freeze. Protect from direct heat and light. FlexTouch: Room temperature <30°C (86°F) for 42 days; do not refrigerate after initial use or store w/ the needle in place. Protect from direct heat and light. Always remove the needle after each inj and use a new needle for each inj.

LEVITRA – vardenafil hydrochloride

RX

Class: Phosphodiesterase-5 (PDE-5) inhibitor

ADULT DOSAGE

Erectile Dysfunction

Initial: 10mg prn, 60 min prior to sexual activity

Titrate: May decrease to 5mg or increase to max of 20mg based on efficacy and side effects

Max: 1 dose/day

PEDIATRIC DOSAGE

Pediatric use may not have been established

DOSING CONSIDERATIONS

Concomitant Medications

Ritonavir:
Max: 2.5mg/72 hrs

Indinavir/Saquinavir/Atazanavir/Clarithromycin/Ketoconazole (400mg/day)/Itraconazole (400mg/day):
Max: 2.5mg/24 hrs

Ketoconazole (200mg/day)/Itraconazole (200mg/day)/Erythromycin:
Max: 5mg/24 hrs

Stable on α-Blocker:
Initial: 5mg; 2.5mg when used w/ certain CYP3A4 inhibitors
Consider a time interval between dosing

Renal Impairment
Dialysis: Avoid use

Hepatic Impairment
Moderate (Child-Pugh B):
Initial: 5mg
Max: 10mg
Severe (Child-Pugh C): Avoid use

Elderly
≥65 Years:
Initial: 5mg

ADMINISTRATION

Oral route

Take w/ or w/o food.

HOW SUPPLIED

Tab: 2.5mg, 5mg, 10mg, 20mg

CONTRAINDICATIONS

Concomitant use w/ guanylate cyclase stimulators and regular or intermittent use w/ nitrates and nitric oxide donors.

WARNINGS/PRECAUTIONS

Avoid if sexual activity is not recommended due to underlying cardiovascular (CV) status, or if w/ severe hepatic impairment (Child-Pugh C)/congenital QT prolongation, or if on renal dialysis. Patients w/ left ventricular outflow obstruction (eg, aortic stenosis, idiopathic hypertrophic subaortic stenosis) may be sensitive to vasodilation. Has vasodilatory properties resulting in transient decreases in supine BP. Not recommended w/ unstable angina, hypotension (resting systolic BP <90mmHg), uncontrolled HTN (>170/110mmHg), recent history of stroke, life-threatening arrhythmia, or MI (w/in last 6 months), severe cardiac failure, or hereditary degenerative retinal disorders, including retinitis pigmentosa. Rare reports of prolonged erections >4 hrs and priapism. Caution w/ bleeding disorders, significant active peptic ulceration, anatomical deformation of the penis (eg, angulation, cavernosal fibrosis, Peyronie's disease) or conditions that predispose to priapism (eg, sickle cell anemia, multiple myeloma, leukemia). Non-arteritic anterior ischemic optic neuropathy (NAION) reported (rare); d/c if sudden loss of vision occurs. Caution in patients w/ underlying NAION risk factors; increased risk w/ previous history of NAION and individuals w/ "crowded" optic disc. Sudden decrease or loss of hearing accompanied by tinnitus and dizziness reported; d/c if this occurs. QT prolongation may occur.

ADVERSE REACTIONS

Headache, flushing, rhinitis, dyspepsia, sinusitis, flu syndrome.

DRUG INTERACTIONS

See Contraindications. Avoid w/ Class IA (eg, quinidine, procainamide) or Class III (eg, amiodarone, sotalol) antiarrhythmics and other agents for ED. Caution w/ medications known to prolong QT interval. Increased levels w/ CYP3A4 inhibitors (eg, ritonavir, ketoconazole, clarithromycin). Caution when coadministering α-blockers; additive effect on BP may be anticipated. CYP3A4/5 or CYP2C9 inhibitors may reduce clearance.

PATIENT CONSIDERATIONS

Assessment: Assess for CV disease, left ventricular outflow obstruction, congenital or history of QT prolongation, hereditary degenerative retinal disorders, bleeding disorders, active peptic ulceration, anatomical deformation of the penis, conditions that predispose to priapism, renal/hepatic impairment, potential underlying causes of ED, risk for NAION, and for possible drug interactions. Obtain baseline BP.

Monitoring: Monitor for priapism, changes in vision/hearing, QT prolongation, and other adverse reactions.

Counseling: Instruct to take ud. Inform that regular and/or intermittent use of nitrates may cause BP to suddenly drop to an unsafe level. Inform that use is contraindicated w/ guanylate cyclase stimulators (eg, riociguat). Inform patients w/ preexisting CV risk factors of the potential cardiac risk of sexual activity. Inform that concomitant use of α-blockers may lower BP significantly. Instruct to contact physician for dose modification if not satisfied w/ quality of sexual performance or in case of an unwanted effect. Instruct to seek immediate medical assistance if erection persists >4 hrs; inform that penile tissue damage and permanent loss of potency may result. Instruct to d/c and seek medical attention in the event of sudden loss of vision in 1 or both eyes; inform of the increased risk of NAION w/ history of NAION in 1 eye and in patients w/ a "crowded" optic disc. Instruct to d/c treatment and seek prompt medical attention in the event of sudden decrease or loss of hearing that may be accompanied by tinnitus and dizziness. Counsel about protective measures necessary to guard against STDs, including HIV; inform that drug does not protect against STDs.

STORAGE: 25°C (77°F); excursions permitted to 15-30°C (59-86°F).

LEVOPHED – norepinephrine bitartrate

RX

Class: Alpha-adrenergic agonist

To prevent sloughing and necrosis in area of extravasation, area should be infiltrated with 10-15mL saline sol containing 5-10mg of Regitine (brand of phentolamine), an adrenergic blocking agent. Sympathetic blockade with phentolamine causes immediate and conspicuous local hyperemic changes if infiltrated within 12 hrs. Give phentolamine as soon as possible after the extravasation is noted.

ADULT DOSAGE

Acute Hypotension

For BP control in certain acute hypotensive states (eg, pheochromocytomectomy, sympathectomy, poliomyelitis, spinal anesthesia, MI, septicemia, blood transfusion, and drug reactions)

Average Dosage:
Initial: 8-12mcg/min (2-3mL) as IV infusion until low normal BP (80-100mmHg systolic) is established and maintained by adjusting rate of flow
Maint: 2-4mcg/min (0.5-1mL)

High Dosage:
Individualize dose (as high as 68mg/day)

Continue infusion until adequate BP and tissue perfusion are maintained w/o therapy
Reduce dose gradually, avoiding abrupt withdrawal

Adjunct Treatment of Cardiac Arrest and Profound Hypotension:
Average Dosage:
Initial: 8-12mcg/min (2-3mL) as IV infusion until low normal BP (80-100mmHg systolic) is established and maintained by adjusting rate of flow
Maint: 2-4mcg/min (0.5-1mL)

PEDIATRIC DOSAGE

Pediatric use may not have been established

DOSING CONSIDERATIONS

Elderly
Start at lower end of dosing range

ADMINISTRATION

IV route
Inj is a concentrated, potent drug that must be diluted in dextrose containing sol prior to infusion
An infusion should be given into a large vein
Avoid contact w/ iron salts, alkalis, or oxidizing agents

Diluent
Dilute in D5 inj or D5 and NaCl inj
Whole blood or plasma, if indicated to increase blood volume, should be administered separately (eg, Y-tube and individual containers if given simultaneously)

HOW SUPPLIED

Inj: 4mg/4mL

CONTRAINDICATIONS
Hypotension from blood volume deficits, except as an emergency measure to maintain coronary and cerebral artery perfusion until blood volume replacement therapy can be completed, mesenteric or peripheral vascular thrombosis (unless administration is necessary as a life-saving procedure in the opinion of the attending physician), profound hypoxia or hypercarbia, concomitant use of cyclopropane and halothane anesthetics.

WARNINGS/PRECAUTIONS
Contains sodium metabisulfite; may cause allergic-type reactions (eg, anaphylactic symptoms, life-threatening or less severe asthmatic episodes). May produce dangerously high BP with overdoses due to potency and varying response; monitor BP every 2 min from initial administration until desired BP is obtained, then every 5 min if administration is to be continued. Headache may be a symptom of HTN due to overdosage; monitor rate of flow constantly. Infusions should be given into a large vein, particularly an antecubital vein whenever possible. Avoid a catheter tie-in technique if possible. Occlusive vascular diseases (eg, atherosclerosis, arteriosclerosis, diabetic endarteritis, Buerger's disease) more likely to occur in the lower than in the upper extremity; avoid leg veins in elderly or in those suffering from such disorders. Gangrene in lower extremity reported when given in an ankle vein. Check infusion site frequently for free flow. Avoid extravasation into the tissues; local necrosis might ensue. Blanching may occur; consider changing the infusion site at intervals to allow effects of local vasoconstriction to subside. Caution in elderly.

ADVERSE REACTIONS
Ischemic injury, bradycardia, arrhythmias, anxiety, headache, respiratory difficulty, extravasation necrosis at inj site.

DRUG INTERACTIONS
See Contraindications. Caution with MAOI or triptyline/imipramine antidepressants; severe, prolonged HTN may result.

PATIENT CONSIDERATIONS

Assessment: Assess hypotension and need for blood volume replacement. Assess use as emergency measure or life-saving procedure (eg, hypotension from blood volume deficits to maintain coronary and cerebral artery perfusion until blood volume replacement therapy can be completed, mesenteric or peripheral vascular thrombosis). Assess for profound hypoxia or hypercarbia, sulfite sensitivity, pregnancy/nursing status, and possible drug interactions. Assess use in elderly and occlusive vascular diseases. Obtain baseline BP.

Monitoring: Monitor for HTN, headache, gangrene, extravasation, blanching, and hypersensitivity/allergic reactions. Monitor infusion site, rate of flow, BP, and central venous pressure.

Counseling: Inform of risks/benefits of therapy. Advise to inform physician if headache occurs.

STORAGE: 20-25°C (68-77°F); (vial) excursions permitted to 15-30° (59-86°F). Protect from light.

LEVOXYL – levothyroxine sodium

RX

Class: Thyroid replacement hormone

Do not use for the treatment of obesity or weight loss; doses within range of daily hormonal requirements are ineffective for weight reduction in euthyroid patients. Serious or life-threatening manifestations of toxicity may occur when given in larger doses, particularly when given in association with sympathomimetic amines.

ADULT DOSAGE

Hypothyroidism

Replacement/supplemental therapy in hypothyroidism of any etiology, except transient hypothyroidism during the recovery phase of subacute thyroiditis

Adjust dose based on periodic assessment of patient's clinical response and lab parameters

Usual: 1.7mcg/kg/day; >200mcg/day seldom required

Severe Hypothyroidism:
Initial: 12.5-25mcg/day
Titrate: Increase by 25mcg/day every 2-4 weeks until TSH level normalized

Secondary (Pituitary)/Tertiary (Hypothalamic) Hypothyroidism: Titrate until euthyroid and serum free-T4 level is restored to the upper 1/2 of the normal range

PEDIATRIC DOSAGE

Hypothyroidism

Replacement/supplemental therapy in hypothyroidism of any etiology, except transient hypothyroidism during the recovery phase of subacute thyroiditis

Adjust dose based on periodic assessment of patient's clinical response and lab parameters

Usual:
0-3 Months of Age: 10-15mcg/kg/day
3-6 Months of Age: 8-10mcg/kg/day
6-12 Months of Age: 6-8mcg/kg/day
1-5 Years: 5-6mcg/kg/day
6-12 Years: 4-5mcg/kg/day
>12 Years: 2-3mcg/kg/day
Growth/Puberty Complete: 1.7mcg/kg/day

Infants w/ Serum T4 <5mcg/dL or Undetectable T4:
Initial: 50mcg/day

Subclinical Hypothyroidism: Lower doses may be adequate to normalize TSH level (eg, 1mcg/kg/day)

Pituitary TSH Suppressant

Used to treat/prevent various types of euthyroid goiters (eg, thyroid nodules, subacute or chronic lymphocytic thyroiditis, multinodular goiter) and to manage thyroid cancer

Well-Differentiated (Papillary and Follicular) Thyroid Cancer:

Usual: >2mcg/kg/day, w/ target TSH level <0.1 mU/L
High-Risk Tumors: Target TSH level <0.01 mU/L

Benign Nodules and Nontoxic Multinodular Goiter:
Suppressed to a higher TSH target than that used for treatment of thyroid cancer (eg, 0.1-0.5 mU/L for nodules, 0.5-1.0 mU/L for multinodular goiter)

Chronic/Severe Hypothyroidism:
Children:
Initial: 25mcg/day
Titrate: Increase by 25mcg increments every 2-4 weeks until desired effect is achieved

DOSING CONSIDERATIONS

Pregnancy

May increase levothyroxine requirements

Elderly

Hypothyroidism:
>50 Years:
Initial: 25-50mcg/day
Titrate: Increase by 12.5-25mcg increments every 6-8 weeks prn
W/ Underlying Cardiac Disease:
Initial: 12.5-25mcg/day
Titrate: Increase by 12.5-25mg increments every 4-6 weeks

Adverse Reactions

Minimize Hyperactivity in Older Children:
Initial: Give 1/4 of full replacement dose
Titrate: Increase on a weekly basis by 1/4 the full recommended replacement dose until the full recommended replacement dose is reached

Other Important Considerations

Hypothyroidism w/ Underlying Cardiac Disease:

Infants (Risk for Cardiac Failure):
Initial: Consider lower dose (eg, 25mcg/day)
Titrate: Increase dose in 4-6 weeks prn
<50 Years:
Initial: 25-50mcg/day
Titrate: Increase by 12.5-25mcg increments every 6-8 weeks prn

ADMINISTRATION

Oral route

Take in the am on an empty stomach at least 30 min before food
Take w/ water
Take at least 4 hrs apart from drugs that are known to interfere w/ its absorption

Pediatrics

May crush tab and mix w/ 5-10mL of water

HOW SUPPLIED

Tab: 25mcg, 50mcg, 75mcg, 88mcg, 100mcg, 112mcg, 125mcg, 137mcg, 150mcg, 175mcg, 200mcg

CONTRAINDICATIONS

Untreated subclinical (suppressed serum TSH level w/ normal T3 and T4 levels) or overt thyrotoxicosis of any etiology, acute MI, uncorrected adrenal insufficiency, hypersensitivity to any of the inactive ingredients in the formulation.

WARNINGS/PRECAUTIONS

Should not be used in the treatment of male or female infertility unless associated with hypothyroidism. Contraindicated in patients with nontoxic diffuse goiter or nodular thyroid disease, particularly in elderly or with underlying cardiovascular (CV) disease if serum TSH level is already suppressed; use with caution if TSH level is not suppressed and carefully monitor thyroid function. Has narrow therapeutic index; carefully titrate dose to avoid over- or under-treatment. May decrease bone mineral density (BMD) with long term use; give minimum dose necessary to achieve desired clinical and biochemical response. Caution with CV disorders and the elderly. If cardiac symptoms develop or worsen, reduce or withhold dose for 1 week and then restart at lower dose. Overtreatment may produce CV effects (eg, increase in HR, increase in cardiac wall thickness, increase in cardiac contractility, precipitation of angina or arrhythmias). Monitor patients with coronary artery disease (CAD) closely during surgical procedures; may precipitate cardiac arrhythmias. Caution in patients with diabetes mellitus (DM). Patients with concomitant adrenal insufficiency should be treated with replacement glucocorticoids prior to therapy.

ADVERSE REACTIONS

Fatigue, increased appetite, weight loss, heat intolerance, headache, hyperactivity, irritability, insomnia, palpitations, arrhythmias, dyspnea, hair loss, menstrual irregularities, pseudotumor cerebri (children), slipped capital femoral epiphysis (children).

DRUG INTERACTIONS

Concurrent sympathomimetics may increase effects of sympathomimetics or thyroid hormone; may increase risk of coronary insufficiency with CAD. Upward dose adjustments may be needed for insulin and oral hypoglycemic agents. May decrease absorption with soybean flour, cottonseed meal, walnuts, and dietary fiber. May increase oral anticoagulant activity; adjust dose of anticoagulant and monitor PT. May decrease levels and effects of digitalis glycosides. Transient reduction in TSH secretion with dopamine/dopamine agonists, glucocorticoids, octreotide. Decreased thyroid hormone secretion with aminoglutethimide, amiodarone, iodide (including iodine-containing radiographic contrast agents), lithium, methimazole, propylthiouracil (PTU), sulfonamides, and tolbutamide. May increase thyroid hormone secretion with amiodarone and iodide. May decrease T4 absorption with antacids (aluminum and magnesium hydroxides), simethicone, bile acid sequestrants (cholestyramine, colestipol), calcium carbonate, cation exchange resins (kayexalate), ferrous sulfate, orlistat, and sucralfate; administer at least 4 hrs apart. May increase serum thyroxine-binding globulin (TBG) concentrations with clofibrate, estrogen-containing oral contraceptives, oral estrogens, heroin/methadone, 5-fluorouracil, mitotane, and tamoxifen. May decrease serum TBG concentrations with androgens/anabolic steroids, asparaginase, glucocorticoids, and slow-release nicotinic acid. May cause protein-binding site displacement with furosemide (>80mg IV), heparin, hydantoins, NSAIDs (fenamates, phenylbutazone), and salicylates (>2g/day). May alter T4 and T3 metabolism with carbamazepine, hydantoins, phenobarbital, and rifampin. May decrease T4 5'-deiodinase activity with amiodarone, β-adrenergic antagonists (eg, propranolol >160mg/day), glucocorticoids (eg, dexamethasone >4mg/day), and PTU. Concurrent use with tricyclic (eg, amitriptyline) and tetracyclic (eg, maprotiline) antidepressants may increase the therapeutic and toxic effects of both drugs. Coadministration with sertraline in patients stabilized on levothyroxine may result in increased levothyroxine requirements. Interferon-α may cause development of antithyroid microsomal antibodies and transient hypothyroidism, hyperthyroidism, or both. Interleukin-2 has been associated with transient painless thyroiditis. Excessive use with growth hormones (eg, somatropin, somatrem) may accelerate epiphyseal closure. Ketamine may produce marked HTN and tachycardia. May reduce uptake of radiographic agents. Decreased theophylline clearance may occur in hypothyroid patients. Altered levels of thyroid hormone and/or TSH levels with choral hydrate, diazepam, ethionamide, lovastatin, metoclopramide, 6-mercaptopurine, nitroprusside, para-aminosalicylate sodium, perphenazine, resorcinol (excessive topical use), and thiazide diuretics.

PATIENT CONSIDERATIONS

Assessment: Assess for untreated subclinical or overt thyrotoxicosis, acute MI, uncorrected adrenal insufficiency, CAD, CV disorders, nontoxic diffuse goiter, nodular thyroid disease, DM, hypersensitivity, pregnancy/nursing status, and possible drug interactions. In patients with secondary or tertiary hypothyroidism, assess for additional hypothalamic/pituitary hormone deficiencies. Assess TSH levels. In infants with congenital hypothyroidism, assess for other congenital anomalies.

Monitoring: Monitor for CV effects. In patients on long-term therapy, monitor for signs/symptoms of decreased BMD. In patients with nontoxic diffuse goiter or nodular thyroid disease, monitor for precipitation of thyrotoxicosis. In adults with primary hypothyroidism, perform periodic monitoring of serum TSH levels. In pediatric patients with congenital hypothyroidism, perform periodic monitoring of serum TSH levels and total or free T4 levels. In patients with secondary and tertiary hypothyroidism, perform periodic monitoring of serum free T4 levels. Refer to PI for TSH and T4 monitoring parameters. Closely monitor PT if coadministered with an oral anticoagulant.

Counseling: Instruct to notify physician if allergic to any foods or medicines, pregnant or plan to become pregnant, breastfeeding or taking any other drugs, including prescriptions and OTC preparations. Instruct to notify physician of any other medical conditions, particularly heart disease, diabetes, clotting disorders, and adrenal or pituitary gland problems. Instruct not to stop or change dose unless directed by physician. Instruct to take on empty stomach, at least 1/2 hr before eating any food. Advise that partial hair loss may occur during the 1st few months of therapy, but is usually temporary. Instruct to notify physician or dentist prior to surgery about levothyroxine therapy.

Inform that drug should not be used for weight control. Inform patients that tabs may rapidly swell and disintegrate, resulting in choking, gagging, tab getting stuck in throat, or difficulty swallowing; advise to take with a full glass of water. Instruct to notify physician if rapid or irregular heartbeat, chest pain, SOB, leg cramps, headache, or any other unusual medical event occurs. Inform that dose may be increased during pregnancy. Inform that drug should not be administered within 4 hrs of agents such as iron/calcium supplements and antacids.

STORAGE: 20-25°C (68-77°F); excursions permitted to 15-30°C (59-86°F). Store away from heat, moisture, and light.

LEXAPRO – escitalopram oxalate RX

Class: Selective serotonin reuptake inhibitor (SSRI)

Antidepressants increased the risk of suicidal thinking and behavior (suicidality) in children, adolescents, and young adults in short-term studies of major depressive disorder (MDD) and other psychiatric disorders. Monitor and observe closely for clinical worsening, suicidality, or unusual changes in behavior in patients who are started on antidepressant therapy. Advise families and caregivers of the need for close observation and communication with the prescriber. Not approved for use in pediatric patients <12 yrs of age.

ADULT DOSAGE

Major Depressive Disorder

Initial: 10mg qd

Titrate: May increase to 20mg after a minimum of 1 week

Generalized Anxiety Disorder

Initial: 10mg qd

Titrate: May increase to 20mg after a minimum of 1 week

Dosing Considerations with MAOIs

Switching to/from an MAOI for Psychiatric Disorders:

Allow at least 14 days between discontinuation of an MAOI and initiation of treatment, and allow at least 14 days between discontinuation of treatment and initiation of an MAOI

W/ Other MAOIs (eg, Linezolid, IV Methylene Blue):

Do not start escitalopram in a patient being treated w/ linezolid or IV methylene blue

In patients already receiving escitalopram, if acceptable alternatives are not available and benefits outweigh risks, d/c escitalopram and administer linezolid or IV methylene blue; monitor for serotonin syndrome for 2 weeks or until 24 hrs after the last dose of linezolid or IV methylene blue, whichever comes 1st. May resume escitalopram therapy 24 hrs after the last dose of linezolid or IV methylene blue

PEDIATRIC DOSAGE

Major Depressive Disorder

≥12 Years:

Initial: 10mg qd

Titrate: May increase to 20mg after a minimum of 3 weeks

Dosing Considerations with MAOIs

Switching to/from an MAOI for Psychiatric Disorders:

Allow at least 14 days between discontinuation of an MAOI and initiation of treatment, and allow at least 14 days between discontinuation of treatment and initiation of an MAOI

W/ Other MAOIs (eg, Linezolid, IV Methylene Blue):

Do not start escitalopram in a patient being treated w/ linezolid or IV methylene blue

In patients already receiving escitalopram, if acceptable alternatives are not available and benefits outweigh risks, d/c escitalopram and administer linezolid or IV methylene blue; monitor for serotonin syndrome for 2 weeks or until 24 hrs after the last dose of linezolid or IV methylene blue, whichever comes 1st. May resume escitalopram therapy 24 hrs after the last dose of linezolid or IV methylene blue

DOSING CONSIDERATIONS

Hepatic Impairment

10mg/day

Elderly

10mg/day

Discontinuation

Gradually reduce dose; if intolerable symptoms occur following a decrease in dose or upon discontinuation, consider resuming previously prescribed dose or continue decreasing dose at a more gradual rate

ADMINISTRATION

Oral route

Administer in the am or pm, w/ or w/o food

HOW SUPPLIED

Sol: 5mg/5mL [240mL]; **Tab:** 5mg, 10mg*, 20mg* *scored

CONTRAINDICATIONS

Use of MAOIs intended to treat psychiatric disorders w/ escitalopram oxalate or w/in 14 days of stopping treatment w/ escitalopram oxalate. Use of escitalopram oxalate w/in 14 days of stopping an MAOI intended to treat psychiatric disorders. Starting escitalopram oxalate in a patient being treated w/ MAOIs (eg, linezolid or IV methylene blue). Concomitant use w/ pimozide. Hypersensitivity to escitalopram or citalopram or any of the inactive ingredients in this product.

WARNINGS/PRECAUTIONS

Not approved for the treatment of bipolar depression. Serotonin syndrome reported; d/c immediately and initiate supportive symptomatic treatment. Avoid abrupt discontinuation; gradual dose reduction is recommended whenever possible. Convulsions reported; caution with history of seizure disorder. Activation of mania/hypomania reported; caution with history of mania. Hyponatremia may occur; caution in elderly and volume-depleted patients. Consider discontinuation in patients with symptomatic hyponatremia and institute appropriate medical intervention. May increase the risk of bleeding events. May impair mental/physical abilities. Pupillary dilation that occurs following use may trigger an angle-closure attack in a patient with anatomically narrow angles who does not have a patent iridectomy. May precipitate mixed/manic episode in patients at risk for bipolar disorder; screen for risk for bipolar disorder prior to initiating treatment. Caution with diseases/conditions that produce altered metabolism or hemodynamic responses, and with severe renal impairment.

ADVERSE REACTIONS

N/V, insomnia, ejaculation disorder, increased sweating, somnolence, fatigue, diarrhea, dry mouth, headache, constipation, decreased appetite, neck/shoulder pain, decreased libido, anorgasmia.

DRUG INTERACTIONS

See Contraindications. Not recommended for use with alcohol. May cause serotonin syndrome with other serotonergic drugs (eg, triptans, TCAs, fentanyl) and with drugs that impair metabolism of serotonin; d/c immediately if this occurs. Caution with other centrally acting drugs, and drugs metabolized by CYP2D6 (eg, desipramine). Increased risk of bleeding with aspirin, NSAIDs, warfarin, and other drugs that affect coagulation. May increase levels with cimetidine. Rare reports of weakness, hyperreflexia, and incoordination with sumatriptan. Possible increased clearance with carbamazepine. May decrease levels of ketoconazole. May increase levels of metoprolol. Increased risk of hyponatremia with diuretics. Monitor lithium levels and adjust its dose appropriately.

PATIENT CONSIDERATIONS

Assessment: Assess for drug hypersensitivity, risk for bipolar disorder, history of seizure disorder, history of mania, volume depletion, diseases/conditions that produce altered metabolism or hemodynamic response, susceptibility to angle-closure glaucoma, hepatic/renal impairment, pregnancy/nursing status, and possible drug interactions. Obtain detailed psychiatric history.

Monitoring: Monitor for signs/symptoms of clinical worsening, serotonin syndrome, bleeding events, hyponatremia, seizures, cognitive and motor impairment, activation of mania/hypomania, angle-closure glaucoma, and other adverse reactions. If therapy is abruptly discontinued, monitor for discontinuation symptoms. Regularly monitor weight and growth in pediatrics. Periodically reassess the need for maintenance treatment.

Counseling: Inform about the benefits and risks of therapy. Counsel on the appropriate use of the drug. Advise to look for emergence of symptoms associated with an increased risk for suicidal thinking and behavior; instruct to report such symptoms, especially if severe, abrupt in onset, or not part of presenting symptoms. Caution about risk of serotonin syndrome with other serotonergic agents (eg, triptans, buspirone, St. John's wort) and about risk of bleeding with ASA, warfarin, or other drugs that affect coagulation. Caution about risk of angle-closure glaucoma. Instruct to notify physician if taking or planning to take any prescription or OTC drugs. Inform that improvement may be noticed in 1-4 weeks; instruct to continue therapy ud. Caution about operating hazardous machinery, including automobiles. Instruct to avoid alcohol. Instruct to notify physician if pregnant, intending to become pregnant, or if breastfeeding. Inform of the need for comprehensive treatment program.

STORAGE: 25°C (77°F); excursions permitted to 15-30°C (59-86°F).

LIALDA — mesalamine

RX

Class: 5-aminosalicylic acid derivative

ADULT DOSAGE

Ulcerative Colitis

Induction of Remission:
Active, Mild to Moderate: 2-4 tabs qd

Maint of Remission:
2 tabs qd

PEDIATRIC DOSAGE

Pediatric use may not have been established

DOSING CONSIDERATIONS

Elderly

Start at lower end of dosing range

ADMINISTRATION

Oral route

Take w/ a meal

Swallow tab whole

HOW SUPPLIED

Tab, Delayed-Release: 1.2g

CONTRAINDICATIONS

Known hypersensitivity to salicylates or aminosalicylates or to any of the ingredients in this product.

WARNINGS/PRECAUTIONS

Renal impairment, including minimal change nephropathy, acute/chronic interstitial nephritis, and, rarely, renal failure reported; evaluate renal function prior to therapy and periodically thereafter. Caution with known renal impairment or history of renal disease. Has been associated with an acute intolerance syndrome that may be difficult to distinguish from an exacerbation of ulcerative colitis (UC); observe closely for worsening of symptoms and d/c therapy if acute intolerance syndrome is suspected. Patients with sulfasalazine hypersensitivity may have similar reaction to therapy. Mesalamine-induced cardiac hypersensitivity reactions (eg, myocarditis, pericarditis) reported; caution with conditions that predispose to the development of myocarditis or pericarditis. Hepatic failure reported in patients with preexisting liver disease; caution with liver disease. Pyloric stenosis or other organic/functional obstruction in the upper GI tract may cause prolonged gastric retention of therapy, which could delay drug release in the colon. Caution with sulfasalazine hypersensitivity and in elderly. May interfere with lab tests.

ADVERSE REACTIONS

Headache, flatulence, UC, abnormal LFTs, abdominal pain.

DRUG INTERACTIONS

Nephrotoxic agents, including NSAIDs, may increase risk of renal reactions. Azathioprine or 6-mercaptopurine may increase risk for blood disorders.

L

PATIENT CONSIDERATIONS

Assessment: Assess for hypersensitivity to the drug, salicylates/aminosalicylates, or sulfasalazine, conditions that predispose to the development of myocarditis or pericarditis, pyloric stenosis or other organic/functional upper GI tract obstruction, hepatic impairment, pregnancy/nursing status, and possible drug interactions. Evaluate renal function prior to initiation of therapy.

Monitoring: Monitor for acute intolerance syndrome, hypersensitivity reactions, hepatic failure, and other adverse reactions. Perform periodic monitoring of renal function. Monitor blood cell counts in elderly.

Counseling: Instruct not to take drug if hypersensitive to salicylates (eg, aspirin) or other mesalamines. Inform to notify physician of all medications being taken and if pregnant, planning to become pregnant, or breastfeeding. Instruct to inform physician if allergic to sulfasalazine, if taking NSAIDs or other nephrotoxic agents, azathioprine, or 6-mercaptopurine, and if experiencing cramping, abdominal pain, bloody diarrhea, fever, headache, or rash. Inform to notify physician of history of myocarditis/pericarditis or stomach blockage, and if patient has kidney/liver disease.

STORAGE: 15-25°C (59-77°F); excursions permitted to 30°C (86°F).

LIBRAX — chlordiazepoxide hydrochloride/clidinium bromide RX

Class: Anticholinergic/benzodiazepine

ADULT DOSAGE

Acute Enterocolitis

Adjunctive Therapy:

Maint: 1-2 caps tid-qid ac and hs

Peptic Ulcer

Adjunctive Therapy:

Maint: 1-2 caps tid-qid ac and hs

Irritable Bowel Syndrome

Adjunctive Therapy:

Maint: 1-2 caps tid-qid ac and hs

PEDIATRIC DOSAGE

Pediatric use may not have been established

DOSING CONSIDERATIONS

Elderly/Debilitated

Initial: Not more than 2 caps/day

Titrate: Increase gradually prn and as tolerated

ADMINISTRATION

Oral route

HOW SUPPLIED

Cap: (Chlordiazepoxide/Clidinium) 5mg/2.5mg

CONTRAINDICATIONS

Glaucoma, prostatic hypertrophy, benign bladder neck obstruction, known hypersensitivity to chlordiazepoxide HCl and/or clidinium bromide.

WARNINGS/PRECAUTIONS

Use lowest effective dose in debilitated patients. May impair mental/physical abilities. Caution with renal/hepatic impairment and in elderly. Chlordiazepoxide: Increased risk of congenital malformations during 1st trimester of pregnancy; avoid use. Paradoxical reactions (eg, excitement, stimulation, acute rage) reported in psychiatric patients. Caution in the treatment of anxiety states with evidence of impending depression; suicidal tendencies may be present. Avoid abrupt withdrawal after extended therapy; withdrawal symptoms reported following discontinuation. Clidinium: Inhibition of lactation may occur.

ADVERSE REACTIONS

Drowsiness, ataxia, confusion, skin eruptions, edema, extrapyramidal symptoms, dry mouth, nausea, constipation, altered libido, blood dyscrasias, jaundice, hepatic dysfunction, blurred vision, urinary hesitancy.

DRUG INTERACTIONS

Additive effects with alcohol and other CNS depressants. Coadministration with other psychotropic agents is not recommended; caution with MAOIs and phenothiazines. Constipation has occurred more often when coadministered with other spasmolytic agents. Chlordiazepoxide: Altered coagulation effects reported with oral anticoagulants.

PATIENT CONSIDERATIONS

Assessment: Assess for glaucoma, prostatic hypertrophy, benign bladder neck obstruction, anxiety, renal/hepatic dysfunction, alcohol intake, history of drug abuse, drug hypersensitivity, pregnancy/nursing status, and possible drug interactions.

Monitoring: Monitor for ataxia, oversedation, drowsiness, confusion, and other adverse reactions. Monitor for paradoxical reactions (eg, excitement, stimulation, acute rage) in psychiatric patients. Periodic blood counts and LFTs are advisable when treatment is protracted. Monitor for signs of impending depression, or any suicidal tendencies.

Counseling: Inform that psychological and physical dependence may develop, and advise to consult physician before increasing dose or discontinuing abruptly. Advise to observe caution when performing hazardous tasks (eg, operating machinery/driving). Advise to notify physician if pregnant/breastfeeding or planning to become pregnant. Inform of potential additive effects with alcohol and other CNS depressants.

STORAGE: 25°C (77°F); excursions permitted to 15-30°C (59-86°F).

LIDODERM PATCH – lidocaine

RX

Class: Acetamide local anesthetic

ADULT DOSAGE

Postherpetic Neuralgia

Relief of Pain:

Apply to intact skin to cover the most painful area

Apply up to 3 patches, only once for up to 12 hrs w/in 24-hr period

PEDIATRIC DOSAGE

Pediatric use may not have been established

DOSING CONSIDERATIONS

Concomitant Medications

Consider total amount absorbed from all formulations when used concomitantly w/ other local anesthetics

Adverse Reactions

Remove patch if irritation or burning occurs; may reapply when irritation subsides

Other Important Considerations
Debilitated/Impaired Elimination:
Treat smaller areas

ADMINISTRATION

Transdermal route

May cut patches into smaller sizes before removal of the release liner
Avoid contact with water (eg, bathing, swimming, or showering)
Wash hands after handling and avoid eye contact
Apply immediately after removal from protective envelope
May wear clothing over the area of application
Fold used patches and discard patches or pieces of patches

HOW SUPPLIED

Patch: 5% [30[s]]

CONTRAINDICATIONS

Known history of sensitivity to local anesthetics of the amide type, or to any other component of the product.

WARNINGS/PRECAUTIONS

Serious adverse events may occur in children or pets if ingested; keep out of reach. Excessive dosing by applying to larger areas or for longer than the recommended wearing time may result in serious adverse effects. Increased risk of toxicity in patients with severe hepatic disease. Caution with history of drug sensitivities, smaller patients, and patients with impaired elimination. Avoid broken or inflamed skin, placement of external heat (eg, heating pads, electric blankets) and eye contact.

ADVERSE REACTIONS

Application-site reactions (eg, erythema, edema, bruising, papules, vesicles, discoloration, depigmentation, burning sensation, pruritus, dermatitis, petechia, blisters, exfoliation, abnormal sensation).

DRUG INTERACTIONS

Additive toxic effects with concomitant Class I antiarrhythmics (eg, tocainide, mexiletine); use caution. Consider total amount absorbed from all formulations containing other local anesthetics.

PATIENT CONSIDERATIONS

Assessment: Assess for history of drug sensitivities to local anesthetics of the amide type and para-aminobenzoic acid derivatives, hepatic disease, pregnancy/nursing status, and for possible drug interactions.

Monitoring: Monitor for local skin reactions, allergic/anaphylactoid reactions, liver function, pain intensity, pain relief (periodically), and other adverse reactions.

Counseling: Instruct to remove patch if irritation or burning sensation occurs during application and not to reapply until irritation subsides. If eye contact occurs, instruct to immediately wash with water or saline and protect eye until sensation returns. Counsel to avoid application to larger areas and for longer than recommended wearing time. Advise to avoid applying to broken or inflamed skin. Instruct to wash hands after handling patch and to fold used patches so adhesive side sticks to itself. Instruct to keep out of reach of children and pets.

STORAGE: Store at 25°C (77°F); excursions permitted to 15-30°C (59-86°F).

LINZESS – linaclotide

RX

Class: Guanylate cyclase-C (GC-C) agonist

Contraindicated in pediatric patients up to 6 yrs of age. Avoid use in pediatric patients 6-17 yrs of age; safety and efficacy has not been established in pediatric patients <18 yrs of age.

ADULT DOSAGE

Irritable Bowel Syndrome with Constipation

290mcg qd

Chronic Idiopathic Constipation

145mcg qd

PEDIATRIC DOSAGE

Pediatric use may not have been established

ADMINISTRATION

Oral route

Take PO on an empty stomach, at least 30 min prior to 1st meal of the day.
Swallow cap whole; do not crush or chew cap or contents.
For adult patients with swallowing difficulties, administer in applesauce or water.

Administration in Applesauce:
Place one tsp of applesauce at room temperature into a clean container.
Open cap and sprinkle entire contents in applesauce.
Consume entire contents immediately; do not chew beads.
Do not store the applesauce and beads for later use.

Administration in Water:
Pour approx 30mL of bottled water at room temperature into a clean cup.
Open cap and sprinkle entire contents into water.
Gently swirl beads and water for at least 10 sec.
Swallow entire mixture of beads and water immediately.
Add another 30mL of water to any beads remaining in cup, swirl for 10 sec, and swallow immediately.
It is not necessary to consume all beads to deliver complete dose.
Do not store the bead-water mixture for future use.

NG or Gastric Feeding Tube:
Draw-up the beads and water mixture to an appropriately sized catheter-tipped syringe and apply rapid and steady pressure (10mL/10 sec) to dispense the syringe contents into the tube.
After administering the bead-water mixture, flush NG/gastric tube with a min of 10mL of water.
It is not necessary to flush all the beads through to deliver the complete dose.

HOW SUPPLIED
Cap: 145mcg, 290mcg

CONTRAINDICATIONS
Pediatric patients <6 yrs of age, known or suspected mechanical GI obstruction.

WARNINGS/PRECAUTIONS
Diarrhea commonly reported; consider dose suspension and rehydration if severe diarrhea occurs.

ADVERSE REACTIONS
Diarrhea, abdominal pain, flatulence, abdominal distension, viral gastroenteritis, headache, URTI, sinusitis.

PATIENT CONSIDERATIONS
Assessment: Assess for known or suspected mechanical GI obstruction and pregnancy/nursing status.

Monitoring: Monitor for diarrhea and other adverse reactions.

Counseling: Advise to seek medical attention if experiencing unusual or severe abdominal pain and/or severe diarrhea, especially if in combination w/ hematochezia or melena; instruct to d/c treatment and contact physician if severe diarrhea occurs. Instruct to skip dose if the dose is missed, and take next dose at the regular time; advise not to take 2 doses at the same time.

STORAGE: 25°C (77°F); excursions permitted between 15-30°C (59-86°F). Keep caps in the original container. Do not subdivide or repackage. Protect from moisture. Do not remove desiccant from the container.

LIPITOR – atorvastatin calcium

RX

Class: HMG-CoA reductase inhibitor (statin)

ADULT DOSAGE
Hyperlipidemia/Mixed Dyslipidemia

Initial: 10mg or 20mg qd (or 40mg qd for LDL reduction >45%)
Range: 10-80mg qd

After initiation and/or upon titration, analyze lipid levels w/in 2-4 weeks and adjust dose accordingly

Homozygous Familial Hypercholesterolemia

10-80mg qd

Prevention of Cardiovascular Disease

Dose based on current clinical practice

PEDIATRIC DOSAGE
Heterozygous Familial Hypercholesterolemia

10-17 Years (Boys and Postmenarchal Girls):
Initial: 10mg/day
Titrate: Adjust dose at intervals of ≥4 weeks
Max: 20mg/day

DOSING CONSIDERATIONS
Concomitant Medications

Cyclosporine/Tipranavir plus Ritonavir/Telaprevir:
Avoid use

Lopinavir plus Ritonavir:
Use lowest dose necessary

Clarithromycin/Itraconazole/Fosamprenavir/Ritonavir plus Saquinavir, Darunavir, or Fosamprenavir:
Limit to 20mg/day; use lowest dose necessary

Nelfinavir or Boceprevir:
Limit to 40mg/day; use lowest dose necessary

ADMINISTRATION

Oral route

Take as a single dose at any time of the day, w/ or w/o food.

HOW SUPPLIED

Tab: 10mg, 20mg, 40mg, 80mg

CONTRAINDICATIONS

Active liver disease, which may include unexplained persistent elevations in hepatic transaminase levels; hypersensitivity to any component of this medication; women who are pregnant or may become pregnant; nursing mothers.

WARNINGS/PRECAUTIONS

Has not been studied in conditions where the major lipoprotein abnormality is elevation of chylomicrons (Fredrickson Types I and V). Rare cases of rhabdomyolysis w/ acute renal failure secondary to myoglobinuria reported. Increased risk of rhabdomyolysis w/ history of renal impairment; closely monitor for skeletal muscle effects. May cause myopathy (including immune-mediated necrotizing myopathy [IMNM]); d/c if markedly elevated CPK levels occur or if myopathy is diagnosed or suspected. Temporarily withhold or d/c in any patient w/ an acute, serious condition suggestive of myopathy or having a risk factor predisposing to development of renal failure secondary to rhabdomyolysis. Persistent increases in serum transaminases reported. Fatal and nonfatal hepatic failure reported (rare); promptly interrupt therapy if serious liver injury w/ clinical symptoms and/or hyperbilirubinemia or jaundice occurs and do not restart if no alternate etiology found. Caution in patients who consume substantial quantities of alcohol and/or have history of liver disease. Increases in HbA1c and FPG levels reported. May blunt adrenal and/or gonadal steroid production. Increased risk of hemorrhagic stroke in patients w/ recent stroke or transient ischemic attack (TIA). Caution in elderly.

ADVERSE REACTIONS

Nasopharyngitis, arthralgia, diarrhea, pain in extremity, UTI, dyspepsia, nausea, musculoskeletal pain, muscle spasms, myalgia, insomnia.

DRUG INTERACTIONS

See Dosing Considerations. Avoid w/ gemfibrozil. Caution w/ fibrates and drugs that decrease levels or activity of endogenous steroid hormones (eg, ketoconazole, spironolactone, cimetidine). Increased risk of myopathy w/ fibric acid derivatives, erythromycin, lipid-modifying doses of niacin, strong CYP3A4 inhibitors (eg, clarithromycin, HIV protease inhibitors), and azole antifungals; consider lower initial and maintenance doses. Strong CYP3A4 inhibitors and grapefruit juice may increase levels. CYP3A4 inducers (eg, efavirenz, rifampin) may decrease levels. Delayed atorvastatin administration after rifampin administration associated w/ a significant reduction in atorvastatin levels; simultaneous coadministration w/ rifampin is recommended. May increase digoxin levels; monitor appropriately. May increase exposure for norethindrone and ethinyl estradiol; consider such increases when selecting an oral contraceptive for a woman taking atorvastatin. Myopathy, including rhabdomyolysis, reported w/ colchicine; use w/ caution. OATP1B1 inhibitors (eg, cyclosporine) may increase bioavailability.

PATIENT CONSIDERATIONS

Assessment: Assess for active or history of liver disease, unexplained and persistent elevations in serum transaminase levels, pregnancy/nursing status, history of renal impairment, risk factors predisposing to the development of renal failure secondary to rhabdomyolysis, alcohol intake, recent stroke or TIA, hypersensitivity to the drug, and possible drug interactions. Obtain baseline LFTs.

Monitoring: Monitor for signs/symptoms of rhabdomyolysis and myopathy (including IMNM). Monitor lipid profile and CPK levels. Perform LFTs as clinically indicated.

Counseling: Advise to adhere to the National Cholesterol Education Program-recommended diet, a regular exercise program, and periodic testing of a fasting lipid panel. Inform of the substances that should not be taken concomitantly w/ the drug. Advise to inform other healthcare professionals that they are taking the drug. Inform of the risk of myopathy; instruct to report promptly any unexplained muscle pain, tenderness, or weakness, particularly if accompanied by malaise or fever or if these muscle signs or symptoms persist after discontinuation. Inform that liver function will be checked prior to initiation and if signs or symptoms of liver injury occur; instruct to report promptly any symptoms that may indicate liver injury. Instruct women of childbearing age to use effective method of birth control to prevent pregnancy. Advise to d/c therapy and contact physician if pregnancy occurs. Instruct not to use the drug if breastfeeding.

STORAGE: 20-25°C (68-77°F).

Lithium 450mg ER Tablets – lithium carbonate

RX

Class: Antimanic agent

Lithium toxicity is closely related to serum levels, and can occur at doses close to therapeutic levels. Facilities for prompt and accurate serum lithium determinations should be available before initiating therapy.

ADULT DOSAGE

Manic-Depressive Illness

Individualize dose according to serum levels and clinical response

Acute Mania:
1800mg/day in divided doses to achieve desired serum levels of 1-1.5mEq/L

Monitor serum levels 2X/week, and until serum level and clinical condition have been stabilized

Long-Term Control:
Usual: 900-1200mg/day in divided doses to maintain desirable serum levels of 0.6-1.2mEq/L

Monitor serum lithium levels in uncomplicated cases at least every 2 months

Patients unusually sensitive to lithium may exhibit toxic signs at serum levels <1mEq/L

Conversions

Switching from Immediate-Release (IR) Caps to Extended-Release (ER) Tabs:
Give the same total daily dose when possible

When previous dosage of IR lithium is not a multiple of 450mg (eg, 1500mg), initiate ER tab at the multiple of 450mg nearest to, but below, the original daily dose (eg, 1350mg)

When the 2 doses are unequal, give larger dose in pm (eg, 1350mg/day [450mg am and 900mg pm]); if desired, give total daily dose tid (eg, 1350mg/day [450mg tid])

Monitor at 1- to 2-week intervals and adjust dose if necessary, until stable and satisfactory serum levels and clinical state achieved

When closer titration is required than that available w/ doses of ER tabs in increments of 450mg, use IR caps

Most patients on maint therapy are stabilized on 900mg daily (eg, 450mg bid ER tab)

PEDIATRIC DOSAGE

Manic-Depressive Illness

≥12 Years:
Individualize dose according to serum levels and clinical response

Acute Mania:
1800mg/day in divided doses to achieve desired serum levels of 1-1.5mEq/L

Monitor serum levels 2X/week, and until serum level and clinical condition have been stabilized

Long-Term Control:
Usual: 900-1200mg/day in divided doses to maintain desirable serum levels of 0.6-1.2mEq/L

Monitor serum lithium levels in uncomplicated cases at least every 2 months

Patients unusually sensitive to lithium may exhibit toxic signs at serum levels <1mEq/L

Conversions

Switching from Immediate-Release (IR) Caps to Extended-Release (ER) Tabs:
Give the same total daily dose when possible

When previous dosage of IR lithium is not a multiple of 450mg (eg, 1500mg), initiate ER tab at the multiple of 450mg nearest to, but below, the original daily dose (eg, 1350mg)

When the 2 doses are unequal, give larger dose in pm (eg, 1350mg/day [450mg am and 900mg pm]); if desired, give total daily dose tid (eg, 1350mg/day [450mg tid])

Monitor at 1- to 2-week intervals and adjust dose if necessary, until stable and satisfactory serum levels and clinical state achieved

When closer titration is required than that available w/ doses of ER tabs in increments of 450mg, use IR caps

Most patients on maint therapy are stabilized on 900mg daily (eg, 450mg bid ER tab)

DOSING CONSIDERATIONS

Elderly
May require lower dosages to achieve therapeutic serum levels

ADMINISTRATION

Oral route

Doses are usually given bid (approx 12-hr intervals)

HOW SUPPLIED

Tab, Extended-Release: 450mg* *scored

WARNINGS/PRECAUTIONS

Avoid w/ significant renal or cardiovascular disease (CVD), severe debilitation/dehydration, or Na^+ depletion. Use extreme caution if psychiatric indication is life-threatening, and if such patient fails to respond to other measures. May be associated w/ the unmasking of Brugada syndrome; avoid w/ known or suspected Brugada syndrome. Chronic therapy may be associated w/ diminution of renal concentrating ability; carefully manage to avoid dehydration w/ resulting lithium retention and toxicity. Morphologic changes w/ glomerular and interstitial fibrosis and nephron atrophy reported.

L

Assess kidney function prior to and during therapy. May decrease Na+ reabsorption, which could lead to Na+ depletion; maintain normal diet, including salt, and an adequate fluid intake at least during the initial stabilization period. Decreased tolerance reported to ensue from protracted sweating or diarrhea; if this occurs, administer supplemental fluid and salt. Temporarily reduce dose or d/c therapy w/ sweating, diarrhea, or concomitant infection w/ elevated temperature. Caution w/ thyroid disorders; monitor thyroid function. May impair mental/physical abilities.

ADVERSE REACTIONS

Fine hand tremor, polyuria, mild thirst, general discomfort, diarrhea, N/V, drowsiness, lithium toxicity, blackout spells, ataxia, dry mouth, alopecia, oliguria, albuminuria.

DRUG INTERACTIONS

Encephalopathic syndrome (eg, weakness, lethargy, fever) followed by irreversible brain damage w/ neuroleptics reported; monitor for evidence of neurological toxicity and d/c therapy if such signs appear. May prolong effects of neuromuscular blockers; use w/ caution. Caution w/ diuretics; monitor lithium levels and adjust lithium dose if necessary. Caution w/ calcium channel blockers; may increase risk of neurotoxicity. Increased levels w/ indomethacin, piroxicam, and other NSAIDs (eg, selective COX-2 inhibitors); monitor levels closely when initiating or discontinuing NSAID use. Acetazolamide, urea, xanthine preparations, and alkalinizing agents (eg, sodium bicarbonate) may decrease levels. May provoke lithium toxicity w/ metronidazole; monitor closely. Risk of lithium toxicity w/ ACE inhibitors (eg, enalapril, captopril) and angiotensin II receptor antagonists (eg, losartan); may need to reduce lithium dose and monitor lithium levels more often. Caution w/ SSRIs. May interact w/ methyldopa, phenytoin, and carbamazepine.

PATIENT CONSIDERATIONS

Assessment: Assess for CVD, severe debilitation, dehydration, Na^+ depletion, life-threatening psychiatric indication, thyroid disorders, Brugada syndrome or risk factors, pregnancy/nursing status, and for possible drug interactions. Assess baseline renal function (eg, tubular function, glomerular function).

Monitoring: Monitor for diminution of renal concentrating ability (eg, nephrogenic diabetes insipidus), glomerular and interstitial fibrosis, nephron atrophy, decreased tolerance to therapy, decreased Na^+ reabsorption, signs of lithium toxicity, and other adverse reactions. Monitor for renal or thyroid function. Monitor patient's clinical state and serum lithium levels regularly.

Counseling: Inform of the risks and benefits of therapy. Counsel about clinical signs of lithium toxicity (eg, diarrhea, vomiting, tremor); advise to d/c therapy and notify physician if any of these signs occur. Advise to seek immediate emergency assistance if fainting, lightheadedness, abnormal heartbeats, SOB, or other adverse reactions develop. Advise to use caution w/ activities requiring alertness.

STORAGE: 25°C (77°F); excursions permitted to 15-30°C (59-86°F).

L

LIVALO – pitavastatin

RX

Class: HMG-CoA reductase inhibitor (statin)

ADULT DOSAGE

Primary Hypercholesterolemia/Mixed Dyslipidemia

Initial: 2mg qd
Range: 1-4mg qd
Max: 4mg qd

After initiation or upon titration, analyze lipid levels after 4 weeks and adjust dose accordingly

PEDIATRIC DOSAGE

Pediatric use may not have been established

DOSING CONSIDERATIONS

Concomitant Medications

Erythromycin:
Max: 1mg qd

Rifampin:
Max: 2mg qd

Renal Impairment

Moderate/Severe (GFR 30-59mL/min/1.73m² and GFR 15-29mL/min/1.73m² Not Receiving Hemodialysis, Respectively)/ESRD Receiving Hemodialysis:
Initial: 1mg qd
Max: 2mg qd

ADMINISTRATION

Oral route

Take PO at any time of the day w/ or w/o food

HOW SUPPLIED

Tab: 1mg, 2mg, 4mg

CONTRAINDICATIONS

Active liver disease, including unexplained persistent elevations of hepatic transaminase levels, women who are pregnant or may become pregnant, nursing mothers, and coadministration with cyclosporine. Known hypersensitivity to any component of this product.

WARNINGS/PRECAUTIONS

Increased risk for severe myopathy with doses >4mg qd. Myopathy (including immune-mediated necrotizing myopathy [IMNM]) and rhabdomyolysis with acute renal failure secondary to myoglobinuria reported. Caution with predisposing factors for myopathy (eg, advanced age [≥65 yrs], renal impairment, and inadequately treated hypothyroidism). D/C if markedly elevated creatine kinase (CK) levels occur or myopathy is diagnosed/suspected and temporarily withhold in any patient experiencing an acute or serious condition suggestive of myopathy or predisposing to the development of renal failure secondary to rhabdomyolysis (eg, sepsis, hypotension, dehydration). Increases in serum transaminases (eg, AST, ALT) reported; perform LFTs before the initiation of treatment and if signs or symptoms of liver injury occur. Fatal and nonfatal hepatic failure reported (rare); promptly interrupt therapy if serious liver injury with clinical symptoms and/or hyperbilirubinemia or jaundice occurs; do not restart if no alternative etiology found. Increases in HbA1c and fasting serum glucose levels reported. Caution with substantial alcohol consumption.

ADVERSE REACTIONS

Back pain, constipation, myalgia.

DRUG INTERACTIONS

See Contraindications. Erythromycin and rifampin may increase exposure. Due to an increased risk of myopathy/rhabdomyolysis, avoid coadministration with gemfibrozil and use caution when coadministered with fibrates and colchicine. May enhance risk of skeletal muscle effects with niacin; consider dose reduction with lipid-modifying doses of niacin. Monitor PT and INR with warfarin.

L

PATIENT CONSIDERATIONS

Assessment: Assess for hepatic/renal impairment, inadequately treated hypothyroidism, substantial alcohol consumption, pregnancy/nursing status, possible drug interactions, and other conditions where treatment is cautioned/contraindicated. Obtain baseline lipid profile.

Monitoring: Monitor signs/symptoms of myopathy, rhabdomyolysis, IMNM, acute renal failure, hypersensitivity reactions, and other adverse reactions. Monitor for increases in HbA1c and fasting serum glucose levels. Perform periodic monitoring of lipid profile and CK levels. Analyze lipid levels 4 weeks after initiation/titration. Perform LFTs with signs or symptoms of liver injury. Monitor PT and INR when using warfarin.

Counseling: Advise to promptly notify physician of any unexplained muscle pain, tenderness, or weakness, particularly if accompanied by malaise or fever, or if these muscle signs/symptoms persist after discontinuing treatment. Advise to discuss all medications, both prescription and OTC, with physician. Counsel women of childbearing age to use effective method of birth control to prevent pregnancy during therapy. Instruct pregnant or breastfeeding women to d/c therapy and consult physician. Inform that liver enzymes will be checked before therapy and if signs/symptoms of liver injury occur (eg, fatigue, anorexia, right upper abdominal discomfort, dark urine, or jaundice). Advise to report promptly any symptoms that may indicate liver injury.

STORAGE: 15-30°C (59-86°F). Protect from light.

Lo/Ovral-28 – ethinyl estradiol/norgestrel

RX

Class: Estrogen/progestogen combination

Cigarette smoking increases the risk of serious cardiovascular side effects. Risk increases with age (>35 yrs of age) and extent of smoking (≥15 cigarettes/day). Women who use oral contraceptives should be strongly advised not to smoke.

OTHER BRAND NAMES

Low-Ogestrel, Cryselle

ADULT DOSAGE

Contraception

1 tab qd at the same time each day for 28 days, then repeat

Start 1st Sunday after menses begin or on 1st day of menses

PEDIATRIC DOSAGE

Contraception

Not indicated for use premenarche; refer to adult dosing

Conversions

Lo/Ovral:

Switching from 21-Day Regimen:
Wait 7 days after last tab before starting therapy

Switching from 28-Day Regimen:
Start therapy on the day after her last tab; do not wait any days between packs

Switching from Progestin-Only Pill:
Start therapy next day; use a nonhormonal backup method of birth control for first 7 days of therapy

Switching from an Implant or Inj:
Start therapy on the day of implant removal or day the next inj is due; use a nonhormonal backup method of birth control for first 7 days of therapy

Missed Dose

Cryselle:
If ≥2 white tabs are missed, another method of contraception should be used until a white tab is taken for 7 consecutive days
If ≥1 light-green tabs are missed, no other method of contraception is needed

DOSING CONSIDERATIONS

Other Important Considerations

Lo/Ovral:
Postpartum Women Who Do Not Breastfeed/After 2nd Trimester Abortion: Start therapy no earlier than 28 days postpartum; advise to use a nonhormonal backup method for the first 7 days of therapy
1st Trimester Abortion/Miscarriage: May be initiated immediately; backup contraception is not needed if therapy started immediately

Cryselle:
Nonlactating Mother: May initiate postpartum

Lo-Ogestrel:
Postpartum Women After Full-Term Delivery: Do not initiate earlier than 4-6 weeks postpartum
Termination of Pregnancy in the First 12 Weeks: Start therapy immediately or w/in 7 days
Termination of Pregnancy After 12 Weeks: Start therapy after 2 weeks

ADMINISTRATION

Oral route

Take dose at intervals not exceeding 24 hrs
Cryselle: Take preferably after pm meal or at hs

HOW SUPPLIED

Tab: (Ethinyl Estradiol [EE]/Norgestrel) 0.03mg/0.3mg

CONTRAINDICATIONS

Thrombophlebitis, thromboembolic disorders, history of deep vein thrombophlebitis/thromboembolic disorders, cerebrovascular disease or coronary artery disease (CAD), known or suspected carcinoma of the breast, carcinoma of the endometrium or other known or suspected estrogen-dependent neoplasia, undiagnosed abnormal genital bleeding, cholestatic jaundice of pregnancy or jaundice with prior pill use, known or suspected pregnancy, hepatic adenomas or carcinomas or (Low-Ogestrel) benign liver tumors. (Lo/Ovral) Past history of cerebrovascular disease or CAD, active liver disease, valvular heart disease with thrombogenic complications, thrombogenic rhythm disorders, hereditary or acquired thrombophilias, major surgery with prolonged immobilization, diabetes with vascular involvement, headaches with focal neurological symptoms, uncontrolled HTN, personal history of breast cancer, hypersensitivity to any of the components of the product.

WARNINGS/PRECAUTIONS

Increased risk of myocardial infarction (MI), vascular disease, thromboembolism, stroke, hepatic neoplasia, and gallbladder disease. Increased risk of morbidity and mortality if other risk factors (eg, certain inherited or acquired thrombophilia, HTN, hyperlipidemia, obesity, diabetes) are present. If feasible, d/c at least 4 weeks prior to and for 2 weeks after elective surgery of a type associated with an increased risk of thromboembolism and during and following prolonged immobilization. Start use no earlier than 4-6 weeks after delivery in women who elect not to breastfeed, or a midtrimester pregnancy termination. May increase risk of breast cancer and cancer of the reproductive organs. Retinal thrombosis reported; d/c if there is unexplained partial or complete loss of vision; onset of proptosis or diplopia; papilledema; or if retinal vascular lesions develop. Contact lens wearers who develop visual changes or changes in lens tolerance should be assessed by an ophthalmologist. Should not be used to induce withdrawal bleeding as a test for pregnancy, nor to treat threatened or habitual abortion during pregnancy. Rule out pregnancy if 2 consecutive periods are missed. May cause glucose intolerance; monitor prediabetic and diabetic patients. May elevate serum TG and LDL levels and may render the control of hyperlipidemias more difficult. Elevations of plasma TGs may lead to pancreatitis and other complications. May elevate BP; monitor closely and d/c use if significant BP elevation occurs. New onset/exacerbation of migraine or recurrent, persistent, severe headache may develop; d/c and evaluate the cause if this occurs. Women with migraine may be at increased risk of stroke. Breakthrough bleeding and spotting reported; rule out malignancy or pregnancy. Post-pill amenorrhea or oligomenorrhea may occur. D/C if jaundice develops. May cause fluid retention. Caution with history of depression; d/c if depression recurs to serious degree. Diarrhea and/or vomiting may reduce hormone absorption. May affect certain endocrine function tests, LFTs, and blood components in lab tests. (Lo/Ovral) Ectopic and intrauterine pregnancy may occur in contraceptive failures. If using Sunday Start method, during the first cycle, contraceptive reliance should not be placed on therapy until a white tab has been taken daily for 7 consecutive days. (Low-Ogestrel) Use an additional method of protection until after the first 7 days of administration in the initial cycle. (Cryselle) During the first cycle, contraceptive reliance should not be placed on therapy until a white tab has been taken daily for 7 consecutive days.

ADVERSE REACTIONS

N/V, breakthrough bleeding, spotting, amenorrhea, migraine, depression, vaginal candidiasis, edema, weight changes, change in cervical erosion and secretion, menstrual flow changes, GI symptoms (eg, abdominal pain, cramps, bloating), rash (allergic).

DRUG INTERACTIONS

(Lo/Ovral) Reduced effects resulting in pregnancy or breakthrough bleeding may occur with antibiotics, anticonvulsants, and other drugs that increase the metabolism of contraceptive steroids (eg, rifabutin, primidone, dexamethasone, modafinil); consider back up nonhormonal method of birth control. Significant changes (increase or decrease) in estrogen and progestin levels noted in some cases with anti-HIV protease inhibitors. Herbal products containing St. John's wort may induce hepatic enzymes (cytochrome P450) and p-glycoprotein transporter and may reduce the effectiveness of contraceptive steroids, and may also result in breakthrough bleeding. Atorvastatin increases EE exposure; ascorbic acid and acetaminophen (APAP) increases EE bioavailability. CYP3A4 inhibitors (eg, indinavir, itraconazole, ketoconazole) increase levels. Troleandomycin may increase risk of intrahepatic cholestasis. Increased plasma concentrations of cyclosporine, prednisolone and other corticosteroids, and theophylline. Decreased plasma concentrations of APAP. Increased clearance of temazepam, salicylic acid, morphine, and clofibric acid. (Cryselle/Low-Ogestrel) Reduced efficacy and increased incidence of breakthrough bleeding and menstrual irregularities with rifampin, barbiturates, phenylbutazone, phenytoin sodium, and possibly with griseofulvin, ampicillin, and tetracyclines.

PATIENT CONSIDERATIONS

Assessment: Assess for hypersensitivity to drug, breast cancer, estrogen-dependent neoplasia, abnormal genital bleeding, thrombophlebitis, thromboembolic disorders, past history of deep vein thrombophlebitis or thromboembolic disorders, cerebrovascular disease or CAD, known/suspected pregnancy, or any other conditions where treatment is cautioned/contraindicated. Assess nursing status and for possible drug interactions.

Monitoring: Monitor for MI, stroke, hepatic neoplasia, bleeding irregularities, thromboembolism, onset or exacerbation of headaches or migraines, and other adverse reactions. Monitor serum glucose levels in diabetic and prediabetic patients, BP with history of HTN, lipid levels with history of hyperlipidemia, and for signs of worsening depression with previous history of the disorder. Monitor liver function. Monitor women with strong family history of breast cancer or with breast nodules. Refer contact lens wearers to an ophthalmologist if visual changes develop. Perform periodic medical history and physical exam.

Counseling: Inform of the benefits and risks of therapy. Inform that drug does not protect against HIV infection (AIDS) and other sexually transmitted diseases. Advise to avoid smoking. Instruct to take exactly ud at intervals not exceeding 24 hrs. Advise about risks of pregnancy if dose is missed. Instruct that if one dose is missed, to take as soon as possible and take next pill at regular scheduled time. Inform that spotting, light bleeding, or nausea may occur during the first 1-3 packs of pills; advise not to d/c medication and if symptoms persist, to notify physician. Instruct to d/c if pregnancy is confirmed/suspected. Inform that certain drugs may make therapy less effective and the possible need to use additional contraception. Instruct to notify physician if breastfeeding. If scheduled for any lab test, advise patient to inform physician that taking birth control pills.

STORAGE: 20-25°C (68-77°F). (Low-Ogestrel) 15-25°C (59-77°F).

LOESTRIN 21 – ethinyl estradiol/norethindrone acetate

RX

Class: Estrogen/progestogen combination

Cigarette smoking increases the risk of serious cardiovascular (CV) side effects. Risk increases w/ age and w/ heavy smoking (≥15 cigarettes/day) and is quite marked in women >35 yrs of age. Women who use oral contraceptives are strongly advised not to smoke.

OTHER BRAND NAMES

Junel 1.5/30, Gildess 1/20, Junel 1/20, Microgestin 1.5/30, Gildess 1.5/30, Microgestin 1/20, Loestrin 21 1.5/30, Loestrin 21 1/20

ADULT DOSAGE

Contraception

1 tab qd for 21 days, stop for 7 days, and then repeat

Start 1st Sunday after menses begin or 1st day of menses

Missed Dose

Miss 1 Tab: Take as soon as dose is remembered; take next tab at regular time

Miss 2 Consecutive Tabs in Week 1 or 2: Take 2 tabs as soon as remembered and 2 tabs the next day; use another birth control method for 7 days following the missed tabs

Miss 2 Consecutive Tabs in Week 3 or Miss ≥3 Consecutive Tabs: (Sunday Start) Take 1 tab qd until Sunday, then discard remaining tabs and start a new pack of tabs immediately on Sunday. (Day 1 Start) Throw out rest of the pack and start new pack that same day. (Sunday/Day 1 Start) Use another birth control method for 7 days following missed tabs

PEDIATRIC DOSAGE

Contraception

Not indicated for use premenarche; refer to adult dosing

ADMINISTRATION

Oral route

Take regularly w/ a meal or hs

Take exactly ud and at intervals not exceeding 24 hrs

Use an additional method of protection until after the 1st week of administration in the initial cycle when utilizing the Sunday Start regimen

HOW SUPPLIED

Tab: (Norethindrone-Ethinyl Estradiol [EE]) (1/20) 1mg-0.02mg, (1.5/30) 1.5mg-0.03mg

CONTRAINDICATIONS

Thrombophlebitis, thromboembolic disorders, past history of deep vein thrombophlebitis or thromboembolic disorders, cerebral vascular or coronary artery disease, known or suspected carcinoma of the breast, carcinoma of the endometrium or other known or suspected estrogen-dependent neoplasia, undiagnosed abnormal genital bleeding, cholestatic jaundice of pregnancy or jaundice w/ prior pill use, hepatic adenomas or carcinomas, known/suspected pregnancy.

WARNINGS/PRECAUTIONS

Increased risk of MI, thromboembolism, stroke, hepatic neoplasia, gallbladder disease, and vascular disease. If feasible, d/c at least 4 weeks prior to and for 2 weeks after elective surgery of a type associated w/ an increased risk of thromboembolism, and during and following prolonged immobilization. Start use no earlier than 4-6 weeks after delivery in women who elect not to breastfeed. May increase risk of breast cancer and increase the risk of cervical intraepithelial neoplasia. Retinal thrombosis reported; d/c if unexplained partial or complete loss of vision occurs, or if onset of proptosis or diplopia, papilledema, or retinal vascular lesions develop. Rule out pregnancy before continuing therapy in any patient who has missed 2 consecutive periods; consider possibility of pregnancy at the first missed period if patient has not adhered to the prescribed dosing schedule. May cause glucose intolerance; monitor prediabetic and diabetic patients. May elevate serum TG and LDL levels and may render the control of hyperlipidemias more difficult. May cause increased BP and fluid retention; monitor closely and d/c use if significant BP elevation occurs. D/C and evaluate the cause if onset/exacerbation of a migraine or development of a headache w/ a new pattern which is recurrent, persistent, or severe develops. Breakthrough bleeding and spotting reported; rule out malignancy or pregnancy. Post-pill amenorrhea or oligomenorrhea may occur. D/C if jaundice develops. Carefully observe women w/ history of depression; d/c if depression recurs to a serious degree. Contact lens wearers who develop visual changes or changes in lens tolerance should be assessed by an ophthalmologist. May affect certain endocrine function tests, LFTs, and blood components in lab tests.

ADVERSE REACTIONS

N/V, GI symptoms, breakthrough bleeding, spotting, amenorrhea, migraine, mental depression, vaginal candidiasis, edema, weight changes, menstrual flow changes, melasma, breast changes, changes in cervical erosion and secretion, rash (allergic).

DRUG INTERACTIONS

Reduced effects, increased breakthrough bleeding, and menstrual irregularities w/ rifampin. Increased metabolism and possibly reduced contraceptive effectiveness w/ anticonvulsants (eg, phenobarbital, phenytoin, carbamazepine). Reduced plasma levels w/ troglitazone, resulting in possible reduced contraceptive effectiveness. Pregnancy reported w/ antimicrobials (eg, ampicillin, tetracycline, griseofulvin). Atorvastatin may increase norethindrone and EE exposure. Ascorbic acid and acetaminophen (APAP) may increase EE levels. Increased plasma levels of cyclosporine, prednisolone, and theophylline reported w/ concomitant use. Decreased levels of APAP and increased clearance of temazepam, salicylic acid, morphine, and clofibric acid reported w/ concomitant use. A reduction in contraceptive effectiveness and increased incidence of breakthrough bleeding may occur w/ phenylbutazone.

PATIENT CONSIDERATIONS

Assessment: Assess for hypersensitivity to drug, thrombophlebitis or thromboembolic disorders, HTN, hyperlipidemia, diabetes, breast cancer, endometrial cancer or other estrogen-dependent neoplasia, undiagnosed abnormal genital bleeding, cholestatic jaundice of pregnancy or jaundice w/ prior pill use, pregnancy/nursing status, and for any other conditions where treatment is contraindicated/cautioned. Assess for possible drug interactions.

Monitoring: Monitor for MI, thromboembolism, stroke, hepatic neoplasia, and other adverse effects. Monitor BP w/ history of HTN, serum glucose levels in diabetic or prediabetic patients, lipid levels w/ hyperlipidemia, and for signs of worsening depression w/ previous history. Monitor liver function. Monitor women who have breast nodules or a strong family history of breast cancer. Perform annual history and physical exam including special reference to BP, breasts, abdomen and pelvic organs, including cervical cytology, and relevant laboratory tests.

Counseling: Counsel about potential adverse effects. Inform that drug does not protect against HIV infection (AIDS) and other sexually transmitted diseases. Counsel that cigarette smoking increases the risk of serious CV effects and that women who use oral contraceptives should not smoke. Instruct to take exactly ud and at intervals not exceeding 24 hrs. Instruct on what to do if pills are missed. Instruct to use additional method of protection until after the 1st week of administration in the initial cycle when utilizing the Sunday Start regimen. Inform that spotting or breakthrough bleeding may occur; advise not to d/c medication and instruct to notify physician if symptoms persist. Instruct to d/c if pregnancy is confirmed/suspected during treatment. If scheduled for any lab test, advise to inform physician of use of birth control pills. Instruct to notify physician if breastfeeding. Inform that certain drugs may make therapy less effective and that additional contraception may be needed.

STORAGE: 20-25°C (68-77°F).

LOMOTIL — atropine sulfate/diphenoxylate hydrochloride

CV

Class: Anticholinergic/opioid

ADULT DOSAGE

Diarrhea

Adjunctive Therapy:
Initial: 2 tabs or 10mL qid
Titrate: Reduce dose after symptoms are controlled
Maint: 2 tabs or 10mL qd
Max: 20mg/day diphenoxylate

D/C if symptoms not controlled after 10 days at max dose of 20mg/day (diphenoxylate)

PEDIATRIC DOSAGE

Diarrhea

Adjunctive Therapy:
2-12 Years:
Initial: 0.3-0.4mg/kg/day of sol in four divided doses
Titrate: Reduce dose after symptoms are controlled
Maint: May be as low as 25% of initial dose

D/C if no improvement w/in 48 hrs

ADMINISTRATION

Oral route

Plastic dropper should be used when measuring liquid for administration to children

HOW SUPPLIED

(Diphenoxylate-Atropine) Sol: 2.5mg-0.025mg/5mL [60mL]; **Tab:** 2.5mg-0.025mg

CONTRAINDICATIONS

Known hypersensitivity to diphenoxylate or atropine, obstructive jaundice, diarrhea associated w/ pseudomembranous enterocolitis or enterotoxin-producing bacteria.

WARNINGS/PRECAUTIONS

Avoid in children <2 yrs. Overdosage may result in severe respiratory depression and coma, leading to brain damage or death. Avoid use with severe dehydration or electrolyte imbalance until corrective therapy is initiated. May induce toxic megacolon with acute ulcerative colitis; d/c if abdominal distention occurs or untoward symptoms develop. May cause intestinal fluid retention. Avoid with diarrhea associated with organisms that penetrate the intestinal mucosa, and with pseudomembranous enterocolitis. Extreme caution with advanced hepatorenal disease and liver dysfunction. Caution in pediatrics, especially with Down's syndrome.

ADVERSE REACTIONS

Numbness of extremities, dizziness, anaphylaxis, drowsiness, toxic megacolon, N/V, urticaria, pruritus, anorexia, pancreatitis, paralytic ileus, euphoria, malaise/lethargy.

DRUG INTERACTIONS

MAOIs may precipitate hypertensive crisis. (Diphenoxylate) May potentiate barbiturates, tranquilizers, and alcohol. Potential to prolong $T_{1/2}$ of drugs for which the rate of elimination is dependent on the microsomal drug metabolizing enzyme system.

PATIENT CONSIDERATIONS

Assessment: Assess for hypersensitivity, obstructive jaundice, diarrhea associated with pseudomembranous enterocolitis or enterotoxin-producing bacteria, severe dehydration, electrolyte imbalance, hepatic dysfunction, hepatorenal disease, ulcerative colitis, Down's syndrome, diarrhea (caused by *Escherichia coli*, *Salmonella*, *Shigella*), pregnancy/nursing status, and possible drug interactions.

Monitoring: Monitor for severe dehydration, electrolyte imbalance, renal function, toxic megacolon in ulcerative colitis, abdominal distention, signs of atropinism, and other adverse reactions.

Counseling: Instruct to take ud and not to exceed the recommended dosage. Inform of consequences of overdosage, including severe respiratory depression and coma, possibly leading to permanent brain damage or death. Instruct to exercise caution while operating machinery/driving. Advise to avoid alcohol and other CNS depressants. Advise to keep medicines out of reach of children. Inform patient that drowsiness or dizziness may occur.

L

STORAGE: Dispense liquids in original container.

LONSURF – tipiracil/trifluridine RX

Class: Thymidine phosphorylase inhibitor/nucleoside metabolic inhibitor

ADULT DOSAGE

Metastatic Colorectal Cancer

Treatment of patients who have been previously treated w/ fluoropyrimidine-, oxaliplatin- and irinotecan-based chemotherapy, an anti-VEGF biological therapy, and if RAS wild-type, an anti-EGFR therapy

Initial: 35mg/m²/dose bid on Days 1-5 and Days 8-12 of each 28-day cycle until disease progression or unacceptable toxicity

Max: 80mg/dose (based on the trifluridine component)

Round dose to the nearest 5mg increment

PEDIATRIC DOSAGE

Pediatric use may not have been established

DOSING CONSIDERATIONS

Obtain CBC counts prior to and on Day 15 of each cycle

Do Not Initiate the Cycle Until:

ANC ≥1500/mm³ or febrile neutropenia is resolved

Platelets are ≥75,000/mm³

Grade 3 or 4 nonhematological adverse reactions are resolved to Grade 0 or 1

W/in a Treatment Cycle, Withhold for Any of the Following:

ANC <500/mm³ or febrile neutropenia

Platelets <50,000/mm³

Grade 3 or 4 nonhematological adverse reactions

After Recovery, Resume Therapy After Reducing the Dose by 5mg/m²/dose from the Previous Dose Level, if the Following Occur:

Febrile neutropenia

Uncomplicated Grade 4 neutropenia (which has recovered to ≥1500/mm³) or thrombocytopenia (which has recovered to ≥75,000/mm³) that results in >1 week delay in start of next cycle

Nonhematologic Grade 3 or Grade 4 adverse reaction except for Grade 3 nausea and/or vomiting controlled by antiemetic therapy or Grade 3 diarrhea responsive to antidiarrheal medication

Max of 3 dose reductions are permitted to a minimum dose of 20mg/m^2 bid. Do not escalate dose after it has been reduced.

ADMINISTRATION

Oral route

Take w/in 1 hr of completion of morning and evening meals.

HOW SUPPLIED

Tab: (Trifluridine/Tipiracil) 15mg/6.14mg, 20mg/8.19mg.

WARNINGS/PRECAUTIONS

Severe and life-threatening myelosuppression consisting of anemia, neutropenia, thrombocytopenia, and febrile neutropenia reported; obtain CBC counts prior to and on Day 15 of each cycle of therapy and more frequently as clinically indicated. May cause fetal harm. Females of reproductive potential should use effective contraception during treatment.

ADVERSE REACTIONS

Anemia, neutropenia, asthenia/fatigue, N/V, thrombocytopenia, decreased appetite, diarrhea, abdominal pain, pyrexia.

PATIENT CONSIDERATIONS

Assessment: Assess pregnancy/nursing status. Obtain CBC counts prior to each cycle.

Monitoring: Monitor for adverse reactions. Obtain CBC counts on Day 15 of each cycle and more frequently as clinically indicated.

Counseling: Advise to immediately contact healthcare provider if patients experience signs/symptoms of infection and advise to keep all appointments for blood tests. Advise not to take additional doses to make up for missed or held doses. Instruct to contact healthcare provider for severe or persistent N/V, diarrhea, or abdominal pain. Instruct to take w/in 1 hr after eating am and pm meals. Inform patient that anyone else who handles the medication should wear gloves. Advise pregnant women of the potential risk to the fetus. Instruct females of reproductive potential to use effective contraception during treatment. Instruct males w/ female partners of reproductive potential to use condoms during treatment and for at least 3 months after the final dose. Advise women not to breastfeed during treatment and for 1 day following the final dose.

STORAGE: 20-25°C (68-77°F); excursions permitted to 15-30°C (59-86°F). If stored outside original bottle, discard after 30 days.

LOPERAMIDE HCL – loperamide hydrochloride

RX

Class: Antidiarrheal

ADULT DOSAGE

Diarrhea

Control and symptomatic relief of diarrhea associated w/ inflammatory bowel disease. Also indicated for reducing the volume of discharge from ileostomies

Acute Nonspecific Diarrhea:

Initial: 4mg then 2mg after each unformed stool

Max: 16mg/day

Chronic Diarrhea:

4mg then 2mg after each unformed stool until diarrhea is controlled; reduce dose to meet the individual requirements. When optimal daily dosage has been established, may give as single or divided doses

Maint: 4-8mg. If no clinical improvements after 16mg/day for at least 10 days, symptoms are unlikely to be controlled by further administration

May continue administration if diarrhea cannot be adequately controlled w/ diet or specific treatment

PEDIATRIC DOSAGE

Diarrhea

Control and symptomatic relief of diarrhea associated w/ inflammatory bowel disease. Also indicated for reducing the volume of discharge from ileostomies

Acute Diarrhea:

1st Day Dosage Schedule:

2-5 Years:

13-20kg: Use OTC liquid formulation

6-8 Years:

20-30kg:

Initial: 2mg bid

Max: 4mg/day

8-12 Years:

>30kg:

Initial: 2mg tid

Max: 6mg/day

Subsequent Daily Dosage:

After 1st treatment day, give subsequent doses (1mg/10kg) only after a loose stool

ADMINISTRATION

Oral route

HOW SUPPLIED

Cap: 2mg

CONTRAINDICATIONS

Known hypersensitivity to loperamide HCl or to any of the excipients, abdominal pain in the absence of diarrhea, infants <24 months of age. As primary therapy for acute dysentery (characterized by blood in stool and high fever), acute ulcerative colitis, bacterial enterocolitis caused by invasive organism (including *Salmonella, Shigella, Campylobacter*), pseudomembranous colitis associated with broad-spectrum antibiotics.

WARNINGS/PRECAUTIONS

Use of drug does not preclude the need for appropriate fluid and electrolyte therapy. Do not use when inhibition of peristalsis is to be avoided due to possible risk of significant sequelae, including ileus, megacolon, and toxic megacolon. D/C promptly if constipation, abdominal distention, or ileus develop. Symptomatic treatment only; determine underlying etiology and treat when appropriate/indicated. AIDS patients treated for diarrhea should d/c therapy at earliest signs of abdominal distention; toxic megacolon reported with infectious colitis from viral/bacterial pathogens. Caution in young children; dehydration may influence variability of response to the drug. Extremely rare allergic reactions, including anaphylaxis and anaphylactic shock, reported. In acute diarrhea, d/c therapy if no improvement is observed in 48 hrs. Caution with hepatic impairment; monitor closely for signs of CNS toxicity.

ADVERSE REACTIONS

Constipation, nausea, abdominal cramps.

DRUG INTERACTIONS

Increased plasma levels with quinidine or ritonavir; caution when coadministered with P-gp inhibitors. Decreased saquinavir exposure; monitor closely for therapeutic efficacy of saquinavir.

PATIENT CONSIDERATIONS

L

Assessment: Assess for known hypersensitivity, abdominal pain in absence of diarrhea, acute dysentery, acute ulcerative colitis, bacterial enterocolitis, pseudomembranous colitis, fluid and electrolyte depletion, hepatic dysfunction, pregnancy/nursing status, and possible drug interactions.

Monitoring: Monitor for allergic reactions, constipation, abdominal distention, ileus, megacolon, and other adverse reactions.

Counseling: Counsel patient to notify physician if diarrhea does not improve in 48 hrs, has blood in stool, or if fever or abdominal distention develops. Advise that tiredness, dizziness, or drowsiness may occur in the setting of diarrheal syndromes; use caution when driving or operating machinery.

STORAGE: 20-25°C (68-77°F).

Lopid – gemfibrozil

RX

Class: Fibric acid derivative

ADULT DOSAGE

Coronary Heart Disease

Adjunctive therapy to diet to reduce risk of developing coronary heart disease only in Type IIb patients w/o history of or symptoms of existing coronary heart disease who have had an inadequate response to weight loss, dietary therapy, exercise, and other pharmacologic agents and who have the triad of low HDL, elevated LDL, and elevated TG levels

1200mg in 2 divided doses 30 min before am and pm meals

Hypertriglyceridemia

Adjunctive therapy to diet for treatment of adults w/ very high elevations of serum TG levels (Types IV and V hyperlipidemia) who present a risk of pancreatitis and who do not respond adequately to diet

1200mg in 2 divided doses 30 min before am and pm meals

PEDIATRIC DOSAGE

Pediatric use may not have been established

ADMINISTRATION

Oral route

Take 30 min before am and pm meals

HOW SUPPLIED

Tab: 600mg* *scored

CONTRAINDICATIONS

Hepatic or severe renal dysfunction, including primary biliary cirrhosis; preexisting gallbladder disease; hypersensitivity to gemfibrozil; combination therapy w/ repaglinide or simvastatin.

WARNINGS/PRECAUTIONS

Cholelithiasis reported; perform gallbladder studies if cholelithiasis is suspected and d/c therapy if gallstones are found. May be associated with myositis; d/c if myositis is suspected/diagnosed. Control any medical problems (eg, diabetes mellitus [DM], hypothyroidism) that contribute to lipid abnormalities before initiating therapy. D/C if lipid response is inadequate after 3 months of therapy. Mild Hgb, Hct, and WBC decreases, and severe anemia, leukopenia, thrombocytopenia, and bone marrow hypoplasia reported; periodically monitor blood counts during the first 12 months of therapy. Abnormal LFTs reported; periodically monitor LFTs and d/c if abnormalities persist. Worsening renal insufficiency reported upon the addition of therapy in patients with baseline plasma creatinine >2mg/dL. Estrogen therapy is associated with massive rises in plasma TGs; discontinuation of estrogen therapy may obviate the need for specific drug therapy of hypertriglyceridemia.

ADVERSE REACTIONS

Dyspepsia, abdominal pain, diarrhea, fatigue.

DRUG INTERACTIONS

See Contraindications. Caution with anticoagulants; reduce anticoagulant dose and frequently monitor prothrombin until it has been definitely determined that prothrombin level has stabilized. Increased risk of myopathy and rhabdomyolysis with HMG-CoA reductase inhibitors. Reduced exposure with resin-granule drugs (eg, colestipol); administer ≥2 hrs apart. May potentiate myopathy with colchicine; caution when prescribing with colchicine, especially in elderly patients or patients with renal dysfunction.

PATIENT CONSIDERATIONS

Assessment: Assess for hepatic/renal dysfunction, gallbladder disease, other medical conditions (eg, DM, hypothyroidism), hypersensitivity to drug, pregnancy/nursing status, and possible drug interactions. Obtain lipid levels.

Monitoring: Monitor for signs/symptoms of cholelithiasis, myositis, worsening renal insufficiency, and other adverse reactions. Periodically monitor serum lipids levels, CBC, and LFTs. Frequently monitor prothrombin with anticoagulants. Closely observe patients with significantly elevated TGs during therapy.

Counseling: Inform about potential risks/benefits of therapy. Advise to report to physician any muscle pain/tenderness/weakness, or other adverse reactions. Instruct to notify physician if pregnant/nursing or planning to become pregnant.

STORAGE: 20-25°C (68-77°F). Protect from light and humidity.

LORZONE – chlorzoxazone

RX

Class: Muscular analgesic (centrally acting)

ADULT DOSAGE

Musculoskeletal Conditions

Adjunct to rest, physical therapy, and other measures for relief of discomfort associated w/ acute, painful musculoskeletal conditions

375mg Tab:

Usual: 1 tab tid or qid

Titrate: May increase to 2 tabs (750mg) tid or qid if adequate response is not obtained

Dosage can be reduced as improvement occurs

750mg Tab:

Usual: 1/3 tab (250mg) tid or qid. Give 2/3 tab (500mg) tid or qid for painful musculoskeletal conditions

PEDIATRIC DOSAGE

Pediatric use may not have been established

Titrate: May increase to 1 tab (750mg) tid or qid if adequate response is not obtained

Dosage can be reduced as improvement occurs

ADMINISTRATION

Oral route

HOW SUPPLIED

Tab: 375mg, 750mg

CONTRAINDICATIONS

Known intolerance to the drug.

WARNINGS/PRECAUTIONS

Serious (including fatal) hepatocellular toxicity reported rarely; d/c immediately if any signs/symptoms of hepatotoxicity or abnormal liver enzymes develop. Caution w/ known allergies or w/ history of allergic reactions to drugs; d/c if a sensitivity reaction occurs.

ADVERSE REACTIONS

Drowsiness, dizziness, lightheadedness, malaise, overstimulation.

DRUG INTERACTIONS

May have additive effect w/ alcohol or other CNS depressants.

PATIENT CONSIDERATIONS

Assessment: Assess for intolerance to chlorzoxazone, known allergies or history of allergic reactions to drugs, hepatic impairment, pregnancy/nursing status, and possible drug interactions.

Monitoring: Monitor for signs/symptoms of hepatotoxicity, sensitivity reactions, and other adverse reactions. Monitor LFTs.

Counseling: Inform of the risks and benefits of therapy. Instruct to d/c immediately and contact physician if signs/symptoms of hepatotoxicity (eg, fever, rash, right upper quadrant pain, dark urine) or a sensitivity reaction (eg, urticaria, redness, itching of the skin) occur.

STORAGE: 20-25°C (68-77°F).

LOTEMAX SUSPENSION – loteprednol etabonate RX

Class: Corticosteroid

ADULT DOSAGE

Steroid-Responsive Inflammatory Ocular Conditions

Treatment of palpebral and bulbar conjunctiva, cornea, and anterior segment of the globe, such as allergic conjunctivitis, acne rosacea, superficial punctate keratitis, herpes zoster keratitis, iritis, cyclitis, and selected infective conjunctivitides

Apply 1-2 drops into the conjunctival sac of the affected eye(s) qid; may increase up to 1 drop qh, if necessary, during initial treatment w/in the 1st week

Reevaluate if signs/symptoms fail to improve after 2 days

Postoperative Inflammation

Apply 1-2 drops into the conjunctival sac of the operated eye(s) qid beginning 24 hrs after surgery, and continuing throughout the first 2 weeks of the postoperative period

PEDIATRIC DOSAGE

Pediatric use may not have been established

ADMINISTRATION

Ocular route

Shake vigorously before use

HOW SUPPLIED

Sus: 0.5% [5mL, 10mL, 15mL]

CONTRAINDICATIONS
Most viral diseases of the cornea and conjunctiva (eg, epithelial herpes simplex keratitis [dendritic keratitis], vaccinia, varicella), mycobacterial infection of the eye, fungal diseases of ocular structures, known or suspected hypersensitivity to any of the ingredients of this preparation and to other corticosteroids.

WARNINGS/PRECAUTIONS
For ophthalmic use only. Prolonged use may result in glaucoma with damage to the optic nerve, defects in visual acuity and fields of vision, and in posterior subcapsular cataract formation; caution with glaucoma. Prolonged use may suppress host response and increase hazard of secondary ocular infections. Perforations reported with diseases causing thinning of cornea/sclera. May mask or enhance existing infection in acute purulent conditions of the eye. Caution with history of herpes simplex; may prolong course and exacerbate severity of many viral infections of the eye. May delay healing and increase incidence of bleb formation after cataract surgery. Initial prescription and renewal of medication order beyond 14 days should only be made after examination of the patient with aid of magnification (eg, slit-lamp biomicroscopy) and, where appropriate, fluorescein staining. Monitor IOP if used for ≥10 days. Fungal infections of the cornea may develop coincidentally with long-term use; consider fungal invasion in any persistent corneal ulceration and take fungal cultures when appropriate. For steroid-responsive diseases, caution not to d/c therapy prematurely. Should not be used for acute anterior uveitis in patients who require a more potent corticosteroid.

ADVERSE REACTIONS
Abnormal vision/blurring, burning on instillation, chemosis, discharge, dry eyes, epiphora, foreign body sensation, itching, photophobia, headache, rhinitis, pharyngitis.

PATIENT CONSIDERATIONS

Assessment: Assess for previous drug hypersensitivity, viral diseases of the cornea and conjunctiva, mycobacterial infection of the eye, fungal diseases of ocular structures, glaucoma, thinning of the cornea/sclera, history of herpes simplex, and pregnancy/nursing status. Perform examination of patient with the aid of magnification (eg, slit-lamp biomicroscopy, fluorescein staining). Assess use in patients who have undergone recent cataract surgery.

Monitoring: Monitor for glaucoma and its complications, defects in visual acuity and fields of vision, posterior subcapsular cataract formation, perforation of the cornea/sclera, secondary ocular infections, fungal infections, masking of existing infections, and other adverse reactions. Reevaluate if signs/symptoms fail to improve after 2 days. Monitor IOP during prolonged use (≥10 days). Perform examination of patient with the aid of magnification (eg, slit-lamp biomicroscopy, fluorescein staining) before renewal of medication order beyond 14 days.

Counseling: Advise not to allow dropper tip to touch any surface to avoid contamination of sus. Instruct to consult physician if pain develops or if redness, itching, or inflammation becomes aggravated. Inform not to wear soft contact lenses during treatment.

STORAGE: 15-25°C (59-77°F); store upright. Do not freeze.

LOTENSIN HCT – benazepril hydrochloride/hydrochlorothiazide RX

Class: ACE inhibitor/thiazide diuretic

D/C when pregnancy is detected. Drugs that act directly on the renin-angiotensin system (RAS) can cause injury/death to the developing fetus.

ADULT DOSAGE

Hypertension

Uncontrolled BP on Benazepril or HCTZ Alone:
Initial: 10mg/12.5mg qd
Titrate: May increase after 2-3 weeks prn to help achieve BP goals
Max: 20mg/25mg
Replacement Therapy: May be substituted for the titrated individual components

PEDIATRIC DOSAGE

Pediatric use may not have been established

ADMINISTRATION
Oral route

HOW SUPPLIED
Tab: (Benazepril/HCTZ) 5mg/6.25mg*, 10mg/12.5mg*, 20mg/12.5mg*, 20mg/25mg* *scored

CONTRAINDICATIONS

Anuria; hypersensitivity to benazepril, to any other ACE inhibitor, to hydrochlorothiazide, or to other sulfonamide-derived drugs; history of angioedema w/ or w/o previous ACE inhibitor treatment. Coadministration w/ aliskiren in patients w/ diabetes.

WARNINGS/PRECAUTIONS

Not for initial therapy of HTN. Head/neck angioedema reported; d/c and institute appropriate therapy immediately. Higher incidence of angioedema in blacks than nonblacks. Intestinal angioedema reported; monitor for abdominal pain. Anaphylactoid reactions reported during desensitization with hymenoptera venom, dialysis with high-flux membranes, and LDL apheresis with dextran sulfate absorption. Symptomatic hypotension may occur, most likely in patients with volume and/or salt depletion; correct depletion before initiating therapy. Enhanced effects in postsympathectomy patients. Excessive hypotension, which may be associated with oliguria, azotemia, and (rarely) with acute renal failure and death, may occur in patients with CHF; monitor closely during first 2 weeks of therapy and whenever dose is increased. May cause changes in renal function, including renal failure; consider withholding or discontinuing therapy if clinically significant decrease in renal function develops. May increase BUN or SrCr in patients with renal artery stenosis. May cause agranulocytosis and bone marrow depression. Associated with syndrome that starts with cholestatic jaundice and progresses to fulminant hepatic necrosis and sometimes death (rare); d/c if jaundice or marked hepatic enzyme elevations develop. May cause exacerbation or activation of systemic lupus erythematosus (SLE). May cause idiosyncratic reaction, resulting in acute transient myopia and acute angle-closure glaucoma; d/c as rapidly as possible. May cause serum electrolyte abnormalities. Persistent nonproductive cough reported. Hypotension may occur with surgery or during anesthesia. May decrease serum protein-bound iodine levels without signs of thyroid disturbance. D/C before testing for parathyroid function. HCTZ: May alter glucose tolerance and raise serum cholesterol and TG levels. May cause or exacerbate hyperuricemia and precipitate gout. May elevate serum Ca^{2+}; avoid with hypercalcemia. May precipitate hepatic coma in patients with hepatic impairment or progressive liver disease.

ADVERSE REACTIONS

Dizziness, fatigue, postural dizziness, headache.

DRUG INTERACTIONS

See Contraindications. Caution with other antihypertensives. May affect K^+ levels with K^+ supplements and K^+-sparing diuretics; monitor K^+ periodically. Increased lithium levels and lithium toxicity reported; monitor lithium levels. Dual blockade of the RAS is associated with increased risks of hypotension, hyperkalemia, and changes in renal function (including acute renal failure); closely monitor BP, renal function, and electrolytes with concomitant agents that also affect the RAS. Avoid aliskiren in patients with renal impairment (GFR <60mL/min). NSAIDs, including selective COX-2 inhibitors, may attenuate antihypertensive effect and may cause deterioration of renal function. Benazepril: Nitritoid reactions reported with injectable gold. HCTZ: May potentiate action of other antihypertensives, especially ganglionic/peripheral adrenergic-blocking drugs. Cholestyramine and colestipol resins reduce absorption from GI tract; administer at least 4 hrs before or 4-6 hrs after administration of resins. Drug-induced hypokalemia or hypomagnesemia may predispose patient to digoxin toxicity. May increase responsiveness to skeletal muscle relaxants (eg, curare derivatives). Dosage adjustment of antidiabetic drugs may be required. May reduce renal excretion of cytotoxic agents (eg, cyclophosphamide, methotrexate) and enhance their myelosuppressive effects. Anticholinergics (eg, atropine, biperiden) may increase bioavailability due to decrease in GI motility and stomach emptying rate. Prokinetic drugs may decrease bioavailability. Increased risk of hyperuricemia and gout-type complications with cyclosporine. May potentiate orthostatic hypotension with alcohol, barbiturates, or narcotics. May reduce response to pressor amines (eg, noradrenaline).

PATIENT CONSIDERATIONS

Assessment: Assess for anuria, sulfonamide-derived drug hypersensitivity, history of angioedema/allergy/asthma, risk factors for angle-closure glaucoma, volume/salt depletion, CHF, collagen vascular diseases, SLE, hypercalcemia, diabetes, renal/hepatic impairment, postsympathectomy status, pregnancy/nursing status, and possible drug interactions.

Monitoring: Monitor for angioedema, anaphylactoid reactions, exacerbation/activation of SLE, myopia, angle-closure glaucoma, hyperuricemia or precipitation of gout, and other adverse reactions. Monitor BP, LFTs, renal function, serum electrolytes, cholesterol, and TG levels. Monitor WBCs in patients with collagen vascular disease and renal impairment.

Counseling: Inform about fetal risks if taken during pregnancy and discuss treatment options in women planning to become pregnant; instruct to report pregnancy as soon as possible. Instruct to d/c therapy and to immediately report signs/symptoms of angioedema. Instruct to report lightheadedness, especially during the 1st days of therapy; advise to d/c and consult with a physician if syncope occurs. Inform that inadequate fluid intake, excessive perspiration, diarrhea, or vomiting may lead to excessive fall in BP, with the same consequences of lightheadedness and possible syncope. Advise not to use K^+ supplements or salt substitutes containing K^+ without consulting physician. Advise to promptly report any indication of infection.

STORAGE: ≤30°C (86°F). Protect from moisture and light.

LOTREL – amlodipine besylate/benazepril hydrochloride

RX

Class: ACE inhibitor/calcium channel blocker (CCB) (dihydropyridine)

D/C when pregnancy is detected. Drugs that act directly on the renin-angiotensin system (RAS) can cause injury/death to the developing fetus.

ADULT DOSAGE

Hypertension

Not Adequately Controlled on Monotherapy w/ Either Agent:

Initial: 2.5mg/10mg qd

Titrate: May increase up to 10mg/40mg qd if BP remains uncontrolled

Replacement Therapy: May substitute for titrated components

PEDIATRIC DOSAGE

Pediatric use may not have been established

DOSING CONSIDERATIONS

Renal Impairment

CrCl ≤30mL/min: Not recommended for use

Hepatic Impairment

Consider using lower doses

Elderly

Consider lower initial doses

ADMINISTRATION

Oral route

HOW SUPPLIED

Cap: (Amlodipine/Benazepril) 2.5mg/10mg, 5mg/10mg, 5mg/20mg, 5mg/40mg, 10mg/20mg, 10mg/40mg

CONTRAINDICATIONS

Coadministration w/ aliskiren in patients w/ diabetes. History of angioedema, w/ or w/o previous ACE inhibitor treatment; hypersensitivity to benazepril, to any other ACE inhibitor, to amlodipine, or to any of the excipients of this product.

WARNINGS/PRECAUTIONS

Symptomatic hypotension may occur, most likely in patients w/ volume- or salt-depletion; correct volume and/or salt depletion before starting therapy. Symptomatic hypotension may occur in patients w/ severe aortic stenosis. Benazepril: Head and neck angioedema reported; d/c and treat immediately if laryngeal stridor or angioedema of face/tongue/glottis occurs. Black patients have a higher incidence of angioedema compared to nonblacks. Intestinal angioedema reported; monitor for abdominal pain. Anaphylactoid reactions reported during desensitization w/ hymenoptera (wasp sting) venom, in patients dialyzed w/ high-flux membranes, and in patients undergoing LDL apheresis w/ dextran sulfate absorption. Excessive hypotension, which may be associated w/ oliguria, azotemia, and (rarely) acute renal failure and death, may occur in CHF patients; monitor patients during first 2 weeks of therapy and whenever dose is increased or a diuretic is added or its dose increased. Cholestatic hepatitis and acute liver failure reported rarely; d/c if jaundice or marked elevation of hepatic enzymes develops. May cause changes in renal function, including acute renal failure; patients whose renal function depends on the RAS (eg, renal artery stenosis, severe heart failure, post MI) may be at particular risk; consider withholding or discontinuing therapy if clinically significant decrease in renal function develops. Hyperkalemia and persistent nonproductive cough reported. Hypotension may occur w/ surgery or during anesthesia. Amlodipine: Worsening angina and acute MI (AMI) may develop after starting or increasing the dose, particularly in patients w/ severe obstructive coronary artery disease (CAD). Caution w/ aortic/mitral stenosis, or obstructive hypertrophic cardiomyopathy.

ADVERSE REACTIONS

Cough, headache, dizziness, edema, angioedema.

DRUG INTERACTIONS

See Contraindications. Benazepril: Increased risk for angioedema w/ mammalian target of rapamycin inhibitor (eg, temsirolimus, sirolimus, everolimus). Coadministration w/ NSAIDs, including selective COX-2 inhibitors, may result in deterioration of renal function and attenuation of antihypertensive effect. Diabetic patients receiving concomitant insulin or oral antidiabetics may develop hypoglycemia. Dual blockade of the RAS is associated w/ increased risks of hypotension, hyperkalemia, and changes in renal function (including acute renal failure); avoid combined use of RAS inhibitors, and closely monitor BP, renal function, and electrolytes w/ concomitant agents that also block the RAS. Avoid w/ aliskiren in patients w/ renal impairment (GFR <60mL/min). K^+

supplements, K^+-sparing diuretics (eg, spironolactone, amiloride, triamterene), or K^+-containing salt substitutes may increase risk of hyperkalemia; frequently monitor serum K^+. May attenuate K^+ loss caused by thiazide diuretics. Increased lithium levels and symptoms of lithium toxicity reported; frequently monitor lithium levels. Nitritoid reactions (eg, facial flushing, N/V, hypotension) reported w/ injectable gold. Amlodipine: May increase exposure of simvastatin; limit dose of simvastatin to 20mg daily. Increased systemic exposure w/ moderate and strong CYP3A inhibitors; monitor for symptoms of hypotension and edema. Monitor BP when coadministered w/ CYP3A4 inducers.

PATIENT CONSIDERATIONS

Assessment: Assess for history of angioedema, diabetes, hypersensitivity to drug, aortic/mitral stenosis, obstructive hypertrophic cardiomyopathy, CHF, severe obstructive CAD, volume/salt depletion, hepatic/renal impairment, pregnancy/nursing status, and possible drug interactions.

Monitoring: Monitor for signs/symptoms of hypotension, anaphylactoid or hypersensitivity reactions, head/neck and intestinal angioedema, worsening angina or AMI, and other adverse reactions. Monitor BP, hepatic/renal function, and serum K^+ levels.

Counseling: Inform of the consequences of exposure to the medication during pregnancy and of treatment options in women planning to become pregnant. Advise to report pregnancies as soon as possible. Advise diabetic patients about the possibility of hypoglycemic reactions when drug is used concomitantly w/ insulin or oral antidiabetics. Advise to seek medical attention if symptoms of hypotension, anaphylactoid or hypersensitivity reactions, angioedema, infection, trouble swallowing, breathing problems, or hepatic dysfunction occurs

STORAGE: 25°C (77°F); excursions permitted to 15-30°C (59-86°F). Protect from moisture.

LOTRISONE – betamethasone dipropionate/clotrimazole RX

Class: Azole antifungal/corticosteroid

L

ADULT DOSAGE

Tinea Corporis (Ringworm)

≥17 Years:
Apply a thin film into affected skin areas bid for 1 week
Max: 45g/week

Reevaluate if no improvement seen after 1 week; do not use for >2 weeks

Tinea Cruris (Jock Itch)

≥17 Years:
Apply a thin film into affected skin areas bid for 1 week
Max: 45g/week

Reevaluate if no improvement seen after 1 week; do not use for >2 weeks

Tinea Pedis (Athlete's Foot)

≥17 Years:
Gently massage sufficient amount into affected skin areas bid for 2 weeks
Max: 45g/week

Reevaluate if no improvement seen after 2 weeks; do not use for >4 weeks

PEDIATRIC DOSAGE

Pediatric use may not have been established

ADMINISTRATION

Topical route

Do not use w/ occlusive dressings unless directed by a physician

HOW SUPPLIED

Cre: (Betamethasone/Clotrimazole) 0.05%/1% [15g, 45g]

WARNINGS/PRECAUTIONS

Not for oral, ophthalmic, or intravaginal use. Avoid use with occlusive dressings. May cause reversible hypothalamic-pituitary-adrenal (HPA) axis suppression with the potential for glucocorticosteroid insufficiency during and after withdrawal of treatment. Cushing's syndrome and hyperglycemia may occur. Factors predisposing to HPA axis suppression include use of high-potency steroids, large treatment surface areas, prolonged use, use of occlusive dressings, altered skin barrier, liver failure, and young age. Evaluate periodically for evidence of HPA axis suppression.

Gradually withdraw drug, reduce frequency of application, or substitute a less potent corticosteroid if HPA axis suppression is documented. Pediatric patients may be more susceptible to systemic toxicity. Not recommended for treatment of diaper dermatitis. Caution in elderly.

ADVERSE REACTIONS

Paresthesia, rash, edema, secondary infection.

PATIENT CONSIDERATIONS

Assessment: Assess for hypersensitivity to drug, predisposing factors to HPA axis suppression, and pregnancy/nursing status.

Monitoring: Monitor for signs/symptoms of HPA axis suppression, Cushing's syndrome, hyperglycemia, and other adverse reactions. Perform periodic monitoring for HPA axis suppression using adrenocorticotropic hormone stimulation test. Review diagnosis if no clinical improvement seen after 1 week of treatment for tinea corporis or tinea cruris, and 2 weeks for tinea pedis.

Counseling: Inform to use externally ud. Advise to avoid intravaginal contact or contact with the eyes or mouth. Advise not to use on the face or underarms. When using in the groin area, counsel to use only for 2 weeks and apply the cream sparingly; advise to wear loose-fitting clothing and to notify physician if condition persists after 2 weeks. Instruct not to bandage, cover, or wrap the treatment area unless directed by physician. Advise to avoid use in the diaper area. Instruct to report any signs of local adverse reactions to physician. Instruct to notify physician if no improvement seen after 1 week of treatment for tinea cruris or tinea corporis, or 2 weeks for tinea pedis.

STORAGE: 20-25°C (68-77°F); excursions permitted to 15-30°C (59-86°F).

LOVAZA — omega-3-acid ethyl esters

RX

Class: Lipid-regulating agent

ADULT DOSAGE

Severe Hypertriglyceridemia (≥500mg/dL)

4g/day (4 caps qd or 2 caps bid)

PEDIATRIC DOSAGE

Pediatric use may not have been established

ADMINISTRATION

Oral route

Swallow caps whole; do not break open, crush, dissolve, or chew

HOW SUPPLIED

Cap: 1g

CONTRAINDICATIONS

Known hypersensitivity (eg, anaphylactic reaction) to Lovaza or any of its components.

WARNINGS/PRECAUTIONS

Increases in ALT levels without a concurrent increase in AST levels reported. May increase LDL levels; monitor LDL levels periodically during therapy. Contains ethyl esters of omega-3 fatty acids (eicosapentaenoic acid [EPA] and docosahexaenoic acid [DHA]), obtained from oil of several fish sources; caution with known hypersensitivity to fish and/or shellfish. Recurrent symptomatic atrial fibrillation/flutter (A-fib/flutter) reported in patients with paroxysmal or persistent A-fib, particularly within the first 2-3 months of initiating therapy. Assess TG levels carefully before initiating therapy and monitor TG levels periodically during therapy.

ADVERSE REACTIONS

Eructation, taste perversion, dyspepsia.

DRUG INTERACTIONS

Periodically monitor patients receiving concomitant treatment with an anticoagulant or other drugs affecting coagulation (eg, antiplatelet agents). D/C or change medications known to exacerbate hypertriglyceridemia (eg, β-blockers, thiazides, estrogens), if possible, prior to consideration of therapy.

PATIENT CONSIDERATIONS

Assessment: Assess for hypersensitivity to drug, fish and/or shellfish; hepatic impairment; A-fib/flutter; pregnancy/nursing status; and possible drug interactions. Attempt to control serum lipids with appropriate diet, exercise, weight loss in obese patients, and control of any medical problems that are contributing to lipid abnormalities (eg, diabetes mellitus, hypothyroidism). Assess TG and LDL levels.

Monitoring: Monitor for recurrent symptomatic A-fib/flutter in patients with paroxysmal or persistent A-fib. Monitor for allergic reactions and other adverse reactions. Periodically monitor ALT and AST levels in patients with hepatic impairment. Periodically monitor LDL and TG levels.

Counseling: Instruct to notify physician if allergic to fish and/or shellfish. Advise that the use of lipid-regulating agents does not reduce the importance of adhering to diet. Advise not to alter caps in any way and to ingest intact caps only. Instruct to take as prescribed.

STORAGE: 25°C (77°F); excursions permitted to 15-30°C (59-86°F). Do not freeze.

LOVENOX — enoxaparin sodium

RX

Class: Low molecular weight heparin (LMWH)

Epidural or spinal hematomas resulting in long-term or permanent paralysis may occur in patients anticoagulated with low molecular weight heparins (LMWHs) or heparinoids and are receiving neuraxial anesthesia or undergoing spinal puncture. Increased risk with indwelling epidural catheters, concomitant use of other drugs that affect hemostasis (eg, NSAIDs, platelet inhibitors, other anticoagulants), history of traumatic or repeated epidural or spinal punctures, a history of spinal deformity or spinal surgery, or when optimal timing between the administration of enoxaparin and neuraxial procedures is not known. Monitor frequently for signs/symptoms of neurological impairment; if neurological compromise noted, urgent treatment is necessary. Consider benefit and risks before neuraxial intervention in patients anticoagulated or to be anticoagulated for thromboprophylaxis.

ADULT DOSAGE

Deep Vein Thrombosis

Prophylaxis:

Abdominal Surgery:
40mg SQ qd w/ initial dose given 2 hrs prior to surgery for 7-10 days (up to 12 days in clinical trials)

Hip Replacement Surgery:
Twice-Daily Dosing: 30mg SQ q12h w/ initial dose given 12-24 hrs after surgery for 7-10 days (up to 14 days in clinical trials)
Once-Daily Dosing: 40mg SQ qd w/ initial dose given 12 hrs prior to surgery for 7-10 days (up to 14 days in clinical trials)

Continue prophylaxis w/ 40mg SQ qd for 3 weeks following initial phase

Knee Replacement Surgery:
30mg SQ q12h w/ initial dose given 12-24 hrs after surgery for 7-10 days (up to 14 days in clinical trials)

Acute Illness w/ Severely Restricted Mobility:
40mg SQ qd for 6-11 days (up to 14 days in clinical trials)

Acute Treatment:
Outpatient (w/o Pulmonary Embolism):
1mg/kg SQ q12h for 7 days (up to 17 days in clinical trials)
Inpatient (w/ or w/o Pulmonary Embolism):
1mg/kg SQ q12h, or 1.5mg/kg SQ qd at the same time every day for 7 days (up to 17 days in clinical trials)

Outpatient and Inpatient Treatments:
Initiate warfarin therapy when appropriate (usually w/in 72 hrs of enoxaparin); continue enoxaparin for at least 5 days and until therapeutic oral anticoagulant effect has been achieved

Unstable Angina

Prophylaxis:
1mg/kg SQ q12h in conjunction w/ oral aspirin therapy (100-325mg qd) for 2-8 days (up to 12.5 days in clinical trials)

Myocardial Infarction

Non-Q-Wave:
Prophylaxis:
1mg/kg SQ q12h in conjunction w/ oral aspirin therapy (100-325mg qd) for 2-8 days (up to 12.5 days in clinical trials)

PEDIATRIC DOSAGE

Pediatric use may not have been established

L

Acute ST- Segment Elevation:
Treatment:
<75 Years:
Initial: 30mg single IV bolus plus a 1mg/kg SQ dose, followed by 1mg/kg SQ q12h
Max: 100mg for the first 2 SQ doses only

All patients should receive aspirin (75-325mg qd) as soon as they are identified as having ST-segment elevation MI unless contraindicated

Concomitant Thrombolytic (Fibrin-Specific or Non-Fibrin Specific):
Administer enoxaparin between 15 min before and 30 min after the start of fibrinolytic therapy

Percutaneous Coronary Intervention:
Last SQ Enoxaparin Dose Given <8 hrs Before Balloon Inflation: No additional dosing needed
Last SQ Enoxaparin Dose Given >8 hrs Before Balloon Inflation: Administer 0.3mg/kg IV bolus

DOSING CONSIDERATIONS

Renal Impairment
Severe (CrCl <30mL/min):
Prophylaxis in Abdominal Surgery: 30mg SQ qd
Prophylaxis in Hip/Knee Replacement Surgery: 30mg SQ qd
Prophylaxis in Acute Illness: 30mg SQ qd
Outpatient Treatment of Acute DVT w/o Pulmonary Embolism (w/ Warfarin): 1mg/kg SQ qd
Inpatient Treatment of Acute DVT w/ or w/o Pulmonary Embolism (w/ Warfarin): 1mg/kg SQ qd
Ischemic Prophylaxis in Unstable Angina/Non-Q-Wave MI (w/ Aspirin): 1mg/kg SQ qd
Treatment of Acute ST-Segment Elevation MI in Patients <75 Years (w/ Aspirin): 30mg single IV bolus plus a 1mg/kg SQ dose, followed by 1mg/kg SQ qd
Treatment of Acute ST-Segment Elevation MI in Patients ≥75 Years (w/ Aspirin): 1mg/kg SQ qd (no initial bolus)

Elderly
≥75 Years:
Acute ST-Segment Elevation MI:
Do not use initial IV bolus
Initial: 0.75mg/kg SQ q12h
Max: 75mg for the first 2 doses only

ADMINISTRATION

SQ or IV (for multidose vial) route

Use tuberculin syringe or equivalent when using multidose vials
Prefilled syringes and graduated prefilled syringes are for single, one-time use only and are available w/ a system that shields the needle after inj

SQ Inj Technique
Remove the prefilled syringe from the blister packaging by peeling at the arrow as directed on the blister; do not remove by pulling on the plunger as this may damage the syringe
Patients should be lying down and enoxaparin administered by deep SQ inj
Do not expel the air bubble from the prefilled syringe before the inj
Administration should be alternated between the left and right anterolateral and left and right posterolateral abdominal wall
The whole length of the needle should be introduced into a skin fold held between the thumb and forefinger; the skin fold should be held throughout the inj
Do not rub the inj site after completion of the inj

IV (Bolus) Inj
Use multiple-dose vial and administer through an IV line
Do not mix or coadminister w/ other medications
Flush the chosen IV access w/ a sufficient amount of saline or dextrose sol prior to and following the IV bolus administration of enoxaparin to clear the port of drug; enoxaparin may be safely administered w/ normal saline sol (0.9%) or D5W

HOW SUPPLIED

Inj: (Multidose Vial) 300mg/3mL; (Prefilled Syringe) 30mg/0.3mL, 40mg/0.4mL, 60mg/0.6mL, 80mg/0.8mL, 100mg/mL, 120mg/0.8mL, 150mg/mL

CONTRAINDICATIONS

Active major bleeding, thrombocytopenia associated with a positive in vitro test for antiplatelet antibody in the presence of enoxaparin sodium, hypersensitivity to heparin or pork products, hypersensitivity to benzyl alcohol (only with the multidose formulation), Known hypersensitivity to enoxaparin sodium (eg, pruritus, urticaria, anaphylactic/anaphylactoid reactions).

WARNINGS/PRECAUTIONS

Consider pharmacokinetic profile of enoxaparin to reduce the potential risk of bleeding associated with concurrent use with epidural or spinal anesthesia/analgesia or spinal puncture. Placement or removal of catheter should be delayed for at least 12 hrs after administration of lower doses and at least 24 hrs after higher doses. Extreme caution with increased risk of hemorrhage (eg, bacterial endocarditis, congenital or acquired bleeding disorders) and with history of heparin-induced thrombocytopenia. Major hemorrhages, including retroperitoneal and intracranial bleeding, reported. To minimize the risk of bleeding following vascular instrumentation during treatment of unstable angina, non-Q-wave MI, and acute STEMI, adhere precisely to the intervals recommended between doses. Observe for signs of bleeding or hematoma formation at the site of the procedure. Caution in patients with bleeding diathesis, uncontrolled arterial HTN or history of recent GI ulceration, diabetic retinopathy, renal dysfunction, and hemorrhage. Thrombocytopenia reported; d/c if platelet count <100,000/mm^3. Cannot be used interchangeably (unit for unit) with heparin or other LMWH. Pregnant women with mechanical prosthetic heart valves may be at higher risk for thromboembolism and have a higher rate of fetal loss; monitor anti-factor Xa levels, and adjust dosage prn. Multidose vial contains benzyl alcohol that crosses the placenta and has been associated with fatal "gasping syndrome" in premature neonates; use with caution or only when clearly needed in pregnant women. Periodic CBC, including platelet count and stool occult blood tests are recommended during course of treatment. Anti-factor Xa may be used to monitor anticoagulant activity in patients with significant renal impairment or if abnormal coagulation parameters or bleeding occurs. Hyperkalemia reported in patients with renal failure. Increase in exposure with prophylactic dosages (non-weight adjusted) observed in low-weight women (<45kg) and low-weight men (<57kg). Higher risk for thromboembolism in obese patients; observe for signs/symptoms of thromboembolism. Caution with hepatic impairment.

ADVERSE REACTIONS

Epidural or spinal hematoma, hemorrhage, ecchymosis, anemia, peripheral edema, fever, dyspnea, nausea, ALT/AST elevations.

DRUG INTERACTIONS

See Boxed Warning. D/C agents that may enhance the risk of hemorrhage prior to therapy (eg, anticoagulants, platelet inhibitors, such as acetylsalicylic acid, salicylates, NSAIDs [including ketorolac tromethamine], dipyridamole, or sulfinpyrazone). If coadministration is essential, conduct close monitoring. May increase risk of hyperkalemia with K^+-sparing drugs, and administration of K^+.

PATIENT CONSIDERATIONS

Assessment: Assess for presence of active major bleeding, thrombocytopenia, hypersensitivity to heparin or pork products, hypersensitivity to benzyl alcohol, renal dysfunction, obesity, any other conditions where treatment is cautioned, nursing/pregnancy status, and for possible drug interactions.

Monitoring: Monitor for signs/symptoms of hemorrhage, thrombocytopenia, hyperkalemia, thromboembolism, and other adverse reactions. Monitor for epidural or spinal hematomas, and for neurological impairment if used concomitantly with spinal/epidural anesthesia or spinal puncture. Periodically monitor CBC, including platelet count, and stool occult blood tests. If bleeding occurs, monitor anti-factor Xa levels.

Counseling: Inform of the benefits and risks of therapy. Instruct to watch for signs/symptoms of spinal or epidural hematoma (tingling, numbness, muscular weakness) if patients have had neuraxial anesthesia or spinal puncture, particularly, if they are taking concomitant NSAIDs, platelet inhibitors, or other anticoagulants; instruct to contact physician if these occur. Advise to seek medical attention if unusual bleeding, bruising, signs of thrombocytopenia, or allergic reactions develop. Counsel that it will take longer than usual to stop bleeding; explain that patient may bruise and/or bleed more easily when treated with enoxaparin. Inform of administration instructions if therapy is to continue after discharge. Instruct to notify physicians and dentists of enoxaparin therapy prior to surgery or taking a new drug.

STORAGE: 25°C (77°F); excursions permitted to 15-30°C (59-86°F). Do not store multidose vials for >28 days after first use.

LUCENTIS – ranibizumab

RX

Class: Monoclonal antibody/vascular endothelial growth factor (VEGF)-A blocker

ADULT DOSAGE

Neovascular (Wet) Age-Related Macular Degeneration

0.5mg (0.05mL of 10mg/mL sol) once a month (approx 28 days)

May administer 3 monthly doses followed by less frequent dosing (eg, 4-5 doses on average in 9 months)

May also administer 1 dose every 3 months after 4 monthly doses

Macular Edema

Following Retinal Vein Occlusion:
0.5mg (0.05mL of 10mg/mL sol) once a month (approx 28 days)

Diabetic Macular Edema

0.3mg (0.05mL of 6mg/mL sol) once a month (approx 28 days)

Diabetic Retinopathy

Non-Proliferative/Proliferative Diabetic Retinopathy w/ Diabetic Macular Edema:

0.3mg (0.05mL of 6mg/mL sol) once a month (approx 28 days)

PEDIATRIC DOSAGE

Pediatric use may not have been established

ADMINISTRATION

Intravitreal route

Preparation

1. All of vial contents are withdrawn through a 5-micron, 19-gauge filter needle attached to a 1-cc tuberculin syringe
2. Discard filter needle after withdrawal of the vial contents and do not use for intravitreal inj
3. Replace filter needle w/ a sterile 30-gauge x 1/2-inch needle for intravitreal inj
4. Contents should be expelled until plunger tip is aligned w/ line that marks 0.05mL on the syringe

Administration

1. Adequate anesthesia and a broad-spectrum microbicide should be given prior to inj
2. Each vial should only be used for treatment of a single eye; if contralateral eye requires treatment, a new vial should be used and the sterile field, syringe, gloves, drapes, eyelid speculum, filter, and inj needles should be changed before administration to other eye

HOW SUPPLIED

Inj: 6mg/mL, 10mg/mL

CONTRAINDICATIONS

Ocular or periocular infections. Known hypersensitivity to ranibizumab or any of the excipients in the medication.

WARNINGS/PRECAUTIONS

Endophthalmitis and retinal detachments may occur; always use proper aseptic inj technique. Increases in IOP reported both preinj and postinj (at 60 min); monitor IOP prior to/following inj and manage appropriately. Potential risk of arterial thromboembolic events (ATEs) (eg, nonfatal stroke, nonfatal MI, vascular death). Fatal events may occur in patients w/ DME and DR at baseline.

ADVERSE REACTIONS

Conjunctival hemorrhage, eye pain, vitreous floaters/detachment, increased IOP, intraocular inflammation, cataract, nasopharyngitis, foreign body sensation in eyes, eye irritation, lacrimation increased, visual disturbance/vision blurred, ocular hyperemia, dry eye, influenza, headache.

DRUG INTERACTIONS

Serious intraocular inflammation may develop when used adjunctively w/ verteporfin photodynamic therapy (PDT); incidence reported when drug was administered 7 days after verteporfin PDT.

PATIENT CONSIDERATIONS

Assessment: Assess for ocular or periocular infections, hypersensitivity to the drug, pregnancy/nursing status, and possible drug interactions.

Monitoring: Monitor for signs/symptoms of endophthalmitis, retinal detachments, ATEs, hypersensitivity reactions, and other adverse reactions. Monitor IOP prior to and 30 min following inj using tonometry. Check for perfusion of the optic nerve head immediately after inj. Monitor following inj to permit early treatment should an infection occur.

Counseling: Inform about the risk of developing endophthalmitis following administration. Instruct to seek immediate care from an ophthalmologist if the eye becomes red, sensitive to light, painful, or develops a change in vision.

STORAGE: 2-8°C (36-46°F). Do not freeze. Protect from light. Store in the original carton until time of use.

LUMIGAN – bimatoprost

RX

Class: Prostaglandin analogue

ADULT DOSAGE

Elevated Intraocular Pressure

Open-Angle Glaucoma/Ocular HTN:
1 drop in the affected eye(s) qpm

PEDIATRIC DOSAGE

Elevated Intraocular Pressure

Open-Angle Glaucoma/Ocular HTN:
≥16 Years:
1 drop in the affected eye(s) qpm

DOSING CONSIDERATIONS

Concomitant Medications

Space dosing by at least 5 min if using >1 topical ophthalmic drug

L

ADMINISTRATION

Ocular route

HOW SUPPLIED

Sol: 0.01% [2.5mL, 5mL, 7.5mL]

WARNINGS/PRECAUTIONS

Changes to pigmented tissues, including increased pigmentation of iris (may be permanent), eyelid, and eyelashes (may be reversible) reported. Regularly examine patients with noticeably increased iris pigmentation. May cause changes to eyelashes and vellus hair in the treated eye. Intraocular inflammation reported; caution with active intraocular inflammation (eg, uveitis). Macular edema, including cystoid macular edema, reported; caution with aphakic patients, pseudophakic patients with a torn posterior lens capsule, or patients at risk of macular edema. Bacterial keratitis reported with multidose containers. Remove contact lenses prior to instillation; may reinsert 15 min after administration.

ADVERSE REACTIONS

Conjunctival hyperemia/edema/hemorrhage, eye irritation/pain/pruritus, reduced visual acuity, blurred vision, skin hyperpigmentation, eyelid erythema/pruritus, growth of eyelashes, hypertrichosis, instillation site irritation, punctate keratitis.

PATIENT CONSIDERATIONS

Assessment: Assess for active intraocular inflammation, risk of macular edema, contact lens use, and pregnancy/nursing status. Assess use in aphakic patients, and in pseudophakic patients with a torn posterior lens capsule.

Monitoring: Monitor for changes to pigmented tissue, changes in eyelashes and vellus hair, intraocular inflammation, exacerbation of intraocular inflammation, macular edema, bacterial keratitis, and other adverse reactions.

Counseling: Advise about the potential for increased brown pigmentation of iris (may be permanent) and the possibility of darkening of eyelid skin (may be reversible after discontinuation). Inform about the possibility of eyelash and vellus hair changes in the treated eye during treatment. Instruct to avoid touching tip of dispensing container to the eye, surrounding structures, fingers, or any other surface in order to avoid contamination of the sol. Advise to consult physician if having ocular surgery, if an intercurrent ocular condition (eg, trauma or infection) develops, or if any ocular reactions develop. Instruct to remove contact lenses prior to instillation and reinsert 15 min after administration. Instruct to administer at least 5 min apart if using more than 1 topical ophthalmic drug.

STORAGE: 2-25°C (36-77°F).

LUNESTA – eszopiclone

CIV

Class: Nonbenzodiazepine hypnotic agent

ADULT DOSAGE

Insomnia

Initial: 1mg immediately hs

Titrate: May increase to 2mg or 3mg if clinically indicated

Max: 3mg qd immediately hs

Use lowest effective dose

PEDIATRIC DOSAGE

Pediatric use may not have been established

DOSING CONSIDERATIONS

Concomitant Medications

Potent CYP3A4 Inhibitors:

Max: 2mg

Concomitant CNS Depressants: Dose adjustments may be necessary

Hepatic Impairment

Severe:

Max: 2mg

Elderly

Elderly/Debilitated:

Max: 2mg

ADMINISTRATION

Oral route

Take immediately hs with at least 7-8 hrs remaining before planned time of awakening

Do not administer with or immediately after a meal

HOW SUPPLIED

Tab: 1mg, 2mg, 3mg

CONTRAINDICATIONS

Known hypersensitivity to eszopiclone.

WARNINGS/PRECAUTIONS

May impair daytime function at the higher dose (2mg or 3mg), even when used as prescribed; monitor for excess depressant effects. May impair physical/mental abilities. Increased risk of next-day psychomotor impairment if taken with less than a full night of sleep remaining (7-8 hrs) or if higher than recommended dose is taken. Initiate only after careful evaluation; failure of insomnia to remit after 7-10 days of treatment may indicate presence of a primary psychiatric and/or medical illness. Use the lowest possible effective dose, especially in elderly. Severe anaphylactic/anaphylactoid reactions reported; do not rechallenge if angioedema develops. Abnormal thinking and behavioral changes (eg, bizarre behavior, agitation, hallucinations, depersonalization) reported. Amnesia and other neuropsychiatric symptoms may occur unpredictably. Worsening of depression, including suicidal thoughts and actions (including completed suicides), reported in primarily depressed patients. Complex behaviors (eg, sleep-driving) reported; consider discontinuation if a sleep-driving episode occurs. Withdrawal signs/symptoms reported following rapid dose decrease or abrupt discontinuation. Should be taken immediately hs; taking medication while still up and about may result in short-term memory impairment, hallucinations, impaired coordination, dizziness, and lightheadedness. Caution with severe hepatic impairment, elderly/debilitated patients, patients with diseases/conditions that could affect metabolism/hemodynamic responses, compromised respiratory function, history of alcohol/drug abuse, history of psychiatric disorders, and in patients exhibiting signs and symptoms of depression.

ADVERSE REACTIONS

Headache, unpleasant taste, somnolence, dry mouth, dizziness, infection, rash, pain, N/V, diarrhea, hallucinations, dyspepsia, nervousness, depression, anxiety.

DRUG INTERACTIONS

See Dosage. Not recommended with other sedative-hypnotics hs or in the middle of the night. Additive effects may occur with other CNS depressants (eg, benzodiazepines, opioids, TCAs, alcohol), including daytime use; consider downward dose adjustment of both drugs. Increased risk of next-day psychomotor impairment if coadministered with other CNS depressants and other drugs that increase blood levels of eszopiclone. Increased risk of complex behaviors with alcohol and other CNS depressants. May produce additive effect on psychomotor performance with ethanol. Decreased digit symbol substitution test scores with olanzapine. Decreased exposure and effects with CYP3A4 inducers (eg, rifampicin). Increased exposure with ketoconazole and other strong CYP3A4 inhibitors (eg, clarithromycin, nefazodone, ritonavir); dose reduction needed.

PATIENT CONSIDERATIONS

Assessment: Assess for psychiatric or physical disorder, depression, severe hepatic impairment, diseases/conditions that could affect metabolism/hemodynamic responses, compromised respiratory function, history of alcohol/drug abuse, history of psychiatric disorders, drug hypersensitivity, pregnancy/nursing status, and possible drug interactions.

Monitoring: Monitor for excessive depressant effects, anaphylactic/anaphylactoid reactions, emergence of any new behavioral signs/symptoms, withdrawal symptoms, abnormal thinking, and other adverse reactions.

Counseling: Inform of the risks and benefits of therapy. Inform that therapy may cause next-day impairment even when used as prescribed. Caution patients taking the 3mg dose against driving and other activities requiring complete mental alertness the day after use; inform that impairment may be present despite feeling fully awake. Advise to seek medical attention immediately if any adverse reactions (eg, severe anaphylactic/anaphylactoid reactions, sleep-driving, other complex behaviors) develop. Advise to immediately report any suicidal thoughts. Advise not to use therapy if patient drank alcohol that pm or hs.

STORAGE: 25°C (77°F); excursions permitted to 15-30°C (59-86°F).

Luvox CR – fluvoxamine maleate

RX

Class: Selective serotonin reuptake inhibitor (SSRI)

Antidepressants increased the risk of suicidal thinking and behavior (suicidality) in children, adolescents, and young adults in short-term studies of major depressive disorder and other psychiatric disorders. Monitor and observe closely for clinical worsening, suicidality, or unusual changes in behavior.

ADULT DOSAGE

Obsessive Compulsive Disorder

Initial: 100mg qhs

Titrate: Increase by 50mg every week, as tolerated, until max therapeutic benefit is achieved

Max: 300mg/day

Maint/Continuation of Extended Treatment:
Adjust to lowest effective dose; periodically reassess need for continued treatment

Dosing Considerations with MAOIs

Switching to/from an MAOI for Psychiatric Disorders:
Allow at least 14 days between discontinuation of an MAOI and initiation of treatment, and allow at least 14 days between discontinuation of treatment and initiation of an MAOI

W/ Other MAOIs (eg, Linezolid, IV Methylene Blue):
Do not start fluvoxamine in patients being treated w/ linezolid or IV methylene blue
In patients already receiving fluvoxamine, if acceptable alternatives are not available and benefits outweigh risks, d/c fluvoxamine and administer linezolid or IV methylene blue; monitor for serotonin syndrome for 2 weeks or until 24 hrs after the last dose of linezolid or IV methylene blue, whichever comes 1st. May resume fluvoxamine therapy 24 hrs after the last dose of linezolid or IV methylene blue

PEDIATRIC DOSAGE

Pediatric use may not have been established

DOSING CONSIDERATIONS

Hepatic Impairment
Titrate slowly

Elderly
Titrate slowly

Discontinuation
Gradually reduce dose whenever possible

If intolerable symptoms occur following a decrease in dose or upon discontinuation of treatment, may resume the previously prescribed dose; subsequently, may continue decreasing dose but at a more gradual rate

ADMINISTRATION

Oral route

Do not crush or chew caps

HOW SUPPLIED

Cap, Extended-Release: 100mg, 150mg

CONTRAINDICATIONS

Use of an MAOI for psychiatric disorders either concomitantly or within 14 days of stopping treatment. Treatment within 14 days of stopping an MAOI for psychiatric disorders. Starting treatment in patients being treated with MAOIs (eg, linezolid, IV methylene blue). Concomitant use of thioridazine, tizanidine, pimozide, alosetron, or ramelteon.

WARNINGS/PRECAUTIONS

Not approved for the treatment of bipolar depression. May precipitate mixed/manic episode in patients at risk for bipolar disorder; screen for risk of bipolar disorder prior to initiating therapy. Serotonin syndrome reported; d/c immediately and initiate supportive symptomatic treatment. Pupillary dilation that occurs following use may trigger an angle-closure attack in a patient with anatomically narrow angles who does not have a patent iridectomy. Adverse events reported upon discontinuation; gradually reduce dose. May increase risk of bleeding events. Activation of mania/hypomania reported. Avoid with unstable epilepsy and monitor patients with controlled epilepsy; d/c if seizures occur or seizure frequency increases. Hyponatremia may occur; caution in the elderly, volume-depleted patients, and patients taking a diuretic. Consider discontinuation in patients with symptomatic hyponatremia and institute appropriate medical intervention. Caution with diseases/conditions that affect metabolism or hemodynamic responses, and in pregnancy (3rd trimester).

ADVERSE REACTIONS

Insomnia, N/V, headache, somnolence, asthenia, diarrhea, anorexia, dizziness, abnormal ejaculation, dry mouth, dyspepsia, sweating, anxiety, tremor, decreased libido.

DRUG INTERACTIONS

See Contraindications. Inhibits several CYP450 enzymes that are known to be involved in metabolism of other drugs, such as CYP1A2 (eg, theophylline, propranolol, tizanidine), CYP3A4 (eg, alprazolam), CYP2C9 (eg, warfarin), and CYP2C19 (eg, omeprazole). Caution with CYP450 inhibitors (eg, quinidine), and in patients with reduced levels of CYP2D6 activity. Clinically significant interactions possible with drugs that have a narrow therapeutic ratio (eg, pimozide, omeprazole, phenytoin). Avoid with alcohol and diazepam. May increase levels of TCAs, carbamazepine, warfarin, clozapine, methadone, tacrine, propranolol, amitriptyline, clomipramine, or imipramine. Bradycardia reported with diltiazem. Orthostatic hypotension, hypotension, and bradycardia reported with metoprolol. May reduce clearance of mexiletine, theophylline, and benzodiazepines metabolized by hepatic oxidation (eg, alprazolam, midazolam, triazolam). Increased risk of bleeding with aspirin, NSAIDs, and other drugs that affect coagulation. May increase PT with warfarin; monitor PT and adjust dose of oral anticoagulants. Caution with lithium; may enhance serotonergic effects and cause seizures. May cause serotonin syndrome with other serotonergic drugs (eg, triptans, TCAs, fentanyl, tryptophan) and with drugs that impair metabolism of serotonin; d/c immediately if this occurs. Smoking increases metabolism. Refer to PI for dosing modifications when used with certain concomitant therapies.

PATIENT CONSIDERATIONS

Assessment: Assess for susceptibility to angle-closure glaucoma, risk/presence of bipolar disorder, volume depletion, history of mania, seizures, history of drug abuse, disease/condition that affects metabolism or hemodynamic response, hepatic impairment, pregnancy/nursing status, and possible drug interactions.

Monitoring: Monitor for signs/symptoms of clinical worsening, suicidality, unusual changes in behavior, serotonin syndrome, angle-closure glaucoma, bleeding events, hyponatremia, seizures, activation of mania/hypomania, discontinuation symptoms, hepatic dysfunction, and other adverse reactions. Monitor height and weight periodically in children. Monitor PT with warfarin and other oral anticoagulants. Periodically reassess the need for continued treatment.

Counseling: Inform of risks, benefits, and appropriate use of therapy. Counsel to be alert for the emergence of suicidality, unusual changes in behavior, or worsening of depression, especially early during treatment and when the dose is adjusted up or down; instruct to report such symptoms especially if severe, abrupt in onset, or not part of presenting symptoms. Advise to inform physician if taking or planning to take any prescription or OTC drugs. Advise that drug may increase the risk of bleeding events. Inform that drug may cause mild pupillary dilation, which in susceptible individuals, may lead to an episode of angle-closure glaucoma. Caution about operating hazardous machinery. Instruct to notify physician if pregnant, intending to become pregnant, or breastfeeding. Instruct to avoid alcohol. Advise to notify physician if allergic reactions develop during therapy.

STORAGE: Store at 25°C (77°F); excursions permitted to 15-30°C (59-86°F). Avoid exposure to >30°C (86°F). Protect from high humidity.

Luxiq — betamethasone valerate

RX

Class: Corticosteroid

ADULT DOSAGE

Inflammatory and Pruritic Manifestations of Corticosteroid-Responsive Dermatoses

Apply small amounts to affected scalp area bid (am and pm)

D/C when control is achieved

Reassess diagnosis if no improvement w/in 2 weeks

PEDIATRIC DOSAGE

Pediatric use may not have been established

ADMINISTRATION

Topical route

Avoid use w/ occlusive dressing unless directed

Application

Invert can and dispense a small amount of foam onto a saucer or other cool surface; do not dispense directly onto hands as foam will begin to melt immediately upon contact w/ warm skin

Pick up small amounts of foam w/ fingers and gently massage into affected area until foam disappears

Repeat until entire affected scalp area is treated

L

HOW SUPPLIED

Foam: 0.12% [50g, 100g]

CONTRAINDICATIONS

Hypersensitivity to betamethasone valerate, other corticosteroids, or to any ingredient in the preparation.

WARNINGS/PRECAUTIONS

Systemic absorption may produce reversible hypothalamic-pituitary-adrenal (HPA) axis suppression, manifestations of Cushing's syndrome, hyperglycemia, and glucosuria. Evaluate periodically for evidence of HPA axis suppression when applying to large surface area or to areas under occlusion; d/c treatment, reduce frequency of application, or substitute a less potent steroid if HPA axis suppression is noted. D/C and institute appropriate therapy if irritation develops. Use appropriate antifungal or antibacterial agent in the presence of dermatological infections; if favorable response does not occur promptly, d/c until infection is controlled. Pediatric patients may be more susceptible to systemic toxicity from equivalent doses.

ADVERSE REACTIONS

Application-site burning/itching/stinging.

PATIENT CONSIDERATIONS

Assessment: Assess for hypersensitivity to the drug, dermatological infections, and pregnancy/nursing status.

Monitoring: Monitor for signs/symptoms of HPA axis suppression, Cushing's syndrome, hyperglycemia, glucosuria, skin irritation, allergic contact dermatitis, and other adverse reactions. Monitor for signs of glucocorticosteroid insufficiency after withdrawal. Monitor clinical improvement; if no improvement seen within 2 weeks, reassess diagnosis.

Counseling: Advise to use externally and ud, to avoid contact with eyes, and not to use for any disorder other than that for which it was prescribed. Instruct not to bandage, cover, or wrap treated scalp area unless directed by physician. Advise to report any signs of local adverse reactions to physician. Advise to d/c use when control is achieved, and to notify physician if no improvement is seen within 2 weeks. Instruct to avoid fire, flame, or smoking during and immediately following application.

STORAGE: 20-25°C (68-77°F). Do not expose to heat or store at >49°C (120°F).

LYNPARZA – olaparib

RX

Class: PARP inhibitor

ADULT DOSAGE

Advanced Ovarian Cancer

Monotherapy in Patients w/ Deleterious/ Suspected Deleterious Germline BRCA Mutation Who Have Been Treated w/ ≥3 Prior Lines of Chemotherapy:

Usual: 400mg bid; continue until disease progression or unacceptable toxicity

Missed Dose

If patient misses a dose, instruct to take next dose at its scheduled time

PEDIATRIC DOSAGE

Pediatric use may not have been established

DOSING CONSIDERATIONS

Concomitant Medications

CYP3A Inhibitors:

Avoid concomitant use of strong/moderate inhibitors and consider alternatives w/ less CYP3A inhibition.

If Inhibitor Cannot Be Avoided:

Strong CYP3A Inhibitor: Reduce dose to 150mg bid

Moderate CYP3A Inhibitor: Reduce dose to 200mg bid

Adverse Reactions

To manage adverse reactions, consider dose interruption of treatment or dose reduction

Usual: 200mg bid; may reduce to 100mg bid if further dose reduction is required

ADMINISTRATION

Oral route

Swallow whole; do not chew, dissolve, or open

Do not take if cap appears deformed or shows evidence of leakage

HOW SUPPLIED

Cap: 50mg

WARNINGS/PRECAUTIONS

Myelodysplastic syndrome/acute myeloid leukemia (MDS/AML) reported. Do not start therapy until patients have recovered from hematological toxicity caused by previous chemotherapy (≤CTCAE Grade 1). For prolonged hematological toxicities, interrupt therapy and monitor blood counts weekly until recovery; if the levels have not recovered to ≤CTCAE Grade 1 after 4 weeks, refer to a hematologist for further investigations. D/C if MDS/AML is confirmed. Pneumonitis (including fatal cases) reported; interrupt treatment and initiate prompt investigation if new or worsening respiratory symptoms (eg, dyspnea, fever, cough, wheezing, radiological abnormality) occur. D/C if pneumonitis is confirmed. May cause fetal harm; avoid pregnancy while taking therapy. If contraceptive methods are being considered, use highly effective contraception during treatment and for at least 1 month following the last dose of therapy.

ADVERSE REACTIONS

Anemia, N/V, dyspepsia, abdominal pain/discomfort, decreased appetite, diarrhea, fatigue/asthenia, nasopharyngitis/URI, arthralgia/musculoskeletal pain, myalgia, lab abnormalities.

DRUG INTERACTIONS

Potentiation and prolongation of myelosuppressive toxicity w/ other myelosuppressive anticancer agents, including DNA damaging agents. Avoid w/ strong CYP3A inhibitors (eg, itraconazole, telithromycin, clarithromycin) and moderate CYP3A inhibitors (eg, amprenavir, ciprofloxacin, imatinib); if strong or moderate CYP3A inhibitors must be coadministered, reduce dose of olaparib. Avoid grapefruit and Seville oranges. Avoid w/ strong CYP3A inducers (eg, phenytoin, carbamazepine, St. John's wort) and moderate CYP3A4 inducers (eg, bosentan, efavirenz, modafinil); if a moderate CYP3A inducer cannot be avoided, be aware of a potential for decreased efficacy of olaparib.

PATIENT CONSIDERATIONS

Assessment: Assess pregnancy/nursing status, and for possible drug interactions. Assess for presence of deleterious or suspected deleterious germline BRCA-mutations. Obtain baseline CBC.

Monitoring: Monitor for MDS/AML, pneumonitis, and for other adverse reactions. For prolonged hematological toxicities, monitor blood counts weekly until recovery. Monitor CBC monthly.

Counseling: Instruct to take ud and to not take w/ grapefruit or Seville oranges. Advise to contact physician if experiencing any new or worsening respiratory symptoms, or signs of hematological

L

toxicity or MDS/AML. Instruct to inform physician if patient is pregnant or becomes pregnant. Inform female patients of the risk to a fetus and potential loss of pregnancy. Advise females of reproductive potential to use effective contraception during therapy and for at least 1 month after receiving the last dose. Advise not to breastfeed while on therapy. Counsel that mild or moderate N/V is very common in patients receiving olaparib and that patients should contact their physician who will advise on available antiemetic treatment options.

STORAGE: 25°C (77°F); excursions permitted to 15-30°C (59-86°F). Do not expose to >40°C (104°F); do not take the drug if it is suspected of having been exposed to >40°C (104°F).

LYRICA – pregabalin CV

Class: GABA analogue

ADULT DOSAGE

Neuropathic Pain

Associated w/ Diabetic Peripheral Neuropathy:
Initial: 50mg tid (150mg/day)
Titrate: May increase to 300mg/day w/in 1 week prn
Max: 100mg tid (300mg/day)

Associated w/ Spinal Cord Injury:
Initial: 75mg bid
Titrate: May increase to 150mg bid (300mg/day) w/in 1 week prn
Max: 300mg bid (600mg/day) if no sufficient pain relief experienced following 2-3 weeks of treatment w/ 150mg bid

Postherpetic Neuralgia

Initial: 75mg bid or 50mg tid (150mg/day)
Titrate: May increase to 300mg/day w/in 1 week prn
Max: 600mg/day divided bid or tid if no sufficient pain relief experienced following 2-4 weeks of treatment w/ 300mg/day

Partial Onset Seizures

Adjunctive Therapy:
Initial: 150mg/day divided bid-tid
Titrate: May increase up to max dose of 600mg/day

Fibromyalgia

Initial: 75mg bid
Titrate: May increase to 150mg bid (300mg/day) w/in 1 week prn
Max: 225mg bid (450mg/day)

PEDIATRIC DOSAGE

Pediatric use may not have been established

DOSING CONSIDERATIONS

Renal Impairment

Recommended Dose of 150mg/day BID or TID w/ Normal Renal Function:
CrCl 30-60mL/min: 75mg/day bid or tid
CrCl 15-30mL/min: 25-50mg/day qd or bid
CrCl <15mL/min: 25mg/day qd

Recommended Dose of 300mg/day BID or TID w/ Normal Renal Function:
CrCl 30-60mL/min: 150mg/day bid or tid
CrCl 15-30mL/min: 75mg/day qd or bid
CrCl <15mL/min: 25-50mg/day qd

Recommended Dose of 450mg/day BID or TID w/ Normal Renal Function:
CrCl 30-60mL/min: 225mg/day bid or tid
CrCl 15-30mL/min: 100-150mg/day qd or bid
CrCl <15mL/min: 50-75mg/day qd

Recommended Dose of 600mg/day BID or TID w/ Normal Renal Function:
CrCl 30-60mL/min: 300mg/day bid or tid
CrCl 15-30mL/min: 150mg/day qd or bid
CrCl <15mL/min: 75mg/day qd

Hemodialysis:
25mg qd Regimen: Take 1 supplemental dose of 25mg or 50mg
25-50mg qd Regimen: Take 1 supplemental dose of 50mg or 75mg
50-75mg qd Regimen: Take 1 supplemental dose of 75mg or 100mg
75mg qd Regimen: Take 1 supplemental dose of 100mg or 150mg

Discontinuation
Taper over minimum of 1 week

ADMINISTRATION
Oral route

HOW SUPPLIED
Cap: 25mg, 50mg, 75mg, 100mg, 150mg, 200mg, 225mg, 300mg; **Sol:** 20mg/mL [16 fl oz]

CONTRAINDICATIONS
Known hypersensitivity to pregabalin or any of its components.

WARNINGS/PRECAUTIONS
Angioedema reported; d/c immediately if symptoms of angioedema with respiratory compromise occur. Caution in patients who had a previous episode of angioedema. Hypersensitivity reactions reported; d/c immediately if symptoms occur. Avoid abrupt withdrawal; gradually taper over a minimum of 1 week. Increased risk of suicidal thoughts/behavior; monitor for emergence or worsening of depression, suicidal thought/behavior, and/or unusual changes in mood/behavior. May cause weight gain and peripheral edema; caution with CHF. May cause dizziness and somnolence; may impair physical/mental abilities. New or worsening of preexisting tumors reported. Blurred vision, decreased visual acuity, visual field changes, and funduscopic changes reported. Creatine kinase (CK) elevations and rhabdomyolysis reported; d/c if myopathy is diagnosed or suspected or if markedly elevated CK levels occur. Associated with a decrease in platelet counts and PR interval prolongation. Caution in patients with renal impairment.

ADVERSE REACTIONS
Somnolence, dizziness, peripheral edema, ataxia, weight gain, dry mouth, fatigue, asthenia, blurred vision, diplopia, edema, nasopharyngitis, constipation, abnormal thinking, tremor.

DRUG INTERACTIONS
May increase risk of angioedema with other drugs associated with angioedema (eg, ACE inhibitors). Additive effects on cognitive and gross motor functioning with oxycodone, lorazepam, and ethanol. Caution with thiazolidinedione class of antidiabetic drugs; higher frequencies of weight gain and peripheral edema reported. Gabapentin reported to cause a small reduction in absorption rate. Reduced lower GI tract function (eg, intestinal obstruction, paralytic ileus, constipation) reported with medications that have the potential to produce constipation, such as opioid analgesics.

PATIENT CONSIDERATIONS

Assessment: Assess for hypersensitivity, renal impairment, preexisting tumors, history of drug abuse, history of depression, previous episode of angioedema, CHF, pregnancy/nursing status, and possible drug interactions. Obtain baseline weight.

Monitoring: Monitor for angioedema, hypersensitivity reactions, peripheral edema, weight gain, new tumors or worsening of preexisting tumors, ophthalmological effects, rhabdomyolysis, dizziness, somnolence, emergence or worsening of depression, suicidal thoughts or behavior, and/or changes in behavior. Monitor CK levels and platelet counts. Monitor ECG for PR interval prolongation.

Counseling: Instruct to d/c therapy and seek medical attention if hypersensitivity reactions or symptoms of angioedema occur. Inform patients and caregivers to be alert for the emergence or worsening of depression, unusual changes in mood or behavior, or the emergence of suicidal thoughts or behavior; immediately report behaviors of concern to physician. Counsel that dizziness, somnolence, blurred vision, and other CNS signs and symptoms may occur; advise to use caution when operating machinery/driving. Inform that weight gain and edema may occur. Instruct not to abruptly/rapidly d/c therapy. Instruct to report unexplained muscle pain, tenderness, or weakness, particularly if accompanied by malaise or fever, to physician. Instruct not to consume alcohol while on therapy. Instruct to notify physician if pregnant, intending to become pregnant, breastfeeding or intending to breastfeed. Inform men on therapy who plan to father a child of the potential risk of male-mediated teratogenicity. Instruct diabetic patients to pay attention to skin integrity while on therapy.

STORAGE: 25°C (77°F); excursions permitted to 15-30°C (59-86°F).

M-M-R II – measles, mumps, and rubella virus vaccine live RX

Class: Vaccine

ADULT DOSAGE

Measles, Mumps, and Rubella Vaccine

0.5mL SQ

Refer to PI for vaccination considerations

PEDIATRIC DOSAGE

Measles, Mumps, and Rubella Vaccine

≥12 Months of Age:

0.5mL SQ; recommended age for primary vaccination is 12-15 months; revaccinate prior to elementary school entry

If vaccinated when <12 months of age, give another dose between 12-15 months of age followed by revaccination before elementary school entry

Refer to PI for measles outbreak schedule and other vaccination considerations

ADMINISTRATION

SQ route

Inject preferably into the outer aspect of upper arm.
A 25-gauge, 5/8" needle is recommended.

Reconstitution

1. Use only diluent supplied.
2. Withdraw entire volume of diluent into syringe to be used for reconstitution.
3. Inject all diluent in syringe into vial of lyophilized vaccine; agitate to mix thoroughly.
4. Withdraw entire contents into a syringe and inject total volume of restored vaccine SQ.

HOW SUPPLIED

Inj: 0.5mL

CONTRAINDICATIONS

Hypersensitivity to any component of the vaccine (including gelatin), pregnancy, anaphylactic/anaphylactoid reactions to neomycin, febrile respiratory illness or other active febrile infection, immunosuppressive therapy (except corticosteroids as replacement therapy), blood dyscrasias, leukemia, lymphomas of any type, malignant neoplasms affecting bone marrow or lymphatic systems, primary and acquired immunodeficiency states (including immunosuppression associated w/ AIDS or other clinical manifestations of HIV infection, cellular immune deficiencies, hypogammaglobulinemic and dysgammaglobulinemic states), family history of congenital or hereditary immunodeficiency.

WARNINGS/PRECAUTIONS

Caution w/ history of cerebral injury, individual or family histories of convulsions or any other condition in which stress due to fever should be avoided. Extreme caution w/ history of anaphylactic/anaphylactoid, or other immediate reactions (eg, hives, swelling of mouth and throat, difficulty breathing, hypotension, shock) subsequent to egg ingestion; may be at an enhanced risk of immediate-type hypersensitivity reactions. Neomycin allergy often manifests as a contact dermatitis; a history of contact dermatitis to neomycin is not a contraindication. Severe thrombocytopenia may develop in individuals w/ current thrombocytopenia; individuals who experienced thrombocytopenia w/ 1st dose may also develop thrombocytopenia w/ repeat doses. Evaluate serologic status to determine need for additional doses. Have adequate treatment provisions, including epinephrine inj (1:1000), available for immediate use should an anaphylactic/anaphylactoid reaction occur. HIV infected children and young adults who are not immunosuppressed may be vaccinated, but vaccine may be less effective than for uninfected persons; monitor closely for vaccine-preventable diseases. Ensure that inj does not enter a blood vessel. Excretion of small amounts of the live attenuated rubella virus from the nose or throat 7-28 days after vaccination reported. Avoid w/ active untreated tuberculosis (TB). May not result in protection in 100% of vaccinees. Persons vaccinated w/ inactivated vaccine followed w/in 3 months by live vaccine should be revaccinated w/ 2 doses of live vaccine. May result in temporary depression of tuberculin skin sensitivity; administer tuberculin test either before or simultaneously w/ vaccine.

ADVERSE REACTIONS

Panniculitis, atypical measles, fever, syncope, headache, dizziness, malaise, diarrhea, N/V, irritability, arthralgia, arthritis, pneumonia, sore throat, Stevens-Johnson syndrome.

DRUG INTERACTIONS

See Contraindications. Do not give w/ immune globulin (IG); may interfere w/ expected immune response. Give vaccine 1 month before or after administration of other live viral vaccines. Defer vaccination for ≥3 months following administration of IG (human), or blood/plasma transfusions. Concurrent administration w/ diphtheria, tetanus, pertussis (DTP), and/or oral poliovirus vaccines is not recommended.

PATIENT CONSIDERATIONS

Assessment: Assess for hypersensitivity to any component of the vaccine, current health/medical status, vaccination history, thrombocytopenia, active untreated TB, any other conditions where treatment is contraindicated or cautioned, pregnancy/nursing status, and possible drug interactions.

Monitoring: Monitor for anaphylactic/anaphylactoid reactions, thrombocytopenia, vaccine-preventable diseases in HIV patients, and other adverse reactions.

Counseling: Inform of benefits/risks of vaccination. Instruct to report any serious adverse reactions. Instruct to avoid pregnancy for 3 months after vaccination and inform of the reasons for this precaution.

STORAGE: Protect from light. **Unreconstituted Vaccine:** -50 to +8°C (-58 to +46°F). **Before Reconstitution:** 2-8°C (36-46°F). May refrigerate diluent or store separately at room temperature; do not freeze diluent. **Reconstituted Vaccine:** 2-8°C (36-46°F) in a dark place; discard if not used w/in 8 hrs.

MACROBID – nitrofurantoin macrocrystals/nitrofurantoin monohydrate RX

Class: Imidazolidinedione antibacterial

ADULT DOSAGE

Urinary Tract Infections

Caused by susceptible strains of *Escherichia coli* or *Staphylococcus saprophyticus*

Acute Uncomplicated (Acute Cystitis): 100mg q12h for 7 days

PEDIATRIC DOSAGE

Urinary Tract Infections

Caused by susceptible strains of *Escherichia coli* or *Staphylococcus saprophyticus*

>12 Years:

Acute Uncomplicated (Acute Cystitis): 100mg q12h for 7 days

ADMINISTRATION

Oral route

Take with food

HOW SUPPLIED

Cap: 100mg

CONTRAINDICATIONS

Anuria, oliguria, significant impairment of renal function (CrCl <60mL/min or clinically significant elevated SrCr), pregnancy at term (38-42 weeks' gestation), during labor and delivery or when onset of labor is imminent, and neonates <1 month of age, previous history of cholestatic jaundice/hepatic dysfunction associated w/ nitrofurantoin, known hypersensitivity to nitrofurantoin.

WARNINGS/PRECAUTIONS

Not for treatment of pyelonephritis or perinephric abscesses. Many patients who undergo treatment are predisposed to persistence/reappearance of bacteriuria; if this occurs after treatment, select other therapeutic agents with broader tissue distribution. Acute, subacute, or chronic pulmonary reactions (diffuse interstitial pneumonitis, pulmonary fibrosis, or both) reported; d/c and take appropriate measures if these occur. Closely monitor pulmonary condition if on long-term therapy. Hepatic reactions (eg, hepatitis, cholestatic jaundice, chronic active hepatitis, hepatic necrosis) occur rarely. Monitor periodically for changes in biochemical tests that would indicate liver injury; withdraw immediately and take appropriate measures if hepatitis occurs. Peripheral neuropathy, which may become severe or irreversible, reported; risk may be enhanced with renal impairment, anemia, diabetes mellitus (DM), electrolyte imbalance, vitamin B deficiency, and debilitating disease. Monitor periodically for renal function changes with long-term therapy. Optic neuritis reported rarely. May induce hemolytic anemia of the primaquine-sensitivity type; d/c therapy if hemolysis occurs. *Clostridium difficile*-associated diarrhea (CDAD) reported; d/c therapy is CDAD is suspected/confirmed. Use in the absence of a proven or strongly suspected bacterial infection or prophylactic indication is unlikely to provide benefit and increases the risk of the development of drug-resistant bacteria. Lab test interactions may occur. Caution with impaired renal function and in elderly.

ADVERSE REACTIONS

Nausea, headache.

DRUG INTERACTIONS

Antacids containing magnesium trisilicate reduce both the rate and extent of absorption. Uricosuric drugs (eg, probenecid, sulfinpyrazone) may inhibit renal tubular secretion of nitrofurantoin; resulting increased nitrofurantoin serum levels may increase toxicity, and the decreased urinary levels could lessen its efficacy.

PATIENT CONSIDERATIONS

Assessment: Assess for anuria, oliguria, significant renal impairment, history of cholestatic jaundice/hepatic dysfunction associated with nitrofurantoin, G6PD deficiency, DM, anemia, electrolyte imbalance, vitamin B deficiency, debilitating disease, drug hypersensitivity, pregnancy/nursing status, and possible drug interactions. Obtain urine specimens for culture and susceptibility testing prior to therapy.

Monitoring: Monitor for persistence or reappearance of bacteriuria, acute/subacute/chronic pulmonary reactions, hepatic reactions, peripheral neuropathy, optic neuritis, hematologic manifestations, and CDAD. Monitor LFTs periodically. Monitor renal and pulmonary function periodically during long-term therapy. Obtain urine specimens for culture and susceptibility testing after completion of therapy.

Counseling: Inform of the potential risks and benefits of therapy. Advise to take with food (ideally breakfast and dinner) to further enhance tolerance and improve drug absorption. Instruct to complete the full course of therapy and advise to contact physician if any unusual symptoms occur during therapy. Advise not to take antacids containing magnesium trisilicate while on therapy. Inform that therapy treats bacterial, not viral, infections. Advise to take exactly ud; skipping doses or not completing full course may decrease effectiveness and increase drug resistance. Inform that diarrhea is a common problem that usually ends when antibiotic is discontinued. Inform that watery and bloody stools (with/without stomach cramps and fever) may develop even as late as 2 or more months after having taken the last dose; instruct to contact physician as soon as possible if this occurs.

STORAGE: 15-30°C (59-86°F).

MACRODANTIN — nitrofurantoin macrocrystals

RX

Class: Imidazolidinedione antibacterial

M

ADULT DOSAGE

Urinary Tract Infections

Due to susceptible *Escherichia coli*, enterococci, *Staphylococcus aureus*, and certain susceptible *Klebsiella* and *Enterobacter* species

50-100mg qid for 1 week or for at least 3 days after sterility of the urine obtained

Long-Term Suppressive Therapy:
Reduce dose to 50-100mg qhs

PEDIATRIC DOSAGE

Urinary Tract Infections

Due to susceptible *Escherichia coli*, enterococci, *Staphylococcus aureus*, and certain susceptible *Klebsiella* and *Enterobacter* species

≥1 Month of Age:
5-7mg/kg/day given in 4 divided doses for 1 week or for at least 3 days after sterility of the urine obtained

Long-Term Suppressive Therapy:
1mg/kg/day given in a single dose or in 2 divided doses

ADMINISTRATION

Oral route

Take with food

HOW SUPPLIED

Cap: 25mg, 50mg, 100mg

CONTRAINDICATIONS

Anuria, oliguria, significant impairment of renal function (CrCl <60mL/min or clinically significant elevated SrCr), pregnancy at term (38-42 weeks' gestation), during labor and delivery, or when the onset of labor is imminent, neonates <1 month of age, previous history of cholestatic jaundice/hepatic dysfunction associated w/ nitrofurantoin, known hypersensitivity to nitrofurantoin.

WARNINGS/PRECAUTIONS

Not for the treatment of pyelonephritis or perinephric abscesses. Many patients who undergo treatment are predisposed to persistence/reappearance of bacteriuria; if this occurs after treatment, select other therapeutic agents with broader tissue distribution. Acute, subacute, or chronic pulmonary reactions (diffuse interstitial pneumonitis, pulmonary fibrosis, or both) reported; d/c and take appropriate measures if these occur. Closely monitor pulmonary condition if on long-term therapy. Hepatic reactions (eg, hepatitis, cholestatic jaundice, chronic active hepatitis, hepatic necrosis) occur rarely. Monitor periodically for changes in biochemical tests that would indicate liver injury; withdraw immediately and take appropriate measures if hepatitis occurs. Peripheral neuropathy, which may become severe or irreversible, reported; risk may be enhanced with renal impairment, anemia, diabetes mellitus (DM), electrolyte imbalance, vitamin B deficiency, and debilitating disease. Monitor periodically for renal function changes with long-term therapy.

Optic neuritis reported rarely. May induced hemolytic anemia of the primaquine-sensitivity type; d/c therapy if hemolysis occurs. *Clostridium difficile*-associated diarrhea (CDAD) reported; d/c therapy if CDAD is suspected/confirmed. Use in the absence of a proven or strongly suspected bacterial infection or prophylactic indication is unlikely to provide benefit and increases the risk of the development of drug-resistant bacteria. Lab test interactions may occur. Caution with impaired renal function and in elderly.

ADVERSE REACTIONS

Pulmonary hypersensitivity reactions, hepatic reactions, peripheral neuropathy, exfoliative dermatitis, erythema multiforme, lupus-like syndrome, nausea, emesis, anorexia, asthenia, vertigo, nystagmus, dizziness, headache, drowsiness.

DRUG INTERACTIONS

Antacids containing magnesium trisilicate reduce both the rate and extent of absorption. Uricosuric drugs (eg, probenecid, sulfinpyrazone) may inhibit renal tubular secretion of nitrofurantoin; resulting increased nitrofurantoin serum levels may increase toxicity, and the decreased urinary levels could lessen its efficacy.

PATIENT CONSIDERATIONS

Assessment: Assess for anuria, oliguria, significant renal impairment, history of cholestatic jaundice/hepatic dysfunction associated with nitrofurantoin, G6PD deficiency, DM, anemia, electrolyte imbalance, vitamin B deficiency, debilitating disease, drug hypersensitivity, pregnancy/nursing status, and possible drug interactions. Obtain urine specimen for culture and susceptibility testing prior to therapy.

Monitoring: Monitor for persistence or reappearance of bacteriuria, acute/subacute/chronic pulmonary reactions, hepatic reactions, peripheral neuropathy, optic neuritis, hematologic manifestations, and CDAD. Monitor LFTs periodically. Monitor renal and pulmonary function periodically during long-term therapy. Obtain urine specimens for culture and susceptibility testing after completion of therapy.

Counseling: Inform of the potential risks and benefits of therapy. Advise to take with food to further enhance tolerance and improve drug absorption. Instruct to complete full course of therapy and advise to contact physician if any unusual symptoms occur during therapy. Advise not to take antacid preparations containing magnesium trisilicate while on therapy. Inform that therapy treats bacterial, not viral, infections. Advise to take exactly ud; skipping doses or not completing full course may decrease effectiveness and increase drug resistance. Inform that diarrhea is a common problem that usually ends when antibiotic is discontinued. Inform that watery and bloody stools (with/without stomach cramps and fever) may develop even as late as ≥2 months after having taken the last dose; instruct to contact physician as soon as possible if this occurs.

STORAGE: 20-25°C (68-77°F).

M

MALARONE – atovaquone/proguanil hydrochloride

RX

Class: Antiprotozoal agent/dihydrofolate reductase inhibitor

OTHER BRAND NAMES

Malarone Pediatric

ADULT DOSAGE

Malaria

Prophylaxis of *Plasmodium falciparum* Malaria, Including in Areas Resistant to Chloroquine:

1 adult strength tab (250mg/100mg) qd; start 1 or 2 days before entering a malaria-endemic area and continue daily during stay and for 7 days after return

Treatment of Acute, Uncomplicated *P. falciparum* Malaria:

4 adult strength tabs (1g/400mg) qd for 3 consecutive days

PEDIATRIC DOSAGE

Malaria

Prophylaxis of *Plasmodium falciparum* Malaria, Including in Areas Resistant to Chloroquine:

11-20kg:

1 pediatric tab (62.5mg/25mg) qd

21-30kg:

2 pediatric tabs (125mg/50mg) qd

31-40kg:

3 pediatric tabs (187.5mg/75mg) qd

>40kg:

1 adult strength tab (250mg/100mg) qd

Start 1 or 2 days before entering a malaria-endemic area and continue daily during stay and for 7 days after return

Treatment of Acute, Uncomplicated *P. falciparum* Malaria:

5-8kg:

2 pediatric tabs (125mg/50mg) qd

9-10kg:
3 pediatric tabs (187.5mg/75mg) qd
11-20kg:
1 adult strength tab (250mg/100mg) qd
21-30kg:
2 adult strength tabs (500mg/200mg) qd
31-40kg:
3 adult strength tabs (750mg/300mg) qd
>40kg:
4 adult strength tabs (1g/400mg) qd
Treat for 3 consecutive days

ADMINISTRATION
Oral route

Take at the same time each day w/ food or a milky drink
Repeat dose in the event of vomiting w/in 1 hr after dosing
May crush and mix w/ condensed milk just prior to administration for patients who may have difficulty swallowing tabs

HOW SUPPLIED
Tab: (Atovaquone/Proguanil) 250mg/100mg (adult), 62.5mg/25mg (pediatric)

CONTRAINDICATIONS
Known hypersensitivity reactions to atovaquone or proguanil hydrochloride or any component of the formulation. For prophylaxis in patients w/ severe renal impairment (CrCl <30mL/min).

WARNINGS/PRECAUTIONS
Reduced atovaquone absorption in patients with diarrhea or vomiting; monitor for parasitemia and consider use of an antiemetic if vomiting occurs. Alternative antimalarial therapy may be required in patients with severe or persistent diarrhea or vomiting. In mixed *P. falciparum* and *Plasmodium vivax* infections, *P. vivax* parasite relapse occurred commonly when patients were treated with atovaquone-proguanil alone. Treat with a different blood schizonticide in the event of recrudescent *P. falciparum* infections after treatment or failure of chemoprophylaxis. Elevated liver lab tests and cases of hepatitis and hepatic failure requiring liver transplantation reported with prophylactic use. Patients with severe malaria are not candidates for oral therapy. Caution for the treatment of malaria in patients with severe renal impairment. Caution in elderly.

M

ADVERSE REACTIONS
Abdominal pain, headache, N/V, diarrhea, asthenia, anorexia, dizziness, dreams, insomnia, oral ulcers, cough, pruritus.

DRUG INTERACTIONS
Atovaquone: Decreased levels with rifampin or rifabutin; not recommended with rifampin or rifabutin. Decreased levels with tetracycline; monitor for parasitemia. Reduced bioavailability with metoclopramide; use only if other antiemetics are not available. Decreased indinavir trough concentrations; use caution. Proguanil: May potentiate anticoagulant effect of warfarin and other coumarin-based anticoagulants; use caution when initiating or withdrawing in patients on continuous treatment with coumarin-based anticoagulants, and closely monitor coagulation tests with concomitant use.

PATIENT CONSIDERATIONS

Assessment: Assess for severity of malaria, drug hypersensitivity, renal dysfunction, diarrhea, vomiting, pregnancy/nursing status, and possible drug interactions.

Monitoring: Monitor for clinical response, N/V, diarrhea, hepatic/renal dysfunction, hypersensitivity, and other adverse reactions. Monitor parasitemia in patients who are vomiting. Monitor for relapse of infection when patients are treated with atovaquone-proguanil alone. Closely monitor coagulation tests when concomitant use with warfarin and other coumarin-based anticoagulants.

Counseling: Instruct that if a dose is missed, to take a dose as soon as possible and then to return to normal dosing schedule. Advise not to double the next dose if a dose is skipped. Counsel about serious adverse events associated with therapy (eg, hepatitis, severe skin reactions, neurological and hematological events). Instruct to consult physician regarding alternative forms of prophylaxis if prophylaxis is prematurely discontinued for any reason. Inform that protective clothing, insect repellents, and bednets are important components of malaria prophylaxis. Instruct to seek medical attention for any febrile illness that occurs during or after return from a malaria-endemic area. Discuss with pregnant women anticipating travel to malarious areas about the risks/benefits of such travel.

STORAGE: 25°C (77°F); excursions permitted to 15-30°C (59-86°F).

Mavik – trandolapril

RX

Class: ACE inhibitor

D/C when pregnancy is detected. Drugs that act directly on the renin-angiotensin system (RAS) can cause injury/death to the developing fetus.

ADULT DOSAGE

Hypertension

Not Receiving Diuretics:
Initial:
1mg qd in nonblack patients
2mg qd in black patients
Titrate: Adjust dose at intervals of at least 1 week based on BP response
Usual: 2-4mg qd

May treat w/ bid dosing if inadequately treated w/ 4mg qd
May add diuretic if not adequately controlled

Receiving Diuretics:
If possible d/c diuretic 2-3 days prior to therapy to avoid hypotension. If BP is not controlled w/ trandolapril alone, then diuretic therapy should be resumed
Initial: 0.5mg
Titrate: Adjust to the optimal response

Heart Failure Post-Myocardial Infarction

Initial: 1mg qd
Titrate: Increase to target dose of 4mg qd as tolerated
If not tolerated, continue w/ the greatest tolerated dose

Left Ventricular Dysfunction Post-Myocardial Infarction

Initial: 1mg qd
Titrate: Increase to target dose of 4mg qd as tolerated
If not tolerated, continue w/ the greatest tolerated dose

PEDIATRIC DOSAGE

Pediatric use may not have been established

DOSING CONSIDERATIONS

Renal Impairment
CrCl <30mL/min:
Initial: 0.5mg qd
Titrate: Adjust to optimal response

Hepatic Impairment
Cirrhosis:
Initial: 0.5mg qd
Titrate: Adjust to optimal response

ADMINISTRATION

Oral route

HOW SUPPLIED

Tab: 1mg*, 2mg, 4mg *scored

CONTRAINDICATIONS

Hypersensitivity to this product, hereditary/idiopathic angioedema, history of ACE inhibitor-associated angioedema. Coadministration w/ aliskiren in patients w/ diabetes.

WARNINGS/PRECAUTIONS

Anaphylactoid reactions reported during desensitization w/ hymenoptera venom, dialysis w/ high-flux membranes, and LDL apheresis w/ dextran sulfate absorption. Angioedema reported; d/c, treat appropriately, and monitor until swelling disappears if laryngeal stridor or angioedema of the face, tongue, or glottis occurs. Intestinal angioedema reported; monitor for abdominal pain. Higher rate of angioedema in blacks than nonblacks. Symptomatic hypotension may occur w/ volume and/or salt depletion, major surgery, or during anesthesia. Excessive hypotension associated w/ oliguria and/or azotemia, and rarely w/ acute renal failure and/or death, may occur in patients

M

w/ CHF; monitor during first 2 weeks of therapy and w/ dosage increases. Caution w/ ischemic heart disease, aortic stenosis, or cerebrovascular disease; avoid hypotension. Consider lower doses of drug or concomitant diuretic if transient hypotension occurs. May cause agranulocytosis and bone marrow depression; consider periodic monitoring of WBCs in patients w/ collagen vascular disease (eg, systemic lupus erythematosus, scleroderma) and/or renal disease. Rarely associated w/ syndrome of cholestatic jaundice, fulminant hepatic necrosis, and death; d/c if jaundice develops. May cause changes in renal function. Increases in BUN and SrCr reported; dosage reduction and/or discontinuation may be required. Hyperkalemia reported; caution w/ renal insufficiency and diabetes mellitus (DM). Persistent nonproductive cough reported.

ADVERSE REACTIONS

Cough, dizziness, hypotension, elevated serum uric acid, elevated BUN, dyspepsia, syncope, hyperkalemia, bradycardia, hypocalcemia, myalgia, elevated creatinine, gastritis, cardiogenic shock, intermittent claudication.

DRUG INTERACTIONS

See Contraindications. Dual blockade of the RAS is associated w/ increased risks of hypotension, hyperkalemia, and changes in renal function (including acute renal failure); closely monitor BP, renal function, and electrolytes w/ concomitant agents that also affect the RAS. Avoid w/ aliskiren in patients w/ renal impairment (GFR <60mL/min). Excessive BP reduction reported w/ diuretics. K^+-sparing diuretics (spironolactone, triamterene, amiloride), K^+ supplements, or K^+-containing salt substitutes may increase risk of hyperkalemia; use w/ caution and monitor serum K^+. May increase blood glucose lowering effect of antidiabetic medications (insulin, oral hypoglycemic agents). Increased lithium levels and symptoms of lithium toxicity reported; use w/ caution and frequently monitor serum lithium levels. Increased risk of lithium toxicity if a diuretic is also used. Coadministration w/ NSAIDs, including selective COX-2 inhibitors, may result in deterioration of renal function; monitor renal function periodically. Antihypertensive effect may be attenuated by NSAIDs. Nitritoid reactions (eg, facial flushing, N/V, hypotension) reported rarely w/ injectable gold. May enhance hypotensive effect of certain inhalation anesthetics.

PATIENT CONSIDERATIONS

Assessment: Assess for hereditary/idiopathic angioedema, history of ACE inhibitor-associated angioedema, volume/salt depletion, CHF, ischemic heart disease, aortic stenosis, cerebrovascular disease, collagen vascular disease, DM, renal/hepatic impairment, hypersensitivity to the drug, pregnancy/nursing status, and possible drug interactions.

Monitoring: Monitor for anaphylactoid reactions, angioedema, hypotension, jaundice, hyperkalemia, cough, and other adverse reactions. Consider periodic monitoring of WBCs in patients w/ collagen vascular disease and/or renal disease. Monitor BP and renal/hepatic function.

Counseling: Advise to d/c and to consult physician if any signs/symptoms of angioedema (eg, swelling of the face, extremities, eyes, lips, or tongue, or difficulty in swallowing or breathing) develop or if syncope occurs. Inform that lightheadedness may occur, especially during the 1st days of therapy; instruct to report to physician if this occurs. Inform that inadequate fluid intake, excessive perspiration, diarrhea, or vomiting may lead to an excessive fall in BP w/ the same consequences of lightheadedness and possible syncope. Advise to inform physician of therapy prior to surgery and/or anesthesia. Advise not to use K^+ supplements or salt substitutes containing K^+ w/o consulting physician. Instruct to immediately report any signs/symptoms of infection (eg, sore throat, fever). Inform females of childbearing age about the consequences of exposure during pregnancy. Instruct to report pregnancy to physician as soon as possible.

STORAGE: 20-25°C (68-77°F).

MAXALT — rizatriptan benzoate

RX

Class: 5-$HT_{1B/1D}$ agonist (triptans)

OTHER BRAND NAMES

Maxalt-MLT

ADULT DOSAGE

Migraine

W/ or w/o Aura:

Initial: 5mg or 10mg single dose; separate repeat doses by at least 2 hrs if migraine returns

Max: 30mg/24 hrs

PEDIATRIC DOSAGE

Migraine

W/ or w/o Aura:

6-17 Years:

<40kg: 5mg single dose

≥40kg: 10mg single dose

DOSING CONSIDERATIONS

Concomitant Medications

Propranolol:

6-17 Years:

≥40kg:

5mg single dose

Max: 5mg/24 hrs

≥18 Years:

5mg single dose

Max: 3 doses/24 hrs

Elderly

Start at lower end of dosing range

ADMINISTRATION

Oral route

Tab, Disintegrating

Do not remove blister from outer pouch until just prior to dosing

Peel open w/ dry hands and place tab on tongue, where it will dissolve and be swallowed w/ saliva

HOW SUPPLIED

Tab: 5mg, 10mg; **Tab, Disintegrating:** (MLT) 5mg, 10mg

CONTRAINDICATIONS

Ischemic coronary artery disease (CAD) (angina pectoris, history of MI, or documented silent ischemia) or other significant underlying cardiovascular (CV) disease, coronary artery vasospasm (eg, Prinzmetal's angina), history of stroke or transient ischemic attack (TIA), peripheral vascular disease (PVD), ischemic bowel disease, uncontrolled HTN, hemiplegic/basilar migraine. Recent use (within 24 hrs) of another 5-HT_1 agonist or ergotamine-containing/ergot-type medication (eg, dihydroergotamine, methysergide). Concurrent use or recent discontinuation (within 2 weeks) of an MAO-A inhibitor. Hypersensitivity to rizatriptan benzoate.

WARNINGS/PRECAUTIONS

Use only when diagnosis of migraine has been clearly established. If no response after the 1st migraine attack, reconsider diagnosis before treating subsequent attacks. Not indicated for prevention of migraine attacks. Serious cardiac adverse reactions, including acute MI, reported. May cause coronary artery vasospasm (Prinzmetal's angina). Perform CV evaluation prior to therapy with multiple CV risk factors; consider administering 1st dose in a medically supervised setting and perform ECG immediately following administration in patients with a negative CV evaluation. Consider periodic CV evaluation in intermittent long-term users who have CV risk factors. Life-threatening cardiac rhythm disturbances (eg, ventricular tachycardia/fibrillation leading to death) reported; d/c if these occur. Sensations of tightness, pain, pressure, and heaviness in precordium, throat, neck, and jaw, usually of noncardiac origin, commonly occur after treatment; evaluate if cardiac origin is suspected. Cerebral/subarachnoid hemorrhage and stroke reported; d/c if cerebrovascular event occurs. Evaluate for other potentially serious neurological conditions before treatment. May cause noncoronary vasospastic reactions (eg, peripheral vascular ischemia, GI vascular ischemia, splenic infarction, Raynaud's syndrome); rule out before administering additional doses if experiencing signs/symptoms of noncoronary vasospasms. Transient and permanent blindness and significant partial vision loss reported. Overuse of acute migraine drugs may lead to exacerbation of headache (medication overuse headache); detoxification, including withdrawal of the overused drugs, and treatment of withdrawal symptoms may be necessary. Serotonin syndrome may occur; d/c if serotonin syndrome is suspected. Significant elevation in BP, including hypertensive crisis with acute impairment of organ systems, reported. Caution in elderly. (Tab, Disintegrating) Contains phenylalanine.

ADVERSE REACTIONS

Paresthesia, dry mouth, nausea, dizziness, somnolence, asthenia/fatigue, pain/pressure sensation.

DRUG INTERACTIONS

See Contraindications. Increased plasma area under the curve with propranolol; adjust dose. Serotonin syndrome reported with SSRIs, SNRIs, and TCAs.

PATIENT CONSIDERATIONS

Assessment: Assess for ischemic CAD or other significant underlying CV disease, history of stroke or TIA, PVD, ischemic bowel disease, uncontrolled HTN, hemiplegic/basilar migraine, neurological conditions, phenylketonuria, drug hypersensitivity, pregnancy/nursing status, and possible drug interactions. Perform CV evaluation with multiple CV risk factors.

Monitoring: Monitor for coronary artery vasospasm, cardiac rhythm disturbances, cerebrovascular event, noncoronary vasospastic reactions, serotonin syndrome, BP elevation, and other adverse reactions. Consider periodic CV evaluation in intermittent long-term users who have CV risk factors.

Counseling: Inform of possible serious CV side effects, including chest pain, SOB, weakness, and slurring of speech, and to seek medical advice in the presence of such symptoms. Caution about the risk of serotonin syndrome. Advise to notify physician if pregnant, breastfeeding, or planning to breastfeed. Instruct to evaluate their ability to perform complex tasks during migraine attacks and after administration. Inform that overuse (≥10 days/month) may lead to exacerbation of headache; encourage to record headache frequency and drug use. (Tab, Disintegrating) Inform phenylketonuric patients that tab contains phenylalanine.

STORAGE: 15-30°C (59-86°F).

MAXITROL – dexamethasone/neomycin sulfate/polymyxin B sulfate RX

Class: Antibacterial/corticosteroid combination

ADULT DOSAGE

Steroid-Responsive Inflammatory Ocular Conditions

For which a corticosteroid is indicated and where bacterial infection or risk of bacterial infection exists

Oint:

Apply small amount (1/2 inch) in conjunctival sac(s) up to 3-4X daily

Not more than 8g should be prescribed initially

Sus:

Instill 1-2 drops in conjunctival sac(s) up to 4-6X daily in mild disease and hourly in severe disease; taper to d/c as inflammation subsides

Not more than 20mL should be prescribed initially

PEDIATRIC DOSAGE

Steroid-Responsive Inflammatory Ocular Conditions

For which a corticosteroid is indicated and where bacterial infection or risk of bacterial infection exists

Sus:

≥2 Years:

Instill 1-2 drops in conjunctival sac(s) up to 4-6X daily in mild disease and hourly in severe disease; taper to d/c as inflammation subsides

Not more than 20mL should be prescribed initially

ADMINISTRATION

Ocular route

Oint

Tilt head back. Place finger on cheek just under the eye and gently pull down until a "V" pocket is formed between eyeball and lower lid. Place small amount of oint in the "V" pocket. Look downward before closing eye

HOW SUPPLIED

Oint: (Dexamethasone/Neomycin Sulfate/Polymyxin Sulfate) (0.1%/3.5mg/10,000 U)/g [3.5g]; **Sus:** (Dexamethasone/Neomycin Sulfate/Polymyxin Sulfate) (0.1%/3.5mg/10,000 U)/mL [5mL]

CONTRAINDICATIONS

Epithelial herpes simplex keratitis (dendritic keratitis), vaccinia, varicella, and other viral diseases of the cornea and conjunctiva; mycobacterial infection of the eye; fungal diseases of ocular structures; known or suspected hypersensitivity to any of the ingredients of this preparation and to other corticosteroids.

WARNINGS/PRECAUTIONS

For topical ophthalmic use only. Prolonged use may cause glaucoma with damage to the optic nerve, defects in visual acuity and fields of vision, posterior subcapsular cataract formation, suppressed host response, increased risk of secondary ocular infections, or persistent corneal fungal infections. May cause perforations when used with diseases causing thinning of cornea or sclera. May mask infection or enhance existing infection in acute purulent conditions of the eye. Monitor intraocular pressure (IOP) if used for ≥10 days. May cause cutaneous sensitization. Caution in the treatment of herpes simplex. Perform eye exam prior to therapy and renewal of medication. (Sus) Usage after cataract surgery may delay healing and increase incidence of bleb formation. May prolong course and exacerbate severity of ocular viral infections (eg, herpes simplex). Do not inject subconjunctivally, nor directly introduce into anterior chamber of the eye. Reevaluate patient if no improvement seen after 2 days. Suspect fungal invasion in any persistent corneal ulceration during or after therapy; take fungal cultures when appropriate.

ADVERSE REACTIONS

Allergic sensitizations, elevated IOP, posterior subcapsular cataract formation, delayed wound healing, secondary infections.

PATIENT CONSIDERATIONS

Assessment: Assess for active viral diseases of the cornea and conjunctiva, epithelial herpes simplex keratitis, vaccinia, varicella, mycobacterial infection of the eye, fungal disease of ocular structures, diseases causing thinning of sclera or cornea, acute purulent conditions, history of cataract surgery, hypersensitivity to the drug or its components, and pregnancy/nursing status. Perform eye exam (eg, slit-lamp biomicroscopy, fluorescein staining) prior to therapy.

Monitoring: Monitor for signs/symptoms of glaucoma, optic nerve damage, visual acuity and visual field defects, subcapsular cataract, ocular/corneal perforations, cutaneous sensitizations, and for bacterial, viral, and fungal infections. Monitor IOP and perform eye exams (eg, slit-lamp biomicroscopy, fluorescein staining) prior to renewal of medication. (Sus) Monitor use after cataract surgery. Perform fungal cultures when fungal invasion is suspected.

Counseling: Advise not to touch dropper tip to any surface; may contaminate drug. Instruct to keep out of reach of children. Instruct to use medication as prescribed. Inform that medication is for topical ophthalmic use only. Instruct to inform physician if pregnant or breastfeeding. (Oint) Advise not to wear contact lenses if signs and symptoms of bacterial ocular infection are present. Instruct not to use product if the imprinted carton seals have been damaged or removed. (Sus) Advise to d/c and consult physician if inflammation or pain persists >48 hrs or becomes aggravated. Warn that use of the same bottle by more than one person may spread infection. Instruct to shake well before use and keep bottle tightly closed when not in use.

STORAGE: (Oint) 2-25°C (36-77°F). (Sus) 8-27°C (46-80°F). Store upright.

MEDROL – methylprednisolone

RX

Class: Glucocorticoid

ADULT DOSAGE

Steroid-Responsive Disorders

Initial: 4-48mg/day, depending on disease and response

Maint: Decrease dose by small amounts to lowest effective dose

Withdraw gradually after long-term therapy

Acute Exacerbations of Multiple Sclerosis:

200mg/day for 1 week followed by 80mg qod for 1 month

Alternate Day Therapy (ADT):

Twice the usual daily dose administered every other am

Refer to PI for detailed information on ADT

PEDIATRIC DOSAGE

Steroid-Responsive Disorders

Initial: 4-48mg/day, depending on disease and response

Maint: Decrease dose by small amounts to lowest effective dose

Withdraw gradually after long-term therapy

Acute Exacerbations of Multiple Sclerosis:

200mg/day for 1 week followed by 80mg qod for 1 month

ADT:

Twice the usual daily dose administered every other am

Refer to PI for detailed information on ADT

ADMINISTRATION

Oral route

HOW SUPPLIED

Tab: 2mg*, 4mg*, 8mg*, 16mg*, 32mg*; (Dose-Pak) 4mg* [21^s] *scored

CONTRAINDICATIONS

Systemic fungal infections, known hypersensitivity to components.

WARNINGS/PRECAUTIONS

May need to increase dose before, during, and after stressful situations. May mask signs of infection or cause new infections. Possible benefits should be weighed against potential hazards if used during pregnancy/nursing. Prolonged use may produce glaucoma, optic nerve damage, and secondary ocular infections. May cause BP elevation, increased K^+ excretion, and salt/water retention. More severe/fatal course of infections reported with chickenpox and measles. Caution with *Strongyloides*, latent tuberculosis (TB), hypothyroidism, cirrhosis, ocular herpes simplex, HTN, diverticulitis, fresh intestinal anastomoses, ulcerative colitis, osteoporosis, myasthenia gravis, renal insufficiency, and peptic ulcer disease. Kaposi's sarcoma reported. Growth and development of children on prolonged therapy should be monitored. Monitor for psychic disturbances. Avoid abrupt withdrawal.

ADVERSE REACTIONS

Fluid and electrolyte disturbances, HTN, osteoporosis, muscle weakness, cushingoid state, menstrual irregularities, impaired wound healing, convulsions, ulcerative esophagitis, excessive sweating, increased intracranial pressure, glaucoma, abdominal distention, headache, decreased carbohydrate tolerance.

DRUG INTERACTIONS

Reduced efficacy with hepatic enzyme inducers (eg, phenobarbital, phenytoin, rifampin). Increases clearance of chronic high-dose aspirin (ASA). Caution with ASA in hypoprothrombinemia. Effects on oral anticoagulants are variable; monitor PT. Increased insulin and oral hypoglycemic requirements in diabetics. Avoid live vaccines with immunosuppressive doses. Possible decreased vaccine response with killed or inactivated vaccines with immunosuppressive doses. Mutual inhibition of metabolism with cyclosporine; convulsions reported. Potentiated by ketoconazole and troleandomycin. Concomitant administration with immunosuppressive agents may be associated with development of infections.

PATIENT CONSIDERATIONS

Assessment: Assess for systemic fungal infections, current infections, active TB, vaccination history, ulcerative colitis, diverticulitis, peptic ulcer with impending perforation, renal/hepatic insufficiency, septic arthritis/unstable joint, HTN, osteoporosis, myasthenia gravis, thyroid status, psychotic tendencies, drug hypersensitivity, and possible drug interactions.

Monitoring: Monitor for adrenocortical insufficiency, occurrence of infection, psychic derangement, cataracts, acute myopathy, Kaposi's sarcoma, and fluid retention. Monitor serum electrolytes, TSH, LFTs, intraocular pressure, and BP. Monitor urinalysis, blood sugar, weight, chest x-ray, and upper GI x-ray (if ulcer history) regularly during prolonged therapy. Monitor growth and development of infants and children on prolonged corticosteroids therapy.

Counseling: Advise not to d/c abruptly or without medical supervision. Inform that susceptibility to infections may increase. Instruct to avoid exposure to chickenpox or measles and to seek medical advice immediately if exposed. Recommend dietary salt restriction and K^+ supplementation.

STORAGE: 20-25°C (68-77°F).

MEGACE ES – megestrol acetate

RX

Class: Progesterone

OTHER BRAND NAMES

Megace

ADULT DOSAGE

Weight Loss

Anorexia, Cachexia or Unexplained Significant Weight Loss in AIDS Patients:

Megace ES:
Initial: 625mg/day (5mL/day)

Megace:
Initial: 800mg/day (20mL/day)
Daily doses of 400mg/day and 800mg/day found to be effective

PEDIATRIC DOSAGE

Pediatric use may not have been established

DOSING CONSIDERATIONS

Elderly
Start at lower end of dosing range

ADMINISTRATION

Oral route

Shake well before use

HOW SUPPLIED

Sus: (ES) 125mg/mL [150mL]; (Megace) 40mg/mL [240mL]

CONTRAINDICATIONS

History of hypersensitivity to megestrol acetate or any component of the formulation, known or suspected pregnancy.

WARNINGS/PRECAUTIONS

Institute only after treatable causes of weight loss are sought and addressed. 125mg/mL strength is not substitutable with other strengths (eg, 40mg/mL). Overt Cushing's syndrome and asymptomatic pituitary-adrenal suppression reported with chronic use. Adrenal insufficiency reported in patients receiving or being withdrawn from chronic therapy; consider use of replacement or stress doses of a rapidly acting glucocorticoid. New onset diabetes mellitus (DM) and exacerbation of preexisting DM reported with chronic use. Breakthrough bleeding reported in women. Caution with history of thromboembolic disease and in elderly.

ADVERSE REACTIONS

Diarrhea, rash, flatulence, N/V, HTN, headache, pain, asthenia, insomnia, anemia, fever, decreased libido, impotence, hyperglycemia.

DRUG INTERACTIONS

(ES) May decrease exposure of indinavir; consider higher dose of indinavir.

PATIENT CONSIDERATIONS

Assessment: Assess for preexisting DM, history of thromboembolic disease, hypersensitivity to drug, pregnancy/nursing status, and possible drug interactions.

Monitoring: Monitor for adrenal insufficiency, new onset/exacerbation of DM, vaginal bleeding, and other adverse reactions.

Counseling: Inform about product differences to avoid overdosing or underdosing. Instruct to use ud. Advise to report any adverse reactions. Advise women of childbearing potential to use contraception while on therapy, and to notify physician if pregnancy occurs.

STORAGE: 15-25°C (59-77°F). Protect from heat.

MEKINIST – trametinib

RX

Class: Kinase inhibitor

ADULT DOSAGE

Unresectable or Metastatic Melanoma with BRAF V600E or V600K Mutations

2mg qd, at the same time each day, as a single agent or in combination w/ dabrafenib until disease progression or unacceptable toxicity occurs

Missed Dose

Do not take a missed dose w/in 12 hrs of the next dose

PEDIATRIC DOSAGE

Pediatric use may not have been established

DOSING CONSIDERATIONS

Adverse Reactions

Dose Reductions for Trametinib:
First Dose Reduction: 1.5mg qd
Second Dose Reduction: 1mg qd
Subsequent Modification: Permanently d/c if unable to tolerate 1mg qd

Febrile Drug Reaction:
Fever >104°F or Fever Complicated by Rigors, Hypotension, Dehydration, or Renal Failure: Withhold until fever resolves, then resume at same or lower dose level

Cutaneous:
Grade 3 or 4 Skin Toxicity or Intolerable Grade 2 Skin Toxicity: Withhold for up to 3 weeks; resume at a lower dose level if improved or permanently d/c if not improved

Cardiac:
Asymptomatic, Absolute Decrease in Left Ventricular Ejection Fraction (LVEF) of 10% or Greater from Baseline and Below Lower Limits of Normal (LLN) from Pretreatment Value: Withhold for up to 4 weeks. If improved to normal LVEF value, resume at a lower dose level. If not improved to normal LVEF value, permanently d/c
Symptomatic CHF/Absolute Decrease in LVEF >20% from Baseline that is Below LLN: Permanently d/c

Venous Thromboembolism (VTE):
Uncomplicated Deep Vein Thrombosis (DVT) or Pulmonary Embolism (PE): Withhold for up to 3 weeks; resume at a lower dose level if improved to Grade 0-1 or permanently d/c if not improved
Life-Threatening PE: Permanently d/c

Ocular Toxicities:
Retinal Pigment Epithelial Detachments: Withhold for up to 3 weeks. If improved, resume at same or lower dose level. If not improved, d/c or resume at a lower dose
Retinal Vein Occlusion (RVO): Permanently d/c

Pulmonary:
Interstitial Lung Disease (ILD)/Pneumonitis: Permanently d/c

Other:
Any Grade 3 Adverse Reactions or Intolerable Grade 2 Adverse Reactions: Withhold; resume at a lower dose level if improved to Grade 0-1 or permanently d/c if not improved
First Occurrence of Any Grade 4 Adverse Reaction: Withhold until adverse reaction improves to Grade 0-1, then resume at a lower dose level; or permanently d/c
Recurrent Grade 4 Adverse Reaction: Permanently d/c
Refer to dabrafenib PI for recommended dose modifications

M

ADMINISTRATION
Oral route
Take at least 1 hr ac or 2 hrs pc.

HOW SUPPLIED
Tab: 0.5mg, 2mg

WARNINGS/PRECAUTIONS
See Dosing Considerations. Not indicated for treatment of patients who have received prior BRAF-inhibitor therapy. New primary malignancies, cutaneous and noncutaneous, may occur when therapy is administered w/ dabrafenib. Perform dermatologic evaluations prior to initiation of therapy when used w/ dabrafenib, every 2 months while on therapy, and for up to 6 months following discontinuation of the combination. Hemorrhages (eg, major hemorrhages defined as symptomatic bleeding in a critical area or organ) and VTE may occur. Cardiomyopathy, including cardiac failure, may occur; assess LVEF by echocardiogram or multigated acquisition (MUGA) scan before initiation of therapy as a single agent or w/ dabrafenib, 1 month after initiation, and then at 2- to 3-month intervals while on treatment. RVO reported and may lead to macular edema, decreased visual function, neovascularization, and glaucoma; urgently (w/in 24 hrs), perform ophthalmological evaluation for patient-reported loss of vision or other visual disturbances. Retinal pigment epithelial detachments may occur; retinal detachments may be bilateral and multifocal, occurring in the central macular region of the retina or elsewhere in the retina. Perform ophthalmological evaluation periodically and at any time a patient reports visual disturbances. ILD or pneumonitis reported; withhold therapy in patients presenting w/ new/progressive pulmonary symptoms and findings (eg, cough, dyspnea, hypoxia, pleural effusion, infiltrates) pending clinical investigations. Serious febrile reactions and fever of any severity accompanied by hypotension, rigors or chills, dehydration, or renal failure may occur when therapy is administered w/ dabrafenib. Monitor SrCr and other evidence of renal function during and following severe pyrexia. Administer antipyretics as secondary prophylaxis when resuming therapy if patient had a prior episode of severe febrile reaction or fever associated w/ complications. Administer corticosteroids (eg, prednisone 10mg daily) for at least 5 days for second or subsequent pyrexia if temperature does not return to baseline w/in 3 days of onset of pyrexia, or for pyrexia associated w/ complications (eg, dehydration, hypotension, renal failure, severe chills/rigors), and there is no evidence of active infection. Serious skin toxicity may occur. Hyperglycemia may occur when therapy is administered w/ dabrafenib; monitor serum glucose levels upon initiation and as clinically appropriate in patients w/ preexisting diabetes or hyperglycemia. May cause fetal harm.

ADVERSE REACTIONS
Single Agent Trametinib: Rash, diarrhea, lymphedema, acneiform dermatitis, dry skin, pruritus, paronychia, stomatitis, abdominal pain, HTN, hemorrhage.
W/ Dabrafenib: Pyrexia, N/V, rash, chills, diarrhea, HTN, and peripheral edema.

PATIENT CONSIDERATIONS
Assessment: Assess for diabetes, hyperglycemia, and pregnancy/nursing status. Confirm the presence of BRAF V600E or V600K mutation in tumor specimens. Assess if patient has received prior BRAF-inhibitor therapy. Perform dermatologic evaluations prior to initiation of therapy when used w/ dabrafenib. Assess LVEF by echocardiogram or MUGA scan before initiation of therapy as a single agent or w/ dabrafenib.

Monitoring: Monitor for new primary malignancies, hemorrhagic events, VTE, cardiomyopathy, retinal pigment epithelial detachment, RVO, ILD, pneumonitis, febrile reactions, skin toxicity, and other adverse reactions. When used w/ dabrafenib, perform dermatologic evaluations every 2 months while on therapy, and for up to 6 months following discontinuation of the combination. When therapy is given as a single agent or w/ dabrafenib, assess LVEF by echocardiogram or MUGA scan 1 month after initiation, and then at 2- to 3-month intervals while on treatment. Perform ophthalmological evaluation periodically and at any time a patient reports visual disturbances. Monitor serum glucose levels when therapy is used in combination w/ dabrafenib upon initiation and as clinically appropriate in patients w/ preexisting diabetes or hyperglycemia.

Counseling: Inform that evidence of BRAF V600E or V600K mutation w/in the tumor specimen is necessary to identify patients for whom treatment is indicated. Inform that combined use w/ dabrafenib may result in development of new primary cutaneous and noncutaneous malignancies, increase risk of intracranial and GI hemorrhage, increase risk of PE/DVT, and cause serious febrile reactions; advise to contact physician for signs/symptoms of malignancies, unusual bleeding/hemorrhage, venous thrombosis, or if fever develops. Advise to immediately report any signs/symptoms of heart failure, visual changes, cough or dyspnea, progressive or intolerable rash, and severe diarrhea. Advise of the need to undergo BP monitoring and to notify physician if symptoms of HTN develop. Inform of the risk of fetal harm if taken during pregnancy; instruct females of reproductive potential to use highly effective contraception during treatment and for 4 months after the last dose. Advise to contact physician if patient becomes pregnant, or if pregnancy is suspected. Instruct not to breastfeed during treatment and for 4 months after the last dose. Inform of the potential risk for impaired fertility. Instruct to take ud.

STORAGE: 2-8°C (36-46°F). Do not freeze. Protect from moisture and light. Do not place in pill boxes.

Metadate CD – methylphenidate hydrochloride

CII

Class: CNS stimulant

Caution with history of drug dependence or alcoholism. Chronic abuse may lead to marked tolerance and psychological dependence with varying degrees of abnormal behavior. Frank psychotic episodes may occur, especially with parenteral abuse. Careful supervision is required during withdrawal from abusive use since severe depression may occur. Withdrawal following chronic use may unmask symptoms of underlying disorder that may require follow-up.

ADULT DOSAGE

Attention-Deficit Hyperactivity Disorder

Refer to pediatric dosing

PEDIATRIC DOSAGE

Attention-Deficit Hyperactivity Disorder

≥6 Years:

Initial: 20mg qam

Titrate: May adjust in weekly 10-20mg increments, depending upon tolerability and degree of efficacy observed

Max: 60mg/day

DOSING CONSIDERATIONS

Adverse Reactions

Reduce dose or d/c if paradoxical aggravation of symptoms or other adverse events occur

D/C if no improvement seen after appropriate dosage adjustment over 1 month

ADMINISTRATION

Oral route

Administer qam before breakfast

May be swallowed whole w/ the aid of liquids, or alternatively, may open caps and sprinkle contents onto a small amount (tbsp) of applesauce and consume immediately

Drinking some fluids (eg, water) should follow the intake of sprinkles w/ applesauce

Do not crush or chew cap or cap contents

HOW SUPPLIED

Cap, Extended-Release: 10mg, 20mg, 30mg, 40mg, 50mg, 60mg

M

CONTRAINDICATIONS

Marked anxiety, tension, agitation, glaucoma, motor tics, family history or diagnosis of Tourette's syndrome, severe HTN, angina pectoris, cardiac arrhythmias, heart failure, recent myocardial infarction (MI), hyperthyroidism, or thyrotoxicosis. Known hypersensitivity to methylphenidate or other components of the product. Rare hereditary problems of fructose intolerance, glucose-galactose malabsorption, or sucrase-isomaltase insufficiency. On the day of surgery. Treatment w/ MAOIs or w/in a minimum of 14 days following discontinuation of an MAOI.

WARNINGS/PRECAUTIONS

Avoid with known serious structural cardiac abnormalities, cardiomyopathy, serious heart rhythm abnormalities, coronary artery disease, or other serious cardiac problems. Sudden death reported in children and adolescents with structural cardiac abnormalities or other serious heart problems. Sudden deaths, stroke, and MI reported in adults. May increase BP and HR; caution with conditions that might be compromised by increases in BP/HR. Prior to treatment, obtain medical history (including assessment for family history of sudden death or ventricular arrhythmia) and perform physical exam to assess for presence of cardiac disease. Promptly perform cardiac evaluation if symptoms of cardiac disease develop. May exacerbate symptoms of behavior disturbance and thought disorder in patients with preexisting psychotic disorder. Caution in patients with comorbid bipolar disorder; may induce mixed/manic episodes. May cause treatment-emergent psychotic or manic symptoms (eg, hallucinations, delusional thinking, mania) in children and adolescents without prior history of psychotic illness or mania; consider discontinuation if such symptoms occur. Aggressive behavior or hostility reported in children and adolescents. May cause long-term suppression of growth in children; monitor growth, and may need to interrupt treatment in patients not growing or gaining height or weight as expected. May lower convulsive threshold; d/c if seizures occur. Priapism, sometimes requiring surgical intervention, reported. Associated with peripheral vasculopathy, including Raynaud's phenomenon; carefully observe for digital changes. Difficulties with accommodation and blurring of vision reported. May produce a positive result during drug testing.

ADVERSE REACTIONS

Headache, abdominal pain, anorexia, insomnia.

DRUG INTERACTIONS

See Contraindications. Caution with pressor agents. May inhibit metabolism of coumarin anticoagulants, anticonvulsants (eg, phenobarbital, phenytoin, primidone), phenylbutazone, and some antidepressants (eg, TCAs, SSRIs); downward dose adjustment and monitoring of plasma drug concentrations (or coagulation times for coumarin) of these drugs may be necessary when initiating or discontinuing methylphenidate. Clearance might be affected by urinary pH, either being increased with acidifying agents or decreased with alkalinizing agents; caution with agents that alter urinary pH. Avoid with alcohol.

PATIENT CONSIDERATIONS

Assessment: Assess for hypersensitivity to the drug, hereditary problems of fructose intolerance, glucose-galactose malabsorption, or sucrase-isomaltase insufficiency, marked anxiety, tension, agitation, glaucoma, motor tics, family history or diagnosis of Tourette's syndrome, cardiovascular conditions, history of drug dependence or alcoholism, psychotic disorder, comorbid bipolar disorder, any other conditions where treatment is contraindicated or cautioned, pregnancy/nursing status, and possible drug interactions.

Monitoring: Monitor for changes in HR and BP, signs/symptoms of cardiac disease, exacerbation of behavior disturbance and thought disorder, psychosis, mania, appearance of or worsening of aggressive behavior or hostility, seizures, priapism, peripheral vasculopathy (including Raynaud's phenomenon), visual disturbances, and other adverse reactions. In pediatric patients, monitor growth. Perform periodic monitoring of CBC, differential, and platelet counts during prolonged therapy. Periodically reevaluate long-term usefulness of drug.

Counseling: Advise to avoid alcohol while taking the drug. Inform about the benefits and risks of therapy. Counsel on the appropriate use of the medication. Instruct to seek immediate medical attention in the event of priapism. Instruct to report to physician any new numbness, pain, skin color change, or sensitivity to temperature in fingers or toes; instruct to contact physician immediately with any signs of unexplained wounds appearing on fingers or toes while taking the drug.

STORAGE: 25°C (77°F); excursions permitted to 15-30°C (59-86°F).

METOCLOPRAMIDE – metoclopramide

RX

Class: Dopamine antagonist/prokinetic

May cause tardive dyskinesia (TD); d/c if signs/symptoms of TD develop. Avoid use for >12 weeks of therapy unless benefit outweighs risk.

M

OTHER BRAND NAMES

Reglan

ADULT DOSAGE

Gastroesophageal Reflux Disease

Oral:
10-15mg up to qid 30 min ac and hs

Intermittent Symptoms:
Single doses up to 20mg prior to the provoking situation

Esophageal Erosions/Ulcerations:
15mg/dose qid

Therapy should not exceed 12 weeks in duration

Diabetic Gastroparesis

Oral:
10mg 30 min ac and hs for 2-8 weeks

Inj:
10mg IV over 1-2 min for up to 10 days, then initiate oral administration

Initial route of administration should be determined by the severity of the presenting symptoms

Postoperative Nausea/Vomiting

Inj:
10mg or 20mg IM near end of surgery

Chemotherapy-Induced Nausea/Vomiting

Inj:
IV infused over at least 15 min, 30 min before chemotherapy and repeated q2h for two doses, then q3h for 3 doses

PEDIATRIC DOSAGE

Small Bowel Intubation

Inj:
Administer as a single dose (undiluted) IV over 1-2 min if the tube has not passed the pylorus w/ conventional maneuvers in 10 min

<6 Years: 0.1mg/kg
6-14 Years: 2.5-5mg
>14 Years: 10mg

Initial Two Doses:
Highly Emetogenic Drugs (eg, Cisplatin, Dacarbazine): 2mg/kg
Less Emetogenic Regimens: 1mg/kg

Small Bowel Intubation

Inj:
10mg single dose (undiluted) IV over 1-2 min if the tube has not passed the pylorus w/ conventional maneuvers in 10 min

Aid in Radiological Exam

Inj:
When Delayed Gastric Emptying Interferes w/ Examination of the Stomach/Small Intestine:
10mg single dose (undiluted) IV over 1-2 min

DOSING CONSIDERATIONS

Renal Impairment
Oral/Inj:
CrCl <40mL/min:
Initial: 1/2 the recommended dose; adjust dose as appropriate

Elderly
Oral: 5mg/dose

Adverse Reactions
Inj:
Acute Dystonic Reactions: Inject 50mg diphenhydramine IM

ADMINISTRATION

Oral, IV/IM route

Inj
Doses >10mg: Dilute in 50mL of a parenteral sol; preferred sol is normal saline
Refer to PI for Admixture Compatibilities
Admixture Incompatibilities:
Cephalothin Sodium
Chloramphenicol Sodium
Sodium Bicarbonate

HOW SUPPLIED

Inj (Reglan): 5mg/mL [2mL, 10mL, 30mL]; **Sol:** 5mg/5mL [473mL]; **Tab (Reglan):** 5mg, 10mg*
*scored

CONTRAINDICATIONS

When GI motility stimulation is dangerous (eg, GI hemorrhage, mechanical obstruction, perforation), pheochromocytoma, known sensitivity or intolerance to the drug, epilepsy, concomitant drugs that cause extrapyramidal symptoms (EPS).

WARNINGS/PRECAUTIONS

Mental depression may occur; caution with prior history of depression. EPS, primarily as acute dystonic reactions, may occur. May cause parkinsonian-like symptoms; caution with preexisting Parkinson's disease. May suppress signs of TD; do not use for symptomatic control of TD. Neuroleptic malignant syndrome reported; d/c, monitor, and institute intensive symptomatic treatment. Risk of developing fluid retention and volume overload, especially in patients with cirrhosis or CHF; d/c if these occur. Caution with HTN, renal impairment, and/or in elderly. May increase risk of developing methemoglobinemia and/or sulfhemoglobinemia with NADH-cytochrome b_5 reductase deficiency. May experience withdrawal symptoms after discontinuation. (Inj) Undiluted IV inj should be given slowly since rapid administration may cause anxiety, restlessness, and drowsiness. May increase pressure on suture lines after a gut anastomosis or closure; use caution with PONV.

ADVERSE REACTIONS

TD, restlessness, drowsiness, fatigue, lassitude.

DRUG INTERACTIONS

See Contraindications. GI motility effect antagonized by anticholinergics and narcotic analgesics. Additive sedation with alcohol, sedatives, hypnotics, narcotics, or tranquilizers. Caution with MAOIs. May diminish absorption of drugs from stomach (eg, digoxin) and increase rate and/or extent of absorption of drugs from small bowel (eg, acetaminophen, tetracycline, levodopa, ethanol, cyclosporine). Insulin dose or timing of dose may require adjustment. Rare cases of hepatotoxicity reported with drugs with hepatotoxic potential. Inhibits central and peripheral effects of apomorphine.

PATIENT CONSIDERATIONS

Assessment: Assess for conditions when GI motility stimulation is dangerous, pheochromocytoma, epilepsy, sensitivity or tolerance to the drug, CHF, cirrhosis, history of depression, Parkinson's disease, HTN, NADH-cytochrome b_5 reductase and G6PD deficiency, diabetes mellitus, renal impairment, pregnancy/nursing status, and possible drug interactions.

Monitoring: Monitor for signs/symptoms of depression, EPS, parkinsonian-like symptoms, TD, NMS, HTN, fluid retention/volume overload, withdrawal symptoms, hypersensitivity reactions, and other adverse reactions.

Counseling: Inform that drug may impair mental and physical abilities; advise to use caution while operating machinery/driving. Discuss the risks and benefits of treatment.

STORAGE: 20-25°C (68-77°F). (Inj) If diluted with NaCl, may be stored frozen for up to 4 weeks. Diluted sol may be stored up to 48 hrs (without freezing) if protected from light; 24 hrs in normal lighting conditions.

METOLAZONE – metolazone

RX

Class: Quinazoline diuretic

OTHER BRAND NAMES

Zaroxolyn

ADULT DOSAGE

Edema

Accompanying Congestive Heart Failure/ Renal Disease (Nephrotic Syndrome and States of Diminished Renal Function):
Initial: 5-20mg qd
May be advisable to give a larger dose for patients who experience paroxysmal nocturnal dyspnea

Hypertension

Mild-Moderate:
Initial: 2.5-5mg qd
Adjust dose at appropriate intervals to achieve max therapeutic effect

PEDIATRIC DOSAGE

Pediatric use may not have been established

M

ADMINISTRATION

Oral route

HOW SUPPLIED

Tab: 10mg; (Zaroxolyn) 2.5mg, 5mg

CONTRAINDICATIONS

Anuria, hepatic coma or precoma, known allergy or hypersensitivity to metolazone.

WARNINGS/PRECAUTIONS

Do not interchange metolazone tabs, Zaroxolyn tabs, and other formulations of metolazone that share their slow/incomplete bioavailability and are not therapeutically equivalent at the same doses to Mykrox tabs, a more rapidly available and completely bioavailable metolazone product. Formulations bioequivalent to Zaroxolyn or to Mykrox should not be interchanged for one another. May cause rapid onset of severe hyponatremia and/or hypokalemia following initial doses; d/c and initiate supportive measures immediately when symptoms of severe electrolyte imbalance appear rapidly. Monitor serum K^+ at regular and appropriate intervals, and institute dose reduction, K^+ supplementation, or addition of a K^+-sparing diuretic whenever indicated. Cross-allergy may occur in patients allergic to sulfonamide-derived drugs, thiazides, or quinethazone. Sensitivity reactions (eg, angioedema, bronchospasm) may occur with 1st dose. Observe for signs of fluid and/or electrolyte imbalance (eg, hyponatremia, hypochloremic alkalosis, hypokalemia). May produce low-salt syndrome in patients with severe edema accompanying cardiac failure or renal disease, especially with hot weather and a low-salt diet. Monitor serum and urine electrolytes in patients with protracted vomiting, severe diarrhea, or who are receiving parenteral fluids. Increased risk of hypokalemia with rapid diuresis, severe liver disease, inadequate oral intake, or when excess K^+ is being lost extrarenally. May increase urinary excretion of Mg^{2+}, which may result in hypomagnesemia. May cause hyperglycemia and glycosuria in patients with diabetes or latent diabetes. Increases serum uric acid and may occasionally precipitate gouty attacks. May precipitate azotemia; d/c if azotemia and oliguria worsen during treatment in patients with severe renal disease. Caution with severe renal impairment and in elderly. Orthostatic hypotension may occur. Hypercalcemia may occur, especially in patients with high bone turnover states, and may signify hidden hyperparathyroidism; d/c before tests for parathyroid function are performed. May exacerbate/activate systemic lupus erythematosus (SLE).

ADVERSE REACTIONS
Chest pain, orthostatic hypotension, syncope, neuropathy, toxic epidermal necrolysis, Stevens-Johnson syndrome, necrotizing angiitis, hepatitis, intrahepatic cholestatic jaundice, pancreatitis, joint pain, aplastic anemia, blurred vision, chills, dry mouth.

DRUG INTERACTIONS
Concomitant administration with furosemide and other loop diuretics may result in unusually large/prolonged fluid and electrolyte losses. Caution to avoid excessive reduction of BP, especially during initial therapy with other antihypertensives; dose adjustments of other antihypertensives may be necessary. Orthostatic hypotension may be potentiated with alcohol, barbiturates, narcotics, or other antihypertensives. Drug-induced hypokalemia may increase sensitivity of myocardium to digitalis. May reduce lithium clearance and increase risk of its toxicity; avoid concomitant use. Hypercalcemia may occur with high doses of vitamin D. Corticosteroids or adrenocorticotropic hormone may increase salt/water retention and increase risk of hypokalemia. Drug-induced hypokalemia may enhance neuromuscular blocking effects of curariform drugs (eg, tubocurarine); may be advisable to d/c metolazone 3 days before elective surgery. Salicylates or other NSAIDs may decrease antihypertensive effects. May decrease arterial responsiveness to norepinephrine. May decrease methenamine efficacy. May affect hypoprothrombinemic response to anticoagulants; dose adjustments may be necessary.

PATIENT CONSIDERATIONS

Assessment: Assess for hypersensitivity to drug, thiazides, quinethazone, or sulfonamide-derived drugs. Assess for anuria, hepatic coma or precoma, diabetes, high bone turnover states, hepatic/renal impairment, any other conditions where treatment is cautioned, pregnancy/nursing status, and possible drug interactions.

Monitoring: Monitor for exacerbation or activation of SLE, hyperglycemia, glycosuria, hyperuricemia or precipitation of gout, hypersensitivity reactions, orthostatic hypotension, azotemia, and other adverse reactions. Monitor serum electrolytes periodically.

Counseling: Advise to take ud. Inform of possible adverse effects; advise to promptly report any adverse reactions to physician.

STORAGE: 25°C (77°F); excursions permitted to 15-30°C (59-86°F). Protect from light.

METOPROLOL – metoprolol tartrate

RX

Class: Selective β_1 blocker

Do not abruptly d/c therapy in patients w/ coronary artery disease (CAD). Severe exacerbation of angina, MI, and ventricular arrhythmias reported in patients w/ CAD following abrupt discontinuation of therapy w/ β-blockers. When discontinuing chronically administered metoprolol, particularly in patients w/ CAD, gradually reduce dose over a period of 1-2 weeks w/ careful monitoring. If angina markedly worsens or acute CAD develops, promptly reinstate metoprolol administration, at least temporarily, and take other measures appropriate for management of unstable angina. CAD may be unrecognized; may be prudent not to d/c therapy abruptly even in patients treated only for HTN.

OTHER BRAND NAMES
Lopressor

ADULT DOSAGE

Hypertension

Tab:

Initial: 100mg/day PO in single or divided doses, whether used alone or added to a diuretic

Titrate: May increase at weekly (or longer) intervals until optimum BP reduction is achieved

Effective Range: 100-450mg/day

Doses >450mg/day not studied

Angina Pectoris

Long-Term Treatment:

Tab:

Initial: 100mg/day PO in 2 divided doses

Titrate: Gradually increase at weekly intervals until optimum clinical response is achieved or there is pronounced slowing of HR

PEDIATRIC DOSAGE

Pediatric use may not have been established

Effective Range: 100-400mg/day

Doses >400mg/day not studied

If treatment is to be discontinued, gradually decrease dose over 1-2 weeks

Myocardial Infarction

Treatment of hemodynamically stable patients w/ definite or suspected acute MI to reduce cardiovascular mortality

Early Phase:
5mg IV bolus every 2 min for 3 doses (monitor BP, HR, and ECG); initiate treatment as soon as possible after patient's arrival in the hospital
In Patients Who Tolerate Full IV Dose (15mg): Initiate tabs, 50mg q6h, 15 min after last IV dose and continue for 48 hrs; thereafter, maint dose is 100mg bid
In Patients Who Cannot Tolerate Full IV Dose: Initiate tabs, either 25mg or 50mg q6h (depending on the degree of intolerance) 15 min after the last IV dose or as soon as clinical condition allows; d/c w/ severe intolerance

Late Phase:
Initiate tabs, 100mg bid, as soon as clinical condition allows, for ≥3 months; start in patients w/ contraindications to early phase treatment, patients intolerant to the full early treatment, and patients in whom the physician wishes to delay therapy for any other reason

DOSING CONSIDERATIONS

M

<u>Hepatic Impairment</u>
Initiate at low doses w/ cautious gradual dose titration according to clinical response

<u>Elderly</u>
>65 Years:
Start at lower end of dosing range

ADMINISTRATION
Oral/IV route

<u>Tab</u>
Swallow unchewed w/ a glass of water.
Always take in standardized relation w/ meals; continue taking w/ the same schedule during the course of therapy.

<u>Inj</u>
Parenteral administration should be done in a setting w/ intensive monitoring.

HOW SUPPLIED
Tab: 25mg*; (Lopressor) 50mg*, 100mg*; **Inj:** (Lopressor) 5mg/5mL *scored

CONTRAINDICATIONS
Hypersensitivity to metoprolol tartrate and related derivatives, to any of the excipients, or to other β-blockers. HR <45 beats/min, 2nd- and 3rd-degree heart block, significant 1st-degree heart block, systolic BP <100mmHg, moderate to severe cardiac failure. **Tab:** Sinus bradycardia, >1st-degree heart block, cardiogenic shock, overt cardiac failure, sick sinus syndrome, severe peripheral arterial circulatory disorders.

WARNINGS/PRECAUTIONS
May cause depression of myocardial contractility and may precipitate heart failure (HF) and cardiogenic shock. May be necessary to lower the dose or d/c if signs/symptoms of HF develop. Chronically administered therapy should not be routinely withdrawn prior to major surgery; however, may augment risks of general anesthesia and surgical procedures. Bradycardia, including sinus pause, heart block, and cardiac arrest reported; increased risk in patients w/ 1st degree atrioventricular block, sinus node dysfunction, or conduction disorders. Reduce dose or d/c if severe bradycardia develops. Avoid w/ bronchospastic diseases; may be used in patients w/ bronchospastic disease who do not respond to or cannot tolerate other antihypertensive treatment. May mask tachycardia occurring w/ hypoglycemia; other manifestations (eg, dizziness, sweating) may not be significantly affected. If used in the setting of pheochromocytoma, should be given in combination w/ an α-blocker, and only after the α-blocker has been initiated; may cause a paradoxical increase in BP if administered alone. May mask certain clinical signs (eg, tachycardia) of

hyperthyroidism and may precipitate thyroid storm w/ abrupt withdrawal. Patients w/ a history of severe anaphylactic reaction to a variety of allergens may be more reactive to repeated challenge and may be unresponsive to usual doses of epinephrine.

ADVERSE REACTIONS

Bradycardia, tiredness, dizziness, depression, SOB, diarrhea, pruritus, rash, heart block, HF, hypotension.

DRUG INTERACTIONS

Additive effects w/ catecholamine-depleting drugs (eg, reserpine). May increase risk of bradycardia w/ digitalis glycosides; monitor HR and PR interval. May produce an additive reduction in myocardial contractility w/ calcium channel blockers. Potent CYP2D6 inhibitors (eg, fluvoxamine, chlorpromazine, quinidine) may increase levels. Hydralazine may inhibit presystemic metabolism, leading to increased levels. May potentiate antihypertensive effects of α-blockers (eg, guanethidine, betanidine, reserpine). May potentiate the postural hypotensive effect of 1st dose of prazosin. May potentiate hypertensive response to withdrawal of clonidine; when given concomitantly w/ clonidine, d/c several days before clonidine is withdrawn. May enhance vasoconstrictive action of ergot alkaloids. Withhold therapy before dipyridamole testing, w/ careful monitoring of HR following the dipyridamole inj. **Inj:** Some inhalational anesthetics may enhance cardiodepressant effect.

PATIENT CONSIDERATIONS

Assessment: Assess for hypersensitivity to the drug, sinus bradycardia, heart block, cardiogenic shock, HF, CAD, bronchospastic diseases, hypoglycemia, hyperthyroidism, hepatic impairment, any other conditions where treatment is contraindicated or cautioned, pregnancy/nursing status, and possible drug interactions. Obtain baseline ECG.

Monitoring: Monitor for signs/symptoms of HF, cardiogenic shock, bradycardia, thyroid storm, hypersensitivity reactions, and other adverse reactions. Monitor BP, HR, ECG, and hemodynamic status.

Counseling: Advise to take tabs regularly and continuously, ud, w/ or immediately following meals. Warn against interruption or discontinuation of therapy w/o physician's advice. Advise to avoid operating automobiles and machinery or engaging in other tasks requiring alertness until response to therapy has been determined. Instruct to contact physician if difficulty in breathing or other adverse reactions occur, and to inform physician/dentist of therapy before undergoing any type of surgery.

STORAGE: 20-25°C (68-77°F). Protect from moisture. (Lopressor) 25°C (77°F); excursions permitted to 15-30°C (59-86°F). **Tab:** Protect from moisture and heat. **Inj:** Protect from light and heat.

METOPROLOL TARTRATE/HCTZ – hydrochlorothiazide/metoprolol tartrate

RX

Class: Selective beta$_1$ blocker/thiazide diuretic

Exacerbation of angina and, in some cases, myocardial infarction (MI) reported following abrupt discontinuation. When discontinuing therapy, avoid abrupt withdrawal even without overt angina pectoris. Caution patients against interruption of therapy without physician's advice.

OTHER BRAND NAMES

Lopressor HCT

ADULT DOSAGE

Hypertension

If fixed combination represents dose titrated to patient's needs; therapy with combination may be more convenient than with separate components

Combination Therapy:

100-200mg of metoprolol and hydrochlorothiazide (HCTZ) 25-50mg per day given qd or in divided doses

Max HCTZ: 50mg/day

May gradually add another antihypertensive when necessary, beginning with 50% of the usual recommended starting dose

PEDIATRIC DOSAGE

Pediatric use may not have been established

DOSING CONSIDERATIONS

Elderly

Start at lower end of dosing range

ADMINISTRATION

Oral route

HOW SUPPLIED

Tab: (Metoprolol/HCTZ) 50mg/25mg*, 100mg/25mg*, 100mg/50mg*; (Lopressor HCT) 50mg/25mg*, 100mg/25mg* *scored

CONTRAINDICATIONS

Metoprolol Tartrate: Sinus bradycardia; >1st-degree heart block; cardiogenic shock; overt cardiac failure; hypersensitivity to metoprolol tartrate and related derivatives, any of the excipients, or to other β-blockers; sick sinus syndrome; severe peripheral arterial circulatory disorders. **HCTZ:** Anuria, hypersensitivity to HCTZ or sulfonamide-derived drugs.

WARNINGS/PRECAUTIONS

Not for initial therapy. Caution with hepatic dysfunction and in elderly. Metoprolol: May cause/precipitate heart failure; d/c if cardiac failure continues despite adequate treatment. Avoid with bronchospastic diseases, but may use with caution if unresponsive to/intolerant of other antihypertensives. Avoid withdrawal of chronically administered therapy prior to major surgery; however, may augment risks of general anesthesia and surgical procedures. Caution with diabetic patients; may mask tachycardia occurring with hypoglycemia. Paradoxical BP increase reported with pheochromocytoma; give in combination with and only after initiating α-blocker therapy. May mask hyperthyroidism. Avoid abrupt withdrawal in suspected thyrotoxicosis; may precipitate thyroid storm. HCTZ: Caution with severe renal disease; may precipitate azotemia. If progressive renal impairment becomes evident, d/c therapy. May precipitate hepatic coma in patients with liver dysfunction/disease. Sensitivity reactions are more likely to occur with history of allergy or bronchial asthma. May exacerbate/activate systemic lupus erythematosus (SLE). May cause idiosyncratic reaction, resulting in acute transient myopia and acute angle-closure glaucoma; d/c HCTZ as rapidly as possible. Fluid/electrolyte imbalance (eg, hyponatremia, hypochloremic alkalosis, hypokalemia) may develop. May cause hyperuricemia and precipitation of frank gout. Latent diabetes mellitus (DM) may manifest during therapy. Enhanced effects seen in postsympathectomy patients. D/C prior to parathyroid function test. Decreased Ca^{2+} excretion observed. Altered parathyroid gland, with hypercalcemia and hypophosphatemia observed with prolonged therapy. May increase urinary excretion of Mg^{2+}, resulting in hypomagnesemia.

ADVERSE REACTIONS

Fatigue, lethargy, dizziness, vertigo, flu syndrome, drowsiness, somnolence, hypokalemia, headache, bradycardia.

DRUG INTERACTIONS

Metoprolol: May exhibit additive effect with catecholamine-depleting drugs (eg, reserpine). Digitalis glycosides may increase risk of bradycardia. Some inhalation anesthetics may enhance cardiodepressant effect. May be unresponsive to usual doses of epinephrine. Potent CYP2D6 inhibitors (eg, certain antidepressants, antipsychotics, antiarrhythmics, antiretrovirals, antihistamines, antimalarials, antifungals, stomach ulcer drugs) may increase levels. Increased risk for rebound HTN following clonidine withdrawal; d/c metoprolol several days before withdrawing clonidine. Effects can be reversed by β-agonists (eg, dobutamine, isoproterenol). HCTZ: Hypokalemia can sensitize/exaggerate cardiac response to toxic effects of digitalis. Risk of hypokalemia with steroids or adrenocorticotropic hormone. Insulin requirements may change in diabetic patients. May decrease arterial responsiveness to norepinephrine. May increase responsiveness to tubocurarine. May increase risk of lithium toxicity. Rare reports of hemolytic anemia with methyldopa. NSAIDs may reduce diuretic, natriuretic, and antihypertensive effects. Impaired absorption reported with cholestyramine and colestipol. Alcohol, barbiturates, and narcotics may potentiate orthostatic hypotension. May potentiate other antihypertensive drugs (eg, ganglionic or peripheral adrenergic-blocking drugs).

PATIENT CONSIDERATIONS

Assessment: Assess for history of heart failure, sulfonamide hypersensitivity, SLE, hyperthyroidism, DM, pheochromocytoma, hepatic/renal impairment, any other conditions where treatment is contraindicated/cautioned, pregnancy/nursing status, and possible drug interactions. Obtain baseline serum electrolytes.

Monitoring: Monitor for signs/symptoms of cardiac failure, hypoglycemia, thyrotoxicosis, electrolyte imbalance, exacerbation/activation of SLE, hyperuricemia or precipitation of gout, hypersensitivity reactions, hepatic/renal dysfunction, myopia, angle-closure glaucoma, and other adverse reactions. Monitor serum electrolytes.

Counseling: Instruct to take regularly and continuously, ud, with or immediately following meals. If dose is missed, instruct to take next dose at scheduled time (without doubling the dose) and not to d/c without consulting physician. Instruct to avoid driving, operating machinery, or engaging in tasks requiring alertness until response to therapy is determined. Advise to contact physician if difficulty in breathing or other adverse reactions occur, and to inform physician/dentist of drug therapy before undergoing any type of surgery.

STORAGE: (Lopressor HCT) 25°C (77°F); excursions permitted to 15-30°C (59-86°F). (Metoprolol/HCTZ) 20-25°C (68-77°F). Protect from moisture.

MICARDIS – telmisartan

RX

Class: Angiotensin II receptor blocker (ARB)

D/C when pregnancy is detected. Drugs that act directly on the renin-angiotensin system (RAS) can cause injury/death to the developing fetus.

ADULT DOSAGE

Hypertension

Initial: 40mg qd
Range: 40-80mg/day
May add diuretic if BP not controlled w/ 80mg

Risk Reduction of Myocardial Infarction, Stroke, Cardiovascular Death

For use in patients ≥55 years of age at high risk of developing major CV events who are unable to take ACE inhibitors

80mg qd

PEDIATRIC DOSAGE

Pediatric use may not have been established

DOSING CONSIDERATIONS

Hepatic Impairment
Including Biliary Obstructive Disorders:
Start at low doses and titrate slowly

ADMINISTRATION

Oral route

Take w/ or w/o food

HOW SUPPLIED

Tab: 20mg, 40mg, 80mg

CONTRAINDICATIONS

Known hypersensitivity (eg, anaphylaxis, angioedema) to telmisartan or any other component of this product, coadministration w/ aliskiren in patients w/ diabetes.

WARNINGS/PRECAUTIONS

May develop orthostatic hypotension in patients on dialysis. Symptomatic hypotension may occur in patients with an activated RAS (eg, volume- and/or salt-depleted patients receiving high doses of diuretics); correct this condition before therapy or monitor closely. Hyperkalemia may occur, particularly in patients with advanced renal impairment, HF, and on renal replacement therapy; monitor serum electrolytes periodically. Caution in patients with hepatic impairment (eg, biliary obstructive disorders); reduced clearance may be expected. Oliguria and/or progressive azotemia and (rarely) acute renal failure and/or death may occur in patients whose renal function is dependent on the RAS (eg, severe CHF). May increase SrCr/BUN in patients with renal artery stenosis.

ADVERSE REACTIONS

URTI, back pain, sinusitis, diarrhea, intermittent claudication, skin ulcer.

DRUG INTERACTIONS

See Contraindications. Dual blockade of the RAS is associated with increased risk of hypotension, hyperkalemia, and changes in renal function (eg, acute renal failure); avoid combined use of RAS inhibitors. Closely monitor BP, renal function, and electrolytes with concomitant agents that also affect the RAS. Avoid with aliskiren in patients with renal impairment (GFR <60mL/min). Avoid with an ACE inhibitor. Coadministration with ramipril may increase ramipril/ramiprilat levels and decrease telmisartan levels; not recommended with ramipril. Hyperkalemia may occur with K^+ supplements, K^+-sparing diuretics, K^+-containing salt substitutes, or other drugs that increase K^+ levels. May increase digoxin levels; monitor digoxin levels upon initiating, adjusting, and discontinuing therapy. May increase serum lithium levels/toxicity; monitor lithium levels during concomitant use. NSAIDs, including selective COX-2 inhibitors, may attenuate antihypertensive effect and may deteriorate renal function; monitor renal function periodically.

M

PATIENT CONSIDERATIONS

Assessment: Assess for known hypersensitivity to drug, biliary obstructive disorders, CHF, renal artery stenosis, hepatic/renal impairment, volume/salt depletion, dialysis patients, pregnancy/nursing status, and possible drug interactions.

Monitoring: Monitor for symptomatic hypotension and other adverse reactions. Monitor BP, ECG, renal function, and serum electrolytes.

Counseling: Inform women of childbearing age about the consequences of exposure to the medication during pregnancy. Discuss treatment options with women planning to become pregnant. Instruct to report pregnancies to the physician as soon as possible.

STORAGE: 25°C (77°F); excursions permitted to 15-30°C (59-86°F).

MICARDIS HCT – hydrochlorothiazide/telmisartan **RX**

Class: Angiotensin II receptor blocker (ARB)/thiazide diuretic

D/C when pregnancy is detected. Drugs that act directly on the renin-angiotensin system (RAS) can cause injury/death to the developing fetus.

ADULT DOSAGE

Hypertension

Patients whose BP is not adequately controlled w/ telmisartan monotherapy 80mg, or is not adequately controlled by 25mg qd hydrochlorothiazide (HCTZ), or is controlled but experience hypokalemia

Initial: 80mg/12.5mg qd
Titrate: May increase up to 160mg/25mg after 2-4 weeks

Patients titrated to the individual components may instead receive the corresponding dose of Micardis HCT

PEDIATRIC DOSAGE

Pediatric use may not have been established

M

DOSING CONSIDERATIONS

Renal Impairment
Severe (CrCl ≤30mL/min): Not recommended

Hepatic Impairment
Severe: Not recommended

Biliary Obstructive Disorders/Hepatic Insufficiency:
Initial: 40mg/12.5mg qd under close medical supervision

Elderly
Start at lower end of dosing range

ADMINISTRATION

Oral route

Do not remove tab from blister until immediately before administration.
May be administered w/ other antihypertensive drugs.

HOW SUPPLIED

Tab: (Telmisartan/HCTZ) 40mg/12.5mg, 80mg/12.5mg, 80mg/25mg

CONTRAINDICATIONS

Hypersensitivity to any component of the medication, anuria, coadministration w/ aliskiren in patients w/ diabetes.

WARNINGS/PRECAUTIONS

Not for initial therapy. Symptomatic hypotension may occur in patients w/ an activated RAS (eg, volume- or salt-depleted patients). Correct volume or salt depletion prior to administration of therapy. Changes in renal function (eg, acute renal failure) may occur. Patients whose renal function may depend in part on the activity of the RAS may be at risk of developing oliguria, progressive azotemia, or acute renal failure. Consider withholding or discontinuing therapy in patients who develop a clinically significant decrease in renal function. **HCTZ:** May cause hypokalemia, hyponatremia, and hypomagnesemia. Decreases urinary calcium excretion and may cause elevations of serum calcium. May alter glucose tolerance and raise serum levels of cholesterol and TGs. Hyperuricemia may occur or frank gout may be precipitated. Hypersensitivity reactions may occur; more likely to occur in patients w/ history of allergy or bronchial asthma. May cause an idiosyncratic reaction, resulting in acute transient myopia and acute angle-closure glaucoma;

d/c as rapidly as possible. May cause exacerbation or activation of systemic lupus erythematosus (SLE). The antihypertensive effects of the drug may be enhanced in the postsympathectomy patient. **Telmisartan:** May cause hyperkalemia, particularly in patients w/ renal insufficiency or diabetes.

ADVERSE REACTIONS

URTI, dizziness, sinusitis, fatigue, diarrhea.

DRUG INTERACTIONS

See Contraindications. Increases in serum lithium concentrations and lithium toxicity reported; monitor serum lithium levels during concomitant use. NSAIDs, including selective COX-2 inhibitors, may decrease effects of diuretics and ARBs and may deteriorate renal function (possible acute renal failure). Avoid w/ aliskiren in patients w/ renal impairment (GFR <60mL/min). **HCTZ:** Dosage adjustment of antidiabetic drugs (eg, oral agents, insulin) may be required. Anionic exchange resins (eg, cholestyramine, colestipol) may impair absorption; stagger the dose of HCTZ and the resin such that HCTZ is administered at least 4 hrs before or 4-6 hrs after the administration of the resin. **Telmisartan:** Use w/ other drugs that raise serum K^+ may result in hyperkalemia; monitor serum K^+. Dual blockade of the RAS is associated w/ increased risks of hypotension, hyperkalemia, and renal impairment; avoid combined use of RAS inhibitors. Closely monitor BP, renal function, and electrolytes in patients on concomitant agents that affect the RAS. May increase digoxin peak plasma concentration and digoxin trough concentrations; monitor digoxin levels.

PATIENT CONSIDERATIONS

Assessment: Assess for hypersensitivity to the drugs and their components, anuria, sulfonamide-derived hypersensitivity, history of penicillin allergy, volume/salt depletion, SLE, diabetes, CHF, hepatic/renal impairment, biliary obstructive disorder, renal artery stenosis, postsympathectomy status, pregnancy/nursing status, and possible drug interactions. Obtain baseline BP.

Monitoring: Monitor for signs/symptoms of fluid/electrolyte imbalance, exacerbation/activation of SLE, idiosyncratic reaction, precipitation of gout, hypersensitivity reactions, and other adverse reactions. Monitor BP, serum electrolytes, renal/hepatic function, Ca^{2+} levels, cholesterol, and TG levels periodically.

Counseling: Inform women of childbearing age about the consequences of exposure to the medication during pregnancy. Discuss treatment options w/ women planning to become pregnant. Instruct to report pregnancies to the physician as soon as possible. Caution that lightheadedness may occur, especially during the 1st days of therapy. Inform that inadequate fluid intake, excessive perspiration, diarrhea, or vomiting can lead to an excessive fall in BP, w/ the same consequences of lightheadedness and possible syncope. Instruct to contact physician if syncope occurs. Advise not to use K^+ supplements or salt substitutes that contain K^+ w/o consulting physician. Advise to d/c therapy and seek immediate medical attention if the patient experiences symptoms of acute myopia or secondary angle-closure glaucoma.

STORAGE: 25°C (77°F); excursions permitted to 15-30°C (59-86°F).

MICROZIDE — hydrochlorothiazide

RX

Class: Thiazide diuretic

ADULT DOSAGE

Hypertension

Initial: 12.5mg qd
Max: 50mg/day

PEDIATRIC DOSAGE

Pediatric use may not have been established

DOSING CONSIDERATIONS

Elderly

Start at lower end of dosing range, utilizing 12.5mg increments for further titration

ADMINISTRATION

Oral route

HOW SUPPLIED

Cap: 12.5mg

CONTRAINDICATIONS

Anuria, hypersensitivity to this product or other sulfonamide-derived drugs.

WARNINGS/PRECAUTIONS

May cause idiosyncratic reaction, resulting in acute transient myopia and acute angle-closure glaucoma; d/c as rapidly as possible. May manifest latent diabetes mellitus (DM). May precipitate azotemia with renal impairment. Hypokalemia reported; monitor serum electrolytes and for sign/symptoms of fluid/electrolyte disturbances. Dilutional hyponatremia may occur in edematous patients in hot weather. Hyperuricemia or acute gout may be precipitated. Caution with hepatic impairment; hepatic coma may occur with severe liver disease. Decreased Ca^{2+} excretion and changes in parathyroid glands with hypercalcemia and hypophosphatemia reported during prolonged use. D/C prior to parathyroid test.

ADVERSE REACTIONS

Weakness, hypotension, pancreatitis, jaundice, diarrhea, vomiting, hematologic abnormalities, anaphylactic reactions, electrolyte imbalance, muscle spasm, vertigo, renal failure, erythema multiforme, transient blurred vision, impotence.

DRUG INTERACTIONS

Potentiation of orthostatic hypotension with alcohol, barbiturates, narcotics. Additive effect or potentiation with antihypertensive drugs. Dose adjustment of antidiabetic drugs (oral agents or insulin) may be required. Reduced absorption with cholestyramine or colestipol. Increased risk of electrolyte depletion (eg, hypokalemia) with corticosteroids and adrenocorticotropic hormone. May decrease response to pressor amines (eg, norepinephrine). May increase responsiveness to nondepolarizing skeletal muscle relaxants (eg, tubocurarine). Increased risk of lithium toxicity; avoid with lithium. NSAIDs may reduce diuretic, natriuretic, and antihypertensive effects. May cause hypokalemia, which can sensitize or exaggerate the response of the heart to the toxic effects of digitalis.

PATIENT CONSIDERATIONS

Assessment: Assess for anuria, known hypersensitivity to sulfonamide-derived drugs, history of penicillin allergy, DM, risk for developing hypokalemia, impaired renal/hepatic function, edema, pregnancy/nursing status, and for possible drug interactions. Obtain baseline serum electrolytes.

Monitoring: Monitor for signs/symptoms of decreased visual acuity, ocular pain, azotemia, hypokalemia, fluid/electrolyte disturbances, dilutional hyponatremia, hyperuricemia or acute gout, and hepatic coma. Periodically monitor serum electrolytes in patients with risk for developing hypokalemia.

Counseling: Counsel about signs/symptoms of fluid and electrolyte imbalance and advise to seek prompt medical attention.

STORAGE: 20-25°C (68-77°F). Protect from light, moisture, freezing, -20°C (-4°F). Keep container tightly closed.

MINIPRESS — prazosin hydrochloride RX

Class: $Alpha_1$ blocker (quinazoline)

ADULT DOSAGE

Hypertension

Initial: 1mg bid-tid
Titrate: May slowly increase to a total of 20mg/day in divided doses
Maint: 6-15mg/day in divided doses
Doses >20mg usually do not increase efficacy; however, some may benefit from further increases up to 40mg/day in divided doses
May maintain adequately on a bid dose regimen

PEDIATRIC DOSAGE

Pediatric use may not have been established

DOSING CONSIDERATIONS

Concomitant Medications

Use w/ a Diuretic or Other Antihypertensive Agent:
Reduce to 1mg or 2mg tid, then retitrate

Use w/ a PDE-5 Inhibitor:
Initiate PDE-5 inhibitor at the lowest dose

ADMINISTRATION

Oral route

HOW SUPPLIED

Cap: 1mg, 2mg, 5mg

CONTRAINDICATIONS

Known sensitivity to quinazolines, prazosin, or any of the inert ingredients.

WARNINGS/PRECAUTIONS

May cause syncope w/ sudden loss of consciousness; minimize syncopal episodes by limiting initial dose to 1mg, by subsequently increasing the dose slowly, and by introducing any additional antihypertensive w/ caution. Prolonged erections and priapism reported; penile tissue damage and permanent loss of potency may result if priapism is not treated immediately. Intraoperative floppy iris syndrome observed during cataract surgery. False (+) results may occur in screening tests for pheochromocytoma; d/c w/ elevated urinary vanillylmandelic acid levels and retest after 1 month.

ADVERSE REACTIONS

Dizziness, headache, drowsiness, lack of energy, weakness, palpitations, N/V, edema, orthostatic hypotension, dyspnea, syncope, depression, urinary frequency, diarrhea.

DRUG INTERACTIONS

See Dosing Considerations. Additive hypotensive effects w/ diuretics, β-blockers (eg, propranolol), or other antihypertensives. Additive BP-lowering effects and symptomatic hypotension w/ PDE-5 inhibitors.

PATIENT CONSIDERATIONS

Assessment: Assess for previous hypersensitivity to drug/quinazolines, pregnancy/nursing status, and for possible drug interactions. Obtain baseline BP.

Monitoring: Monitor for signs/symptoms of hypotension, dizziness, lightheadedness, syncope, priapism, and other adverse reactions.

Counseling: Inform that dizziness or drowsiness may occur after 1st dose; instruct to avoid driving or performing hazardous tasks for first 24 hrs after taking the drug or when dose is increased. Advise that dizziness, lightheadedness, or fainting may occur, especially when rising from a lying or sitting position; inform that getting up slowly may lessen these problems. Inform that these problems may also occur if taking alcohol, standing for long periods, exercising, or during hot weather, and advise caution during these situations. Instruct to seek immediate medical attention if an erection persists >4 hrs.

STORAGE: <30°C (86°F).

MINIVELLE – estradiol

RX

Class: Estrogen

Increased risk of endometrial cancer in a woman with a uterus who uses unopposed estrogens. Adding a progestin to estrogen therapy has been shown to reduce risk of endometrial hyperplasia. Adequate diagnostic measures should be undertaken to rule out malignancy in postmenopausal women with undiagnosed persistent or recurring abnormal genital bleeding. Should not be used for the prevention of cardiovascular (CV) disease or dementia. Increased risk of stroke and deep vein thrombosis (DVT) reported in postmenopausal women (50-79 yrs of age) treated with daily oral conjugated estrogens (CEs) alone and when combined with medroxyprogesterone acetate (MPA). Increased risk of developing probable dementia reported in postmenopausal women ≥65 yrs of age treated with daily CEs alone and when combined with MPA. Increased risks of pulmonary embolism (PE), myocardial infarction (MI), and invasive breast cancer reported in postmenopausal women (50-79 yrs of age) treated with daily oral CEs combined with MPA. Should be prescribed at the lowest effective dose and for the shortest duration consistent with treatment goals and risks.

ADULT DOSAGE

Postmenopausal Osteoporosis

Prevention:

Initial: 0.025mg/day 2X weekly

Titrate: Adjust dose as necessary

Menopausal Vasomotor Symptoms

Moderate to Severe:

Initial: 0.0375mg/day 2X weekly

Titrate: Adjust dose based on response.

Attempts to taper or d/c therapy should be made at 3- to 6-month intervals

PEDIATRIC DOSAGE

Pediatric use may not have been established

ADMINISTRATION

Transdermal route

Patch Application Instructions

Place adhesive side on a clean, dry area on the lower abdomen (below the umbilicus) or buttocks

Replace 2X weekly (every 3-4 days)

Rotate application sites, with an interval of at least 1 week allowed between applications to a particular site

Refer to PI for further application instructions

HOW SUPPLIED

Patch: 0.025mg/day, 0.0375mg/day, 0.05mg/day, 0.075mg/day, 0.1mg/day [8[S]]

CONTRAINDICATIONS

Undiagnosed abnormal genital bleeding, known/suspected/history of breast cancer, known/suspected estrogen-dependent neoplasia, active/history of DVT/PE/arterial thromboembolic disease (eg, stroke, MI), known anaphylactic reaction/angioedema/hypersensitivity w/ estradiol, known liver impairment/disease, known protein C/protein S/antithrombin deficiency or other known thrombophilic disorders, known/suspected pregnancy.

WARNINGS/PRECAUTIONS

D/C immediately if PE, DVT, stroke, or MI occurs or is suspected. If feasible, d/c at least 4-6 weeks before surgery of the type associated with an increased risk of thromboembolism, or during periods of prolonged immobilization. May increase risk of gallbladder disease requiring surgery and risk of ovarian cancer. May lead to severe hypercalcemia in patients with breast cancer and bone metastases; d/c and take appropriate measures if hypercalcemia occurs. Retinal vascular thrombosis reported; d/c therapy pending exam if sudden partial/complete loss of vision, or sudden onset of proptosis, diplopia, or migraine occurs. D/C permanently if exam reveals papilledema or retinal vascular lesions. May increase BP and thyroid-binding globulin levels. May be associated with elevations of plasma TGs leading to pancreatitis in patients with preexisting hypertriglyceridemia; consider discontinuation if pancreatitis occurs. Caution with history of cholestatic jaundice associated with past estrogen use or with pregnancy; d/c in case of recurrence. May cause fluid retention. Caution with hypoparathyroidism; hypocalcemia may occur. Cases of malignant transformation of residual endometrial implants reported in women treated posthysterectomy with estrogen therapy alone; consider addition of progestin for patients known to have residual endometriosis posthysterectomy. Anaphylactic/anaphylactoid reactions, and angioedema involving eye/eyelid, face, larynx, pharynx, tongue, and extremity with or without urticaria requiring medical intervention reported; do not reapply in patients who develop angioedema anytime during the course of treatment. May exacerbate symptoms of angioedema in women with hereditary angioedema. May exacerbate asthma, diabetes mellitus, epilepsy, migraines, porphyria, systemic lupus erythematosus, and hepatic hemangiomas. May affect certain endocrine and blood components in lab tests.

ADVERSE REACTIONS

M

Constipation, dyspepsia, nausea, influenza-like illness, pain, nasopharyngitis, sinusitis, upper respiratory tract infection, back pain, headache, depression, insomnia, breast tenderness, intermenstrual bleeding, sinus congestion.

DRUG INTERACTIONS

CYP3A4 inducers (eg, St. John's wort preparations, phenobarbital, carbamazepine) may decrease levels, possibly resulting in a decrease in therapeutic effects and/or changes in the uterine bleeding profile. CYP3A4 inhibitors (eg, erythromycin, ketoconazole, grapefruit juice) may increase levels, and may result in side effects. Patients concomitantly receiving thyroid hormone replacement therapy and estrogens may require increased doses of thyroid replacement therapy; monitor thyroid function.

PATIENT CONSIDERATIONS

Assessment: Assess for abnormal genital bleeding, presence/history of breast cancer, estrogen-dependent neoplasia, active/history of DVT/PE/arterial thromboembolic disease, liver impairment/disease, thrombophilic disorders, known anaphylactic reaction or angioedema/hypersensitivity to the drug, pregnancy/nursing status, any other conditions where treatment is contraindicated or cautioned, need for progestin therapy, and for possible drug interactions.

Monitoring: Monitor for signs/symptoms of CV disorders, malignant neoplasms, dementia, gallbladder disease, hypercalcemia, visual abnormalities, BP and plasma TG elevations, pancreatitis, cholestatic jaundice, hypothyroidism, fluid retention, exacerbation of endometriosis, anaphylactic/anaphylactoid reactions, angioedema, and other adverse reactions. Perform adequate diagnostic measures (eg, endometrial sampling) in patients with undiagnosed, persistent or recurring abnormal genital bleeding. Perform annual breast exam; schedule mammography based on patient's age, risk factors, and prior mammogram results. Monitor thyroid function if on thyroid hormone replacement therapy. Perform periodic evaluation to determine treatment need.

Counseling: Inform of the importance of reporting unusual vaginal bleeding to physician as soon as possible. Inform of possible serious adverse reactions of therapy (eg, CV disorders, malignant neoplasms, probable dementia) and of possible less serious but common adverse reactions (eg, headache, breast pain and tenderness, N/V). Instruct to have yearly breast exams by a physician and to perform monthly breast self-exams.

STORAGE: 20-25°C (68-77°F); excursions permitted between 15-30°C (59-86°F). Do not store unpouched; apply immediately upon removal from the protective pouch.

MINOCIN – minocycline

RX

Class: Tetracyclines

ADULT DOSAGE

General Dosing

Cap:
Initial: 200mg
Maint: 100mg q12h
Alternate Dosing:
Initial: If more frequent doses are preferred, give two or four 50mg caps
Maint: One 50mg cap qid

Inj:
Initial: 200mg
Maint: 100mg q12h
Max: 400mg/24 hrs

Parenteral therapy is indicated only when oral therapy is not adequate or tolerated; institute oral therapy as soon as possible

Gonococcal Infections

Uncomplicated Infections Other Than Urethritis and Anorectal Infections in Men:
Cap:
Initial: 200mg
Maint: 100mg q12h for a minimum of 4 days, w/ post-therapy cultures w/in 2-3 days

Urethral Infections

Cap:
Uncomplicated Gonococcal Urethritis in Men When Penicillin is Contraindicated:
100mg q12h for 5 days

Uncomplicated Infections Caused by *Chlamydia trachomatis/Ureaplasma urealyticum*:
100mg q12h for at least 7 days

Syphilis

When Penicillin is Contraindicated:
Cap:
Initial: 200mg
Maint: 100mg q12h over a period of 10-15 days

Meningococcal Carrier State

Cap:
Usual: 100mg q12h for 5 days

Mycobacterial Infections

***Mycobacterium marinum* Infections:**
Cap:
Optimal doses have not been established; 100mg q12h for 6-8 weeks have been successfully used

Endocervical Infections

Uncomplicated Infections Caused by *Chlamydia trachomatis/Ureaplasma urealyticum*:
Cap:
100mg q12h for at least 7 days

Rectal Infections

Uncomplicated Infections Caused by *Chlamydia trachomatis/Ureaplasma urealyticum*:
Cap:
100mg q12h for at least 7 days

PEDIATRIC DOSAGE

General Dosing

>8 Years:
Cap/Inj:
Initial: 4mg/kg
Maint: 2mg/kg q12h, not to exceed usual adult dose

M

Other Indications

Treatment of the Following Infections Caused by Susceptible Microorganisms:
Rocky Mountain spotted fever
Typhus fever and the typhus group
Q fever
Rickettsialpox
Tick fevers
Respiratory tract infections
Lymphogranuloma venereum
Psittacosis (ornithosis)
Trachoma
Inclusion conjunctivitis
Relapsing fever
Chancroid (cap)
Plague
Tularemia
Cholera
Campylobacter fetus infections
Brucellosis (in conjunction w/ streptomycin)
Bartonellosis
Granuloma inguinale
UTIs
Skin and skin structure infections

Treatment of Infections Caused by Susceptible Strains:
Escherichia coli
Enterobacter aerogenes
Shigella species
Acinetobacter species

Treatment of the following infections caused by susceptible microorganisms When Penicillin is Contraindicated:
Infections in women caused by *Neisseria gonorrhoeae* (cap)
Meningitis (inj)
Yaws
Listeriosis
Anthrax
Vincent's infection
Actinomycosis
Clostridium species infection

Adjunctive therapy in acute intestinal amebiasis and severe acne

M

DOSING CONSIDERATIONS

Renal Impairment

CrCl <80mL/min:
Max Dose: 200mg/24 hrs

Elderly

Start at lower end of dosing range

ADMINISTRATION

Oral/IV routes

Cap

Take w/ or w/o food
Swallow whole w/ adequate amounts of fluids

IV

Administer as an IV infusion over 60 min
Avoid rapid administration

Reconstitution:
Reconstitute w/ 5mL of sterile water for inj and immediately further dilute in 100-1000mL w/ NaCl inj, dextrose inj, or dextrose and NaCl inj, or in 250-1000mL lactated Ringer's inj, but not w/ other sol containing Ca^{2+}

Incompatibilities:
Do not add additives or other medications or infuse simultaneously through the same IV line including Y-connectors; if the same IV line is used for sequential infusion of additional medications,

the line should be flushed before and after infusion of minocycline w/ NaCl inj, dextrose inj, dextrose and NaCl inj, or lactated Ringer's inj

HOW SUPPLIED

Cap: 50mg, 75mg, 100mg; **Inj:** 100mg

CONTRAINDICATIONS

Hypersensitivity to any of the tetracyclines or to any of the components of the product formulation.

WARNINGS/PRECAUTIONS

May cause fetal harm. May cause permanent discoloration of the teeth (yellow-gray-brown) if used during tooth development (last 1/2 of pregnancy, infancy, and childhood to 8 yrs of age); do not use during tooth development. Enamel hypoplasia reported. May decrease fibula growth rate in premature infants. Drug rash w/ eosinophilia and systemic symptoms (DRESS), including fatal cases, reported; d/c immediately if this syndrome is recognized. May cause an increase in BUN; w/ significant impaired renal function, high levels of therapy may lead to azotemia, hyperphosphatemia, and acidosis. Photosensitivity manifested by an exaggerated sunburn reaction reported. CNS side effects reported; may impair mental/physical abilities. *Clostridium difficile*-associated diarrhea (CDAD) reported; may need to d/c if CDAD is suspected or confirmed. Associated w/ intracranial HTN (pseudotumor cerebri); increased risk in women of childbearing age who are overweight or have a history of intracranial HTN. If visual disturbance occurs, prompt ophthalmologic evaluation is warranted. Intracranial pressure can remain elevated for weeks after drug cessation; monitor patients until they stabilize. May result in bacterial resistance if used in the absence of proven or suspected bacterial infection, or a prophylactic indication; take appropriate measures if superinfection develops. Hepatotoxicity reported. False elevations of urinary catecholamine levels may occur due to interference w/ the fluorescence test. (Cap) Not indicated for the treatment of meningococcal infection; reserve prophylactic use for situations in which the risk of meningococcal meningitis is high. (Inj) Contains magnesium sulfate heptahydrate; caution in patients w/ heart block or myocardial damage.

ADVERSE REACTIONS

Neutropenia, agranulocytosis, lupus-like syndrome, serum sickness-like syndrome, fever, N/V, diarrhea, increased liver enzymes, thyroid cancer, anaphylaxis, exfoliative dermatitis, Stevens-Johnson syndrome, skin and mucous membrane pigmentation, headache.

DRUG INTERACTIONS

Caution w/ other hepatotoxic drugs. Depresses plasma prothrombin activity; may require downward adjustment of anticoagulant dosage. May interfere w/ bactericidal action of PCN; avoid concurrent use. Fatal renal toxicity reported w/ methoxyflurane. May decrease effectiveness of oral contraceptives. Avoid isotretinoin shortly before, during, and after therapy; each drug alone is associated w/ pseudotumor cerebri. Increased risk of ergotism w/ ergot alkaloids or their derivatives. (Cap) Impaired absorption w/ antacids containing aluminum, Ca^{2+}, or Mg^{2+}, and iron-containing preparations. (Inj) Potentially serious drug interactions may occur when IV magnesium sulfate heptahydrate is given concomitantly w/ CNS depressants, neuromuscular blocking agents, and cardiac glycosides.

PATIENT CONSIDERATIONS

Assessment: Assess for hypersensitivity to drug, risk for intracranial HTN, hepatic/renal impairment, pregnancy/nursing status, and possible drug interactions. Perform culture and susceptibility tests. (Cap) In venereal disease when coexistent syphilis is suspected, perform a dark-field examination and blood serology. (Inj) Assess for heart block or myocardial damage. Perform serologic test for syphilis (if treating gonorrhea). Obtain baseline serum Mg^{2+} levels in patients w/ renal impairment.

Monitoring: Monitor for DRESS, photosensitivity, CNS effects, CDAD, intracranial HTN, superinfection, and other adverse reactions. Perform periodic lab evaluations of organ systems, including hematopoietic, renal, and hepatic studies. (Cap) In venereal disease when coexistent syphilis is suspected, repeat blood serology monthly for at least 4 months. (Inj) In patients w/ gonorrhea, perform a follow-up serologic test for syphilis after 3 months. Monitor serum Mg^{2+} levels in patients w/ renal impairment. Closely monitor patients w/ heart block or myocardial damage.

Counseling: Apprise of the potential hazard to fetus if used during pregnancy; instruct to notify physician if pregnant. Counsel that therapy should only be used to treat bacterial, not viral, infections. Instruct to take exactly ud even if the patient feels better early in the course of therapy. Inform that skipping doses or not completing the full course of therapy may decrease effectiveness of treatment and increase bacterial resistance. Inform that diarrhea may be experienced; instruct to immediately contact physician if watery and bloody stools (w/ or w/o stomach cramps and fever) occur, even as late as ≥2 months after the last dose. Advise that photosensitivity manifested by an exaggerated sunburn reaction may occur; instruct to d/c treatment at the 1st evidence of skin erythema. Caution patients who experience CNS symptoms about driving vehicles or using hazardous machinery while on therapy. Inform that drug may render oral contraceptives less effective.

STORAGE: 20-25°C (68-77°F). (Cap) Protect from light, moisture, and excessive heat. (Inj) Once diluted into an IV bag, store either at room temperature for up to 4 hrs or refrigerated at 2-8°C (36-46°F) for up to 24 hrs; discard any unused portions after that period.

MINOCYCLINE EXTENDED-RELEASE TABLETS – minocycline hydrochloride RX

Class: Tetracyclines

OTHER BRAND NAMES
Solodyn

ADULT DOSAGE

Acne Vulgaris

Treatment of Inflammatory Lesions of Non-Nodular Moderate to Severe Acne:
1mg/kg qd for 12 weeks

Body Weight and Strength to Achieve Approximately 1mg/kg:
45-49kg: 45mg (1-0.92mg/kg)
50-59kg: 55mg (1.10-0.93mg/kg)
60-71kg: 65mg (1.08-0.92mg/kg)
72-84kg: 80mg (1.11-0.95mg/kg)
85-96kg: 90mg (1.06-0.94mg/kg)
97-110kg: 105mg (1.08-0.95mg/kg)
111-125kg: 115mg (1.04-0.92mg/kg)
126-136kg: 135mg (1.07-0.99mg/kg)

PEDIATRIC DOSAGE

Acne Vulgaris

Treatment of Inflammatory Lesions of Non-Nodular Moderate to Severe Acne:
≥12 Years:
1mg/kg qd for 12 weeks

Body Weight and Strength to Achieve Approximately 1mg/kg:
45-49kg: 45mg (1-0.92mg/kg)
50-59kg: 55mg (1.10-0.93mg/kg)
60-71kg: 65mg (1.08-0.92mg/kg)
72-84kg: 80mg (1.11-0.95mg/kg)
85-96kg: 90mg (1.06-0.94mg/kg)
97-110kg: 105mg (1.08-0.95mg/kg)
111-125kg: 115mg (1.04-0.92mg/kg)
126-136kg: 135mg (1.07-0.99mg/kg)

DOSING CONSIDERATIONS

Renal Impairment
Decrease total dosage by either reducing the recommended individual doses and/or by extending time intervals between doses

Elderly
Start at lower end of dosing range

ADMINISTRATION
Oral route
Swallow tab whole; do not chew, crush, or split.
May take w/ or w/o food; ingestion w/ food may help reduce the risk of esophageal irritation and ulceration.

HOW SUPPLIED
Tab, Extended-Release: 45mg, 90mg, 135mg; (Solodyn) 55mg, 65mg, 80mg, 105mg, 115mg

CONTRAINDICATIONS
Hypersensitivity to any of the tetracyclines.

WARNINGS/PRECAUTIONS
Higher doses may be associated w/ more acute vestibular side effects. May cause fetal harm; avoid use during pregnancy or by individuals of either gender who are attempting to conceive a child. Avoid use during tooth development (last 1/2 of pregnancy, infancy, childhood up to 8 yrs of age); may cause permanent discoloration (yellow-gray-brown) of the teeth. Enamel hypoplasia reported. May decrease fibula growth rate in premature infants. *Clostridium difficile* associated diarrhea (CDAD) reported; may need to d/c if CDAD is suspected or confirmed. Serious liver injury, including irreversible drug-induced hepatitis and fulminant hepatic failure (sometimes fatal) reported. May cause an increase in BUN; w/ significant renal impairment, higher levels of therapy may lead to azotemia, hyperphosphatemia, and acidosis. CNS side effects reported; may impair mental/physical abilities. Pseudotumor cerebri (benign intracranial HTN) reported; if visual disturbance occurs during treatment, check for papilledema. Associated w/ development of autoimmune syndromes; d/c immediately and perform LFTs, antinuclear antibody (ANA) test, CBC, and other appropriate tests. Photosensitivity manifested by an exaggerated sunburn reaction reported. Cases of anaphylaxis, serious skin reactions (eg, Stevens-Johnson syndrome), erythema multiforme, and drug rash w/ eosinophilia and systemic symptoms (DRESS) syndrome reported; d/c immediately if DRESS occurs. May induce hyperpigmentation in many organs. Drug-resistant bacteria may develop; use only as indicated. May result in overgrowth of nonsusceptible organisms, including fungi; d/c and institute appropriate therapy if superinfection occurs. False elevations of urinary catecholamine levels may occur due to interference with the fluorescence test.

ADVERSE REACTIONS
Headache, fatigue, dizziness, pruritus, malaise, mood alteration.

DRUG INTERACTIONS
Avoid w/ isotretinoin; may also cause pseudotumor cerebri. Depresses plasma prothrombin activity; may require downward adjustment of anticoagulant dosage. May interfere w/ bactericidal

action of penicillin; avoid concomitant use. Fatal renal toxicity reported w/ methoxyflurane. Antacids containing aluminum, Ca^{2+}, or Mg^{2+}, and iron-containing preparations may impair absorption. May cause changes in estradiol, progestinic hormone, follicle-stimulating hormone and luteinizing hormone levels, of breakthrough bleeding, or of contraceptive failure w/ low dose oral contraceptives.

PATIENT CONSIDERATIONS

Assessment: Assess for renal impairment, visual disturbances, hypersensitivity to any tetracyclines, pregnancy/nursing status, and possible drug interactions.

Monitoring: Monitor for signs/symptoms of CDAD, hepatotoxicity, superinfection, pseudotumor cerebri, visual disturbance, papilledema, DRESS syndrome, CNS side effects, autoimmune syndrome, photosensitivity, and other adverse reactions. Periodically monitor hematopoietic/renal/hepatic function. Perform LFTs, ANA test, and CBC in patients showing symptoms of an autoimmune syndrome. Perform drug serum level determinations w/ prolonged therapy in patients w/ renal impairment.

Counseling: Instruct to avoid use if pregnant, or if planning to conceive a child (patients of either gender). Inform that pseudomembranous colitis may occur; instruct to seek medical attention if watery/bloody stools develop. Inform of the possibility of hepatotoxicity; instruct to seek medical advice if loss of appetite, tiredness, diarrhea, skin turning yellow, bleeding easily, confusion, or sleepiness occurs. Instruct patients who experience CNS symptoms to use caution in driving or operating machinery and advise to seek medical help for persistent headaches/blurred vision. Inform that drug may render oral contraceptives less effective; advise to use 2nd form of contraception during therapy. Inform that autoimmune syndromes may occur; instruct to d/c immediately and seek medical help if symptoms (eg, arthralgia, fever, rash, malaise) are experienced. Counsel about discoloration of skin, scars, teeth, or gums that may arise from therapy. Inform that photosensitivity reactions may occur; advise to minimize/avoid exposure to natural/artificial sunlight (tanning beds, UVA/B treatment), to wear loose-fitting clothes when outdoors, and to d/c at 1st evidence of skin erythema. Instruct to take exactly ud; inform that skipping doses or not completing full course of therapy may decrease effectiveness and increase likelihood of bacterial resistance.

STORAGE: 20-25°C (68-77°F). Protect from light, moisture, and excessive heat. **Solodyn:** 25°C (77°F); excursions permitted to 15-30°C (59-86°F). Protect from light, moisture, and excessive heat.

MIRAPEX – pramipexole dihydrochloride

RX

Class: Dopamine receptor agonist

ADULT DOSAGE

Parkinson's Disease

Initial: 0.375mg/day given in 3 divided doses
Titrate: May increase gradually not more frequently than every 5-7 days
Maint: 1.5-4.5mg/day administered in equally divided doses tid w/ or w/o levodopa; consider reduction of levodopa dose when used in combination w/ therapy

Suggested Ascending Dosage Schedule:
Week 1: 0.125mg tid
Week 2: 0.25mg tid
Week 3: 0.5mg tid
Week 4: 0.75mg tid
Week 5: 1mg tid
Week 6: 1.25mg tid
Week 7: 1.5mg tid

If a significant interruption in therapy has occurred, retitration may be warranted

Restless Legs Syndrome

Moderate to Severe Primary Restless Legs Syndrome (RLS):
Initial: 0.125mg qd
Titrate: May increase dose every 4-7 days; no evidence that the 0.75mg dose provides additional benefit beyond the 0.5mg dose

PEDIATRIC DOSAGE

Pediatric use may not have been established

Ascending Dosage Schedule:
Titration Step 1: 0.125mg qd
Titration Step 2 (If Needed): 0.25mg qd
Titration Step 3 (If Needed): 0.5mg qd

Administer 2-3 hrs before hs
If a significant interruption in therapy has occurred, retitration may be warranted

DOSING CONSIDERATIONS

Renal Impairment

Parkinson's Disease:

Mild (CrCl >50mL/min):
Initial: 0.125mg tid
Max: 1.5mg tid

Moderate (CrCl 30-50mL/min):
Initial: 0.125mg bid
Max: 0.75mg tid

Severe (CrCl 15 to <30mL/min):
Initial: 0.125mg qd
Max: 1.5mg qd

Very Severe (CrCl <15mL/min and Hemodialysis Patients):
Has not been adequately studied in this group of patients

RLS:

Moderate and Severe Renal Impairment (CrCl 20-60mL/min):
Increase duration between titration steps to 14 days

Discontinuation

Parkinson's Disease:
May be tapered off at a rate of 0.75mg/day until daily dose has been reduced to 0.75mg; thereafter, may reduce dose by 0.375mg/day

ADMINISTRATION

Oral route

Take w/ or w/o food.

HOW SUPPLIED

Tab: 0.125mg, 0.25mg*, 0.5mg*, 0.75mg, 1mg*, 1.5mg* *scored

WARNINGS/PRECAUTIONS

Falling asleep during activities of daily living and somnolence reported; should ordinarily be discontinued if significant daytime sleepiness or episodes of falling asleep during activities that require active participation develop. May impair mental/physical abilities. May cause orthostatic hypotension; monitor for signs/symptoms, especially during dose escalation. May cause intense urges (eg, to gamble/spend money, increased sexual urges, binge eating) and patients may experience the inability to control these urges while on therapy; consider dose reduction or discontinuation of therapy. Hallucinations reported; risk increases w/ age. May experience new or worsening mental status and behavioral changes, which may be severe, including psychotic-like behavior during treatment or after starting/increasing the dose. Avoid w/ major psychotic disorder. May cause or exacerbate preexisting dyskinesia. Rhabdomyolysis and retinal deterioration may occur. Symptom complex resembling the neuroleptic malignant syndrome reported w/ rapid dose reduction, withdrawal of, or changes in dopaminergic therapy; if possible, avoid sudden discontinuation/rapid dose reduction, and if a decision is made to d/c therapy, taper to reduce the risk of hyperpyrexia and confusion. May cause fibrotic complications (eg, retroperitoneal fibrosis, pulmonary infiltrates, pleural effusion, pleural thickening, pericarditis, cardiac valvulopathy). Monitor for melanomas frequently and regularly; perform periodic skin examinations. Rebound and augmentation in RLS reported.

ADVERSE REACTIONS

Early Parkinson's Disease (w/o Levodopa): Nausea, dizziness, somnolence, insomnia, constipation, asthenia, hallucinations.

Advanced Parkinson's Disease (w/ Levodopa): Postural (orthostatic) hypotension, dyskinesia, extrapyramidal syndrome, insomnia, dizziness, hallucinations, dream abnormalities, confusion, constipation, asthenia, somnolence, dystonia, gait abnormality, hypertonia, dry mouth, amnesia, urinary frequency.

RLS: Nausea, somnolence.

DRUG INTERACTIONS

Sedating medications or alcohol, and medications that increase plasma levels of pramipexole (eg, cimetidine) may increase risk of drowsiness. Dopamine antagonists, (eg, neuroleptics [phenothiazines, butyrophenones, thioxanthenes] or metoclopramide) may diminish effectiveness. May potentiate dopaminergic side effects of levodopa.

PATIENT CONSIDERATIONS

Assessment: Assess for preexisting dyskinesia, major psychotic disorder, sleep disorders, renal impairment, pregnancy/nursing status, and possible drug interactions.

Monitoring: Monitor for drowsiness or sleepiness, orthostatic hypotension, impulse control/compulsive behaviors, hallucinations, new/worsening mental status and behavioral changes, signs/symptoms of rhabdomyolysis, retinal deterioration, fibrotic complications, melanomas, and other adverse reactions.

Counseling: Instruct to take as prescribed. If a dose is missed, advise not to double the next dose. Advise that the occurrence of nausea may be reduced if taken w/ food. Instruct not to take both immediate-release pramipexole and extended-release pramipexole. Advise and alert about the potential sedating effects, including somnolence and the possibility of falling asleep while engaged in activities of daily living; instruct not to drive a car or engage in other potentially dangerous activities until the patient has gained sufficient experience w/ pramipexole tabs to gauge whether or not it affects the patient's mental and/or motor performance adversely. Advise to inform physician if taking alcohol or other sedating medications. Inform of the possibility to experience intense urges and the inability to control these urges. Inform that hallucinations and other psychotic-like behavior may occur. Advise that postural (orthostatic) hypotension may develop w/ or w/o symptoms. Advise to monitor for melanomas frequently and regularly. Instruct to notify physician if pregnant/intending to become pregnant during therapy or breastfeeding/intending to breastfeed.

STORAGE: 25°C (77°F); excursions permitted to 15-30°C (59-86°F). Protect from light.

MIRAPEX ER – pramipexole dihydrochloride

RX

Class: Dopamine receptor agonist

ADULT DOSAGE

Parkinson's Disease

Initial: 0.375mg qd

Titrate: Based on efficacy and tolerability, may increase gradually not more frequently than every 5-7 days, 1st to 0.75mg/day and then by 0.75mg increments

Max: 4.5mg/day

If a significant interruption in therapy occurs, retitration may be warranted

Conversions

Switching from Immediate-Release Pramipexole Tabs:

May switch overnight at the same daily dose; monitor to determine if dosage adjustment is necessary

PEDIATRIC DOSAGE

Pediatric use may not have been established

DOSING CONSIDERATIONS

Renal Impairment

Moderate (CrCl 30-50mL/min):

Initial: Administer qod; carefully assess therapeutic response and tolerability before increasing to daily dosing after 1 week, and before any additional titration in 0.375mg increments

Titrate: Dose adjustment should occur no more frequently than at weekly intervals

Max: 2.25mg/day

Severe (CrCl <30mL/min)/Hemodialysis:

Not recommended

Discontinuation

May taper off at a rate of 0.75mg/day until daily dose has been reduced to 0.75mg; thereafter, may reduce dose by 0.375mg/day

ADMINISTRATION

Oral route

Take w/ or w/o food.

Swallow whole; do not chew, crush, or divide tab.

HOW SUPPLIED

Tab, Extended-Release (ER): 0.375mg, 0.75mg, 1.5mg, 2.25mg, 3mg, 3.75mg, 4.5mg

WARNINGS/PRECAUTIONS

Falling asleep during activities of daily living and somnolence reported; should ordinarily be discontinued if significant daytime sleepiness or episodes of falling asleep during activities that require active participation develop. May impair mental/physical abilities. May cause orthostatic hypotension; monitor for signs/symptoms, especially during dose escalation. May cause intense urges (eg, to gamble/spend money, increased sexual urges, binge eating) and patients may experience the inability to control these urges while on therapy; consider dose reduction or discontinuation of therapy. Hallucinations (visual, auditory, or mixed) reported; risk increases w/ age. May experience new or worsening mental status and behavioral changes, which may be severe, including psychotic-like behavior during treatment or after starting/increasing the dose. Avoid w/ major psychotic disorder. May cause or exacerbate preexisting dyskinesia. Rhabdomyolysis and retinal deterioration may occur. Symptom complex resembling the neuroleptic malignant syndrome may occur w/ rapid dose reduction, withdrawal of, or changes in dopaminergic therapy; if possible, avoid sudden discontinuation/rapid dose reduction, and if a decision is made to d/c therapy, taper to reduce the risk of hyperpyrexia and confusion. May cause fibrotic complications (eg, retroperitoneal fibrosis, pulmonary infiltrates, pleural effusion, pleural thickening, pericarditis, cardiac valvulopathy). Monitor for melanomas frequently and regularly; perform periodic skin examinations.

ADVERSE REACTIONS

Early Parkinson's Disease (w/o Levodopa): Somnolence, nausea, constipation, dizziness, fatigue, hallucinations, dry mouth, muscle spasms, peripheral edema.

Advanced Parkinson's Disease (w/ Levodopa): Dyskinesia, nausea, constipation, hallucinations, headache, anorexia.

DRUG INTERACTIONS

Sedating medications or alcohol, and medications that increase plasma levels of pramipexole (eg, cimetidine) may increase risk of drowsiness. May potentiate dopaminergic side effects of levodopa. Dopamine antagonists (eg, neuroleptics [phenothiazines, butyrophenones, thioxanthenes] or metoclopramide) may diminish effectiveness.

PATIENT CONSIDERATIONS

Assessment: Assess for preexisting dyskinesia, major psychotic disorder, renal impairment, sleep disorders, pregnancy/nursing status, and possible drug interactions.

Monitoring: Monitor for drowsiness or sleepiness, orthostatic hypotension, impulse control/compulsive behaviors, hallucinations, new or worsening mental status and behavioral changes, signs/symptoms of rhabdomyolysis, melanomas, fibrotic complications, retinal deterioration, and other adverse reactions. Monitor therapeutic response/tolerability at a minimal interval of 5 days or longer after each dose increment.

Counseling: Instruct to take therapy as prescribed. Advise that if a dose is missed, to take it as soon as possible, but no later than 12 hrs after the regularly scheduled time. Instruct that if 12 hrs have passed, to skip the missed dose and take the next dose on the following day at the regularly scheduled time. Advise that nausea may be reduced if taken w/ food. Instruct not to take both immediate-release and ER pramipexole. Advise and alert about the potential sedating effects; instruct not to drive a car or engage in other dangerous activities until gaining sufficient experience w/ therapy. Advise to inform physician if taking alcohol or other sedating medications. Inform of the possibility to experience intense urges and the inability to control these urges. Inform that hallucinations and other psychotic-like behavior may occur. Advise that postural (orthostatic) hypotension may develop w/ or w/o symptoms. Advise to monitor for melanomas frequently and regularly. Instruct to notify physician if pregnant/intending to be pregnant during therapy or if breastfeeding/intending to breastfeed.

STORAGE: 25°C (77°F); excursions permitted to 15-30°C (59-86°F). Protect from exposure to high humidity.

MIRCETTE — desogestrel/ethinyl estradiol

RX

Class: Estrogen/progestogen combination

Cigarette smoking increases the risk of serious cardiovascular (CV) side effects. Risk increases with age and with heavy smoking (≥15 cigarettes/day) and is quite marked in women >35 yrs. Women who use oral contraceptives should be strongly advised not to smoke.

OTHER BRAND NAMES

Kariva

ADULT DOSAGE

Contraception

1 tab qd for 28 days, then repeat

Start 1st Sunday after menses begins or 1st day of menses

PEDIATRIC DOSAGE

Contraception

Not indicated for use premenarche; refer to adult dosing

Missed Dose

Miss 1 Active Tab: Take missed tab as soon as remembered

Miss 2 Consecutive Active Tabs in Week 1 or 2: Take 2 tabs the day remembered and 2 tabs the next day; thereafter, resume taking 1 tab qd until pack is finished. Use backup method of birth control if having intercourse in the 7 days after missing pills

Miss 2 Consecutive Active Tabs in Week 3 or Miss ≥3 Active Tabs in a Row at Any Time: (Sunday Start) Continue to take 1 tab qd until Sunday, then throw out the rest of the pack and start a new pack of pills that same day. (Day 1 Start) Throw out rest of the pack and start new pack the same day. (Sunday/Day 1 Start) Use backup method of birth control if having intercourse in the 7 days after missing pills

Conversions

Switching from a Sunday Start Oral Contraceptive:

Sunday Start:

Take 1st tab on the 2nd Sunday after last tab of a 21-day regimen or take on the 1st Sunday after last inactive tab of a 28-day regimen

Switching Directly from Another Oral Contraceptive:

Day 1 Start:

Take 1st tab on the 1st day of menstruation which begins after last active tab of previous product

ADMINISTRATION

Oral route

Take exactly ud and at intervals not exceeding 24 hrs

Use another method of contraception until after the first 7 consecutive days of administration when initiating a Sunday Start regimen

HOW SUPPLIED

Tab: (Ethinyl Estradiol-Desogestrel) 0.02mg-0.15mg, (Ethinyl Estradiol) 0.01mg

CONTRAINDICATIONS

Thrombophlebitis or past history of deep vein thrombophlebitis, thromboembolic disorders (current or past history), suspected/known pregnancy, cerebral vascular or coronary artery disease, undiagnosed abnormal genital bleeding, cholestatic jaundice of pregnancy or jaundice with prior pill use, known/suspected breast carcinoma, carcinoma of the endometrium or other known/suspected estrogen-dependent neoplasia, hepatic adenomas or carcinomas.

WARNINGS/PRECAUTIONS

Increased risk of MI, vascular disease, thromboembolism, stroke, hepatic neoplasia, and gallbladder disease. Increased risk of morbidity and mortality with HTN, hyperlipidemias, obesity, and diabetes mellitus (DM). D/C at least 4 weeks prior to and for 2 weeks after elective surgery associated with an increased risk of thromboembolism and during and following prolonged immobilization, if feasible. Start use no earlier than 4 weeks after delivery in women who elect not to breastfeed. Caution in women with CV disease risk factors. May develop visual changes or changes in lens tolerance in contact lens wearers. Retinal thrombosis reported; d/c if unexplained partial or complete loss of vision, onset of proptosis or diplopia, papilledema, or retinal vascular lesions develop. Should not be used to induce withdrawal bleeding as a test for pregnancy, or to treat threatened or habitual abortion during pregnancy. May decrease glucose tolerance; monitor prediabetic and diabetic patients. May elevate BP; monitor closely and d/c use if significant BP elevation occurs. New onset/exacerbation of migraine, or recurrent, persistent, severe headache may develop; d/c if these occur. Breakthrough bleeding and spotting reported; rule out malignancy or pregnancy. D/C if jaundice develops. May be poorly metabolized in patients with impaired liver function. May cause fluid retention; caution with conditions that aggravate fluid retention. Caution with history of depression; d/c if depression recurs to a serious degree. Does not protect against HIV infection (AIDS) and other STDs. Perform annual history/physical exam; monitor women with history of breast cancer. Not for use before menarche. May affect certain endocrine, LFTs, and blood components in laboratory tests.

ADVERSE REACTIONS

N/V, breakthrough bleeding, spotting, amenorrhea, migraine, mental depression, vaginal candidiasis, edema, weight changes, abdominal cramps/bloating, menstrual flow changes, pulmonary embolism, MI, HTN.

DRUG INTERACTIONS

Reduced efficacy and increased breakthrough bleeding and menstrual irregularities with rifampin, barbiturates, phenylbutazone, phenytoin sodium, carbamazepine, and possibly with griseofulvin, ampicillin, and tetracyclines. May decrease lamotrigine levels; dosage adjustment of lamotrigine may be necessary.

PATIENT CONSIDERATIONS

Assessment: Assess for current or history of thrombophlebitis or thromboembolic disorders, history of HTN, hyperlipidemia, DM, obesity, breast cancer, nursing status, or any other conditions where treatment is contraindicated/cautioned, and possible drug interactions.

Monitoring: Monitor for MI, thromboembolism, stroke, hepatic neoplasia, and other adverse effects. Monitor BP with history of HTN, serum glucose levels in diabetic or prediabetic patients, lipid levels with hyperlipidemia, and for signs of worsening depression with previous history. Refer contact lens wearer to ophthalmologist if ocular changes develop. Perform annual history and physical exam. Monitor women with strong family history of breast cancer or who have breast nodules. Monitor LFTs, PT, thyroxine binding-globulin, T3 and T4, and serum folate levels.

Counseling: Counsel about potential adverse effects, and to avoid smoking while on therapy. Inform that drug does not protect against HIV infection and other STDs. Inform about pregnancy risk if pills are missed. Instruct to take at the same time every day and that intervals between doses should not exceed 24 hrs. Instruct that when initiating a Sunday Start regimen, to use another method of contraception until after first 7 consecutive days of administration. Instruct if one "active" pill is missed to take as soon as remembered, and take next pill at regular time.

STORAGE: 20-25°C (68-77°F).

M

MIRENA – levonorgestrel

RX

Class: Progestin contraceptive

ADULT DOSAGE

Contraception

Recommended for females who have had at least 1 child

Contraception for Up to 5 Years:
Insert into the uterine cavity during the first 7 days of the menstrual cycle

Following 1st Trimester Abortion: Insert immediately after a 1st trimester abortion

Following 2nd Trimester Abortion/ Postpartum: Postpone insertion by a minimum of 6 weeks or until the uterus is fully involuted; wait until involution is complete before insertion

Timing of Removal:
Should not remain in the uterus after 5 yrs
If pregnancy is not desired, removal should be carried out during menstruation, provided the woman is still experiencing regular menses
If removal will occur at other times during the cycle, consider starting a new contraceptive method a week prior to removal

Heavy Menstrual Bleeding

Recommended for females who have had at least 1 child

In Women Who Choose to Use Intrauterine Contraception as their Method of Contraception:
Insert into the uterine cavity during the first 7 days of the menstrual cycle

Following 1st Trimester Abortion: Insert immediately after a 1st trimester abortion

PEDIATRIC DOSAGE

Contraception

Not indicated for use premenarche; refer to adult dosing

Heavy Menstrual Bleeding

Not indicated for use premenarche; refer to adult dosing

Following 2nd Trimester Abortion/ Postpartum: Postpone insertion by a minimum of 6 weeks or until the uterus is fully involuted; wait until involution is complete before insertion

Timing of Removal:
Should not remain in the uterus after 5 yrs
If pregnancy is not desired, removal should be carried out during menstruation, provided the woman is still experiencing regular menses
If removal will occur at other times during the cycle, consider starting a new contraceptive method a week prior to removal

Conversions

Switching to a Different Birth Control Method:
Patients w/ Regular Cycles:
Time removal and initiation of new method to ensure continuous contraception. Either remove Mirena during the first 7 days of the menstrual cycle and start the new method immediately, or start the new method at least 7 days prior if removal is to occur at other times during the cycle
Patients w/ Irregular Cycles/Amenorrhea:
Start the new method at least 7 days before removal

ADMINISTRATION

Intrauterine route

Should be inserted by a trained healthcare provider.
Back-up contraception is not needed if inserted as directed.
Consider administering analgesics prior to insertion.
Remove Mirena if it is not positioned completely w/in the uterus; do not reinsert once it is removed.
Must be removed by the end of the 5th year.
Refer to PI for additional insertion and removal instructions.

HOW SUPPLIED

Intrauterine Insert: 52mg

CONTRAINDICATIONS

Pregnancy or suspicion of pregnancy, congenital or acquired uterine anomaly (including fibroids if they distort the uterine cavity), acute or history of pelvic inflammatory disease (PID) (unless there has been a subsequent intrauterine pregnancy), postpartum endometritis or infected abortion in the past 3 months, known/suspected uterine or cervical neoplasia, known/suspected or history of breast cancer or other progestin-sensitive cancer, uterine bleeding of unknown etiology, untreated acute cervicitis or vaginitis (including bacterial vaginosis or other lower genital tract infections until infection is controlled), acute liver disease or liver tumor (benign or malignant), conditions associated w/ increased susceptibility to pelvic infections, and previously inserted IUD that has not been removed. Hypersensitivity to any component of this product.

WARNINGS/PRECAUTIONS

Not for post-coital contraception. Should be inserted by a trained healthcare provider. Evaluate for ectopic pregnancy and remove device if pregnancy occurs. Increased risk of septic abortion, miscarriage, sepsis, premature delivery/labor, and possible congenital anomalies if pregnancy occurs and device is left in place. Severe infection or sepsis, including Group A streptococcal sepsis (GAS) reported; use aseptic technique during insertion of device. Associated w/ increased risk of PID and actinomycosis. May alter bleeding pattern and result in spotting, irregular bleeding, heavy bleeding, oligomenorrhea, and amenorrhea; perform appropriate diagnostic measures to rule out endometrial pathology if bleeding irregularities develop during prolonged use. Perforation may occur and may reduce contraceptive effectiveness; risk increased if inserted in lactating women and may be increased if inserted when the uterus is fixed retroverted or not completely involuted during postpartum. Partial or complete expulsion may occur; may be replaced w/in 7 days after the onset of a menstrual period after ruling out pregnancy. Ovarian cysts and breast cancer reported. Caution in patients w/ coagulopathy, migraine, focal migraine w/ asymmetrical visual loss or other symptoms indicating transient cerebral ischemia, exceptionally severe headache, marked increase in BP, and in patients w/ severe arterial disease. Consider removing device if uterine/cervical malignancy or jaundice arises during use. Consider possibility that device may have been displaced (eg, expelled or perforated the uterus) if the threads are not visible or are significantly shortened; exclude pregnancy and verify location of device. If device is displaced, remove it.

ADVERSE REACTIONS
Alterations of menstrual bleeding patterns (eg, unscheduled uterine bleeding, decreased uterine bleeding, increased scheduled uterine bleeding, female genital tract bleeding), abdominal/pelvic pain, amenorrhea, headache/migraine, genital discharge, vulvovaginitis.

DRUG INTERACTIONS
Drugs or herbal products that induce enzymes, including CYP3A4, that metabolize progestins (eg, barbiturates, bosentan, carbamazepine) may decrease levels. HIV protease inhibitors or non-nucleoside reverse transcriptase inhibitors may significantly increase or decrease plasma levels. CYP3A4 inhibitors (eg, itraconazole, ketoconazole) may increase plasma hormone levels. Caution w/ use of anticoagulants.

PATIENT CONSIDERATIONS

Assessment: Assess for congenital or acquired uterine anomaly, acute or history of PID, known/suspected or history of breast cancer or other progestin-sensitive cancer, acute liver disease or liver tumor, pregnancy/nursing status, any other conditions where treatment is contraindicated or cautioned, and for possible drug interactions. Perform a complete medical and social history and if indicated, a physical examination, and appropriate tests for any forms of genital or other STIs.

Monitoring: Monitor for intrauterine/ectopic pregnancy, severe infection/sepsis, GAS, PID, actinomycosis, bleeding pattern alterations, perforation, expulsion, migraine/exceptionally severe headache, jaundice, marked BP increase, and other adverse reactions. Reexamine and evaluate 4-6 weeks after insertion and once a yr thereafter, or more frequently if clinically indicated. Monitor if threads are still visible and for length of threads.

Counseling: Inform that product does not protect against HIV infection (AIDS) and other STIs. Explain the risks/benefits/side effects of the device. Inform of the risk of ectopic pregnancy, including loss of fertility; instruct to promptly report symptoms of ectopic pregnancy to physician. Inform of the possibility of PID and of its symptoms; instruct to promptly notify physician if any symptoms of PID develop. Inform that irregular/prolonged bleeding and spotting, and/or cramps may occur during the 1st few weeks after insertion; instruct to report to physician if symptoms continue or are severe. Instruct on how to check if the device's threads still protrude from the cervix and caution not to pull on the threads and displace device. Inform that no contraceptive protection exists if device is displaced or expelled. Instruct to contact physician if any adverse reactions develop, if pregnancy is suspected or occurs, if HIV positive seroconversion occurs in the patient or her partner, or if possible exposure to STIs occurs.

M

STORAGE: 25°C (77°F); excursions permitted to 15-30°C (59-86°F).

MIRTAZAPINE – mirtazapine

RX

Class: $Alpha_2$ antagonist

Antidepressants increased the risk of suicidal thinking and behavior (suicidality) in children, adolescents, and young adults in short-term studies of major depressive disorder and other psychiatric disorders. Monitor and observe closely for clinical worsening, suicidality, or unusual changes in behavior in patients who are started on antidepressant therapy. Not approved for use in pediatric patients.

OTHER BRAND NAMES
Remeron, RemeronSolTab

ADULT DOSAGE

Major Depressive Disorder

Initial: 15mg qhs
Titrate: Dose changes should not be made at intervals of <1-2 weeks
Max: 45mg/day

Dosing Considerations with MAOIs

Switching to/from an MAOI for Psychiatric Disorders:
Allow at least 14 days between discontinuation of an MAOI and initiation of mirtazapine, and allow at least 14 days between discontinuation of mirtazapine and initiation of an MAOI

W/ Other MAOIs (eg, Linezolid, IV Methylene Blue):
Do not start mirtazapine in patients being treated w/ linezolid or IV methylene blue. In patients already receiving mirtazapine,

PEDIATRIC DOSAGE
Pediatric use may not have been established

if acceptable alternatives are not available and benefits outweigh risks, d/c mirtazapine promptly and administer linezolid or IV methylene blue; monitor for serotonin syndrome for 2 weeks or until 24 hrs after the last dose of linezolid or IV methylene blue, whichever comes 1st. May resume mirtazapine therapy 24 hrs after the last dose of linezolid or IV methylene blue

DOSING CONSIDERATIONS

Discontinuation

Gradually reduce dose over several weeks whenever possible

ADMINISTRATION

Oral route

RemeronSolTab

Open blister pack w/ dry hands and place tab on the tongue.
Use immediately after removal from blister; once removed, it cannot be stored.
Tab will disintegrate rapidly on the tongue and can be swallowed w/ saliva; no water is needed.
Do not split the tab.

HOW SUPPLIED

Tab: 7.5mg; (Remeron) 15mg*, 30mg*, 45mg; **Tab, Disintegrating:** (RemeronSolTab) 15mg, 30mg, 45mg *scored

CONTRAINDICATIONS

Known hypersensitivity to mirtazapine or to any of the excipients. Use of an MAOI for psychiatric disorders either concomitantly or w/in 14 days of stopping treatment. Treatment w/in 14 days of stopping an MAOI for psychiatric disorders. Starting treatment in patients being treated w/ other MAOIs (eg, linezolid, IV methylene blue).

WARNINGS/PRECAUTIONS

Not approved for treatment of bipolar depression. May precipitate a mixed/manic episode in patients at risk for bipolar disorder; screen for risk of bipolar disorder prior to initiating treatment. Agranulocytosis and severe neutropenia reported; d/c if sore throat, fever, stomatitis, or other signs of infection develop, along w/ low WBC counts. Serotonin syndrome reported; d/c immediately if symptoms occur and initiate supportive symptomatic treatment. Pupillary dilation that occurs following use may trigger an angle-closure attack in a patient w/ anatomically narrow angles who does not have a patent iridectomy. Akathisia/psychomotor restlessness reported; increasing the dose may be detrimental in patients who develop these symptoms. May impair mental/physical abilities. Hyponatremia, mania/hypomania, somnolence, dizziness, increased appetite, weight gain, and elevation in cholesterol/TG/ALT levels reported. May cause seizures. Caution w/ hepatic/renal impairment, diseases/conditions affecting metabolism or hemodynamic responses, and in the elderly. May cause orthostatic hypotension; caution w/ cardiovascular (CV) or cerebrovascular disease that could be exacerbated by hypotension and conditions that predispose to hypotension. Decreased clearance in elderly patients and in patients w/ moderate to severe renal or hepatic impairment.

ADVERSE REACTIONS

Somnolence, increased appetite, weight gain, dizziness, dry mouth, constipation, asthenia, flu syndrome, abnormal dreams, abnormal thinking.

DRUG INTERACTIONS

See Dosage and Contraindications. May cause serotonin syndrome w/ other serotonergic drugs (eg, triptans, TCAs, fentanyl) and w/ drugs that impair metabolism of serotonin; d/c immediately if this occurs. Caution w/ antihypertensives and drugs known to cause hyponatremia. Phenytoin, carbamazepine, and other hepatic metabolism inducers (eg, rifampicin) may decrease levels; may need to increase mirtazapine dose or if such inducers are discontinued, may need to reduce mirtazapine. Cimetidine and ketoconazole may increase levels; may need to decrease mirtazapine dose when concomitant treatment w/ cimetidine is started, or increase dose when cimetidine treatment is discontinued. Avoid alcohol and diazepam or drugs similar to diazepam while on therapy. Caution w/ potent CYP3A4 inhibitors, HIV protease inhibitors, azole antifungals, erythromycin, or nefazodone. Increased INR w/ warfarin; monitor INR.

PATIENT CONSIDERATIONS

Assessment: Assess for risk of bipolar disorder or hyponatremia, susceptibility to angle-closure glaucoma, CV or cerebrovascular diseases, history of mania/hypomania/seizure, conditions that predispose to hypotension, renal/hepatic impairment, diseases/conditions affecting metabolism or hemodynamic response, hypersensitivity to drug, pregnancy/nursing status, and possible drug interactions.

Monitoring: Monitor for signs/symptoms of clinical worsening, suicidality, unusual changes in behavior, agranulocytosis, neutropenia, serotonin syndrome, angle-closure glaucoma, akathisia, somnolence, dizziness, increased appetite, weight gain, elevation in cholesterol/TG/ALT levels, hyponatremia, seizures, orthostatic hypotension, and other adverse reactions. Monitor INR w/ warfarin. Periodically re-evaluate long-term usefulness of the drug.

Counseling: Inform about the risks, benefits, and appropriate use of therapy. Advise families and caregivers of the need for close observation for signs of clinical worsening and suicidal risks and to report such signs to physician. Warn about risk of developing agranulocytosis and instruct to contact physician if signs of infection (eg, fever, chills, sore throat) develop. Advise to use caution when engaging in hazardous activities. Advise that improvement may be noticed in 1-4 weeks of therapy; instruct to continue therapy ud. Advise to inform physician if taking or intending to take any prescription or OTC drugs. Instruct to avoid alcohol while on therapy. Instruct to notify physician if pregnant, intending to become pregnant, or breastfeeding. Caution about the risk of angle-closure glaucoma. **RemeronSolTab:** Inform phenylketonuric patients that the tab contains phenylalanine.

STORAGE: 25°C (77°F); excursions permitted to 15-30°C (59-86°F). Protect from light and moisture.

MITIGARE – colchicine RX

Class: Miscellaneous gout agent

ADULT DOSAGE

Gout Flares

Prophylaxis: 0.6mg qd or bid
Max: 1.2mg/day

PEDIATRIC DOSAGE

Pediatric use may not have been established

DOSING CONSIDERATIONS

Concomitant Medications

CYP3A4 or P-gp Inhibitors: If concomitant use cannot be avoided, reduce daily dose or frequency and monitor for colchicine toxicity

M

Renal Impairment

Severe: Consider dose reduction or alternative therapy
Hemodialysis: Monitor carefully for colchicine toxicity

Hepatic Impairment

Severe: Consider dose reduction or alternative therapy

Elderly

Consider dose reduction

ADMINISTRATION

Oral route

Take w/o regard to meals.

HOW SUPPLIED

Cap: 0.6mg

CONTRAINDICATIONS

Concomitant use w/ drugs that inhibit both P-gp and CYP3A4 inhibitors in patients w/ renal or hepatic impairment. Patients w/ both renal and hepatic impairment.

WARNINGS/PRECAUTIONS

Not an analgesic medication and should not be used to treat pain from other causes. Fatal overdoses reported. Myelosuppression, leukopenia, granulocytopenia, thrombocytopenia, pancytopenia, and aplastic anemia reported. Neuromuscular toxicity and rhabdomyolysis reported w/ chronic use; increased risk w/ drugs known to cause these effects and in patients w/ impaired renal function and in the elderly.

ADVERSE REACTIONS

Abdominal pain, diarrhea, N/V.

DRUG INTERACTIONS

See Contraindications and Dosing Considerations. Inhibition of both CYP3A4 and P-gp by dual inhibitors (eg, clarithromycin) reported to produce life-threatening or fatal colchicine toxicity. Toxicities reported w/ CYP3A4 inhibitors (eg, grapefruit juice, erythromycin, verapamil) or P-gp inhibitors (eg, cyclosporine); avoid use. May increase risk of myopathy w/ HMG-CoA reductase inhibitors and fibrates.

PATIENT CONSIDERATIONS

Assessment: Assess for renal/hepatic impairment, pregnancy/nursing status, and possible drug interactions

Monitoring: Monitor for myelosuppression, leukopenia, granulocytopenia, thrombocytopenia, pancytopenia, aplastic anemia, neuromuscular toxicity, rhabdomyolysis, and other adverse reactions. Monitor patients on hemodialysis for colchicine toxicity.

Counseling: If a dose is missed, advise to take dose as soon as possible and return to normal dosing schedule; advise not to double the next dose if a dose is skipped. Advise that fatal overdoses have been reported; instruct to keep out of the reach of children. Advise that bone marrow depression w/ agranulocytosis, aplastic anemia, and thrombocytopenia may occur. Advise that many drugs or other substances may interact w/ treatment; instruct to provide all healthcare providers w/ a list of current medications (including nonprescription medications or herbal products) patients are taking and to check w/ healthcare provider before starting new medications. Advise to avoid grapefruit and grapefruit juice. Advise patients that muscle pain or weakness, tingling or numbness in fingers or toes may occur; instruct to d/c and seek medical evaluation immediately.

STORAGE: 20-25°C (68-77°F). Protect from light and moisture.

MOBIC – meloxicam RX

Class: NSAID

NSAIDs may cause an increased risk of serious cardiovascular (CV) thrombotic events, MI, stroke, and serious GI adverse events, including bleeding, ulceration, and perforation of the stomach or intestines. Elderly patients at greater risk for serious GI events. Contraindicated for the treatment of perioperative pain in the setting of CABG surgery.

ADULT DOSAGE

Osteoarthritis

Initial/Maint: 7.5mg qd
Max: 15mg/day

Rheumatoid Arthritis

Initial/Maint: 7.5mg qd
Max: 15mg/day

PEDIATRIC DOSAGE

Juvenile Rheumatoid Arthritis

Pauciarticular or Polyarticular Course:
≥2 Years:
0.125mg/kg qd
Max: 7.5mg/day

Use of the oral sus is recommended to improve dosing accuracy in smaller weight children

DOSING CONSIDERATIONS

Renal Impairment

Hemodialysis:
Max: 7.5mg/day

ADMINISTRATION

Oral route

Take w/o regard to time of meals.
7.5mg/5mL or 15mg/10mL oral sus may be substituted for 7.5mg or 15mg tab, respectively.

Sus

Shake gently before using.

HOW SUPPLIED

Sus: 7.5mg/5mL; **Tab:** 7.5mg, 15mg

CONTRAINDICATIONS

Known hypersensitivity to meloxicam. ASA or other NSAID allergy that precipitates asthma, urticaria, or allergic-type reactions. Treatment of perioperative pain in the setting of CABG surgery.

WARNINGS/PRECAUTIONS

Use lowest effective dose for the shortest duration possible. Extreme caution with history of ulcer disease or GI bleeding. May cause elevations of LFTs; d/c if liver disease develops, or if systemic manifestations occur. May lead to onset of new HTN, or worsening of preexisting HTN. Fluid retention and edema reported. Renal papillary necrosis, renal insufficiency, acute renal failure, and other renal injury reported after long-term use. Not recommended for use with severe renal impairment (CrCl <20mL/min). Caution in patients with considerable dehydration; rehydrate 1st, then start therapy. Caution in debilitated patients, with preexisting kidney disease, and asthma. Closely monitor patients with significant renal impairment. Avoid with ASA triad/ASA-sensitive asthma. May cause anaphylactoid reactions and serious skin adverse events (eg, exfoliative dermatitis, Stevens-Johnson syndrome, toxic epidermal necrolysis); d/c at 1st appearance of rash or other signs of hypersensitivity. Avoid use starting at 30 weeks gestation; may cause premature closure of ductus arteriosus. Not a substitute for corticosteroids or for treatment of corticosteroid insufficiency. May mask signs of inflammation and fever. Anemia may occur; with long-term use, monitor Hgb/Hct if symptoms of anemia develop. May inhibit platelet aggregation and prolong bleeding time. May be associated with a reversible delay in ovulation; not recommended in women with difficulties conceiving, or who are undergoing investigation of infertility.

ADVERSE REACTIONS
Abdominal pain, diarrhea, dyspepsia, nausea, headache, anemia, arthralgia, insomnia, URTI, UTI, dizziness, pain, pharyngitis, edema, influenza-like symptoms.

DRUG INTERACTIONS
Patients taking ACE inhibitors, thiazides, and loop diuretics (eg, furosemide) may have impaired response to these therapies. Risk of renal toxicity when coadministered with diuretics, ACE inhibitors, and angiotensin II receptor antagonists. Increased risk of GI bleeding with anticoagulants (eg, warfarin), smoking, alcohol, and oral corticosteroids. May diminish antihypertensive effect of ACE inhibitors. Not recommended with ASA; increased rate of GI ulceration or other complications with low-dose ASA. May elevate lithium plasma levels; observe for signs of lithium toxicity. May increase cyclosporine and MTX toxicities. (Sus) Not recommended with sodium polystyrene sulfonate (Kayexalate).

PATIENT CONSIDERATIONS

Assessment: Assess for cardiovascular disease (CVD), risk factors for CVD, ASA triad, coagulation disorders, any other conditions where treatment is contraindicated or cautioned, renal/hepatic dysfunction, pregnancy/nursing status, and possible drug interactions. Assess use in elderly and debilitated patients.

Monitoring: Monitor for signs/symptoms of CV thrombotic events, HTN, GI events, fluid retention, edema, and anaphylactoid/skin reactions. Monitor BP, renal function, and LFTs. Perform periodic monitoring of CBC and chemistry profile with long-term use.

Counseling: Advise to seek medical attention if symptoms of CV events (eg, chest pain, SOB, weakness, slurring of speech), GI ulceration and bleeding (eg, epigastric pain, dyspepsia, melena, hematemesis), hepatotoxicity (eg, nausea, fatigue, lethargy, pruritus, jaundice, right upper quadrant tenderness, flu-like symptoms), anaphylactoid reaction (eg, difficulty breathing, swelling of face/throat), skin rash, blisters, fever, hypersensitivity reaction (eg, itching), weight gain, or edema occur. Instruct to avoid use starting at 30 weeks gestation. Advise females of reproductive potential who desire pregnancy that drug may be associated with a reversible delay in ovulation.

STORAGE: 25°C (77°F); excursions permitted to 15-30°C (59-86°F). Keep tabs in a dry place.

M

MODERIBA – ribavirin

RX

Class: Nucleoside analogue

Not for monotherapy treatment of chronic hepatitis C (CHC) virus infection. Primary toxicity is hemolytic anemia. Anemia associated w/ therapy may result in worsening of cardiac disease and lead to fatal and nonfatal MIs. Avoid w/ history of significant/unstable cardiac disease. Contraindicated in women who are pregnant and in male partners of pregnant women. Extreme care must be taken to avoid pregnancy during therapy and for 6 months after completion of therapy in both female patients and in female partners of male patients who are taking therapy. Use at least 2 reliable forms of effective contraception during treatment and for 6 months after discontinuation.

ADULT DOSAGE

Chronic Hepatitis C with Compensated Liver Disease

Combination w/ Peginterferon Alfa-2a:
Not Previously Treated w/ Interferon Alpha:
Monoinfection:
Genotypes 1, 4:
<75kg: 1000mg/day in 2 divided doses
≥75kg: 1200mg/day in 2 divided doses
Treatment Duration: 48 weeks

Genotypes 2, 3:
800mg/day in 2 divided doses
Treatment Duration: 24 weeks

HIV Coinfection:
800mg/day
Treatment Duration: 48 weeks (regardless of genotype)

PEDIATRIC DOSAGE

Chronic Hepatitis C with Compensated Liver Disease

Combination w/ Peginterferon Alfa-2a:
Not Previously Treated w/ Interferon Alpha:
Monoinfection:
5-17 Years:
23-33kg: 200mg qam and 200mg qpm
34-46kg: 200mg qam and 400mg qpm
47-59kg: 400mg qam and 400mg qpm
60-74kg: 400mg qam and 600mg qpm
≥75kg: 600mg qam and 600 mg qpm

Patients who reach their 18th birthday while receiving combination therapy should remain on the pediatric dosing regimen through the completion of therapy

Treatment Duration:
Genotypes 2, 3: 24 weeks
Other Genotypes: 48 weeks

DOSING CONSIDERATIONS

Renal Impairment

Adults:

CrCl 30-50mL/min: Alternating doses, 200mg and 400mg qod

CrCl<30mL/min or Hemodialysis: 200mg/day

Adverse Reactions

W/O Cardiac Disease:

Hgb <10g/dL:

Adults: 200mg qam and 400mg qpm

Pediatrics:

23-33kg: 200mg qam

34-46kg: 200mg qam and 200mg qpm

47-59kg: 200mg qam and 200mg qpm

60-74kg: 200mg qam and 400mg qpm

≥75kg: 200mg qam and 400mg qpm

Hgb <8.5g/dL:

Adults and Pediatrics: D/C ribavirin

W/ History of Stable Cardiac Disease:

Hgb Decrease of ≥2g/dL During any 4-Week Treatment Period:

Adults: 200mg qam and 400mg qpm

Pediatrics:

23-33kg: 200mg qam

34-46kg: 200mg qam and 200mg qpm

47-59kg: 200mg qam and 200mg qpm

60-74kg: 200mg qam and 400mg qpm

≥75kg: 200mg qam and 400mg qpm

Hgb <12g/dL After 4 Weeks at Reduced Dose:

Adults and Pediatrics: D/C ribavirin

Adults:

If ribavirin has been withheld due to either a lab abnormality or clinical adverse reaction, may attempt to restart at 600mg/day and further increase to 800mg/day; not recommended to increase to the original assigned dose (1000-1200mg)

Pediatrics:

Upon resolution of a lab abnormality or clinical adverse reaction, may attempt to increase ribavirin dose to the original dose. If ribavirin has been withheld due to a lab abnormality or clinical adverse reaction, may make attempt to restart ribavirin at 1/2 the full dose

Discontinuation

Consider if at least a 2 $\log_{10}$ HCV RNA reduction from baseline by Week 12 is not achieved
Consider if HCV RNA levels remain detectable after treatment Week 24
D/C if hepatic decompensation develops during treatment

ADMINISTRATION

Oral route

Take w/ food
Refer to peginterferon alfa-2a labeling for dosage and administration instructions

HOW SUPPLIED

Tab: 200mg, 400mg, 600mg

CONTRAINDICATIONS

Women who are or may become pregnant, men whose female partners are pregnant, hemoglobinopathies (eg, thalassemia major, sickle cell anemia), and in combination w/ didanosine. When used w/ peginterferon alfa-2a, refer to the individual monograph.

WARNINGS/PRECAUTIONS

Combination therapy is associated w/ significant adverse reactions (eg, severe depression and suicidal ideation, hemolytic anemia, suppression of bone marrow function, autoimmune/infectious/ophthalmologic/cerebrovascular disorders, pulmonary dysfunction, colitis, pancreatitis, diabetes). Do not start therapy unless a negative pregnancy test has been obtained immediately prior to therapy. Caution w/ baseline risk of severe anemia (eg, spherocytosis, history of GI bleeding). Caution w/ preexisting cardiac disease; suspend or d/c therapy if cardiovascular status deteriorates. Risk of hepatic decompensation and death in CHC patients w/ cirrhosis. Severe acute hypersensitivity reactions and serious skin reactions reported. D/C w/ hepatic decompensation, confirmed pancreatitis, severe hypersensitivity, or if signs/symptoms of severe skin reactions develop. Pulmonary disorders (eg, dyspnea, pulmonary infiltrates, pneumonitis, pulmonary HTN, pneumonia) reported. Closely monitor if pulmonary infiltrates/function impairment develop and d/c if appropriate. Decreases in height and weight reported in pediatric patients.

M

ADVERSE REACTIONS
Hemolytic anemia, fatigue/asthenia, neutropenia, headache, pyrexia, myalgia, irritability/anxiety/nervousness, insomnia, alopecia, rigors, N/V, anorexia.

DRUG INTERACTIONS
See Contraindications. Closely monitor for treatment associated toxicities (eg, hepatic decompensation) w/ nucleoside reverse transcriptase inhibitors; consider dose reduction or discontinuation of peginterferon alfa-2a and/or ribavirin. Severe neutropenia and severe anemia reported w/ zidovudine; consider discontinuation of zidovudine if appropriate. Severe pancytopenia and bone marrow suppression reported w/ azathioprine; monitor CBC, including platelet counts, weekly for the 1st month, twice monthly for the 2nd and 3rd months of treatment, then monthly or more frequently if dosage or other therapy changes are necessary; d/c peginterferon alfa-2a, ribavirin, and azathioprine if pancytopenia develops.

PATIENT CONSIDERATIONS

Assessment: Assess for hemoglobinopathies, autoimmune hepatitis, hepatic decompensation, baseline risk of severe anemia, history of or preexisting cardiac disease, nursing status, and possible drug interactions. Conduct pregnancy test (including in female partners of male patients), standard hematological and biochemical lab tests, ECG in patients w/ preexisting cardiac abnormalities, renal/thyroid function test, and CD4 count in HIV patients. Assess baseline height and weight in pediatric patients.

Monitoring: Monitor for hemolytic anemia, hepatic decompensation, pancreatitis, hypersensitivity/skin reactions, pulmonary infiltrates/function impairment, and other adverse reactions. Monitor cardiac status, TSH, and HCV RNA. Perform hematological tests at Weeks 2 and 4 and biochemical tests at Week 4; perform additional testing periodically. Perform pregnancy testing monthly and for 6 months after discontinuation (including female partners of male patients). Monitor height and weight in pediatric patients. In patients on concomitant therapy w/ azathioprine, monitor CBC, including platelet counts, weekly for the 1st month, twice monthly for the 2nd and 3rd months of treatment, then monthly or more frequently if dosage or other therapy changes are necessary.

Counseling: Counsel on risks/benefits associated w/ treatment. Inform of pregnancy risks; instruct to use at least 2 forms of effective contraception during therapy and for 6 months after discontinuation of therapy (including female partners of male patients). Advise to notify physician immediately in the event of pregnancy. Advise that lab evaluations are required prior to starting therapy and periodically thereafter. Advise to be well-hydrated, especially during the initial stages of treatment. Caution to avoid driving/operating machinery if dizziness, confusion, somnolence, or fatigue develops. Instruct not to drink alcohol; inform that alcohol may exacerbate CHC infection. Inform to take appropriate precautions to prevent HCV transmission.

STORAGE: 25°C (77°F); excursions permitted between 15-30°C (59-86°F).

MONODOX — doxycycline monohydrate

RX

Class: Tetracyclines

ADULT DOSAGE

General Dosing

Initial: 100mg q12h or 50mg q6h on 1st day
Maint: 100mg qd or 50mg q12h

More Severe Infections (eg, Chronic UTIs):
100mg q12h

Streptococcal Infections:
Continue therapy for 10 days

Gonococcal Infections

Uncomplicated Infections (Except Anorectal Infections in Men):
100mg bid for 7 days

Alternate Dosing:
Single visit dose of 300mg stat followed in 1 hr by a second 300mg dose

Acute Epididymo-Orchitis

Caused by *Neisseria gonorrhoeae/Chlamydia trachomatis*:
100mg bid for at least 10 days

Syphilis

Primary and Secondary:
300mg/day in divided doses for at least 10 days

PEDIATRIC DOSAGE

General Dosing

>8 Years:

≤100 lbs:
2mg/lb divided into 2 doses on 1st day, followed by 1mg/lb qd or as 2 divided doses, on subsequent days
More Severe Infections: Up to 2mg/lb

>100 lbs:
Initial: 100mg q12h or 50mg q6h on 1st day
Maint: 100mg qd or 50mg q12h
More Severe Infections (eg, Chronic UTIs):
100mg q12h

Streptococcal Infections:
Continue therapy for 10 days

Inhalational Anthrax (Postexposure)

<100 lbs:
1mg/lb bid for 60 days
≥100 lbs:
100mg bid for 60 days

Chlamydia trachomatis Infections

Uncomplicated Urethral/Endocervical/Rectal Infections:
100mg bid for at least 7 days

Nongonococcal Urethritis

Caused by *Chlamydia trachomatis* and *Ureaplasma urealyticum*:
100mg bid for at least 7 days

Inhalational Anthrax (Postexposure)

100mg bid for 60 days

Other Indications

Treatment of the Following Infections Caused by Susceptible Microorganisms:
Rocky Mountain spotted fever
Typhus fever and the typhus group
Q fever
Rickettsialpox
Tick fevers
Respiratory tract infections
Lymphogranuloma venereum
Psittacosis (ornithosis)
Trachoma
Inclusion conjunctivitis
Relapsing fever
Chancroid
Plague
Tularemia
Cholera
Campylobacter fetus infections
Brucellosis (in conjunction w/ streptomycin)
Bartonellosis
Granuloma inguinale
UTIs

Treatment of Infections Caused by the Following Susceptible Strains:
Escherichia coli
Enterobacter aerogenes
Shigella species
Acinetobacter species

Treatment of the Following Infections Caused by Susceptible Microorganisms When Penicillin is Contraindicated:
Uncomplicated gonorrhea
Yaws
Listeriosis
Vincent's infection
Actinomycosis
Clostridium species

Adjunctive therapy in acute intestinal amebiasis and severe acne

ADMINISTRATION

Oral route

Administer w/ adequate amounts of fluid
May be given w/ food if gastric irritation occurs

HOW SUPPLIED

Cap: 50mg, 75mg, 100mg

CONTRAINDICATIONS

Hypersensitivity to any of the tetracyclines.

WARNINGS/PRECAUTIONS

May cause permanent discoloration of the teeth (yellow-gray-brown) if used during tooth development (last 1/2 of pregnancy, infancy, and childhood to 8 yrs of age); do not use in this age group, except for anthrax. Enamel hypoplasia reported. *Clostridium difficile*-associated diarrhea (CDAD) reported; d/c if CDAD is suspected or confirmed. May decrease fibula growth rate in prematures. May cause an increase in BUN. Photosensitivity, manifested by an exaggerated sunburn reaction, reported; d/c at the 1st evidence of skin erythema. May result in bacterial resistance if used in the absence of proven or suspected bacterial infection, or a prophylactic indication; take appropriate measures if superinfection develops. Associated w/ intracranial HTN (pseudotumor cerebri); increased risk in women of childbearing age who are overweight or have a history of intracranial HTN. If visual disturbance occurs, prompt ophthalmologic evaluation is warranted. Intracranial pressure can remain elevated for weeks after drug cessation; monitor patients until they stabilize. Incision and drainage or other surgical procedures should be performed in conjunction w/ antibacterial therapy when indicated. False elevations of urinary catecholamine levels may occur due to interference w/ the fluorescence test.

ADVERSE REACTIONS

Diarrhea, hepatotoxicity, maculopapular/erythematous rash, Stevens-Johnson syndrome, toxic epidermal necrolysis, anorexia, N/V, urticaria, serum sickness, pericarditis, hemolytic anemia, thrombocytopenia, neutropenia, eosinophilia.

DRUG INTERACTIONS

Avoid concomitant use w/ isotretinoin; may increase risk of intracranial HTN. Depresses plasma prothrombin activity; may require downward adjustment of anticoagulant dose. May interfere w/ bactericidal action of PCN; avoid concurrent use. Impaired absorption w/ antacids containing aluminum, Ca^{2+}, or Mg^{2+}, and iron-containing preparations. Decreased $T_{1/2}$ w/ barbiturates, carbamazepine, and phenytoin. Fatal renal toxicity reported w/ methoxyflurane. May render oral contraceptives less effective.

PATIENT CONSIDERATIONS

Assessment: Assess for hypersensitivity to drug or any tetracyclines, risk for intracranial HTN, pregnancy/nursing status, and possible drug interactions. Perform culture and susceptibility tests. In venereal disease when coexistent syphilis is suspected, perform a dark-field examination and blood serology.

Monitoring: Monitor for CDAD, photosensitivity, skin erythema, superinfection, intracranial HTN, visual disturbance, and other adverse reactions. In long-term therapy, perform periodic lab evaluations of organ systems, including hematopoietic, renal, and hepatic studies. In venereal disease when coexistent syphilis is suspected, repeat blood serology monthly for at least 4 months.

Counseling: Apprise of the potential hazard to fetus if used during pregnancy. Advise to avoid excessive sunlight or artificial UV light, and to d/c therapy if phototoxicity (eg, skin eruptions) occurs; advise to consider use of sunscreen or sunblock. Inform that absorption of drug is reduced when taken w/ bismuth subsalicylate, or w/ foods, especially those that contain Ca^{2+}. Inform that drug may increase incidence of vaginal candidiasis. Inform that diarrhea is a common problem caused by therapy, which usually ends when therapy is discontinued. Instruct to immediately contact physician if watery and bloody stools (w/ or w/o stomach cramps and fever) occur, even as late as ≥2 months after the last dose. Counsel that therapy should only be used to treat bacterial, not viral, infections. Instruct to take exactly ud, even if patient feels better early in the course of therapy. Inform that skipping doses or not completing the full course of therapy may decrease effectiveness of treatment and increase bacterial resistance.

STORAGE: 20-25°C (68-77°F); excursions permitted to 15-30°C (59-86°F).

MORPHINE ORAL SOLUTION AND TABLETS – morphine sulfate CII

Class: Opioid analgesic

Oral sol is available in 10mg/5mL, 20mg/5mL, and 100mg/5mL concentrations. The 100mg/5mL (20mg/mL) concentration is indicated for use in opioid-tolerant patients only. Use caution when prescribing and administering to avoid dosing errors due to confusion between different concentrations and between mg and mL, which could result in accidental overdose and death. Ensure the proper dose is communicated and dispensed. Keep sol out of reach of children. Seek emergency medical help immediately in case of accidental ingestion.

ADULT DOSAGE

Moderate to Severe Pain

Acute and Chronic:

Opioid-Naive Patients:

Initial: 10-20mg (sol) or 15-30mg (tab) q4h prn

Titrate: Adjust dose based on response to the initial dose

Opioid-Tolerant Patients:

Use the 100mg/5mL sol only for patients who have already been titrated to a stable analgesic regimen using lower strengths of

PEDIATRIC DOSAGE

Pediatric use may not have been established

morphine sulfate and who can benefit from use of a smaller volume of sol

Conversions

From Parenteral Morphine to Oral Morphine Sulfate:
Anywhere from 3-6mg of oral morphine sulfate may be required to provide pain relief equivalent to 1mg of parenteral morphine

From Parenteral/Oral Non-Morphine Opioids to Oral Morphine Sulfate:
Adjust based on response to oral morphine sulfate; refer to published relative potency information

From Controlled-Release Oral Morphine to Oral Morphine Sulfate:
The same total amount of morphine sulfate is available from oral sol, tabs, and controlled-release and extended-release capsules; the extended duration of release of morphine sulfate results in reduced maximum and increased minimum plasma concentrations as compared to shorter acting morphine sulfate products. Dosage adjustment w/ close observation is necessary

DOSING CONSIDERATIONS

Renal Impairment
Start w/ lower doses and titrate slowly

Hepatic Impairment
Start w/ lower doses and titrate slowly

Elderly
Start at lower end of dosing range

Discontinuation
Gradually taper dose

ADMINISTRATION
Oral route

100mg/5mL Sol
Always use the enclosed calibrated oral syringe

HOW SUPPLIED
Sol: 10mg/5mL [15mL, 100mL, 500mL], 20mg/5mL [100mL, 500mL], 100mg/5mL [15mL, 30mL, 120mL]; **Tab:** 15mg*, 30mg* *scored

CONTRAINDICATIONS
Known hypersensitivity to morphine, morphine salts, or any components of the product; respiratory depression in absence of resuscitative equipment; acute or severe bronchial asthma or hypercarbia; confirmed/suspected paralytic ileus.

WARNINGS/PRECAUTIONS
Respiratory depression occurs more frequently in elderly or debilitated patients and in those w/ conditions accompanied by hypoxia, hypercapnia, or upper airway obstruction. Caution and consider alternative nonopioid analgesics w/ COPD or cor pulmonale, and in patients having substantially decreased respiratory reserve (eg, severe kyphoscoliosis), hypoxia, hypercapnia, or preexisting respiratory depression; use only under careful medical supervision at the lowest effective dose. High potential for abuse; is subject to misuse, abuse, or diversion. Possible respiratory depressant effects and potential to elevate CSF pressure may be markedly exaggerated in the presence of head injury, intracranial lesions, or a preexisting increase in intracranial pressure (ICP); may produce effects on pupillary response and consciousness which may obscure neurologic signs of further increases in ICP in patients w/head injuries. May cause severe hypotension in patients whose ability to maintain BP has already been compromised by a depleted blood volume or concurrent administration of drugs (eg, phenothiazines, general anesthetics). May produce orthostatic hypotension and syncope in ambulatory patients. Caution w/ circulatory shock. Avoid w/GI obstruction, especially paralytic ileus; may prolong the obstruction. May obscure diagnosis or clinical course w/ acute abdominal conditions. Caution w/ biliary tract disease, including acute pancreatitis; may cause spasm of the sphincter of Oddi and diminish biliary and pancreatic secretions. Caution w/and reduce dose in patients w/ severe renal or hepatic impairment, Addison's disease, hypothyroidism, prostatic hypertrophy, or urethral stricture, and in elderly or debilitated

patients. Caution w/ CNS depression, toxic psychosis, acute alcoholism, and delirium tremens. May aggravate convulsions in patients w/ convulsive disorders and may induce/aggravate seizures. May impair mental/physical abilities. (100mg/5mL Sol) May cause fatal respiratory depression when administered to patients who are not tolerant to the respiratory depressant effects of opioids. Use only for patients who have already been titrated to a stable analgesic regimen using lower strengths and who can benefit from use of a smaller volume of oral sol.

ADVERSE REACTIONS

Respiratory depression, apnea, circulatory depression, respiratory arrest, shock, cardiac arrest, lightheadedness, dizziness, sedation, N/V, sweating, constipation, somnolence.

DRUG INTERACTIONS

Caution w/ CNS depressants (eg, sedatives, hypnotics, general anesthetics, antiemetics, phenothiazines, alcohol); may increase risk of respiratory depression, hypotension, profound sedation, or coma. May enhance neuromuscular-blocking action of skeletal muscle relaxants and produce an increased degree of respiratory depression. Do not administer mixed agonist/antagonist analgesics (eg, pentazocine, nalbuphine, butorphanol) to patients who have received or are receiving a course of therapy w/ morphine; may reduce analgesic effect and/or may precipitate withdrawal symptoms. Apnea, confusion, and muscle twitching reported w/ cimetidine; monitor for increased respiratory and CNS depression. MAOIs potentiate action of morphine; allow at least 14 days after stopping MAOIs before initiating treatment. Anticholinergics or other medications w/ anticholinergic activity may increase risk of urinary retention and/or severe constipation, which may lead to paralytic ileus. Absorption/exposure may be increased w/ P-gp inhibitors (eg, quinidine); use w/ caution.

PATIENT CONSIDERATIONS

Assessment: Assess for hypersensitivity to the drug or to any components of the product, drug abuse/addiction risk, prior opioid therapy, opioid tolerance, respiratory depression, or any other conditions where treatment is contraindicated or cautioned, pregnancy/nursing status, and for possible drug interactions.

Monitoring: Monitor for respiratory depression, CSF pressure elevation, orthostatic hypotension, syncope, aggravation of convulsions/seizures, and other adverse reactions. During chronic therapy, especially for noncancer-related pain, periodically reassess the continued need for the use of therapy.

Counseling: Advise to take only ud and not to adjust dose w/o consulting a physician. Inform that the drug may impair the ability to perform potentially hazardous activities (eg, operating machinery/driving); advise to refrain from any potentially dangerous activity until it is established that patient is not adversely affected. Advise to avoid CNS depressants except by the orders of the prescribing physician, and to avoid alcohol during therapy. Instruct women of childbearing potential who become or are planning to become pregnant to consult physician prior to therapy; advise that prolonged use during pregnancy may cause fetal-neonatal physical dependence and neonatal withdrawal may also occur. Counsel on the importance of safely tapering the dose if patient has been receiving therapy for more than a few weeks and cessation of therapy is indicated. Inform that drug has a potential for abuse and should be protected from theft and never be given to anyone other than for whom it was prescribed. Instruct to keep in a secure place out of reach of children, and that when no longer needed, destroy the unused sol/tabs by flushing down the toilet. Inform of the most common adverse events that may occur during therapy and the potential for severe constipation.

STORAGE: 20-25°C (68-77°F). Protect from moisture.

MOVANTIK — naloxegol

CII

Class: Opioid antagonist

ADULT DOSAGE

Opioid-Induced Constipation

In Patients W/ Chronic Non-Cancer Pain:

Usual: 25mg qd in am; reduce dose to 12.5mg qd if not tolerated

D/C all maint laxative therapy prior to initiation of therapy

Laxative(s) can be used prn, if suboptimal response to therapy after 3 days

PEDIATRIC DOSAGE

Pediatric use may not have been established

DOSING CONSIDERATIONS

Concomitant Medications

Moderate CYP3A4 Inhibitors: Avoid use; reduce dose to 12.5mg qd and monitor for adverse reactions if use is unavoidable

Renal Impairment

CrCl <60mL/min:

Initial: 12.5mg qd

Titrate: If dosage is well tolerated but opioid-induced constipation symptoms continue, may increase dose to 25mg qd taking into consideration potential for markedly increased exposures in some patients w/ renal impairment and increased risk of adverse reactions w/ higher exposures

Hepatic Impairment

Severe (Child-Pugh Class C): Avoid use

Discontinuation

D/C therapy if treatment w/ the opioid pain medication is also discontinued

Other Important Considerations

Shown to be efficacious in patients who have taken opioids for at least 4 weeks
Avoid consumption of grapefruit or grapefruit juice during treatment

ADMINISTRATION

Oral route

Take on an empty stomach at least 1 hr prior to or 2 hrs after the 1st meal of the day
Swallow tab whole, do not crush or chew

HOW SUPPLIED

Tab: 12.5mg, 25mg

CONTRAINDICATIONS

Known/suspected GI obstruction and patients at increased risk of recurrent obstruction, concomitant use of strong CYP3A4 inhibitors (eg, clarithromycin, ketoconazole), known serious or severe hypersensitivity reaction to naloxegol or any of its excipients.

WARNINGS/PRECAUTIONS

GI perforation may occur in patients w/ conditions that may be associated w/ localized or diffuse reduction of structural integrity in the wall of the GI tract (eg, peptic ulcer disease, Ogilvie's syndrome, diverticular disease, infiltrative GI tract malignancies); caution in patients w/ these conditions and in patients w/ other conditions which might result in impaired integrity of the GI tract wall (eg, Crohn's disease). D/C in patients who develop severe, persistent, or worsening abdominal pain. Clusters of symptoms consistent w/ opioid withdrawal (eg, hyperhidrosis, chills, diarrhea) reported. Patients receiving methadone as therapy for pain were reported to have higher frequency of GI adverse reactions that may have been related to opioid withdrawal than patients receiving other opioids. May be at increased risk for opioid withdrawal or reduced analgesia in patients w/ disruptions to the blood-brain barrier; use w/ caution.

ADVERSE REACTIONS

Abdominal pain, diarrhea, N/V, flatulence, headache, hyperhidrosis.

DRUG INTERACTIONS

See Dosing Considerations and Contraindications. Potential for additive effect of opioid receptor antagonism and increased risk of opioid withdrawal w/ other opioid antagonists; avoid use w/ another opioid antagonist. Strong CYP3A4 inducers (eg, rifampin, carbamazepine, St. John's wort) may significantly decrease plasma levels and efficacy; not recommended for use w/ strong CYP3A4 inducers. Grapefruit or grapefruit juice may increase plasma levels.

PATIENT CONSIDERATIONS

Assessment: Assess for serious/severe hypersensitivity reaction to the drug or any of its excipients, GI obstruction, increased risk of recurrent GI obstruction, conditions associated w/ localized or diffuse reduction of structural integrity in the wall of the GI tract, conditions which might result in impaired integrity of GI tract wall, disruptions to the blood-brain barrier, renal/hepatic impairment, pregnancy/nursing status, and other possible drug interactions.

Monitoring: Monitor for signs/symptoms of GI perforation, severe/persistent/worsening abdominal pain, opioid withdrawal symptoms, and other adverse reactions.

Counseling: Advise to take exactly ud. Counsel to inform physician when starting or stopping any concomitant medication. Advise to d/c therapy and to promptly seek medical attention if unusually severe, persistent, or worsening abdominal pain develops. Inform that clusters of symptoms consistent w/ opioid withdrawal may occur while taking therapy. Counsel that taking methadone as therapy for pain condition may increase likelihood of having GI adverse reactions that may be related to opioid withdrawal. Advise females of reproductive potential that the use of drug during pregnancy may precipitate opioid withdrawal in a fetus. Advise females who are nursing against breastfeeding during treatment due to potential for opioid withdrawal in nursing infants.

STORAGE: 20-25°C (68-77°F); excursions permitted to 15-30°C (59-86°F).

MOVIPREP — ascorbic acid/polyethylene glycol 3350/ potassium chloride/sodium ascorbate/sodium chloride/sodium sulfate

RX

Class: Bowel cleanser

ADULT DOSAGE

Bowel Cleansing

Prior to Colonoscopy:

Split-Dose (2-Day) Regimen (Preferred Method):

Take Dose 1 the pm before the colonoscopy (10-12 hrs before Dose 2), then take Dose 2 the next morning on the day of the colonoscopy, starting at least 3.5 hrs prior to colonoscopy

Evening-Only (1-Day) Regimen (Alternative Method):

Take Dose 1 at least 3.5 hrs before hs the pm before the colonoscopy, then take Dose 2 about 1.5 hrs after starting Dose 1 on the pm before the colonoscopy

PEDIATRIC DOSAGE

Pediatric use may not have been established

ADMINISTRATION

Oral route

Take 2 separate doses in conjunction w/ fluids

Drink only clear liquids up to 2 hrs before the colonoscopy or as prescribed by healthcare provider, then stop drinking liquids until after the colonoscopy

Take w/in 24 hrs after it is mixed in water; do not add other ingredients to the sol

Split-Dose (2-Day) Regimen (Preferred Method)

Dose 1:

1. Empty the contents of 1 pouch A and 1 pouch B into the container
2. Add lukewarm water to the fill line on the container and mix
3. Drink one 8-oz glass (240mL) every 15 min; be sure to drink all of the sol. This should take about 1 hr
4. Fill the container w/ 16-oz (two 8-oz glasses) of clear liquid and drink all of this liquid before going to bed

Dose 2:

1. Repeat steps 1 through 3 from Dose 1 instructions
2. Fill the container w/ 16-oz (two 8-oz glasses) of clear liquid and drink all of this liquid at least 2 hrs before the colonoscopy

Evening only (1-Day) Regimen (Alternative Method)

Dose 1:

1. Empty the contents of 1 pouch A and 1 pouch B into the container
2. Add lukewarm water to the fill line on the container and mix
3. Drink one 8-oz glass (240mL) every 15 min; be sure to drink all of the sol. This should take about 1 hr

Dose 2:

1. Repeat Steps 1 through 3 from Dose 1 instructions
2. Fill the container again to the fill line w/ clear liquid and drink all of this liquid before going to bed

HOW SUPPLIED

Sol (Powder): Pouch A (Polyethylene Glycol 3350/Sodium Sulfate/Sodium Chloride/Potassium Chloride) 100g/7.5g/2.691g/1.015g; Pouch B (Ascorbic Acid/Sodium Ascorbate) 4.7g/5.9g

CONTRAINDICATIONS

GI obstruction, bowel perforation, gastric retention, ileus, toxic colitis, toxic megacolon, hypersensitivity to any components of MoviPrep.

WARNINGS/PRECAUTIONS

Consume only clear liquids (no solid food) from the start of treatment until after the colonoscopy. Do not consume any clear liquids at least 2 hrs before the colonoscopy. Adequately hydrate before, during, and after use. If significant vomiting or signs of dehydration develop, consider performing postcolonoscopy lab tests (electrolytes, SrCr, and BUN). Correct electrolyte abnormalities before treatment. Consider performing predose and postcolonoscopy lab tests in patients with known or suspected hyponatremia. Serious arrhythmias reported (rare); use with caution and consider predose and postcolonoscopy ECGs in patients at increased risk of serious cardiac arrhythmias. Generalized tonic-clonic seizures and/or loss of consciousness reported (rare); caution in patients with a history of or at increased risk of seizures (eg, with known/suspected hyponatremia). Caution with impaired renal function. May produce colonic mucosal aphthous ulcerations; consider this when interpreting colonoscopy findings in patients with known/suspected inflammatory bowel disease. Serious cases of ischemic colitis reported. If severe bloating, abdominal distention/pain occurs, slow administration or temporarily d/c until symptoms abate. Caution with severe ulcerative colitis; impaired gag reflex; in patients prone to regurgitation/aspiration; or with G6PD deficiency, especially in G6PD-deficient patients with an active infection, history of hemolysis, or taking concomitant medications known to precipitate hemolytic reactions. Contains phenylalanine.

ADVERSE REACTIONS

Abdominal distension, anal discomfort, thirst, N/V, abdominal pain, sleep disorder, rigors, hunger, malaise, dizziness.

DRUG INTERACTIONS

Increased risk of colonic mucosal aphthous ulcerations with stimulant laxatives; concurrent use not recommended. Caution with drugs that increase risk of electrolyte abnormalities (eg, diuretics, ACE inhibitors, ARBs) or affect renal function (eg, NSAIDs). Caution with drugs that lower seizure threshold (eg, TCAs) and in patients withdrawing from alcohol or benzodiazepines. Caution with drugs that increase the risk of arrhythmias and prolonged QT in the setting of fluid and electrolyte abnormalities. Consider additional patient evaluations as appropriate. Oral medication administered within 1 hr of the start of administration may be flushed from GI tract and may not be absorbed.

PATIENT CONSIDERATIONS

Assessment: Assess for GI obstruction, bowel perforation, gastric retention, ileus, toxic colitis, toxic megacolon, electrolyte abnormalities, G6PD deficiency, renal impairment, drug hypersensitivity, any other conditions where treatment is cautioned, pregnancy/nursing status, and possible drug interactions. Consider performing predose lab tests (electrolytes, SrCr, and BUN) in patients with electrolyte abnormalities or renal impairment. Consider predose ECGs in patients at increased risk of serious cardiac arrhythmias.

Monitoring: Monitor for arrhythmias, generalized tonic-clonic seizures, loss of consciousness, colonic mucosal aphthous ulceration, ischemic colitis, bloating, abdominal distention/pain, and other adverse reactions. Monitor patients with impaired gag reflex and patients prone to regurgitation/aspiration. Consider performing postcolonoscopy lab tests (electrolytes, SrCr, BUN) in patients who develop significant vomiting or signs of dehydration after taking therapy, in patients with electrolyte abnormalities, and in patients with renal impairment. Consider postcolonoscopy ECGs in patients at increased risk of serious cardiac arrhythmias.

Counseling: Inform patients who require a low phenylalanine diet that the product contains a max of 233mg aspartame/treatment (provides 131mg phenylalanine). Instruct to inform physician if patient has trouble swallowing or is prone to regurgitation/aspiration. Inform that each pouch needs to be diluted in water before ingestion and instruct to drink additional clear liquid. Inform that oral medications may not be absorbed properly if taken within 1 hr of starting each dose of the drug. Instruct not to take other laxatives during therapy. Advise to adequately hydrate before, during, and after use. Counsel that clear soup and/or plain yogurt may be taken for dinner, finishing at least 1 hr prior to treatment. Inform that the 1st bowel movement may occur 1 hr after the start of administration, and abdominal bloating and distention may occur before the 1st bowel movement. If severe abdominal discomfort or distention occurs, advise to stop treatment temporarily or drink each portion at longer intervals until symptoms diminish; if severe symptoms persist, instruct to notify physician. Instruct to consume only clear liquids (no solid food) from the start of treatment until after the colonoscopy. Instruct to not consume any clear liquids at least 2 hrs before the colonoscopy.

STORAGE: 20-25°C (68-77°F); excursions permitted to 15-30°C (59-86°F). Reconstituted Sol: Store upright and keep refrigerated. Use within 24 hrs.

MOXATAG – amoxicillin

RX

Class: Semisynthetic ampicillin derivative

ADULT DOSAGE

Tonsillitis and/or Pharyngitis

Secondary to *Streptococcus pyogenes*:
775mg qd for 10 days

PEDIATRIC DOSAGE

Tonsillitis and/or Pharyngitis

Secondary to *Streptococcus pyogenes*:
≥12 Years:
775mg qd for 10 days

DOSING CONSIDERATIONS

Renal Impairment

Severe (CrCl <30mL/min)/Hemodialysis: Not recommended

ADMINISTRATION

Oral route

Take w/in 1 hr of finishing a meal
Do not chew or crush

HOW SUPPLIED
Tab, Extended-Release: 775mg

CONTRAINDICATIONS
Known serious hypersensitivity to amoxicillin or to other drugs in the same class or anaphylactic reactions to β-lactams.

WARNINGS/PRECAUTIONS
Serious, occasionally fatal, hypersensitivity (anaphylactic) reactions may occur; increased risk w/ a history of penicillin hypersensitivity and/or history of sensitivity to multiple allergens. D/C if allergic reaction occurs and institute appropriate therapy. *Clostridium difficile*-associated diarrhea (CDAD) reported; may need to d/c if CDAD is suspected or confirmed. May result in bacterial resistance w/ use in the absence of a proven/suspected bacterial infection or a prophylactic indication; d/c and institute appropriate therapy if superinfection develops. Avoid w/ mononucleosis; may cause erythematous skin rash. Lab test interactions may occur. Caution in elderly.

ADVERSE REACTIONS
Vulvovaginal mycotic infection, diarrhea, N/V, abdominal pain, headache.

DRUG INTERACTIONS
Concurrent use w/ probenecid may increase/prolong levels; decreases renal tubular secretion of amoxicillin. Chloramphenicol, macrolides, sulfonamides, and tetracyclines may interfere w/ bactericidal effects. Lowers estrogen reabsorption and potentially reduces efficacy of combined oral estrogen/progesterone contraceptives.

PATIENT CONSIDERATIONS

Assessment: Assess for known serious hypersensitivity reactions to the drug or to other drugs in the same class, anaphylactic reactions to β-lactams, mononucleosis, renal impairment, pregnancy/nursing status, and for possible drug interactions.

Monitoring: Monitor for serious anaphylactic and hypersensitivity reactions, erythematous skin rash, development of drug resistance or superinfection, signs/symptoms of CDAD, and other adverse reactions. Monitor renal function, particularly in elderly.

Counseling: Instruct to take w/in 1 hr of finishing a meal and at approx the same time every day. Instruct not to chew or crush tab. Inform that no other forms of immediate-release amoxicillin can be substituted for this therapy. Instruct to take exactly ud; explain that skipping doses or not completing full course may decrease effectiveness and increase resistance. Advise to notify physician immediately if serious hypersensitivity reactions occur. Instruct to notify physician as soon as possible if watery and bloody stools (w/ or w/o stomach cramps and fever) develop, even as late as 2 or more months after the last dose of therapy.

STORAGE: 25°C (77°F); excursions permitted to 15-30°C (59-86°).

MS Contin – morphine sulfate — CII

Class: Opioid analgesic

Exposes users to the risks of opioid addiction, abuse, and misuse, leading to overdose and death; assess each patient's risk prior to prescribing therapy and monitor regularly for the development of these behaviors/conditions. Serious, life-threatening, or fatal respiratory depression may occur; monitor during initiation or following a dose increase. Crushing, chewing, or dissolving tab can cause rapid release and absorption of a potentially fatal dose; instruct to swallow tab whole. Accidental ingestion, especially in children, can result in fatal overdose. Prolonged use during pregnancy can result in neonatal opioid withdrawal syndrome; advise pregnant women of the risk and ensure availability of appropriate treatment.

ADULT DOSAGE

Severe Pain (Daily, Around-the-Clock Management)

Use as 1st Opioid Analgesic:
Initial: 15mg q8h or q12h
Titrate: Dose adjustments may be done every 1-2 days

Opioid Intolerant Patients:
Initial: 15mg q12h
Titrate: Dose adjustments may be done every 1-2 days

Breakthrough Pain:
May require a dose increase, or may need rescue medication w/ an immediate-release analgesic

PEDIATRIC DOSAGE
Pediatric use may not have been established

Conversions

From Other Oral Morphine:
Administer 1/2 of 24 hr requirement on an q12h schedule or administer 1/3 of the daily requirement on an q8h schedule

From Other Opioids:
D/C all other around-the-clock opioids when therapy is initiated and initiate dosing at 15mg q8-12h

From Parenteral Morphine:
Ratio: 2-6mg of oral morphine may be required to provide analgesia equivalent to 1mg of parenteral morphine; typically, a dose of morphine that is approximately 3X the previous daily parenteral morphine requirement is sufficient

From Other Non-Morphine Opioids (Parenteral or Oral):
Begin w/ 1/2 the estimated daily morphine requirement as initial dose, managing inadequate analgesia by supplementation w/ immediate-release morphine

DOSING CONSIDERATIONS

Discontinuation
Use a gradual downward titration of the dose; do not abruptly d/c

ADMINISTRATION

Oral route

Swallow tab whole; do not crush, dissolve, or chew

HOW SUPPLIED

Tab, Extended-Release: 15mg, 30mg, 60mg, 100mg, 200mg

CONTRAINDICATIONS

Significant respiratory depression, acute or severe bronchial asthma in an unmonitored setting or in the absence of resuscitative equipment, known or suspected paralytic ileus, hypersensitivity (eg, anaphylaxis) to morphine.

WARNINGS/PRECAUTIONS

Reserve for use in patients for whom alternative treatment options are ineffective, not tolerated, or would be otherwise inadequate to provide sufficient management of pain. Should be prescribed only by healthcare professionals who are knowledgeable in the use of potent opioids for the management of chronic pain. Life-threatening respiratory depression is more likely to occur in elderly, cachectic, or debilitated patients. Consider alternative nonopioid analgesics in patients with significant COPD or cor pulmonale, and in patients having a substantially decreased respiratory reserve, hypoxia, hypercapnia, or preexisting respiratory depression. May cause severe hypotension, orthostatic hypotension, and syncope; increased risk in patients whose ability to maintain BP has already been compromised by a reduced blood volume or concurrent administration of certain CNS depressants. Avoid with circulatory shock, impaired consciousness, or coma. Monitor patients who may be susceptible to intracranial effects of carbon dioxide retention for signs of sedation and respiratory depression, particularly when initiating therapy. Therapy may obscure clinical course in patients with head injury. Avoid with GI obstruction. May cause spasm of sphincter of Oddi and increase in serum amylase; monitor for worsening symptoms with biliary tract disease (eg, acute pancreatitis). May aggravate convulsions in patients with convulsive disorders and may induce or aggravate seizures. May impair mental/physical abilities. Caution in elderly. Not recommended for use during or immediately prior to labor.

ADVERSE REACTIONS

Respiratory depression, constipation, dizziness, sedation, N/V, sweating, dysphoria, euphoric mood.

DRUG INTERACTIONS

Respiratory depression, hypotension, profound sedation, or coma may occur with CNS depressants (eg, sedatives, hypnotics, neuroleptics, alcohol); if coadministration is considered, reduce dose of one or both agents. Mixed agonist/antagonist (eg, pentazocine, nalbuphine, butorphanol) and partial agonist (buprenorphine) may reduce analgesic effect or precipitate withdrawal symptoms; avoid coadministration. May enhance neuromuscular-blocking action of skeletal muscle relaxants and produce increased respiratory depression. MAOIs have been reported to potentiate the effects of morphine anxiety, confusion, and significant depression of respiration or coma; avoid use or within 14 days of MAOI use. Cimetidine may potentiate morphine-induced respiratory depression. May reduce efficacy of diuretics. May lead to acute urine retention, particularly in men with enlarged prostates. Anticholinergics or other drugs with anticholinergic activity may increase risk of urinary retention and/or severe constipation, which may lead to paralytic ileus. Absorption/exposure may be increased with P-gp inhibitors (eg, quinidine) by about 2-fold; monitor for signs of respiratory and CNS depression.

PATIENT CONSIDERATIONS

Assessment: Assess for drug abuse/addiction risk, prior opioid therapy, opioid tolerance, respiratory depression, drug hypersensitivity, COPD or other respiratory complications, GI obstruction, paralytic ileus, head injury, history of seizure, pregnancy/nursing status, possible drug interactions, and any other conditions where treatment is contraindicated or cautioned.

Monitoring: Monitor for signs/symptoms of respiratory depression (especially within first 24-72 hrs of initiation), hypotension, symptoms of worsening biliary tract disease, aggravation/induction of seizures, tolerance, physical dependence, mental/physical impairment, and other adverse reactions. Routinely monitor for signs of misuse, abuse, and addiction. Periodically reassess the continued need for therapy.

Counseling: Inform that use of drug can result in addiction, abuse, and misuse; instruct not to share drug with others and to take steps to protect from theft or misuse. Inform about risk of life-threatening respiratory depression; advise how to recognize respiratory depression and to seek medical attention if breathing difficulties develop. Advise to store drug securely; accidental exposure, especially in children, can result in serious harm/death. Instruct to dispose unused drug by flushing down the toilet. Inform females of reproductive potential that prolonged use during pregnancy may result in neonatal opioid withdrawal syndrome. Inform that potentially serious additive effects may occur when used with alcohol or other CNS depressants, and advise not to use such drugs unless supervised by physician. Instruct on how to take the medication properly. Inform that drug may cause orthostatic hypotension and syncope, and may impair the ability to perform potentially hazardous activities; advise to not perform such tasks until they know how they will react to medication. Advise of the potential for severe constipation (including management instructions), on how to recognize anaphylaxis, and when to seek medical attention. Inform females that drug can cause fetal harm; instruct to notify physician if pregnant/planning to become pregnant.

STORAGE: 25°C (77°F); excursions permitted between 15-30°C (59-86°F).

M

MULTAQ – dronedarone

RX

Class: Class III antiarrhythmic

Doubles the risk of death in patients with symptomatic heart failure (HF), with recent decompensation, requiring hospitalization or NYHA Class IV HF; contraindicated in these patients. Doubles the risk of death, stroke, and hospitalization for HF in patients with permanent A-fib; contraindicated in patients in A-fib who will not or cannot be cardioverted into normal sinus rhythm.

ADULT DOSAGE

Atrial Fibrillation

Reduce Risk of Hospitalization for Patients in Sinus Rhythm w/ History of Paroxysmal/ Persistent A-Fib:
400mg bid (w/ am and pm meal)

PEDIATRIC DOSAGE

Pediatric use may not have been established

ADMINISTRATION

Oral route

Take once w/ am meal and again w/ pm meal

HOW SUPPLIED

Tab: 400mg

CONTRAINDICATIONS

Permanent A-fib, symptomatic HF with recent decompensation requiring hospitalization or NYHA Class IV symptoms, 2nd- or 3rd-degree atrioventricular block or sick sinus syndrome (except when used with a functioning pacemaker), bradycardia <50 bpm, liver or lung toxicity related to previous use of amiodarone, QTc Bazett interval ≥500 msec or PR interval >280 msec, severe hepatic impairment, women who are or may become pregnant, nursing mothers. Concomitant use of strong CYP3A inhibitors (eg, ketoconazole, clarithromycin, nefazodone), drugs or herbal products that prolong QT interval and might increase risk of torsades de pointes (eg, phenothiazine antipsychotics, TCAs, certain oral macrolide antibiotics, Class I and III antiarrhythmics). Hypersensitivity to the active substance or to any of the excipients.

WARNINGS/PRECAUTIONS

Monitor cardiac rhythm no less than every 3 months. Cardiovert patients or d/c drug if patients are in A-fib. Only initiate in patients who are receiving appropriate antithrombotic therapy. New onset or worsening of HF reported; d/c if HF develops or worsens and requires hospitalization. Hepatocellular liver injury (including acute liver failure requiring transplant) reported; d/c if hepatic injury is suspected and test serum enzymes, AST, ALT, alkaline phosphatase, and serum bilirubin. Do not restart therapy without another explanation for observed liver injury. Interstitial lung disease (including pneumonitis and pulmonary fibrosis) reported. Onset of dyspnea or nonproductive cough may be related to pulmonary toxicity; evaluate patients carefully. D/C if pulmonary toxicity is confirmed. K^+ levels should be within normal range prior to and during therapy. May induce moderate QTc (Bazett) prolongation. Increase in SrCr, prerenal azotemia, and acute renal failure often in the setting of HF or hypovolemia reported. Premenopausal women who have not undergone hysterectomy/oophorectomy must use effective contraception while on therapy.

ADVERSE REACTIONS

QT prolongation, SrCr increase, diarrhea, N/V, abdominal pain, asthenic conditions, bradycardia, rashes, pruritus, eczema, dermatitis, allergic dermatitis.

DRUG INTERACTIONS

See Contraindications. Hypokalemia/hypomagnesemia may occur with K^+-depleting diuretics. May increase exposure to digoxin. Digoxin may also potentiate electrophysiologic effects; consider discontinuing or 1/2 the dose of digoxin and closely monitor serum levels and for toxicity if digoxin treatment is continued. Calcium channel blockers (CCBs) may potentiate effects on conduction and may increase exposure. Bradycardia more frequently observed with β-blockers. Give a low dose of CCBs or β-blockers initially and increase only after ECG verification of good tolerability. Avoid grapefruit juice, rifampin, or other CYP3A inducers (eg, phenobarbital, carbamazepine, St. John's wort). May increase exposure of simvastatin/simvastatin acid, CCBs, dabigatran, P-glycoprotein substrates, and CYP2D6 substrates (eg, β-blockers, TCAs, SSRIs). Avoid doses >10mg qd of simvastatin. May increase plasma levels of tacrolimus, sirolimus, and other CYP3A substrates with a narrow therapeutic range; monitor concentrations and adjust dosage appropriately. Clinically significant INR elevations with oral anticoagulants and increased S-warfarin exposure reported; monitor INR after initiating therapy in patients taking warfarin.

PATIENT CONSIDERATIONS

Assessment: Assess for recent HF decompensation, permanent A-fib, hepatic impairment, any other conditions where treatment is contraindicated/cautioned, pregnancy/nursing status, and possible drug interactions. Assess serum K^+ levels.

Monitoring: Monitor for signs/symptoms of new/worsening HF, hepatic injury, pulmonary toxicity, and QT interval prolongation. Monitor cardiac rhythm no less than every 3 months, hepatic serum enzymes periodically, especially during first 6 months, and renal function periodically.

Counseling: Instruct to take with meals and not to take with grapefruit juice. If a dose is missed, advise to take next dose at the regularly scheduled time and not to double the dose. Counsel to consult physician if signs/symptoms of HF or potential liver injury occur and before stopping the treatment. Advise to inform physician of any history of HF, rhythm disturbance other than A-fib or atrial flutter, or predisposing conditions, such as uncorrected hypokalemia. Advise to report any use of other prescription, nonprescription medication, or herbal products, particularly St. John's wort. Counsel patients of childbearing potential about appropriate contraceptive choices while on therapy.

STORAGE: 25°C (77°F); excursions permitted to 15-30°C (59-86°F).

MYALEPT — metreleptin

RX

Class: Leptin analogue

Anti-metreleptin antibodies w/ neutralizing activity have been identified; consequences may include inhibition of endogenous leptin action and/or loss of drug efficacy. Severe infection and/or worsening metabolic control reported; test for anti-metreleptin antibodies w/ neutralizing activity if severe infections or signs suspicious for loss of drug efficacy during treatment develop. T-cell lymphoma reported in patients w/ acquired generalized lipodystrophy; carefully consider the benefits and risks of treatment in patients w/ significant hematologic abnormalities and/or acquired generalized lipodystrophy. Available only through a restricted program under a Risk Evaluation and Mitigation Strategy (REMS) called the Myalept REMS Program.

ADULT DOSAGE

Leptin Deficiency

Adjunct to diet as replacement therapy to treat the complications of leptin deficiency in patients w/ congenital or acquired generalized lipodystrophy

≤40kg:

Initial:

Males and Females: 0.06mg/kg (0.012mL/kg)

PEDIATRIC DOSAGE

Leptin Deficiency

Adjunct to diet as replacement therapy to treat the complications of leptin deficiency in patients w/ congenital or acquired generalized lipodystrophy

≤40kg:

Initial:

Males and Females: 0.06mg/kg (0.012mL/kg)

Dose Adjustment: 0.02mg/kg (0.004mL/kg)
Max Daily Dose: 0.13mg/kg (0.026mL/kg)

>40kg:
Initial:
Male: 2.5mg (0.5mL)
Female: 5mg (1mL)
Dose Adjustment: 1.25-2.5mg (0.25-0.5mL)
Max Daily Dose: 10mg (2mL)

Dose Adjustment: 0.02mg/kg (0.004mL/kg)
Max Daily Dose: 0.13mg/kg (0.026mL/kg)

>40kg:
Initial:
Male: 2.5mg (0.5mL)
Female: 5mg (1mL)
Dose Adjustment: 1.25-2.5mg (0.25-0.5mL)
Max Daily Dose: 10mg (2mL)

DOSING CONSIDERATIONS

Elderly

Start at lower end of dosing range

Discontinuation

Patients at Risk for Pancreatitis:

Taper dose over a 1-week period. During tapering, monitor TG levels and consider initiating or adjusting dose of lipid-lowering medications prn

Other Important Considerations

Dose adjustments, including possible large reductions, of insulin or insulin secretagogue (eg, sulfonylurea) may be necessary; monitor blood glucose in patients on concomitant insulin therapy, especially those on high doses, or insulin secretagogue

ADMINISTRATION

SQ route

Should be administered at the same time every day.

May administer at any time of the day, w/o regard to the timing of meals.

Administer into the SQ tissue of the abdomen, thigh or upper arm; use different inj site each day when injecting in the same region.

After choosing an inj site, pinch the skin and at a 45° angle, inject the sol.

Avoid IM inj, especially in patients w/ minimal SQ adipose tissue.

Doses exceeding 1mL can be administered as 2 inj (the total daily dose divided equally) to minimize potential inj-site discomfort due to volume; when dividing doses due to volume, doses can be administered one after the other.

Reconstitution

Reconstitute w/ 2.2mL of sterile bacteriostatic water for inj (0.9% benzyl alcohol), or w/ 2.2mL of sterile water for inj.

Use w/in 3 days when stored refrigerated between 2-8°C (36-46°F) and protected from light.

For neonates and infants, reconstitute w/ preservative-free sterile water for inj and administer immediately.

Compatibility

Do not mix w/, or transfer into, the contents of another vial of metreleptin.

Do not add other medications, including insulin; use a separate syringe for insulin inj.

HOW SUPPLIED

Inj: 5mg/mL [11.3mg]

CONTRAINDICATIONS

General obesity not associated w/ congenital leptin deficiency, prior severe hypersensitivity reactions to metreleptin or to any of the product components.

WARNINGS/PRECAUTIONS

Not indicated for use w/ HIV-related lipodystrophy, or in patients w/ metabolic disease, including diabetes mellitus and hypertriglyceridemia, w/o concurrent evidence of congenital or acquired generalized lipodystrophy. Case of anaplastic large cell lymphoma reported. Cases of progression of autoimmune hepatitis and membranoproliferative glomerulonephritis (associated w/ massive proteinuria and renal failure) reported in patients w/ acquired generalized lipodystrophy; carefully consider the potential benefits and risks of treatment in patients w/ autoimmune disease. Generalized hypersensitivity reported; consider discontinuing if a hypersensitivity reaction occurs. Contains benzyl alcohol when reconstituted w/ Bacteriostatic Water for Inj; preservative-free Water for Inj is recommended for use in neonates and infants. Caution in elderly.

ADVERSE REACTIONS

Headache, hypoglycemia, decreased weight, abdominal pain, arthralgia, dizziness, ear infection, fatigue, nausea, ovarian cyst, URTI, anemia, back pain, diarrhea, paresthesia.

DRUG INTERACTIONS

See Dosing Considerations. Caution w/ drugs metabolized by CYP450 (eg, oral contraceptives, drugs w/ a narrow therapeutic index); effect of metreleptin on CYP450 enzymes may be clinically relevant for CYP450 substrates w/ a narrow therapeutic index, where dose is individually adjusted. Upon initiation or discontinuation of metreleptin, in patients being treated w/ CYP450 substrates w/ a narrow therapeutic index, perform therapeutic monitoring of effect (eg, warfarin) or drug concentration (eg, cyclosporine, theophylline) and adjust the individual dose of the agent PRN.

PATIENT CONSIDERATIONS

Assessment: Assess for hypersensitivity to the drug, general obesity not associated w/ congenital leptin deficiency, risk factors of pancreatitis, hematologic abnormalities, pregnancy/nursing status, and possible drug interactions.

Monitoring: Monitor for severe infections, worsening metabolic control, T-cell lymphoma in patients w/ acquired generalized lipodystrophy, hypersensitivity reactions, and other adverse events. Test for anti-metreleptin antibodies w/ neutralizing activity in patients who develop severe infections or show signs suspicious for loss of metreleptin efficacy during treatment. When discontinuing therapy in patients w/ risk factors for pancreatitis, monitor TG levels. Closely monitor blood glucose levels in patients on concomitant insulin or insulin secretagogue therapy.

Counseling: Inform about the risks/benefits of therapy. Instruct that if a dose is missed, administer dose as soon as noticed, and resume the normal dosing schedule the next day. Inform on the signs/symptoms that would warrant antibody testing. Inform on the signs/symptoms that indicate changes in hematologic status and the importance of routine lab assessment and physician monitoring. Advise that the risk of hypoglycemia is increased w/ insulin or an insulin secretagogue; instruct to closely monitor blood glucose levels. Advise patients w/ history of autoimmune disease on signs/symptoms that indicate exacerbation of underlying autoimmune disease and the importance of routine lab assessments and physician monitoring. Instruct to seek medical advice if symptoms of hypersensitivity occur. Advise nursing mothers that breastfeeding is not recommended. Inform patients/caregivers about proper preparation and administration of drug; advise that 1st dose should be administered under the supervision of a qualified healthcare professional. Instruct patients w/ a history of pancreatitis and/or severe hypertriglyceridemia to taper dose over a 1-week period when discontinuing therapy; advise that additional monitoring of TG levels and possible initiation or dose adjustment of lipid-lowering medications may be considered.

STORAGE: 2-8°C (36-46°F). Do not freeze. Protect from light. Do not shake or vigorously agitate reconstituted vial. Refer to PI for further storage and handling instructions.

M

MYFORTIC – mycophenolic acid

RX

Class: Inosine monophosphate dehydrogenase (IMPDH) inhibitor

Use during pregnancy is associated w/ increased risks of pregnancy loss and congenital malformations; counsel females of reproductive potential regarding pregnancy prevention and planning. Immunosuppression may lead to increased risk of development of lymphoma and other malignancies, particularly of the skin. Increased susceptibility to infections (bacterial, viral, fungal, protozoal, opportunistic). Only physicians experienced in immunosuppressive therapy and management of organ transplant patients should prescribe mycophenolic acid (MPA). Manage patients in facilities equipped and staffed w/ adequate lab and supportive medical resources. Physician responsible for maintenance therapy should have complete information requisite for patient follow-up.

ADULT DOSAGE

Organ Rejection Prophylaxis

Kidney Transplant:
720mg bid (1440mg/day)

Use in combination w/ cyclosporine and corticosteroids

PEDIATRIC DOSAGE

Organ Rejection Prophylaxis

≥5 Years:
At Least 6 Months Post Kidney Transplant:
400mg/m^2 bid
Max: 720mg bid
BSA 1.19-1.58m^2: Dose either w/ three 180mg tabs, or one 180mg tab plus one 360mg tab bid (1080mg/day)
BSA >1.58m^2: Dose either w/ four 180mg tabs, or two 360mg tabs bid (1440mg/day)

Use in combination w/ cyclosporine and corticosteroids

ADMINISTRATION

Oral route

Take on an empty stomach, 1 hr before or 2 hrs after food intake.
Swallow whole; do not crush, chew, or cut tabs.

HOW SUPPLIED

Tab, Delayed-Release: 180mg, 360mg

CONTRAINDICATIONS

Hypersensitivity to mycophenolate sodium, mycophenolic acid, mycophenolate mofetil, or to any of its excipients.

WARNINGS/PRECAUTIONS

Should not be used interchangeably w/ mycophenolate mofetil (MMF) tabs and caps w/o medical supervision. Limit exposure to sunlight and UV light in patients at increased risk for skin cancer. Polyomavirus-associated nephropathy (PVAN), JC virus associated progressive multifocal leukoencephalopathy (PML), cytomegalovirus (CMV) infections, reactivation of hepatitis B (HBV) or hepatitis C (HCV) reported; consider reduction in immunosuppression for patients who develop evidence of new or reactivated viral infections. PVAN, especially due to BK virus infection, is associated w/ serious outcomes, including deteriorating renal function and renal graft loss. Consider PML in differential diagnosis in patients reporting neurological symptoms and consider consultation w/ a neurologist as clinically indicated. Cases of pure red cell aplasia (PRCA) reported when used w/ other immunosuppressive agents; monitor CBC weekly during the 1st month, twice monthly for the 2nd and 3rd month of therapy, and then monthly through 1st yr. Interrupt dosing or reduce dose, perform appropriate tests, and manage accordingly, if blood dyscrasias occur (neutropenia [ANC $<1.3 \times 10^3/\mu L$] or anemia). GI bleeding (requiring hospitalization), intestinal perforations, gastric ulcers, and duodenal ulcers reported; caution w/ active serious digestive system disease. Avoid w/ rare hereditary deficiency of hypoxanthine-guanine phosphoribosyl-transferase (HGPRT) (eg, Lesch-Nyhan and Kelley-Seegmiller syndromes). Caution in elderly.

ADVERSE REACTIONS

Anemia, leukopenia, constipation, N/V, diarrhea, dyspepsia, UTI, CMV infection, insomnia, postoperative pain.

DRUG INTERACTIONS

Caution w/ combination immunosuppressant therapy. Avoid live attenuated vaccines. Mg^{2+}- and aluminum-containing antacids may decrease levels; do not administer simultaneously. Azathioprine and MMF inhibit purine metabolism; avoid concomitant use w/ azathioprine or MMF. Cholestyramine or other agents that may interfere w/ enterohepatic recirculation or drugs that may bind bile acids (eg, bile acid sequestrates or oral activated charcoal) may reduce efficacy; avoid concomitant use. Sevelamer may decrease levels; do not administer simultaneously w/ sevelamer and other Ca^{2+}-free phosphate binders. Cyclosporine may decrease levels; there is a potential change of MPA levels after switching from cyclosporine to other immunosuppressive drugs or from other immunosuppressive drugs to cyclosporine. Concomitant norfloxacin and metronidazole may decrease levels; avoid w/ the combination of norfloxacin and metronidazole. Rifampin may decrease levels; avoid concomitant use unless the benefit outweighs the risk. May decrease levels and effects of hormonal contraceptives; coadminister w/ caution, and additional barrier contraceptive methods must be used. Drugs that undergo renal tubular secretion (eg, acyclovir/valacyclovir, ganciclovir/valganciclovir) may increase levels of both drugs; monitor blood cell counts. Drugs that alter the GI flora (eg, ciprofloxacin or amoxicillin plus clavulanic acid) may interact w/ MMF by disrupting enterohepatic recirculation.

PATIENT CONSIDERATIONS

Assessment: Assess for hypersensitivity to the drug, HBV or HCV infected patients, hereditary deficiency of HGPRT (eg, Lesch-Nyhan and Kelley-Seegmiller syndromes), active digestive disease, pregnancy/nursing status, and for possible drug interactions. Females of reproductive potential should have a serum or urine pregnancy test (sensitivity of at least 25 mIU/mL) immediately before starting therapy.

Monitoring: Monitor for signs/symptoms of lymphomas and other malignancies (eg, skin cancer), infections including reactivation of HBV or HCV, blood dyscrasias (eg, PRCA), GI complications, and other adverse reactions. Monitor CBC weekly during the 1st month, twice monthly for the 2nd and 3rd month of therapy, and then monthly through 1st yr. Monitor pregnancy status by doing a pregnancy test (sensitivity of at least 25 mIU/mL) 8-10 days after initiation of therapy and repeatedly during follow-up visits.

Counseling: Inform that use in pregnancy is associated w/ an increased risk of 1st trimester pregnancy loss and congenital malformation; discuss pregnancy testing, prevention (including acceptable contraception methods), and planning. Discuss appropriate alternative immunosuppressants w/ less potential for embryofetal toxicity in patients who are considering pregnancy. Advise not to breastfeed during therapy. Inform about increased risk of developing lymphomas and other malignancies; advise to limit exposure to sunlight and UV light by wearing protective clothing and using sunscreen w/ high protection factor. Inform about increased risk of developing a variety of infections, including opportunistic infections, due to immunosuppression. Inform about risk for developing blood dyscrasias. Instruct to report if experiencing any symptoms of infection, unexpected bruising, bleeding, or any other manifestation of bone marrow suppression. Inform that therapy may cause GI tract complications, including bleeding, intestinal perforations, and gastric or duodenal ulcers; advise to contact healthcare provider if symptoms of GI bleeding or sudden onset or persistent abdominal pain occurs. Inform that therapy may interfere w/ the usual response to immunizations and to avoid live vaccines. Advise to report to physician the use of any other medications while on therapy. Encourage to enroll in the pregnancy registry if patient becomes pregnant while on therapy.

STORAGE: 25°C (77°F); excursions permitted to 15-30°C (59-86°F). Protect from moisture.

MYRBETRIQ – mirabegron

RX

Class: Beta-3 adrenergic agonist

ADULT DOSAGE

Overactive Bladder

Initial: 25mg qd

Titrate: May increase to 50mg qd based on individual efficacy and tolerability

PEDIATRIC DOSAGE

Pediatric use may not have been established

DOSING CONSIDERATIONS

Renal Impairment

Severe (CrCl 15-29mL/min or eGFR 15-29mL/min/1.73m^2):
Max: 25mg qd

ESRD: Not recommended

Hepatic Impairment

Moderate (Child-Pugh Class B):
Max: 25mg qd

Severe (Child-Pugh Class C): Not recommended

ADMINISTRATION

Oral route

Take w/ or w/o food.
Swallow whole w/ water; do not chew, divide, or crush.

HOW SUPPLIED

Tab, Extended-Release: 25mg, 50mg

CONTRAINDICATIONS

Known hypersensitivity reactions to mirabegron or any component of the tab.

WARNINGS/PRECAUTIONS

May increase BP; not recommended in patients w/ severe uncontrolled HTN. Worsening of preexisting HTN reported infrequently. Urinary retention in patients w/ bladder outlet obstruction (BOO) reported. Angioedema of the face, lips, tongue, and/or larynx reported; if involvement of the tongue, hypopharynx, or larynx occurs, promptly d/c therapy and initiate appropriate therapy and/or measures necessary to ensure a patent airway.

ADVERSE REACTIONS

HTN, nasopharyngitis, UTI, headache.

DRUG INTERACTIONS

Increases systemic exposure of CYP2D6 substrates (eg, metoprolol, desipramine); monitoring and dose adjustment may be necessary, especially w/ narrow therapeutic index CYP2D6 substrates (eg, thioridazine, flecainide, propafenone). Increases digoxin levels; consider lowest dose for digoxin initially and monitor digoxin levels. May increase warfarin levels. Caution w/ antimuscarinic medications for overactive bladder (OAB); urinary retention reported w/ concomitant use.

PATIENT CONSIDERATIONS

Assessment: Assess for HTN, BOO, renal/hepatic impairment, pregnancy/nursing status, and possible drug interactions.

Monitoring: Monitor for urinary retention in patients w/ BOO, angioedema, and other adverse reactions. Monitor BP periodically, especially in hypertensive patients.

Counseling: Inform that therapy may increase BP and has also been associated w/ infrequent UTI, rapid heartbeat, rash, and pruritus. Inform that urinary retention has been reported when therapy was taken w/ antimuscarinic drugs used in the treatment of OAB. Instruct to contact physician if these effects are experienced.

STORAGE: 25°C (77°F); excursions permitted from 15-30°C (59-86°F).

M

MYSOLINE – primidone

RX

Class: Pyrimidinedione derivative

ADULT DOSAGE

Seizures

Grand Mal, Psychomotor, and Focal Epileptic Seizures (Alone or w/ Other Anticonvulsants):

No Prior Antiepileptic Therapy:

Initial:

Days 1-3: 100-125mg qhs

Days 4-6: 100-125mg bid

Days 7-9: 100-125mg tid

Days 10/Maint: 250mg tid

Usual Maint: 250mg tid or qid

Max: 500mg qid

Already Receiving Other Anticonvulsants:

Initial: 100-125mg qhs

Titrate: Increase gradually to maint dose as other drug is gradually decreased. Continue until satisfactory dosage level achieved or other medication is completely withdrawn. When therapy w/ primidone alone is the objective, transition from concomitant therapy should not be completed in <2 weeks

Max: 2g/day

May also control grand mal seizures refractory to other anticonvulsant therapy

PEDIATRIC DOSAGE

Seizures

Grand Mal, Psychomotor, and Focal Epileptic Seizures (Alone or w/ Other Anticonvulsants):

<8 Years:

Days 1-3: 50mg qhs

Days 4-6: 50mg bid

Days 7-9: 100mg bid

Days 10/Maint: 125-250mg tid

Usual Maint: 125-250mg tid or 10-25mg/kg/day in divided doses

≥8 Years:

No Prior Antiepileptic Therapy:

Initial:

Days 1-3: 100-125mg qhs

Days 4-6: 100-125mg bid

Days 7-9: 100-125mg tid

Days 10/Maint: 250mg tid

Usual Maint: 250mg tid or qid

Max: 500mg qid

Already Receiving Other Anticonvulsants:

Initial: 100-125mg qhs

Titrate: Increase gradually to maint dose as other drug is gradually decreased. Continue until satisfactory dosage level achieved or other medication is completely withdrawn. When therapy w/ primidone alone is the objective, transition from concomitant therapy should not be completed in <2 weeks

Max: 2g/day

May also control grand mal seizures refractory to other anticonvulsant therapy

M

ADMINISTRATION

Oral route

HOW SUPPLIED

Tab: 50mg*, 250mg* *scored

CONTRAINDICATIONS

Porphyria, phenobarbital hypersensitivity.

WARNINGS/PRECAUTIONS

Avoid abrupt withdrawal; may precipitate status epilepticus. Increased risk of suicidal thoughts or behavior; monitor for emergence or worsening of depression, suicidal thoughts/behavior, or any unusual changes in mood or behavior. Increased incidence of birth defects reported; encourage pregnant patients to enroll in the North American Antiepileptic Drug (NAAED) Pregnancy Registry. Neonatal hemorrhage reported in newborns; give pregnant women prophylactic vitamin K1 therapy for 1 month prior to, and during, delivery.

ADVERSE REACTIONS

Ataxia, vertigo, granulocytopenia, agranulocytosis, red-cell hypoplasia, aplasia.

PATIENT CONSIDERATIONS

Assessment: Assess for porphyria, hypersensitivity to phenobarbital, prior anticonvulsant therapy, depression, and pregnancy/nursing status.

Monitoring: Monitor for status epilepticus, emergence or worsening of depression, suicidal thoughts/behavior, and any unusual changes in mood or behavior. Monitor CBC, drug serum blood level, and sequential multiple analysis-12 test every 6 months.

Counseling: Counsel patients, their caregivers, and families that the therapy may increase risk of suicidal thoughts and behavior and advise to be alert for the emergence or worsening of symptoms of depression, any unusual changes in mood or behavior, or the emergence of suicidal thoughts, behavior, or thoughts about self-harm. Instruct to immediately report behaviors of concern to healthcare providers. Encourage pregnant patients to enroll in the NAAED Pregnancy Registry (1-888-233-2334).

STORAGE: 20-25°C (68-77°F).

NABUMETONE – nabumetone

RX

Class: NSAID

NSAIDs cause an increased risk of serious cardiovascular (CV) thrombotic events (eg, MI, stroke), which can be fatal; risk may occur early in treatment and may increase w/ duration of use. Contraindicated in the setting of CABG surgery. NSAIDs cause an increased risk of serious GI adverse events (eg, bleeding, ulceration, perforation of the stomach/intestines), which can be fatal and can occur at any time during use and w/o warning symptoms; elderly patients are at greater risk.

ADULT DOSAGE

Osteoarthritis

Initial: 1000mg qd

Titrate: Adjust dose/frequency based on individual needs after observing response to initial therapy; some patients may obtain relief from 1500-2000mg/day

Max: 2000mg/day

May be given qd-bid; use lowest effective dose for chronic treatment

Rheumatoid Arthritis

Initial: 1000mg qd

Titrate: Adjust dose/frequency based on individual needs after observing response to initial therapy; some patients may obtain relief from 1500-2000mg/day

Max: 2000mg/day

May be given qd-bid; use lowest effective dose for chronic treatment

PEDIATRIC DOSAGE

Pediatric use may not have been established

DOSING CONSIDERATIONS

Renal Impairment

Moderate (CrCl 30-49mL/min):

Initial: ≤750mg qd

Max: 1500mg/day

Severe (CrCl <30mL/min):

Initial: ≤500mg qd

Max: 1000mg/day

ADMINISTRATION

Oral route

Take w/ or w/o food.

HOW SUPPLIED

Tab: 500mg, 750mg

CONTRAINDICATIONS

Known hypersensitivity to nabumetone or product excipients; history of asthma, urticaria, or allergic-type reactions after taking aspirin (ASA) or other NSAIDs; in the setting of CABG surgery.

WARNINGS/PRECAUTIONS

Use lowest effective dose for shortest duration possible. Increased CV thrombotic risk reported at higher doses. Avoid in patients w/ a recent MI unless benefits outweigh the risks; if used, monitor for signs of cardiac ischemia. May cause HTN or worsen preexisting HTN. Fluid retention and edema reported. Avoid in patients w/ severe heart failure (HF) unless benefits outweigh the risks; if used, monitor for signs of worsening HF. Use w/ extreme caution in patients w/ history of ulcer disease or GI bleeding, or risk factors for GI bleeding (eg, longer duration of NSAID therapy, older age, poor general health status). D/C if a serious GI adverse event is suspected, until event is ruled out; for high-risk patients, consider alternate therapies that do not involve NSAIDs. Renal papillary necrosis and other renal injury reported after long-term use. Renal toxicity also reported in patients in whom renal prostaglandins have a compensatory role in the maintenance of renal perfusion; increased risk w/ renal/hepatic impairment, HF, and in elderly. Not recommended w/ advanced renal disease; if therapy must be initiated, closely monitor renal function. D/C if renal disease develops. Anaphylactoid reactions may occur; avoid w/ ASA triad. May cause serious skin reactions (eg, exfoliative dermatitis, Stevens-Johnson syndrome, toxic epidermal necrolysis); d/c at 1st appearance of skin rash or any other sign of hypersensitivity. Avoid in late pregnancy; may cause premature closure of ductus arteriosus. Not a substitute for corticosteroids or for the treatment of corticosteroid insufficiency. May mask signs of inflammation and fever. May cause elevation of LFTs or severe hepatic reactions (eg, jaundice, fatal fulminant hepatitis, liver necrosis, hepatic failure);

d/c if liver disease develops, systemic manifestations occur, or abnormal LFTs persist/worsen. Anemia may occur; monitor Hgb/Hct if anemia develops. May inhibit platelet aggregation and prolong bleeding time; carefully monitor patients w/ coagulation disorders. Caution w/ preexisting asthma. May be associated w/ more reactions to sun exposure than might be expected based on skin tanning types.

ADVERSE REACTIONS

Diarrhea, dyspepsia, abdominal pain, constipation, flatulence, N/V, positive stool guaiac, dizziness, headache, pruritus, rash, tinnitus, edema.

DRUG INTERACTIONS

May diminish the antihypertensive effect of ACE inhibitors. Increased risk of renal toxicity w/ diuretics. Not recommended w/ ASA due to potential for increased adverse effects. May reduce the natriuretic effect of thiazide and loop diuretics. May increase lithium levels; monitor for lithium toxicity. May enhance methotrexate toxicity; caution w/ concomitant use. Synergistic effect on GI bleeding w/ warfarin. Monitor patients receiving anticoagulants. Increased risk of GI bleeding w/ oral corticosteroids, anticoagulants, smoking, and alcohol use. May blunt the CV effects of several therapeutic agents used to treat fluid retention and edema (eg, diuretics, ACE inhibitors, ARBs).

PATIENT CONSIDERATIONS

Assessment: Assess for history of asthma, urticaria, or allergic-type reactions w/ ASA or other NSAIDs, ASA triad, HTN, severe HF, history of ulcer disease or GI bleeding, coagulation disorders, renal/hepatic function, pregnancy/nursing status, any other conditions where treatment is contraindicated or cautioned, and possible drug interactions. Obtain baseline BP.

Monitoring: Monitor BP, CBC, bleeding time, LFTs, renal function, and chemistry profile periodically. Monitor for GI bleeding/ulceration/perforation, CV thrombotic events, MI, stroke, HTN, fluid retention, edema, skin/allergic reactions, photosensitivity, and other adverse reactions.

Counseling: Instruct to notify physician immediately if symptoms of CV thrombotic events, GI ulceration/bleeding, skin/hypersensitivity reactions, congestive HF, hepatotoxicity, or anaphylactoid reactions occur. Instruct to avoid in late pregnancy.

STORAGE: 20-25°C (68-77°F).

NAMENDA – memantine hydrochloride

RX

Class: NMDA receptor antagonist

OTHER BRAND NAMES

Namenda XR

ADULT DOSAGE

Alzheimer's Disease

Moderate to Severe Dementia:

Sol, Tab:
Initial: 5mg qd
Titrate: Increase in 5mg increments to 10mg/day (5mg bid), 15mg/day (5mg and 10mg as separate doses), and 20mg/day (10mg bid) at ≥1-week intervals

Cap, ER:
Initial: 7mg qd
Titrate: Increase in 7mg increments to 28mg qd at ≥1-week intervals
Max/Target Dose: 28mg qd

Conversions

Switching from Tabs to Cap, ER: Switch from 10mg bid tabs to 28mg qd caps the day following last dose of 10mg tab
Severe Renal Impairment: Switch from 5mg bid tabs to 14mg qd caps the day following last dose of 5mg tab

Missed Dose

Sol, Tab
If a single dose is missed, take next dose as scheduled and do not double dose; if missed for several days, resume dose at lower dose and retitrate

PEDIATRIC DOSAGE

Pediatric use may not have been established

DOSING CONSIDERATIONS

Renal Impairment

Severe (CrCl 5-29mL/min):

Target Dose:

Sol, Tab: 5mg bid

Cap, ER: 14mg/day

ADMINISTRATION

Oral route

May take w/ or w/o food

Sol

Do not mix w/ any other liquid

Administer w/ a dosing device (syringe, syringe adaptor cap, tubing, other supplies needed) that comes w/ the drug

Use syringe to withdraw correct volume of oral sol and squirt slowly into the corner of the mouth

Cap, ER

Swallow cap whole; do not divide, chew, or crush

May be opened, sprinkled on applesauce, and swallowed

HOW SUPPLIED

Sol: 2mg/mL [360mL]; **Tab:** 5mg, 10mg; **Titration-Pack:** 5mg [28[s]], 10mg [21[s]]. **Cap, ER:** 7mg, 14mg, 21mg, 28mg; **Titration Pack:** 7mg [7[s]], 14mg [7[s]], 21mg [7[s]], 28mg [7[s]].

CONTRAINDICATIONS

Known hypersensitivity to memantine HCl or to any excipients used in the formulation.

WARNINGS/PRECAUTIONS

Conditions that raise urine pH may decrease urinary elimination, resulting in increased plasma levels. Caution in patients with severe renal/hepatic impairment.

ADVERSE REACTIONS

Dizziness, headache, constipation, confusion, HTN, coughing, somnolence, hallucination, vomiting, back pain, (Sol, Tab) pain, (Cap, ER) diarrhea, influenza, weight gain, anxiety.

DRUG INTERACTIONS

Caution with other N-methyl-D-aspartate (NMDA) antagonists (eg, amantadine, ketamine, dextromethorphan) and drugs that alter urine pH towards the alkaline condition (eg, carbonic anhydrase inhibitors, sodium bicarbonate). (Cap, ER) Coadministration with drugs eliminated via renal (cationic system) mechanism (eg, HCTZ, triamterene, metformin, cimetidine, ranitidine) may result in altered plasma levels of both agents.

PATIENT CONSIDERATIONS

Assessment: Assess for hypersensitivity to drug, conditions that raise urine pH, renal/hepatic impairment, pregnancy/nursing status, and possible drug interactions.

Monitoring: Monitor for hypersensitivity reactions and other adverse reactions. Monitor renal/hepatic function.

Counseling: Instruct to take as prescribed. Inform about possible side effects and instruct to notify physician if any develop. (Sol, Tab) Instruct to follow dose titration schedule and not to resume dosing without consulting physician if there has been a failure to take the medication for several days. (Tab) Instruct not to use any damaged or tampered tabs. (Sol) Instruct on how to use the oral sol dosing device.

STORAGE: 25°C (77°F); excursions permitted to 15-30°C (59-86°F).

NAMZARIC — donepezil hydrochloride/memantine hydrochloride RX

Class: Acetylcholinesterase (AChE) inhibitor/NMDA receptor antagonist

ADULT DOSAGE

Alzheimer's Disease

Moderate to Severe Dementia of the Alzheimer's Type Stabilized on Memantine 10mg bid or 28mg ER qd and Donepezil 10mg:

Switch to 28mg-10mg qpm; start the day following the last dose of memantine and donepezil administered separately

Missed Dose

If a dose is missed, the next dose should be taken as scheduled, w/o doubling up the dose

PEDIATRIC DOSAGE

Pediatric use may not have been established

DOSING CONSIDERATIONS

Renal Impairment

Severe (CrCl 5-29mL/min):

Stabilized on Memantine 5mg bid or 14mg ER qd and Donepezil 10mg: Switch to 14mg-10mg qd

ADMINISTRATION

Oral route

May take w/ or w/o food
Swallow cap whole and intact; do not divide, chew, or crush
May be opened, sprinkled on applesauce, and swallowed w/o chewing
Consume entire contents of each cap; the dose should not be divided

HOW SUPPLIED

Cap, ER: (Memantine-Donepezil) 14mg-10mg, 28mg-10mg

CONTRAINDICATIONS

Known hypersensitivity to memantine HCl, donepezil HCl, piperidine derivatives, or to any excipients used in the formulation.

WARNINGS/PRECAUTIONS

Memantine: Conditions that raise urine pH may decrease urinary elimination, resulting in increased plasma levels. Donepezil: May exaggerate succinylcholine-type muscle relaxation during anesthesia. May have vagotonic effects on sinoatrial (SA) and AV nodes, manifesting as bradycardia or heart block. Syncopal episodes reported. May increase gastric acid secretion; monitor closely for symptoms of active or occult GI bleeding, especially in patients at increased risk for developing ulcers (eg, history of ulcer disease, concomitant use of NSAIDs). May produce diarrhea and N/V; observe closely at the initiation of treatment. May cause bladder outflow obstruction and generalized convulsions. Caution w/ history of asthma or obstructive pulmonary disease.

ADVERSE REACTIONS

Headache, diarrhea, dizziness, anorexia, N/V, ecchymosis, insomnia, muscle cramp, fatigue.

DRUG INTERACTIONS

Memantine: Caution w/ other N-methyl-D-aspartate (NMDA) antagonists (eg, amantadine, ketamine, dextromethorphan) and drugs that alter urine pH towards the alkaline condition (eg, carbonic anhydrase inhibitors, sodium bicarbonate). Donepezil: Inhibitors of CYP3A4 (eg, ketoconazole) and CYP2D6 (eg, quinidine) inhibit metabolism in vitro. CYP3A4 inducers (eg, phenytoin, carbamazepine, dexamethasone, rifampin, phenobarbital) may increase elimination rate. May interfere w/ the activity of anticholinergic medications. Synergistic effect w/ similar neuromuscular blocking agents (eg, succinylcholine) or cholinergic agonists (eg, bethanechol).

PATIENT CONSIDERATIONS

Assessment: Assess for hypersensitivity to the drug or piperidine derivatives, underlying cardiac conduction abnormalities, risk for developing ulcers, conditions that raise urine pH, history of asthma or obstructive pulmonary disease, renal impairment, pregnancy/nursing status, and possible drug interactions.

Monitoring: Monitor for vagotonic effects on SA and AV nodes, syncopal episodes, active/occult GI bleeding, diarrhea, N/V, bladder outflow obstruction, generalized convulsions, and other adverse reactions.

Counseling: Instruct to take as prescribed. Inform that drug may cause headache, diarrhea, dizziness, anorexia, N/V, and ecchymosis.

STORAGE: 25°C (77°F); excursions permitted between 15-30°C (59-86°F).

NAPRELAN — naproxen sodium

RX

Class: NSAID

NSAIDs may increase risk of serious cardiovascular (CV) thrombotic events, MI, and stroke; increased risk w/ duration of use and w/ CV disease (CVD) or risk factors for CVD. Contraindicated for the treatment of perioperative pain in the setting of CABG surgery. May increase risk of serious GI adverse events (eg, bleeding, ulceration, and stomach/intestinal perforation), which can be fatal and can occur at any time during use and w/o warning symptoms; elderly patients are at greater risk.

ADULT DOSAGE

Rheumatoid Arthritis

Initial: 750mg or 1000mg qd

Titrate:

Adjust dose/frequency depending on clinical response
In patients who tolerate lower doses well, may increase to two 750mg tabs or three 500mg tabs once daily for limited periods, as needed

PEDIATRIC DOSAGE

Pediatric use may not have been established

Osteoarthritis

Initial: 750mg or 1000mg qd

Titrate:

Adjust dose/frequency depending on clinical response

In patients who tolerate lower doses well, may increase to two 750mg tabs or three 500mg tabs once daily for limited periods, as needed

Ankylosing Spondylitis

Initial: 750mg or 1000mg qd

Titrate:

Adjust dose/frequency depending on clinical response

In patients who tolerate lower doses well, may increase to two 750mg tabs or three 500mg tabs once daily for limited periods, as needed

Mild to Moderate Pain

Initial: 1000mg qd; may give 1500mg qd for a limited period in patients requiring greater analgesia

Max: 1000mg/day after limited period of 1500mg qd

Primary Dysmenorrhea

Initial: 1000mg qd; may give 1500mg qd for a limited period in patients requiring greater analgesia

Max: 1000mg/day after limited period of 1500mg qd

Bursitis/Tendinitis

Acute:

Initial: 1000mg qd; may give 1500mg qd for a limited period in patients requiring greater analgesia

Max: 1000mg/day after limited period of 1500mg qd

Gout

Acute:

Day 1: 1000-1500mg qd

Succeeding Days: 1000mg qd until attack subsides

DOSING CONSIDERATIONS

Renal Impairment

Start at lower end of dosing range

Hepatic Impairment

Start at lower end of dosing range

Elderly

Start at lower end of dosing range

ADMINISTRATION

Oral route

HOW SUPPLIED

Tab, Controlled-Release: 375mg, 500mg, 750mg

CONTRAINDICATIONS

Known hypersensitivity to naproxen; history of asthma, urticaria, or allergic-type reactions w/ aspirin (ASA) or other NSAIDs; treatment of perioperative pain in the setting of CABG surgery.

WARNINGS/PRECAUTIONS

Use lowest effective dose for the shortest duration possible. May cause HTN or worsen preexisting HTN; monitor BP closely. Fluid retention and edema reported; caution w/ fluid retention or heart failure (HF). Caution w/ history of ulcer disease, GI bleeding, or risk factors for GI bleeding; monitor for GI ulceration/bleeding and d/c if serious GI event occurs. Renal injury reported w/ long-term use; increased risk w/ renal/hepatic impairment, HF, and elderly. Not recommended w/ advanced renal disease or moderate to severe or severe renal impairment (CrCl <30mL/min); monitor renal function closely if therapy is initiated. Anaphylactoid reactions may occur. Caution w/ asthma and avoid w/ ASA-sensitive asthma and the ASA triad. May cause serious skin reactions (eg, exfoliative dermatitis, Stevens-Johnson syndrome, toxic epidermal necrolysis); d/c at 1st appearance of skin rash/hypersensitivity. Avoid in late pregnancy; may cause premature closure of ductus arteriosus. Not a substitute for corticosteroids nor treatment for corticosteroid insufficiency. May mask signs of inflammation and fever. May cause elevated LFTs or severe hepatic reactions; d/c if liver disease or systemic manifestations occur, and if abnormal LFTs persist/worsen. Anemia reported; monitor Hgb/Hct if anemia develops. May inhibit platelet aggregation and prolong bleeding time; monitor patients w/ coagulation disorders.

ADVERSE REACTIONS

CV thrombotic events, MI, stroke, GI events, headache, dyspepsia, flu syndrome, pain, infection, nausea, diarrhea, constipation, rhinitis, sinusitis, UTI.

DRUG INTERACTIONS

Increased risk of GI bleeding w/ oral corticosteroids, anticoagulants, alcohol use, and smoking. Risk of renal toxicity w/ diuretics and ACE inhibitors. Monitor patients receiving anticoagulants. May diminish antihypertensive effect of ACE inhibitors. Not recommended w/ ASA. May reduce natriuretic effect of loop (eg, furosemide) or thiazide diuretics; monitor for signs of renal failure and diuretic efficacy. May increase lithium levels; monitor for lithium toxicity. May enhance methotrexate toxicity; caution w/ concomitant use. Synergistic effect on GI bleeding w/ warfarin.

PATIENT CONSIDERATIONS

Assessment: Assess for history of asthma, urticaria, or allergic-type reactions w/ ASA or other NSAIDs, ASA triad, CVD, risk factors for CVD, HTN, fluid retention, HF, history of ulcer disease, history of/risk factors for GI bleeding, general health status, renal/hepatic function, coagulation disorders, pregnancy/nursing status, and possible drug interactions. Obtain baseline CBC and BP.

Monitoring: Monitor BP, CBC, bleeding time, LFTs, renal function, and chemistry profile periodically. Monitor for GI bleeding/ulceration/perforation, CV thrombotic events, MI, stroke, HTN, fluid retention, edema, and skin/allergic reactions.

Counseling: Inform to seek medical advice if symptoms of CV events, GI ulceration/bleeding, skin/hypersensitivity reactions, unexplained weight gain or edema, hepatotoxicity, or anaphylactoid reactions occur. Instruct to avoid in late pregnancy.

STORAGE: 20-25°C (68-77°F).

NAPROSYN – naproxen

RX

Class: NSAID

NSAIDs may increase risk of serious cardiovascular thrombotic events, MI, and stroke; increased risk with duration of use and with cardiovascular disease (CVD) or risk factors for CVD. Increased risk of serious GI adverse events (eg, bleeding, ulceration, and stomach/intestinal perforation) that can be fatal and occur anytime during use without warning symptoms; elderly patients are at a greater risk. Contraindicated for treatment of perioperative pain in the setting of CABG surgery.

OTHER BRAND NAMES

EC-Naprosyn, Anaprox, Anaprox DS

ADULT DOSAGE

Gout

Acute Attack:

Naprosyn:

Initial: 750mg, then 250mg q8h until attack subsides

Anaprox:

Initial: 825mg, then 275mg q8h until attack subsides

Bursitis

Anaprox/Anaprox DS:

Initial: 550mg, then 550mg q12h or 275mg q6-8h as required

Max: 1375mg/day initially, 1100mg/day thereafter

Rheumatoid Arthritis

Naprosyn:

250mg, 375mg, or 500mg bid

EC-Naprosyn:

375mg or 500mg bid

PEDIATRIC DOSAGE

Juvenile Arthritis

≥2 Years:

Sus:

Usual: 5mg/kg bid

Anaprox:
275mg bid

Anaprox DS:
550mg bid

Titrate: Adjust dose/frequency up or down depending on clinical response; may increase to 1500mg/day for ≤6 months if patient can tolerate lower doses well

Ankylosing Spondylitis

Naprosyn:
250mg, 375mg, or 500mg bid

EC-Naprosyn:
375mg or 500mg bid

Anaprox:
275mg bid

Anaprox DS:
550mg bid

Titrate: Adjust dose/frequency up or down depending on clinical response; may increase to 1500mg/day for ≤6 months if patient can tolerate lower doses well

Pain

Anaprox/Anaprox DS:
Initial: 550mg, then 550mg q12h or 275mg q6-8h as required
Max: 1375mg/day initially, 1100mg/day thereafter

Primary Dysmenorrhea

Anaprox/Anaprox DS:
Initial: 550mg, then 550mg q12h or 275mg q6-8h as required
Max: 1375mg/day initially, 1100mg/day thereafter

Osteoarthritis

Naprosyn:
250mg, 375mg, or 500mg bid

EC-Naprosyn:
375mg or 500mg bid

Anaprox:
275mg bid

Anaprox DS:
550mg bid

Titrate: Adjust dose/frequency up or down depending on clinical response; may increase to 1500mg/day for ≤6 months if patient can tolerate lower doses well

DOSING CONSIDERATIONS

Renal Impairment
Start w/ lower end of dosing range
Moderate to Severe (CrCl <30mL/min): Not recommended

Hepatic Impairment
Start w/ lower end of dosing range

Elderly
Start w/ lower end of dosing range

ADMINISTRATION

Oral route

EC-Naprosyn
Do not chew, crush, or break

HOW SUPPLIED

Sus: (Naprosyn) 125mg/5mL [473mL]; **Tab:** (Naprosyn) 250mg*, 375mg, 500mg*, (Anaprox [naproxen sodium]) 275mg, (Anaprox DS [naproxen sodium]) 550mg*; **Tab, Delayed-Release:** (EC-Naprosyn) 375mg, 500mg *scored

CONTRAINDICATIONS

Known hypersensitivity to naproxen and naproxen sodium; history of asthma, urticaria, or other allergic-type reactions w/ ASA or other NSAIDs; treatment of perioperative pain in the setting of CABG surgery.

WARNINGS/PRECAUTIONS

Use lowest effective dose for the shortest duration possible. May cause HTN or worsen preexisting HTN; monitor BP closely. Fluid retention and edema reported; caution with fluid retention, HTN, or HF. Caution with prior history of ulcer disease, GI bleeding, and risk factors for GI bleeding; monitor for GI ulceration/bleeding and d/c if serious GI event occurs. May exacerbate inflammatory bowel disease. Renal injury reported with long-term use; increased risk with renal/hepatic impairment, hypovolemia, HF, salt depletion, and in elderly. Not recommended with advanced renal disease or moderate to severe renal impairment (CrCl <30mL/min); monitor renal function closely and hydrate adequately. D/C if signs and symptoms consistent with renal disease develop. Anaphylactoid reactions may occur. Caution with asthma and avoid with ASA-sensitive asthma and the ASA triad. May cause serious skin adverse events (eg, exfoliative dermatitis, Stevens-Johnson syndrome, toxic epidermal necrolysis); d/c at 1st appearance of skin rash/hypersensitivity. Avoid in late pregnancy; may cause premature closure of ductus arteriosus. Not a substitute for corticosteroids or for the treatment of corticosteroid insufficiency. May mask signs of inflammation and fever. Periodically monitor Hgb if initial Hgb ≤10g and receiving long-term therapy. Perform ophthalmic studies if visual changes/disturbances occur. May cause elevations of LFTs or severe hepatic reactions; d/c if liver disease or systemic manifestations occur, or if abnormal LFTs persist/worsen. Caution with chronic alcoholic liver disease and other diseases with decreased/abnormal plasma proteins if high doses are administered; dosage adjustment may be required. Anemia reported; monitor Hgb/Hct if anemia develops. May inhibit platelet aggregation and prolong bleeding time; monitor patients with coagulation disorders. Monitor CBC and chemistry profile periodically with long-term treatment. (Sus, Anaprox/Anaprox DS) Contains Na^+; caution with severely restricted Na^+ intake. (EC-Naprosyn) Not recommended for initial treatment of acute pain.

ADVERSE REACTIONS

Cardiovascular (CV) thrombotic events, MI, stroke, GI adverse events, edema, drowsiness, dizziness, constipation, heartburn, abdominal pain, nausea, headache, tinnitus, dyspnea, pruritus.

DRUG INTERACTIONS

Avoid with other naproxen products. Not recommended with ASA. Risk of renal toxicity with diuretics, ACE inhibitors, and ARBs. May reduce natriuretic effect of loop (eg, furosemide) or thiazide diuretics; monitor for signs of renal failure and diuretic efficacy. May diminish antihypertensive effect of ACE inhibitors, ARBs, or β-blockers (eg, propranolol); monitor changes in BP. May result in deterioration of renal function, including possible acute renal failure with ACE inhibitors or ARBs; monitor closely for signs of worsening renal function. May enhance methotrexate toxicity; caution with concomitant use. May increase lithium levels and reduce renal lithium clearance; monitor for lithium toxicity. Increased risk of GI bleeding with SSRIs, oral corticosteroids, anticoagulants, alcohol, and smoking; monitor carefully. Synergistic effect on GI bleeding with warfarin. Potential for interaction with other albumin-bound drugs (eg, coumarin-type anticoagulants, sulfonylureas, hydantoins, other NSAIDs, ASA); dose adjustment with hydantoin, sulfonamide, or sulfonylurea may be required. Probenecid significantly increases plasma levels and extends $T_{1/2}$. Antacids, sucralfate, and cholestyramine can delay absorption. (EC-Naprosyn) Not recommended with H_2-blockers, sucralfate, or intensive antacid therapy.

PATIENT CONSIDERATIONS

Assessment: Assess for history of asthma, urticaria, or allergic-type reactions with ASA or other NSAIDs, ASA triad, CVD, risk factors for CVD, HTN, fluid retention, HF, salt restriction, history of ulcer disease, history of/risk factors for GI bleeding, general health status, history of IBD, renal/hepatic impairment, hypovolemia, decreased/abnormal plasma proteins, coagulation disorders, pregnancy/nursing status, and for possible drug interactions. Obtain baseline CBC and BP.

Monitoring: Monitor for GI bleeding/ulceration/perforation, CV thrombotic events, MI, stroke, HTN, fluid retention, edema, and skin/allergic reactions. Monitor BP, CBC, LFTs, renal function, and chemistry profile periodically.

Counseling: Inform to seek medical advice if symptoms of CV events, GI ulceration/bleeding, skin/hypersensitivity reactions, unexplained weight gain or edema, hepatotoxicity, or anaphylactoid reactions occur. Instruct to avoid use in late pregnancy. Instruct to use caution when performing activities that require alertness if drowsiness, dizziness, vertigo, or depression occurs.

STORAGE: 15-30°C (59-86°F). (Sus) Avoid excessive heat, >40°C (104°F). Shake gently before use.

N

NASONEX – mometasone furoate monohydrate

RX

Class: Corticosteroid

ADULT DOSAGE

Seasonal/Perennial Allergic Rhinitis

2 sprays/nostril qd

Prophylaxis:

May start 2-4 weeks before pollen season

Nasal Congestion:

2 sprays/nostril qd

Nasal Polyps

2 sprays/nostril qd-bid

PEDIATRIC DOSAGE

Seasonal/Perennial Allergic Rhinitis

2-11 Years:

1 spray/nostril qd

≥12 Years:

2 sprays/nostril qd

Prophylaxis:

May start 2-4 weeks before pollen season (≥12 years)

Nasal Congestion:

2-11 Years:

1 spray/nostril qd

≥12 Years:

2 sprays/nostril qd

ADMINISTRATION

Intranasal route

HOW SUPPLIED

Spray: 50mcg/spray [17g]

CONTRAINDICATIONS

Known hypersensitivity to mometasone furoate or any of its ingredients.

WARNINGS/PRECAUTIONS

Local nasal effects (eg, epistaxis, *Candida* infections of nose and pharynx, nasal septum perforation, impaired wound healing) may occur; d/c when infection occurs. Glaucoma and/or cataracts may develop; monitor closely in patients with change in vision, history of increased intraocular pressure (IOP), glaucoma, and/or cataracts. D/C if hypersensitivity reactions, including instances of wheezing, occur. May increase susceptibility to infections; caution with active/quiescent tuberculosis (TB), ocular herpes simplex, or untreated bacterial, fungal, and systemic viral infections. Hypercorticism and adrenal suppression may appear when used at higher than recommended doses or in susceptible individuals at recommended doses; d/c slowly if such changes occur. May reduce growth velocity of pediatrics; monitor growth routinely.

ADVERSE REACTIONS

Headache, viral infection, pharyngitis, epistaxis/blood-tinged mucus, cough, upper respiratory tract infection, dysmenorrhea, musculoskeletal pain, sinusitis, N/V.

DRUG INTERACTIONS

May increase plasma concentrations with ketoconazole.

PATIENT CONSIDERATIONS

Assessment: Assess for previous hypersensitivity, active/quiescent TB, infections, ocular herpes simplex, change in vision, history of IOP, glaucoma or cataracts, recent nasal septum ulcers, nasal surgery/trauma, pregnancy/nursing status, and possible drug interactions.

Monitoring: Monitor for acute adrenal insufficiency, hypercorticism, nasal or pharyngeal *Candida* infections, suppression of growth velocity in children, hypersensitivity reactions, wheezing, nasal septum perforation, changes in vision, glaucoma, cataracts, increased IOP, epistaxis, wound healing, worsening of infections, and other adverse reactions.

Counseling: Advise to take ud at regular intervals and not to increase prescribed dosage. Inform patients that treatment may be associated with adverse reactions (eg, epistaxis, nasal septum perforation, *Candida* infection). Inform that glaucoma and/or cataracts may develop. Counsel to avoid exposure to chickenpox or measles and to immediately consult a physician if exposed. Contact physician if symptoms worsen or do not improve. Supervise young children during administration. Advise patient to take missed dose as soon as remembered. Counsel on proper priming and administration techniques.

STORAGE: 25°C (77°F); excursions permitted to 15-30°C (59-86°F). Protect from light.

N

NATESTO – testosterone

CIII

Class: Androgen

ADULT DOSAGE

Testosterone Replacement Therapy

Congenital/Acquired Primary Hypogonadism or Hypogonadotropic Hypogonadism in Males:

Usual: 11mg (2 pump actuations; 1 actuation/nostril) tid for a total dose of 33mg/day

Consider alternative treatment if total testosterone concentration is consistently <300ng/dL; if total testosterone concentration is consistently >1050ng/dL, d/c therapy

PEDIATRIC DOSAGE

Pediatric use may not have been established

DOSING CONSIDERATIONS

Concomitant Medications

Use w/ other nasally administered drugs other than sympathomimetic decongestants (eg, oxymetazoline) is not recommended

Discontinuation

Severe Rhinitis: If patient experiences an episode of severe rhinitis, temporarily d/c therapy pending resolution of the severe rhinitis symptoms. If severe rhinitis symptoms persist, alternative testosterone replacement therapy is recommended

ADMINISTRATION

Intranasal route

Administer tid (in the am, afternoon, and pm) (6-8 hrs apart) preferably at the same time each day
Completely depress pump 1X in each nostril to receive total dose
Do not administer to other parts of the body
Replace dispenser when the top of the piston inside dispenser reaches the arrow at the top of the inside label

Preparing the Pump

Prime pump by inverting pump, and depressing pump 10X; discard any amount of product dispensed directly into a sink and thoroughly wash away the gel w/ warm water
Wipe tip w/ a clean, dry tissue
If gel gets on to the hands, wash hands w/ warm water and soap
Priming should be done only prior to the 1st use of each dispenser

Administering the Dose

1. Blow nose, then remove cap from dispenser
2. Place the right index finger on the pump of the actuator while in front of a mirror; slowly advance the tip of the actuator into the left nostril upwards until the finger on the pump reaches the base of the nose
3. Tilt actuator so that opening on the tip of the actuator is in contact w/ lateral wall of nostril to ensure application of gel to the nasal wall
4. Slowly depress pump until it stops
5. Remove actuator from nose while wiping the tip along the inside of the lateral nostril wall to fully transfer the gel
6. Using left index finger, repeat steps 2-5 for the right nostril
7. Use a clean, dry tissue to wipe tip of actuator and replace cap on dispenser
8. Press on nostrils at a point just below the bridge of the nose and lightly massage
9. Refrain from blowing nose or sniffing for 1 hr after administration

HOW SUPPLIED

Gel: 5.5mg/actuation [60 actuations]

CONTRAINDICATIONS

Breast carcinoma or known/suspected prostate carcinoma in men; women who are or may become pregnant, or are breastfeeding.

WARNINGS/PRECAUTIONS

Nasal adverse reactions (eg, nasopharyngitis, rhinorrhea, epistaxis) reported; determine whether further evaluation or discontinuation of therapy is appropriate. Not recommended for use in patients w/ mucosal inflammatory disorders (eg, Sjogren's syndrome), sinus disease, and those w/ a history of nasal disorders, nasal/sinus surgery, or nasal fracture w/in the previous 6 months or nasal fracture that caused a deviated anterior nasal septum. Patients w/ BPH and geriatric patients may be at increased risk of worsening of signs/symptoms of BPH. May increase risk for prostate cancer. Increases in Hct, reflective of increases in RBC mass, may require discontinuation of therapy. If Hct becomes elevated, d/c until Hct decreases to an acceptable level. Increase in RBC mass may increase risk of thromboembolic events. Venous thromboembolic events (eg, deep vein thrombosis, pulmonary embolism) reported; d/c and initiate workup and management if a venous thromboembolic event is suspected. Increased risk of major adverse cardiovascular events (MACE) reported. Not indicated for use in women. Suppression of spermatogenesis may occur w/ large doses. Prolonged use of high doses of orally active 17-α-alkyl androgens has been associated w/ serious hepatic effects (eg, peliosis hepatis, hepatic neoplasms, cholestatic hepatitis); d/c promptly if any signs/symptoms of hepatic dysfunction occur. May promote retention of Na^+ and water. Risk of edema w/ or w/o CHF in patients w/ preexisting cardiac, renal, or hepatic disease; diuretic therapy, in addition to discontinuation of therapy, may be required. Gynecomastia may develop and persist. May potentiate sleep apnea, especially in those w/ risk factors (eg, obesity, chronic lung disease). Changes in serum lipid profile may occur and may require discontinuation of therapy. Caution in cancer patients at risk of hypercalcemia and associated hypercalciuria. May decrease levels of thyroxine-binding globulins, resulting in decreased total T4 serum levels and increased resin uptake of T3 and T4.

ADVERSE REACTIONS

Prostate-specific antigen increased, headache, rhinorrhea, epistaxis, nasal discomfort, nasopharyngitis, bronchitis, URTI, sinusitis, nasal scab, nasal dryness, nasal congestion, parosmia, pain in extremity.

DRUG INTERACTIONS

See Dosing Considerations. Changes in insulin sensitivity or glycemic control may occur; may decrease blood glucose and, therefore, may necessitate a dose reduction of anti-diabetic medication in diabetic patients. Changes in anticoagulant activity may occur; frequently monitor PT/INR in patients taking warfarin, especially at initiation and termination of androgen therapy. Concurrent use w/ corticosteroids may increase fluid retention; monitoring required, particularly in patients w/ cardiac, renal, or hepatic disease. Oxymetazoline given 30 min prior to therapy may decrease total testosterone levels.

PATIENT CONSIDERATIONS

Assessment: Assess for mucosal inflammatory disorders; sinus disease, history of nasal disorders, nasal/sinus surgery, or nasal fracture w/in the previous 6 months or nasal fracture that caused a deviated anterior nasal septum; BPH; prostate cancer; cardiac/renal/hepatic disease; obesity; chronic lung disease, any other conditions where treatment is contraindicated or cautioned; and for possible drug interactions. Obtain baseline Hct and lipid levels. Confirm diagnosis of hypogonadism by measuring testosterone levels in am on at least 2 separate days prior to initiation.

Monitoring: Monitor for nasal adverse reactions, worsening of signs/symptoms of BPH, venous thromboembolic events, signs/symptoms of hepatic dysfunction, edema w/ or w/o CHF, gynecomastia, sleep apnea, MACE, and other adverse reactions. Monitor lipid profile periodically. Check serum testosterone levels periodically, starting as soon as 1 month after initiation of therapy. In cancer patients at risk for hypercalcemia, regularly monitor serum Ca^{2+} levels. Evaluate Hct level 3-6 months after starting therapy, then annually. Evaluate for prostate cancer 3-6 months after initiation of treatment, then in accordance w/ prostate cancer screening practices.

Counseling: Advise about possible adverse reactions, including risk of MACE. Inform that men w/ known/suspected prostate or breast cancer should not use therapy. Instruct to report to physician any nasal signs/symptoms or any signs/symptoms of hepatic dysfunction (eg, jaundice). Counsel to use ud, to report any changes in state of health to physician, and to never share medication w/ anyone.

STORAGE: 20-25°C (68-77°F); excursions permitted to 15-30°C (59-86°F). Discard used dispensers in household trash in a manner that prevents accidental exposure of children or pets.

NATPARA – parathyroid hormone

RX

Class: Parathyroid hormone analogue

Potential risk of osteosarcoma; use only in patients who cannot be well-controlled on Ca^{2+} and active forms of vitamin D alone and for whom the potential benefits are considered to outweigh this risk. Avoid use w/ increased baseline risk for osteosarcoma such as patients w/ Paget's disease of bone or unexplained elevations of alkaline phosphatase, pediatric and young adult patients w/ open epiphyses, patients w/ hereditary disorders predisposing to osteosarcoma, or patients w/ a prior history of external beam or implant radiation therapy involving the skeleton. Available only through a restricted program under a Risk Evaluation and Mitigation Strategy (REMS) called the Natpara REMS program.

N

ADULT DOSAGE

Hypocalcemia with Hypoparathyroidism

Adjunct to Ca^{2+} and Vitamin D to Control Hypocalcemia:

Before Initiating and During Therapy:
Confirm 25-hydroxyvitamin D stores are sufficient; if insufficient, replace to sufficient levels
Confirm serum Ca^{2+} is >7.5mg/dL before initiating therapy

Initiating Therapy:
1. Initiate at 50mcg qd
2. In patients using active forms of vitamin D, decrease dose of active vitamin D by 50%, if serum Ca^{2+} >7.5mg/dL
3. In patients using Ca^{2+} supplements, maintain Ca^{2+} supplement dose
4. Measure serum Ca^{2+} concentration w/in 3-7 days
5. Adjust dose of active vitamin D or Ca^{2+} supplement or both based on serum Ca^{2+} value and clinical assessment; refer to PI for suggested adjustments
6. Repeat steps 4 and 5 until target serum Ca^{2+} levels are w/in the lower 1/2 of the normal range (8-9mg/dL), active vitamin D has been discontinued, and Ca^{2+} supplementation is sufficient to meet daily requirements

Titration:
Dose Increase: May increase in increments of 25mcg every 4 weeks up to a max of 100mcg/day if serum Ca^{2+} cannot be maintained >8mg/dL w/o an active form of vitamin D and/or oral Ca^{2+} supplementation
Dose Decrease: May decrease to as low as 25mcg/day if total serum Ca^{2+} is repeatedly >9mg/dL after active form of vitamin D has been discontinued and Ca^{2+} supplement has been decreased to a dose sufficient to meet daily requirements
After a dose change, monitor clinical response as well as serum Ca^{2+}; adjust active vitamin D and Ca^{2+} supplements per steps 4-6 above if indicated

Maint Dose:
Use lowest dose that achieves total serum Ca^{2+} (albumin-corrected) w/in the lower 1/2 of normal total serum Ca^{2+} range, w/o the need for active forms of vitamin D and w/ Ca^{2+} supplementation sufficient to meet daily requirements; monitor serum Ca^{2+} and 24 hr urinary calcium once maint dose is achieved

Missed Dose

Next dose should be administered as soon as reasonably feasible and additional exogenous Ca^{2+} should be taken in the event of hypocalcemia

PEDIATRIC DOSAGE

Pediatric use may not have been established

DOSING CONSIDERATIONS

Elderly
Start at low end of dosing range

Dose Interruption or Discontinuation
Abrupt interruption or discontinuation can result in severe hypocalcemia; resume treatment w/, or increase the dose of, an active form of vitamin D and Ca^{2+}supplements if indicated in patients interrupting or discontinuing therapy

N

ADMINISTRATION
SQ route

Administer in thigh; alternate thigh every day
Refer to PI for the instructions to reconstitute using the mixing device for reconstitution and to administer using the pen delivery device (Q-Cliq pen)

HOW SUPPLIED
Inj: 25mcg/dose, 50mcg/dose, 75mcg/dose, 100mcg/dose

WARNINGS/PRECAUTIONS
Severe hypercalcemia reported; risk is highest when starting or increasing dose of parathyroid hormone. Treat hypercalcemia per standard practice and consider holding and/or lowering parathyroid hormone dose if severe hypercalcemia occurs. Severe hypocalcemia reported; risk is highest when parathyroid hormone is withheld, missed, or abruptly discontinued. Resume treatment w/, or increase dose of, an active form of vitamin D or Ca^{2+} supplements or both if indicated in patients interrupting or discontinuing therapy. Caution in elderly.

ADVERSE REACTIONS
Paresthesia, hypo/hypercalcemia, headache, N/V, hypoaesthesia, diarrhea, arthralgia, hypercalciuria, pain in extremity, URTI, upper abdominal pain, sinusitis, HTN, neck pain.

DRUG INTERACTIONS
Not recommended w/ alendronate. Concomitant use w/ cardiac glycosides (eg, digoxin) may predispose patients to digitalis toxicity if hypercalcemia develops; carefully monitor serum Ca^{2+} and digoxin levels, and for signs/symptoms of digoxin toxicity. Adjustment of digoxin and/ or parathyroid hormone may be needed.

PATIENT CONSIDERATIONS

Assessment: Assess for increased baseline risk for osteosarcoma, pregnancy/nursing status, and for possible drug interactions. Assess serum Ca^{2+} levels, and 25-hydroxyvitamin D stores.

Monitoring: Monitor for signs and symptoms of osteosarcoma, hypo/hypercalcemia, and other adverse reactions. Monitor serum Ca^{2+} levels and 25-hydroxyvitamin D stores.

Counseling: Inform of the risks/benefits of therapy. Inform that the drug is available only through a restricted program called the Natpara REMS program. Advise of potential risk of osteosarcoma and to promptly report signs/symptoms of possible osteosarcoma (eg, persistent localized pain, occurrence of a new tissue mass that is tender to palpation). Advise that severe hypercalcemia may occur when initiating/adjusting dose and/or making changes to coadministered drugs known to raise serum Ca^{2+}; instruct to report symptoms promptly, report any changes to coadministered drugs known to influence Ca^{2+} levels, and follow recommended serum Ca^{2+} monitoring. Inform that severe hypocalcemia may occur when therapy is abruptly interrupted/discontinued; instruct to report symptoms of severe hypocalcemia promptly, report interruption in dosing, follow recommended serum Ca^{2+} monitoring, and to contact physician in the event of dose interruption as doses of active vitamin D and Ca^{2+} supplementation may need adjustment. Instruct to report use of digoxin-containing medication, and follow recommended serum Ca^{2+} monitoring. Counsel patient or caregiver on the proper technique for administering SQ inj using the mixing device and the Q-Cliq pen, including the use of aseptic technique.

STORAGE: (Cartridge) Prior to Reconstitution: 2-8°C (36-46°F). After Reconstitution: Store in the Q-Cliq pen at 2-8°C (36-46°F) and may be used for up to 14 days under these conditions; discard after 14 days. Store away from heat and light. Avoid exposure to elevated temperatures. Do not freeze or shake. (Mixing Device/Empty Q-Cliq Pen) Room temperature.

NATURE-THROID – thyroid

RX

Class: Thyroid replacement hormone

ADULT DOSAGE

Hypothyroidism

Replacement/supplemental therapy in hypothyroidism of any etiology, except transient hypothyroidism during the recovery phase of subacute thyroiditis

Initial: 32.5mg/day; 16.25mg/day is recommended in patients w/ myxedema, particularly if cardiovascular impairment is suspected
Titrate: Increase by 16.25mg every 2-3 weeks
Maint: 65-130mg/day

PEDIATRIC DOSAGE

Hypothyroidism

Congenital:
0-6 Months of Age: 4.8-6mg/kg/day (16.25-32.5mg/day)
6-12 Months of Age: 3.6-4.8mg/kg/day (32.5-48.75mg/day)
1-5 Years: 3-3.6mg/kg/day (48.75-65mg/day)
6-12 Years: 2.4-3mg/kg/day (65-97.5mg/day)
>12 Years: 1.2-1.8mg/kg/day (>97.5mg/day)

N

Myxedema Coma:
Initial: 400mcg (100mcg/mL) of levothyroxine sodium (T4) given rapidly; follow by daily supplements of 100-200mcg given IV

Pituitary TSH Suppressant

Used to treat/prevent various types of euthyroid goiters (eg, thyroid nodules, subacute or chronic lymphocytic thyroiditis [Hashimoto's], multinodular goiter) and to manage thyroid cancer

1.56mg/kg/day of levothyroxine (T4) for 7-10 days

Diagnostic Aid

In Suppression Tests to Differentiate Suspected Mild Hyperthyroidism or Thyroid Gland Anatomy:
1.56mg/kg/day of levothyroxine (T4) for 7-10 days

DOSING CONSIDERATIONS

Adverse Reactions
Hypothyroidism:
Angina: Reduce dose if angina occurs

Elderly
Start at lower end of dosing range

ADMINISTRATION

Oral route

HOW SUPPLIED

Tab: 16.25mg, 32.5mg, 48.75mg, 65mg, 81.25mg, 97.5mg, 113.75mg, 130mg, 146.25mg, 162.5mg, 195mg, 260mg, 325mg

CONTRAINDICATIONS

Uncorrected adrenal cortical insufficiency, untreated thyrotoxicosis, hypersensitivity to any of their active or extraneous constituents.

WARNINGS/PRECAUTIONS

Not for treatment of obesity; larger doses in euthyroid patients can cause serious or even life-threatening toxicity. Not for the treatment of male or female infertility unless accompanied by hypothyroidism. Caution with cardiovascular (CV) disorders (eg, angina pectoris) and elderly with risk of occult cardiac disease; initiate at low doses and reduce dose if aggravation of CV disease suspected. May aggravate diabetes mellitus (DM), diabetes insipidus (DI), or adrenal cortical insufficiency. Treatment of myxedema coma requires simultaneous administration of glucocorticoids. Excessive doses in infants may cause craniosynostosis. Caution with strong suspicion of thyroid gland autonomy. Androgens, corticosteroids, estrogens, iodine-containing preparations, and salicylates may interfere with lab tests.

DRUG INTERACTIONS

Large doses in euthyroid patients may cause serious or even life-threatening toxicity particularly with sympathomimetic amines. Closely monitor PT in patients on oral anticoagulants; dose reduction of anticoagulant may be required. May increase insulin or oral hypoglycemic requirements. Potentially impaired absorption with cholestyramine and colestipol; space dosing by 4-5 hrs. Estrogens may decrease free T4; increase in thyroid dose may be needed.

PATIENT CONSIDERATIONS

Assessment: Assess for adrenal cortical insufficiency, thyrotoxicosis, apparent hypersensitivity to the drug, CV disorders (CAD, angina pectoris), DM/DI, myxedema coma, nursing status, and possible drug interactions.

Monitoring: Monitor response to treatment, urinary glucose levels in patients with DM, PT in patients receiving anticoagulants, and for aggravation of CV disease. Monitor thyroid function periodically.

Counseling: Inform that replacement therapy is taken essentially for life except in transient hypothyroidism. Instruct to immediately report to physician any signs/symptoms of thyroid hormone toxicity (eg, chest pain, increased pulse rate, palpitations, excessive sweating, heat intolerance, nervousness). Inform the importance of frequent/close monitoring of PT and urinary glucose and the need for dose adjustment of antidiabetic and/or oral anticoagulant medication. Inform that partial loss of hair may be seen in children in 1st few months of therapy.

STORAGE: 15-30°C (59-86°F).

NEORAL – cyclosporine

RX

Class: Calcineurin-inhibitor immunosuppressant

Should only be prescribed by physicians experienced in management of systemic immunosuppressive therapy for indicated diseases. Manage patients in facilities equipped and staffed w/ adequate lab and supportive medical resources. Increased susceptibility to infection and development of neoplasia (eg, lymphoma) may result from immunosuppression. May be coadministered w/ other immunosuppressive agents in kidney, liver, and heart transplant patients. Not bioequivalent to Sandimmune and cannot be used interchangeably w/o physician supervision. Caution in switching from Sandimmune. Monitor cyclosporine blood concentrations in transplant and rheumatoid arthritis (RA) patients to avoid toxicity due to high concentrations. Dose adjustments should be made to minimize possible organ rejection due to low concentrations in transplant patients. Increased risk of developing skin malignancies in psoriasis patients previously treated w/ PUVA, methotrexate (MTX) or other immunosuppressive agents, UVB, coal tar, or radiation therapy. May cause systemic HTN and nephrotoxicity. Monitor for renal dysfunction, including structural kidney damage, during therapy.

ADULT DOSAGE

Organ Transplant

Organ Rejection Prophylaxis in Kidney, Liver, and Heart Allogeneic Transplants:
Newly Transplanted Patients:
Initial dose may be given 4-12 hrs prior to transplant or given postoperatively; dose varies depending on transplanted organ and other immunosuppressive agents included in protocol

Suggested Initial Doses:
Renal Transplant: 9mg/kg/day ± 3mg/kg/day
Liver Transplant: 8mg/kg/day ± 4mg/kg/day
Heart Transplant: 7mg/kg/day ± 3mg/kg/day

Give bid

Subsequently adjust dose to achieve a predefined blood concentration

Adjunct therapy w/ adrenal corticosteroids is recommended initially

Conversion from Sandimmune:
Start w/ same daily dose as was previously used w/ Sandimmune (1:1 dose conversion); subsequently adjust dose to attain the pre-conversion blood trough concentration.
After conversion, monitor blood trough concentration every 4-7 days while adjusting to trough levels until concentration attains pre-conversion value.

Transplant Patients w/ Poor Sandimmune Absorption:
Patients tend to have higher cyclosporine concentrations after conversion to therapy; caution when converting patients at doses >10mg/kg/day.
Titrate dose individually based on trough concentrations, tolerability, and clinical response and measure blood trough concentration at least 2X a week (daily if initial dose >10mg/kg/day) until stabilized w/in desired range.

Rheumatoid Arthritis

Severe, active rheumatoid arthritis where the disease has not adequately responded to methotrexate (MTX)

W/ or w/o MTX:
Initial: 2.5mg/kg/day, taken bid
Titrate: May increase by 0.5-0.75mg/kg/day after 8 weeks and again after 12 weeks
Max: 4mg/kg/day

Salicylates, NSAIDs, and oral corticosteroids may be continued

D/C if no benefit is seen by 16 weeks

PEDIATRIC DOSAGE

Organ Rejection Prophylaxis

Transplant recipients as young as 1 year of age have received Neoral with no unusual adverse effects

N

Combination w/ MTX:
Most patients can be treated w/ doses of ≤3mg/kg/day when combined w/ MTX doses of up to 15mg/week

Plaque Psoriasis

In immunocompetent patients w/ severe, recalcitrant, plaque psoriasis who failed to respond to at least 1 systemic therapy (eg, PUVA, retinoids, methotrexate) or for whom other systemic therapies are contraindicated, or cannot be tolerated

Initial: 2.5mg/kg/day, taken bid, for at least 4 weeks
Titrate: If clinical improvement does not occur, increase dose at 2-week intervals by approx 0.5mg/kg/day
Max: 4mg/kg/day

D/C if satisfactory response cannot be achieved after 6 weeks at 4mg/kg/day or the patient's max tolerated dose

DOSING CONSIDERATIONS

Renal Impairment
In Kidney, Liver, and Heart Transplant:
Reduce dose if indicated
In Rheumatoid Arthritis/Plaque Psoriasis:
Not recommended for use

Hepatic Impairment
Severe: Dose reduction may be necessary

Elderly
Start at lower end of dosing range

Adverse Events
Rheumatoid Arthritis/Plaque Psoriasis:
Reduce dose by 25-50% to control adverse events; d/c therapy if dose reduction is not effective or if adverse event or abnormality is severe

Other Important Considerations
Avoid consumption of grapefruit or grapefruit juice during therapy

ADMINISTRATION

Oral route

Always administer daily dose in 2 divided doses (bid); administer on a consistent schedule w/ regard to time of day and relation to meals.

Sol

1. Dilute w/ room temperature orange or apple juice to make sol more palatable; avoid switching diluents frequently or diluting w/ grapefruit juice.
2. Take the prescribed amount of sol from the container using supplied dosing syringe, after removal of protective cover, and transfer sol to a glass of orange or apple juice (do not use a plastic container).
3. Stir well and drink at once; do not allow diluted oral sol to stand before drinking.
4. Rinse the glass w/ more diluent to ensure that the total dose is consumed.
5. After use, dry the outside of dosing syringe w/ a clean towel and replace protective cover.
6. Do not rinse dosing syringe w/ water or other cleaning agents; if syringe requires cleaning, it must be completely dry before resuming use.

HOW SUPPLIED

Cap: 25mg, 100mg; **Sol:** 100mg/mL [50mL]

CONTRAINDICATIONS

Hypersensitivity to cyclosporine or to any of the ingredients of the formulation. **RA/Psoriasis:** Abnormal renal function, uncontrolled HTN, malignancies. **Psoriasis:** Concomitant PUVA or UVB therapy, MTX, other immunosuppressants, coal tar, or radiation therapy.

WARNINGS/PRECAUTIONS

May cause hepatotoxicity and liver injury (eg, cholestasis, jaundice, hepatitis, liver failure). Elevations of SrCr and BUN may occur and reflect a reduction in GFR; closely monitor renal function and frequent dose adjustments may be indicated. Elevations in SrCr and BUN levels do not necessarily indicate rejection; evaluate patient before initiating dose adjustment. Thrombocytopenia and microangiopathic hemolytic anemia, resulting in graft failure, significant hyperkalemia (sometimes associated w/ hyperchloremic metabolic acidosis) and hyperuricemia

N

reported. Avoid excessive ultraviolet light exposure. Oversuppression of the immune system may result in an increased risk of infection/malignancy; caution w/ a multiple immunosuppressant regimen. Increased risk of developing bacterial, viral, fungal, protozoal, and opportunistic infections (eg, polyomavirus infections). JC virus-associated progressive multifocal leukoencephalopathy and polyomavirus-/BK virus-associated nephropathy reported; consider reduction in immunosuppression if either develops. Convulsions, encephalopathy including posterior reversible encephalopathy syndrome, and rarely, optic disc edema reported. Evaluate before and during treatment for development of malignancies. In RA patients, monitor BP on at least 2 occasions and obtain 2 baseline SrCr levels before treatment, then monitor BP and SrCr every 2 weeks for the first 3 months of therapy, and then monthly if the patient is stable or more frequently during dose adjustments. In psoriasis patients, assess BP on at least 2 occasions and obtain baseline SrCr, BUN, CBC, Mg^{2+}, K^+, uric acid, and lipids before treatment, then monitor every 2 weeks for the first 3 months of therapy, and then monthly if the patient is stable or more frequently during dose adjustments. Monitor CBC and LFTs monthly w/ MTX. Monitor SrCr and BP after initiation or increases in NSAID dose for RA. Consider the alcohol content of the drug when given to patients in whom alcohol intake should be avoided or minimized (eg, pregnant or breastfeeding women, patients presenting w/ liver disease or epilepsy, alcoholic patients, or pediatric patients). HTN may occur and persist, and may require antihypertensive therapy.

ADVERSE REACTIONS

Increased susceptibility to infection, neoplasia, renal dysfunction, HTN, hirsutism/hypertrichosis, tremor, headache, gum hyperplasia, diarrhea, N/V, paresthesia, hypertriglyceridemia, hyperesthesia.

DRUG INTERACTIONS

See Boxed Warning, Dosing Considerations, and Contraindications. Avoid w/ K^+-sparing diuretics, aliskiren, orlistat, bosentan, or dabigatran. Vaccinations may be less effective; avoid live vaccines during therapy. Frequent gingival hyperplasia reported w/ nifedipine; avoid concomitant use w/ nifedipine in patients in whom gingival hyperplasia develops as a side effect of cyclosporine. Caution w/ rifabutin, nephrotoxic drugs, HIV protease inhibitors (eg, indinavir, nelfinavir, ritonavir, saquinavir), K^+-sparing drugs (eg, ACE inhibitors, ARBs), K^+-containing drugs, and K^+-rich diet. Ciprofloxacin, gentamicin, tobramycin, vancomycin, trimethoprim w/ sulfamethoxazole, melphalan, amphotericin B, ketoconazole, azapropazon, colchicine, diclofenac, naproxen, sulindac, cimetidine, ranitidine, tacrolimus, fibric acid derivatives (eg, bezafibrate, fenofibrate), MTX, and NSAIDs may potentiate renal dysfunction; closely monitor renal function and reduce dose of coadministered drug or consider alternative treatment if significant renal impairment occurs. Diltiazem, nicardipine, verapamil, fluconazole, itraconazole, ketoconazole, voriconazole, azithromycin, clarithromycin, erythromycin, quinupristin/dalfopristin, methylprednisolone, allopurinol, amiodarone, bromocriptine, colchicine, danazol, imatinib, metoclopramide, nefazodone, oral contraceptives, grapefruit, grapefruit juice, HIV protease inhibitors, boceprevir, and telaprevir may increase levels. Nafcillin, rifampin, carbamazepine, oxcarbazepine, phenobarbital, phenytoin, bosentan, octreotide, orlistat, sulfinpyrazone, terbinafine, ticlopidine, and St. John's wort may decrease levels. May increase levels of bosentan, dabigatran, and CYP3A4, P-gp, or organic anion transporter protein substrates. May increase levels of ambrisentan; do not titrate ambrisentan dose to the recommended max daily dose. CYP3A4 and/or P-gp inducers and inhibitors may alter levels; may require dose adjustments of cyclosporine if cyclosporine concentrations are significantly altered. May reduce clearance of digoxin, colchicine, prednisolone, HMG-CoA reductase inhibitors (statins), aliskiren, bosentan, dabigatran, repaglinide, NSAIDs, sirolimus, and etoposide. Digitalis toxicity reported when used w/ digoxin; monitor digoxin levels. May increase levels and enhance toxic effects (eg, myopathy, neuropathy) of colchicine; may reduce colchicine dose. Myotoxicity cases seen w/ lovastatin, simvastatin, atorvastatin, pravastatin, and, rarely fluvastatin; temporarily withhold or d/c statin therapy if signs of myopathy develop or w/ risk factors predisposing to severe renal injury, including renal failure, secondary to rhabdomyolysis. May increase levels of repaglinide, thereby increasing the risk of hypoglycemia; closely monitor blood glucose levels. High doses of cyclosporine may increase the exposure to anthracycline antibiotics (eg, doxorubicin, mitoxantrone, daunorubicin) in cancer patients. May double diclofenac blood levels; dose of diclofenac should be in the lower end of the therapeutic range. May increase MTX levels and decrease levels of active metabolite of MTX. May elevate SrCr and increase levels of sirolimus; give 4 hrs after cyclosporine administration. Convulsions reported w/ high-dose methylprednisolone. Calcium antagonists may interfere w/ cyclosporine metabolism. Avoid in psoriasis patients receiving other immunosuppressive agents or radiation therapy (including PUVA and UVB).

PATIENT CONSIDERATIONS

Assessment: Assess for hypersensitivity to the drug, renal dysfunction, uncontrolled HTN, presence of malignancies, pregnancy/nursing status, and possible drug interactions. RA: Before initiating treatment, assess BP (on at least 2 occasions) and obtain 2 SrCr levels. Psoriasis: Prior to treatment, perform a dermatological and physical examination, including measuring BP. Assess for presence of occult infections and for the presence of tumors. Assess for atypical skin lesions and biopsy them. Obtain baseline SrCr (at least twice), BUN, LFTs, bilirubin, CBC, Mg^{2+}, K^+, uric acid, and lipid levels.

Monitoring: Monitor for signs/symptoms of hepatotoxicity, liver injury, nephrotoxicity, thrombocytopenia, microangiopathic hemolytic anemia, HTN, hyperkalemia, lymphomas and other malignancies, serious/polyoma virus infections, convulsions and other neurotoxicities, and other adverse reactions. Monitor cyclosporine blood concentrations routinely in transplant patients and periodically in RA patients. RA: Monitor BP and SrCr every 2 weeks during the initial 3 months of treatment, then monthly if patient is stable. Monitor SrCr and BP after an increase of the dose of NSAIDs and after initiation of new NSAID therapy. If coadministered w/ MTX, monitor CBC and LFTs monthly. Psoriasis: Monitor for occult infections and tumors. Monitor SrCr, BUN, BP, CBC, uric acid, K^+, lipids, and Mg^{2+} levels every 2 weeks during first 3 months of treatment, then monthly if stable.

Counseling: Instruct to contact physician before changing formulations of cyclosporine, which may require dose changes. Inform that repeated lab tests are required while on therapy. Advise of the potential risks if used during pregnancy and inform of the increased risk of neoplasia, HTN, and renal dysfunction. Inform that vaccinations may be less effective and to avoid live vaccines during therapy. Advise to take the medication on a consistent schedule w/ regard to time and meals, and to avoid grapefruit and grapefruit juice. Inform to avoid excessive sun exposure.

STORAGE: 20-25°C (68-77°F). (Sol) Use w/in 2 months upon opening. Do not refrigerate. At <20°C (68°F) may form gel; light flocculation, or formation of light sediment may occur; allow to warm to 25°C (77°F) to reverse changes.

NESINA — alogliptin

RX

Class: Dipeptidyl peptidase-4 (DPP-4) inhibitor

ADULT DOSAGE	PEDIATRIC DOSAGE
Type 2 Diabetes Mellitus 25mg qd	Pediatric use may not have been established

DOSING CONSIDERATIONS

Renal Impairment

Moderate (CrCl ≥30 to <60mL/min): 12.5mg qd

Severe (CrCl ≥15 to <30mL/min): 6.25mg qd

ESRD (CrCl <15mL/min or Requiring Hemodialysis): 6.25mg qd

ADMINISTRATION

Oral route

N

May be taken w/ or w/o food.

May be administered w/o regard to timing of hemodialysis.

HOW SUPPLIED

Tab: 6.25mg, 12.5mg, 25mg

CONTRAINDICATIONS

History of a serious hypersensitivity reaction (eg, anaphylaxis, angioedema, severe cutaneous adverse reactions) to alogliptin-containing products.

WARNINGS/PRECAUTIONS

Not for use in type 1 diabetes mellitus (DM) or for treatment of diabetic ketoacidosis. Acute pancreatitis reported; d/c if pancreatitis is suspected and initiate appropriate management. Serious hypersensitivity reactions reported; d/c if suspected, assess for other potential causes and institute alternative treatment. Caution w/ history of angioedema w/ another DPP-4 inhibitor. Fatal/nonfatal hepatic failure and serum ALT >3X ULN reported; initiate w/ caution in patients w/ abnormal LFTs. Interrupt treatment and investigate probable cause if clinically significant liver enzyme elevations and abnormal LFTs persist/worsen; do not restart w/o another explanation for abnormal LFTs. Severe and disabling arthralgia has been reported in patients taking DPP-4 inhibitors. Consider as a possible cause for severe joint pain and d/c therapy if appropriate.

ADVERSE REACTIONS

Hypoglycemia, nasopharyngitis, headache, URTI.

DRUG INTERACTIONS

Lower dose of insulin therapy or insulin secretagogue (eg, sulfonylurea) may be required to reduce risk of hypoglycemia.

PATIENT CONSIDERATIONS

Assessment: Assess renal/hepatic function, previous hypersensitivity to the drug, history of pancreatitis, type of DM, diabetic ketoacidosis, history of angioedema w/ another DPP-4 inhibitor, pregnancy/nursing status, and possible drug interactions. Obtain baseline FPG and HbA1c.

Monitoring: Monitor for pancreatitis, arthralgia, and hypersensitivity reactions. Monitor FPG, HbA1c, and renal/hepatic function periodically.

Counseling: Inform of risks/benefits of therapy. Inform of signs/symptoms of pancreatitis; instruct to d/c promptly and contact physician if persistent severe abdominal pain occurs. Inform that allergic reactions and liver injury have been reported; instruct to d/c and seek medical advice promptly if these occur. Inform that hypoglycemia can occur, particularly when therapy is used in combination w/ insulin or sulfonylurea; explain risks/symptoms/appropriate management of hypoglycemia. Inform patients that severe and disabling joint pain may occur. The time to onset of symptoms can range from one day to years. Instruct patients to seek medical advice if severe joint pain occurs. Instruct to take only ud; if a dose is missed, advise not to double next dose. Instruct to inform physician if unusual symptom develops or if a symptom persists/worsens.

STORAGE: 25°C (77°C); excursions permitted to 15-30°C (59-86°F).

NEULASTA – pegfilgrastim RX

Class: Granulocyte colony-stimulating factor (G-CSF)

ADULT DOSAGE

Chemotherapy-Associated Neutropenia

To decrease the incidence of infection in patients w/ nonmyeloid malignancies receiving myelosuppressive anticancer drugs associated w/ febrile neutropenia

6mg SQ once per chemotherapy cycle; do not administer between 14 days before and 24 hrs after administration of cytotoxic chemotherapy

Hematopoietic Subsyndrome of Acute Radiation Syndrome

To increase survival in patients acutely exposed to myelosuppressive doses of radiation

Two doses of 6mg SQ, administered 1 week apart

Administer first dose as soon as possible after suspected or confirmed exposure to radiation levels >2 gray (Gy)

Obtain a baseline CBC; do not delay administration if a CBC is not readily available. Estimate a patient's absorbed radiation dose (eg, level of radiation exposure) based on information from public health authorities, biodosimetry if available, or clinical findings (eg, time to onset of vomiting, lymphocyte depletion kinetics)

PEDIATRIC DOSAGE

Chemotherapy-Associated Neutropenia

To decrease the incidence of infection in patients w/ nonmyeloid malignancies receiving myelosuppressive anticancer drugs associated w/ febrile neutropenia

<10kg: 0.1mg/kg (0.01mL/kg)
10-20kg: 1.5mg (0.15mL)
21-30kg: 2.5mg (0.25mL)
31-44kg: 4mg (0.40mL)
≥45kg: Refer to adult dosing

Administer once per chemotherapy cycle; do not administer between 14 days before and 24 hrs after administration of cytotoxic chemotherapy

Hematopoietic Subsyndrome of Acute Radiation Syndrome

To increase survival in patients acutely exposed to myelosuppressive doses of radiation

<10kg: 0.1mg/kg (0.01mL/kg)
10-20kg: 1.5mg (0.15mL)
21-30kg: 2.5mg (0.25mL)
31-44kg: 4mg (0.40mL)
≥45kg: Refer to adult dosing

Administer first dose as soon as possible after suspected or confirmed exposure to radiation levels >2 Gy

Administer second dose 1 week after the first dose

Obtain a baseline CBC; do not delay administration if a CBC is not readily available. Estimate a patient's absorbed radiation dose (eg, level of radiation exposure) based on information from public health authorities, biodosimetry if available, or clinical findings (eg, time to onset of vomiting, lymphocyte depletion kinetics)

ADMINISTRATION

SQ route

Administer via a single prefilled syringe for manual use or w/ the On-body Injector.
Use of the On-body Injector has not been studied in pediatric patients.
Prefilled syringe is not designed to allow for direct administration of doses <0.6mL (6mg).

Instructions for On-body Injector

For Physicians:

- Fill the On-body Injector w/ pegfilgrastim using prefilled syringe and apply to patient's skin (abdomen or back of arm).
- Use back of the arm only if a caregiver is available to monitor the status of the On-body Injector.
- Approx 27 hrs after the application, pegfilgrastim will be delivered over approx 45 min.

- May initiate administration on the same day as the administration of cytotoxic chemotherapy, as long as On-body Injector delivers pegfilgrastim no less than 24 hrs after administration of cytotoxic chemotherapy.
- Do not use On-body Injector to deliver any other drug product except pegfilgrastim prefilled syringe co-packaged w/ On-body Injector.
- Apply to intact, non-irritated skin on the arm or abdomen.
- Missed dose may occur due to an On-body Injector failure/leakage; if a dose is missed, administer new dose by single prefilled syringe for manual use, as soon as possible after detection.
- Refer to Healthcare Provider Instructions for Use for the On-body Injector for Neulasta for full administration information.

HOW SUPPLIED

Inj: 6mg/0.6mL [prefilled syringe for manual use, Onpro Kit]

CONTRAINDICATIONS

History of serious allergic reactions to pegfilgrastim or filgrastim.

WARNINGS/PRECAUTIONS

Not indicated for the mobilization of peripheral blood progenitor cells for hematopoietic stem cell transplantation. Splenic rupture, including fatal cases, may occur; evaluate for an enlarged spleen or splenic rupture if left upper abdominal or shoulder pain occurs. Acute respiratory distress syndrome (ARDS) may occur; evaluate for ARDS if fever and lung infiltrates or respiratory distress develops, and d/c if ARDS develops. Serious allergic reactions (eg, anaphylaxis) may occur; permanently d/c if a serious allergic reaction occurs. Use of On-body Injector may result in a significant reaction in patients who have reactions to acrylic adhesives. Severe and sometimes fatal sickle cell crises may occur in patients w/ sickle cell disorders. Glomerulonephritis reported; evaluate for cause if glomerulonephritis is suspected and consider dose reduction or interruption of pegfilgrastim if causality is likely. WBC counts of ≥100 x 10^9/L reported; monitor WBC counts during therapy. May act as a growth factor for any tumor type. Capillary leak syndrome reported; closely monitor patients who develop symptoms of capillary leak syndrome and administer standard symptomatic treatment, which may include a need for intensive care. Needle cap on prefilled syringe contains latex; do not administer to persons w/ latex allergies. Increased hematopoietic activity of the bone marrow in response to therapy may result in transiently positive bone imaging changes; consider this when interpreting bone-imaging results.

ADVERSE REACTIONS

Bone pain, pain in extremity.

N

PATIENT CONSIDERATIONS

Assessment: Assess for history of hypersensitivity to pegfilgrastim or filgrastim, acrylic/latex allergy, sickle cell disorders, and pregnancy/nursing status. In patients w/ hematopoietic subsyndrome of acute radiation syndrome, obtain CBC.

Monitoring: Monitor for enlarged spleen/splenic rupture, ARDS, serious allergic reactions, sickle cell crises (in patients w/ sickle cell disorders), glomerulonephritis, capillary leak syndrome, and other adverse reactions. Monitor CBC.

Counseling: Advise on the proper administration of pegfilgrastim and how to use the On-body Injector. Advise of the risks of therapy (eg, splenic rupture, ARDS, serious allergic reactions, sickle cell crisis, glomerulonephritis, capillary leak syndrome). Advise to avoid activities (eg, traveling, driving, operating heavy machinery) during 26-29 hrs following application of On-body Injector (this includes the 45-min delivery period plus 1 hr post-delivery). Advise female patients to notify physician if pregnant or nursing.

STORAGE: 2-8°C (36-46°F). **Prefilled Syringe for Manual Use:** Protect from light. Do not shake. Discard syringes stored at room temperature for >48 hrs. Avoid freezing; if frozen, thaw in the refrigerator before administration. Discard syringe if frozen more than once. **Onpro Kit:** Do not hold Kit at room temperature >12 hrs prior to use; discard if stored at room temperature for >12 hrs.

NEUPOGEN — filgrastim

RX

Class: Granulocyte colony-stimulating factor (G-CSF)

ADULT DOSAGE

Myelosuppressive Chemotherapy

Decrease the incidence of infection, as manifested by febrile neutropenia, in patients w/ nonmyeloid malignancies receiving myelosuppressive anti-cancer drugs associated w/ a significant incidence of severe neutropenia w/ fever

PEDIATRIC DOSAGE

General Dosing

Studied in pediatric patients w/ chemotherapy-associated neutropenia and in pediatric patients w/ severe chronic neutropenia; refer to PI

Initial: 5mcg/kg/day; administer as a single SQ inj, by short IV infusion (15-30 min), or by continuous IV infusion
Titrate: May increase in increments of 5mcg/kg for each chemotherapy cycle, according to duration and severity of ANC nadir

D/C if ANC increases beyond 10,000/mm^3

Administer at least 24 hrs after cytotoxic chemotherapy; do not administer w/in the 24-hr period prior to chemotherapy

Administer daily for up to 2 weeks or until the ANC has reached 10,000/mm^3 following the expected chemotherapy-induced neutrophil nadir

Induction or Consolidation Chemotherapy

To reduce the time to neutrophil recovery and the duration of fever, following induction or consolidation chemotherapy treatment of patients w/ acute myeloid leukemia (AML)

Initial: 5mcg/kg/day; administer as a single SQ inj, by short IV infusion (15-30 min), or by continuous IV infusion
Titrate: May increase in increments of 5mcg/kg for each chemotherapy cycle, according to duration and severity of ANC nadir

D/C if ANC increases beyond 10,000/mm^3

Administer at least 24 hrs after cytotoxic chemotherapy; do not administer w/in the 24-hr period prior to chemotherapy

Administer daily for up to 2 weeks or until the ANC has reached 10,000/mm^3 following the expected chemotherapy-induced neutrophil nadir

Bone Marrow Transplantation

To reduce the duration of neutropenia and neutropenia-related clinical sequelae (eg, febrile neutropenia) in patients w/ nonmyeloid malignancies undergoing myeloablative chemotherapy followed by bone marrow transplantation

10mcg/kg/day administered as an IV infusion no longer than 24 hrs; administer the first dose at least 24 hrs after cytotoxic chemotherapy and at least 24 hrs after bone marrow infusion

Dose Adjustments During Neutrophil Recovery:
When ANC >1000/mm^3 for 3 Consecutive Days: Reduce to 5mcg/kg/day*
If ANC Remains >1000/mm^3 for 3 More Consecutive Days: D/C therapy
If ANC Decreases to <1000/mm^3: Resume at 5mcg/kg/day

*If ANC decreases to <1000/mm^3 at any time during the 5mcg/kg/day administration, increase dose to 10mcg/kg/day, and follow the above steps

Hematopoietic Progenitor Cell Mobilization

Mobilization of autologous hematopoietic progenitor cells into the peripheral blood for collection by leukapheresis

10mcg/kg/day SQ inj; administer for ≥4 days before the 1st leukapheresis procedure and continue until the last leukapheresis

Administration of therapy for 6-7 days w/ leukapheresis on Days 5, 6, and 7 was found to be safe and effective

Monitor neutrophil counts after 4 days of therapy, and d/c if WBC count rises to >100,000/mm^3

Severe Chronic Neutropenia

For chronic administration to reduce the incidence and duration of sequelae of neutropenia in symptomatic patients w/ congenital neutropenia, cyclic neutropenia, or idiopathic neutropenia

Initial:

Congenital Neutropenia: 6mcg/kg SQ bid

Idiopathic/Cyclic Neutropenia: 5mcg/kg SQ qd

Individualize dose based on the patient's clinical course as well as ANC; in rare instances, patients w/ congenital neutropenia have required doses ≥100mcg/kg/day

During the initial 4 weeks of therapy and during the 2 weeks following any dosage adjustment, monitor CBCs w/ differential and platelet counts. Once a patient is clinically stable, monitor CBCs w/ differential and platelet counts monthly during the first year of treatment. Thereafter, if the patient is clinically stable, less frequent routine monitoring is recommended

Hematopoietic Syndrome of Acute Radiation Syndrome

To increase survival in patients acutely exposed to myelosuppressive doses of radiation

10mcg/kg SQ qd; administer as soon as possible after suspected/confirmed exposure to radiation doses >2 gray

Obtain a baseline CBC and then serial CBCs approx every third day until the ANC remains >1000/mm^3 for 3 consecutive CBCs; do not delay administration if a CBC is not readily available

Continue administration of therapy until the ANC remains >1000/mm^3 for 3 consecutive CBCs or exceeds 10,000/mm^3 after a radiation-induced nadir

DOSING CONSIDERATIONS

Concomitant Medications

Cytotoxic Chemotherapy: Do not use Neupogen in the period 24 hrs before through 24 hrs after the administration of cytotoxic chemotherapy

ADMINISTRATION

SQ/IV route

Prior to use, remove the vial or prefilled syringe from the refrigerator and allow Neupogen to reach room temperature for a minimum of 30 min and a max of 24 hrs; discard any vial or prefilled syringe left at room temperature for >24 hrs.

Discard unused portion in vials or prefilled syringes; do not re-enter the vial or save unused drug for later administration.

SQ Inj

Inject in the outer area of upper arms, abdomen, thighs, or upper outer areas of buttocks.

Instructions for Prefilled Syringe

Persons w/ latex allergies should not administer the prefilled syringe, because the needle cap contains dry natural rubber (derived from latex).

Dilution Instructions (Vial Only)

If required for IV administration, vials may be diluted in D5 inj from a concentration of 300mcg/mL to 5mcg/mL; do not dilute to a final concentration <5mcg/mL.

Sol diluted to concentrations from 5mcg/mL to 15mcg/mL should be protected from adsorption to plastic materials by the addition of albumin (human) to a final concentration of 2mg/mL.

When diluted in D5 inj or D5 plus albumin (human), Neupogen is compatible w/ glass bottles, polyvinylchloride and polyolefin IV bags, and polypropylene syringes.

Do not dilute w/ saline; product may precipitate.

Store diluted sol at room temperature for up to 24 hrs; this 24-hr time period includes the time during room temperature storage of the infusion sol and the duration of the infusion.

HOW SUPPLIED

Inj: 300mcg/mL, 480mcg/1.6mL [vial]; 300mcg/0.5mL, 480mcg/0.8mL [prefilled syringe]

CONTRAINDICATIONS

History of serious allergic reactions to human granulocyte colony-stimulating factors (eg, filgrastim, pegfilgrastim).

WARNINGS/PRECAUTIONS

Splenic rupture, including fatal cases, reported. Acute respiratory distress syndrome (ARDS) reported; d/c in patients w/ ARDS. Serious allergic reactions, including anaphylaxis, reported; permanently d/c in patients w/ serious allergic reactions. Sickle cell crisis, in some cases fatal, reported in patients w/ sickle cell trait/disease. Glomerulonephritis has occurred, generally resolving after dose reduction or discontinuation. If glomerulonephritis is suspected, evaluate for cause; if causality is likely, consider dose-reduction or interruption of therapy. Not approved for peripheral blood progenitor cell mobilization in healthy donors. Capillary leak syndrome (CLS) reported. Myelodysplastic syndrome (MDS) and AML reported to occur in the natural history of congenital neutropenia w/o cytokine therapy. Cytogenetic abnormalities, transformation to MDS, and AML observed in patients treated for severe chronic neutropenia (SCN); carefully consider the risks and benefits of continuing therapy if a patient w/ SCN develops abnormal cytogenetics or myelodysplasia. Thrombocytopenia and leukocytosis reported. Cutaneous vasculitis reported. Hold therapy in patients w/ cutaneous vasculitis; treatment may be started at a reduced dose when the symptoms resolve and ANC has decreased. May act as a growth factor for any tumor type. Increased hematopoietic activity of the bone marrow in response to growth factor therapy has been associated w/ transient positive bone-imaging changes; consider this when interpreting bone-imaging results.

ADVERSE REACTIONS

Nausea, pyrexia, thrombocytopenia, bone/back/chest pain, dizziness, pain, fatigue, dyspnea, headache, cough, rash, pain in extremity, arthralgia, increased blood lactate dehydrogenase, increased blood alkaline phosphatase.

DRUG INTERACTIONS

Avoid simultaneous use w/ chemotherapy and radiation therapy.

PATIENT CONSIDERATIONS

Assessment: Assess for hypersensitivity to the drug, latex allergy, sickle cell disorder, pregnancy/nursing status, and possible drug interactions. Obtain baseline CBC and platelet count. Confirm diagnosis of SCN prior to therapy.

Monitoring: Monitor for splenic rupture, ARDS, serious allergic reactions, sickle cell crisis, glomerulonephritis, CLS, cutaneous vasculitis, thrombocytopenia, leukocytosis, and other adverse reactions. Monitor for cytogenetic abnormalities, transformation to MDS, and AML in patients w/ SCN. In patients receiving myelosuppressive chemotherapy or induction and/or consolidation chemotherapy for AML, monitor CBC and platelet count twice weekly. Monitor CBCs and platelet counts frequently following marrow transplantation. In patients w/ SCN, monitor CBCs w/ differential and platelet counts during the initial 4 weeks of therapy and during the 2 weeks following any dose adjustment. Once patient is clinically stable, monitor CBCs w/ differential and platelet counts monthly during the 1st yr of treatment; thereafter, if clinically stable, less frequent routine monitoring is recommended. Monitor serial CBCs approx every 3rd day until the ANC remains >1000/mm^3 for 3 consecutive CBCs in patients acutely exposed to myelosuppressive doses of radiation.

Counseling: Inform that rupture or enlargement of the spleen may occur; advise to immediately report to physician if symptoms develop. Advise to seek immediate medical attention if signs/symptoms of hypersensitivity reaction occur. Advise to immediately report to physician if dyspnea develops. Discuss potential risks and benefits for patients w/ sickle cell disease prior to administration. Advise to immediately report signs/symptoms of glomerulonephritis to physician. Advise to immediately report to physician signs/symptoms of vasculitis. Advise females of reproductive potential that therapy should be used during pregnancy only if the potential benefit justifies the potential risk to the fetus. Advise patients acutely exposed to myelosuppressive doses of radiation that efficacy studies of therapy for this indication could not be conducted in humans for ethical and feasibility reasons; approval of this use was based on efficacy studies conducted in animals.

STORAGE: 2-8°C (36-46°F). Protect from light. Avoid freezing; if frozen, thaw in the refrigerator before administration. Discard if frozen more than once. Avoid shaking.

NEURONTIN – gabapentin

RX

Class: GABA analogue

ADULT DOSAGE

Postherpetic Neuralgia

Initial: 300mg single dose on Day 1, then 300mg bid (600mg/day) on Day 2, and 300mg tid (900mg/day) on Day 3
Titrate: May subsequently increase prn up to 600mg tid (1800mg/day)

Partial Seizures

Adjuvant Therapy for Partial Onset Seizures w/ Epilepsy, w/ and w/o Secondary Generalization:

Initial: 300mg tid
Maint: 300-600mg tid
Doses up to 2400mg/day (long-term) and 3600mg/day (short-term) have been well tolerated
Administer tid using 300mg or 400mg caps, or 600mg or 800mg tabs
Dosing intervals should not exceed 12 hrs

PEDIATRIC DOSAGE

Partial Seizures

Adjuvant Therapy for Partial Onset Seizures w/ Epilepsy, w/ and w/o Secondary Generalization:

3-11 Years:
Initial: 10-15mg/kg/day in 3 divided doses
Titrate: Increase to recommended maint dose over a period of approx 3 days

3-4 Years:
Maint: 40mg/kg/day in 3 divided doses

5-11 Years:
Maint: 25-35mg/kg/day in 3 divided doses
Doses up to 50mg/kg/day have been well tolerated
Dosing intervals should not exceed 12 hrs

≥12 Years:
Initial: 300mg tid
Maint: 300-600mg tid
Doses up to 2400mg/day (long-term) and 3600mg/day (short-term) have been well tolerated
Administer tid using 300mg or 400mg caps, or 600mg or 800mg tabs
Dosing intervals should not exceed 12 hrs

DOSING CONSIDERATIONS

Renal Impairment

≥12 Years:
CrCl ≥60mL/min: 900-3600mg/day in 3 divided doses
CrCl >30-59mL/min: 400-1400mg/day in 2 divided doses
CrCl >15-29mL/min: 200-700mg single daily dose
CrCl 15mL/min: 100-300mg single daily dose
CrCl <15mL/min: Reduce daily dose in proportion to CrCl
Hemodialysis: Dose adjustment is necessary; see PI

Discontinuation

Dose Reduction/Substitution/Discontinuation: Should be done gradually over a minimum of 1 week

ADMINISTRATION

Oral route
Take w/ or w/o food.
Swallow caps whole w/ water.
If the scored tab is broken to administer a half-tab, take the unused half-tab as the next dose; discard half-tabs that are not used w/in 28 days of breaking the scored tab.

HOW SUPPLIED

Cap: 100mg, 300mg, 400mg; **Sol:** 250mg/5mL [470mL]; **Tab:** 600mg*, 800mg* *scored

CONTRAINDICATIONS

Hypersensitivity to the drug or its ingredients.

WARNINGS/PRECAUTIONS

Drug reaction w/ eosinophilia and systemic symptoms (DRESS)/multiorgan hypersensitivity reported; evaluate immediately if signs/symptoms (eg, fever, lymphadenopathy) are present and d/c if an alternative etiology cannot be established. May cause anaphylaxis and angioedema; d/c and seek immediate medical care if experience signs/symptoms of anaphylaxis or angioedema. May cause significant driving impairment. Somnolence/sedation and dizziness reported. May impair mental/physical abilities. Do not abruptly d/c; may increase seizure frequency. Increases the risk of suicidal thoughts/behavior. Use in pediatric patients w/ epilepsy 3-12 yrs of age is associated w/ the occurrence of CNS-related adverse events. May have tumorigenic potential. Sudden and unexplained deaths reported in patients w/ epilepsy. Lab test interactions may occur. Caution in elderly.

ADVERSE REACTIONS

Dizziness, somnolence, fatigue, peripheral edema, hostility, diarrhea, asthenia, infection, dry mouth, nystagmus, constipation, N/V, ataxia, fever, amblyopia.

DRUG INTERACTIONS

Decreases hydrocodone exposure; consider the potential for alteration in hydrocodone exposure and effect when gabapentin is started or discontinued in a patient taking hydrocodone. Morphine may increase gabapentin concentrations; dose adjustment may be required. Observe for signs of CNS depression (eg, somnolence, sedation, respiratory depression) when used w/ other drugs w/ sedative properties (eg, morphine) because of potential synergy. Decreased bioavailability w/ Maalox; take gabapentin at least 2 hrs following Maalox administration.

PATIENT CONSIDERATIONS

Assessment: Assess for hypersensitivity to the drug, renal impairment, depression, pregnancy/nursing status, and possible drug interactions.

Monitoring: Monitor for DRESS, anaphylaxis, angioedema, somnolence/sedation, dizziness, emergence/worsening of depression, suicidal thoughts/behavior, unusual changes in mood/behavior, development/worsening of tumors, increased seizure frequency (upon abrupt discontinuation), and other adverse reactions.

Counseling: Instruct to immediately report to physician any rash or other signs/symptoms of hypersensitivity/anaphylaxis, angioedema, emergence/worsening of depression symptoms, any unusual changes in mood/behavior, emergence of suicidal thoughts/behavior, or thoughts of self-harm. Inform that therapy may cause a significant driving impairment, dizziness, somnolence, and other signs/symptoms of CNS depression; advise not to drive a car or operate other complex machinery until patient has gained sufficient experience on therapy. Instruct to notify physician if pregnant/breastfeeding or intending to become pregnant or to breastfeed during therapy; encourage enrollment in the North American Antiepileptic Drug Pregnancy Registry if patient becomes pregnant.

STORAGE: **Cap/Tab:** 25°C (77°F); excursions permitted to 15-30°C (59-86°F). **Sol:** 2-8°C (36-46°F).

NEXAVAR – sorafenib

RX

Class: Kinase inhibitor

ADULT DOSAGE

Hepatocellular Carcinoma

Unresectable:

400mg (two 200mg tabs) bid

Continue until patient is no longer clinically benefiting from therapy or until unacceptable toxicity occurs

Advanced Renal Cell Carcinoma

400mg (two 200mg tabs) bid

Continue until patient is no longer clinically benefiting from therapy or until unacceptable toxicity occurs

Differentiated Thyroid Carcinoma

Locally recurrent or metastatic, progressive, differentiated thyroid carcinoma that is refractory to radioactive iodine treatment

400mg (two 200mg tabs) bid

Continue until patient is no longer clinically benefiting from therapy or until unacceptable toxicity occurs

PEDIATRIC DOSAGE

Pediatric use may not have been established

DOSING CONSIDERATIONS

Adverse Reactions

Dermatologic Toxicities:

Hepatocellular/Renal Cell Carcinoma:

Grade 1 (Numbness/Dysesthesia/Paresthesia/Tingling/Painless Swelling/Erythema/Discomfort of Hands or Feet That Does Not Disrupt Normal Activities):

Any Occurrence: Continue treatment and consider topical therapy for symptomatic relief

Grade 2 (Painful Erythema and Swelling of Hands or Feet and/or Discomfort Affecting Normal Activities):

1st Occurrence: Continue treatment and consider topical therapy for symptomatic relief

No Improvement w/in 7 Days or 2nd/3rd Occurrence: Interrupt treatment until toxicity resolves to Grade 0-1; when resuming treatment, decrease dose by 1 dose level (400mg/day or 400mg qod)

4th Occurrence: D/C treatment

Grade 3 (Moist Desquamation/Ulceration/Blistering/Severe Pain of Hands or Feet, or Severe Discomfort That Causes Inability to Work or Perform Activities of Daily Living):
1st/2nd Occurrence: Interrupt treatment until toxicity resolves to Grade 0-1; when resuming treatment, decrease dose by 1 dose level (400mg/day or 400mg qod)
3rd Occurrence: D/C treatment

Differentiated Thyroid Carcinoma:
Grade 1:
Any Occurrence: Continue treatment

Grade 2:
1st Occurrence: Decrease dose to 600mg/day
No Improvement w/in 7 Days or 2nd/3rd Occurrence: Interrupt treatment until toxicity resolves or improves to Grade 1; if treatment is resumed, decrease dose as follows:
1st Dose Reduction: 600mg/day (400mg and 200mg 12 hrs apart)
2nd Dose Reduction: 400mg/day (200mg bid)
3rd Dose Reduction: 200mg qd
4th Occurrence: D/C treatment permanently

Grade 3:
1st Occurrence: Interrupt treatment until toxicity resolves or improves to Grade 1; if treatment is resumed, decrease dose to 600mg/day (400mg and 200mg 12 hrs apart)
2nd Occurrence: Interrupt treatment until toxicity resolves or improves to Grade 1; if treatment is resumed, decrease dose to 400mg/day (200mg bid)
3rd Occurrence: D/C treatment

Discontinuation
Temporary interruption or permanent discontinuation may be required for the following:
1. Cardiac ischemia or infarction
2. Hemorrhage requiring medical intervention
3. Severe or persistent HTN despite adequate anti-hypertensive therapy
4. GI perforation
5. QTc prolongation
6. Severe drug-induced liver injury

Other Important Considerations
Patients Undergoing Major Surgical Procedures: Temporarily interrupt therapy

Dose Reductions:
Hepatocellular Carcinoma/Renal Cell Carcinoma:
When dose reduction is necessary, reduce to 400mg qd; if additional dose reduction is required, reduce to a single 400mg dose qod

Differentiated Thyroid Carcinoma:
1st Dose Reduction: 600mg/day (400mg and 200mg 12 hrs apart)
2nd Dose Reduction: 400mg/day (200mg bid)
3rd Dose Reduction: 200mg qd

ADMINISTRATION
Oral route

Take w/o food (at least 1 hr ac or 2 hrs pc)

HOW SUPPLIED
Tab: 200mg

CONTRAINDICATIONS
Known severe hypersensitivity to sorafenib or any other component of this medication, concomitant use w/ carboplatin and paclitaxel in patients w/ squamous cell lung cancer.

WARNINGS/PRECAUTIONS
HTN, cardiac ischemia, and/or infarction reported; consider temporary or permanent discontinuation. Increased risk of bleeding may occur; consider permanent discontinuation if bleeding necessitates medical intervention. Hand-foot skin reaction and rash reported; may require topical treatment, temporary interruption, and/or dose modification, or permanent discontinuation in severe or persistent cases. Severe dermatologic toxicities, including Stevens-Johnson syndrome (SJS) and toxic epidermal necrolysis (TEN) reported; d/c if SJS or TEN are suspected. D/C if GI perforation occurs. Temporarily interrupt therapy when undergoing major surgical procedures. May prolong the QT/QTc interval; avoid in patients w/ congenital long QT syndrome. Monitor electrolytes and ECG in patients w/ congestive heart failure (CHF), bradyarrhythmias, and in patients taking drugs known to prolong the QT interval (eg, Class Ia and III antiarrhythmics). Correct electrolyte abnormalities (Mg^{2+}, K^+, Ca^{2+}). Interrupt treatment if QTc interval is >500 msec or for an increase from baseline ≥60 msec. Drug-induced hepatitis, and increased bilirubin and INR may occur; d/c in case of significantly increased transaminases w/o alternative explanation (eg, viral hepatitis, progressing underlying malignancy). May impair exogenous thyroid suppression; monitor TSH levels monthly and adjust thyroid replacement medication as needed in patients w/ DTC. May cause fetal harm.

ADVERSE REACTIONS

HTN, fatigue, weight loss, rash, hand-foot skin reaction, alopecia, pruritus, diarrhea, N/V, abdominal pain, anorexia, constipation, hemorrhage, infection, decreased appetite.

DRUG INTERACTIONS

See Contraindications. Avoid w/ gemcitabine/cisplatin in squamous cell lung cancer patients. Avoid w/ strong CYP3A4 inducers (eg, carbamazepine, dexamethasone, St. John's wort); strong CYP3A4 inducers may decrease systemic exposure. Infrequent bleeding or increased INR w/ warfarin; monitor for changes in PT, INR, or bleeding episodes. Decreased exposure w/ oral neomycin.

PATIENT CONSIDERATIONS

Assessment: Assess for bleeding disorders, upcoming major surgical procedures, CHF, bradyarrhythmias, electrolyte abnormalities, congenital long QT syndrome, drug hypersensitivity, pregnancy/nursing status, and possible drug interactions.

Monitoring: Monitor for cardiac ischemia/infarction, hemorrhage, HTN, dermatologic toxicities, GI perforation, QT/QTc prolongation, and other adverse reactions. Monitor BP weekly during the first 6 weeks and periodically thereafter. Monitor electrolytes (eg, Mg^{2+}, Ca^{2+}, K^{+}) and ECG in patients w/ CHF, bradyarrhythmias, and in patients taking drugs known to prolong the QT interval. Monitor LFTs regularly, and TSH levels monthly. Monitor patients taking concomitant warfarin for changes in PT, INR, or clinical bleeding episodes.

Counseling: Inform about risks and benefits of therapy. Instruct to report to physician any episodes of bleeding or cardiac ischemia (eg, chest pain). Inform that HTN may develop, especially during the first 6 weeks; advise that BP should be monitored regularly during therapy. Inform of possible occurrence of hand-foot skin reaction and rash during therapy and appropriate countermeasures. Advise that GI perforation and drug-induced hepatitis may occur and to report signs/symptoms of hepatitis. Inform that temporary interruption of therapy is recommended in patients undergoing major surgical procedures. Counsel patients w/ a history of prolonged QT interval that drug can worsen the condition. Inform that the drug may cause birth defects or fetal loss during pregnancy; instruct both males and females to use effective birth control during treatment and for at least 2 weeks after stopping therapy. Instruct to notify physician if patient becomes pregnant while on therapy. Advise against breastfeeding while on therapy.

STORAGE: 25°C (77°F); excursions permitted to 15-30°C (59-86°F). Store in a dry place.

NEXIUM ORAL — esomeprazole magnesium

RX

Class: Proton pump inhibitor (PPI)

N

ADULT DOSAGE

Gastroesophageal Reflux Disease

Healing of Erosive Esophagitis:
20mg or 40mg qd for 4-8 weeks; may consider an additional 4-8 weeks of treatment if not healed

Maint of Healing of Erosive Esophagitis:
20mg qd for up to 6 months

Symptomatic GERD:
20mg qd for 4 weeks; may consider an additional 4 weeks of treatment if symptoms do not resolve completely

NSAID-Associated Gastric Ulcer

Risk Reduction of NSAID-Associated Gastric Ulcer:
20mg or 40mg qd for up to 6 months

***Helicobacter pylori* Eradication**

Triple Therapy:
40mg qd + amoxicillin 1000mg bid + clarithromycin 500mg bid, all for 10 days

Pathological Hypersecretory Conditions

Eg, Zollinger-Ellison Syndrome:
40mg bid; adjust dose to individual patient needs

Doses up to 240mg/day have been administered

PEDIATRIC DOSAGE

Gastroesophageal Reflux Disease

Symptomatic GERD

1-11 Years:
10mg qd for up to 8 weeks
Max: 1mg/kg/day

12-17 Years:
20mg qd for 4 weeks

Healing of Erosive Esophagitis:

1-11 Years:
<20kg: 10mg qd for 8 weeks
≥20kg: 10mg or 20mg qd for 8 weeks
Max: 1mg/kg/day

12-17 Years:
20mg or 40mg qd for 4-8 weeks

Erosive Esophagitis Due to Acid-Mediated GERD:

1 Month to <1 Year:
3-5kg: 2.5mg qd for up to 6 weeks
>5-7.5kg: 5mg qd for up to 6 weeks
>7.5-12kg: 10mg qd for up to 6 weeks
Max: 1.33mg/kg/day

DOSING CONSIDERATIONS

Hepatic Impairment

Severe (Child-Pugh Class C):

Max Dose: 20mg/day

ADMINISTRATION

Oral route

Take at least 1 hr ac.

Cap

Swallow whole, or alternatively, open cap and add granules on 1 tbsp of applesauce, then swallow immediately; do not chew or crush the granules.

NG Tube:

1. Open and empty the intact granules into a 60mL catheter tipped syringe and mix w/ 50mL of water.
2. Replace the plunger and shake the syringe vigorously for 15 sec.
3. Attach the syringe to a NG tube and deliver the contents of the syringe into the stomach.
4. Flush the NG tube w/ additional water after use.

Sus

1. Empty the contents of a 2.5mg or 5mg pkt into 5mL of water. For the 10mg, 20mg, and 40mg pkts, empty into 15mL of water.
2. Stir and leave 2-3 min to thicken.
3. Stir and drink w/in 30 min. If any medicine remains after drinking, add more water, stir, and drink immediately.
4. In cases where 2 pkts need to be used, may mix in a similar way by adding twice the required amount of water or follow mixing instructions provided.

NG/Gastric Tube:

1. Add 5mL of water to a catheter tipped syringe, then add contents of a 2.5mg or 5mg pkt. For 10mg, 20mg, and 40mg pkts, volume of water in the syringe should be 15mL.
2. Immediately shake syringe and leave 2-3 min to thicken.
3. Shake syringe and inject through NG or gastric tube, French size ≥6, into the stomach w/in 30 min.
4. Refill the syringe w/ an equal amount of water (5mL or 15mL).
5. Shake and flush any remaining contents from NG or gastric tube into stomach.

HOW SUPPLIED

Cap, Delayed-Release: 20mg, 40mg; **Oral Sus, Delayed-Release:** 2.5mg, 5mg, 10mg, 20mg, 40mg (granules/pkt)

CONTRAINDICATIONS

Known hypersensitivity to substituted benzimidazoles or to any component of the medication. When used w/ clarithromycin and amoxicillin, refer to the individual monographs.

WARNINGS/PRECAUTIONS

Symptomatic response does not preclude the presence of gastric malignancy. Atrophic gastritis reported w/ long-term omeprazole use. Acute interstitial nephritis reported; d/c if this develops. Cyanocobalamin (vitamin B12) deficiency may occur due to malabsorption, w/ daily long-term treatment (eg, >3 yrs) w/ any acid-suppressing medications. May increase risk of *Clostridium difficile* associated diarrhea (CDAD), especially in hospitalized patients. May increase risk for osteoporosis-related fractures of the hip, wrist, or spine, especially w/ high-dose and long-term therapy. Use lowest dose and shortest duration possible. Hypomagnesemia reported and may require Mg^{2+} replacement and discontinuation of therapy. Drug-induced decrease in gastric acidity results in enterochromaffin-like cell hyperplasia and increased chromogranin A (CgA) levels, which may interfere w/ investigations for neuroendocrine tumors; d/c treatment for at least 14 days before assessing CgA levels and consider repeating test if initial CgA levels are high.

ADVERSE REACTIONS

Adults: Headache, diarrhea, abdominal pain.

Pediatrics: (1-11 years) Diarrhea, headache, somnolence. (12-17 years) Headache, abdominal pain, diarrhea, nausea.

DRUG INTERACTIONS

CYP2C19 or CYP3A4 inducers may decrease levels; avoid w/ St. John's wort or rifampin. Reduces pharmacological activity of clopidogrel; avoid concomitant use. May reduce atazanavir and nelfinavir levels; concomitant use not recommended. May change absorption or levels of antiretrovirals. May increase levels of saquinavir, cilostazol, and tacrolimus; consider saquinavir and cilostazol dose reduction. May reduce the absorption of drugs where gastric pH is an important determinant of bioavailability; ketoconazole, atazanavir, iron salts, erlotinib, and mycophenolate mofetil (MMF) absorption may decrease, while digoxin absorption may increase. Caution in transplant patients receiving MMF. Monitor for increases in INR and PT w/ warfarin. Decreases clearance of diazepam. Increased exposure w/ combined inhibitors of CYP2C19 and CYP3A4 (eg, voriconazole); consider dose adjustment w/ Zollinger-Ellison syndrome. Increased levels of esomeprazole and 14-hydroxyclarithromycin w/ amoxicillin and clarithromycin. Caution w/ digoxin or other drugs that may cause hypomagnesemia (eg, diuretics). May elevate and prolong levels of methotrexate (MTX) and/or its metabolite, possibly leading to toxicities; consider temporary withdrawal of therapy w/ high-dose MTX.

PATIENT CONSIDERATIONS

Assessment: Assess for hypersensitivity to substituted benzimidazoles or to any component of the formulation, hepatic dysfunction, risk for osteoporosis-related fractures, pregnancy/nursing status, and possible drug interactions. Obtain Mg^{2+} levels in patients expected to be on prolonged therapy.

Monitoring: Monitor for signs/symptoms of atrophic gastritis, acute interstitial nephritis, cyanocobalamin deficiency, bone fractures, hypomagnesemia, CDAD, and other adverse reactions.

Counseling: Advise to notify physician if taking or beginning to take other medications. Inform that antacids may be used while on therapy. Instruct not to chew or crush cap; if opening cap to mix granules w/ food, mix w/ applesauce only. Inform about proper technique for administration of opened cap or oral sus. Inform regarding the correct amount of water to use when mixing dose of oral sus. Advise to immediately report and seek care for diarrhea that does not improve and for any cardiovascular/neurological symptoms.

STORAGE: 25°C (77°F); excursions permitted to 15-30°C (59-86°F).

NEXPLANON — etonogestrel

RX

Class: Progestin contraceptive

ADULT DOSAGE

Contraception

No Preceding Hormonal Contraceptive Use in the Past Month:
Insert subdermally in the upper arm between Day 1 (1st day of menstrual bleeding) and Day 5 of menstrual cycle, even if patient is still bleeding

Following Abortion or Miscarriage:
1st Trimester: Insert w/in 5 days following 1st trimester abortion or miscarriage
2nd Trimester: Insert between 21-28 days following 2nd trimester abortion or miscarriage

Postpartum:
Not Breastfeeding: Insert between 21-28 days postpartum
Breastfeeding: Insert after the 4th postpartum week

Remove by the end of the 3rd year; if continued contraceptive protection is desired, may replace by a new implant at the time of removal using the same incision of the previous implant

Conversions

Switching from Combination Hormonal Contraceptives:
Insert implant on the day after the last active tab of the previous combined oral contraceptive or on the day of the removal of the vaginal ring or transdermal patch. At the latest, insert implant on the day following the usual tab-free, ring-free, patch-free or placebo tab interval of the previous combined hormonal contraceptive

Switching from Progestin-Only Contraceptives:
Injectable Contraceptives: Insert implant on the day the next inj is due
Minipill: Insert implant on any day of the month, w/in 24 hrs after taking the last tab
Contraceptive Implant or Intrauterine System (IUS): Insert implant on the same day as the previous contraceptive implant or IUS is removed

PEDIATRIC DOSAGE

Contraception

Not indicated for use premenarche; refer to adult dosing

ADMINISTRATION

Subdermal route

Insert implant at the inner side of the non-dominant upper arm about 8-10 cm (3-4 inches) above the medial epicondyle of the humerus, to reduce the risk of neural or vascular injury.
If inserted as recommended, backup contraception is not necessary.
If deviating from the recommended timing of insertion, advise to use a barrier method until 7 days after insertion; if intercourse has already occurred, pregnancy should be excluded.
In postpartum/breastfeeding women, advise to use a barrier method until 7 days after insertion; if intercourse has already occurred, pregnancy should be excluded.

Insertion Procedure

1. Anesthetize the insertion area (eg, w/ anesthetic spray or by injecting 2mL of 1% lidocaine).
2. Remove the transparent protection cap by sliding it horizontally in the direction of the arrow away from the needle.
3. Do not touch the purple slider until the needle is fully inserted subdermally.
4. Puncture the skin w/ the tip of the needle slightly angled <30°.
5. Lower the applicator to a horizontal position and insert needle to its full length.
6. Unlock the purple slider by pushing it slightly down and move the slider fully back until it stops.
7. Remove the applicator.
8. Verify the presence of the implant by palpation.

Refer to PI for further administration details and for removal procedure.

HOW SUPPLIED

Implant: 68mg

CONTRAINDICATIONS

Known or suspected pregnancy, current/history of thrombosis or thromboembolic disorders, benign or malignant liver tumors, active liver disease, undiagnosed abnormal genital bleeding, known/suspected/personal history of breast cancer, current/history of other progestin-sensitive cancer, or allergic reaction to any of the components.

WARNINGS/PRECAUTIONS

Confirm by palpation immediately after insertion; failure to insert implant properly may lead to an unintended pregnancy. Complications related to insertion or removal procedures (eg, pain, paresthesias, bleeding, hematoma, scarring, infection) may occur. If infection develops at the insertion site, start suitable treatment; if infection persists, remove implant. Incomplete insertions or infections may lead to expulsion. Neural or vascular injury may occur if inserted too deeply. Implant removal may be difficult/impossible if inserted incorrectly, inserted too deeply, not palpable, if it is encased in fibrous tissue, or if it has migrated. Implant migration w/in the arm from the insertion site reported; may be related to a deep insertion. Reports of implants located w/in vessels of the arm and the pulmonary artery (rare); may be related to deep insertions or intravascular insertion. If at any time the implant cannot be palpated, it should be localized and removed. Failure to remove may result in continued effects of etonogestrel. May cause changes in menstrual bleeding patterns, ectopic pregnancy, thrombotic/vascular events, ovarian cysts, breast cancer, cervical cancer or intraepithelial neoplasia, hepatic adenomas, weight gain, gallbladder disease, and fluid retention. Perform appropriate measures to rule out malignancy if undiagnosed, persistent, or recurrent abnormal vaginal bleeding occurs. Carefully monitor women w/ a family history of breast cancer and those who develop breast nodules. Do not use prior to 21 days postpartum. Evaluate for retinal vein thrombosis immediately if there is unexplained loss of vision, proptosis, diplopia, papilledema, or retinal vascular lesions. Consider removal of implant if significant depression develops or in case of long-term immobilization due to surgery or illness. Remove implant in the event of thrombosis or if jaundice develops. Women w/ a history of HTN-related diseases or renal disease should be discouraged from using hormonal contraception. Remove implant if a significant increase in BP unresponsive to antihypertensive therapy or sustained HTN occurs. May induce mild insulin resistance and small changes in glucose levels; monitor prediabetic and diabetic women. May elevate LDL levels. Restart contraception immediately after removal for continued contraceptive protection. Contact lens wearers who develop visual changes or changes in lens tolerance should be assessed by an ophthalmologist. Broken or bent implants while in the patient's arm reported; broken or bent implant may slightly increase the release rate of etonogestrel. Remove implant in its entirety when it is removed. May decrease sex hormone-binding globulin (SHBG) and thyroxine levels initially, followed by gradual recovery. May be less effective in overweight women.

ADVERSE REACTIONS

Headache, vaginitis, weight increase, acne, breast pain, abdominal pain, pharyngitis, leukorrhea, influenza-like symptoms, dizziness, dysmenorrhea, back pain, emotional lability, nausea, pain.

DRUG INTERACTIONS

Drugs or herbal products that induce enzymes, including CYP3A4 that metabolize progestins (eg, barbiturates, bosentan, carbamazepine), may decrease levels of progestins and decrease the effectiveness therapy; recommended to remove implant if on long-term treatment w/ hepatic enzyme-inducing drugs. HIV protease inhibitors or non-nucleoside reverse transcriptase inhibitors have been reported in some cases to cause significant changes (increase or decrease) in plasma levels of progestins. CYP3A4 inhibitors (eg, itraconazole, ketoconazole) may increase levels of etonogestrel. May affect metabolism of other drugs and consequently may either increase (eg, cyclosporine) or decrease (eg, lamotrigine) plasma concentrations of coadministered drugs.

PATIENT CONSIDERATIONS

Assessment: Assess for current or past history of thrombosis or thromboembolic disorders, benign or malignant liver tumors, active liver disease, undiagnosed abnormal genital bleeding, known/suspected/history of breast cancer or current or past history of other progestin-sensitive cancer, history of HTN-related diseases or renal disease, history of depressed mood, diabetes, hyperlipidemia, conditions that might be aggravated by fluid retention, pregnancy status, or for any other conditions where treatment is contraindicated or cautioned. Assess nursing status and for possible drug interactions.

Monitoring: Monitor for complications of insertion/removal of implant, changes in menstrual bleeding pattern, ectopic pregnancy, thrombotic/other vascular events, ovarian cysts, breast/cervical cancer, intraepithelial neoplasia, liver dysfunction, weight gain, gallbladder disease, fluid retention, and other adverse events. Monitor for visual changes or changes in lens tolerance in patients who wear contact lens and refer to an ophthalmologist if changes occur. Monitor glucose levels in diabetic and prediabetic patients, BP w/ history of HTN, lipid levels w/ a history of hyperlipidemia. Monitor for signs of depression w/ previous history. In cases of undiagnosed, persistent, or recurrent abnormal vaginal bleeding, perform appropriate measures to rule out malignancy. Perform BP check and other indicated healthcare annually.

Counseling: Inform of the risks and benefits of therapy. Counsel about insertion and removal procedure of the implant. Provide patient w/ a copy of the Patient Labeling and ensure information is understood before insertion and removal. Inform that consent form is included in the package and advise to complete consent form. Provide patient w/ the user card after insertion in order to have a record of the location of the implant in the upper arm and when it should be removed. Inform that the implant does not protect against HIV infection (AIDS) or other STDs. Advise that use may be associated w/ changes in normal menstrual bleeding patterns.

STORAGE: 25°C (77°F); excursions permitted to 15-30°C (59-86°F). Avoid storing at temperatures >30°C (86°F).

NIASPAN – niacin

RX

Class: Nicotinic acid

N

ADULT DOSAGE

Hyperlipidemia

For use in patients w/ primary hyperlipidemia and mixed dyslipidemia. To reduce the risk of recurrent nonfatal MI in patients w/ a history of MI and hyperlipidemia. To slow progression or promote regression of atherosclerotic disease in patients w/ a history of coronary artery disease and hyperlipidemia in combination w/ a bile acid binding resin. To reduce elevated total cholesterol and LDL levels in patients w/ primary hyperlipidemia in combination w/ a bile acid binding resin. Adjunctive therapy in patients w/ severe hypertriglyceridemia who present a risk of pancreatitis and who do not respond adequately to a determined dietary effort to control them

>16 Years:

Initial: 500mg qhs after a low-fat snack

Titrate: Increase by 500mg every 4 weeks; after Week 8, titrate to patient response and tolerance; increase to 1500mg qd if response to 1000mg qd is inadequate and may subsequently increase to 2000mg qd

Do not increase daily dose by >500mg in any 4-week period

Maint: 1000-2000mg qhs

Max: 2000mg/day

Women may respond at lower doses than men

If therapy is discontinued for an extended period, reinstitution should include a titration phase

PEDIATRIC DOSAGE

Pediatric use may not have been established

DOSING CONSIDERATIONS

Renal Impairment

Use caution

ADMINISTRATION

Oral route

Take at hs after a low-fat snack.

Swallow tab whole; do not break, crush, or chew.

Avoid administration on an empty stomach and slowly increase niacin dose to reduce flushing, pruritus, and GI distress.

May take aspirin (ASA) (up to 325mg) 30 min prior to treatment to reduce flushing.

Two of the 500mg tabs and one of the 1000mg tabs are interchangeable; do not interchange three 500mg tabs w/ two 750mg tabs.

Equivalent doses of niacin ER should not be substituted for sustained-release (modified-release, timed-release) niacin preparations or immediate-release (IR) (crystalline) niacin.

HOW SUPPLIED

Tab, Extended-Release: 500mg, 750mg, 1000mg

CONTRAINDICATIONS

Active liver disease or unexplained persistent elevations in hepatic transaminases, active peptic ulcer disease (PUD), arterial bleeding. Hypersensitivity to niacin or any component of this medication.

WARNINGS/PRECAUTIONS

Do not substitute for equivalent doses of sustained-release (modified-release, timed-release) niacin or IR (crystalline) niacin; severe hepatic toxicity, including fulminant hepatic necrosis, have occurred in patients who have substituted sustained-release (modified-release, timed-release) niacin products for IR (crystalline) niacin at equivalent doses. If switching from IR niacin, initiate w/ low doses (eg, 500mg at hs) and titrate to desired therapeutic response. Caution in patients w/ unstable angina or in the acute phase of MI, particularly if also receiving vasoactive drugs (eg, nitrates, calcium channel blockers, adrenergic blocking agents). Caution in patients w/ renal impairment, or who consume substantial quantities of alcohol, and/or have history of liver disease. Closely observe patients w/ history of jaundice, hepatobiliary disease, or peptic ulcer. Has not been shown to reduce cardiovascular morbidity or mortality among patients already treated w/ a statin. Associated w/ abnormal LFTs; monitor LFTs (eg, AST, ALT) before treatment, every 6-12 weeks for the 1st yr, and periodically thereafter (eg, 6-month intervals). If elevated serum transaminase levels develop, measurements should be repeated promptly and then performed more frequently. D/C if transaminase levels progress, particularly if they rise to 3X ULN and are persistent, or if associated w/ nausea, fever, and/or malaise. May increase FPG; closely monitor diabetic/potentially diabetic patients (particularly during 1st few months of therapy or dose adjustment), and adjust diet and/or hypoglycemic therapy if necessary. Associated w/ dose-related reductions in platelet count and phosphorus (P) levels; periodically monitor P levels in patients at risk for hypophosphatemia. Associated w/ increases in PT; carefully evaluate patients undergoing surgery. Elevated uric acid levels reported; caution in patients predisposed to gout. Lab test interactions may occur.

ADVERSE REACTIONS

Flushing (warmth, redness, itching, and/or tingling), diarrhea, N/V, increased cough, pruritus, rash.

DRUG INTERACTIONS

Avoid ingestion of alcohol, hot drinks, or spicy foods around the time of administration; may increase flushing and pruritus. Use caution when prescribing niacin (≥1g/day) w/ statins; may increase risk of myopathy and rhabdomyolysis; consider performing periodic serum CPK and K^+ determinations if used concomitantly w/ a statin. Separate dosing from bile acid-binding resins by at least 4-6 hrs. ASA may decrease the metabolic clearance of nicotinic acid. May potentiate the effects of ganglionic blocking agents and vasoactive drugs, resulting in postural hypotension. Vitamins or other nutritional supplements containing large doses of niacin or related compounds (eg, nicotinamide) may potentiate adverse effects. Use caution w/ anticoagulants; monitor platelet counts and PT.

PATIENT CONSIDERATIONS

Assessment: Assess for history of/active liver disease or PUD, unexplained persistent hepatic transaminase elevations, predisposure to gout, arterial bleeding, history of jaundice or hepatobiliary disease, renal impairment, risk for hypophosphatemia, drug hypersensitivity, any other conditions where treatment is contraindicated or cautioned, pregnancy/nursing status, and possible drug interactions. Obtain baseline LFTs and lipid levels.

Monitoring: Monitor for signs/symptoms of liver dysfunction, decreases in platelet counts and P levels, increases in PT and uric acid levels, and other adverse reactions. Monitor LFTs every 6-12 weeks for the 1st yr, and periodically thereafter. Monitor lipid levels. Frequently monitor blood glucose levels. Periodically monitor P levels in patients at risk for hypophosphatemia. Monitor PT and platelet counts in patients on concomitant therapy w/ anticoagulants. Monitor patients on concomitant therapy w/ statins for any signs/symptoms of muscle pain, tenderness, or weakness, particularly during the initial months of therapy and during any periods of upward dosage titration; consider performing periodic serum CPK and K^+ determinations in such situations.

Counseling: Advise to adhere to the National Cholesterol Education Program-recommended diet, a regular exercise program, and periodic testing of a fasting lipid panel. Instruct to contact physician before restarting therapy if dosing is interrupted for any length of time. Instruct to notify physician of any unexplained muscle pain, tenderness or weakness, dizziness, changes in blood glucose if diabetic, and all medications being taken (eg, vitamins or other nutritional supplements containing niacin or nicotinamide). Inform that flushing may occur and may subside after several weeks of consistent use of therapy. Instruct that if awakened by flushing at night, to get up slowly, especially if feeling dizzy or faint, or taking BP medications. Advise of the symptoms of flushing and how they differ from the symptoms of MI. Instruct to avoid ingestion of alcohol, hot beverages, and spicy foods around the time of administration to minimize flushing. Advise to d/c use and contact physician if pregnant. Instruct not to use niacin if breastfeeding.

STORAGE: 20-25°C (68-77°F).

NINLARO – ixazomib

RX

Class: Proteasome inhibitor

ADULT DOSAGE

Multiple Myeloma

Use in combination w/ lenalidomide and dexamethasone for the treatment of patients w/ multiple myeloma who have received at least one prior therapy; continue treatment until disease progression or unacceptable toxicity

Ixazomib:

Initial: 4mg once a week on Days 1, 8, and 15 of a 28-day treatment cycle

Lenalidomide:

Initial: 25mg qd on Days 1-21 of a 28-day treatment cycle

Dexamethasone:

Initial: 40mg on Days 1, 8, 15, and 22 of a 28-day treatment cycle

Prior to Initiation of a New Cycle of Therapy:

- ANC should be ≥1000/mm³
- Platelet count should be ≥75,000/mm³
- Non-hematologic toxicities should, at the physician's discretion, generally be recovered to patient's baseline condition or ≤Grade 1

Missed Dose

If a dose is delayed or missed, take only if the next scheduled dose is ≥72 hrs away. A missed dose should not be taken w/in 72 hrs of the next scheduled dose. A double dose should not be taken to make up for the missed dose.

If vomiting occurs after taking a dose, do not repeat dose; resume dosing at the time of the next scheduled dose

PEDIATRIC DOSAGE

Pediatric use may not have been established

DOSING CONSIDERATIONS

Renal Impairment

Severe Renal Impairment (CrCl <30mL/min)/ESRD Requiring Dialysis: Reduce starting dose to 3mg; administer w/o regard to the timing of dialysis

Hepatic Impairment

Moderate (Total Bilirubin >1.5-3X ULN) or Severe (Total Bilirubin >3X ULN): Reduce starting dose to 3mg

Adverse Reactions

Ixazomib Dose Reductions:

Recommended Starting Dose: 4mg

First Dose Reduction: 3mg

Second Dose Reduction: 2.3mg

Hematological Toxicities:
Thrombocytopenia (Platelet Count <30,000/mm³): Withhold ixazomib and lenalidomide until platelet count is ≥30,000/mm³; following recovery, resume lenalidomide at the next lower dose and resume ixazomib at its most recent dose. If platelet count falls to <30,000/mm³ again, withhold ixazomib and lenalidomide until platelet count is ≥30,000/mm³; following recovery, resume ixazomib at the next lower dose and resume lenalidomide at its most recent dose. For additional occurrences, alternate dose modification of lenalidomide and ixazomib

Neutropenia (ANC <500/mm³): Withhold ixazomib and lenalidomide until ANC is ≥500/mm³. Consider adding G-CSF as per guidelines. Following recovery, resume lenalidomide at the next lower dose and resume ixazomib at its most recent dose. If ANC falls to <500/mm³ again, withhold ixazomib and lenalidomide until ANC is at least 500/mm³; following recovery, resume ixazomib at the next lower dose and resume lenalidomide at its most recent dose. For additional occurrences, alternate dose modification of lenalidomide and ixazomib

Non-Hematological Toxicities:
Rash:
Grade 2 or 3: Withhold lenalidomide until rash recovers to ≤Grade 1; following recovery, resume lenalidomide at the next lower dose. If Grade 2 or 3 rash occurs again, withhold ixazomib and lenalidomide until rash recovers to ≤Grade 1; following recovery, resume ixazomib at the next lower dose and resume lenalidomide at its most recent dose. For additional occurrences, alternate dose modification of lenalidomide and ixazomib
Grade 4: D/C treatment regimen

Peripheral Neuropathy:
Grade 1 Peripheral Neuropathy w/ Pain or Grade 2 Peripheral Neuropathy: Withhold ixazomib until peripheral neuropathy recovers to ≤Grade 1 w/o pain or patient's baseline; following recovery, resume ixazomib at its most recent dose
Grade 2 Peripheral Neuropathy w/ Pain or Grade 3 Peripheral Neuropathy: Withhold ixazomib. Toxicities should generally recover to baseline condition or ≤Grade 1 prior to resuming; following recovery, resume ixazomib at the next lower dose
Grade 4 Peripheral Neuropathy: D/C treatment regimen

Other Non-Hematological Toxicities:
Other Grade 3 or 4 Non-Hematological Toxicities: Withhold ixazomib. Toxicities should generally recover to baseline condition or ≤Grade 1 prior to resuming; if attributable to ixazomib, resume at the next lower dose following recovery

Refer to the individual monographs for lenalidomide and dexamethasone for additional information

N

ADMINISTRATION
Oral route

Take once a week on the same day and at approx the same time for the first 3 weeks of a 4-week cycle.
Take at least 1 hr ac or at least 2 hrs pc.
Swallow whole w/ water; do not crush, chew, or open.

HOW SUPPLIED
Cap: 2.3mg, 3mg, 4mg

WARNINGS/PRECAUTIONS
See Dosing Considerations. Thrombocytopenia reported; platelet nadirs typically occurring between Days 14-21 of each 28-day cycle and recovery to baseline by the start of the next cycle. Monitor platelet counts at least monthly during treatment; consider more frequent monitoring during the first three cycles. Rash, peripheral edema, diarrhea, constipation, and N/V reported. Peripheral neuropathy reported; monitor for symptoms of neuropathy. Drug-induced liver injury, hepatocellular injury, hepatic steatosis, hepatitis cholestatic, and hepatotoxicity reported; monitor hepatic enzymes regularly and adjust dosing for Grade 3 or 4 symptoms. May cause fetal harm.

ADVERSE REACTIONS
Diarrhea, constipation, thrombocytopenia, peripheral neuropathy, N/V, peripheral edema, back pain.

DRUG INTERACTIONS
Avoid w/ strong CYP3A inducers (eg, rifampin, phenytoin, carbamazepine).

PATIENT CONSIDERATIONS

Assessment: Assess for hypersensitivity to drug, preexisting renal or hepatic dysfunction, and pregnancy/nursing status. Obtain baseline platelet counts and ANC and assess non-hematologic toxicities.

Monitoring: Monitor platelet counts at least monthly during treatment; consider more frequent monitoring during the first three cycles. Monitor hepatic enzymes regularly. Monitor for signs/symptoms of neuropathy, edema, cutaneous reaction, and other adverse reactions. Monitor ANC, platelet counts, and non-hematologic toxicities before each new cycle of therapy. Monitor pregnancy status for females of reproductive potential.

Counseling: Instruct to take ud. Advise that ixazomib and dexamethasone should not be taken at the same time, because dexamethasone should be taken w/ food. Inform that direct contact w/ the cap contents should be avoided and instruct to avoid direct contact of cap contents w/ the skin or eyes, in case of cap breakage. If contact occurs w/ the skin, advise to wash thoroughly w/ soap and water; if contact occurs w/ the eyes, instruct to flush thoroughly w/ water. Advise to store caps in original packaging, and not to remove the cap from the packaging until just prior to administration. Advise patient that they may experience low platelet counts, diarrhea, constipation, N/V, new or worsening symptoms of peripheral neuropathy, unusual swelling of their extremities or weight gain due to swelling, new or worsening rash, jaundice, or right upper quadrant abdominal pain; advise to report any related symptoms to physician. Advise women of the potential risk to a fetus and to avoid becoming pregnant while on treatment and for 90 days following final dose; advise to contact physician immediately if patient becomes pregnant during treatment or w/in 90 days of the final dose. Advise to inform physician about other medications currently being taken and before starting any new medications.

STORAGE: Room temperature. Do not store >30°C (86°F). Do not freeze. Store in original packaging until immediately prior to use.

NITRO-DUR – nitroglycerin

RX

Class: Nitrate vasodilator

OTHER BRAND NAMES

Minitran

ADULT DOSAGE

Angina Pectoris

Prevention:

Initial: 0.2-0.4mg/hr patch for 12-14 hrs/day, remove patch for 10-12 hrs/day

PEDIATRIC DOSAGE

Pediatric use may not have been established

DOSING CONSIDERATIONS

Elderly

Start at lower end of dosing range

ADMINISTRATION

Transdermal route

HOW SUPPLIED

Patch: 0.1mg/hr, 0.2mg/hr, 0.3mg/hr, 0.4mg/hr, 0.6mg/hr, 0.8mg/hr [30^{s}]; (Minitran) 0.1mg/hr, 0.2mg/hr, 0.4mg/hr, 0.6mg/hr [30^{s}]

CONTRAINDICATIONS

Allergy to nitroglycerin or the adhesives used in the patches, concomitant use w/ phosphodiesterase inhibitors (eg, sildenafil, tadalafil, vardenafil) for erectile dysfunction or pulmonary arterial HTN, or the soluble guanylate cyclase stimulator riociguat.

WARNINGS/PRECAUTIONS

Use careful clinical or hemodynamic monitoring to avoid the hazards of hypotension and tachycardia if treating patients w/ acute MI or CHF. Do not discharge a cardioverter/defibrillator through a paddle electrode that overlies the patch; the arcing that may be seen in this situation is harmless in itself, but it may be associated w/ local current concentration that can cause damage to the paddles and burns to the patient. Severe hypotension, particularly w/ upright posture, may occur w/ even small doses, particularly in elderly; caution in elderly patients w/ volume depletion, hypotension, or on multiple medications. Nitroglycerin-induced hypotension may be accompanied by paradoxical bradycardia and increased angina pectoris. May aggravate the angina caused by hypertrophic cardiomyopathy, particularly in elderly. Tolerance and physical dependence may occur.

ADVERSE REACTIONS

Headache, lightheadedness, hypotension, syncope.

DRUG INTERACTIONS

See Contraindications. Vasodilating effects may be additive w/ those of other vasodilators (eg, alcohol).

PATIENT CONSIDERATIONS

Assessment: Assess for hypersensitivity to drug, acute MI, CHF, volume depletion, hypotension, angina caused by hypertrophic cardiomyopathy, pregnancy/nursing status, and possible drug interactions.

Monitoring: Monitor for hypotension, paradoxical bradycardia, increased/aggravated angina pectoris, tolerance, physical dependence, and other adverse reactions. Perform careful clinical or hemodynamic monitoring in patients w/ acute MI or CHF.

Counseling: Inform that daily headaches sometimes accompany treatment and that the headaches may be a marker of the activity of the drug; advise to resist the temptation to avoid headaches by altering the schedule of treatment, since loss of headache may be associated w/ simultaneous loss of antianginal efficacy. Inform that therapy may be associated w/ lightheadedness on standing, especially just after rising from a recumbent or seated position; counsel that lightheadedness may be more frequent in patients who have consumed alcohol. Instruct to properly discard patches.

STORAGE: 25°C (77°F); excursions permitted to 15-30°C (59-86°F). Do not refrigerate.

NITROSTAT – nitroglycerin

RX

Class: Nitrate vasodilator

ADULT DOSAGE

Angina Pectoris

Acute Relief:

1 tab SL or in the buccal pouch at the 1st sign of an acute attack

May repeat approx every 5 min until relief is obtained

If pain persists after a total of 3 tabs in 15 min, or if pain is different than is typically experienced, prompt medical attention is recommended

Acute Prophylaxis:

May be used 5-10 min prior to engaging in activities that might precipitate an acute attack

PEDIATRIC DOSAGE

Pediatric use may not have been established

DOSING CONSIDERATIONS

Elderly

Start at lower end of dosing range

ADMINISTRATION

SL or buccal route

Dissolve under tongue or in buccal pouch; do not chew, crush, or swallow tabs

During administration the patient should rest, preferably in the sitting position

HOW SUPPLIED

Tab, SL: 0.3mg, 0.4mg, 0.6mg

CONTRAINDICATIONS

Early MI, severe anemia, increased intracranial pressure (ICP), patients who are using a PDE-5 inhibitor (eg, sildenafil citrate, tadalafil, vardenafil hydrochloride), known hypersensitivity to nitroglycerin.

WARNINGS/PRECAUTIONS

Use careful clinical or hemodynamic monitoring in patients with acute MI (AMI) or CHF. Excessive use may lead to tolerance; use only the smallest dose required for effective relief of the acute anginal attack. Severe hypotension, particularly with upright posture, may occur with small doses; caution with volume depletion or hypotension. Nitroglycerin-induced hypotension may be accompanied by paradoxical bradycardia and increased angina pectoris. May aggravate angina caused by hypertrophic cardiomyopathy. As tolerance to other forms of nitroglycerin develops, effect on exercise tolerance is blunted. Physical dependence may occur. D/C if blurring of vision or drying of the mouth occurs. Excessive dosage may produce severe headaches. Lab test interactions may occur. Caution in elderly.

ADVERSE REACTIONS

Headache, vertigo, dizziness, weakness, palpitation, N/V, diaphoresis, pallor, collapse/syncope, flushing, drug rash, exfoliative dermatitis.

DRUG INTERACTIONS

See Contraindications. Hypotension may occur with alcohol. Enhanced vasodilatory and hemodynamic effects with ASA. Caution with alteplase therapy. IV nitroglycerin reduces the anticoagulant effect of heparin. TCAs (eg, amitriptyline, desipramine, doxepin) and anticholinergics may make SL tab dissolution difficult. Avoid ergotamine and related drugs or monitor for ergotism symptoms if unavoidable. Long-acting nitrates may decrease therapeutic effect.

PATIENT CONSIDERATIONS

Assessment: Assess for early MI, severe anemia, increased ICP, AMI, CHF, volume depletion, hypotension, angina caused by hypertrophic cardiomyopathy, drug hypersensitivity, pregnancy/nursing status, and possible drug interactions.

Monitoring: Monitor for hypotension, paradoxical bradycardia, increased/aggravated angina pectoris, tolerance, physical dependence, blurring of vision, drying of mouth, headache, and other adverse reactions. Perform careful clinical or hemodynamic monitoring in patients with AMI or CHF.

Counseling: Counsel on the proper dosage and administration of the drug. Advise to sit down when taking the drug and to use caution when returning to standing position. Inform about side effects of the drug (eg, burning or tingling sensation when administered SL, headaches, lightheadedness upon standing). Counsel that lightheadedness may be more frequent in patients who have consumed alcohol. Instruct to keep in original glass container and to tightly cap after each use to prevent loss of potency.

STORAGE: 20-25°C (68-77°F).

NORCO – acetaminophen/hydrocodone bitartrate CII

Class: Opioid analgesic

Associated w/ cases of acute liver failure, at times resulting in liver transplant and death. Most cases of liver injury are associated w/ APAP use at doses >4000mg/day, and often involve >1 APAP-containing product.

ADULT DOSAGE

Moderate to Moderately Severe Pain

5mg/325mg:
Usual: 1 or 2 tabs q4-6h prn
Max: 8 tabs/day

7.5mg/325mg, 10mg/325mg:
Usual: 1 tab q4-6h prn
Max: 6 tabs/day

PEDIATRIC DOSAGE

Pediatric use may not have been established

DOSING CONSIDERATIONS

Elderly
Start at lower end of dosing range

ADMINISTRATION

Oral route

HOW SUPPLIED

Tab: (Hydrocodone/APAP) 5mg/325mg*, 7.5mg/325mg*, 10mg/325mg* *scored

CONTRAINDICATIONS

Hypersensitivity to hydrocodone or acetaminophen.

WARNINGS/PRECAUTIONS

Increased risk of acute liver failure in patients w/ underlying liver disease. May cause serious skin reactions (eg, acute generalized exanthematous pustulosis, Stevens-Johnson syndrome, toxic epidermal necrolysis); d/c at the 1st appearance of skin rash or any other sign of hypersensitivity. Hypersensitivity and anaphylaxis reported; d/c immediately if signs/symptoms occur. May produce dose-related respiratory depression and irregular/periodic breathing. Respiratory depressant effects and CSF pressure elevation capacity may be markedly exaggerated in the presence of head injury, other intracranial lesions, or a preexisting increase in intracranial pressure. May obscure clinical course of head injuries and acute abdominal conditions. Caution w/ hypothyroidism, Addison's disease, prostatic hypertrophy, urethral stricture, severe hepatic/renal impairment, or in elderly/debilitated. Suppresses cough reflex; caution w/ pulmonary disease and in postoperative use. Lab test interactions may occur. May be habit-forming.

ADVERSE REACTIONS

Acute liver failure, lightheadedness, dizziness, sedation, N/V.

DRUG INTERACTIONS

Increased risk of acute liver failure w/ alcohol. Additive CNS depression w/ other narcotics, antihistamines, antipsychotics, antianxiety agents, or other CNS depressants (eg, alcohol); reduce dose of one or both agents. Concomitant use w/ MAOIs or TCAs may increase the effect of either the antidepressant or hydrocodone.

PATIENT CONSIDERATIONS

Assessment: Assess for history of hypersensitivity to drug, level of pain intensity, type of pain, patient's general condition and medical status, renal/hepatic impairment, pregnancy/nursing status, any other conditions where treatment is cautioned, and possible drug interactions.

Monitoring: Monitor for signs/symptoms of hypersensitivity or anaphylaxis, serious skin reactions, acute liver failure, respiratory depression, elevations in CSF pressure, drug abuse/dependence/

N

tolerance, and other adverse reactions. In patients w/ severe hepatic/renal disease, monitor effects w/ serial hepatic and/or renal function tests.

Counseling: Instruct to look for APAP on package labels and not to use >1 APAP-containing product. Instruct to seek medical attention immediately upon ingestion of >4000mg/day of APAP, even if feeling well. Advise to d/c use and contact physician immediately if signs of allergy develop. Inform about signs of serious skin reactions. Inform that drug may impair mental/physical abilities, and to use caution if performing potentially hazardous tasks (eg, driving, operating machinery). Instruct to avoid alcohol and other CNS depressants. Inform that drug may be habit-forming; instruct to take only ud.

STORAGE: (5mg-325mg) 15-30°C (59-86°F). (7.5mg-325mg, 10mg-325mg) 20-25°C (68-77°F).

NORPACE — disopyramide phosphate

RX

Class: Class I antiarrhythmic

In a long-term clinical study in patients with asymptomatic non-life-threatening ventricular arrhythmias who had a myocardial infarction, an excessive mortality or non-fatal cardiac arrest rate was seen in patients treated with encainide or flecainide compared to placebo. Considering the known proarrhythmic properties of Norpace or Norpace CR and the lack of evidence of improved survival, its use should be reserved for patients with life-threatening ventricular arrhythmias.

OTHER BRAND NAMES

Norpace CR

ADULT DOSAGE

Ventricular Arrhythmias

Treatment of Documented Ventricular Arrhythmias (eg, sustained ventricular tachycardia)

Individualize dose based on response and tolerance

Usual: 400-800mg/day in divided dose

Recommended:

<110 lbs: 100mg q6h immediate-release (IR) or 200mg q12h extended-release (CR)

≥110 lbs: 150mg q6h (600mg/day) IR or 300mg q12h CR

Rapid Control of Ventricular Arrhythmia:

LD: 300mg IR (200mg if <110 lbs)

Follow w/ maint dose

Titrate:

If no response/evidence of toxicity w/in 6 hrs of LD, may give 200mg q6h IR

If no response to 200mg q6h of IR w/in 48 hrs; d/c disopyramide or consider hospitalizing patient for monitoring while subsequent 250mg or 300mg q6h IR is given

Patients w/ cardiomyopathy/cardiac decompensation, limit initial dose to 100mg q6-8h IR and adjust gradually; do not give LD

Switching from IR to CR:

Maint schedule of CR may be started 6 hrs after last dose of IR

Transferring to Norpace or Norpace CR from Quinidine Sulfate or Procainamide:

Norpace or Norpace CR should be started using the regular maint schedule w/o a LD 6-12 hrs after the last dose of quinidine sulfate or 3-6 hrs after the last dose of procainamide

PEDIATRIC DOSAGE

Ventricular Arrhythmias

Treatment of Documented Ventricular Arrhythmias (eg, sustained ventricular tachycardia)

<1 Year: 10-30mg/kg/day

1-4 Years: 10-20mg/kg/day

4-12 Years: 10-15mg/kg/day

12-18 Years: 6-15mg/kg/day

Give in equally divided doses q6h

Hospitalize patient during initial therapy

Start dose titration at lower end of range

DOSING CONSIDERATIONS

Renal Impairment

CrCl >40mL/min: 100mg q6h IR or 200mg q12h CR

CrCl 30-40mL/min: 100mg q8h IR, w/ or w/o initial 150mg LD

CrCl 15-30mL/min: 100mg q12h IR, w/ or w/o initial 150mg LD

CrCl <15mL/min: 100mg q24h IR, w/ or w/o initial 150mg LD

Hepatic Impairment
Moderate: 100mg q6h IR or 200mg q12h CR
Elderly
Start at low end of dosing range
Adverse Reactions
Anticholinergic Side Effects:
Adjust dose based on side effects
Reduce recommended dose by 1/3 from 600mg/day to 400mg/day w/o changing the dosing interval

ADMINISTRATION
Oral route
Preparation of a 1mg/mL to 10mg/mL Liquid Sus
Add the entire contents of Norpace caps to cherry syrup (100mg caps contain 100mg of disopyramide base)
Prepare cherry syr as follows: cherry juice, 475mL; sucrose 800g; alcohol, 20mL; purified water, a sufficient quantity to make 1000mL
The resulting sus, when refrigerated, is stable for 1 month and should be thoroughly shaken before the measurement of each dose
The sus should be dispensed in an amber glass bottle with a child-resistant closure
Norpace CR caps should not be used to prepare the above sus

HOW SUPPLIED
Cap: (Norpace) 100mg, 150mg; **Cap, Extended-Release:** (Norpace CR) 100mg, 150mg

CONTRAINDICATIONS
Known hypersensitivity to disopyramide, cardiogenic shock, 2nd- or 3rd-degree atrioventricular block (if no pacemaker present), congenital QT prolongation.

WARNINGS/PRECAUTIONS
May cause or worsen congestive heart failure (CHF) and produce hypotension due to negative inotropic properties. Reduce dose if 1st-degree heart block occurs. Avoid with urinary retention, glaucoma, and myasthenia gravis unless adequate overriding measures taken. Atrial flutter/fibrillation; digitalize 1st. Monitor closely or withdraw if QT prolongation >25% occurs and ectopy continues. D/C if QRS widening >25% occurs. Avoid LD with cardiomyopathy or cardiac decompensation. Correct K^+ abnormalities before therapy. Reduce dose with renal/hepatic dysfunction; monitor ECG. Avoid CR formulation with CrCl <=40mL/min. Caution with sick sinus syndrome, Wolff-Parkinson-White syndrome, bundle branch block, or elderly. May significantly lower blood glucose.

ADVERSE REACTIONS
Dry mouth, urinary retention/frequency/urgency, constipation, blurred vision, GI effects, dizziness, fatigue, headache.

DRUG INTERACTIONS
Avoid type IA and IC antiarrhythmics, and propranolol except in unresponsive, life-threatening arrhythmias. Hepatic enzyme inducers may lower levels. Avoid within 48 hrs before or 24 hrs after verapamil. Possible fatal interactions with CYP3A4 inhibitors. Monitor blood glucose with β-blockers, alcohol.

PATIENT CONSIDERATIONS
Assessment: Prior to therapy, patients with atrial flutter/fibrillation should be digitalized and K^+ abnormalities should be corrected. Assess for cardiogenic shock, preexisting 2nd- or 3rd-degree heart block, presence of functioning pacemaker, sick sinus syndrome (bradycardia/tachycardia syndrome), Wolff-Parkinson-White syndrome, bundle branch block, congenital QT prolongation, myocardial infarction, life-threatening arrhythmia, CHF, cardiomyopathy or myocarditis, chronic malnutrition, hepatic/renal impairment, alcohol intake, glaucoma, myasthenia gravis, urinary retention or BPH, pregnancy/nursing status, and possible drug interactions.

Monitoring: Monitor for hypotension, HF, PR interval prolongation, widening of QRS, hypoglycemia, heart block, urinary retention, and myasthenia crisis.

Counseling: Inform about risks/benefits; report adverse reactions. Instruct to notify physician if pregnant/nursing.

STORAGE: 25°C (77°F); excursions permitted to 15-30°C (59-86°F).

NORTRIPTYLINE – nortriptyline hydrochloride
RX

Class: Tricyclic antidepressant (TCA)

Antidepressants increased the risk of suicidal thinking and behavior (suicidality) in short-term studies in children, adolescents, and young adults with major depressive disorder and other psychiatric disorders. Monitor and observe closely for clinical worsening, suicidality, or unusual changes in behavior in patients who are started on antidepressant therapy. Not approved for use in pediatric patients.

OTHER BRAND NAMES
Pamelor

ADULT DOSAGE
Depression
Usual: 25mg tid or qid; initiate at a low level and increase as required
Alternate Regimen: Total daily dose may be given qd
Max: 150mg/day
Monitor plasma levels w/ doses >100mg/day and maintain in the optimum range of 50-150ng/mL
Following remission, maintenance medication may be required for a longer period of time at the lowest dose that will maintain remission
Dosing Considerations with MAOIs
Switching to/from an MAOI for Psychiatric Disorders:
Allow at least 14 days between discontinuation of an MAOI and initiation of treatment, and allow at least 14 days between discontinuation of treatment and initiation of an MAOI
Use w/ Other MAOIs (eg, Linezolid, IV Methylene Blue):
Do not start nortriptyline in a patient being treated w/ linezolid or IV methylene blue
In patients already receiving nortriptyline, if acceptable alternatives are not available and benefits outweigh risks, d/c nortriptyline and administer linezolid or IV methylene blue; monitor for serotonin syndrome for 2 weeks or until 24 hrs after the last dose of linezolid or IV methylene blue, whichever comes 1st. May resume nortriptyline therapy 24 hours after the last dose of linezolid or IV methylene blue

PEDIATRIC DOSAGE
Depression
Cap:
Adolescents:
30-50mg/day in single or divided doses
Following remission, maintenance medication may be required for a longer period of time at the lowest dose that will maintain remission
Dosing Considerations with MAOIs
Switching to/from an MAOI for Psychiatric Disorders:
Allow at least 14 days between discontinuation of an MAOI and initiation of treatment, and allow at least 14 days between discontinuation of treatment and initiation of an MAOI
Use w/ Other MAOIs (eg, Linezolid, IV Methylene Blue):
Do not start nortriptyline in a patient being treated w/ linezolid or IV methylene blue
In patients already receiving nortriptyline, if acceptable alternatives are not available and benefits outweigh risks, d/c nortriptyline and administer linezolid or IV methylene blue; monitor for serotonin syndrome for 2 weeks or until 24 hrs after the last dose of linezolid or IV methylene blue, whichever comes 1st. May resume nortriptyline therapy 24 hours after the last dose of linezolid or IV methylene blue

N

DOSING CONSIDERATIONS
Elderly
30-50mg/day in single or divided doses
Adverse Reactions
Reduce dose if a patient develops minor side effects and promptly d/c if adverse effects of a serious nature or allergic manifestations occur

ADMINISTRATION
Oral route

HOW SUPPLIED
Cap: 10mg, 25mg, 50mg, 75mg; **Sol:** 10mg/5mL [16 fl oz]

CONTRAINDICATIONS
Use of an MAOI for psychiatric disorders either concomitantly or within 14 days of stopping treatment. Treatment within 14 days of stopping an MAOI for psychiatric disorders. Starting treatment in a patient being treated with other MAOIs (eg, linezolid, IV methylene blue). Hypersensitivity to nortriptyline HCl or other tricyclic antidepressants. During the acute recovery period following MI.

WARNINGS/PRECAUTIONS
Not approved for the treatment of bipolar depression. May precipitate mixed/manic episode in patients at risk for bipolar disorder. May produce sinus tachycardia and prolong conduction time; MI, arrhythmia, and strokes reported. Caution with cardiovascular disease (CVD), glaucoma, history of urinary retention, and hyperthyroidism. May lower seizure threshold, exacerbate psychosis or activate schizophrenia, or alter glucose levels. D/C several days prior to elective surgery. May impair mental/physical abilities. Serotonin syndrome reported; d/c immediately and initiate supportive symptomatic treatment. Pupillary dilation that occurs following use may trigger an angle-closure attack in a patient with anatomically narrow angles who does not have a patent iridectomy.

ADVERSE REACTIONS
Arrhythmias, hypotension, HTN, tachycardia, MI, heart block, stroke, confusion, hallucination, insomnia, tremors, ataxia, dry mouth, blurred vision, skin rash.

DRUG INTERACTIONS

See Contraindications. May cause serotonin syndrome with other serotonergic drugs (eg, triptans, TCAs, fentanyl) and with drugs that impair metabolism of serotonin; d/c immediately if this occurs. May block antihypertensive effect of guanethidine and similar agents. Caution in patients on thyroid medications. Alcohol may potentiate effects. May produce "stimulating" effect with reserpine. Monitor and adjust dose with anticholinergic and sympathomimetic drugs. Increased plasma levels with cimetidine. Hypoglycemia reported with chlorpropamide. Drugs that inhibit CYP2D6 (eg, quinidine, cimetidine, many CYP2D6 substrates [eg, other antidepressants, phenothiazines, propafenone, flecainide]) may increase plasma concentrations and may require lower doses for either TCA or the other drug and monitoring of TCA plasma levels. Caution with SSRI coadministration and when switching between TCAs and SSRIs; sufficient time must elapse before starting therapy when switching from fluoxetine (at least 5 weeks may be necessary). Longer $T_{1/2}$, higher exposure, and decreased clearance with quinidine.

PATIENT CONSIDERATIONS

Assessment: Assess for recent MI, known hypersensitivity to drug, bipolar disorder risk, susceptibility to angle-closure glaucoma, CVD, hyperthyroidism, history of urinary retention/seizure disorder/mania/schizophrenia, any other conditions where treatment is cautioned or contraindicated, pregnancy/nursing status, and possible drug interactions.

Monitoring: Monitor for signs/symptoms of clinical worsening, suicidality, unusual changes in behavior, mixed manic episodes, arrhythmias, psychosis, serotonin syndrome, angle-closure glaucoma, changes in blood glucose levels, seizures, cognitive/motor impairment, and other adverse reactions.

Counseling: Advise to avoid alcohol. Instruct to seek medical attention for symptoms of activation of mania, seizures, clinical worsening, cardiovascular events, increasing psychosis, increasing anxiety/agitation, and hypo/hyperglycemia. Inform that physical/mental abilities may be impaired. Advise about the risk of angle-closure glaucoma in susceptible individuals.

STORAGE: 20-25°C (68-77°F).

NORVASC – amlodipine besylate

RX

Class: Calcium channel blocker (CCB) (dihydropyridine)

ADULT DOSAGE

Hypertension

Alone or in combination w/ other antihypertensive agents

Initial: 5mg qd

Titrate: Adjust according to BP goals

Wait 7-14 days between titration steps; if clinically warranted, titrate more rapidly and assess patient frequently

Max: 10mg qd

Angina

Chronic stable angina or confirmed or suspected vasospastic (Prinzmetal's/variant) angina, alone or in combination w/ other antianginals

Usual: 5-10mg qd

Coronary Artery Disease

Reduces the risk of hospitalization due to angina and reduces risk of coronary revascularization procedures in patients w/ recently documented coronary artery disease by angiography and w/o heart failure or an ejection fraction <40%

Usual: 5-10mg qd

PEDIATRIC DOSAGE

Hypertension

Alone or in combination w/ other antihypertensive agents

6-17 Years:

Usual: 2.5-5mg qd

Max: 5mg qd

DOSING CONSIDERATIONS

Concomitant Medications

HTN:

Other Antihypertensives: 2.5mg qd

Hepatic Impairment

HTN:

Initial: 2.5mg qd

Angina: Give lower dose

Elderly

HTN:

Initial: 2.5mg qd

Angina: Give lower dose

Other Important Considerations

HTN:

Small/Fragile Patients:

Initial: 2.5mg qd

ADMINISTRATION

Oral route

HOW SUPPLIED

Tab: 2.5mg, 5mg, 10mg

CONTRAINDICATIONS

Known sensitivity to amlodipine.

WARNINGS/PRECAUTIONS

May cause symptomatic hypotension, particularly in patients w/ severe aortic stenosis. Worsening angina and acute MI may develop after starting or increasing the dose, particularly w/ severe obstructive CAD. Titrate slowly in patients w/ severe hepatic impairment.

ADVERSE REACTIONS

Edema, palpitations, dizziness, fatigue, flushing.

DRUG INTERACTIONS

Increased systemic exposure w/ moderate and strong CYP3A inhibitors and may require dose reduction; monitor for symptoms of hypotension and edema to determine the need for dose adjustment. Closely monitor BP if coadministered w/ CYP3A inducers. Monitor for hypotension when coadministered w/ sildenafil. May increase simvastatin exposure; limit dose of simvastatin to 20mg daily. May increase systemic exposure of cyclosporine or tacrolimus; monitor trough blood levels of cyclosporine and tacrolimus frequently and adjust dose when appropriate.

PATIENT CONSIDERATIONS

Assessment: Assess for hypersensitivity to the drug, severe aortic stenosis, severe obstructive CAD, hepatic impairment, pregnancy/nursing status, and possible drug interactions. Obtain baseline BP.

Monitoring: Monitor for worsening of angina, MI, and other adverse reactions. Monitor BP.

Counseling: Inform of the risks/benefits of therapy. Advise to seek medical attention if any adverse effects develop. Instruct to take as prescribed.

STORAGE: 15-30°C (59-86°F).

NORVIR — ritonavir

RX

Class: Protease inhibitor

Coadministration w/ several classes of drugs, including sedative hypnotics, antiarrhythmics, or ergot alkaloid preparations, may result in potentially serious and/or life-threatening adverse events due to possible effects of ritonavir (RTV) on the hepatic metabolism of certain drugs. Review medications taken by patients prior to prescribing RTV or when prescribing other medications to patients already taking RTV.

ADULT DOSAGE

HIV-1 Infection

In Combination w/ Other Antiretrovirals:

600mg bid; initiate at no less than 300mg bid and increase at 2- to 3-day intervals by 100mg bid

Max: 600mg bid

PEDIATRIC DOSAGE

HIV-1 Infection

In Combination w/ Other Antiretrovirals:

>1 Month of Age:

Initial: 250mg/m^2 bid

Titrate: Increase at 2- to 3-day intervals by 50mg/m^2 bid

Maint: 350-400mg/m^2 bid or highest tolerated dose

Max: 600mg bid

DOSING CONSIDERATIONS

Concomitant Medications

Reduce dose when used w/ other protease inhibitors

Hepatic Impairment

Severe (Child-Pugh Class C): Not recommended

Elderly
Start at lower end of dosing range

Other Important Considerations
Do not administer oral sol to neonates before a postmenstrual age (1st day of the mother's last menstrual period to birth plus the time elapsed after birth) of 44 weeks has been attained

ADMINISTRATION

Oral route

Take w/ meals

Tab
Swallow tab whole; do not chew, break, or crush tab

Sol
May improve the taste by mixing w/ chocolate milk, Ensure, or Advera, w/in 1 hr of dosing

HOW SUPPLIED

Cap: 100mg; **Sol:** 80mg/mL [240mL]; **Tab:** 100mg

CONTRAINDICATIONS

Coadministration w/ voriconazole or St. John's wort. Coadministration of RTV w/ several classes of drugs (including sedative hypnotics, antiarrhythmics, or ergot alkaloid preparations) is contraindicated and may result in potentially serious and/or life-threatening adverse events due to possible effects of RTV on the hepatic metabolism of these drugs (eg, alfuzosin HCl, amiodarone, flecainide, propafenone, quinidine, dihydroergotamine, ergotamine, methylergonovine, cisapride, lovastatin, simvastatin, pimozide, sildenafil when used for treatment of pulmonary arterial HTN, triazolam, oral midazolam). Known hypersensitivity (eg, toxic epidermal necrolysis or Stevens-Johnson syndrome) to ritonavir or any of its components.

WARNINGS/PRECAUTIONS

Hepatic transaminase elevations >5X ULN, clinical hepatitis, and jaundice reported; increased risk w/ underlying hepatitis B or C. Caution w/ preexisting liver diseases, liver enzyme abnormalities, or hepatitis; consider increased AST/ALT monitoring, especially during first 3 months of therapy. Pancreatitis observed; d/c if diagnosed. Allergic reactions, anaphylaxis, Stevens-Johnson syndrome, and toxic epidermal necrolysis reported; d/c if severe reactions develop. Prolonged PR interval and 2nd- or 3rd-degree atrioventricular (AV) block may occur; caution w/ underlying structural heart disease, preexisting conduction system abnormalities, ischemic heart disease, and cardiomyopathies. May elevate TG and total cholesterol levels. New onset or exacerbation of diabetes mellitus (DM), hyperglycemia, diabetic ketoacidosis, immune reconstitution syndrome, autoimmune disorders (eg, Graves' disease, polymyositis, Guillain-Barre syndrome) in the setting of immune reconstitution, and redistribution/accumulation of body fat reported. Increased bleeding in patients w/ hemophilia type A and B reported. Various degrees of cross-resistance observed. Lab test interactions may occur. (Sol) Contains alcohol and propylene glycol; do not use in preterm neonates in the immediate postnatal period because of possible toxicities. If benefit of treating infants immediately after birth outweighs potential risk, monitor closely for increases in serum osmolality and SrCr, and for drug-related toxicity.

ADVERSE REACTIONS

Diarrhea, N/V, abdominal pain, dizziness, dysgeusia, paresthesia, peripheral neuropathy, rash, fatigue/asthenia, arthralgia, back pain, coughing, oropharyngeal pain, pruritus, flushing.

DRUG INTERACTIONS

See Boxed Warning and Contraindications. Coadministration w/ CYP3A substrates for which elevated plasma concentrations are associated w/ serious and/or life-threatening reactions is contraindicated. May increase exposure of CYP2D6 substrates. Not recommended w/ fluticasone, other glucocorticoids that are metabolized by CYP3A, salmeterol, high doses of itraconazole or ketoconazole, and simeprevir. Avoid w/ colchicine in patients w/ renal/hepatic impairment, saquinavir/rifampin/RTV combination, avanafil, and rivaroxaban. Delavirdine may increase levels and rifampin may decrease levels. May increase levels of CYP3A substrates, atazanavir, darunavir, amprenavir, saquinavir, tipranavir, maraviroc, normeperidine, disopyramide, lidocaine, mexiletine, dasatinib, nilotinib, vincristine, vinblastine, rivaroxaban, carbamazepine, clonazepam, ethosuximide, nefazodone, SSRIs, TCAs, desipramine, trazodone, dronabinol, ketoconazole, itraconazole, colchicine, clarithromycin, rifabutin, quinine, quetiapine, β-blockers, calcium channel blockers, digoxin, bosentan, simeprevir, atorvastatin, rosuvastatin, cyclosporine, tacrolimus, sirolimus, fluticasone, budesonide, salmeterol, fentanyl, perphenazine, risperidone, thioridazine, avanafil, sildenafil, tadalafil, vardenafil, diazepam, estazolam, flurazepam, zolpidem, parenteral midazolam, dexamethasone, prednisone, and methamphetamine. May decrease levels of raltegravir, meperidine, divalproex, lamotrigine, bupropion, voriconazole, atovaquone, theophylline, methadone, and ethinyl estradiol. Caution w/ other drugs that prolong the PR interval, particularly w/ those drugs metabolized by CYP3A. May alter concentrations of warfarin (monitor INR) and indinavir. May need to decrease dose of tramadol and propoxyphene. RTV formulations contain alcohol; may produce disulfiram-like reactions w/ disulfiram or metronidazole. Refer to PI for dosing modifications when used w/ certain concomitant therapies.

PATIENT CONSIDERATIONS

Assessment: Assess for previous hypersensitivity to the drug, preexisting liver diseases, hepatitis, DM, hemophilia type A or B, underlying cardiac problems, lipid disorders, pregnancy/nursing status, and possible drug interactions. Obtain baseline ECG, LFTs, and CPK, uric acid, TG, and cholesterol levels.

Monitoring: Monitor for signs/symptoms of anaphylaxis or allergic reactions, hepatitis, jaundice, hepatic dysfunction, new onset or exacerbation of DM, hyperglycemia, pancreatitis, AV block, cardiac conduction abnormalities, immune reconstitution syndrome, fat redistribution/accumulation, and for other adverse reactions. Monitor for increased bleeding in patients w/ hemophilia type A or B. Monitor ECG, LFTs, and CPK, uric acid, TG, and cholesterol levels. Frequently monitor INR during coadministration w/ warfarin.

Counseling: Instruct to take prescribed dose ud. Instruct to inform physician if weight changes in children occur. Inform that therapy is not a cure for HIV-1 infection and illnesses associated w/ HIV-1 infection may still be experienced. Advise to practice safe sex; to use latex or polyurethane condoms; not to share personal items (eg, toothbrush, razor blades), needles, or other inj equipment; and not to breastfeed. Advise to notify physician of any use of prescription, OTC, or herbal products, particularly St. John's wort. Advise to use additional or alternative contraceptive measures if receiving estrogen-based hormonal contraceptives. Counsel about potential adverse effects; instruct to report signs/symptoms of worsening liver disease, pancreatitis, Stevens-Johnson syndrome, PR prolongation, and DM.

STORAGE: Cap: 2-8°C (36-46°F). May not require refrigeration if used w/in 30 days and stored below 25°C (77°F). Protect from light. Avoid exposure to excessive heat. Sol: 20-25°C (68-77°F). Do not refrigerate. Avoid exposure to excessive heat. Tab: ≤30°C (86°F). Exposure up to 50°C (122°F) for 7 days permitted. Exposure to high humidity outside the original or USP equivalent tight container (≤60mL) for >2 weeks is not recommended.

Novolin 70/30 – NPH, human insulin isophane (rDNA origin)/ regular, human insulin (rDNA origin) OTC

Class: Insulin (combination)

N

ADULT DOSAGE

Diabetes Mellitus

Individualize dose

PEDIATRIC DOSAGE

Diabetes Mellitus

Individualize dose

ADMINISTRATION

SQ route

To mix, roll gently and use right away.
Do not use if the liquid in the vial remains clear after the vial has been rolled gently.
Use only if cloudy or milky; there may be air bubbles.
Inject in stomach area, upper arms, buttocks, or upper legs.
Rotate inj site w/in the chosen area w/ each dose.
Do not mix w/ any insulins.

HOW SUPPLIED

Inj: (Isophane/Regular) (70 U/30 U)/mL [10mL]

WARNINGS/PRECAUTIONS

Avoid in patients w/ hypoglycemia. Any change of insulin should be made cautiously and only under medical supervision. Hyperglycemia may occur if dosage is not taken, which may lead to diabetic ketoacidosis if not treated. May need to change dosage w/ illness, stress, diet change, change in physical activity/exercise, other medicines, or surgery. Hypoglycemia may occur; monitor for symptoms of hypoglycemia (eg, sweating, dizziness, blurred vision). May impair physical and mental abilities. Serious allergic reaction, inj-site reaction, hands/feet swelling, vision changes, and hypokalemia may occur. May cause lipodystrophy; rotate inj site. May cause or worsen heart failure (HF) w/ thiazolidinediones (TZDs); may need to adjust or d/c insulin and TZD if this occurs.

ADVERSE REACTIONS

Hypoglycemia, allergic reaction, inj-site reaction, lipodystrophy, hands/feet swelling, vision changes, hypokalemia.

DRUG INTERACTIONS

Avoid w/ alcohol (eg, beer, wine); may affect blood glucose.

PATIENT CONSIDERATIONS

Assessment: Assess for medical conditions, hypoglycemia, drug hypersensitivity, pregnancy/nursing status, and possible drug interactions. Obtain baseline blood glucose levels.

Monitoring: Monitor for signs and symptoms of hypoglycemia, lipodystrophy, allergic reactions, vision changes, hypokalemia, and other adverse effects. Monitor blood glucose levels. Monitor for HF if taking a TZD concomitantly.

Counseling: Inform about potential risks and benefits of taking insulin and possible adverse reactions. If taking a TZD concomitantly, advise to notify physician if any new or worsening symptoms of HF (eg, SOB, swelling of the ankles/feet, sudden weight gain) occur. Inform about proper administration techniques, lifestyle management, regular blood glucose monitoring, signs and symptoms of hypoglycemia/hyperglycemia, management of hypoglycemia/hyperglycemia, and proper storage of insulin. Advise to consult physician if pregnant/nursing, stressed, ill, changing diet/physical activity, or having surgery, because changes in insulin dosage may be needed. Instruct to exercise caution when driving or operating machinery. Advise to always check carefully for correct type of insulin before administering. Instruct to notify physician of all medicines that are being taken.

STORAGE: **Unopened:** 2-8°C (36-46°F) or if refrigeration is not possible, ≤25°C (77°F) for ≤6 weeks. Do not freeze. Protect from light. **Opened:** <25°C (77°F) for ≤6 weeks; discard unused portion after 6 weeks. Keep away from direct heat/light. Do not refrigerate an opened vial.

Novolin N – NPH, human insulin isophane (rDNA origin) OTC

Class: Insulin (intermediate-acting)

ADULT DOSAGE

Diabetes Mellitus

Individualize dose

PEDIATRIC DOSAGE

Diabetes Mellitus

Individualize dose

ADMINISTRATION

SQ route

To mix, roll gently and use right away.

Do not use if the liquid in the vial remains clear after the vial has been rolled gently.

Use only if cloudy or milky; there may be air bubbles.

Do not use if precipitate becomes lumpy, granular in appearance, or has formed deposit of solid particles on the wall of the vial.

Inject in stomach area, upper arms, buttocks, or upper legs; rotate inj site w/in chosen area w/ each dose.

Do not mix w/ any insulin other than regular human insulin in same syringe.

HOW SUPPLIED

Inj: 100 U/mL [10mL]

WARNINGS/PRECAUTIONS

Avoid in patients w/ hypoglycemia. Any change of insulin should be made cautiously and only under medical supervision. Hyperglycemia may occur if dosage is not taken. Hyperglycemia may lead to diabetic ketoacidosis if not treated; may cause loss of consciousness, coma, or death. May need to change dosage w/ illness, stress, change in diet, change in physical activity/exercise, other medicines, or surgery. May impair mental/physical abilities. Hypoglycemia may occur; monitor for symptoms of hypoglycemia (eg, sweating, dizziness, blurred vision). Serious allergic reaction, inj-site reactions, hands/feet swelling, vision changes, and hypokalemia may occur. May cause lipodystrophy; rotate inj site. May cause or worsen heart failure (HF) w/ thiazolidinediones (TZDs); may need to adjust or d/c insulin and TZD if this occurs.

ADVERSE REACTIONS

Hypoglycemia, allergic reaction, inj-site reaction, lipodystrophy, hands/feet swelling, vision changes, hypokalemia.

DRUG INTERACTIONS

Avoid w/ alcohol (eg, beer, wine); may affect blood glucose.

PATIENT CONSIDERATIONS

Assessment: Assess for medical conditions, hypoglycemia, drug hypersensitivity, pregnancy/nursing status, and possible drug interactions. Obtain baseline blood glucose levels.

Monitoring: Monitor for signs of hypoglycemia, hypokalemia, vision changes, lipodystrophy, allergic reactions, and other adverse reactions. Monitor blood glucose levels. Monitor for HF if taking a TZD concomitantly.

Counseling: Inform about potential risks and benefits of taking insulin and possible adverse reactions. If taking a TZD concomitantly, advise to notify physician if any new or worsening symptoms of HF (eg, SOB, swelling of the ankles/feet, sudden weight gain) occur. Counsel on proper administration techniques, lifestyle management, regular blood glucose monitoring, signs and symptoms of hypoglycemia/hyperglycemia, management of hypoglycemia/hyperglycemia, and proper storage of insulin. Advise to consult physician if pregnant/nursing, stressed, ill, changing diet/physical activity, or having surgery, because changes in insulin dosage may be needed. Instruct to exercise caution when driving or operating machinery. Advise to always check carefully for correct type of insulin before administering. Instruct to notify physician of all medicines that are being taken.

STORAGE: Unopened: 2-8°C (36-46°F) or if refrigeration is not possible, ≤25°C (77°F) for ≤6 weeks. Do not freeze; do not use if frozen. Protect from light. **Opened:** <25°C (77°F) for ≤6 weeks; discard unused portion after 6 weeks. Keep away from direct heat/light. Do not refrigerate an opened vial.

NOVOLIN R – regular, human insulin (rDNA origin) OTC

Class: Insulin (short-acting)

ADULT DOSAGE

Diabetes Mellitus

Individualize dose and timing of administration

Total Daily Insulin Requirement:
Usual: 0.5-1 U/kg/day

PEDIATRIC DOSAGE

Type 1 Diabetes Mellitus

≥2 Years:
Individualize dose and timing of administration

Total Daily Insulin Requirement:
Usual: 0.5-1 U/kg/day

DOSING CONSIDERATIONS

Renal Impairment
Dose requirements may be reduced

Hepatic Impairment
Dose requirements may be reduced

ADMINISTRATION

SQ/IV route

Do not use in insulin pumps.
If Novolin R is mixed w/ NPH human insulin, Novolin R should be drawn into the syringe first and the mixture should be injected immediately after mixing.
Do not administer insulin mixtures IV.

SQ
Inject approx 30 min prior to the start of a meal.
Use w/ an intermediate or long-acting insulin.
Inject in abdominal region, buttocks, thigh, or upper arm; rotate inj sites w/in the same region.

IV
Use at concentrations from 0.05-1 U/mL in infusion systems using polypropylene infusion bags.
May be used w/ the following infusion fluids: 0.9% NaCl, D5, D10 w/ 40mmol/L potassium chloride.

HOW SUPPLIED

Inj: 100 U/mL [10mL]

CONTRAINDICATIONS

During episodes of hypoglycemia or w/ hypersensitivity to Novolin R or one of its excipients.

WARNINGS/PRECAUTIONS

Any change of insulin dose should be made cautiously and only under medical supervision. Changing from one insulin product to another or changing the strength may result in the need for a change in dosage. May require dose adjustments in patients who change level of physical activity or meal plan. Stress, illness, or emotional disturbances may alter insulin requirements. Hypoglycemia may occur and may impair ability to concentrate and react; caution in patients w/ hypoglycemia unawareness and who may be predisposed to hypoglycemia (eg, patients who are fasting or have erratic food intake, pediatric patients, elderly). Hypokalemia may occur; caution in patients who may be at risk. Hyperglycemia, diabetic ketoacidosis, or hyperosmolar hyperglycemic non-ketotic syndrome may develop if taken less than needed. Redness, swelling, or itching at inj site may occur. Localized reactions and generalized myalgias reported w/ metacresol, an excipient in Novolin R. Severe, life-threatening, generalized allergy, including anaphylaxis, may occur. Increases in titers of anti-insulin antibodies reported. May be administered IV under medical supervision w/ close monitoring of blood glucose and K^+ concentrations. Caution in elderly.

ADVERSE REACTIONS

Hypoglycemia, allergic reactions, lipodystrophy, weight gain, peripheral edema, transitory reversible ophthalmologic refraction disorder.

DRUG INTERACTIONS

May require dose adjustment and close monitoring w/ drugs that may increase blood glucose-lowering effect and susceptibility to hypoglycemia (eg, oral antidiabetic medications, ACE inhibitors, MAOIs), drugs that may reduce blood glucose-lowering effect leading to worsening of glycemic control (eg, corticosteroids, sympathomimetic agents, atypical antipsychotics), or drugs that may either potentiate or weaken blood glucose-lowering effect (eg, β-blockers, clonidine, lithium salts). Alcohol may increase susceptibility to hypoglycemia. Pentamidine may cause hypoglycemia, sometimes followed by hyperglycemia. Hypoglycemic signs may be reduced or absent w/ sympatholytics (eg, β-blockers, clonidine, guanethidine). Caution w/ K^+-lowering medications or medications sensitive to serum K^+ concentrations. Thiazolidinediones (TZDs) may cause dose-related fluid retention and heart failure (HF); observe for signs and symptoms of HF and consider dose reduction or discontinuation of TZDs if HF develops.

PATIENT CONSIDERATIONS

Assessment: Assess for drug hypersensitivity, hypoglycemia unawareness, predisposal to hypoglycemia, risk of hypokalemia, renal/hepatic impairment, pregnancy/nursing status, and possible drug interactions. Obtain baseline blood glucose and HbA1c levels.

Monitoring: Monitor for signs and symptoms of hypoglycemia, lipodystrophy, hypersensitivity, allergic reactions, dose-related fluid retention, HF, and other adverse effects. Monitor blood glucose, HbA1c, and K^+ concentrations (frequently during IV).

Counseling: Inform about potential risks and benefits of therapy, including possible adverse reactions. Offer continued education and advise on insulin therapies, inj technique, lifestyle management, regular glucose monitoring, periodic HbA1c testing, recognition and management of hypo/hyperglycemia, adherence to meal planning, complications of therapy, timing of dose, instruction in the use of inj devices, and proper storage. Inform that frequent, patient-performed blood glucose measurements are needed to achieve optimal glycemic control and to avoid both hyper/hypoglycemia. Advise to use caution when driving or operating machinery. Instruct to inform physician if patients intend to become pregnant, or if they become pregnant. Instruct to always carefully check that they are administering the correct insulin to avoid medication errors.

STORAGE: **Unopened:** 2-8°C (36-46°F) or if carried as a spare or if refrigeration not possible, ≤25°C (77°F) for 42 days. Do not freeze. Protect from light. Do not expose to heat/light. **Opened:** <25°C (77°F) for 42 days, away from heat/light. Do not refrigerate after 1st use.

NOVOLOG – insulin aspart (rDNA origin)

RX

Class: Insulin (rapid-acting)

N

ADULT DOSAGE

Diabetes Mellitus

SQ/IV:

Total Daily Insulin Requirement:

Usual: 0.5-1 U/kg/day; generally used w/ an intermediate- or long-acting insulin

Meal-Related SQ Regimen:

50-70% of total requirement may be provided by insulin aspart; remainder provided by an intermediate- or long-acting insulin

PEDIATRIC DOSAGE

Type 1 Diabetes Mellitus

≥2 Years:

SQ:

Total Daily Insulin Requirement:

Usual: 0.5-1 U/kg/day; generally used w/ an intermediate- or long-acting insulin

Meal-Related SQ Regimen:

50-70% of total requirement may be provided by insulin aspart; remainder provided by an intermediate- or long-acting insulin

ADMINISTRATION

SQ/IV route

SQ

Administer in the abdominal region, buttocks, thigh, or upper arm; rotate inj sites w/in the same region

Administer immediately (w/in 5-10 min) ac

May be diluted w/ insulin diluting medium

If mixed w/ NPH insulin, draw insulin aspart into syringe first and inject immediately after mixing

Continuous SQ Insulin Infusion by External Pump

Infuse premeal boluses immediately (w/in 5-10 min) ac

Rotate infusion sites w/in the same region

Do not use diluted or mixed insulins w/ external pump

Initial Programming of External Insulin Infusion Pump:

Base on total daily insulin dose of previous regimen

Approx 50% of total dose given as meal-related boluses; remainder given as basal infusion

Change insulin in the reservoir at least every 6 days; change infusion sets and infusion set insertion site at least every 3 days

IV

Use at concentrations 0.05-1.0 U/mL in infusion systems using polypropylene infusion bags; stable in infusion fluids such as 0.9% NaCl

Do not administer insulin mixtures IV

HOW SUPPLIED

Inj: 100 U/mL [3mL, PenFill cartridge, FlexPen, FlexTouch; 10mL, vial]

CONTRAINDICATIONS

During episodes of hypoglycemia, in patients with hypersensitivity to Novolog or one of its excipients.

WARNINGS/PRECAUTIONS

Insulin delivery devices should never be shared between patients, even if needle is changed; may carry a risk for transmission of blood-borne pathogens. Any change of insulin dose should be made cautiously and under medical supervision. Changing from 1 insulin product to another or changing the insulin strength may result in the need for a change in dosage. May require dosage adjustment w/ change in physical activity or meal plan. Illness, emotional disturbances, or other stresses may alter insulin requirements. Hypoglycemia may occur and may impair ability to concentrate and react; caution in patients w/ hypoglycemia unawareness and who may be predisposed to hypoglycemia. Hypokalemia, inj-site redness/swelling/itching, and severe, life-threatening, generalized allergy may occur. Contains metacresol as excipient; localized reactions and generalized myalgias reported. Increases in anti-insulin antibodies observed; may need to adjust insulin dose to correct a tendency towards hyper/hypoglycemia. Malfunction of the insulin pump or infusion set or insulin degradation can lead to a rapid onset of hyperglycemia and ketosis; prompt identification and correction of the cause is necessary. Train patients using continuous SQ infusion pump therapy to administer by inj and have alternate insulin therapy available in case of pump failure. IV administration should be under medical supervision w/ close monitoring of blood glucose and K^+ levels. Caution w/ renal/hepatic impairment.

ADVERSE REACTIONS

Hypoglycemia, headache, hyporeflexia, onychomycosis, sensory disturbance, UTI, nausea, diarrhea, chest pain, abdominal pain, skin disorder, sinusitis.

DRUG INTERACTIONS

May require dose adjustment and increased frequency of glucose monitoring w/ drugs that may increase the risk of hypoglycemia (eg, ACE inhibitors, MAOIs, salicylates), drugs that may decrease the glucose-lowering effect (eg, atypical antipsychotics [eg, olanzapine, clozapine], corticosteroids, oral contraceptives), or drugs that may increase or decrease the glucose-lowering effect (eg, alcohol, β-blockers, clonidine, lithium salts). Pentamidine may cause hypoglycemia, sometimes followed by hyperglycemia. Signs and symptoms of hypoglycemia may be blunted w/ β-blockers, clonidine, guanethidine, and reserpine. Caution w/ K^+-lowering drugs or drugs sensitive to serum K^+ concentrations. Observe for signs/symptoms of heart failure (HF) if treated concomitantly w/ a peroxisome proliferator-activated receptor (PPAR)-gamma agonist (eg, thiazolidinedione); consider discontinuation or dose reduction of the PPAR-gamma agonist if HF develops.

N

PATIENT CONSIDERATIONS

Assessment: Assess for predisposition to hypoglycemia, risk of hypokalemia, hypersensitivity, renal/hepatic impairment, pregnancy/nursing status, and possible drug interactions. Obtain baseline blood glucose and HbA1c levels.

Monitoring: Monitor for signs/symptoms of hypoglycemia, hypokalemia, allergic reactions, and other adverse effects. Monitor blood glucose, HbA1c, K^+ levels, and renal/hepatic function.

Counseling: Advise to never share insulin delivery device w/ another person, even if needle is changed. Inform about potential risks and benefits of therapy. Counsel on proper inj technique, lifestyle management, regular glucose monitoring, periodic HbA1c testing, recognition and management of hypo/hyperglycemia, adherence to meal planning, complications of insulin therapy, timing of dose, instruction in the use of inj or SQ insulin infusion pump, and proper storage of insulin. Inform that the ability to concentrate and react may be impaired as a result of hypoglycemia; advise to use caution when driving or operating machinery. Instruct to always carefully check that appropriate insulin is administered to avoid medication errors. Advise to inform physician if pregnant or intending to become pregnant.

STORAGE: Unused: 2-8°C (36-46°F) until expiration date. Do not freeze or store directly adjacent to the refrigerator cooling element; do not use if it has been frozen. Should not be drawn into a syringe and stored for later use. Opened: <30°C (86°F) for up to 28 days. (Vials) May refrigerate. (PenFill/FlexPen/FlexTouch) Do not refrigerate. Pump: Discard insulin in reservoir after exposure to >37°C (98.6°F). Diluted Sol: <30°C (86°F) for 28 days. Sol in Infusion Fluids: Stable at room temperature for 24 hrs. Protect from direct heat and light.

Novolog Mix 70/30 – insulin aspart protamine (rDNA origin)/ insulin aspart (rDNA origin) RX

Class: Insulin (combination)

ADULT DOSAGE

Type 1 Diabetes Mellitus

Individualize dose; inject w/in 15 min ac

Typically dosed bid (w/ each dose intended to cover 2 meals or a meal and snack)

Type 2 Diabetes Mellitus

Individualize dose; inject w/in 15 min ac or pc

Typically dosed bid (w/ each dose intended to cover 2 meals or a meal and snack)

PEDIATRIC DOSAGE

Pediatric use may not have been established

DOSING CONSIDERATIONS

Elderly

Start at lower end of dosing range

ADMINISTRATION

SQ route

Administer in the abdominal region, buttocks, thigh, or upper arm; rotate inj sites w/in the same region

Do not use in insulin infusion pump; do not mix w/ any other insulin product

Always use a new needle for each inj and always remove needle after each inj to prevent contamination

Resuspension

Resuspension is easier when the insulin has reached room temperature

Vial:

1. Roll vial gently between hands in a horizontal position 10X to mix it
2. Repeat rolling procedure until the sus appears uniformly white and cloudy
3. Inject immediately

FlexPen:

1. Roll 10X gently between hands in a horizontal position
2. Turn FlexPen upside down so that the glass ball moves from 1 end of the reservoir to the other at least 10X
3. Repeat rolling and turning procedure until the sus appears uniformly white and cloudy
4. Inject immediately
5. Repeat turning procedure at least 10X before each subsequent inj

HOW SUPPLIED

Inj: (Insulin Aspart Protamine/Insulin Aspart) (70 U/30 U)/mL [3mL, FlexPen; 10mL, vial]

CONTRAINDICATIONS

During episodes of hypoglycemia, hypersensitivity to Novolog Mix 70/30 or one of its excipients.

WARNINGS/PRECAUTIONS

FlexPens must never be shared between patients, even if needle is changed; may carry a risk for transmission of blood-borne pathogens. Any change of insulin dose should be made cautiously and under medical supervision. Changing from 1 insulin product to another or changing the insulin strength may result in the need for a change in dosage; changes may also be necessary during illness, emotional stress, and other physiologic stress in addition to changes in meals and exercise. Hypoglycemia may occur and may impair ability to concentrate and react. Hypokalemia, inj-site reactions (eg, erythema, edema, pruritus), and severe, life-threatening, generalized allergy may occur. Contains metacresol as excipient; localized reactions and generalized myalgias reported. Changes in cross-reactive anti-insulin antibodies reported; may need to adjust dose in order to correct a tendency towards hyper/hypoglycemia. Caution w/ renal/hepatic impairment.

ADVERSE REACTIONS

Hypoglycemia, headache, influenza-like symptoms, dyspepsia, back pain, diarrhea, pharyngitis, rhinitis, skeletal pain, URTI, neuropathy, abdominal pain.

DRUG INTERACTIONS

May require insulin dose adjustment and close monitoring w/ drugs that may increase blood glucose-lowering effect and susceptibility to hypoglycemia (eg, oral antidiabetic products, pramlintide, ACE inhibitors), drugs that may reduce blood glucose-lowering effect (eg, corticosteroids, niacin, danazol), or drugs that may potentiate or weaken blood glucose-lowering effect (β-blockers, clonidine, lithium salts, alcohol). Pentamidine may cause hypoglycemia, sometimes followed by hyperglycemia. Signs of hypoglycemia may be reduced or absent w/ sympatholytics (eg, β-blockers, clonidine, guanethidine). Caution w/ K^+-lowering drugs or drugs sensitive to K^+ concentrations. Observe for signs/symptoms of heart failure (HF) if treated concomitantly w/ a peroxisome proliferator-activated receptor (PPAR)-gamma agonist (eg, thiazolidinediones); consider discontinuation or dose reduction of the PPAR-gamma agonist if HF develops.

PATIENT CONSIDERATIONS

Assessment: Assess for predisposition to hypoglycemia, risk of hypokalemia, renal/hepatic impairment, drug hypersensitivity, pregnancy/nursing status, and possible drug interactions. Obtain baseline blood glucose and HbA1c levels.

Monitoring: Monitor for signs/symptoms of hypoglycemia, hypokalemia, allergic reactions, and other adverse effects. Monitor blood glucose, HbA1c, K^+ levels, and renal/hepatic function.

Counseling: Advise to never share FlexPen w/ another person, even if the needle is changed. Inform about potential risks and benefits of therapy. Counsel on proper inj technique, lifestyle management, regular glucose monitoring, periodic HbA1c testing, recognition and management of hypo/hyperglycemia, adherence to meal planning, complications of insulin therapy, timing of dose, instruction in the use of inj devices, and proper storage of insulin. Inform that the ability to concentrate and react may be impaired as a result of hypoglycemia; advise to use caution when driving or operating machinery. Instruct to always carefully check that appropriate insulin is administered to avoid medication errors. Advise to inform physician if pregnant/intending to become pregnant.

STORAGE: Unopened: 2-8°C (36-46°F) until expiration date, or room temperature (<30°C [86°F]) for 28 days (vial) or 14 days (FlexPen). Do not freeze; do not use if it has been frozen. Do not store directly adjacent to the refrigerator cooling element. Opened: <30°C (86°F) for 28 days (vial) or 14 days (FlexPen). Do not refrigerate FlexPen; store w/o a needle attached. Protect from excessive heat or sunlight.

NOVOSEVEN RT – coagulation factor VIIa (recombinant) RX

Class: Antihemophilic agent

N

Serious arterial and venous thrombotic events reported. Monitor for signs/symptoms of activation of the coagulation system and for thrombosis.

ADULT DOSAGE

Congenital Hemophilia

Congenital Hemophilia A or B w/ Inhibitors:

Acute Bleeding Episodes:

Hemostatic: 90mcg/kg IV q2h until hemostasis is achieved, or until treatment has been judged to be inadequate; adjust dose based on severity of bleeding

Post-Hemostatic: 90mcg/kg IV q3-6h for severe bleeds until after homeostasis is achieved to maintain the hemostatic plug; monitor and minimize duration

Perioperative Management:

Minor Surgery:

Initial: 90mcg/kg IV immediately before surgery and repeat q2h for the duration of surgery

Postsurgical: 90mcg/kg IV q2h for 48 hrs, then q2-6h until healing occurs

Major Surgery:

Initial: 90mcg/kg IV immediately before surgery and repeat q2h for the duration of surgery

Postsurgical: 90mcg/kg IV q2h for 5 days, then q4h until healing occurs

Administer additional bolus doses if required

Acquired Hemophilia

Acute Bleeding Episodes:

70-90mcg/kg IV q2-3h until hemostasis is achieved

PEDIATRIC DOSAGE

Congenital Hemophilia

Congenital Hemophilia A or B w/ Inhibitors:

Acute Bleeding Episodes:

Hemostatic: 90mcg/kg IV q2h until hemostasis is achieved, or until treatment has been judged to be inadequate; adjust dose based on severity of bleeding

Post-Hemostatic: 90mcg/kg IV q3-6h for severe bleeds until after homeostasis is achieved to maintain the hemostatic plug; monitor and minimize duration

Perioperative Management:

Minor Surgery:

Initial: 90mcg/kg IV immediately before surgery and repeat q2h for the duration of surgery

Postsurgical: 90mcg/kg IV q2h for 48 hrs, then q2-6h until healing occurs

Major Surgery:

Initial: 90mcg/kg IV immediately before surgery and repeat q2h for the duration of surgery

Postsurgical: 90mcg/kg IV q2h for 5 days, then q4h until healing occurs

Administer additional bolus doses if required

Factor VII Deficiency

Congenital:

Acute Bleeding Episodes:

Perioperative Management:
Minor/Major Surgery: 70-90mcg/kg IV immediately before surgery and repeat q2-3h for the duration of surgery, and until hemostasis is achieved

Factor VII Deficiency

Congenital:
Acute Bleeding Episodes:
15-30mcg/kg IV q4-6h until hemostasis is achieved

Perioperative Management:
Minor/Major Surgery: 15-30mcg/kg IV immediately before surgery and repeat q4-6h for the duration of surgery and until hemostasis is achieved

Effective treatment has been achieved w/ doses as low as 10mcg/kg

Glanzmann's Thrombasthenia

Refractory to platelet transfusions, w/ or w/o antibodies to platelets

Acute Bleeding Episodes:
90mcg/kg IV q2-6h in severe bleeding episodes requiring systemic hemostatic therapy until hemostasis is achieved

Perioperative Management:
Minor/Major Surgery:
Initial: 90mcg/kg IV immediately before surgery and repeat q2h for the duration of the procedure
Postsurgical: 90mcg/kg IV q2-6h to prevent postoperative bleeding

Higher average infused doses (median dose of 100mcg/kg) were noted for surgical patients who had clinical refractoriness w/ or w/o platelet-specific antibodies compared to those w/ neither

15-30mcg/kg IV q4-6h until hemostasis is achieved

Perioperative Management:
Minor/Major Surgery: 15-30mcg/kg IV immediately before surgery and repeat q4-6h for the duration of surgery and until hemostasis is achieved

Effective treatment has been achieved w/ doses as low as 10mcg/kg

Glanzmann's Thrombasthenia

Refractory to platelet transfusions, w/ or w/o antibodies to platelets

Acute Bleeding Episodes:
90mcg/kg IV q2-6h in severe bleeding episodes requiring systemic hemostatic therapy until hemostasis is achieved

Perioperative Management:
Minor/Major Surgery:
Initial: 90mcg/kg IV immediately before surgery and repeat q2h for the duration of the procedure
Postsurgical: 90mcg/kg IV q2-6h to prevent postoperative bleeding

Higher average infused doses (median dose of 100mcg/kg) were noted for surgical patients who had clinical refractoriness w/ or w/o platelet-specific antibodies compared to those w/ neither

ADMINISTRATION

IV route

For IV bolus only; administer as a slow bolus inj over 2-5 min, depending on the dose administered.
Do not mix w/ other infusion sol.
Use 0.9% NaCl inj if line needs to be flushed before/after administration.
Administer w/in 3 hrs after reconstitution and discard any unused sol.

Reconstitution

Bring the powder and diluent to room temperature but not >37°C (98.6°F).

Powder and Vial of Diluent:
Add 1.1mL, 2.1mL, 5.2mL, or 8.1mL of the histidine diluent to 1mg, 2mg, 5mg, or 8mg vial of the powder respectively.
Use syringe needles w/ 20-/26-gauge size.
Do not inject the diluent directly on the powder but aim the needle against the side so that the stream of liquid runs down the vial wall.
Gently swirl until all the material dissolves.

Powder and Prefilled Diluent Syringe:
Use the 1mL, 2mL, 5mL, or 8mL of the prefilled diluent syringe for the 1mg, 2mg, 5mg, or 8mg vial respectively.
Refer to PI for further administration instructions.

HOW SUPPLIED

Inj: 1mg, 2mg, 5mg, 8mg

WARNINGS/PRECAUTIONS

Coagulation parameters do not necessarily correlate w/ or predict effectiveness of therapy.
Increased risk of developing thromboembolic events due to circulating tissue factor or predisposing coagulopathy in patients w/ disseminated intravascular coagulation (DIC), advanced atherosclerotic disease, crush injury, septicemia, and uncontrolled postpartum hemorrhage. Caution w/

administration to patients w/ an increased risk of thromboembolic complications (eg, history of coronary artery disease [CAD], liver disease, DIC, postoperative immobilization, elderly, neonates). Reduce dose or d/c treatment depending on patient's condition if there is lab confirmation of intravascular coagulation or presence of clinical thrombosis. Hypersensitivity reactions, including anaphylaxis, reported. Administer only if clearly needed in patients w/ known hypersensitivity to the drug or any of its components, or in patients w/ known hypersensitivity to mouse, hamster, or bovine proteins; if symptoms occur, d/c treatment, administer appropriate treatment, and weigh the benefit/risks prior to restarting treatment. Antibody formation may be suspected if FVIIa activity fails to reach expected level, PT is not corrected, or bleeding is not controlled after treatment w/ recommended doses; perform analysis for antibodies. Lab test interactions may occur.

ADVERSE REACTIONS

Arterial and venous thrombotic events, fever, pain, deep thrombophlebitis, pulmonary embolism, cerebrovascular disorder, angina pectoris, anaphylactic shock, abnormal hepatic function.

DRUG INTERACTIONS

Avoid simultaneous use w/ activated prothrombin complex concentrates or prothrombin complex concentrates. Thrombosis may occur if administered concomitantly w/ coagulation factor XIII.

PATIENT CONSIDERATIONS

Assessment: Assess for risk of thromboembolic complications (eg, DIC, history of CAD, liver disease, postoperative immobilization), hypersensitivity to drug, mouse, hamster, or bovine proteins, pregnancy/nursing status, and for possible drug interactions. Obtain baseline PT and FVII coagulant activity in FVII-deficient patients.

Monitoring: Monitor for development of signs/symptoms of activation of the coagulation system or thrombosis. Monitor PT, FVII activity, and for antibody formation in FVII-deficient patients. Monitor for hypersensitivity reactions, including anaphylaxis, and other adverse reactions.

Counseling: Advise to immediately seek medical help if early signs of hypersensitivity reactions (eg, hives, urticaria, tightness of chest) and signs of thrombosis (eg, new onset swelling and pain in the limbs or abdomen, new onset chest pain, SOB) occur.

STORAGE: 2-25°C (36-77°F). Do not freeze. Protect from light. **Reconstituted Sol:** Room temperature or refrigerated for up to 3 hrs. Do not freeze or store in syringes.

N

NUCALA – mepolizumab

RX

Class: Monoclonal antibody/interleukin-5 (IL-5) receptor antagonist

ADULT DOSAGE

Asthma

Add-on maint treatment of severe asthma in patients w/ an eosinophilic phenotype

100mg SQ every 4 weeks into the upper arm, thigh, or abdomen

PEDIATRIC DOSAGE

Asthma

Add-on maint treatment of severe asthma in patients w/ an eosinophilic phenotype

≥12 Years:

100mg SQ every 4 weeks into the upper arm, thigh, or abdomen

ADMINISTRATION

SQ route

Reconstitution Instructions

1. Reconstitute mepolizumab in the vial w/ 1.2mL sterile water for inj (SWFI), preferably using a 2 or 3mL syringe and a 21-gauge needle; the reconstituted sol will contain a concentration of 100mg/mL. Do not mix w/ other medications.
2. Direct the stream of SWFI vertically onto the center of the lyophilized cake. Gently swirl the vial for 10 sec w/ a circular motion at 15-sec intervals until the powder is dissolved. Do not shake the reconstituted sol.
3. If a mechanical reconstitution device (swirler) is used, swirl at 450 rpm for no longer than 10 min. Alternatively, swirling at 1000 rpm for no longer than 5 min is acceptable.
4. If the reconstituted sol is not used immediately, store at <30°C (86°F), do not freeze, and discard if not used w/in 8 hrs of reconstitution.

Administration

1. For SQ administration, preferably using a 1mL polypropylene syringe fitted w/ a disposable 21- to 27-gauge x 0.5-inch (13mm) needle.
2. Just before administration, remove 1mL of reconstituted mepolizumab. Do not shake the reconstituted sol.
3. Administer the 1mL inj (equivalent to 100mg mepolizumab) SQ into the upper arm, thigh, or abdomen.

HOW SUPPLIED

Inj: 100mg

CONTRAINDICATIONS

History of hypersensitivity to mepolizumab or excipients in the formulation.

WARNINGS/PRECAUTIONS

Not indicated for treatment of other eosinophilic conditions or relief of acute bronchospasm or status asthmaticus. D/C in the event of a hypersensitivity reaction. Herpes zoster reported; consider varicella vaccination if medically appropriate prior to starting therapy. Do not d/c systemic or inhaled corticosteroids abruptly upon initiation of therapy; reductions in corticosteroid dose, if appropriate, should be gradual and performed under the direct supervision of a physician. Reduction in corticosteroid dose may be associated w/ systemic withdrawal symptoms and/or unmask conditions previously suppressed by systemic corticosteroid therapy. Treat patients w/ preexisting helminth infections before initiating therapy; if patients become infected while receiving treatment and do not respond to anti-helminth treatment, d/c mepolizumab until infection resolves.

ADVERSE REACTIONS

Headache, inj-site reactions, back pain, fatigue, influenza, UTI, upper abdominal pain, pruritus, eczema, muscle spasms.

PATIENT CONSIDERATIONS

Assessment: Assess for other eosinophilic conditions, acute bronchospasm or status asthmaticus, preexisting helminth infections, hypersensitivity to drug or excipients in the formulation, and pregnancy/nursing status.

Monitoring: Monitor for hypersensitivity reactions, acute asthma symptoms or acute exacerbations, herpes zoster, parasitic infection, and other adverse reactions.

Counseling: Inform that hypersensitivity reactions have occurred after administration and instruct to contact physician if such reactions occur. Inform that mepolizumab does not treat acute asthma symptoms or acute exacerbations. Instruct to seek medical advice if asthma remains uncontrolled or worsens after initiation of treatment. Inform that herpes zoster infections have occurred and where medically appropriate, varicella vaccination should be considered before starting treatment. Instruct not to d/c systemic or inhaled corticosteroids except under the direct supervision of a physician. Inform women there is a pregnancy exposure registry that monitors pregnancy outcomes in women exposed to mepolizumab during pregnancy.

STORAGE: <25°C (77°F). Do not freeze. Store in the original package to protect from light.

N

NUCYNTA — tapentadol

CII

Class: Centrally acting analgesic

ADULT DOSAGE

Acute Pain

Moderate to Severe:

Usual: 50mg, 75mg, or 100mg q4-6h depending upon pain intensity

Day 1: May give 2nd dose 1 hr after 1st dose if pain relief is inadequate, then 50mg, 75mg, or 100mg q4-6h

Adjust dose to maintain adequate analgesia w/ acceptable tolerability

Max: 700mg on Day 1, then 600mg/day thereafter

Periodically reassess continued need for use during chronic therapy, especially for noncancer-related pain

PEDIATRIC DOSAGE

Pediatric use may not have been established

DOSING CONSIDERATIONS

Hepatic Impairment

Moderate (Child-Pugh Score 7-9):

Initial: 50mg no more frequently than once q8h

Max: 3 doses/24 hrs

Elderly

Start at lower end of dosing range

Discontinuation

Taper dose gradually

ADMINISTRATION
Oral route

Take w/ or w/o food

HOW SUPPLIED
Tab: 50mg, 75mg, 100mg

CONTRAINDICATIONS
Significant respiratory depression, acute or severe bronchial asthma or hypercarbia in an unmonitored setting or in the absence of resuscitative equipment, known or suspected paralytic ileus, and patients receiving MAOIs or who have taken them within the last 14 days. Hypersensitivity (eg, anaphylaxis, angioedema) to tapentadol or to any other ingredients of the product.

WARNINGS/PRECAUTIONS
Abuse liability similar to other opioid agonists legal or illicit; assess each patient's risk for opioid abuse or addiction prior to prescribing. Routinely monitor all patients for signs of misuse, abuse, and addiction; misuse or abuse by crushing, chewing, snorting, or injecting will pose a significant risk that could result in overdose and death. Respiratory depression, if not immediately recognized and treated, may lead to respiratory arrest and death. Accidental ingestion, especially in children, can result in fatal overdose. Respiratory depression is more likely to occur in elderly, cachectic, or debilitated patients; monitor closely, particularly when given with drugs that depress respiration. Monitor for respiratory depression and consider use of alternative nonopioid analgesics in patients with significant COPD or cor pulmonale, and in patients with a substantially decreased respiratory reserve, hypoxia, hypercarbia, or preexisting respiratory depression. May cause severe hypotension. Monitor for signs of sedation and respiratory depression in patients susceptible to the intracranial effects of carbon dioxide retention (eg, those with evidence of increased intracranial pressure or brain tumors). May obscure clinical course in patients with a head injury. Avoid with circulatory shock, impaired consciousness, or coma. May aggravate convulsions in patients with convulsive disorders and may induce or aggravate seizures; monitor for worsened seizure control in patients with history of seizure disorders. May cause spasm of sphincter of Oddi; monitor for worsening symptoms in patients with biliary tract disease (eg, acute pancreatitis). Withdrawal symptoms may occur if discontinued abruptly. May impair mental/physical abilities. Monitor for respiratory/CNS depression with moderate hepatic impairment. Avoid use with severe renal/hepatic impairment. Not for use during and immediately prior to labor.

ADVERSE REACTIONS
N/V, dizziness, somnolence, constipation, pruritus, dry mouth, hyperhidrosis, fatigue.

DRUG INTERACTIONS
See Contraindications. Avoid use with alcoholic beverages or medications containing alcohol, other opioids, or drugs of abuse; may have additive effects. CNS depressants (eg, sedatives or hypnotics, general anesthetics, phenothiazines, tranquilizers, alcohol, anxiolytics, neuroleptics, muscle relaxants, other opioids, illicit drugs) may increase risk of respiratory depression, hypotension, profound sedation, or coma; start tapentadol at 1/3 to 1/2 of the usual dose and consider using a lower dose of concomitant CNS depressant. Serotonin syndrome may occur with serotonergic drugs (eg, SSRIs, SNRIs, TCAs, triptans, drugs that affect the serotonergic neurotransmitter system [eg, mirtazapine, trazodone, tramadol]), and drugs that may impair metabolism of serotonin (eg, MAOIs); use with caution. Avoid use with mixed agonist/antagonist analgesics (eg, butorphanol, nalbuphine, pentazocine), and partial agonists (eg, buprenorphine); may precipitate withdrawal symptoms. Anticholinergics may increase risk of urinary retention and/or severe constipation, which may lead to paralytic ileus.

PATIENT CONSIDERATIONS

Assessment: Assess for personal/family history or risk factors for drug abuse or addiction, general condition and medical status, opioid experience/tolerance, pain type/severity, previous opioid daily dose, potency and type of prior analgesics used, respiratory depression, COPD or other respiratory complications, GI obstruction, paralytic ileus, renal/hepatic impairment, pregnancy/nursing status, possible drug interactions, and any other condition where treatment is contraindicated or cautioned.

Monitoring: Monitor for improvement of pain, signs/symptoms of respiratory depression, hypotension, symptoms of worsening biliary tract disease, aggravation/induction of seizure, tolerance, physical dependence, mental/physical impairment, serotonin syndrome, and other adverse reactions. Routinely monitor for signs of misuse, abuse, and addiction. Periodically reassess continued need for use during chronic therapy, especially for noncancer-related pain.

Counseling: Instruct to take only as prescribed and not to d/c without first discussing the need for a tapering regimen with prescriber. Inform that drug has potential for abuse; instruct not to share drug with others and to take steps to protect from theft or misuse. Discuss the risks of respiratory depression, orthostatic hypotension, syncope, severe constipation, and anaphylaxis; counsel on how to recognize symptoms and when to seek medical attention. Inform that accidental exposure may result in serious harm or death; advise to dispose unused tabs by flushing them down the toilet. Inform about risks of concomitant use of alcohol, other CNS depressants, MAOIs, and serotonergic drugs; instruct to notify physician if taking/planning to take additional medications. Instruct to not consume alcoholic beverages, or take prescription and OTC products that contain alcohol, during treatment. Counsel that drug may cause seizures if at risk for seizures or if patient has epilepsy; advise to d/c therapy and seek medical attention if seizures occur during therapy. Inform that drug may impair the ability to perform potentially hazardous activities (eg, driving a car or operating heavy machinery); advise not to perform such tasks until patients know how they will react to the medication. Advise females that drug can cause fetal harm; instruct to notify physician if pregnant/planning to become pregnant.

STORAGE: ≤25°C (77°F); excursions permitted to 15-30°C (59-86°F). Protect from moisture.

NUCYNTA ER – tapentadol

CII

Class: Centrally acting analgesic

Exposes users to risks of addiction, abuse, and misuse, which can lead to overdose and death; assess each patient's risk prior to prescribing and monitor regularly for development of these behaviors/conditions. Serious, life-threatening, or fatal respiratory depression may occur; monitor during initiation or following a dose increase. Crushing, dissolving, or chewing tab can cause rapid release and absorption of potentially fatal dose; instruct patients to swallow tab whole. Accidental ingestion, especially by children, can result in a fatal overdose. Prolonged use during pregnancy can result in neonatal opioid withdrawal syndrome; advise pregnant women of the risk and ensure availability of appropriate treatment. Avoid use with alcoholic beverages or medications containing alcohol; may result in increased levels and potentially fatal overdose of tapentadol.

ADULT DOSAGE

Severe Pain (Daily, Around-the-Clock Management)

Pain severe enough to require daily, around-the-clock, long-term opioid treatment and for which alternative treatment options are inadequate

1st Opioid Analgesic/Opioid Intolerant Patients:

Initial: 50mg bid (q12h)

Titrate: Increase by 50mg no more than twice daily every 3 days

Diabetic Peripheral Neuropathy

Neuropathic pain severe enough to require daily, around-the-clock, long-term opioid treatment and for which alternative treatment options are inadequate

1st Opioid Analgesic/Opioid Intolerant Patients:

Initial: 50mg bid (q12h)

Titrate: Increase by 50mg no more than twice daily every 3 days

Conversions

From Immediate-Release (IR) to (Extended-Release) ER Tapentadol:

Use the equivalent total daily dose of IR tapentadol and divide it into 2 equal doses of ER tapentadol separated by approx 12-hr intervals

From Other Opioids:

D/C all other around-the-clock opioids when therapy is initiated; begin w/ 1/2 of the estimated daily tapentadol requirement as the initial dose, managing inadequate analgesia by supplementation w/ IR rescue medication

PEDIATRIC DOSAGE

Pediatric use may not have been established

DOSING CONSIDERATIONS

Renal Impairment

Severe: Not recommended

Hepatic Impairment

Moderate (Child-Pugh Score 7-9):

Initial: 50mg qd

Max: 100mg/day

N

Severe (Child-Pugh Score 10-15):
Not recommended

Elderly
Start at lower end of dosing range

Discontinuation
Use gradual downward titration

ADMINISTRATION

Oral route

Swallow tab whole; do not cut, crush, dissolve, or chew
Take 1 tab at a time w/ enough water to ensure complete swallowing

HOW SUPPLIED

Tab, ER: 50mg, 100mg, 150mg, 200mg, 250mg

CONTRAINDICATIONS

Significant respiratory depression, acute or severe bronchial asthma or hypercarbia in an unmonitored setting or in the absence of resuscitative equipment, known or suspected paralytic ileus, patients receiving MAOIs or who have taken them within the last 14 days. Hypersensitivity (eg, anaphylaxis, angioedema) to tapentadol or to any other ingredients of the product.

WARNINGS/PRECAUTIONS

Reserve for use in patients for whom alternative treatment options are ineffective, not tolerated, or would be otherwise inadequate to provide sufficient management of pain. Should only be prescribed by healthcare professionals who are knowledgeable in the use of potent opioids for management of chronic pain. D/C all other tapentadol and tramadol products when initiating and during therapy. Life-threatening respiratory depression is more likely to occur in elderly, cachectic, or debilitated patients. Consider alternative nonopioid analgesics in patients with significant COPD or cor pulmonale, and in patients having a substantially decreased respiratory reserve, hypoxia, hypercarbia, or preexisting respiratory depression. May cause severe hypotension; increased risk in patients whose ability to maintain BP is compromised by a reduced blood volume or concurrent administration of certain CNS depressants. Avoid with circulatory shock, impaired consciousness, or coma. Monitor patients who may be susceptible to intracranial effects of carbon dioxide retention for signs of sedation and respiratory depression when initiating therapy. May obscure clinical course in patients with head injury. May aggravate convulsions and induce/aggravate seizures. May cause spasm of sphincter of Oddi; monitor patients with biliary tract disease (eg, acute pancreatitis). May impair mental/physical abilities. Monitor for respiratory/CNS depression with moderate hepatic impairment. Not recommended with severe renal/hepatic impairment.

ADVERSE REACTIONS

Respiratory depression, N/V, dizziness, constipation, headache, somnolence, fatigue, dry mouth, hyperhidrosis, pruritus, insomnia, dyspepsia, diarrhea, decreased appetite, anxiety.

DRUG INTERACTIONS

See Boxed Warning and Contraindications. Hypotension, profound sedation, coma, and respiratory depression may occur with CNS depressants (eg, sedatives, anxiolytics, hypnotics); if coadministration is required, consider dose reduction of one or both agents. Serotonin syndrome may occur with serotonergic drugs (eg, SSRIs, SNRIs, TCAs, triptans, drugs that affect serotonergic neurotransmitter system) and drugs that may impair metabolism of serotonin (eg, MAOIs). Avoid use of mixed agonist/antagonist (eg, nalbuphine, pentazocine, butorphanol) and partial agonists (eg, buprenorphine) analgesics; may reduce analgesic effects and/or precipitate withdrawal symptoms. Enhanced neuromuscular blocking action and increased degree of respiratory depression with skeletal muscle relaxants. Anticholinergics may increase risk of urinary retention and/or severe constipation, which may lead to paralytic ileus.

PATIENT CONSIDERATIONS

Assessment: Assess for abuse/addiction risk, opioid experience/tolerance, pain type/severity, pregnancy/nursing status, possible drug interactions, and any other condition where treatment is contraindicated or cautioned.

Monitoring: Monitor for signs/symptoms of respiratory depression, hypotension, symptoms of worsening biliary tract disease, aggravation/induction of seizure, mental/physical impairment, serotonin syndrome, and other adverse reactions. Routinely monitor for signs of misuse, abuse, and addiction.

Counseling: Inform that drug has potential for abuse and addiction; instruct not to share drug with others and to take steps to protect from theft or misuse. Inform about risk of accidental exposure and advise to store securely and to dispose unused tabs by flushing them down the toilet. Inform about the risks of life-threatening respiratory depression, orthostatic hypotension, and syncope. Inform about risks of concomitant use of alcohol, other CNS depressants, MAOIs, and serotonergic drugs; instruct to notify physician if taking/planning to take additional medications. Instruct to not consume alcoholic beverages or take prescription/OTC products that contain alcohol during treatment. Counsel on the risk for seizures and advise to d/c therapy and seek medical attention if seizures occur. Advise to use ud. Inform that drug may impair the ability to perform potentially hazardous activities; advise not to perform such tasks until patients know how they will react to medication. Advise of potential for severe constipation, including management instructions. Advise how to recognize anaphylaxis and when to seek medical attention. Advise females that drug can cause fetal harm; instruct to notify physician if pregnant/planning to become pregnant.

STORAGE: ≤25°C (77°F); excursions permitted to 15-30°C (59-86°F). Protect from moisture.

NuLYTELY – polyethylene glycol 3350/potassium chloride/sodium bicarbonate/sodium chloride

RX

Class: Bowel cleanser

OTHER BRAND NAMES

Trilyte

ADULT DOSAGE

Bowel Cleansing

Prior to Colonoscopy:

Oral:

240mL (8 oz) every 10 min until 4L consumed or rectal effluent is clear

NG Tube:

20-30mL/min (1.2-1.8L/hr)

PEDIATRIC DOSAGE

Bowel Cleansing

Prior to Colonoscopy:

≥6 Months of Age:

Oral/NG Tube:

25mL/kg/hr until rectal effluent is clear

ADMINISTRATION

Oral/NG Tube route

May be used w/ or w/o flavor pack
Rapid drinking of each portion is preferred to drinking small amounts continuously
First bowel movement should occur approx 1 hr after the start of administration

Nulytely

Sol is more palatable if chilled prior to administration
Patients may consume water or clear liquids during and after completion of the bowel preparation up until 2 hrs before the time of the colonoscopy

Instructions Prior to Dosage:

On the day prior to colonoscopy, instruct patients to:
1. Take only clear liquids, but avoid red and purple liquids. Patients may consume a light breakfast
2. If adding a flavor pack, pour the contents of the 2g flavor powder into the container prior to reconstitution. No additional flavorings should be added. Discard unused flavor packs. The flavor packs are for use only in combination w/ the contents of the accompanying 4L container
3. Early in the pm prior to colonoscopy, fill the supplied container containing the powder (and if applicable, a flavor powder) w/ lukewarm water to the 4L fill line. The sol is clear and colorless when reconstituted to a final volume of 4L
4. After capping the container, shake vigorously several times to ensure that the ingredients are dissolved

Trilyte

Sol is more palatable if chilled prior to administration; chilled sol is not recommended for infants
No solid food should be consumed during the 3- to 4-hr period before drinking the sol, but in no case should solid foods be eaten w/in 2 hr of taking Trilyte w/ flavor packs

Preparation of Sol:

1. If adding a flavor pack, tear open 1 flavor pack at the indicated marking and pour contents into the bottle before reconstitution; discard unused flavor packs
2. Shake well to incorporate flavoring into the powder
3. Add tap water to fill line marked 4L
4. Replace cap tightly and shake well until all ingredients have dissolved; no additional ingredients should be added to the sol

HOW SUPPLIED

Sol (Powder): (Polyethylene Glycol (PEG) 3350/Potassium Chloride/Sodium Bicarbonate/Sodium Chloride) 420g/1.48g/5.72g/11.2g [4L]

CONTRAINDICATIONS

GI obstruction, ileus, or gastric retention; bowel perforation; toxic colitis or toxic megacolon; known allergy or hypersensitivity to any component of NuLYTELY.

WARNINGS/PRECAUTIONS

Slow administration or temporarily d/c if severe bloating, distention, or abdominal pain develops; caution w/ severe ulcerative colitis. Monitor for occurrence of possible hypoglycemia in children <2 years of age as the sol has no caloric substrate. Dehydration and hypokalemia reported in

N

children. Caution in patients w/ impaired gag reflex, unconscious or semiconscious patients, and patients prone to regurgitation or aspiration; observe during administration especially if administered via NG tube. (Nulytely) Adequately hydrate before, during, and after use; caution w/ CHF when replacing fluids. Consider performing postcolonoscopy lab tests (electrolytes, SrCr, BUN) and treat accordingly if significant vomiting or signs of dehydration develop. Correct fluid and electrolyte abnormalities before treatment. Caution w/ conditions that increase risk for fluid and electrolyte disturbances or may increase risk of adverse events (eg, seizures, arrhythmias, and renal impairment). Serious arrhythmias reported rarely; caution in patients at increased risk of arrhythmias and consider predose and postcolonoscopy ECGs. Generalized tonic-clonic seizures and/or loss of consciousness reported; caution in patients w/ a history of or at increased risk of seizures (eg, w/ known/suspected hyponatremia). Caution w/ impaired renal function; consider performing baseline and postcolonoscopy lab tests. May produce colonic mucosal aphthous ulcerations; consider this when interpreting colonoscopy findings in patients w/ known/suspected inflammatory bowel disease. Serious cases of ischemic colitis reported. Not for direct ingestion; direct ingestion of undissolved powder may increase risk of N/V, dehydration, and electrolyte disturbances.

ADVERSE REACTIONS

Nausea, abdominal fullness, abdominal bloating.

DRUG INTERACTIONS

Oral medication administered w/in 1 hr of start of administration may be flushed from GI tract and may not be absorbed properly. (Nulytely) Caution w/ medications that increase risk for fluid and electrolyte disturbances or may increase risk of adverse events (eg, seizures, arrhythmias, prolonged QT, renal impairment). Caution w/ drugs that lower seizure threshold (eg, TCAs) and in patients withdrawing from alcohol or benzodiazepines. Caution w/ drugs that may affect renal function (eg, diuretics, ACE inhibitors, ARBs, NSAIDs). Avoid w/ stimulant laxatives (eg, bisacodyl, sodium picosulfate); may increase the risk of mucosal ulceration or ischemic colitis.

PATIENT CONSIDERATIONS

Assessment: Assess for drug hypersensitivity, GI obstruction, bowel perforation, gastric retention, ileus, toxic colitis, toxic megacolon, fluid and electrolyte abnormalities, renal impairment, any other conditions where treatment is cautioned, pregnancy/nursing status, and possible drug interactions. Consider predose ECG in patients at increased risk of serious cardiac arrhythmias.

Monitoring: Monitor arrhythmias, generalized tonic-clonic seizures, loss of consciousness, colonic mucosal aphthous ulceration, ischemic colitis, and other adverse reactions. Monitor patients w/ impaired gag reflex, unconscious or semiconscious patients, and patients prone to regurgitation/ aspiration, especially if administered via NG tube. Monitor for hypoglycemia, dehydration, and hypokalemia in children. Consider performing postcolonoscopy lab tests (electrolytes, SrCr, BUN) in patients w/ dehydration or renal impairment.

Counseling: Inform that sol is more palatable if chilled. Instruct to inform physician if patient has trouble swallowing or is prone to regurgitation or aspiration. Instruct not to take other laxatives. Instruct to consume water or clear liquids during the bowel preparation and after completion of the bowel preparation up until 2 hrs before the time of the colonoscopy. If severe bloating, distention, or abdominal pain occurs, instruct to slow or temporarily d/c administration until symptoms abate; advise to report these events to physician. Instruct to d/c and contact physician if hives, rashes, or any allergic reaction develops. Instruct to notify physician if signs/symptoms of dehydration develop. Inform that oral medication administered w/in 1 hr of the start of administration may be flushed from the GI tract and the medication may not be absorbed completely. Counsel that rapid drinking of each portion is preferred rather than drinking small amounts continuously. Inform that 1st bowel movement should occur approximately 1 hr after start of administration and to continue drinking until the watery stool is clear and free of solid matter.

STORAGE: 25°C (77°F); excursions permitted between 15-30°C (59-86°F). Reconstituted Sol: Keep refrigerated. Use w/in 48 hrs.

NUTROPIN – somatropin (rDNA origin) RX

Class: Recombinant human growth hormone (hGH)

OTHER BRAND NAMES

Nutropin AQ

ADULT DOSAGE

Growth Hormone Deficiency

Adult or Childhood-Onset Etiology:
Weight-Based:
Initial: ≤0.006mg/kg qd SQ
Titrate: May increase based on individual requirements

PEDIATRIC DOSAGE

Growth Hormone Deficiency

Due to an inadequate secretion of endogenous growth hormone

Individualize dose

Usual: Up to 0.3mg/kg/week

Maint: Individualize dose
Max:
≤35 Years: 0.025mg/kg qd
>35 Years: 0.0125mg/kg qd

Non-Weight-Based:
Initial: 0.2mg/day SQ (range, 0.15-0.30mg/day)
Titrate: May increase gradually every 1-2 months by increments of 0.1-0.2mg/day based on clinical response and serum insulin-like growth factor-I (IGF-I) concentrations
Maint: Individualize dose

Pubertal Patients: May use up to 0.7mg/kg/week
Divide weekly dose into daily SQ inj

Idiopathic Short Stature

Treatment of idiopathic short stature defined by height standard deviation score ≤-2.25, and associated w/ growth rates unlikely to permit attainment of adult height in the normal range, in pediatric patients whose epiphyses are not closed and for whom diagnostic evaluation excludes other causes associated w/ short stature that should be observed or treated by other means
Individualize dose
Usual: Up to 0.3mg/kg/week
May use up to 0.7mg/kg/week in pubertal patients w/ growth hormone deficiency
Divide weekly dose into daily SQ inj

Growth Failure Secondary to Chronic Kidney Disease

Individualize dose
Usual: Up to 0.35mg/kg/week
Continue therapy up to the time of renal transplantation
Divide weekly dose into daily SQ inj
Hemodialysis: Give at hs or at least 3-4 hrs after dialysis
Chronic Cycling Peritoneal Dialysis: Give in am after completion of dialysis
Chronic Ambulatory Peritoneal Dialysis: Give in pm during overnight exchange

Turner Syndrome

Treatment of short stature associated w/ Turner syndrome
Individualize dose
Usual: Up to 0.375mg/kg/week divided into equal doses 3-7X/week SQ

DOSING CONSIDERATIONS

Concomitant Medications

Oral Estrogen: May increase the dose requirements in women

Elderly

Consider lower starting dose and smaller dose increments

ADMINISTRATION

SQ route
Rotate inj sites to avoid lipodystrophy

Reconstitution

Vial:
After the dose has been determined, reconstitute as follows:
1. Each 10 mg vial should be reconstituted w/ 1-10mL of bacteriostatic water for inj (benzyl alcohol preserved) only. The pH of Nutropin after reconstitution w/ bacteriostatic water for inj (benzyl alcohol preserved) is approx 7.4
2. For use in newborns or if sensitivity to the diluents occurs, may reconstitute w/ sterile water for inj; use immediately and discard unused portion
3. Following reconstitution, swirl the vial w/ a gentle rotary motion until contents are completely dissolved; do not shake, and use it only if it is clear

Cartridge:
1. The Nutropin AQ Pen 10 and 20mg cartridges are color-banded to help ensure appropriate use w/ the Nutropin AQ Pen delivery device. Each cartridge must be used w/ its corresponding color-coded Nutropin AQ Pen
2. Follow the directions provided in the Nutropin AQ Pen and Nutropin AQ NuSpin 5, 10, or 20 instructions for use

HOW SUPPLIED

Inj: 10mg; (AQ) 10mg/2mL, 20mg/2mL [pen cartridge], 5mg/2mL, 10mg/2mL, 20mg/2mL [NuSpin]

CONTRAINDICATIONS

Acute critical illness due to complications following open-heart surgery, abdominal surgery, multiple accidental trauma, or with acute respiratory failure. Pediatric patients with Prader-Willi syndrome (PWS) who are severely obese, have a history of upper airway obstruction or sleep apnea, or have severe respiratory impairment. Pediatric patients who have growth failure due to genetically confirmed PWS. Active malignancy, or evidence of progression or recurrence of an underlying intracranial tumor. Active proliferative or severe nonproliferative diabetic retinopathy. Growth promotion in pediatric patients with closed epiphysis. Known hypersensitivity to somatropin, excipients, or diluent.

WARNINGS/PRECAUTIONS

Reevaluate adults who were treated with somatropin for GHD in childhood and whose epiphyses are closed. Treatment for short stature should be discontinued when epiphyses are fused. Implement effective weight control in patients with PWS and treat respiratory infections aggressively. Increased risk of developing malignancies in children with certain rare genetic causes of short stature; monitor for development of neoplasms if treatment is initiated. Monitor for increased growth, or potential malignant changes, of preexisting nevi. Undiagnosed impaired glucose tolerance and overt diabetes mellitus (DM) may be unmasked, and new-onset type 2 DM reported. Intracranial HTN with papilledema, visual changes, headache, N/V reported; d/c therapy if papilledema occurs. Fluid retention in adults may occur. Monitor other hormonal replacement treatments in patients with hypopituitarism. Undiagnosed/untreated hypothyroidism may prevent optimal response. Hypothyroidism may become evident or worsen. Slipped capital femoral epiphysis (SCFE) and progression of scoliosis may occur in pediatric patients. Increased risk of ear/hearing disorders and cardiovascular (CV) disorders in TS patients. Periodically examine children with growth failure secondary to CKD for evidence of renal osteodystrophy progression. Tissue atrophy may occur; rotate inj site. Allergic reactions may occur. Serum levels of inorganic phosphorus, alkaline phosphatase, parathyroid hormone, and IGF-I may increase. Pancreatitis reported rarely. Bacteriostatic water for inj diluent contains benzyl alcohol, which has been associated with serious adverse events and death, particularly in pediatric patients. Obese individuals are more likely to manifest adverse effects when treated with a weight based regimen. Estrogen replete women may need higher doses than men. Caution in elderly.

ADVERSE REACTIONS

Arthralgia, edema, joint disorders, otitis media, ear disorders, glucose intolerance, fluid retention.

DRUG INTERACTIONS

May inhibit 11β-hydroxysteroid dehydrogenase type 1, resulting in reduced serum cortisol concentrations; may need glucocorticoid replacement or dose adjustments of glucocorticoid therapy. Glucocorticoid therapy may attenuate growth-promoting effects in children; carefully adjust glucocorticoid replacement therapy. May increase clearance of antipyrine. May alter clearance of compounds metabolized by CYP450 liver enzymes (eg, corticosteroids, sex steroids, anticonvulsants, cyclosporine); monitor carefully. May need to adjust dose of insulin and/or oral/injectable hypoglycemic agents, and thyroid hormone replacement therapy.

PATIENT CONSIDERATIONS

Assessment: Assess for PWS, preexisting DM or impaired glucose tolerance, hypothyroidism, hypopituitarism, history of scoliosis, hypersensitivity, any other conditions where treatment is contraindicated or cautioned, pregnancy/nursing status, and possible drug interactions. Perform funduscopic exam. Obtain x-rays of the hip in CKD patients.

Monitoring: Monitor for growth, clinical response, compliance, neoplasm, increased growth or malignant changes of preexisting nevi, fluid retention, intracranial HTN, allergic reactions, pancreatitis, and SCFE and progression of scoliosis in pediatric patients (eg, onset of limp, hip or knee pain). Perform periodic thyroid function tests, funduscopic exam, and monitoring glucose levels. In patients with PWS, monitor weight as well as for signs of respiratory infection, sleep apnea, and upper airway obstruction. Monitor patients with a history of GHD secondary to an intracranial neoplasm routinely for progression/recurrence of the tumor. In patients with TS, monitor for ear/CV disorders.

Counseling: Inform about potential benefits and risks of therapy, proper administration, and usage and disposal. Caution against any reuse of needles and syringes.

STORAGE: 2-8°C (36-46°F). Avoid freezing. After Reconstitution with Bacteriostatic Water for Inj: 2-8°C (36-46°F) for 14 days. Avoid freezing. (AQ) 2-8°C (36-46°F) for 28 days after initial use. Avoid freezing. Protect from light.

NuvaRing – ethinyl estradiol/etonogestrel

RX

Class: Estrogen/progestogen combination

Cigarette smoking increases the risk of serious cardiovascular (CV) events. Risk increases with age and with number of cigarettes smoked. Not for use by women who are >35 yrs of age and smoke.

ADULT DOSAGE

Contraception

1 ring, inserted in the vagina and left in place continuously for 3 weeks, then removed for 1 week. Insert new ring 1 week after the last ring was removed

No Hormonal Contraceptive Use in the Preceding Cycle:
May insert ring on Days 1-5 of menstrual bleeding; if inserted on Days 2-5 of cycle, use an additional barrier method of contraception (eg, male condom w/ spermicide) for the first 7 days

Changing from a Combination Hormonal Contraceptive:
May switch on any day, but at the latest on the day following the usual hormone-free interval

Changing from Progestin-Only Method (Progestin-Only Pill, Implant, Inj, or Progestin-Releasing Intrauterine System):
May switch on any day from the progestin-only pill; start using ring on the day after taking last progestin-only pill
May switch from an implant or intrauterine system on the day of its removal and from an injectable on the day when the next inj is due
In all cases, additional barrier method (eg, male condom w/ spermicide) should be used for the first 7 days

Use After Abortion/Miscarriage:
May start w/in the first 5 days following a complete 1st trimester abortion/miscarriage; no additional method of contraception needed
If not started w/in 5 days, follow instructions for "No Hormonal Contraceptive Use in the Preceding Cycle" and use a non-hormonal contraceptive method in the meantime

Following Childbirth or 2nd Trimester Abortion/Miscarriage:
Use may be initiated no earlier than 4 weeks postpartum in women who elect not to breastfeed, or 4 weeks after a 2nd trimester abortion/miscarriage
If use is begun postpartum, use an additional method of contraception (eg, male condom w/ spermicide) for the first 7 days

PEDIATRIC DOSAGE

Contraception

Not indicated for use premenarche; refer to adult dosing

DOSING CONSIDERATIONS

Other Important Considerations

Inadvertent Removal/Expulsion:

Ring is Left Outside of Vagina for <3 Hrs: Rinse and reinsert as soon as possible, but at the latest w/in 3 hrs. If ring is lost, insert new vaginal ring and continue regimen w/o alteration

Ring is Left Outside of Vagina for >3 Hrs During Weeks 1 and 2: Reinsert ring as soon as remembered and use barrier method (eg, condoms w/ spermicides) until ring has been used continuously for 7 days

Ring is Left Outside of Vagina for >3 Hrs During Week 3: Discard that ring and insert new ring immediately which will start the next 3-week use period. Alternatively, insert new ring no later than 7 days from the time the previous ring was removed/expelled if previous ring was used continuously for at least 7 days. In either case, use a barrier method (eg, condoms w/ spermicides) until new ring has been used continuously for 7 days

Prolonged Ring-Free Interval:
If ring-free interval has been extended beyond 1 week, must use additional method of contraception until ring has been used continuously for 7 days

Prolonged Use of Ring:
Left in Place for Up to 1 Extra Week (up to 4 Weeks Total): Remove ring and insert new ring after 1-week ring-free interval

Left in Place for >4 Weeks: Remove ring, and if pregnancy is ruled out, may restart ring w/ additional method of contraception until ring has been used continuously for 7 days

Ring Breakage:
Discard ring and replace w/ new ring

Use w/ Other Vaginal Products:
Use of diaphragm is not recommended as backup method w/ ring use; ring may interfere w/ correct placement/position of a diaphragm

ADMINISTRATION

Intravaginal route

Compress ring and insert into the vagina; exact position of ring inside the vagina is not critical for its function
Ring must be inserted on the appropriate day and left in place for 3 consecutive weeks
Remove ring 3 weeks later, on the same day of the week and at about the same time as it was inserted

Removal/Reinsertion
Remove by hooking index finger under the forward rim or by grasping the rim between index and middle finger and pulling out
Used ring should be placed in the sachet (foil pouch) and discarded in a waste receptacle; do not flush in toilet
Reinsert new ring exactly 1 week after previous ring was removed, even if menstrual bleeding has not finished

HOW SUPPLIED

Vaginal ring: (Ethinyl Estradiol/Etonogestrel) (0.015mg/0.120mg)/day

CONTRAINDICATIONS

A high risk of arterial or venous thrombotic diseases (eg, women who are known to smoke [if >35 yrs of age]), current or history of deep vein thrombosis or pulmonary embolism, cerebrovascular disease, coronary artery disease, thrombogenic valvular or thrombogenic rhythm diseases of the heart (eg, subacute bacterial endocarditis with valvular disease, or atrial fibrillation), inherited or acquired hypercoagulopathies, uncontrolled HTN, diabetes mellitus with vascular disease, headaches with focal neurological symptoms or migraine headaches with aura, >35 yrs of age with any migraine headaches. Benign or malignant liver tumors or liver disease, undiagnosed abnormal uterine bleeding, pregnancy, current or history of breast cancer or other estrogen- or progestin-sensitive cancer. Hypersensitivity to any of the components of NuvaRing.

WARNINGS/PRECAUTIONS

Consider possibility of ovulation and conception prior to 1st use. Increased risk of a venous thromboembolic event (VTE) and arterial thromboses; d/c if these occur. D/C if unexplained loss of vision, proptosis, diplopia, papilledema, or retinal vascular lesions develop; evaluate for retinal vein thrombosis immediately. D/C at least 4 weeks prior to and 2 weeks after major surgery associated with an elevated risk of thromboembolism and during and following prolonged immobilization, if feasible. Caution in women with CV disease risk factors. If patient exhibits signs/symptoms of toxic shock syndrome (TSS), consider possibility of this diagnosis and initiate appropriate medical evaluation and treatment. Acute or chronic disturbances of liver function may necessitate discontinuation until LFTs return to normal and CHC causation has been excluded. D/C if jaundice develops. May increase risk of cervical cancer or intraepithelial neoplasia, hepatic adenoma, hepatocellular carcinoma, and gallbladder disease. Increase in BP reported; monitor BP and d/c if BP rises significantly. May not be suitable for women with conditions that make the vagina more susceptible to vaginal irritation or ulceration; vaginal/cervical erosion or ulceration reported. May increase risk of cholestasis with subsequent CHC use in patients with a history of CHC-related or pregnancy-related cholestasis. May decrease glucose tolerance; monitor prediabetic and diabetic women. Consider alternative contraception with uncontrolled dyslipidemia. May increase risk of pancreatitis with hypertriglyceridemia or a family history thereof. D/C if indicated and evaluate cause if new headaches that are recurrent, persistent, or severe develop. Consider discontinuation in case of increased frequency or severity of migraine during use. Unscheduled (breakthrough or intracyclic) bleeding and spotting reported; check for causes (eg, pregnancy, malignancy) if bleeding persists or occurs after previously regular cycles. Consider possibility of pregnancy if scheduled (withdrawal) bleeding does not occur and patient has not adhered to prescribed dosing schedule or has adhered to prescribed regimen and misses 2 consecutive periods; d/c if pregnancy confirmed. Caution with history of depression; d/c if it recurs to a serious degree. May induce or exacerbate angioedema in patients with hereditary angioedema. Chloasma may occur; avoid exposure to sun or UV radiation in women with a tendency to chloasma. Inadvertent insertion into urinary bladder reported; assess for ring insertion into urinary bladder with persistent urinary symptoms and if unable to locate ring. Cases of disconnection of the ring at the weld joint reported; discard the ring and replace it with a new ring if this occurs. May interfere with correct placement and position of a diaphragm. May influence results of certain lab tests.

ADVERSE REACTIONS

Vaginitis, headache, mood changes, device-related events, vaginal discharge, increased weight, N/V, vaginal discomfort, breast pain, dysmenorrhea, abdominal pain.

DRUG INTERACTIONS

May decrease plasma concentrations and potentially diminish effectiveness or increase breakthrough bleeding when used concomitantly with drugs or herbal products that induce CYP3A4 (eg, phenytoin, barbiturates, products containing St. John's wort); use an alternative method of contraception or a backup method when used concomitantly with enzyme inducers, and continue backup contraception for 28 days after discontinuing enzyme inducers. Atorvastatin, ascorbic acid, acetaminophen, CYP3A4 inhibitors (eg, itraconazole, grapefruit juice, ketoconazole), and vaginal miconazole nitrate may increase plasma hormone levels. HIV protease inhibitors (eg, nelfinavir, ritonavir, indinavir), hepatitis C virus protease inhibitors (eg, boceprevir, telaprevir), and non-nucleoside reverse transcriptase inhibitors (eg, nevirapine, etravirine) may cause significant changes in plasma levels. May inhibit the metabolism of other compounds (eg, cyclosporine, prednisolone, theophylline, tizanidine, voriconazole) and increase their plasma concentrations. May decrease levels of acetaminophen, clofibric acid, morphine, salicylic acid, and temazepam. May decrease levels of lamotrigine and reduce seizure control; dosage adjustments of lamotrigine may be necessary. May raise serum concentrations of thyroxine-binding globulin and cortisol-binding globulin; may need to increase dose of replacement thyroid hormone or cortisol therapy.

PATIENT CONSIDERATIONS

Assessment: Assess for high risk of arterial or venous thrombotic diseases; benign or malignant liver tumors; liver disease; undiagnosed, abnormal uterine bleeding; presence or history of breast cancer or other estrogen- or progestin-sensitive cancer; pregnancy; and any other conditions where treatment is contraindicated/cautioned. Assess nursing status and for possible drug interactions.

Monitoring: Monitor for arterial thromboses or VTEs, TSS, hepatic adenomas, hepatocellular carcinoma, gallbladder disease, and other adverse effects. Monitor lipid levels with hyperlipidemia, BP, serum glucose levels in diabetic or prediabetic patients, and for signs of worsening depression with previous history. Have a yearly visit with patient for a BP check and for other indicated healthcare.

Counseling: Inform of risks and benefits of therapy. Inform that cigarette smoking increases risk of serious CV events. Inform of increased risk of VTE. Counsel that therapy does not protect against HIV infection (AIDS) or other STDs. Instruct not to use during pregnancy and to d/c if pregnancy is planned or occurs during use. Instruct to use a barrier method of contraception when ring is out for >3 continuous hrs until ring has been used continuously for at least 7 days. Counsel to use a backup or alternative method of contraception when enzyme inducers are concomitantly used. Inform that breast milk production may be reduced with use. Instruct postpartum women who have not yet had a normal period, to use an additional nonhormonal method of contraception for the first 7 days. Instruct on proper usage and what to do if not compliant with timing of insertion and removal. Inform that ring may be expelled while removing a tampon, during intercourse, or with straining during a bowel movement. Inform that amenorrhea may occur. Advise that pregnancy should be ruled out in the event of amenorrhea, if ring has been out of the vagina for >3 consecutive hrs, if ring-free interval was extended >1 week, if a period was missed for ≥2 consecutive cycles, or if ring has been retained for >4 weeks.

STORAGE: 2-8°C (36-46°F). After dispensing, store up to 4 months at 25°C (77°F); excursions permitted to 15-30°C (59-86°F). Avoid direct sunlight or >30°C (86°F).

NUVIGIL – armodafinil

CIV

Class: Wakefulness-promoting agent

ADULT DOSAGE

Narcolepsy

Excessive Sleepiness Associated w/ Narcolepsy:
Usual: 150-250mg taken as a single dose qam

Shift Work Disorder

Excessive Sleepiness Associated w/ Shift Work Disorder:
Usual: 150mg qd taken as a single dose approx 1 hr prior to start of work shift

Obstructive Sleep Apnea

Excessive Sleepiness Associated w/ Obstructive Sleep Apnea:
Usual: 150-250mg taken as a single dose qam

PEDIATRIC DOSAGE

Pediatric use may not have been established

DOSING CONSIDERATIONS

Hepatic Impairment

Severe Impairment: Reduce dose

Elderly

Consider lower doses

ADMINISTRATION

Oral route

HOW SUPPLIED

Tab: 50mg, 150mg, 200mg, 250mg

CONTRAINDICATIONS

Known hypersensitivity to modafinil or armodafinil or its inactive ingredients.

WARNINGS/PRECAUTIONS

Not indicated as treatment for underlying obstruction in OSA; if continuous positive airway pressure (CPAP) is the treatment of choice, treat w/ CPAP for an adequate period of time prior to initiation of therapy. Rare cases of serious or life-threatening rash, including Stevens-Johnson syndrome (SJS), toxic epidermal necrolysis (TEN), and drug rash w/ eosinophilia and systemic symptoms (DRESS) reported; d/c treatment at 1st sign of rash, unless rash is clearly not drug-related. Angioedema, anaphylaxis reactions, multiorgan hypersensitivity reactions, and psychiatric adverse reactions reported; d/c treatment if symptoms develop. Caution w/ cardiovascular disease (CVD) or history of psychosis, depression, or mania. Avoid in patients w/ history of left ventricular hypertrophy or w/ mitral valve prolapse who have experienced mitral valve prolapse syndrome (eg, ischemic ECG changes, chest pain, arrhythmia) w/ CNS stimulants. May impair mental/physical abilities. Level of wakefulness may not return to normal in patients w/ abnormal levels of sleepiness. Potential for abuse.

ADVERSE REACTIONS

Headache, nausea, dizziness, insomnia, diarrhea, dry mouth, anxiety, depression, rash.

DRUG INTERACTIONS

Reduced exposure of CYP3A4/5 substrates (eg, cyclosporine, midazolam, triazolam); consider dose adjustment of these drugs. Effectiveness of steroidal contraceptives may be reduced during and for 1 month after discontinuation of therapy; alternative or concomitant methods of contraception are recommended. Cyclosporine levels may be reduced; monitor levels and consider dosage adjustment. Increased exposure of CYP2C19 substrates (eg, omeprazole, diazepam, phenytoin); dosage reduction of these drugs may be required. Frequently monitor PT/INR w/ warfarin. Caution w/ MAOIs.

N

PATIENT CONSIDERATIONS

Assessment: Assess for hypersensitivity to modafinil or to drug, hepatic impairment, psychosis, depression, mania, left ventricular hypertrophy, mitral valve prolapse, other CVDs, pregnancy/nursing status, and possible drug interactions.

Monitoring: Monitor for serious rash, SJS, TEN, DRESS, angioedema, anaphylaxis, hypersensitivity reactions, multiorgan hypersensitivity reactions, psychiatric adverse symptoms, and other adverse reactions. Monitor for signs of misuse or abuse. Monitor HR and BP. Frequently reassess degree of sleepiness. Consider close monitoring in elderly. Monitor PT/INR frequently w/ warfarin.

Counseling: Inform that drug is not a replacement for sleep. Inform that therapy may improve but not eliminate the abnormal tendency to fall asleep; instruct not to alter previous behavior w/ regard to potentially dangerous activities or other activities requiring appropriate levels of wakefulness, until and unless treatment has shown to produce levels of wakefulness that permit such activities. Inform of importance of continuing previously prescribed treatments. Advise to avoid alcohol during therapy. Advise to notify physician if pregnant, intending to become pregnant, or nursing. Caution about increased risk of pregnancy when using steroidal contraceptives and for 1 month after discontinuation of therapy. Instruct to inform physician if taking/planning to take any prescribed or OTC drugs. Instruct to d/c and notify physician if rash, hives, mouth sores, blisters, peeling skin, trouble swallowing or breathing or related allergic phenomenon, depression, anxiety, or signs of psychosis or mania develop.

STORAGE: 20-25°C (68-77°F).

NYSTATIN/TRIAMCINOLONE – nystatin/triamcinolone acetonide RX

Class: Corticosteroid/polyene antifungal

ADULT DOSAGE

Cutaneous Candidiasis

Apply gently bid (am and pm)

D/C after 25 days if symptoms persist

PEDIATRIC DOSAGE

Cutaneous Candidiasis

Apply gently bid (am and pm)

D/C after 25 days if symptoms persist

ADMINISTRATION
Topical route

Avoid use with occlusive dressings

HOW SUPPLIED
Cre, Oint: (Nystatin-Triamcinolone) 100,000 U/g-0.1% [15g, 30g, 60g]

CONTRAINDICATIONS
History of hypersensitivity to any of the components.

WARNINGS/PRECAUTIONS
Avoid occlusive dressing. Monitor periodically for hypothalamic-pituitary-adrenal (HPA) axis suppression with prolonged use or when applied over a large area. D/C if hypersensitivity or irritation develops. Systemic absorption with topical corticosteroids reported; children are more prone to systemic toxicity. May cause Cushing's syndrome, hyperglycemia, and glucosuria.

ADVERSE REACTIONS
Acneiform eruption, burning, itching, irritation, secondary infection.

PATIENT CONSIDERATIONS

Assessment: Assess proper diagnosis (eg, KOH smears, cultures), pregnancy/status.

Monitoring: Monitor for signs/symptoms of reversible HPA axis suppression, impaired thermal homeostasis, Cushing's syndrome, hyperglycemia, glucosuria, irritation at treatment site, and hypersensitivity reactions. If applying large doses to large surface area, monitor for HPA-axis suppression by using urinary free cortisol and ACTH stimulation tests. In pediatric patients, monitor for signs/symptoms of systemic toxicity, HPA-axis suppression, Cushing's syndrome, and intracranial HTN. Monitor for response to therapy; if lack of response, repeat appropriate microbiological studies.

Counseling: Instruct to use exactly ud, topically. Avoid contact with eyes. Treatment area should not be bandaged or wrapped as to be occluded. Advise to contact physician if any adverse events develop. Inform that if applying to inguinal area, apply sparingly and wear loose clothing. Parents of pediatric patients should be instructed to avoid using tight fitting diapers or plastic pants when treating diaper area. Instruct to take preventative measures to avoid reinfection.

STORAGE: Room temperature; avoid freezing.

NYSTOP – nystatin

RX

Class: Polyene antifungal

ADULT DOSAGE
Candida Infections

Cutaneous or Mucocutaneous Mycotic Infections Caused by *Candida albicans* and Other Susceptible *Candida* Species:
Apply to lesions bid-tid until healing is complete

***Candida* Infection of the Feet:**
Dust the powder on the feet and in all footwear

PEDIATRIC DOSAGE
Candida Infections

Cutaneous or Mucocutaneous Mycotic Infections Caused by *Candida albicans* and Other Susceptible *Candida* Species:
Apply to lesions bid-tid until healing is complete

***Candida* Infection of the Feet:**
Dust the powder on the feet and in all footwear

ADMINISTRATION
Topical route

HOW SUPPLIED
Powder: 100,000 U/g [15g, 30g, 60g]

CONTRAINDICATIONS
History of hypersensitivity to any of the components.

WARNINGS/PRECAUTIONS
Not for systemic, PO, intravaginal, or ophthalmic use. D/C if irritation or sensitization develops and institute appropriate measures. Confirm diagnosis of *Candida* infection using potassium hydroxide smears, cultures, or other diagnostic methods; repeat test if there is a lack of therapeutic response.

ADVERSE REACTIONS
Allergic reactions, burning, itching, rash, eczema, pain on application site.

PATIENT CONSIDERATIONS

Assessment: Assess for history of hypersensitivity to the drug or any of its components and pregnancy/nursing status. Confirm diagnosis of *Candida* infection using appropriate diagnostic methods.

Monitoring: Monitor for irritation or sensitization, other adverse reactions, and therapeutic response. Reassess diagnosis if there is a lack of therapeutic response.

Counseling: Instruct to use exactly ud, including replacement of missed dose. Advise not to use the medication for any disorder other than prescribed. Instruct not to interrupt or d/c therapy until treatment is completed, even if symptomatic relief occurs within the first few days of treatment. Advise to notify physician promptly if skin irritation develops.

STORAGE: 15-30°C (59-86°F). Avoid excessive heat (40°C [104°F]).

ODOMZO — sonidegib

RX

Class: Hedgehog pathway inhibitor

May cause embryo-fetal death or severe birth defects when administered to a pregnant woman. Verify the pregnancy status of females of reproductive potential prior to initiating therapy. Advise females of reproductive potential to use effective contraception during treatment and for at least 20 months after the last dose. Advise males of the potential risk of exposure through semen and to use condoms w/ a pregnant partner or a female partner of reproductive potential during treatment and for at least 8 months after the last dose.

ADULT DOSAGE

Basal Cell Carcinoma

Locally advanced basal cell carcinoma that has recurred following surgery or radiation therapy, or for those who are not candidates for surgery or radiation therapy

200mg qd until disease progression or unacceptable toxicity

PEDIATRIC DOSAGE

Pediatric use may not have been established

DOSING CONSIDERATIONS

Adverse Reactions

Interrupt Therapy for:

1. Severe or intolerable musculoskeletal adverse reactions
2. First occurrence of serum creatine kinase (CK) elevation between 2.5 and 10X ULN
3. Recurrent serum CK elevation between 2.5 and 5X ULN

Resume at 200mg/day upon resolution of clinical signs and symptoms

O

Permanently D/C Therapy for:

1. Serum CK elevation >2.5X ULN w/ worsening renal function
2. Serum CK elevation >10X ULN
3. Recurrent serum CK elevation >5X ULN
4. Recurrent severe or intolerable musculoskeletal adverse reactions

ADMINISTRATION

Oral route

Take on an empty stomach, at least 1 hr ac or 2 hrs pc.

HOW SUPPLIED

Cap: 200mg

WARNINGS/PRECAUTIONS

Advise not to donate blood or blood products while taking sonidegib and for at least 20 months after the last dose. Musculoskeletal adverse reactions, which may be accompanied by serum CK elevations reported; advise to report promptly any new unexplained muscle pain, tenderness or weakness occurring during treatment or that persists after discontinuing therapy. Obtain baseline serum CK and creatinine levels prior to initiating therapy, periodically during treatment, and as clinically indicated (eg, if muscle symptoms are reported). Obtain SrCr and CK levels at least weekly in patients w/ musculoskeletal adverse reactions w/ concurrent serum CK elevation >2.5X ULN until resolution of clinical signs and symptoms.

ADVERSE REACTIONS

Muscle spasms, alopecia, dysgeusia, fatigue, abdominal pain, N/V, musculoskeletal pain, decreased weight, myalgia, diarrhea, decreased appetite, headache, pain, pruritus.

DRUG INTERACTIONS

Avoid w/ strong CYP3A inhibitors (eg, saquinavir, ketoconazole, nefazodone), and w/ moderate CYP3A inhibitors (eg, atanazavir, diltiazem, fluconazole). If a moderate CYP3A inhibitor must be used, administer the moderate CYP3A inhibitor for <14 days and monitor closely for adverse reactions, particularly musculoskeletal adverse reactions. Avoid w/ strong and moderate CYP3A inducers (eg, carbamazepine, efavirenz, modafinil).

PATIENT CONSIDERATIONS

Assessment: Assess for hypersensitivity to drug, pregnancy/nursing status, and for possible drug interactions. Obtain baseline CK levels and renal function tests.

Monitoring: Monitor for musculoskeletal adverse reactions (eg, rhabdomyolysis, muscle spasms, musculoskeletal pain) and for other adverse reactions. Monitor CK and SrCr levels periodically and as clinically indicated. Obtain SrCr and CK levels at least weekly in patients w/ musculoskeletal adverse reactions w/ concurrent serum CK elevations >2.5X ULN until clinical signs/symptoms are resolved.

Counseling: Inform females of reproductive potential that drug may cause fetal harm and to use effective contraception during treatment and for at least 20 months after the last dose. Inform males, even those w/ prior vasectomy, to use condoms, to avoid potential drug exposure in both pregnant partners and female partners of reproductive potential during treatment and for at least 8 months after the last dose. Counsel female patients and female partners of male patients to contact their healthcare provider if they become pregnant or suspect that they may be pregnant. Inform females who may have been exposed to sonidegib during pregnancy, either directly or through seminal fluid, to contact the Novartis Pharmaceuticals Corporation. Instruct not to donate blood or blood products while taking sonidegib and for 20 months after stopping treatment. Advise to contact healthcare provider immediately if new or worsening signs/symptoms of muscle toxicity, dark urine, decreased urine output, or the inability to urinate develops. Instruct to take on an empty stomach, at least 1 hr ac or 2 hrs pc. Advise women not to breastfeed during treatment and for up to 20 months after the last dose.

STORAGE: 25°C (77°F); excursions permitted to 15-30°C (59-86°F).

OFEV – nintedanib

RX

Class: Kinase inhibitor

ADULT DOSAGE

Idiopathic Pulmonary Fibrosis

Recommended: 150mg bid approx 12 hrs apart

Max: 300mg/day

Missed Dose

If a dose is missed, the next dose should be taken at the next scheduled time; do not make up for a missed dose

PEDIATRIC DOSAGE

Pediatric use may not have been established

DOSING CONSIDERATIONS

Hepatic Impairment

Mild (Child Pugh A):
100mg bid approx 12 hrs apart

Moderate (Child Pugh B) or Severe (Child Pugh C):
Not recommended

Adverse Reactions

In addition to symptomatic treatment, if applicable, dose reduction or temporary interruption may be required until the specific adverse reaction resolves to levels that allow continuation of therapy

Treatment may be resumed at the full dosage (150mg bid), or at the reduced dosage (100mg bid), which subsequently may be increased to the full dosage. If 100mg bid is not tolerated, d/c treatment

Liver Enzyme Elevations:

AST/ALT >3X to <5X ULN w/o Signs of Severe Liver Damage:
Interrupt treatment or reduce dose to 100mg bid; once LFTs return to baseline, may reintroduce at a reduced dosage (100mg bid), which subsequently may be increased to the full dosage (150mg bid)

AST/ALT Elevations >5X ULN or >3X ULN w/ Signs/Symptoms of Severe Liver Damage:
D/C treatment

Mild Hepatic Impairment (Child Pugh A):
Consider treatment interruption/discontinuation for management of adverse reactions

ADMINISTRATION

Oral route

Take w/ food.
Swallow whole w/ liquid; do not chew or crush caps.

HOW SUPPLIED

Cap: 100mg, 150mg

WARNINGS/PRECAUTIONS

See Dosing Considerations. Associated w/ elevations of liver enzymes and bilirubin; conduct LFTs prior to treatment, monthly for 3 months, and every 3 months thereafter, and as clinically indicated. Diarrhea reported; treat at 1st signs w/ adequate hydration and antidiarrheal medication (eg, loperamide) and consider treatment interruption if diarrhea continues. D/C treatment if severe diarrhea persists despite symptomatic treatment. N/V reported; may require dose reduction or treatment interruption if N/V persists despite appropriate supportive care including antiemetic therapy. D/C treatment if severe N/V does not resolve. Can cause fetal harm. Arterial thromboembolic events (eg, myocardial infarction) reported; caution when treating patients at higher cardiovascular (CV) risk including known coronary artery disease. Consider treatment interruption in patients who develop signs or symptoms of acute myocardial ischemia. May increase the risk of bleeding and GI perforation. Caution in patients who have had recent abdominal surgery, and d/c therapy in patients who develop GI perforation.

ADVERSE REACTIONS

Diarrhea, N/V, abdominal pain, liver enzyme elevation, decreased appetite, weight decreased, headache, HTN.

DRUG INTERACTIONS

P-gp and CYP3A4 inhibitors (eg, erythromycin, ketoconazole) may increase exposure; monitor closely for tolerability. P-gp and CYP3A4 inducers (eg, carbamazepine, phenytoin, St. John's wort, rifampicin) may decrease exposure; avoid coadministration. Monitor closely for bleeding if on full anticoagulation therapy and adjust anticoagulation treatment as necessary. Smoking was associated w/ decreased exposure, which may alter the efficacy profile of nintedanib.

PATIENT CONSIDERATIONS

Assessment: Assess for CV risk, hepatic impairment, risk of bleeding/GI perforation, recent abdominal surgery, pregnancy/nursing status, possible drug interactions, and if smoking. Conduct LFTs and a pregnancy test prior to treatment.

Monitoring: Monitor for GI disorders, arterial thromboembolic events, bleeding events, GI perforation, and other adverse reactions. Monitor for liver enzyme elevations; conduct LFTs (ALT, AST, bilirubin) monthly for 3 months, and every 3 months thereafter, and as clinically indicated.

Counseling: Advise that liver function testing will be needed periodically. Advise to immediately report any symptoms of a liver problem. Inform that GI disorders such as diarrhea or N/V were the most commonly reported GI events; advise that physician may recommend hydration, antidiarrheal medications (eg, loperamide), or antiemetic medications to treat these side effects. Instruct to contact physician at the 1st signs of diarrhea or for any severe or persistent diarrhea or N/V. Counsel on pregnancy planning and prevention. Advise females of childbearing potential of the potential hazard to a fetus, to avoid becoming pregnant while receiving treatment, and to use effective contraception during treatment and for at least 3 months after taking the last dose of the drug. Advise to notify physician if pregnancy occurs during therapy. Advise that breastfeeding is not recommended. Advise about the signs and symptoms of acute myocardial ischemia and other arterial thromboembolic events and the urgency to seek immediate medical care for these conditions. Advise to report unusual bleeding or any signs and symptoms of GI perforation. Encourage to stop smoking prior to treatment and to avoid smoking during treatment. If a dose is missed, instruct to take the next dose at the next scheduled time and to not make up for a missed dose.

STORAGE: 25°C (77°F); excursions permitted to 15-30°C (59-86°F). Protect from exposure to high humidity and avoid excessive heat. If repackaged, use tight container.

OFIRMEV – acetaminophen

RX

Class: Analgesic

Caution when prescribing, preparing, and administering therapy to avoid dosing errors that could result in accidental overdose and death. Ensure that the dose in mg and mL is not confused, the dosing is based on weight for patients <50kg, infusion pumps are properly programmed, and the total daily dose of acetaminophen (APAP) from all sources does not exceed max daily limits. Associated w/ cases of acute liver failure, at times resulting in liver transplant and death. Most cases of liver injury are associated w/ APAP use at doses that exceed the max daily limits, and often involve >1 APAP-containing product.

ADULT DOSAGE

Moderate to Severe Pain

Adjunct to Opioid Analgesics:

<50kg:

Usual: 12.5mg/kg q4h or 15mg/kg q6h

Max: 15mg/kg (up to 750mg)/dose or 75mg/kg (up to 3750mg)/day

PEDIATRIC DOSAGE

Moderate to Severe Pain

Adjunct to Opioid Analgesics:

2-12 Years:

Usual: 12.5mg/kg q4h or 15mg/kg q6h

Max: 15mg/kg (up to 750mg)/dose or 75mg/kg (up to 3750mg)/day

≥50kg:
Usual: 650mg q4h or 1000mg q6h
Max: 1000mg/dose or 4000mg/day

Mild to Moderate Pain

<50kg:
Usual: 12.5mg/kg q4h or 15mg/kg q6h
Max: 15mg/kg (up to 750mg)/dose or 75mg/kg (up to 3750mg)/day

≥50kg:
Usual: 650mg q4h or 1000mg q6h
Max: 1000mg/dose or 4000mg/day

Fever

<50kg:
Usual: 12.5mg/kg q4h or 15mg/kg q6h
Max: 15mg/kg (up to 750mg)/dose or 75mg/kg (up to 3750mg)/day

≥50kg:
Usual: 650mg q4h or 1000mg q6h
Max: 1000mg/dose or 4000mg/day

≥13 Years:
<50kg:
Usual: 12.5mg/kg q4h or 15mg/kg q6h
Max: 15mg/kg (up to 750mg)/dose or 75mg/kg (up to 3750mg)/day

≥50kg:
Usual: 650mg q4h or 1000mg q6h
Max: 1000mg/dose or 4000mg/day

Mild to Moderate Pain

2-12 Years:
Usual: 12.5mg/kg q4h or 15mg/kg q6h
Max: 15mg/kg (up to 750mg)/dose or 75mg/kg (up to 3750mg)/day

≥13 Years:
<50kg:
Usual: 12.5mg/kg q4h or 15mg/kg q6h
Max: 15mg/kg (up to 750mg)/dose or 75mg/kg (up to 3750mg)/day

≥50kg:
Usual: 650mg q4h or 1000mg q6h
Max: 1000mg/dose or 4000mg/day

Fever

2-12 Years:
Usual: 12.5mg/kg q4h or 15mg/kg q6h
Max: 15mg/kg (up to 750mg)/dose or 75mg/kg (up to 3750mg)/day

≥13 Years:
<50kg:
Usual: 12.5mg/kg q4h or 15mg/kg q6h
Max: 15mg/kg (up to 750mg)/dose or 75mg/kg (up to 3750mg)/day

≥50kg:
Usual: 650mg q4h or 1000mg q6h
Max: 1000mg/dose or 4000mg/day

DOSING CONSIDERATIONS

Renal Impairment

Severe (CrCl ≤30mL/min): May need to give at longer dosing intervals and a reduced total daily dose

Hepatic Impairment

May need to reduce total daily dose

ADMINISTRATION

IV route

Minimum dosing interval should be 4 hrs

Adults and Adolescents ≥50kg Requiring 1000mg Doses

Administer the dose by inserting a vented IV set through the septum of the 100mL vial
May be administered w/o further dilution
Administer contents of the vial IV over 15 min

Doses <1000mg

Withdraw appropriate dose from vial and place into a separate empty, sterile container (eg, glass bottle, plastic IV container, syringe) for IV infusion
The entire 100mL vial is not intended for use in patients weighing <50kg; discard the unused portion
Place small volume pediatric doses up to 60mL in volume in a syringe and administer over 15 min using syringe pump

Once vacuum seal of vial is penetrated, or contents transferred to another container, administer dose w/in 6 hrs
Do not add other medications to sol; diazepam and chlorpromazine are physically incompatible

HOW SUPPLIED

Inj: 10mg/mL [100mL]

CONTRAINDICATIONS

Known hypersensitivity to acetaminophen or to any of the excipients in the IV formulation, severe hepatic impairment or severe active liver disease.

WARNINGS/PRECAUTIONS

Caution w/ alcoholism, chronic malnutrition, or severe hypovolemia (eg, due to dehydration or blood loss). May cause hypersensitivity, anaphylaxis, and serious skin reactions (eg, acute generalized exanthematous pustulosis, Stevens-Johnson syndrome, toxic epidermal necrolysis); d/c at the 1st appearance of signs/symptoms.

ADVERSE REACTIONS

Liver failure, N/V, headache, insomnia, constipation, pruritus, agitation, atelectasis.

DRUG INTERACTIONS

Substances that induce or regulate CYP2E1 may alter the metabolism and increase hepatotoxic potential. Excessive alcohol use may induce hepatic cytochromes, but ethanol may also inhibit metabolism. Increased INR in some patients stabilized on sodium warfarin; more frequent assessment of INR may be appropriate.

PATIENT CONSIDERATIONS

Assessment: Assess for previous hypersensitivity, alcoholism, chronic malnutrition, severe hypovolemia, hepatic/renal impairment, pregnancy/nursing status, and possible drug interactions.

Monitoring: Monitor for signs/symptoms of hypersensitivity and anaphylaxis, acute liver failure, serious skin reactions, and other adverse reactions. Monitor the end of infusion to prevent the possibility of air embolism, especially in cases where therapy is the primary infusion. Monitor INR frequently in patients stabilized on sodium warfarin.

Counseling: Inform about the risks and benefits of therapy. Instruct not to exceed the recommended dose. Instruct to notify physician if any adverse reactions occur or if pregnant/nursing or planning to become pregnant. Counsel about possible drug interactions.

STORAGE: 20-25°C (68-77°F). Do not refrigerate or freeze.

Ofloxacin Otic – ofloxacin

RX

Class: Fluoroquinolone

OTHER BRAND NAMES

Floxin Otic (Discontinued)

ADULT DOSAGE

Otitis Externa

Usual: 10 drops (0.5mL) into affected ear qd for 7 days

Otitis Media

Chronic Suppurative Otitis Media w/ Perforated Tympanic Membranes:

Usual: 10 drops (0.5mL) into affected ear bid for 14 days

PEDIATRIC DOSAGE

Otitis Externa

6 Months-13 Years:

Usual: 5 drops (0.25mL) into affected ear qd for 7 days

≥13 Years:

Usual: 10 drops (0.5mL) into affected ear qd for 7 days

Otitis Media

Chronic Suppurative Otitis Media w/ Perforated Tympanic Membranes:

≥12 Years:

Usual: 10 drops (0.5mL) into affected ear bid for 14 days

Acute Otitis Media w/ Tympanostomy Tubes:

1-12 Years:

Usual: 5 drops (0.25mL) into affected ear bid for 10 days

ADMINISTRATION

Otic route

Instillation

1. Warm sol by holding bottle in hand for 1-2 min
2. Lie w/ affected ear upward then instill drops; maintain position for 5 min
3. For acute otitis media w/ tympanostomy tubes and chronic suppurative otitis media w/ perforated tympanostomy tubes, pump tragus 4X by pushing inward to facilitate penetration into the middle ear
4. Repeat for opposite ear if necessary

HOW SUPPLIED

Sol: 0.3% [5mL, 10mL]

CONTRAINDICATIONS

History of hypersensitivity to ofloxacin, to other quinolones, or to any of the components in the medication.

WARNINGS/PRECAUTIONS

D/C if hypersensitivity reaction occurs. Prolonged use may result in overgrowth of nonsusceptible organisms; reevaluate if no improvement after one week. If otorrhea persists after a full course, or if two or more episodes occur within 6 months, further evaluation is recommended. Not for injection or ophthalmic use.

ADVERSE REACTIONS

Pruritus, application-site reaction, taste perversion.

PATIENT CONSIDERATIONS

Assessment: Assess for drug hypersensitivity, preexisting cholesteatoma, foreign body or tumor, pregnancy/nursing status.

Monitoring: Monitor for anaphylactic reactions, cardiovascular collapse, loss of consciousness, angioedema, airway obstruction, dyspnea, urticaria and itching, overgrowth of nonsusceptible organisms, for improvement/persistence of otorrhea.

Counseling: Counsel to avoid touching applicator tip to fingers or other surfaces to avoid contamination. D/C and instruct to contact physician if signs of allergy occur. Instruct patients to warm bottle by holding for 1-2 min, to avoid dizziness that may result from instillation of a cold solution. Instruct to lie with affected ear upward, before instilling the drops; maintain position for 5 min. Instruct to repeat if necessary, for opposite ear.

STORAGE: 20-25°C (68-77°F). Protect from light.

OLEPTRO – trazodone hydrochloride

RX

Class: Triazolopyridine derivative

Antidepressants increased the risk of suicidal thinking and behavior (suicidality) in children, adolescents, and young adults in short-term studies of major depressive disorder (MDD) and other psychiatric disorders. Monitor and observe closely for clinical worsening, suicidality, or unusual changes in behavior. Not approved for use in pediatric patients.

ADULT DOSAGE

Major Depressive Disorder

Initial: 150mg qhs

Titrate: May increase by 75mg/day every 3 days (eg, start 225mg on Day 4 of therapy)

Max: 375mg/day

Maint: Generally recommended to continue treatment for several months after an initial response; maintain on the lowest effective dose

Once adequate response is achieved, may reduce dose gradually, w/ subsequent adjustment depending on therapeutic response

Dosing Considerations with MAOIs

Switching to/from an MAOI for Psychiatric Disorders:

Allow at least 14 days between discontinuation of an MAOI and initiation of treatment, and conversely allow at least 14 days between discontinuing treatment before starting an MAOI

Use w/ Other MAOIs (eg, Linezolid, IV Methylene Blue):

Do not start trazodone in patients being treated w/ linezolid or IV methylene blue

If acceptable alternatives are not available and benefits outweigh risks of serotonin syndrome, d/c trazodone promptly and administer linezolid or IV methylene blue; monitor for serotonin syndrome for 2 weeks or until 24 hrs after last dose of linezolid or IV methylene blue, whichever comes 1st. May resume trazodone therapy 24 hrs after last dose of linezolid or IV methylene blue

PEDIATRIC DOSAGE

Pediatric use may not have been established

DOSING CONSIDERATIONS

Discontinuation

Gradually reduce dose whenever possible

ADMINISTRATION

Oral route

Take at the same time every day, in the late pm preferably hs, on an empty stomach
May swallow whole or as a 1/2 tab by breaking the tab along the score line; do not chew or crush

HOW SUPPLIED

Tab, Extended Release: 150mg*, 300mg* *scored

CONTRAINDICATIONS

Use of an MAOI for psychiatric disorders either concomitantly or within 14 days of stopping treatment. Treatment within 14 days of stopping an MAOI for psychiatric disorders. Starting treatment in patients being treated with other MAOIs (eg, linezolid, IV methylene blue).

WARNINGS/PRECAUTIONS

Monitor for withdrawal symptoms when discontinuing treatment; reduce dose gradually. Serotonin syndrome reported; d/c immediately and initiate supportive symptomatic treatment. Pupillary dilation that occurs following use may trigger an angle-closure attack in a patient with anatomically narrow angles who does not have a patent iridectomy. May precipitate mixed/manic episode in patients at risk for bipolar disorder; screen for risk of bipolar disorder prior to initiating treatment. Not approved for treatment of bipolar depression. May cause QT/QTc interval prolongation, torsades de pointes, cardiac arrhythmias, and hypotension, including orthostatic hypotension and syncope. Not recommended for use during the initial recovery phase of myocardial infarction (MI). May increase risk of bleeding events. Priapism reported; caution in men with conditions that may predispose to priapism (eg, sickle cell anemia, multiple myeloma, leukemia) or with penile anatomical deformation; d/c with erection lasting >6 hrs (painful or not). Hyponatremia may occur; caution in elderly and volume-depleted patients. Consider discontinuation in patients with symptomatic hyponatremia and institute appropriate medical intervention. May cause somnolence or sedation and may impair mental/physical abilities. Caution with cardiac disease, hepatic/renal impairment, and in elderly.

ADVERSE REACTIONS

Somnolence, sedation, headache, dry mouth, dizziness, nausea, fatigue, diarrhea, constipation, back pain, blurred vision, sexual dysfunction.

DRUG INTERACTIONS

See Contraindications. May cause serotonin syndrome with other serotonergic drugs (eg, triptans, TCAs, fentanyl) and with drugs that impair serotonin metabolism; d/c immediately if this occurs. May enhance response to alcohol, barbiturates, and other CNS depressants. Increased risk of cardiac arrhythmia with drugs that prolong QT interval or CYP3A4 inhibitors. CYP3A4 inhibitors (eg, ritonavir, ketoconazole, indinavir) may increase levels with the potential for adverse effects. Potent CYP3A4 inhibitors may increase risk of cardiac arrhythmia; consider lower dose of trazodone. Carbamazepine (CYP3A4 inducer) may decrease levels; monitor to determine if a trazodone dose increase is required. Increased serum digoxin or phenytoin levels reported; monitor serum levels and adjust dosages PRN. Concomitant use with an antihypertensive may require a dose reduction of the antihypertensive drug. Monitor for potential risk of bleeding and use caution with NSAIDs, aspirin, and other drugs that affect coagulation or bleeding. Increased risk of hyponatremia with diuretics. Altered PT reported in patients on warfarin.

PATIENT CONSIDERATIONS

Assessment: Assess for drug hypersensitivity, risk for bipolar disorder, cardiac disease (eg, recent MI), conditions that may predispose to priapism, penile anatomical deformation, susceptibility to angle-closure glaucoma, volume depletion, hepatic/renal impairment, pregnancy/nursing status, and possible drug interactions.

Monitoring: Monitor for clinical worsening, suicidality, unusual changes in behavior, mania/hypomania, serotonin syndrome, angle-closure glaucoma, QT/QTc interval prolongation, cardiac arrhythmias, hypotension, syncope, bleeding events, priapism, hyponatremia, withdrawal symptoms, and other adverse reactions. Periodically reassess to determine the continued need for maintenance treatment.

Counseling: Inform of the risks, benefits, and appropriate use of therapy. Instruct patients and caregivers to notify physician if signs of clinical worsening, changes in behavior, or suicidality occur. Instruct to report to physician the occurrence of anxiety, agitation, panic attacks, insomnia, irritability, hostility, aggressiveness, impulsivity, akathisia, hypomania, or mania. Instruct to inform physician if patient has history of bipolar disorder, cardiac disease, or MI. Caution about the risks of serotonin syndrome, angle-closure glaucoma, priapism, hypotension, syncope, bleeding, and withdrawal symptoms. Instruct men to immediately d/c use and contact physician if erection lasts >6 hrs, whether painful or not. Caution against performing potentially hazardous tasks (eg, operating machinery) until reasonably certain that treatment does not affect them. Inform that therapy may enhance response to alcohol. Instruct to notify physician if intending to become pregnant, or nursing.

STORAGE: 15-30°C (59-86°F).

Omeclamox-Pak – amoxicillin/clarithromycin/omeprazole RX

Class: *H. pylori* treatment combination

ADULT DOSAGE

***Helicobacter pylori* Eradication**

***Helicobacter Pylori* Infection and Duodenal Ulcer Disease:**

Usual: 20mg omeprazole + 500mg clarithromycin + 1000mg amoxicillin, each given bid (am and pm) ac for 10 days

Ulcer Present When Initiating Therapy: Give an additional 18 days of omeprazole 20mg qd

PEDIATRIC DOSAGE

Pediatric use may not have been established

DOSING CONSIDERATIONS

Renal Impairment

Severe: Prolong clarithromycin dosing intervals

Hepatic Impairment

Avoid use

ADMINISTRATION

Oral route

Take each dose of 4 pills in the am and 4 pills in the pm ac

Swallow whole; do not crush or chew

HOW SUPPLIED

Cap: (Amoxicillin) 500mg; **Cap, Delayed-Release:** (Omeprazole) 20mg; **Tab:** (Clarithromycin) 500mg

CONTRAINDICATIONS

Concomitant use with ergotamine or dihydroergotamine and pimozide, known hypersensitivity to omeprazole, any macrolide antibiotic, any penicillin, or any component of the formulations.

WARNINGS/PRECAUTIONS

Avoid use in Asian patients unless benefits outweigh risks. Lab test interactions may occur. Amoxicillin: Serious and occasionally fatal hypersensitivity (anaphylactic) reactions reported in patients on PCN therapy; caution with history of PCN hypersensitivity and/or a history of sensitivity to multiple allergens. Not recommended in patients with mononucleosis; may develop erythematosus skin rash. Caution in elderly. Clarithromycin: Use in pregnancy only when there is no appropriate alternative therapy. Exacerbation of symptoms of myasthenia gravis and new onset of myasthenic syndrome reported. Amoxicillin/Clarithromycin: *Clostridium difficile*-associated diarrhea (CDAD) reported; may need to d/c if CDAD is suspected or confirmed. May result in bacterial resistance with prolonged use in the absence of proven or suspected bacterial infection, or a prophylactic indication; d/c if superinfections occur and institute appropriate therapy. Omeprazole: Symptomatic response does not preclude the presence of gastric malignancy. Acute interstitial nephritis (AIN) reported; d/c if AIN develops.

ADVERSE REACTIONS

Diarrhea, taste perversion, headache.

DRUG INTERACTIONS

See Contraindications. Amoxicillin: May decrease renal tubular secretion when coadministered with probenecid. Clarithromycin: May lead to increased exposure to colchicine when coadministered; monitor for colchicine toxicity. May increase levels of drugs metabolized by CYP3A, digoxin, theophylline, carbamazepine, and statins (eg, lovastatin, simvastatin). May potentiate antiarrhythmic effects with concurrent use of antiarrhythmic drugs. Torsades de pointes may occur with quinidine or disopyramide. May increase systemic exposure of sildenafil; consider a reduction in sildenafil dose. May alter the effect of triazolobenziodidiazepines/related benzodiazepines. CNS effects (eg, somnolence, confusion) reported with concomitant triazolam. Omeprazole: Monitor patients taking drugs metabolized by CYP450 (eg, cyclosporine, disulfiram, benzodiazepines). May reduce levels of atazanavir and nelfinavir; concomitant use not recommended. May increase levels of saquinavir and tacrolimus; consider dose reduction of saquinavir. May increase systemic exposure of cilostazol; consider a reduction in cilostazol dose. May reduce absorption of drugs where gastric pH is an important determinant of bioavailability; absorption of ketoconazole, atazanavir, iron salts, erlotinib, and mycophenolate mofetil may decrease, while absorption of digoxin may increase. Monitor patients when digoxin is taken concomitantly. Caution with mycophenolate mofetil in transplant patients. Clarithromycin/Omeprazole: May alter the anticoagulant effects of warfarin and other anticoagulants; monitor PT and INR. May alter the antiretroviral effects of antiretrovirals.

PATIENT CONSIDERATIONS

Assessment: Assess for hypersensitivity to the drug, macrolides, PCNs, cephalosporins, or other allergens. Assess for myasthenia gravis, mononucleosis, renal/hepatic impairment, gastric malignancy, pregnancy/nursing status, and possible drug interactions.

Monitoring: Monitor for hypersensitivity reactions, drug interactions, exacerbation of symptoms of myasthenia gravis and new onset of myasthenic syndrome, CDAD, superinfections, development of drug-resistant bacteria, erythematosus skin rash, AIN, and other adverse reactions. Monitor PT/INR with warfarin and other anticoagulants.

Counseling: Inform about risks/benefits of therapy. Advise that diarrhea may occur and will usually end when therapy is discontinued. Instruct to contact physician as soon as possible if watery/blood stools (w/ or w/o stomach cramps and fever) develop even as late as 2 or more months after having taken the last dose of therapy. Counsel that therapy should only be used to treat bacterial, not viral, infections. Instruct to take exactly ud; inform that skipping doses or not completing full course may decrease effectiveness and increase antibiotic resistance.

STORAGE: 20-25°C (68-77°F). Protect from light and moisture.

OMNARIS – ciclesonide

RX

Class: Non-halogenated glucocorticoid

ADULT DOSAGE

Seasonal/Perennial Allergic Rhinitis

2 sprays/nostril qd
Max: 2 sprays/nostril/day (200mcg/day)

PEDIATRIC DOSAGE

Perennial Allergic Rhinitis

≥12 Years:
2 sprays/nostril qd
Max: 2 sprays/nostril/day (200mcg/day)

Seasonal Allergic Rhinitis

≥6 Years:
2 sprays/nostril qd
Max: 2 sprays/nostril/day (200mcg/day)

DOSING CONSIDERATIONS

Elderly
Start at low end of dosing range

ADMINISTRATION

Intranasal route

Priming
Shake bottle gently and prime pump by actuating 8X before initial use.
Reprime w/ 1 spray or until fine mist appears if not used for 4 consecutive days.

HOW SUPPLIED

Spray: 50mcg/spray [12.5g]

CONTRAINDICATIONS

Known hypersensitivity to ciclesonide or any of the ingredients of the nasal spray.

WARNINGS/PRECAUTIONS

Epistaxis reported. *Candida albicans* infections of the nose or pharynx may occur; examine periodically and treat accordingly. Nasal septal perforation may occur; avoid spraying directly onto nasal septum. May impair wound healing; avoid w/ recent nasal septal ulcers, nasal surgery, or nasal trauma until healing has occurred. Glaucoma and/or cataracts may develop. Risk for more severe/fatal course of infections (eg, chickenpox, measles); avoid exposure in patients who have not had these diseases or have not been properly immunized. May increase susceptibility to infections; caution w/ active or quiescent tuberculosis (TB), untreated local or systemic fungal/bacterial infections, systemic viral or parasitic infections, or ocular herpes simplex. D/C slowly if hypercorticism and adrenal suppression occur. Risk of adrenal insufficiency and withdrawal symptoms when replacing systemic corticosteroids w/ topical corticosteroids. May exacerbate symptoms of asthma and other conditions requiring long-term systemic corticosteroid use w/ rapid dose decrease. May reduce growth velocity in pediatric patients. Caution in elderly.

ADVERSE REACTIONS

Headache, epistaxis, nasopharyngitis, back pain, pharyngolaryngeal pain, sinusitis, influenza, nasal discomfort, bronchitis, UTI, cough.

DRUG INTERACTIONS

Ketoconazole may increase exposure of the active metabolite des-ciclesonide.

PATIENT CONSIDERATIONS

Assessment: Assess for drug hypersensitivity, TB, any infections, ocular herpes simplex, history of increased IOP, glaucoma, cataracts, recent nasal septal ulcers, nasal surgery/trauma, use of other inhaled or systemic corticosteroids, pregnancy/nursing status, and possible drug interactions. Assess if patients have not been immunized or exposed to infections, such as measles or chickenpox.

Monitoring: Monitor for hypercorticism, adrenal suppression, TB, infections, ocular herpes simplex, chickenpox, and measles. Monitor for epistaxis, nasal septal perforation, growth velocity in children, wound healing, visual changes, hypoadrenalism in infants born to mothers receiving corticosteroids during pregnancy, and hypersensitivity reactions. Monitor for adrenal insufficiency and withdrawal symptoms when replacing systemic w/ topical corticosteroids.

Counseling: Counsel on appropriate priming and administration of spray; avoid spraying in eyes or directly onto nasal septum. Instruct to take ud at regular intervals; not to exceed prescribed dosage. Instruct to contact physician if symptoms do not improve by a reasonable time (over 1-2 weeks in seasonal allergic rhinitis and 5 weeks in perennial allergic rhinitis) or if condition worsens. Counsel about risks of epistaxis, nasal ulceration, *Candida* infections, and other adverse reactions. Instruct to avoid exposure to chickenpox or measles and to consult physician if exposed to chickenpox or measles. Inform that worsening of existing TB infections, fungal/bacterial/viral/parasitic infections, or ocular herpes simplex may occur. Instruct to inform physician if change in vision occurs.

STORAGE: 25°C (77°F); excursions permitted to 15-30°C (59-86°F). Do not freeze. Discard after 4 months after removal from pouch or after 120 actuations following initial priming, whichever comes 1st.

OMNIPRED — prednisolone acetate

RX

Class: Corticosteroid

ADULT DOSAGE

Steroid-Responsive Inflammatory Ocular Conditions

Treatment of palpebral and bulbar conjunctiva, cornea, and anterior segment of globe, such as allergic conjunctivitis, acne rosacea, superficial punctate keratitis, herpes zoster keratitis, iritis, cyclitis, or selected infective conjunctivitides

Instill 2 drops in eye(s) qid

Reevaluate if signs/symptoms do not improve after 2 days

Corneal Injury

Chemical, Radiation, or Thermal Burns, or Penetration of Foreign Bodies:

Instill 2 drops in eye(s) qid

Reevaluate if signs/symptoms do not improve after 2 days

PEDIATRIC DOSAGE

Pediatric use may not have been established

ADMINISTRATION

Ocular route

Shake well before use

Use concomitantly with an anti-infective agent in cases of bacterial infections

HOW SUPPLIED

Sus: 1% [5mL, 10mL]

CONTRAINDICATIONS

Viral diseases of the cornea and conjunctiva (eg, epithelial herpes simplex keratitis, vaccinia, varicella); mycobacterial infection of the eye, and fungal diseases of ocular structures; known/suspected hypersensitivity to any of the ingredients of this preparation and to other corticosteroids.

WARNINGS/PRECAUTIONS

Prolonged use may result in glaucoma with damage to the optic nerve, defects in visual acuity and fields of vision, and in posterior subcapsular cataract formation. Prolonged use may suppress host immune response and increase hazard of secondary ocular infections. Use in the presence of thin corneal or scleral tissue, which may be caused by various ocular diseases or long-term use of topical corticosteroids, may lead to perforation. May enhance activity of or mask acute purulent infections of the eye. Routinely monitor intraocular pressure (IOP) if used for ≥10 days. Caution with glaucoma.

Use after cataract surgery may delay healing and increase incidence of bleb formation. May prolong course and exacerbate severity of many viral infections of the eye; use with extreme caution with history of herpes simplex. Not effective in mustard gas keratitis and Sjogren's keratoconjunctivitis. Fungal infections of the cornea may develop coincidentally with long-term use; suspect fungal invasion in any persistent corneal ulceration. In chronic conditions, withdraw treatment by gradually decreasing frequency of application. Caution not to d/c therapy prematurely.

ADVERSE REACTIONS
Elevation of IOP, glaucoma, optic nerve damage, posterior subcapsular cataract formation, delayed wound healing, acute anterior uveitis, globe perforation.

PATIENT CONSIDERATIONS

Assessment: Assess for viral diseases of cornea and conjunctiva, mycobacterial infection of the eye, fungal diseases of ocular structures, hypersensitivity to drug or other corticosteroids, history of herpes simplex, thin corneal or scleral tissue, glaucoma, cataract surgery, and pregnancy/nursing status.

Monitoring: Monitor for glaucoma, optic nerve damage, visual acuity and fields of vision defects, posterior subcapsular cataracts, secondary ocular infections, perforation of the cornea/sclera, exacerbation of viral infections of eye, fungal invasion, and other adverse reactions. Routinely monitor IOP if used for ≥10 days. Monitor for improvement of signs/symptoms.

Counseling: Advise to d/c use and consult physician if inflammation or pain persists >48 hrs or becomes aggravated. Instruct to use caution to avoid touching the bottle tip to eyelids or to any other surfaces to prevent contamination. Instruct to keep bottle tightly closed when not in use and to keep it out of reach of children.

STORAGE: 8-24°C (46-75°F); upright position.

ONDANSETRON — ondansetron

RX

Class: 5-HT_3 receptor antagonist

OTHER BRAND NAMES
Zofran, Zofran ODT

ADULT DOSAGE

Chemotherapy-Induced Nausea/Vomiting

Inj:

Prevention of N/V Associated w/ Initial and Repeat Courses of Emetogenic Chemotherapy (Including High-Dose Cisplatin):
Three 0.15mg/kg IV doses (diluted) up to a max of 16mg/dose; infuse over 15 min. Give 1st dose 30 min before the start of chemotherapy, then give subsequent doses 4 and 8 hrs after the 1st dose

Oral:

Prevention of N/V Associated w/ Highly Emetogenic Chemotherapy (Including Cisplatin ≥50mg/m²):
24mg (given as three 8mg tabs) 30 min before start of single-day chemotherapy

Prevention of N/V Associated w/ Moderately Emetogenic Chemotherapy:
8mg bid; give 1st dose 30 min before chemotherapy, then give subsequent dose 8 hrs after 1st dose, then administer 8mg q12h for 1-2 days after completion of chemotherapy

Postoperative Nausea/Vomiting

Prevention:

Inj:
4mg IM/IV undiluted immediately before induction of anesthesia or postoperatively if prophylactic antiemetic was not received and N/V occurs w/in 2 hrs after surgery; infuse IV in not less than 30 sec, preferably over 2-5 min

Oral:
16mg given 1 hr before induction of anesthesia

PEDIATRIC DOSAGE

Chemotherapy-Induced Nausea/Vomiting

Inj:

Prevention of N/V Associated w/ Initial and Repeat Courses of Emetogenic Chemotherapy (Including High-Dose Cisplatin):

6 Months-18 Years:
Three 0.15mg/kg IV doses (diluted) up to a max of 16mg/dose; infuse over 15 min. Give 1st dose 30 min before the start of chemotherapy, then give subsequent doses 4 and 8 hrs after the 1st dose

Oral:

Prevention of N/V Associated w/ Moderately Emetogenic Cancer Chemotherapy:

4-11 Years:
4mg tid; give 1st dose 30 min before chemotherapy, then give subsequent doses 4 and 8 hrs after 1st dose, then administer 4mg q8h for 1-2 days after completion of chemotherapy

≥12 Years:
8mg bid; give 1st dose 30 min before chemotherapy, then give subsequent dose 8 hrs after 1st dose, then administer 8mg q12h for 1-2 days after completion of chemotherapy

Postoperative Nausea/Vomiting

Prevention:

1 Month-12 Years:

Inj:
≤40kg: 0.1mg/kg IV single dose
>40kg: 4mg IV single dose

Radiotherapy Associated Nausea/Vomiting

Oral:

Prevention in Patients Receiving Either Total Body Irradiation, Single High-Dose Fraction to the Abdomen, or Daily Fractions to the Abdomen:

Usual: 8mg tid

Total Body Irradiation:

8mg should be administered 1-2 hrs before each fraction of radiotherapy administered each day

Single High-Dose Fraction Radiotherapy to the Abdomen:

8mg should be administered 1-2 hrs before radiotherapy, w/ subsequent doses q8h after 1st dose for 1-2 days after completion of radiotherapy

Daily Fractionated Radiotherapy to the Abdomen:

8mg should be administered 1-2 hrs before radiotherapy, w/ subsequent doses q8h after 1st dose for each day radiotherapy is given

Infuse in not less than 30 sec, preferably over 2-5 min immediately before or after induction of anesthesia or postoperatively if prophylactic antiemetic was not received and N/V occurs shortly after surgery

DOSING CONSIDERATIONS

Hepatic Impairment

Severe (Child-Pugh Score ≥10):

Oral:

Max: 8mg/day

Inj:

Max: 8mg/day infused over 15 min beginning 30 min prior to emetogenic chemotherapy

ADMINISTRATION

IV/IM/Oral routes

ODT

Do not attempt to push tabs through the foil backing
Peel back the foil backing of 1 blister and gently remove tab
Immediately place tab on top of the tongue where it will dissolve in seconds, then swallow w/ saliva

Inj

Should be diluted in 50mL of D5 or NaCl before administration
Do not mix w/ alkaline sol as a precipitate may form

HOW SUPPLIED

Tab: 24mg; **(Zofran) Inj:** 2mg/mL [20mL], **Sol:** 4mg base/5mL [50mL], **Tab/Tab, Disintegrating (ODT):** 4mg, 8mg

CONTRAINDICATIONS

Concomitant use w/ apomorphine, known hypersensitivity to ondansetron or any of its components.

WARNINGS/PRECAUTIONS

Hypersensitivity reactions reported in patients hypersensitive to other selective 5-HT_3 receptor antagonists. ECG changes, including QT interval prolongation and torsades de pointes, reported; avoid in patients w/ congenital long QT syndrome. Monitor ECG in patients with electrolyte abnormalities (eg, hypokalemia, hypomagnesemia), CHF, bradyarrhythmias, and in patients taking other medications that lead to QT prolongation. Serotonin syndrome reported; d/c and initiate supportive treatment if symptoms occur. Use in patients following abdominal surgery or w/ chemotherapy-induced N/V may mask a progressive ileus and/or gastric distension. Does not stimulate gastric/intestinal peristalsis; do not use instead of NG suction. (ODT) Contains phenylalanine; caution in phenylketonuric patients.

ADVERSE REACTIONS

Headache, diarrhea, constipation, fever, pruritus, dizziness, bradycardia, drowsiness/sedation. (Inj) Inj-site reaction. (PO) Malaise/fatigue, anxiety/agitation, urinary retention.

DRUG INTERACTIONS

See Contraindications. Inducers or inhibitors of CYP3A4, CYP2D6, and CYP1A2 may change the clearance and $T_{1/2}$. Potent CYP3A4 inducers (eg, phenytoin, carbamazepine, rifampin) may significantly increase clearance and decrease blood levels. May reduce analgesic activity of tramadol. May cause serotonin syndrome w/ other serotonergic drugs (eg, SSRIs, SNRIs, MAOIs, mirtazapine, fentanyl, lithium, tramadol, IV methylene blue); d/c and initiate supportive treatment if symptoms occur.

PATIENT CONSIDERATIONS

Assessment: Assess for previous hypersensitivity to the drug, congenital long QT syndrome, electrolyte abnormalities, CHF, bradyarrhythmias, hepatic impairment, pregnancy/nursing status, and possible drug interactions. (ODT) Assess for phenylketonuria.

Monitoring: Monitor for QT interval prolongation, torsades de pointes, hypersensitivity reactions, serotonin syndrome, and other adverse reactions. Monitor ECG in patients w/ electrolyte abnormalities, CHF, bradyarrhythmias, and in patients taking other medications that lead to QT prolongation. In patients who recently underwent abdominal surgery or in patients w/ chemotherapy-induced N/V, monitor for masking of a progressive ileus and/or gastric distension.

Counseling: Inform about potential benefits/risks of therapy. Inform that drug may cause serious cardiac arrhythmias (eg, QT prolongation); instruct patients to contact physician if they perceive a change in their HR, if they feel lightheaded, or have a syncopal episode. Inform that chances of developing severe cardiac arrhythmias are higher in patients w/ a personal/family history of abnormal heart rhythms (eg, congenital long QT syndrome), patients taking medications (eg, diuretics) that may cause electrolyte abnormalities, and in patients w/ hypokalemia or hypomagnesemia. Advise of the possibility of serotonin syndrome; instruct to seek immediate medical attention if changes in mental status, autonomic instability, neuromuscular symptoms w/ or w/o GI symptoms occur. Inform that drug may cause hypersensitivity reactions, some as severe as anaphylaxis and bronchospasm; instruct to report any signs/symptoms of hypersensitivity reactions to physician. Advise to report the use of all medications to physician. Inform that drug may cause headache, drowsiness/sedation, constipation, fever, and diarrhea. Inform phenylketonuric patients that ODT contains phenylalanine.

STORAGE: 20-25°C (68-77°F); excursions permitted to 15-30°C (59-86°F). Protect from light. Zofran: (Inj/ODT/Tab) 2-30°C (36-86°F). (Sol) 15-30°C (59-86°F); store bottles upright in cartons. (Inj/Sol/Tab) Protect from light. (Inj) Diluted Sol: Do not use beyond 24 hrs. Refer to PI for further information on stability and handling.

ONGLYZA – saxagliptin

RX

Class: Dipeptidyl peptidase-4 (DPP-4) inhibitor

ADULT DOSAGE

Type 2 Diabetes Mellitus

2.5mg or 5mg qd

PEDIATRIC DOSAGE

Pediatric use may not have been established

O

DOSING CONSIDERATIONS

Concomitant Medications

Strong CYP3A4/5 Inhibitors: 2.5mg qd

Insulin Secretagogue (eg, Sulfonylurea)/Insulin: May require a lower dose of insulin secretagogue or insulin

Renal Impairment

Moderate or Severe/ESRD Requiring Hemodialysis (CrCl ≤50mL/min): 2.5mg qd

Administer following hemodialysis

ADMINISTRATION

Oral route

Take regardless of meals.
Do not split or cut tab.

HOW SUPPLIED

Tab: 2.5mg, 5mg

CONTRAINDICATIONS

History of a serious hypersensitivity reaction to saxagliptin (eg, anaphylaxis, angioedema, or exfoliative skin conditions).

WARNINGS/PRECAUTIONS

Not for treatment of type 1 diabetes mellitus (DM) or diabetic ketoacidosis. Acute pancreatitis reported; d/c if pancreatitis is suspected and initiate appropriate management. Serious hypersensitivity reactions reported; if suspected, d/c therapy, assess for other potential causes, and institute alternative treatment. Caution in patients w/ history of angioedema to another DPP-4 inhibitor and in elderly. Severe and disabling arthralgia reported; d/c if appropriate.

ADVERSE REACTIONS

URTI, UTI, headache, peripheral edema.

DRUG INTERACTIONS

See Dosing Considerations. Increased incidence of hypoglycemia reported w/ a sulfonylurea or insulin. Ketoconazole and other strong CYP3A4/5 inhibitors (eg, atazanavir, clarithromycin, itraconazole) may increase plasma levels.

PATIENT CONSIDERATIONS

Assessment: Assess for previous hypersensitivity to the drug, history of pancreatitis, type of DM, diabetic ketoacidosis, history of angioedema to another DPP-4 inhibitor, pregnancy/nursing status, and possible drug interactions. Obtain baseline renal function, and FPG and HbA1c levels.

Monitoring: Monitor for pancreatitis, hypersensitivity reactions, and other adverse reactions. Monitor FPG, HbA1c, and renal function periodically.

Counseling: Inform of the potential risks, benefits, and alternative modes of therapy. Advise on the importance of adherence to dietary instructions, regular physical activity, periodic blood glucose monitoring and HbA1c testing, recognition and management of hypo/hyperglycemia, and assessment of diabetic complications. Instruct to seek medical advice promptly during periods of stress as medication requirements may change. Instruct to d/c use and notify physician if signs and symptoms of pancreatitis or allergic reactions occur. Counsel to inform physician if any unusual symptom develops, or if any existing symptom persists or worsens. Inform that severe and disabling joint pain may occur; instruct to seek medical advice if severe joint pain occurs. Inform that if a dose was missed, to take the next dose as prescribed, unless otherwise instructed by physician; instruct not to take an extra dose the next day.

STORAGE: 20-25°C (68-77°F); excursions permitted to 15-30°C (59-86°F).

OPANA – oxymorphone hydrochloride CII

Class: Opioid analgesic

ADULT DOSAGE

Moderate to Severe Pain

Acute:
Opioid-Naive:
Initial: 10-20mg q4-6h depending on pain intensity; doses >20mg is not recommended
Titrate: Adjust dose to adequate pain relief (generally mild or no pain)

Maint:
Continually reevaluate; if level of pain increases, identify source of pain while adjusting the dose

Conversions

From Parenteral Oxymorphone:
Give 10X the total daily parenteral oxymorphone dose in 4-6 equally divided doses

From Other Oral Opioids:
Initial: 1/2 the calculated total daily dose in 4-6 equally divided doses, given q4-6h
Titrate: Gradually adjust until adequate pain relief and acceptable side effects achieved

PEDIATRIC DOSAGE

Pediatric use may not have been established

DOSING CONSIDERATIONS

Concomitant Medications

CNS Depressants (Sedatives/Hypnotics, General Anesthetics, Phenothiazines, Tranquilizers, and Alcohol):
Initial: 1/3 to 1/2 of the usual dose

MAOIs: Not recommended

Renal Impairment
<50mL/min:
Initial: 5mg; use caution
Titrate: Slowly adjust dose while monitoring side effects

Hepatic Impairment
Mild:
Initial: 5mg; use caution
Titrate: Slowly adjust to an acceptable level of analgesia based on response to initial dose

Elderly
Initial: Start at low end of dosing range (eg, 5mg)

Discontinuation
Taper doses gradually to prevent signs/symptoms of withdrawal

ADMINISTRATION

Oral route

HOW SUPPLIED

Tab: 5mg, 10mg

CONTRAINDICATIONS

Known hypersensitivity to oxymorphone, morphine analogues (eg, codeine), or to any other ingredients in the product; respiratory depression (except in monitored settings with resuscitative equipment); acute/severe bronchial asthma or hypercarbia; paralytic ileus; moderate/severe hepatic impairment.

WARNINGS/PRECAUTIONS

Respiratory depression may occur; extreme caution in elderly or debilitated, or with conditions accompanied by hypoxia, hypercapnia, or decreased respiratory reserve (eg, asthma, chronic obstructive pulmonary disease or cor pulmonale, severe obesity, sleep apnea syndrome, myxedema, kyphoscoliosis, CNS depression, coma). May be abused in a manner similar to other opioid agonists. Respiratory depressant effects and potential to elevate CSF pressure may be markedly exaggerated in the presence of head injury, intracranial lesions, or preexisting increased intracranial pressure (ICP). May produce effects on papillary response and consciousness, which may obscure neurologic signs of further increases in ICP in patients with head injuries; extreme caution with increased ICP or impaired consciousness. May cause severe hypotension; caution with circulatory shock. Caution with adrenocortical insufficiency (eg, Addison's disease), prostatic hypertrophy or urethral stricture, severe pulmonary impairment, moderate/severe renal dysfunction, mild hepatic impairment, and toxic psychosis. May induce or aggravate convulsions/seizures. May diminish propulsive peristaltic waves in the GI tract; monitor for decreased bowel motility in postoperative patients. May obscure diagnosis or clinical course in patients with acute abdominal conditions. May cause spasm of the sphincter of Oddi; caution with biliary tract disease, including acute pancreatitis. May impair physical/mental abilities. Not recommended for use during and immediately prior to labor. Physical dependence and tolerance may occur. Avoid abrupt discontinuation.

ADVERSE REACTIONS

Constipation, N/V, pyrexia, somnolence, headache, dizziness, pruritus, confusion.

DRUG INTERACTIONS

Additive CNS depression with other CNS depressants (eg, sedatives, hypnotics, tranquilizers, general anesthetics, phenothiazines, other opioids, alcohol). Avoid with ethanol. Caution with MAOI; not recommended within 14 days of MAOI use. Anticholinergics may increase risk of urinary retention and/or severe constipation, which may lead to paralytic ileus. CNS side effects (eg, confusion, disorientation, respiratory depression, apnea, seizures) reported with cimetidine. Mixed agonist/antagonist analgesics (pentazocine, nalbuphine, butorphanol, buprenorphine) may reduce analgesic effect and/or precipitate withdrawal symptoms; use with caution. May cause severe hypotension with phenothiazines or other agents that compromise vasomotor tone.

PATIENT CONSIDERATIONS

Assessment: Assess for level of pain intensity, type of pain, degree of opioid tolerance, patient's general condition and medical status, history of or risk factors for abuse and addiction, renal/hepatic impairment, pregnancy/nursing status, any other conditions where treatment is contraindicated or cautioned, and possible drug interactions.

Monitoring: Monitor for signs/symptoms of respiratory depression, hypotension, convulsions/seizures, decreased bowel motility in postoperative patients, spasm of sphincter of Oddi, physical dependence, tolerance, abuse/addiction, and other adverse reactions.

Counseling: Instruct to take drug ud. Inform that drug has potential for abuse and should be protected from theft. Instruct to dispose of any unused tabs by flushing down the toilet. Advise to contact physician if experiencing adverse events or inadequate pain control during therapy. Instruct not to adjust dose without consulting physician. Inform that drug may impair mental/physical abilities. Advise to avoid alcohol or other CNS depressants. Advise of the potential for severe constipation. Advise to consult physician if pregnant or planning to become pregnant. Inform that if taking medication for more than a few weeks, to avoid abrupt withdrawal; dosing will need to be tapered.

STORAGE: 25°C (77°F); excursions permitted to 15-30°C (59-86°F).

OPANA ER – oxymorphone hydrochloride CII

Class: Opioid analgesic

Exposes users to risks of addiction, abuse, and misuse, leading to overdose and death; assess each patient's risk prior to prescribing and monitor regularly for development of these behaviors/conditions. Serious, life-threatening, or fatal respiratory depression may occur; monitor upon initiation or following a dose increase. Crushing, chewing, or dissolving tab can cause rapid release and absorption of potentially fatal dose; instruct patients to swallow tab whole. Accidental ingestion of even 1 dose, especially by children, can result in a fatal overdose. Prolonged use during pregnancy can result in neonatal opioid withdrawal syndrome; advise pregnant women of the risk and ensure availability of appropriate treatment. Avoid use with alcoholic beverages or medications containing alcohol; co-ingestion may result in increased plasma levels and potentially fatal overdose.

ADULT DOSAGE

Severe Pain (Daily, Around-the-Clock Management)

1st Opioid Analgesic/Opioid Intolerant Patients:
Initial: 5mg q12h
Titrate: May adjust dose every 3-7 days in increments of 5-10mg q12h

Conversions

From Immediate-Release (IR) to Extended-Release (ER) Oxymorphone:
Administer 1/2 the total daily IR dose as ER, q12h

From Parenteral Oxymorphone:
Administer 10X the total daily parenteral oxymorphone dose as ER in 2 equally divided doses

From Other Oral Opioids:
D/C all other around-the-clock opioids when therapy is initiated; refer to PI for conversion factors and dose calculations

PEDIATRIC DOSAGE

Pediatric use may not have been established

DOSING CONSIDERATIONS

Renal Impairment
CrCl <50mL/min:
Opioid-Naive: Initiate treatment w/ 5mg dose
On Prior Opioid Therapy: Initiate at 50% lower than the starting dose for a patient w/ normal renal function on prior opioids and titrate slowly

Hepatic Impairment
Mild:
Opioid-Naive: Initiate treatment w/ 5mg dose
On Prior Opioid Therapy: Initiate at 50% lower than the starting dose for a patient w/ normal hepatic function on prior opioids and titrate slowly

Elderly
Opioid-Naive: Initiate treatment w/ 5mg dose
On Prior Opioid Therapy: Initiate at 50% lower than the starting dose for a younger patient on prior opioids and titrate slowly

Discontinuation
Use gradual downward dose titration every 2-4 days

O

ADMINISTRATION

Oral route

Do not presoak, lick, or otherwise wet tab prior to placing in mouth
Swallow tab whole; do not crush, dissolve, or chew
Take 1 tab at a time w/ enough water to ensure complete swallowing
Take on an empty stomach, at least 1 hr ac or 2 hrs pc

HOW SUPPLIED

Tab, ER: 5mg, 7.5mg, 10mg, 15mg, 20mg, 30mg, 40mg

CONTRAINDICATIONS

Significant respiratory depression, acute/severe bronchial asthma or hypercarbia, known or suspected paralytic ileus and GI obstruction, moderate or severe hepatic impairment, hypersensitivity (eg, anaphylaxis) to oxymorphone, any other ingredients in the product, or to morphine analogs (eg, codeine).

WARNINGS/PRECAUTIONS

Reserve use in patients for whom alternative treatment options are ineffective, not tolerated, or would be otherwise inadequate to provide sufficient management of pain. Should only be prescribed by healthcare professionals who are knowledgeable in the use of potent opioids for management of chronic pain. Life-threatening respiratory depression is more likely to occur in elderly, cachectic, or debilitated patients. Consider alternative nonopioid analgesics in patients with significant COPD or cor pulmonale, and in patients having a substantially decreased respiratory reserve, hypoxia, hypercapnia, or preexisting respiratory depression. May cause severe hypotension, orthostatic hypotension, and syncope; increased risk in patients whose ability to maintain BP has already been compromised by a reduced blood volume or concurrent administration of certain CNS depressants. Avoid with circulatory shock. Monitor patients who may be susceptible to intracranial effects of carbon dioxide retention for signs of sedation and respiratory depression when initiating therapy. May obscure clinical course in a patient with head injury. Avoid with impaired consciousness or coma. Difficulty in swallowing tab, and intestinal obstruction reported; consider alternative analgesic in patients who have difficulty swallowing or have underlying GI disorders that may predispose them to obstruction. May cause spasm of sphincter of Oddi and increase in serum amylase; monitor patients for worsening symptoms with biliary tract disease. May aggravate convulsions and induce/aggravate seizures. May impair mental/physical abilities. Not for use during and immediately prior to labor.

ADVERSE REACTIONS

Respiratory depression, constipation, N/V, diarrhea, somnolence, headache, dizziness, pruritus, increased sweating, dry mouth, sedation, insomnia, fatigue, decreased appetite, abdominal pain.

DRUG INTERACTIONS

See Boxed Warning. Hypotension, profound sedation, coma, respiratory depression, and death may occur with CNS depressants (eg, sedatives, anxiolytics, neuroleptics); if coadministration is considered, reduce dose of 1 or both agents. Monitor use in elderly, cachectic, and debilitated patients when coadministered with other drugs that depress respiration. Mixed agonist/antagonist analgesics (pentazocine, nalbuphine, butorphanol) and partial agonists (buprenorphine) may reduce analgesic effect or precipitate withdrawal symptoms; avoid concomitant use. May enhance neuromuscular blocking action of skeletal muscle relaxants and increase degree of respiratory depression. Cimetidine may potentiate opioid-induced respiratory depression. Anticholinergics or other drugs with anticholinergic activity may increase risk of urinary retention and/or severe constipation, which may lead to paralytic ileus.

PATIENT CONSIDERATIONS

Assessment: Assess for abuse/addiction risk, pain intensity, prior opioid therapy, opioid tolerance, respiratory depression, renal/hepatic impairment, GI obstruction, drug hypersensitivity, pregnancy/nursing status, possible drug interactions, or any other conditions where treatment is contraindicated or cautioned.

Monitoring: Monitor for sedation, respiratory depression (especially within first 24-72 hrs of initiation or following a dose increase), hypotension, seizures/convulsions, and other adverse reactions. Monitor BP and serum amylase levels. Routinely monitor for signs of misuse, abuse, and addiction. Periodically reassess the continued need for therapy.

Counseling: Inform that use of drug can result in addiction, abuse, and misuse; instruct not to share with others and to take steps to protect from theft or misuse. Inform about risk and signs/symptoms of respiratory depression. Advise to store securely and dispose of unused tabs by flushing down the toilet. Inform female patients of reproductive potential that prolonged use during pregnancy may result in neonatal opioid withdrawal syndrome. Advise that drug may cause fetal harm and instruct to inform physician if pregnant/planning to become pregnant. Instruct not to consume alcoholic beverages or prescription and OTC products that contain alcohol during treatment. Inform that potentially serious additive effects may occur when used with alcohol or other CNS depressants, and not to use such drugs unless supervised by physician. Instruct to take drug exactly as prescribed, and not to d/c without 1st discussing the need for a tapering regimen with the physician. Inform that occasionally, inactive ingredients may be eliminated as a soft mass in stool that may resemble the original tab; inform that the active medication has already been absorbed by the time they see the soft mass. Inform that drug may cause orthostatic hypotension and syncope. Inform that drug may impair the ability to perform potentially hazardous activities; advise not to perform such tasks until they know how they will react to medication. Advise of potential for severe constipation, including management instructions. Advise how to recognize anaphylaxis and when to seek medical attention.

STORAGE: 25°C (77°F); excursions permitted to 15-30°C (59-86°F).

OPDIVO — nivolumab

RX

Class: Monoclonal antibody/programmed death receptor-1 (PD-1) blocker

ADULT DOSAGE

Unresectable or Metastatic Melanoma

BRAF V600 Wild-Type Unresectable/Metastatic Melanoma or BRAF V600 Mutation-Positive Unresectable/Metastatic Melanoma:

3mg/kg IV every 2 weeks until disease progression or unacceptable toxicity

PEDIATRIC DOSAGE

Pediatric use may not have been established

Unresectable/Metastatic Melanoma, in Combination w/ Ipilimumab:
1mg/kg IV, followed by ipilimumab on the same day, every 3 weeks for 4 doses; the subsequent dose of nivolumab is 3mg/kg IV every 2 weeks until disease progression or unacceptable toxicity, as a single agent

Metastatic Non-Small Cell Lung Cancer

W/ Progression On or After Platinum-Based Chemotherapy:
Patients w/ EGFR or ALK genomic aberrations should have disease progression on FDA-approved therapy for these aberrations prior to receiving nivolumab

3mg/kg IV every 2 weeks until disease progression or unacceptable toxicity

Advanced Renal Cell Carcinoma

In Patients Who Have Received Prior Anti-Angiogenic Therapy:
3mg/kg IV every 2 weeks until disease progression or unacceptable toxicity

---

DOSING CONSIDERATIONS

Adverse Reactions

Infusion Reactions:
Mild or Moderate: Interrupt or slow infusion rate
Severe or Life-Threatening: D/C

Colitis:
Grade 2 Diarrhea or Colitis: Withhold dose*
Grade 3 Diarrhea or Colitis: Withhold dose* (single-agent nivolumab) or permanently d/c (in combination w/ ipilimumab)
Grade 4 Diarrhea or Colitis: Permanently d/c

Pneumonitis:
Grade 2: Withhold dose*
Grade 3 or 4: Permanently d/c

Hepatitis:
AST or ALT >3 and up to 5X ULN or Total Bilirubin >1.5 and up to 3X ULN: Withhold dose*
AST or ALT >5X ULN or Total Bilirubin >3X ULN: Permanently d/c

Hypophysitis:
Grade 2 or 3: Withhold dose*
Grade 4: Permanently d/c

Adrenal Insufficiency:
Grade 2: Withhold dose*
Grade 3 or 4: Permanently d/c

Type 1 Diabetes Mellitus (DM):
Grade 3 Hyperglycemia: Withhold dose*
Grade 4 Hyperglycemia: Permanently d/c

Nephritis and Renal Dysfunction:
SrCr >1.5 and up to 6X ULN: Withhold dose*
SrCr >6X ULN: Permanently d/c

Rash:
Grade 3: Withhold dose*
Grade 4: Permanently d/c

Encephalitis:
New Onset Moderate or Severe Neurologic Signs or Symptoms: Withhold dose*
Immune-Mediated Encephalitis: Permanently d/c

Other:
Other Grade 3 Adverse Reaction:
1st Occurrence: Withhold dose*
Recurrence of Same Grade 3 Adverse Reactions: Permanently d/c
Life-Threatening or Grade 4 Adverse Reactions: Permanently d/c
Requirement for ≥10mg/day Prednisone or Equivalent for >12 Weeks: Permanently d/c
Persistent Grade 2 or 3 Adverse Reactions Lasting ≥12 Weeks: Permanently d/c

When administered w/ ipilimumab, if nivolumab is withheld, ipilimumab should also be withheld

*Resume treatment when adverse reaction returns to Grade 0 or 1

O

ADMINISTRATION

IV route

Preparation

1. Withdraw required volume of product and transfer into an IV container.
2. Dilute w/ either 0.9% NaCl inj or D5 inj to prepare an infusion w/ a final concentration ranging from 1-10mg/mL.
3. Mix diluted sol by gentle inversion; do not shake.
4. Discard partially used or empty vials.
5. After preparation, store infusion either at room temperature for ≤4 hrs from time of preparation (including room temperature storage of infusion in IV container and time for infusion administration) or at 2-8°C (36-46°F) for ≤24 hrs from time of infusion preparation; do not freeze.

Administration

Administer over 60 min through IV line containing a sterile, non-pyrogenic, low protein binding in-line filter (pore size 0.2-1.2μm).

Do not coadminister other drugs through the same IV line.

Flush IV line at end of infusion.

When administered w/ ipilimumab, infuse nivolumab 1st followed by ipilimumab on the same day. Use separate infusion bags and filters for each infusion.

HOW SUPPLIED

Inj: 10mg/mL [4mL, 10mL]

WARNINGS/PRECAUTIONS

Refer to Dosing Considerations for recommendations to withhold or d/c therapy for the following adverse reactions. Refer to PI for corticosteroid dose in the management of the following adverse reactions. Immune-mediated pneumonitis, including fatal cases, reported; administer corticosteroids for ≥Grade 2 pneumonitis, followed by corticosteroid taper. Immune-mediated colitis may occur. Administer corticosteroids followed by corticosteroid taper for Grade 3 or 4 colitis. Administer corticosteroids followed by corticosteroid taper for Grade 2 colitis lasting >5 days; if worsening or no improvement occurs, increase corticosteroid dose. Permanently d/c therapy for recurrent colitis upon restarting therapy. Immune-mediated hepatitis may occur; administer corticosteroids for ≥Grade 2 transaminase elevations, w/ or w/o concomitant elevation in total bilirubin. Hypophysitis may occur; administer corticosteroids for ≥Grade 2 hypophysitis. Adrenal insufficiency may occur; administer corticosteroids for Grade 3 or 4 adrenal insufficiency. Thyroid disorders may occur; administer hormone replacement therapy for hypothyroidism and initiate medical management for control of hyperthyroidism. Type 1 DM may occur; administer insulin for type 1 diabetes. Immune-mediated nephritis and renal dysfunction may occur. For Grade 2 or 3 SrCr elevation, withhold therapy and administer corticosteroids followed by corticosteroid taper; if worsening or no improvement occurs, increase corticosteroid dose and permanently d/c therapy. Permanently d/c therapy and administer corticosteroids followed by corticosteroid taper for Grade 4 SrCr elevation. Immune-mediated rash may occur; administer corticosteroids for Grade 3 or 4 rash. Severe rash, including rare cases of fatal toxic epidermal necrolysis, reported. Immune-mediated encephalitis may occur; if other etiologies are ruled out, administer corticosteroids followed by corticosteroid taper. Other clinically significant immune-mediated adverse reactions (eg, uveitis, pancreatitis, abducens nerve paresis, demyelination, polymyalgia rheumatica, autoimmune neuropathy) may occur during therapy and after discontinuation of therapy; exclude other causes. Based on severity of the adverse reaction, permanently d/c or withhold therapy, administer high-dose corticosteroids, and if appropriate, initiate hormone replacement therapy. Upon improvement to ≤Grade 1, initiate corticosteroid taper and continue to taper over at least 1 month. Consider restarting therapy after completion of corticosteroid taper based on the severity of the event. Severe infusion reactions reported. May cause fetal harm.

ADVERSE REACTIONS

Melanoma: (Single Agent) Fatigue, rash, musculoskeletal pain, pruritus, diarrhea, nausea. (W/ Ipilimumab) Fatigue, rash, diarrhea, nausea, pyrexia, vomiting, dyspnea.

Metastatic Non-Small Cell Lung Cancer: Fatigue, musculoskeletal pain, cough, decreased appetite, constipation.

Advanced Renal Cell Carcinoma: Asthenic conditions, cough, nausea, rash, dyspnea, diarrhea, constipation, decreased appetite, back pain, arthralgia.

PATIENT CONSIDERATIONS

Assessment: Assess pregnancy/nursing status. Obtain baseline liver/renal (eg, SrCr)/thyroid function.

Monitoring: Monitor for signs w/ radiographic imaging and symptoms of pneumonitis. Monitor for signs/symptoms of immune-mediated colitis, hypophysitis, adrenal insufficiency, rash, encephalitis, hyperglycemia, and other adverse reactions. Monitor for abnormal liver tests, elevated SrCr, and thyroid function periodically.

Counseling: Inform of the risk of immune-mediated adverse reactions that may require corticosteroid treatment and withholding or discontinuation of therapy (eg, pneumonitis, colitis, hepatitis, endocrinopathies, nephritis and renal dysfunction, rash, encephalitis); instruct to immediately contact healthcare provider if signs/symptoms of an immune-mediated adverse reaction occur. Advise of the potential risk of infusion reaction. Advise females of reproductive potential of the potential risk to a fetus and instruct to inform their healthcare provider of known/ suspected pregnancy and to use effective contraception during treatment and for at least 5 months following the last dose of therapy. Advise women not to breastfeed while on therapy.

STORAGE: 2-8°C (36-46°F). Protect from light. Do not freeze or shake.

ORACEA – doxycycline

RX

Class: Tetracyclines

ADULT DOSAGE

Rosacea

Inflammatory Lesions (Papules/Pustules):
Usual: 40mg qam

PEDIATRIC DOSAGE

Pediatric use may not have been established

DOSING CONSIDERATIONS

Elderly

Start at lower end of dosing range

ADMINISTRATION

Oral route

Take on an empty stomach, preferably at least 1 hr ac or 2 hrs pc

Administer w/ adequate amounts of fluid to reduce the risk of esophageal irritation and ulceration

HOW SUPPLIED

Cap: 40mg

CONTRAINDICATIONS

Hypersensitivity to doxycycline or any of the other tetracyclines.

WARNINGS/PRECAUTIONS

Do not use for treating bacterial infections, providing antibacterial prophylaxis, or reducing the numbers of (or eliminating) microorganisms associated w/ any bacterial disease. May cause fetal harm. May cause permanent discoloration of the teeth (yellow-gray-brown) if used during tooth development (last half of pregnancy, infancy, childhood up to 8 yrs of age). Enamel hypoplasia reported. Do not use during tooth development unless other drugs are not likely to be effective or are contraindicated. May decrease fibula growth rate in premature infants. *Clostridium difficile*-associated diarrhea (CDAD) reported; d/c if CDAD is suspected or confirmed. May result in overgrowth of non-susceptible microorganisms, including fungi; d/c and institute appropriate therapy if superinfection occurs. Caution in patients w/ a history of or predisposition to *Candida* overgrowth. Bacterial resistance may develop; use only as indicated and do not exceed recommended dosage. Photosensitivity manifested by an exaggerated sunburn reaction reported. Development of autoimmune syndromes reported; d/c immediately and perform LFTs, antinuclear antibody (ANA), CBC, and other appropriate tests in symptomatic patients. Tissue hyperpigmentation reported. May increase BUN. Caution in patients w/ renal impairment; may lead to excessive systemic accumulations and possible liver toxicity. Lower than usual total dosages are indicated and if therapy is prolonged, serum drug level determinations may be advisable. Associated w/ pseudotumor cerebri (benign intracranial HTN) in adults and bulging fontanels in infants. Lab test interactions may occur.

ADVERSE REACTIONS

Nasopharyngitis, sinusitis, diarrhea, HTN.

DRUG INTERACTIONS

Depresses plasma prothrombin activity; may require downward adjustment of anticoagulant dosage. May interfere w/ bactericidal action of penicillin; avoid concurrent use. Fatal renal toxicity reported w/ methoxyflurane. Bismuth subsalicylate, proton pump inhibitors, antacids containing aluminum, Ca^{2+}, or Mg^{2+}, and iron-containing preparations may impair absorption. May interfere w/ the effectiveness of low dose oral contraceptives. Avoid concurrent use w/ oral retinoids (eg, isotretinoin, acitretin); pseudotumor cerebri reported. Barbiturates, carbamazepine, and phenytoin decrease the $T_{1/2}$ of doxycycline.

PATIENT CONSIDERATIONS

Assessment: Assess for hypersensitivity to drug and other tetracyclines, renal impairment, history of or predisposition to *Candida* overgrowth, visual disturbances, pregnancy/nursing status, and possible drug interactions.

Monitoring: Monitor for signs/symptoms of CDAD, superinfection, photosensitivity, autoimmune syndromes, tissue hyperpigmentation, and other adverse reactions. Monitor serum drug levels in patients w/ renal impairment if therapy is prolonged. Routinely check for papilledema while on treatment. Perform periodic lab evaluations of organ systems, including hematopoietic, renal, and hepatic studies. If symptoms of autoimmune syndrome occur, perform LFTs, ANA, CBC, and other appropriate tests.

Counseling: Instruct to take exactly ud. Inform that drug should not be used by pregnant or breastfeeding women nor by individuals of either gender who are attempting to conceive a child. Inform that drug may render oral contraceptives less effective; advise females to use a 2nd form of contraception. Inform that pseudomembranous colitis and pseudotumor cerebri may occur; instruct to seek immediate medical attention if watery/bloody stools, or headache or blurred vision occur. Instruct to minimize/avoid exposure to natural or artificial sunlight and d/c at 1st evidence of sunburn, advise to wear loose-fitting clothes, and discuss other sun protection measures. Instruct to d/c and contact physician if arthralgia, fever, rash, or malaise develops. Inform that drug may cause discoloration of skin, scars, teeth, or gums.

STORAGE: 15-30°C (59-86°F).

ORAPRED – prednisolone sodium phosphate

RX

Class: Glucocorticoid

ADULT DOSAGE

Steroid-Responsive Disorders

Initial: 5-60mg/day (1.67-20mL), depending on disease and response

Maint: Decrease initial dose in small decrements to lowest effective dose

Multiple Sclerosis

Acute Exacerbations:
200mg/day for a week, followed by 80mg qod for 1 month

PEDIATRIC DOSAGE

Steroid-Responsive Disorders

Initial: 0.14-2mg/kg/day in 3 or 4 divided doses (4-60mg/m^2/day)

Nephrotic Syndrome

>2 Years:
60mg/m^2/day given in 3 divided doses for 4 weeks, followed by 4 weeks of single dose alternate-day therapy at 40mg/m^2/day

Asthma

Uncontrolled by Inhaled Corticosteroids and Long-Acting Bronchodilators:
1-2mg/kg/day in single or divided doses; continue short course ("burst") therapy until peak expiratory flow rate of 80% of personal best is achieved or symptoms resolve (usually 3-10 days)

O

DOSING CONSIDERATIONS

Elderly
Start at lower end of dosing range

Discontinuation
Withdraw gradually after long-term therapy

ADMINISTRATION

Oral route

HOW SUPPLIED

Sol: 15mg/5mL [237mL]

CONTRAINDICATIONS

Systemic fungal infections, hypersensitivity to the drug or any of its components.

WARNINGS/PRECAUTIONS

May need to increase dose before, during, and after stressful situations. May produce reversible hypothalamic-pituitary-adrenal (HPA) axis suppression with the potential for glucocorticosteroid insufficiency after withdrawal; gradually reduce dose. May impair mineralocorticoid secretion; administer salt and/or mineralocorticoid concurrently. Metabolic clearance is decreased in hypothyroidism and increased in hyperthyroidism; changes in thyroid status may necessitate dose adjustment. May increase susceptibility to infections, mask signs of current infection, activate latent disease, or exacerbate intercurrent infections. Rule out latent or active amebiasis before initiating therapy. May cause more serious/fatal course of chickenpox and measles; avoid exposure, and if exposed, consider prophylaxis/treatment. Caution with *Strongyloides* infestation, active/latent tuberculosis (TB) or tuberculin reactivity, HTN, CHF, and renal insufficiency. May cause BP elevation, salt/water retention, and increased K^+ and Ca^{2+} excretion; dietary salt restriction and K^+ supplementation may be necessary. Not for use in cerebral malaria and active ocular herpes simplex. Signs of GI perforation (eg, peritoneal irritation) may be masked, minimal, or absent. Caution with nonspecific ulcerative colitis; probable impending perforation, abscess, or other pyogenic infections; diverticulitis; fresh intestinal anastomoses; and active/latent peptic ulcers. Psychic derangements may appear and existing emotional instability or psychotic tendencies may be aggravated. May decrease bone formation and increase bone resorption, and may lead to inhibition of bone growth in children/adolescents and the development of osteoporosis at any age; caution with increased risk of osteoporosis. May produce posterior subcapsular cataracts, glaucoma with possible optic nerve damage, and may enhance the establishment of secondary ocular infections; not recommended in optic neuritis treatment. Acute myopathy with high doses reported, most often in patients with disorders of neuromuscular transmission (eg, myasthenia gravis). Elevation of CK or IOP may occur. May suppress reactions to skin tests. Kaposi's sarcoma reported. Enhanced effect in patients with cirrhosis and hypothyroidism. Caution in elderly.

ADVERSE REACTIONS

Fluid retention, HTN, decreased carbohydrate tolerance, abdominal distention, increased appetite, weight gain, glaucoma, osteoporosis, muscle weakness, development of cushingoid state, menstrual irregularities, convulsions, headache, impaired wound healing, increased sweating.

DRUG INTERACTIONS

Live or live, attenuated vaccines are contraindicated with immunosuppressive doses. Killed or inactivated vaccines may be administered, although response is unpredictable. May exhibit a diminished response to toxoids and live or inactivated vaccines. May potentiate replication of some organisms contained in live, attenuated vaccines. Hepatic enzyme inducers (eg, barbiturates, phenytoin, ephedrine) may enhance metabolism and require corticosteroid dosage increase. Increased activity of both drugs may occur with cyclosporine; convulsions reported with concurrent use. Estrogens may decrease hepatic metabolism and increase effect. Ketoconazole may decrease metabolism leading to an increased risk of corticosteroid side effects. May inhibit response to warfarin. ASA or other NSAIDs may increase risk of GI side effects; caution with ASA in hypoprothrombinemia patients. May increase clearance of salicylates. Closely monitor for hypokalemia with K^+-depleting agents (eg, amphotericin B, diuretics). May increase risk of arrhythmias with digitalis glycosides. Concomitant use with anticholinesterase agents may produce severe weakness in patients with myasthenia gravis; d/c anticholinesterase agents at least 24 hrs before initiating therapy. May increase blood glucose levels; dosage adjustments of antidiabetic agents may be required. Acute myopathy reported with neuromuscular blocking drugs (eg, pancuronium).

PATIENT CONSIDERATIONS

Assessment: Assess for hypersensitivity to drug or any of its components, unusual stress, current infections, systemic fungal infections, latent/active amebiasis, peptic ulcer and TB, cerebral malaria, ocular herpes simplex, CHF, HTN, renal insufficiency, diverticulitis, intestinal anastomoses, ulcerative colitis, cirrhosis, psychotic tendencies, myasthenia gravis, thyroid disorders, any other conditions where treatment is contraindicated or cautioned, pregnancy/nursing status, and possible drug interactions.

Monitoring: Monitor for HPA axis suppression, infections, changes in thyroid status, cataracts, glaucoma, Kaposi's sarcoma, growth/development (in pediatric patients), osteoporosis, acute myopathy, psychic derangements, emotional instability or psychotic tendencies aggravation, and other adverse reactions. Monitor BP, serum electrolytes, and CK. Monitor IOP if used for >6 weeks. Frequently monitor coagulation indices with warfarin.

Counseling: Instruct not to d/c therapy abruptly or without medical supervision. Instruct to inform any physician of intake of corticosteroids and to seek medical advice at once if fever or other signs of infection develop. Instruct to avoid exposure to chickenpox or measles; instruct to seek medical advice without delay if exposed.

STORAGE: 2-8°C (36-46°F). Keep tightly closed.

O

ORBACTIV – oritavancin

RX

Class: Lipoglycopeptide

ADULT DOSAGE

Skin and Skin Structure Infections

Acute bacterial infections caused by *Staphylococcus aureus* (including methicillin-susceptible and methicillin-resistant isolates), *Streptococcus pyogenes, Streptococcus agalactiae, Streptococcus dysgalactiae, Streptococcus anginosus* group (includes *S. anginosus, S. intermedius,* and *S. constellatus*), and *Enterococcus faecalis* (vancomycin-susceptible isolates only)

Single 1200mg dose by IV infusion over 3 hrs

PEDIATRIC DOSAGE

Pediatric use may not have been established

ADMINISTRATION

IV route

Preparation

Three 400mg vials need to be reconstituted and diluted to prepare a single 1200mg dose.

Reconstitution:

1. Add 40mL of sterile water for inj to reconstitute each vial to provide a 10mg/mL sol per vial.
2. Gently swirl each vial to avoid foaming and ensure that all powder is completely reconstituted in sol.

Dilution:

1. Use only D5W for dilution; do not use normal saline, as it is incompatible and may cause precipitation of the drug.
2. Withdraw and discard 120mL from a 1000mL IV bag of D5W.
3. Withdraw 40mL from each of the 3 reconstituted vials and add to D5W IV bag to bring the bag volume to 1000mL; this yields a concentration of 1.2mg/mL.

Diluted IV sol in an infusion bag should be used w/in 6 hrs when stored at room temperature, or w/in 12 hrs when refrigerated at 2-8°C (36-46°F). Combined storage time (reconstituted sol in the vial and diluted sol in the bag) and 3-hr infusion time should not exceed 6 hrs at room temperature or 12 hrs if refrigerated.

Incompatibilities

1. IV substances, additives, or other medications mixed in normal saline should not be added to oritavancin single-use vials or infused simultaneously through the same IV line or through a common IV port.
2. Drugs formulated at a basic or neutral pH may be incompatible.
3. Do not administer simultaneously w/ commonly used IV drugs through a common IV port; if the same IV line is used for sequential infusion of additional medications, the line should be flushed w/ D5W before and after infusion of oritavancin.

HOW SUPPLIED

Inj: 400mg

CONTRAINDICATIONS

Use of IV unfractionated heparin sodium for 120 hrs (5 days) after administration of therapy. Known hypersensitivity to oritavancin.

WARNINGS/PRECAUTIONS

May artificially prolong certain laboratory coagulation tests. Artificially prolongs activated PTT (aPTT) for 120 hrs, PT and INR for up to 12 hrs, and activated clotting time for up to 24 hrs by binding to and preventing action of the phospholipid reagents commonly used in lab coagulation tests. Has been shown to elevate D dimer concentrations up to 72 hrs after administration of therapy. For patients who require aPTT monitoring w/in 120 hrs of dosing, a non-phospholipid dependent coagulation test (eg, Factor Xa [chromogenic] assay) or an alternative anticoagulant not requiring aPTT monitoring may be considered. Serious hypersensitivity reactions reported; d/c immediately and institute appropriate supportive care if an acute hypersensitivity reaction occurs. Infusion-related reactions (eg, pruritus, urticaria, flushing) reported; consider slowing or interrupting drug infusion. *Clostridium difficile*-associated diarrhea (CDAD) reported; d/c if CDAD is suspected or confirmed. Osteomyelitis reported; institute appropriate alternate antibacterial therapy if suspected or diagnosed. May result in bacterial resistance if used in the absence of proven or suspected bacterial infection.

ADVERSE REACTIONS

Headache, N/V, limb and SQ abscesses, diarrhea.

DRUG INTERACTIONS

See Contraindications. Nonspecific, weak inhibitor (CYP2C9 and CYP2C19) or inducer (CYP3A4 and CYP2D6) of several CYP isoforms. Use caution when concomitantly administering w/ drugs w/ a narrow therapeutic window that are predominantly metabolized by 1 of the affected CYP450 enzymes (eg, warfarin); coadministration may increase (eg, CYP2C9 substrates) or decrease (eg, CYP2D6 substrates) concentrations of the narrow therapeutic range drug. Coadministration w/ warfarin may result in higher exposure of warfarin, which may increase the risk of bleeding. Use oritavancin in patients on chronic warfarin therapy only when the benefits can be expected to outweigh the risk of bleeding; frequently monitor for signs of bleeding.

PATIENT CONSIDERATIONS

Assessment: Assess for hypersensitivity to drug or other glycopeptides, pregnancy/nursing status, and for possible drug interactions. Perform culture and susceptibility testing.

Monitoring: Monitor for hypersensitivity reactions, infusion-related reactions, CDAD, osteomyelitis, development of drug-resistant bacteria, and other adverse reactions. Frequently monitor for signs of bleeding w/ warfarin.

Counseling: Advise that allergic reactions may occur and that serious allergic reactions require immediate treatment. Advise to inform the physician about any previous hypersensitivity reactions to the drug, other glycopeptides, or other allergens. Inform that diarrhea is a common problem caused by therapy and usually resolves when therapy is discontinued; instruct to contact physician if severe watery or bloody diarrhea develops.

STORAGE: 20-25°C (68-77°F); excursions permitted to 15-30°C (59-86°F). **Diluted Sol in Infusion Bag:** Use w/in 6 hrs when stored at room temperature or use w/in 12 hrs when refrigerated at 2-8°C (36-46°F). Combined storage time (reconstituted sol in the vial and the diluted sol in the bag) and 3-hr infusion time should not exceed 6 hrs at room temperature or 12 hrs if refrigerated.

ORENCIA – abatacept

RX

Class: Selective costimulation modulator

ADULT DOSAGE

Rheumatoid Arthritis

To reduce signs and symptoms, induce major clinical response, inhibit progression of structural damage, and improve physical function in adults w/ moderate to severe active rheumatoid arthritis; may be used as monotherapy or concomitantly w/ disease-modifying antirheumatic drugs other than TNF antagonists

IV Regimen:

Initial:

<60kg: 500mg

60-100kg: 750mg

>100kg: 1000mg

Maint: Give succeeding infusions at 2 and 4 weeks after the 1st infusion and every 4 weeks thereafter

SQ Regimen:

125mg SQ inj once weekly w/ or w/o an IV LD

If initiating w/ an IV LD, initiate w/ a single IV infusion (as per body weight categories listed in the IV regimen), followed by the first 125mg SQ inj w/in a day of the IV infusion

Switching from IV to SQ Regimen:

Give the 1st SQ dose instead of the next scheduled IV dose

PEDIATRIC DOSAGE

Juvenile Idiopathic Arthritis

To reduce signs and symptoms of moderately to severely active polyarticular juvenile idiopathic arthritis; may be used as monotherapy or concomitantly w/ methotrexate

6-17 Years:

IV Regimen:

Initial:

<75kg: 10mg/kg

≥75kg: Follow adult IV dosing regimen; not to exceed 1000mg

Maint: Give succeeding infusions at 2 and 4 weeks after the 1st infusion and every 4 weeks thereafter

ADMINISTRATION

IV/SQ route

IV

Give as an IV infusion over 30 min

Do not infuse in the same IV line w/ other agents

IV Infusion Preparation

Reconstitute w/ 10mL of sterile water for inj; only use silicone-free disposable syringe provided w/ each vial and an 18- to 21-gauge needle

Rotate vial w/ gentle swirling until contents are completely dissolved; do not shake, and avoid prolonged/vigorous agitation

Vent vial w/ needle to dissipate any foam after complete dissolution of powder

Further dilute reconstituted sol w/ 0.9% NaCl inj using the same silicone-free disposable syringe to a total volume of 100mL

Final concentration of abatacept in the bag or bottle will depend upon the amount of drug added, but will be ≤10mg/mL

Do not shake bag or bottle

May store fully diluted sol at room temperature or at 2-8°C (36-46°F) before use

Infusion of fully diluted sol must be completed w/in 24 hrs of reconstitution; discard if not administered w/in 24 hrs

SQ

Administer inj to front thigh or abdomen (except for the 2-inch area around navel) for self-inj, or outer area of the upper arm if a caregiver is administering dose

Rotate inj site (at least 1 inch away from last inj site)

Do not inject into areas where the skin is tender, bruised, red, or hard

HOW SUPPLIED

Inj: 125mg/mL [prefilled syringe], 250mg [vial]

WARNINGS/PRECAUTIONS
Anaphylaxis or anaphylactoid reactions reported w/ IV use; permanently d/c and institute appropriate therapy if an anaphylactic or other serious allergic reaction occurs. Serious infections, including sepsis and pneumonia, reported; caution in patients w/ history of recurrent infections, underlying conditions that may predispose to infections, or chronic, latent, or localized infections. D/C if a serious infection develops. Screen for latent tuberculosis (TB) infection and viral hepatitis prior to initiation of therapy; treat patients testing (+) for TB prior to therapy. Hepatitis B reactivation may occur. JIA patients should be brought up-to-date w/ all immunizations prior to initiation of therapy. Caution in patients w/ COPD; monitor for worsening of respiratory status. May affect host defenses against infections and malignancies. Caution in elderly. (IV) Contains maltose that may react w/ glucose dehydrogenase pyrroloquinoline quinone-based glucose monitoring and may result in falsely elevated blood glucose readings on the day of infusion; consider methods that do not react w/ maltose in patients requiring blood glucose monitoring.

ADVERSE REACTIONS
Headache, URTI, nasopharyngitis, nausea, sinusitis, UTI, influenza, bronchitis, dizziness, cough, back pain, HTN, dyspepsia, rash, pain in extremities.

DRUG INTERACTIONS
May experience more infections and serious infections w/ TNF antagonists; concurrent use is not recommended. Monitor for signs of infection while transitioning from TNF antagonist to abatacept. Concomitant use w/ other biologic RA therapy (eg, anakinra) is not recommended. Do not give live vaccines concurrently w/ therapy or w/in 3 months of its discontinuation.

PATIENT CONSIDERATIONS

Assessment: Assess for previous hypersensitivity to drug, history of recurrent infections, chronic/latent/localized infections, underlying conditions that may predispose to infection, COPD, pregnancy/nursing status, and possible drug interactions. Assess immunization history in pediatric patients. Screen for latent TB infection w/ a tuberculin skin test and for viral hepatitis.

Monitoring: Monitor for signs/symptoms of hypersensitivity, infection, hepatitis B reactivation, worsening of respiratory status in COPD patients, immunosuppression, malignancies, and other adverse reactions.

Counseling: Instruct to immediately contact physician if an allergic reaction or infection occurs. Inform that may be tested for TB prior to therapy. Counsel not to receive live vaccines during therapy or w/in 3 months of its discontinuation. Inform caregivers that patients w/ JIA should be brought up-to-date w/ all immunizations prior to therapy and discuss how to best handle future immunizations once therapy has been initiated. Instruct to inform physician if pregnant/nursing or planning to become pregnant. Inform that the formulation for IV administration contains maltose, which can give falsely elevated blood glucose readings on the day of administration w/ certain blood glucose monitors; advise to discuss methods that do not react w/ maltose.

O

STORAGE: 2-8°C (36-46°F). Protect from light; store in original package until time of use. Do not allow prefilled syringe to freeze. Fully Diluted Sol: May store at room temperature or at 2-8°C (36-46°F); discard if not administered w/in 24 hrs.

ORKAMBI – ivacaftor/lumacaftor RX

Class: CFTR potentiator

ADULT DOSAGE

Cystic Fibrosis

Treatment of cystic fibrosis in patients who are homozygous for the *F508del* mutation in the *CFTR* gene

2 tabs q12h w/ fat-containing food

Missed Dose

Take missed dose w/in 6 hrs, w/ fat-containing food. If >6 hrs have passed, skip missed dose and resume at normal schedule

PEDIATRIC DOSAGE

Cystic Fibrosis

Treatment of cystic fibrosis in patients who are homozygous for the *F508del* mutation in the *CFTR* gene

≥12 Years:
2 tabs q12h w/ fat-containing food

Missed Dose

Take missed dose w/in 6 hrs, w/ fat-containing food. If >6 hrs have passed, skip missed dose and resume at normal schedule

DOSING CONSIDERATIONS

Concomitant Medications

In patients currently taking strong CYP3A inhibitors, reduce Orkambi dose to 1 tab daily for the 1st week of treatment; following this period, continue w/ the recommended dose

If Orkambi is interrupted for more than 1 week and then reinitiated while taking strong CYP3A inhibitors, patients should reduce Orkambi dose to 1 tab daily for the 1st week of treatment reinitiation; following this period, continue w/ the recommended dose

Hepatic Impairment

Moderate (Child-Pugh Class B): 2 tabs in the am and 1 tab in the pm

Severe (Child-Pugh Class C): Max dose of 1 tab in the am and 1 tab in the pm or less

ADMINISTRATION

Oral route

Appropriate fat-containing foods include eggs, avocados, nuts, butter, peanut butter, cheese pizza, and whole-milk dairy products.

HOW SUPPLIED

Tab: (Lumacaftor/Ivacaftor) 200mg/125mg

WARNINGS/PRECAUTIONS

Worsening of liver function (eg, hepatic encephalopathy) in patients w/ advanced liver disease reported; use w/ caution, and monitor closely. Elevated transaminases/serum bilirubin levels reported. Monitor closely if increased transaminase/bilirubin levels develop, until abnormalities resolve, and interrupt dosing w/ ALT or AST >5X ULN or w/ ALT or AST >3X ULN and bilirubin >2X ULN; consider benefits and risks of resuming dosing. Respiratory events observed more commonly during initiation of therapy; perform additional monitoring during initiation of therapy in patients w/ percent predicted FEV_1 ($ppFEV_1$) <40. Non-congenital lens opacities reported in pediatric patients; baseline and follow-up ophthalmological exams are recommended in pediatric patients. Use FDA-cleared cystic fibrosis mutation test to detect the presence of *F580del* mutation on both alleles of the *CFTR* gene if patient's genotype is unknown. Caution in patients w/severe renal impairment (CrCl ≤30mL/min) or ESRD.

ADVERSE REACTIONS

Dyspnea, nasopharyngitis, nausea, diarrhea, URTI, fatigue, abnormal respiration, blood creatine phosphokinase increased, rash, flatulence, rhinorrhea, influenza.

DRUG INTERACTIONS

See Dosing Considerations. Increased ivacaftor exposure w/ concomitant itraconazole. May decrease systemic exposure of CYP3A substrates which may decrease the therapeutic effect; co-administration is not recommended w/ sensitive CYP3A substrates or CYP3A substrates w/ a narrow therapeutic index. May alter exposure of CYP2B6, CYP2C8, CYP2C9, CYP2C19, and P-gp substrates. Strong CYP3A inducers (eg, rifampin, St. John's wort) may significantly reduce ivacaftor exposure which may reduce therapeutic effectiveness; co-administration w/ strong CYP3A inducers is not recommended. Monitor serum concentration of digoxin and titrate digoxin dose as needed. May decrease the exposure of montelukast. May reduce the exposure/effectiveness of prednisone, methylprednisolone, ibuprofen, citalopram, escitalopram, and sertraline; may require higher doses. May decrease the exposure of clarithromycin, erythromycin, and telithromycin, which may reduce the effectiveness of these antibiotics; consider an alternative to these antibiotics (eg, ciprofloxacin, azithromycin, levofloxacin). May reduce exposure/effectiveness of itraconazole, ketoconazole, posaconazole, and voriconazole; concomitant use not recommended. Monitor patients closely for breakthrough fungal infections if use is necessary; consider an alternative (eg, fluconazole). May decrease hormonal contraceptive exposure/effectiveness and increase menstrual abnormality events; avoid concomitant use. Hormonal contraceptives should not be relied upon as an effective method of contraception when co-administered. May reduce exposure/effectiveness of repaglinide and alter the exposure of sulfonylurea; a dose adjustment may be required. May reduce exposure/effectiveness of proton pump inhibitors (eg, omeprazole, esomeprazole, lansoprazole), and may alter the exposure of ranitidine; a dose adjustment may be required. May alter the exposure of warfarin; monitor INR.

PATIENT CONSIDERATIONS

Assessment: Assess for history of transaminase elevations, renal/hepatic impairment, pregnancy/nursing status, and possible drug interactions. Assess baseline ALT, AST, and bilirubin levels. Obtain baseline ophthalmological examinations in pediatric patients. Use an FDA-cleared CF mutation test to detect the presence of *F508del* mutation on both alleles of the *CFTR* gene if patient's genotype is unknown.

Monitoring: Monitor for respiratory events, cataracts in pediatric patients, and other adverse reactions. Monitor ALT/AST/bilirubin levels every 3 months during the 1st yr of therapy and annually thereafter. Perform follow-up ophthalmological examinations in pediatric patients. Monitor patients w/ $ppFEV_1$<40 during treatment initiation.

Counseling: Inform that treatment may worsen liver function in patients w/ advanced liver disease. Advise that abnormalities in liver function have occurred and that blood tests will be performed prior to initiating therapy, every 3 months during the 1st yr, and annually thereafter. Explain that chest discomfort, dyspnea, and abnormal respiration may occur. Instruct to notify physician of all medications currently being taking, including herbal supplements or vitamins; instruct how to properly take concomitant drugs. Instruct patients on alternative methods of birth control. Inform that drug is best absorbed by the body when taken w/ fat-containing food. Inform about missed dosing instructions. Advise that abnormality of the eye lens has been noted in some children and adolescents receiving therapy and that baseline and follow-up ophthalmological exam and follow-up exams are recommended in pediatric patients initiating therapy.

STORAGE: 20-25°C (68-77°F); excursions permitted to 15-30°C (59-86°F).

ORTHO TRI-CYCLEN – ethinyl estradiol/norgestimate RX

Class: Estrogen/progestogen combination

Cigarette smoking increases risk of serious cardiovascular (CV) events. Risk increases w/ age (>35 yrs of age) and w/ the number of cigarettes smoked. Contraindicated in women who are >35 yrs of age and smoke.

ADULT DOSAGE

Contraception

1 tab qd at the same time each day, for 28 days, then repeat

Start 1st Sunday after menses begin or 1st day of menses

Acne Vulgaris

Moderate Acne in Females Who Desire Oral Contraception:
1 tab qd at the same time each day, for 28 days, then repeat

Start 1st Sunday after menses begin or 1st day of menses

Missed Dose

Miss 1 Active Tab in Weeks 1, 2, or 3:
Take as soon as possible. Continue taking 1 tab qd until the pack is finished

Miss 2 Active Tabs in Weeks 1 or 2:
Take 2 missed tabs as soon as possible and the next 2 active tabs the next day. Continue taking 1 tab qd until pack is finished. Use additional nonhormonal contraception (eg, condom, spermicide) as backup if the patient has intercourse w/in 7 days after missing tabs

Miss 2 Active Tabs in Week 3 or Miss ≥3 Active Tabs in a Row in Weeks 1, 2, or 3:
(Day 1 Start) Throw out the rest of the pack and start a new pack that same day. (Sunday Start) Continue to take 1 tab qd until Sunday, then throw out the rest of the pack and start a new pack that same day. (Day 1 Start/Sunday Start) Use additional nonhormonal contraception as backup if the patient has intercourse w/in 7 days after missing tabs

Conversions

Switching from Another Oral Contraceptive:
Start on the same day that a new pack of the previous oral contraceptive would have started

Switching from Another Contraceptive Method:

Transdermal Patch/Vaginal Ring/Inj:
Start therapy on the day when next application would have been scheduled

Intrauterine Contraceptive:
Start on the day of removal; if the intrauterine device is not removed on the 1st day of menstrual cycle, additional nonhormonal contraceptive is needed for the first 7 days of the 1st cycle pack

Implant:
Start therapy on the day of removal

PEDIATRIC DOSAGE

Contraception

Not indicated for use premenarche; refer to adult dosing

Acne Vulgaris

Moderate Acne in Postpubertal Females ≥15 Years of Age Who Desire Oral Contraception:
1 tab qd at the same time each day, for 28 days, then repeat

Start 1st Sunday after menses begin or 1st day of menses

O

DOSING CONSIDERATIONS

Adverse Reactions

GI Disturbances: If vomiting/diarrhea occurs w/in 3-4 hrs after taking an active tab, handle this as a missed tab

Other Important Considerations

Starting Therapy after Abortion or Miscarriage:

1st Trimester: May start immediately; if starting therapy immediately, additional contraception is not needed. If therapy is not started w/in 5 days after termination of the pregnancy, use additional nonhormonal contraception for the first 7 days of 1st cycle pack

2nd Trimester: Do not start until 4 weeks after a 2nd trimester abortion or miscarriage

Starting Therapy after Childbirth:

Do not start until 4 weeks after delivery

ADMINISTRATION

Oral route

Take w/o regard to meals.

Sunday Start Regimen

Use additional nonhormonal contraception for the first 7 days of 1st cycle pack.

HOW SUPPLIED

Tab: (Ethinyl Estradiol [EE]/Norgestimate) 0.035mg/0.18mg, 0.035mg/0.215mg, 0.035mg/0.25mg

CONTRAINDICATIONS

High risk of arterial/venous thrombotic diseases (eg, smoking [if >35 yrs of age], presence/history of deep vein thrombosis [DVT]/pulmonary embolism [PE], inherited or acquired hypercoagulopathies, cerebrovascular disease, coronary artery disease [CAD], thrombogenic valvular/ thrombogenic rhythm diseases of the heart [eg, subacute bacterial endocarditis w/ valvular disease or A-fib], uncontrolled HTN, diabetes mellitus [DM] w/ vascular disease, headaches w/ focal neurological symptoms or migraine headaches w/ aura [women >35 yrs of age w/ any migraine headaches]), benign/malignant liver tumors, liver disease, undiagnosed abnormal uterine bleeding, pregnancy, presence/history of breast cancer or other estrogen- or progestin-sensitive cancer.

WARNINGS/PRECAUTIONS

D/C if an arterial thrombotic event or venous thromboembolic event (VTE) occurs. D/C if there is unexplained loss of vision, proptosis, diplopia, papilledema, or retinal vascular lesions; evaluate for retinal vein thrombosis immediately. If feasible, d/c at least 4 weeks before and through 2 weeks after major surgery or other surgeries known to have an elevated risk of VTE as well as during and following prolonged immobilization. In women who are not breastfeeding, initiate therapy no earlier than 4 weeks after delivery; risk of postpartum VTE decreases after the 3rd postpartum week, whereas the risk of ovulation increases after the 3rd postpartum week. Increased risk of VTE and arterial thromboses (eg, strokes, MI). Caution w/ CV disease risk factors. D/C if jaundice develops. May increase risk of developing hepatocellular carcinoma. Increased BP reported; d/c if BP rises significantly. May worsen existing gallbladder disease. May increase risk of cholestasis in women w/ history of pregnancy-related cholestasis. May increase risk of cervical cancer or intraepithelial neoplasia, and gallbladder disease. May decrease glucose tolerance. Consider alternative contraception w/ uncontrolled dyslipidemia. Increased risk of pancreatitis w/ hypertriglyceridemia or family history of hypertriglyceridemia. Evaluate the cause of new headaches that are recurrent, persistent, or severe, and d/c if indicated; consider discontinuation in the case of increased frequency or severity of migraine during use. Unscheduled bleeding and spotting may occur; rule out pregnancy or malignancy. May cause amenorrhea; if scheduled bleeding does not occur, consider possibility of pregnancy. Administration of therapy to induce withdrawal bleeding should not be used as a test for pregnancy. Caution w/ history of depression; d/c if depression recurs to a serious degree. May interfere w/ lab tests (eg, coagulation factors, lipids, glucose tolerance, binding proteins). Chloasma may occur, especially w/ history of chloasma gravidarum; avoid exposure to the sun or UV radiation. **EE:** In women w/ hereditary angioedema, may induce/exacerbate angioedema.

ADVERSE REACTIONS

Irregular uterine bleeding, nausea, headache/migraine, abdominal/GI pain, vaginal infection, genital discharge, breast issues (eg, breast pain, discharge, and enlargement), mood disorders.

DRUG INTERACTIONS

Drugs or herbal products that induce certain enzymes, including CYP3A4 (eg, phenytoin, barbiturates, carbamazepine) may decrease levels and potentially diminish effectiveness of therapy or increase breakthrough bleeding; use an alternative or back-up method of contraception and continue back-up contraception for 28 days after discontinuing the enzyme inducer. CYP3A4 inhibitors (eg, itraconazole, voriconazole, grapefruit juice) may increase levels. Significant changes in levels when coadministered w/ HIV protease inhibitors; decreased levels w/ nelfinavir, ritonavir, darunavir/ritonavir, (fos)amprenavir/ritonavir, lopinavir/ritonavir, and tipranavir/ritonavir, and increased levels w/ indinavir and atazanavir/ritonavir. Decreased levels w/ boceprevir, telaprevir, and nevirapine, and increased levels w/ etravirine. May decrease levels of acetaminophen (APAP), clofibric acid, morphine, salicylic acid, and temazepam. May significantly decrease levels of lamotrigine and may reduce seizure control; dosage adjustment of lamotrigine may be needed. May need to increase dose of thyroid hormone in patients on thyroid hormone replacement therapy due to increased thyroid-binding globulin. **EE:** Colesevelam reported to significantly decrease EE exposure; decreased drug interaction reported when the 2 drug products are given 4 hrs apart. Atorvastatin or rosuvastatin may increase EE exposure; ascorbic acid and APAP may increase EE levels. May inhibit metabolism and increase levels of other compounds (eg, cyclosporine, prednisolone, theophylline, tizanidine, voriconazole).

PATIENT CONSIDERATIONS

Assessment: Assess for DVT, PE, cerebrovascular disease, CAD, DM w/ vascular disease, headaches w/ focal neurological symptoms or migraine headaches w/ aura, pregnancy/nursing status, any other conditions where treatment is contraindicated or cautioned, and possible drug interactions.

Monitoring: Monitor for bleeding irregularities, venous/arterial thrombotic events, cervical cancer or intraepithelial neoplasia, retinal vein thrombosis or any other ophthalmic changes, jaundice, new/worsening headaches or migraines, depression, cholestasis w/ history of pregnancy-related cholestasis, pancreatitis, and other adverse reactions. Monitor BP in patients w/ HTN, glucose levels in diabetic or prediabetic patients, and lipid levels w/ dyslipidemia. Conduct a yearly visit in all patients for a BP check and for other indicated healthcare.

Counseling: Inform of risk/benefits of therapy. Advise to take ud. Counsel that cigarette smoking increases the risk of serious CV events and women who are >35 yrs of age and smoke should not use combination oral contraceptives (COCs). Inform of the risk of VTE. Inform that the drug does not protect against HIV infection (AIDS) and other sexually transmitted infections. Advise not to use during pregnancy; if pregnancy occurs during use, instruct to stop further use. Instruct on what to do in the event tabs are missed. Counsel to use a back-up or alternative method of contraception when enzyme inducers are used w/ therapy. Inform that COCs may reduce breast milk production. Counsel women who start COCs postpartum and have not yet had a period, to use an additional method of contraception until an active pill has been taken for 7 consecutive days. Inform that amenorrhea may occur; consider pregnancy in the event of amenorrhea at the time of 1st missed period, and rule out pregnancy in the event of amenorrhea in 2 or more consecutive cycles.

STORAGE: 20-25°C (68-77°F); excursions permitted to 15-30°C (59-86°F). Protect from light.

Ortho Tri-Cyclen Lo – ethinyl estradiol/norgestimate RX

Class: Estrogen/progestogen combination

O

Cigarette smoking increases risk of serious cardiovascular (CV) events. Risk increases w/ age (>35 yrs of age) and w/ the number of cigarettes smoked. Contraindicated in women who are >35 yrs of age and smoke.

ADULT DOSAGE

Contraception

1 tab qd at the same time each day, for 28 days, then repeat

Start either on 1st day of menses or on 1st Sunday after onset of menses

Conversions

Switching from Another Oral Contraceptive:
Start on the same day that a new pack of the previous oral contraceptive would have been started

Switching from Another Contraceptive Method:
Transdermal Patch/Vaginal Ring/Inj:
Start therapy on the day when the next application/insertion/inj would have been scheduled

Intrauterine Contraceptive:
Start on the day of removal; if the intrauterine device is not removed on the 1st day of menstrual cycle, additional nonhormonal contraceptive (eg, condom, spermicide) is needed for the first 7 days of the 1st cycle pack

Implant:
Start therapy on the day of removal

PEDIATRIC DOSAGE

Contraception

Not indicated for use premenarche; refer to adult dosing

Missed Dose

Miss 1 Active Tab in Weeks 1, 2, or 3: Take tab as soon as possible. Continue taking 1 tab qd until the pack is finished

Miss 2 Active Tabs in Weeks 1 or 2: Take the 2 missed tabs as soon as possible and the next 2 active tabs the next day. Continue taking 1 tab qd until pack is finished. Use additional nonhormonal contraception as backup if the patient has intercourse w/in 7 days after missing tabs

Miss 2 Active Tabs in Week 3 or Miss ≥3 Active Tabs in a Row in Weeks 1, 2, or 3: (Day 1 Start) Throw out the rest of the pack and start a new pack that same day. (Sunday Start) Continue taking 1 tab qd until Sunday, then throw out the rest of the pack and start a new pack that same day. (Day 1 Start/Sunday Start) Use additional nonhormonal contraception as backup if the patient has intercourse w/in 7 days after missing tabs

DOSING CONSIDERATIONS

Adverse Reactions

GI Disturbances: In case of severe vomiting/diarrhea, absorption may not be complete and additional contraceptive measures should be taken; if vomiting/diarrhea occurs w/in 3-4 hrs after taking an active tab, handle this as a missed tab

Other Important Considerations

Starting Therapy after Abortion or Miscarriage:

1st Trimester: May start immediately; if therapy is started immediately, additional method of contraception is not needed. If therapy is not started w/in 5 days after termination of the pregnancy, use additional nonhormonal contraception for the first 7 days of 1st cycle pack

2nd Trimester: Do not start until 4 weeks after a 2nd trimester abortion or miscarriage

Starting Therapy after Childbirth:

Do not start until 4 weeks after delivery; consider possibility of ovulation and conception in women who have not yet had a period postpartum

ADMINISTRATION

Oral route

Take w/o regard to meals.

Take tabs in the order directed on the blister pack.

Sunday Start Regimen

For the 1st cycle, use additional nonhormonal method of contraception for the first 7 consecutive days of administration.

HOW SUPPLIED

Tab: (Ethinyl Estradiol [EE]/Norgestimate) 0.025mg/0.18mg, 0.025mg/0.215mg, 0.025mg/0.25mg

CONTRAINDICATIONS

High risk of arterial/venous thrombotic diseases (eg, smoking [if >35 yrs of age], presence/history of deep vein thrombosis [DVT]/pulmonary embolism [PE], inherited or acquired hypercoagulopathies, cerebrovascular disease, coronary artery disease [CAD], thrombogenic valvular/thrombogenic rhythm diseases of the heart [eg, subacute bacterial endocarditis w/ valvular disease or A-fib], uncontrolled HTN, diabetes mellitus [DM] w/ vascular disease, headaches w/ focal neurological symptoms or migraine headaches w/ aura [women >35 yrs of age w/ any migraine headaches]), benign/malignant liver tumors, liver disease, undiagnosed abnormal uterine bleeding, pregnancy, presence/history of breast cancer or other estrogen- or progestin-sensitive cancer.

WARNINGS/PRECAUTIONS

D/C if an arterial thrombotic event or venous thromboembolic event (VTE) occurs. D/C if there is unexplained loss of vision, proptosis, diplopia, papilledema, or retinal vascular lesions; evaluate for retinal vein thrombosis immediately. If feasible, d/c at least 4 weeks before and through 2 weeks after major surgery or other surgeries known to have an elevated risk of VTE as well as during and following prolonged immobilization. In women who are not breastfeeding, initiate therapy no earlier than 4 weeks after delivery; risk of postpartum VTE decreases after the 3rd postpartum week, whereas the risk of ovulation increases after the 3rd postpartum week. Increased risk of VTE and arterial thromboses (eg, strokes, MI). D/C if jaundice develops. Hepatic adenomas may occur; increased risk of hepatocellular carcinoma reported in long-term users. Increased BP reported;

d/c if BP rises significantly. May increase risk of gallbladder disease or worsen existing gallbladder disease. May increase risk of cholestasis in women w/ history of pregnancy-related cholestasis. May decrease glucose tolerance. Consider alternative contraception w/ uncontrolled dyslipidemia. May increase risk of pancreatitis in women w/ hypertriglyceridemia or family history thereof. Evaluate the cause of new headaches that are recurrent, persistent, or severe, and d/c therapy if indicated; consider discontinuation in the case of increased frequency or severity of migraine during use. Unscheduled bleeding and spotting may occur; rule out pregnancy or malignancy. May cause amenorrhea; amenorrhea or oligomenorrhea after discontinuation may occur. Caution w/ history of depression; d/c if depression recurs to a serious degree. May increase risk of cervical cancer or intraepithelial neoplasia. Chloasma may occur, especially w/ history of chloasma gravidarum; women w/ a tendency to chloasma should avoid exposure to the sun or UV radiation while on therapy. May interfere w/ lab tests (eg, coagulation factors, lipids, glucose tolerance, binding proteins). **EE:** In women w/ hereditary angioedema, may induce/exacerbate angioedema.

ADVERSE REACTIONS

Headache/migraine, N/V, breast issues (including tenderness, pain, enlargement, discharge), abdominal pain, menstrual disorders (including dysmenorrhea, menstrual discomfort, menstrual disorder), mood disorders (including mood alteration and depression), acne, vulvovaginal infection.

DRUG INTERACTIONS

Drugs or herbal products that induce certain enzymes, including CYP3A4 (eg, phenytoin, barbiturates, carbamazepine) may decrease levels and potentially diminish effectiveness of therapy or increase breakthrough bleeding; use an alternative or back-up method of contraception when using enzyme inducers and continue back-up contraception for 28 days after discontinuing the enzyme inducer. CYP3A4 inhibitors (eg, itraconazole, voriconazole, grapefruit juice) may increase levels. Significant changes (increase/decrease) in estrogen and/or progestin levels reported w/ HIV/hepatitis C virus protease inhibitors or non-nucleoside reverse transcriptase inhibitors. May decrease levels of acetaminophen (APAP), clofibric acid, morphine, salicylic acid, and temazepam. May significantly decrease levels of lamotrigine and may reduce seizure control; dosage adjustment of lamotrigine may be necessary. Women on thyroid hormone replacement therapy may need to increase dose of thyroid hormone due to increased levels of thyroid-binding globulin. **EE:** Colesevelam reported to significantly decrease EE exposure; decreased drug interaction when the 2 drug products are given 4 hrs apart. Atorvastatin or rosuvastatin may increase EE exposure; ascorbic acid and APAP may increase EE levels. May inhibit metabolism and increase levels of other compounds (eg, cyclosporine, prednisolone, theophylline, tizanidine, voriconazole).

PATIENT CONSIDERATIONS

Assessment: Assess for DVT, PE, cerebrovascular disease, CAD, DM w/ vascular disease, headaches w/ focal neurological symptoms or migraine headaches w/ aura, pregnancy/nursing status, any other conditions where treatment is contraindicated or cautioned, and possible drug interactions.

Monitoring: Monitor for venous/arterial thrombotic events, cervical cancer or intraepithelial neoplasia, bleeding irregularities, retinal vein thrombosis or any other ophthalmic changes, jaundice, new/worsening headaches or migraines, depression, cholestasis w/ history of pregnancy-related cholestasis, pancreatitis, and other adverse reactions. Monitor BP in women w/ HTN, glucose levels in diabetic or prediabetic women, and lipid levels w/ dyslipidemia. Conduct a yearly visit in all patients for a BP check and for other indicated healthcare.

Counseling: Inform of risks/benefits of therapy. Advise to take ud. Explain that cigarette smoking increases the risk of serious CV events and women who are >35 yrs of age and smoke should not use combination oral contraceptives (COCs). Inform of the risk of VTE. Inform that the drug does not protect against HIV infection (AIDS) and other sexually transmitted infections. Advise not to use during pregnancy; if pregnancy occurs during use, instruct to stop further use. Instruct on what to do in the event tabs are missed. Instruct to use a back-up or alternative method of contraception when enzyme inducers are used w/ therapy. Inform that COCs may reduce breast milk production. Instruct women who start COCs postpartum and have not yet had a period to use an additional method of contraception until an active pill has been taken for 7 consecutive days. Inform that amenorrhea may occur; explain that patient and healthcare providers should consider pregnancy in the event of amenorrhea at the time of 1st missed period, and rule out pregnancy in the event of amenorrhea in ≥2 consecutive cycles.

STORAGE: 20-25°C (68-77°F); excursions permitted to 15-30°C (59-86°F). Protect from light.

OSENI — alogliptin/pioglitazone

RX

Class: Dipeptidyl peptidase-4 (DPP-4) inhibitor/thiazolidinedione (glitazone)

Thiazolidinediones, including pioglitazone, cause or exacerbate CHF in some patients. After initiation and dose increases, monitor carefully for signs and symptoms of heart failure (HF); manage accordingly and consider discontinuation or dose reduction if HF develops. Not recommended w/ symptomatic HF. Contraindicated w/ established NYHA Class III or IV HF.

ADULT DOSAGE

Type 2 Diabetes Mellitus

Adjunct to diet and exercise to improve glycemic control when treatment w/ both alogliptin and pioglitazone is appropriate

Initial:

Inadequately Controlled on Diet and Exercise:
25mg/15mg qd or 25mg/30mg qd

Inadequately Controlled on Metformin Monotherapy:
25mg/15mg qd or 25mg/30mg qd

On Alogliptin and Requiring Additional Glycemic Control:
25mg/15mg qd or 25mg/30mg qd

On Pioglitazone and Requiring Additional Glycemic Control:
25mg/15mg qd, 25mg/30mg qd, or 25mg/45mg qd as appropriate based upon current therapy

Switching from Alogliptin Coadministered w/ Pioglitazone:
Initiate at the dose of alogliptin and pioglitazone based upon current therapy

Patients w/ CHF (NYHA Class I or II):
25mg/15mg qd

Max: 25mg/45mg qd

PEDIATRIC DOSAGE

Pediatric use may not have been established

DOSING CONSIDERATIONS

Concomitant Medications

Strong CYP2C8 Inhibitors (eg, Gemfibrozil):
Max: 25mg/15mg qd

Renal Impairment

Moderate (CrCl ≥30 to <60mL/min): 12.5mg/15mg qd, 12.5mg/30mg qd, or 12.5mg/45mg qd
Severe or ESRD: Not recommended for use; coadministration of pioglitazone and alogliptin 6.25mg qd based on individual requirements may be considered

ADMINISTRATION

Oral route

May be taken w/ or w/o food.
Do not split tabs before swallowing.

HOW SUPPLIED

Tab: (Alogliptin/Pioglitazone) 12.5mg/15mg, 12.5mg/30mg, 12.5mg/45mg, 25mg/15mg, 25mg/30mg, 25mg/45mg

CONTRAINDICATIONS

Hypersensitivity reaction (eg, anaphylaxis, angioedema, severe cutaneous adverse reactions) to Oseni or its components, NYHA Class III or IV HF.

WARNINGS/PRECAUTIONS

Not for use w/ type 1 diabetes mellitus (DM) or for treatment of diabetic ketoacidosis. Fatal and nonfatal hepatic events reported; obtain baseline LFTs, and initiate w/ caution in patients w/ abnormal LFTs. Measure LFTs promptly in patients who report symptoms that may indicate liver injury; if results are abnormal (ALT >3X ULN), interrupt treatment and investigate for the probable cause, and do not restart therapy w/o another explanation for the LFT abnormalities. **Alogliptin:** Acute pancreatitis reported; d/c if suspected and initiate appropriate management. Serious hypersensitivity reactions reported; d/c if suspected, assess for other potential causes, and institute alternative treatment for diabetes. Caution w/ history of angioedema to another DPP-4 inhibitor. Severe and disabling arthralgia reported in patients taking DPP-4 inhibitors; d/c if appropriate. **Pioglitazone:** May cause dose-related fluid retention when used alone or in combination w/ other antidiabetic medications; most common when used w/ insulin. Dose-related edema reported. Increased incidence of bone fractures reported in females. Not for use in patients w/ active bladder cancer; consider benefits versus risks in patients w/ a prior history of bladder cancer. Macular edema reported; promptly refer to an ophthalmologist if visual symptoms occur. May result in ovulation in some premenopausal anovulatory women, which may increase risk for pregnancy; adequate contraception is recommended in all premenopausal women.

ADVERSE REACTIONS

Nasopharyngitis, back pain, URTI, influenza, hypoglycemia.

DRUG INTERACTIONS

See Dosing Considerations. May require lower dose of insulin or insulin secretagogue to minimize risk of hypoglycemia. **Pioglitazone:** Increased exposure and $T_{1/2}$ w/ strong CYP2C8 inhibitors (eg, gemfibrozil). CYP2C8 inducers (eg, rifampin) may decrease exposure; if a CYP2C8 inducer is started or stopped during treatment, dose may need to be adjusted based on clinical response.

PATIENT CONSIDERATIONS

Assessment: Assess for HF or risk of HF, edema, renal/hepatic function, bone health, history of pancreatitis, diabetic ketoacidosis, active/history of bladder cancer, history of angioedema to another DPP-4 inhibitor, pregnancy/nursing status, and possible drug interactions. Obtain FPG and HbA1c.

Monitoring: Monitor for signs/symptoms of CHF, pancreatitis, hypersensitivity reactions, fractures, visual symptoms, severe and disabling arthralgia, and other adverse reactions. Monitor LFTs, FPG, and HbA1c. Monitor renal function periodically.

Counseling: Inform of the potential risks and benefits of therapy. Instruct to immediately report to physician any symptoms that may indicate HF. Inform that pancreatitis may occur; instruct to promptly d/c use and contact physician if persistent severe abdominal pain occurs. Instruct to d/c use and seek medical advice promptly if signs/symptoms of allergic reactions, liver injury, or bladder cancer occur. Inform that hypoglycemia can occur; explain the risks, symptoms, and appropriate management. Counsel premenopausal women to use adequate contraception during treatment. Instruct to seek medical advice if severe joint pain occurs. Advise not to double the next dose if a dose is missed. Instruct to inform physician if an unusual symptom develops or if a symptom persists or worsens.

STORAGE: 25°C (77°F); excursions permitted to 15-30°C (59-86°F). Protect from moisture and humidity.

OSPHENA — ospemifene

RX

Class: Estrogen agonist/antagonist

Has estrogen agonistic effects in the endometrium. Increased risk of endometrial cancer in a woman w/ a uterus who uses unopposed estrogens. Adding a progestin to estrogen therapy reduces the risk of endometrial hyperplasia. Perform adequate diagnostic measures to rule out malignancy in postmenopausal women w/ undiagnosed persistent/recurring abnormal genital bleeding. Increased risk of stroke and deep vein thrombosis (DVT) reported in postmenopausal women (50-79 yrs of age) who received daily oral conjugated estrogens-alone. Should be prescribed for the shortest duration consistent w/ treatment goals and risks.

ADULT DOSAGE

Dyspareunia

Moderate to Severe Dyspareunia, a Symptom of Vulvar and Vaginal Atrophy, Due to Menopause:

Usual: 60mg qd

Reevaluate periodically as clinically appropriate to determine if treatment is still necessary

PEDIATRIC DOSAGE

Pediatric use may not have been established

O

DOSING CONSIDERATIONS

Hepatic Impairment

Severe (Child-Pugh Class C): Should not be used

ADMINISTRATION

Oral route

Take w/ food

HOW SUPPLIED

Tab: 60mg

CONTRAINDICATIONS

Undiagnosed abnormal genital bleeding; known or suspected estrogen-dependent neoplasia; active DVT, pulmonary embolism (PE) or a history of these conditions; active arterial thromboembolic disease (eg, stroke, MI) or history of these conditions; hypersensitivity (eg, angioedema, urticaria, rash, pruritus) to ospemifene or any of the ingredients of the product; women who are or may become pregnant.

WARNINGS/PRECAUTIONS

Manage risk factors for cardiovascular disorders, arterial vascular disease (eg, HTN, diabetes mellitus, tobacco use, hypercholesterolemia, obesity), and/or venous thromboembolism (VTE) (eg, personal/family history of VTE, obesity, systemic lupus erythematosus) appropriately. MI reported. D/C immediately if thromboembolic/hemorrhagic stroke or VTE occurs or is suspected. If feasible, d/c therapy at least 4-6 weeks before surgery of the type associated w/ an increased risk of thromboembolism, or during periods of prolonged immobilization. Avoid w/ known/suspected breast cancer or w/ a history of breast cancer. Avoid w/ severe hepatic impairment.

ADVERSE REACTIONS

Hot flush, vaginal discharge, muscle spasms.

DRUG INTERACTIONS

Avoid w/ estrogens and estrogen agonists/antagonists. Fluconazole increases systemic exposure and may increase ospemifene-related adverse reactions; avoid concomitant use. Rifampin, a strong

CYP3A4/moderate CYP2C9/moderate CYP2C19 inducer, decreases systemic exposure; coadministration w/ CYP3A4, CYP2C9, and/or CYP2C19 inducers would be expected to decrease systemic exposure, which may decrease clinical effect. Ketoconazole increases systemic exposure; chronic ketoconazole administration may increase risk of ospemifene-related adverse reactions. Use w/ other drug products that are highly protein bound may increase exposure of either that drug or ospemifene. May increase risk of ospemifene-related adverse reactions w/ CYP3A4 and CYP2C9 inhibitors.

PATIENT CONSIDERATIONS

Assessment: Assess for drug hypersensitivity, undiagnosed abnormal genital bleeding, known/suspected estrogen-dependent neoplasia, active/history of DVT, active/history of PE, active/history of arterial thromboembolic disease, known/suspected or history of breast cancer, hepatic impairment, pregnancy/nursing status, possible drug interactions, or any other condition where treatment is cautioned or contraindicated.

Monitoring: Monitor for endometrial cancer, thromboembolic/hemorrhagic stroke, DVT, and other adverse reactions. Reevaluate periodically as clinically appropriate to determine if treatment is still necessary. Perform adequate diagnostic measures, including directed and random endometrial sampling when indicated, to rule out malignancy in postmenopausal women w/ undiagnosed persistent/recurring abnormal genital bleeding.

Counseling: Advise of risks and benefits of therapy. Inform that therapy may initiate/increase occurrence of hot flashes in some women. Inform postmenopausal women who have had hypersensitivity reactions to therapy not to take the drug. Inform postmenopausal women of the importance of reporting unusual vaginal bleeding to healthcare provider as soon as possible.

STORAGE: 20-25°C (68-77°F); excursions permitted to 15-30°C (59-86°F).

OTEZLA — apremilast

Class: Phosphodiesterase-4 (PDE-4) inhibitor

RX

ADULT DOSAGE

Psoriatic Arthritis

Initial Dosage Titration:
Day 1: 10mg (am)
Day 2: 10mg bid (am and pm)
Day 3: 10mg (am) and 20mg (pm)
Day 4: 20mg bid (am and pm)
Day 5: 20mg (am) and 30mg (pm)

Maint:
Day 6 and Thereafter: 30mg bid (am and pm)

Plaque Psoriasis

Patients w/ Moderate to Severe Plaque Psoriasis Who Are Candidates for Phototherapy or Systemic Therapy:

Initial Dosage Titration:
Day 1: 10mg (am)
Day 2: 10mg bid (am and pm)
Day 3: 10mg (am) and 20mg (pm)
Day 4: 20mg bid (am and pm)
Day 5: 20mg (am) and 30mg (pm)

Maint:
Day 6 and Thereafter: 30mg bid (am and pm)

PEDIATRIC DOSAGE

Pediatric use may not have been established

DOSING CONSIDERATIONS

Renal Impairment

Severe (CrCl <30mL/min):
Initial Dosage Titration:
Days 1-3: 10mg qam
Days 4 and 5: 20mg qam
Maint:
Day 6 and Thereafter: 30mg qam

ADMINISTRATION

Oral route

May be administered w/o regard to meals.
Do not crush, split, or chew.

HOW SUPPLIED

Tab: 10mg, 20mg, 30mg

CONTRAINDICATIONS

Known hypersensitivity to apremilast or to any excipients in the formulation.

WARNINGS/PRECAUTIONS

Depression or depressed mood, and suicidal ideation and behavior reported; carefully evaluate the risks and benefits of continuing treatment if such events occur. Weight decrease reported; consider discontinuation if unexplained or clinically significant weight loss occurs.

ADVERSE REACTIONS

Diarrhea, headache/tension headache, N/V, URTI.

DRUG INTERACTIONS

Decreased exposure w/ strong CYP450 inducers (eg, rifampin), which may result in loss of efficacy; not recommended w/ CYP450 inducers (eg, rifampin, phenobarbital, carbamazepine).

PATIENT CONSIDERATIONS

Assessment: Assess for history of depression and/or suicidal thoughts or behavior, drug hypersensitivity, renal impairment, pregnancy/nursing status, and possible drug interactions.

Monitoring: Monitor for emergence or worsening of depression, suicidal thoughts, or other mood changes, and for other adverse reactions. Monitor weight regularly and monitor renal function.

Counseling: Inform of the risks and benefits of therapy. Advise patients, their caregivers, and families to be alert for emergence or worsening of depression, suicidal thoughts, or other mood changes, and to contact physician if such changes occur. Counsel to monitor weight regularly and to notify physician if unexplained or clinically significant weight loss occurs. Instruct to take only as prescribed.

STORAGE: <30°C (86°F).

OVACE WASH – sodium sulfacetamide RX

Class: Sulfonamide

OTHER BRAND NAMES

Ovace Plus Wash

ADULT DOSAGE

Scaling Dermatoses

Seborrheic Dermatitis and Seborrhea Sicca (Dandruff):

Wash affected area bid (am and pm) or ud; repeat application for 8-10 days or ud

May rinse cleanser off sooner or use less frequently if skin dryness occurs

May lengthen interval between applications as condition subsides; may apply once or twice weekly, or every other week to prevent recurrence

If condition recurs after discontinuing therapy, reinitiate application as at the beginning of treatment

Secondary Infections

Secondary Bacterial Infections of Skin Due to Organisms Susceptible to Sulfonamides:

Wash affected area bid (am and pm) or ud

Repeat application for 8-10 days or ud

May rinse cleanser off sooner or use less frequently if skin dryness occurs

PEDIATRIC DOSAGE

Scaling Dermatoses

Seborrheic Dermatitis and Seborrhea Sicca (Dandruff):

≥12 Years:

Wash affected area bid (am and pm) or ud; repeat application for 8-10 days or ud

May rinse cleanser off sooner or use less frequently if skin dryness occurs

May lengthen interval between applications as condition subsides; may apply once or twice weekly, or every other week to prevent recurrence

If condition recurs after discontinuing therapy, reinitiate application as at the beginning of treatment

Secondary Infections

≥12 Years:

Secondary Bacterial Infections of Skin Due to Organisms Susceptible to Sulfonamides:

Wash affected area bid (am and pm) or ud

Repeat application for 8-10 days or ud

May rinse cleanser off sooner or use less frequently if skin dryness occurs

ADMINISTRATION

Topical route

Seborrheic Dermatitis/Dandruff:

Wet skin and liberally apply to areas to be cleansed, massage gently into skin working into a full lather, rinse thoroughly, pat dry, and repeat after 10-20 sec.

Rinse w/ plain water to remove excess medication.
Shampoo hair at least once a week.

Secondary Infections:
Wet skin and liberally apply to areas to be cleansed, massage gently into skin for 10-20 sec working into a full lather, rinse thoroughly, and pat dry.
Rinse w/ plain water to remove excess medication.

HOW SUPPLIED
Wash: 10% [180mL, 355mL, 480mL], (Plus) 10% [473mL]

CONTRAINDICATIONS
Known or suspected hypersensitivity to any ingredients of the product, kidney disease.

WARNINGS/PRECAUTIONS
Stevens-Johnson syndrome (SJS) and drug-induced systemic lupus erythematosus (SLE) reported. May cause proliferation of nonsusceptible organisms, including fungi. Caution in patients who may be prone to hypersensitivity to topical sulfonamides; d/c if signs of hypersensitivity or other untoward reaction occurs. Local irritation or sensitization may occur during long-term therapy. Systemic toxic reactions (eg, agranulocytosis, acute hemolytic anemia, purpura hemorrhagica) indicate hypersensitivity to sulfonamides. Employ particular caution if areas of denuded or abraded skin are involved; systemic absorption is greater following application to large, infected, abraded, denuded, or severely burned areas.

ADVERSE REACTIONS
Irritation, hypersensitivity.

DRUG INTERACTIONS
Incompatible w/ silver preparations.

PATIENT CONSIDERATIONS

Assessment: Assess for hypersensitivity to any of the ingredients of the product, kidney disease, pregnancy/nursing status, and possible drug interactions.
Assess if treatment area contains denuded or abraded skin.

Monitoring: Monitor for signs/symptoms of hypersensitivity reactions, SJS, drug-induced SLE, systemic toxic reactions, and other adverse reactions. Monitor for local irritation or sensitization if used for long-term therapy. When applying to large, infected, abraded, denuded, or severely burned areas, monitor for occurrence of adverse events produced by systemic administration of sulfonamides and perform appropriate lab testing.

Counseling: Counsel to d/c therapy if condition worsens or if rash develops in the area being treated or elsewhere. Instruct to d/c promptly and notify physician if any signs of arthritis, fever, or mouth sores develop. Instruct to avoid contact w/ eyes, lips, and mucous membranes. Inform that a slight discoloration may occasionally occur when an excessive amount of the product is used and comes in contact w/ white fabrics; inform that this discoloration is readily removed by ordinary laundering w/o bleaches.

STORAGE: 20-25°C (68-77°F); excursions permitted between 15-30°C (59-86°F). Brief exposure up to 40°C (104°F) may be tolerated provided the mean kinetic temperature does not exceed 25°C (77°F); minimize such exposure. Protect from freezing and excessive heat. Product may tend to darken slightly on storage; slight discoloration does not impair efficacy or safety of product. Keep tightly closed.

Ovcon-35 – ethinyl estradiol/norethindrone

RX

Class: Estrogen/progestogen combination

Cigarette smoking increases the risk of serious cardiovascular side effects. Risk increases w/ age and w/ heavy smoking (≥15 cigarettes/day) and is quite marked in women >35 yrs of age. Women who use oral contraceptives should be strongly advised not to smoke.

OTHER BRAND NAMES
Balziva

ADULT DOSAGE

Contraception

1 tab qd for 28 days, then repeat regimen on the next day after the last tab

Start on the 1st day of menses or 1st Sunday after menses begin

PEDIATRIC DOSAGE

Contraception

Not indicated for use premenarche; refer to adult dosing

DOSING CONSIDERATIONS

Adverse Reactions

GI Disturbances: Use a back-up method of contraception for the remainder of that cycle if significant GI disturbance occurs

ADMINISTRATION

Oral route

Take at the same time every day

Use a nonhormonal contraceptive as backup during the 1st 7 days of therapy of initiating therapy (Sunday starter) or restarting after ≥2 missed doses

HOW SUPPLIED

Tab: (Ethinyl Estradiol/Norethindrone) 0.035mg/0.4mg

CONTRAINDICATIONS

Thrombophlebitis, current or history of thromboembolic disorders, past history of deep vein thrombophlebitis, cerebrovascular or coronary artery disease, known or suspected carcinoma of the breast, endometrial carcinoma or other known or suspected estrogen-dependent neoplasia, undiagnosed abnormal genital bleeding, cholestatic jaundice of pregnancy or jaundice w/ prior pill use, hepatic adenomas or carcinomas, known or suspected pregnancy.

WARNINGS/PRECAUTIONS

Increased risk of MI, thromboembolism, cerebrovascular events, gallbladder disease, and hepatic neoplasia. May increase risk of vascular disease. If feasible, d/c at least 4 weeks prior to and for 2 weeks after elective surgery of a type associated with an increase in risk of thromboembolism and during and following prolonged immobilization. Start therapy no earlier than 4-6 weeks after delivery in women who elect not to breastfeed. May increase risk of breast cancer and cervical intraepithelial neoplasia. Retinal thrombosis reported; d/c if unexplained partial or complete loss of vision, onset of proptosis or diplopia, papilledema, or retinal vascular lesions develop. Increased risk of gallbladder surgery reported. May cause glucose intolerance. Changes in serum TG and lipoprotein levels reported. May cause fluid retention and increase BP; d/c if significant elevation of BP occurs. D/C and evaluate the cause if onset/exacerbation of migraine or headache w/ a new pattern that is recurrent, persistent, or severe develops. Breakthrough bleeding and spotting reported; rule out malignancy or pregnancy. D/C if jaundice develops. Monitor closely w/ depression and d/c if depression recurs to serious degree. Contact lens wearers who develop visual changes or changes in lens tolerance should be assessed by an ophthalmologist. May affect certain endocrine function tests, LFTs, and blood components in lab tests.

ADVERSE REACTIONS

N/V, breakthrough bleeding, GI symptoms, spotting, menstrual flow changes, amenorrhea, migraine, mental depression, vaginal candidiasis, edema, weight changes, cervical ectropion and secretion changes, melasma, breast changed (tenderness, enlargement, secretion), rash.

DRUG INTERACTIONS

Reduced effects, increased breakthrough bleeding, and menstrual irregularities w/ rifampin, barbiturates, phenylbutazone, phenytoin sodium, and possibly w/ griseofulvin, ampicillin, and tetracyclines.

PATIENT CONSIDERATIONS

Assessment: Assess for thrombophlebitis or thromboembolic disorders, HTN, hyperlipidemia, diabetes, breast cancer, undiagnosed abnormal genital bleeding, pregnancy/nursing status, possible drug interactions, and any other conditions where treatment is contraindicated or cautioned.

Monitoring: Monitor for signs/symptoms of thromboembolism, stroke, MI, and other adverse reactions. Monitor BP in patients w/ a history of HTN, HTN-related disease, or renal disease; for signs of depression in patients w/ a history of depression; serum glucose levels in prediabetic and diabetic patients; and lipid levels in patients w/ a history of hyperlipidemia. Perform annual history and physical exam including special reference to BP, breasts, abdomen and pelvic organs, including cervical cytology, and relevant laboratory tests. Monitor women w/ a strong family history of breast cancer or who have breast nodules.

Counseling: Inform that medication does not protect against HIV infection (AIDS) and other STDs. Counsel about possible serious side effects. Advise to avoid smoking while on therapy. Inform that if spotting, light bleeding, or nausea occurs during first 1-3 packs of pills, to not d/c medication, and if symptoms persist, to notify physician. Inform that if vomiting or diarrhea occurs, efficacy may decrease; instruct to use backup method of contraception and to contact physician. Advise to notify physician of all prescription/nonprescription medications currently taking. Instruct patients w/ contact lenses to notify physician if changes in vision or lens tolerance develop. Instruct to use additional method of protection until after patient has taken seven pills if using the Sunday-start method. Inform on what to do if pills are missed.

STORAGE: 20-25°C (68-77°F).

Oxaydo – oxycodone hydrochloride

CII

Class: Opioid analgesic

ADULT DOSAGE

Moderate to Severe Pain

Acute:

Patients Not Currently Receiving Opioid Analgesics:
Initial: 5-15mg q4-6h prn
Titrate: Adjust based on response to initial dose

Chronic:
Dose at lowest level that will achieve acceptable analgesia and tolerable adverse reactions, on an around-the-clock basis

Conversions

From Fixed-Ratio Oral Opioid/Nonopioid Combinations:
Determine whether or not to continue nonopioid analgesic. Titrate dose in response to the level of analgesia and adverse reactions afforded by dosing regimen regardless of whether nonopioid is continued

From Other Oral Opioid Therapy:
Closely observe and adjust dose based on patient's response to therapy

PEDIATRIC DOSAGE

Pediatric use may not have been established

DOSING CONSIDERATIONS

Renal Impairment
Initial: Follow conservative approach and adjust according to clinical situation

Hepatic Impairment
Initial: Follow conservative approach and adjust according to clinical situation

Elderly
Start at low end of the dosing range

Discontinuation
Gradually taper over time to prevent development of withdrawal; generally can decrease therapy by 25% to 50% per day w/ careful monitoring

ADMINISTRATION

Oral route
Swallow tab whole.
Take each tab w/ enough water to ensure complete swallowing immediately after placing in the mouth.
Not for crushing and dissolution.
Do not administer via NG, gastric, or other feeding tubes.

HOW SUPPLIED

Tab: 5mg, 7.5mg

CONTRAINDICATIONS

Respiratory depression in unmonitored settings and in the absence of resuscitative equipment; known or suspected paralytic ileus; acute or severe bronchial asthma or hypercarbia; known hypersensitivity to oxycodone, oxycodone salts, or any components of the product.

WARNINGS/PRECAUTIONS

Respiratory depression may occur; increased risk in elderly/debilitated patients, in those suffering from conditions accompanied by hypoxia, hypercapnia, or upper airway obstruction, or w/ large initial doses given to nontolerant patients. Extreme caution w/ COPD or cor pulmonale, in patients having substantially decreased respiratory reserve (eg, severe kyphoscoliosis), hypoxia, hypercapnia, or preexisting respiratory depression; consider alternative nonopioid analgesics. Potential for misuse and abuse. Respiratory depressant effects and its potential to elevate CSF pressure may be exaggerated in the presence of head injury, intracranial lesions, or preexisting increased intracranial pressure (ICP). May produce effects on pupillary response and consciousness. May cause severe hypotension in patients whose ability to maintain blood pressure has been compromised by a depleted intravascular volume. Orthostatic hypotension in ambulatory patients may occur. Caution w/ circulatory shock. Do not administer to patients w/ GI obstruction; may result in prolonged obstruction. May obscure diagnosis or clinical course of acute abdominal conditions. Caution w/ biliary tract disease; may cause spasm of sphincter of Oddi and diminish biliary/pancreatic secretions. Caution and reduce dose w/ severe renal/hepatic impairment, Addison's disease, hypothyroidism, prostatic hypertrophy, urethral stricture, and in elderly/debilitated patients. May induce/aggravate seizures. Caution in CNS depression, toxic psychosis, acute alcoholism, and delirium tremens. May impair mental/physical abilities.

ADVERSE REACTIONS

N/V, constipation, headache, pruritus, insomnia, dizziness, asthenia, somnolence.

DRUG INTERACTIONS

Caution and reduce dose w/ other CNS depressants (eg, sedatives, hypnotics, general anesthetics, antiemetics, phenothiazines, tranquilizers, alcohol); may increase risk of respiratory depression, hypotension, profound sedation, or coma. Avoid alcoholic beverages/alcohol-containing medications. Risk of severe hypotension w/ phenothiazines, general anesthetics, or other agents that compromise vasomotor tone. May enhance neuromuscular blocking action of skeletal muscle relaxants and may increase respiratory depression. Mixed agonist/antagonist analgesics (eg, pentazocine, nalbuphine, butorphanol, buprenorphine) may reduce effect and/or precipitate withdrawal; do not administer mixed agonist/antagonist analgesics to patients who have received or are receiving a course of therapy w/ a pure opioid agonist. Not recommended in patients taking MAOIs or w/in 14 days of stopping treatment; may intensify effects causing anxiety, confusion, and significant respiratory depression or coma. Increased levels w/ voriconazole. Caution w/ CYP3A4 inhibitors (eg, macrolide antibiotics, azole-antifungal agents, protease inhibitors); may prolong opioid effects. May decrease levels/efficacy or result in development of abstinence syndrome w/ rifampin and other CYP3A4 inducers (eg, carbamazepine, phenytoin); use w/ caution. Urinary retention/severe constipation potentially leading to paralytic ileus may occur w/ anticholinergics. Caution w/ CYP2D6 inhibitors.

PATIENT CONSIDERATIONS

Assessment: Assess for level of pain intensity, type of pain, respiratory depression, COPD, hypoxia, hypercarbia, asthma, GI obstruction, renal/hepatic impairment, or any other conditions where treatment is contraindicated or cautioned. Assess for pregnancy/nursing status and possible drug interactions.

Monitoring: Monitor for signs/symptoms of respiratory depression, CNS depression, seizures/convulsions, CSF pressure elevation, hypotension, and other adverse reactions. Monitor BP. Monitor for tolerance, physical dependence, and signs of misuse, abuse, and addiction.

Counseling: Advise to take ud and to take each tab w/ enough water to ensure complete swallowing. Instruct to swallow whole and not to crush/dissolve tab or pre-soak, lick, or otherwise wet the tablet prior to placing in the mouth. Advise to not adjust the dose w/o consulting healthcare provider. Advise that drowsiness, dizziness, or lightheadedness may occur. Inform that therapy may impair mental/physical abilities; instruct to refrain from potentially dangerous activities. Instruct to not combine w/ alcohol or other CNS depressants. Instruct to inform physician if pregnant or planning to become pregnant. Inform that dosing will need to be tapered if taking medication for more than a few weeks. Advise that medication has potential for abuse; protect from theft. Advise to not share or permit use by other individuals. Instruct to dispose of any unused medication by flushing down the toilet. Advise of possible occurrence of severe constipation and other adverse reactions.

STORAGE: 25°C (77°F); excursions permitted to 15-30°C (59-86°F). Protect from moisture.

OXYBUTYNIN – oxybutynin chloride

RX

Class: Anticholinergic

OTHER BRAND NAMES

Ditropan (Discontinued)

ADULT DOSAGE

Uninhibited Neurogenic or Reflex Neurogenic Bladder

Relief of Symptoms of Bladder Instability Associated with Voiding:

Usual: 5mg bid-tid

Max: 5mg qid

PEDIATRIC DOSAGE

Uninhibited Neurogenic or Reflex Neurogenic Bladder

Relief of Symptoms of Bladder Instability Associated with Voiding:

≥5 Years:

Usual: 5mg bid

Max: 5mg tid

DOSING CONSIDERATIONS

Elderly

Start at lower end of doing range

Frail Elderly:

Initial: 2.5mg bid-tid

ADMINISTRATION

Oral route

HOW SUPPLIED

Syrup: 5mg/5mL [118mL, 473mL]; **Tab:** 5mg* *scored

CONTRAINDICATIONS

Urinary retention, gastric retention and other severe decreased GI motility conditions, uncontrolled narrow-angle glaucoma, and in patients at risk for these conditions. Hypersensitivity to the drug substance or other components of the product.

WARNINGS/PRECAUTIONS

Angioedema of the face, lips, tongue, and/or larynx reported; d/c if involvement of the tongue, hypopharynx, or larynx occurs. Variety of CNS anticholinergic effects reported; consider dose reduction or discontinuation. May aggravate symptoms of hyperthyroidism, coronary heart disease (CHD), congestive heart failure (CHF), cardiac arrhythmias, hiatal hernia, tachycardia, HTN, myasthenia gravis, and prostatic hypertrophy. Caution with preexisting dementia treated with cholinesterase inhibitors, hepatic/renal impairment, myasthenia gravis, clinically significant bladder outflow obstruction, GI obstructive disorders, ulcerative colitis, intestinal atony, gastroesophageal reflux disorder, and in frail elderly.

ADVERSE REACTIONS

Dry mouth, dizziness, constipation, somnolence, nausea, blurred vision, urinary hesitation, headache, urinary tract infection, nervousness, dyspepsia, urinary retention, insomnia.

DRUG INTERACTIONS

May increase frequency and/or severity of adverse effects with other anticholinergics or with other agents that produce dry mouth, constipation, somnolence, and/or other anticholinergic effects. May alter GI absorption of other drugs due to GI motility effects; caution with drugs with narrow therapeutic index. Increased levels with ketoconazole. CYP3A4 inhibitors (eg, antimycotics, macrolides) may alter mean pharmacokinetic parameters; caution when coadministered. Caution with drugs that can cause or exacerbate esophagitis (eg, bisphosphonates).

PATIENT CONSIDERATIONS

Assessment: Assess for urinary and gastric retention, other severe decreased GI motility conditions, uncontrolled narrow-angle glaucoma, preexisting dementia, hepatic/renal impairment, myasthenia gravis, hyperthyroidism, CHD, CHF, hypersensitivity to the drug, other conditions where treatment is contraindicated or cautioned, pregnancy/nursing status, and possible drug interactions.

Monitoring: Monitor for aggravation of myasthenia gravis, hyperthyroidism, CHD, CHF, cardiac arrhythmias, hiatal hernia, tachycardia, HTN, and prostatic hypertrophy symptoms. Monitor for signs of anticholinergic CNS effects, hypersensitivity reactions, and other adverse reactions.

Counseling: Inform that angioedema may occur and could result in life-threatening airway obstruction; advise to promptly d/c therapy and seek medical attention if tongue/laryngopharynx edema or difficulty breathing occurs. Inform that heat prostration may occur when administered in high environmental temperature. Inform that drug may produce drowsiness or blurred vision; advise to exercise caution. Inform that alcohol may enhance drowsiness.

STORAGE: (Tab) 20-25°C (68-77°F). (Syrup) 15-30°C (59-86°F).

OxyContin – oxycodone hydrochloride

CII

Class: Opioid analgesic

Exposes users to risks of addiction, abuse, and misuse, leading to overdose and death; assess each patient's risk prior to prescribing and monitor regularly for development of these behaviors/conditions. Serious, life-threatening, or fatal respiratory depression may occur; monitor during initiation or following a dose increase. Crushing, dissolving, or chewing tab can cause rapid release and absorption of potentially fatal dose; instruct patients to swallow tab whole. Accidental ingestion, especially by children, can result in a fatal overdose. Prolonged use during pregnancy can result in neonatal opioid withdrawal syndrome; advise pregnant women of the risk and ensure availability of appropriate treatment. Concomitant use of CYP3A4 inhibitors or discontinuation of CYP3A4 inducers can result in oxycodone overdose; monitor patients receiving concomitant CYP3A4 inhibitors/inducers.

ADULT DOSAGE

Severe Pain (Daily, Around-the-Clock Management)

1st Opioid Analgesic/Opioid-Intolerant Patients:
Initial: 10mg q12h
Titrate: Increase total daily dose by 25-50% every 1-2 days when clinically indicated

Conversions

From Other Oral Oxycodone Formulations:
Administer 1/2 of total daily dose q12h

From Other Opioids:
D/C all other around-the-clock opioids when therapy is initiated and initiate dosing using 10mg q12h

From Transdermal Fentanyl:
Initiate treatment 18 hrs following removal of patch; 10mg q12h should be initially substituted for each 25mcg/hr fentanyl transdermal patch

PEDIATRIC DOSAGE

Severe Pain (Daily, Around-the-Clock Management)

Use in patients ≥11 yrs already receiving and tolerating opioids for at least 5 consecutive days; for the 2 days immediately preceding dosing w/ Oxycontin, patients must be taking a minimum of 20mg/day of oxycodone or its equivalent

Do not use if opioid requirement is <20mg/day; d/c all other opioids when initiating therapy

Conversion Formula:
Mg/Day of Prior Opioid x Conversion Factor = Mg/Day of Oxycontin

Divide the calculated total daily dose by 2 to get the q12h dose

Conversion Factors:
Oxycodone: 1
Hydrocodone: 0.9
Hydromorphone: 4 (oral), 20 (parenteral)
Morphine: 0.5 (oral), 3 (parenteral)
Tramadol: 0.17 (oral), 0.2 (parenteral)

For patients receiving high-dose parenteral opioids, a more conservative conversion is warranted; for high-dose parenteral morphine, use 1.5 instead of 3 as a multiplication factor

For patients taking ≥1 opioid, calculate the approx oxycodone dose for each opioid and sum the totals to obtain the approx Oxycontin daily dosage

For patients on a regimen of fixed-ratio opioid/nonopioid analgesic products, use only the opioid component of these products in the conversion

If using asymmetric dosing, give higher dose in the am and the lower dose in the pm

Conversion from Transdermal Fentanyl:
Initiate treatment 18 hrs following removal of patch; 10mg q12h should be initially substituted for each 25mcg/hr fentanyl transdermal patch

Initial: Round down to the nearest Oxycontin dose; if the rounded calculated dose is <20mg, do not initiate
Titrate: Increase total daily dose by 25% every 1-2 days when clinically indicated

DOSING CONSIDERATIONS

Concomitant Medications
If patient is currently on a CNS depressant, initiate Oxycontin at 1/3 to 1/2 the recommended starting dose and monitor

Hepatic Impairment
Initiate at 1/3 to 1/2 the recommended starting dose, followed by careful dose titration

Elderly
Reduce starting dose to 1/3 to 1/2 the recommended dose in debilitated, opioid-intolerant patients

Discontinuation
Use gradual downward titration

ADMINISTRATION

Oral route
Do not presoak, lick, or otherwise wet tab prior to placing in mouth.
Swallow tab whole; do not crush, dissolve, or chew.
Take 1 tab at a time w/ enough water to ensure complete swallowing.

HOW SUPPLIED

Tab, Extended-Release: 10mg, 15mg, 20mg, 30mg, 40mg, 60mg, 80mg

CONTRAINDICATIONS

Significant respiratory depression, acute or severe bronchial asthma in unmonitored settings or in the absence of resuscitative equipment, known or suspected paralytic ileus and GI obstruction, hypersensitivity (eg, anaphylaxis) to oxycodone.

WARNINGS/PRECAUTIONS

Reserve use in patients for whom alternative treatment options are ineffective, not tolerated, or would be otherwise inadequate to provide sufficient management of pain. Should only be prescribed by healthcare professionals who are knowledgeable in the use of potent opioids for management of chronic pain. 60mg and 80mg tabs, a single dose >40mg, or a total daily dose >80mg are only for use in opioid-tolerant patients. Life-threatening respiratory depression is more likely to occur in elderly, cachectic, or debilitated patients. Consider alternative nonopioid analgesics in patients w/ significant COPD or cor pulmonale, and in patients having a substantially decreased respiratory reserve, hypoxia, hypercapnia, or preexisting respiratory depression. May cause severe hypotension, orthostatic hypotension, and syncope; increased risk in patients whose ability to maintain BP has already been compromised by a reduced blood volume or concurrent administration of certain CNS depressants. Avoid w/ circulatory shock. Monitor patients who may be susceptible to intracranial effects of carbon dioxide retention for signs of sedation and respiratory depression when initiating therapy. Therapy may obscure clinical course in patient w/ head injury. Avoid w/ impaired consciousness or coma. Difficulty in swallowing tab, intestinal obstruction, and exacerbation of diverticulitis reported; consider alternative analgesic in patients who have difficulty swallowing or have underlying GI disorders that may predispose them to obstruction. May cause spasm of sphincter of Oddi and increase in serum amylase; monitor patients w/ biliary tract disease. May aggravate convulsions and induce/aggravate seizures. May impair mental or physical abilities. Urine drug test may not detect oxycodone reliably. Not recommended for use immediately prior to labor.

ADVERSE REACTIONS

Respiratory depression, constipation, N/V, somnolence, dizziness, pruritus, headache, dry mouth, asthenia, sweating, apnea, respiratory arrest, circulatory depression, hypotension.

DRUG INTERACTIONS

See Boxed Warning. Respiratory depression, hypotension, and profound sedation or coma may occur w/ CNS depressants (eg, sedatives, anxiolytics, neuroleptics); if coadministration is required, consider dose reduction of one or both agents. Monitor use in elderly, cachectic, and debilitated patients when coadministered w/ other drugs that depress respiration. May enhance neuromuscular blocking action of true skeletal muscle relaxants and increase respiratory depression. CYP3A4 inhibitors (eg, erythromycin, ketoconazole, ritonavir) may increase levels of oxycodone and prolong opioid effects; these effects could be more pronounced w/ concomitant use of CYP2D6 and 3A4 inhibitors. CYP3A4 inducers (eg, rifampin, carbamazepine, phenytoin) may decrease levels and cause lack of efficacy, or development of abstinence syndrome. If coadministration is necessary, use w/ caution when initiating oxycodone treatment in patients currently taking or discontinuing CYP3A4 inhibitors/inducers. Mixed agonist/antagonists (eg, pentazocine, nalbuphine, butorphanol) or partial agonists (buprenorphine) may reduce analgesic effect or precipitate withdrawal symptoms; avoid coadministration. May reduce efficacy of diuretics and lead to acute urinary retention. Anticholinergics or other medications w/ anticholinergic activity may increase risk of urinary retention and/or severe constipation and lead to paralytic ileus.

PATIENT CONSIDERATIONS

Assessment: Assess for abuse/addiction risk, pain intensity, prior opioid therapy, opioid tolerance, respiratory depression, drug hypersensitivity, pregnancy/nursing status, possible drug interactions, or any other conditions where treatment is contraindicated or cautioned.

Monitoring: Monitor for respiratory depression (especially w/in first 24-72 hrs of initiation), hypotension, seizures/convulsions, and other adverse reactions. Monitor BP and serum amylase levels. Routinely monitor for signs of misuse, abuse, and addiction. Periodically reassess the continued need for therapy.

Counseling: Inform that use of drug can result in addiction, abuse, and misuse; instruct not to share w/ others and to take steps to protect from theft or misuse. Inform patients about risk of respiratory depression. Advise to store securely and dispose unused tabs by flushing down the toilet. Inform female patients of reproductive potential that prolonged use during pregnancy may result in neonatal opioid withdrawal syndrome and instruct to inform physician if pregnant or planning to become pregnant. Inform that potentially serious additive effects may occur when used w/ CNS depressants, and not to use such drugs unless supervised by healthcare provider. Instruct about proper administration instructions. Inform that drug may cause orthostatic hypotension, syncope, or may impair the ability to perform potentially hazardous activities; advise to not perform such tasks until they know how they will react to medication. Advise of potential for severe constipation, including management instructions. Advise how to recognize anaphylaxis and when to seek medical attention. Advise caregivers to strictly adhere to dosing when giving to pediatric patients.

STORAGE: 25°C (77°F); excursions permitted to 15-30°C (59-86°F).

PAXIL – paroxetine hydrochloride

RX

Class: Selective serotonin reuptake inhibitor (SSRI)

Antidepressants increased the risk of suicidal thinking and behavior (suicidality) in children, adolescents, and young adults in short-term studies of major depressive disorder and other psychiatric disorders. Monitor and observe closely for clinical worsening, suicidality, or unusual changes in behavior in patients who are started on antidepressants. Not approved for use in pediatric patients.

ADULT DOSAGE

Major Depressive Disorder

Initial: 20mg/day
Titrate: May increase in 10mg/day increments at intervals of at least 1 week
Maint: Efficacy is maintained for periods of up to 1 yr w/ doses that averaged about 30mg
Max: 50mg/day

Obsessive Compulsive Disorder

Initial: 20mg/day
Titrate: May increase in 10mg/day increments at intervals of at least 1 week
Recommended: 40mg/day
Max: 60mg/day

Panic Disorder

W/ or w/o Agoraphobia:
Initial: 10mg/day
Titrate: May increase in 10mg/day increments at intervals of at least 1 week
Target Dose: 40mg/day
Max: 60mg/day

Anxiety Disorders

Social Anxiety Disorder:
Initial/Usual: 20mg/day
Titrate: May increase in 10mg/day increments at intervals of at least 1 week
Range: 20-60mg/day; no additional benefit for doses >20mg/day

Generalized Anxiety Disorder:
Initial/Usual: 20mg/day
Titrate: May increase in 10mg/day increments at intervals of at least 1 week
Range: 20-50mg/day

Post-traumatic Stress Disorder

Initial: 20mg/day
Titrate: May increase in 10mg/day increments at intervals of at least 1 week
Range: 20-50mg/day

Dosing Considerations with MAOIs

Switching to/from an MAOI for Psychiatric Disorders:
Allow at least 14 days between discontinuation of an MAOI and initiation of treatment, and conversely allow at least 14 days between discontinuing treatment before starting an MAOI

Use w/ Other MAOIs (eg, Linezolid, IV Methylene Blue):
If acceptable alternatives are not available and benefits outweigh risks of serotonin syndrome, d/c paroxetine promptly and administer linezolid or IV methylene blue; monitor for serotonin syndrome for 2 weeks or until 24 hrs after last dose of linezolid or IV methylene blue, whichever comes 1st.
May resume paroxetine therapy 24 hrs after last dose of linezolid or IV methylene blue

PEDIATRIC DOSAGE

Pediatric use may not have been established

DOSING CONSIDERATIONS

Severe Renal Impairment

Initial: 10mg/day
Max: 40mg/day

Severe Hepatic Impairment

Initial: 10mg/day
Max: 40mg/day

Elderly

Elderly/Debilitated:
Initial: 10mg/day
Max: 40mg/day

Discontinuation

Reduce gradually; consider resuming previously prescribed dose if intolerable symptoms occur following a decrease in dose or upon discontinuation. Subsequently, may continue to decrease the dose, but at a more gradual rate

ADMINISTRATION

Oral route

Take w/ or w/o food
Give qd, usually in the am

Tab

Swallow whole; do not chew or crush

Sus

Shake well before use

HOW SUPPLIED

Sus: 10mg/5mL [250mL]; **Tab:** 10mg*, 20mg*, 30mg, 40mg *scored

CONTRAINDICATIONS

Use of an MAOI for psychiatric disorders either concomitantly or within 14 days of stopping treatment. Treatment within 14 days of stopping an MAOI for psychiatric disorders. Starting treatment in a patient being treated with other MAOIs (eg, linezolid, IV methylene blue). Concomitant use with thioridazine or pimozide. Hypersensitivity to paroxetine or any of the inactive ingredients in this medication.

WARNINGS/PRECAUTIONS

May precipitate mixed/manic episode in patients at risk for bipolar disorder. Not approved for treatment of bipolar depression. Serotonin syndrome reported; d/c immediately and initiate supportive symptomatic treatment. Pupillary dilation that occurs following use may trigger an angle-closure attack in a patient with anatomically narrow angles who does not have a patent iridectomy. Increased risk of congenital malformations reported in 1st trimester of pregnancy; neonates exposed to therapy late in the 3rd trimester have developed complications. Activation of mania/hypomania reported; caution with history of mania. Seizures reported; d/c if seizures develop. Adverse reactions reported upon discontinuation; avoid abrupt withdrawal. Akathisia may develop. Hyponatremia may occur; caution in elderly and volume-depleted patients. Consider discontinuation in patients with symptomatic hyponatremia and institute appropriate medical intervention. May increase risk of bleeding events. Bone fracture risk following exposure to some antidepressants reported. Caution with diseases/conditions affecting hemodynamic responses or metabolism, severe hepatic/renal impairment, and in elderly/debilitated patients. Mydriasis reported; caution with narrow-angle glaucoma.

ADVERSE REACTIONS

Asthenia, nausea, somnolence, headache, insomnia, abnormal ejaculation, dry mouth, constipation, dizziness, diarrhea, decreased libido, sweating, decreased appetite, tremor, impotence.

DRUG INTERACTIONS

See Contraindications. Not recommended with SSRIs, SNRIs, tryptophan, and alcohol. May cause serotonin syndrome with other serotonergic drugs (eg, triptans, TCAs, fentanyl) and with drugs that impair metabolism of serotonin; d/c immediately if this occurs. Metabolism and pharmacokinetics may be affected by the induction or inhibition of drug-metabolizing enzymes. Increased risk of bleeding with aspirin, NSAIDs, warfarin, and other anticoagulants. Increased risk of hyponatremia with diuretics. Increased levels with cimetidine. Decreased levels with phenobarbital, phenytoin, and fosamprenavir/ritonavir. Caution with drugs that are metabolized by CYP2D6 (eg, phenothiazines, risperidone, type 1C antiarrhythmics) and with drugs that inhibit CYP2D6 (eg, quinidine). May increase levels of desipramine, risperidone, procyclidine and theophylline. May increase levels of atomoxetine; may require dose adjustments of atomoxetine. May inhibit metabolism of TCAs. May displace or be displaced by other highly protein-bound drugs. May reduce efficacy of tamoxifen. Caution with warfarin, TCAs, lithium, and digoxin. Severe hypotension reported when added to chronic metoprolol treatment.

PATIENT CONSIDERATIONS

Assessment: Assess for drug hypersensitivity, risk of bipolar disorder, history of seizures or mania, volume depletion, diseases/conditions that affect metabolism or hemodynamic responses, hepatic/renal impairment, susceptibility to angle-closure glaucoma or narrow-angle glaucoma, pregnancy/nursing status, and for possible drug interactions.

Monitoring: Monitor for signs/symptoms of clinical worsening, suicidality, unusual changes in behavior, serotonin syndrome, angle-closure glaucoma, seizures, activation of mania/hypomania, akathisia, bone fracture, hyponatremia especially in the elderly, abnormal bleeding, and other adverse reactions. Periodically reevaluate long-term usefulness of therapy.

Counseling: Inform about benefits, risks, and appropriate use of therapy. Caution about risk of serotonin syndrome, angle-closure glaucoma, and bleeding. Counsel to be alert for emergence of unusual changes in behavior, worsening of depression, and suicidal ideation, especially during drug initiation or dose adjustment. Caution against operating hazardous machinery (including automobiles) until reasonably certain that therapy does not adversely affect ability to engage in such activities. Inform that improvement may be noticed in 1-4 weeks; instruct to continue therapy ud. Inform physician if taking, or planning to take, any prescription or OTC drugs. Instruct to notify physician if pregnant/intending to become pregnant, or if breastfeeding. Advise to avoid alcohol.

STORAGE: Tab: 15-30°C (59-86°F). Sus: ≤25°C (77°F).

PAXIL CR – paroxetine hydrochloride

RX

Class: Selective serotonin reuptake inhibitor (SSRI)

Antidepressants increased the risk of suicidal thinking and behavior (suicidality) in short-term studies in children, adolescents, and young adults with major depressive disorder and other psychiatric disorders. Monitor and observe closely for clinical worsening, suicidality, or unusual changes in behavior in patients who are started on antidepressants. Not approved for use in pediatric patients.

ADULT DOSAGE

Major Depressive Disorder

Initial: 25mg/day
Titrate: May increase by 12.5mg/day increments at intervals of at least 1 week
Max: 62.5mg/day

Panic Disorder

W/ or w/o Agoraphobia:
Initial: 12.5mg/day
Titrate: May increase by 12.5mg/day increments at intervals of at least 1 week
Max: 75mg/day

Social Anxiety Disorder

Initial: 12.5mg/day
Titrate: May increase by 12.5mg/day increments at intervals of at least 1 week
Max: 37.5mg/day

Premenstrual Dysphoric Disorder

Initial: 12.5mg/day; give either qd throughout menstrual cycle or limit to luteal phase of menstrual cycle
Titrate: May increase to 25mg/day at intervals of at least 1 week

Dosing Considerations with MAOIs

Switching to/from an MAOI for Psychiatric Disorders:
Allow at least 14 days between discontinuation of an MAOI and initiation of treatment, and allow at least 14 days between discontinuation of treatment and initiation of an MAOI

Use w/ Other MAOIs (eg, Linezolid, IV Methylene Blue):
Do not start paroxetine in a patient being treated w/ linezolid or IV methylene blue
In patients already receiving paroxetine, if

PEDIATRIC DOSAGE

Pediatric use may not have been established

P

acceptable alternatives are not available and benefits outweigh risks, d/c paroxetine and administer linezolid or IV methylene blue; monitor for serotonin syndrome for 2 weeks or until 24 hrs after the last dose of linezolid or IV methylene blue, whichever comes 1st. May resume paroxetine therapy 24 hrs after the last dose of linezolid or IV methylene blue

DOSING CONSIDERATIONS

Renal Impairment

Severe (CrCl <30mL/min):
Initial: 12.5mg/day
Max: 50mg/day

Hepatic Impairment

Severe:
Initial: 12.5mg/day
Max: 50mg/day

Elderly

Elderly/Debilitated:
Initial: 12.5mg/day
Max: 50mg/day

Discontinuation

Gradually reduce dose whenever possible; consider resuming previously prescribed dose if intolerable symptoms occur following a decrease in dose or upon discontinuation. Subsequently, may continue to decrease the dose, but at a more gradual rate

ADMINISTRATION

Oral route

Administer as a single daily dose, usually in the am
Take w/ or w/o food
Swallow whole; do not chew or crush

HOW SUPPLIED

Tab, Controlled-Release: 12.5mg, 25mg, 37.5mg

CONTRAINDICATIONS

Use of MAOIs intended to treat psychiatric disorders either concomitantly or within 14 days of stopping treatment. Treatment within 14 days of stopping an MAOI intended to treat psychiatric disorders. Starting treatment in patients being treated with MAOIs (eg, linezolid, IV methylene blue). Concomitant use with thioridazine or pimozide. Hypersensitivity to paroxetine or any of the inactive ingredients in this medication.

WARNINGS/PRECAUTIONS

May precipitate mixed/manic episode in patients at risk for bipolar disorder. Not approved for treatment of bipolar depression. Serotonin syndrome reported; d/c immediately and initiate supportive symptomatic treatment. Pupillary dilation that occurs following use may trigger an angle-closure attack in a patient with anatomically narrow angles who does not have a patent iridectomy. Increased risk of congenital malformations reported in 1st trimester of pregnancy; neonates exposed to therapy late in the 3rd trimester have developed complications. Activation of mania/hypomania reported; caution with history of mania. Seizures reported; d/c if seizures occur. Adverse reactions upon discontinuation (eg, dysphoric mood, irritability) reported; avoid abrupt withdrawal. Akathisia may develop. Hyponatremia reported; caution in elderly and volume-depleted patients. Consider discontinuation in patients with symptomatic hyponatremia and institute appropriate medical intervention. May increase risk of bleeding events. Bone fracture risk following exposure to some antidepressants reported. Caution with disease/conditions that could affect metabolism or hemodynamic responses, severe renal/hepatic impairment, pregnancy (3rd trimester), and in elderly/debilitated patients. May impair mental/physical abilities. Mydriasis reported; caution with narrow-angle glaucoma.

ADVERSE REACTIONS

Suicidality, somnolence, insomnia, nausea, asthenia, abnormal ejaculation, dry mouth, constipation, dizziness, diarrhea, decreased libido, sweating, abnormal vision, headache, tremor.

DRUG INTERACTIONS

See Contraindications. Serotonin syndrome reported with other serotonergic drugs (eg, triptans, TCAs, fentanyl, lithium, tramadol, tryptophan, buspirone, St. John's wort) and with drugs that impair serotonin metabolism. Use with other SSRIs, SNRIs, or tryptophan is not recommended. Avoid alcohol. Concomitant use with aspirin (ASA), NSAIDs, warfarin, and other anticoagulants may increase risk of bleeding events. Use with diuretics may increase risk of developing hyponatremia. Increased levels with cimetidine. Reduced levels with phenobarbital, phenytoin, and fosamprenavir/

ritonavir. Caution with drugs that are metabolized by CYP2D6 (eg, nortriptyline, phenothiazines, risperidone, type 1C antiarrhythmics) and with drugs that inhibit CYP2D6 (eg, quinidine). May increase levels of desipramine, risperidone, atomoxetine, and theophylline. May reduce efficacy of tamoxifen. May displace or be displaced by other highly protein-bound drugs. May increase procyclidine levels; reduce dose if anticholinergic effects are seen. May inhibit metabolism of TCAs. Caution with digoxin, TCAs, and lithium.

PATIENT CONSIDERATIONS

Assessment: Assess for drug hypersensitivity, risk of bipolar disorder, history of seizures or mania, volume depletion, diseases/conditions that affect metabolism or hemodynamic response, hepatic/renal impairment, narrow-angle glaucoma, susceptibility to angle-closure glaucoma, pregnancy/nursing status, and for possible drug interactions.

Monitoring: Monitor for signs/symptoms of clinical worsening, suicidality, unusual changes in behavior, serotonin syndrome, seizures, activation of mania/hypomania, akathisia, bone fracture, hyponatremia especially in the elderly, abnormal bleeding, angle-closure glaucoma, and other adverse reactions. Upon discontinuation, monitor for symptoms. Periodically reassess need for continued therapy.

Counseling: Inform about the risks, benefits, and appropriate use of therapy. Advise to avoid alcohol use. Instruct to notify physician of all prescription or OTC drugs currently taking or planning to take. Caution about risk of serotonin syndrome, angle-closure glaucoma, and bleeding. Instruct patient, families, and caregivers to report emergence of anxiety, agitation, panic attacks, insomnia, irritability, hostility, aggressiveness, impulsivity, akathisia, hypomania, mania, unusual changes in behavior, worsening of depression, and suicidal ideation, especially during drug initiation or dose adjustment. Caution operating hazardous machinery (including automobiles) until reasonably certain that therapy does not adversely affect ability to engage in such activities. Inform that improvement may be noticed in 1-4 weeks; instruct to continue therapy ud. Instruct to notify physician if pregnant/intending to become pregnant, or if breastfeeding.

STORAGE: ≤25°C (77°F).

PEDIARIX – diphtheria and tetanus toxoids and acellular pertussis adsorbed, hepatitis B (recombinant) and inactivated poliovirus vaccine

RX

Class: Toxoid/vaccine combination

P

PEDIATRIC DOSAGE

Active Immunization Against Diphtheria, Tetanus, Pertussis, Hepatitis B Virus, and Poliomyelitis

For Use in Infants Born of Hepatitis B Surface Antigen (HBsAg)-Negative Mothers:

6 Weeks to 6 Years (Prior to 7th Birthday):

0.5mL IM dose as a 3-dose series at 2, 4, and 6 months (at intervals of 6-8 weeks, preferably 8 weeks); 1st dose may be given as early as 6 weeks of age

Modified Schedules in Previously Vaccinated Children:

Children Previously Vaccinated w/ Diphtheria and Tetanus Toxoids and Acellular Pertussis Vaccine Adsorbed (DTaP):

May use to complete the first 3 doses of the DTaP series in children who have received 1 or 2 doses of Infanrix and are also scheduled to receive the other vaccine components of Pediarix

Children Previously Vaccinated w/ Hepatitis B Vaccine:

May be used to complete the hepatitis B vaccination series following 1 or 2 doses of another hepatitis B vaccine (monovalent or as part of a combination vaccine), including vaccines from other manufacturers, in children born of HBsAg-negative mothers who are also scheduled to receive the other vaccine components of Pediarix

A 3-dose series may be administered to infants born of HBsAg-negative mothers and who received a dose of hepatitis B vaccine at or shortly after birth

Children Previously Vaccinated w/ Inactivated Poliovirus Vaccine (IPV): May be used to complete the first 3 doses of the IPV series in children who have received 1 or 2 doses of IPV from a different manufacturer and are also scheduled to receive the other vaccine components of Pediarix

Booster Immunization Following Pediarix: Children who have received a 3-dose series w/ Pediarix should complete the DTaP and IPV series according to the recommended schedule; children should receive Infanrix as their 4th dose of DTaP and either Infanrix or Kinrix as their 5th dose of DTaP; Kinrix or another manufacturer's IPV may be used to complete the 4-dose IPV series

ADMINISTRATION

IM route

Administer in the anterolateral aspect of the thigh (children <1 yr) and in the deltoid muscle (older children); do not inject in the gluteal area or areas where there may be a major nerve trunk

Shake vigorously; do not use if resuspension does not occur w/ vigorous shaking

Do not mix w/ any other vaccine in the same syringe or vial

Administer other vaccines separately, at different inj site

HOW SUPPLIED

Inj: 0.5mL [prefilled syringe]

CONTRAINDICATIONS

Severe allergic reaction (eg, anaphylaxis) after a previous dose of diphtheria toxoid-, tetanus toxoid-, pertussis antigen-, hepatitis B-, or poliovirus-containing vaccine or any component of this vaccine (eg, yeast, neomycin, polymyxin B). Encephalopathy (eg, coma, decreased level of consciousness, prolonged seizures) within 7 days of administration of a previous pertussis-containing vaccine that is not attributable to another identifiable cause. Progressive neurologic disorder (eg, infantile spasms, uncontrolled epilepsy, progressive encephalopathy).

WARNINGS/PRECAUTIONS

Use in infants is associated with higher risk of fever relative to separately administered vaccines. Evaluate potential benefits and risks of vaccine administration if Guillain-Barre syndrome occurs within 6 weeks of receipt of a prior tetanus toxoid-containing vaccine. Tip caps of prefilled syringes may contain natural rubber latex; may cause allergic reactions in latex-sensitive individuals. Syncope may occur and can be accompanied by transient neurological signs. Evaluate the potential benefits and risks of vaccine administration if any of the following events occur in temporal relation to receipt of a pertussis-containing vaccine: temperature ≥40.5°C (105°F) within 48 hrs not due to another identifiable cause; collapse or shock-like state occurring within 48 hrs; persistent, inconsolable crying lasting ≥3 hrs, occurring within 48 hrs; or seizures with or without fever occurring within 3 days. May administer an antipyretic at the time of vaccination and for the ensuing 24 hrs in children at higher risk for seizures. Apnea following IM administration observed in premature infants; consider infant's medical status, and the potential benefits and possible risks of vaccination. Review immunization history for possible vaccine sensitivity; appropriate treatment should be available for possible allergic reactions.

ADVERSE REACTIONS

Local inj-site reactions (pain, redness, swelling), fever, irritability/fussiness, drowsiness, loss of appetite.

DRUG INTERACTIONS

Immunosuppressive therapies, including irradiation, antimetabolites, alkylating agents, cytotoxic drugs, and corticosteroids (used in greater than physiologic doses), may reduce immune response to vaccine.

PATIENT CONSIDERATIONS

Assessment: Assess for history of encephalopathy, development of Guillain-Barre syndrome following a prior tetanus toxoid-containing vaccine, progressive neurologic disorder, immunosuppression, risk for seizures, possible drug interactions, and hypersensitivity to latex, yeast, neomycin, or polymyxin B. Review immunization history for possible vaccine sensitivity and previous vaccination-related adverse reactions. Assess use in premature infants.

Monitoring: Monitor for signs/symptoms of Guillain-Barre syndrome, allergic reactions, syncope, neurological signs, apnea in premature infants, and other adverse reactions.

Counseling: Inform parents/guardians about potential benefits/risks of immunization, and of the importance of completing the immunization series. Counsel parents/guardians about potential adverse reactions; instruct to report any adverse events to physician.

STORAGE: 2-8°C (36-46°F). Do not freeze. Discard if frozen.

PEGASYS – peginterferon alfa-2a — RX

Class: Biological response modifier

May cause or aggravate fatal or life-threatening neuropsychiatric, autoimmune, ischemic, and infectious disorders. Monitor closely w/ periodic clinical and lab evaluations. D/C w/ persistently severe or worsening signs/symptoms of these conditions.

ADULT DOSAGE

Chronic Hepatitis C with Compensated Liver Disease

W/O HIV Coinfection:
Monotherapy:
180mcg once weekly for 48 weeks

Combination Treatment:
Genotypes 1, 4:
180mcg once weekly for 48 weeks (if used w/ ribavirin only)

Genotypes 2, 3:
180mcg once weekly for 24 weeks (if used w/ ribavirin only)

W/ HIV Coinfection:
180mcg once weekly for 48 weeks (if used w/ ribavirin only)

Chronic Hepatitis B with Compensated Liver Disease

HBeAg-Positive and HBeAg-Negative:
180mcg once weekly for 48 weeks

PEDIATRIC DOSAGE

Chronic Hepatitis C with Compensated Liver Disease

≥5 Years:
Combination w/ Ribavirin:
180mcg/1.73m^2 x BSA once weekly
Max Dose: 180mcg

Treatment Duration:
Genotypes 2, 3: 24 weeks
Other Genotypes: 48 weeks

Treatment Initiation Prior to 18 Years:
Maintain pediatric dosing through the completion of therapy

DOSING CONSIDERATIONS

Renal Impairment
Adults:
CrCl <30mL/min and/or Hemodialysis: 135mcg once weekly
If severe adverse reactions or lab abnormalities develop, dose can be reduced to 90mcg once weekly until reactions abate; d/c if intolerance persists after dosage adjustment

Hepatic Impairment
Child Pugh-Score >6 (Class B and C): D/C Pegasys

Adverse Reactions
Neutropenia:
Adults:
ANC <750 cells/mm^3: Reduce dose to 135mcg once weekly
ANC <500 cells/mm^3: D/C until ANC values return to >1000 cells/mm^3; restart at 90mcg once weekly

Pediatrics:
ANC 750-999 cells/mm^3:
Weeks 1-2: Reduce dose to 135mcg/1.73m^2 x BSA
Weeks 3-48: No dose modification

ANC 500-749 cells/mm^3:
Weeks 1-2: Hold dose until >750 cells/mm^3 then resume at 135mcg/1.73m^2 x BSA
Weeks 3-48: Reduce dose to 135mcg/1.73m^2 x BSA

ANC 250-499 cells/mm^3:
Weeks 1-2: Hold dose until >750 cells/mm^3 then resume at 90mcg/1.73m^2 x BSA
Weeks 3-48: Hold dose until >750 cells/mm^3 then resume at 135mcg/1.73m^2 x BSA

ANC <250 cells/mm^3 (or Febrile Neutropenia): D/C treatment

Thrombocytopenia:
Adults:

Platelets <50,000 cells/mm³: Reduce dose to 90mcg once weekly
Platelets <25,000 cells/mm³: D/C treatment

Pediatrics:
Platelets <50,000 cells/mm³: 90mcg/1.73m² x BSA

Transaminase Elevations:
Adults:
Progressive ALT Increases After Dose Reduction: D/C therapy
ALT Increases w/ Increased Bilirubin/Evidence of Hepatic Decompensation: D/C therapy

Chronic Hepatitis C Patients:
Progressive ALT Increases Above Baseline: Reduce dose to 135mcg; resume therapy after flares subside

Chronic Hepatitis B Patients:
ALT Elevations >5X ULN: Reduce dose to 135mcg or temporarily d/c; resume therapy after flares subside
Persistent, Severe Flares (ALT >10X Above ULN): Consider discontinuation

Pediatrics:
Persistent/Increasing ALT Elevations ≥5 but <10X ULN: Modify dose to 135mcg/1.73m² x BSA; reduce dose further if necessary
Persistent ALT Elevations ≥10X ULN: D/C treatment

Depression:
Initial Management (4-8 Weeks):
Adults:
Moderate: Decrease dose to 135mcg or 90mcg once weekly
Severe: Permanently d/c treatment

Pediatrics:
Moderate: Decrease dose to 135mcg/1.73m² x BSA or 90mcg/1.73m² x BSA once weekly
Severe: Permanently d/c treatment

Worsening of Depression Severity After 8 Weeks:
Adults:
Mild: Decrease dose to 135mcg or 90mcg once weekly or d/c
Moderate: Permanently d/c treatment

Pediatrics:
Mild: Decrease dose to 135mcg/1.73m² x BSA or 90mcg/1.73m² x BSA once weekly
Moderate: Permanently d/c treatment
Refer to PI for psychiatric visit schedule

Discontinuation

Chronic Hepatic C Genotype 1 in Combination w/ Ribavirin or Alone:
D/C if at least a 2 $\log_{10}$ HCV RNA reduction from baseline is not achieved by Week 12
D/C if undetectable HCV RNA is not achieved after 24 weeks

ADMINISTRATION

SQ route

Administer in abdomen or thigh
Discard unused portion in single-use vials or prefilled syringes in excess of the labeled volume

Recommended Volume to be Administered for Different Dosages

180mcg/mL in a Vial:
90mcg Dose: Use 0.5mL
135mcg Dose: Use 0.75mL
180mcg Dose: Use entire 1mL

180mcg/0.5mL in a Prefilled Syringe:
90mcg: Use 0.25mL
135mcg: Use 0.375mL
180mcg: Use entire 0.5mL

180mcg/0.5mL in an Autoinjector:
90mcg: Do not use
135mcg: Do not use
180mcg: May use

135mcg/0.5mL in an Autoinjector:
90mcg: Do not use
135mcg: May use
180mcg: Do not use

HOW SUPPLIED

Inj: 180mcg/0.5mL [prefilled syringe]; 180mcg/0.5mL, 135mcg/0.5mL [ProClick autoinjector]; 180mcg/mL [vial]

CONTRAINDICATIONS

Known hypersensitivity reactions (eg, urticaria, angioedema, bronchoconstriction, anaphylaxis, Stevens-Johnson syndrome) to alpha interferons or any component of this medication. autoimmune hepatitis, hepatic decompensation (Child-Pugh score >6 [Class B and C]) in cirrhotic patients before treatment, hepatic decompensation w/ Child-Pugh score ≥6 in cirrhotic CHC patients coinfected w/ HIV before treatment, neonates and infants (contains benzyl alcohol). When used with other HCV antiviral drugs, including ribavirin, refer to the individual monograph(s).

WARNINGS/PRECAUTIONS

Not recommended, alone or in combination w/ ribavirin w/o additional HCV antiviral drugs, in CHC patients who previously failed therapy w/ an interferon-alfa, and in CHC patients who have had a solid organ transplantation. Avoid in combination w/ ribavirin in pregnant women or men whose female partners are pregnant. Extreme caution w/ history of depression; d/c immediately in severe cases and institute psychiatric intervention. HTN, supraventricular arrhythmias, chest pain, and MI reported; caution w/ preexisting cardiac disease. May cause bone marrow suppression and severe cytopenias; d/c, at least temporarily, if severe decrease in neutrophil or platelet count develops. May cause or aggravate hypo/hyperthyroidism, ophthalmologic disorders, and pulmonary disorders. Hypo/hyperglycemia, diabetes mellitus, and ischemic and hemorrhagic cerebrovascular events reported. CHC patients w/ cirrhosis may be at risk for hepatic decompensation and death; d/c immediately w/ hepatic decompensation. Exacerbation of hepatitis B reported; d/c immediately if hepatic decompensation, progressive ALT increases, or increased bilirubin occurs. Ulcerative or hemorrhagic/ischemic colitis, pancreatitis, and severe acute hypersensitivity reactions reported; d/c if any of these develop. Consider discontinuation of treatment and immediately start appropriate anti-infective therapy if serious and severe infections occur. D/C w/ new or worsening ophthalmologic disorders, pulmonary infiltrates or pulmonary function impairment. Peripheral neuropathy reported in combination w/ telbivudine. May inhibit growth in pediatric patients. May impair fertility in women. Caution in renal impairment and in the elderly.

ADVERSE REACTIONS

Neuropsychiatric/autoimmune/ischemic/infectious disorders, inj-site reactions, fatigue/asthenia, diarrhea, pyrexia, rigors, N/V, anorexia, myalgia, headache, irritability/anxiety/nervousness.

DRUG INTERACTIONS

May inhibit CYP1A2 and increase exposure of theophylline; monitor theophylline serum levels and consider dose adjustments. May increase levels of methadone; monitor for toxicity. Hepatic decompensation can occur w/ peginterferon alfa-2a/ribavirin in combination w/ other HCV antiviral drugs and nucleoside reverse transcriptase inhibitors (NRTIs); refer to PI for other HCV antiviral drugs and the respective NRTIs for guidance regarding toxicity management. Concomitant use of peginterferon alfa-2a/ribavirin w/ zidovudine may cause severe neutropenia and severe anemia; consider discontinuation of zidovudine as medically appropriate and also consider dose reduction or discontinuation of peginterferon alfa-2a, ribavirin or both if worsening clinical toxicities are observed, including hepatic decompensation (eg, Child-Pugh >6). Pancytopenia and bone marrow suppression reported to occur w/in 3-7 weeks after the concomitant administration of pegylated interferon/ribavirin and azathioprine; d/c peginterferon alfa-2a, ribavirin, and azathioprine for pancytopenia, and do not re-introduce pegylated interferon/ribavirin w/ concomitant azathioprine.

PATIENT CONSIDERATIONS

Assessment: Assess for neuropsychiatric, autoimmune, ischemic or infectious disorders, hepatic/renal impairment, known hypersensitivity reactions, history of treatment failure w/ interferon alfa in CHC patients, history of solid organ transplantation in CHC patients, nursing status, possible drug interactions, or any other conditions where treatment is contraindicated or cautioned. Obtain baseline CBC, TSH, $CD4^+$ (HIV), and eye exam. Perform ECG for preexisting cardiac diseases. Obtain pregnancy test in women of childbearing potential.

Monitoring: Monitor for signs/symptoms of neuropsychiatric, autoimmune, ischemic, infectious, cardiovascular, cerebrovascular, endocrine, and pulmonary disorders; bone marrow toxicities; colitis; pancreatitis; delayed growth in pediatric patients; and other adverse reactions. Monitor hematological (Weeks 2, 4, and periodically thereafter) and biochemical tests (Week 4 and periodically thereafter), and TSH (every 12 weeks). Perform periodic eye exams in patients w/ preexisting ophthalmologic disorders. Perform monthly pregnancy tests if on combination therapy w/ ribavirin and for 6 months after discontinuation. Monitor clinical status and hepatic/renal function.

Counseling: Counsel on benefits and risks of therapy. Advise not to use drug in combination w/ ribavirin for pregnant women or men whose female partners are pregnant. Inform of the teratogenic/embryocidal risks w/ ribavirin; instruct to use 2 forms of effective contraception during ribavirin therapy and for 6 months post-therapy. Inform that drug is not known if drug will prevent transmission of HCV/HBV infection to others. Advise that it is not known if therapy will prevent cirrhosis, liver failure or liver cancer in HBV patients. Advise that laboratory evaluations are required prior to therapy, and periodically thereafter. Counsel to avoid alcohol, and avoid driving or operating machinery if dizziness, confusion, somnolence, or fatigue occurs. Instruct to remain well hydrated, and not to switch to another brand of interferon w/o consulting physician. Instruct on the proper preparation and administration, and disposal techniques for therapy.

STORAGE: 2-8°C (36-46°F). Do not leave out of the refrigerator for >24 hrs. Do not freeze or shake. Protect from light.

PENICILLIN VK – penicillin V potassium

RX

Class: Penicillin (PCN)

ADULT DOSAGE

Fusospirochetosis

Mild to Moderately Severe Infections of the Oropharynx:

Usual: 250-500mg q6-8h

Streptococcal Infections

Mild to Moderately Severe URTIs, Scarlet Fever, and Mild Erysipelas:

Usual: 125-250mg q6-8h for 10 days

Respiratory Tract Infections

Mild to Moderately Severe Pneumococcal Infections:

Usual: 250-500mg q6h until patient has been afebrile for at least 2 days

Otitis Media

Mild to Moderately Severe Pneumococcal Infections:

Usual: 250-500mg q6h until patient has been afebrile for at least 2 days

Skin and Skin Structure Infections

Mild Staphylococcal Infections of the Skin and Soft Tissues:

Usual: 250-500mg q6-8h

Culture and sensitivity tests should be performed

Endocarditis

Prophylaxis against bacterial endocarditis in patients w/ congenital heart disease/ rheumatic/other acquired valvular heart disease when undergoing dental procedures or surgical procedures of the upper respiratory tract

Usual: 2g 1 hr before the procedure, then 1g 6 hrs later

Other Indications

Prevention of Recurrence Following Rheumatic Fever and/or Chorea:

Usual: 125-500mg bid on a continuing basis

PEDIATRIC DOSAGE

Otitis Media

Mild to Moderately Severe Pneumococcal Infections:

≥12 Years:

Usual: 250-500mg q6h until patient has been afebrile for at least 2 days

Skin and Skin Structure Infections

Mild Staphylococcal Infections of the Skin and Soft Tissues:

≥12 Years:

Usual: 250-500mg q6h

Culture and sensitivity tests should be performed

Fusospirochetosis

Mild to Moderately Severe Infections of the Oropharynx:

≥12 Years:

Usual: 250-500mg q6-8h

Streptococcal Infections

Mild to Moderately Severe URTIs, Scarlet Fever, and Mild Erysipelas:

≥12 Years:

Usual: 125-250mg q6-8h for 10 days

Respiratory Tract Infections

Mild to Moderately Severe Pneumococcal Infections:

≥12 Years:

Usual: 250-500mg q6h until patient has been afebrile for at least 2 days

Other Indications

≥12 Years:

Prevention of Recurrence Following Rheumatic Fever and/or Chorea:

Usual: 125-500mg bid on a continuing basis

Prophylaxis Against Bacterial Endocarditis:

In patients w/ congenital heart disease/ rheumatic/other acquired valvular heart disease when undergoing dental procedures or surgical procedures of the upper respiratory tract

<60 lbs:

Usual: 1g 1 hr before the procedure, then 500mg 6 hrs later

ADMINISTRATION

Oral route

Directions for Mixing Sol

125mg/mL Sol: Reconstitute 100mL or 200mL bottle size w/ 75mL or 150mL of water, respectively

250mg/5mL Sol: Reconstitute 100mL or 200mL bottle size w/ 75mL or 150mL of water, respectively

Add water in 2 portions, shaking vigorously between each aliquot

HOW SUPPLIED
Sol: 125mg/5mL [100mL, 200mL], 250mg/5mL [100mL, 200mL]; **Tab:** 250mg, 500mg

CONTRAINDICATIONS
Previous hypersensitivity reaction to any penicillin.

WARNINGS/PRECAUTIONS
Not for treatment of severe pneumonia, empyema, bacteremia, pericarditis, meningitis, and arthritis during the acute stage. Necessary dental care should be accomplished in infections involving the gum tissue. Oral penicillin should not be used in patients at particularly high risk for endocarditis (eg, those w/ prosthetic heart valves or surgically constructed systemic pulmonary shunts). Should not be used as adjunctive prophylaxis for genitourinary instrumentation/surgery, lower intestinal tract surgery, sigmoidoscopy, and childbirth. Serious and fatal anaphylactic reactions reported; caution w/ a history of hypersensitivity to PCN, cephalosporins, and/or multiple allergens. Caution w/ history of significant allergies and/or asthma. D/C if an allergic reaction occurs and institute appropriate therapy. *Clostridium difficile*-associated diarrhea (CDAD) reported; d/c therapy if CDAD is suspected/confirmed. Use in the absence of a proven/strongly suspected bacterial infection or a prophylactic indication is unlikely to provide benefit and increases the risk of drug-resistant bacteria. Prolonged use may promote overgrowth of nonsusceptible organisms; take appropriate measures if superinfection develops. Oral route of administration should not be relied upon w/ severe illness, N/V, gastric dilatation, cardiospasm, or intestinal hypermotility. Obtain cultures following completion of treatment for streptococcal infections.

ADVERSE REACTIONS
Epigastric distress, N/V, diarrhea, black hairy tongue, hypersensitivity reactions (skin eruptions, urticaria, other serum-sickness like reactions, laryngeal edema, anaphylaxis), fever, eosinophilia.

PATIENT CONSIDERATIONS

Assessment: Assess for previous hypersensitivity reactions to PCNs/cephalosporins or other allergens, history of asthma, N/V, gastric dilatation, severe illness, cardiospasm, intestinal hypermotility, and pregnancy/nursing status. Obtain cultures and sensitivity tests, especially in suspected staphylococcal infections.

Monitoring: Monitor for signs/symptoms of hypersensitivity reactions, CDAD, superinfections, and other adverse reactions. Obtain cultures following completion of treatment of streptococcal infections.

Counseling: Counsel that therapy only treats bacterial, not viral, infections. Instruct to take ud; inform that skipping doses or not completing the full course of therapy may decrease effectiveness and increase resistance. Inform that diarrhea may occur. Instruct to seek medical attention if watery and bloody stools (w/ or w/o stomach cramps and fever) occur even after ≥2 months of discontinuing therapy.

STORAGE: 20-25°C (68-77°F). (Reconstituted Sol) Store in a refrigerator. Discard any unused portion after 14 days.

PENLAC – ciclopirox RX

Class: Broad-spectrum antifungal

ADULT DOSAGE

Onychomycosis

Mild to Moderate Onychomycosis w/o Lunula Involvement Due to *Trichophyton rubrum*:
Apply evenly over the entire plate qd (preferably at hs or 8 hrs before washing); when nail plate is free of nail bed (eg, onychomycosis), apply to the nail bed, hyponychium, and under the surface of the nail plate

Repeat regimen for up to 48 weeks

PEDIATRIC DOSAGE

Onychomycosis

Mild to Moderate Onychomycosis w/o Lunula Involvement Due to *Trichophyton rubrum*:
≥12 Years:
Apply evenly over the entire plate qd (preferably at hs or 8 hrs before washing); when nail plate is free of nail bed (eg, onychomycosis), apply to the nail bed, hyponychium, and under the surface of the nail plate

Repeat regimen for up to 48 weeks

ADMINISTRATION
Topical route
Sol should not be removed on a daily basis; apply daily over previous coat and remove w/ alcohol every 7 days
Removal of the unattached, infected nail, as frequently as monthly, by a healthcare professional, weekly trimming by the patient, and daily application of the medication are all integral parts of this therapy

HOW SUPPLIED
Sol: 8% [6.6mL]

CONTRAINDICATIONS
Hypersensitivity to any of the components.

WARNINGS/PRECAUTIONS
Not for ophthalmic, oral, or intravaginal use; for use on nails and immediately adjacent skin only. Should be used as a component of a comprehensive management program for onychomycosis and should be used only under medical supervision by a healthcare professional who has special competence in the diagnosis and treatment of nail disorders, including minor nail procedures. D/C and treat appropriately if sensitivity reaction or chemical irritation occurs. Caution with removal of infected nail in patients with a history of insulin-dependent diabetes mellitus (DM) or diabetic neuropathy.

ADVERSE REACTIONS
Periungual erythema, erythema of the proximal nail fold, nail shape change, nail irritation, ingrown toenail, nail discoloration.

DRUG INTERACTIONS
Avoid with systemic antifungal agents for onychomycosis.

PATIENT CONSIDERATIONS

Assessment: Assess for insulin-dependent DM, diabetic neuropathy, drug hypersensitivity, pregnancy/nursing status, and possible drug interactions.

Monitoring: Monitor for sensitivity reactions, chemical irritation, and other adverse reactions. Perform frequent (eg, monthly) removal of unattached infected nails, trimming of onycholytic nail, and filing of any excess horny material.

Counseling: Advise to avoid contact with the eyes and mucous membranes. Instruct to apply medication evenly over entire nail plate and 5mm of surrounding skin. Advise that if possible, the medication should be applied to the nail bed, hyponychium, and the under surface of the nail plate when it is free of the nail bed (eg, onycholysis). Instruct to notify physician if signs of increased irritation at the application site develop. Instruct to inform physician if patient has diabetes or problems with numbness in toes or fingers for consideration of appropriate nail management program. Instruct to file away (with emery board) loose nail material and trim nails as required or ud. Advise to not use nail polish or other nail cosmetic products on the treated nails. Instruct not to use medication near open flame. Inform that it may take up to 48 weeks of daily application of the medication (including monthly professional removal of unattached infected nails) to achieve a clear or almost clear nail.

STORAGE: 15-30°C (59-86°F). Flammable; keep away from heat and flame. Protect from light.

PERCOCET – acetaminophen/oxycodone

CII

Class: Opioid analgesic

Associated with cases of acute liver failure, at times resulting in liver transplant and death. Most cases of liver injury are associated with APAP use at doses >4000mg/day, and often involve >1 APAP-containing product.

OTHER BRAND NAMES
Endocet

ADULT DOSAGE

Moderate to Moderately Severe Pain

2.5mg/325mg Strength:
Usual: 1 or 2 tabs q6h prn
Max: 12 tabs/day

5mg/325mg Strength:
Usual: 1 tab q6h prn
Max: 12 tabs/day

7.5mg/325mg Strength:
Usual: 1 tab q6h prn
Max: 8 tabs/day

10mg/325mg Strength:
Usual: 1 tab q6h prn
Max: 6 tabs/day

If pain is constant, administer at regular intervals on an around-the-clock schedule
Max APAP Dose: 4g/day

PEDIATRIC DOSAGE
Pediatric use may not have been established

DOSING CONSIDERATIONS

Discontinuation

Taper dose gradually in patients treated for more than a few weeks

ADMINISTRATION

Oral route

HOW SUPPLIED

Tab: (Oxycodone/APAP) 2.5mg/325mg, 5mg/325mg*, 7.5mg/325mg, 10mg/325mg *scored

CONTRAINDICATIONS

Known hypersensitivity to oxycodone, acetaminophen, or any other component of the product. **Oxycodone:** Significant respiratory depression (in unmonitored settings or absence of resuscitative equipment), acute or severe bronchial asthma or hypercarbia, suspected/known paralytic ileus.

WARNINGS/PRECAUTIONS

May be abused in a manner similar to other opioid agonists. Respiratory depression may occur; use extreme caution and consider alternative nonopioid analgesics in patients with acute asthma, chronic obstructive pulmonary disorder, cor pulmonale, preexisting respiratory impairment, or in the elderly or debilitated. Respiratory depressant effects may be markedly exaggerated in the presence of head injury, other intracranial lesions or preexisting increase in intracranial pressure. Produces effects on pupillary response and consciousness that may obscure neurologic signs of worsening in patients with head injuries. May cause severe hypotension; caution with circulatory shock. May produce orthostatic hypotension in ambulatory patients. Increased risk of acute liver failure in patients with underlying liver disease. May cause serious skin reactions (eg, acute generalized exanthematous pustulosis, Stevens-Johnson syndrome, toxic epidermal necrolysis), which can be fatal; d/c at the 1st appearance of skin rash or any other sign of hypersensitivity. Hypersensitivity and anaphylaxis reported; d/c immediately if signs/symptoms occur. May obscure diagnosis or clinical course in patients with acute abdominal conditions. Caution with CNS depression, hypothyroidism, Addison's disease, prostatic hypertrophy, urethral stricture, acute alcoholism, delirium tremens, kyphoscoliosis with respiratory depression, myxedema, toxic psychosis, hepatic/renal/pulmonary impairment, and in elderly/debilitated. May aggravate convulsions with convulsive disorders and may induce or aggravate seizures in some clinical settings. Monitor for decreased bowel motility in postoperative patients. May cause spasm of the sphincter of Oddi; caution with biliary tract disease, including acute pancreatitis. May cause increases in serum amylase level. Physical dependence and tolerance may occur. Do not abruptly d/c. Lab test interactions may occur. Not recommended for use during and immediately prior to labor and delivery.

ADVERSE REACTIONS

Lightheadedness, dizziness, drowsiness/sedation, N/V, respiratory depression, apnea, respiratory arrest, circulatory depression, hypotension, shock.

DRUG INTERACTIONS

Oxycodone: May cause severe hypotension after coadministration with drugs that compromise vasomotor tone (eg, phenothiazines). May enhance neuromuscular-blocking action of skeletal muscle relaxants and increase respiratory depression. Additive CNS depression with CNS depressants (eg, general anesthetics, phenothiazines, tranquilizers, alcohol); use in reduced dosages. Coadministration with anticholinergics may produce paralytic ileus. Agonist/antagonist analgesics (eg, pentazocine, nalbuphine, naltrexone, butorphanol) may reduce the analgesic effect or precipitate withdrawal symptoms; use with caution. APAP: Increased risk of acute liver failure with alcohol; hepatotoxicity reported in chronic alcoholics. Increase in glucuronidation, resulting in increased plasma clearance and decreased $T_{1/2}$ with oral contraceptives. Propranolol and probenecid may increase pharmacologic/therapeutic effects. May decrease effects of loop diuretics, lamotrigine, and zidovudine.

PATIENT CONSIDERATIONS

Assessment: Assess for level of pain intensity, type of pain, patient's general condition and medical status, or any other conditions where treatment is contraindicated or cautioned. Assess for drug hypersensitivity, renal/hepatic/pulmonary impairment, pregnancy/nursing status, and possible drug interactions.

Monitoring: Monitor for acute liver failure, respiratory depression, hypotension, skin/hypersensitivity/anaphylactic reactions, convulsions/seizures, decreased bowel motility in postoperative patients, spasm of sphincter of Oddi, increases in serum amylase levels, physical dependence, tolerance, and other adverse reactions.

Counseling: Advise to d/c use and contact physician immediately if signs of allergy develop. Instruct to look for APAP on package labels and not to use >1 APAP-containing product. Instruct to seek medical attention immediately upon ingestion of >4000mg/day of APAP, even if patient is feeling well. Inform about the signs of serious skin reactions. Advise to destroy unused tabs by flushing down the toilet. Inform that drug may impair mental/physical abilities required to perform hazardous tasks. Instruct to avoid alcohol or other CNS depressants. Advise not to adjust dose without consulting physician and not to abruptly d/c if on treatment for more than a few weeks. Inform that drug has potential for abuse and should be protected from theft. Instruct to consult physician if pregnant, planning to become pregnant, or breastfeeding.

STORAGE: 20-25°C (68-77°F).

PERIDEX – chlorhexidine gluconate

RX

Class: Antimicrobial

ADULT DOSAGE

Gingivitis

For Use Between Dental Visits:
Rinse w/ 15mL (undiluted) for 30 sec bid (am and pm) after toothbrushing; initiate directly following a dental prophylaxis

Reevaluate and give a thorough prophylaxis at intervals no longer than 6 months

PEDIATRIC DOSAGE

Pediatric use may not have been established

DOSING CONSIDERATIONS

Oral route

Not intended for ingestion; should be expectorated after rinsing
Instruct to not rinse w/ water or other mouthwashes, brush teeth, or eat immediately after using

ADMINISTRATION

Oral route.

HOW SUPPLIED

Sol: 0.12% [15mL, 118mL, 473mL, 1893mL]

CONTRAINDICATIONS

Hypersensitivity to chlorhexidine gluconate or other formula ingredients.

WARNINGS/PRECAUTIONS

Has not been tested among patients with acute necrotizing ulcerative gingivitis (ANUG). Effect on periodontitis has not been determined. Presence or absence of gingival inflammation following treatment should not be used as a major indicator of underlying periodontitis in patients having coexisting gingivitis and periodontitis. Increase in supragingival calculus reported. Calculus deposits should be removed by a dental prophylaxis at intervals not greater than six months. Anaphylaxis, as well as serious allergic reactions, reported. May stain oral surfaces (eg, tooth surfaces, restorations, dorsum of tongue), and alter taste perception. Caution in patients with anterior facial restorations with rough surfaces or margins.

ADVERSE REACTIONS

Increase in staining of teeth and other oral surfaces, increase in calculus formation, alteration in taste perception, oral irritation, local allergy-type symptoms.

PATIENT CONSIDERATIONS

Assessment: Assess for drug hypersensitivity, ANUG, coexisting periodontitis and gingivitis, anterior facial restorations with rough surfaces or margins, and pregnancy/nursing status.

Monitoring: Monitor for staining of oral surfaces, alteration of taste, anaphylaxis and serious allergic reactions, and other adverse reactions.

Counseling: Advise to use the oral rinse bid (am and pm) for 30 sec after brushing. Instruct to not rinse with water or other mouthwashes, brush teeth, or eat immediately afterward. Instruct to expectorate after rinsing and not to ingest.

STORAGE: 20-25°C (68-77°F); excursions permitted to 15-30°C (59-86°F).

PERPHENAZINE – perphenazine

RX

Class: Piperazine phenothiazine

Increased mortality in elderly patients with dementia-related psychosis reported; most deaths appeared to be either cardiovascular (eg, heart failure, sudden death) or infectious (eg, pneumonia) in nature. Not approved for the treatment of dementia-related psychosis.

ADULT DOSAGE

Schizophrenia

Moderately Disturbed Non-Hospitalized Patients:
Initial: 4-8mg tid
Maint: Reduce to minimum effective dose, as soon as possible

PEDIATRIC DOSAGE

Schizophrenia

≥12 Years:
Moderately Disturbed Non-Hospitalized Patients:
Initial: 4-8mg tid
Maint: Reduce to minimum effective dose, as soon as possible

Hospitalized Patients:
Usual: 8-16mg bid-qid
Max: 64mg/day

Nausea/Vomiting

Severe:
Usual: 8-16mg/day in divided doses; may need 24mg/day

Hospitalized Patients:
Usual: 8-16mg bid-qid
Max: 64mg/day

DOSING CONSIDERATIONS

Elderly

Start at lower end of dosing range

ADMINISTRATION

Oral route

HOW SUPPLIED

Tab: 2mg, 4mg, 8mg, 16mg

CONTRAINDICATIONS

Comatose or greatly obtunded patients; coadministration w/ large doses of CNS depressants (eg, barbiturates, alcohol, narcotics, analgesics, antihistamines); blood dyscrasias, bone marrow depression, or liver damage; hypersensitivity to perphenazine products, their components, or related compounds; subcortical brain damage w/ or w/o hypothalamic damage.

WARNINGS/PRECAUTIONS

Not effective for the management of behavioral complications in patients with mental retardation. Tardive dyskinesia reported; d/c if signs/symptoms appear. Neuroleptic Malignant Syndrome (NMS) reported; d/c therapy and carefully monitor for recurrences if therapy is reintroduced. Hypotension may occur; caution in patients with mitral insufficiency or pheochromocytoma. Rebound HTN may occur with pheochromocytoma. May lower convulsive threshold; caution with alcohol withdrawal and convulsive disorders. Caution with psychic depression. May impair mental/physical abilities. Increased risk of extrapyramidal and/or withdrawal symptoms in neonates if administered during the 3rd trimester. Leukopenia/neutropenia and agranulocytosis have been reported. Caution with preexisting low WBC or history of drug induced leukopenia/neutropenia; monitor CBC frequently and d/c at 1st sign of decline in WBC. Monitor for fever or infection with neutropenia; d/c if severe neutropenia (absolute neutrophil count <1000/mm^3) develops. Increased risk of suicide in depressed patients; avoid access to large quantities of the drug. May elevate prolactin levels; caution with previously detected breast cancer. Antiemetic effect may mask signs of overdosage of other drugs and obscure diagnosis of intestinal obstruction or brain tumor. D/C if significant rise in body temperature occurs; suggestive of intolerance. Monitor renal/hepatic function periodically; d/c therapy if abnormal LFTs/BUN. Caution with renal impairment, respiratory impairment due to acute pulmonary infections, or chronic respiratory disorders (eg, severe asthma, emphysema). Avoid abrupt cessation of high-dose therapy. Possibility of liver damage, corneal and lenticular deposits, and irreversible dyskinesias with long-term use. Avoid sun exposure; photosensitivity reported. Caution in elderly. Not recommended for pediatrics <12 yrs of age.

P

ADVERSE REACTIONS

Extrapyramidal reactions, cerebral edema, seizures, drowsiness, dry mouth, salivation, N/V, diarrhea, anorexia, constipation, urticaria, skin reactions, eczema, postural hypotension, tachycardia.

DRUG INTERACTIONS

See Contraindications. Additive effects with CNS depressants (eg, opiates, analgesics, antihistamines, barbiturates); use with caution and in reduced dosage. Avoid coadministration with alcohol; additive effects, hypotension and increased risk of suicide/overdose may occur. Additive anticholinergic effects with atropine/atropine-like drugs and phosphorous insecticide exposure; use with caution. Cytochrome P450 2D6 inhibitors (TCAs, SSRIs) may increase levels; monitor closely; lower doses may be required. May lower convulsive threshold; increased dosage of anticonvulsants may be required. May reverse effects of epinephrine; do not administer if hypotension develops. Hypotensive phenomena may occur in patients undergoing surgery receiving large doses of the drug; reduce dosage of anesthetics and CNS depressants.

PATIENT CONSIDERATIONS

Assessment: Assess for dementia-related psychosis, mental retardation with behavioral complications, state of consciousness, blood dyscrasia, bone marrow depression, respiratory/hepatic/renal impairment, subcortical brain damage with/without hypothalamic damage, mitral insufficiency, pheochromocytoma, alcohol withdrawal, convulsive disorder, psychic depression, low WBC count, history of drug-induced leukopenia/neutropenia, suicidal ideation, breast cancer, heat/sun exposure, alcohol use, hypersensitivity to drug, pregnancy/nursing status, and possible drug interactions.

Monitoring: Monitor for hypersensitivity reactions, tardive dyskinesia, NMS, hypotension, leukopenia/neutropenia/agranulocytosis, fever, infection, renal function, corneal and lenticular deposits, dyskinesias, and photosensitivity reactions. Monitor for hypotensive phenomena in patients undergoing surgery. Monitor temperature, CBC, LFTs, BUN, and prolactin levels periodically.

Counseling: Inform about benefits and risks of the drug. Advise to avoid hazardous tasks (operating machinery/driving) and sun exposure. Caution about additive effects with alcohol.

STORAGE: 20-25°C (68-77°F); tight, light-resistant container.

PHENOBARBITAL – phenobarbital

CIV

Class: Barbiturate

ADULT DOSAGE

Sedation

Sedative:

Tab (15mg, 30mg, 60mg, 100mg):
30-120mg in 2-3 divided doses

Tab (16.2mg, 32.4mg, 64.8mg, 97.2mg):
30-120mg in 2-3 divided doses; individualize frequency by patient response
Doses >400mg/24 hrs not recommended

Elixir:
30-120mg in 2-3 divided doses; individualize dose based on patient response
Doses >400mg/24 hrs not recommended

Hypnotic:

Tab (15mg, 30mg, 60mg, 100mg):
100-320mg

Tab (16.2mg, 32.4mg, 64.8mg, 97.2mg):
100-200mg

Elixir:
100-200mg

Seizures

Generalized/Partial Seizures:

Tab (16.2mg, 32.4mg, 64.8mg, 97.2mg):
60-200mg/day

Elixir:
60-200mg/day

Anticonvulsant:

Tab (15mg, 30mg, 60mg, 100mg):
50-100mg bid or tid

PEDIATRIC DOSAGE

Sedation

Tab (15mg, 30mg, 60mg, 100mg):
6mg/kg/day in 3 divided doses

Seizures

Generalized/Partial Seizures:

Tab (16.2mg, 32.4mg, 64.8mg, 97.2mg):
3-6mg/kg/day

Elixir:
3-6mg/kg/day

Also used in the treatment/prophylaxis of febrile seizures

Anticonvulsant:

Tab (15mg, 30mg, 60mg, 100mg):
15-50mg bid or tid

DOSING CONSIDERATIONS

Renal Impairment
Reduce dose

Hepatic Impairment
Reduce dose

Elderly
Elderly/Debilitated: Reduce dose

ADMINISTRATION
Oral route

HOW SUPPLIED
Elixir: 20mg/5mL [473mL]; **Tab:** 15mg, 16.2mg*, 30mg*, 32.4mg*, 60mg, 64.8mg*, 97.2mg*, 100mg*
*scored

CONTRAINDICATIONS
Hypersensitivity to barbiturates, marked impairment of liver function or respiratory disease in which dyspnea or obstruction is evident. (Elixir/16.2mg, 32.4mg, 64.8mg, 97.2mg Tab) History of manifest/latent porphyria. (15mg, 30mg, 60mg, 100mg Tab) Personal or familial history of acute intermittent porphyria, known previous addiction to sedative/hypnotic group.

WARNINGS/PRECAUTIONS
Caution w/ borderline hypoadrenal function and history of drug abuse or dependence. Caution in patients who are mentally depressed or w/ suicidal tendencies. Caution when prescribing large amounts to patients w/ a history of emotional disturbances. Elderly or debilitated patients may

react w/ marked excitement, depression, or confusion. (15mg, 30mg, 60mg, 100mg Tab) May increase reaction to painful stimuli in small doses; cannot be relied upon to relieve pain or even produce sedation or sleep in the presence of severe pain if taken alone. Caution w/ decreased liver function. (Elixir/16.2mg, 32.4mg, 64.8mg, 97.2mg Tab) Caution w/ acute or chronic pain; may induce paradoxical excitement or mask important symptoms. Some persons, especially children, may repeatedly produce excitement rather than depression. Avoid in patients showing premonitory signs of hepatic coma. May cause fetal damage. Use during labor may result in respiratory depression in the newborn. Cognitive deficits reported in children taking drug for complicated febrile seizures. May be habit-forming; limit prescription and dispensing to amount required for the interval until the next appointment. Withdraw gradually in patients taking excessive doses over long periods of time.

ADVERSE REACTIONS

Respiratory/CNS depression, apnea, circulatory collapse, hypersensitivity reactions, N/V, headache, somnolence.

DRUG INTERACTIONS

May produce additive depressant effects w/ other CNS depressants (eg, other sedatives/hypnotics, antihistamines, tranquilizers, alcohol). May diminish systemic effects of exogenous corticosteroids (eg, hydrocortisone). Decreased anticoagulant response of oral anticoagulants (eg, warfarin, acenocoumarol, dicumarol, phenprocoumon); determine PT frequently. Dose adjustments of anticoagulants may be required if barbiturates are added to or withdrawn from the dosage regimen. (Elixir/16.2mg, 32.4mg, 64.8mg, 97.2mg Tab) Dose adjustments of corticosteroids may be required if barbiturates are added to or withdrawn from the dosage regimen. May decrease griseofulvin levels; avoid concomitant use. May shorten $T_{1/2}$ of doxycycline for as long as 2 weeks after barbiturate therapy is discontinued; monitor response to doxycycline closely if given concurrently. Monitor phenytoin and barbiturate blood levels frequently when given concurrently. Increased levels w/ sodium valproate and valproic acid; closely monitor barbiturate blood levels and adjust dose as indicated. MAOIs may prolong effects. May decrease effect of estradiol w/ pretreatment or w/ concurrent use. Pregnancy reported w/ oral contraceptives; may suggest use of alternative contraceptive method.

PATIENT CONSIDERATIONS

Assessment: Assess for known barbiturate hypersensitivity, history of porphyria, respiratory disease w/ evident dyspnea or obstruction, hypoadrenal function, suicidal tendencies, history of drug abuse or dependence, mental depression, hepatic impairment, debilitation, pain, pregnancy/nursing status, and possible drug interactions. (Elixir/16.2mg, 32.4mg, 64.8mg, 97.2mg Tab) Assess for renal impairment.

Monitoring: Monitor for marked excitement, depression, and confusion in elderly and debilitated patients. Monitor for tolerance, psychological and physical dependence, and withdrawal symptoms. Monitor PT frequently if used w/ coumarin anticoagulants. (Elixir/16.2mg, 32.4mg, 64.8mg, 97.2mg Tab) Monitor for paradoxical excitement and for masking of symptoms in patients w/ acute/chronic pain. Monitor for cognitive deficits in children w/ complicated febrile seizures. Perform periodic lab evaluation of hematopoietic, renal, and hepatic systems during prolonged therapy.

Counseling: Inform that medication may impair mental/physical abilities required for the performance of potentially hazardous tasks (eg, driving/operating machinery); advise to use caution. (Elixir/16.2mg, 32.4mg, 64.8mg, 97.2mg Tab) Inform of the risk of psychological and/or physical dependence; instruct not to increase dose w/o consulting physician. Instruct to avoid alcohol while on therapy; inform that use of other CNS depressants (eg, alcohol, narcotics, tranquilizers, antihistamines) may result in additional CNS depressant effects.

STORAGE: 20-25°C (68-77°F). (15mg, 30mg, 60mg, 100mg Tab) Protect from light and moisture.

PHOSLYRA – calcium acetate

RX

Class: Phosphate binder

ADULT DOSAGE

Hyperphosphatemia

In Patients w/ ESRD:

Initial: 10mL w/ each meal

Titrate: Increase dose gradually to lower serum phosphorus (P) levels to the target range, every 2-3 weeks until acceptable serum P level is reached, as long as hypercalcemia does not develop

Usual: 15-20mL w/ each meal

PEDIATRIC DOSAGE

Pediatric use may not have been established

DOSING CONSIDERATIONS

Elderly

Start at lower end of dosing range

ADMINISTRATION

Oral route

HOW SUPPLIED

Sol: 667mg (169mg Ca^{2+} base)/5mL [473mL]

CONTRAINDICATIONS

Hypercalcemia.

WARNINGS/PRECAUTIONS

May develop hypercalcemia. If hypercalcemia develops, reduce dose or d/c immediately depending on severity. Chronic hypercalcemia may lead to vascular calcification and other soft-tissue calcification; radiographic evaluation of suspected anatomical regions may be helpful in early detection of soft-tissue calcification. Maintain serum calcium-phosphorus (Ca x P) product $<55mg^2/dL^2$.

ADVERSE REACTIONS

Hypercalcemia, diarrhea, dizziness, edema, weakness.

DRUG INTERACTIONS

Avoid w/ other Ca^{2+} supplements, including Ca^{2+}-based nonprescription antacids. Hypercalcemia may aggravate digitalis toxicity. May induce a laxative effect w/ other products containing maltitol. Fluoroquinolones must be taken at least 2 hrs before or 6 hrs after therapy. Tetracyclines must be taken at least 1 hr before therapy. Levothyroxine must be taken at least 4 hrs before or 4 hrs after therapy. Consider separating the timing of the administration of oral medications where a reduction in the bioavailability of a medication would have a clinically significant effect on its safety/efficacy. Consider monitoring clinical responses or blood levels of concomitant medications that have a narrow therapeutic range.

PATIENT CONSIDERATIONS

Assessment: Assess for hypercalcemia, pregnancy/nursing status, and for possible drug interactions.

Monitoring: Monitor for hypercalcemia, confusion, delirium, stupor, coma, anorexia, N/V, vascular/other soft-tissue calcification, and other adverse reactions. Monitor serum Ca^{2+} twice weekly early in treatment, during dose adjustment, and periodically thereafter. Monitor for serum P levels periodically.

Counseling: Instruct to take w/ meals, adhere to prescribed diets, and to avoid use of Ca^{2+} supplements including nonprescription antacids. Inform about symptoms of hypercalcemia. Advise patients who are taking an oral medication to take the drug 1 hr before or 3 hrs after calcium acetate.

STORAGE: 25°C (77°F); excursions permitted to 15-30°C (59-86°F).

P

PLAQUENIL — hydroxychloroquine sulfate

RX

Class: Quinine derivative

Before prescribing, physicians should be completely familiar w/ the complete prescribing information.

ADULT DOSAGE

Rheumatoid Arthritis

Initial: 400-600mg/day

Some patients may require temporary reduction of initial dose due to troublesome side effects; later (usually from 5-10 days), dose may be gradually increased to optimum response level

Maint: When a good response is obtained (usually in 4-12 weeks), reduce dose by 50% and continue at 200-400mg/day

May resume therapy or continue on an intermittent schedule if relapse occurs after drug withdrawal if there are no ocular contraindications

D/C if objective improvement (eg, reduced joint swelling, increased mobility) does not occur w/in 6 months

PEDIATRIC DOSAGE

Malaria

Suppression:

5mg base/kg weekly; begin 2 weeks prior to exposure

Max: 400mg (310mg base)/dose

If Unable to Begin 2 Weeks Prior to Exposure:

10mg base/kg in 2 divided doses, 6 hrs apart

Continue suppressive therapy for 8 weeks after leaving endemic area

Treatment of Acute Attack:

1st Dose: 10mg base/kg, not exceeding a single dose of 620mg

2nd Dose: 5mg base/kg 6 hrs after 1st dose, not exceeding a single dose of 310mg base

3rd Dose: 5mg base/kg 18 hrs after 2nd dose

4th Dose: 5mg base/kg 24 hrs after 3rd dose

Malaria

Suppression:
400mg on exactly the same day of each week; begin 2 weeks prior to exposure

If Unable to Begin 2 Weeks Prior to Exposure:
800mg in 2 divided doses, 6 hrs apart

Continue suppressive therapy for 8 weeks after leaving endemic area

Treatment of Acute Attack:
800mg, followed by 400mg 6-8 hrs later, then 400mg on each of 2 consecutive days

Alternative Dosing:
800mg single dose, or calculate on the basis of body weight (total of 25mg base/kg administered in 3 days)

Lupus Erythematosus

Chronic Discoid and Systemic:
Initial: 400mg qd-bid for several weeks or months
Prolonged Maint: 200-400mg/day

ADMINISTRATION

Oral route

Rheumatoid Arthritis (RA)

Take w/ a meal or glass of milk.

HOW SUPPLIED

Tab: 200mg (200mg tab=155mg base)

CONTRAINDICATIONS

In the presence of retinal/visual field changes attributable to any 4-aminoquinoline compound, known hypersensitivity to 4-aminoquinoline compounds, for long-term therapy in children.

WARNINGS/PRECAUTIONS

Not effective against chloroquine-resistant strains of *Plasmodium falciparum*. Carefully examine for visual acuity, central visual field, and color vision, including fundoscopy, prior to long-term therapy; repeat exam at least annually. Increased risk of retinal toxicity if recommended daily dose is exceeded sharply. D/C immediately if any visual disturbance occurs and closely observe for possible progression of the abnormality. Retinal and visual disturbances may progress even after discontinuation of therapy. Suicidal behavior reported. Extrapyramidal disorders may occur. May precipitate a severe attack of psoriasis and may exacerbate porphyria; avoid use in these conditions unless benefits outweigh possible hazard. Avoid in pregnancy except in the suppression/treatment of malaria if benefit outweighs the risk. Caution w/ hepatic disease, alcoholism, and G6PD deficiency. Perform periodic blood cell counts w/ prolonged therapy; d/c therapy if any severe blood disorder appears that is not attributable to the disease under treatment. **Lupus Erythematosus/RA:** Irreversible retinal damage reported w/ long-term or high dosage of 4-aminoquinoline therapy. Perform baseline and periodic (every 3 months) ophthalmologic exams w/ prolonged therapy. Examine all patients periodically including testing of knee and ankle reflexes; d/c treatment if muscular weakness occurs. Dermatologic reactions may occur. Caution w/ impaired renal function and/or metabolic acidosis.

ADVERSE REACTIONS

Malaria: Headache, dizziness, GI complaints, nervousness, tremor, retinopathy w/ changes in pigmentation, visual field defects.

Lupus Erythematosus/RA: Irritability, nervousness, emotional changes, headache, dizziness, skeletal muscle palsies, abnormal nerve conduction, blurred vision, corneal changes, abnormal retina pigmentation, pruritus, photosensitivity, N/V, urticaria.

DRUG INTERACTIONS

Caution w/ hepatotoxic drugs. **Lupus Erythematosus/RA:** Caution w/ drugs w/ a significant tendency to produce dermatitis.

PATIENT CONSIDERATIONS

Assessment: Assess for retinal or visual field defects, psoriasis, porphyria, hep[illegible]/renal disease, alcoholism, G6PD deficiency, chloroquine-resistant strains of *P. falciparum*, an[illegible] conditions where treatment is contraindicated or cautioned, pregnancy/nursing status, [illegible]ble drug interactions. Perform baseline ophthalmologic exams w/ prolonged therapy.

Monitoring: Monitor for retinal/visual disturbances, severe psoriasis attack, exacerbation of porphyria, dermatologic reactions, extrapyramidal disorders, and other adverse reactions. Perform periodic (every 3 months) ophthalmologic exams w/ prolonged therapy and monitor CBC w/ differential and platelet count. Periodically test for knee and ankle reflexes in RA patients.

Counseling: Inform about adverse effects and instruct to seek medical attention if any signs/ symptoms develop. Advise about need for periodic follow-up.

STORAGE: Room temperature up to 30°C (86°F).

PLAVIX – clopidogrel bisulfate

RX

Class: Antiplatelet agent

Effectiveness is dependent on activation to an active metabolite via CYP2C19. Poor metabolizers of CYP2C19 w/ acute coronary syndrome (ACS) or undergoing percutaneous coronary intervention treated w/ clopidogrel at recommended doses exhibit higher cardiovascular (CV) event rates than patients w/ normal CYP2C19 function. Tests are available to identify a patient's CYP2C19 genotype; these tests can be used as an aid in determining therapeutic strategy. Consider alternative treatment or treatment strategies in patients identified as CYP2C19 poor metabolizers.

ADULT DOSAGE

Acute Coronary Syndrome

Unstable Angina/Non-ST-Elevation MI:
LD: 300mg
Maint: 75mg qd. Initiate aspirin (ASA) (75-325mg qd) and continue in combination w/ clopidogrel

ST-Elevation MI:
75mg qd w/ ASA (75-325mg qd), w/ or w/o thrombolytics
May initiate w/ or w/o a LD

Recent Myocardial Infarction/Recent Stroke/ Peripheral Arterial Disease

75mg qd

PEDIATRIC DOSAGE

Pediatric use may not have been established

ADMINISTRATION

Oral route

May be administered w/ or w/o food.

HOW SUPPLIED

Tab: 75mg, 300mg

CONTRAINDICATIONS

Active pathological bleeding (eg, peptic ulcer, intracranial hemorrhage), hypersensitivity (eg, anaphylaxis) to clopidogrel or any component of the product.

WARNINGS/PRECAUTIONS

Increases the risk of bleeding; d/c 5 days prior to surgery if an antiplatelet effect is not desired. Avoid lapses in therapy; if therapy must be temporarily discontinued, restart as soon as possible. Premature discontinuation may increase risk of CV events. Thrombotic thrombocytopenic purpura (TTP) reported. Hypersensitivity (eg, rash, angioedema, hematologic reaction) reported, including in patients w/ a history of hypersensitivity or hematologic reaction to other thienopyridines.

ADVERSE REACTIONS

Bleeding.

DRUG INTERACTIONS

Reduced antiplatelet activity w/ omeprazole or esomeprazole; avoid concomitant use, or consider using another acid-reducing agent w/ minimal or no CYP2C19 inhibitory effect on the formation of clopidogrel active metabolite. Certain CYP2C19 inhibitors may reduce platelet inhibition. NSAIDs, warfarin, SSRIs, SNRIs, and ASA may increase risk of bleeding.

PATIENT CONSIDERATIONS

Assessment: Assess for active pathological bleeding, hypersensitivity to drug or another thienopyridine, CYP2C19 genotype, pregnancy/nursing status, and possible drug interactions. Assess use in patients at risk for increased bleeding (eg, undergoing surgery).

Monitoring: Monitor for bleeding, TTP, hypersensitivity, and other adverse reactions.

Counseling: Inform about the benefits and risks of treatment. Instruct to take exactly as prescribed and not to d/c w/o consulting the prescribing physician. Inform that they will bruise and bleed more easily and that bleeding will take longer than usual to stop. Advise to report any unanticipated, prolonged, or excessive bleeding, or blood in stool or urine. Instruct to seek prompt medical

P

attention if unexplained fever, weakness, extreme skin paleness, purple skin patches, yellowing of the skin or eyes, or neurological changes occur. Instruct to notify physician or dentist about therapy before scheduling any invasive procedure. Advise to inform physician of all medications, including OTC medications and dietary supplements, they are taking or planning to take.

STORAGE: 25°C (77°F); excursions permitted to 15-30°C (59-86°F).

PLEGRIDY — peginterferon beta-1a

RX

Class: Biological response modifier

ADULT DOSAGE

Multiple Sclerosis

Treatment of Relapsing Forms:

Day 1: 63mcg SQ

Day 15: 94mcg SQ

On Day 29 and Thereafter: 125mcg SQ every 14 days

Premedication

Prophylactic and concurrent use of analgesics and/or antipyretics may prevent or ameliorate flu-like symptoms sometimes experienced during treatment

PEDIATRIC DOSAGE

Pediatric use may not have been established

ADMINISTRATION

SQ route

Rotate inj sites; usual sites are abdomen, back of the upper arm, and thigh.

Prefilled pens and syringes are for a single dose only; discard after use.

HOW SUPPLIED

Inj: 125mcg/0.5mL [prefilled pen, prefilled syringe]; (Starter Pack) 63mcg/0.5mL, 94mcg/0.5mL [prefilled pen, prefilled syringe]

CONTRAINDICATIONS

History of hypersensitivity to natural or recombinant interferon beta or peginterferon, or any other component of the formulation.

WARNINGS/PRECAUTIONS

Elevations in hepatic enzymes and hepatic injury reported. Depression and suicidal ideation reported; consider discontinuation if depression or other severe psychiatric symptoms develop. Seizures reported. Anaphylaxis and other serious allergic reactions (eg, angioedema, urticaria) reported; d/c if a serious allergic reaction occurs. Inj-site reactions reported; decision to d/c therapy following necrosis at a single inj site should be based on the extent of the necrosis. If therapy is continued after inj-site necrosis has occurred, avoid administration near the affected area until it is fully healed; if multiple lesions occur, d/c until healing occurs. Cardiovascular (CV) events reported; monitor patients w/ significant cardiac disease for worsening of their cardiac condition during initiation and continuation of treatment. Decreased peripheral blood counts reported; monitor for infections, bleeding, and symptoms of anemia. Cases of thrombotic microangiopathy (TMA) (eg, thrombotic thrombocytopenia purpura, hemolytic uremic syndrome), some fatal, reported w/ interferon β products; d/c and manage if TMA occurs. Autoimmune disorders reported; consider discontinuation if a new autoimmune disorder develops. Monitor for adverse reactions due to increased drug exposure in patients w/ severe renal impairment.

ADVERSE REACTIONS

Inj-site erythema/pain/pruritus, influenza-like illness, pyrexia, headache, myalgia, chills, asthenia, arthralgia, N/V, ALT/AST increased.

PATIENT CONSIDERATIONS

Assessment: Assess for seizure disorder, cardiac disease, myelosuppression, renal/hepatic impairment, history of hypersensitivity to drug, and pregnancy/nursing status.

Monitoring: Monitor for signs/symptoms of hepatic injury; depression, suicidal ideation, or other severe psychiatric symptoms; seizures; serious allergic reactions; inj-site reactions/necrosis; CV events or worsening of cardiac condition; TMA, autoimmune disorders; and other adverse reactions. Monitor for infections, bleeding, and symptoms of anemia. Monitor CBCs, differential WBC count, and platelet counts; patients w/ myelosuppression may require more intensive monitoring.

Counseling: Advise not to change the dose or schedule of administration w/o medical consultation. Instruct on how to self-inject therapy and inform of the proper procedures to follow. Advise to rotate areas of inj w/ each dose, and not to inject into an area of the body where the skin is irritated, reddened, bruised, infected, or scarred in any way. Instruct to check the inj site after 2 hrs for redness, swelling, and tenderness, and to contact physician if a skin reaction occurs and does not clear up in a few days. Advise to inform physician if pregnant/breastfeeding. Inform of the symptoms of hepatic dysfunction, depression, suicidal ideation, seizures, and worsening cardiac condition, and instruct to immediately report any of these symptoms to physician. Instruct to seek immediate medical attention if symptoms of allergic reactions and anaphylaxis occur. Advise that inj-site reactions may occur and to promptly report any signs of necrosis at inj site. Inform that flu-like symptoms are common following initiation of therapy.

STORAGE: 2-8°C (36-46°F). Protect from light. Do not freeze; discard if frozen. Once removed from the refrigerator, allow to warm to room temperature (about 30 min) prior to inj; do not use external heat sources (eg, hot water) to warm the product. If refrigeration is unavailable, may store at 2-25°C (36-77°F) for up to 30 days; protect from light. May be removed from, and returned to, a refrigerator if necessary. The total combined time out of refrigeration, w/in a temperature range of 2-25°C (36-77°F), should not exceed 30 days.

PLETAL – cilostazol

RX

Class: Phosphodiesterase-3 (PDE-3) inhibitor

Contraindicated in patients w/ heart failure (HF) of any severity. Cilostazol and several of its metabolites are PDE3 inhibitors; several drugs w/ this pharmacologic effect have caused decreased survival compared to placebo in patients w/ class III-IV HF.

ADULT DOSAGE

Intermittent Claudication

Reduction of Symptoms:

100mg bid

D/C if symptoms have not improved after 3 months

PEDIATRIC DOSAGE

Pediatric use may not have been established

DOSING CONSIDERATIONS

Concomitant Medications

Strong or Moderate CYP3A4 or CYP2C19 Inhibitors: Reduce dose to 50mg bid

ADMINISTRATION

Oral route

Take at least 1/2 hr before or 2 hrs after breakfast and dinner.

HOW SUPPLIED

Tab: 50mg, 100mg

CONTRAINDICATIONS

HF of any severity, hypersensitivity (eg, anaphylaxis, angioedema) to cilostazol or any components of the product.

WARNINGS/PRECAUTIONS

May induce tachycardia, palpitation, tachyarrhythmia, or hypotension; patients w/ a history of ischemic heart disease may be at risk for exacerbations of angina pectoris or MI. Cases of thrombocytopenia or leukopenia progressing to agranulocytosis reported. Avoid in patients w/ hemostatic disorders or active pathologic bleeding.

ADVERSE REACTIONS

Headache, diarrhea, abnormal stools, palpitation, dizziness, pharyngitis, infection, peripheral edema, rhinitis, dyspepsia, abdominal pain, tachycardia.

DRUG INTERACTIONS

See Dosing Considerations. Coadministration of strong (eg, ketoconazole) and moderate (eg, erythromycin, diltiazem, grapefruit juice) CYP3A4 inhibitors may increase exposure. Coadministration w/ CYP2C19 inhibitors (eg, ticlopidine, fluconazole, omeprazole) may increase exposure of active metabolites.

PATIENT CONSIDERATIONS

Assessment: Assess for hypersensitivity to drug, HF of any severity, hemostatic disorders, active pathologic bleeding, history of ischemic heart disease, renal/hepatic impairment, pregnancy/nursing status, and possible drug interactions.

Monitoring: Monitor for tachycardia, palpitation, tachyarrhythmia, hypotension, and other adverse reactions. Periodically monitor platelets and WBC counts.

Counseling: Advise to take at least 1/2 hr ac or 2 hrs pc. Instruct to discuss w/ physician before taking any other medication. Inform that the beneficial effects of therapy may not be immediate;

P

although benefit may be experienced in 2-4 weeks after initiation of therapy, advise that treatment for up to 12 weeks may be required before a beneficial effect is experienced. Instruct to d/c if symptoms do not improve after 3 months.

STORAGE: 25°C (77°F); excursions permitted to 15-30°C (59-86°F).

PNEUMOVAX 23 – pneumococcal vaccine polyvalent RX

Class: Vaccine

ADULT DOSAGE

Prevention of Pneumococcal Disease

Active immunization against serotypes 1, 2, 3, 4, 5, 6B, 7F, 8, 9N, 9V, 10A, 11A, 12F, 14, 15B, 17F, 18C, 19F, 19A, 20, 22F, 23F, and 33F

≥50 Years:
Single 0.5mL dose

PEDIATRIC DOSAGE

Prevention of Pneumococcal Disease

Active immunization against serotypes 1, 2, 3, 4, 5, 6B, 7F, 8, 9N, 9V, 10A, 11A, 12F, 14, 15B, 17F, 18C, 19F, 19A, 20, 22F, 23F, and 33F

≥2 Years and at Increased Risk for Pneumococcal Disease:
Single 0.5mL dose

ADMINISTRATION

IM/SQ route

Administer into the deltoid muscle or lateral mid-thigh
Do not mix w/ other vaccines in the same syringe or vial

Single-Dose and Multidose Vials
Withdraw 0.5mL from the vial using a sterile needle and syringe

Single-Dose, Prefilled Syringe
Package does not contain a needle; attach a sterile needle to prefilled syringe by twisting in a clockwise direction until the needle fits securely on the syringe

Revaccination
Advisory Committee on Immunization Practices has recommendations for revaccination against pneumococcal disease for persons at high risk who were previously vaccinated w/ Pneumovax 23; routine revaccination of immunocompetent persons previously vaccinated w/ a 23-valent vaccine is not recommended

HOW SUPPLIED

Inj: 0.5mL [prefilled syringe, single-dose vial, multidose vial]

CONTRAINDICATIONS

History of anaphylactic/anaphylactoid or severe allergic reaction to any component of the vaccine.

WARNINGS/PRECAUTIONS

Do not inject intravascularly or intradermally. Defer vaccination in patients with moderate or severe acute illness. Caution with severely compromised cardiovascular (CV) and/or pulmonary function in whom a systemic reaction would pose a significant risk. Does not replace the need for antibiotic prophylaxis (eg, PCN) against pneumococcal infection; antibiotic prophylaxis should not be discontinued after vaccination in patients who require antibiotic prophylaxis. Response to vaccine may be diminished in immunocompromised individuals. May not be effective in preventing pneumococcal meningitis in patients with chronic CSF leakage resulting from congenital lesions, skull fractures, or neurosurgical procedures. Will not prevent disease caused by capsular types of pneumococcus other than those contained in the vaccine. Caution in elderly.

ADVERSE REACTIONS

Local inj-site reactions (eg, pain, soreness, tenderness, swelling, induration, erythema), asthenia, fatigue, myalgia, headache.

DRUG INTERACTIONS

Persons receiving immunosuppressive therapies may have a diminished immune response to the vaccine. Reduced immune response to zoster vaccine live reported; consider separation of vaccinations by at least 4 weeks.

PATIENT CONSIDERATIONS

Assessment: Assess for moderate/severe acute illness, severely compromised CV and/or pulmonary function, chronic CSF leakage, vaccination history, history of anaphylactic/anaphylactoid or severe allergic reaction to any component of the vaccine, immunocompromised conditions, pregnancy/nursing status, and for possible drug interactions.

Monitoring: Monitor for hypersensitivity reactions and other adverse reactions.

Counseling: Inform of potential benefits/risks of vaccination. Inform that the vaccine may not offer 100% protection from pneumococcal infection. Instruct to report any serious adverse reactions to physician.

STORAGE: 2-8°C (36-46°F).

POLYTRIM – polymyxin B sulfate/trimethoprim

RX

Class: Antibiotic/dihydrofolate reductase inhibitor

ADULT DOSAGE

Ocular Infections

Mild-Moderate Surface Bacterial Infections:
(eg, blepharoconjunctivitis, acute bacterial conjunctivitis)

Instill 1 drop in affected eye(s) q3h for 7-10 days
Max: 6 doses/day

PEDIATRIC DOSAGE

Ocular Infections

Mild-Moderate Surface Bacterial Infections:
(eg, blepharoconjunctivitis, acute bacterial conjunctivitis)

≥2 Months of Age:
Instill 1 drop in affected eye(s) q3h for 7-10 days
Max: 6 doses/day

ADMINISTRATION
Ocular route

HOW SUPPLIED
Sol: (Trimethoprim-Polymyxin B) 1mg-10,000 U/mL [10mL]

CONTRAINDICATIONS
Known hypersensitivity to any of the components.

WARNINGS/PRECAUTIONS
Do not inject into eye. Not indicated for the prophylaxis or treatment of ophthalmia neonatorum.

ADVERSE REACTIONS
Local irritation, lid edema, itching, increased redness, tearing, burning, stinging, circumocular rash, superinfection (prolonged use).

PATIENT CONSIDERATIONS

Assessment: Assess proper diagnosis of causative organisms, that medication is not being used as treatment for patients with ophthalmia neonatorum, and use in pregnant/nursing females.

Monitoring: Monitor for signs/symptoms of hypersensitivity reactions (eg, lid edema, itching, increased redness, tearing, and circumocular rash). For patients on prolonged therapy, monitor for overgrowth of nonsusceptible organisms (eg, fungi) and for the development of a superinfection.

Counseling: Advise to avoid contaminating applicator tip with material from eye, fingers, or other sources. Instruct to d/c therapy if redness, irritation, swelling, or pain persists or worsens. Advise not to wear contact lenses if there are signs/symptoms of ocular bacterial infections.

STORAGE: 15-25°C (59-77°F). Protect from light.

PORTRAZZA – necitumumab

RX

Class: Monoclonal antibody/EGFR blocker

Cardiopulmonary arrest and/or sudden death reported. Closely monitor serum electrolytes, including serum Mg^+, K^+, and Ca^+ w/ aggressive replacement when warranted during and after administration. Hypomagnesemia reported; monitor patients for hypomagnesemia, hypocalcemia, and hypokalemia prior to each dose during treatment and for at least 8 weeks following completion. Withhold for Grade 3 or 4 electrolyte abnormalities. Replete electrolytes as medically appropriate.

ADULT DOSAGE

Metastatic Squamous Non-Small Cell Lung Cancer

1st-Line Treatment in Combination w/ Gemcitabine and Cisplatin:
800mg IV over 60 min on Days 1 and 8 of each 3-week cycle prior to gemcitabine and cisplatin infusion

Continue until disease progression or unacceptable toxicity

PEDIATRIC DOSAGE

Pediatric use may not have been established

Premedication

Previous Grade 1 or 2 Infusion-Related Reaction (IRR):
Premedicate w/ diphenhydramine hydrochloride (or equivalent) prior to all subsequent infusions

2nd Grade 1 or 2 Occurrence of IRR:
Premedicate for all subsequent infusions, w/ diphenhydramine hydrochloride (or equivalent), acetaminophen (or equivalent), and dexamethasone (or equivalent) prior to each infusion

DOSING CONSIDERATIONS

Adverse Reactions

IRR:
Grade 1: Reduce the infusion rate by 50%
Grade 2: Stop the infusion until signs and symptoms have resolved to Grade 0 or 1; resume at 50% reduced rate for all subsequent infusions
Grade 3 or 4: Permanently d/c

Dermatologic Toxicity:
Grade 3 Rash or Acneiform Rash: Withhold until symptoms resolve to Grade ≤2, then resume at reduced dose of 400mg for at least 1 treatment cycle. If symptoms do not worsen, may increase dose to 600mg and 800mg in subsequent cycles

Permanently D/C If:
- Grade 3 rash or acneiform rash does not resolve to Grade ≤2 w/in 6 weeks
- Reactions worsen or become intolerable at a dose of 400mg
- Patient experiences Grade 3 skin induration/fibrosis
- Patient experiences Grade 4 dermatologic toxicity

ADMINISTRATION

IV route

Administer via infusion pump over 60 min through a separate infusion line; flush the line w/ 0.9% NaCl inj at the end of infusion.

Preparation for Administration

1. Dilute the required volume of necitumumab w/ 0.9% NaCl inj, in an IV infusion container to a final volume of 250mL; do not use sol containing dextrose.
2. Gently invert the container to ensure adequate mixing.
3. Do not freeze or shake the infusion sol. Do not dilute w/ other sol or co-infuse w/ other electrolytes or medication.
4. Store diluted infusion sol for no >24 hrs at 2-8°C (36-46°F), or no >4 hrs at room temperature (up to 25°C [77°F]).
5. Discard vial w/ any unused portion.

HOW SUPPLIED

Inj: 800mg/50mL

WARNINGS/PRECAUTIONS

See Dosing Considerations. Once electrolyte abnormalities and hypomagnesemia improve to Grade ≤2, subsequent cycles may be administered. Venous thromboembolic events (VTEs) and arterial thromboembolic events (ATEs) reported w/ combination treatment; d/c in patients w/ serious/life-threatening VTE or ATE. The most common ATEs were cerebral stroke, ischemia, and MI. Dermatologic toxicities, including rash, dermatitis acneiform, acne, dry skin, pruritus, generalized rash, skin fissures, maculopapular rash, and erythema reported; limit sun exposure. IRR reported; d/c for serious or life-threatening IRR. Not indicated for the treatment of patients w/ non-squamous non-small cell lung cancer. May cause fetal harm.

ADVERSE REACTIONS

Rash, vomiting, diarrhea, dermatitis acneiform.

PATIENT CONSIDERATIONS

Assessment: Assess for presence or history of cardiopulmonary and dermatologic disease, pregnancy/nursing status, and for possible drug interactions. Obtain serum electrolyte levels (Mg^{2+}, K^+, Ca^{2+}).

Monitoring: Monitor for signs/symptoms of cardiopulmonary arrest, dermatologic toxicities, IRR, VTEs/ATEs, and other adverse reactions. Monitor electrolytes (eg, hypomagnesemia, hypokalemia, hypocalcemia) periodically during and for up to 8 weeks after completion of therapy.

Counseling: Advise patients of risk of decreased blood levels of Mg^{2+}, K^+, and Ca^{2+} and instruct to take medicines to replace the electrolytes exactly as advised. Inform of the increased risk of VTEs/

ATEs. Instruct to minimize sun exposure w/ protective clothing and use of sunscreen. Advise to report if signs/symptoms of an infusion reaction develop. Instruct to notify physician if pregnant or nursing; inform of the potential risk to a fetus and instruct to not breastfeed during treatment and for 3 months following final dose. Advise of the need for adequate contraception in females during therapy and for 3 months after the last dose.

STORAGE: 2-8°C (36-46°F). Protect from light. Do not freeze or shake the vial.

PRADAXA — dabigatran etexilate mesylate

RX

Class: Direct thrombin inhibitor (DTI)

Premature discontinuation of therapy increases the risk of thrombotic events. If therapy is discontinued for a reason other than pathological bleeding or completion of a course of therapy, consider coverage w/ another anticoagulant. Epidural or spinal hematomas may occur in patients treated w/ dabigatran who are receiving neuraxial anesthesia or undergoing spinal puncture; may result in long-term or permanent paralysis. Consider these risks when scheduling for spinal procedures. Increased risk of developing epidural or spinal hematomas w/ the use of indwelling epidural catheters, concomitant use of other drugs that affect hemostasis (eg, NSAIDs, platelet inhibitors, other anticoagulants), history of traumatic or repeated epidural or spinal punctures, history of spinal deformity or spinal surgery, or unknown optimal timing between the administration of therapy and neuraxial procedures. Monitor frequently for signs/symptoms of neurological impairment; if noted, urgent treatment is necessary. Consider benefits and risks before neuraxial intervention in patients anticoagulated or to be anticoagulated.

ADULT DOSAGE

Reduce Risk of Stroke and Systemic Embolism in Nonvalvular Atrial Fibrillation

150mg bid

Deep Vein Thrombosis/Pulmonary Embolism

Treatment in Patients Treated w/ a Parenteral Anticoagulant for 5-10 Days:
150mg bid

Reduce Risk of Recurrent Deep Vein Thrombosis (DVT)/Pulmonary Embolism (PE) in Previously Treated Patients:
150mg bid

Prophylaxis of DVT and PE Following Hip Replacement Surgery:
110mg taken 1-4 hrs after surgery and after hemostasis has been achieved, then 220mg taken qd for 28-35 days; if therapy is not started on the day of surgery, after hemostasis has been achieved, initiate treatment w/ 220mg qd

Conversions

Conversion from Warfarin:
D/C warfarin and start therapy when INR <2.0

Conversion to Warfarin:
CrCl ≥50mL/min: Start warfarin 3 days before discontinuing therapy
CrCl 30-50mL/min: Start warfarin 2 days before discontinuing therapy
CrCl 15-30mL/min: Start warfarin 1 day before discontinuing therapy
CrCl <15mL/min: No recommendations can be made

Conversion from Parenteral Anticoagulants:
Start 0-2 hrs before the time that the next dose of the parenteral drug was to have been administered, or at time of discontinuation of a continuously administered parenteral drug (eg, IV unfractionated heparin)

Conversion to Parenteral Anticoagulant:
CrCl ≥30mL/min: Wait 12 hrs after last dose before initiating treatment w/ a parenteral anticoagulant

PEDIATRIC DOSAGE

Pediatric use may not have been established

CrCl <30mL/min: Wait 24 hrs after last dose before initiating treatment w/ a parenteral anticoagulant

Missed Dose

Take missed dose as soon as possible on the same day; skip the missed dose if it cannot be taken at least 6 hrs before the next scheduled dose

DOSING CONSIDERATIONS

Concomitant Medications

Reduction in Risk of Stroke and Systemic Embolism in Nonvalvular A-Fib:
CrCl 30-50mL/min w/ Concomitant P-gp Inhibitors: Reduce dose to 75mg bid if given w/ P-gp inhibitors dronedarone or systemic ketoconazole
CrCl <30mL/min w/ Concomitant P-gp Inhibitors: Avoid coadministration

Treatment and Reduction in Risk of Recurrent DVT/PE:
CrCl <50mL/min w/ Concomitant P-gp Inhibitors: Avoid coadministration

Prophylaxis of DVT and PE Following Hip Replacement Surgery:
CrCl <50mL/min w/ Concomitant P-gp Inhibitors: Avoid coadministration

Renal Impairment

Reduction in Risk of Stroke and Systemic Embolism in Nonvalvular A-Fib:
CrCl 15-30mL/min: 75mg bid
CrCl <15mL/min or on Dialysis: Dosing recommendations cannot be provided

Treatment and Reduction in the Risk of Recurrent DVT/PE:
CrCl ≤30mL/min or on Dialysis: Dosing recommendations cannot be provided

Prophylaxis of DVT and PE Following Hip Replacement Surgery:
CrCl ≤30mL/min or on Dialysis: Dosing recommendations cannot be provided

Other Important Considerations

Surgery/Other Interventions:
CrCl ≥50mL/min: D/C 1-2 days before invasive or surgical procedures, if possible
CrCl <50mL/min: D/C 3-5 days before invasive or surgical procedures, if possible

Consider longer times for patients undergoing major surgery, spinal puncture, or placement of spinal/epidural catheter or port.
Use a specific reversal agent (idarucizumab) in case of emergency surgery or urgent procedures when reversal of dabigatran is needed; refer to idarucizumab PI for additional information. Restart dabigatran as soon as medically appropriate.

ADMINISTRATION

Oral route

Take w/ or w/o food w/ a full glass of water.
Swallow cap whole.

P

HOW SUPPLIED

Cap: 75mg, 110mg, 150mg

CONTRAINDICATIONS

Active pathological bleeding, mechanical prosthetic heart valve, serious hypersensitivity reaction to dabigatran (eg, anaphylactic reaction or anaphylactic shock).

WARNINGS/PRECAUTIONS

Renal impairment may increase anticoagulant activity and $T_{1/2}$. D/C therapy in patients who develop acute renal failure and consider alternative anticoagulant therapy. Increases risk of bleeding and may cause significant and, sometimes, fatal bleeding; promptly evaluate for any signs/symptoms of blood loss. D/C therapy in patients w/ active pathological bleeding. Consider administration of platelet concentrates in cases where thrombocytopenia is present or long-acting antiplatelet drugs have been used. Use for the prophylaxis of thromboembolic events in patients w/ A-fib in the setting of other forms of valvular heart disease (including the presence of a bioprosthetic heart valve) is not recommended.

ADVERSE REACTIONS

GI reactions (eg, dyspepsia, gastritis-like symptoms), bleeding events.

DRUG INTERACTIONS

See Boxed Warning and Dosing Considerations. **Reduction of Risk of Stroke and Systemic Embolism in Non-valvular A-Fib:** P-gp inducers (eg, rifampin) may reduce exposure to dabigatran; should generally avoid concomitant use. Concomitant use w/ P-gp inhibitors in patients w/ renal impairment may produce increased exposure of dabigatran compared to that seen with either factor alone. **Prophylaxis of DVT and PE Following Hip Replacement Surgery:** May be helpful to separate timing of administration of dabigatran and the P-gp inhibitor by several hours, in patients w/ CrCl ≥50mL/min who have concomitant administration of P-gp inhibitors (eg, dronedarone, systemic ketoconazole).

PATIENT CONSIDERATIONS

Assessment: Assess for history of serious hypersensitivity reaction to drug, active pathological bleeding, mechanical prosthetic heart valve, A-fib in the setting of other forms of valvular heart disease, risk factors for bleeding and epidural or spinal hematomas, renal impairment, pregnancy/nursing status, and possible drug interactions.

Monitoring: Monitor for bleeding, GI adverse reactions, hypersensitivity reactions, and other adverse events. Periodically monitor renal function as clinically indicated. When necessary, monitor anticoagulant activity by using activated PTT or ecarin clotting time, and not INR. Monitor for signs/symptoms of neurological impairment (eg, midline back pain, sensory/motor deficits [numbness, tingling, weakness in lower limbs], bowel/bladder dysfunction) frequently in patients receiving neuraxial anesthesia or undergoing spinal puncture.

Counseling: Instruct to take exactly as prescribed and not to d/c w/o talking to physician. Instruct to keep drug in original bottle to protect from moisture and not to put it in pill boxes/organizers. When >1 bottle is dispensed, instruct to open only 1 bottle at a time. Instruct to remove only 1 cap from the opened bottle at the time of use and to immediately and tightly close bottle. Inform that bleeding may be longer and occur more easily. Instruct to call physician if any signs/symptoms of bleeding, dyspepsia, or gastritis occur. Advise patients who have had neuraxial anesthesia or spinal puncture to watch for signs and symptoms of spinal/epidural hematoma, particularly if concomitantly taking NSAIDs or platelet inhibitors; instruct to contact physician immediately if symptoms occur. Instruct to inform physician of intake of dabigatran before any invasive procedure (including dental procedures) is scheduled. Advise patients to list all prescription/OTC medications or dietary supplements they may be taking or planning to take. Instruct to inform healthcare provider if planning to undergo surgery or already had surgery to place a prosthetic heart valve.

STORAGE: 25°C (77°F); excursions permitted to 15-30°C (59-86°F). Store in original package to protect from moisture. Once bottle is opened, use w/in 4 months; keep tightly closed.

PRALUENT – alirocumab

RX

Class: Proprotein Convertase Subtilisin Kexin Type 9 (PCSK9) Inhibitor

ADULT DOSAGE

Primary Hyperlipidemia

Adjunct to diet and maximally tolerated statin therapy for the treatment of patients w/ heterozygous familial hypercholesterolemia or clinical atherosclerotic cardiovascular disease, who require additional lowering of LDL-C

Initial: 75mg SQ once every 2 weeks
Titrate: May increase to max dose if LDL-C response is inadequate
Max: 150mg every 2 weeks

Missed Dose

If a dose is missed, administer the inj w/in 7 days from the missed dose and then resume the original schedule. If the missed dose is not administered w/in 7 days, wait until the next dose on the original schedule

PEDIATRIC DOSAGE

Pediatric use may not have been established

P

ADMINISTRATION

SQ route

Allow alirocumab to warm to room temperature for 30-40 min prior to use; use as soon as possible after it has warmed up. Do not use if it has been at room temperature for ≥24 hrs.
Administer in the thigh, abdomen, or upper arm; rotate inj site w/ each inj.
Do not inject into areas of active skin disease or injury (eg, sunburns, skin rashes, inflammation, skin infections).
Do not coadminister w/ other injectable drugs at the same inj site.

HOW SUPPLIED

Inj: 75mg/mL, 150mg/mL [prefilled pen, prefilled syringe]

CONTRAINDICATIONS

History of a serious hypersensitivity reaction to alirocumab.

WARNINGS/PRECAUTIONS
Hypersensitivity reactions, including some serious events (eg, hypersensitivity vasculitis and hypersensitivity reactions requiring hospitalization), reported; if signs/symptoms of serious allergic reactions occur, d/c treatment, treat according to the standard of care, and monitor until signs/symptoms resolve.

ADVERSE REACTIONS
Nasopharyngitis, inj-site reactions, influenza, UTI, diarrhea, bronchitis, myalgia, muscle spasms, sinusitis.

PATIENT CONSIDERATIONS

Assessment: Assess for drug hypersensitivity and pregnancy/nursing status. Obtain baseline lipid levels.

Monitoring: Monitor for hypersensitivity reactions. Measure LDL-C levels w/in 4-8 weeks of initiating or titrating therapy.

Counseling: Instruct on proper inj technique, including aseptic technique, and how to use the prefilled pen/syringe correctly; inform that it may take up to 20 sec to inject alirocumab. Caution that the prefilled pen/syringe must not be reused and inform about the proper technique of disposal in a puncture-resistant container. Advise to d/c therapy and seek prompt medical attention if any signs/symptoms of serious allergic reactions occur.

STORAGE: 2-8°C (36-46°F). Store in the outer carton in order to protect from light. Do not freeze. Do not expose to extreme heat. Do not shake.

PRANDIMET — metformin hydrochloride/repaglinide

RX

Class: Biguanide/meglitinide

Lactic acidosis may occur due to metformin accumulation; risk increases with conditions such as sepsis, dehydration, excess alcohol intake, hepatic impairment, renal impairment, and acute CHF. If acidosis is suspected, d/c and hospitalize patient immediately.

ADULT DOSAGE

Type 2 Diabetes Mellitus

In patients who are already treated w/ a meglitinide and metformin or who have inadequate glycemic control on a meglitinide alone or metformin alone

May administer bid-tid

Inadequately Controlled w/ Metformin Monotherapy:
Initial: 1mg/500mg bid w/ meals
Titrate: Gradually escalate dose based on glycemic response

Inadequately Controlled w/ Meglitinide Monotherapy:
Initial: 500mg of metformin component bid
Titrate: Gradually escalate dose based on glycemic response

Currently Using Repaglinide and Metformin Concomitantly:
Initial: Initiate at a dose similar to, but not exceeding, doses of current repaglinide and metformin therapy
Titrate: Increase as necessary to achieve targeted glycemic control

Max: (10mg/2500mg)/day or (4mg/1000mg)/meal

PEDIATRIC DOSAGE

Pediatric use may not have been established

ADMINISTRATION
Oral route

Take dose w/in 15 min ac; timing may vary from immediately preceding meal up to 30 min before meal
If meal is skipped, skip dose for that meal

HOW SUPPLIED
Tab: (Repaglinide/Metformin) 1mg/500mg, 2mg/500mg

CONTRAINDICATIONS
Renal impairment (eg, SrCr ≥1.5mg/dL [males], ≥1.4mg/dL [females], or abnormal CrCl), acute or chronic metabolic acidosis, including diabetic ketoacidosis, concomitant gemfibrozil, known hypersensitivity to PrandiMet or any inactive ingredients in the product.

WARNINGS/PRECAUTIONS
Do not initiate in patients ≥80 yrs of age unless renal function is normal. Temporarily d/c at the time of or prior to intravascular contrast studies with iodinated materials, and withhold for 48 hrs subsequent to the procedure and reinstitute only if renal function is normal. Avoid with hepatic impairment. May cause hypoglycemia; risk increased in elderly, debilitated, or malnourished patients, or with adrenal or pituitary insufficiency. May decrease vitamin B12 levels; measure hematologic parameters annually. Suspend temporarily for any surgical procedure (except minor procedures not associated with restricted food and fluid intake); restart when oral intake is resumed and renal function is normal. Temporary loss of glycemic control may occur when exposed to stress; may need to withhold therapy and temporarily administer insulin. D/C promptly in hypoxic states (eg, acute CHF, shock, acute myocardial infarction). Evaluate promptly for evidence of ketoacidosis or lactic acidosis if laboratory abnormalities or clinical illness develops; d/c immediately if acidosis occurs.

ADVERSE REACTIONS
Lactic acidosis, GI system disorder, symptomatic hypoglycemia, headache, diarrhea, nausea, upper respiratory tract infection.

DRUG INTERACTIONS
See Contraindications. May increase C_{max} of fenofibrate. Metformin: Alcohol potentiates effect of metformin on lactate metabolism. Caution with drugs that may affect renal function or result in significant hemodynamic change or may interfere with the disposition of metformin, such as cationic drugs eliminated by renal tubular secretion (eg, amiloride, digoxin, morphine). Cimetidine, furosemide, nifedipine, and ibuprofen may increase levels. Propranolol may decrease levels. May decrease levels of furosemide. Repaglinide: Not for use in combination with NPH-insulin. Risk of hypoglycemia increased with alcohol. Hypoglycemia may be difficult to recognize with β-adrenergic blocking drugs. CYP2C8 inhibitors, CYP3A4 inhibitors, or CYP2C8/3A4 inducers may alter pharmacokinetics and pharmacodynamics. Clarithromycin, deferasirox, fenofibrate, gemfibrozil, itraconazole, ketoconazole, simvastatin, trimethoprim, and OATP1B1 inhibitors (eg, cyclosporine) may increase levels. Levonorgestrel/ethinyl estradiol combination may decrease area under the curve and increase C_{max}. Nifedipine and rifampin may decrease levels. May increase levels of ethinyl estradiol.

PATIENT CONSIDERATIONS

Assessment: Assess for metabolic acidosis, diabetic ketoacidosis, type of DM, renal/hepatic function, risk factors for lactic acidosis, susceptibility to hypoglycemia, drug hypersensitivity, pregnancy/nursing status, and possible drug interactions. Assess if patient is planning to undergo any surgical procedure or is under any form of stress. Obtain baseline FPG and HbA1c.

Monitoring: Monitor for lactic acidosis, clinical illness, hypoxic states, and other adverse reactions. Monitor renal function, especially in elderly patients, at least annually. Monitor vitamin B12 levels in patients predisposed to develop subnormal vitamin B12 levels. Monitor FPG, HbA1c, and hematologic parameters periodically.

Counseling: Inform of potential risks/advantages of therapy, alternative modes of therapy, the importance of adherence to dietary instructions, regular exercise program, and regular testing of blood glucose, HbA1c, renal function, and hematologic parameters. Inform about risks of hypoglycemia and lactic acidosis, their symptoms and treatment, and predisposing conditions. Instruct to seek medical advice during periods of stress as medication needs may change. Advise to d/c drug immediately and notify physician if unexplained hyperventilation, myalgia, malaise, unusual somnolence, or other nonspecific symptoms occur. Instruct to take drug with meals; if a meal is skipped, instruct to skip the dose for that meal. Counsel against excessive alcohol intake.

STORAGE: ≤25°C (77°F). Protect from moisture.

PRANDIN – repaglinide

RX

Class: Meglitinide

ADULT DOSAGE

Type 2 Diabetes Mellitus

Administer dose w/in 15-30 min ac, bid-qid in response to changes in meal pattern

Initial:

Not Previously Treated or HbA1c <8%: 0.5mg w/ each meal preprandially

Previously Treated and HbA1c ≥8%: 1mg or 2mg w/ each meal preprandially

PEDIATRIC DOSAGE

Pediatric use may not have been established

Titrate: May double preprandial dose up to 4mg until satisfactory blood glucose response; at least 1 week should elapse to assess response after each dose adjustment
Range: 0.5-4mg w/ meals preprandially
Max: 16mg/day

Replacing Other Oral Hypoglycemics:
Repaglinide may be started on the day after the final dose is given; observe carefully for hypoglycemia due to potential overlapping drug effects. Close monitoring for up to 1 week or longer may be indicated when transferred from longer half-life sulfonylurea agents (eg, chlorpropamide)

Combination Therapy:
May add metformin or a thiazolidinedione if repaglinide monotherapy does not result in adequate glycemic control; may add repaglinide if metformin or thiazolidinedione monotherapy does not provide adequate control
Starting dose and dose adjustments for repaglinide combination therapy is the same as for repaglinide monotherapy

DOSING CONSIDERATIONS

Concomitant Medications
W/ Thiazolidinedione or w/ Metformin:
If hypoglycemia occurs in patients taking a combination of repaglinide and a thiazolidinedione or repaglinide and metformin, reduce dose of repaglinide

Renal Impairment
Severe (CrCl 20-40mL/min):
Initial: 0.5mg ac; titrate carefully

Hepatic Impairment
Utilize longer intervals between dose adjustments to fully assess response

ADMINISTRATION

Oral route

Take w/in 15-30 min ac

HOW SUPPLIED

Tab: 0.5mg, 1mg, 2mg

CONTRAINDICATIONS

Diabetic ketoacidosis w/ or w/o coma, type 1 DM, concomitant gemfibrozil, known hypersensitivity to the drug or its inactive ingredients.

WARNINGS/PRECAUTIONS

May cause hypoglycemia; risk increased in elderly, debilitated or malnourished patients, or with adrenal, pituitary, hepatic, or severe renal insufficiency. Loss of glycemic control may occur when exposed to stress; may need to d/c therapy and administer insulin. Secondary failure may occur; assess adequate dose adjustment and adherence to diet before classifying a patient as a secondary failure. Caution with hepatic impairment.

ADVERSE REACTIONS

Hypoglycemia, upper respiratory infection, headache, rhinitis, sinusitis, bronchitis, arthralgia, back pain, N/V, diarrhea, dyspepsia, constipation, paresthesia, chest pain.

DRUG INTERACTIONS

See Contraindications. Not for use in combination with NPH-insulin. CYP3A4 and/or CYP2C8 inducers (eg, barbiturates, carbamazepine), CYP3A4 inhibitors (eg, erythromycin), and CYP2C8 inhibitors (eg, montelukast) may alter metabolism; use with caution. OATP1B1 inhibitors (eg, cyclosporine), itraconazole, ketoconazole, clarithromycin, trimethoprim, and deferasirox may increase levels. Rifampin may decrease levels. NSAIDs, highly protein-bound drugs, salicylates, sulfonamides, cyclosporine, chloramphenicol, coumarins, probenecid, MAOIs, β-blockers, alcohol, and >1 glucose-lowering drug may potentiate hypoglycemic action. Thiazides and other diuretics, corticosteroids, phenothiazines, thyroid products, estrogens, oral contraceptives, phenytoin, nicotinic acid, sympathomimetics, calcium channel blockers, and isoniazid tend to produce hyperglycemia and may lead to loss of glycemic control. β-blockers may mask hypoglycemia. May increase ethinyl estradiol levels and levonorgestrel C_{max}. Levonorgestrel/ethinyl estradiol combination and simvastatin may increase C_{max}.

PATIENT CONSIDERATIONS

Assessment: Assess for diabetic ketoacidosis, type 1 DM, adrenal/pituitary/hepatic/severe renal insufficiency, drug hypersensitivity, pregnancy/nursing status, and possible drug interactions. Assess FPG, postprandial glucose (PPG), and HbA1c.

Monitoring: Monitor for hypo/hyperglycemia, secondary failure, and other adverse events. Monitor FPG, PPG, HbA1c, and renal/hepatic function.

Counseling: Inform of potential risks/benefits of therapy, alternative modes of therapy, the importance of adherence to dietary instructions, regular exercise program, and regular blood glucose and HbA1c testing. Inform about risks of hypoglycemia, its symptoms and treatment, and predisposing conditions. Instruct to take drug ac (bid-qid preprandially); if a meal is skipped (or an extra meal is added), instruct to skip (or add) a dose for that meal.

STORAGE: ≤25°C (77°F). Protect from moisture.

PRAVASTATIN – pravastatin sodium

RX

Class: HMG-CoA reductase inhibitor (statin)

OTHER BRAND NAMES

Pravachol

ADULT DOSAGE

Hyperlipidemia

Primary Hypercholesterolemia/Mixed Dyslipidemia/Primary Dysbetalipoproteinemia:

Initial: 40mg qd

Titrate: Increase to 80mg qd if 40mg qd does not achieve desired cholesterol levels

Maximal effect of a given dose is seen w/in 4 weeks; perform periodic lipid determinations at this time and adjust dose accordingly

Prevention of Cardiovascular Disease

Dose based on current clinical practice

PEDIATRIC DOSAGE

Heterozygous Familial Hypercholesterolemia

8-13 Years:

20mg qd

Doses >20mg have not been studied in this patient population

14-18 Years:

Initial: 40mg qd

Doses >40mg have not been studied in this patient population

DOSING CONSIDERATIONS

Concomitant Medications

Bile Acid Resins:

Administer pravastatin either 1 hr or more before or at least 4 hrs following the resin

Clarithromycin:

Limit pravastatin dose to 40mg qd

Immunosuppressive Drugs (eg, Cyclosporine):

Initial: 10mg qhs

Titrate: Increase dose cautiously

Max: 20mg/day

Renal Impairment

Significant:

Initial: 10mg qd

ADMINISTRATION

Oral route

Administer as a single dose at any time of the day, w/ or w/o food.

HOW SUPPLIED

Tab: 10mg; (Pravachol) 20mg, 40mg, 80mg

CONTRAINDICATIONS

Hypersensitivity to any component of the medication; active liver disease or unexplained, persistent elevations of serum transaminases; pregnancy; nursing mothers.

WARNINGS/PRECAUTIONS

Rare cases of rhabdomyolysis w/ acute renal failure secondary to myoglobinuria reported. Increased risk of rhabdomyolysis w/ history of renal impairment; closely monitor for skeletal muscle effects. Uncomplicated myalgia and myopathy (including immune-mediated necrotizing myopathy [IMNM]) reported; d/c if markedly elevated CPK levels occur or myopathy is diagnosed/suspected. Temporarily withhold in any patient experiencing an acute or serious condition predisposing to development of renal failure secondary to rhabdomyolysis. May cause biochemical liver function abnormalities; perform LFTs prior to initiation of therapy and when clinically indicated. Caution in patients who have recent (<6 months) history of liver disease, have signs that may suggest liver disease, or are heavy alcohol users, or are elderly. Fatal and nonfatal hepatic failure reported (rare); promptly interrupt therapy if serious liver injury w/ clinical symptoms and/or hyperbilirubinemia or jaundice occurs and do not restart if no alternate etiology found. May blunt adrenal or gonadal steroid hormone production. Evaluate patients who display clinical evidence of endocrine dysfunction. Not studied in conditions where the major lipoprotein abnormality is elevation of chylomicrons (Fredrickson Types I and V). Not evaluated in patients w/ rare homozygous familial hypercholesterolemia; statins reported to be less effective because patients lack functional LDL receptors.

ADVERSE REACTIONS

Musculoskeletal pain/traumatism, URTI, chest pain, influenza, fatigue, cough, N/V, dizziness, sinus abnormality, rash, diarrhea, headache, muscle cramp, anxiety/nervousness.

DRUG INTERACTIONS

See Dosing Considerations. Increased risk of myopathy/rhabdomyolysis w/ cyclosporine, fibrates, niacin (nicotinic acid), erythromycin, clarithromycin, colchicine, and gemfibrozil; avoid w/ gemfibrozil and use caution w/ colchicine and other fibrates. Niacin may enhance risk of skeletal muscle effects; consider dose reduction of pravastatin. Caution w/ drugs that may diminish levels or activity of steroid hormones (eg, ketoconazole, spironolactone, cimetidine).

PATIENT CONSIDERATIONS

Assessment: Assess for history of or active liver disease, unexplained persistent serum transaminase elevations, predisposing factors for myopathy, alcohol consumption, renal impairment, hypersensitivity to the drug, pregnancy/nursing status, and possible drug interactions. Obtain baseline lipid profile and LFTs.

Monitoring: Monitor for signs/symptoms of rhabdomyolysis, myopathy (including IMNM), liver/ endocrine dysfunction, and other adverse reactions. Monitor lipid profile, LFTs when clinically indicated, and CPK levels.

Counseling: Advise to report promptly any unexplained muscle pain, tenderness, or weakness, particularly if accompanied by malaise or fever or if these muscle signs or symptoms persist after discontinuation, or any symptoms that may indicate liver injury. Counsel females of childbearing potential on appropriate contraceptive methods while on therapy.

STORAGE: 20-25°C (68-77°F); excursions permitted to 15-30°C (59-86°F). Protect from light and moisture. **Pravachol:** 25°C (77°F); excursions permitted to 15-30°C (59-86°F). Protect from light and moisture.

PRAXBIND – idarucizumab

RX

Class: Antidote

P

ADULT DOSAGE

Dabigatran Reversal

For use in emergency surgery/urgent procedures, or in the event of life-threatening or uncontrolled bleeding, to reverse the anticoagulant effects of dabigatran

5g IV, provided as 2 separate vials each containing 2.5g/50mL; limited data to support administration of an additional 5g

If reappearance of bleeding w/ elevated coagulation parameters occurs after 1 dose of 5g, may give another 5g dose

Similarly, patients who require a 2nd emergency surgery/urgent procedure and have elevated coagulation parameters may receive an additional 5g dose

Dabigatran treatment can be initiated 24 hrs after administration

PEDIATRIC DOSAGE

Pediatric use may not have been established

ADMINISTRATION

IV route

Do not mix w/ other products.

Administer w/in 1 hr after withdrawing from vial.

Administer dose as 2 consecutive infusions or a bolus inj by injecting both vials consecutively. A preexisting IV line may be used for administration; the line must be flushed w/ 0.9% NaCl prior to infusion.

HOW SUPPLIED

Inj: 2.5g/50mL

WARNINGS/PRECAUTIONS

Reversing dabigatran therapy exposes patients to the thrombotic risk of their underlying disease; consider resuming anticoagulant therapy as soon as medically appropriate. Elevated coagulation parameters (eg, aPTT, ECT) have been observed. If an anaphylactic reaction or other serious allergic reaction occurs, immediately d/c. Serious adverse reactions reported in patients w/ hereditary fructose intolerance due to sorbitol excipient. Recommended dose of idarucizumab contains 4g of sorbitol; consider the combined daily metabolic load of sorbitol/fructose from all sources, including idarucizumab and other drugs containing sorbitol when prescribing.

ADVERSE REACTIONS

Headache, hypokalemia, delirium, constipation, pyrexia, pneumonia.

PATIENT CONSIDERATIONS

Assessment: Assess for thromboembolic risk, hereditary fructose intolerance, and pregnancy/nursing status.

Monitoring: Monitor for allergic/anaphylactic reaction, signs/symptoms of thromboembolism, coagulation parameters (aPTT, ECT), bleeding, and other adverse reactions.

Counseling: Inform patients that reversing dabigatran therapy exposes them to the thromboembolic risk of their underlying disease. Instruct to get immediate medical attention for any signs/symptoms of bleeding. Inform of signs/symptoms of allergic hypersensitivity reactions. Inform patients w/ hereditary fructose intolerance that drug contains sorbitol.

STORAGE: 2-8°C (36-46°F). Do not freeze. Do not shake. Unopened vial may be kept at 25°C (77°F) for ≤48 hrs if stored in the original package to protect from light, or ≤6 hrs when exposed to light.

PREDNISOLONE – prednisolone

Class: Glucocorticoid

RX

ADULT DOSAGE

Steroid-Responsive Disorders

Syr/Tab:

Initial: 5-60mg/day depending on disease and response

Maint: Decrease initial dose in small decrements to lowest effective dose

Tab:

Alternate-Day Therapy: Administer twice the usual daily dose every other am; refer to PI for more detailed information

PEDIATRIC DOSAGE

Steroid-Responsive Disorders

Syr/Tab:

Initial: 5-60mg/day depending on disease and response

Maint: Decrease dose by small amounts to lowest effective dose

Tab:

Alternate-Day Therapy: Administer twice the usual daily dose every other am; refer to PI for more detailed information

DOSING CONSIDERATIONS

Discontinuation

Withdraw gradually after long-term therapy

ADMINISTRATION

Oral route

HOW SUPPLIED

Syrup: 5mg/5mL [120mL], 15mg/5mL [240mL, 480mL]; **Tab:** 5mg* *scored

CONTRAINDICATIONS

Systemic fungal infections.

WARNINGS/PRECAUTIONS

May need to increase dose before, during, and after stressful situation. May mask signs of infection or cause new infections. May decrease resistance and inability to localize infection. Possible benefits should be weighed against potential hazards if used during pregnancy/nursing. Prolonged use may produce posterior subcapsular cataracts, glaucoma, optic nerve damage, and secondary ocular infections. May cause BP elevation, increased K^+/Ca^{2+} excretion, and salt/water retention. Dietary salt restriction and K^+ supplementation may be necessary when used in large doses. More serious/fatal course of infections reported with chickenpox and measles; avoid exposure. Reactivation of disease may occur with latent TB or tuberculin reactivity. Caution with hypothyroidism, cirrhosis,

P

ocular herpes simplex, HTN, diverticulitis, fresh intestinal anastomoses, nonspecific ulcerative colitis, osteoporosis, myasthenia gravis, renal insufficiency, and active or latent peptic ulcer. Growth and development of children on prolonged therapy should be monitored. May cause psychic derangements or aggravate existing emotional instability or psychotic tendencies. Avoid abrupt withdrawal. (Syrup) D/C treatment if a period of spontaneous remission occurs in a chronic condition.

ADVERSE REACTIONS

Fluid and electrolyte disturbances, osteoporosis, muscle weakness, cushingoid state, menstrual irregularities, facial erythema, convulsions, impaired wound healing, increased sweating, decreased carbohydrate tolerance, glaucoma, posterior subcapsular cataracts, vertigo, headache, abdominal distention.

DRUG INTERACTIONS

Caution with ASA in hypoprothrombinemia. Avoid smallpox vaccination and other immunization procedures, especially if on high doses of corticosteroids. Increased insulin and PO hypoglycemic requirements in diabetics.

PATIENT CONSIDERATIONS

Assessment: Assess for systemic fungal infections/other current infections, active TB, vaccination history, hypothyroidism, cirrhosis, renal insufficiency, HTN, ocular herpes simplex, ulcerative colitis, diverticulitis, fresh intestinal anastomoses, active or latent peptic ulcer, osteoporosis, myasthenia gravis, psychotic tendencies, pregnancy/nursing status, and for possible drug interactions.

Monitoring: Monitor for adrenocortical insufficiency, salt/water retention, new infections, psychic derangements, posterior subcapsular cataracts, glaucoma, optic nerve damage, and secondary ocular infections. Monitor BP, serum K^+ and Ca^{2+} levels. Monitor growth and development of infants/children on prolonged therapy (including bone growth) and for hypoadrenalism in infants born to mothers who received substantial doses. (Syrup) Obtain BP, weight, routine lab studies (including 2-hr postprandial blood glucose and serum K^+), chest x-ray, and upper GI x-rays (with known/suspected peptic ulcer disease) at regular intervals during prolonged therapy.

Counseling: Advise not to d/c abruptly. Counsel to avoid exposure to chickenpox or measles if on an immunosuppressant dose of corticosteroids; instruct to report immediately if exposed.

STORAGE: 20-25°C (68-77°F). (Syrup) Do not refrigerate.

PREDNISONE – prednisone

RX

Class: Glucocorticoid

OTHER BRAND NAMES

Prednisone Intensol

P

ADULT DOSAGE

Steroid-Responsive Disorders

Initial: 5-60mg/day, depending on disease and response

Maint: Decrease initial dose in small decrements to lowest effective dose

Alternate-Day Therapy: Administer twice the usual daily dose every other am; refer to PI for more detailed information

Multiple Sclerosis

Acute Exacerbations:

200mg/day for 1 week, followed by 80mg qod for 1 month

PEDIATRIC DOSAGE

Steroid-Responsive Disorders

Initial: 5-60mg/day, depending on disease and response

Maint: Decrease initial dose in small decrements to lowest effective dose

Alternate-Day Therapy: Administer twice the usual daily dose every other am; refer to PI for more detailed information

Multiple Sclerosis

Acute Exacerbations:

200mg/day for 1 week, followed by 80mg qod for 1 month

DOSING CONSIDERATIONS

Elderly

Start at lower end of dosing range

Discontinuation

Withdraw gradually after long-term therapy

ADMINISTRATION

Oral route

Take before, during, or immediately pc or w/ food or milk to reduce gastric irritation
Administer in the am prior to 9 am; when large doses are given, administer antacids between meals
Multiple dose therapy should be evenly distributed in evenly spaced intervals throughout the day

HOW SUPPLIED
Sol: (Intensol) 5mg/mL [30mL]; 5mg/5mL [120mL, 500mL]; **Tab:** 1mg*, 2.5mg*, 5mg*, 10mg*, 20mg*, 50mg* *scored

CONTRAINDICATIONS
Systemic fungal infections, known hypersensitivity to the components of the medication.

WARNINGS/PRECAUTIONS
Monitor for situations that may make dosage adjustments necessary (eg, change in clinical status secondary to remissions/exacerbations in the disease process, individual drug responsiveness, effect of patient exposure to stress). Anaphylactoid reactions may occur. May need to increase dose before, during, and after stressful situation. May cause BP elevation, salt/water retention, and increased K^+ and Ca^{2+} excretion; dietary salt restriction and K^+ supplementation may be necessary. Caution in patients w/ a recent MI. May produce reversible hypothalamic-pituitary-adrenal (HPA) axis suppression w/ the potential for corticosteroid insufficiency after withdrawal of treatment. Metabolic clearance is decreased in hypothyroid patients and increased in hyperthyroid patients; changes in thyroid status may necessitate dose adjustment. May increase susceptibility to infections, mask signs of current infection, activate latent disease, or exacerbate intercurrent infections. Avoid use in the presence of systemic fungal infections unless needed to control life-threatening drug reactions. Rule out latent or active amebiasis before initiating therapy. Caution w/ *Strongyloides* infestation, active/latent TB or tuberculin reactivity, HTN, CHF, and renal insufficiency. Caution w/ active or latent peptic ulcers, diverticulitis, fresh intestinal anastomoses, and nonspecific ulcerative colitis; may increase risk of perforation. Signs of peritoneal irritation following GI perforation may be minimal/absent. Not for use in cerebral malaria and active ocular herpes simplex. May cause more serious/fatal course of chickenpox and measles; avoid exposure, and if exposed, consider prophylaxis/treatment. May produce posterior subcapsular cataracts, glaucoma w/ possible optic nerve damage, and may enhance the establishment of secondary ocular infections due to bacteria, fungi, or viruses. Kaposi's sarcoma reported. Not recommended in optic neuritis treatment. Drug-induced secondary adrenocortical insufficiency may be minimized by gradual dose reduction. Enhanced effect in patients w/ hypothyroidism and cirrhosis. May decrease bone formation and increase bone resorption, and may lead to inhibition of bone growth in pediatric patients and development of osteoporosis at any age; caution w/ increased risk of osteoporosis. Acute myopathy w/ high doses reported, most often in patients w/ neuromuscular transmission disorders (eg, myasthenia gravis). Psychiatric derangements may appear and existing emotional instability or psychotic tendencies may be aggravated. Elevation of creatine kinase (CK) may occur. May elevate IOP; monitor IOP if used for >6 weeks. May suppress reactions to skin tests.

ADVERSE REACTIONS
Anaphylactoid reactions, HTN, osteoporosis, muscle weakness, menstrual irregularities, insomnia, impaired wound healing, ulcerative esophagitis, increased sweating, decreased carbohydrate tolerance, glaucoma, weight gain, nausea, malaise, anemia.

DRUG INTERACTIONS
Live or live, attenuated vaccines are contraindicated w/ immunosuppressive doses. May diminish response to toxoids and live or inactivated vaccines. Closely monitor for hypokalemia when administered w/ K^+-depleting agents (eg, amphotericin B, diuretics). Cardiac enlargement and CHF may occur w/ concomitant use of amphotericin B. Macrolide antibiotics may decrease clearance. Concomitant use w/ anticholinesterase agents (eg, neostigmine, pyridostigmine) may produce severe weakness in myasthenia gravis patients; d/c anticholinesterase agents at least 24 hrs before start of therapy. May inhibit response to warfarin; frequently monitor coagulation indices. May increase blood glucose levels; dose adjustment of antidiabetic agents may be required. May decrease serum concentration of isoniazid. Extreme caution w/ bupropion; employ low initial dosing and small gradual increases. Cholestyramine may increase clearance. Increased activity of both drugs may occur w/ cyclosporine; convulsions reported w/ concurrent use. May increase risk of arrhythmias due to hypokalemia w/ digitalis glycosides. Estrogens, including oral contraceptives, may decrease hepatic metabolism and increase effect. Increased risk of tendon rupture, especially in elderly, w/ concomitant fluoroquinolones. CYP3A4 inducers (eg, barbiturates, phenytoin, carbamazepine, rifampin) may enhance metabolism and may require increase in corticosteroid dose. CYP3A4 inhibitors (eg, ketoconazole, ritonavir, macrolide antibiotics such as erythromycin) may increase plasma levels. May increase clearance of other drugs that are metabolized by CYP3A4 (eg, indinavir, erythromycin), resulting in decreased plasma levels. Increased risk of corticosteroid side effects w/ ketoconazole. Aspirin (ASA) or other NSAIDs may increase risk of GI side effects. Caution w/ ASA in hypoprothrombinemia patients. May increase clearance of salicylates. Decreased therapeutic effect w/ phenytoin. Increased doses of quetiapine may be required to maintain control of schizophrenia symptoms. Caution w/ thalidomide; toxic epidermal necrolysis reported w/ concomitant use. Acute myopathy reported w/ neuromuscular blocking drugs (eg, pancuronium).

PATIENT CONSIDERATIONS
Assessment: Assess for hypersensitivity to drug, CHF, HTN, renal impairment, systemic fungal infections, other current infections, active TB, latent/active amebiasis, cerebral malaria, active ocular herpes simplex, emotional instability or psychotic tendencies, recent MI, vaccination history,

thyroid status, any other conditions where treatment is cautioned, pregnancy/nursing status, and for possible drug interactions.

Monitoring: Monitor for anaphylactoid reactions, HPA axis suppression, adrenocortical insufficiency, salt/water retention, infections, change in thyroid status, cataracts, glaucoma, Kaposi's sarcoma, emotional instability or psychotic tendencies aggravation, and other adverse reactions. Monitor IOP, BP, CK, and serum electrolytes. Monitor growth and development of infants/children on prolonged therapy. Frequently monitor coagulation indices w/ warfarin.

Counseling: Instruct not to d/c therapy abruptly or w/o medical supervision. Instruct to inform any medical attendants of intake of corticosteroids and to seek medical advice at once if fever or other signs of infection develop. Advise to avoid exposure to chickenpox or measles; instruct to seek medical advice w/o delay if exposed.

STORAGE: 20-25°C (68-77°F). (Tab) Protect from moisture. (Intensol) Discard opened bottle after 90 days.

PREMARIN TABLETS – conjugated estrogens

RX

Class: Estrogen

Estrogens increase the risk of endometrial cancer. Perform adequate diagnostic measures, including endometrial sampling, to rule out malignancy in postmenopausal women w/ undiagnosed persistent or recurring abnormal genital bleeding. Should not be used for the prevention of cardiovascular (CV) disease or dementia. Increased risks of MI, stroke, invasive breast cancer, pulmonary embolism (PE), and deep vein thrombosis (DVT) in postmenopausal women (50-79 yrs of age) reported. Increased risk of developing probable dementia in postmenopausal women ≥65 yrs of age reported. Should be prescribed at the lowest effective dose and for the shortest duration consistent w/ treatment goals and risks.

ADULT DOSAGE

Postmenopausal Osteoporosis

Prevention:

Initial: 0.3mg qd continuously or cyclically (eg, 25 days on, 5 days off)

Titrate: Adjust subsequent dose based on clinical and bone mineral density responses

Use lowest effective dose and for the shortest duration consistent w/ treatment goals and risk

Menopausal Vasomotor Symptoms

Moderate to Severe:

Initial: 0.3mg/day continuously or cyclically (eg, 25 days on followed by 5 days off)

Titrate: Subsequent dose adjustment may be made based on response

Use lowest effective dose for the shortest duration; reevaluate periodically

Menopausal Vulvar/Vaginal Atrophy

Moderate to Severe:

Initial: 0.3mg/day continuously or cyclically (eg, 25 days on followed by 5 days off)

Titrate: Subsequent dose adjustment may be made based on response

Use lowest effective dose for the shortest duration; reevaluate periodically

Hypoestrogenism

Female Hypogonadism:

0.3 or 0.625mg qd cyclically (eg, 3 weeks on and 1 week off)

Titrate: Adjust dose based on severity of symptoms and response of the endometrium

Female Castration/Primary Ovarian Failure:

Usual: 1.25mg qd cyclically

Titrate: Adjust dose based on severity of symptoms and response

Use lowest effective dose and for the shortest duration consistent w/ treatment goals and risk

PEDIATRIC DOSAGE

Pediatric use may not have been established

Metastatic Breast Cancer

Palliative Treatment in Appropriately Selected Women and Men:
10mg tid for a minimum of 3 months

Use lowest effective dose and for the shortest duration consistent w/ treatment goals and risk

Prostate Carcinoma

Palliative Treatment of Advanced Androgen-Dependent Carcinoma:
1.25-2.5mg (two 1.25mg tabs) tid

Use lowest effective dose and for the shortest duration consistent w/ treatment goals and risk

ADMINISTRATION

Oral route

May take w/o regard to meals

HOW SUPPLIED

Tab: 0.3mg, 0.45mg, 0.625mg, 0.9mg, 1.25mg

CONTRAINDICATIONS

Undiagnosed abnormal genital bleeding; known/suspected/history of breast cancer except in appropriately selected patients being treated for metastatic disease; known/suspected estrogen-dependent neoplasia; active/history of DVT/PE/arterial thromboembolic disease (eg, stroke, MI); known anaphylactic reaction/angioedema w/ conjugated estrogens; liver impairment/disease; known protein C, protein S, antithrombin deficiency, or other known thrombophilic disorders; known/suspected pregnancy.

WARNINGS/PRECAUTIONS

D/C immediately if stroke, DVT, PE, and MI occurs or is suspected. Caution in patients w/ risk factors for arterial vascular disease and/or venous thromboembolism. If feasible, d/c at least 4-6 weeks before surgery of the type associated w/ an increased risk of thromboembolism, or during periods of prolonged immobilization. May increase risk of ovarian cancer and gallbladder disease requiring surgery. May lead to severe hypercalcemia in patients w/ breast cancer and bone metastases; d/c and take appropriate measures if hypercalcemia occurs. Retinal vascular thrombosis reported; if visual abnormalities or migraine occurs, d/c pending examination. If examination reveals papilledema or retinal vascular lesions, d/c permanently. Anaphylaxis and angioedema involving tongue, larynx, face, hands, and feet requiring medical intervention reported; d/c if anaphylactic reaction w/ or w/o angioedema occurs. Cases of malignant transformation of residual endometrial implants reported in women treated post-hysterectomy w/ estrogen-alone therapy; consider addition of progestin for women known to have residual endometriosis post-hysterectomy. May elevate BP and thyroid-binding globulin levels. May elevate plasma TGs leading to pancreatitis in patients w/ preexisting hypertriglyceridemia; consider discontinuation if pancreatitis occurs. Caution w/ history of cholestatic jaundice associated w/ past estrogen use or w/ pregnancy; d/c in case of recurrence. May cause fluid retention; caution w/ cardiac/renal dysfunction. Caution w/ hypoparathyroidism; estrogen-induced hypocalcemia may occur. May exacerbate symptoms of angioedema in women w/ hereditary angioedema. May exacerbate asthma, diabetes mellitus, epilepsy, migraine, porphyria, systemic lupus erythematosus, and hepatic hemangiomas; use w/ caution. May affect certain endocrine and blood components in lab tests.

ADVERSE REACTIONS

Abdominal pain, asthenia, back pain, headache, pain, depression, insomnia, dizziness, leukorrhea, breast pain, vaginal hemorrhage, vaginitis, flatulence, nausea, weight gain.

DRUG INTERACTIONS

CYP3A4 inducers (eg, St. John's wort, phenobarbital, carbamazepine, rifampin) may decrease levels, which may decrease therapeutic effects and/or change uterine bleeding profile. CYP3A4 inhibitors (eg, erythromycin, clarithromycin, ketoconazole) may increase levels, which may result in side effects. Women concomitantly receiving thyroid hormone replacement therapy may require increased doses of their thyroid replacement therapy; monitor thyroid function.

PATIENT CONSIDERATIONS

Assessment: Assess for undiagnosed abnormal genital bleeding, estrogen-dependent neoplasia, presence or history of breast cancer, active/history of DVT/PE/arterial thromboembolic disease, thrombophilic disorders, pregnancy/nursing status, any other conditions where treatment is contraindicated or cautioned, need for progestin therapy, and possible drug interactions.

Monitoring: Monitor for signs/symptoms of CV events, malignant neoplasms, dementia, gallbladder disease, hypercalcemia, visual abnormalities, anaphylaxis, angioedema, BP and serum TG elevations, fluid retention, exacerbation of endometriosis and other conditions, and other adverse reactions.

Perform annual breast exam; schedule mammography based on age, risk factors, and prior mammogram results. Monitor thyroid function in women on thyroid replacement therapy. In cases of undiagnosed persistent or recurring genital bleeding, perform adequate diagnostic measures (eg, endometrial sampling) to rule out malignancies. Periodically reevaluate to determine the need of therapy.

Counseling: Inform of the risks/benefits of therapy. Inform of the importance of reporting vaginal bleeding to physician as soon as possible. Inform of possible serious adverse reactions and of possible less serious but common adverse reactions of estrogen therapy.

STORAGE: 20-25°C (68-77°F); excursions permitted to 15-30°C (59-86°F).

PREMARIN VAGINAL – conjugated estrogens RX

Class: Estrogen

Increased risk of endometrial cancer in a woman w/ a uterus who uses unopposed estrogens. Adding a progestin to estrogen therapy reduces the risk of endometrial hyperplasia. Adequate diagnostic measures (eg, directed or random endometrial sampling) should be undertaken to rule out malignancy in postmenopausal women w/ undiagnosed, persistent or recurring abnormal genital bleeding. Should not be used for the prevention of cardiovascular disease (CVD) or dementia. Increased risk of stroke and deep vein thrombosis (DVT) reported in postmenopausal women (50-79 yrs of age) treated w/ daily oral conjugated estrogens (CEs) alone and when combined w/ medroxyprogesterone acetate (MPA). Increased risk of developing probable dementia reported in postmenopausal women ≥65 yrs of age treated w/ daily CEs alone and when combined w/ MPA. Increased risks of pulmonary embolism (PE), MI, and invasive breast cancer reported in postmenopausal women (50-79 yrs of age) treated w/ daily oral CEs combined w/ MPA. Should be prescribed at the lowest effective dose and for the shortest duration consistent w/ treatment goals and risks.

ADULT DOSAGE

Atrophic Vaginitis and Kraurosis Vulvae

Initial: 0.5g intravaginally in a cyclic regimen (daily for 21 days, and then off for 7 days)
Titrate: Dose adjustments (0.5-2g) may be made based on individual response

Dyspareunia

Moderate to Severe Dyspareunia Due to Menopause:
0.5g intravaginally 2X/week (eg, Monday and Thursday) continuously or in a cyclic regimen (21 days of therapy followed by 7 days off of therapy)

PEDIATRIC DOSAGE

Pediatric use may not have been established

P

ADMINISTRATION

Intravaginal route

HOW SUPPLIED

Vaginal Cre: 0.625mg/g [30g]

CONTRAINDICATIONS

Undiagnosed abnormal genital bleeding; known/suspected/history of breast cancer; known/suspected estrogen-dependent neoplasia; active or history of DVT/PE; active or history of arterial thromboembolic disease (eg, stroke, MI); known anaphylactic reaction or angioedema to CEs vaginal cream; known liver dysfunction/disease; known protein C, protein S, or antithrombin deficiency or other known thrombophilic disorders; known/suspected pregnancy.

WARNINGS/PRECAUTIONS

Systemic absorption reported. D/C therapy immediately if stroke, DVT, PE, or MI occurs or is suspected. Caution in patients w/ risk factors for arterial vascular disease and/or venous thromboembolism. If feasible, d/c at least 4-6 weeks before surgery of the type associated w/ an increased risk of thromboembolism, or during periods of prolonged immobilization. May increase risk of gallbladder disease requiring surgery and risk of ovarian cancer. May lead to severe hypercalcemia in patients w/ breast cancer and bone metastases; d/c and take appropriate measures if hypercalcemia occurs. Retinal vascular thrombosis reported; d/c pending examination if sudden partial/complete loss of vision or sudden onset of proptosis, diplopia, or migraine occurs. If examination reveals papilledema or retinal vascular lesions, d/c therapy permanently. May elevate BP and thyroid-binding globulin levels. May be associated w/ elevations of plasma TGs, leading to pancreatitis in patients w/ preexisting hypertriglyceridemia; consider discontinuation if pancreatitis occurs. Caution w/ history of cholestatic jaundice associated w/ past estrogen use or pregnancy; d/c in case of recurrence. May cause fluid retention. Caution in patients w/ hypoparathyroidism; estrogen-induced hypocalcemia may occur. Cases of malignant transformation of residual endometrial implants reported in women treated posthysterectomy w/ estrogen-alone therapy; consider addition of progestin for these patients. Anaphylaxis and angioedema reported w/ orally administered Premarin. May exacerbate symptoms of angioedema in women w/ hereditary angioedema. May exacerbate asthma, diabetes mellitus (DM), epilepsy, migraine, porphyria, systemic lupus erythematosus, and hepatic hemangiomas; use w/ caution. May weaken latex condoms; consider potential for CEs vaginal cream to weaken and contribute to the failure of condoms, diaphragms, or cervical caps made of latex or rubber. May affect certain endocrine function tests, HDL, LDL, TG levels, and blood components in lab tests. Consider addition of progestin for postmenopausal women w/ a uterus to reduce the risk of endometrial cancer.

ADVERSE REACTIONS

Headache, pelvic pain, vasodilation, breast pain, leukorrhea, vaginitis, vulvovaginal disorder.

DRUG INTERACTIONS

CYP3A4 inducers (eg, St. John's wort preparations, phenobarbital, carbamazepine) may decrease levels, which may result in a decrease in therapeutic effects and/or changes in the uterine bleeding profile. CYP3A4 inhibitors (eg, erythromycin, ketoconazole, grapefruit juice) may increase levels and may result in side effects. Patients dependent on thyroid hormone replacement therapy who are also receiving estrogens may require increased doses of thyroid replacement therapy; monitor thyroid function.

PATIENT CONSIDERATIONS

Assessment: Assess for abnormal genital bleeding, estrogen-dependent neoplasia, presence/history of breast cancer, arterial thromboembolic disease, DVT/PE, hereditary angioedema, previous hypersensitivity, thrombophilic disorders, or any other conditions where treatment is contraindicated or cautioned. Assess use in women ≥65 yrs of age and in those w/ DM, asthma, epilepsy, migraines or porphyria, SLE, or hepatic hemangiomas. Assess for cardiac or renal dysfunction, pregnancy/nursing status, need for progestin therapy, and possible drug interactions.

Monitoring: Monitor for signs/symptoms of cardiovascular events, malignant neoplasms, dementia, gallbladder disease, hypercalcemia, visual abnormalities, pancreatitis, hypertriglyceridemia, cholestatic jaundice, hypothyroidism, fluid retention, exacerbation of endometriosis and other conditions. Perform annual breast exam; schedule mammography based on age, risk factors, and prior mammogram results. Regularly monitor BP, thyroid function in women on thyroid replacement therapy, and periodically evaluate to determine need for treatment. Perform adequate diagnostic measures (eg, endometrial sampling) to rule out malignancies if undiagnosed persistent or recurring genital bleeding occurs.

Counseling: Advise to notify physician if signs/symptoms of unusual vaginal bleeding occur. Inform about possible serious adverse reactions (eg, CVD, malignant neoplasms, and probable dementia) and possible less serious but common adverse reactions (eg, headache, breast pain/tenderness, N/V). Instruct to perform monthly breast self-examination. Inform that medication may weaken barrier contraceptives (eg, latex or rubber condoms, diaphragms, cervical caps).

STORAGE: 20-25°C (68-77°F); excursions permitted to 15-30°C (59-86°F).

PREMPHASE – conjugated estrogens/medroxyprogesterone acetate RX

Class: Estrogen/progestogen combination

Estrogens increase the risk of endometrial cancer. Perform adequate diagnostic measures, including endometrial sampling, to rule out malignancy in postmenopausal women w/ undiagnosed persistent or recurring abnormal genital bleeding. Should not be used for the prevention of cardiovascular disease (CVD) or dementia. Increased risk of MI, stroke, invasive breast cancer, PE, and DVT in postmenopausal women (50-79 yrs of age) reported. Increased risk of developing probable dementia in postmenopausal women ≥65 yrs of age reported. Should be prescribed at the lowest effective dose and for the shortest duration consistent w/ treatment goals and risks.

OTHER BRAND NAMES

Prempro

ADULT DOSAGE

Menopausal Vasomotor Symptoms

Moderate to Severe:

Prempro:

1 tab qd

Premphase:

Days 1-14: One maroon 0.625mg conjugated estrogens (CE) tab qd

Days 15-28: One light-blue tab containing 0.625mg CE and 5mg medroxyprogesterone acetate qd

PEDIATRIC DOSAGE

Pediatric use may not have been established

Use lowest effective dose for the shortest duration; reevaluate periodically

Menopausal Vulvar/Vaginal Atrophy

Moderate to Severe:
Prempro:
1 tab qd

Premphase:
Days 1-14: One maroon 0.625mg conjugated estrogens (CE) tab qd
Days 15-28: One light-blue tab containing 0.625mg CE and 5mg medroxyprogesterone acetate qd

Use lowest effective dose for the shortest duration; reevaluate periodically

Postmenopausal Osteoporosis

Prevention:
Prempro:
1 tab qd

Premphase:
Days 1-14: One maroon 0.625mg conjugated estrogens (CE) tab qd
Days 15-28: One light-blue tab containing 0.625mg CE and 5mg medroxyprogesterone acetate qd

Use lowest effective dose for the shortest duration; reevaluate periodically

ADMINISTRATION

Oral route

HOW SUPPLIED

Tab: (Premphase) (Conjugated Estrogens [CE]) 0.625mg, (CE/Medroxyprogesterone) 0.625mg/5mg; (Prempro) (CE/Medroxyprogesterone) 0.3mg/1.5mg, 0.45mg/1.5mg, 0.625mg/2.5mg, 0.625mg/5mg

CONTRAINDICATIONS

Undiagnosed abnormal genital bleeding; known/suspected/history of breast cancer; known/suspected estrogen-dependent neoplasia; active or history of DVT/PE/arterial thromboembolic disease (eg, stroke, MI); known anaphylactic reaction/angioedema to Prempro/Premphase; known liver dysfunction/disease; known protein C, protein S, antithrombin deficiency, or other known thrombophilic disorders; known/suspected pregnancy.

P

WARNINGS/PRECAUTIONS

D/C immediately if PE, DVT, stroke, or MI occurs or is suspected. If feasible, d/c at least 4-6 weeks before surgery of the type associated w/ an increased risk of thromboembolism, or during periods of prolonged immobilization. May increase risk of ovarian cancer. May increase risk of gallbladder disease requiring surgery. May lead to severe hypercalcemia in patients w/ breast cancer and bone metastases; d/c and take appropriate measures if hypercalcemia occurs. Retinal vascular thrombosis reported; d/c pending examination if sudden partial/complete loss of vision or sudden onset of proptosis, diplopia, or migraine occurs. D/C permanently if examination reveals papilledema or retinal vascular lesions. May increase BP and thyroid-binding globulin levels. May be associated w/ elevations of plasma TGs; consider discontinuation if pancreatitis occurs. Caution w/ history of cholestatic jaundice associated w/ past estrogen use or w/ pregnancy; d/c in case of recurrence. May cause fluid retention. Caution w/ hypoparathyroidism; hypocalcemia may occur. Anaphylaxis and angioedema reported. May exacerbate symptoms of angioedema in women w/ hereditary angioedema. May exacerbate endometriosis, asthma, diabetes mellitus, epilepsy, migraine, porphyria, systemic lupus erythematosus, and hepatic hemangiomas. May affect certain endocrine and blood components in lab tests.

ADVERSE REACTIONS

Headache, breast pain, abdominal pain, back pain, depression, nausea, flatulence, peripheral edema, weight gain, pruritus, breast enlargement, dysmenorrhea, leukorrhea, vaginitis, asthenia.

DRUG INTERACTIONS

CYP3A4 inducers (eg, St. John's wort, phenobarbital, carbamazepine) may decrease levels, which may decrease therapeutic effects and/or cause changes in the uterine bleeding profile. CYP3A4 inhibitors (eg, erythromycin, ketoconazole, grapefruit juice) may increase levels and may result in side effects. Aminoglutethimide may significantly depress bioavailability of medroxyprogesterone acetate (MPA). Patients concomitantly receiving thyroid hormone replacement therapy and estrogens may require increased doses of their thyroid replacement therapy; monitor thyroid function.

PATIENT CONSIDERATIONS

Assessment: Assess for abnormal genital bleeding, presence/history of breast cancer, estrogen-dependent neoplasia, active or history of DVT/PE/arterial thromboembolic disease, liver dysfunction/disease, thrombophilic disorders, known anaphylactic reaction or angioedema to the drug, cardiac or renal dysfunction, other conditions where treatment is contraindicated or cautioned, pregnancy/nursing status, and possible drug interactions.

Monitoring: Monitor for signs/symptoms of CVD, malignant neoplasms, dementia, gallbladder disease, hypercalcemia, visual abnormalities, BP and plasma TG elevations, pancreatitis, cholestatic jaundice, hypothyroidism, fluid retention, anaphylaxis, angioedema, exacerbation of endometriosis, and for other adverse reactions. Perform annual breast examinations; schedule mammography based on patient age, risk factors, and prior mammogram results. Perform adequate diagnostic measures (eg, endometrial sampling) in patients w/ undiagnosed persistent or recurring genital bleeding. Perform periodic evaluation to determine treatment need.

Counseling: Inform of the importance of reporting abnormal vaginal bleeding to physician as soon as possible. Advise of possible serious adverse reactions of therapy (eg, CVD, malignant neoplasms, probable dementia) and of possible less serious but common adverse reactions (eg, headache, breast pain and tenderness, N/V). Instruct to have yearly breast examinations by a healthcare provider and to perform monthly breast self-examinations.

STORAGE: 20-25°C (68-77°F); excursions permitted to 15-30°C (59-86°F).

PREPOPIK – anhydrous citric acid/magnesium oxide/sodium picosulfate RX

Class: Bowel cleanser

ADULT DOSAGE

Bowel Cleansing

Prior to Colonoscopy:

Split-Dose Regimen (Preferred Method):

1st Dose: Take during the pm before colonoscopy (eg, 5-9 pm), followed by five 8-oz drinks (upper line on dosing cup) of clear liquids hs. Consume clear liquids w/in 5 hrs

2nd Dose: Take the next day, approx 5 hrs before colonoscopy, followed by at least three 8-oz drinks of clear liquids before the colonoscopy. Consume clear liquids w/in 5 hrs up until 2 hrs before time of the colonoscopy

Day-Before Regimen (Alternative Method):

1st Dose: Take in afternoon or early pm (eg, 4-6 pm) before colonoscopy, followed by five 8-oz drinks of clear liquids before next dose. Consume clear liquids w/in 5 hrs

2nd Dose: Take approx 6 hrs later in the late pm (eg, 10 pm-12 am) the night before colonoscopy, followed by three 8-oz drinks of clear liquids hs. Consume clear liquids w/in 5 hrs

PEDIATRIC DOSAGE

Pediatric use may not have been established

DOSING CONSIDERATIONS

Adverse Reactions

Severe Bloating/Distention/Abdominal Pain Following 1st Dose: Delay 2nd dose until symptoms resolve

ADMINISTRATION

Oral route

Only clear liquids (no solid food or milk) should be consumed on the day before the colonoscopy up until 2 hrs before the time of the colonoscopy

Reconstitution

1. Reconstitute the powder right before each administration; do not prepare sol in advance
2. Fill the supplied dosing cup w/ cold water up to the lower (5 oz) line on the cup and pour in the contents of 1 pkt of powder
3. Stir for 2-3 min; reconstituted sol may become slightly warm as the powder dissolves

HOW SUPPLIED

Sol (Powder): (Sodium Picosulfate/Magnesium Oxide/Anhydrous Citric Acid) 10mg/3.5g/12g [16.1g, 16.2g]

CONTRAINDICATIONS

Severely reduced renal function (CrCl <30mL/min); GI obstruction or ileus, bowel perforation; toxic colitis or toxic megacolon; gastric retention; allergy to any of the ingredients in the product.

WARNINGS/PRECAUTIONS

May cause fluid/electrolyte disturbances, arrhythmias, and generalized tonic-clonic seizures; correct fluid and electrolyte abnormalities prior to treatment. Caution with CHF when replacing fluids. If vomiting or signs of dehydration (including signs of orthostatic hypotension) develop after treatment, perform postcolonoscopy lab tests (eg, electrolytes, SrCr, BUN) and treat accordingly. Caution with patients at risk of seizure (eg, known/suspected hyponatremia). Caution with impaired renal function and severe active ulcerative colitis. May produce colonic mucosal aphthous ulceration. Serious cases of ischemic colitis reported. Caution in patients prone to regurgitation/aspiration or with impaired gag reflex. Direct ingestion of undissolved powder may increase risk of N/V, dehydration, and electrolyte disturbance. Rule out GI obstruction/perforation before administration.

ADVERSE REACTIONS

Headache, N/V.

DRUG INTERACTIONS

Increased risk of colonic mucosal aphthous ulceration with stimulant laxatives. Caution with drugs that increase the risk of fluid and electrolyte abnormalities, drugs that affect renal function (eg, diuretics, ACE inhibitors, ARBs, NSAIDs), drugs associated with hypokalemia (eg, corticosteroid, cardiac glycosides) or hyponatremia, drugs that lower seizure threshold (eg, TCAs), drugs known to induce antidiuretic hormone secretion (eg, SSRIs, antipsychotics, carbamazepine), and in patients withdrawing from alcohol or benzodiazepines. Caution with drugs that increase the risk for arrhythmias and prolonged QT in the setting of fluid and electrolyte abnormalities. Oral medications given within 1 hr of administration may be flushed from GI tract and may not be absorbed. Take tetracycline and fluoroquinolone antibiotics, iron, digoxin, chlorpromazine, and penicillamine at least 2 hrs before and not <6 hrs after administration. Reduced efficacy with antibiotics.

PATIENT CONSIDERATIONS

Assessment: Assess for previous hypersensitivity to any of the components, electrolyte abnormalities, risk for arrhythmias, CHF, risk/history of seizures, renal impairment, ileus, GI obstruction/perforation, gastric retention, toxic colitis/megacolon, ulcerative colitis, impaired gag reflex, regurgitation or aspiration tendencies, pregnancy/nursing status, and possible drug interactions. Perform predose lab tests (eg, electrolytes, SrCr, BUN) and ECG.

Monitoring: Monitor for fluid/electrolyte disturbances, arrhythmias, seizures, GI ulceration, colitis, bloating, abdominal distention/pain, and other adverse reactions. Perform postcolonoscopy lab tests and ECG.

Counseling: Advise to adequately hydrate before, during, and after use. Instruct not to take other laxatives during therapy. Inform patients that if they experience severe bloating, distention or abdominal pain following the 1st pkt, delay the 2nd administration until the symptoms resolve. Instruct patients to contact their healthcare provider if they develop signs/symptoms of dehydration, have trouble swallowing, or are prone to regurgitation or aspiration. Inform that product is not for direct ingestion.

STORAGE: 25°C (77°F); excursions permitted to 15-30°C (59-86°F).

PREVACID — lansoprazole

RX

Class: Proton pump inhibitor (PPI)

OTHER BRAND NAMES

Prevacid SoluTab

ADULT DOSAGE

Pathological Hypersecretory Conditions

Treatment Including Zollinger-Ellison Syndrome:

Initial: 60mg qd
Titrate: Individualize dose

Doses up to 90mg bid have been administered
Divide dose if >120mg/day

Active Duodenal Ulcer

Treatment:
15mg qd for 4 weeks

Maint of Healing of Duodenal Ulcer:
15mg qd

PEDIATRIC DOSAGE

Gastroesophageal Reflux Disease

Symptomatic GERD:
1-11 Years:
≤30kg: 15mg qd for up to 12 weeks; may increase up to 30mg bid after ≥2 weeks if still symptomatic
>30kg: 30mg qd for up to 12 weeks; may increase up to 30mg bid after ≥2 weeks if still symptomatic

Symptomatic Nonerosive GERD:
12-17 Years:
15mg qd for up to 8 weeks

NSAID-Associated Gastric Ulcer

Healing:
30mg qd for 8 weeks

Risk Reduction:
15mg qd for up to 12 weeks

Helicobacter pylori Eradication

W/ Duodenal Ulcer Disease to Reduce the Risk of Duodenal Ulcer Recurrence:

Triple Therapy:
30mg cap + clarithromycin 500mg + amoxicillin 1000mg, all bid for 10 or 14 days

Dual Therapy:
Allergic/Intolerant/Resistant to Clarithromycin:
30mg cap + amoxicillin 1000mg, all tid w/ for 14 days

Gastroesophageal Reflux Disease

Symptomatic GERD:
15mg qd for up to 8 weeks

Treatment of Erosive Esophagitis:
30mg qd for up to 8 weeks; may give for 8 more weeks if healing does not occur
May consider an additional 8-week course if there is a recurrence of erosive esophagitis

Maint of Healing of Erosive Esophagitis:
15mg qd

Gastric Ulcers

Benign:
30mg qd for up to 8 weeks

Treatment of Erosive Esophagitis:
1-11 Years:
≤30kg: 15mg qd for up to 12 weeks; may increase up to 30mg bid after ≥2 weeks if still symptomatic
>30kg: 30mg qd for up to 12 weeks; may increase up to 30mg bid after ≥2 weeks if still symptomatic
12-17 Years:
30mg qd for up to 8 weeks

DOSING CONSIDERATIONS

Hepatic Impairment
Severe: Consider dose adjustment

ADMINISTRATION

Oral route

Take ac.

Cap
Swallow whole; do not crush or chew
If trouble swallowing, may sprinkle intact granules on 1 tbsp of either applesauce, Ensure pudding, cottage cheese, yogurt or strained pears, or into 60mL of either apple juice, orange juice, or tomato juice and swallow immediately.
NG Tube (≥16 French):
Mix intact granules into 40mL of apple juice; do not use other liquids.
Inject through the NG tube into the stomach.
Flush w/ additional apple juice to clear the tube.

Disintegrating SoluTab
Do not break, crush, chew, or cut.
Allow tab to disintegrate on tongue, w/ or w/o water, until particles can be swallowed.
Oral Syringe:
Place a 15mg tab in oral syringe and draw up 4mL of water, or place a 30mg tab w/ 10mL of water.
Shake gently to allow for a quick dispersal.
After the tab has dispersed, administer w/in 15 min.
Refill the syringe w/ approx 2mL (5mL for the 30mg tab) of water, shake gently, and administer any remaining contents.
NG Tube (≥8 French):
Place a 15mg tab in a syringe and draw up 4mL of water, or place a 30mg tab w/ 10mL of water.
Shake gently to allow for a quick dispersal.
After the tab has dispersed, inject through the NG tube into the stomach w/in 15 min.
Refill the syringe w/ approx 5mL of water, shake gently, and flush the NG tube.

HOW SUPPLIED

Cap, Delayed-Release: 15mg, 30mg; **Tab, Disintegrating (SoluTab):** 15mg, 30mg

CONTRAINDICATIONS

Known severe hypersensitivity to any component of the formulation. When used w/ clarithromycin and/or amoxicillin, refer to the individual monographs.

P

WARNINGS/PRECAUTIONS

Symptomatic response does not preclude the presence of gastric malignancy. Acute interstitial nephritis reported; d/c if this develops. Cyanocobalamin (vitamin B12) deficiency may occur due to malabsorption with daily long-term treatment (eg, >3 yrs) with any acid-suppressing medications. May increase risk for *Clostridium difficile*-associated diarrhea (CDAD), especially in hospitalized patients. May increase risk for osteoporosis-related fractures of the hip, wrist, or spine, especially with high-dose and long-term therapy. Use lowest dose and shortest duration appropriate to the condition being treated. Hypomagnesemia reported; Mg^{2+} replacement and discontinuation of therapy may be required. (Tab, Disintegrating) Contains phenylalanine.

ADVERSE REACTIONS

Abdominal pain, constipation, diarrhea, nausea, dizziness, headache.

DRUG INTERACTIONS

May reduce the absorption of drugs where gastric pH is an important determinant of bioavailability; ampicillin esters, ketoconazole, atazanavir, nelfinavir, iron salts, erlotinib and mycophenolate mofetil (MMF) absorption may decrease, while digoxin absorption may increase. May substantially decrease concentrations of HIV protease inhibitors (eg, atazanavir, nelfinavir); avoid coadministration. Caution in transplant patients receiving MMF. May increase theophylline clearance; may require theophylline dose titration when lansoprazole is started or stopped. Monitor for increases in INR and PT with warfarin. May increase tacrolimus levels. May elevate and prolong levels of MTX leading to toxicities; consider temporary withdrawal of therapy with high-dose MTX. Caution with digoxin or other drugs that may cause hypomagnesemia (eg, diuretics).

PATIENT CONSIDERATIONS

Assessment: Assess for hepatic insufficiency, risk for osteoporosis, phenylketonuria, previous hypersensitivity to the drug, pregnancy/nursing status, and possible drug interactions. Obtain baseline Mg^{2+} levels in patients expected to be on prolonged treatment.

Monitoring: Monitor for signs/symptoms of acute interstitial nephritis, cyanocobalamin deficiency, bone fractures, CDAD, hypersensitivity reactions, and other adverse reactions. Monitor Mg^{2+} levels periodically in patients expected to be on prolonged treatment.

Counseling: Advise to seek immediate medical attention if diarrhea does not improve or cardiovascular/neurological symptoms (eg, palpitations, dizziness, seizures, tetany) develop. Instruct to take exactly ud. Inform of alternative methods of administration if patient has swallowing difficulties.

STORAGE: 25°C (77°F); excursions permitted to 15-30°C (59-86°F).

PREVIDENT – sodium fluoride

RX

Class: Fluoride preparation

P

OTHER BRAND NAMES

PreviDent 5000 Plus, Denta 5000 Plus

ADULT DOSAGE

Dental Caries Prevention

Apply a thin ribbon to toothbrush and brush thoroughly qd for 2 min, preferably at hs; expectorate after use

PEDIATRIC DOSAGE

Prevention and Control of Dental Caries

6-16 Years:
Apply a thin ribbon to toothbrush and brush thoroughly qd for 2 min, preferably at hs; expectorate and rinse mouth thoroughly after use

ADMINISTRATION

Topical route (teeth)

For best results, do not eat, drink, or rinse for 30 min

HOW SUPPLIED

Gel: (PreviDent) 1.1% [2 oz (56g)]; **Cre:** (PreviDent 5000 Plus/Denta 5000 Plus) 1.1% [1.8 oz (51g)]

CONTRAINDICATIONS

Not for pediatrics <6 yrs unless recommended by dentist or physician.

WARNINGS/PRECAUTIONS

Prolonged ingestion may lead to dental fluorosis in pediatrics <6 yrs. Not for systemic treatment. Do not swallow.

ADVERSE REACTIONS

Allergic reactions.

PATIENT CONSIDERATIONS

Assessment: Assess for dental caries, dental fluorosis, patient age, and pregnancy/nursing status.

Monitoring: Monitor for allergic reactions and other idiosyncrasies.

Counseling: Instruct patient not to swallow after use. Adults should not eat, drink, or rinse for 30 min after use; however, pediatrics 6-16 yrs should rinse mouth thoroughly after use. Keep out of reach of children.

STORAGE: 20-25°C (68-77°F).

PREVNAR 13 – pneumococcal 13-valent conjugate vaccine (diphtheria CRM197 protein) RX

Class: Vaccine

ADULT DOSAGE

***Streptococcus pneumoniae* Immunization**

Active immunization for the prevention of pneumonia and invasive disease caused by *S. pneumoniae* serotypes 1, 3, 4, 5, 6A, 6B, 7F, 9V, 14, 18C, 19A, 19F, and 23F

≥50 Years:
0.5mL IM as a single dose

PEDIATRIC DOSAGE

***Streptococcus pneumoniae* Immunization**

6 Weeks-5 Years (Prior to 6th Birthday):
Active immunization for the prevention of invasive disease caused by *S. pneumoniae* serotypes 1, 3, 4, 5, 6A, 6B, 7F, 9V, 14, 18C, 19A, 19F, and 23F. Also indicated for active immunization for the prevention of otitis media caused by *S. pneumoniae* serotypes 4, 6B, 9V, 14, 18C, 19F, and 23F

Vaccination Schedule for Infants and Toddlers:
0.5mL IM as a 4-dose series at 2, 4, and 6 months of age (at intervals of 4-8 weeks), and then at 12-15 months of age (at least 2 months after 3rd dose); 1st dose may be given as early as 6 weeks of age

Vaccination Schedule for Unvaccinated Children 7 Months-5 Years:
7-11 Months: Three 0.5mL IM doses; administer first 2 doses at least 4 weeks apart, and 3rd dose after 1st birthday, at least 2 months after 2nd dose
12-23 Months: Two 0.5mL IM doses at least 2 months apart
24 Months-5 Years (Prior to 6th Birthday): One 0.5mL IM dose

Vaccination Schedule for Children 15 Months-5 Years Previously Vaccinated w/ Prevnar Pneumococcal 7-Valent Conjugate Vaccine:
May give 1 dose of Prevnar 13 to elicit immune response to the 6 additional serotypes; this catch-up dose should be administered at least 8 weeks after the final dose of Prevnar

6-17 Years (Prior to 18th Birthday):
Active immunization for the prevention of invasive disease caused by *S. pneumoniae* serotypes 1, 3, 4, 5, 6A, 6B, 7F, 9V, 14, 18C, 19A, 19F, and 23F

Vaccination Schedule:
0.5mL IM as a single dose; if Prevnar was previously administered, at least 8 weeks should elapse before receiving Prevnar 13

ADMINISTRATION

IM route

Shake vigorously immediately prior to use; do not use if the vaccine cannot be resuspended
Do not mix w/ other vaccines/products in the same syringe

When administered at the same time as another injectable vaccine(s), administer w/ different syringes and at different inj sites

Preferred Sites for Inj:
Infants: Anterolateral aspect of the thigh
Toddlers/Children/Adults: Deltoid muscle of the upper arm
Do not inject in the gluteal area or areas where there may be a major nerve trunk and/or blood vessel

HOW SUPPLIED

Inj: 0.5mL

CONTRAINDICATIONS

Severe allergic reaction (eg, anaphylaxis) to any component of Prevnar 13 or any diphtheria toxoid-containing vaccine.

WARNINGS/PRECAUTIONS

Epinephrine and other appropriate agents must be immediately available should an acute anaphylactic reaction occur following administration. Individuals w/ altered immunocompetence, including those at higher risk for invasive pneumococcal disease (eg, individuals w/ congenital or acquired splenic dysfunction, HIV infection, malignancy, hematopoietic stem cell transplant, nephrotic syndrome, preterm infants, children w/ sickle cell disease), may have reduced antibody responses to immunization. Apnea following IM vaccination observed in some premature infants; consider infant's medical status, and the potential benefits and possible risks of vaccination.

ADVERSE REACTIONS

Pain/redness/tenderness/swelling at inj site, irritability, decreased appetite, fever, increased/decreased sleep, limitation of arm movement, fatigue, headache, chills, muscle/joint pain, rash, vomiting.

DRUG INTERACTIONS

Patients receiving immunosuppressive therapy (eg, irradiation, corticosteroids, antimetabolites, alkylating agents, cytotoxic agents) may not respond optimally to active immunization. Prior receipt of Pneumovax 23 w/in 1 yr results in diminished immune responses to therapy.

PATIENT CONSIDERATIONS

Assessment: Assess for altered immunocompetence, hypersensitivity/vaccination history, pregnancy/nursing status, and possible drug interactions.

Monitoring: Monitor for anaphylactic/hypersensitivity reactions, inj-site reactions, and other possible adverse reactions.

Counseling: Inform of the potential benefits/risks of vaccination, and of the importance of completing the immunization series unless contraindicated. Instruct to report any suspected adverse reactions to physician.

STORAGE: After Shipping: May arrive at 2-25°C (36-77°F). Upon Receipt: 2-8°C (36-46°F). Do not freeze; discard if frozen.

PREVPAC – amoxicillin/clarithromycin/lansoprazole

RX

Class: H. pylori treatment combination

ADULT DOSAGE

Helicobacter pylori **Eradication**

***H. pylori* Infection and Duodenal Ulcer Disease (Active or 1-Year History):**
Usual: 30mg lansoprazole, 1g amoxicillin, and 500mg clarithromycin administered together bid (am and pm) for 10 or 14 days

PEDIATRIC DOSAGE

Pediatric use may not have been established

DOSING CONSIDERATIONS

Renal Impairment

Severe (w/ or w/o Coexisting Hepatic Impairment): May need to decrease dosage or prolong dosing intervals of clarithromycin
CrCl <30mL/min: Not recommended

Hepatic Impairment

Severe: Consider reduction of lansoprazole dosage

ADMINISTRATION

Oral route

Take each dose ac
Swallow each pill whole

HOW SUPPLIED

Cap: (Amoxicillin) 500mg; **Cap, Delayed-Release:** (Lansoprazole) 30mg; **Tab:** (Clarithromycin) 500mg

CONTRAINDICATIONS

Lansoprazole: Known severe hypersensitivity to any component of the formulation. **Amoxicillin:** History of severe hypersensitivity reactions (eg, anaphylaxis, Stevens-Johnson syndrome) to amoxicillin or other beta-lactam antibiotics (eg, penicillins, cephalosporins). **Clarithromycin:** Known hypersensitivity to clarithromycin, erythromycin, or any of the macrolide antibiotics. History of cholestatic jaundice/hepatic dysfunction associated w/ prior use of clarithromycin. History of QT prolongation or ventricular cardiac arrhythmia, including torsades de pointes. Concomitant administration w/ cisapride, pimozide, astemizole, terfenadine, ergotamine, dihydroergotamine, or HMG-CoA reductase inhibitors (statins) that are extensively metabolized by CYP3A4 (lovastatin or simvastatin). Concomitant administration w/ colchicine in patients w/ renal/hepatic impairment.

WARNINGS/PRECAUTIONS

Not recommended with CrCl <30mL/min. Lab test interactions may occur. Caution in elderly. **Amoxicillin:** Serious and occasionally fatal hypersensitivity (anaphylactic) reactions reported in patients on penicillin (PCN) therapy; caution with history of PCN hypersensitivity and/or a history of sensitivity to multiple allergens. Immediately d/c therapy and initiate appropriate treatment if severe acute hypersensitivity reactions occur. **Clarithromycin:** Use in pregnancy only when there is no appropriate alternative therapy. Exacerbation of symptoms of myasthenia gravis and new onset of myasthenic syndrome reported. Hepatic dysfunction reported; d/c immediately if signs/symptoms of hepatitis occur. May cause QT interval prolongation, arrhythmia, and torsades de pointes; avoid with ongoing proarrhythmic conditions (eg, uncorrected hypokalemia or hypomagnesemia), and clinically significant bradycardia. **Lansoprazole:** Symptomatic response does not preclude the presence of gastric malignancy. Acute interstitial nephritis (AIN) reported; d/c if AIN develops. Amoxicillin/Clarithromycin: *Clostridium difficile*-associated diarrhea (CDAD) reported; d/c if CDAD is suspected or confirmed. May result in bacterial resistance with prolonged use in the absence of proven or suspected bacterial infection, or a prophylactic indication; d/c if superinfections occur and institute appropriate therapy.

ADVERSE REACTIONS

Diarrhea, taste perversion, headache.

DRUG INTERACTIONS

See Contraindications. **Amoxicillin:** Probenecid decreases renal tubular secretion. Chloramphenicol, macrolides, sulfonamides, and tetracyclines may interfere with bactericidal effects of PCN. May affect the gut flora, leading to lower estrogen reabsorption and reduced efficacy of combined oral estrogen/progesterone contraceptives. **Clarithromycin:** Avoid with class IA (quinidine, procainamide) or class III (dofetilide, amiodarone, sotalol) antiarrhythmic agents. Hypotension may occur with calcium channel blockers metabolized by CYP3A4 (eg, verapamil, amlodipine, diltiazem). Concomitant use with oral hypoglycemic agents and/or insulin may result in significant hypoglycemia; monitor glucose levels. May increase theophylline, carbamazepine, digoxin, colchicine, tolterodine, itraconazole, and saquinavir levels. Tolterodine 1mg bid is recommended in patients deficient in CYP2D6 activity (poor metabolizers). Bradyarrhythmias and lactic acidosis observed with verapamil. May decrease zidovudine levels; separate administration by at least 2 hrs. Fluconazole, itraconazole, and saquinavir may increase levels. Ritonavir and atazanavir may increase clarithromycin exposure and significantly decrease 14-OH clarithromycin exposure; consider alternative antibacterial therapy for indications other than infections due to *Mycobacterium avium* complex. Do not coadminister doses >1000mg/day with protease inhibitors. Decrease dose by 50% when coadministered with atazanavir. May increase concentrations of CYP3A substrates, which may lead to increased/prolonged therapeutic and adverse effects; caution with CYP3A substrates, especially those with narrow safety margin (eg, carbamazepine) and/or extensively metabolized by CYP3A enzyme. CYP3A inducers (eg, efavirenz, nevirapine, rifampicin, rifabutin, rifapentine) may decrease clarithromycin levels and increase 14-OH clarithromycin levels; consider alternative antibacterial treatment. May increase exposure of sildenafil, tadalafil, and vardenafil; coadministration is not recommended. May increase midazolam exposure; dose adjustments may be necessary when oral midazolam is coadministered. Caution and consider appropriate dose adjustments with triazolam or alprazolam. CNS effects reported with triazolam. Torsades de pointes reported with quinidine or disopyramide; monitor ECG. Interactions with drugs not thought to be metabolized by CYP3A (eg, hexobarbital, phenytoin, valproate) reported. **Lansoprazole:** May elevate and prolong levels of methotrexate (MTX) and/or its metabolite, possibly leading to toxicities; consider temporary withdrawal of therapy with high-dose MTX. May reduce absorption of drugs where gastric pH is an important determinant of bioavailability (eg, absorption of ampicillin esters, ketoconazole, atazanavir, iron salts, erlotinib, and mycophenolate mofetil may decrease, while absorption of digoxin may increase). Caution with mycophenolate mofetil in transplant patients. May interact with drugs metabolized by CYP450 enzymes (CYP1A2, CYP2C9, CYP2C19, CYP2D6, CYP3A). May increase theophylline clearance; may require additional titration of theophylline dosage when lansoprazole is started or stopped. May increase tacrolimus levels, especially in transplant patients who are intermediate or poor metabolizers of CYP2C19. Delayed absorption and reduced bioavailability with sucralfate; give at least 30 min prior to sucralfate. **Clarithromycin/Lansoprazole:** May alter the anticoagulant effects of warfarin and other anticoagulants; monitor PT and INR. Refer to PI for additional drug interaction information.

PATIENT CONSIDERATIONS

Assessment: Assess for history of hypersensitivity to drug, macrolides, β-lactam antibiotics (PCNs, cephalosporins), or other allergens. Assess for ongoing proarrhythmic conditions, bradycardia, myasthenia gravis, renal/hepatic impairment, any other conditions where treatment is contraindicated or cautioned, pregnancy/nursing status, and possible drug interactions.

Monitoring: Monitor for hypersensitivity reactions, hepatic dysfunction, QT prolongation, CDAD, superinfections, exacerbation of myasthenia gravis symptoms, new onset of symptoms of myasthenic syndrome, AIN, and other adverse reactions. Periodically monitor renal/hepatic/hematopoietic function during prolonged therapy. Monitor PT/INR with warfarin and other anticoagulants.

Counseling: Inform about risks/benefits of therapy. Advise to report the use of any other medications. Advise that diarrhea may occur and will usually end if therapy is discontinued. Instruct to contact physician as soon as possible if watery/bloody stools (with/without stomach cramps and fever) develop even as late as 2 or more months after having taken the last dose of therapy. Counsel that therapy should only be used to treat bacterial, not viral, infections. Instruct to take exactly ud; inform that skipping doses or not completing full course may decrease effectiveness and increase antibiotic resistance. Instruct to immediately report and seek care for any cardiovascular/neurological symptoms.

STORAGE: 20-25°C (68-77°F). Protect from light and moisture.

PREZISTA — darunavir

RX

Class: Protease inhibitor

ADULT DOSAGE

HIV-1 Infection

Combination w/ Ritonavir (RTV) and Other Antiretrovirals:

Treatment-Naive:
800mg (8mL) + RTV 100mg (1.25mL) qd

Treatment-Experienced:

No Darunavir Resistance Associated Substitutions:
800mg (8mL) + RTV 100mg (1.25mL) qd

≥1 Darunavir Resistance Associated Substitution:
600mg (6mL) + RTV 100mg (1.25mL) bid

When Genotypic Testing is Not Feasible:
600mg (6mL) + RTV 100mg (1.25mL) bid

PEDIATRIC DOSAGE

HIV-1 Infection

Combination w/ Ritonavir (RTV) and Other Antiretrovirals:

3-<18 Years:

Treatment-Naive/Treatment-Experienced w/ No Darunavir Resistance Associated Substitutions:

≥10-<11kg: 350mg (3.6mL) + RTV 64mg (0.8mL) qd

≥11-<12kg: 385mg (4mL) + RTV 64mg (0.8mL) qd

≥12-<13kg: 420mg (4.2mL) + RTV 80mg (1mL) qd

≥13-<14kg: 455mg (4.6mL) + RTV 80mg (1mL) qd

≥14-<15kg: 490mg (5mL) + RTV 96mg (1.2mL) qd

≥15-<30kg: 600mg (6mL) + RTV 100mg (1.25mL) qd

≥30-<40kg: 675mg (6.8mL) + RTV 100mg (1.25mL) qd

≥40kg: 800mg (8mL) + RTV 100mg (1.25mL) qd

Treatment-Experienced w/ ≥1 Darunavir Resistance Associated Substitution:

≥10-<11kg: 200mg (2mL) + RTV 32mg (0.4mL) bid

≥11-<12kg: 220mg (2.2mL) + RTV 32mg (0.4mL) bid

≥12-<13kg: 240mg (2.4mL) + RTV 40mg (0.5mL) bid

≥13-<14kg: 260mg (2.6mL) + RTV 40mg (0.5mL) bid

≥14-<15kg: 280mg (2.8mL) + RTV 48mg (0.6mL) bid

≥15-<30kg: 375mg (3.8mL) + RTV 48mg (0.6mL) bid

≥30-<40kg: 450mg (4.6mL) + RTV 60mg (0.75mL) bid

≥40kg: 600mg (6mL) + RTV 100mg (1.25mL) bid

DOSING CONSIDERATIONS

Hepatic Impairment

Severe: Not recommended for use

ADMINISTRATION

Oral route

Take w/ food

Tab

Swallow whole w/ a drink

Sus

Shake well before each use

8mL darunavir dose should be taken as two 4mL administrations w/ the included oral dosing syringe

HOW SUPPLIED

Sus: 100mg/mL [200mL]; **Tab:** 75mg, 150mg, 600mg, 800mg

CONTRAINDICATIONS

Concomitant use w/ drugs that are highly dependent on CYP3A for clearance and for which elevated plasma concentrations are associated w/ serious and/or life-threatening events, and w/ certain other drugs that may lead to reduced efficacy of darunavir (eg, alfuzosin, dronedarone, colchicine, ranolazine, pimozide, dihydroergotamine, ergotamine, methylergonovine, cisapride, oral midazolam, triazolam, St. John's wort, lovastatin, simvastatin, rifampin, sildenafil [when used to treat pulmonary arterial HTN]).

WARNINGS/PRECAUTIONS

Must be coadministered w/ RTV and food to achieve desired effect. Drug-induced hepatitis and liver injury reported; consider performing increased AST/ALT monitoring in patients w/ underlying chronic hepatitis, cirrhosis, or those w/ pretreatment transaminase elevations. Consider interruption or discontinuation of therapy if evidence of new/worsening liver dysfunction occurs. Increased risk for liver function abnormalities in patients w/ preexisting liver dysfunction, including chronic active hepatitis B or C. Severe skin reactions sometimes accompanied by fever and/or transaminase elevations, Stevens-Johnson syndrome (rare), toxic epidermal necrolysis, drug rash w/ eosinophilia and systemic symptoms, and acute generalized exanthematous pustulosis reported; d/c if severe skin reactions develop. Caution in patients w/ a known sulfonamide allergy. New onset diabetes mellitus (DM), exacerbation of preexisting DM, hyperglycemia, and diabetic ketoacidosis reported. Immune reconstitution syndrome, autoimmune disorders (eg, Graves' disease, polymyositis, Guillain-Barre syndrome) in the setting of immune reconstitution, redistribution/accumulation of body fat, and increased bleeding in hemophilia type A and B reported. Caution in elderly.

ADVERSE REACTIONS

Diarrhea, N/V, headache, abdominal pain, rash, asthenia, anorexia, pruritus, fatigue, decreased appetite.

DRUG INTERACTIONS

See Contraindications. Avoid w/ tadalafil during initiation. Not recommended w/ lopinavir/RTV, saquinavir, apixaban, dabigatran etexilate, rivaroxaban, rifapentine, simeprevir, boceprevir, telaprevir, everolimus, salmeterol, avanafil, and other protease inhibitors. Not recommended w/ voriconazole unless an assessment comparing predicted benefit to risk ratio justifies use of voriconazole. May increase levels of indinavir, maraviroc, antiarrhythmics, digoxin, carbamazepine, trazodone, amitriptyline, desipramine, imipramine, nortriptyline, clarithromycin, anticoagulant, ketoconazole, itraconazole, rifabutin, antineoplastics, quetiapine, antipsychotics, β-blockers, calcium channel blockers, systemic corticosteroids, inhaled/nasal corticosteroid, bosentan, simeprevir, HMG-CoA reductase inhibitors, immunosuppressants, salmeterol, norbuprenorphine, avanafil, sildenafil for erectile dysfunction, vardenafil, tadalafil, sedatives/hypnotics, and CYP3A, CYP2D6, and P-gp substrates. May decrease levels of phenytoin, phenobarbital, warfarin, methadone, boceprevir, telaprevir, ethinyl estradiol, norethindrone, sertraline, and paroxetine. CYP3A inhibitors, P-gp inhibitors, ketoconazole, itraconazole, indinavir, simeprevir, and rifabutin may increase levels. CYP3A inducers, systemic dexamethasone, lopinavir/RTV, saquinavir, antineoplastics, boceprevir, and telaprevir may decrease levels. Give didanosine 1 hr before or 2 hrs after administration. Increased lumefantrine exposure may increase the risk of QT prolongation; caution w/ artemether/lumefantrine. May require initiation or dose adjustments of insulin or oral hypoglycemics for treatment of DM. May increase risk for development of systemic corticosteroid effects including Cushing's syndrome and adrenal suppression w/ corticosteroids metabolized by CYP3A. Refer to PI for dosing modifications when used w/ certain concomitant therapies.

PATIENT CONSIDERATIONS

Assessment: Assess for sulfonamide allergy, liver dysfunction, hemophilia, preexisting DM, pregnancy/nursing status, and possible drug interactions. Assess ability to swallow tab in children ≥15kg. In treatment-experienced patients, assess treatment history and perform phenotypic or genotypic testing.

Monitoring: Monitor for signs/symptoms of hepatotoxicity, severe skin reactions, new onset/exacerbation of DM, diabetic ketoacidosis, fat redistribution/accumulation, immune reconstitution syndrome, autoimmune disorders, and other adverse reactions. In patients w/ hemophilia, monitor

P

for bleeding events. Consider performing increased AST/ALT monitoring in patients w/ underlying chronic hepatitis, cirrhosis, or those w/ pretreatment transaminase elevations. Monitor INR during coadministration w/ warfarin.

Counseling: Inform that therapy is not a cure for HIV and that illnesses associated w/ HIV may continue. Advise to avoid doing things that can spread HIV infection to others. Instruct not to alter dose or d/c w/o consulting physician. Counsel to take drug immediately for missed dose <6 hrs and <12 hrs, for bid and qd dosing respectively, and to take the next dose at regular scheduled time. Instruct that if a dose is missed by >6 hrs or >12 hrs, for bid and qd dosing respectively, take the next dose as scheduled; instruct not to double the dose. Advise about the signs/symptoms of liver problems. Inform that mild to severe skin reactions may develop; advise to d/c immediately if signs/symptoms of severe skin reactions develop. Instruct to notify physician if taking any other prescription, OTC, or herbal medication. Instruct to use alternative contraceptive measures if on estrogen-based contraceptive during therapy. Inform that redistribution and accumulation of body fat may occur.

STORAGE: 25°C (77°F); excursions permitted to 15-30°C (59-86°F). (Sus) Do not refrigerate or freeze. Avoid exposure to excessive heat.

PRILOSEC – omeprazole

RX

Class: Proton pump inhibitor (PPI)

ADULT DOSAGE

***Helicobacter pylori* Eradication**

To Reduce the Risk of Duodenal Ulcer Recurrence:

Triple Therapy:
Omeprazole 20mg + clarithromycin 500mg + amoxicillin 1000mg, each given bid x 10 days. Give additional 18 days of omeprazole 20mg qd if ulcer is present at the time of initiation of therapy

Dual Therapy:
Omeprazole 40mg qd + clarithromycin 500mg tid x 14 days. Give additional 14 days of omeprazole 20mg qd if ulcer is present at the time of initiation of therapy

Active Duodenal Ulcer

20mg qd for 4 weeks; some patients may require an additional 4 weeks

Gastroesophageal Reflux Disease

Symptomatic Treatment:
20mg qd for up to 4 weeks

Erosive Esophagitis

Treatment Due to Acid-Mediated GERD:
20mg qd for 4-8 weeks. Efficacy used for >8 weeks has not been established. If a patient does not respond to 8 weeks of treatment, an additional 4 weeks may be given; if there is recurrence of erosive esophagitis or GERD symptoms, additional 4- to 8-week courses may be considered

Maint of Healing Due to Acid-Mediated GERD:
20mg qd. Controlled studies do not extend beyond 12 months

Gastric Ulcers

Active Benign:
40mg qd for 4-8 weeks

Pathological Hypersecretory Conditions

Long-Term Treatment:
Initial: 60mg qd
Titrate: Individualize and continue for as long as clinically indicated. Doses up to 120mg tid have been administered

Doses >80mg/day should be administered in divided doses

PEDIATRIC DOSAGE

Erosive Esophagitis

Treatment Due to Acid-Mediated GERD:
1 Month to <1 Year of Age:
3 to <5kg: 2.5mg qd for up to 6 weeks
5 to <10kg: 5mg qd for up to 6 weeks
≥10kg: 10mg qd for up to 6 weeks

1-16 Years:
5 to <10kg: 5mg qd for 4-8 weeks
10 to <20kg: 10mg qd for 4-8 weeks
≥20kg: 20mg qd for 4-8 weeks
Efficacy used for >8 weeks has not been established. If a patient does not respond to 8 weeks of treatment, an additional 4 weeks may be given; if there is recurrence of erosive esophagitis or GERD symptoms, additional 4- to 8-week courses may be considered

Maint of Healing Due to Acid-Mediated GERD:
1-16 Years:
5 to <10kg: 5mg qd
10 to <20kg: 10mg qd
≥20kg: 20mg qd
Controlled studies do not extend beyond 12 months

Gastroesophageal Reflux Disease

Symptomatic Treatment:
1-16 Years:
5 to <10kg: 5mg qd for up to 4 weeks
10 to <20kg: 10mg qd for up to 4 weeks
≥20kg: 20mg qd for up to 4 weeks

DOSING CONSIDERATIONS

Hepatic Impairment

Child-Pugh Class A, B, or C:

Reduce dose to 10mg qd when used for the maint of healing of erosive esophagitis

Other Important Considerations

Asian Population:

Reduce dose to 10mg qd when used for the maint of healing of erosive esophagitis

ADMINISTRATION

Oral route

Take ac.

May be used concomitantly w/ antacids.

Cap, Delayed-Release

Swallow whole; do not chew.

May also be opened and administered as follows if unable to swallow intact capsule:

1. Place 1 tablespoon of applesauce in a clean container; the applesauce used should not be hot and should be soft enough to be swallowed w/o chewing.
2. Open the cap and carefully empty all of the pellets inside the cap on the applesauce.
3. Mix the pellets w/ the applesauce and swallow applesauce and pellets immediately w/ a glass of cool water to ensure complete swallowing of the pellets. Do not chew/crush the pellets, and do not save for future use.

Oral Sus, Delayed-Release

Oral Administration in Water:

1. Empty the contents of a 2.5mg pkt into 5mL of water or 10mg pkt into 15mL of water.
2. Stir and leave 2-3 min to thicken.
3. Stir and drink w/in 30 min.
4. If any material remains after drinking, add more water, stir, and drink immediately.

Administration w/ Water via NG or Gastric Tube (Size 6 or Larger):

1. Add 5mL of water to a catheter-tipped syringe and then add the contents of a 2.5mg pkt (or 15mL of water for the 10mg pkt).
2. Immediately shake the syringe and leave 2-3 min to thicken.
3. Shake the syringe and inject through the NG or gastric tube into the stomach w/in 30 min.
4. Refill the syringe w/ an equal amount of water; shake and flush any remaining contents into the stomach.

HOW SUPPLIED

Cap, Delayed-Release: 10mg, 20mg, 40mg; **Oral Sus, Delayed-Release:** 2.5mg, 10mg (granules/pkt)

CONTRAINDICATIONS

Known hypersensitivity to substituted benzimidazoles or to any component of the formulation. Concomitant use w/ rilpivirine-containing products. When used w/ clarithromycin and amoxicillin, refer to the individual monographs.

WARNINGS/PRECAUTIONS

Symptomatic response to therapy does not preclude the presence of gastric malignancy. Atrophic gastritis reported w/ long-term use. Acute interstitial nephritis reported; d/c if this develops. Cyanocobalamin (vitamin B12) deficiency may occur due to malabsorption w/ daily long-term treatment (eg, >3 yrs) w/ any acid-suppressing medications. May increase risk of *Clostridium difficile*-associated diarrhea (CDAD), especially in hospitalized patients. May increase risk for osteoporosis-related fractures of the hip, wrist, or spine, especially w/ high-dose and long-term therapy. Use lowest dose and shortest duration appropriate to the condition being treated. Hypomagnesemia reported and may require Mg^{2+} replacement and discontinuation of therapy.

ADVERSE REACTIONS

Headache, abdominal pain, N/V, diarrhea, flatulence.

DRUG INTERACTIONS

See Contraindications. Decreased exposure of some antiretroviral drugs (eg, rilpivirine, atazanavir, nelfinavir) when used concomitantly w/ omeprazole may reduce antiviral effect and promote development of drug resistance. Increased exposure of other antiretroviral drugs (eg, saquinavir) may increase toxicity. Avoid concomitant use w/ atazanavir and nelfinavir. Increased INR and PT w/ concomitant warfarin; monitor INR and PT and adjust dose of warfarin, if needed. Concomitant use w/ methotrexate (MTX) may elevate and prolong serum levels of MTX and/or its metabolite, possibly leading to MTX toxicities; may consider temporary withdrawal of omeprazole in patients receiving high-dose MTX. Concomitant use of omeprazole 80mg reduced levels of active metabolite of clopidogrel and reduced platelet inhibition; avoid concomitant use and consider alternative antiplatelet therapy. Increased exposure of citalopram leading to increased risk of QT prolongation. Increased exposure of one of the active metabolites of cilostazol. Potential for increased exposure of phenytoin; monitor phenytoin levels and adjust dose as needed. Increased exposure of diazepam; monitor for increased sedation and reduce diazepam dose as needed. Potential for increased exposure of digoxin; monitor digoxin levels and adjust dose as needed. May reduce absorption of other drugs dependent on gastric pH for absorption (eg, iron salts, erlotinib, mycophenolate mofetil, ketoconazole) due to its effect on reducing intragastric acidity. Use w/ caution in transplant patients receiving mycophenolate mofetil. Potential for increased exposure of tacrolimus, especially in transplant patients who are intermediate or poor metabolizers of CYP2C19; monitor tacrolimus whole blood concentration and adjust dose as needed. Serum chromogranin A (CgA) levels increase secondary to PPI-induced decreases in gastric acidity and may cause false positive results in diagnostic investigations for neuroendocrine tumors; temporarily stop omeprazole treatment at least 14 days before assessing CgA levels and consider repeating the test if initial CgA levels are high. May cause hyper-response in gastrin secretion in response to secretin stimulation test, falsely suggesting gastrinoma; temporarily stop omeprazole treatment at least 14 days before assessing. False positive urine screening tests for tetrahydrocannabinol reported; consider alternative confirmatory method to verify positive results. Interactions w/ other drugs metabolized via CYP450 (eg, cyclosporine, disulfiram) reported; monitor and determine if necessary to adjust dose of these other drugs. Decreased exposure of omeprazole when used concomitantly w/ strong CYP2C19 or CYP3A4 inducers; avoid concomitant use w/ St. John's wort and rifampin. Increased exposure of omeprazole w/ CYP2C19 or CYP3A4 inhibitors; consider dose adjustment of omeprazole in patients w/ Zollinger-Ellison syndrome who may require higher doses and are taking voriconazole. Monitor Mg^{2+} levels prior to initiation and periodically during treatment in patients who take PPIs w/ medications such as digoxin or drugs that may cause hypomagnesemia (eg, diuretics). Refer to PI for further information on drug interactions.

PATIENT CONSIDERATIONS

Assessment: Assess for hypersensitivity to the drug or to substituted benzimidazoles, risk for osteoporosis-related fractures, hepatic impairment, pregnancy/nursing status, and possible drug interactions. Obtain baseline Mg^{2+} levels in patients expected to be on prolonged therapy.

Monitoring: Monitor for signs/symptoms of atrophic gastritis, acute interstitial nephritis, cyanocobalamin deficiency, bone fractures, hypersensitivity reactions, CDAD, and other adverse reactions. Monitor Mg^{2+} levels periodically in patients expected to be on prolonged therapy. Monitor INR and PT when given w/ warfarin.

Counseling: Inform to take exactly ud. Advise to report to physician if experiencing any signs/symptoms consistent w/ hypersensitivity reactions, acute interstitial nephritis, cyanocobalamin deficiency, CDAD, bone fracture, or hypomagnesemia. Advise to report to physician if starting treatment w/ clopidogrel, St. John's wort, or rifampin. Advise to notify physician if taking high-dose methotrexate.

STORAGE: Cap: 15-30°C (59-86°F). Protect from light and moisture. **Oral Sus:** 25°C (77°F); excursions permitted to 15-30°C (59-86°F).

PRINIVIL – lisinopril

RX

Class: ACE inhibitor

P

D/C when pregnancy is detected. Drugs that act directly on the renin-angiotensin system (RAS) can cause injury and death to the developing fetus.

ADULT DOSAGE

Hypertension

Initial: 10mg qd or 5mg qd in patients taking diuretics

Usual Range: 20-40mg qd. Doses up to 80mg have been used but do not appear to give a greater effect

May add a low-dose diuretic (eg, hydrochlorothiazide 12.5mg) if BP is not controlled

Heart Failure

Reduce Signs/Symptoms in Patients Not Responding Adequately to Diuretics and Digitalis:

Adjunct w/ Diuretics and (Usually) Digitalis:

Initial: 5mg qd; 2.5mg qd w/ hyponatremia (serum Na^+ <130mEq/L)

Max: 40mg qd

Diuretic dose may need to be adjusted to help minimize hypovolemia

Acute Myocardial Infarction

PEDIATRIC DOSAGE

Hypertension

≥6 Years:

GFR >30mL/min/1.73m²:

Initial: 0.07mg/kg qd (up to 5mg total)

Titrate: Adjust dose according to BP response

Max: 0.61mg/kg (up to 40mg) qd

Reduction of Mortality in Treatment of Hemodynamically Stable Patients w/in 24 Hrs of Acute MI (AMI):
5mg w/in 24 hrs of onset of symptoms, followed by 5mg after 24 hrs, 10mg after 48 hrs, and then 10mg qd for at least 6 weeks

In patients w/ low systolic BP (SBP) (100-120mmHg) during the first 3 days after infarct, initiate therapy w/ 2.5mg. If hypotension occurs (SBP ≤100mmHg) consider doses of 2.5mg or 5mg. D/C therapy if prolonged hypotension occurs (SBP <90mmHg for >1 hr)

DOSING CONSIDERATIONS

Renal Impairment

CrCl 10-30mL/min:
Reduce initial dose to 1/2 of the usual recommended dose (eg, HTN, 5mg; heart failure or AMI, 2.5mg)

Hemodialysis or CrCl <10mL/min:
Initial: 2.5mg qd

Pediatric Patients:
GFR <30mL/min/1.73m²: Not recommended

ADMINISTRATION

Oral route

HOW SUPPLIED

Tab: 5mg*, 10mg*, 20mg* *scored

CONTRAINDICATIONS

History of ACE inhibitor-associated angioedema or hypersensitivity, hereditary or idiopathic angioedema. Coadministration w/ aliskiren in patients w/ diabetes.

WARNINGS/PRECAUTIONS

Head/neck angioedema reported; d/c and administer appropriate therapy. Patients w/ a history of angioedema unrelated to ACE inhibitor therapy may be at increased risk of angioedema during therapy. Higher rate of angioedema in blacks than nonblacks. Intestinal angioedema reported; monitor for abdominal pain. Anaphylactoid reactions reported during desensitization w/ hymenoptera venom, dialysis w/ high-flux membranes, and LDL apheresis w/ dextran sulfate absorption. May cause changes in renal function, including acute renal failure, especially in patients whose renal function may depend in part on the activity of the RAS; consider withholding or discontinuing therapy if a clinically significant decrease in renal function develops. May cause symptomatic hypotension, sometimes complicated by oliguria, progressive azotemia, acute renal failure, or death; closely monitor patients at risk of excessive hypotension for the first 2 weeks of treatment and whenever therapy and/or diuretic dose is increased. Avoid in patients who are hemodynamically unstable after an AMI. Symptomatic hypotension may occur in patients w/ severe aortic stenosis or hypertrophic cardiomyopathy. Hypotension may occur w/ major surgery or during anesthesia. May cause hyperkalemia; periodically monitor serum K^+ during therapy. Associated w/ a syndrome that starts w/ cholestatic jaundice or hepatitis and progresses to fulminant hepatic necrosis and sometimes death; d/c therapy if jaundice or marked hepatic enzyme elevations develop.

ADVERSE REACTIONS

Headache, dizziness, cough, hypotension, chest pain, increased creatinine, hyperkalemia, syncope.

DRUG INTERACTIONS

See Contraindications. Initiation of therapy in patients on diuretics may result in excessive reduction of BP. Decrease or d/c diuretic or increase the salt intake prior to initiation of therapy; if this is not possible, reduce the starting dose of lisinopril. Attenuates K^+ loss caused by thiazide-type diuretics. K^+-sparing diuretics (eg, spironolactone, amiloride, triamterene) may increase hyperkalemia risk; frequently monitor serum K^+ if concomitant use of such agents is indicated. Increased risk of hyperkalemia w/ K^+ supplements or K^+-containing salt substitutes. May cause an increased blood-glucose-lowering effect w/ risk of hypoglycemia w/ antidiabetic medicines (insulins, oral hypoglycemic agents). NSAIDs, including selective COX-2 inhibitors, may result in deterioration of renal function, including possible acute renal failure in elderly, volume depleted or patients w/ compromised renal function. Antihypertensive effect may be attenuated by NSAIDs. Dual blockade of the RAS is associated w/ increased risks of hypotension, syncope, hyperkalemia, and changes in renal function (including acute renal failure); avoid combined use of RAS inhibitors, and monitor BP, renal function, and electrolytes w/ other agents that affect the RAS. Avoid w/ aliskiren in patients w/ renal impairment (GFR <60mL/min). Lithium toxicity reported; monitor serum lithium levels during concurrent use. Nitritoid reactions reported w/ injectable gold. Increased BUN and SrCr w/ diuretics. Coadministration w/ mTOR inhibitors (eg, temsirolimus, sirolimus, everolimus) may increase risk for angioedema.

PATIENT CONSIDERATIONS

Assessment: Assess for hypersensitivity to the drug, hereditary or idiopathic angioedema, history of ACE inhibitor-associated angioedema, risk factors for hyperkalemia, risk of excessive hypotension, renal artery stenosis, severe aortic stenosis or hypertrophic cardiomyopathy, renal impairment, pregnancy/nursing status, and possible drug interactions.

Monitoring: Monitor for angioedema, anaphylactoid reactions, hyperkalemia, and other adverse reactions. Monitor BP, LFTs, serum K^+, and renal function.

Counseling: Inform of pregnancy risks and discuss treatment options for women planning to become pregnant; instruct to report pregnancy to physician as soon as possible. Instruct to immediately report signs/symptoms of angioedema and to avoid drug until they have consulted w/ prescribing physician. Instruct to report lightheadedness, especially during 1st few days of therapy; if syncope occurs, advise to d/c therapy until physician is consulted. Advise that excessive perspiration, dehydration, and other causes of volume depletion (eg, vomiting, diarrhea) may lead to excessive fall in BP; instruct to consult w/ a physician. Advise not to use salt substitutes containing K^+ w/o consulting physician. Advise diabetic patients treated w/ oral antidiabetic agents or insulin to closely monitor for hypoglycemia, especially during the 1st month of combined use. Instruct to report promptly any indication of infection, which may be a sign of leukopenia/ neutropenia.

STORAGE: 15-30°C (59-86°F). Protect from moisture.

PRISTIQ – desvenlafaxine

RX

Class: Serotonin and norepinephrine reuptake inhibitor (SNRI)

Antidepressants increased the risk of suicidal thoughts and behavior in children, adolescents, and young adults in short-term studies. Monitor and observe closely for worsening, and emergence of suicidal thoughts and behaviors. Not approved for use in pediatric patients.

ADULT DOSAGE

Major Depressive Disorder

50mg qd

50-400mg/day were effective; no additional benefit at doses >50mg/day and more frequent adverse reactions reported at higher doses

Switching from Other Antidepressants:

May need to taper initial antidepressant

Dosing Considerations with MAOIs

Switching to/from an MAOI for Psychiatric Disorders:

Allow at least 14 days between discontinuation of an MAOI and initiation of desvenlafaxine, and allow at least 7 days between discontinuation of desvenlafaxine and initiation of an MAOI

W/ Other MAOIs (eg, Linezolid, IV Methylene Blue):

Do not start desvenlafaxine in a patient being treated w/ linezolid or IV methylene blue

In patients already receiving desvenlafaxine, if acceptable alternatives are not available and benefits outweigh risks, d/c desvenlafaxine promptly and administer linezolid or IV methylene blue; monitor for serotonin syndrome for 7 days or until 24 hrs after the last dose of linezolid or IV methylene blue, whichever comes 1st. May resume desvenlafaxine therapy 24 hrs after the last dose of linezolid or IV methylene blue

PEDIATRIC DOSAGE

Pediatric use may not have been established

P

DOSING CONSIDERATIONS

Renal Impairment

Moderate (CrCl 30-50mL/min):

Max: 50mg/day

Severe (CrCl <30mL/min)/ESRD:

Max: 25mg qd or 50mg qod; do not give supplemental doses after dialysis

Hepatic Impairment

Moderate to Severe:

Usual: 50mg/day

Max: Dose escalation >100mg/day not recommended

Discontinuation

Gradually reduce dose; if intolerable symptoms occur following a decrease in dose or upon discontinuation, consider resuming the previously prescribed dose and continue decreasing the dose at a more gradual rate. The 25mg dose is available for discontinuing therapy

ADMINISTRATION

Oral route

Take at approx the same time each day, w/ or w/o food.
Swallow tab whole w/ fluid; do not divide, crush, chew, or dissolve.

HOW SUPPLIED

Tab, Extended-Release: 25mg, 50mg, 100mg

CONTRAINDICATIONS

Hypersensitivity to desvenlafaxine succinate, venlafaxine HCl, or to any excipients in the formulation. Use of an MAOI intended to treat psychiatric disorders either concomitantly or w/in 7 days of stopping treatment. Treatment w/in 14 days of stopping an MAOI to treat psychiatric disorders. Starting treatment in patients being treated w/ other MAOIs (eg, linezolid, IV methylene blue).

WARNINGS/PRECAUTIONS

Not approved for the treatment of bipolar depression. Serotonin syndrome reported; d/c immediately if symptoms occur and initiate supportive symptomatic treatment. Caution w/ preexisting HTN or cardiovascular (CV)/cerebrovascular conditions that might be compromised by increases in BP. Consider dose reduction or discontinuation of therapy if sustained increases in BP occur. May increase risk of bleeding events. Pupillary dilation that occurs following use may trigger an angle-closure attack in a patient w/ anatomically narrow angles who does not have a patent iridectomy. Activation of mania/hypomania reported. Discontinuation symptoms reported. Avoid abrupt discontinuation. Seizures reported. Hyponatremia may occur; caution in elderly and volume-depleted patients. Consider discontinuation in patients w/ symptomatic hyponatremia. Interstitial lung disease and eosinophilic pneumonia may occur; consider diagnosis for either in patients w/ progressive dyspnea, cough, or chest discomfort, and consider discontinuing therapy. False (+) urine immunoassay screening tests for phencyclidine and amphetamines reported.

ADVERSE REACTIONS

N/V, dry mouth, dizziness, insomnia, somnolence, hyperhidrosis, constipation, anxiety, decreased appetite, tremor, mydriasis, erectile dysfunction, anorgasmia, fatigue, vision blurred.

DRUG INTERACTIONS

See Contraindications. Avoid w/ other desvenlafaxine-containing products or venlafaxine products; may increase levels and increase dose-related adverse reactions. Avoid alcohol consumption. May cause serotonin syndrome w/ other serotonergic drugs (eg, triptans, TCAs, fentanyl) and w/ drugs that impair metabolism of serotonin; d/c desvenlafaxine and any concomitant serotonergic agent immediately if serotonin syndrome occurs. Caution w/ NSAIDs, aspirin (ASA), warfarin, and other drugs that affect coagulation or bleeding, due to increased risk of bleeding. May increase risk of hyponatremia w/ diuretics. Potent CYP3A4 inhibitors (eg, ketoconazole) may increase levels. CYP2D6 substrates (eg, desipramine, atomoxetine, dextromethorphan) should be dosed at the original level when coadministered w/ 100mg desvenlafaxine or lower, or when desvenlafaxine is discontinued; reduce the dose of these substrates by up to 1/2 if coadministered w/ 400mg of desvenlafaxine.

PATIENT CONSIDERATIONS

Assessment: Assess for risk for bipolar disorder, history of mania/hypomania, seizure disorders, HTN, CV/cerebrovascular conditions, susceptibility to angle-closure glaucoma, volume depletion, hypersensitivity to the drug, hepatic/renal impairment, pregnancy/nursing status, and possible drug interactions.

Monitoring: Monitor for signs/symptoms of clinical worsening (eg, suicidality, unusual changes in behavior), serotonin syndrome, abnormal bleeding, angle-closure glaucoma, activation of mania/hypomania, seizures, hyponatremia, interstitial lung disease, eosinophilic pneumonia, and other adverse reactions. Monitor BP, LFTs, and renal function. Monitor for discontinuation symptoms (eg, dysphoric mood, irritability, agitation) when discontinuing therapy. Carefully monitor patients receiving concomitant warfarin therapy when treatment w/ desvenlafaxine is initiated or discontinued. Periodically reassess to determine the need for continued treatment.

Counseling: Advise patients, families, and caregivers about the benefits and risks of treatment and counsel on its appropriate use. Counsel patients, families, and caregivers to look for the emergence of suicidality, especially early during treatment and when the dose is adjusted up or down. Caution about the risk of serotonin syndrome, particularly w/ the concomitant use w/ other serotonergic agents. Inform that concomitant use w/ ASA, NSAIDs, warfarin, or other drugs that affect coagulation may increase the risk of bleeding. Advise to monitor BP regularly, to observe for signs/symptoms of activation of mania/hypomania, to avoid alcohol, and not to d/c therapy w/o notifying physician. Inform that discontinuation effects may occur when stopping treatment and a dose of 25mg/day is available for discontinuing therapy. Caution about risk of angle-closure glaucoma. Caution against operating hazardous machinery (including automobiles) until reasonably certain that therapy does not adversely affect ability to engage in such activities. Advise to notify physician if allergic phenomena develop, if pregnant, intending to become pregnant, or if breastfeeding. Inform that an inert matrix tab may pass in the stool or via colostomy.

STORAGE: 20-25°C (68-77°F); excursions permitted to 15-30°C (59-86°F).

ProAir HFA – albuterol sulfate

RX

Class: $Beta_2$ agonist

ADULT DOSAGE

Bronchospasm

Treatment/Prevention of Bronchospasm w/ Reversible Obstructive Airway Disease:
2 inh q4-6h; 1 inh q4h may be sufficient in some patients

Exercise-Induced Bronchospasm

Prevention:
2 inh 15-30 min prior to exercise

PEDIATRIC DOSAGE

Bronchospasm

Treatment/Prevention of Bronchospasm w/ Reversible Obstructive Airway Disease:
≥4 Years:
2 inh q4-6h; 1 inh q4h may be sufficient in some patients

Exercise-Induced Bronchospasm

Prevention:
≥4 Years:
2 inh 15-30 min prior to exercise

DOSING CONSIDERATIONS

Elderly
Start at lower end of dosing range

ADMINISTRATION

Oral inh route

Shake well before each spray.

Priming
Prime inhaler before using for the 1st time and when inhaler has not been used for >2 weeks by releasing 3 sprays into the air, away from the face.

HOW SUPPLIED

MDI: 90mcg of albuterol base/inh [200 actuations]

CONTRAINDICATIONS

History of hypersensitivity to albuterol or any components of the medication.

WARNINGS/PRECAUTIONS

May produce paradoxical bronchospasm; d/c immediately and institute alternative therapy if this occurs. More doses than usual may be a marker of destabilization of asthma and may require reevaluation of the patient and treatment regimen; anti-inflammatory treatment (eg, corticosteroids) may be needed. May produce clinically significant cardiovascular (CV) effects; may need to d/c. ECG changes and immediate hypersensitivity reactions may occur. Fatalities reported w/ excessive use. Caution w/ CV disorders (eg, coronary insufficiency, arrhythmias, HTN), convulsive disorders, hyperthyroidism, diabetes mellitus (DM), and in patients unusually responsive to sympathomimetic amines. May produce significant hypokalemia and BP changes. Aggravation of preexisting DM and ketoacidosis reported w/ large doses of IV albuterol. Caution w/ renal impairment.

ADVERSE REACTIONS

Pharyngitis, headache, rhinitis, dizziness, musculoskeletal pain, tachycardia.

DRUG INTERACTIONS

Avoid w/ other short-acting sympathomimetic aerosol bronchodilators; caution w/ additional adrenergic drugs administered by any route. Use w/ β-blockers may block pulmonary effect and produce severe bronchospasm in asthmatic patients; avoid concomitant use. If needed, consider cardioselective β-blockers and use w/ caution. ECG changes and/or hypokalemia caused by non-K^+-sparing diuretics (eg, loop, thiazide) may be acutely worsened; use caution and consider monitoring K^+ levels. May decrease digoxin levels; monitor serum digoxin levels. Use extreme caution w/ MAOIs and TCAs, or w/in 2 weeks of discontinuation of such agents; consider alternative therapy in patients taking MAOIs or TCAs.

PATIENT CONSIDERATIONS

Assessment: Assess for history of hypersensitivity to drug, CV disorders, convulsive disorders, hyperthyroidism, DM, renal impairment, pregnancy/nursing status, and possible drug interactions. Assess use in patients unusually responsive to sympathomimetic amines.

Monitoring: Monitor for paradoxical bronchospasm, deterioration of asthma, CV effects, ECG changes, hypokalemia, immediate hypersensitivity reactions, and other adverse reactions. Monitor BP, HR, and ECG changes. Monitor renal function in elderly.

Counseling: Inform not to increase dose/frequency of doses w/o consulting physician. Advise to seek immediate medical attention if treatment becomes less effective for symptomatic relief, symptoms become worse, and/or there is a need to use product more frequently than usual. Instruct to keep plastic mouthpiece clean to prevent medication build-up and blockage; advise to wash, shake to remove excess water, and air dry mouthpiece thoroughly at least once a week. Inform that inhaler may cease to deliver medication if not cleaned properly. Inform that drug may cause paradoxical bronchospasm; instruct to d/c if this occurs. Instruct to take concurrent inhaled drugs and other asthma medications only ud. Inform of the common adverse effects of treatment (eg, palpitations, chest pain, rapid HR, tremor, nervousness). Instruct to notify physician if pregnant/nursing. Instruct to use only w/ supplied actuator and not to use actuator w/ other aerosol medications.

STORAGE: 15-25°C (59-77°F). Protect from freezing and direct sunlight. Contents under pressure; do not puncture or incinerate. Exposure to temperatures >49°C (120°F) may cause bursting.

PROBENECID/COLCHICINE — colchicine/probenecid

RX

Class: Uricosuric

ADULT DOSAGE

Gouty Arthritis

Treatment of chronic gouty arthritis when complicated by frequent, recurrent acute attacks of gout

Usual: 1 tab qd for 1 week, then 1 tab bid thereafter

Titrate: Daily dose may be increased by 1 tab every 4 weeks w/in tolerance (and usually not >4 tabs/day) if symptoms are not controlled or the 24-hr uric acid excretion is <700mg

When acute attacks have been absent for ≥6 months and serum urate levels remain w/in normal limits, the daily dose may be decreased by 1 tab every 6 months

PEDIATRIC DOSAGE

Pediatric use may not have been established

DOSING CONSIDERATIONS

Renal Impairment

2 tabs/day may be adequate

Chronic Renal Insufficiency (GFR ≤30mL/min): Probenecid may not be effective

Adverse Reactions

Gastric Intolerance: May be indicative of overdose; correct by decreasing the dose

ADMINISTRATION

Oral route

Do not initiate therapy until an acute gouty attack has subsided; however, if an acute attack is precipitated during therapy, probenecid and colchicine may be continued w/o changing the dose, and additional colchicine or other appropriate therapy should be given to control the acute attack

A liberal fluid intake is recommended, as well as sufficient sodium bicarbonate (3-7.5g/day) or potassium citrate (7.5g/day) to maintain an alkaline urine

HOW SUPPLIED

Tab: (Probenecid/Colchicine) 500mg/0.5mg

CONTRAINDICATIONS

Hypersensitivity to this product or to probenecid or colchicine. Blood dyscrasias, uric acid kidney stones, children <2 yrs of age, pregnancy, initiating therapy before acute gout attack subsides, coadministration with salicylates.

WARNINGS/PRECAUTIONS

Exacerbation of gout may occur. Severe allergic reactions and anaphylaxis reported rarely; d/c if hypersensitivity occurs. Caution with history of peptic ulcer. Hematuria, renal colic, costovertebral pain, and formation of uric acid stones reported; maintain liberal fluid intake and alkalization of urine. May not be effective in chronic renal insufficiency (GFR ≤30mL/min). Reversible azoospermia reported. Colchicine is an established mutagen; may be carcinogenic.

ADVERSE REACTIONS

Headache, dizziness, fever, pruritus, acute gouty arthritis, purpura, leukopenia, peripheral neuritis, muscular weakness, N/V, urticaria, anemia, dermatitis, alopecia.

DRUG INTERACTIONS

See Contraindications. Salicylates and pyrazinamide antagonize uricosuric effects; use acetaminophen (APAP) if mild analgesic is needed. Probenecid increases plasma levels of penicillin and other β-lactams; psychic disturbances reported. Methotrexate levels increased with coadministration; reduce dose and monitor levels. May prolong/enhance effects of sulfonylureas; increased risk of hypoglycemia. Increased $T_{1/2}$ and levels of indomethacin, naproxen, ketoprofen, meclofenamate, lorazepam, APAP, and rifampin. Increased levels of sulindac and sulfonamides; monitor sulfonamide levels with prolonged use. Inhibits renal transport of amino hippuric acid, aminosalicylic acid, indomethacin, sodium iodomethamate and related iodinated organic acids, 17-ketosteroids, pantothenic acid, phenolsulfonphthalein, sulfonamides, and sulfonylureas. Possible falsely high plasma levels of theophylline. Decreases hepatic/renal excretion of sulfobromophthalein. May require significantly less thiopental for induction of anesthesia.

PATIENT CONSIDERATIONS

Assessment: Assess for known blood dyscrasias, uric acid kidney stones, acute/chronic gout attack, history of peptic ulcer, renal function, hypersensitivity to drug, pregnancy/nursing status, and possible drug interactions.

Monitoring: Monitor for signs/symptoms of gout exacerbation, allergic reactions, hematuria, renal colic, costovertebral pain, and uric acid stone formation. Monitor serum uric acid levels.

Counseling: Inform about the risks and benefits of therapy and importance of liberal fluid intake. Advise to seek medical attention if symptoms of allergic reaction, hematuria, renal colic, or costovertebral pain occur.

STORAGE: 20-25°C (68-77°F). Protect from light.

P

PROCARDIA XL – nifedipine

RX

Class: Calcium channel blocker (CCB) (dihydropyridine)

OTHER BRAND NAMES

Nifedical XL

ADULT DOSAGE

Angina

Vasospastic Angina/Chronic Stable Angina (Effort-Associated Angina)

Initial: 30 or 60mg qd

Titrate: Adjust dose over a 7- to 14-day period, but may proceed more rapidly if symptoms warrant

Max: 120mg/day; caution w/ doses >90mg

Use nearest equivalent total daily dose when switching to extended-release tab from nifedipine caps alone or in combination w/ other antianginal medications; titrate as clinically warranted

Hypertension

Initial: 30 or 60mg qd

Titrate: Adjust dose over a 7- to 14-day period, but may proceed more rapidly if symptoms warrant

PEDIATRIC DOSAGE

Pediatric use may not have been established

Max: 120mg/day

May use alone or in combination w/ other antihypertensive agents

DOSING CONSIDERATIONS

Discontinuation

Gradually decrease w/ close supervision

Other Important Considerations

Avoid w/ grapefruit juice

ADMINISTRATION

Oral route

Swallow tab whole; do not crush, divide, or chew.

HOW SUPPLIED

Tab, Extended-Release: 30mg, 60mg, 90mg; (Nifedical XL) 30mg, 60mg

CONTRAINDICATIONS

Known hypersensitivity reaction to nifedipine.

WARNINGS/PRECAUTIONS

May cause excessive hypotension; monitor BP initially and w/ titration. May increase frequency, duration, and/or severity of angina or acute MI (AMI), particularly w/ severe obstructive coronary artery disease (CAD). May develop heart failure (HF) after beginning therapy, w/ a higher risk in patients w/ tight aortic stenosis. GI obstruction and bezoars reported rarely; caution w/ altered GI anatomy (eg, severe GI narrowing, colon cancer, small bowel obstruction), hypomotility disorders, and concomitant medications (eg, H_2-histamine blockers, NSAIDs, laxatives). Tab adherence to GI wall w/ ulceration reported. Mild to moderate peripheral edema, typically associated w/ arterial vasodilation, may occur; differentiate peripheral edema from the effects of increasing left ventricular dysfunction in patients w/ angina or HTN complicated by CHF. Transient elevations of enzymes (eg, alkaline phosphatase, creatine phosphokinase, lactate dehydrogenase, AST, ALT), cholestasis w/ or w/o jaundice, and allergic hepatitis reported (rare). May decrease platelet aggregation and increase bleeding time. Positive direct Coombs test w/ or w/o hemolytic anemia reported. Reversible elevation in BUN and SrCr reported rarely in patients w/ chronic renal insufficiency. Decreased clearance resulting in higher exposure reported in the elderly.

ADVERSE REACTIONS

Edema, headache.

DRUG INTERACTIONS

β-blockers may increase the likelihood of CHF, severe hypotension, or angina exacerbation; avoid abrupt β-blocker withdrawal. Severe hypotension and/or increased fluid volume reported together w/ β-blockers and fentanyl or other narcotic analgesics; if condition permits, allow sufficient time (at least 36 hrs) for nifedipine to be washed out prior to surgery w/ fentanyl. May increase digoxin levels; monitor digoxin when initiating, adjusting, and discontinuing nifedipine to avoid possible over- or under-digitalization. May increase PT w/ coumarin anticoagulants. Cimetidine may increase levels; caution during titration. Monitor w/ other medications known to lower BP. Phenytoin may lower systemic exposure to nifedipine; avoid w/ phenytoin or any known CYP3A4 inducer. CYP3A inhibitors (eg, fluconazole, itraconazole, clarithromycin) may result in increased exposure to nifedipine when coadministered; monitor carefully and consider initiating nifedipine at the lowest dose available. Grapefruit juice increases levels; avoid ingestion of grapefruit/grapefruit juice while on therapy.

PATIENT CONSIDERATIONS

Assessment: Assess for acute coronary syndrome, severe obstructive CAD, aortic stenosis, recent β-blocker withdrawal, renal impairment, altered GI anatomy, hypomotility disorders, hypersensitivity to the drug, pregnancy/nursing status, and possible drug interactions.

Monitoring: Monitor for excessive hypotension, increased frequency, duration, and/or severity of angina and/or AMI, HF, signs/symptoms of GI obstruction, bezoars, peripheral edema, cholestasis w/ or w/o jaundice, allergic hepatitis, and other adverse reactions. Monitor BP, BUN, SrCr, and for decreased platelet aggregation and increased bleeding time.

Counseling: Inform about potential risks/benefits of drug. Instruct to notify physician if pregnant/nursing or if any adverse reactions occur. Inform that it is normal to occasionally observe a tab-like material in the stool.

STORAGE: Protect from moisture and humidity. **Procardia XL:** <30°C (86°F). **Nifedical XL:** 25°C (77°F); excursions permitted to 15-30°C (59-86°F).

ProCentra — dextroamphetamine sulfate

CII

Class: CNS stimulant

High potential for abuse. Prolonged use may lead to drug dependence and must be avoided. Misuse may cause sudden death and serious cardiovascular (CV) adverse events.

ADULT DOSAGE

Narcolepsy

Initial: 10mg/day

Titrate: May increase in increments of 10mg at weekly intervals until optimal response is obtained

Usual: 5-60mg/day in divided doses

Give 1st dose on awakening; additional doses (1 or 2) at intervals of 4-6 hrs

PEDIATRIC DOSAGE

Narcolepsy

Usual: 5-60mg/day in divided doses

Give 1st dose on awakening; additional doses (1 or 2) at intervals of 4-6 hrs

6-12 Years:

Initial: 5mg/day

Titrate: May increase in increments of 5mg at weekly intervals until optimal response is obtained

≥12 Years:

Initial: 10mg/day

Titrate: May increase in increments of 10mg at weekly intervals until optimal response is obtained

Attention-Deficit Hyperactivity Disorder

3-5 Years:

Initial: 2.5mg/day

Titrate: May increase in increments of 2.5mg at weekly intervals until optimal response is obtained

≥6 Years:

Initial: 5mg qd or bid

Titrate: May increase in increments of 5mg at weekly intervals until optimal response is obtained. Only in rare cases will it be necessary to exceed a total of 40mg/day

Give 1st dose on awakening; additional doses (1 or 2) at intervals of 4-6 hrs

P

DOSING CONSIDERATIONS

Adverse Reactions

Narcolepsy:

Reduce dose if bothersome adverse reactions appear (eg, insomnia, anorexia)

ADMINISTRATION

Oral route

Avoid late pm doses.

HOW SUPPLIED

Oral Sol: 5mg/5mL (473mL)

CONTRAINDICATIONS

Advanced arteriosclerosis, symptomatic CV disease (CVD), moderate to severe HTN, hyperthyroidism, known hypersensitivity or idiosyncrasy to the sympathomimetic amines, glaucoma, agitated states, and history of drug abuse. During or w/in 14 days following MAOI use.

WARNINGS/PRECAUTIONS

Sudden death reported in children and adolescents w/ structural cardiac abnormalities or other serious heart problems. Sudden death, stroke, and MI reported in adults. Avoid w/ known serious structural cardiac abnormalities, cardiomyopathy, serious heart rhythm abnormalities, coronary artery disease, or other serious cardiac problems. May cause a modest increase in average BP and HR. Prior to treatment, obtain medical history and perform physical exam to assess for presence of cardiac disease. Promptly perform cardiac evaluation if symptoms of cardiac disease develop during treatment. May exacerbate symptoms of behavior disturbance and thought disorder in patients w/ preexisting psychotic disorder. May induce mixed/manic episodes in patients w/ comorbid bipolar disorder. May cause treatment-emergent psychotic or manic symptoms in children and adolescents w/o a prior history of psychotic illness or mania; consider discontinuation if such symptoms occur. Aggressive behavior or hostility reported in children and adolescents w/ ADHD. May cause long-term suppression of growth in children; monitor growth, and may need to interrupt treatment in patients not growing or gaining height or weight as expected. May lower convulsive threshold; d/c if seizures occur. Associated w/ peripheral vasculopathy, including Raynaud's phenomenon. Difficulties w/ accommodation and blurring of vision reported. May exacerbate motor and phonic tics and Tourette's syndrome. May elevate plasma corticosteroid levels and interfere w/ urinary steroid determinations.

ADVERSE REACTIONS

Palpitations, tachycardia, BP elevation, dizziness, insomnia, euphoria, tremor, headache, dryness of mouth, diarrhea, constipation, urticaria, impotence, changes in libido, rhabdomyolysis.

DRUG INTERACTIONS

See Contraindications. GI acidifying agents (eg, guanethidine, reserpine, glutamic acid) and urinary acidifying agents (eg, ammonium chloride, sodium acid phosphate) lower blood levels and efficacy. Inhibits adrenergic blockers. GI alkalinizing agents (eg, sodium bicarbonate) and urinary alkalinizing agents (eg, acetazolamide, some thiazides) increase blood levels and therefore potentiate actions. May enhance activity of TCAs or sympathomimetic agents. Desipramine or protriptyline and possibly other TCAs cause striking and sustained increases in the concentration of *d*-amphetamine in the brain; CV effects can be potentiated. May counteract sedative effects of antihistamines. May antagonize effect of antihypertensives. Chlorpromazine and haloperidol block dopamine and norepinephrine reuptake, thus inhibiting central stimulant effects. May delay intestinal absorption of ethosuximide, phenobarbital, and phenytoin; coadministration w/ phenobarbital or phenytoin may produce a synergistic anticonvulsant action. Lithium carbonate may inhibit stimulatory effects. Potentiates analgesic effect of meperidine. Acidifying agents used in methenamine therapy increase urinary excretion and reduce efficacy. Enhances adrenergic effect of norepinephrine. In cases of propoxyphene overdosage, CNS stimulation is potentiated and fatal convulsions can occur. Inhibits hypotensive effect of veratrum alkaloids.

PATIENT CONSIDERATIONS

Assessment: Assess for hypersensitivity/idiosyncrasy to sympathomimetic amines, advanced arteriosclerosis, symptomatic CVD, moderate to severe HTN, hyperthyroidism, glaucoma, agitated states, history of drug abuse, tics, Tourette's syndrome, preexisting psychotic disorder, risk for/comorbid bipolar disorder, cardiac disease, medical conditions that might be compromised by increases in BP or HR, any other conditions where treatment is cautioned, pregnancy/nursing status, and possible drug interactions.

Monitoring: Monitor for changes in HR and BP, signs/symptoms of cardiac disease, exacerbation of behavioral disturbance and thought disorder, psychosis, mania, appearance or worsening of aggressive behavior or hostility, seizures, visual disturbances, exacerbation of motor and phonic tics or Tourette's syndrome, and other adverse reactions. Monitor growth and weight in pediatric patients. Observe carefully for signs and symptoms of peripheral vasculopathy; further clinical evaluation (eg, rheumatology referral) may be appropriate for certain patients.

Counseling: Inform about benefits and risks of treatment. Inform that drug has high potential for abuse. Caution against engaging in potentially hazardous activities. Instruct patients beginning treatment about the risk of peripheral vasculopathy and associated signs/symptoms. Instruct to report any new numbness, pain, skin color change, or sensitivity to temperature in fingers/toes, and to call physician immediately w/ any signs of unexplained wounds appearing on fingers/toes.

STORAGE: 20-25°C (68-77°F).

PROCHLORPERAZINE — prochlorperazine edisylate; prochlorperazine maleate RX

Class: Phenothiazine derivative

Elderly patients with dementia-related psychosis treated with antipsychotic drugs are at an increased risk of death; most deaths appeared to be cardiovascular (CV) (eg, heart failure, sudden death) or infectious (eg, pneumonia) in nature. Treatment with conventional antipsychotic drugs may similarly increase mortality. Not approved for the treatment of patients with dementia-related psychosis.

OTHER BRAND NAMES

Compazine (Discontinued)

ADULT DOSAGE

Nausea/Vomiting

Tab:

Usual: 5mg or 10mg tid-qid

Daily dose >40mg should only be used in resistant cases

IM:

Initial: 5-10mg q3-4h prn

PEDIATRIC DOSAGE

Nausea/Vomiting

≥2 Years:

Tab:

20-29 lbs:

Usual: 2.5mg qd-bid

Max: 7.5mg/day

30-39 lbs:

Max: 40mg/day

IV:
2.5-10mg slow inj or infusion at rate ≤5mg/min
Max: 10mg single dose and 40mg/day

N/V w/ Surgery:

IM:
5-10mg 1-2 hrs before induction of anesthesia (repeat once in 30 min if necessary)

IV:
5-10mg as slow inj or infusion 15-30 min before induction of anesthesia. To control acute symptoms during or after surgery, repeat once if necessary
Max: 40mg/day

Psychotic Disorders

Tab:

Nonpsychotic Anxiety
Usual: 5mg tid-qid
Max: 20mg/day, not longer than 12 weeks

Mild Conditions Including Schizophrenia:
Usual: 5 or 10mg tid-qid

Moderate-Severe Conditions (Hospitalized/ Supervised):
Initial: 10mg tid-qid.
Titrate: Increase gradually until controlled or bothersome side effects

More Severe Disturbances:
Usual: 100-150mg/day

IM:
Start w/ lowest recommended dose and adjust based on severity

Schizophrenia w/ Severe Symptomatology:
Initial: 10-20mg, may repeat q2-4h if necessary (or, in resistant cases, every hr)
Switch to PO after obtaining control at the same dosage level or higher

Prolonged Parenteral Therapy:
10-20mg IM q4-6h

Usual: 2.5mg bid-tid
Max: 10mg/day

40-85 lbs:
Usual: 2.5mg tid or 5mg bid
Max: 15mg/day

Severe N/V:

IM:
Usual: 0.06mg/lb; control is usually obtained w/ 1 dose

Schizophrenia

Tab:

2-12 Years:
Initial: 2.5mg bid-tid; do not give >10mg on the 1st day
Titrate: Increase according to response
Max:
2-5 Years: 20mg/day
6-12 Years: 25mg/day

IM:

<12 Years:
Usual: 0.06mg/lb. Control is usually obtained with 1 dose. Switch to PO after obtaining control at the same dosage level or higher

P

DOSING CONSIDERATIONS

Elderly

Start at lower end of dosing range and increase more gradually

Other Important Considerations

Debilitated or Emaciated Adults:
Increase more gradually

ADMINISTRATION

IV, IM, Oral route

Inj

Inject deeply into upper, outer quadrant of the buttock
SQ is not advisable because of local irritation
May be administered either undiluted or diluted in isotonic sol
When given IV, do not use bolus inj
Do not mix w/ other agents in the syringe
Avoid getting injection sol on hands or clothing because of potential contact dermatitis

HOW SUPPLIED

Inj: (Edisylate) 5mg/mL [2mL, 10mL]; **Tab:** (Maleate) 5mg, 10mg

CONTRAINDICATIONS

Known hypersensitivity to phenothiazines, comatose states, concomitant large doses of CNS depressants (eg, alcohol, barbiturates, narcotics), pediatric surgery, pediatrics <2 yrs of age or <20 lbs.

WARNINGS/PRECAUTIONS

Secondary extrapyramidal symptoms can occur. Tardive dyskinesia (TD) may develop, especially in elderly and during long-term use. Neuroleptic malignant syndrome (NMS) reported; d/c if it occurs and institute appropriate treatment. Caution during reintroduction of therapy as NMS recurrence reported. Avoid in patients with bone marrow depression, previous hypersensitivity reaction, and in pregnant women. May impair mental and/or physical abilities, especially during the 1st few days of therapy. May mask symptoms of overdose of other drugs, and obscure diagnosis of intestinal obstruction, brain tumor, and Reye's syndrome; avoid in children/adolescents whose signs and symptoms suggest Reye's syndrome. May cause hypotension; caution with large doses and parenteral administration in patients with impaired CV system. May interfere with thermoregulation; caution in patients exposed to extreme heat. Evaluate therapy periodically with prolonged use. Leukopenia/neutropenia/agranulocytosis reported; monitor during 1st few months of therapy, and d/c at 1st sign of leukopenia or if severe neutropenia (absolute neutrophil count <1000/mm^3) occurs. Caution with glaucoma, in children with dehydration or acute illness, and in elderly. May produce α-adrenergic blockade, lower seizure threshold, or elevate prolactin levels. D/C 48 hrs before myelography; may resume after 24 hrs postprocedure.

ADVERSE REACTIONS

NMS, cholestatic jaundice, leukopenia, agranulocytosis, drowsiness, dizziness, amenorrhea, blurred vision, skin reactions, hypotension, motor restlessness, extrapyramidal symptoms, TD, dystonia, pseudoparkinsonism.

DRUG INTERACTIONS

See Contraindications. May intensify and prolong action of CNS depressants (eg, alcohol, anesthetics, narcotics), atropine, and organophosphorus insecticides. May decrease oral anticoagulant effects. Thiazide diuretics accentuate orthostatic hypotension. Increased levels of both drugs with propranolol. Anticonvulsants may need dosage adjustment; may lower convulsive threshold. May interfere with metabolism of phenytoin and precipitate toxicity. Risk of encephalopathic syndrome occurs with lithium. May antagonize antihypertensive effects of guanethidine and related compounds. Avoid use prior to myelography with metrizamide; vomiting as a sign of toxicity of cancer chemotherapeutic drugs may be obscured by the antiemetic effect. May reverse effect of epinephrine. May cause paradoxical further lowering of BP with epinephrine and other pressor agents (excluding norepinephrine bitartrate and phenylephrine HCl).

PATIENT CONSIDERATIONS

Assessment: Assess for Reye's syndrome, TD, pregnancy/nursing status, possible drug interactions, impaired CV system, breast cancer, glaucoma, bone marrow depression, preexisting low WBC count, history of drug-induced leukopenia/neutropenia, history of psychosis, and seizure disorder. Assess use in children with acute illness or dehydration, elderly, debilitated, or emaciated patients.

Monitoring: Monitor for extrapyramidal symptoms, signs/symptoms of TD, NMS, hypotension, fever, sore throat, infection, jaundice, motor restlessness, dystonia, pseudoparkinsonism, and hypersensitivity reactions. Monitor CBC, WBC, and prolactin levels. Conduct liver studies if fever with grippe-like symptoms occur.

Counseling: Inform about the risks and benefits of therapy. Instruct to avoid engaging in hazardous activities and exposure to extreme heat. Counsel to seek medical attention if symptoms of TD, NMS, hypotension, mydriasis, encephalopathic syndrome, sore throat, infection, deep sleep, or hypersensitivity reactions occur.

STORAGE: Tab, Inj: 20-25°C (68-77°F). Protect from light. (Inj) Do not freeze.

P

PROCRIT — epoetin alfa

RX

Class: Erythropoiesis stimulator

Increased risk of death, MI, stroke, venous thromboembolism (VTE), thrombosis of vascular access, and tumor progression or recurrence. Use the lowest dose sufficient to reduce/avoid the need for RBC transfusions. Chronic Kidney Disease (CKD): Greater risks for death, serious adverse cardiovascular (CV) reactions, and stroke when administered to target Hgb level >11g/dL. Cancer: Shortened overall survival and/or increased risk of tumor progression or recurrence in patients w/ breast, non-small cell lung, head and neck, lymphoid, and cervical cancers. Must enroll in and comply w/ the ESA APPRISE Oncology Program to prescribe and/or dispense drug to patients. Use only for anemia from myelosuppressive chemotherapy. Not indicated for patients receiving myelosuppressive chemotherapy when anticipated outcome is cure. D/C following completion of chemotherapy course. Perisurgery: Due to increased risk of deep venous thrombosis (DVT), DVT prophylaxis is recommended.

ADULT DOSAGE

Anemia

Chronic Kidney Disease Associated Anemia: Patients on Dialysis:

Initiate treatment when Hgb is <10g/dL

If Hgb approaches/exceeds 11g/dL, reduce or interrupt dose

Initial: 50-100 U/kg IV/SQ 3X weekly; IV recommended for hemodialysis patients

PEDIATRIC DOSAGE

Anemia

Chronic Kidney Disease Associated Anemia: 1 Month-16 Years on Dialysis:

Initiate treatment when Hgb is <10g/dL

If Hgb approaches/exceeds 11g/dL, reduce or interrupt dose

Initial: 50 U/kg IV/SQ 3X weekly; IV recommended for hemodialysis patients

Patients Not on Dialysis:
Consider initiating treatment when Hgb is <10g/dL AND the following considerations apply:
1. Rate of Hgb decline indicates likelihood of requiring a RBC transfusion AND,
2. Reducing the risk of alloimmunization and/or other RBC transfusion-related risks is a goal
If Hgb exceeds 10g/dL, reduce or interrupt dose and use lowest dose sufficient to reduce the need for RBC transfusion
Initial: 50-100 U/kg IV/SQ 3X weekly
All Patients:
Do not increase dose more frequently than once every 4 weeks; decreases in dose may occur more frequently
If Hgb Rises Rapidly (eg, >1g/dL in any 2-Week Period): Reduce dose by ≥25% prn to reduce rapid responses
If Hgb Has Not Increased by >1g/dL After 4 Weeks: Increase dose by 25%
If adequate response is not achieved over a 12-week escalation period, use lowest dose that will maintain a Hgb level sufficient to reduce need for RBC transfusions and evaluate other causes of anemia; d/c if responsiveness does not improve
Zidovudine Associated Anemia in HIV-Infected Patients:
Initial: 100 U/kg IV/SQ 3X weekly
Titrate:
No Hgb Increase After 8 Weeks: Increase dose by approx 50-100 U/kg at 4- to 8-week intervals until Hgb reaches level needed to avoid RBC transfusions or 300 U/kg
Hgb >12g/dL: Withhold therapy until Hgb <11g/dL; then resume at a dose 25% below previous dose
D/C therapy if an increase in Hgb is not achieved at 300 U/kg for 8 weeks
Chemotherapy Associated Anemia:
Initiate if Hgb <10g/dL and if there is a minimum of 2 additional months of planned chemotherapy
Initial: 150 U/kg SQ 3X weekly or 40,000 U SQ weekly until completion of a chemotherapy course
Dose Reduction: Reduce by 25% if:
1. Hgb increases >1g/dL in any 2-week period
2. Hgb reaches a level needed to avoid a RBC transfusion
Withhold dose if Hgb exceeds level needed to avoid RBC transfusion; reinitiate at a dose 25% below previous dose when Hgb approaches a level where RBC transfusions may be required
Dose Increase: After initial 4 weeks of therapy, if Hgb increases by <1g/dL and remains below 10g/dL increase dose to 300 U/kg 3X weekly or 60,000 U weekly
D/C therapy if there is no response in Hgb levels or if RBC transfusions are still required after 8 weeks
Surgery Patients:
300 U/kg/day SQ for 10 days before, on the day of, and for 4 days after surgery; or 600 U/kg SQ in 4 doses administered 21, 14, and 7 days before surgery and on the day of surgery
DVT prophylaxis is recommended

Do not increase dose more frequently than once every 4 weeks; decreases in dose may occur more frequently
If Hgb Rises Rapidly (eg, >1g/dL in any 2-Week Period): Reduce dose by ≥25% prn to reduce rapid responses
If Hgb Has Not Increased by >1g/dL After 4 Weeks: Increase dose by 25%
If adequate response is not achieved over a 12-week escalation period, use lowest dose that will maintain a Hgb level sufficient to reduce need for RBC transfusions and evaluate other causes of anemia; d/c if responsiveness does not improve
Chemotherapy Associated Anemia:
5-18 Years:
Initiate if Hgb <10g/dL and if there is a minimum of 2 additional months of planned chemotherapy
Initial: 600 U/kg IV weekly until completion of a chemotherapy course
Dose Reduction: Reduce by 25% if
1. Hgb increases >1g/dL in any 2-week period
2. Hgb reaches a level needed to avoid a RBC transfusion
Withhold dose if Hgb exceeds level needed to avoid RBC transfusion; reinitiate at a dose 25% below previous dose when Hgb approaches a level where RBC transfusions may be required
Dose Increase: After initial 4 weeks of therapy, if Hgb increases by <1g/dL and remains below 10g/dL increase dose to 900 U/kg (max 60,000 U) weekly
D/C therapy if there is no response in Hgb levels or if RBC transfusions are still required after 8 weeks

P

ADMINISTRATION

IV/SQ route

Do not shake; do not use if shaken or frozen
Discard unused portions in preservative-free vials; do not re-enter preservative-free vials
Do not dilute
Preservative-free vials may be admixed in a syringe w/ bacteriostatic 0.9% NaCl inj, w/ benzyl alcohol 0.9% in a 1:1 ratio

HOW SUPPLIED

Inj: 2000 U/mL, 3000 U/mL, 4000 U/mL, 10,000 U/mL, 40,000 U/mL [single-dose vial]; 10,000 U/mL [2mL], 20,000 U/mL [1mL] [multidose vial]

CONTRAINDICATIONS

Uncontrolled HTN, pure red cell aplasia (PRCA) that begins after treatment w/ epoetin alfa or other erythropoietin protein drugs, serious allergic reactions to epoetin alfa. (Multidose Vials) Neonates, infants, pregnant women, and nursing mothers.

WARNINGS/PRECAUTIONS

Not indicated for use in patients w/ cancer receiving hormonal agents, biologic products, or radiotherapy, unless also receiving concomitant myelosuppressive chemotherapy; in patients scheduled for surgery who are willing to donate autologous blood; in patients undergoing cardiac/vascular surgery, or as a substitute for RBC transfusions in patients requiring immediate correction of anemia. Evaluate transferrin saturation and serum ferritin prior to and during treatment; administer supplemental iron when serum ferritin is <100mcg/L or serum transferrin saturation is <20%. Correct/exclude other causes of anemia (eg, vitamin deficiency, metabolic/chronic inflammatory conditions, bleeding) before initiating therapy. Hypertensive encephalopathy and seizures reported in patients w/ CKD. Appropriately control HTN prior to initiation of and during treatment; reduce/withhold therapy if BP becomes difficult to control. PRCA and severe anemia, w/ or w/o other cytopenias that arise following development of neutralizing antibodies to erythropoietin reported. Withhold and evaluate for neutralizing antibodies to erythropoietin if severe anemia and low reticulocyte count develop; d/c permanently if PRCA develops, and do not switch to other erythropoiesis-stimulating agents. Serious allergic reactions may occur; immediately and permanently d/c therapy. Contains albumin; may carry an extremely remote risk for transmission of viral diseases or Creutzfeldt-Jakob disease. Patients may require adjustments in their dialysis prescriptions after initiation of therapy, or require increased anticoagulation w/ heparin to prevent clotting of extracorporeal circuit during hemodialysis. Multidose vial contains benzyl alcohol; benzyl alcohol is associated w/ serious adverse events and death, particularly in pediatric patients.

ADVERSE REACTIONS

MI, stroke, VTE, thrombosis of vascular access, tumor progression/recurrence, pyrexia, N/V, HTN, cough, arthralgia, pruritus, rash, headache, dizziness.

PATIENT CONSIDERATIONS

Assessment: Assess for uncontrolled HTN, previous hypersensitivity to the drug, causes of anemia, pregnancy/nursing status, and other conditions where treatment is contraindicated or cautioned. Obtain baseline Hgb levels, transferrin saturation, and serum ferritin.

Monitoring: Monitor for signs/symptoms of an allergic reaction, CV/thromboembolic events, stroke, premonitory neurologic symptoms, PRCA, severe anemia, progression/recurrence of tumor, and other adverse reactions. Monitor BP, transferrin saturation, and serum ferritin. Following initiation of therapy and after each dose adjustment, monitor Hgb weekly until Hgb is stable and sufficient to minimize need for RBC transfusion.

Counseling: Inform of the risks/benefits of therapy and of the increased risks of mortality, serious CV reactions, thromboembolic reactions, stroke, and tumor progression. Advise of the need to have regular lab tests for Hgb. Inform cancer patients that they must sign the patient-physician acknowledgment form prior to therapy. Instruct to undergo regular BP monitoring, adhere to prescribed antihypertensive regimen, and follow recommended dietary restrictions. Advise to contact physician for new-onset neurologic symptoms or change in seizure frequency. Instruct regarding proper disposal of used syringes and caution against the reuse of needles, syringes, or unused portions of single-dose vials.

STORAGE: 2-8°C (36-46°F). Do not freeze; do not use if it has been frozen. Protect from light. Discard unused portions of multidose vials 21 days after initial entry.

PROCTOFOAM-HC – hydrocortisone acetate/pramoxine hydrochloride RX

Class: Anesthetic/corticosteroid

ADULT DOSAGE

Inflammatory and Pruritic Manifestations of Corticosteroid-Responsive Dermatoses

Anal Region:

Apply to affected area tid-qid

D/C if no evidence of improvement w/in 2 or 3 weeks after starting therapy, or if condition worsens

PEDIATRIC DOSAGE

Inflammatory and Pruritic Manifestations of Corticosteroid-Responsive Dermatoses

Anal Region:

Apply to affected area tid-qid; use least amount effective for condition

D/C if no evidence of improvement w/in 2 or 3 weeks after starting therapy, or if condition worsens

ADMINISTRATION

Topical route

For anal administration, use the applicator supplied

For perianal use, transfer a small quantity to a tissue and rub in gently

Directions for Use

1. Shake foam container vigorously for 5-10 sec before each use; do not remove container cap during use of the product
2. Hold container upright on a level surface and gently place the tip of the applicator onto the nose of the container cap; pull plunger past the fill line on the applicator barrel
3. To fill applicator barrel, press down firmly on cap flanges, hold for 1-2 sec, and release
4. Wait 5-10 sec to allow foam to expand in applicator barrel; repeat until foam reaches fill line. It usually requires 3-4 pumps for foam to reach fill line
5. Remove applicator from container cap; if foam goes beyond fill line, it will continue to expand and flow backwards, resulting in foam build-up under cap
6. Gently insert tip into anus; once in place, push plunger to expel foam, then withdraw applicator
7. After each use, applicator parts should be pulled apart for thorough cleaning w/ warm water. Since some foam will appear under the cap, the cap and underlying tip should be pulled apart and rinsed to help prevent build-up of foam and possible blockage

Priming

Prime the container by pressing down firmly on flanges and then release. W/ initial priming, a burst of air may come out of the container; it usually requires 1-2 pumps for foam to appear

HOW SUPPLIED

Foam: (Hydrocortisone/Pramoxine) 1%/1% [10g]

CONTRAINDICATIONS

P

History of hypersensitivity to any components of the preparation.

WARNINGS/PRECAUTIONS

Do not insert any part of the aerosol container directly into the anus. Avoid contact with eyes. Contents of the container are under pressure; do not burn or puncture. Systemic absorption may produce reversible hypothalamic-pituitary-adrenal (HPA) axis suppression, manifestations of Cushing's syndrome, hyperglycemia, and glucosuria. Application of more potent steroids, use over large surface areas, prolonged use, and the addition of occlusive dressings may augment systemic absorption. Periodically evaluate for evidence of HPA axis suppression when a large dose is applied to a large surface area or under an occlusive dressing; if noted, withdraw the drug, reduce frequency of application, or substitute with a less potent steroid. Infrequently, signs and symptoms of steroid withdrawal may occur, requiring supplemental systemic corticosteroids. D/C and institute appropriate therapy if irritation develops. Use appropriate antifungal or antibacterial agent in the presence of dermatological infections; if a favorable response does not occur promptly, d/c until infection has been adequately controlled. Pediatric patients may be more susceptible to systemic toxicity. Chronic therapy may interfere with growth and development of pediatric patients. Caution in elderly.

ADVERSE REACTIONS

Burning, itching, irritation, dryness, folliculitis, hypertrichosis, acneiform eruptions, hypopigmentation, perioral dermatitis, allergic contact dermatitis, skin maceration, secondary infection, skin atrophy, striae, miliaria.

PATIENT CONSIDERATIONS

Assessment: Assess for drug hypersensitivity, conditions that augment systemic absorption, dermatological infections, and pregnancy/nursing status.

Monitoring: Monitor for signs/symptoms of HPA axis suppression, Cushing's syndrome, hyperglycemia, glucosuria, steroid withdrawal, irritation, dermatological infections, systemic toxicity in pediatric patients, and other adverse reactions. When a large dose is applied to a large surface area or under an occlusive dressing, monitor for HPA axis suppression by using urinary free cortisol and adrenocorticotropic hormone stimulation tests. Monitor for improvement or worsening of condition.

Counseling: Instruct to use ud (anal or perianal use only) and to avoid contact with eyes. Advise not to use for any disorder other than for which it was prescribed. Instruct to report any signs of adverse reactions.

STORAGE: 20-25°C (68-77°F). Do not store at temperatures >49°C (120°F). Do not refrigerate.

PROGRAF – tacrolimus

RX

Class: Calcineurin-inhibitor immunosuppressant

Immunosuppression may lead to increased risk of lymphoma and other malignancies, particularly of the skin. Increased susceptibility to infections (bacterial, viral, fungal, protozoal, opportunistic). Should only be prescribed by physicians experienced in immunosuppressive therapy and management of organ transplant patients. Manage patients in facilities equipped and staffed w/ adequate lab and supportive medical resources. Physician responsible for maintenance therapy should have complete information requisite for patient follow-up.

ADULT DOSAGE

Hepatic Transplant

Prophylaxis of organ rejection in patients receiving allogeneic liver transplant; recommended to be used concomitantly w/ adrenal corticosteroids early post-transplant

Cap:
Initial: 0.1-0.15mg/kg/day as 2 divided doses, q12h; administer no sooner than 6 hrs after liver transplant
Titrate: Based on clinical assessments of rejection and tolerability
Maint: Lower dosages than the initial dosage may be sufficient

Observed Tacrolimus Whole Blood Trough Concentrations w/ Liver Transplant:
Months 1-12: 5-20ng/mL

IV:
Initial: 0.03-0.05mg/kg/day

If receiving tacrolimus IV infusion, give 1st oral dose 8-12 hrs after discontinuing the IV infusion

Renal Transplant

Prophylaxis of organ rejection in patients receiving allogeneic kidney transplant; recommended to be used concomitantly w/ azathioprine or mycophenolate mofetil (MMF) and adrenal corticosteroids (early post-transplant)

Cap:
Initial: 0.2mg/kg/day in combination w/ azathioprine or 0.1mg/kg/day in combination w/ MMF/Interleukin (IL)-2 receptor antagonist; give as 2 divided doses, q12h. May administer w/in 24 hrs of kidney transplant, but should be delayed until renal function has recovered
Titrate: Based on clinical assessments of rejection and tolerability
Maint: Lower dosages than the initial dosage may be sufficient

Observed Tacrolimus Whole Blood Trough Concentrations w/ Kidney Transplant:
W/ Azathioprine:
Months 1-3: 7-20ng/mL
Months 4-12: 5-15ng/mL

PEDIATRIC DOSAGE

Hepatic Transplant

Prophylaxis of organ rejection in patients receiving allogeneic liver transplant; recommended to be used concomitantly w/ adrenal corticosteroids early post-transplant

Cap:
Initial: 0.15-0.2mg/kg/day as 2 divided doses, q12h; administer no sooner than 6 hrs after liver transplant

Observed Tacrolimus Whole Blood Trough Concentrations w/ Liver Transplant:
Months 1-12: 5-20ng/mL

IV:
Initial: 0.03-0.05mg/kg/day

P

W/ MMF/IL-2 Receptor Antagonist:
Months 1-12: 4-11ng/mL

IV:
Initial: 0.03-0.05mg/kg/day

If receiving tacrolimus IV infusion, give 1st oral dose 8-12 hrs after discontinuing the IV infusion

Cardiac Transplant

Prophylaxis of organ rejection in patients receiving allogeneic heart transplant; recommended to be used concomitantly w/ azathioprine or mycophenolate mofetil (MMF) and adrenal corticosteroids (early post-transplant)

Cap:
Initial: 0.075mg/kg/day as 2 divided doses, q12h; administer no sooner than 6 hrs after heart transplant
Titrate: Based on clinical assessments of rejection and tolerability
Maint: Lower dosages than the initial dosage may be sufficient

Observed Tacrolimus Whole Blood Trough Concentrations w/ Heart Transplant:
Months 1-3: 10-20ng/mL
Months ≥4: 5-15ng/mL

IV:
Initial: 0.01mg/kg/day

If receiving tacrolimus IV infusion, give 1st oral dose 8-12 hrs after discontinuing the IV infusion

DOSING CONSIDERATIONS

Concomitant Medications
Cyclosporine: Do not use simultaneously; d/c tacrolimus or cyclosporine at least 24 hrs before initiating the other

Renal Impairment
Liver/Heart Transplant:
Preexisting Renal Impairment: Start at lower end of dosing range
Kidney Transplant:
Postoperative Oliguria: Initial dose should be administered no sooner than 6 hrs and w/in 24 hrs of transplantation, but may be delayed until renal function shows evidence of recovery

Hepatic Impairment
Severe (Child-Pugh ≥10): May require lower doses

Elderly
Start at lower end of dosing range

Other Important Considerations
Black patients may require higher doses
Do not eat grapefruit or drink grapefruit juice

ADMINISTRATION

Oral/IV route

Inj should be used only as a continuous IV infusion and when the patient cannot tolerate oral administration of cap

Cap
Take consistently, either w/ or w/o food

IV
Dilute product w/ 0.9% NaCl inj or D5 inj to concentration between 0.004mg/mL and 0.02mg/mL prior to use
Diluted infusion sol should be stored in glass or polyethylene containers and should be discarded after 24 hrs; do not store in PVC container due to decreased stability and potential for extraction of phthalates; in situations where more dilute sol are utilized (eg, pediatric dosing), PVC-free tubing should likewise be used to minimize the potential for significant drug adsorption onto tubing
Should not be mixed or co-infused w/ sol of pH ≥9 (eg, ganciclovir, acyclovir)

HOW SUPPLIED

Cap: 0.5mg, 1mg, 5mg; **Inj:** 5mg/mL [1mL]

CONTRAINDICATIONS

Hypersensitivity to tacrolimus. **Inj:** Hypersensitivity to polyoxyl 60 hydrogenated castor oil (HCO-60).

WARNINGS/PRECAUTIONS

Limit exposure to sunlight and UV light in patients at increased risk for skin cancer. Increased risk for polyoma virus infections, CMV viremia, and CMV disease. Polyoma virus-associated nephropathy (PVAN) reported; may lead to renal function deterioration and kidney graft loss. Progressive multifocal leukoencephalopathy (PML) reported; consider PML in differential diagnosis in patients reporting neurological symptoms and consider consultation w/ a neurologist. Consider reductions in immunosuppression if CMV viremia, CMV disease, or if evidence of PVAN or PML develops. May cause new onset diabetes mellitus; closely monitor blood glucose concentrations. May cause acute/chronic nephrotoxicity; closely monitor patients w/ renal dysfunction. Consider changing to another immunosuppressive therapy in patients w/ persistent SrCr elevations unresponsive to dose adjustments. May cause neurotoxicity (eg, posterior reversible encephalopathy syndrome [PRES], delirium, coma); if PRES is suspected or diagnosed, maintain BP control and immediately reduce immunosuppression. Hyperkalemia and HTN reported. May prolong the QT/QTc interval and may cause torsades de pointes; avoid in patients w/ congenital long QT syndrome and consider obtaining ECGs and monitoring electrolytes (Mg^{2+}, K^+, Ca^{2+}) periodically in patients w/ CHF, bradyarrhythmias, those taking certain antiarrhythmic medications or other medicinal products that lead to QT prolongation, and those w/ electrolyte disturbances. Myocardial hypertrophy reported; consider dose reduction or discontinuation if diagnosed and consider echocardiographic evaluation in patients who develop renal failure or clinical manifestations of ventricular dysfunction. Pure red cell aplasia (PRCA) reported; consider discontinuation if diagnosed. GI perforation reported; institute appropriate medical/surgical management promptly. (Inj) Anaphylactic reactions may occur; should be reserved for patients unable to take cap orally. Patients should be under continuous observation for at least the first 30 min following the start of infusion and at frequent intervals thereafter; d/c infusion if signs/symptoms of anaphylaxis occur.

ADVERSE REACTIONS

Lymphoma, malignancies, infections, tremor, HTN, abnormal renal function, headache, insomnia, hyperglycemia, hyperkalemia, hypomagnesemia, diarrhea, N/V, paresthesia.

DRUG INTERACTIONS

See Dosing Considerations. Not recommended w/ sirolimus in liver or heart transplants; safety and efficacy not established in kidney transplant. Due to potential for additive/synergistic renal impairment, caution w/ drugs that may be associated w/ renal dysfunction (eg, aminoglycosides, ganciclovir, amphotericin B). Increased whole blood concentrations w/ CYP3A inhibitors (eg, antifungals, calcium channel blockers [CCBs], macrolide antibiotics), and magnesium and aluminum hydroxide antacids. Decreased whole blood concentrations w/ CYP3A inducers. May increase mycophenolic acid (MPA) exposure after crossover from cyclosporine to tacrolimus in patients concomitantly receiving MPA-containing products. Avoid w/ nelfinavir unless the benefits outweigh the risks. Monitor whole blood concentrations and adjust tacrolimus dose if used concomitantly w/ protease inhibitors (eg, ritonavir, telaprevir, boceprevir), CCBs (eg, verapamil, diltiazem, nifedipine), erythromycin, clarithromycin, troleandomycin, chloramphenicol, rifampin, rifabutin, phenytoin, carbamazepine, phenobarbital, St. John's wort, magnesium and aluminum hydroxide antacids, bromocriptine, nefazodone, metoclopramide, danazol, ethinyl estradiol, amiodarone, methylprednisolone, herbal products containing *Schisandra sphenanthera* extracts, or CYP3A inhibitors/inducers. Monitor whole blood concentrations and adjust tacrolimus dose when concomitant use of antifungal drugs (eg, azoles, caspofungin) w/ tacrolimus is initiated or discontinued; initially reduce tacrolimus dose to 1/3 of the original dose when initiating therapy w/ voriconazole or posaconazole. May increase levels of phenytoin; monitor phenytoin levels and adjust phenytoin dose as needed. Caution w/ antihypertensive agents (eg, K^+-sparing diuretics, ACE inhibitors, ARBs) or other agents associated w/ hyperkalemia. Reduce tacrolimus dose, closely monitor tacrolimus whole blood concentrations, and monitor for QT prolongation when coadministered w/ CYP3A4 substrates and/or inhibitors that also have the potential to prolong the QT interval. Amiodarone may increase whole blood concentrations w/ or w/o concurrent QT prolongation. Avoid live vaccines during therapy. Caution w/ concomitant immunosuppressants.

PATIENT CONSIDERATIONS

Assessment: Assess for drug hypersensitivity, congenital long QT syndrome, CHF, bradyarrhythmias, electrolyte disturbances, renal/hepatic impairment, pregnancy/nursing status, and possible drug interactions. (Inj) Assess for hypersensitivity to HCO-60.

Monitoring: Monitor tacrolimus blood concentrations in conjunction w/ other laboratory and clinical parameters. Monitor for lymphomas and other malignancies, infections, neurotoxicity, HTN, QT prolongation, PRCA, GI perforation, and other adverse reactions. Monitor serum K^+ and glucose concentrations. (Inj) Monitor for anaphylactic reactions.

Counseling: Inform of the risks and benefits of therapy. Advise to take medicine at the same 12-hr interval every day and not to eat grapefruit or drink grapefruit juice in combination w/ the drug. Advise to limit exposure to sunlight and UV light by wearing protective clothing and to use a sunscreen w/ a high protection factor. Instruct to contact physician if frequent urination, increased thirst or hunger, vision changes, deliriums, tremors, or any symptoms of infection develop. Advise to attend all visits and complete all blood tests ordered by medical team. Inform that therapy may cause high BP, which may require treatment w/ antihypertensive therapy. Instruct to inform physician if planning to become pregnant or breastfeed or when starting or stopping any medication (prescription and nonprescription medicines, natural/herbal remedies, nutritional supplements, vitamins). Inform that therapy may interfere w/ the usual response to immunizations and that live vaccines should be avoided.

STORAGE: (Cap) 25°C (77°F); excursions permitted to 15-30°C (59-86°F). (Inj) 5-25°C (41-77°F).

PROLIA – denosumab

RX

Class: IgG_2 monoclonal antibody

ADULT DOSAGE

Osteoporosis

Postmenopausal Osteoporosis:
Postmenopausal women at high risk for fracture, or patients who have failed or are intolerant to other available osteoporosis therapy

Usual: 60mg as a single SQ inj once every 6 months

To Increase Bone Mass in Men w/ Osteoporosis:
Men at high risk for fracture, or patients who have failed or are intolerant to other available osteoporosis therapy

Usual: 60mg as a single SQ inj once every 6 months

Calcium and Vitamin D Supplementation:
All patients should receive Ca^{2+} 1000mg/day and ≥400 IU vitamin D daily

Bone Loss

In Men Receiving Androgen Deprivation Therapy for Nonmetastatic Prostate Cancer:

Usual: 60mg as a single SQ inj once every 6 months

In Women Receiving Adjuvant Aromatase Inhibitor Therapy for Breast Cancer:

Usual: 60mg as a single SQ inj once every 6 months

Calcium and Vitamin D Supplementation:
All patients should receive Ca^{2+} 1000mg/day and ≥400 IU vitamin D daily

Missed Dose

If a dose is missed, administer as soon as patient is available, then schedule inj every 6 months from date of last inj

PEDIATRIC DOSAGE

Pediatric use may not have been established

ADMINISTRATION

SQ route

Administer in the upper arm/thigh or abdomen

Avoid vigorous shaking

People sensitive to latex should not handle the grey needle cap on the single-use prefilled syringe, which contains dry natural rubber (a derivative of latex)

Prior to administration, remove from the refrigerator and bring to room temperature by standing in the original container for 15-30 min

Instructions for Prefilled Syringe w/ Needle Safety Guard:
Do not slide the green safety guard forward over the needle before administering the inj; it will lock in place and prevent inj

Instructions for Single-Use Vial:
Use a 27-gauge needle to withdraw and inject the 1mL dose
Do not re-enter the vial; discard vial and any liquid remaining in the vial

HOW SUPPLIED

Inj: 60mg/mL [prefilled syringe, vial]

CONTRAINDICATIONS

Hypocalcemia, pregnancy, history of systemic hypersensitivity to any component of the product.

WARNINGS/PRECAUTIONS

Should be administered by a healthcare professional. Do not give w/ other drugs that contain the same active ingredient (eg, Xgeva). Hypersensitivity, including anaphylaxis, reported; d/c further use and initiate appropriate therapy if an anaphylactic or other clinically significant allergic reaction occurs. Hypocalcemia may be exacerbated; correct preexisting hypocalcemia prior to initiating therapy. Monitor Ca^{2+} and mineral levels (phosphorus [P] and Mg^{2+}) w/in 14 days of inj in patients predisposed to hypocalcemia and disturbances of mineral metabolism (eg, history of hypoparathyroidism, malabsorption syndromes, excision of the small intestine). Significant risk of hypocalcemia following administration w/ severe renal impairment (CrCl <30mL/min) or receiving dialysis; marked elevations of serum parathyroid hormone (PTH) may develop. Osteonecrosis of the jaw (ONJ) may occur; a dental examination is recommended w/ appropriate preventive dentistry prior to treatment in patients w/ risk factors for ONJ (eg, invasive dental procedures, diagnosis of cancer, concomitant therapies [eg, chemotherapy, corticosteroids, angiogenesis inhibitors]). Atypical low-energy or low-trauma fractures of the femoral shaft reported; evaluate patients w/ thigh/groin pain to rule out an incomplete femur fracture and consider interruption of therapy. Endocarditis and serious skin, abdomen, urinary tract, and ear infections leading to hospitalization reported; assess need for continued therapy if serious infections develop. Increased risk for serious infections in patients w/ an impaired immune system. Epidermal and dermal adverse events may occur; consider discontinuing therapy if severe symptoms develop. Severe and occasionally incapacitating bone, joint, and/or muscle pain reported; consider discontinuing use if severe symptoms develop. Significant suppression of bone remodeling as evidenced by markers of bone turnover and bone histomorphometry reported.

ADVERSE REACTIONS

Back pain, anemia, vertigo, upper abdominal pain, peripheral edema, cystitis, URTI, pneumonia, hypercholesterolemia, pain in extremity, musculoskeletal pain, bone pain, sciatica, arthralgia, nasopharyngitis.

DRUG INTERACTIONS

Immunosuppressant agents may increase the risk of serious infections. Concomitant administration of drugs associated w/ ONJ may increase risk of developing ONJ.

P

PATIENT CONSIDERATIONS

Assessment: Assess for drug hypersensitivity, preexisting hypocalcemia, history of hypoparathyroidism, thyroid/parathyroid surgery, malabsorption syndromes, excision of the small intestine, renal impairment, impairment of the immune system, risk factors for ONJ, pregnancy/nursing status, and possible drug interactions. Perform routine oral exam, and dental examination w/ appropriate preventive dentistry in patients w/ risk factors for ONJ.

Monitoring: Monitor for signs/symptoms of hypocalcemia, infections, hypersensitivity, dermatological reactions, serum PTH elevation, ONJ, atypical femoral fractures, delayed fracture healing, musculoskeletal pain, and other adverse reactions. Monitor Ca^{2+} and mineral levels (P and Mg^{2+}) w/in 14 days of inj in patients predisposed to hypocalcemia and disturbances of mineral metabolism.

Counseling: Counsel not to take w/ other drugs w/ the same active ingredient. Inform about the importance of maintaining Ca^{2+} levels w/ adequate Ca^{2+} and vitamin D supplementation. Advise to seek prompt medical attention if signs/symptoms of hypocalcemia, infections, dermatological reactions, or hypersensitivity reactions develop. Advise to maintain good oral hygiene during treatment and to inform dentist prior to dental procedures of current treatment. Instruct to inform physician or dentist if patient experiences persistent pain and/or slow healing of the mouth or jaw after dental surgery. Advise to report new or unusual thigh, hip, or groin pain. Inform that severe bone, joint, and/or muscle pain reported during therapy; instruct to report development of severe symptoms. Inform that therapy should not be used if pregnant or nursing. Counsel to adhere to proper schedule of administration.

STORAGE: 2-8°C (36-46°F). Do not freeze. Use w/in 14 days. Protect from direct light and heat. Avoid vigorous shaking.

PROMETHAZINE – promethazine hydrochloride

RX

Class: Phenothiazine derivative

Do not be use in pediatric patients <2 yrs of age; potential for fatal respiratory depression. Caution when administering to patients ≥2 yrs of age; use lowest effective dose and avoid concomitant administration of other drugs w/ respiratory depressant effects.

OTHER BRAND NAMES

Promethegan, Phenadoz

ADULT DOSAGE

Nausea/Vomiting

Active Therapy:
12.5-25mg q4-6h, prn

Prophylaxis During Surgery and Postoperative Period:
25mg q4-6h, prn

Sedation

Nighttime, Presurgical, or Obstetrical Sedation:
25-50mg

Pre- and Postoperative Use

Preoperative Medication:
50mg in combination w/ reduced dose of narcotic or barbiturate and the required amount of a belladonna alkaloid

Postoperative Sedation/Adjunctive Use w/ Analgesics:
25-50mg

Allergies

25mg qhs or 12.5mg ac and hs; may give 6.25-12.5mg tid

Adjust to lowest effective dose

Motion Sickness

Initial: 25mg 30-60 min before travel and repeat after 8-12 hrs, if necessary
Maint: 25mg bid (on arising and before pm meal)

Other Indications

Perennial and seasonal allergic rhinitis, vasomotor rhinitis, allergic conjunctivitis due to inhalant allergens and foods, mild uncomplicated allergic skin manifestations of urticaria and angioedema, amelioration of allergic reactions to blood or plasma, and dermographism. Adjunct therapy in anaphylactic reactions. Pre/postoperative or obstetric sedation. Prevention and control of N/V associated w/ certain types of anesthesia and surgery. Adjunct therapy w/ meperidine or other analgesics for control of postoperative pain. Sedation, relief of apprehension, and production of light sleep. Active and prophylactic treatment of motion sickness. Antiemetic in postoperative patients.

PEDIATRIC DOSAGE

Allergies

≥2 Years:
25mg qhs or 12.5mg ac and hs; may give 6.25-12.5mg tid

Adjust to lowest effective dose

Nausea/Vomiting

≥2 Years:
Active Therapy:
Usual: 0.5mg/lb; adjust dose based on patient age/weight and severity of condition

Prophylaxis During Surgery and the Postoperative Period:
25mg q4-6h, prn

Sedation

≥2 Years:
12.5-25mg qhs

Pre- and Postoperative Use

≥2 Years:
Preoperative Medication:
0.5mg/lb in combination w/ reduced dose of narcotic or barbiturate and the appropriate dose of an atropine-like drug

Postoperative Sedation/Adjunctive Use w/ Analgesics:
12.5-25mg

Motion Sickness

≥2 Years:
12.5-25mg bid

Other Indications

Perennial and seasonal allergic rhinitis, vasomotor rhinitis, allergic conjunctivitis due to inhalant allergens and foods, mild uncomplicated allergic skin manifestations of urticaria and angioedema, amelioration of allergic reactions to blood or plasma, and dermographism. Adjunct therapy in anaphylactic reactions. Pre/postoperative or obstetric sedation. Prevention and control of N/V associated w/ certain types of anesthesia and surgery. Adjunct therapy w/ meperidine or other analgesics for control of postoperative pain. Sedation, relief of apprehension, and production of light sleep. Active and prophylactic treatment of motion sickness. Antiemetic in postoperative patients.

DOSING CONSIDERATIONS

Elderly
Start at lower end of dosing range

ADMINISTRATION

Oral/rectal route

HOW SUPPLIED

Sup: (Phenadoz) 12.5mg, 25mg, (Promethegan) 50mg; **Syrup:** 6.25mg/5mL [118mL, 237mL, 473mL] **Tab:** 12.5mg*, 25mg*, 50mg *scored

CONTRAINDICATIONS

Pediatric patients <2 yrs of age; comatose states; known hypersensitivity or idiosyncratic reaction to promethazine or to other phenothiazines; treatment of lower respiratory tract symptoms, including asthma.

WARNINGS/PRECAUTIONS

Not recommended for uncomplicated vomiting in pediatric patients; should be limited to prolonged vomiting of known etiology. Avoid in pediatric patients whose signs and symptoms may suggest Reye's syndrome or other hepatic diseases. May impair mental/physical abilities. May lead to potentially fatal respiratory depression; avoid w/ compromised respiratory function. May lower seizure threshold. Caution w/ bone marrow depression; leukopenia and agranulocytosis reported. Neuroleptic malignant syndrome (NMS) reported alone or w/ antipsychotics; d/c immediately and monitor. Hallucinations and convulsions may occur in pediatric patients. Acutely ill pediatric patients associated w/ dehydration may have an increased susceptibility to dystonias. Cholestatic jaundice reported. Caution w/ narrow-angle glaucoma, prostatic hypertrophy, stenosing peptic ulcer, bladder-neck or pyloroduodenal obstruction, cardiovascular disease, and liver function impairment. Lab test interactions may occur. Caution in elderly patients.

ADVERSE REACTIONS

Drowsiness, sedation, blurred vision, dizziness, increased or decreased BP, urticaria, dry mouth, N/V, hallucination, leukopenia, asthma, apnea, photosensitivity, angioneurotic edema.

DRUG INTERACTIONS

See Boxed Warning. May increase incidence of extrapyramidal effects w/ MAOIs. May increase, prolong, or intensify the sedative action of other CNS depressants, (eg, alcohol, sedatives/ hypnotics, narcotics, TCAs); avoid such agents or reduce dosage. Reduce dose of barbiturates by at least 50% if given concomitantly. Reduce dose of narcotics by 25-50% if given concomitantly. May reverse vasopressor effect of epinephrine; do not use to treat hypotension associated w/ promethazine overdose. Caution w/ anticholinergics. Caution w/ medications that may affect seizure threshold (eg, narcotics, local anesthetics). Leukopenia and agranulocytosis reported when used w/ other known marrow-toxic agents.

PATIENT CONSIDERATIONS

Assessment: Assess for drug hypersensitivity or past idiosyncratic reaction to phenothiazines, bone marrow depression, narrow-angle glaucoma, pregnancy/nursing status, possible drug interactions, or any other conditions where treatment is contraindicated or cautioned. Assess for signs/ symptoms of hepatic diseases, and for Reye's syndrome in pediatric patients.

Monitoring: Monitor for signs/symptoms of CNS/respiratory depression, NMS, seizures, cholestatic jaundice, leukopenia, agranulocytosis, and other adverse reactions. Monitor for hallucinations, convulsions, extrapyramidal symptoms, and respiratory depression, and for dystonias in pediatric patients.

Counseling: Inform that therapy may cause drowsiness and impairment of mental and/or physical abilities. Counsel to report any involuntary muscle movements. Instruct to avoid alcohol use, prolonged sun exposure, and concomitant use of other CNS depressants.

STORAGE: Keep tightly closed. (Syrup/Tab) 20-25°C (68-77°F). (Sup) 2-8°C (36-46°F). (Syrup/ Tab) Protect from light.

PROMETHAZINE DM – dextromethorphan hydrobromide/ promethazine hydrochloride

RX

Class: Antitussive/phenothiazine derivative

Promethazine HCl should not be used in patients <2 yrs; potential for fatal respiratory depression. Caution when administering to patients ≥2 yrs; use lowest effective dose and avoid concomitant administration of respiratory depressants.

ADULT DOSAGE

Antihistamine/Cough Suppressant

Temporary relief of coughs and upper respiratory symptoms associated with allergy or the common cold

5mL q4-6h
Max: 30mL/24 hrs

PEDIATRIC DOSAGE

Antihistamine/Cough Suppressant

Temporary relief of coughs and upper respiratory symptoms associated with allergy or the common cold

2 to <6 Years:
1.25-2.5mL q4-6h

P

Max: 10mL/24 hrs

6 to <12 Years:
2.5-5mL q4-6h
Max: 20mL/24 hrs

≥12 Years:
5mL q4-6h
Max: 30mL/24 hrs

DOSING CONSIDERATIONS

Elderly

Start at lower end of dosing range

ADMINISTRATION

Oral route

HOW SUPPLIED

Syrup: (Dextromethorphan-Promethazine) 15mg-6.25mg/5mL

CONTRAINDICATIONS

Dextromethorphan: Concomitant MAOIs. **Promethazine:** Comatose states; known hypersensitivity or idiosyncratic reaction to promethazine or to other phenothiazines; treatment of lower respiratory tract symptoms, including asthma.

WARNINGS/PRECAUTIONS

Should be given to a pregnant woman only if clearly needed. Avoid prolonged exposure to sunlight. Promethazine: Caution in pediatrics ≥2 yrs. Respiratory depression and apnea, sometimes associated with death, are strongly associated with promethazine products and are not directly related to individualized weight-based dosing. Avoid in pediatric patients whose signs and symptoms may suggest Reye's syndrome or hepatic diseases. May impair mental/physical abilities. May lower seizure threshold; caution with seizure disorders. May lead to potentially fatal respiratory depression; avoid with compromised respiratory function (eg, COPD, sleep apnea). Caution with bone marrow depression; leukopenia and agranulocytosis reported. Neuroleptic malignant syndrome (NMS) reported; d/c immediately. Hallucinations and convulsions may occur in pediatrics with therapeutic doses or overdoses. Acutely ill, dehydrated pediatric patients may have increased susceptibility to dystonias. Caution with narrow-angle glaucoma, prostatic hypertrophy, stenosing peptic ulcer, bladder neck or pyloroduodenal obstruction, CV disease, hepatic impairment. Cholestatic jaundice reported. May increase blood glucose. Dextromethorphan: Caution in atopic children, sedated, or debilitated patients, and patients confined to supine position.

ADVERSE REACTIONS

Drowsiness, dizziness, sedation, blurred vision, dry mouth, increased or decreased BP, rash, N/V, respiratory depression, apnea, leukopenia, agranulocytosis, NMS.

DRUG INTERACTIONS

P

See Boxed Warning and Contraindications. Promethazine: May increase, prolong, or intensify the sedative action of other CNS depressants, such as alcohol, sedatives/hypnotics (including barbiturates), narcotics, narcotic analgesics, general anesthetics, TCAs, and tranquilizers; avoid such agents or administer in reduced dosages. Reduce barbiturate dose by at least 1/2 and narcotic analgesics by 1/4 to 1/2. May reverse vasopressor effect of epinephrine. Caution with concomitant medications that may also affect seizure threshold (eg, narcotics, local anesthetics). Caution with concomitant use of other agents with anticholinergic properties. Leukopenia and agranulocytosis reported, usually when used in association with other marrow-toxic agents. NMS reported alone or in combination with antipsychotic drugs. Dextromethorphan: Hyperpyrexia, hypotension, and death have been reported coincident with the coadministration of MAOIs and products containing dextromethorphan.

PATIENT CONSIDERATIONS

Assessment: Assess for drug hypersensitivity or idiosyncrasy, or any other conditions where treatment is contraindicated or cautioned. Assess for pregnancy/nursing status and possible drug interactions. Assess use in atopic children, elderly, debilitated, and for signs/symptoms of Reye's syndrome, hepatic diseases, or encephalopathy in pediatrics.

Monitoring: Monitor for signs/symptoms of CNS/respiratory depression, NMS, seizures, cholestatic jaundice, leukopenia, and agranulocytosis. Monitor children for hallucinations, convulsions, extrapyramidal symptoms, and dystonias. Monitor for false positive and false negative pregnancy tests, blood glucose levels, and BP.

Counseling: Inform that therapy may cause marked drowsiness or may impair mental and/or physical abilities required for performing hazardous tasks (eg, operating machinery, driving). Instruct to report involuntary muscle movements. Counsel to avoid the use of alcohol and other CNS depressants while on therapy. Instruct to avoid prolonged exposure to the sun.

STORAGE: 20-25°C (68-77°F). Protect from light. Keep bottle tightly closed. Dispense in a tight, light-resistant container with a child-resistant closure.

PROMETHAZINE VC WITH CODEINE – codeine phosphate/phenylephrine hydrochloride/promethazine hydrochloride

CV

Class: Antitussive/phenothiazine derivative/sympathomimetic

Contraindicated in pediatric patients <6 yrs of age. Concomitant administration of promethazine products with other respiratory depressants is associated with respiratory depression, and sometimes death, in pediatric patients. Respiratory depression, including fatalities, have been reported with use of promethazine in patients <2 yrs of age. Respiratory depression and death reported in children who received codeine following tonsillectomy and/or adenoidectomy and had evidence of being ultra-rapid metabolizers of codeine due to a CYP2D6 polymorphism.

ADULT DOSAGE

Antihistamine/Cough Suppressant/Nasal Decongestant

Temporary relief of coughs and upper respiratory symptoms (eg, nasal congestion) associated with allergy or the common cold

5mL q4-6h

Max: 30mL/24 hrs

PEDIATRIC DOSAGE

Antihistamine/Cough Suppressant/Nasal Decongestant

Temporary relief of coughs and upper respiratory symptoms (eg, nasal congestion) associated with allergy or the common cold

6 to <12 Years:
2.5-5mL q4-6h
Max: 30mL/24 hrs

≥12 Years:
5mL q4-6h
Max: 30mL/24 hrs

DOSING CONSIDERATIONS

Elderly

Start at lower end of dosing range

ADMINISTRATION

Oral route

Measure w/ an accurate measuring device

HOW SUPPLIED

Syrup: (Codeine/Promethazine/Phenylephrine) 10mg/6.25mg/5mg/5mL [118mL, 237mL, 473mL]

CONTRAINDICATIONS

Pediatric patients <6 yrs of age. **Codeine:** Postoperative pain management in children who have undergone tonsillectomy and/or adenoidectomy, known hypersensitivity to the drug, treatment of lower respiratory tract symptoms (eg, asthma). **Promethazine:** Comatose states, known hypersensitivity or idiosyncratic reaction to promethazine or to other phenothiazines, treatment of lower respiratory tract symptoms (eg, asthma). **Phenylephrine:** HTN, peripheral vascular insufficiency, known hypersensitivity to the drug, concomitant use w/ MAOIs.

P

WARNINGS/PRECAUTIONS

Should only be given to a pregnant woman if clearly needed. Caution in elderly. Lab test interactions may occur. Codeine: Do not increase dose if cough fails to respond to treatment. May cause/aggravate constipation. May release histamine; caution in atopic children. Capacity to elevate CSF pressure and respiratory depressant effects may be markedly exaggerated in head injury, intracranial lesions, or with preexisting increase in intracranial pressure. May obscure clinical course in patients with head injuries. Avoid with acute febrile illness with productive cough or in chronic respiratory disease. May produce orthostatic hypotension in ambulatory patients. Give with caution and reduce initial dose with acute abdominal conditions, convulsive disorders, significant hepatic/renal impairment, fever, hypothyroidism, Addison's disease, ulcerative colitis, prostatic hypertrophy, recent GI or urinary tract surgery, and in very young, elderly, or debilitated patients. Use lowest effective dose for the shortest period of time. Potential for abuse and dependence. Promethazine: May impair mental/physical abilities. May lead to potentially fatal respiratory depression; avoid with compromised respiratory function (eg, COPD, sleep apnea). May lower seizure threshold; caution with seizure disorders. Leukopenia and agranulocytosis reported, especially when given with other marrow-toxic agents; caution with bone-marrow depression. Neuroleptic malignant syndrome (NMS) reported; d/c immediately if NMS occurs. Hallucinations and convulsions reported in pediatric patients. Acutely ill pediatric patients who are dehydrated may have increased susceptibility to dystonias. Cholestatic jaundice reported. Caution with narrow-angle glaucoma, prostatic hypertrophy, stenosing peptic ulcer, pyloroduodenal/bladder-neck obstruction, cardiovascular disease, or impaired liver function. Increased blood glucose reported. Phenylephrine: Caution with diabetes mellitus and thyroid/heart diseases. May cause urinary retention in men with symptomatic BPH. May decrease cardiac output; use extreme caution with arteriosclerosis, in elderly, and/or patients with initially poor cerebral or coronary circulation.

ADVERSE REACTIONS
Respiratory depression, drowsiness, dizziness, somnolence, anxiety, sedation, tremor, blurred vision, dry mouth, increased or decreased BP, N/V, urinary retention, NMS, constipation.

DRUG INTERACTIONS
See Boxed Warning and Contraindications. Promethazine: May increase, prolong, or intensify the sedative action of other CNS depressants (eg, alcohol, narcotics, general anesthetics, tranquilizers); avoid such agents or administer in reduced doses. Reduce dose of barbiturate by at least 1/2 and narcotic analgesics by 1/4 to 1/2; individualize dose. Do not use epinephrine to treat hypotension associated with promethazine overdose; may reverse vasopressor effect of epinephrine. Caution with other agents with anticholinergic properties and drugs that also affect seizure threshold (eg, narcotics, local anesthetics). Phenylephrine: Pressor response increased with TCAs and decreased with prior administration of phentolamine or other α-adrenergic blockers. Ergot alkaloids may cause excessive rise in BP. Tachycardia or other arrhythmias may occur with bronchodilator sympathomimetics, epinephrine, or other sympathomimetics. Reflex bradycardia blocked and pressor response enhanced with atropine sulfate. Cardiostimulating effects blocked with prior administration of propranolol or other β-adrenergic blockers. Synergistic adrenergic response with diet preparations (eg, amphetamines, phenylpropanolamine).

PATIENT CONSIDERATIONS
Assessment: Assess for drug hypersensitivity or idiosyncrasy, history of drug abuse/dependence, head injury, compromised respiratory function, poor cerebral/coronary circulation, or any other conditions where treatment is contraindicated or cautioned, pregnancy/nursing status, and for possible drug interactions.

Monitoring: Monitor for signs/symptoms of CNS and respiratory depression, constipation, leukopenia, agranulocytosis, cholestatic jaundice, seizures, NMS, orthostatic hypotension, abuse/dependence, increased blood glucose levels, and other adverse reactions. Monitor for urinary retention in men with BPH. Monitor pediatric patients for hallucinations, convulsions, and dystonias. Reevaluate 5 days or sooner if cough is unresponsive to treatment.

Counseling: Inform that therapy may cause marked drowsiness and may impair mental and/or physical abilities required for performing hazardous tasks; advise to avoid such activities until it is known that they do not become drowsy or dizzy with therapy. Instruct to avoid the use or reduce dose of alcohol and other CNS depressants while on therapy. Advise to report any involuntary muscle movements, and to avoid prolonged sun exposure. Inform that therapy may produce orthostatic hypotension. Advise patients that some people have a genetic variation that results in codeine changing into morphine more rapidly and completely than other people; instruct caregivers of children receiving codeine for other reasons to monitor for signs of respiratory depression. Inform about risks and the signs of morphine overdose. Instruct nursing mothers to notify pediatrician immediately, or get emergency medical attention, if signs of morphine toxicity (eg, increased sleepiness, difficulty breastfeeding, breathing difficulties, limpness) are noticed in their infants.

STORAGE: 20-25°C (68-77°F).

PROPAFENONE – propafenone hydrochloride RX

Class: Class IC antiarrhythmic

Increased rate of death or reversed cardiac arrest rate reported in patients treated with encainide or flecainide (Class 1C antiarrhythmics) in a study of patients with asymptomatic non-life-threatening ventricular arrhythmias who had a MI >6 days but <2 yrs previously. Consider any 1C antiarrhythmic to have a significant proarrhythmic risk in patients with structural heart disease. Avoid in patients with non-life-threatening ventricular arrhythmias, even if experiencing unpleasant, but not life-threatening signs/symptoms.

OTHER BRAND NAMES
Rythmol

ADULT DOSAGE
Paroxysmal Atrial Fibrillation/Flutter

Associated w/ Disabling Symptoms in Patients w/o Structural Heart Disease:

Initial: 150mg q8h (450mg/day)
Titrate: May increase at a minimum of 3 to 4 day intervals to 225mg q8h (675mg/day). May increase to 300mg q8h (900mg/day) if additional therapeutic effect is needed
Max: 900mg/day

PEDIATRIC DOSAGE
Pediatric use may not have been established

Paroxysmal Supraventricular Tachycardia

Associated w/ Disabling Symptoms in Patients w/o Structural Heart Disease:

Initial: 150mg q8h (450mg/day)
Titrate: May increase at a minimum of 3 to 4 day intervals to 225mg q8h (675mg/day). May increase to 300mg q8h (900mg/day) if additional therapeutic effect is needed
Max: 900mg/day

Ventricular Arrhythmias

Initial: 150mg q8h (450mg/day)
Titrate: May increase at a minimum of 3 to 4 day intervals to 225mg q8h (675mg/day). May increase to 300mg q8h (900mg/day) if additional therapeutic effect is needed
Max: 900mg/day

Initiate therapy in the hospital for patients w/ sustained ventricular tachycardia

DOSING CONSIDERATIONS

Hepatic Impairment

Consider reducing dose

Elderly

Start at lower end of dosing range. Increase more gradually during initial phase

Other Important Considerations

Significant QRS Widening/2nd- or 3rd-Degree Atrioventricular Block: Consider reducing dose

Ventricular Arrhythmia w/ Marked Previous Myocardial Damage: Increase more gradually during initial phase

ADMINISTRATION

Oral route

HOW SUPPLIED

Tab: 300mg*; (Rythmol) 150mg*, 225mg* *scored

CONTRAINDICATIONS

Heart failure (HF), cardiogenic shock, known Brugada syndrome, bradycardia, marked hypotension, bronchospastic disorders or severe obstructive pulmonary disease, marked electrolyte imbalance, and sinoatrial, AV, and intraventricular disorders of impulse generation or conduction (eg, sick sinus node syndrome, AV block) in the absence of an artificial pacemaker.

WARNINGS/PRECAUTIONS

Do not use to control ventricular rate during atrial fibrillation. Concomitant treatment with drugs that increase the functional AV nodal refractory period is recommended. May cause new or worsened arrhythmias; evaluate ECG prior to and during therapy to determine if response supports continued treatment. Brugada syndrome may be unmasked after exposure to therapy; perform ECG after initiation of treatment and d/c if changes are suggestive of Brugada syndrome. May provoke overt HF. Conduction disturbances (eg, 1st to 3rd-degree AV block, bundle branch block, intraventricular conduction delay, bradycardia), agranulocytosis, positive antinuclear antibody (ANA) titers, and exacerbation of myasthenia gravis reported. D/C if persistent or worsening elevation of ANA titers detected. May alter pacing and sensing thresholds of implanted pacemakers and defibrillators; monitor and reprogram devices accordingly during and after therapy. Reversible, short-term drop (within normal range) in sperm count may occur. Treatment of ventricular arrhythmias should be initiated in the hospital. Caution in patients with renal/hepatic dysfunction and in elderly.

ADVERSE REACTIONS

Unusual taste, N/V, dizziness, constipation, headache, fatigue, blurred vision, weakness.

DRUG INTERACTIONS

Avoid with Class IA and III antiarrhythmics (eg, quinidine, amiodarone) and withhold these agents for at least 5 half-lives prior to therapy. Inhibitors of CYP2D6 (eg, desipramine, paroxetine, ritonavir) and CYP3A4 (eg, ketoconazole, saquinavir, erythromycin) may increase levels; avoid simultaneous use with both a CYP2D6 and a CYP3A4 inhibitor. Amiodarone can affect conduction and repolarization; coadministration is not recommended. Fluoxetine may increase levels in extensive metabolizers. Rifampin may decrease levels and may increase norpropafenone (active metabolite) levels. May increase levels of digoxin, propranolol, metoprolol, and warfarin; monitor digoxin levels and INR. May result in severe adverse events (eg, convulsions, AV block, acute circulatory failure) with abrupt cessation of orlistat. May increase risk of CNS side effects of lidocaine. CYP1A2 inhibitors (eg, amiodarone, tobacco smoke) and cimetidine may increase levels.

P

PATIENT CONSIDERATIONS

Assessment: Assess for HF, cardiogenic shock, sinoatrial/AV/intraventricular disorders, implanted pacemaker/defibrillator, bradycardia, marked hypotension, bronchospastic disorders or severe obstructive pulmonary disease, marked electrolyte imbalance, MI, renal/hepatic dysfunction, known Brugada syndrome, pregnancy/nursing status, and possible drug interactions. Evaluate ECG prior to therapy.

Monitoring: Monitor for proarrhythmic effects, signs/symptoms of conduction disturbances, agranulocytosis, HF, unmasking of Brugada syndrome, exacerbation of myasthenia gravis, and other adverse reactions. Monitor implanted pacemakers and defibrillators during and after therapy and reprogram accordingly. Evaluate ECG during therapy. Monitor ANA titers and renal/hepatic function. Monitor INR when given with warfarin.

Counseling: Inform about risks/benefits of therapy. Advise to report symptoms that may be associated with electrolyte imbalance to physician. Inform to notify physician of all Rx, herbal/natural preparations, and OTC medications currently being taken or of any changes with these products. Instruct not to double the next dose if a dose is missed and to take next dose at the usual time.

STORAGE: 20-25°C (68-77°F). (Rythmol) 25°C (77°F); excursions permitted to 15-30°C (59-86°F).

PROPECIA – finasteride RX

Class: Type II 5 alpha-reductase inhibitor (5-ARI)

ADULT DOSAGE

Male Pattern Hair Loss

Androgenetic Alopecia:

1 tab (1mg) qd for ≥3 months

Continued use is recommended to sustain benefit; reevaluate periodically

PEDIATRIC DOSAGE

Pediatric use may not have been established

ADMINISTRATION

Oral route

Take w/ or w/o meals

HOW SUPPLIED

Tab: 1mg

CONTRAINDICATIONS

Pregnancy, women of childbearing potential, hypersensitivity to any component of this medication.

P

WARNINGS/PRECAUTIONS

Withdrawal of treatment may lead to reversal of effect within 12 months. Potential risk to male fetus; broken or crushed tabs should not be handled by pregnant women or women who may potentially be pregnant. May decrease serum prostate specific antigen (PSA) levels during therapy or in the presence of prostate cancer; any confirmed increase from lowest PSA value during treatment may signal presence of prostate cancer and should be evaluated. May increase risk of high-grade prostate cancer. Caution with liver dysfunction.

ADVERSE REACTIONS

Decreased libido, erectile dysfunction, ejaculation disorder.

PATIENT CONSIDERATIONS

Assessment: Assess for liver dysfunction and previous hypersensitivity to the drug and its components. Obtain baseline PSA levels.

Monitoring: Monitor for hypersensitivity reactions or other adverse reactions. Monitor PSA levels.

Counseling: Instruct pregnant or potentially pregnant women not to handle crushed or broken tabs due to possible absorption and potential risk to male fetus; advise to immediately wash contact area with soap and water if contact occurs. Inform that there was an increase in high-grade prostate cancer in men treated with 5α-reductase inhibitors indicated for BPH treatment. Instruct to promptly report any changes in breasts (eg, lumps, pain, nipple discharge) to physician.

STORAGE: 15-30°C (59-86°F). Protect from moisture.

PROPRANOLOL – propranolol hydrochloride

RX

Class: Nonselective beta blocker

OTHER BRAND NAMES

Inderal (Discontinued)

ADULT DOSAGE

Hypertension

Sol/Tab:
Initial: 40mg bid
Titrate: May increase gradually until adequate BP control is achieved
Maint: 120-240mg/day

In some instances, 640mg/day may be required

If control is not adequate w/ bid dosing, a larger dose, or tid therapy may achieve better control

Angina Pectoris

Due to coronary atherosclerosis to decrease angina frequency and increase exercise tolerance

Sol/Tab:
80-320mg/day given bid, tid or qid

Reduce dose gradually over a period of a few weeks if therapy is to be discontinued

Atrial Fibrillation

Sol/Tab:
10-30mg tid or qid ac and hs

Myocardial Infarction

To reduce cardiovascular mortality in patients who have survived the acute phase of MI and are clinically stable

Sol/Tab:
Initial: 40mg tid
Titrate: Increase to 60-80mg tid after 1 month as tolerated
Maint: 180-240mg/day in divided doses (either bid or tid)
Max: 240mg/day

Migraine

Prophylaxis:
Sol/Tab:
Initial: 80mg/day in divided doses
Usual: 160-240mg/day
Titrate: May increase gradually for optimum prophylaxis

D/C gradually if a satisfactory response is not obtained w/in 4-6 weeks after reaching max dose

Essential Tremor

Familial or Hereditary:
Sol/Tab:
Initial: 40mg bid
Usual: 120mg/day
May be necessary to give 240-320mg/day

Hypertrophic Subaortic Stenosis

Sol/Tab:
Usual: 20-40mg tid or qid ac and hs

Pheochromocytoma

PEDIATRIC DOSAGE

Pediatric use may not have been established

P

Sol/Tab:
Usual: 60mg/day in divided doses for 3 days before surgery w/ α-adrenergic blocker

Inoperable Tumor:
Usual: 30mg/day in divided doses w/ α-adrenergic blocker

Arrhythmias

Life-threatening or those occurring under anesthesia (supraventricular/ventricular tachycardia, tachyarrhythmia of digitalis intoxication, resistant tachyarrhythmia due to excessive catecholamine action during anesthesia)

Inj:
Usual: 1-3mg IV at ≤1mg/min
May give a 2nd dose if necessary after 2 min then do not give additional drug in <4 hrs

Do not give additional dose when desired alteration in rate/rhythm is achieved

Transfer to oral therapy as soon as possible

DOSING CONSIDERATIONS

Hepatic Insufficiency
Inj:
Consider lower dose

Elderly
Start at lower end of dosing range

ADMINISTRATION

Oral/IV route

HOW SUPPLIED

Inj: 1mg/mL; **Sol:** 20mg/5mL, 40mg/5mL [500mL]; **Tab:** 10mg*, 20mg*, 40mg*, 60mg*, 80mg*
*scored

CONTRAINDICATIONS

Cardiogenic shock, sinus bradycardia and >1st-degree block, bronchial asthma, known hypersensitivity to propranolol HCl.

WARNINGS/PRECAUTIONS

Exacerbation of angina and MI following abrupt discontinuation reported; when discontinuation is planned, reduce dose gradually over at least a few weeks. Reinstitute therapy if exacerbation of angina occurs upon interruption and take other measures for management of angina pectoris; follow same procedure in patients at risk of occult atherosclerotic heart disease who are given propranolol for other indication since coronary artery disease may be unrecognized. May precipitate more severe failure in patients w/ CHF; avoid w/ overt CHF and caution in patients w/ history of heart failure (HF) who are well-compensated and are receiving additional therapies. Caution w/ bronchospastic lung disease, hepatic/renal impairment, Wolff-Parkinson-White (WPW) syndrome, and tachycardia. Chronically administered therapy should not be routinely withdrawn prior to major surgery; however, may augment risks of general anesthesia and surgical procedures. May mask acute hypoglycemia and hyperthyroidism signs/symptoms. May be more difficult to adjust insulin dose in labile insulin-dependent diabetics. Abrupt withdrawal may be followed by an exacerbation of symptoms of hyperthyroidism, including thyroid storm. May reduce IOP. Hypersensitivity/anaphylactic/cutaneous reactions reported. Patients w/ history of severe anaphylactic reaction to a variety of allergens may be more reactive to repeated accidental/diagnostic/therapeutic challenge; may be unresponsive to usual doses of epinephrine. Elevated serum K+, transaminases, and alkaline phosphatase levels reported. Increases in BUN reported in patients w/ severe HF. Not for treatment of hypertensive emergencies. (Oral) Not indicated for migraine attack that has started and tremor associated w/ parkinsonism. Continued use in patients w/o history of HF may lead to cardiac failure.

ADVERSE REACTIONS

Bradycardia, CHF, hypotension, lightheadedness, mental depression, N/V, agranulocytosis, respiratory distress.

DRUG INTERACTIONS

Administration w/ CYP450 (2D6, 1A2, 2C19) substrates, inducers, and inhibitors may lead to clinically relevant drug interactions. Increased levels and/or toxicity w/ substrates/inhibitors of CYP2D6 (eg, amiodarone, cimetidine, fluoxetine, ritonavir), CYP1A2 (eg, imipramine, ciprofloxacin, isoniazid, theophylline), and CYP2C19 (eg, fluconazole, teniposide, tolbutamide). Decreased blood levels w/ hepatic enzyme inducers (eg, rifampin, ethanol, phenytoin, phenobarbital). May increase levels of propafenone, lidocaine, nifedipine, zolmitriptan, rizatriptan, diazepam and its metabolites. Increased levels w/ nisoldipine, nicardipine, and chlorpromazine. May decrease theophylline clearance. Increased thioridazine plasma and metabolite (mesoridazine) concentrations w/ doses ≥160mg/day. Decreased levels w/ aluminum hydroxide gel, cholestyramine, and colestipol. May decrease levels of lovastatin and pravastatin. Increased warfarin levels and PT; monitor PT. Additive effect w/ propafenone and amiodarone. Caution w/ drugs that slow atrioventricular (AV) nodal conduction (eg, digitalis, lidocaine, calcium channel blockers); increased risk of bradycardia w/ digitalis. Significant bradycardia, HF, and CV collapse reported w/ concomitant verapamil. Bradycardia, hypotension, high-degree heart block, and HF reported w/ concomitant diltiazem. Concomitant ACE inhibitors may cause hypotension. May antagonize effects of clonidine; administer cautiously to patients withdrawing from clonidine. Prolongation of 1st dose hypotension may occur w/ concomitant prazosin. Postural hypotension reported w/ concomitant terazosin or doxazosin. Monitor for excessive reduction of resting sympathetic nervous activity w/ catecholamine-depleting drugs (eg, reserpine). Patients on long-term therapy may experience uncontrolled HTN w/ concomitant epinephrine. β-receptor agonists (eg, dobutamine, isoproterenol) may reverse effects. NSAIDs (eg, indomethacin) may blunt the antihypertensive effect. Coadministration w/ methoxyflurane and trichloroethylene may depress myocardial contractility. Hypotension and cardiac arrest reported w/ concomitant haloperidol. Thyroxine may result in a lower than expected T3 concentration when coadministered w/ propranolol. May exacerbate hypotensive effects of MAOIs or TCAs. (Inj) Severe bradycardia, asystole, and HF reported w/ concomitant disopyramide. Increased bronchial hyperreactivity w/ ACE inhibitors. (Oral) Increased levels w/ alcohol.

PATIENT CONSIDERATIONS

Assessment: Assess for cardiogenic shock, sinus bradycardia, AV heart block, bronchial asthma, CHF, bronchospastic lung disease, hyperthyroidism, diabetes, WPW syndrome, tachycardia, hepatic/renal impairment, history/presence of HF, risk for occult atherosclerotic heart disease, hypersensitivity to drug, pregnancy/nursing status, and possible drug interactions.

Monitoring: Monitor for signs/symptoms of cardiac failure, hypoglycemia, decreased IOP, hyperthyroidism, withdrawal symptoms, hypersensitivity reactions, and other adverse reactions. (Inj) Monitor ECG and central venous pressure. (Oral) For HTN (bid dosing), measure BP near the end of dosing interval to determine satisfactory BP control.

Counseling: Inform of the risk/benefits of therapy. Instruct not to interrupt or d/c therapy w/o physician's advice. Inform that therapy may interfere w/ glaucoma screening test.

STORAGE: 20-25°C (68-77°F); (Sol) excursions permitted to 15-30°C (59-86°F). (Inj) Protect from freezing and excessive heat. (Tab) Protect from light.

PROSCAR – finasteride

RX

Class: Type II 5 alpha-reductase inhibitor (5-ARI)

P

ADULT DOSAGE

Benign Prostatic Hyperplasia

Monotherapy or in Combination w/ Doxazosin:

1 tab (5mg) qd

PEDIATRIC DOSAGE

Pediatric use may not have been established

ADMINISTRATION

Oral route

Take w/ or w/o meals

HOW SUPPLIED

Tab: 5mg

CONTRAINDICATIONS

Hypersensitivity to any component of this medication. Women who are or may potentially be pregnant.

WARNINGS/PRECAUTIONS

Not approved for the prevention of prostate cancer. May decrease serum prostate specific antigen (PSA) concentration during therapy or in the presence of prostate cancer; establish a new baseline PSA at least 6 months after starting treatment and monitor PSA periodically thereafter. Any confirmed increase from lowest PSA value during treatment may signal presence of prostate cancer. May increase risk of high-grade prostate cancer. Potential risk to male fetus; broken or crushed tabs should not be handled by pregnant women or women who may potentially be pregnant. May decrease ejaculate volume and total sperm per ejaculate. Prior to treatment initiation, consider other urological conditions that may cause similar symptoms; BPH and prostate cancer may coexist. Monitor for obstructive uropathy in patients with large residual urinary volume and/or severely diminished urinary flow; such patients may not be candidates for therapy. Caution with liver dysfunction.

ADVERSE REACTIONS

Impotence, decreased libido, decreased ejaculate volume, asthenia, postural hypotension, dizziness, abnormal ejaculation.

PATIENT CONSIDERATIONS

Assessment: Assess for liver dysfunction, previous hypersensitivity to the drug, other urological conditions that may cause similar symptoms, residual urinary volume, and diminished urinary flow.

Monitoring: Monitor for obstructive uropathy in patients with large residual urinary volume and/or severely diminished urinary flow. Monitor for signs/symptoms of prostate cancer, hypersensitivity reactions, and other adverse reactions. Obtain baseline PSA levels at least 6 months after starting treatment and monitor PSA periodically thereafter.

Counseling: Inform that therapy may increase risk of high-grade prostate cancer. Instruct pregnant or potentially pregnant females not to handle crushed or broken tabs due to possible absorption and potential risk to male fetus; advise to immediately wash contact area with soap and water if contact occurs. Advise that the volume of ejaculate may be decreased and impotence/decreased libido may occur. Instruct to promptly report to physician any changes in breasts (eg, lumps, pain, nipple discharge).

STORAGE: Room temperature <30°C (86°F). Protect from light.

PROTONIX – pantoprazole sodium

RX

Class: Proton pump inhibitor (PPI)

OTHER BRAND NAMES

Protonix IV

ADULT DOSAGE

Gastroesophageal Reflux Disease

Short-Term Treatment of Erosive Esophagitis Associated w/ GERD:
40mg qd for up to 8 weeks; may consider additional 8-week course if not healed after 8 weeks of treatment

Maint of Healing of Erosive Esophagitis:
40mg qd; no controlled studies beyond 12 months

GERD Associated w/ History of Erosive Esophagitis:
40mg qd by IV infusion for 7-10 days; d/c as soon as patient is able to receive oral formulation

Pathological Hypersecretory Conditions

Long-term treatment of pathological hypersecretory conditions, including Zollinger-Ellison syndrome

40mg bid
Titrate: Adjust to individual needs and continue for as long as clinically indicated; doses up to 240mg have been administered

Refer to PI for IV dosing

PEDIATRIC DOSAGE

Gastroesophageal Reflux Disease

Short-Term Treatment of Erosive Esophagitis Associated w/ GERD:

≥5 Years:
≥15kg-<40kg: 20mg qd for up to 8 weeks
≥40kg: 40mg qd for up to 8 weeks

ADMINISTRATION

Oral/IV route

Tab/Sus
Do not split, chew, or crush.

Tab
Swallow whole, w/ or w/o food.
If patients are unable to swallow a 40mg tab, two 20mg tabs may be taken.

Sus
Administer approx 30 min ac via oral administration in apple juice or applesauce or NG tube in apple juice only; do not administer in other liquids/foods.

Do not divide the 40mg pkt to create a 20mg dosage.

Oral Administration in Applesauce:

Sprinkle granules on 1 tsp of applesauce and take w/in 10 min of preparation.

Take sips of water to ensure granules are washed down.

Oral Administration in Apple Juice:

Empty granules into a small cup or tsp containing 1 tsp of apple juice.

Stir for 5 sec and swallow immediately.

Rinse container once or twice w/ apple juice and swallow immediately to ensure entire dose is taken.

NG Tube/Gastrostomy Tube Administration:

Connect the catheter tip of the syringe to a 16 French (or larger) tube.

Empty the contents of the pkt into the barrel of the syringe.

Add 10mL (2 tsp) of apple juice and gently tap and/or shake the barrel of the syringe to help rinse the syringe and tube.

Repeat at least twice more using the same amount of apple juice each time; no granules should remain in the syringe.

IV

Flush IV line before and after administration.

GERD Associated w/ History of Erosive Esophagitis:

15-Min Infusion:

Reconstitute w/ 10mL of 0.9% NaCl and further dilute w/ 100mL of D5 inj, 0.9% NaCl, or lactated Ringer's inj to a final concentration of approx 0.4mg/mL.

May store reconstituted sol for up to 6 hrs at room temperature prior to further dilution.

Admixed sol must be used w/in 24 hrs from the time of initial reconstitution.

Administer over approx 15 min at a rate of approx 7mL/min.

2-Min Infusion:

Reconstitute w/ 10mL of 0.9% NaCl to a final concentration of approx 4mg/mL.

The reconstituted sol may be stored for up to 24 hrs at room temperature prior to IV infusion.

Administer over at least 2 min.

HOW SUPPLIED

Inj: 40mg; **Sus, Delayed-Release:** 40mg (granules/pkt); **Tab, Delayed-Release:** 20mg, 40mg

CONTRAINDICATIONS

Known hypersensitivity reactions (eg, anaphylaxis) to any component of the formulation or any substituted benzimidazole.

WARNINGS/PRECAUTIONS

Symptomatic response does not preclude the presence of gastric malignancy. Acute interstitial nephritis reported; d/c if this develops. May increase risk of *Clostridium difficile*-associated diarrhea (CDAD), especially in hospitalized patients. May increase risk for osteoporosis-related fractures of the hip, wrist, or spine, especially w/ high-dose and long-term therapy. Use lowest dose and shortest duration appropriate to the condition being treated. Hypomagnesemia reported and may require Mg^{2+} replacement and discontinuation of therapy; consider monitoring Mg^{2+} levels prior to and periodically during therapy w/ prolonged treatment. Anaphylaxis and other serious reactions (eg, erythema multiforme, Stevens-Johnson syndrome, toxic epidermal necrolysis) reported; may require emergency medical treatment. Lab test interactions may occur. (Oral) Atrophic gastritis noted w/ long-term therapy, particularly in patients who were *Helicobacter pylori* positive. Vitamin B12 deficiency caused by hypo- or achlorhydria may occur w/ long-term use (eg, >3 yrs). (IV) Thrombophlebitis reported. Contains EDTA, a chelator of metal ions including zinc; consider zinc supplementation in patients prone to zinc deficiency. Mild, transient transaminase elevations observed in clinical studies.

ADVERSE REACTIONS

Headache, diarrhea, N/V, abdominal pain, flatulence, dizziness, rash, fever, URI, arthralgia.

DRUG INTERACTIONS

Concomitant use w/ atazanavir or nelfinavir is not recommended; may substantially decrease atazanavir or nelfinavir concentrations. Monitor for increases in INR and PT w/ warfarin. May reduce the absorption of drugs where gastric pH is an important determinant of bioavailability; ketoconazole, ampicillin esters, atazanavir, iron salts, erlotinib, mycophenolate mofetil (MMF) absorption may decrease. Caution in transplant patients receiving MMF. Caution w/ digoxin or other drugs that may cause hypomagnesemia (eg, diuretics). May elevate and prolong levels of MTX and/or its metabolite, possibly leading to toxicities; consider temporary withdrawal of therapy w/ high-dose MTX. (IV) Use caution when other EDTA-containing products are also coadministered IV.

PATIENT CONSIDERATIONS

Assessment: Assess for hypersensitivity to the drug, risk for osteoporosis-related fractures, pregnancy/nursing status, and possible drug interactions. Obtain baseline Mg^{2+} levels. (IV) Assess if prone to zinc deficiency.

Monitoring: Monitor for signs/symptoms of acute interstitial nephritis, CDAD, bone fractures, hypersensitivity reactions, and other adverse reactions. Monitor Mg^{2+} levels periodically. Monitor INR and PT when given w/ warfarin. (Oral) Monitor for signs/symptoms of atrophic gastritis

P

and vitamin B12 deficiency. (IV) Monitor for thrombophlebitis, zinc deficiency, and transaminase elevations.

Counseling: Instruct to take ud. Inform of the most frequently occurring adverse reactions. Instruct to inform physician if any unusual symptom develops, or if any known symptom persists or worsens; advise to immediately report and seek care for any cardiovascular or neurological symptoms (eg, palpitation, dizziness, seizures, tetany) and for diarrhea that does not improve. Instruct to inform physician of all medications currently being taken, including OTC medications, as well as allergies to any medications. Inform that concomitant administration of antacids does not affect the absorption of the tabs. Advise that oral sus pkt is a fixed dose and cannot be divided to make smaller dose.

STORAGE: 20-25°C (68-77°F); excursions permitted to 15-30°C (59-86°F). (IV) Protect from light.

PROVENTIL HFA – albuterol sulfate

RX

Class: $Beta_2$ agonist

ADULT DOSAGE

Bronchospasm

Treatment/Prevention:
Usual: 2 inh q4-6h; 1 inh q4h may be sufficient in some patients

Exercise-Induced Bronchospasm

Prevention:
Usual: 2 inh 15-30 min before exercise

PEDIATRIC DOSAGE

Bronchospasm

≥4 Years:
Treatment/Prevention:
Usual: 2 inh q4-6h; 1 inh q4h may be sufficient in some patients

Exercise-Induced Bronchospasm

≥4 Years:
Prevention:
Usual: 2 inh 15-30 min before exercise

ADMINISTRATION

Oral inh route

Shake well before use.
Discard canister after 200 sprays have been used.

Priming
Prime inhaler before using for 1st time or if inhaler has not been used for >2 weeks by releasing 4 test sprays into air, away from the face.

HOW SUPPLIED

MDI: 90mcg of albuterol base/inh [200 inh]

CONTRAINDICATIONS

History of hypersensitivity to albuterol or any other components in this medication.

WARNINGS/PRECAUTIONS

May produce paradoxical bronchospasm that may be life threatening; d/c immediately and institute alternative therapy if this occurs. More doses than usual may be a marker of destabilization of asthma and may require reevaluation of the patient and treatment regimen; give special consideration to the possible need for anti-inflammatory treatment (eg, corticosteroids). May produce clinically significant cardiovascular (CV) effects; may need to d/c. ECG changes reported. Immediate hypersensitivity reactions may occur. Fatalities reported w/ excessive use. Caution w/ CV disorders (eg, coronary insufficiency, arrhythmias, HTN), convulsive disorders, hyperthyroidism, diabetes mellitus (DM), and in patients unusually responsive to sympathomimetic amines. May cause significant BP changes and hypokalemia. Aggravation of preexisting DM and ketoacidosis reported w/ large doses of IV albuterol. Caution in elderly.

ADVERSE REACTIONS

Tachycardia, tremor, rhinitis, URTI, fever, inhalation-site sensation, inhalation-taste sensation, nervousness, allergic reaction, respiratory disorder, N/V.

DRUG INTERACTIONS

Use w/ β-blockers may block pulmonary effects and produce severe bronchospasm in asthmatic patients; avoid concomitant use. If needed, consider cardioselective β-blockers and use w/ caution. ECG changes and/or hypokalemia caused by non-K^+-sparing diuretics (eg, loop or thiazide diuretics) may be acutely worsened; use caution during coadministration. May decrease serum digoxin levels. Use extreme caution w/ MAOIs and TCAs, or w/in 2 weeks of discontinuation of such agents.

PATIENT CONSIDERATIONS

Assessment: Assess for history of hypersensitivity to the drug, CV disorders, convulsive disorders, hyperthyroidism, DM, pregnancy/nursing status, and possible drug interactions. Assess use in patients unusually responsive to sympathomimetic amines.

Monitoring: Monitor for paradoxical bronchospasm, deterioration of asthma, CV effects, ECG changes, hypokalemia, immediate hypersensitivity reactions, and other adverse effects. Monitor BP and HR.

Counseling: Instruct not to increase dose/frequency of doses w/o consulting physician. Advise to seek immediate medical attention if treatment becomes less effective for symptomatic relief, symptoms become worse, and/or there is a need to use the product more frequently than usual. Instruct to keep plastic mouthpiece clean to prevent medication build-up and blockage; advise to wash, shake to remove excess water, and air dry mouthpiece thoroughly at least once a week. Inform that inhaler may cease to deliver medication if not cleaned properly. Instruct to take concurrent inhaled drugs/asthma medications only as directed. Inform of the common side effects of treatment, such as chest pain, palpitations, rapid HR, tremor, or nervousness. Advise to notify physician if pregnant/nursing. Advise to avoid spraying in eyes. Instruct to use only w/ supplied actuator and not to use actuator w/ other aerosol medications.

STORAGE: 15-25°C (59-77°F). Store inhaler w/ the mouthpiece down. Contents under pressure; do not puncture or incinerate. Exposure to temperatures >49°C (120°F) may cause bursting.

PROVERA – medroxyprogesterone acetate

RX

Class: Progestogen

Estrogen plus progestin therapy should not be used for the prevention of cardiovascular disease (CVD) or dementia. Increased risk of deep vein thrombosis (DVT), pulmonary embolism (PE), stroke, and MI reported in postmenopausal women (50-79 yrs of age) treated w/ daily oral conjugated estrogens (CEs) combined w/ medroxyprogesterone acetate (MPA). Increased risk of developing probable dementia reported in postmenopausal women ≥65 yrs of age treated w/ daily CEs combined w/ MPA. Increased risk of invasive breast cancer reported w/ estrogen plus progestin. Should be prescribed at the lowest effective dose and for the shortest duration consistent w/ treatment goals and risks.

ADULT DOSAGE

Abnormal Uterine Bleeding

Due to Hormonal Imbalance in the Absence of Organic Pathology (eg, Fibroids, Uterine Cancer):
5 or 10mg/day for 5-10 days beginning on Day 16 or 21 of cycle; 10mg/day for 10 days, beginning on Day 16 of the cycle is recommended to produce an optimum secretory transformation of an endometrium that has been adequately primed w/ either endogenous or exogenous estrogen

Endometrial Hyperplasia

Reduce Incidence in Non-Hysterectomized Postmenopausal Women Receiving Daily Oral CEs 0.625mg Tabs:
5 or 10mg/day for 12-14 consecutive days/month, beginning on Day 1 or 16 of cycle

Secondary Amenorrhea

5 or 10mg/day for 5-10 days. 10mg/day for 10 days is a dose for inducing an optimum secretory transformation of an endometrium that has been adequately primed w/ either endogenous or exogenous estrogen. May start therapy at any time

PEDIATRIC DOSAGE

Pediatric use may not have been established

ADMINISTRATION

Oral route

HOW SUPPLIED

Tab: 2.5mg*, 5mg*, 10mg* *scored

CONTRAINDICATIONS

Undiagnosed abnormal genital bleeding, known/suspected/history of breast cancer, known/suspected estrogen- or progesterone-dependent neoplasia, active/history of DVT/PE or arterial thromboembolic disease (eg, stroke, MI), known anaphylactic reaction or angioedema to medroxyprogesterone acetate, known liver impairment or disease, known/suspected pregnancy.

P

WARNINGS/PRECAUTIONS

D/C estrogen plus progestin therapy immediately if PE, DVT, stroke, or MI occurs or is suspected. If feasible, d/c estrogen plus progestin therapy at least 4-6 weeks before surgery of the type associated w/ an increased risk of thromboembolism, or during periods of prolonged immobilization. Increased risk of endometrial cancer reported w/ use of unopposed estrogen therapy in women w/ a uterus; adding a progestin to estrogen therapy has been shown to reduce risk of endometrial hyperplasia, which may be a precursor to endometrial cancer. Estrogen plus progestin therapy may increase risk of ovarian cancer. D/C estrogen plus progestin therapy pending exam if there is sudden partial or complete loss of vision, or a sudden onset of proptosis, diplopia or migraine; d/c permanently if exam reveals papilledema or retinal vascular lesions. In cases of unexpected abnormal vaginal bleeding, perform adequate diagnostic measures. Monitor BP at regular intervals w/ estrogen plus progestin therapy. Estrogen plus progestin therapy may increase plasma TGs, leading to pancreatitis in women w/ preexisting hypertriglyceridemia; consider discontinuation of treatment if pancreatitis occurs. Caution w/ history of cholestatic jaundice associated w/ past estrogen use or w/ pregnancy; d/c in case of recurrence. May cause fluid retention; caution in cardiac or renal impairment. Caution in women w/ hypoparathyroidism as estrogen-induced hypocalcemia may occur. Estrogen plus progestin therapy may exacerbate asthma, diabetes mellitus, epilepsy, migraine, porphyria, systemic lupus erythematosus, and hepatic hemangiomas. Withdrawal bleeding may occur w/in 3-7 days after discontinuing therapy. May affect LFTs and certain endocrine and blood components in lab tests.

ADVERSE REACTIONS

Abnormal uterine bleeding, breast tenderness, galactorrhea, urticaria, pruritus, edema, rash, menstrual changes, change in weight, mental depression, insomnia, somnolence, dizziness, headache, nausea.

DRUG INTERACTIONS

Women on thyroid replacement therapy may require higher doses of thyroid hormone.

PATIENT CONSIDERATIONS

Assessment: Assess for abnormal genital bleeding, cardiac or renal impairment, presence or history of breast cancer, estrogen- or progesterone-dependent neoplasias, active/history of DVT/PE or arterial thromboembolic disease, any other conditions where treatment is contraindicated or cautioned, and for possible drug interactions.

Monitoring: Monitor for signs/symptoms of CVD, malignant neoplasms, visual abnormalities, hypertriglyceridemia, fluid retention, exacerbation of asthma, and other adverse reactions. Perform annual breast exam; schedule mammography based on age, risk factors, and prior mammogram results. Regularly monitor BP in patients on estrogen plus progestin therapy. Monitor thyroid function in patients on thyroid replacement therapy. Periodically reevaluate (every 3-6 months) need for therapy. In cases of undiagnosed, persistent, or recurrent genital bleeding in women w/ a uterus, perform adequate diagnostic measures (eg, endometrial sampling) to rule out malignancy.

Counseling: Advise of risks and benefits of therapy. Instruct to have annual breast exams and perform monthly breast self-exams. Advise to schedule mammography exams based on age, risk factors, and prior mammogram results. Inform of possible increased risk of minor birth defects in children whose mothers are exposed to progestins during the 1st trimester of pregnancy; inform of the importance of reporting exposure of therapy in early pregnancy.

STORAGE: 20-25°C (68-77°F).

PROVIGIL – modafinil

CIV

Class: Wakefulness-promoting agent

ADULT DOSAGE

Excessive Sleepiness

Associated w/ Narcolepsy/Obstructive Sleep Apnea/Shift Work Disorder:
200mg qd
Max: 400mg/day as a single dose

PEDIATRIC DOSAGE

Pediatric use may not have been established

DOSING CONSIDERATIONS

Hepatic Impairment

Severe: 100mg qd

Elderly

Consider using lower doses

ADMINISTRATION
Oral route

Narcolepsy/Obstructive Sleep Apnea
Take as single dose in am

Shift Work Disorder
Take 1 hr prior to start of work shift

HOW SUPPLIED
Tab: 100mg, 200mg* *scored

CONTRAINDICATIONS
Known hypersensitivity to modafinil or armodafinil or its inactive ingredients.

WARNINGS/PRECAUTIONS
Not indicated as treatment for underlying obstruction in OSA; if continuous positive airway pressure (CPAP) is the treatment of choice, treat w/ CPAP for an adequate period of time prior to initiating and during treatment. Rare cases of serious or life-threatening rash, including Stevens-Johnson syndrome (SJS), toxic epidermal necrolysis (TEN), and drug rash w/ eosinophilia and systemic symptoms (DRESS), reported; d/c at the 1st sign of rash, unless the rash is clearly not drug-related. Angioedema reported; d/c if angioedema or anaphylaxis occurs. Multiorgan hypersensitivity reactions reported; d/c if suspected. Level of wakefulness may not return to normal in patients w/ abnormal levels of sleepiness. Psychiatric adverse reactions reported; caution w/ history of psychosis, depression, or mania. Consider discontinuation if psychiatric symptoms develop in association w/ drug administration. May impair mental and/or physical abilities. Cardiovascular (CV) adverse reactions reported; not recommended in patients w/ a history of left ventricular hypertrophy (LVH) or in patients w/ mitral valve prolapse who have experienced mitral valve prolapse syndrome (eg, ischemic ECG changes, chest pain, arrhythmia) when previously receiving CNS stimulants. Caution w/ known CV disease (CVD). Caution in elderly. Potential for abuse.

ADVERSE REACTIONS
Headache, nausea, nervousness, anxiety, insomnia, rhinitis, diarrhea, back pain, dizziness, dyspepsia, anorexia, dry mouth, pharyngitis, chest pain, HTN.

DRUG INTERACTIONS
May reduce exposure of CYP3A4/5 substrates (eg, midazolam, triazolam); consider dose adjustment of these drugs. Effectiveness of steroidal contraceptives (eg, ethinyl estradiol) may be reduced when used w/ therapy and for 1 month after discontinuation of therapy; alternative or concomitant methods of contraception are recommended. May reduce levels of cyclosporine; consider dose adjustment for cyclosporine. May increase exposure of CYP2C19 substrates (eg, phenytoin, diazepam, propranolol). In individuals deficient in the CYP2D6 enzyme, levels of CYP2D6 substrates, which have ancillary routes of elimination through CYP2C19 (eg, TCAs, SSRIs) may be increased; dose adjustments of these drugs and other drugs that are substrates for CYP2C19 may be necessary. Consider more frequent monitoring of PT/INR w/ warfarin. Caution w/ MAOIs.

PATIENT CONSIDERATIONS

Assessment: Assess for hypersensitivity to the drug, history of psychosis, depression, mania, or LVH, mitral valve prolapse, other CVD, hepatic impairment, pregnancy/nursing status, and possible drug interactions.

Monitoring: Monitor for rash, SJS, TEN, DRESS, angioedema, anaphylaxis, multiorgan hypersensitivity reactions, psychiatric symptoms, CV events (especially in patients w/ a history of MI or unstable angina), and other adverse reactions. Monitor for signs of misuse or abuse. Monitor HR and BP. Frequently reassess degree of sleepiness. Monitor PT/INR frequently w/ warfarin.

Counseling: Instruct to d/c use and notify physician immediately if allergic reactions and other adverse reactions (eg, chest pain, rash, depression, anxiety, signs of psychosis/mania) develop. Advise not to alter previous behavior w/ regard to potentially dangerous activities (eg, driving, operating machinery) or other activities requiring appropriate levels of wakefulness, until and unless treatment has been shown to produce levels of wakefulness that permit such activities. Inform that drug is not a replacement for sleep. Counsel patients that it may be critical that they continue to take their previously prescribed treatments (eg, patients w/ OSA receiving CPAP). Advise to notify physician if pregnancy occurs, if intending to become pregnant, or if breastfeeding. Caution regarding the potential increased risk of pregnancy when using steroidal contraceptives w/ therapy and for 1 month after discontinuation of therapy. Instruct to inform physician if taking/planning to take any prescription/OTC drugs, and to avoid alcohol.

STORAGE: 20-25°C (68-77°F).

PROZAC — fluoxetine hydrochloride

RX

Class: Selective serotonin reuptake inhibitor (SSRI)

Antidepressants increased the risk of suicidal thoughts and behavior in children, adolescents, and young adults in short-term studies. Monitor closely for worsening and for emergence of suicidal thoughts and behaviors in patients who are started on antidepressant therapy. Not approved for use in children <7 yrs of age.

OTHER BRAND NAMES

Prozac Weekly

ADULT DOSAGE

Major Depressive Disorder

Initial: 20mg/day qam
Titrate: Consider a dose increase after several weeks if improvement is insufficient; administer doses >20mg/day qam or bid (am and noon)
Max: 80mg/day

Prozac Weekly:
Initiate 7 days after the last daily dose of 20mg cap
Consider reestablishing a daily dosing regimen if satisfactory response is not maintained

Switching to a TCA:
May need to reduce TCA dose and monitor plasma concentrations temporarily w/ coadministration or when fluoxetine has been recently discontinued

Obsessive Compulsive Disorder

Initial: 20mg/day qam
Titrate: Consider a dose increase after several weeks if improvement is insufficient; administer doses >20mg/day qam or bid (am and noon)
Range: 20-60mg/day
Max: 80mg/day

Bulimia Nervosa

Initial: 60mg/day qam; may titrate up to this target dose over several days
Max: 60mg/day

P

Panic Disorder

W/ or w/o Agoraphobia:
Initial: 10mg/day
Titrate: Increase to 20mg/day after 1 week; consider a dose increase after several weeks if no improvement
Max: 60mg/day

Bipolar I Disorder

Depressive Episodes:
In Combination w/ Olanzapine:
Initial: 20mg fluoxetine + 5mg olanzapine qpm
Range: 20-50mg fluoxetine + 5-12.5mg olanzapine
Max: 75mg fluoxetine + 18mg olanzapine

Major Depressive Disorder

Use in patients who do not respond to 2 separate trials of different antidepressants of adequate dose and duration in the current episode

In Combination w/ Olanzapine:
Initial: 20mg fluoxetine + 5mg olanzapine qpm
Range: 20-50mg fluoxetine + 5-20mg olanzapine
Max: 75mg fluoxetine + 18mg olanzapine

PEDIATRIC DOSAGE

Major Depressive Disorder

≥8 Years:
Initial: 10 or 20mg/day
Titrate: After 1 week at 10mg/day, increase to 20mg/day

Lower Weight Children:
Initial/Target: 10mg/day
Titrate: Consider a dose increase to 20mg/day after several weeks if improvement is insufficient

Switching to a TCA:
May need to reduce TCA dose and monitor plasma concentrations temporarily w/ coadministration or when fluoxetine has been recently discontinued

Obsessive Compulsive Disorder

≥7 Years:
Initial: 10mg/day
Titrate: Increase to 20mg/day after 2 weeks; consider additional dose increases after several more weeks if improvement is insufficient
Range: 20-60mg/day

Lower Weight Children:
Initial: 10mg/day
Titrate: Consider additional dose increases after several weeks if improvement is insufficient
Range: 20-30mg/day
Max: 60mg/day

Bipolar I Disorder

Depressive Episodes:
In Combination w/ Olanzapine:
10-17 Years:
Initial: 20mg fluoxetine + 2.5mg olanzapine qpm
Max: 50mg fluoxetine + 12mg olanzapine

Dosing Considerations with MAOIs

Switching to/from an MAOI for Psychiatric Disorders:
Allow at least 14 days between discontinuation of an MAOI and initiation of treatment, and allow at least 5 weeks between discontinuation of treatment and initiation of an MAOI

W/ Other MAOIs (eg, Linezolid, IV Methylene Blue):
Do not start fluoxetine in patients being treated w/ linezolid or IV methylene blue
In patients already receiving fluoxetine, if acceptable alternatives are not available and benefits outweigh risks, d/c fluoxetine and administer linezolid or IV methylene blue; monitor for serotonin syndrome for 5 weeks or until 24 hrs after the last dose of linezolid or

Dosing Considerations with MAOIs

Switching to/from an MAOI for Psychiatric Disorders:
Allow at least 14 days between discontinuation of an MAOI and initiation of treatment, and allow at least 5 weeks between discontinuation of treatment and initiation of an MAOI

W/ Other MAOIs (eg, Linezolid, IV Methylene Blue):
Do not start fluoxetine in patients being treated w/ linezolid or IV methylene blue
In patients already receiving fluoxetine, if acceptable alternatives are not available and benefits outweigh risks, d/c fluoxetine and administer linezolid or IV methylene blue; monitor for serotonin syndrome for 5 weeks or until 24 hrs after the last dose of linezolid or IV methylene blue, whichever comes 1st. May resume fluoxetine therapy 24 hrs after the last dose of linezolid or IV methylene blue

IV methylene blue, whichever comes 1st. May resume fluoxetine therapy 24 hrs after the last dose of linezolid or IV methylene blue

DOSING CONSIDERATIONS

Concomitant Medications

Combination w/ Olanzapine:

Patients Predisposed to Hypotensive Reactions w/ Hepatic Impairment, Slow Metabolizers, Pharmacodynamic Olanzapine Sensitivity:

Initial: 20mg fluoxetine + 2.5-5mg olanzapine
Titrate slowly and adjust dosage prn

Hepatic Impairment

Use lower or less frequent dosage

Elderly

Consider lower or less frequent dosage

Other Important Considerations

Concomitant Illness: May require dose adjustments

ADMINISTRATION

Oral route

Take w/ or w/o food

HOW SUPPLIED

Cap: 10mg, 20mg, 40mg; **Cap, Delayed-Release (Prozac Weekly):** 90mg

CONTRAINDICATIONS

Use of an MAOI for psychiatric disorders either concomitantly or within 5 weeks of stopping treatment. Treatment within 14 days of stopping an MAOI for psychiatric disorders. Starting treatment in patients being treated with other MAOIs (eg, linezolid, IV methylene blue). Concomitant use with pimozide or thioridazine.

WARNINGS/PRECAUTIONS

Serotonin syndrome reported; d/c immediately and initiate supportive symptomatic treatment. Anaphylactoid and pulmonary reactions reported; d/c if unexplained allergic reaction or rash occurs. May precipitate mixed/manic episode in patients at risk for bipolar disorder. Weight loss and anorexia reported. May increase risk of bleeding reactions. Pupillary dilation that occurs following use may trigger an angle-closure attack in a patient with anatomically narrow angles who does not have a patent iridectomy. Hyponatremia may occur; caution in elderly and volume-depleted patients. Consider discontinuation in patients with symptomatic hyponatremia and institute appropriate medical intervention. Convulsions, mania/hypomania, anxiety, insomnia, and nervousness reported. QT interval prolongation and ventricular arrhythmia (eg, torsades de pointes) reported. Caution in patients with congenital long QT syndrome, previous history of QT prolongation, family history of long QT syndrome or sudden cardiac death, and other conditions that predispose to QT prolongation and ventricular arrhythmia. Consider discontinuing treatment and obtaining cardiac evaluation if signs or symptoms of ventricular arrhythmia develop. Caution in patients with diseases/conditions that could affect hemodynamic responses or metabolism. May alter glycemic control in patients with diabetes. May impair mental/physical abilities. Long elimination $T_{1/2}$; changes in dose may not be fully reflected in plasma for several weeks. Adverse reactions reported upon discontinuation; avoid abrupt withdrawal.

ADVERSE REACTIONS

Somnolence, anorexia, anxiety, asthenia, diarrhea, dry mouth, dyspepsia, headache, insomnia, tremor, pharyngitis, flu syndrome, dizziness, nausea, nervousness.

DRUG INTERACTIONS

See Contraindications. Do not use thioridazine within 5 weeks of discontinuing therapy. Caution with CNS-active drugs. Avoid with other drugs that cause QT prolongation (eg, ziprasidone, erythromycin, quinidine). May cause serotonin syndrome with other serotonergic drugs (eg, triptans, TCAs, fentanyl) and with drugs that impair metabolism of serotonin; d/c immediately if this occurs. Increased risk of bleeding with aspirin, NSAIDs, warfarin, and other anticoagulants. Rare reports of prolonged seizures with electroconvulsive therapy. Drugs that are tightly bound to plasma proteins (eg, warfarin, digitoxin) may cause a shift in plasma concentrations, resulting in an adverse effect. Caution with CYP2D6 substrates, including antidepressants (eg, TCAs), antipsychotics (eg, phenothiazines and most atypicals), and antiarrhythmics (eg, propafenone, flecainide). Consider decreasing dose of drugs metabolized by CYP2D6, especially drugs with a narrow therapeutic index (eg, flecainide, propafenone, vinblastine). May prolong $T_{1/2}$ of diazepam. May increase levels of phenytoin, carbamazepine, haloperidol, clozapine, imipramine, and desipramine. Coadministration with alprazolam resulted in increased alprazolam levels and further psychomotor performance decrement. Anticonvulsant toxicity reported with phenytoin and carbamazepine. Antidiabetic drugs (eg, insulin, oral hypoglycemics) may require dose adjustment. May cause lithium toxicity; monitor lithium levels. Increased risk of hyponatremia with diuretics. Increased levels with CYP2D6 inhibitors.

PATIENT CONSIDERATIONS

Assessment: Assess for volume depletion, history of seizures, risk for/presence of bipolar disorder, diseases/conditions that affect metabolism or hemodynamic responses, diabetes, susceptibility to angle-closure glaucoma, congenital long QT syndrome, previous history of QT prolongation, family history of long QT syndrome or sudden cardiac death, other conditions that predispose to QT prolongation and ventricular arrhythmia, pregnancy/nursing status, and possible drug interactions. Consider ECG assessment if initiating treatment in patients with risk factors for QT prolongation and ventricular arrhythmia.

Monitoring: Monitor for clinical worsening, suicidality, unusual changes in behavior, allergic reactions, serotonin syndrome, bleeding reactions, angle-closure glaucoma, altered appetite and weight, hyponatremia, seizures, activation of mania/hypomania, hypoglycemia/hyperglycemia, QT interval prolongation, ventricular arrhythmia, and other adverse reactions. Monitor height and weight in children periodically. Consider periodic ECG monitoring if initiating treatment in patients with risk factors for QT prolongation and ventricular arrhythmia. Periodically reassess need for continued/maintenance treatment.

Counseling: Inform of risks, benefits, and appropriate use of therapy. Counsel to be alert for the emergence of suicidality, unusual changes in behavior, or worsening of depression, especially early during treatment and when the dose is adjusted up or down. Inform about risk of serotonin syndrome with concomitant use with other serotonergic agents. Counsel to seek medical care immediately if rash/hives or unusual bruising/bleeding develops, or if experiencing signs/symptoms associated with serotonin syndrome or hyponatremia. Inform that drug may cause mild pupillary dilation, which in susceptible individuals, may lead to an episode of angle-closure glaucoma. Inform that QT interval prolongation and ventricular arrhythmia (eg, torsades de pointes) have been reported. Advise to avoid operating hazardous machinery or driving a car until effects of drug are known. Advise to inform physician if taking or planning to take any prescription or OTC drugs, if pregnant/intending to become pregnant, or if breastfeeding. Instruct to take ud, not to stop taking medication without consulting physician, and to consult physician if symptoms do not improve.

STORAGE: 15-30°C (59-86°F). (Cap) Protect from light.

PULMICORT – budesonide

RX

Class: Corticosteroid

OTHER BRAND NAMES

Pulmicort Respules, Pulmicort Flexhaler

ADULT DOSAGE

Asthma

Flexhaler:
Maint:
Initial: 180-360mcg bid
Max: 720mcg bid

PEDIATRIC DOSAGE

Asthma

1-8 Years:
Respules:
Maint/Prophylaxis:
Previously on Bronchodilators Alone:
Initial: 0.5mg qd or 0.25mg bid
Max: 0.5mg/day

Previously on Inhaled Corticosteroids:
Initial: 0.5mg qd or 0.25mg bid
Max: 1mg/day
Previously on Oral Corticosteroids:
Initial: 1mg qd or 0.5mg bid
Max: 1mg/day
Symptomatic Children Not Responding to Nonsteroidal Therapy:
Initial: 0.25mg qd
≥6 Years:
Flexhaler:
Prophylaxis:
Initial: 180-360mcg bid
Max: 360mcg bid

DOSING CONSIDERATIONS

Elderly

Flexhaler:

Start at lower end of dosing range

ADMINISTRATION

Oral inhalation route

Patients should rinse mouth w/ water w/o swallowing after inh

Flexhaler

Priming is required prior to initial use

Respules

Administer via jet nebulizer connected to air compressor w/ adequate air flow (eg, Pari-LC-Jet Plus Nebulizer [w/ face mask or mouthpiece] connected to a Pari Master compressor)
Administer separately from other nebulizable medications in the nebulizer

HOW SUPPLIED

Powder, Inhalation: (Flexhaler) 90mcg/dose, 180mcg/dose. **Sus, Inhalation:** (Respules) 0.25mg/2mL, 0.5mg/2mL, 1mg/2mL [2mL]

CONTRAINDICATIONS

Primary treatment of status asthmaticus or other acute episodes of asthma where intensive measures are required. Hypersensitivity to budesonide or any components of the medication. (Flexhaler) Severe hypersensitivity to milk proteins.

WARNINGS/PRECAUTIONS

Candida albicans infections of mouth and pharynx reported; treat and/or d/c if needed. Not indicated for the rapid relief of bronchospasm or other acute episodes of asthma; may require oral corticosteroids. Increased susceptibility to infections (eg, chickenpox, measles), may lead to serious/fatal course; if exposed, consider prophylaxis/treatment. Caution w/ tuberculosis, untreated systemic fungal, bacterial, viral or parasitic infections, and ocular herpes simplex. Deaths due to adrenal insufficiency reported w/ transfer from systemic to inhaled corticosteroids (ICS); if oral corticosteroids are required, wean slowly from systemic steroid use after transferring to ICS. Transfer from systemic to inhalation therapy may unmask allergic conditions (eg, rhinitis, conjunctivitis). Observe for systemic corticosteroid withdrawal effects. Hypercorticism and adrenal suppression may appear; reduce dose slowly. Decreases in bone mineral density (BMD) reported; caution w/ chronic use of drugs that can reduce bone mass (eg, anticonvulsants, corticosteroids). May cause reduction in growth velocity in pediatrics. Glaucoma, increased IOP, and cataracts reported. Bronchospasm, w/ immediate increase in wheezing, may occur; d/c immediately. Rare cases of systemic eosinophilic conditions and vasculitis consistent w/ Churg-Strauss syndrome reported. Hypersensitivity reactions reported; d/c if signs and symptoms occur. (Flexhaler) Caution in elderly.

ADVERSE REACTIONS

Respiratory infection. (Flexhaler) Nasopharyngitis, headache, fever, sinusitis, pain, N/V, insomnia, dry mouth, weight gain. (Respules) Rhinitis, otitis media, coughing, viral infection, ear infection, gastroenteritis.

DRUG INTERACTIONS

Oral ketoconazole increases plasma levels of oral budesonide. Inhibition of metabolism and increased exposure w/ CYP3A4 inhibitors. Caution w/ ketoconazole and other known strong CYP3A4 inhibitors (eg, ritonavir, clarithromycin, itraconazole, nefazodone).

PATIENT CONSIDERATIONS

Assessment: Assess for concomitant diseases (eg, status asthmaticus, acute bronchospasm, other acute episodes of asthma), infections, major risk factors for decreased bone mineral

P

content, history of eye disorders, hypersensitivity, pregnancy/nursing status, and possible drug interactions. Obtain baseline cortisol production levels. Assess lung function in oral corticosteroids withdrawal. (Flexhaler) Assess for severe milk protein hypersensitivity and hepatic disease.

Monitoring: Monitor for localized oral infections w/ *C. albicans*, worsening or acutely deteriorating asthma, systemic corticosteroid effects, decreased BMD, height in children, vision change, bronchospasm, and hypersensitivity reactions. (Flexhaler) Monitor for hepatic disease.

Counseling: Advise to use at regular intervals and rinse mouth after inhalation; effectiveness depends on regular use. Instruct to d/c if oral candidiasis or hypersensitivity reactions occur. Inform that medication is not meant to relieve acute asthma symptoms and extra doses should not be used for that purpose. Instruct not to d/c w/o physician's guidance; symptoms may recur after discontinuation. Warn to avoid exposure to chickenpox or measles; if exposed, consult physician. Counsel that max benefit may not be achieved for ≥1-2 weeks (Flexhaler) or ≥4-6 weeks (Respules); instruct to notify physician if symptoms worsen or do not improve in that time frame. (Flexhaler) Instruct not to repeat inhalation even if the patient did not feel medication when inhaling; discard whole device after labeled number of inhalations have been used. Advise to carry a warning card indicating need for supplemental systemic corticosteroid during periods of stress or severe asthma attack if chronic systemic corticosteroids have been reduced or withdrawn. Instruct to consult physician if pregnant/breastfeeding or intend to become pregnant.

STORAGE: (Flexhaler): 20-25°C (68-77°F). Cover tightly. Store in a dry place. (Respules): 20-25°C (68-77°F). Protect from light. Do not freeze. After aluminum foil opened, unused ampules stable for 2 weeks. Once opened, use promptly.

PULMOZYME – dornase alfa

RX

Class: Enzyme

ADULT DOSAGE

Cystic Fibrosis

Improves pulmonary function in conjunction with standard therapies

2.5mg qd via nebulizer/compressor system (may benefit with bid dosing)

PEDIATRIC DOSAGE

Cystic Fibrosis

Improves pulmonary function in conjunction with standard therapies

≥5 Years:

2.5mg qd via nebulizer/compressor system (may benefit with bid dosing)

P

ADMINISTRATION

Inhalation route

Should not be diluted or mixed with other drugs in the nebulizer

Squeeze each ampule prior to use to check for leaks

Once opened, entire contents of the ampule must be used or discarded

Refer to PI for the recommended nebulizer/compressor systems

HOW SUPPLIED

Sol: 2.5mg/2.5mL

CONTRAINDICATIONS

Known hypersensitivity to dornase alfa, Chinese Hamster ovary cell products, or any component of the product.

WARNINGS/PRECAUTIONS

May consider use for pediatric patients younger than 5 years of age who may experience potential benefit in pulmonary function or who may be at risk of RTI.

ADVERSE REACTIONS

Voice alteration, pharyngitis, rash, laryngitis, chest pain, conjunctivitis, rhinitis, fever, dyspnea, dyspepsia, antibodies development.

PATIENT CONSIDERATIONS

Assessment: Assess for hypersensitivity to the drug, Chinese hamster ovary cell products, or any component of the drug, and nursing status.

Monitoring: Monitor for worsening of the condition and other adverse reactions.

Counseling: Instruct on the proper techniques to store and handle therapy. Advise to squeeze each ampule prior to use in order to check for leaks. Instruct to discard sol if cloudy or discolored. Inform that entire contents of ampule must be used or discarded once opened. Instruct on the proper use and maintenance of the nebulizer and compressor system. Instruct to not dilute or mix with other drugs in the nebulizer.

STORAGE: Store in the protective foil pouch at 2-8°C (36-46°F). Protect from light. Refrigerate during transport and do not expose to room temperatures for a total time of 24 hrs.

PURIXAN – mercaptopurine

RX

Class: Purine analogue

ADULT DOSAGE

Acute Lymphoblastic Leukemia

Component of a Multi-agent Combination Chemotherapy Maint Regimen:

Initial: 1.5-2.5mg/kg (50-75mg/m^2) as a single daily dose

Continuation of appropriate dosing requires periodic monitoring of absolute neutrophil count and platelet count to assure sufficient drug exposure and to adjust for excessive hematological toxicity

PEDIATRIC DOSAGE

Acute Lymphoblastic Leukemia

Component of a Multi-agent Combination Chemotherapy Maint Regimen:

Initial: 1.5-2.5mg/kg (50-75mg/m^2) as a single daily dose

Continuation of appropriate dosing requires periodic monitoring of absolute neutrophil count and platelet count to assure sufficient drug exposure and to adjust for excessive hematological toxicity

DOSING CONSIDERATIONS

Renal Impairment

Consider starting at lower end of dosing range or increasing the dosing interval to 36-48 hrs

Hepatic Impairment

Consider starting at lower end of dosing range

Elderly

Consider starting at lower end of dosing range

Thiopurine S-Methyltransferase (TPMT) Deficiency

Homozygous TPMT Deficiency: May require up to a 90% dosage reduction

Heterozygous TPMT Deficiency: May require dose reduction based on toxicities

ADMINISTRATION

Oral route

Shake vigorously for at least 30 sec

Once opened, use within 6 weeks

HOW SUPPLIED

Sus: 20mg/mL [100mL]

WARNINGS/PRECAUTIONS

Increased risk for severe mercaptopurine toxicity in patients with inherited little or no TPMT activity; evaluate TPMT status in patients with evidence of severe bone marrow toxicity or with repeated episodes of myelosuppression. Dose-related bone marrow suppression may occur; adjust dose for severe neutropenia and thrombocytopenia. Hepatotoxicity reported; interrupt therapy in patients with evidence of hepatotoxicity. Monitor LFTs more frequently in patients who are receiving mercaptopurine with other hepatotoxic drugs or with known pre-existing liver disease. Therapy is immunosuppressive and may impair the immune response to infectious agents. May cause fetal harm. May increase risk of secondary malignancies. Caution with renal/hepatic impairment and in elderly.

ADVERSE REACTIONS

Myelosuppression, anorexia, N/V, diarrhea, malaise, rash.

DRUG INTERACTIONS

Allopurinol inhibits 1st-pass oxidative metabolism, leading to mercaptopurine toxicity (bone marrow suppression, N/V); avoid concomitant use. May decrease anticoagulant effectiveness of warfarin; monitor PT/INR and adjust warfarin dose if necessary. Drugs that inhibit TPMT (eg, aminosalicylate derivatives [eg, olsalazine, mesalamine, sulfasalazine]), drugs whose primary or secondary toxicity is myelosuppression, and trimethoprim-sulfamethoxazole may exacerbate myelosuppression; if coadministration with aminosalicylate derivatives is necessary, use the lowest possible doses of each drug and closely monitor for bone marrow suppression. May impair the immune response to vaccines; response to all vaccines may be diminished and there is a risk of infection with live virus vaccines.

PATIENT CONSIDERATIONS

Assessment: Assess for TPMT deficiency, renal/hepatic impairment, pregnancy/nursing status, and possible drug interactions.

Monitoring: Monitor for myelosuppression, hepatotoxicity, immunosuppression, secondary malignancies, and other adverse reactions. Monitor serum transaminase levels, alkaline phosphatase, and bilirubin levels at weekly intervals when first beginning therapy and at monthly intervals thereafter. Monitor CBC. Evaluate bone marrow in patients with prolonged or repeated marrow suppression to assess leukemia status and marrow cellularity. Evaluate TPMT status in patients with clinical or lab evidence of severe bone marrow toxicity, or with repeated episodes of myelosuppression.

Counseling: Instruct on proper handling, storage, administration, disposal and clean-up of accidental spillage of the medication; counsel regarding which syringe to use and how to administer a specified dose. Inform that the major toxicities of therapy are related to myelosuppression, hepatotoxicity, and GI toxicity; instruct to contact physician if patient experiences fever, sore throat, jaundice, N/V, signs of local infection, bleeding from any site, or symptoms suggestive of anemia. Advise women of childbearing potential to avoid becoming pregnant. Inform that the oral dispensing syringe is intended for multiple use; instruct on how to clean the syringe.

STORAGE: 15-25°C (59-77°F) in a dry place. Do not store >25°C.

PYRIDIUM – phenazopyridine hydrochloride RX

Class: Urinary tract analgesic

ADULT DOSAGE

Irritation of Lower Urinary Tract Mucosa

Symptomatic Relief of Pain, Burning, Urgency, Frequency, and Other Discomforts Caused by Infection, Trauma, Surgery, Endoscopic Procedures, or Passage of Sounds/Catheters:
Usual: 200mg tid
Max Duration: 2 days, when used concomitantly w/ an antibacterial agent for treatment of UTI

PEDIATRIC DOSAGE

Pediatric use may not have been established

ADMINISTRATION

Oral route

Take pc

HOW SUPPLIED

Tab: 100mg, 200mg

CONTRAINDICATIONS

Hypersensitivity to phenazopyridine HCl, renal insufficiency.

WARNINGS/PRECAUTIONS

D/C when symptoms are controlled. A yellowish tinge of the skin/sclera may indicate accumulation due to impaired renal excretion and the need to d/c therapy. Produces a reddish-orange discoloration of the urine and may stain fabric; staining of contact lenses reported. May interfere with urinalysis based on spectrometry or color reactions.

ADVERSE REACTIONS

Headache, rash, pruritus, GI disturbance, anaphylactoid-like reaction.

PATIENT CONSIDERATIONS

Assessment: Assess for previous hypersensitivity to the drug, renal insufficiency, cause of urinary pain, and pregnancy/nursing status.

Monitoring: Monitor for control of symptoms, development of yellowish tinge of the skin/sclera, and other adverse reactions.

Counseling: Inform that drug produces a reddish-orange discoloration of urine and may stain fabric and contact lenses.

STORAGE: 20-25°C (68-77°F); excursions permitted to 15-30°C (59-86°F).

QNASL – beclomethasone dipropionate

RX

Class: Corticosteroid

ADULT DOSAGE

Seasonal/Perennial Allergic Rhinitis

Nasal Symptoms:
Usual: 2 actuations/nostril qd
Max: 4 actuations/day

PEDIATRIC DOSAGE

Seasonal/Perennial Allergic Rhinitis

Nasal Symptoms:
4-11 Years:
Usual: 1 actuation/nostril qd
Max: 2 actuations/day
≥12 Years:
Usual: 2 actuations/nostril qd
Max: 4 actuations/day

ADMINISTRATION
Intranasal route

Priming
Spray 4X into the air, away from eyes and face
The dose counter should read 120 after initial priming
If not used for 7 consecutive days it should be primed by spraying 2X

HOW SUPPLIED
Aerosol: 40mcg/actuation, 80mcg/actuation [8.7g]

CONTRAINDICATIONS
History of hypersensitivity to beclomethasone dipropionate and/or any other ingredients of the product.

WARNINGS/PRECAUTIONS
Epistaxis, nasal erosions, nasal ulcerations reported; d/c if these occur. *Candida albicans* infections of the nose and pharynx may occur; treat and, if needed, d/c therapy. Monitor for evidence of *Candida* infection or possible changes in the nasal mucosa periodically during prolonged use. Nasal septal perforation may occur. May impair wound healing; avoid with recent nasal septal ulcers, nasal surgery, or nasal trauma until healed. Glaucoma and/or cataracts may develop; monitor patients with a change in vision or with a history of increased intraocular pressure (IOP), glaucoma, and/or cataracts. Hypersensitivity reactions (eg, anaphylaxis, angioedema, urticaria, rash) may occur; d/c if such reactions develop. May lead to serious/fatal course of chickenpox or measles; avoid exposure and if exposed, consider prophylaxis/treatment. Caution with active or quiescent tuberculous infections, untreated local or systemic fungal or bacterial infections, systemic viral or parasitic infections, or ocular herpes simplex. Risk of adrenal insufficiency and withdrawal symptoms when replacing systemic corticosteroid with topical corticosteroid; monitor closely. D/C slowly if symptoms of hypercorticism and adrenal suppression occur. May reduce growth velocity in pediatric patients. Caution in elderly.

ADVERSE REACTIONS
Nasal discomfort, epistaxis, headache.

Q

PATIENT CONSIDERATIONS

Assessment: Assess for drug hypersensitivity, active or quiescent tuberculous infections, local/systemic infections, ocular herpes simplex, recent nasal ulcers/surgery/trauma, history of increased IOP, glaucoma, cataracts, immunization status, and pregnancy/nursing status.

Monitoring: Monitor for systemic corticosteroid effects (eg, hypercorticism, adrenal suppression), epistaxis, nasal discomfort/ulceration, nasal septal perforation, infections, nasal or pharyngeal *C. albicans* infections, hypersensitivity reactions, growth velocity in children, hypoadrenalism (in infants born to mothers receiving corticosteroids during pregnancy), and other adverse reactions. Monitor for adrenal insufficiency and withdrawal symptoms in the event of replacing systemic corticosteroid with topical corticosteroid.

Counseling: Counsel on appropriate priming and administration. Counsel about risks of epistaxis, nasal ulceration, nasal discomfort, *Candida* infections, and other adverse reactions. Inform that glaucoma and cataracts may develop; instruct to inform physician if visual changes occur. Advise to d/c therapy if hypersensitivity reactions occur. Advise to avoid exposure to chickenpox or measles and to consult physician if exposed. Inform of potential worsening of existing tuberculosis, fungal/bacterial/viral/parasitic infections, or ocular herpes simplex. Instruct to contact physician immediately if symptoms do not improve, or if the condition worsens. Advise to avoid spraying in the eyes or mouth.

STORAGE: 25°C (77°F); excursions permitted between 15-30°C (59-86°F). Do not puncture. Do not store near heat or open flame.

QSYMIA – phentermine/topiramate CIV

Class: Anorectic sympathomimetic amine/sulfamate-substituted monosaccharide

ADULT DOSAGE

Weight Loss

Adjunct to a reduced-calorie diet and increased physical activity for chronic weight management in patients w/ initial BMI ≥30kg/m^2, or ≥27kg/m^2 in the presence of ≥1 weight-related comorbidity

Initial: 3.75mg/23mg qd for 14 days
Titrate: After 14 days, increase to 7.5mg/46mg qd; d/c or escalate dose if patient has not lost at least 3% of baseline weight after 12 weeks
Dose Escalation: Increase to 11.25mg/69mg qd for 14 days, followed by 15mg/92mg qd; d/c if patient has not lost at least 5% of baseline weight after 12 weeks on 15mg/92mg

Use 3.75mg/23mg and 11.25mg/69mg strengths for titration purposes only

Discontinuation: D/C 15mg/92mg gradually by taking a dose qod for at least 1 week prior to stopping treatment

PEDIATRIC DOSAGE

Pediatric use may not have been established

DOSING CONSIDERATIONS

Renal Impairment

Moderate (CrCl ≥30-<50mL/min) to Severe (CrCl <30mL/min):
Max: 7.5mg/46mg qd

ESRD on Dialysis:
Avoid use

Hepatic Impairment

Moderate (Child-Pugh Score 7-9):
Max: 7.5mg/46mg qd

Severe (Child-Pugh Score 10-15):
Avoid use

Elderly

Start at lower end of dosing range

ADMINISTRATION

Oral route

Take w/ or w/o food

Take qam; avoid pm dosing due to the possibility of insomnia

HOW SUPPLIED

Cap, Extended-Release: (Phentermine/Topiramate) 3.75mg/23mg, 7.5mg/46mg, 11.25mg/69mg, 15mg/92mg

CONTRAINDICATIONS

Pregnancy, glaucoma, hyperthyroidism, during or w/in 14 days of administration of MAOIs, known hypersensitivity or idiosyncrasy to the sympathomimetic amines.

WARNINGS/PRECAUTIONS

May cause fetal harm; use effective contraception to prevent pregnancy. Available through a limited program under the Risk Evaluation and Mitigation Strategy. May increase resting HR; monitor resting HR regularly in all patients, especially those with cardiac or cerebrovascular disease or when initiating or increasing dose. Reduce dose or d/c if sustained increase in resting HR or persistent SrCr elevations occur. Increased risk of suicidal thoughts/behavior; monitor for emergence/worsening of depression, suicidal thoughts/behavior, and/or any unusual changes in mood or behavior, and d/c if these occur. Avoid with history of suicidal attempts or active suicidal ideation. Acute myopia associated with secondary angle-closure glaucoma reported; d/c immediately to reverse symptoms. Mood/sleep disorders, including anxiety and insomnia, may occur; consider dose reduction or withdrawal for clinically significant or persistent symptoms. May impair physical/mental abilities; consider dose reduction or withdrawal if cognitive dysfunction persists. Hyperchloremic, non-anion gap, metabolic acidosis reported. Conditions that predispose to acidosis (eg, renal disease, severe respiratory disorders, status epilepticus, diarrhea, surgery, ketogenic diet) may be additive to the bicarbonate lowering effects of topiramate. Weight loss may increase risk of hypoglycemia in patients with type 2 DM treated with insulin and/or insulin secretagogues (eg, sulfonylureas), and risk of hypotension in those treated with antihypertensives; appropriate changes should be made to antidiabetic or antihypertensive therapy if hypoglycemia or hypotension develops. Seizures associated with abrupt withdrawal in individuals without history of seizures or epilepsy; taper dose gradually if using 15mg/92mg and monitor for seizures in situations where immediate termination of therapy is required. Avoid with ESRD on dialysis or severe hepatic impairment (Child-Pugh 10-15). Associated with kidney stone formation; increase fluid intake to increase urine output. Oligohidrosis reported; monitor for decreased sweating and increased body temperature during physical activity, especially in hot weather. May increase risk of hypokalemia. Potential for abuse. Lab test interactions may occur. Caution in elderly.

ADVERSE REACTIONS

Paresthesia, dry mouth, constipation, URTI, headache, dysgeusia, insomnia, nasopharyngitis, dizziness, sinusitis, bronchitis, nausea, back pain, diarrhea, blurred vision.

DRUG INTERACTIONS

See Contraindications. May decrease exposure of ethinyl estradiol and increase exposure of norethindrone with single dose of oral contraceptive. Alcohol or CNS depressants (eg, barbiturates, benzodiazepines, sleep medications) may potentiate CNS depression. May potentiate the K^+ wasting action of non-K^+-sparing diuretics; monitor for hypokalemia. Avoid with other drugs that inhibit carbonic anhydrase (eg, zonisamide, acetazolamide, methazolamide, dichlorphenamide); may increase severity of metabolic acidosis and kidney stone formation. Caution with other drugs that predispose patients to heat-related disorders (eg, other carbonic anhydrase inhibitors, drugs with anticholinergic activity). Phenytoin or carbamazepine may decrease plasma levels. Concurrent administration of valproic acid has been associated with hyperammonemia with or without encephalopathy, and hypothermia.

PATIENT CONSIDERATIONS

Assessment: Assess for known hypersensitivity or idiosyncrasy to sympathomimetic amines, glaucoma, hyperthyroidism, cardiac and cerebrovascular disease, history of behavioral/mood disorders, history of seizures, renal/hepatic dysfunction, any other conditions where treatment is contraindicated or cautioned, pregnancy/nursing status, and possible drug interactions. Obtain baseline HR and blood chemistry profile (eg, bicarbonate, creatinine, K^+, glucose).

Monitoring: Monitor for acute myopia, secondary angle-closure glaucoma, emergence/worsening of depression, suicidal thoughts or behavior, mood/sleep disorders, cognitive dysfunction, hyperchloremic metabolic acidosis, seizures, kidney stone formation, oligohidrosis, and hyperthermia. Monitor HR regularly and blood chemistry profile (eg, bicarbonate, creatinine, K^+, glucose) periodically. Assess pregnancy status monthly during therapy.

Counseling: Inform that therapy is for chronic weight management in conjunction with a reduced-calorie diet and increased physical activity. Inform that drug is only available through certified pharmacies. Instruct to inform physician about all medications, nutritional supplements, and vitamins (including any weight loss products) taken while on therapy. Instruct on how to properly take the medication. Instruct to avoid pregnancy/breastfeeding while on therapy and to notify physician immediately if patient becomes pregnant during treatment. Advise to report symptoms of sustained periods of heart pounding or racing while at rest, suicidal behavior/ideation, mood changes, depression, severe/persistent eye pain or significant visual changes, any changes in attention/concentration/memory, and/or difficulty finding words. Advise not to drive/operate machinery until reaction to the medication is known. Instruct to notify physician about any factors that can increase the risk of acidosis (eg, prolonged diarrhea, surgery, high protein/low carbohydrate diet, and/or concomitant medications such as other carbonic anhydrase inhibitors) and to avoid alcohol while on therapy. Instruct diabetic patients to monitor blood glucose levels and to report symptoms of hypoglycemia to physician. Advise not to abruptly d/c therapy without notifying physician. Advise to increase fluid intake and report symptoms of severe side or back pain, and/or blood in urine to physician. Advise to monitor for decreased sweating and increased body temperature during physical activity, especially in hot weather.

STORAGE: 15-25°C (59-77°F). Protect from moisture.

QUDEXY XR – topiramate

RX

Class: Sulfamate-substituted monosaccharide antiepileptic

ADULT DOSAGE

Epilepsy

Monotherapy:

Partial Onset Seizures or Primary Generalized Tonic-Clonic Seizures:

Usual: 400mg qd

PEDIATRIC DOSAGE

Epilepsy

Monotherapy:

Partial Onset Seizures or Primary Generalized Tonic-Clonic Seizures:

Q

Titration Schedule:
Week 1: 50mg qd
Week 2: 100mg qd
Week 3: 150mg qd
Week 4: 200mg qd
Week 5: 300mg qd
Week 6: 400mg qd

Adjunctive Therapy:
Partial Onset Seizures, Primary Generalized Tonic-Clonic Seizures, or Lennox-Gastaut Syndrome:

≥17 Years:
Initial: 25-50mg qd
Titrate: Increase in increments of 25-50mg every week to achieve effective dose
Usual:
Partial Onset Seizures or Lennox-Gastaut Syndrome: 200-400mg qd
Primary Generalized Tonic-Clonic Seizures: 400mg qd

2-<10 Years:
Initial: 25mg qpm for the 1st week
Titrate: May increase to 50mg qd in the 2nd week, then by 25-50mg qd each subsequent week. Titration to the minimum maint dose should be attempted over 5-7 weeks; additional titration to a higher dose (up to the max maint dose) can be attempted in weekly increments by 25-50mg qd, up to the max recommended maint dose for each range of body weight
Up to 11kg:
Minimum Maint Dose: 150mg/day
Max Maint Dose: 250mg/day
12-22kg:
Minimum Maint Dose: 200mg/day
Max Maint Dose: 300mg/day
23-31kg:
Minimum Maint Dose: 200mg/day
Max Maint Dose: 350mg/day
32-38kg:
Minimum Maint Dose: 250mg/day
Max Maint Dose: 350mg/day
>38kg:
Minimum Maint Dose: 250mg/day
Max Maint Dose: 400mg/day

≥10 Years:
Usual: 400mg qd
Titration Schedule:
Week 1: 50mg qd
Week 2: 100mg qd
Week 3: 150mg qd
Week 4: 200mg qd
Week 5: 300mg qd
Week 6: 400mg qd

Adjunctive Therapy:
Partial Onset Seizures, Primary Generalized Tonic-Clonic Seizures, or Lennox-Gastaut Syndrome:

2-16 Years:
Usual: 5-9mg/kg qd
Titrate: Begin titration at 25mg qpm (based on a range of 1-3mg/kg/day) for 1st week. Subsequently, increase at 1- or 2-week intervals by increments of 1-3mg/kg to achieve optimal clinical response; longer intervals between dose adjustments may be used if required

Q

DOSING CONSIDERATIONS

Concomitant Medications

Phenytoin and/or Carbamazepine:
May require an adjustment of the dose of phenytoin to achieve optimal clinical outcome
Addition or withdrawal of phenytoin and/or carbamazepine during adjunctive therapy may require dose adjustment of topiramate

Renal Impairment

CrCl <70mL/min: Use 1/2 the usual starting and maint dose
Hemodialysis: Supplemental dose may be required

ADMINISTRATION

Oral route

May take w/o regard to meals
May swallow whole or carefully open and sprinkle entire contents on a small amount (tsp) of soft food; swallow drug/food mixture immediately and do not chew/crush

HOW SUPPLIED

Cap, Extended-Release: 25mg, 50mg, 100mg, 150mg, 200mg

CONTRAINDICATIONS

Patients w/ metabolic acidosis taking concomitant metformin.

WARNINGS/PRECAUTIONS

Acute myopia associated w/ secondary angle-closure glaucoma reported; d/c as rapidly as possible to reverse symptoms. Visual field defects reported in patients independent of elevated IOP; consider discontinuing therapy if visual problems occur. Oligohydrosis and hyperthermia reported, mostly in pediatric patients; monitor for decreased sweating and increased body temperature. Hyperchloremic, non-anion gap, metabolic acidosis reported; conditions or therapies that predispose to acidosis may be additive to the bicarbonate lowering effects. Consider discontinuing or reducing dose if metabolic acidosis develops/persists. If decision is to continue therapy, consider alkali treatment. Increased risk of suicidal thoughts/behavior; monitor for the emergence/worsening of depression, suicidal thoughts/behavior, and/or any unusual changes in mood or behavior. Cognitive-related dysfunction, psychiatric/behavioral disturbances, and somnolence or fatigue reported. May cause fetal harm; increased risk for cleft lip and/or palate in infants if used during pregnancy. Gradually withdraw therapy to minimize the potential for seizures or increased seizure frequency; appropriate monitoring is recommended when rapid withdrawal is required. Patients w/ inborn errors of metabolism or reduced hepatic mitochondrial activity may be at an increased risk for hyperammonemia w/ or w/o encephalopathy; consider hyperammonemic encephalopathy and measure ammonia levels in patients who develop unexplained lethargy, vomiting, or changes in mental status associated w/ therapy. Kidney stone formation reported; hydration is recommended to reduce new stone formation. Paresthesia may occur.

ADVERSE REACTIONS

Anorexia, anxiety, dizziness, fatigue, fever, infection, weight decrease, cognitive problems, paresthesia, somnolence, psychomotor slowing, mood problems, difficulty w/ memory, nervousness, confusion.

DRUG INTERACTIONS

See Dosing Considerations and Contraindications. May decrease contraceptive efficacy and increase breakthrough bleeding w/ combination oral contraceptives. Phenytoin or carbamazepine may decrease levels. Concomitant administration of valproic acid has been associated w/ hyperammonemia w/ or w/o encephalopathy and hypothermia. Concomitant administration w/ other CNS depressants or alcohol can result in significant CNS depression; use w/ extreme caution and avoid w/ alcohol. Concomitant use w/ other carbonic anhydrase inhibitors (eg, zonisamide, acetazolamide, dichlorphenamide) may increase the severity of metabolic acidosis and may also increase the risk of kidney stone formation; monitor for appearance or worsening of metabolic acidosis. Increase in systemic exposure of lithium observed following topiramate doses of ≤600mg/day; monitor lithium levels. Caution w/ agents that predispose patients to heat-related disorders (eg, carbonic anhydrase inhibitors, anticholinergics).

PATIENT CONSIDERATIONS

Assessment: Assess for metabolic acidosis in patients taking concomitant metformin, predisposing factors for metabolic acidosis, renal dysfunction, inborn errors of metabolism, reduced hepatic mitochondrial activity, pregnancy/nursing status, and possible drug interactions. Obtain baseline serum bicarbonate, CrCl, and blood ammonia levels.

Monitoring: Monitor for signs/symptoms of acute myopia, secondary angle-closure glaucoma, visual field defects, oligohydrosis, hyperthermia, depression or suicidal thoughts/behavior, cognitive or neuropsychiatric adverse reactions, kidney stones, renal dysfunction, metabolic acidosis, paresthesia, hyperammonemia, and other adverse reactions. Monitor serum bicarbonate and blood ammonia levels.

Counseling: Instruct to take only as prescribed. Instruct to seek immediate medical attention if blurred vision, visual disturbances, periorbital pain, high or persistent fever, or decreased sweating occurs. Inform about the risk for metabolic acidosis that may be asymptomatic and may be associated w/ adverse effects on kidneys, bones, and growth in pediatric patients, and on the fetus. Instruct to immediately report to the physician if emergence or worsening of depression, unusual changes in mood/behavior, emergence of suicidal thoughts, or behavior/thoughts about self-harm occur. Advise to use caution when engaging in activities where loss of consciousness may result in serious danger. Inform of pregnancy risks; encourage pregnant women to enroll in the North American Antiepileptic Drug Pregnancy Registry. Warn about possible development of hyperammonemia w/ or w/o encephalopathy; instruct to contact physician if unexplained lethargy, vomiting, or mental status changes develop. Instruct to maintain adequate fluid intake to minimize risk of kidney stones. Inform that therapy may cause reduction in body temperature that can lead to alterations in mental status; if changes are noted, instruct to measure body temperature and contact physician. Instruct to consult physician if tingling in the arms and legs occurs.

STORAGE: 20-25°C (68-77°F); excursions permitted to 15-30°C (59-86°F). Protect from moisture.

QUILLIVANT XR – methylphenidate hydrochloride

CII

Class: CNS stimulant

High potential for abuse and dependence. Assess the risk of abuse prior to prescribing, and monitor for signs of abuse and dependence while on therapy.

ADULT DOSAGE

Attention-Deficit Hyperactivity Disorder

Initial: 20mg qam
Titrate: May be titrated weekly in increments of 10mg to 20mg
Max: 60mg/day

Maint/Extended Treatment:
Periodically reevaluate long-term usefulness w/ trials off medication to assess functioning w/o pharmacotherapy

D/C if no improvement observed after appropriate dosage adjustments over 1 month

PEDIATRIC DOSAGE

Attention-Deficit Hyperactivity Disorder

≥6 Years:
Initial: 20mg qam
Titrate: May be titrated weekly in increments of 10mg to 20mg
Max: 60mg/day

Maint/Extended Treatment:
Periodically reevaluate long-term usefulness w/ trials off medication to assess functioning w/o pharmacotherapy

D/C if no improvement observed after appropriate dosage adjustments over 1 month

DOSING CONSIDERATIONS

Adverse Reactions
Reduce dose or d/c if necessary, if paradoxical aggravation of symptoms or other adverse events occur

ADMINISTRATION

Oral route

Take w/ or w/o food
Vigorously shake bottle for at least 10 sec before each dose to ensure that the proper dose is administered
Use only w/ the oral dosing dispenser provided

Reconstitution Instructions for Pharmacist
Reconstitute 300mg bottle w/ 53mL water; reconstitute 600mg bottle w/ 105mL water; reconstitute 750mg bottle w/ 131mL water; reconstitute 900mg bottle w/158mL water
Shake vigorously for at least 10 sec to prepare sus

Refer to PI for further administration instructions

HOW SUPPLIED

Sus, Extended-Release: 5mg/mL [60mL, 120mL, 150mL, 180mL]

CONTRAINDICATIONS

Known hypersensitivity to methylphenidate, or other components of the product. Treatment w/ or w/in 14 days following discontinuation of treatment w/ an MAOI.

Q

WARNINGS/PRECAUTIONS

Sudden death reported in children and adolescents with structural cardiac abnormalities and other serious cardiac problems. Sudden death, stroke, and MI reported in adults. Avoid with known structural cardiac abnormalities, cardiomyopathy, serious cardiac arrhythmias, coronary artery disease, or other serious cardiac problems. May increase BP and HR. May exacerbate symptoms of behavior disturbance and thought disorder in patients with a preexisting psychotic disorder. May induce a manic or mixed episode in patients with bipolar disorder. May cause psychotic or manic symptoms in patients without a prior history of psychotic illness or mania at recommended doses; consider discontinuation if such symptoms occur. Priapism reported; seek immediate medical attention if abnormally sustained or frequent and painful erections develop. Associated with peripheral vasculopathy, including Raynaud's phenomenon; monitor for digital changes. May cause long-term suppression of growth in pediatric patients; may need to interrupt treatment in patients not growing or gaining height or weight as expected.

ADVERSE REACTIONS

Affect lability, excoriation, initial insomnia, tic, decreased appetite, vomiting, motion sickness, eye pain, rash.

DRUG INTERACTIONS

See Contraindications.

PATIENT CONSIDERATIONS

Assessment: Assess for drug hypersensitivity, cardiac problems, psychotic disorders, bipolar disorder, pregnancy/nursing status, and for possible drug interactions. Obtain baseline height/

weight in children. Screen patients for risk factors for developing a manic episode and the risk of abuse before starting therapy.

Monitoring: Monitor for stroke, MI, HTN, tachycardia, exacerbations of behavior disturbances and thought disorders, psychotic or manic symptoms, digital changes, priapism, and other adverse reactions. Monitor growth in children. Monitor for signs of abuse and dependence. Periodically reevaluate long-term usefulness.

Counseling: Inform about risks, benefits, and appropriate use of treatment. Counsel that drug has potential for abuse or dependence; instruct to keep medication in a safe place to prevent abuse. Advise of the potential for serious cardiovascular risks, including sudden death, MI, and stroke; instruct to contact physician immediately if symptoms, such as exertional chest pain, unexplained syncope, or other symptoms suggestive of cardiac disease develop. Advise that the drug can elevate BP and HR, can cause psychotic or manic symptoms even in patients without a prior history of psychotic symptoms or mania, and in pediatric patients can cause slowing of growth and weight loss. Advise of the possibility of priapism; instruct to seek immediate medical attention in the event of priapism. Inform about the risk of peripheral vasculopathy, including Raynaud's phenomenon; instruct to report to the physician any numbness, pain, skin color change, sensitivity to temperature in fingers or toes, and any signs of unexplained wounds appearing on fingers or toes. Instruct to inform physician if pregnant/intending to become pregnant during therapy. Advise of the potential fetal effects from use during pregnancy.

STORAGE: 25°C (77°F); excursions permitted from 15-30°C (59-86°F). Stable for up to 4 months after reconstitution.

QVAR – beclomethasone dipropionate

RX

Class: Corticosteroid

ADULT DOSAGE

Asthma

Previously on Bronchodilators Alone:
Initial: 40-80mcg bid
Max: 320mcg bid

Previously on Inhaled Corticosteroids:
Initial: 40-160mcg bid
Max: 320mcg bid

PEDIATRIC DOSAGE

Asthma

5-11 Years:
Previously on Bronchodilators Alone or Inhaled Corticosteroids:
Initial: 40mcg bid
Max: 80mcg bid

≥12 Years:
Previously on Bronchodilators Alone:
Initial: 40-80mcg bid
Max: 320mcg bid

Previously on Inhaled Corticosteroids:
Initial: 40-160mcg bid
Max: 320mcg bid

DOSING CONSIDERATIONS

Concomitant Medications

Systemic Corticosteroids (eg, Prednisone):
Slowly wean patient beginning after at least 1 week of therapy

Elderly

Start at lower end of dosing range

ADMINISTRATION

Oral inh route

Advise patient to rinse mouth after inh

Priming

Actuate into the air twice before using for the 1st time or if not used for >10 days

HOW SUPPLIED

MDI: 40mcg/inh, 80mcg/inh [120 actuations]

CONTRAINDICATIONS

Primary treatment of status asthmaticus or other acute episodes of asthma where intensive measures are required. Known hypersensitivity to beclomethasone dipropionate or any of the ingredients in the product.

WARNINGS/PRECAUTIONS

Candida albicans infections of mouth and pharynx may occur; treat and/or interrupt therapy if needed. Not indicated for relief of acute bronchospasm. Deaths due to adrenal insufficiency have occurred during and after transfer from systemic to inhaled corticosteroids; wean slowly from systemic corticosteroid use after transferring to therapy. Resume oral corticosteroids (in large doses) immediately during periods of stress or a severe asthmatic attack in patients previously withdrawn from systemic corticosteroids. Transfer from systemic to inhaled corticosteroids may unmask allergic conditions previously suppressed by systemic therapy (eg, rhinitis, conjunctivitis, eczema). Increased susceptibility to infections. May lead to more serious/fatal course of chickenpox or measles; avoid exposure, and if exposed, consider prophylaxis/treatment. Caution w/ active or quiescent tuberculosis (TB), untreated systemic fungal/bacterial/parasitic/viral infections, or ocular herpes simplex. Paradoxical bronchospasm, w/ immediate increase in wheezing, may occur after dosing; treat immediately w/ a short-acting inhaled bronchodilator; d/c and institute alternative therapy. Hypersensitivity reactions (eg, urticaria, angioedema, rash) may occur; d/c if these occur. Monitor for systemic corticosteroid effects; reduce dose slowly if hypercorticism and adrenal suppression occur. Caution should be taken in observing patients postoperatively or during periods of stress for evidence of inadequate adrenal response. May cause reduction in growth velocity in pediatric patients; monitor growth. Decreases in bone mineral density (BMD) reported w/ long-term use; monitor in patients w/ major risk factors (eg, prolonged immobilization, family history of osteoporosis, chronic use of drugs that can reduce bone mass). Glaucoma, increased intraocular pressure (IOP), and cataracts reported w/ long-term use. Caution in elderly.

ADVERSE REACTIONS

Headache, pharyngitis, URTI, rhinitis, increased asthma symptoms, oral symptoms (inhalation route), sinusitis, dysphonia, dysmenorrhea, coughing.

PATIENT CONSIDERATIONS

Assessment: Assess for status asthmaticus, acute asthma episodes, acute bronchospasm, active/quiescent TB, untreated systemic infections, ocular herpes simplex, known hypersensitivity to drug or to any of the ingredients, risk factors for BMD, history of increased IOP/glaucoma/cataracts, and pregnancy/nursing status.

Monitoring: Monitor for paradoxical bronchospasm, hypercorticism, adrenal suppression/insufficiency, BMD, changes in vision, glaucoma, increased IOP, cataracts, infections, hypersensitivity reactions, asthma instability, and other adverse reactions. Monitor growth in pediatric patients.

Counseling: Advise to contact physician if oropharyngeal candidiasis develops. Instruct to avoid exposure to chickenpox or measles, and, if exposed, to consult physician w/o delay. Inform about risks of immunosuppression, hypercorticism, adrenal suppression, reduction in bone mineral density, reduced growth velocity in pediatric patients, glaucoma, and cataracts. Advise that drug is not intended for use in the treatment of acute asthma; instruct to immediately contact physician if asthma deteriorates. Advise to use medication at regular intervals since its effectiveness depends on regular use. Instruct to contact physician if symptoms do not improve after 2 weeks of therapy or if condition worsens. Counsel about the proper priming/use of inhaler. Instruct not to stop abruptly and to immediately contact physician if drug is discontinued.

STORAGE: 25°C (77°F); excursions permitted to 15-30°C (59-86°F). For optimal results, canister should be at room temperature when used. Do not puncture, use/store near heat or open flame, or throw container into fire/incinerator. Exposure to temperatures >49°C (120°F) may cause bursting.

RANEXA – ranolazine

RX

Class: Miscellaneous antianginal

ADULT DOSAGE

Chronic Angina

Initial: 500mg bid
Titrate: Increase to 1000mg bid prn
Max: 1000mg bid

May be used w/ β-blockers, nitrates, calcium channel blockers, antiplatelet therapy, lipid-lowering therapy, ACE inhibitors, and ARBs

Missed Dose

If a dose is missed, take the prescribed dose at the next scheduled time; do not double the next dose

PEDIATRIC DOSAGE

Pediatric use may not have been established

DOSING CONSIDERATIONS

Concomitant Medications

Moderate CYP3A Inhibitors (eg, Diltiazem, Verapamil, Erythromycin):
Max Dose: 500mg bid

P-gp Inhibitors (eg, Cyclosporine):
Titrate ranolazine based on clinical response

Elderly
Start at lower end of dosing range

ADMINISTRATION
Oral route

Take w/ or w/o meals.
Swallow tab whole; do not crush, break, or chew.

HOW SUPPLIED
Tab, Extended-Release: 500mg, 1000mg

CONTRAINDICATIONS
Liver cirrhosis, concomitant use w/ CYP3A inducers (eg, rifampin, phenobarbital, phenytoin) or strong CYP3A inhibitors (eg, ketoconazole, itraconazole, clarithromycin).

WARNINGS/PRECAUTIONS
May prolong QTc interval in a dose-related manner. Acute renal failure reported in patients w/ severe renal impairment (CrCl <30mL/min); d/c and treat appropriately if acute renal failure develops. Monitor renal function after initiation and periodically in patients w/ moderate to severe renal impairment (CrCl <60mL/min) for increases in SrCr accompanied by an increase in BUN.

ADVERSE REACTIONS
Dizziness, headache, constipation, nausea.

DRUG INTERACTIONS
See Contraindications and Dosing Considerations. P-gp inhibitors (eg, cyclosporine) may increase concentrations. May increase levels of simvastatin; limit simvastatin dose to 20mg qd. May increase concentrations of other sensitive CYP3A substrates (eg, lovastatin) and CYP3A substrates w/ a narrow therapeutic range (eg, cyclosporine, tacrolimus, sirolimus); may require dose adjustment of these drugs. May increase exposure to digoxin and CYP2D6 substrates (eg, TCAs, antipsychotics); may require digoxin dose adjustment and lower doses of CYP2D6 substrates. May increase levels of metformin; do not exceed 1700mg/day of metformin if coadministered w/ ranolazine 1000mg bid and monitor blood glucose levels and risks associated w/ high metformin exposure.

PATIENT CONSIDERATIONS

Assessment: Assess for liver cirrhosis, QT interval prolongation, renal impairment, pregnancy/nursing status, and possible drug interactions.

Monitoring: Monitor for ECG changes (eg, QT interval prolongation) and other adverse reactions. Monitor renal function (eg, SrCr, BUN) after initiation and periodically in patients w/ moderate to severe renal impairment.

Counseling: Inform that drug will not abate an acute angina episode. Inform that drug should not be used w/ drugs that are strong CYP3A inhibitors or CYP3A inducers. Inform that drug should not be used in patients w/ liver cirrhosis. Advise to inform physician if receiving drugs that are moderate CYP3A inhibitors or P-gp inhibitors. Advise to limit grapefruit juice or grapefruit products. Inform that drug may produce QTc interval prolongation, and to inform physician of any personal or family history of QTc prolongation, congenital long QT syndrome, or if receiving drugs that prolong QTc interval. Advise to inform physician of any renal function impairment before or while taking drug. Inform that drug may cause dizziness and lightheadedness, and instruct to contact physician if experiencing fainting spells; instruct patients to know how they react to the drug before engaging in activities requiring mental alertness or coordination (eg, operating machinery, driving). Instruct to take exactly ud.

STORAGE: 25°C (77°F); excursions permitted to 15-30°C (59-86°F).

R

RANITIDINE – ranitidine hydrochloride

RX

Class: H_2 blocker

OTHER BRAND NAMES
Zantac Oral, Zantac Injection

ADULT DOSAGE

General Dosing

Inj:
For hospitalized patients w/ pathological hypersecretory conditions or intractable duodenal ulcers, or as an alternative to the oral dosage form for short-term use in patients who are unable to take oral medication

IM:
50mg q6-8h

PEDIATRIC DOSAGE

Erosive Esophagitis

Endoscopically Diagnosed:
1 Month-16 Years:
PO:
5-10mg/kg/day given as 2 divided doses

Duodenal Ulcers

Short-Term Treatment of Active Ulcers:
1 Month-16 Years:

IV:
50mg q6-8h as intermittent bolus/infusion or 6.25mg/hr continuous IV infusion
Max: 400mg/day

Gastric Ulcers

Short-Term Treatment of Active, Benign Ulcers:
PO:
150mg bid
Maint: 150mg hs

Gastroesophageal Reflux Disease

PO:
150mg bid

Erosive Esophagitis

Endoscopically Diagnosed:
PO:
150mg qid
Maint: 150mg bid

Duodenal Ulcers

Short-Term Treatment of Active Ulcers:
PO:
150mg bid or 300mg qd after pm meal or hs
Maint: 150mg hs

Pathological Hypersecretory Conditions

Treatment of pathological hypersecretory conditions (eg, Zollinger-Ellison syndrome, systemic mastocytosis)

PO:
150mg bid; adjust dose according to patient needs and continue as long as clinically indicated. Doses up to 6g/day have been employed w/ severe disease

Continuous IV Infusion:
Zollinger-Ellison Syndrome:
Initial: 1mg/kg/hr
Titrate: May increase after 4 hrs by 0.5mg/kg/hr increments if gastric acid output is >10mEq/hr or patient becomes symptomatic
Doses up to 2.5mg/kg/hr and infusion rates as high as 220mg/hr have been used

PO:
2-4mg/kg bid
Maint: 2-4mg/kg qd
Max: 300mg/day (treatment), 150mg/day (maint)

Inj:
2-4mg/kg/day IV given q6-8h
Max: 50mg IV q6-8h

Gastric Ulcers

Short-Term Treatment of Active, Benign Ulcers:
1 Month-16 Years:
PO:
2-4mg/kg bid
Maint: 2-4mg/kg qd
Max: 300mg/day (treatment), 150mg/day (maint)

Gastroesophageal Reflux Disease

1 Month-16 Years:
PO:
5-10mg/kg/day given as 2 divided doses

Other Indications

Inj:
<1 Month of Age:
Limited data in neonatal patients receiving extracorporeal membrane oxygenation suggest that ranitidine may be useful and safe for increasing gastric pH for patients at risk of GI hemorrhage

2mg/kg given q12-24h or as a continuous infusion should be considered

DOSING CONSIDERATIONS

Renal Impairment

CrCl <50mL/min: 150mg PO q24h or 50mg IV/IM q18-24h; may increase dosing frequency to q12h or even further, w/ caution
Hemodialysis: Give dose at the end of treatment

ADMINISTRATION

Oral/IM/IV routes

PO

Administer concomitant antacids prn for pain relief to patients w/ active duodenal ulcer; active, benign gastric ulcer; hypersecretory states; GERD; or erosive esophagitis

Inj
IV:
Intermittent Bolus:
Dilute ranitidine 50mg inj in 0.9% NaCl inj or other compatible IV sol to a concentration ≤2.5mg/mL (20mL)
Inject at a rate ≤4mL/min (5 min)
Intermittent Infusion:
Dilute ranitidine 50mg inj in D5 inj or other compatible IV sol to a concentration ≤0.5mg/mL (100mL)
Infuse at a rate ≤5-7mL/min (15-20 min)
Continuous Infusion:
Add ranitidine inj to D5 inj or other compatible IV sol; deliver at a rate of 6.25mg/hr (eg, 150mg of ranitidine inj in 250mL of D5 inj at 10.7mL/hr)

For Zollinger-Ellison patients, dilute ranitidine inj in D5 inj or other compatible IV sol to a concentration ≤2.5mg/mL

IM:
No dilution necessary

Stability:
Stable for 48 hrs at room temperature when added to or diluted w/ most commonly used IV sol (eg, 0.9% NaCl inj, D5 inj, 10% dextrose inj, lactated Ringer's inj, 5% sodium bicarbonate inj)

HOW SUPPLIED
Cap: 150mg, 300mg; **Syrup:** 15mg/mL [16 fl oz]; **(Zantac) Inj:** 25mg/mL [2mL, 6mL]; **Tab:** 150mg, 300mg

CONTRAINDICATIONS
Hypersensitivity to ranitidine or any of the ingredients.

WARNINGS/PRECAUTIONS
Symptomatic response does not preclude the presence of gastric malignancy. Caution w/ hepatic/renal dysfunction. May precipitate acute porphyric attacks in patients w/ acute porphyria; avoid w/ history of acute porphyria. False (+) tests for urine protein w/ Multistix may occur. Caution in elderly. D/C immediately if hepatocellular, cholestatic, or mixed hepatitis occurs. (Inj) Do not exceed recommended administration rates; bradycardia reported w/ rapid infusion. ALT elevations may occur; monitor if on IV therapy for ≥5 days at doses ≥100mg qid.

ADVERSE REACTIONS
Headache, constipation, diarrhea, N/V, abdominal discomfort/pain, rash.

DRUG INTERACTIONS
Affects bioavailability of other drugs through several mechanisms (eg, competition for renal tubular secretion, alteration of gastric pH, CYP450 inhibition). Increased plasma levels of procainamide w/ high doses of ranitidine; monitor for procainamide toxicity when administered w/ oral ranitidine at a dose >300mg/day. Altered PT w/ warfarin; closely monitor PT. May alter absorption of drugs in which gastric pH is an important determinant of bioavailability; may increase absorption of triazolam, midazolam, and glipizide and decrease absorption of ketoconazole, atazanavir, delavirdine, and gefitinib. Monitor for excessive/prolonged sedation w/ oral midazolam and triazolam. Chronic use w/ delavirdine is not recommended.

PATIENT CONSIDERATIONS
Assessment: Assess for hypersensitivity to the drug, renal/hepatic impairment, history of acute porphyria, pregnancy/nursing status, and possible drug interactions.

Monitoring: Monitor for signs/symptoms of hepatic effects (eg, hepatitis, elevations in ALT values), hypersensitivity reactions, and other adverse reactions. Monitor PT in patients receiving warfarin.

Counseling: Inform that antacids may be taken prn for relief of pain. Instruct to notify physician if any adverse events develop.

STORAGE: Cap: 20-25°C (68-77°F) in a dry place. Protect from light. Tab: 15-30°C (59-86°F) in a dry place. Protect from light. Syrup: 4-25°C (39-77°F). Do not freeze. Inj: 4-25°C (39-77°F); excursions permitted to 30°C (86°F). Protect from light. Avoid excessive heat; brief exposure up to 40°C (104°F) does not adversely affect the product. Protect from freezing.

R

RAPAFLO – silodosin

RX

Class: $Alpha_1$ antagonist

ADULT DOSAGE
Benign Prostatic Hyperplasia
8mg qd w/ a meal

PEDIATRIC DOSAGE
Pediatric use may not have been established

DOSING CONSIDERATIONS
Renal Impairment
CrCl 30-50mL/min: 4mg qd w/ a meal

ADMINISTRATION
Oral route

Take w/ a meal
Patients who have difficulty swallowing caps may sprinkle the cap powder on a tbsp of applesauce (should not be hot)
Swallow immediately (w/in 5 min) w/o chewing and follow with 8 oz of cool water
Do not subdivide the contents of cap or store any powder/applesauce mixture for future use

HOW SUPPLIED
Cap: 4mg, 8mg

CONTRAINDICATIONS

Severe renal impairment (CrCl <30mL/min), severe hepatic impairment (Child-Pugh score ≥10), concomitant administration w/ strong CYP3A4 inhibitors (eg, ketoconazole, clarithromycin, itraconazole, ritonavir), history of hypersensitivity to silodosin or any of the ingredients of the product.

WARNINGS/PRECAUTIONS

Not for treatment of HTN. Postural hypotension and syncope may occur; may impair mental/physical abilities. Caution in patients with moderate renal impairment. Examine patients prior to therapy to rule out prostate cancer. Intraoperative floppy iris syndrome (IFIS) observed during cataract surgery in some patients on α_1-blockers or previously treated with α_1-blockers.

ADVERSE REACTIONS

Retrograde ejaculation, dizziness, diarrhea, orthostatic hypotension, headache, nasopharyngitis, nasal congestion.

DRUG INTERACTIONS

See Contraindications. Avoid with other α-blockers and strong P-glycoprotein (P-gp) inhibitors (eg, cyclosporine). Caution with antihypertensives. Coadministration with PDE-5 inhibitors may cause symptomatic hypotension; caution with use. Increased concentrations with P-gp inhibitors and moderate CYP3A4 inhibitors (eg, diltiazem, erythromycin, verapamil). UGT2B7 inhibitors (eg, probenecid, valproic acid, fluconazole) may potentially increase exposure.

PATIENT CONSIDERATIONS

Assessment: Assess for drug hypersensitivity, renal/hepatic impairment, prostate cancer, and possible drug interactions.

Monitoring: Monitor for signs/symptoms of postural hypotension, syncope, IFIS during cataract surgery, and other adverse reactions.

Counseling: Counsel about possible occurrence of symptoms related to postural hypotension (eg, dizziness); advise to use caution when driving, operating machinery, or performing hazardous tasks, particularly in patients with low BP or taking antihypertensives. Inform that most common side effect seen is an orgasm with reduced or no semen; inform that this side effect does not pose a safety concern and is reversible when drug is discontinued. Advise to notify ophthalmologist about the use of the drug before cataract surgery or other eye procedures, even if no longer taking silodosin.

STORAGE: 25°C (77°F); excursions permitted to 15-30°C (59-86°F). Protect from light and moisture.

RAPIVAB – peramivir

RX

Class: Neuraminidase inhibitor

ADULT DOSAGE

Influenza

Treatment of Acute Uncomplicated Influenza:
Single 600mg dose, via IV infusion for 15-30 min

PEDIATRIC DOSAGE

Pediatric use may not have been established

R

DOSING CONSIDERATIONS

Renal Impairment

CrCl 30-49mL/min: 200mg
CrCl 10-29mL/min: 100mg

ADMINISTRATION

IV route

Administer w/in 2 days of onset of symptoms of influenza
In patients w/ chronic renal impairment maintained on hemodialysis, administer after dialysis

Dilute an appropriate dose of peramivir 10mg/mL sol in 0.9% or 0.45% NaCl, D5, or lactated Ringer's to a max volume of 100mL
Administer diluted sol via IV infusion for 15-30 min

Compatible w/ 0.9% or 0.45% NaCl, D5, or lactated Ringer's
Do not mix or coinfuse w/ other IV medications
If diluted sol refrigerated, allow to reach room temperature then administer immediately
Refer to PI for further administration instructions

HOW SUPPLIED

Inj: 10mg/mL [20mL]

WARNINGS/PRECAUTIONS

Emergence of resistance substitutions can decrease drug effectiveness; consider available information on influenza drug susceptibility patterns and treatment effects when deciding whether to use peramivir. Rare cases of serious skin reactions (eg, erythema multiforme, Stevens-Johnson syndrome) reported; institute appropriate treatment if a serious skin reaction occurs or is suspected. Neuropsychiatric events (eg, hallucinations, delirium, abnormal behavior), in some cases resulting in fatal outcomes, reported; monitor for signs of abnormal behavior. Serious bacterial infections may begin with influenza-like symptoms or may coexist with or occur during the course of influenza; peramivir does not prevent these complications.

ADVERSE REACTIONS

Diarrhea, increased alanine aminotransferase/serum glucose/CPK, decreased neutrophils.

DRUG INTERACTIONS

Avoid use of live attenuated influenza vaccine within 2 weeks before or 48 hrs after administration of peramivir, unless medically indicated.

PATIENT CONSIDERATIONS

Assessment: Assess for renal impairment, pregnancy/nursing status, and possible drug interactions.

Monitoring: Monitor for signs/symptoms of serious skin/hypersensitivity reactions, neuropsychiatric events, and other adverse reactions.

Counseling: Advise of the risk of serious skin reactions and to seek immediate medical attention if a skin reaction occurs. Advise of the risk of neuropsychiatric events in patients with influenza and to contact physician if experiencing signs of abnormal behavior after receiving treatment.

STORAGE: 20-25°C (68-77°F); excursions permitted to 15-30°C (59-86°F). Diluted Sol: 2-8°C (36-46°F) for up to 24 hrs.

REBIF — interferon beta-1a

RX

Class: Biological response modifier

ADULT DOSAGE

Multiple Sclerosis

Treatment of Relapsing Forms:
22mcg or 44mcg 3X/week

Titration Schedule for 22mcg Prescribed Dose:
Week 1: 4.4mcg (half of 8.8mcg syringe)
Week 2: 4.4mcg (half of 8.8mcg syringe)
Week 3: 11mcg (half of 22mcg syringe)
Week 4: 11mcg (half of 22mcg syringe)
Week 5 and After: 22mcg
Use only prefilled syringes to titrate to the 22mcg prescribed dose

Titration Schedule for 44mcg Prescribed Dose:
Week 1: 8.8mcg
Week 2: 8.8mcg
Week 3: 22mcg
Week 4: 22mcg
Week 5 and After: 44mcg
Prefilled syringes or autoinjectors can be used to titrate to the 44mcg prescribed dose

Premedication

Concurrent use of analgesics and/or antipyretics may help ameliorate flu-like symptoms on treatment days

PEDIATRIC DOSAGE

Pediatric use may not have been established

DOSING CONSIDERATIONS

Elderly

Start at lower end of dosing range

Adverse Reactions

Decreased Peripheral Blood Counts: May necessitate dose reduction or discontinuation until toxicity is resolved

Elevated LFTs: May necessitate dose reduction or discontinuation until toxicity is resolved

ADMINISTRATION

SQ route

Administer at the same time (preferably late afternoon or pm) on the same 3 days at least 48 hrs apart each week.
Rotate site of inj w/ each dose.
Refer to PI for additional instructions.

HOW SUPPLIED

Inj: 22mcg/0.5mL, 44mcg/0.5mL [prefilled syringe, Rebidose autoinjector]; (Titration Pack) 8.8mcg/0.2mL, 22mcg/0.5mL [prefilled syringe, Rebidose autoinjector]

CONTRAINDICATIONS

History of hypersensitivity to natural or recombinant interferon beta, human albumin, or any other component of the formulation.

WARNINGS/PRECAUTIONS

Depression, suicidal ideation, and suicide attempts reported; consider cessation of treatment if depression develops. Severe liver injury reported rarely; d/c immediately if jaundice or other symptoms of liver dysfunction appear. Asymptomatic elevation of hepatic transaminases (particularly ALT) may occur; caution w/ active liver disease, alcohol abuse, increased serum ALT (>2.5X ULN), or history of significant liver disease. Consider dose reduction if ALT rises >5X ULN; may gradually re-escalate dose when enzyme levels have normalized. Anaphylaxis (rare) and other allergic reactions (eg, skin rash, urticaria) reported; d/c if anaphylaxis occurs. Inj-site reactions (eg, necrosis), decreased peripheral blood counts in all cell lines (including pancytopenia), thrombotic microangiopathy (including thrombotic thrombocytopenic purpura and hemolytic uremic syndrome), seizures, and new or worsening thyroid abnormalities reported. D/C if clinical symptoms and lab findings consistent w/ thrombotic microangiopathy occur. Caution in patients w/ preexisting seizure disorders.

ADVERSE REACTIONS

Inj-site disorders, headache, fatigue, fever, rigors, chest pain, back pain, myalgia, abdominal pain, depression, elevation of liver enzymes, hematologic abnormalities.

DRUG INTERACTIONS

Consider the potential for hepatic injury when used in combination w/ known hepatotoxic products, or when new agents are added to the regimen.

PATIENT CONSIDERATIONS

Assessment: Assess for depression, history of or active liver disease, alcohol abuse, preexisting seizure disorder, thyroid dysfunction, myelosuppression, history of hypersensitivity to drug or to human albumin, pregnancy/nursing status, and possible drug interactions.

Monitoring: Monitor for depression, suicidal ideation, jaundice, anaphylaxis, allergic reactions, inj-site reactions, seizures, thrombotic microangiopathy, and other adverse reactions. Perform CBC and LFTs at regular intervals (1, 3, and 6 months) following initiation of therapy and then periodically thereafter in the absence of clinical symptoms; patients w/ myelosuppression may require more intensive monitoring of CBC, w/ differential and platelet counts. Perform thyroid function tests every 6 months in patients w/ a history of thyroid dysfunction, or as clinically indicated.

Counseling: Inform of the symptoms of depression, suicidal ideation, hepatic injury, decreased peripheral blood counts, and seizures, and instruct to immediately report any of these symptoms to physician. Instruct to seek immediate medical attention if symptoms of allergic reactions and anaphylaxis occur. Advise patients that inj-site reactions may occur and to promptly report any signs of necrosis at inj site. Inform that flu-like symptoms are common following initiation of therapy; advise on concurrent use of analgesics and/or antipyretics to help reduce flu-like symptoms on treatment days. Instruct on the use of aseptic technique when self-administering the drug and on the importance of rotating inj sites. Explain the importance of proper disposal of prefilled syringes and autoinjectors, and caution against reuse of these items. Inform about the risks/benefits of treatment during pregnancy.

STORAGE: 2-8°C (36-46°F). Do not freeze. If needed, may store at 2-25°C (36-77°F) for up to 30 days and away from heat and light, but refrigeration is preferred.

RECLAST – zoledronic acid

RX

Class: Bisphosphonate

ADULT DOSAGE

Osteoporosis

Treatment in Men and Postmenopausal Women:

5mg IV once a yr

PEDIATRIC DOSAGE

Pediatric use may not have been established

Prevention in Postmenopausal Women:
5mg IV once every 2 yrs

Glucocorticoid-Induced Osteoporosis:
In men and women who are either initiating or continuing systemic glucocorticoids in a daily dosage ≥7.5mg of prednisone and who are expected to remain on glucocorticoids for ≥12 months

Treatment/Prevention:
5mg IV once a yr

Paget's Disease

5mg IV

May consider retreatment in patients who have relapsed (based on increases in serum alkaline phosphatase), failed to achieve normalization of serum alkaline phosphatase, or those w/ symptoms

DOSING CONSIDERATIONS

Other Important Considerations

Recommended Intake of Ca^{2+} and Vitamin D:
In Osteoporosis: At least 1200mg of Ca^{2+} daily and 800-1000 IU of vitamin D daily
In Paget's Disease: 1500mg of Ca^{2+} daily in divided doses (750mg bid or 500mg tid) and 800 IU of vitamin D daily, particularly in the 2 weeks following administration

ADMINISTRATION

IV route

Infuse IV over ≥15 min at a constant rate
Hydrate patients appropriately prior to administration
IV infusion should be followed by a 10mL normal saline flush of the IV line
Do not allow sol to come in contact with any Ca^{2+} or other divalent cation-containing sol
Administer as a single IV sol through a separate vented infusion line
May give acetaminophen following administration to reduce incidence of acute-phase reaction symptoms

HOW SUPPLIED

Inj: 5mg/100mL

CONTRAINDICATIONS

Hypocalcemia, CrCl <35mL/min, acute renal impairment. Known hypersensitivity to zoledronic acid or any components of this medication.

WARNINGS/PRECAUTIONS

Consider discontinuation after 3-5 yrs of use in patients at low-risk for fracture; periodically reevaluate risk for fracture in patients who d/c therapy. Contains same active ingredient as Zometa; do not treat w/ Reclast if on concomitant therapy w/ Zometa. Treat preexisting hypocalcemia and disturbances of mineral metabolism prior to treatment. Risk of hypocalcemia in Paget's disease. Withhold therapy until normovolemic status has been achieved if history or physical signs suggest dehydration. Caution w/ chronic renal impairment. Acute renal impairment, including renal failure, reported, especially in patients w/ preexisting renal compromise, advanced age, concomitant nephrotoxic medications or diuretic therapy, or severe dehydration. Transient increase in SrCr may be greater w/ impaired renal function; interim monitoring or CrCl should be performed in at-risk patients. Assess fluid status in patients at increased risk of acute renal failure (ARF) (eg, elderly, concomitant diuretic therapy). Osteonecrosis of the jaw (ONJ) reported; risk may increase w/ duration of exposure to drug or w/ concomitant administration of drugs associated w/ ONJ. Consider a dental examination w/ appropriate preventive dentistry prior to treatment in patients w/ a history of concomitant risk factors (eg, cancer, chemotherapy, angiogenesis inhibitors, radiotherapy, corticosteroids, poor oral hygiene, preexisting dental disease or infection, anemia, coagulopathy) and if possible, avoid invasive dental procedures while on treatment. Atypical, low-energy, or low-trauma fractures of the femoral shaft reported; evaluate any patient w/ a history of bisphosphonate exposure who presents w/ thigh/groin pain to rule out an incomplete femur fracture, and consider interruption of therapy. Avoid use in pregnancy; may cause fetal harm. Severe and occasionally incapacitating bone, joint, and/or muscle pain reported; consider withholding future treatment if severe symptoms develop. Caution w/ ASA sensitivity; bronchoconstriction reported.

ADVERSE REACTIONS

Pain, chills, dizziness, osteoarthritis, fatigue, dyspnea, headache, HTN, influenza-like illness, myalgia, arthralgia, pyrexia, N/V.

DRUG INTERACTIONS
Caution w/ aminoglycosides; may have an additive effect to lower serum Ca^{2+} levels for prolonged periods. Caution w/ loop diuretics; may increase risk of hypocalcemia. Caution w/ other potentially nephrotoxic drugs (eg, NSAIDs). In patients w/ renal impairment, exposure to concomitant medications that are primarily renally excreted (eg, digoxin) may increase.

PATIENT CONSIDERATIONS

Assessment: Assess for hypocalcemia, disturbances of mineral metabolism, risk factors for developing renal impairment and ONJ, ASA sensitivity, previous hypersensitivity to the drug, pregnancy/nursing status, and possible drug interactions. Obtain SrCr and calculate CrCl based on actual body weight before each dose. Assess fluid status in patients at increased risk of ARF. Perform routine oral exam, and consider appropriate preventive dentistry in patients w/ a history of risk factors for ONJ.

Monitoring: Monitor for ONJ, atypical femur fracture, musculoskeletal pain, bronchoconstriction, and other adverse events. Monitor renal function and serum Ca^{2+}/mineral levels. Reevaluate the need for continued therapy on a periodic basis.

Counseling: Inform about benefits/risks of therapy, the symptoms of hypocalcemia, and the importance of Ca^{2+} and vitamin D supplementation. Instruct to notify physician if patient had surgery to remove some or all of parathyroid glands, had sections of intestine removed, takes any other medications, or is unable to take Ca^{2+} supplements. Advise to avoid becoming pregnant during treatment. Advise to eat and drink normally (at least 2 glasses of fluid, such as water, w/in a few hrs prior to infusion) on the day of treatment, w/in a few hrs prior to infusion. Inform of the most commonly associated side effects of therapy and to consult physician if these symptoms persist. Instruct to inform physician or dentist if experiencing persistent pain and/or nonhealing sore of the mouth or jaw.

STORAGE: 25°C (77°F); excursions permitted to 15-30°C (59-86°F). Stable for 24 hrs at 2-8°C (36-46°F) after opening. If refrigerated, allow to reach room temperature before administration.

Rectiv — nitroglycerin

RX

Class: Nitrate vasodilator

ADULT DOSAGE
Moderate to Severe Pain

Associated w/ Chronic Anal Fissure:
Apply 1 inch of oint (375mg) intra-anally q12h for up to 3 weeks

PEDIATRIC DOSAGE
Pediatric use may not have been established

ADMINISTRATION
Intra-anal route

1. Gently squeeze tube until a line of oint the length of the measuring line is expressed onto a covered finger
2. Insert the oint into the anal canal using a covered finger no further than to the 1st finger joint
3. Apply oint around the side of the anal canal; if unable to reach the anal canal due to pain, apply the oint directly to the outside of the anus

HOW SUPPLIED
Oint: 0.4% (4mg/g) [30g tube]

CONTRAINDICATIONS
Concomitant use with phosphodiesterase type 5 (PDE5) (eg, sildenafil, vardenafil, and tadalafil), severe anemia and increased intracranial pressure (ICP), known hypersensitivity to nitroglycerin, other nitrates and nitrites, or any components of the oint.

WARNINGS/PRECAUTIONS
Not for oral, ophthalmic, or intravaginal use. Venous and arterial dilatation reported; may decrease venous blood return and reduce arterial vascular resistance and systolic pressure. Caution with blood volume depletion, existing hypotension, cardiomyopathies, congestive heart failure (CHF), acute MI, or poor cardiac function for other reasons; monitor cardiovascular (CV) status and clinical condition. May produce dose-related headaches, which may be severe.

ADVERSE REACTIONS
Headache, dizziness, hypotension, flushing, allergic reactions, application-site reactions, methemoglobinemia.

DRUG INTERACTIONS
See Contraindications. Marked orthostatic hypotension reported with calcium channel blockers. Additive hypotensive effects with antihypertensive drugs, β-adrenergic blockers, and other nitrates. May increase levels with aspirin. Monitor anticoagulation status when administered with IV heparin.

Decreased 1st-pass metabolism of dihydroergotamine. Consider the possibility of ergotism with ergotamine. Caution with tissue-type plasminogen activator; may decrease thrombolytic effect. May potentiate additive effects with alcohol.

PATIENT CONSIDERATIONS

Assessment: Assess for known hypersensitivity, anemia, ICP, blood volume depletion, existing hypotension, cardiomyopathies, CHF, acute MI, cardiac function, pregnancy/nursing status, and possible drug interactions.

Monitoring: Monitor for CV status, clinical conditions, headaches, and other adverse reactions.

Counseling: Advise patients that treatment may be associated with lightheadedness on standing, especially just after rising from lying or seated position. Inform patient that headaches and dizziness has been reported. Tolerance to headaches occurs. Instruct to avoid driving or operating machinery immediately after applying the ointment. Advise not to use medications for erectile dysfunction (eg, sildenafil, vardenafil, tadalafil); may increase hypotensive effects of nitroglycerin.

STORAGE: 20-25°C (68-77°F); excursions permitted to 15-30°C (59-85°F). Keep tube tightly closed; use within 8 weeks of 1st opening.

RELISTOR – methylnaltrexone bromide

RX

Class: Opioid antagonist

ADULT DOSAGE

Opioid-Induced Constipation

In Patients w/ Chronic Non-Cancer Pain:
Usual: 12mg SQ qd

D/C all maint laxative therapy prior to initiation of therapy
Laxative(s) can be used prn, if suboptimal response to therapy after 3 days

In Patients w/ Advanced Illness Receiving Palliative Care w/ Insufficient Response to Laxative Therapy:

Recommended Dose/Inj Volume Based on Weight:
38-<62kg: 8mg SQ (0.4mL)
62-114kg: 12mg SQ (0.6mL)
<38kg or >114kg: 0.15mg/kg; calculate inj volume by multiplying weight in kg by 0.0075 and rounding up the volume to the nearest 0.1mL

Usual Schedule: 1 dose qod prn
Max: 1 dose/24 hrs

PEDIATRIC DOSAGE

Pediatric use may not have been established

DOSING CONSIDERATIONS

Renal Impairment

Severe (CrCl <30mL/min): Reduce dose by 1/2; only prescribe single-use vials to ensure correct dosing

Discontinuation

D/C if treatment w/ opioid pain medication is also discontinued

Other Important Considerations

Chronic Non-Cancer Pain and Opioid-Induced Constipation:
Shown to be efficacious in patients who have taken opioids for at least 4 weeks; sustained exposure to opioids prior to starting therapy may increase patient's sensitivity to the effects of methylnaltrexone
Reevaluate the continued need for therapy when the opioid regimen is changed to avoid adverse reactions

ADMINISTRATION

SQ route

Inject in the upper arm, abdomen, or thigh; rotate inj sites
Patient should be w/in close proximity to toilet facilities once administered

Single-use Vials

Once drawn into the 1mL syringe w/ a 27-gauge x 1/2-inch needle, if immediate administration is not possible, store at ambient room temperature and administer w/in 24 hrs

Single-use Prefilled Syringes
Prescribe only to patients requiring an 8mg or 12mg dose; do not prescribe prefilled syringes to patients requiring dosing calculated on a mg/kg basis
Do not remove prefilled syringe from the tray until ready to administer

HOW SUPPLIED
Inj: 12mg/0.6mL [vial, prefilled syringe], 8mg/0.4mL [prefilled syringe]

CONTRAINDICATIONS
Known/suspected GI obstruction and at increased risk of recurrent obstruction.

WARNINGS/PRECAUTIONS
Cases of GI perforation reported in patients w/ conditions that may be associated w/ localized or diffuse reduction of structural integrity in the wall of GI tract (eg, peptic ulcer disease, Ogilvie's syndrome, diverticular disease); caution w/ these conditions or w/ other conditions which might result in impaired integrity of the GI tract wall (eg, Crohn's disease). D/C if severe, persistent, or worsening abdominal pain develops. D/C if severe/persistent diarrhea occurs. Symptoms consistent w/ opioid withdrawal (eg, hyperhidrosis, chills, diarrhea) may occur. May be at increased risk for opioid withdrawal and/or reduced analgesia in patients who have disruptions to the blood-brain barrier; use w/ caution.

ADVERSE REACTIONS
Abdominal pain, flatulence, nausea, dizziness, hyperhidrosis, diarrhea.

DRUG INTERACTIONS
Potential for additive effects of opioid receptor antagonism and increased risk of opioid withdrawal if used concomitantly w/ other opioid antagonists; avoid use.

PATIENT CONSIDERATIONS

Assessment: Assess for GI obstruction, increased risk of recurrent GI obstruction, conditions associated w/ localized or diffuse reduction of structural integrity of the GI tract wall, conditions which might result in impaired integrity of GI tract wall, disruptions to the blood-brain barrier, renal impairment, pregnancy/nursing status, and other possible drug interactions.

Monitoring: Monitor for signs/symptoms of GI perforation, severe/persistent/worsening abdominal symptoms, severe/persistent diarrhea, adequacy of analgesia, opioid withdrawal symptoms, and other adverse reactions.

Counseling: Instruct to take ud and inform of proper SQ technique. Instruct to d/c therapy and promptly notify physician if unusually severe, persistent, or worsening abdominal pain develops. Advise patients to d/c treatment if they experience severe/persistent diarrhea. Inform that symptoms consistent w/ opioid withdrawal may occur (eg, sweating, chills, diarrhea) while taking therapy. Advise to be w/in close proximity to toilet facilities once administered. Advise females of reproductive potential who become pregnant or are planning to become pregnant that the use of drug during pregnancy may precipitate opioid withdrawal in a fetus due to the undeveloped blood-brain barrier. Caution females who are nursing against breastfeeding during treatment due to the potential for opioid withdrawal in nursing infants.

STORAGE: 20-25°C (68-77°F); excursions permitted to 15-30°C (59-86°F). Do not freeze. Protect from light.

RELPAX – eletriptan hydrobromide

RX

Class: 5-$HT_{1B/1D}$ agonist (triptans)

ADULT DOSAGE
Migraine
W/ or w/o Aura:
Single Dose: 20mg or 40mg
Max Single Dose: 40mg
May give a 2nd dose at least 2 hrs after 1st dose if migraine has not resolved by 2 hrs or returns after transient improvement
Max Daily Dose: 80mg
Safety of treating >3 migraine attacks/30 days not known

PEDIATRIC DOSAGE
Pediatric use may not have been established

ADMINISTRATION
Oral route
Take w/ or w/o food.

HOW SUPPLIED

Tab: 20mg, 40mg

CONTRAINDICATIONS

Ischemic coronary artery disease (CAD) (eg, angina pectoris, history of MI, documented silent ischemia); coronary artery vasospasm (eg, Prinzmetal's angina); Wolff-Parkinson-White syndrome or arrhythmias associated w/ other cardiac accessory conduction pathway disorders; history of stroke, transient ischemic attack, or hemiplegic/basilar migraine; peripheral vascular disease; ischemic bowel disease; uncontrolled HTN; hypersensitivity to eletriptan hydrobromide. Recent use (w/in 24 hrs) of another 5-HT_1 agonist, ergotamine-containing, or ergot-type medication (eg, dihydroergotamine, methysergide). Recent use (w/in 72 hrs) of the following potent CYP3A4 inhibitors: ketoconazole, itraconazole, nefazodone, troleandomycin, clarithromycin, ritonavir, or nelfinavir.

WARNINGS/PRECAUTIONS

If no treatment response for the 1st migraine attack, reconsider diagnosis before treating any subsequent attacks. Not intended for prevention of migraine attacks. Serious cardiac adverse reactions (eg, acute MI) reported. May cause coronary artery vasospasm (Prinzmetal's angina). Perform cardiovascular (CV) evaluation in triptan-naive patients who have multiple CV risk factors (eg, increased age, diabetes, HTN, smoking, obesity, strong family history of CAD) prior to therapy; if CV evaluation is negative, consider administering 1st dose in a medically-supervised setting and performing an ECG immediately following administration. Consider periodic CV evaluation in long-term intermittent users with risk factors for CAD. Life-threatening cardiac rhythm disturbances, including ventricular tachycardia and ventricular fibrillation leading to death, reported; d/c if these occur. Sensations of tightness, pain, and pressure in the chest, throat, neck, and jaw commonly occur, usually noncardiac in origin. Cerebral/subarachnoid hemorrhage and stroke reported; exclude other potentially serious neurological conditions prior to therapy in patients not previously diagnosed as migraineurs, and in migraineurs who present with atypical symptoms. May cause noncoronary vasospastic reactions (eg, peripheral vascular ischemia, GI vascular ischemia/infarction, Raynaud's syndrome). Overuse of acute migraine drugs may lead to exacerbation of headache; detoxification, including drug withdrawal and treatment of withdrawal symptoms may be necessary. Serotonin syndrome may occur; d/c if suspected. Significant elevation in BP, including hypertensive crisis with acute impairment of organ systems, reported. Anaphylaxis, anaphylactoid, and hypersensitivity reactions reported. Not recommended with severe hepatic impairment.

ADVERSE REACTIONS

Asthenia, dizziness, somnolence, nausea, headache, paresthesia, dry mouth, chest tightness/pain/pressure.

DRUG INTERACTIONS

See Contraindications. Serotonin syndrome reported with SSRIs, SNRIs, TCAs, or MAOIs.

PATIENT CONSIDERATIONS

Assessment: Confirm diagnosis of migraine and exclude other potentially serious neurological conditions prior to therapy. Assess for ischemic CAD, HTN, hemiplegic/basilar migraine, hypersensitivity to drug, or any other conditions where treatment is contraindicated or cautioned. Assess for hepatic dysfunction, pregnancy/nursing status, and possible drug interactions. Perform a CV evaluation for patients who have multiple CV risk factors.

Monitoring: Monitor for signs/symptoms of cardiac events, cerebrovascular events, noncoronary vasospastic reactions, serotonin syndrome, hypersensitivity reactions, HTN, and other adverse reactions. Perform periodic CV evaluation in intermittent long-term users with risk factors for CAD.

Counseling: Inform that therapy may cause serious CV side effects and anaphylactic/anaphylactoid reactions. Instruct to seek medical attention if signs/symptoms of chest pain, SOB, weakness, slurring of speech, or other vasospastic reactions occur. Inform that use of acute migraine drugs for ≥10 days/month may lead to an exacerbation of headache; encourage to record headache frequency and drug use (eg, by keeping a headache diary). Inform about the risk of serotonin syndrome. Inform that medication should not be used during pregnancy and instruct to notify physician if breastfeeding or planning to breastfeed.

STORAGE: 20-25°C (68-77°F); excursions permitted to 15-30°C (59-86°F).

REMICADE – infliximab

RX

Class: Monoclonal antibody/TNF blocker

Increased risk for developing serious infections (eg, active tuberculosis [TB], latent TB reactivation, invasive fungal infections, bacterial/viral infections, opportunistic infections) leading to hospitalization or death, mostly w/ concomitant use w/ immunosuppressants (eg, methotrexate [MTX], corticosteroids). D/C if serious infection or sepsis develops. Active/latent reactivation TB may present w/ disseminated or extrapulmonary disease; test for latent TB before and during therapy and initiate treatment for latent TB prior to infliximab use. Invasive fungal infections reported; consider empiric antifungal therapy in patients at risk who develop severe systemic illness. Consider risks and benefits prior to therapy in patients w/ chronic or recurrent infection. Monitor patients for development of infection during and after treatment, including development of TB in patients who tested (-) for latent TB infection prior to therapy. Lymphoma and other malignancies, some fatal, reported in children and adolescents. Postmarketing cases of aggressive and fatal hepatosplenic T-cell lymphoma (HSTCL) reported, and the majority of cases were in patients w/ Crohn's disease (CD) or ulcerative colitis (UC) and mostly in adolescent and young adult males; almost all of these patients were treated concomitantly w/ azathioprine or 6-mercaptopurine.

ADULT DOSAGE

Rheumatoid Arthritis

Moderately to Severely Active:
For reducing signs/symptoms, inhibiting progression of structural damage, and improving physical function

In Combination w/ MTX:
Induction: 3mg/kg at 0, 2, and 6 weeks
Maint: 3mg/kg every 8 weeks
Incomplete Response: May give up to 10mg/kg or treat every 4 weeks

Ankylosing Spondylitis

Active:
Induction: 5mg/kg at 0, 2, and 6 weeks
Maint: 5mg/kg every 6 weeks

Psoriatic Arthritis

For reducing signs/symptoms of active arthritis, inhibiting progression of structural damage, and improving physical function

W/ or w/o MTX:
Induction: 5mg/kg at 0, 2, and 6 weeks
Maint: 5mg/kg every 8 weeks

Plaque Psoriasis

Chronic Severe (eg, Extensive and/or Disabling):
Induction: 5mg/kg at 0, 2, and 6 weeks
Maint: 5mg/kg every 8 weeks

R

Crohn's Disease

Moderately to Severely Active w/ Inadequate Response to Conventional Therapy:
For reducing signs/symptoms and inducing/maintaining clinical remission

Induction: 5mg/kg at 0, 2, and 6 weeks
Maint: 5mg/kg every 8 weeks

May give 10mg/kg to patients who respond and then lose their response
Consider discontinuation if no response by Week 14

Also indicated for reducing number of draining enterocutaneous and rectovaginal fistulas and maintaining fistula closure in patients w/ fistulizing Crohn's disease

Ulcerative Colitis

Moderately to Severely Active w/ Inadequate Response to Conventional Therapy:
For reducing signs/symptoms, inducing/maintaining clinical remission and

PEDIATRIC DOSAGE

Crohn's Disease

Moderately to Severely Active w/ Inadequate Response to Conventional Therapy:
For reducing signs/symptoms and inducing/maintaining clinical remission

≥6 Years:
Induction: 5mg/kg at 0, 2, and 6 weeks
Maint: 5mg/kg every 8 weeks

Ulcerative Colitis

Moderately to Severely Active w/ Inadequate Response to Conventional Therapy:
For reducing signs/symptoms and inducing/maintaining clinical remission

≥6 Years:
Induction: 5mg/kg at 0, 2, and 6 weeks
Maint: 5mg/kg every 8 weeks

mucosal healing, and eliminating corticosteroid use

Induction: 5mg/kg at 0, 2, and 6 weeks
Maint: 5mg/kg every 8 weeks

ADMINISTRATION

IV route

Do not dilute reconstituted sol w/ any other diluent.
Begin infusion w/in 3 hrs of reconstitution and dilution.
Administer infusion over a period of not less than 2 hrs.
Do not infuse concomitantly in the same IV line w/ other agents.
Refer to PI for further instructions.

HOW SUPPLIED

Inj: 100mg

CONTRAINDICATIONS

Moderate to severe heart failure (HF) (NYHA Class III/IV) w/ doses >5mg/kg, re-administration to patients who have experienced a severe hypersensitivity reaction to infliximab, known hypersensitivity to inactive components of the product or to any murine proteins.

WARNINGS/PRECAUTIONS

Do not initiate w/ an active infection. Increased risk of infection in patients >65 yrs of age and in patients w/ comorbid conditions; consider risks and benefits prior to therapy for those who have resided or traveled in areas of endemic TB or mycoses, and w/ any underlying conditions predisposing to infection. Cases of acute/chronic leukemia, melanoma, and Merkel cell carcinoma reported. Caution in patients w/ moderate to severe COPD, history of malignancy, or in continuing treatment in patients who develop malignancy during therapy. Hepatitis B virus (HBV) reactivation reported; if reactivation occurs, d/c and initiate antiviral therapy w/ appropriate supportive treatment. Severe hepatic reactions (eg, acute liver failure, jaundice, hepatitis, cholestasis) reported; d/c if jaundice or marked elevations of liver enzymes (eg, ≥5X ULN) develop. New onset (rare) HF and worsening of HF reported; d/c if new or worsening symptoms of HF occur. Leukopenia, neutropenia, thrombocytopenia, and pancytopenia reported; consider discontinuation of therapy if significant hematologic abnormalities occur. Caution in patients who have ongoing or history of significant hematologic abnormalities. Hypersensitivity reactions reported; d/c for severe hypersensitivity reactions. CNS manifestation of systemic vasculitis, seizures, and new onset/exacerbation of CNS demyelinating disorders reported (rare); caution in patients w/ these neurologic disorders and consider discontinuation if these disorders develop. Caution when switching from one biologic disease-modifying antirheumatic drug to another; overlapping biological activity may further increase risk of infection. May cause autoantibody formation and, rarely, may develop lupus-like syndrome; d/c if lupus-like syndrome develops. Live vaccines may lead to clinical infections; concurrent administration is not recommended. All pediatric patients should be up to date w/ all vaccinations prior to therapy. Fatal outcome due to disseminated BCG infection reported in infants who received BCG vaccine after in utero exposure to infliximab; wait at least 6 months following birth before administering any live vaccine to infants exposed in utero. Caution in elderly.

ADVERSE REACTIONS

Infusion reactions, nausea, abdominal pain, diarrhea, dyspepsia, URTI, sinusitis, pharyngitis, coughing, bronchitis, rash, headache.

DRUG INTERACTIONS

See Boxed Warning. Avoid w/ live vaccines or therapeutic infectious agents. Avoid use w/ tocilizumab; possible increased immunosuppression and increased risk of infection. Not recommended w/ anakinra or abatacept; may increase risk of serious infections. Not recommended w/ other biological therapeutics used to treat the same conditions. MTX may decrease the incidence of anti-infliximab antibody production and increase infliximab concentrations. Upon initiation or discontinuation of infliximab in patients being treated w/ CYP450 substrates w/ a narrow therapeutic index, monitor therapeutic effect (eg, warfarin) or drug concentration (eg, cyclosporine, theophylline) and adjust individual dose of the drug product as needed.

PATIENT CONSIDERATIONS

Assessment: Assess for active/chronic/recurrent infection (eg, TB, HBV), history of an opportunistic infection, recent travel to areas of endemic TB or endemic mycoses, underlying conditions that may predispose to infection, HF, history of malignancy, moderate to severe COPD, presence or history of significant hematologic abnormalities, neurologic disorders, previous hypersensitivity to drug or to murine proteins, risk factors for skin cancer, pregnancy/nursing status, and for possible drug interactions. Assess vaccination history in pediatric patients. Perform test for latent TB infection.

Monitoring: Monitor for sepsis, TB (active, reactivation, or latent), invasive fungal infections, or bacterial, viral, and other infections caused by opportunistic pathogens during and after therapy. Monitor for development of lymphoma, HSTCL, or other malignancies. Monitor for nonmelanoma skin cancers in psoriasis patients, melanoma and Merkel cell carcinoma, new or worsening symptoms of HF, HBV infection reactivation, hepatotoxicity, hematological events, hypersensitivity reactions, CNS demyelinating disorders, lupus-like syndrome, and other adverse reactions. Monitor LFTs. Perform periodic skin examination, particularly in patients w/ risk factors for skin cancer.

Counseling: Advise of potential risks and benefits of therapy. Inform that therapy may lower the ability of immune system to fight infections; instruct to immediately contact physician if any signs/symptoms of an infection develop, including TB and HBV reactivation. Inform about the risks of lymphoma and other malignancies while on therapy. Advise to report to physician signs of new or worsening medical conditions (eg, heart disease, neurological disease, autoimmune disorders) and symptoms of cytopenia.

STORAGE: 2-8°C (36-46°F). May also be stored up to 30°C (86°F) for a single period of up to 6 months, but not exceeding the original expiration date. Do not return to refrigerated storage after removing from refrigerated storage.

RENVELA – sevelamer carbonate

RX

Class: Phosphate binder

ADULT DOSAGE

Hyperphosphatemia

Chronic Kidney Disease on Dialysis:
Not Taking a Phosphate Binder:
Initial:
800mg Tab:
Serum Phosphorus:
>5.5 and <7.5mg/dL: 1 tab tid
≥7.5mg/dL: 2 tabs tid

Powder:
Serum Phosphorus:
>5.5 and <7.5mg/dL: 0.8g tid
≥7.5mg/dL: 1.6g tid

Dose Titration (All Patients):
Titrate by 0.8g tid w/ meals at 2-week intervals as necessary

Conversions

Switching from Sevelamer HCl Tabs/ Switching Between Sevelamer Carbonate Tabs and Powder:
Use the same dose in grams; further titration may be necessary to achieve desired phosphorus levels

Switching from Calcium Acetate:
Initial:
1 Calcium Acetate 667mg Tab/Meal: 1 sevelamer carbonate 800mg tab/meal
2 Calcium Acetate 667mg Tabs/Meal: 2 sevelamer carbonate 800mg tabs/meal
3 Calcium Acetate 667mg Tabs/Meal: 3 sevelamer carbonate 800mg tabs/meal

1 Calcium Acetate 667mg Tab/Meal: 0.8g sevelamer carbonate powder
2 Calcium Acetate 667mg Tabs/Meal: 1.6g sevelamer carbonate powder
3 Calcium Acetate 667mg Tabs/Meal: 2.4g sevelamer carbonate powder

PEDIATRIC DOSAGE

Pediatric use may not have been established

DOSING CONSIDERATIONS

Elderly
Start at low end of dosing range

ADMINISTRATION

Oral route

Take w/ meals

Powder Preparation Instructions

The entire contents of each pkt should be placed in a cup and mixed thoroughly w/ the appropriate amount of water

Minimum Amount of Water for Dose Preparation:
0.8g Powder Pkt: Use 30mL water
2.4g Powder Pkt: Use 60mL water

Multiple pkt may be mixed together w/ the appropriate amount of water
Stir the mixture vigorously (it does not dissolve) and drink the entire preparation w/in 30 min and resuspend the preparation right before drinking

HOW SUPPLIED

Tab: 800mg; **Powder:** 0.8g/pkt, 2.4g/pkt

CONTRAINDICATIONS

Bowel obstruction.

WARNINGS/PRECAUTIONS

Dysphagia and esophageal tab retention reported with use of tab formulation; consider use of sus formulation in patients with a history of swallowing disorders. Bowel obstruction and perforation reported. Caution in elderly.

ADVERSE REACTIONS

N/V, diarrhea, dyspepsia, abdominal pain, flatulence, constipation.

DRUG INTERACTIONS

Consider separating administration of therapy and an oral medication where a reduction in bioavailability of that medication would have a clinically significant effect on its safety or efficacy (eg, cyclosporine, tacrolimus, levothyroxine). Take oral ciprofloxacin at least 2 hrs before or 6 hrs after therapy. Take oral mycophenolate mofetil at least 2 hrs before therapy. Where possible, consider monitoring clinical response and/or blood levels of concomitant drugs that have a narrow therapeutic range.

PATIENT CONSIDERATIONS

Assessment: Assess for presence of bowel obstruction and other GI disorders (eg, dysphagia, swallowing disorders), pregnancy/nursing status, and possible drug interactions.

Monitoring: Monitor for bowel obstruction and perforation, dysphagia, esophageal tab retention, and other adverse reactions. Monitor bicarbonate and Cl^- levels, and for reduced vitamin D, E, K (clotting factors), and folic acid levels.

Counseling: Advise to take with meals and adhere to prescribed diet. If taking an oral medication where reduced bioavailability would produce a clinically significant effect on safety or efficacy, advise to take medication ≥1 hr before or 3 hrs after dosing. Inform that drug may cause constipation and if left untreated, may lead to severe complications; caution to report new onset or worsening of existing constipation promptly to physician.

STORAGE: 25°C (77°C); excursions permitted to 15-30°C (59-86°F). Protect from moisture.

REPATHA – evolocumab

RX

Class: Proprotein Convertase Subtilisin Kexin Type 9 (PCSK9) Inhibitor

R

ADULT DOSAGE

Primary Hyperlipidemia

Adjunct to diet and maximally tolerated statin therapy for the treatment of adults w/ heterozygous familial hypercholesterolemia or clinical atherosclerotic cardiovascular disease, who require additional lowering of LDL-C

140mg SQ every 2 weeks or 420mg SQ once monthly

Homozygous Familial Hypercholesterolemia

Adjunct to diet and other LDL-lowering therapies (eg, statins, ezetimibe, LDL apheresis) for the treatment of patients w/ homozygous familial hypercholesterolemia who require additional lowering of LDL-C

420mg SQ once monthly

Missed Dose

If a dose is missed, administer as soon as

PEDIATRIC DOSAGE

Homozygous Familial Hypercholesterolemia

Adjunct to diet and other LDL-lowering therapies (eg, statins, ezetimibe, LDL apheresis) for the treatment of patients w/ homozygous familial hypercholesterolemia who require additional lowering of LDL-C

13-17 Years:
420mg SQ once monthly

Missed Dose

If a dose is missed, administer as soon as possible if there are >7 days until the next scheduled dose. If there are <7 days until the next scheduled dose, omit the missed dose and administer the next dose according to the original schedule possible if there are >7 days until the next scheduled dose. If there are <7 days until the next scheduled dose, omit the missed dose and administer the next dose according to the original schedule

ADMINISTRATION

SQ route

Allow to warm to room temperature for >30 min prior to use; do not warm in any other way.

To administer the 420mg dose, give 3 inj consecutively w/in 30 min.

Administer into areas of the abdomen, thigh, or upper arm that are not tender, bruised, red, or indurated; rotate inj site w/ each inj.

Do not coadminister w/ other injectable drugs at the same inj site.

HOW SUPPLIED

Inj: 140mg/mL [prefilled syringe, prefilled autoinjector]

CONTRAINDICATIONS

History of a serious hypersensitivity reaction to evolocumab.

WARNINGS/PRECAUTIONS

Hypersensitivity reactions (eg, rash, urticaria) reported; if signs/symptoms of serious allergic reactions occur, d/c treatment, treat accordingly, and monitor until signs/symptoms resolve.

ADVERSE REACTIONS

Nasopharyngitis, URTI, influenza, back pain, inj-site reactions, cough, UTI, sinusitis, headache, myalgia, dizziness, musculoskeletal pain, HTN, diarrhea, gastroenteritis.

PATIENT CONSIDERATIONS

Assessment: Assess for drug hypersensitivity and pregnancy/nursing status. Assess baseline LDL-C levels.

Monitoring: Monitor for hypersensitivity reactions and for other adverse reactions. Monitor LDL-C levels; measure LDL-C levels w/in 4-8 weeks of initiating therapy in patients w/ homozygous familial hypercholesterolemia.

Counseling: Instruct on proper inj technique; inform that it may take up to 15 sec to inject evolocumab. Advise that needle cover of the prefilled autoinjector and syringe contain dry natural rubber (a derivative of latex) and may cause allergic reactions in individuals sensitive to latex.

STORAGE: Pharmacy: 2-8°C (36-46°F) in the original carton to protect from light. Do not freeze. Do not shake. **Patients/Caregivers:** 2-8°C (36-46°F) in the original carton. Alternatively, can be kept at room temperature (up to 25°C [77°F]) in the original carton; under these conditions, discard if not used w/in 30 days. Protect from direct light and do not expose to temperatures >25°C (77°F).

REQUIP – ropinirole

RX

Class: Dopamine receptor agonist

R

OTHER BRAND NAMES

Requip XL

ADULT DOSAGE

Parkinson's Disease

Tab:

Week 1: 0.25mg tid

Week 2: 0.5mg tid

Week 3: 0.75mg tid

Week 4: 1mg tid

After Week 4: May increase by 1.5mg/day on a weekly basis up to a 9mg/day, and then by up to 3mg/day weekly

Max: 24mg/day (8mg tid)

Discontinuation:

D/C gradually over a 7-day period; reduce frequency of administration from tid to bid for 4 days, then to qd for the remaining 3 days

Tab, Extended-Release (ER):

Initial: 2mg qd for 1-2 weeks

PEDIATRIC DOSAGE

Pediatric use may not have been established

Titrate: May increase by 2mg/day at ≥1-week intervals
Max: 24mg/day

Discontinuation:
D/C gradually over a 7-day period

Restless Legs Syndrome

Moderate to Severe Primary Restless Legs Syndrome:
Tab:
Days 1 and 2: 0.25mg qd 1-3 hrs before hs
Days 3-7: 0.5mg qd 1-3 hrs before hs
Week 2: 1mg qd 1-3 hrs before hs
Week 3: 1.5mg qd 1-3 hrs before hs
Week 4: 2mg qd 1-3 hrs before hs
Week 5: 2.5mg qd 1-3 hrs before hs
Week 6: 3mg qd 1-3 hrs before hs
Week 7: 4mg qd 1-3 hrs before hs
Max: 4mg/day

Conversions

Switching from Immediate-Release (IR) to ER Tabs:
0.75-2.25mg/day IR: 2mg/day ER
3-4.5mg/day IR: 4mg/day ER
6mg/day IR: 6mg/day ER
7.5-9mg/day IR: 8mg/day ER
12mg/day IR: 12mg/day ER
15mg/day IR: 16mg/day ER
18mg/day IR: 18mg/day ER
21mg/day IR: 20mg/day ER
24mg/day IR: 24mg/day ER

DOSING CONSIDERATIONS

Renal Impairment
Tab:
Parkinson's Disease:
ESRD on Hemodialysis:
Initial: 0.25mg tid
Patients Receiving Regular Dialysis:
Max: 18mg/day; supplemental doses after dialysis are not required

Restless Legs Syndrome:
ESRD on Hemodialysis:
Initial: 0.25mg qd
Patients Receiving Regular Dialysis:
Max: 3mg/day; supplemental doses after dialysis are not required

Tab, ER:
ESRD on Hemodialysis:
Initial: 2mg qd
Patients Receiving Regular Dialysis:
Max: 18mg/day; supplemental doses after dialysis are not required

ADMINISTRATION

Oral route

Take w/ or w/o food

If a significant interruption in therapy has occurred, retitration may be warranted

Tab, ER
Swallow whole; do not chew, crush, or divide

HOW SUPPLIED

Tab: 0.25mg, 0.5mg, 1mg, 2mg, 3mg, 4mg, 5mg; **Tab, Extended-Release (XL):** 2mg, 4mg, 6mg, 8mg, 12mg

CONTRAINDICATIONS

Hypersensitivity/allergic reaction (including urticaria, angioedema, rash, pruritus) to ropinirole or to any of the excipients.

WARNINGS/PRECAUTIONS

Falling asleep during activities of daily living and somnolence reported; d/c if significant daytime sleepiness or episodes of falling asleep develop during activities that require active participation.

R

May impair mental/physical abilities. Syncope, sometimes associated with bradycardia reported; caution in patients with significant cardiovascular disease (CVD). May cause orthostatic hypotension. Hallucinations reported; risk increases in the elderly treated with XL tab. May experience new or worsening mental status and behavioral changes, which may be severe, including psychotic-like behavior during treatment or after starting or increasing the dose. Avoid with major psychotic disorder due to risk of exacerbating psychosis. Intense urges to gamble, increased sexual urges, intense urges to spend money, binge or compulsive eating, and/or other intense urges, and the inability to control these urges while on therapy reported; consider dose reduction or stopping medication if such urges develop. May cause or exacerbate preexisting dyskinesia. Symptom complex resembling neuroleptic malignant syndrome (NMS) reported in association with rapid dose reduction, withdrawal of, or changes in dopaminergic therapy; tapering dose at the end of treatment for Parkinson's disease is recommended as a prophylactic measure. Increased risk of developing melanoma. Fibrotic complications (eg, retroperitoneal fibrosis, pulmonary infiltrates, pleural effusion, pleural thickening, pericarditis, cardiac valvulopathy) reported. (Tab) Augmentation or early-am rebound in RLS patients reported; review use of medication and consider dosage adjustment or discontinuation of treatment if this occurs. (Tab, XL) May cause BP elevation and changes in HR; caution in patients with CVD. Risk of incomplete release of medication and medication residue being passed in stool if rapid GI transit occurs.

ADVERSE REACTIONS

N/V, somnolence, abdominal pain, dizziness, headache, constipation, syncope, hallucination, dyskinesia, diarrhea. (Tab) viral infection, dyspepsia, leg edema, confusion, asthenic condition.

DRUG INTERACTIONS

Adjustment of ropinirole dose may be required if estrogen or a potent CYP1A2 inducer/inhibitor is stopped or started during treatment. Increased plasma levels of IR tab with ciprofloxacin. Increased clearance with cigarette smoking. Dopamine antagonists, such as neuroleptics (eg, phenothiazines, butyrophenones, thioxanthenes) or metoclopramide may diminish effectiveness. May potentiate dopaminergic side effects of L-dopa and may cause and/or exacerbate preexisting dyskinesia in patients treated with L-dopa for Parkinson's disease; decreasing dose of the dopaminergic drug may ameliorate this adverse reaction. May increase risk of drowsiness with concomitant sedating medications or medications that increase ropinirole plasma levels.

PATIENT CONSIDERATIONS

Assessment: Assess for presence of sleep disorders (other than RLS), known hypersensitivity/allergic reaction to drug or to any of the excipients, CVD, dyskinesia, major psychotic disorder, renal impairment, pregnancy/nursing status, and possible drug interactions.

Monitoring: Monitor for hypersensitivity reactions, psychotic-like behavior, impulse control/compulsive behaviors, syncope, bradycardia, hallucinations, dyskinesia, fibrotic complications, symptom complex resembling NMS, melanomas, and other adverse reactions. Monitor for signs/symptoms of hypotension, especially during dose escalation. Continually reassess for drowsiness or sleepiness. Perform periodic skin examinations. (Tab) Monitor for augmentation or early-am rebound in RLS patients. (Tab, XL) Monitor for BP elevation and HR changes.

Counseling: Instruct to take only as prescribed. Advise not to double next dose if a dose is missed. Advise about the potential for developing a hypersensitivity/allergic reaction; instruct patients to immediately contact physician if they experience these or similar reactions. Advise and alert about potential sedating effects; instruct patients not to drive a car, operate machinery, or engage in other dangerous activities until they have gained sufficient experience with therapy. Advise of possible additive effects when taking other sedating medications, alcohol, or other CNS depressants concomitantly, or when taking a concomitant medication (eg, ciprofloxacin) that increases ropinirole plasma levels. Advise patients that they may experience syncope and that hypotension/orthostatic hypotension may develop with/without symptoms; caution against standing rapidly after sitting or lying down, especially at treatment initiation. Inform that hallucinations or other psychotic-like behavior may occur; advise patients to promptly report these to physician should they develop. Inform that medication may cause and/or exacerbate preexisting dyskinesia. Advise to inform physician if new or increased gambling urges, sexual urges, uncontrolled spending, binge or compulsive eating, or other urges develop while on therapy. Advise patients to contact physician if they wish to d/c drug or decrease its dose. Advise of the higher risk of developing melanoma; instruct to have skin examined on a regular basis by a qualified healthcare provider when using medication. Instruct to notify physician if pregnant/intending to become pregnant during therapy. Advise that drug may inhibit lactation. (Tab) Inform RLS patients that augmentation and/or rebound may occur after starting treatment. (Tab, XL) Alert to the possibility of increases in BP and that significant increases/decreases in HR may be experienced during treatment.

STORAGE: (Tab) 20-25°C (68-77°F). Protect from light and moisture. (Tab, XL) 25°C (77°F); excursions permitted to 15-30°C (59-86°F).

RESTASIS – cyclosporine

RX

Class: Topical immunomodulator

ADULT DOSAGE

Keratoconjunctivitis Sicca

Instill 1 drop in ou q12h

PEDIATRIC DOSAGE

Keratoconjunctivitis Sicca

≥16 Years:

Instill 1 drop in ou q12h

ADMINISTRATION

Ocular route

Invert unit dose vial a few times to obtain uniform, white, opaque emulsion before using

Can be used concomitantly with artificial tears, allowing 15-min interval between products

HOW SUPPLIED

Emulsion: 0.05% [0.4mL]

CONTRAINDICATIONS

Known or suspected hypersensitivity to any of the ingredients in the formulation.

WARNINGS/PRECAUTIONS

Increased tear production not seen in patients currently taking topical anti-inflammatory drugs or using punctal plugs. Do not touch vial tip to the eye or other surfaces to avoid the potential for eye injury and contamination. Do not administer in patients wearing contact lenses. Remove contact lenses prior to administration; may reinsert 15 min after administration.

ADVERSE REACTIONS

Ocular burning, conjunctival hyperemia, discharge, epiphora, eye pain, foreign body sensation, pruritus, stinging, visual disturbance (eg, blurring).

PATIENT CONSIDERATIONS

Assessment: Assess for hypersensitivity, contact lens use, and pregnancy/nursing status.

Monitoring: Monitor for signs/symptoms of ocular burning and other adverse reactions.

Counseling: Instruct not to allow the vial tip to touch the eye or any surface. Advise to remove contact lenses before administration; inform that lenses may be reinserted 15 min following administration. Advise to use single-use vial immediately after opening and to discard the remaining contents immediately after administration.

STORAGE: 15-25°C (59-77°F).

RESTORIL – temazepam

CIV

Class: Benzodiazepine

ADULT DOSAGE

Insomnia

Short-Term Treatment (Generally 7 to 10 Days):

Usual: 15mg before retiring

7.5mg may be sufficient for some patients and others may need 30mg

Transient Insomnia:

7.5mg before retiring

PEDIATRIC DOSAGE

Pediatric use may not have been established

DOSING CONSIDERATIONS

Elderly

Elderly/Debilitated Patients:

Initial: 7.5mg before retiring

ADMINISTRATION

Oral route

HOW SUPPLIED

Cap: 7.5mg, 15mg, 22.5mg, 30mg

CONTRAINDICATIONS

Women who are or may become pregnant.

R

WARNINGS/PRECAUTIONS

Initiate only after careful evaluation; failure of insomnia to remit after 7-10 days of treatment may indicate primary psychiatric and/or medical illness. Worsening of insomnia and emergence of thinking or behavior abnormalities may occur, especially in elderly; use lowest possible effective dose. Behavioral changes (eg, decreased inhibition, bizarre behavior, agitation, hallucinations, depersonalization) and complex behavior (eg, sleep-driving) reported; strongly consider discontinuation if sleep-driving episode occurs. Amnesia and other neuropsychiatric symptoms may occur unpredictably. Worsening of depression, including suicidal thinking, reported. Withdrawal symptoms may occur after abrupt discontinuation. Rare cases of angioedema and anaphylaxis reported; do not rechallenge. Oversedation, confusion, and/or ataxia may develop w/ large doses in elderly and debilitated patients. Caution w/ hepatic/renal impairment, chronic pulmonary insufficiency, debilitated, severe or latent depression, and in elderly. Abnormal LFTs, renal function tests, and blood dyscrasias reported.

ADVERSE REACTIONS

Drowsiness, headache, fatigue, nervousness, lethargy, dizziness, nausea.

DRUG INTERACTIONS

Increased risk of complex behaviors w/ alcohol and CNS depressants. Potential additive effects w/ hypnotics and CNS depressants. Possible synergistic effect w/ diphenhydramine.

PATIENT CONSIDERATIONS

Assessment: Assess for physical and/or psychiatric disorder, medical illness, severe or latent depression, renal/hepatic dysfunction, chronic pulmonary insufficiency, pregnancy/nursing status, alcohol use, and possible drug interactions.

Monitoring: Monitor for signs/symptoms of withdrawal, tolerance, abuse, dependence, abnormal thinking, behavioral changes, agitation, depersonalization, hallucinations, complex behaviors, amnesia, anxiety, neuropsychiatric symptoms, worsening of depression, suicidal thoughts and actions, angioedema, driving/psychomotor impairment, worsening of insomnia, thinking or behavioral abnormalities, and possible abuse/dependence.

Counseling: Inform about the benefits and risks of treatment. Instruct patient to take as prescribed. Inform about the risks and possibility of physical/psychological dependence, memory problems, and complex behaviors (eg, sleep-driving). Caution against hazardous tasks (eg, operating machinery/driving). Advise not to drink alcohol. Instruct to notify physician if pregnant/planning to become pregnant.

STORAGE: 20-25°C (68-77°F).

Retin-A – tretinoin

RX

Class: Retinoid

OTHER BRAND NAMES

Retin-A Micro

R

ADULT DOSAGE

Acne Vulgaris

Apply qpm/qhs to the skin where acne lesions appear, using enough to cover the entire affected area in a thin layer

PEDIATRIC DOSAGE

Acne Vulgaris

≥12 Years:

Retin-A Micro:

Apply qpm to the skin where acne lesions appear, using enough to cover the entire affected area in a thin layer

ADMINISTRATION

Topical route

Thoroughly cleanse the areas to be treated before applying the medication. To help limit skin irritation, wash treated skin gently, using a mild, non-medicated soap, and pat it dry; avoid washing treated skin too often or scrubbing hard when washing.

Keep away from eyes, mouth, paranasal creases of the nose, and mucous membranes.

Patients treated w/ therapy may use cosmetics.

HOW SUPPLIED

(Retin-A) Cre: 0.025%, 0.05%, 0.1% [20g, 45g]; **Gel:** 0.01%, 0.025% [15g, 45g]; **(Retin-A Micro) Gel:** 0.04%, 0.1% [20g, 45g, 50g], 0.08% [50g]

CONTRAINDICATIONS

Hypersensitivity to any of the ingredients.

WARNINGS/PRECAUTIONS

Severe irritation on eczematous skin reported; use caution in patients w/ this condition. If the degree of local irritation warrants, temporarily reduce the amount/frequency of application, d/c use temporarily, or d/c use all together. D/C therapy if a reaction suggesting sensitivity or chemical irritation occurs. Avoid or minimize unprotected exposure to sunlight, including sunlamps (UV light); avoid use w/ sunburn until fully recovered. Caution in patients who may be required to have considerable sun exposure and those w/ inherent sensitivity to the sun. Use of sunscreen products and protective clothing over treated areas is recommended when exposure cannot be avoided. Weather extremes (eg, cold, wind) may irritate skin. An apparent exacerbation of inflammatory lesions may occur during early weeks of therapy. A transitory feeling of warmth or slight stinging may be noted on application. **Retin-A:** May induce severe local erythema and peeling at application site. Gels are flammable. **Retin-A Micro:** Skin may become excessively dry, red, swollen, or blistered; apply topical moisturizer if dryness is bothersome.

ADVERSE REACTIONS

Skin irritation/burning, erythema, dermatitis, hyper/hypopigmentation.

DRUG INTERACTIONS

Caution w/ topical medications, medicated/abrasive soaps and cleansers, products w/ strong drying effect, and products w/ high concentrations of alcohol, astringents, limes, or spices. Caution w/ medications that cause photosensitivity. Caution w/ preparations containing sulfur, resorcinol, or salicylic acid; allow effects of these agents to subside before initiation of treatment. **Retin-A Micro:** Caution w/ OTC acne preparations containing benzoyl peroxide.

PATIENT CONSIDERATIONS

Assessment: Assess for drug hypersensitivity, sun exposure, sensitivity to sun, sunburn, eczematous skin, pregnancy/nursing status, and possible drug interactions.

Monitoring: Monitor for sensitivity reactions, irritation, local erythema or peeling at application site, and other adverse reactions. Closely monitor alterations of vehicle, drug concentration, or dose frequency by carefully observing therapeutic response and skin tolerance.

Counseling: Instruct to d/c use and consult physician if irritation occurs. Instruct not to use more than the recommended amount and not to apply more than qd. Advise to minimize exposure to sunlight, including sunlamps, and to use sunscreen products and protective clothing over treated areas when exposure to sun cannot be avoided. Inform that weather extremes may be irritating to treated skin. Instruct to use ud, and to keep away from eyes, mouth, angles of the nose, and mucous membranes. Advise to inform physician of other acne preparations being used and if pregnant or breastfeeding. Inform that during the early weeks of therapy, an apparent exacerbation of inflammatory lesions may occur, which should not be considered a reason for discontinuation. **Retin-A Micro:** Advise to apply moisturizer if dryness is bothersome.

STORAGE: (Retin-A) Cre: <27°C (80°F). **Gel:** <30°C (86°F). **(Retin-A Micro) Gel:** 20-25°C (68-77°F); excursions permitted from 15-30°C (59-86°F). Store pump upright.

REVATIO – sildenafil

RX

Class: Phosphodiesterase-5 (PDE-5) inhibitor

ADULT DOSAGE

Pulmonary Arterial Hypertension

Treatment of pulmonary arterial HTN (WHO Group I) to improve exercise ability and delay clinical worsening

PO:

5mg or 20mg tid, 4-6 hrs apart

Max: 20mg tid

IV:

For continued treatment in patients currently taking tabs/sus and who are temporarily unable to take oral medications

2.5mg or 10mg IV bolus tid

PEDIATRIC DOSAGE

Pediatric use may not have been established

ADMINISTRATION

Oral/IV route

Refer to PI for reconstitution of the powder for oral sus

Incompatibilities

Do not mix w/ any other medication or additional flavoring agent

HOW SUPPLIED

Inj: 10mg [12.5mL]; **Sus:** 10mg/mL [112mL]; **Tab:** 20mg

CONTRAINDICATIONS

Concomitant use of organic nitrates in any form, either regularly/intermittently, or riociguat, a guanylate cyclase stimulator. Known hypersensitivity to sildenafil or any component of the tablet, injection, or oral suspension.

WARNINGS/PRECAUTIONS

Adding sildenafil to bosentan therapy does not result in any beneficial effect on exercise capacity. Not recommended in children. Vasodilatory effects may adversely affect patients w/ resting hypotension (BP <90/50), fluid depletion, severe left ventricular outflow obstruction, or autonomic dysfunction. Not recommended w/ pulmonary veno-occlusive disease (PVOD); consider possibility of associated PVOD if signs of pulmonary edema occur. Epistaxis reported in patients w/ pulmonary HTN secondary to connective tissue disorder. When used to treat erectile dysfunction, non-arteritic anterior ischemic optic neuropathy (NAION) was reported. Caution w/ previous NAION in 1 eye and w/ retinitis pigmentosa. Cases of sudden decrease or loss of hearing, possibly accompanied by tinnitus and dizziness, reported. Caution in patients w/ anatomical penile deformation (eg, angulation, cavernosal fibrosis, Peyronie's disease) or w/ predisposition to priapism (eg, sickle-cell anemia, multiple myeloma, leukemia). Penile tissue damage and permanent loss of potency may result if priapism is not immediately treated. Vaso-occlusive crises requiring hospitalization reported in patients w/ pulmonary HTN secondary to sickle-cell disease. Caution in elderly.

ADVERSE REACTIONS

Headache, dyspepsia, gastritis, epistaxis, paresthesia, flushing, diarrhea, insomnia, dyspnea exacerbation, myalgia, nausea, sinusitis, erythema, pyrexia, rhinitis.

DRUG INTERACTIONS

See Contraindications. Vasodilatory effects may adversely affect patients on antihypertensive therapy; monitor BP when given w/ antihypertensives. Reports of epistaxis w/ oral vitamin K antagonists. Avoid w/ other PDE-5 inhibitors. Not recommended w/ ritonavir and other potent CYP3A inhibitors. Symptomatic postural hypotension w/ doxazosin reported. Additional reduction of supine BP w/ oral amlodipine reported.

PATIENT CONSIDERATIONS

Assessment: Assess for hypotension, fluid depletion, left ventricular outflow obstruction, autonomic dysfunction, PVOD, risk factors for developing NAION, previous NAION in 1 eye, retinitis pigmentosa, anatomical deformities of the penis, conditions predisposing to priapism, pulmonary HTN secondary to sickle-cell disease, hypersensitivity to drug, pregnancy/nursing status, and possible drug interactions. Obtain baseline BP.

Monitoring: Monitor for signs of pulmonary edema, decreased/sudden loss of vision or hearing, tinnitus, dizziness, epistaxis, priapism, vaso-occlusive crises, hypersensitivity reactions, and other adverse reactions. Monitor BP.

Counseling: Counsel about risks and benefits of the drug. Inform that drug is also marketed as Viagra for male erectile dysfunction. Advise not to take Viagra or other PDE-5 inhibitors and organic nitrates during therapy. Advise to notify physician if sudden decrease/loss of vision or hearing occurs. Instruct to seek immediate medical attention if an erection persists >4 hrs.

STORAGE: (Tab/Inj) 20-25°C (68-77°F); excursions permitted to 15-30°C (59-86°F). (Sus) <30°C (86°F). Protect from moisture. Constituted: <30°C (86°F) or 2-8°C (36-46°F). Do not freeze. Shelf-life: 60 days.

REVLIMID — lenalidomide

RX

Class: Thalidomide analogue

Do not use during pregnancy; may cause birth defects or embryo-fetal death. Females of reproductive potential should have 2 negative pregnancy tests prior to treatment and must use 2 forms of contraception or continuously abstain from heterosexual sex during and for 4 weeks after treatment. Available only through a restricted distribution program, the Revlimid REMS program. May cause significant neutropenia and thrombocytopenia. Patients on therapy for del 5q myelodysplastic syndrome (MDS) should have their CBC monitored weekly for the first 8 weeks of therapy and at least monthly thereafter; may require dose interruption and/or reduction and use of blood product support and/or growth factors. Increased risk of deep vein thrombosis (DVT) and pulmonary embolism (PE), as well as risk of MI and stroke, reported in patients w/ multiple myeloma (MM) treated w/ lenalidomide and dexamethasone; monitor for and advise patients about signs/symptoms of thromboembolism. Advise patients to seek immediate medical care if symptoms such as SOB, chest pain, or arm or leg swelling develop. Thromboprophylaxis is recommended and the choice of regimen should be based on assessment of individual's underlying risks.

ADULT DOSAGE

Multiple Myeloma

Initial: 25mg qd on Days 1-21 of repeated 28-day cycles in combination w/ dexamethasone; may reduce initial dose of dexamethasone for patients >75 yrs

Continue until disease progression or unacceptable toxicity

In Patients who are not eligible for autologous stem cell transplantation (ASCT), continue treatment until disease progression or unacceptable toxicity. For patients who are ASCT-eligible, hematopoietic stem cell mobilization should occur w/in 4 cycles of a lenalidomide-containing therapy

Myelodysplastic Syndromes

Patients w/ transfusion-dependent anemia due to low- or intermediate-1-risk myelodysplastic syndromes associated w/ a deletion 5q cytogenetic abnormality w/ or w/o additional cytogenetic abnormalities

Initial: 10mg/day

Continue or modify treatment based upon clinical and lab findings

Mantle Cell Lymphoma

Patients whose disease has relapsed or progressed after 2 prior therapies, 1 of which included bortezomib

Initial: 25mg/day on Days 1-21 of repeated 28-day cycles for relapsed or refractory disease

Continue until disease progression or unacceptable toxicity

PEDIATRIC DOSAGE

Pediatric use may not have been established

DOSING CONSIDERATIONS

Renal Impairment

Multiple Myeloma (MM):
Moderate (CrCl 30-50mL/min): Initial: 10mg q24h
Severe (CrCl <30mL/min Not Requiring Dialysis): Initial: 15mg q48h
ESRD (CrCl <30mL/min Requiring Dialysis): Initial: 5mg qd. On dialysis days, administer dose following dialysis

Myelodysplastic Syndromes (MDS):
Moderate (CrCl 30-60mL/min): Initial: 5mg q24h
Severe (CrCl <30mL/min Not Requiring Dialysis): Initial: 2.5mg q24h
ESRD (CrCl <30mL/min Requiring Dialysis): Initial: 2.5mg qd. On dialysis days, administer dose following dialysis

Mantle Cell Lymphoma (MCL):
Moderate (CrCl 30-60mL/min): Initial: 10mg q24h
Severe (CrCl <30mL/min Not Requiring Dialysis): Initial: 15mg q48h
ESRD (CrCl <30mL/min Requiring Dialysis): Initial: 5mg qd. On dialysis days, administer dose following dialysis

Adverse Reactions

MM:
Thrombocytopenia:
Platelets:
Fall to <30,000/μL: Interrupt treatment and follow CBC weekly
Return to ≥30,000/μL: Resume at next lower dose. Do not dose <2.5mg/day
For Each Subsequent Drop <30,000/μL: Interrupt treatment
Return to ≥30,000/μL: Resume at next lower dose; do not dose <2.5mg/day

Neutropenia:
Neutrophils:
Fall to <1000/μL: Interrupt treatment, follow CBC weekly
Return to ≥1000/μL and Neutropenia is Only Toxicity: Resume at 25mg/day or initial starting dose
Return to ≥1000/μL and if Other Toxicity: Resume at next lower dose. Do not dose <2.5mg/day

For Each Subsequent Drop <1000/μL: Interrupt treatment
Return to ≥1000/μL: Resume at next lower dose. Do not dose <2.5mg/day

Other Toxicities in MM:
For other Grade 3/4 toxicities judged to be related to treatment, hold treatment and restart at physician's discretion at next lower dose level when toxicity has resolved to ≤Grade 2

MDS:
Thrombocytopenia w/in 4 Weeks at Starting Dose 10mg/day (Baseline ≥100,000/μL):
Platelets:
Fall to <50,000/μL: Interrupt treatment
Return to ≥50,000/μL: Resume at 5mg/day

Thrombocytopenia w/in 4 Weeks at Starting Dose 10mg/day (Baseline <100,000/μL):
Platelets:
Falls to 50% of Baseline: Interrupt treatment
If Baseline ≥60,000/μL and Return to ≥50,000/μL: Resume at 5mg/day
If Baseline <60,000/μL and Return to ≥30,000/μL: Resume at 5mg/day

Thrombocytopenia after 4 Weeks at Starting Dose 10mg/day:
Platelets:
<30,000/μL or <50,000/μL w/ Platelet Transfusions: Interrupt treatment
Return to ≥30,000/μL (w/o Hemostatic Failure): Resume at 5mg/day

Thrombocytopenia During Treatment at 5mg/day:
Platelets:
<30,000/μL or <50,000/μL w/ Platelet Transfusions: Interrupt treatment
Return to ≥30,000/μL (w/o Hemostatic Failure): Resume at 2.5mg/day

Neutropenia w/in 4 Weeks of Starting Treatment at 10mg/day (Baseline ANC ≥1000/μL):
Neutrophils:
Fall to <750/μL: Interrupt treatment
Return to ≥1000/μL: Resume at 5mg/day

Neutropenia w/in 4 Weeks of Starting Treatment at 10mg/day (Baseline ANC <1000/μL):
Neutrophils:
Fall to <500/μL: Interrupt treatment
Return to ≥500/μL: Resume at 5mg/day

Neutropenia After 4 Weeks of Starting Treatment at 10mg/day:
Neutrophils:
<500/μL for ≥7 days or <500/μL Associated w/ Fever (≥38.5°C): Interrupt treatment
Return to ≥500/μL: Resume at 5mg/day

Neutropenia During Treatment at 5mg/day:
Neutrophils:
<500/μL for ≥7 Days or <500/μL Associated w/ Fever (≥38.5°C): Interrupt treatment
Return to ≥500/μL: Resume at 2.5mg/day

Other Toxicities in MDS:
For other Grade 3/4 toxicities judged to be related to treatment, hold treatment and restart at the physician's discretion at next lower dose level when toxicity has resolved to ≤Grade 2

MCL:
Thrombocytopenia During Treatment:
Platelets:
Fall to <50,000/μL: Interrupt treatment and follow CBC weekly
Return to ≥50,000/μL: Resume at 5mg less than the previous dose. Do not dose <5mg daily

Neutropenia During Treatment:
Neutrophils:
Fall to <1000/μL for at Least 7 Days or Falls to <1000/μL w/ an Associated Temperature ≥38.5°C or Fall to <500/μL:
Interrupt treatment and follow CBC weekly
Return to ≥1000/μL: Resume at 5mg less than previous dose. Do not dose <5mg/day

Other Toxicities in MCL:
For other Grade 3/4 toxicities judged to be related to treatment, hold treatment and restart at next lower dose level when toxicity has resolved to ≤Grade 2

ADMINISTRATION

Oral route

Take at about the same time each day, w/ or w/o food
Swallow cap whole w/ water; do not open, crush, break, or chew

Handling Precautions
Wash skin immediately and thoroughly w/ soap and water if powder from cap contacts the skin. If drug contacts the mucous membranes, flush thoroughly w/ water

R

HOW SUPPLIED

Cap: 2.5mg, 5mg, 10mg, 15mg, 20mg, 25mg

CONTRAINDICATIONS

Pregnancy, hypersensitivity (eg, angioedema, Stevens-Johnson syndrome, toxic epidermal necrolysis) to lenalidomide.

WARNINGS/PRECAUTIONS

Not indicated and not recommended for the treatment of patients w/ chronic lymphocytic leukemia outside of controlled clinical trials; increased risk of death and serious adverse cardiovascular (CV) reactions reported. Avoid pregnancy for at least 4 weeks before beginning therapy, during therapy, during dose interruptions, and for at least 4 weeks after completing therapy. Male patients (including those who had a vasectomy) must always use a latex/synthetic condom during any sexual contact w/ females of reproductive potential during therapy and for up to 28 days after discontinuing therapy. Avoid sperm donation during therapy. Avoid blood donation during treatment and for 1 month following discontinuation. Greater risk of MI or stroke in patients w/ known risk factors, including prior thrombosis; minimize all modifiable factors (eg, hyperlipidemia, HTN, smoking). Increase of invasive 2nd primary malignancies notably acute myelogenous leukemia and MDS reported in patients w/ MM, predominantly in those receiving therapy in combination w/ oral melphalan or immediately following high dose IV melphalan and ASCT. Hepatic failure, including fatal cases, reported in combination w/ dexamethasone. D/C treatment upon elevation of liver enzymes and consider treatment at a lower dose after values return to baseline. Angioedema and serious dermatologic reactions reported; d/c if angioedema, Stevens-Johnson syndrome (SJS), toxic epidermal necrolysis (TEN), Grade 4 rash, or exfoliative or bullous rash is suspected and do not resume following discontinuation for these reactions. Consider treatment interruption or discontinuation for Grade 2-3 skin rash. Avoid w/ a prior history of Grade 4 rash associated w/ thalidomide treatment. Contains lactose. Fatal instances of tumor lysis syndrome reported; caution in patients w/ high tumor burden prior to treatment. Tumor flare reaction (TFR) reported in patients w/ MCL; withhold treatment in patients w/ Grade 3 or 4 TFR until TFR resolves to ≤Grade 1. A decrease in the number of CD34+ cells collected after treatment (>4 cycles) reported; in patients who are ASCT candidates, referral to a transplant center should occur early in treatment to optimize the timing of the stem cell collection. Consider granulocyte-colony stimulating factor (G-CSF) w/ cyclophosphamide or the combination of G-CSF w/ a CXCR4 inhibitor in patients who received >4 cycles of a lenalidomide-containing treatment or for whom inadequate numbers of CD34+ cells have been collected w/ G-CSF alone.

ADVERSE REACTIONS

Thrombocytopenia, neutropenia, PE, pruritus, rash, diarrhea, constipation, nausea, anemia, fatigue, cough, back pain, pyrexia, muscle cramp, asthenia.

DRUG INTERACTIONS

May increase levels of digoxin; monitor digoxin levels periodically. Closely monitor PT and INR w/ warfarin in MM patients. Caution w/ erythropoietic agents or other agents that may increase the risk of thrombosis (eg, estrogen-containing therapies).

PATIENT CONSIDERATIONS

Assessment: Assess for renal/hepatic impairment, history of Grade 4 rash, risk factors for MI and stroke, prior thrombosis, high tumor burden, lactose intolerance, hypersensitivity to the drug, pregnancy/nursing status, and possible drug interactions. Perform pregnancy test 10-14 days before and 24 hrs prior to therapy. Obtain baseline CBC.

Monitoring: Monitor for signs/symptoms of thromboembolism, neutropenia, thrombocytopenia, angioedema, SJS, TEN, tumor lysis syndrome, TFR, 2nd primary malignancies, serious adverse CV reactions, and other adverse reactions. Perform pregnancy test weekly during 1st month, then repeat monthly (regular menstrual cycle) or every 2 weeks (irregular menstrual cycle) and perform pregnancy test if period is missed or if there is any abnormal menstrual bleeding. Monitor CBC periodically; every 7 days (weekly) for the first 2 cycles, on Days 1 and 15 of cycle 3, and every 28 days (4 weeks) thereafter (MM patients taking concomitant dexamethasone); weekly for the first 8 weeks of therapy and at least monthly thereafter (MDS); and weekly for the 1st cycle (28 days), every 2 weeks during cycles 2-4, and monthly thereafter (MCL). Monitor patients w/ neutropenia for signs of infection. Monitor renal/hepatic function. Closely monitor patients w/ high tumor burden. Closely monitor PT and INR w/ warfarin in MM patients.

Counseling: Instruct females of reproductive potential to avoid pregnancy, have monthly pregnancy tests, and to use 2 different forms of contraception, including at least 1 highly effective form, simultaneously during therapy, during dose interruption, and for 4 weeks after completing therapy. Instruct to immediately d/c and contact physician if patient becomes pregnant, misses her menstrual period, experiences unusual menstrual bleeding, stops taking birth control, or believes for any reason that she is pregnant. Instruct males (including those who had a vasectomy) to always use a latex/synthetic condom during any sexual contact w/ females of reproductive potential during therapy and for up to 28 days after discontinuing therapy. Advise males not to donate sperm. Instruct not to donate blood during therapy, during dose interruptions, and for 1 month following discontinuation. Inform of the other risks associated w/ therapy. Instruct that if a dose is missed, may still take dose up to 12 hrs after the time dose is normally taken. Advise that if >12 hrs have elapsed, the dose for that day should be skipped, and the dose for the next day should be taken at the usual time. Advise to observe for bleeding/bruising, especially w/ use of concomitant medication that may increase risk of bleeding.

STORAGE: 20-25°C (68-77°F); excursions permitted to 15-30°C (59-86°F).

Rexulti — brexpiprazole RX

Class: Atypical antipsychotic

Elderly patients w/ dementia-related psychosis treated w/ antipsychotic drugs are at an increased risk of death. Not approved for treatment of patients w/ dementia-related psychosis. Antidepressants increased the risk of suicidal thoughts and behaviors in patients aged 24 years and younger in short-term studies. Monitor closely for clinical worsening and for emergence of suicidal thoughts and behaviors. Safety and efficacy of brexpiprazole have not been established in pediatric patients.

ADULT DOSAGE

Major Depressive Disorder

Adjunctive Treatment:
Initial: 0.5mg or 1mg qd
Titrate: Titrate to 1mg qd, then up to target dose of 2mg qd; increase dose at weekly intervals based on clinical response and tolerability
Max: 3mg/day

Schizophrenia

Initial: 1mg qd on Days 1-4
Titrate: Titrate to 2mg qd on Days 5-7, then to 4mg on Day 8 based on clinical response and tolerability
Target Dose: 2-4mg qd
Max: 4mg/day

PEDIATRIC DOSAGE

Pediatric use may not have been established

DOSING CONSIDERATIONS

Concomitant Medications

Strong CYP2D6 Inhibitors:
Administer 1/2 of brexpiprazole usual dose; adjust to original level if coadministered drug is discontinued. Dose adjustment not needed in patients who are being treated for major depressive disorder (MDD)

Strong CYP3A4 Inhibitors:
Administer 1/2 of brexpiprazole usual dose; adjust to original level if coadministered drug is discontinued

Strong/Moderate CYP2D6 Inhibitors w/ Strong/Moderate CYP3A4 Inhibitors:
Administer 1/4 of brexpiprazole usual dose; adjust to original level if coadministered drug is discontinued

Strong CYP3A4 Inducers:
Double brexpiprazole usual dose over 1-2 weeks; reduce to original level over 1-2 weeks if the coadministered CYP3A4 inducer is discontinued

Renal Impairment

Moderate, Severe, or ESRD (CrCl <60mL/min):
Max Dose:
MDD: 2mg qd
Schizophrenia: 3mg qd

Hepatic Impairment

Moderate to Severe (Child-Pugh Score ≥7):
Max Dose:
MDD: 2mg qd
Schizophrenia: 3mg qd

Elderly

Start at lower end of dosing range

Other Important Considerations

CYP2D6 Poor Metabolizers:
Administer 1/2 of usual dose

Known CYP2D6 Poor Metabolizers Taking Strong/Moderate CYP3A4 Inhibitors:
Administer 1/4 of usual dose

ADMINISTRATION
Oral route

Take w/ or w/o food.

HOW SUPPLIED
Tab: 0.25mg, 0.5mg, 1mg, 2mg, 3mg, 4mg

CONTRAINDICATIONS
Known hypersensitivity to Rexulti or any of its components.

WARNINGS/PRECAUTIONS
Neuroleptic malignant syndrome (NMS) may occur; d/c immediately, institute symptomatic treatment, and monitor. May cause tardive dyskinesia (TD), especially in the elderly; consider discontinuation if signs/symptoms appear. Hyperglycemia, in some cases extreme and associated w/ ketoacidosis or hyperosmolar coma or death, reported w/ atypical antipsychotics. Undesirable alterations in lipids and weight gain have been observed in patients treated w/ atypical antipsychotics. Leukopenia, neutropenia, and agranulocytosis reported w/ atypical antipsychotics. Consider discontinuation at the 1st sign of a clinically significant decline in WBC count in the absence of other causative factors in patients w/ a history of a clinically significant low WBC count/ ANC or drug-induced leukopenia/neutropenia. Monitor patients w/ clinically significant neutropenia for fever or other signs/symptoms of infection and treat promptly if such signs/symptoms occur. D/C in patients w/ severe neutropenia (ANC<1000/mm^3) and follow their WBC count until recovery. May cause orthostatic hypotension and syncope; consider using a lower starting dosage and slower titration, and monitor orthostatic vital signs in patients at increased risk of these adverse reactions or at increased risk of developing complications from hypotension. Caution w/ history of seizures or w/ conditions that potentially lower seizure threshold. May disrupt the body's ability to reduce core body temperature; caution w/ conditions that may contribute to an elevation in core body temperature (eg, exercising strenuously, receiving concomitant medication w/ anticholinergic activity, being subject to dehydration). May cause esophageal dysmotility and aspiration; caution in patients at risk for aspiration pneumonia. May impair physical/mental abilities.

ADVERSE REACTIONS
MDD: Akathisia, headache, somnolence, tremor, dizziness, fatigue, nasopharyngitis, weight increased, increased appetite, anxiety, restlessness.
Schizophrenia: Akathisia, dyspepsia, diarrhea, weight increased, tremor.

DRUG INTERACTIONS
See Dosing Considerations. Strong CYP3A4 inhibitors (eg, itraconazole, clarithromycin, ketoconazole) and strong CYP2D6 inhibitors (eg, paroxetine, fluoxetine, quinidine) may increase exposure. Concomitant use w/ a strong CYP3A4 inhibitor and a strong CYP2D6 inhibitor; or a moderate CYP3A4 inhibitor and a strong CYP2D6 inhibitor; or a strong CYP3A4 inhibitor and a moderate CYP2D6 inhibitor; or a moderate CYP3A4 inhibitor and a moderate CYP2D6 inhibitor, may increase exposure. Strong CYP3A4 inducers (eg, rifampin, St. John's wort) may decrease exposure.

PATIENT CONSIDERATIONS

Assessment: Assess for dementia-related psychosis, drug hypersensitivity, renal/hepatic impairment, history of seizures or conditions that potentially lower the seizure threshold, any other conditions where treatment is cautioned, pregnancy/nursing status, and possible drug interactions. Obtain baseline FPG in patients w/ diabetes mellitus (DM) or at risk for DM. Obtain baseline CBC in patients w/ a history of a clinically significant low WBC count/ANC or drug-induced leukopenia/neutropenia.

Monitoring: Monitor for clinical worsening of depression, emergence of suicidal thoughts and behaviors, NMS, TD, hyperglycemia, dyslipidemia, weight gain, orthostatic hypotension, seizures, esophageal dysmotility, aspiration, and other adverse reactions. Monitor CBC frequently during the 1st few months of therapy in patients w/ a history of a clinically significant low WBC count/ANC or drug-induced leukopenia/neutropenia. Monitor for fever or other signs/symptoms of infection in patients w/ neutropenia. Monitor for worsening of glucose control in patients w/ DM. Monitor FPG periodically during therapy in patients at risk for DM. Periodically reassess to determine the continued need for maintenance treatment.

Counseling: Advise patients and caregivers to look for the emergence of suicidality and instruct them to report such symptoms to the healthcare provider. Advise to contact healthcare provider or report to the emergency room if signs/symptoms of NMS are experienced. Counsel on the signs/symptoms of TD and to contact healthcare provider if these abnormal movements occur. Educate about the risk of metabolic changes, how to recognize symptoms of hyperglycemia and DM, and the need for specific monitoring, including blood glucose, lipids, and weight. Advise patients w/ a preexisting low WBC count or a history of drug induced leukopenia/neutropenia that they should have their CBCs monitored during therapy. Educate about the risk of orthostatic hypotension and syncope. Counsel regarding appropriate care in avoiding overheating and dehydration. Caution about performing activities requiring mental alertness (eg, operating hazardous machinery) until reasonably certain that therapy does not adversely affect ability to engage in such activities. Advise to notify healthcare provider of any changes to prescription/OTC medications currently taking and if pregnant/nursing.

STORAGE: 20-25°C (68-77°F); excursions permitted to 15-30°C (59-86°F).

Reyataz – atazanavir

RX

Class: Protease inhibitor

ADULT DOSAGE

HIV-1 Infection

Treatment-Naive Patients:
300mg + Ritonavir (RTV) 100mg qd, or 400mg qd (w/o RTV) if intolerant to RTV

In Combination w/ Efavirenz for Treatment-Naive Patients:
400mg + RTV 100mg qd

Treatment-Experienced Patients:
300mg + RTV 100mg qd

In Combination w/ H_2-Receptor Antagonist and Tenofovir for Treatment-Experienced Patients:
400mg + RTV 100mg qd

PEDIATRIC DOSAGE

HIV-1 Infection

Powder:
≥3 Months of Age:
Treatment-Naive/Treatment-Experienced Patients:
5 to <15kg: 200mg + RTV 80mg qd
15 to <25kg: 250mg + RTV 80mg qd
≥25kg: 300mg + RTV 100mg qd

Treatment-Naive and Intolerant to 200mg Atazanavir Powder:
5 to <10kg: 150mg + RTV 80mg qd w/ close HIV viral load monitoring

Caps:
6 to <18 Years:
Treatment-Naive/Treatment-Experienced Patients:
15 to <20kg: 150mg + RTV 100mg qd
20 to <40kg: 200mg + RTV 100mg qd
≥40kg: 300mg + RTV 100mg qd

≥13 Years:
Treatment-Naive and Intolerant to RTV:
≥40kg: 400mg qd (w/o RTV)

DOSING CONSIDERATIONS

Concomitant Medications

H_2-Receptor Antagonists/Proton-Pump Inhibitors:
Dose separation may be required

Renal Impairment

ESRD w/ Hemodialysis:
Treatment-Naive: 300mg + RTV 100mg qd
Treatment-Experienced: Not recommended for use

Hepatic Impairment

Coadministration w/RTV is not recommended w/ any degree of hepatic impairment

Treatment-Naive:
Mild (Child-Pugh Class A): 400mg qd (w/o RTV)
Moderate (Child-Pugh Class B): 300mg qd (w/o RTV)
Severe (Child-Pugh Class C): Not recommended for use

Pregnancy

Treatment-Naive and Treatment-Experienced:
300mg + RTV 100mg qd

Treatment-Experienced During 2nd/3rd Trimester w/ Either H_2-Receptor Antagonist or Tenofovir:
400mg + RTV 100mg qd

ADMINISTRATION

Oral route

Take w/ food.

Cap

Do not open.

Use w/o RTV is not recommended for treatment-experienced adults/pediatric patients w/ prior virologic failure.

Powder

Must be taken w/ RTV.

Instructions for Mixing Oral Powder

Preferred Method:

1. Mix the recommended number of pkts w/ a minimum of 1 tbsp of food (eg, applesauce or yogurt).
2. Feed the mixture to the infant or young child.
3. Add an additional 1 tbsp of food to the container, mix, and feed the child the residual mixture.

For Infants Who Can Drink from a Cup:

1. Mix the recommended number of pkts w/ a minimum of 30mL of a beverage (eg, milk or water).

2. Have the child drink the mixture.
3. Add an additional 15mL of beverage to the cup, mix, and have the child drink the residual mixture. If water is used, food should also be taken at the same time.

For Infants <6 Months Who Cannot Eat Solid Food or Drink from a Cup:
1. Mix the recommended number of pkts w/ 10mL of prepared liquid infant formula.
2. Draw up the full amount of the mixture into an oral syringe and administer into either right or left inner cheek of infant.
3. Pour another 10mL of formula into the medicine cup to rinse off remaining oral powder in cup.
4. Draw up residual mixture into the syringe and administer into either inner cheek again.

Administer RTV immediately after powder administration.

Administer the entire dose of oral powder (mixed in the food or beverage) w/in 1 hr (may leave the mixture at room temperature during this 1-hr period).
Ensure that the patient eats or drinks all the food or beverage that contains the powder.
Additional food may be given after consumption of the entire mixture.

HOW SUPPLIED

Cap: 150mg, 200mg, 300mg; **Powder:** 50mg/pkt [30[s]]

CONTRAINDICATIONS

Coadministration w/ drugs that are highly dependent on CYP3A or UGT1A1 for clearance, and for which elevated plasma concentrations are associated w/ serious and/or life-threatening events, and w/ strong CYP3A inducers (eg, alfuzosin, rifampin, irinotecan, triazolam, oral midazolam, dihydroergotamine, ergotamine, ergonovine, methylergonovine, cisapride, St. John's wort, lovastatin, simvastatin, pimozide, sildenafil when used for pulmonary arterial HTN, indinavir, nevirapine). Previously demonstrated clinically significant hypersensitivity (eg, Stevens-Johnson syndrome, erythema multiforme, or toxic skin eruptions) to any of the components of this medication.

WARNINGS/PRECAUTIONS

May prolong PR interval; consider ECG monitoring w/ preexisting conduction system disease. Rash and cases of Stevens-Johnson syndrome, erythema multiforme, and toxic skin eruptions, including drug rash w/ eosinophilia and systemic symptoms (DRESS) syndrome, reported; d/c if severe rash develops. May cause hyperbilirubinemia; dose reduction is not recommended. Powder contains phenylalanine; caution w/ phenylketonuria. Increased risk for further transaminase elevations or hepatic decompensation in patients w/ underlying hepatitis B or C infections or marked transaminase elevations before treatment; obtain LFTs prior to and during treatment. Nephrolithiasis and/or cholelithiasis reported; consider temporary interruption or discontinuation of therapy if signs/symptoms occur. New onset or exacerbation of diabetes mellitus (DM), hyperglycemia, diabetic ketoacidosis, immune reconstitution syndrome, autoimmune disorders (eg, Graves' disease, polymyositis, Guillain-Barre syndrome) in the setting of immune reconstitution, redistribution/accumulation of body fat, and increased bleeding in patients w/ hemophilia A and B reported. Various degrees of cross-resistance observed. Caution in elderly.

ADVERSE REACTIONS

N/V, jaundice/scleral icterus, rash, myalgia, headache, abdominal pain, insomnia, peripheral neurologic symptoms, diarrhea, cough, fever, AST/ALT elevations, neutropenia, hypoglycemia, extremity pain.

DRUG INTERACTIONS

See Contraindications and Dosing Considerations. Not recommended w/ salmeterol. Use w/o RTV not recommended w/ drugs highly dependent on CYP2C8 w/ narrow therapeutic indices (eg, paclitaxel, repaglinide), carbamazepine, phenytoin, phenobarbital, bosentan, and buprenorphine. ATV/RTV is not recommended w/ other protease inhibitors, voriconazole, fluticasone propionate, and boceprevir. Not recommended w/ efavirenz or proton pump inhibitors (PPIs) in treatment-experienced patients. Avoid w/ colchicine in patients w/ renal/hepatic impairment. Caution w/ oral contraceptives. CYP3A4 inducers, tenofovir, carbamazepine, boceprevir, phenytoin, phenobarbital, bosentan, efavirenz, PPIs, antacids, buffered medications, and H_2-receptor antagonists may decrease levels. RTV and clarithromycin may increase levels. Administer 2 hrs before or 1 hr after buffered formulations (eg, didanosine buffered or enteric-coated formulations)/antacids, ≥10 hrs after H_2-receptor antagonists, and 12 hrs after PPIs. May increase levels of CYP3A or UGT1A1 substrates, tenofovir, saquinavir, amiodarone, bepridil, lidocaine (systemic), quinidine, TCAs, trazodone, itraconazole, ketoconazole, colchicine, rifabutin, quetiapine, parenteral midazolam, warfarin (monitor INR), diltiazem and other calcium channel blockers, bosentan, atorvastatin, rosuvastatin, norgestimate, norethindrone, fluticasone propionate, clarithromycin, buprenorphine, norbuprenorphine, immunosuppressants, and PDE-5 inhibitors. ATV/RTV may increase levels of carbamazepine. Rosuvastatin dose should not exceed 10mg/day. May decrease levels of didanosine, and 14-OH clarithromycin (clarithromycin active metabolite). ATV/RTV may decrease levels of phenytoin, phenobarbital, and lamotrigine. Voriconazole may alter levels. May alter levels of ethinyl estradiol. Initiation of medications that inhibit or induce CYP3A may increase or decrease concentrations of ATV/RTV, respectively. Refer to PI for dosing modifications when used w/ certain concomitant therapies.

PATIENT CONSIDERATIONS

Assessment: Assess for treatment history, known hypersensitivity, DM, hemophilia, conduction system disease, phenylketonuria, renal/hepatic impairment, pregnancy/nursing status, and possible drug interactions. Obtain baseline LFTs in patients w/ underlying hepatitis B or C infections or marked transaminase elevations.

Monitoring: Monitor for cardiac conduction abnormalities, PR interval prolongation, rash, DRESS, hyperbilirubinemia, nephrolithiasis, cholelithiasis, new onset or exacerbation of DM, hyperglycemia, diabetic ketoacidosis, autoimmune disorders, immune reconstitution syndrome, fat redistribution/accumulation, cross-resistance among protease inhibitors, and other adverse reactions. Monitor LFTs in patients w/ underlying hepatitis B or C infections or marked transaminase elevations. Monitor for bleeding in patients w/ hemophilia. Closely monitor for adverse events during the first 2 months postpartum.

Counseling: Inform that therapy is not a cure for HIV infection, and patients may continue to experience illnesses associated w/ HIV infections. Advise to avoid doing things that can spread HIV infection to others. Advise to take ud and to take w/ food. Instruct not to alter the dose or d/c therapy w/o consulting physician. Advise caregiver on how to mix oral powder w/ a food or beverage, and to carefully follow the instructions for use and storage of powder formulation. Inform caregivers of patients w/ phenylketonuria that oral powder contains phenylalanine, and advise to call healthcare providers if they have any questions. Instruct to report use of any other medications or herbal products. Advise to consult physician if dizziness or lightheadedness occurs. Inform that mild rashes w/o other symptoms, redistribution or accumulation of body fat, or yellowing of the skin or whites of the eyes may occur. Inform that kidney stones and/or gallstones have been reported. Advise to d/c and seek medical evaluation immediately if signs or symptoms of severe skin reactions or hypersensitivity reactions develop.

STORAGE: Cap: 25°C (77°F); excursions permitted to 15-30°C (59-86°F). **Powder:** <30°C (86°F); may be kept at room temperature 20-30°C (68-86°F) for up to 1 hr prior to administration once powder is mixed w/ food/beverages. Store in original pkt and do not open until ready to use.

RIFADIN – rifampin

RX

Class: Rifamycin derivative

ADULT DOSAGE

Tuberculosis

Treatment of All Forms of Tuberculosis:
10mg/kg qd
Max: 600mg/day
Initial phase of short course therapy consists of rifampin + isoniazid (INH) + pyrazinamide for 2 months; add streptomycin or ethambutol unless the likelihood of INH resistance is very low. Following initial phase, continue treatment w/ rifampin + INH for at least 4 months; treat longer if the patient is still sputum or culture positive, if resistant organisms are present, or if the patient is HIV positive

Meningococcal Carrier State

Treatment of symptomatic carriers of *Neisseria meningitidis* to eliminate meningococci from the nasopharynx

Usual: 600mg bid for 2 days

PEDIATRIC DOSAGE

Tuberculosis

Treatment of All Forms of Tuberculosis:
10-20mg/kg qd
Max: 600mg/day
Initial phase of short course therapy consists of rifampin + isoniazid (INH) + pyrazinamide for 2 months; add streptomycin or ethambutol unless the likelihood of INH resistance is very low. Following initial phase, continue treatment w/ rifampin + INH for at least 4 months; treat longer if the patient is still sputum or culture positive, if resistant organisms are present, or if the patient is HIV positive

Meningococcal Carrier State

Treatment of symptomatic carriers of *Neisseria meningitidis* to eliminate meningococci from the nasopharynx

<1 Month of Age:
5mg/kg q12h for 2 days
≥1 Month of Age:
10mg/kg q12h for 2 days
Max: 600mg/dose

ADMINISTRATION

Oral/IV route

PO

Administer 1 hr ac or 2 hrs pc w/ a full glass of water

IV

Preparation:
Reconstitute lyophilized powder by transferring 10mL of sterile water for inj to a vial containing 600mg of rifampin for inj; swirl vial gently to completely dissolve antibiotic

Prior to administration, withdraw from reconstituted sol a volume equivalent to amount of rifampin calculated to be administered and add to 500mL of infusion medium
Mix well and infuse at a rate allowing for complete infusion w/in 3 hrs
Alternatively, add amount of rifampin calculated to be administered to 100mL of infusion medium and infuse in 30 min
May dilute w/ D5 for inj and normal saline (NS)

Incompatibilities:
Undiluted (5mg/mL) and diluted (1mg/mL in NS) diltiazem hydrochloride and rifampin (6mg/mL in NS) during simulated Y-site administration

Oral Sus
Compound using simple syrup (Syrup NF), simple syrup (Humco Laboratories), Syrpalta syrup (Emerson Laboratories), or raspberry syrup (Humco Laboratories)
Compounding procedure results in a 1% w/v sus containing 10mg/mL of rifampin

Preparation:
Empty contents of four 300mg caps or eight 150mg caps onto a piece of weighing paper and gently crush the contents w/ a spatula to produce a fine powder
Transfer powder blend to a 4 oz amber glass or plastic bottle
Rinse paper and spatula w/ 20mL of 1 of above-mentioned syrups, and add rinse to bottle
Add 100mL of syrup to the bottle and shake vigorously

HOW SUPPLIED

Cap: 150mg, 300mg; **Inj:** 600mg

CONTRAINDICATIONS

History of hypersensitivity to rifampin or any of the components, or to any of the rifamycins. Patients who are taking ritonavir-boosted saquinavir due to an increased risk of severe hepatocellular toxicity. Patients who are receiving atazanavir, darunavir, fosamprenavir, saquinavir, or tipranavir.

WARNINGS/PRECAUTIONS

May produce liver dysfunction; caution with impaired liver function. Monitor LFTs prior to therapy and every 2-4 weeks during therapy; d/c if signs of hepatocellular damage occur. Hyperbilirubinemia and porphyria exacerbation reported. Not for treatment of meningococcal disease. Caution with history of diabetes mellitus (DM); diabetes management may be more difficult. Higher doses than recommended may result in higher incidence of adverse reactions including flu syndrome (fever, chills, and malaise), hematopoietic reactions (leukopenia, thrombocytopenia, or acute hemolytic anemia), cutaneous, GI, and hepatic reactions, SOB, shock, anaphylaxis, and renal failure. Not recommended for intermittent therapy; caution against intentional or accidental interruption of the daily dosage regimen since rare renal hypersensitivity reactions reported when therapy was resumed. IV doses are the same as those for oral. Caution in elderly. (IV) For IV infusion only; do not administer IM or SQ. Avoid extravasation; d/c infusion if local irritation and inflammation occur and restart at another site.

ADVERSE REACTIONS

Heartburn, N/V, headache, fever, drowsiness, dizziness, muscle weakness, visual disturbances, menstrual disturbances, BUN elevation, serum uric acid elevation, flushing, urticaria, rash, edema.

DRUG INTERACTIONS

See Contraindications. Induces certain CYP450 enzymes; dosages of drugs metabolized by these enzymes may require adjustment when starting/stopping therapy. May accelerate the metabolism of anticonvulsants, digitoxin, antiarrhythmics, oral anticoagulants, antifungals, barbiturates, β-blockers, calcium channel blockers, chloramphenicol, clarithromycin, corticosteroids, cyclosporine, cardiac glycoside preparations, clofibrate, oral or other systemic hormonal contraceptives, dapsone, diazepam, doxycycline, fluoroquinolones, haloperidol, oral hypoglycemic agents, levothyroxine, methadone, narcotic analgesics, progestins, quinine, tacrolimus, theophylline, TCAs, and zidovudine; dose adjustments of these drugs may be necessary. May increase requirements for coumarin-type anticoagulants; perform PT daily or as frequently as necessary. Decreased levels of enalaprilat and atovaquone. Increased levels with atovaquone. Concomitant ketoconazole decreases serum levels of both drugs. Antacids may reduce absorption; give daily doses of rifampin at least 1 hr before ingestion of antacids. Increased blood level with probenecid and cotrimoxazole. Increased risk of hepatotoxicity with halothane or isoniazid; avoid concomitant use with halothane and monitor closely for hepatotoxicity when given with isoniazid. Caution with other hepatotoxic agents. Coadministration with sulfasalazine may reduce plasma concentrations of sulfapyridine.

R

PATIENT CONSIDERATIONS

Assessment: Assess for drug hypersensitivity, history of DM, meningococcal disease, hepatic/renal impairment, pregnancy/nursing status, and possible drug interactions. Obtain baseline CBC. Obtain bacteriologic cultures to confirm susceptibility of organism prior to therapy.

Monitoring: Monitor for liver dysfunction, hyperbilirubinemia, porphyria exacerbation, and other adverse reactions. Monitor for LFTs every 2-4 weeks, SrCr, CBC, and platelet count. Monitor treatment response by performing serotyping and susceptibility tests. (IV) Monitor for local irritation and inflammation at infusion site.

Counseling: Counsel that drug treats bacterial and not viral infections. Instruct to take exactly as prescribed. Inform that skipping doses or not completing full course of therapy may decrease effectiveness and increase bacterial resistance. Inform that the drug may produce reddish urine, sweat, sputum, and tears, and that soft contact lenses may be permanently stained. Advise that the reliability of oral or systemic hormonal contraceptives may be affected; instruct to use alternative contraceptive measures. Instruct to notify physician if fever, loss of appetite, malaise, N/V, darkened urine, yellowish discoloration of skin and eyes, and joint pain/swelling occur. Emphasize the compliance with full course of therapy and the importance of not missing any doses.

STORAGE: 25°C (77°F); excursions permitted to 15-30°C (59-86°F). (Cap) Store in dry place. Avoid excessive heat. (IV) Avoid excessive heat (>40°C [104°F]). Protect from light. Reconstituted Sol: Room temperature for 24 hrs. Dilutions in D5W: Room temperature for up to 4 hrs. Dilutions in Normal Saline: Room temperature for up to 24 hrs. Prepare and use within this time.

Risperdal Consta – risperidone

RX

Class: Atypical antipsychotic

Elderly patients w/ dementia-related psychosis treated w/ antipsychotic drugs are at an increased risk of death; most deaths appeared to be cardiovascular (CV) (eg, heart failure, sudden death) or infectious (eg, pneumonia) in nature. Not approved for the treatment of patients w/ dementia-related psychosis.

ADULT DOSAGE

Schizophrenia

Recommended Dose: 25mg IM every 2 weeks
Titrate: May increase to 37.5mg or 50mg if unresponsive to 25mg; upward dose adjustment should not be made more frequently than every 4 weeks
Max: 50mg every 2 weeks

May give a lower initial dose of 12.5mg if clinically warranted (eg, history of poor tolerability to psychotropic medications).
Oral risperidone (or another antipsychotic) should be given w/ the 1st inj of Risperdal Consta, continued for 3 weeks, and then discontinued.
For patients who have never taken oral risperidone, establish tolerability w/ oral risperidone prior to initiating treatment w/ Risperdal Consta.

Bipolar I Disorder

Monotherapy or Adjunctive Therapy to Lithium or Valproate for Maint Treatment:
Recommended Dose: 25mg IM every 2 weeks
Titrate: May increase to 37.5mg or 50mg; upward dose adjustment should not be made more frequently than every 4 weeks
Max: 50mg every 2 weeks

May give a lower initial dose of 12.5mg if clinically warranted (eg, history of poor tolerability to psychotropic medications).
Oral risperidone (or another antipsychotic) should be given w/ the 1st inj of Risperdal Consta, continued for 3 weeks, and then discontinued.
For patients who have never taken oral risperidone, establish tolerability w/ oral risperidone prior to initiating treatment w/ Risperdal Consta.

Conversions

Switching from Other Antipsychotics:
Continue previous antipsychotic for 3 weeks after 1st inj of Risperdal Consta

For patients who have never taken oral risperidone, establish tolerability w/ oral risperidone prior to initiating treatment w/ Risperdal Consta.

PEDIATRIC DOSAGE

Pediatric use may not have been established

DOSING CONSIDERATIONS

Concomitant Medications

Carbamazepine or Other CYP3A4 Inducers (eg, Phenytoin, Rifampin, Phenobarbital):
Initiation of Carbamazepine or Other CYP3A4 Inducers: Closely monitor patients during the first 4-8 weeks; consider dose increase or administration of additional oral risperidone.
Discontinuation of Carbamazepine or Other CYP3A4 Inducers: Reevaluate Risperdal Consta dose and decrease, if necessary. May place patients on lower dose of Risperdal Consta 2-4 weeks before the planned discontinuation of carbamazepine or other CYP3A4 inducers. Patients treated w/ the recommended 25mg dose of Risperdal Consta and discontinuing from carbamazepine or other CYP3A4 inducers should continue 25mg dose unless clinical judgment necessitates a lower dose of 12.5mg or treatment interruption.

CYP2D6 Inhibitors (eg, Fluoxetine, Paroxetine):
Initiation of Risperdal Consta in Patients Receiving Fluoxetine or Paroxetine: Consider a starting dose of 12.5mg.
Initiation of Fluoxetine/Paroxetine: May place patients on a lower dose of Risperdal Consta 2-4 weeks before the planned start of concomitant therapy. When fluoxetine or paroxetine is initiated in patients receiving the recommended 25mg dose of Risperdal Consta, it is recommended to continue treatment w/ 25mg dose unless clinical judgment necessitates a lower dose of 12.5mg or treatment interruption.

Renal Impairment

Titrate w/ oral risperidone prior to initiating treatment w/ Risperdal Consta
Initial: 0.5mg oral risperidone bid during 1st week
Titrate: May increase to 1mg bid or 2mg qd PO during 2nd week. If total daily oral dose of ≥2mg is well tolerated, may administer 25mg IM of Risperdal Consta every 2 weeks (or alternatively, an initial dose of 12.5mg may be appropriate)

Continue oral supplementation for 3 weeks after 1st inj

Hepatic Impairment

Titrate w/ oral risperidone prior to initiating treatment w/ Risperdal Consta
Initial: 0.5mg oral risperidone bid during 1st week
Titrate: May increase to 1mg bid or 2mg qd PO during 2nd week. If total daily oral dose of ≥2mg is well tolerated, may administer 25mg IM of Risperdal Consta every 2 weeks (or alternatively, an initial dose of 12.5mg may be appropriate)

Continue oral supplementation for 3 weeks after 1st inj

Elderly

Recommended Dose: 25mg IM every 2 weeks
Oral risperidone (or another antipsychotic) should be given w/ the 1st inj and continued for 3 weeks

Other Important Considerations

Reinitiation of Treatment After Previous Discontinuation:
Administer supplementation w/ oral risperidone (or another antipsychotic) when restarting patients who have had an interval off treatment w/ Risperdal Consta

ADMINISTRATION

IM route

Administer by deep IM deltoid or gluteal inj only.
Deltoid Administration: Use the 1-inch needle alternating inj between the 2 arms.
Gluteal Administration: Use the 2-inch needle alternating inj between the 2 buttocks.

Do not combine 2 different dose strengths in a single administration.

Instructions for Use

1. Use components provided in dose pack; must reconstitute only in diluent supplied in dose pack.
2. Do not substitute any components of dose pack.
3. Do not store sus after reconstitution; administer dose as soon as possible after reconstitution to avoid settling.
4. Entire contents of vial must be administered to ensure intended dose is delivered.

Refer to PI for further administration instructions.

HOW SUPPLIED

Inj: 12.5mg, 25mg, 37.5mg, 50mg

CONTRAINDICATIONS

Known hypersensitivity to the product.

WARNINGS/PRECAUTIONS

Each inj should be administered by a healthcare professional. Neuroleptic malignant syndrome (NMS) reported; immediately d/c and institute symptomatic treatment and medical monitoring. May cause tardive dyskinesia (TD), especially in the elderly; consider discontinuation if signs/ symptoms appear. Associated w/ metabolic changes (eg, hyperglycemia, dyslipidemia, weight

R

gain) that may increase CV/cerebrovascular risk. Hyperglycemia and diabetes mellitus (DM), in some cases extreme and associated w/ ketoacidosis or hyperosmolar coma or death, reported; monitor for worsening of glucose control in patients w/ DM and FPG in patients at risk for DM. Somnolence, seizures, and hyperprolactinemia reported. May induce orthostatic hypotension; consider dose reduction if hypotension occurs. Caution w/ known CV disease, cerebrovascular disease, and conditions that predispose to hypotension. Elderly patients and those w/ a predisposition to hypotensive reactions should avoid Na^+ depletion or dehydration, and circumstances that accentuate hypotension (alcohol intake, high ambient temperature). Leukopenia, neutropenia, and agranulocytosis reported; consider discontinuation at the 1st sign of a clinically significant decline in WBC count in the absence of other causative factors in patients w/ a history of a clinically significant low WBC count or a drug-induced leukopenia/neutropenia. D/C therapy and follow WBC counts until recovery in patients w/ severe neutropenia (ANC <1000/mm^3). May impair mental/physical abilities. Associated w/ esophageal dysmotility and aspiration; caution in patients at risk for aspiration pneumonia. Priapism and thrombotic thrombocytopenic purpura (TTP) reported. May cause disruption of body temperature regulation; caution when exposed to temperature extremes. May be associated w/ an antiemetic effect and may mask signs/symptoms of overdosage w/ certain drugs or of conditions (eg, intestinal obstruction, Reye's syndrome, brain tumor). Closely supervise patients at high-risk of suicide. Increased sensitivity to antipsychotic medications reported in patients w/ Parkinson's disease or dementia w/ Lewy bodies. Caution w/ diseases/conditions affecting metabolism or hemodynamic responses. Avoid inadvertent inj into a blood vessel.

ADVERSE REACTIONS

Schizophrenia: Headache, parkinsonism, dizziness, akathisia, fatigue, constipation, dyspepsia, sedation, weight increased, pain in extremity, dry mouth.

Bipolar Disorder: (Monotherapy) Weight increased. (Adjunctive Treatment) Tremor, parkinsonism.

DRUG INTERACTIONS

See Dosing Considerations. Caution w/ other centrally-acting drugs or alcohol. May enhance hypotensive effects of other therapeutic agents w/ this potential. May antagonize effects of levodopa and dopamine agonists. Cimetidine or ranitidine may increase bioavailability. Ranitidine may increase exposure. Chronic administration of clozapine may decrease clearance. May increase valproate C_{max}. Fluoxetine, paroxetine, and other CYP2D6 inhibitors may increase levels. Carbamazepine and other CYP3A4 inducers may decrease levels and lead to decreased efficacy.

PATIENT CONSIDERATIONS

Assessment: Assess for known hypersensitivity to drug, dementia-related psychosis, DM, risk for hypotension, history of seizures, hepatic/renal impairment, any other conditions where treatment is cautioned, pregnancy/nursing status, and for possible drug interactions. Obtain baseline FPG in patients at risk for DM.

Monitoring: Monitor for NMS, TD, hyperprolactinemia, orthostatic hypotension, cognitive and motor impairment, seizures, esophageal dysmotility, aspiration, priapism, TTP, metabolic changes, disruption of body temperature, and other adverse reactions. Monitor for glucose control; perform periodic FPG in patients at risk for DM. Monitor for signs/symptoms of leukopenia, neutropenia, and agranulocytosis; perform frequent monitoring of CBC during the 1st few months of therapy in patients w/ history of clinically significant low WBC count or drug-induced leukopenia/neutropenia. Periodically reevaluate long-term risks and benefits of the drug.

Counseling: Advise of risk of orthostatic hypotension and of nonpharmacologic interventions that help to reduce its occurrence. Inform that therapy has the potential to impair judgment, thinking, or motor skills; advise to use caution when operating hazardous machinery, including automobiles. Instruct to notify physician if pregnant/intending to become pregnant during therapy and for at least 12 weeks after last inj. Instruct not to breastfeed while on therapy and for at least 12 weeks after last inj. Advise to inform physician if taking/planning to take any prescription or OTC drugs, and to avoid alcohol during treatment.

STORAGE: 2-8°C (36-46°F). Protect from light. If refrigeration is unavailable, may store at ≤25°C (77°F) for no more than 7 days prior to administration.

RISPERIDONE – risperidone

RX

Class: Atypical antipsychotic

Elderly patients with dementia-related psychosis treated with antipsychotic drugs are at an increased risk of death. Not approved for the treatment of patients with dementia-related psychosis.

OTHER BRAND NAMES
Risperdal, Risperdal M-Tab

ADULT DOSAGE
Schizophrenia

May be administered qd or bid
Initial: 2mg/day
Titrate: May increase at intervals of ≥24 hrs, by 1-2mg/day
Target: 4-8mg/day; efficacy demonstrated in a range of 4-16mg/day
Maint: 2-8mg/day
Max: 16mg/day

If experiencing persistent somnolence, may administer 1/2 daily dose bid

Bipolar Mania

Acute Manic or Mixed Episodes Associated w/ Bipolar I Disorder:
Monotherapy:
Initial: 2-3mg/day
Titrate: May increase at intervals of ≥24 hrs, by 1mg/day
Target: 1-6mg/day
Max: 6mg/day

If experiencing persistent somnolence, may administer 1/2 daily dose bid

Also indicated as adjunctive therapy w/ lithium or valproate for the treatment of acute manic or mixed episodes associated w/ bipolar I disorder

PEDIATRIC DOSAGE
Schizophrenia

13-17 Years:
Initial: 0.5mg qd in am or pm
Titrate: May increase at intervals of ≥24 hrs, by 0.5-1mg/day
Target: 3mg/day; efficacy demonstrated in a range of 1-6mg/day
Max: 6mg/day

If experiencing persistent somnolence, may administer 1/2 daily dose bid

Bipolar Mania

Acute Manic or Mixed Episodes Associated w/ Bipolar I Disorder:
Monotherapy:
10-17 Years:
Initial: 0.5mg qd in am or pm
Titrate: May increase at intervals of ≥24 hrs, by 0.5-1mg/day
Target: 1-2.5mg/day; efficacy demonstrated in range of 0.5-6mg
Max: 6mg/day

If experiencing persistent somnolence, may administer 1/2 daily dose bid

Autistic Disorder

Irritability Associated w/ Autistic Disorder (eg, Symptoms of Aggression Towards Others, Deliberate Self-Injuriousness, Temper Tantrums, Quickly Changing Moods):
5-17 Years:
Total daily dose may be administered qd or divided bid
Initial:
<20kg: 0.25mg/day
≥20kg: 0.5mg/day
Titrate: May increase after a minimum of 4 days
Target:
<20kg: 0.5mg/day
≥20kg: 1mg/day
Maintain target dose for a minimum of 14 days. If not achieving sufficient response, may increase at intervals of ≥2 weeks, by 0.25mg/day (<20kg) or 0.5mg/day (≥20kg)
Range: 0.5-3mg/day

Once sufficient response is achieved and maintained, consider gradually lowering the dose
If experiencing persistent somnolence, may give qd dose hs, divide daily dose bid, or reduce dose

DOSING CONSIDERATIONS
Concomitant Medications
Enzyme Inducers (eg, Carbamazepine, Phenytoin, Rifampin): Increase risperidone dose up to double usual dose when coadministered; may need to decrease dose when enzyme inducers are discontinued

Enzyme Inhibitors (eg, Fluoxetine, Paroxetine): Reduce risperidone dose during coadministration; may need to increase dose when enzyme inhibitors are discontinued
Max: 8mg/day of risperidone in adults during coadministration
Renal Impairment
Adults:

R

Severe (CrCl <30mL/min):
Initial: 0.5mg bid
Titrate: May increase by ≤0.5mg, administered bid. For doses >1.5mg bid, increase in intervals of ≥1 week

Hepatic Impairment
Adults:
10-15 Points on Child-Pugh System:
Initial: 0.5mg bid
Titrate: May increase by ≤0.5mg, administered bid. For doses >1.5mg bid, increase in intervals of ≥1 week

Elderly
Start at lower end of dosing range

Other Important Considerations
Reinitiation of Treatment in Patients Previously Discontinued:
After an interval off risperidone, follow initial titration schedule

ADMINISTRATION

Oral route

May be given w/ or w/o meals

Sol
May be administered directly from calibrated pipette, or may be mixed w/ a beverage prior to administration (not compatible w/ cola or tea)

Tab, Disintegrating
Immediately place the entire tab on the tongue after removing from blister
Swallow w/ or w/o liquid
Do not split or chew

HOW SUPPLIED

Tab, Disintegrating: 0.25mg, (Risperdal M-Tab) 0.5mg, 1mg, 2mg, 3mg, 4mg; **(Risperdal) Sol:** 1mg/mL [30mL]; **Tab:** 0.25mg, 0.5mg, 1mg, 2mg, 3mg, 4mg

CONTRAINDICATIONS

Known hypersensitivity to risperidone.

WARNINGS/PRECAUTIONS

May cause neuroleptic malignant syndrome (NMS); d/c and treat immediately if this occurs. Tardive dyskinesia (TD) may develop; consider discontinuation if signs/symptoms appear. Associated with metabolic changes (eg, hyperglycemia, dyslipidemia, weight gain) that may increase cardiovascular (CV)/cerebrovascular risk. Hyperglycemia and diabetes mellitus (DM), in some cases extreme and associated with ketoacidosis or hyperosmolar coma or death, reported; monitor for worsening of glucose control in patients with DM, and perform FPG testing in patients at risk for DM. Somnolence, seizures, and elevation of prolactin levels reported. May induce orthostatic hypotension; consider dose reduction if hypotension occurs. Caution with known CV disease (CVD), cerebrovascular disease, and conditions that predispose to hypotension. Leukopenia, neutropenia, and agranulocytosis reported; monitor CBC in patients with history of clinically significant low WBC counts or drug-induced leukopenia/neutropenia, and consider discontinuation at 1st sign of clinically significant decline in WBC counts without other causative factors. D/C and follow WBC counts until recovery in patients with severe neutropenia (absolute neutrophil count <1000/mm^3). May impair mental/physical abilities. Esophageal dysmotility and aspiration reported; caution in patients at risk for aspiration pneumonia. Priapism reported. May disrupt body temperature regulation; caution when prescribing for patients who will be exposed to temperature extremes. Patients with Parkinson's disease or dementia with Lewy bodies may experience increased sensitivity. Caution in elderly. (Tab, Disintegrating) Contains phenylalanine.

ADVERSE REACTIONS

Parkinsonism, akathisia, dystonia, tremor, sedation, dizziness, anxiety, blurred vision, N/V, upper abdominal pain, stomach discomfort, salivary hypersecretion, increased appetite, fatigue, constipation.

DRUG INTERACTIONS

Adjust dose when used with CYP2D6 inhibitors (eg, fluoxetine, paroxetine) and enzyme inducers (eg, carbamazepine). May increase valproate peak plasma concentrations. Caution with other centrally-acting drugs and alcohol. May enhance hypotensive effects of other therapeutic agents with this potential. May antagonize effects of levodopa and dopamine agonists. Chronic administration of clozapine may decrease clearance.

PATIENT CONSIDERATIONS

Assessment: Assess for dementia-related psychosis, DM, risk for hypotension, history of seizures, drug hypersensitivity or any other conditions where treatment is cautioned, hepatic/renal function, pregnancy/nursing status, and possible drug interactions. Obtain FPG in patients at risk for DM.

Monitoring: Monitor for NMS, TD, hyperglycemia, hyperprolactinemia, orthostatic hypotension, leukopenia, neutropenia, agranulocytosis, cognitive/motor impairment, seizures, esophageal dysmotility, aspiration, priapism, disruption of body temperature, metabolic changes, and other adverse reactions. Monitor for worsening of glucose control in patients with DM and FPG in patients at risk for DM. Monitor CBC frequently during the 1st few months of therapy in patients with history of clinically significant low WBC count or drug-induced leukopenia/neutropenia. In patients with clinically significant neutropenia, monitor for fever or other symptoms or signs of infection. Periodically reevaluate long-term risks and benefits of the drug.

Counseling: Advise about the risk of orthostatic hypotension, especially during the period of initial dose titration. Inform that therapy has the potential to impair judgment, thinking, or motor skills; advise to use caution when operating hazardous machinery. Instruct to notify physician if pregnant/planning to become pregnant, nursing, and if taking/planning to take any prescription or OTC drugs. Advise to avoid alcohol during treatment. Inform that orally disintegrating tab contains phenylalanine. Inform that treatment can be associated with hyperglycemia and DM, dyslipidemia, and weight gain. Inform about risk of TD.

STORAGE: 20-25°C (68-77°F). (Risperdal/Risperdal M-Tab) 15-25°C (59-77°F). Sol: Protect from light and freezing. Tab: Protect from light and moisture.

RITALIN – methylphenidate hydrochloride

CII

Class: CNS stimulant

Caution w/ history of drug dependence or alcoholism. Chronic abuse may lead to marked tolerance and psychological dependence w/ varying degrees of abnormal behavior. Frank psychotic episodes may occur, especially w/ parenteral abuse. Careful supervision is required during withdrawal from abusive use, since severe depression may occur. Withdrawal following chronic use may unmask symptoms of underlying disorder that may require follow-up.

OTHER BRAND NAMES

Ritalin-SR

ADULT DOSAGE

Attention Deficit Disorders

Tab:
20-30mg/day given in divided doses bid-tid, preferably 30-45 min ac; some patients may require 40-60mg/day and others, 10-15mg/day may be adequate
Last dose should be taken before 6 pm if patient is unable to sleep as a result of taking medication late in the day

Tab, Sustained-Release (SR):
May be used in place of methylphenidate immediate-release (IR) tabs when the 8-hr dosage of SR tab corresponds to the titrated 8-hr dosage of methylphenidate IR tabs

Narcolepsy

Tab:
20-30mg/day given in divided doses bid-tid, preferably 30-45 min ac; some patients may require 40-60mg/day and others, 10-15mg/day may be adequate
Last dose should be taken before 6 pm if patient is unable to sleep as a result of taking medication late in the day

Tab, SR:
May be used in place of methylphenidate IR tabs when the 8-hr dosage of SR tab corresponds to the titrated 8-hr dosage of methylphenidate IR tabs

PEDIATRIC DOSAGE

Attention Deficit Disorders

≥6 Years:
Tab:
Initial: 5mg bid before breakfast and lunch
Titrate: Increase gradually by 5-10mg weekly
Max: 60mg/day

Tab, Sustained-Release (SR):
May be used in place of methylphenidate immediate release (IR) tabs when the 8-hr dosage of SR tab corresponds to the titrated 8-hr dosage of methylphenidate IR tabs

D/C if no improvement seen after appropriate dosage adjustment over 1 month
D/C periodically to assess the child's condition; therapy should not be indefinite

Narcolepsy

≥6 Years:
Tab:
Initial: 5mg bid before breakfast and lunch
Titrate: Increase gradually by 5-10mg weekly
Max: 60mg/day

Tab, SR:
May be used in place of methylphenidate IR tabs when the 8-hr dosage of SR tab corresponds to the titrated 8-hr dosage of methylphenidate IR tabs

D/C if no improvement seen after appropriate dosage adjustment over 1 month
D/C periodically to assess the child's condition; therapy should not be indefinite

DOSING CONSIDERATIONS

Adverse Reactions

Children ≥6 Years:
Reduce dose or, if necessary, d/c if paradoxical aggravation of symptoms or other adverse effects occur

ADMINISTRATION
Oral route

Tab, SR
Swallow tabs whole; do not crush or chew.

HOW SUPPLIED
Tab: (Ritalin) 5mg, 10mg*, 20mg*; **Tab, SR:** (Generic) 10mg, (Ritalin-SR) 20mg *scored

CONTRAINDICATIONS
Marked anxiety, tension, agitation, known hypersensitivity to the drug, glaucoma, motor tics or family history or diagnosis of Tourette's syndrome. Treatment w/ MAOIs or w/in a minimum of 14 days following discontinuation of an MAOI.

WARNINGS/PRECAUTIONS
Avoid w/ known serious structural cardiac abnormalities, cardiomyopathy, serious heart rhythm abnormalities, coronary artery disease, or other serious cardiac problems. Sudden death reported in children and adolescents w/ structural cardiac abnormalities or other serious heart problems. Sudden death, stroke, and MI reported in adults. May increase BP and HR; caution w/ conditions that may be compromised by increases in BP/HR (eg, preexisting HTN, heart failure, recent MI). Prior to treatment, obtain medical history (including assessment for family history of sudden death or ventricular arrhythmia) and perform a physical exam to assess for the presence of cardiac disease. Promptly perform cardiac evaluation if symptoms of cardiac disease develop. May exacerbate symptoms of behavior disturbance and thought disorder in patients w/ preexisting psychotic disorder. Caution in patients w/ comorbid bipolar disorder; may induce mixed/manic episode. May cause treatment-emergent psychotic or manic symptoms (eg, hallucinations, delusional thinking, mania) in children and adolescents w/o prior history of psychotic illness or mania; consider discontinuation if such symptoms occur. Aggressive behavior or hostility reported in children and adolescents. May cause long-term suppression of growth in children; monitor growth, and may need to interrupt treatment in patients not growing or gaining height or weight as expected. May lower convulsive threshold; d/c if seizures occur. Priapism, sometimes requiring surgical intervention, reported. Associated w/ peripheral vasculopathy, including Raynaud's phenomenon. Difficulties w/ accommodation and blurring of vision reported. Patients w/ an element of agitation may react adversely; d/c if necessary.

ADVERSE REACTIONS
Nervousness, insomnia, hypersensitivity reactions, anorexia, nausea, dizziness, palpitations, headache, dyskinesia, drowsiness, BP and pulse changes, tachycardia, angina, cardiac arrhythmia, abdominal pain.

DRUG INTERACTIONS
See Contraindications. Caution w/ pressor agents. May decrease effectiveness of drugs used to treat HTN. May inhibit metabolism of coumarin anticoagulants, anticonvulsants (eg, phenobarbital, phenytoin, primidone), and TCAs (eg, imipramine, clomipramine, desipramine); downward dose adjustment and monitoring of plasma drug concentration (or coagulation times for coumarin) of these drugs may be necessary when initiating or discontinuing methylphenidate.

PATIENT CONSIDERATIONS

R

Assessment: Assess for hypersensitivity to the drug, marked anxiety, tension, agitation, glaucoma, motor tics or family history or diagnosis of Tourette's syndrome, cardiovascular conditions, history of drug dependence or alcoholism, psychotic disorder, comorbid bipolar disorder, any other conditions where treatment is contraindicated or cautioned, pregnancy/nursing status, and possible drug interactions.

Monitoring: Monitor for changes in HR and BP, signs/symptoms of cardiac disease, exacerbation of behavior disturbance and thought disorder, psychosis, mania, appearance of or worsening of aggressive behavior or hostility, seizures, priapism, digital changes, visual disturbances, and other adverse reactions. In pediatric patients, monitor growth. Perform periodic monitoring of CBC, differential, and platelet counts during prolonged therapy.

Counseling: Inform about the benefits and risks of therapy and counsel about appropriate use. Instruct to seek immediate medical attention in the event of priapism. Instruct to report to physician any new numbness, pain, skin color change, or sensitivity to temperature in fingers or toes, and to contact physician immediately if any signs of unexplained wounds appear on fingers or toes while taking the drug.

STORAGE: **Ritalin/Ritalin-SR:** 25°C (77°F); excursions permitted to 15-30°C (59-86°F). **Generic:** 20-25°C (68-77°F). **Tab:** Protect from light. **Tab, SR:** Protect from moisture.

Ritalin LA – methylphenidate hydrochloride

CII

Class: CNS stimulant

Caution w/ history of drug dependence or alcoholism. Chronic abuse may lead to marked tolerance and psychological dependence w/ varying degrees of abnormal behavior. Frank psychotic episodes may occur, especially w/ parenteral abuse. Careful supervision is required during withdrawal from abusive use since severe depression may occur. Withdrawal following chronic use may unmask symptoms of underlying disorder that may require follow-up.

ADULT DOSAGE

Attention-Deficit Hyperactivity Disorder

Refer to pediatric dosing

PEDIATRIC DOSAGE

Attention-Deficit Hyperactivity Disorder

≥6 Years:
Initial: 20mg qam; may begin w/ 10mg when a lower initial dose is appropriate
Titrate: May adjust in weekly 10mg increments
Max: 60mg/day qam

Maint/Extended Treatment:
Periodically reevaluate long-term usefulness of drug for the individual patient w/ trials off medication

D/C if no improvement seen after appropriate dosage adjustment over 1 month

Conversions

Patients Currently Receiving Methylphenidate:
5mg Methylphenidate BID:
10mg Ritalin LA qd
10mg Methylphenidate Bid or 20mg Methylphenidate-SR:
20mg Ritalin LA qd
15mg Methylphenidate BID:
30mg Ritalin LA qd
20mg Methylphenidate Bid or 40mg Methylphenidate-SR:
40mg Ritalin LA qd
30mg Methylphenidate Bid or 60mg Methylphenidate-SR:
60mg Ritalin LA qd

DOSING CONSIDERATIONS

Adverse Reactions

Reduce dose or d/c if paradoxical aggravation of symptoms or other adverse events occur

ADMINISTRATION

Oral route

May be swallowed whole or cap may be opened and cap contents sprinkled over a spoonful of applesauce and consumed immediately, and not stored for future use
Do not crush, chew, or divide cap and/or cap contents

HOW SUPPLIED

Cap, Extended-Release: 10mg, 20mg, 30mg, 40mg, 60mg

CONTRAINDICATIONS

Marked anxiety, tension, agitation, known hypersensitivity to methylphenidate or other components of the product, glaucoma, motor tics, or family history or diagnosis of Tourette's syndrome. Treatment w/ MAOIs or w/in a minimum of 14 days following discontinuation of an MAOI.

WARNINGS/PRECAUTIONS

Sudden death reported in children and adolescents w/ structural cardiac abnormalities or other serious heart problems. Sudden death, stroke, and MI reported in adults. Avoid w/ known serious structural cardiac abnormalities, cardiomyopathy, serious heart rhythm abnormalities, coronary artery disease, or other serious cardiac problems. May increase BP and HR; caution w/ conditions that might be compromised by increases in BP/HR (eg, preexisting HTN, HF, recent MI, ventricular arrhythmia). Promptly perform cardiac evaluation if symptoms of cardiac disease develop. May exacerbate symptoms of behavior disturbance and thought disorder in patients w/ preexisting psychotic disorder. Caution in patients w/ comorbid bipolar disorder; may induce mixed/manic episode. May cause treatment-emergent psychotic or manic symptoms (eg, hallucinations, delusional thinking, mania) in children and adolescents w/o prior history of psychotic illness or

R

mania; consider discontinuation if such symptoms occur. Aggressive behavior or hostility reported in children and adolescents. May cause long-term suppression of growth in children; monitor growth, and may need to interrupt treatment in patients not growing or gaining height or weight as expected. May lower convulsive threshold; d/c if seizures occur. Priapism, sometimes requiring surgical intervention, reported. Associated w/ peripheral vasculopathy, including Raynaud's phenomenon; carefully observe for digital changes. Difficulties w/ accommodation and blurring of vision reported.

ADVERSE REACTIONS

Headache, insomnia, upper abdominal pain, appetite decreased, anorexia, nervousness.

DRUG INTERACTIONS

See Contraindications. Antacids or acid suppressants may alter release. May decrease effectiveness of drugs used to treat HTN. Caution w/ pressor agents. May be associated w/ pharmacodynamic interactions when coadministered w/ direct and indirect dopamine agonists (eg, dihydroxyphenylalanine, TCAs) as well as dopamine antagonists (antipsychotics [eg, haloperidol]). Potential interaction w/ coumarin anticoagulants, anticonvulsants (eg, phenobarbital, phenytoin, primidone), and TCAs (eg, imipramine, clomipramine, desipramine); downward dose adjustment of these drugs and monitoring of plasma drug concentrations (or coagulation times for coumarin) may be necessary when initiating/discontinuing methylphenidate. Avoid w/ alcohol.

PATIENT CONSIDERATIONS

Assessment: Assess for hypersensitivity to the drug, marked anxiety, tension, agitation, glaucoma, motor tics, family history or diagnosis of Tourette's syndrome, history of drug dependence or alcoholism, psychotic disorder, comorbid bipolar disorder, any other conditions where treatment is contraindicated or cautioned, pregnancy/nursing status, and possible drug interactions. Prior to treatment, obtain medical history (including assessment for family history of sudden death or ventricular arrhythmia) and perform physical exam to assess for presence of cardiac disease.

Monitoring: Monitor for changes in HR and BP, signs/symptoms of cardiac disease, exacerbation of behavior disturbance and thought disorder, psychosis, mania, appearance of or worsening of aggressive behavior or hostility, seizures, priapism, peripheral vasculopathy, visual disturbances, and other adverse reactions. In pediatric patients, monitor growth. Perform periodic monitoring of CBC, differential, and platelet counts during prolonged therapy. Periodically reevaluate long-term usefulness of drug.

Counseling: Advise to avoid alcohol while taking the drug. Inform about the benefits and risks of therapy and counsel about appropriate use. Instruct to seek immediate medical attention in the event of priapism. Instruct to report to physician any new numbness, pain, skin color change, or sensitivity to temperature in fingers or toes, and to contact physician immediately if any signs of unexplained wounds appear on fingers or toes while taking the drug.

STORAGE: 25°C (77°F); excursions permitted to 15-30°C (59-86°F).

RITUXAN – rituximab

RX

Class: Monoclonal antibody/CD20 blocker

R

Serious infusion reactions and severe mucocutaneous reactions, some fatal (death has occurred within 24 hrs of infusion), may occur. Monitor patients closely. D/C infusion for severe reaction and treat for Grade 3/4 infusion reactions. Hepatitis B virus (HBV) reactivation can occur, in some cases resulting in fulminant hepatitis, hepatic failure, and death. Screen all patients for HBV infection before treatment initiation; monitor patients during and after treatment. D/C therapy and concomitant medications in the event of HBV reactivation. Fatal progressive multifocal leukoencephalopathy (PML) may occur.

ADULT DOSAGE

Non-Hodgkin's Lymphoma

375mg/m^2 as an IV infusion

Relapsed/Refractory, Low-Grade/Follicular, CD20-Positive, B-Cell Non-Hodgkin's Lymphoma (NHL) as a Single Agent:
Administer once weekly for 4 or 8 doses

Retreatment: Administer once weekly for 4 doses

Previously Untreated Follicular, CD20-Positive, B-Cell NHL:

In Combination w/ Chemotherapy: Administer on Day 1 of each chemotherapy cycle for up to 8 doses

PEDIATRIC DOSAGE

Pediatric use may not have been established

Maint in Complete/Partial Responders:
Administer as a single agent every 8 weeks for 12 doses; initiate 8 weeks following completion of combination treatment w/ chemotherapy

Non-Progressing, Low-Grade, CD20-Positive, B-Cell NHL as a Single Agent After 1st Line Cyclophosphamide, Vincristine, and Prednisone (CVP) Chemotherapy:
Administer once weekly for 4 doses at 6-month intervals following completion of 6-8 CVP chemotherapy cycles
Max: 16 doses

Previously Untreated Diffuse Large B-Cell, CD20-Positive NHL in Combination w/ Cyclophosphamide, Doxorubicin, Vincristine, and Prednisone (CHOP) or Other Anthracycline-Based Chemotherapy:
Administer on Day 1 of each chemotherapy cycle for up to 8 infusions

As a Component of Zevalin:
Infuse 250mg/m^2 w/in 4 hrs prior to the administration of Indium-111 (In-111) Zevalin and w/in 4 hrs prior to the administration of Yttrium-90 (Y-90) Zevalin; administer rituximab and In-111 Zevalin 7-9 days prior to rituximab and Y-90 Zevalin

Refer to the Zevalin PI for additional information

Chronic Lymphocytic Leukemia

In combination w/ fludarabine and cyclophosphamide, for previously untreated and previously treated CD20-positive chronic lymphocytic leukemia

375mg/m^2 the day prior to initiation of fludarabine and cyclophosphamide chemotherapy, then 500mg/m^2 on Day 1 of cycles 2-6 (every 28 days)

Pneumocystis jiroveci pneumonia and anti-herpetic viral prophylaxis is recommended during treatment and for up to 12 months following treatment as appropriate

Rheumatoid Arthritis

In combination w/ methotrexate for moderately to severely active rheumatoid arthritis in patients who have had an inadequate response to ≥1 TNF antagonist therapy

Two 1000mg IV infusions separated by 2 weeks

Administer subsequent courses every 24 weeks or based on evaluation, but not sooner than every 16 weeks

Granulomatosis with Polyangiitis and Microscopic Polyangiitis

In Combination w/ Glucocorticoids:
375mg/m^2 IV infusion once weekly for 4 weeks

Glucocorticoid Administration:
Methylprednisolone 1000mg/day IV for 1-3 days, followed by oral prednisone 1mg/kg/day (not to exceed 80mg/day and tapered per clinical need); begin regimen w/in 14 days prior to or w/ initiation of rituximab and continue during and after the 4-week course of treatment

Pneumocystis jiroveci pneumonia prophylaxis is recommended during treatment and for at least 6 months following the last infusion

Premedication

Premedicate before each infusion w/ acetaminophen and an antihistamine

For patients administered rituximab according to the 90-min infusion rate, the glucocorticoid component of their chemotherapy regimen should be administered prior to infusion

Rheumatoid Arthritis Patients:
Methylprednisolone 100mg IV (or its equivalent) 30 min prior to each infusion

DOSING CONSIDERATIONS

Adverse Reactions

Infusion Reactions: Interrupt or slow the infusion; continue at 1/2 the previous rate upon improvement of symptoms

ADMINISTRATION

IV route

For IV infusion only; do not administer as IV push or bolus
Do not mix or dilute w/ other drugs
Single-use vial; discard any unused portion left in vial

1st Infusion

Initiate at a rate of 50mg/hr; in the absence of infusion toxicity, increase rate by 50mg/hr increments every 30 min, to a max of 400mg/hr

Subsequent Infusions

Standard Infusion: Initiate at a rate of 100mg/hr; in the absence of infusion toxicity, increase by 100mg/hr increments every 30 min, to a max of 400mg/hr

Previously Untreated Follicular and Diffuse Large B-Cell Non-Hodgkin's Lymphoma Patients: Grade 3 or 4 Infusion-Related Adverse Event Not Experienced During Cycle 1:
Administer a 90-min infusion in Cycle 2 w/ a glucocorticoid-containing chemotherapy regimen; initiate at a rate of 20% of the total dose given in the first 30 min and the remaining 80% of the total dose given over the next 60 min. If 90-min infusion is tolerated in cycle 2, use the same rate when administering the remainder of the treatment regimen (through Cycle 6 or 8)

Clinically Significant Cardiovascular Disease/Circulating Lymphocyte Count ≥5000/mm³ Before Cycle 2:
Do not administer the 90-min infusion

Preparation

1. Withdraw the necessary amount of rituximab and dilute to a final concentration of 1-4mg/mL in an infusion bag containing either 0.9% normal saline or D5W
2. Gently invert bag to mix the sol

HOW SUPPLIED

Inj: 100mg/10mL, 500mg/50mL

WARNINGS/PRECAUTIONS

Should only be administered by a healthcare professional with appropriate medical support to manage severe infusion reactions that can be fatal if they occur. Not recommended for use with severe, active infections. *Pneumocystis jiroveci* pneumonia (PCP) and antiherpetic viral prophylaxis is recommended for patients with CLL during treatment and for up to 12 months following treatment as appropriate. PCP prophylaxis is recommended for patients with GPA and MPA during treatment and for at least 6 months following last infusion. Potential for immunogenicity. Acute renal failure, hyperkalemia, hypocalcemia, hyperuricemia, and/or hyperphosphatemia from tumor lysis may occur within 12-24 hrs after the 1st infusion. A high number of circulating malignant cells (≥25,000/mm³) or high tumor burden confers greater risk of tumor lysis syndrome (TLS); administer aggressive IV hydration and antihyperuricemic therapy in patients at high risk of TLS. Correct electrolyte abnormalities, monitor renal function and fluid balance, and administer supportive care, including dialysis as indicated. Serious, including fatal, bacterial, fungal, and new/reactivated viral infections may occur during and following the completion of therapy; d/c for serious infections and institute anti-infective therapy. Infections reported in some patients with prolonged hypogammaglobulinemia (>11 months after rituximab exposure). D/C if severe mucocutaneous reactions, PML, or serious/life-threatening cardiac arrhythmias occur. Perform cardiac monitoring during and after all infusions if arrhythmias develop or with history of arrhythmia/angina. Severe renal toxicity may occur in NHL patients; d/c if SrCr rises or oliguria occurs. Abdominal pain, bowel obstruction, and perforation may occur in combination with chemotherapy. Follow current immunization guidelines and administer non-live vaccines at least 4 weeks prior to therapy for RA patients. Obtain CBC and platelet count prior to each course in lymphoid malignancy patients, at weekly to monthly intervals (more frequently if cytopenia develops) during treatment with rituximab and chemotherapy, and at 2- to 4-month intervals during therapy in RA, GPA, or MPA patients. Not recommended in patients with RA who have not had prior inadequate response to one or more TNF antagonists.

ADVERSE REACTIONS

Infusion reactions, mucocutaneous reactions, hepatitis B reactivation, PML, infections, fever, lymphopenia, chills, asthenia, neutropenia, headache, leukopenia, diarrhea, muscle spasms.

DRUG INTERACTIONS

Renal toxicity reported with cisplatin. Vaccination with live viral vaccines not recommended. Observe closely for signs of infection if biologic agents and/or disease-modifying antirheumatic drugs are used concomitantly.

PATIENT CONSIDERATIONS

Assessment: Assess for severe active infections, preexisting cardiac/pulmonary conditions, prior experience of cardiopulmonary adverse reactions, high number of circulating malignant cells (≥25,000/mm^3), high tumor burden, electrolyte abnormalities, risk/preexisting HBV infection, hypogammaglobulinemia, any other conditions where treatment is cautioned, pregnancy/nursing status, and possible drug interactions. Perform HBsAg and anti-HBc measurement before initiating treatment. Obtain CBC and platelet count.

Monitoring: Monitor fluid and electrolyte balance, cardiac/renal function, CBC, and platelet counts periodically. Monitor for signs/symptoms of infusion reactions, mucocutaneous reactions, hepatitis B reactivation, PML, new-onset neurologic manifestations, TLS, infections, arrhythmias, bowel obstruction/perforation, cytopenias, and other adverse reactions. Closely monitor for infusion reactions in patients with preexisting cardiac/pulmonary conditions, those who experienced prior cardiopulmonary adverse reactions, and those with high numbers of circulating malignant cells. Monitor patients with evidence of current or prior HBV infection for clinical and lab signs of hepatitis or HBV reactivation during and for several months following therapy.

Counseling: Inform of risks of therapy and importance of assessing overall health status at each visit. Inform that drug is detectable in serum for up to 6 months following completion of therapy. Advise to use effective contraception during and for 12 months after therapy.

STORAGE: 2-8°C (36-46°F). Protect from direct sunlight. Do not freeze or shake. Sol for Infusion: 2-8°C (36-46°F) for 24 hrs. Stable for additional 24 hrs at room temperature; however, store diluted solutions at 2-8°C (36-46°F).

ROBAXIN – methocarbamol

RX

Class: Muscular analgesic (centrally acting)

OTHER BRAND NAMES

Robaxin Injection, Robaxin-750

ADULT DOSAGE

Musculoskeletal Conditions

Adjunct for relief of discomfort associated w/ acute, painful musculoskeletal conditions

Oral:

≥16 Years:

Robaxin:

Initial: 3 tabs qid

Maint: 2 tabs qid

Robaxin-750:

Initial: 2 tabs qid

Maint: 1 tab q4h or 2 tabs tid

6g/day are recommended for the first 48-72 hrs; 8g/day may be administered for severe conditions. Thereafter, the dose can usually be reduced to approx 4g/day

Inj:

Moderate Symptoms:

Single 1g (10mL) dose IV/IM; administration of oral form will usually sustain relief initiated by the inj

Max: 3g/day for no more than 3 consecutive days

PEDIATRIC DOSAGE

Tetanus

Inj:

Initial: 15mg/kg or 500mg/m^2; repeat q6h prn

Max: 1.8g/m^2 for 3 consecutive days

Maint dose may be administered by inj into tubing or by IV infusion w/ an appropriate quantity of fluid

R

Severe Cases/Postop Conditions:
Single 1g (10mL) dose IV/IM; may administer additional doses of 1g q8h
Max: 3g/day for no more than 3 consecutive days

Tetanus

Inj:
1 or 2 vials directly into the tubing of the previously inserted indwelling needle; additional 10mL or 20mL may be added to infusion bottle so that a total of up to 30mL (3 vials) is given as initial dose

Repeat q6h until conditions allow for insertion of NG tube; crushed methocarbamol tabs suspended in water or saline may then be given through this tube

Total oral doses up to 24g/day may be required

ADMINISTRATION
Oral/IV/IM route

Directions for IV Use
Inj may be administered undiluted at a max rate of 3mL/min or added to an IV drip of NaCl inj or D5 inj
One vial given as a single dose should not be diluted to more than 250mL for IV infusion
Do not refrigerate after mixing w/ IV infusion fluids
Avoid vascular extravasation of this hypertonic sol, which may result in thrombophlebitis
Patient should be in a recumbent position during and for at least 10-15 min following inj

Directions for IM Use
Not more than 5mL (1/2 vial) should be injected into each gluteal region
Inj may be repeated at 8-hr intervals, if necessary
When satisfactory relief of symptoms is achieved, it can usually be maintained w/ tabs
Not recommended for SQ administration

HOW SUPPLIED
Inj: 100mg/mL [10mL]; **Tab:** 500mg, 750mg

CONTRAINDICATIONS
Hypersensitivity to methocarbamol or to any components in the formulation. **Inj:** Known/suspected renal pathology due to propylene glycol content.

WARNINGS/PRECAUTIONS
May impair mental/physical abilities. May cause color interference in certain screening tests for 5-hydroxy-indoleacetic acid (5-HIAA) and vanillylmandelic acid (VMA). Caution in epilepsy with the inj. Inj rate should not exceed 3mL/min. Avoid extravasation with inj. Avoid use in women who are or may become pregnant and particularly during early pregnancy.

ADVERSE REACTIONS
Lightheadedness, dizziness, drowsiness, nausea, urticaria, pruritus, rash, conjunctivitis, nasal congestion, blurred vision, headache, fever, seizures, syncope, flushing.

DRUG INTERACTIONS
Additive adverse effects with alcohol and other CNS depressants. May inhibit effect of pyridostigmine; caution in patients with myasthenia gravis receiving anticholinergics.

PATIENT CONSIDERATIONS
Assessment: Assess for renal/hepatic impairment, myasthenia gravis, seizures, pregnancy/nursing status, alcohol intake, and drug interactions.

Monitoring: Monitor for congenital and fetal abnormalities if taken during pregnancy, for color interference in certain screening tests for 5-HIAA using nitrosonaphthol reagent, and in screening tests for urinary VMA using Gitlow method.

Counseling: Instruct to use caution while performing hazardous tasks. Warn to avoid alcohol or other CNS depressants. Instruct to notify physician if pregnant/nursing or if planning to become pregnant.

STORAGE: 20-25°C (68-77°F), in tight container; excursions permitted to 15-30°C (59-86°F).

ROTARIX – rotavirus vaccine, live, oral

RX

Class: Vaccine

PEDIATRIC DOSAGE

Rotavirus Gastroenteritis Prevention

Caused by G1 and non-G1 types (G3, G4, and G9):

6-24 Weeks of Age:

Vaccination series consists of two 1mL doses

Administer 1st dose beginning at 6 weeks of age and administer 2nd dose after an interval of at least 4 weeks; the 2-dose series should be completed by 24 weeks of age

If infant spits out or regurgitates most of vaccine dose, may consider a single replacement dose at same vaccination visit

ADMINISTRATION

Oral route

No restrictions on infant's liquid consumption (eg, breast milk), either before or after vaccination

Administer w/in 24 hrs of reconstitution

Reconstitution Instructions for Oral Administration

Reconstitute only w/ accompanying diluents; do not mix w/ other vaccines or sol

1. Remove vial cap and push transfer adapter onto vial (lyophilized vaccine)
2. Shake diluent in oral applicator; connect oral applicator to transfer adapter
3. Push plunger of oral applicator to transfer diluents into vial
4. Withdraw vaccine into oral applicator
5. Twist and remove oral applicator
6. Do not use a needle; not for inj

HOW SUPPLIED

Sus: 1mL

CONTRAINDICATIONS

History of hypersensitivity to any component of the vaccine, severe combined immunodeficiency disease (SCID), history of uncorrected congenital malformation of the GI tract (eg, Meckel's diverticulum) that would predispose infant for intussusception, and history of intussusception.

WARNINGS/PRECAUTIONS

Tip caps of the prefilled oral applicators of diluent may contain natural rubber latex, which may cause allergic reactions in latex-sensitive individuals. Delay administration in infants suffering from acute diarrhea or vomiting. Safety and effectiveness have not been evaluated in infants with chronic GI disorders, with known primary or secondary immunodeficiencies (including HIV), on immunosuppressive therapy, or with malignant neoplasms affecting the bone marrow or lymphatic system, or when administered after exposure to rotavirus. Rotavirus shedding in stool occurs after vaccination. Transmission of vaccine virus from vaccinees to healthy seronegative contacts reported; caution when considering whether to administer to individuals with immunodeficient close contacts. Intussusception reported.

ADVERSE REACTIONS

Fussiness, irritability, cough, runny nose, fever, loss of appetite, vomiting, diarrhea.

DRUG INTERACTIONS

Immunosuppressive therapies, including irradiation, antimetabolites, alkylating agents, cytotoxic drugs, and corticosteroids (used in greater than physiologic doses), may reduce immune response to vaccine.

PATIENT CONSIDERATIONS

Assessment: Assess for previous hypersensitivity to the vaccine, history of uncorrected congenital malformation of the GI tract, history of intussusception, SCID, latex sensitivity, GI disorders, immunocompromised conditions, immunization history, and possible drug interactions.

Monitoring: Monitor for hypersensitivity reactions, intussusception, and other adverse events.

Counseling: Inform parents/guardians of the potential benefits and risks of immunization, and of the importance of completing the immunization series. Inform about the potential for adverse reactions that have been temporally associated with administration of the vaccine or other vaccines containing similar components. Instruct to immediately report any signs and/or symptoms of intussusception.

R

STORAGE: Vials: 2-8°C (36-46°F). Protect from light. Diluent: 2-8°C (36-46°F) or room temperature up to 25°C (77°F). Do not freeze; discard if it has been frozen. Reconstituted Sus: 2-8°C (36-46°F) or room temperature up to 25°C (77°F). Discard if not used within 24 hrs. Do not freeze; discard if it has been frozen.

ROXICET – acetaminophen/oxycodone CII

Class: Opioid analgesic

Associated with cases of acute liver failure, at times resulting in liver transplant and death. Most cases of liver injury are associated with acetaminophen (APAP) use at doses >4000mg/day, and often involve >1 APAP-containing product.

ADULT DOSAGE

Moderate to Moderately Severe Pain

Usual: 1 tab or 5mL (1 tsp) q6h prn
Max: 12 tabs/day or 60mL/day (12 tsp/day)

If pain is constant, give at regular intervals on an around-the-clock schedule

Max: 4g/day of APAP

PEDIATRIC DOSAGE

Pediatric use may not have been established

DOSING CONSIDERATIONS

Discontinuation

Taper dose gradually in patients treated for more than a few weeks

ADMINISTRATION

Oral route

HOW SUPPLIED

(Oxycodone/APAP) **Sol:** 5mg/325mg/5mL [500mL]; **Tab:** 5mg/325mg* *scored

CONTRAINDICATIONS

Known hypersensitivity to oxycodone, acetaminophen, or any other component of this product. **Oxycodone:** Significant respiratory depression (in unmonitored settings or absence of resuscitative equipment), acute or severe bronchial asthma or hypercarbia, suspected/known paralytic ileus.

WARNINGS/PRECAUTIONS

May be abused in a manner similar to other opioid agonists. Respiratory depression may occur; use extreme caution and consider alternative nonopioid analgesics in patients with acute asthma, chronic obstructive pulmonary disorder (COPD), cor pulmonale, preexisting respiratory impairment, or in the elderly or debilitated. Respiratory depressant effects may be markedly exaggerated in the presence of head injury, other intracranial lesions, or preexisting increase in intracranial pressure. Produces effects on pupillary response and consciousness, which may obscure neurologic signs of worsening in patients with head injuries. May cause severe hypotension; caution with circulatory shock. May produce orthostatic hypotension in ambulatory patients. Increased risk of acute liver failure in patients with underlying liver disease. May cause serious skin reactions (eg, acute generalized exanthematous pustulosis, Stevens-Johnson syndrome, toxic epidermal necrolysis), which can be fatal; d/c at the 1st appearance of skin rash or any other sign of hypersensitivity/anaphylaxis. Hypersensitivity and anaphylaxis reported. May obscure diagnosis or clinical course in patients with acute abdominal conditions. Caution with CNS depression, hypothyroidism, Addison's disease, prostatic hypertrophy, urethral stricture, acute alcoholism, delirium tremens, kyphoscoliosis with respiratory depression, myxedema, toxic psychosis, hepatic/renal/pulmonary impairment, and in elderly/debilitated. May aggravate convulsions with convulsive disorders and may induce or aggravate seizures in some clinical settings. Monitor for decreased bowel motility in postoperative patients. May cause spasm of the sphincter of Oddi; caution with biliary tract disease, including acute pancreatitis. May cause increases in serum amylase level. Physical dependence and tolerance may occur. Do not abruptly d/c. Lab test interactions may occur. Not recommended for use during and immediately prior to labor and delivery.

ADVERSE REACTIONS

Acute liver failure, respiratory depression, apnea, respiratory arrest, circulatory depression, hypotension, shock, lightheadedness, dizziness, drowsiness/sedation, N/V.

DRUG INTERACTIONS

Oxycodone: May cause severe hypotension with drugs that compromise vasomotor tone (eg, phenothiazines). May enhance neuromuscular-blocking action of skeletal muscle relaxants and increase respiratory depression. Additive CNS depression with CNS depressants (eg, general anesthetics, phenothiazines, tranquilizers, alcohol); reduce dose of one or both agents. Coadministration with anticholinergics may produce paralytic ileus. Agonist/antagonist analgesics (eg, pentazocine, nalbuphine, butorphanol) may reduce analgesic effect and/or precipitate withdrawal symptoms; use with caution. APAP: Increased risk of acute liver failure with alcohol; hepatotoxicity occurred in chronic alcoholics. Increase in glucuronidation and plasma clearance and decreased $T_{1/2}$ with oral contraceptives. Probenecid and propranolol may increase pharmacologic/therapeutic effects. May decrease effects of loop diuretics, lamotrigine, and zidovudine.

PATIENT CONSIDERATIONS

Assessment: Assess for risks for opioid abuse, addiction, or misuse, patient's general condition and medical status, severity and type of pain, respiratory depression, bronchial asthma, COPD, cor pulmonale, hypercarbia, paralytic ileus, acute alcoholism, drug hypersensitivity, renal/hepatic impairment, pregnancy/nursing status, or any other conditions where treatment is contraindicated or cautioned, and possible drug interactions.

Monitoring: Monitor for development of addiction, abuse, or misuse, physical dependence, tolerance, acute liver failure, respiratory depression, altered consciousness, hypotension, convulsions, hypersensitivity/anaphylactic/serious skin reactions, decreased bowel motility in postoperative patients, spasm of the sphincter of Oddi, and other adverse reactions. Monitor serum amylase levels.

Counseling: Inform that drug contains oxycodone, which is a morphine-like substance. Instruct to keep in a secure place out of reach of children or from theft; advise to seek emergency medical care immediately in case of accidental ingestions. Advise to destroy the unused tabs/oral sol by flushing down the toilet. Advise not to adjust dosing without consulting physician. Inform that drug may impair mental/physical abilities required to perform potentially hazardous tasks (eg, driving, operating heavy machinery). Instruct not to combine with alcohol, opioid analgesics, tranquilizers, sedatives, or other CNS depressants unless under recommendation and guidance of a physician. Inform that drug may cause dangerous additive CNS or respiratory depression if coadministered with another CNS depressant. Instruct to consult physician if pregnant, planning to become pregnant, or if breastfeeding. Advise not to adjust dose without consulting physician and not to abruptly d/c if on treatment for more than a few weeks. Advise to d/c and contact physician immediately if signs of allergy develop. Inform about signs of serious skin reactions. Instruct to look for APAP on package labels and not to use >1 APAP-containing product. Instruct to seek medical attention immediately upon ingestion of >4000mg/day of APAP, even if patient is feeling well.

STORAGE: 20-25°C (68-77°F). (Tab) Protect from moisture.

ROZEREM – ramelteon

RX

Class: Melatonin receptor agonist

ADULT DOSAGE

Insomnia

Difficulty w/ Sleep Onset:
8mg w/in 30 min of hs
Max: 8mg/day

PEDIATRIC DOSAGE

Pediatric use may not have been established

ADMINISTRATION

Oral route

Do not take w/ or immediately after high-fat meal

HOW SUPPLIED

Tab: 8mg

CONTRAINDICATIONS

Rechallenge in patients who developed angioedema after treatment w/ ramelteon. Coadministration w/ fluvoxamine.

WARNINGS/PRECAUTIONS

Angioedema reported; do not rechallenge if angioedema develops. Sleep disturbances may manifest as a physical and/or psychiatric disorder; symptomatic treatment of insomnia should be initiated only after careful evaluation. Failure of insomnia to remit after 7-10 days of therapy may indicate presence of psychiatric and/or medical illness. Cognitive and behavior changes, hallucinations, amnesia, anxiety, other neuropsychiatric symptoms, and complex behaviors reported; d/c if complex sleep behavior occurs. Worsening of depression reported in primarily depressed patients. May impair physical/mental abilities. May affect reproductive hormones (eg, decreased testosterone levels, increased prolactin levels). Not recommended with severe sleep apnea. Do not use with severe hepatic impairment. Caution with moderate hepatic impairment.

ADVERSE REACTIONS

Dizziness, somnolence, fatigue, nausea, exacerbated insomnia.

DRUG INTERACTIONS

See Contraindications. Decreased efficacy with strong CYP inducers (eg, rifampin). Caution with less strong CYP1A2 inhibitors, strong CYP3A4 inhibitors (eg, ketoconazole), and strong CYP2C9 inhibitors (eg, fluconazole). Increased levels with donepezil and doxepin; monitor patients closely. Increased T_{max} of zolpidem; avoid use. Increased risk of complex behaviors with alcohol and other CNS depressants. Additive effect with alcohol; avoid alcohol use.

PATIENT CONSIDERATIONS

Assessment: Assess for hepatic impairment, manifestations of physical and/or psychiatric disorder, depression, sleep apnea, other comorbid diagnoses, hypersensitivity, pregnancy/nursing status, and possible drug interactions.

Monitoring: Monitor for signs/symptoms of angioedema, exacerbations of insomnia, emergence of cognitive or behavioral abnormalities, worsening of depression, complex sleep behaviors, and anaphylactic/anaphylactoid reactions.

Counseling: Inform patients, families, and caregivers about benefits and risks associated with treatment. Counsel for appropriate use and instruct to read Medication Guide. Inform that severe anaphylactic and anaphylactoid reactions may occur; advise to seek immediate medical attention. Instruct to report sleep-driving to doctor immediately. Instruct to consult healthcare provider if cessation of menses, galactorrhea in females, decreased libido, or fertility problems occur. Instruct to take within 30 min prior to hs and confine activities to those necessary to prepare for bed. Instruct to swallow tab whole and to not break tab.

STORAGE: 25°C (77°F); excursions permitted to 15-30°C (59-86°F). Protect from moisture and humidity.

RYTARY — carbidopa/levodopa

RX

Class: Dopa-decarboxylase inhibitor/dopamine precursor

ADULT DOSAGE

Parkinson's Disease

Levodopa Naive:
Initial: 23.75mg/95mg tid for the first 3 days. On the 4th day of treatment, may increase to 36.25mg/145mg tid
Titrate: May increase up to 97.5mg/390mg tid to 5X/day based on clinical response and tolerability
Max: (612.5mg/2450mg)/day

Parkinsonism

Postencephalitic Parkinsonism and Parkinsonism Following Carbon Monoxide/ Manganese Intoxication:
Levodopa Naive:
Initial: 23.75mg/95mg tid for the first 3 days. On the 4th day of treatment, may increase to 36.25mg/145mg tid
Titrate: May increase up to 97.5mg/390mg tid to 5X/day based on clinical response and tolerability
Max: (612.5mg/2450mg)/day

Conversions

From Immediate-Release (IR) Carbidopa-Levodopa:
Total Daily Dose of Levodopa in IR Combination:
400-549mg IR: Three 23.75mg/95mg cap tid
550-749mg IR: Four 23.75mg/95mg cap tid
750-949mg IR: Three 36.25mg/145mg cap tid
950-1249mg IR: Three 48.75mg/195mg cap tid
>1250mg IR: Four 48.7mg/195mg cap tid or three 61.25mg/245mg cap tid

PEDIATRIC DOSAGE

Pediatric use may not have been established

R

DOSING CONSIDERATIONS

Concomitant Medications

Currently Treated w/ Carbidopa and Levodopa Plus Catechol-O-Methyl Transferase Inhibitors:
Initial: May need to increase initial total daily dose of levodopa

Discontinuation

Avoid sudden discontinuation or rapid dose reduction; taper daily dose at time of treatment discontinuation

ADMINISTRATION

Oral route

Swallow whole w/ or w/o food
Do not chew, divide or crush cap
May administer by carefully opening cap and sprinkling entire contents on a small amount of applesauce (1-2 tbsp) and consuming immediately; do not store drug/food mixture for future use

HOW SUPPLIED

Cap, Extended-Release: (Carbidopa/Levodopa) 23.75mg/95mg, 36.25mg/145mg, 48.75mg/195mg, 61.25mg/245mg

CONTRAINDICATIONS

Patients who are currently taking a nonselective MAOI (eg, phenelzine, tranylcypromine) or have recently (within 2 weeks) taken a nonselective MAOI.

WARNINGS/PRECAUTIONS

A symptom complex resembling neuroleptic malignant syndrome (hyperpyrexia and confusion) reported in association with rapid dose reduction, withdrawal of, or changes in dopaminergic therapy; avoid sudden discontinuation/rapid dose reduction, or taper dose if discontinuing therapy. Cardiovascular ischemic events reported; monitor cardiac function in an intensive cardiac care facility during the period of initial dosage adjustment, in patients with a history of MI who have residual atrial, nodal, or ventricular arrhythmias. Increased risk for hallucinations and psychosis; do not use in patients with a major psychotic disorder. Intense urge to gamble, increased sexual urges, intense urges to spend money, binge eating, and/or other intense urges, and the inability to control these urges may occur; consider dose reduction or discontinuation if such urges develop. May cause dyskinesias; may require dose reduction of Rytary or other medications used for the treatment of Parkinson's disease. May increase the possibility of upper GI hemorrhage in patients with history of peptic ulcer. May cause increased intraocular pressure (IOP) in patients with glaucoma. Perform periodic skin examinations to monitor for melanoma. Levodopa: Falling asleep while engaged in activities of daily living and somnolence reported; consider discontinuation if significant daytime sleepiness or episodes of falling asleep during activities that require active participation occur. May impair mental/physical abilities.

ADVERSE REACTIONS

N/V, dizziness, headache, insomnia, abnormal dreams, dry mouth, dyskinesia, anxiety, constipation, orthostatic hypotension.

DRUG INTERACTIONS

See Contraindications. Selective MAO-B inhibitors (eg, rasagiline, selegiline) may be associated with orthostatic hypotension; monitor patients who are taking these drugs concurrently. Iron salts or multivitamins containing iron salts may form chelates and may cause a reduction in bioavailability; monitor patients for worsening Parkinson's symptoms. Levodopa: Caution with concomitant use of sedating medications; may increase the risk for somnolence. Dopamine D2 receptor antagonists (eg, phenothiazines, butyrophenones, risperidone, metoclopramide) and isoniazid may reduce the effectiveness of levodopa; monitor patients for worsening Parkinson's symptoms.

PATIENT CONSIDERATIONS

Assessment: Assess for major psychotic disorder, glaucoma, risk factors that may increase risk for somnolence (eg, presence of sleep disorders), history of peptic ulcer, history of MI with residual atrial, nodal, or ventricular arrhythmias, pregnancy/nursing status, and possible drug interactions.

Monitoring: Monitor for hallucinations, psychosis, control/compulsive behaviors, dyskinesias, drowsiness/sleepiness, somnolence, upper GI hemorrhage in patients with a history of peptic ulcer, increased IOP in patients with glaucoma, and other adverse reactions. Monitor cardiac function in an intensive cardiac care facility during the initial dosage adjustment period in patients with a history of MI who have residual atrial, nodal, or ventricular arrhythmias. Monitor for hyperpyrexia and confusion if sudden discontinuation or rapid dose reduction occurs. Perform periodic skin examinations to monitor for melanoma.

Counseling: Instruct to take ud. Instruct to call physician before stopping therapy and to call physician if withdrawal symptoms (eg, fever, confusion, severe muscle stiffness) develop. Advise that certain side effects (eg, sleepiness and dizziness) that have been reported may affect some patients' ability to drive and operate machinery safely. Inform that hallucinations may occur with levodopa products. Inform of the potential for experiencing intense urges to gamble, increased sexual urges, and other intense urges, and the inability to control these urges while on therapy. Instruct to notify physician if abnormal involuntary movements appear or get worse during treatment. Advise that may develop orthostatic hypotension with or without symptoms (eg, dizziness, nausea, syncope, sweating); advise to rise slowly after sitting or lying down, especially if patient has been doing so for a prolonged period. Advise of the possible additive sedative effects when taking other CNS depressants in combination with therapy. Instruct to notify physician if pregnant/breastfeeding an infant, or intend to breastfeed/become pregnant.

STORAGE: 25°C (77°F); excursions permitted to 15-30°C (59-86°F). Protect from light and moisture.

RYTHMOL SR – propafenone hydrochloride

RX

Class: Class IC antiarrhythmic

Increased rate of death or reversed cardiac arrest rate reported in patients treated with encainide or flecainide (Class 1C antiarrhythmics) in a study of patients with asymptomatic non-life-threatening ventricular arrhythmias who had a MI >6 days but <2 yrs previously. Consider any 1C antiarrhythmics to have significant proarrhythmic risk in patients with structural heart disease. Avoid in patients with non-life-threatening ventricular arrhythmias, even if experiencing unpleasant, but not life-threatening signs/symptoms.

ADULT DOSAGE

Atrial Fibrillation

In Patients w/ No Structural Heart Disease:
Initial: 225mg q12h
Titrate: May increase at a minimum of 5-day intervals to 325mg q12h. May increase to 425mg q12h if additional therapeutic effect is needed

PEDIATRIC DOSAGE

Pediatric use may not have been established

DOSING CONSIDERATIONS

Hepatic Impairment
Reduce dose

Other Important Considerations
Significant QRS Widening/2nd- or 3rd-degree Atrioventricular Block: Reduce dose

ADMINISTRATION

Oral route

Take w/ or w/o food
Do not crush or further divide cap contents

HOW SUPPLIED

Cap, Extended-Release: 225mg, 325mg, 425mg

CONTRAINDICATIONS

Heart failure (HF), cardiogenic shock, known Brugada syndrome, bradycardia, marked hypotension, bronchospastic disorders or severe obstructive pulmonary disease, marked electrolyte imbalance, and sinoatrial, AV and intraventricular disorders of impulse generation or conduction (eg, sick sinus node syndrome, AV block) in the absence of an artificial pacemaker.

WARNINGS/PRECAUTIONS

Do not use to control ventricular rate during A-fib. Concomitant treatment with drugs that increase the functional AV nodal refractory period is recommended. May cause new or worsened arrhythmias; evaluate ECG prior to and during therapy. Brugada syndrome may be unmasked after exposure to therapy; perform ECG after initiation of treatment and d/c if changes are suggestive of Brugada syndrome. May provoke overt HF. Proarrhythmic effects more likely occur in patients with HF or severe MI. Conduction disturbances (eg, 1st-degree AV block), agranulocytosis, positive antinuclear antibody (ANA) titers, and exacerbation of myasthenia gravis reported. D/C if persistent or worsening elevation of ANA titers detected. May alter pacing and sensing thresholds of implanted pacemakers and defibrillators; monitor and reprogram devices accordingly during and after therapy. Reversible, short-term drop (within normal range) in sperm count may occur. Caution with renal/hepatic dysfunction.

ADVERSE REACTIONS

Dizziness, palpitations, chest pain, dyspnea, taste disturbance, nausea, fatigue, anxiety, constipation, URTI, edema, influenza.

DRUG INTERACTIONS

Avoid with Class Ia and III antiarrhythmics (eg, quinidine, amiodarone) and withhold these agents for at least 5 half-lives prior to therapy. Inhibitors of CYP2D6 (eg, desipramine, paroxetine, ritonavir) and CYP3A4 (eg, ketoconazole, ritonavir, erythromycin, grapefruit juice) may increase levels; avoid simultaneous use with both a CYP2D6 and a CYP3A4 inhibitor. Amiodarone can affect conduction and repolarization; coadministration is not recommended. Fluoxetine may increase levels in extensive metabolizers. Rifampin may decrease levels and may increase norpropafenone (active metabolite) levels. May increase levels of digoxin, propranolol, metoprolol, and warfarin; monitor digoxin levels and INR. May result in severe adverse events (eg, convulsions, AV block, acute circulatory failure) with abrupt cessation of orlistat. May increase risk of CNS side effects of lidocaine. CYP1A2 inhibitors (eg, amiodarone, tobacco smoke) and cimetidine may increase levels.

PATIENT CONSIDERATIONS

Assessment: Assess for HF, cardiogenic shock, sinoatrial/AV/intraventricular disorders, implanted pacemaker/defibrillator, bradycardia, marked hypotension, bronchospastic disorders or severe obstructive pulmonary disease, marked electrolyte imbalance, MI, renal/hepatic dysfunction, known Brugada syndrome, pregnancy/nursing status, and possible drug interactions. Evaluate ECG prior to therapy.

Monitoring: Monitor for proarrhythmic effects, signs/symptoms of conduction disturbances, agranulocytosis, HF, unmasking of Brugada syndrome, exacerbation of myasthenia gravis, and other adverse reactions. Monitor implanted pacemakers and defibrillators during and after therapy and reprogram accordingly. Evaluate ECG during therapy. Monitor ANA titers, LFTs, and renal/hepatic function.

Counseling: Inform about risks/benefits of therapy. Advise to report symptoms that may be associated with electrolyte imbalance (eg, excessive/prolonged diarrhea, sweating, vomiting, loss of appetite, thirst). Inform to notify physician of all prescription, herbal/natural preparations, and OTC medications currently being taken or of any changes with these products. Instruct not to double the next dose if a dose is missed and to take next dose at the usual time.

STORAGE: 25°C (77°F); excursions permitted to 15-30°C (59-86°F).

SAFYRAL – drospirenone/ethinyl estradiol/levomefolate calcium RX

Class: Estrogen/progestogen combination

Cigarette smoking increases the risk of serious cardiovascular (CV) events. Risk increases w/ age (>35 yrs of age) and w/ the number of cigarettes smoked. Should not be used by women who are >35 yrs of age and smoke.

ADULT DOSAGE

Contraception

1 tab qd at the same time every day for 28 days, then repeat

Start either on 1st day of menses or on 1st Sunday after onset of menses

Other Indications

May be used to raise folate levels for the purpose of reducing the risk of neural tube defect in a pregnancy conceived while taking the product or shortly after discontinuation

Conversions

Switching from Different Birth Control Pill:
Start on the same day that a new pack of the previous oral contraceptive would have been started

Switching from a Method Other Than a Birth Control Pill:
Transdermal Patch/Vaginal Ring/Inj: Start when next application or dose would have been due
Intrauterine Contraceptive/Implant: Start on day of removal

PEDIATRIC DOSAGE

Contraception

Not indicated for use premenarche; refer to adult dosing

DOSING CONSIDERATIONS

Adverse Reactions

GI Disturbances:
In case of severe vomiting or diarrhea, absorption may not be complete and additional contraceptive measures should be taken. If vomiting occurs w/in 3-4 hrs after taking tab, may regard as missed tab

Other Important Considerations

Postpartum Women Who Do Not Breastfeed/After Second Trimester Abortion: Start therapy no earlier than 4 weeks postpartum; if patient initiates therapy postpartum and has not yet had a period, use an additional method of contraception until patient has taken 7 consecutive days of therapy

ADMINISTRATION

Oral route

Take tabs in the order directed on blister pack, preferably after pm meal or hs

May be taken w/o regard to meals

Take single missed pills as soon as remembered

If 1st taken later than Day 1 of menstrual cycle, use a nonhormonal contraceptive as backup during the first 7 days of therapy

HOW SUPPLIED

Tab: (Drospirenone [DRSP]/Ethinyl Estradiol [EE]/Levomefolate calcium) 3mg/0.03mg/0.451mg; **Tab:** (Levomefolate calcium) 0.451mg

CONTRAINDICATIONS

Renal impairment, adrenal insufficiency, high risk of arterial/venous thrombotic disease (eg, smoking if >35 yrs of age, presence/history of deep vein thrombosis/pulmonary embolism, cerebrovascular disease, coronary artery disease (CAD), thrombogenic valvular or thrombogenic rhythm diseases of the heart [eg, subacute bacterial endocarditis w/ valvular disease, or A-fib], inherited/acquired hypercoagulopathies, uncontrolled HTN, diabetes mellitus [DM] w/ vascular disease, headaches w/ focal neurological symptoms or migraine w/ or w/o aura if >35 yrs of age), undiagnosed abnormal uterine bleeding, presence/history of breast cancer or other estrogen- or progestin-sensitive cancer, benign/malignant liver tumors, liver disease, pregnancy.

WARNINGS/PRECAUTIONS

Increased risk of venous thromboembolism (VTE) and arterial thrombosis (eg, stroke, MI); greatest risk of VTE during the first 6 months of combination oral contraceptive (COC) use and is present after initially starting COC or restarting the same or different COC. D/C if arterial/venous thrombotic event occurs. If feasible, d/c at least 4 weeks before and through 2 weeks after major surgery or other surgeries known to have an elevated risk of thromboembolism. D/C if there is unexplained loss of vision, proptosis, diplopia, papilledema, or retinal vascular lesions; evaluate for retinal vein thrombosis immediately. Potential for hyperkalemia in high-risk patients; contraindicated in patients predisposed to hyperkalemia. May increase risk of cervical cancer, intraepithelial neoplasia, and gallbladder disease. Hepatic adenoma and increased risk of hepatocellular carcinoma reported; d/c if jaundice develops. Cholestasis may occur w/ history of pregnancy-related cholestasis. Increased BP reported; d/c if BP rises significantly. May decrease glucose tolerance; monitor prediabetic and diabetic women. Consider alternative contraception w/ uncontrolled dyslipidemia. May increase risk of pancreatitis w/ hypertriglyceridemia or family history thereof. D/C if new headaches that are recurrent, persistent, or severe develop. Unscheduled bleeding and spotting may occur; rule out pregnancy or malignancy. May encounter post-pill amenorrhea or oligomenorrhea. Caution w/ history of depression; d/c if depression recurs to serious degree. May change results of some lab tests (eg, coagulation factors, lipids, glucose tolerance, binding proteins). Folate may mask vitamin B12 deficiency. May induce/exacerbate angioedema in patients w/ hereditary angioedema. Chloasma may occur; women w/ a tendency to chloasma should avoid sun exposure or UV radiation.

ADVERSE REACTIONS

Premenstrual syndrome, headache/migraine, breast pain/tenderness/discomfort, N/V.

DRUG INTERACTIONS

Consider monitoring serum K^+ levels in high-risk patients who take a strong CYP3A4 inhibitor long-term and concomitantly. Potential for an increase in serum K^+ levels w/ use of other drugs that may increase serum K^+ (eg, ACE inhibitors, heparin, aldosterone antagonists, NSAIDs); monitor K^+ levels during 1st treatment cycle in women receiving daily, long-term treatment for chronic conditions/diseases. Agents that induce certain enzymes, including CYP3A4 (eg, phenytoin, barbiturates, products containing St. John's wort), may decrease COC efficacy or increase breakthrough bleeding; use an alternative contraceptive or a backup method when using inducers and continue backup contraception for 28 days after discontinuation of the inducer. Significant changes (increase or decrease) in plasma estrogen and progestin concentrations reported w/ HIV/hepatitis C virus protease inhibitors or non-nucleoside reverse transcriptase inhibitors. Pregnancy reported w/ antibiotics. Atorvastatin may increase EE exposure. Ascorbic acid and acetaminophen may increase EE concentrations. Moderate or strong CYP3A4 inhibitors such as azole antifungals (eg, ketoconazole, itraconazole, voriconazole, fluconazole), verapamil, macrolides (eg, clarithromycin, erythromycin), diltiazem, and grapefruit juice may increase plasma concentrations of estrogen or progestin or both. May decrease concentrations of lamotrigine and reduce seizure control; dosage adjustments of lamotrigine may be necessary. May increase plasma concentrations of CYP3A4 substrates (eg, midazolam), CYP2C19 substrates (eg, omeprazole, voriconazole), and CYP1A2 substrates (eg, theophylline, tizanidine). Increases thyroid-binding globulin levels; may need to increase dose of thyroid hormone in patients on thyroid hormone replacement therapy.

May decrease pharmacological effect of antifolate drugs (eg, antiepileptics, methotrexate [MTX], pyrimethamine). Reduced folate concentrations via inhibition of dihydrofolate reductase enzyme (eg, MTX, sulfasalazine), reduction of folate absorption (eg, cholestyramine), or via unknown mechanisms (eg, antiepileptics, such as carbamazepine, phenytoin, phenobarbital, primidone, valproic acid).

PATIENT CONSIDERATIONS

Assessment: Assess for renal impairment, abnormal uterine bleeding, adrenal insufficiency, CAD, thrombogenic valvular or thrombogenic rhythm diseases of the heart, pregnancy/nursing status, and for any other conditions where treatment is cautioned or contraindicated. Assess for possible drug interactions. Assess BP levels.

Monitoring: Monitor for bleeding irregularities, venous/arterial thrombotic events, cervical cancer or intraepithelial neoplasia, retinal vein thrombosis, jaundice, new/worsening headaches or migraines, serious depression, cholestasis w/ history of pregnancy-related cholestasis, pancreatitis, and for other adverse reactions. Monitor K^+ levels, thyroid function if receiving thyroid replacement therapy, glucose levels in diabetic and prediabetic patients, depression in patients w/ a history of depression, lipids levels in patients w/ dyslipidemia, and BP in patients w/ HTN. Conduct yearly visit w/ all patients for a BP check and for other indicated healthcare.

Counseling: Inform of benefits and risks of therapy. Counsel that cigarette smoking increases the risk of serious CV events. Inform that drug does not protect against HIV infection and other STDs. Instruct to take at the same time every day preferably after pm meal or hs. Instruct on what to do if pills are missed or vomiting occurs w/in 3-4 hrs after taking tab. Inform that COCs may reduce breast milk production. Inform that amenorrhea may occur and pregnancy should be ruled out if amenorrhea occurs in ≥2 consecutive cycles. Counsel to report if taking folate supplements and advise to maintain folate supplementation upon discontinuation due to pregnancy. Advise to inform physician of preexisting medical conditions and/or drugs currently being taken. Counsel women who start COCs postpartum and have not yet had a period to use additional method of contraception until drug is taken for 7 consecutive days. Instruct to d/c if pregnancy occurs during treatment.

STORAGE: 25°C (77°F); excursions permitted to 15-30°C (59-86°F).

SANDOSTATIN — octreotide acetate

RX

Class: Somatostatin analogue

ADULT DOSAGE

Acromegaly

To reduce blood levels of growth hormone and insulin-like growth factor-1 (IGF-I) (somatomedin C) in acromegaly patients who have had inadequate response to or cannot be treated w/ surgical resection, pituitary irradiation, and bromocriptine mesylate at maximally tolerated doses

Initial: 50mcg tid

Usual: 100mcg tid; some patients require up to 500mcg tid

If an increase in dose fails to provide additional benefit, the dose should be reduced

Withdraw yearly for approx 4 weeks from patients who have received irradiation to assess disease activity; if growth hormone or IGF-I (somatomedin C) levels increase and signs and symptoms recur, therapy may be resumed

Carcinoid Tumors

Symptomatic treatment of patients w/ metastatic carcinoid tumors where it suppresses or inhibits the severe diarrhea and flushing episodes associated w/ the disease

Usual: 100-600mcg/day in 2-4 divided doses (mean dose is 300mcg/day) for the first 2 weeks of therapy

In clinical studies, the median maint dose was approx 450mcg/day, but benefits were

PEDIATRIC DOSAGE

Pediatric use may not have been established

S

obtained in some patients w/ as little as 50mcg, while others required up to 1500mcg/day; experience w/ doses >750mcg/day is limited

Vasoactive Intestinal Peptide-Secreting Tumors

Treatment of the profuse watery diarrhea associated w/ vasoactive intestinal peptide-secreting tumors

Usual: 200-300mcg/day in 2-4 divided doses during the initial 2 weeks of therapy (range 150-750mcg)

Titrate: Adjust dose to achieve a therapeutic response; usually doses >450mcg/day are not required

DOSING CONSIDERATIONS

Elderly

Start at lower end of dosing range

ADMINISTRATION

IV/SQ routes

Avoid multiple SQ inj at the same site w/in short periods of time; rotate sites in a systematic manner
Not compatible in TPN sol
Stable in sterile isotonic saline sol or sterile sol of D5W for 24 hrs

Preparation and Administration

Octreotide may be diluted in volumes of 50-200mL and infused IV over 15-30 min or administered by IV push over 3 min; in emergency situations (eg, carcinoid crisis) it may be given by rapid bolus

HOW SUPPLIED

Inj: 50mcg/mL, 100mcg/mL, 200mcg/mL, 500mcg/mL, 1000mcg/mL

CONTRAINDICATIONS

Sensitivity to this drug or any of its components.

WARNINGS/PRECAUTIONS

May inhibit gallbladder contractility and decrease bile secretion; increased risk of gallbladder abnormalities. May alter balance between the counter-regulatory hormones, insulin, glucagon, and GH and lead to hypo- or hyperglycemia; monitor glucose tolerance periodically. May cause hypothyroidism; monitor thyroid levels periodically. Cardiac conduction and other cardiovascular abnormalities (eg, bradycardia, arrhythmias) may occur; caution in patients at risk. Risk of pregnancy with normalization of IGF-1 and GH in acromegalic women. Pancreatitis, depressed vitamin B12 levels, alteration in fat absorption, and abnormal Schilling's test reported. Caution in elderly.

ADVERSE REACTIONS

Gallbladder abnormalities, cardiac abnormalities, abdominal discomfort, diarrhea, loose stool, N/V, abdominal distention, flatulence, constipation, headache, dizziness, hypoglycemia, hyperglycemia, hypothyroidism.

DRUG INTERACTIONS

May alter absorption of orally administered drugs. May decrease blood levels of cyclosporine and may result in transplant rejection. May require dose adjustments of insulin, oral hypoglycemics, β-blockers, calcium channel blockers, or agents that control fluid and electrolyte balance. Increased availability of bromocriptine. May decrease the metabolic clearance of compounds known to be metabolized by CYP450; caution with other drugs mainly metabolized by CYP3A4 and which have a low therapeutic index (eg, quinidine, terfenadine).

PATIENT CONSIDERATIONS

Assessment: Assess for drug hypersensitivity, renal impairment, diabetes mellitus, cardiac dysfunction, pregnancy/nursing status, and possible drug interactions. Obtain baseline thyroid function tests (TSH, total and/or free T4).

Monitoring: Monitor for biliary tract abnormalities, hypo- and hyperglycemia, hypothyroidism, cardiac conduction abnormalities, and pancreatitis. Monitor GH levels at 1-4 hr intervals for 8-12 hrs post-dose or IGF-1 levels at 2 weeks after drug initiation or dose change with acromegaly. Monitor urinary 5-hydroxyindole acetic acid, plasma serotonin, and plasma Substance P levels with carcinoid tumors. Monitor VIP levels in patients with VIPomas. Monitor thyroid function (periodically) and vitamin B12 levels with chronic therapy.

Counseling: Advise of risks and benefits of treatment. Instruct patients and other persons who may administer the medication about sterile SQ inj technique. Advise female patients of childbearing potential to use contraception during therapy.

STORAGE: 2-8°C (36-46°F) for prolonged storage. Protect from light. Stable for 14 days at 20-30°C (70-86°F) if protected from light. Do not warm artificially; sol can be allowed to come to room temperature prior administration. After initial use, multidose vials should be discarded within 14 days. Open ampuls prior to administration and discard unused portion.

SANDOSTATIN LAR – octreotide acetate

RX

Class: Somatostatin analogue

ADULT DOSAGE

Acromegaly

Long-Term Maint Therapy in Patients Who Have Had an Inadequate Response to Surgery and/or Radiotherapy, or if Surgery and/or Radiotherapy is Not an Option:

Not Currently Receiving Octreotide:
Begin therapy w/ Sandostatin SQ (initial dose of 50mcg tid; most patients require doses of 100-200mcg tid but some patients require up to 500mcg tid) and maintain for at least 2 weeks to determine tolerance

Patients considered to be responders to the drug and who tolerate it may be switched to Sandostatin LAR

Currently Receiving Sandostatin Inj:
Initial: 20mg at 4-week intervals for 3 months

Titrate:
Growth Hormone (GH) ≤2.5ng/mL, Normal Insulin-Like Growth Factor-1 (IGF-1), and Controlled Clinical Symptoms: Maintain at 20mg every 4 weeks
GH >2.5ng/mL, Elevated IGF-1, and/or Uncontrolled Clinical Symptoms: Increase to 30mg every 4 weeks
GH ≤1ng/mL, Normal IGF-1, and Controlled Clinical Symptoms: Reduce to 10mg every 4 weeks
GH, IGF-1, or Symptoms are not Adequately Controlled at 30mg: May increase to 40mg every 4 weeks

Max: 40mg every 4 weeks

In patients who have received pituitary irradiation, withdraw therapy yearly for 8 weeks to assess disease activity; may resume therapy if GH or IGF-1 levels increase and signs/symptoms recur

Carcinoid Tumors

Long-Term Treatment of Severe Diarrhea and Flushing Episodes Associated w/ Metastatic Carcinoid Tumors:

Not Currently Receiving Octreotide:
Begin therapy w/ Sandostatin SQ (100-600mcg/day in 2-4 divided doses; some patients may require doses up to 1500mcg/day) and maintain for at least 2 weeks to determine tolerance

Patients considered to be responders to the drug and who tolerate it may be switched to Sandostatin LAR

Currently Receiving Sandostatin Inj:
Initial: 20mg at 4-week intervals for 2 months; patients should continue to receive Sandostatin SQ for at least 2 weeks in the same dosage taken before the switch

PEDIATRIC DOSAGE

Pediatric use may not have been established

S

Titrate:
If Symptoms are Adequately Controlled:
Consider reducing to 10mg for a trial period; if symptoms recur, then increase to 20mg every 4 weeks
If Symptoms are Not Adequately Controlled:
Increase to 30mg every 4 weeks; lower to 10mg for a trial period if good control is achieved on 20mg dose and if symptoms recur, increase to 20mg every 4 weeks

Max: 30mg every 4 weeks

For exacerbation of symptoms, may give Sandostatin SQ for a few days at the dosage received prior to switching to Sandostatin LAR; d/c when symptoms are again controlled

Vasoactive Intestinal Peptide-Secreting Tumors

Long-Term Treatment of Profuse Watery Diarrhea Associated w/ Vasoactive Intestinal Peptide-Secreting Tumors:

Not Currently Receiving Octreotide:
Begin therapy w/ Sandostatin SQ (200-300mcg in 2-4 divided doses [range 150-750mcg]; doses >450mcg/day are usually not required) and maintain for at least 2 weeks to determine tolerance

Patients considered to be responders to the drug and who tolerate it may be switched to Sandostatin LAR

Currently Receiving Sandostatin Inj:
Initial: 20mg at 4-week intervals for 2 months; patients should continue to receive Sandostatin SQ for at least 2 weeks in the same dosage taken before the switch

Titrate:
If Symptoms are Adequately Controlled:
Consider reducing to 10mg for a trial period; if symptoms recur, then increase to 20mg every 4 weeks
If Symptoms are Not Adequately Controlled:
Increase to 30mg every 4 weeks; lower to 10mg for a trial period if good control is achieved on 20mg dose and if symptoms recur, increase to 20mg every 4 weeks

Max: 30mg every 4 weeks

For exacerbation of symptoms, may give Sandostatin SQ for a few days at the dosage received prior to switching to Sandostatin LAR; d/c when symptoms are again controlled

S

DOSING CONSIDERATIONS

Renal Impairment
Renal Failure Requiring Dialysis:
Initial: 10mg every 4 weeks

Hepatic Impairment
Cirrhotic Patients:
Initial: 10mg every 4 weeks

Elderly
Start at lower end of dosing range

ADMINISTRATION
IM route

Administer in the gluteal region; avoid deltoid inj
Rotate inj sites to avoid irritation

Administer immediately after reconstitution; do not directly inject diluent w/o preparing sus
Refer to PI for further administration instructions

HOW SUPPLIED

Inj, Depot: 10mg, 20mg, 30mg

WARNINGS/PRECAUTIONS

Should be administered by a trained healthcare provider. Rotate inj sites in a systematic manner to avoid irritation. May inhibit gallbladder contractility and decrease bile secretion, which may lead to gallbladder abnormalities or sludge. Alters balance between the counter-regulatory hormones, insulin, glucagon, and GH, which may result in hypo/hyperglycemia. Hypothyroidism may occur. Bradycardia, arrhythmias, and cardiac conduction abnormalities reported. May alter dietary fat absorption. Depressed vitamin B12 levels and abnormal Schilling test reported. Serum zinc may rise excessively when fluid loss is reversed in patients on TPN. Caution in elderly.

ADVERSE REACTIONS

Diarrhea, N/V, abdominal pain, flatulence, constipation, inj-site pain, influenza-like symptoms, fatigue, dizziness, headache, cholelithiasis, back pain, anemia, URTI.

DRUG INTERACTIONS

Associated with nutrient absorption alterations; may alter absorption of orally administered drugs. May decrease cyclosporine levels and result in transplant rejection. May need dose adjustments of insulin, oral hypoglycemics, and drugs with bradycardic effects (eg, β-blockers). Increases availability of bromocriptine. May decrease metabolic clearance of drugs metabolized by CYP450; caution with other drugs mainly metabolized by CYP3A4 and which have a low therapeutic index (eg, quinidine, terfenadine).

PATIENT CONSIDERATIONS

Assessment: Assess for renal/hepatic impairment, cardiac dysfunction, pregnancy/nursing status, and possible drug interactions. Obtain baseline thyroid function tests (TSH, total and/or free T4). Obtain baseline plasma vasoactive intestinal peptide levels with VIPoma.

Monitoring: Monitor for signs/symptoms of gallbladder abnormalities or sludge, hypo/hyperglycemia, hypothyroidism, bradycardia, arrhythmia, cardiac conduction abnormalities, and other adverse reactions. Monitor zinc levels if receiving TPN. Monitor vitamin B12 levels. Monitor thyroid function periodically during chronic therapy. Monitor GH and IGF-1 levels with acromegaly. Monitor urinary 5-hydroxyindole acetic acid, plasma serotonin, and plasma substance P levels with carcinoids.

Counseling: Inform of the risks and benefits of treatment. Advise patients with carcinoid tumors and VIPomas to adhere closely to scheduled return visits for reinjection to minimize exacerbation of symptoms. Instruct patients with acromegaly to adhere to return visit schedule to help assure steady control of GH and IGF-1 levels.

STORAGE: 2-8°C (36-46°F). Protect from light until time of use. Drug product kit should remain at room temperature for 30-60 min prior to preparation of drug sus.

SAPHRIS — asenapine

Class: Atypical antipsychotic

RX

Elderly patients w/ dementia-related psychosis treated w/ antipsychotic drugs are at an increased risk of death. Not approved for treatment of patients w/ dementia-related psychosis.

ADULT DOSAGE

Schizophrenia

5mg bid
Titrate: May increase to 10mg bid after 1 week
Max: 10mg bid

Bipolar I Disorder

Acute Treatment of Manic or Mixed Episodes:
Monotherapy:
Initial: 10mg bid
Titrate: May decrease to 5mg bid if warranted by adverse effects
Max: 10mg bid

Adjunctive Therapy (w/ Lithium or Valproate):
Initial: 5mg bid
Titrate: May increase to 10mg bid
Max: 10mg bid

PEDIATRIC DOSAGE

Bipolar I Disorder

Acute Treatment of Manic or Mixed Episodes:
10-17 Years:
Monotherapy:
Initial: 2.5mg bid
Titrate: May increase to 5mg bid after 3 days, and from 5mg to 10mg bid after 3 additional days
Max: 10mg bid

Pediatric patients appear to be more sensitive to dystonia w/ initial dosing when recommended escalation schedule is not followed

S

ADMINISTRATION

SL route

Place tab under the tongue and allow it to dissolve completely
Do not split, crush, chew, or swallow tabs
Do not eat/drink for 10 min after administration

HOW SUPPLIED

Tab, SL: 2.5mg, 5mg, 10mg

CONTRAINDICATIONS

Severe hepatic impairment (Child-Pugh C), history of hypersensitivity reactions to asenapine.

WARNINGS/PRECAUTIONS

Neuroleptic malignant syndrome (NMS) reported; d/c therapy and institute symptomatic treatment. May cause tardive dyskinesia (TD), especially in the elderly; consider discontinuation of therapy if this occurs. Associated w/ metabolic changes that may increase cardiovascular (CV) and cerebrovascular risk (eg, hyperglycemia sometimes associated w/ ketoacidosis or hyperosmolar coma, dyslipidemia, weight gain). Hypersensitivity reactions reported, usually after the 1st dose. May induce orthostatic hypotension and syncope; consider dose reduction if hypotension occurs. Caution w/ known CV disease, cerebrovascular disease, conditions that predispose to hypotension, and in elderly. Leukopenia, neutropenia, and agranulocytosis may occur; consider discontinuation at 1st sign of a clinically significant decline in WBC count w/o causative factors. D/C therapy and follow WBC count until recovery in patients w/ severe neutropenia (ANC <1000/mm^3). May prolong QTc interval; avoid use w/ history of cardiac arrhythmias and in other circumstances that may increase the risk of torsades de pointes. May elevate prolactin levels. Seizures and somnolence reported. May impair mental/physical abilities. May disrupt body's ability to reduce core body temperature. Caution w/ those at risk for suicide. May cause esophageal dysmotility and aspiration; do not use in patients at risk for aspiration pneumonia.

ADVERSE REACTIONS

Somnolence, insomnia, headache, dizziness, extrapyramidal symptoms, akathisia, vomiting, oral hypoesthesia, constipation, weight increase, fatigue, increased appetite, anxiety, dysgeusia, dyspepsia.

DRUG INTERACTIONS

Avoid use w/ other drugs known to prolong QTc including Class 1A antiarrhythmics (eg, quinidine, procainamide), Class 3 antiarrhythmics (eg, amiodarone, sotalol), antipsychotics (eg, ziprasidone, chlorpromazine, thioridazine), and antibiotics (eg, gatifloxacin, moxifloxacin). Caution w/ other drugs that can induce hypotension/bradycardia/respiratory or CNS depression and drugs w/ anticholinergic activity. May enhance the effects of certain antihypertensive agents; monitor BP and adjust dosage of antihypertensive drug accordingly. May cause greater increase in asenapine exposure when used w/ fluvoxamine; dose reduction of asenapine based on clinical response may be necessary. May enhance the inhibitory effects of paroxetine on its own metabolism and increase exposure of paroxetine; reduce paroxetine dose by 1/2 when used in combination.

PATIENT CONSIDERATIONS

Assessment: Assess for dementia-related psychosis, history of cardiac arrhythmias, factors that may increase risk of torsades de pointes, risk for aspiration pneumonia, hepatic impairment, known hypersensitivity to the drug, history of seizures/conditions that lower seizure threshold, any other conditions where treatment is contraindicated or cautioned, pregnancy/nursing status, and possible drug interactions. Obtain baseline FPG in patients w/ diabetes mellitus (DM) or at risk for DM. Obtain baseline CBC if at risk for leukopenia/neutropenia.

Monitoring: Monitor for QT prolongation, NMS, TD, orthostatic hypotension, seizures, esophageal dysmotility, aspiration, suicidal ideation, hypersensitivity reactions, metabolic changes, and other adverse reactions. Monitor CBC frequently during 1st few months in patients w/ preexisting low WBC count/ANC or drug-induced leukopenia/neutropenia. Monitor for fever or other signs/symptoms of infection in patients w/ clinically significant neutropenia. Monitor worsening of glucose control in patients w/ DM or FPG in patients at risk for DM. Periodically reevaluate long-term risks/benefits if used for extended periods in bipolar patients.

Counseling: Inform of the risks/benefits and appropriate administration instructions of therapy. Inform of the signs/symptoms of serious allergic reaction; instruct to seek immediate medical attention if these develop. Inform that application-site reactions, primarily in the sublingual area, including oral ulcers, blisters, peeling/sloughing, and inflammation have been reported; instruct to monitor for these reactions. Inform that numbness or tingling of the mouth or throat may occur directly after administration and usually resolves w/in 1 hr. Counsel on the signs and symptoms of tardive dyskinesia and advise to contact their physician if these abnormal movements occur. Inform about risk of developing NMS and explain its signs and symptoms. Counsel about the risk of metabolic changes, how to recognize symptoms of hyperglycemia and DM, and the need for specific monitoring. Inform about risk of orthostatic hypotension especially early in treatment, and also at times of reinitiating treatment or increases in dose. Advise patients w/ preexisting low WBC counts or history of drug-induced leukopenia/neutropenia to have their CBC monitored. Caution about performing activities requiring mental alertness. Counsel regarding appropriate care in avoiding overheating and dehydration. Advise to notify physician if taking/planning to take any prescription or OTC medications, or w/ known or suspected pregnancy during therapy. Advise that there is a pregnancy exposure registry that monitors pregnancy outcomes in women exposed during pregnancy.

STORAGE: 15-30°C (59-86°F).

SAVAYSA – edoxaban

RX

Class: Selective factor Xa inhibitor

Reduced efficacy reported in nonvalvular A-fib (NVAF) patients w/ CrCl >95 mL/min; should not be used in NVAF patients w/ CrCl >95mL/min; use another anticoagulant. Increased risk of ischemic events w/ premature discontinuation of any oral anticoagulant in the absence of adequate alternative anticoagulation; consider coverage w/ another anticoagulant if therapy is discontinued for a reason other than pathological bleeding or completion of a course of therapy. Epidural or spinal hematomas may occur in patients treated w/ edoxaban who are receiving neuraxial anesthesia or undergoing spinal puncture; hematomas may result in long-term or permanent paralysis. Increased risk of developing epidural or spinal hematomas in patients using indwelling epidural catheters, concomitant use of other drugs that affect hemostasis (eg, NSAIDs, platelet inhibitors, other anticoagulants), history of traumatic or repeated epidural or spinal punctures, history of spinal deformity or spinal surgery, or unknown optimal timing between the administration of edoxaban and neuraxial procedures. Monitor frequently for signs/symptoms of neurologic impairment; if neurologic compromise noted, urgent treatment is necessary. Consider benefits and risks before neuraxial intervention in patients anticoagulated or to be anticoagulated.

ADULT DOSAGE

Nonvalvular Atrial Fibrillation

Reduce Risk of Stroke and Systemic Embolism:
60mg qd

Deep Vein Thrombosis/Pulmonary Embolism

Treatment:
60mg qd following 5-10 days of initial therapy w/ a parenteral anticoagulant

Conversions

Transition to Edoxaban:
From Warfarin/Other Vitamin K Antagonists:
D/C warfarin and start edoxaban when INR ≤2.5
From Oral Anticoagulants Other Than Warfarin/Other Vitamin K Antagonists: D/C current oral anticoagulant and start edoxaban at the time of next scheduled dose of the other oral anticoagulant
From Low Molecular Weight Heparin (LMWH):
D/C LMWH and start edoxaban at the time of next schedule administration of LMWH
From Unfractionated Heparin: D/C infusion and start edoxaban 4 hrs later

Transition from Edoxaban:
To Warfarin:
Oral Option: For patients taking 60mg, reduce dose to 30mg and begin warfarin concomitantly. For patients taking 30mg, reduce dose to 15mg and begin warfarin concomitantly. INR must be measured at least weekly and just prior to the daily dose of edoxaban to minimize the influence of edoxaban on INR measurements. D/C edoxaban and continue warfarin once a stable INR ≥2 is achieved
Parenteral Option: D/C and administer a parenteral anticoagulant and warfarin at the time of next scheduled edoxaban dose. Once a stable INR ≥2.0 is achieved, d/c parenteral anticoagulant and continue warfarin
To Non-Vitamin-K Dependent Oral Anticoagulants or Parenteral Anticoagulants:
D/C edoxaban and start other PO/parenteral anticoagulant at the time the next dose of edoxaban

PEDIATRIC DOSAGE

Pediatric use may not have been established

S

DOSING CONSIDERATIONS

Concomitant Medications

DVT and PE:

Certain P-gp Inhibitors: 30mg qd

Renal Impairment

Nonvalvular A-Fib:

CrCl >95mL/min: Do not use

CrCl 15-50mL/min: 30mg qd

DVT and PE:

CrCl 15-50mL/min: 30mg qd

Discontinuation

D/C at least 24 hrs before invasive/surgical procedure. May restart edoxaban after the procedure as soon as adequate hemostasis has been established noting that the time to onset of pharmacodynamic effect is 1-2 hrs. Administer a parenteral anticoagulant and then switch to edoxaban if oral medication cannot be taken during/after surgical intervention

Other Important Considerations

DVT and PE:

≤60kg: 30mg qd

ADMINISTRATION

Oral route

May take w/o regard to food.

HOW SUPPLIED

Tab: 15mg, 30mg, 60mg

CONTRAINDICATIONS

Active pathological bleeding.

WARNINGS/PRECAUTIONS

Increases risk of bleeding and can cause serious and potentially fatal bleeding; promptly evaluate any signs or symptoms of blood loss. D/C in patients w/ active pathological bleeding. No established way to reverse anticoagulant effects of edoxaban; effects can be expected to persist for approx 24 hrs after last dose. Indwelling epidural or intrathecal catheters should not be removed earlier than 12 hrs after the last administration of edoxaban; next dose of edoxaban should not be administered earlier than 2 hrs after removal of the catheter. Not recommended w/ mechanical heart valves or moderate to severe mitral stenosis, CrCl <15mL/min, moderate/severe hepatic impairment (Child-Pugh B and C). Increased risk for ischemic stroke in patients w/ NVAF, as renal function improves and edoxaban blood levels decrease.

ADVERSE REACTIONS

Bleeding, rash, abnormal LFTs, anemia.

DRUG INTERACTIONS

See Boxed Warning and Dosing Considerations. May increase risk of bleeding w/ drugs affecting hemostasis (eg, ASA and other antiplatelet agents, anticoagulants, fibrinolytics, thrombolytics, chronic use of NSAIDs); promptly evaluate any signs or symptoms of blood loss if patients are treated concomitantly w/ anticoagulants, ASA, other platelet aggregation inhibitors, and/or NSAIDs. Long-term concomitant treatment w/ other anticoagulants is not recommended; short-term coadministration may be needed for patients transitioning to or from edoxaban. Avoid use w/ rifampin.

PATIENT CONSIDERATIONS

Assessment: Assess for active pathological bleeding, risk factors of developing epidural/spinal hematomas, mechanical heart valves, moderate to severe mitral stenosis, renal/hepatic impairment, pregnancy/nursing status, and possible drug interactions. Assess if patient is receiving neuraxial anesthesia or scheduled to undergo spinal puncture.

Monitoring: Monitor for signs/symptoms of ischemic events w/ premature discontinuation of therapy, bleeding, and other adverse reactions.

Counseling: Inform of the risks and benefits of therapy. Advise that may bleed/bruise more easily or may bleed longer while on therapy. Instruct to report any unusual bleeding immediately to physician. Advise to take exactly as prescribed. Counsel not to d/c therapy w/o talking to physician. Advise to inform all healthcare providers and dentists that patient is taking edoxaban before any surgery, medical or dental procedure is scheduled. Instruct to inform all healthcare providers and dentists if patient is taking/planning to take any prescription medications, OTC drugs, or herbal products. Counsel to inform physician immediately if pregnant/breastfeeding or intending to become pregnant/breastfeed during treatment. Advise patients who are having neuraxial anesthesia or spinal puncture to watch for signs and symptoms of spinal/epidural hematoma; instruct to contact physician immediately if symptoms occur.

STORAGE: 20-25°C (68-77°F); excursions permitted to 15-30°C (59-86°F).

SAVELLA – milnacipran hydrochloride

RX

Class: Serotonin and norepinephrine reuptake inhibitor (SNRI)

Savella is a selective SNRI, similar to some drugs used for the treatment of depression and other psychiatric disorders. Antidepressants increased the risk of suicidal thinking and behavior (suicidality) in children, adolescents, and young adults in short-term studies of major depressive disorder (MDD) and other psychiatric disorders. Monitor appropriately and observe closely for clinical worsening, suicidality, or unusual behavioral changes in patients who are started on milnacipran. Not approved for use in the treatment of MDD and in pediatric patients.

ADULT DOSAGE

Fibromyalgia

Recommended Dose: 50mg bid

Titration Schedule:
Day 1: 12.5mg
Days 2-3: 12.5mg bid
Days 4-7: 25mg bid
After Day 7: 50mg bid
Max: 100mg bid

Dosing Considerations with MAOIs

Switching to/from an MAOI for Psychiatric Disorders:
Allow at least 14 days between discontinuation of an MAOI and initiation of treatment, and allow at least 5 days between discontinuation of treatment and initiation of an MAOI

W/ Other MAOIs (eg, Linezolid, IV Methylene Blue):
Do not start milnacipran in patients being treated w/ linezolid or IV methylene blue
In patients already receiving milnacipran, if acceptable alternatives are not available and benefits outweigh risks, d/c milnacipran and administer linezolid or IV methylene blue; monitor for serotonin syndrome for 5 days or until 24 hrs after the last dose of linezolid or IV methylene blue, whichever comes 1st. May resume milnacipran therapy 24 hrs after the last dose of linezolid or IV methylene blue

PEDIATRIC DOSAGE

Pediatric use may not have been established

DOSING CONSIDERATIONS

Renal Impairment
Moderate: Use w/ caution
Severe (CrCl 5-29mL/min): Reduce maint dose by 50% to 25mg bid; may increase to 50mg bid based on individual response
ESRD: Not recommended

Discontinuation
Taper gradually and do not abruptly d/c after extended use

ADMINISTRATION

Oral route

Take w/ or w/o food
Taking w/ food may improve tolerability

HOW SUPPLIED

Tab: 12.5mg, 25mg, 50mg, 100mg

CONTRAINDICATIONS

Use of an MAOI for psychiatric disorders either concomitantly or w/in 5 days of stopping treatment. Treatment w/in 14 days of stopping an MAOI for psychiatric disorders. Starting treatment in patients being treated w/ other MAOIs (eg, linezolid, IV methylene blue).

WARNINGS/PRECAUTIONS

Serotonin syndrome reported; d/c immediately and initiate supportive symptomatic treatment. Associated w/ increase in BP and HR; treat preexisting HTN, preexisting tachyarrhythmias, and other cardiac diseases before starting therapy. Caution w/ significant HTN or cardiac disease. Consider dose reduction or discontinuation of therapy if sustained increase in BP or HR occurs. Increased liver enzymes and severe liver injury reported; d/c if jaundice or other evidence of liver

S

dysfunction develops. Withdrawal symptoms and physical dependence reported; taper gradually. Hyponatremia may occur; elderly and volume-depleted patients may be at greater risk. Consider discontinuation in patients w/ symptomatic hyponatremia. May increase risk of bleeding events. Caution w/ history of a seizure disorder or mania. May affect urethral resistance and micturition; caution w/ history of dysuria, notably in male patients w/ prostatic hypertrophy, prostatitis, and other lower urinary tract obstructive disorders. Male patients may experience testicular pain or ejaculation disorders. Pupillary dilation that occurs following use may trigger an angle-closure attack in a patient w/ anatomically narrow angles who does not have a patent iridectomy. May aggravate preexisting liver disease; avoid w/ substantial alcohol use or chronic liver disease. Caution in the elderly.

ADVERSE REACTIONS

N/V, headache, constipation, hot flush, insomnia, hyperhidrosis, palpitations, URTI, increased HR, dry mouth, HTN, anxiety, dizziness, migraine, abdominal pain.

DRUG INTERACTIONS

See Contraindications. May cause serotonin syndrome w/ other serotonergic drugs (eg, triptans, TCAs, fentanyl, lithium, tramadol, tryptophan, buspirone, St. John's wort) and w/ drugs that impair metabolism of serotonin; d/c immediately if this occurs. If treatment w/ other serotonergic drugs is clinically warranted, patient should be made aware of potential risk for serotonin syndrome, particularly during dose initiation and dose increases. Paroxysmal HTN and possible arrhythmia may occur w/ epinephrine and norepinephrine. Increase in euphoria and postural hypotension observed in patients who switched from clomipramine; caution w/ other centrally acting drugs. Concomitant use w/ digoxin may potentiate adverse hemodynamic effects. Avoid w/ IV digoxin; postural hypotension and tachycardia reported. May inhibit antihypertensive effect of clonidine. Caution w/ NSAIDs, aspirin (ASA), warfarin, and other drugs that affect coagulation due to potential increased risk of bleeding. Caution w/ drugs that increase BP and HR. May increase risk of hyponatremia w/ diuretics.

PATIENT CONSIDERATIONS

Assessment: Assess for HTN, tachyarrhythmias, cardiac diseases, depression, history of seizure disorder/mania/dysuria, prostatic hypertrophy, prostatitis, lower urinary tract obstructive disorders, volume depletion, susceptibility to angle-closure glaucoma, renal/hepatic impairment, pregnancy/nursing status, and possible drug interactions. Assess alcohol use. Obtain baseline BP and HR.

Monitoring: Monitor for clinical worsening, suicidality, unusual changes in behavior, serotonin syndrome, hyponatremia, bleeding events, withdrawal symptoms, physical dependence, liver dysfunction, angle-closure glaucoma, and other adverse reactions. Monitor for urethral resistance and micturition, testicular pain, and ejaculation disorders in male patients. Monitor BP and HR.

Counseling: Inform about risks/benefits of therapy and counsel on its appropriate use. Advise to look for the emergence of suicidality, especially early during treatment and when the dose is adjusted up or down. Inform about the risk of serotonin syndrome, particularly w/ concomitant use w/ other serotonergic agents. Instruct to consult physician if symptoms of serotonin syndrome and emergence of suicidality occur. Advise to have BP and HR monitored regularly. Caution about the increased risk of abnormal bleeding w/ concomitant use of NSAIDs, ASA, and other drugs that affect coagulation. Caution w/ risk of angle closure glaucoma. Inform that drug may impair mental/physical abilities; caution against operating machinery/driving motor vehicles until effects of drug are known. Instruct to discuss alcohol intake w/ physician prior to initiating therapy. Advise that withdrawal symptoms may occur w/ abrupt discontinuation. Advise that if a dose is missed, to skip the dose and take the next dose at the regular time. Instruct to notify physician if pregnant, intending to become pregnant, or if breastfeeding; encourage to enroll in the Savella Pregnancy Registry if patient becomes pregnant.

S

STORAGE: 25°C (77°F); excursions permitted to 15-30°C (59-86°F).

SAXENDA — liraglutide (rDNA origin) RX

Class: Glucagon-like peptide-1 (GLP-1) receptor agonist

Causes dose-dependent and treatment-duration-dependent thyroid C-cell tumors at clinically relevant exposures in animal studies. It is unknown whether drug causes thyroid C-cell tumors (eg, medullary thyroid carcinoma [MTC]) in humans. Contraindicated in patients w/ a personal or family history of MTC and in patients w/ multiple endocrine neoplasia syndrome type 2 (MEN 2). Counsel patients on the risk of MTC and symptoms of thyroid tumors. Routine monitoring of serum calcitonin or using thyroid ultrasound is of uncertain value for early detection of MTC.

ADULT DOSAGE

Chronic Weight Management

Adjunct to a reduced-calorie diet and increased physical activity in patients w/ BMI $\geq$30kg/m^2 or $\geq$27kg/m^2 w/ at least 1 weight-related comorbid condition

Usual: 3mg daily; dose escalation should be used to reduce the likelihood of GI symptoms

Dose Escalation:
Week 1: 0.6mg/day
Week 2: 1.2mg/day
Week 3: 1.8mg/day
Week 4: 2.4mg/day
Week 5 and Onward: 3mg/day

May delay dose escalation for 1 additional week if unable to tolerate increased dose

D/C if patient is unable to tolerate 3mg dose
D/C if patient has not lost at least 4% of baseline body weight 16 weeks after initiating therapy

Missed Dose

If a dose is missed, resume once-daily regimen w/ next scheduled dose; do not take an extra dose or increase dose to make up for missed dose

If >3 days have elapsed since last dose, reinitiate at 0.6mg/day and retitrate following dose escalation schedule

PEDIATRIC DOSAGE

Pediatric use may not have been established

DOSING CONSIDERATIONS

Concomitant Medications

Insulin Secretagogues: Consider reducing dose of insulin secretagogue (eg, reduce by 1/2

ADMINISTRATION

SQ route

Administer qd at any time of day, w/o regard to timing of meals
May inject in the abdomen, thigh, or upper arm; inj site/timing can be changed w/o dose adjustment

HOW SUPPLIED

Inj: 6mg/mL [3mL]

CONTRAINDICATIONS

MEN 2, personal or family history of MTC, prior serious hypersensitivity reaction to liraglutide or to any of the product components, pregnancy.

WARNINGS/PRECAUTIONS

Should not be used w/ other drugs containing the active ingredient or w/ any other glucagon-like peptide-1 (GLP-1) receptor agonist. Acute pancreatitis, including fatal and nonfatal hemorrhagic or necrotizing pancreatitis, reported; d/c if suspected, and do not restart if confirmed. Acute gallbladder disease reported; if cholelithiasis is suspected, gallbladder studies and appropriate clinical follow up are indicated. May lower blood glucose. Increases in HR reported; d/c if a sustained increase in resting HR develops. Acute renal failure and worsening of chronic renal failure, sometimes requiring hemodialysis, reported. Serious hypersensitivity reactions reported; d/c if a hypersensitivity reaction occurs. Caution w/ history of angioedema w/ another GLP-1 receptor agonist. Suicidal ideation reported; avoid w/ history of suicidal attempts or active suicidal ideation. Monitor for emergence or worsening of depression, suicidal thoughts or behavior, and/or any unusual changes in mood or behavior; d/c if suicidal thoughts/behaviors develop. Slows gastric emptying. Caution w/ renal/hepatic impairment.

ADVERSE REACTIONS

N/V, diarrhea, constipation, hypoglycemia in type 2 DM, decreased appetite, headache, dyspepsia, fatigue, dizziness, abdominal pain, increased lipase, GERD, gastroenteritis, abdominal distention, eructation.

DRUG INTERACTIONS

See Dosage. Do not use w/ insulin. Increased risk for serious hypoglycemia w/ insulin secretagogues (eg, sulfonylureas) in patients w/ type 2 DM. Adjust coadministered antidiabetic drugs, if needed, based on glucose monitoring results and risk of hypoglycemia, in patients w/ type 2 DM. Causes a delay of gastric emptying, and therefore may affect the absorption of concomitantly administered oral medications; use w/ caution.

PATIENT CONSIDERATIONS

Assessment: Assess for previous hypersensitivity to the drug, MEN 2, personal or family history of MTC, history of pancreatitis, type 2 DM, history of angioedema w/ another GLP-1 receptor agonist, history of suicidal attempts or active suicidal ideation, renal/hepatic impairment, pregnancy/nursing status, and possible drug interactions. Obtain blood glucose parameters in patients w/ type 2 DM.

Monitoring: Monitor for thyroid C-cell tumors, elevated serum calcitonin, pancreatitis, acute gallbladder disease, renal impairment, hypersensitivity reactions, emergence or worsening of depression, suicidal thoughts or behavior, any unusual changes in mood or behavior, and other adverse reactions. Monitor blood glucose, especially in patients w/ type 2 DM. Monitor HR at regular intervals.

Counseling: Advise to take exactly as prescribed. Counsel to report symptoms of thyroid tumors (eg, a lump in the neck, hoarseness, dysphagia, dyspnea) to physician. Inform of risk of acute pancreatitis and instruct to d/c therapy and contact physician if persistent severe abdominal pain occurs. Inform that substantial or rapid weight loss can increase the risk of cholelithiasis; advise to contact physician if cholelithiasis is suspected. Advise patients w/ type 2 DM on antidiabetic therapy to monitor blood glucose levels and report symptoms of hypoglycemia to physician. Counsel to report symptoms of sustained periods of heart pounding or racing while at rest to physician, and to d/c therapy if a sustained increase in resting HR occurs. Inform of the potential risk of dehydration due to GI adverse reactions and to take precautions to avoid fluid depletion. Inform of the potential risk of worsening renal function. Instruct to d/c therapy and seek medical advice if symptoms of hypersensitivity reactions occur. Advise to report emergence or worsening of depression, suicidal thoughts or behavior, and/or any unusual changes in mood or behavior, and to d/c therapy if suicidal thoughts or behaviors develop. Instruct to contact physician if jaundice develops. Counsel to never share a pen w/ another person, even if the needle is changed.

STORAGE: 2-8°C (36-46°F). Do not store in the freezer or directly adjacent to the refrigerator cooling element. Do not freeze and do not use if it has been frozen. After Initial Use: 15-30°C (59-86°F) or 2-8°C (36-46°F) for 30 days. Protect from excessive heat and sunlight. Remove and safely discard the needle after each inj; store the pen w/o an inj needle attached.

SEEBRI NEOHALER – glycopyrrolate

RX

Class: Anticholinergic

ADULT DOSAGE

Chronic Obstructive Pulmonary Disease

Long-Term, Maint Treatment of Airflow Obstruction:

Recommended: Orally inhale the contents of 1 cap bid using the Neohaler device

Max: 1 cap bid

PEDIATRIC DOSAGE

Pediatric use may not have been established

ADMINISTRATION

Oral inh route

Caps should only be used w/ Neohaler device.
Do not swallow caps.
Administer at the same time every day.
Store caps in the blister; only remove immediately before use.

HOW SUPPLIED

Cap, Inh: 15.6mcg [60[s]]

CONTRAINDICATIONS

Hypersensitivity to glycopyrrolate or to any of the ingredients.

WARNINGS/PRECAUTIONS

Do not initiate during acutely deteriorating or potentially life-threatening episodes of COPD. Do not use for the relief of acute symptoms (eg, rescue therapy). May produce paradoxical bronchospasm; treat immediately w/ an inhaled, short acting bronchodilator and d/c and institute alternative therapy. Immediate hypersensitivity reactions reported; d/c immediately and institute alternative therapy if signs suggesting an allergic reaction occur. Caution in patients w/ severe hypersensitivity to milk proteins, narrow-angle glaucoma, and urinary retention.

ADVERSE REACTIONS

URTI, nasopharyngitis.

DRUG INTERACTIONS

Avoid w/ other anticholinergic-containing drugs; may lead to an increase in anticholinergic effects.

PATIENT CONSIDERATIONS

Assessment: Assess for hypersensitivity to glycopyrrolate, milk proteins, or any component of the product. Assess for acutely deteriorating COPD, narrow-angle glaucoma, urinary retention, pregnancy/nursing status, and possible drug interactions.

Monitoring: Monitor for deteriorating disease, paradoxical bronchospasm, hypersensitivity reactions, narrow-angle glaucoma, urinary retention, and other adverse reactions.

Counseling: Inform that drug is not for relief of acute symptoms of COPD. Advise that acute symptoms should be treated w/ a rescue inhaler (eg, albuterol). Instruct to seek medical attention immediately if experiencing worsening of symptoms or a need for more inhalations than usual of the rescue inhaler. Advise not to d/c therapy w/o physician guidance. Instruct to d/c therapy if paradoxical bronchospasm occurs. Inform about risks of acute narrow-angle glaucoma and urinary retention associated w/ therapy; instruct to consult physician immediately if any signs/symptoms develop. Instruct on how to correctly administer caps using the Neohaler device. Inform that the contents of the caps are for oral inhalation only and must not be swallowed. Advise to contact physician if pregnancy occurs while on therapy.

STORAGE: 77°F (25°C); excursions permitted to 59-86°F (15-30°C). Do not use the Neohaler device w/ any other caps. Store caps in the blister protected from moisture; remove caps from the blister immediately before use. Always use the new Neohaler inhaler provided w/ each new prescription.

SENSIPAR – cinacalcet

RX

Class: Calcimimetic agent

ADULT DOSAGE

Secondary Hyperparathyroidism

In Patients w/ Chronic Kidney Disease on Dialysis:
Initial: 30mg qd
Titrate: Increase no more frequently than every 2-4 weeks through sequential doses of 30mg, 60mg, 90mg, 120mg, and 180mg qd to target intact parathyroid (iPTH) hormone of 150-300pg/mL

Measure serum Ca^{2+} and phosphorus w/in 1 week and measure iPTH hormone 1-4 weeks after initiation/dose adjustment; serum iPTH levels should be assessed no earlier than 12 hrs after dosing

Once maint dose is established, measure serum Ca^{2+} monthly

May be used alone or in combination w/ vitamin D sterols and/or phosphate binders

Hypercalcemia

In Patients w/ Primary Hyperparathyroidism who are Unable to Undergo Parathyroidectomy and Patients w/ Parathyroid Carcinoma:
Initial: 30mg bid
Titrate: Increase every 2-4 weeks through sequential doses of 30mg bid, 60mg bid, 90mg bid, and 90mg tid-qid as necessary to normalize serum Ca^{2+} levels

Measure serum Ca^{2+} w/in 1 week after initiation/dose adjustment; once maint dose is established, measure serum Ca^{2+} every 2 months

PEDIATRIC DOSAGE

Pediatric use may not have been established

DOSING CONSIDERATIONS

Adverse Reactions

Secondary Hyperparathyroidism in Patients w/ Chronic Kidney Disease on Dialysis:
If serum Ca^{2+} falls <7.5mg/dL, or if hypocalcemia symptoms persist and vitamin D dose cannot be increased, withhold administration until Ca^{2+} levels reach 8.0mg/dL and/or symptoms of hypocalcemia resolve. Treatment should be reinitiated using next lowest dose of cinacalcet

ADMINISTRATION
Oral route

Take whole; do not divide
Take w/ food or shortly after a meal

HOW SUPPLIED
Tab: 30mg, 60mg, 90mg

CONTRAINDICATIONS
Hypocalcemia.

WARNINGS/PRECAUTIONS
Avoid use in patients with CKD not on dialysis. Lowers serum Ca^{2+}; monitor for occurrence of hypocalcemia during treatment. Life-threatening events and fatal outcomes associated with hypocalcemia reported in patients treated with the drug, including pediatric patients. QT prolongation and ventricular arrhythmia secondary to hypocalcemia reported. Seizures reported; monitor serum Ca^{2+}, particularly in patients with history of seizure disorder. Hypotension, worsening HF, and/or arrhythmia reported in patients with impaired cardiac function. Adynamic bone disease may develop with iPTH levels <100pg/mL; reduce dose or d/c therapy if iPTH levels <150pg/mL. Monitor patients with moderate and severe hepatic impairment throughout treatment.

ADVERSE REACTIONS
N/V, diarrhea, myalgia, dizziness, HTN, asthenia, anorexia, paresthesia, fatigue, fracture, hypercalcemia, dehydration, anemia, arthralgia, depression.

DRUG INTERACTIONS
May require dose adjustment with CYP2D6 substrates (eg, desipramine, metoprolol, carvedilol) and particularly those with narrow therapeutic index (eg, flecainide, most TCAs). May require dose adjustment if a patient initiates or discontinues therapy with strong CYP3A4 inhibitors (eg, ketoconazole, itraconazole); closely monitor iPTH and serum Ca^{2+} levels.

PATIENT CONSIDERATIONS

Assessment: Assess for hypocalcemia, history of seizure disorder, hepatic impairment, cardiac function, pregnancy/nursing status, and possible drug interactions. Assess serum Ca^{2+} levels prior to administration.

Monitoring: Monitor for signs/symptoms of hypocalcemia, adynamic bone disease, and other adverse reactions. In patients with impaired cardiac function, monitor for hypotension, worsening HF, and/or arrhythmias. Monitor iPTH/Ca^{2+}/phosphorus levels with moderate and severe hepatic impairment. Monitor serum Ca^{2+} carefully for the occurrence of hypocalcemia during treatment.

Counseling: Inform of the importance of regular blood tests. Advise to report to physician if N/V and potential symptoms of hypocalcemia occur. Advise to report to their physician if taking medication to prevent seizures, have had seizures in the past, and experience any seizure episodes while on therapy. Encourage patients who are nursing during treatment to enroll in Amgen's Lactation Surveillance Program.

STORAGE: 25°C (77°F); excursions permitted to 15-30°C (59-86°F).

SEROQUEL — quetiapine fumarate

RX

Class: Atypical antipsychotic

S

Elderly patients w/ dementia-related psychosis treated w/ antipsychotic drugs are at an increased risk of death. Not approved for the treatment of patients w/ dementia-related psychosis. Antidepressants increased the risk of suicidal thoughts and behavior in children, adolescents, and young adults in short-term studies. Monitor closely for worsening, and for emergence of suicidal thoughts and behaviors in patients who are started on antidepressant therapy. Not approved for use in pediatric patients <10 yrs of age.

ADULT DOSAGE

Schizophrenia

Day 1: 25mg bid
Days 2-3: Increase by 25-50mg divided bid or tid to a range of 300-400mg by Day 4
Titrate: Further adjustments can be made in increments of 25-50mg bid, in intervals of ≥2 days
Recommended Dose: 150-750mg/day
Max: 750mg/day

Maint:
Recommended Dose: 400-800mg/day
Max: 800mg/day

PEDIATRIC DOSAGE

Schizophrenia

13-17 Years:
Day 1: 25mg bid
Day 2: 100mg/day given bid
Day 3: 200mg/day given bid
Day 4: 300mg/day given bid
Day 5: 400mg/day given bid
Titrate: Further adjustments should be in increments ≤100mg/day
Recommended Dose: 400-800mg/day
Max: 800mg/day

May administer tid based on response and tolerability

Switching from Depot Antipsychotics:
Initiate quetiapine therapy in place of the next scheduled inj if medically appropriate

Bipolar I Disorder

Acute Treatment of Manic Episodes:
Monotherapy/Adjunct to Lithium or Divalproex:
Day 1: 100mg/day given bid
Day 2: 200mg/day given bid
Day 3: 300mg/day given bid
Day 4: 400mg/day given bid
Titrate: Further adjustments up to 800mg/day by Day 6 should be in increments of ≤200mg/day
Recommended Dose: 400-800mg/day
Max: 800mg/day

Maint Treatment of Bipolar I Disorder as Adjunct to Lithium or Divalproex:
Recommended Dose: 400-800mg/day given bid
Max: 800mg/day

Bipolar Disorder

Acute Treatment of Depressive Episodes:
Monotherapy:
Day 1: 50mg qhs
Day 2: 100mg qhs
Day 3: 200mg qhs
Day 4: 300mg qhs
Recommended Dose: 300mg/day
Max: 300mg/day

Switching from Depot Antipsychotics:
Initiate quetiapine therapy in place of the next scheduled inj if medically appropriate

Bipolar I Disorder

Acute Treatment of Manic Episodes:
10-17 Years:
Monotherapy:
Day 1: 25mg bid
Day 2: 100mg/day given bid
Day 3: 200mg/day given bid
Day 4: 300mg/day given bid
Day 5: 400mg/day given bid
Titrate: Further adjustments should be in increments ≤100mg/day
Recommended Dose: 400-600mg/day
Max: 600mg/day
May administer tid based on response and tolerability

DOSING CONSIDERATIONS

Concomitant Medications
CYP3A4 Inhibitors:
Reduce quetiapine dose to 1/6 of original dose when coadministered
When CYP3A4 inhibitor is discontinued, increase quetiapine dose by 6-fold

CYP3A4 Inducers:
Increase quetiapine dose up to 5-fold of the original dose when used in combination w/ a chronic treatment (eg, >7-14 days) of a potent CYP3A4 inducer
When CYP3A4 inducer is discontinued, reduce quetiapine dose to original level w/in 7-14 days

Hepatic Impairment
Initial: 25mg/day
Titrate: May increase by 25-50mg/day

Elderly
Initial: 50mg/day
Titrate: May increase by 50mg/day

Other Important Considerations
Debilitated Patients/Predisposed to Hypotension:
Consider slower rate of titration and lower target dose

Reinitiation of Treatment in Patients Previously Discontinued:
Discontinued <1 Week: Reinitiate maint dose
Discontinued >1 Week: Follow initial dosing schedule

ADMINISTRATION

Oral route

Take w/ or w/o food.

HOW SUPPLIED

Tab: 25mg, 50mg, 100mg, 200mg, 300mg, 400mg

CONTRAINDICATIONS

Hypersensitivity to quetiapine or to any excipients in the formulation.

WARNINGS/PRECAUTIONS

Initiate in pediatric patients only after a thorough diagnostic evaluation is conducted and careful consideration is given to the risks of therapy. Neuroleptic malignant syndrome (NMS) reported; d/c and institute symptomatic treatment. Associated w/ metabolic changes that include hyperglycemia/diabetes mellitus (DM), dyslipidemia, and body weight gain. May cause tardive

S

dyskinesia (TD), especially in the elderly; consider discontinuation if this occurs. May induce orthostatic hypotension; caution w/ known cardiovascular/cerebrovascular disease or conditions that predispose patients to hypotension. May increase BP in children and adolescents. Leukopenia, neutropenia, and agranulocytosis reported; d/c at 1st sign of decline in WBC count w/o causative factors in patients w/ preexisting low WBC count or a history of drug induced leukopenia/neutropenia. D/C therapy and follow WBC count until recovery in patients w/ severe neutropenia (ANC <1000/mm^3). Lens changes reported during long-term treatment. May prolong QT interval; avoid in circumstances that may increase the risk of torsades de pointes and/or sudden death. Seizures reported; caution w/ conditions that lower seizure threshold. Decrease in thyroid hormone levels reported; measure TSH and free T4 at baseline and at follow-up in addition to clinical assessment. May elevate prolactin levels. May impair physical/mental abilities. May disrupt body's ability to reduce core body temperature. May cause esophageal dysmotility and aspiration; caution in patients at risk for aspiration pneumonia. Acute withdrawal symptoms (eg, N/V, insomnia) may occur after abrupt cessation; d/c gradually.

ADVERSE REACTIONS

Headache, somnolence, dizziness, dry mouth, constipation, dyspepsia, tachycardia, asthenia, agitation, pain, weight gain, ALT increased, abdominal pain, postural hypotension, N/V.

DRUG INTERACTIONS

See Dosing Considerations. Caution w/ other centrally acting drugs and alcohol. Increased exposure w/ CYP3A4 inhibitors (eg, ketoconazole, ritonavir, nefazodone) and decreased exposure w/ CYP3A4 inducers (eg, phenytoin, carbamazepine, rifampin). May enhance the effects of certain antihypertensives. May antagonize the effects of levodopa and dopamine agonists. QT prolongation reported w/ drugs known to cause electrolyte imbalance. Avoid w/ other drugs that are known to prolong QTc interval (eg, quinidine, amiodarone, ziprasidone). Caution w/ anticholinergic medications.

PATIENT CONSIDERATIONS

Assessment: Assess for history of dementia-related psychosis, risk for hypotension, drug hypersensitivity, psychiatric disorders, hepatic impairment, other conditions where treatment is cautioned, pregnancy/nursing status, and possible drug interactions. Obtain baseline FPG in patients w/ DM or at risk for DM. Obtain baseline CBC if at risk for leukopenia/neutropenia. Obtain baseline TSH and free T4. Obtain baseline BP in children and adolescents. Assess for cataracts by performing lens exam (eg, slit-lamp exam).

Monitoring: Monitor for clinical worsening, suicidality, unusual changes in behavior, NMS, TD, hyperglycemia, orthostatic hypotension, hypothyroidism, seizures, aspiration, and other adverse effects. Monitor CBC frequently during 1st few months in patients w/ preexisting low WBC count or history of drug-induced leukopenia/neutropenia. Monitor for fever or other signs/symptoms of infection in patients w/ neutropenia. Monitor weight regularly, and lipids, hepatic function, and FPG periodically. Monitor for cataract formation shortly after start of treatment, and at 6-month intervals during chronic treatment. Monitor BP periodically during treatment in children and adolescents. Periodically reassess for continued need for maintenance treatment.

Counseling: Inform of the risks and benefits of therapy. Instruct caregivers and patients to contact physician if signs of agitation, anxiety, panic attacks, insomnia, hostility, aggressiveness, impulsivity, akathisia, hypomania, mania, irritability, worsening of depression, changes in behavior, or suicidal ideation develop. Advise about signs/symptoms of NMS, symptoms of hyperglycemia and DM, weight gain, and risk of orthostatic hypotension. Instruct to avoid overheating and dehydration. Caution about performing activities requiring mental alertness. Instruct to notify physician if patient becomes pregnant or intends to become pregnant during therapy, and if patient is taking or plans to take any prescription or OTC drugs.

STORAGE: 25°C (77°F); excursions permitted to 15-30°C (59-86°F).

SEROQUEL XR – quetiapine fumarate

RX

Class: Atypical antipsychotic

Elderly patients w/ dementia-related psychosis treated w/ antipsychotic drugs are at an increased risk of death. Not approved for the treatment of patients w/ dementia-related psychosis. Antidepressants increased the risk of suicidal thoughts and behavior in children, adolescents, and young adults in short-term studies. Monitor closely for worsening, and for emergence of suicidal thoughts and behaviors in patients who are started on antidepressant therapy. Not approved for use in pediatric patients <10 yrs of age.

ADULT DOSAGE

Schizophrenia

Day 1: 300mg/day

Titrate: May increase at intervals as short as 1 day and in increments of up to 300mg/day

PEDIATRIC DOSAGE

Schizophrenia

13-17 Years:

Day 1: 50mg/day

Day 2: 100mg/day

Recommended Dose: 400-800mg/day
Max: 800mg/day

Maint:
Monotherapy:
Recommended Dose: 400-800mg/day
Max: 800mg/day

Bipolar I Disorder

Manic/Mixed Episodes:
Monotherapy or Adjunct to Lithium/ Divalproex:
Day 1: 300mg/day
Day 2: 600mg/day
Day 3 Onward: 400-800mg/day
Max: 800mg/day

Maint:
Adjunct to Lithium/Divalproex:
Recommended Dose: 400-800mg/day
Max: 800mg/day

Bipolar Disorder

Depressive Episodes:
Day 1: 50mg/day
Day 2: 100mg/day
Day 3: 200mg/day
Day 4 Onward: 300mg/day
Max: 300mg/day

Major Depressive Disorder

Adjunct to Antidepressants:
Days 1 & 2: 50mg/day
Day 3: 150mg/day
Recommended Dose: 150-300mg/day
Max: 300mg/day

Conversions

Switching from Immediate-Release to Extended-Release Quetiapine:
Switch at the equivalent total daily dose taken qd

Switching from Depot Antipsychotics:
Initiate quetiapine therapy in place of next scheduled inj if medically appropriate

Day 3: 200mg/day
Day 4: 300mg/day
Day 5: 400mg/day
Recommended Dose: 400-800mg/day
Max: 800mg/day

Bipolar I Disorder

Mania:
10-17 Years:
Monotherapy:
Day 1: 50mg/day
Day 2: 100mg/day
Day 3: 200mg/day
Day 4: 300mg/day
Day 5: 400mg/day
Recommended Dose: 400-600mg/day
Max: 600mg/day

Conversions

Switching from Immediate-Release to Extended-Release Quetiapine:
Switch at the equivalent total daily dose taken qd

Switching from Depot Antipsychotics:
Initiate quetiapine therapy in place of next scheduled inj if medically appropriate

DOSING CONSIDERATIONS

Concomitant Medications

Potent CYP3A4 Inhibitors:
Reduce quetiapine dose to 1/6 of original dose when coadministered
When CYP3A4 inhibitor is discontinued, increase quetiapine dose by 6-fold

Potent CYP3A4 Inducers:
Increase quetiapine dose up to 5-fold of the original dose when used in combination w/ a chronic treatment (eg, >7-14 days) of a potent CYP3A4 inducer
When CYP3A4 inducer is discontinued, reduce quetiapine dose to original level w/in 7-14 days

Hepatic Impairment
Initial: 50mg/day
Titrate: May increase in increments of 50mg/day

Elderly
Initial: 50mg/day
Titrate: May increase in increments of 50mg/day

Other Important Considerations
Debilitated Patients/Predisposed to Hypotension:
Consider slower rate of titration and lower target dose

Reinitiation of Treatment in Patients Previously Discontinued:
Discontinued <1 Week: Reinitiate maint dose
Discontinued >1 Week: Follow initial dosing schedule

ADMINISTRATION

Oral route

S

Swallow tab whole; do not split, crush, or chew
Take w/o food or w/ a light meal (approx 300 calories)
Administer qd, preferably in the pm

HOW SUPPLIED

Tab, Extended-Release: 50mg, 150mg, 200mg, 300mg, 400mg

CONTRAINDICATIONS

Hypersensitivity to quetiapine or to any excipients in the formulation.

WARNINGS/PRECAUTIONS

Initiate in pediatric patients only after a thorough diagnostic evaluation is conducted and careful consideration is given to the risks of therapy. Neuroleptic malignant syndrome (NMS) reported; d/c and institute symptomatic treatment. Associated w/ metabolic changes that include hyperglycemia/diabetes mellitus (DM), dyslipidemia, and body weight gain. May cause tardive dyskinesia (TD), especially in the elderly; consider discontinuation if this occurs. May induce orthostatic hypotension; caution w/ known cardiovascular/cerebrovascular disease or conditions which predispose patients to hypotension. May increase BP in children and adolescents. Leukopenia, neutropenia, and agranulocytosis reported; d/c at 1st sign of decline in WBC count w/o causative factors. D/C therapy and follow WBC count until recovery in patients w/ severe neutropenia (ANC <1000/mm^3). Lens changes reported during long-term treatment. May prolong QT interval; avoid in circumstances that may increase the risk of torsades de pointes and/or sudden death. Seizures reported; caution w/ conditions that lower seizure threshold. Decrease in thyroid hormone levels reported; measure TSH and free T4 at baseline and at follow-up in addition to clinical assessment. May elevate prolactin levels. May impair physical/mental abilities. May disrupt body's ability to reduce core body temperature. May cause esophageal dysmotility and aspiration; caution in patients at risk for aspiration pneumonia. Acute withdrawal symptoms (eg, N/V, insomnia) may occur after abrupt cessation; d/c gradually.

ADVERSE REACTIONS

Dry mouth, constipation, dyspepsia, somnolence, dizziness, orthostatic hypotension, weight gain, fatigue, dysarthria, nasal congestion, extrapyramidal symptoms, increased appetite, increased heart rate, N/V, irritability.

DRUG INTERACTIONS

See Dosing Considerations. Caution w/ other centrally acting drugs and alcohol. Increased exposure w/ CYP3A4 inhibitors (eg, ketoconazole, ritonavir, nefazodone) and decreased exposure w/ CYP3A4 inducers (eg, phenytoin, carbamazepine, rifampin). May enhance the effects of certain antihypertensives. May antagonize the effects of levodopa and dopamine agonists. QT prolongation reported w/ drugs known to cause electrolyte imbalance. Avoid w/ other drugs that are known to prolong QTc interval (eg, quinidine, amiodarone, ziprasidone). Caution w/ anticholinergic medications.

PATIENT CONSIDERATIONS

Assessment: Assess for history of dementia-related psychosis, risk for hypotension, drug hypersensitivity, psychiatric disorders, hepatic impairment, other conditions where treatment is cautioned, pregnancy/nursing status, and possible drug interactions. Obtain baseline FPG in patients w/ DM or at risk for DM. Obtain baseline CBC if at risk for leukopenia/neutropenia. Obtain baseline TSH and free T4. Obtain baseline BP in children and adolescents. Assess for cataracts by performing lens exam (eg, slit-lamp exam).

Monitoring: Monitor for clinical worsening, suicidality, unusual changes in behavior, NMS, TD, hyperglycemia, orthostatic hypotension, hypothyroidism, seizures, aspiration, and other adverse effects. Monitor CBC frequently during 1st few months in patients w/ preexisting low WBC count or history of drug-induced leukopenia/neutropenia. Monitor for fever or other signs/symptoms of infection in patients w/ neutropenia. Monitor weight regularly, and lipids, hepatic function, and FPG periodically. Monitor for cataract formation shortly after start of treatment, and at 6-month intervals during chronic treatment. Monitor BP periodically during treatment in children and adolescents. Periodically reassess for continued need for maintenance treatment.

Counseling: Inform of the risks and benefits of therapy. Instruct caregivers and patients to contact physician if signs of agitation, anxiety, panic attacks, insomnia, hostility, aggressiveness, impulsivity, akathisia, hypomania, mania, irritability, worsening of depression, changes in behavior, or suicidal ideation develop. Advise about signs/symptoms of NMS, symptoms of hyperglycemia and DM, weight gain, or risk of orthostatic hypotension. Instruct to avoid overheating and dehydration. Caution about performing activities requiring mental alertness. Instruct to notify physician if patient becomes pregnant or intends to become pregnant during therapy, and if patient is taking or plans to take any prescription or OTC drugs.

STORAGE: 25°C (77°F); excursions permitted to 15-30°C (59-86°F).

SILENOR – doxepin

Class: H_1 antagonist

RX

ADULT DOSAGE

Insomnia

Difficulty w/ Sleep Maint:

Initial: 6mg qd w/in 30 min of hs; may use 3mg qd if clinically indicated
Max: 6mg/day

PEDIATRIC DOSAGE

Pediatric use may not have been established

DOSING CONSIDERATIONS

Concomitant Medications
Cimetidine:
Max: 3mg

Hepatic Impairment
Initial: 3mg

Elderly
≥65 Years:
Initial: 3mg qd; may increase to 6mg

ADMINISTRATION

Oral route

Do not take w/in 3 hrs of a meal

HOW SUPPLIED

Tab: 3mg, 6mg

CONTRAINDICATIONS

Hypersensitivity to doxepin HCl, any of its inactive ingredients, or other dibenzoxepines; untreated narrow angle glaucoma; severe urinary retention; administration w/ or w/in 2 weeks of MAOIs.

WARNINGS/PRECAUTIONS

Evaluate comorbid diagnoses prior to initiation of treatment. Failure of remission after 7-10 days may indicate the presence of primary psychiatric and/or medical illness that should be evaluated. Complex behaviors (eg, sleep-driving), amnesia, anxiety, and other neuropsychiatric symptoms reported; consider discontinuation if sleep-driving episode occurs. Worsening of depression reported. May impair physical/mental abilities. Caution in patients w/ compromised respiratory function. Avoid in patients w/ severe sleep apnea.

ADVERSE REACTIONS

Somnolence/sedation, URTI/nasopharyngitis, HTN.

DRUG INTERACTIONS

See Contraindications and Dosing Considerations. Sedative effects of alcohol, CNS depressants, and sedating antihistamines may be potentiated w/ concomitant use. Increased exposure w/ inhibitors of CYP2C19, CYP2D6, CYP1A2, and CYP2C9. Exposure doubled w/ cimetidine. Hypoglycemia reported when therapy added to tolazamide regimen.

PATIENT CONSIDERATIONS

Assessment: Assess for drug hypersensitivity, untreated narrow-angle glaucoma, urinary retention, presence of a primary psychiatric and/or medical illness that may cause insomnia, depression, hepatic impairment, sleep apnea, pregnancy/nursing status, and possible drug interactions.

Monitoring: Monitor for treatment response, complex behaviors/neuropsychiatric symptoms, worsening of depression, and other adverse reactions.

Counseling: Inform of benefits and risks associated w/ therapy. Counsel on appropriate use of medication. Instruct to contact physician if sleep-driving occurs or if patient performs other complex behaviors while not fully awake. Instruct to seek medical attention if symptoms of cognitive or behavioral abnormalities or if worsening of insomnia occurs. Inform that medication may cause sedation; caution against operating machinery (eg, automobiles) during therapy. Advise to avoid alcohol consumption during therapy.

STORAGE: 20-25°C (68-77°F). Protect from light.

SILVADENE – silver sulfadiazine

RX

Class: Sulfonamide

OTHER BRAND NAMES

SSD

ADULT DOSAGE

Burns

Adjunct for the Prevention and Treatment of Wound Sepsis in Patients w/ 2nd- and 3rd-Degree Burns:

Apply qd-bid to a thickness of approx 1/16 inch

Whenever necessary, reapply to any areas from which it has been removed due to patient activity

Reapply immediately after hydrotherapy

Continue treatment until satisfactory healing has occurred or until the burn site is ready for grafting; do not withdraw from therapeutic regimen while there remains possibility of infection, except if a significant adverse reaction occurs

PEDIATRIC DOSAGE

Pediatric use may not have been established

ADMINISTRATION

Topical route

Cleanse and debride burn wounds prior to application, under sterile conditions.
Burn areas should be covered w/ cre at all times.
Dressings are not required, however if individual patient requirements make dressings necessary, they may be used.

HOW SUPPLIED

Cre: 1% [50g, 400g, 1000g (jar); 20g, 25g, 50g, 85g (tube)]; (SSD) 1% [50g, 400g (jar); 25g, 50g, 85g (tube)]

CONTRAINDICATIONS

Hypersensitivity to silver sulfadiazine or any of the other ingredients in the preparation. Pregnant women approaching or at term, premature infants, newborn infants during the first 2 months of life.

WARNINGS/PRECAUTIONS

Potential cross-sensitivity w/ other sulfonamides; if allergic reactions attributable to treatment occur, weigh continuation of therapy against potential hazards of the particular allergic reaction. Fungal proliferation in and below the eschar may occur. Caution w/ G6PD deficiency; hemolysis may occur. Drug accumulation may occur if hepatic and renal functions become impaired and elimination of drug decreases; weigh discontinuation of therapy against the therapeutic benefit being achieved. In the treatment of burn wounds involving extensive areas of the body, serum sulfa concentrations may approach adult therapeutic levels (8-12mg%); monitor serum sulfa concentrations in these patients. Monitor renal function and check urine for sulfa crystals. Lab test interactions may occur. Adverse reactions associated w/ sulfonamides (eg, blood dyscrasias, dermatologic and allergic reactions, GI reactions, hepatitis and hepatocellular necrosis, CNS reactions, toxic nephrosis) may occur.

ADVERSE REACTIONS

Transient leukopenia, skin necrosis, erythema multiforme, skin discoloration, burning sensation, rash, interstitial nephritis.

DRUG INTERACTIONS

May inactivate topical proteolytic enzymes.

PATIENT CONSIDERATIONS

Assessment: Assess for hypersensitivity to drug, G6PD deficiency, renal/hepatic impairment, pregnancy/nursing status, and possible drug interactions.

Monitoring: Monitor for allergic reactions, fungal proliferation, renal/hepatic dysfunction, and other adverse reactions. Check urine for sulfa crystals. Monitor serum sulfa concentrations in patients w/ wounds involving extensive areas of the body.

Counseling: Inform of the risks and benefits of therapy. Instruct to use ud. Advise to notify physician if adverse reactions occur.

STORAGE: 20-25°C (68-77°F). **SSD:** 15-30°C (59-86°F).

SIMBRINZA – brimonidine tartrate/brinzolamide

RX

Class: $Alpha_2$ agonist/carbonic anhydrase inhibitor

ADULT DOSAGE

Elevated Intraocular Pressure

Open-Angle Glaucoma/Ocular HTN:
1 drop in the affected eye(s) tid

PEDIATRIC DOSAGE

Elevated Intraocular Pressure

Open-Angle Glaucoma/Ocular HTN:
≥2 Years:
1 drop in the affected eye(s) tid

DOSING CONSIDERATIONS

Concomitant Medications

If >1 topical ophthalmic drug is being used, administer drugs at least 5 min apart

ADMINISTRATION

Ocular route

Shake well before use.

HOW SUPPLIED

Ophthalmic Sus: (Brinzolamide/Brimonidine) 1%/0.2% [8mL]

CONTRAINDICATIONS

Hypersensitivity to any component of this product, neonates and infants (<2 yrs of age).

WARNINGS/PRECAUTIONS

Caution w/ low endothelial cell counts; increased potential for corneal edema. Not recommended w/ severe renal impairment (CrCl <30mL/min). Contains benzalkonium chloride, which may be absorbed by soft contact lenses; contact lenses should be removed during instillation, but may be reinserted 15 min after instillation. Caution w/ severe cardiovascular disease (CVD), severe hepatic impairment, depression, cerebral or coronary insufficiency, Raynaud's phenomenon, orthostatic hypotension, or thromboangiitis obliterans. Bacterial keratitis reported w/ multidose containers. **Brinzolamide:** Systemically absorbed. Fatalities occurred due to severe reactions to sulfonamides, including Stevens-Johnson syndrome, toxic epidermal necrolysis, fulminant hepatic necrosis, agranulocytosis, aplastic anemia, and other blood dyscrasias. Sensitization may recur when a sulfonamide is readministered irrespective of route. D/C if signs of serious reactions or hypersensitivity occur.

ADVERSE REACTIONS

Blurred vision, eye irritation, dysgeusia, dry mouth, eye allergy.

DRUG INTERACTIONS

Potential additive systemic effects w/ oral carbonic anhydrase inhibitors; coadministration is not recommended. Acid-base alterations reported w/ high-dose salicylate therapy in patients treated w/ oral carbonic anhydrase inhibitors. Possible additive or potentiating effect w/ CNS depressants (eg, alcohol, opiates, barbiturates, sedatives, anesthetics). Caution w/ antihypertensives and/or cardiac glycosides. Caution w/ TCAs and MAOIs, which can affect the metabolism and uptake of circulating amines.

PATIENT CONSIDERATIONS

Assessment: Assess for hypersensitivity to drug or to sulfonamides, low endothelial cell counts, renal/hepatic impairment, contact lens use, severe CVD, depression, cerebral or coronary insufficiency, Raynaud's phenomenon, orthostatic hypotension, thromboangiitis obliterans, pregnancy/nursing status, and possible drug interactions.

Monitoring: Monitor for sulfonamide hypersensitivity reactions, potentiation of syndromes associated w/ vascular insufficiency, bacterial keratitis, and other adverse reactions.

Counseling: Advise to d/c use and consult physician if serious or unusual ocular or systemic reactions or signs of hypersensitivity occur. Inform that vision may be temporarily blurred following dosing and fatigue and/or drowsiness may be experienced; instruct to use caution in operating machinery, driving a motor vehicle, and engaging in other hazardous activities. Instruct that ocular sol, if handled improperly or if the tip of dispensing container contacts the eye or surrounding structures, can become contaminated by common bacteria known to cause ocular infections. Advise that using contaminated sol may result in serious eye damage and subsequent loss of vision. Instruct to always replace cap after using. Advise not to use if sol changes color or becomes cloudy. Instruct to consult physician about the continued use of the present multidose container if having ocular surgery or if an intercurrent ocular condition (eg, trauma, infection) develops. If using >1 topical ophthalmic drug, instruct to administer the drugs at least 5 min apart. Advise that contact lenses should be removed during instillation, but may be reinserted 15 min after instillation.

STORAGE: 2-25°C (36-77°F).

SIMCOR – niacin/simvastatin

RX

Class: HMG-CoA reductase inhibitor (statin)/nicotinic acid

ADULT DOSAGE

Hypertriglyceridemia

Not Currently on Niacin ER or Switching from Non-ER Niacin:
Initial: 500mg/20mg qd at hs
Titrate (Niacin ER Component): Increase by no more than 500mg qd every 4 weeks; after Week 8, titrate to patient response and tolerance
Maint: 1000mg/20mg to 2000mg/40mg qd depending on tolerability and lipid levels
Max: 2000mg/40mg qd

If discontinued for >7 days, retitrate as tolerated

Additional Lipid Level Management Needed Despite Simvastatin 20-40mg Only:
Initial: 500mg/40mg qd at hs

Primary Hypercholesterolemia/Mixed Dyslipidemia

Not Currently on Niacin ER or Switching from Non-ER Niacin:
Initial: 500mg/20mg qd at hs
Titrate (Niacin ER Component): Increase by no more than 500mg qd every 4 weeks; after Week 8, titrate to patient response and tolerance
Maint: 1000mg/20mg to 2000mg/40mg qd depending on tolerability and lipid levels
Max: 2000mg/40mg qd

If discontinued for >7 days, retitrate as tolerated

Additional Lipid Level Management Needed Despite Simvastatin 20-40mg Only:
Initial: 500mg/40mg qd at hs

PEDIATRIC DOSAGE

Pediatric use may not have been established

DOSING CONSIDERATIONS

Concomitant Medications
Amiodarone, Amlodipine, or Ranolazine:
Max: 1000mg/20mg/day

Renal Impairment
Severe:
Do not start unless already tolerated ≥10mg simvastatin

S

Other Important Considerations
Chinese Patients:
Caution w/ doses >1000mg/20mg/day

ADMINISTRATION

Oral route

Take at hs w/ a low-fat snack
Swallow whole; do not break, crush, or chew
Avoid administration on an empty stomach to reduce flushing, pruritus, and GI distress
May take aspirin (up to 325mg) 30 min prior to treatment to reduce flushing

HOW SUPPLIED

Tab: (Niacin ER/Simvastatin) 500mg/20mg, 500mg/40mg, 750mg/20mg, 1000mg/20mg, 1000mg/40mg

CONTRAINDICATIONS

Active liver disease or unexplained persistent elevations in hepatic transaminase levels, active peptic ulcer disease (PUD), arterial bleeding, women who are or may become pregnant, and nursing mothers. Concomitant administration with strong CYP3A4 inhibitors (eg, itraconazole, ketoconazole, posaconazole, HIV protease inhibitors, boceprevir, telaprevir, erythromycin, clarithromycin, telithromycin, nefazodone), gemfibrozil, cyclosporine, danazol, verapamil, or diltiazem. Known hypersensitivity to any component of this product.

WARNINGS/PRECAUTIONS

No incremental benefit of Simcor on cardiovascular (CV) morbidity and mortality over and above that demonstrated for simvastatin monotherapy and niacin monotherapy has been established. Niacin ER, at doses of 1500-2000mg/day, in combination with simvastatin, did not reduce the incidence of CV events more than simvastatin in patients with CV disease and mean baseline LDL levels of 74mg/dL. Should be substituted only for equivalent doses of niacin ER (Niaspan); do not substitute for equivalent doses of IR (crystalline) niacin. Dose-related myopathy and/or rhabdomyolysis reported; predisposing factors include advanced age (≥65 yrs of age), female gender, uncontrolled hypothyroidism, and renal impairment. Immune-mediated necrotizing myopathy (IMNM) reported. D/C if markedly elevated CPK levels occur or myopathy is diagnosed/suspected, and temporarily withhold in any patient experiencing an acute or serious condition predisposing to development of renal failure secondary to rhabdomyolysis. Stop treatment for a few days before elective major surgery and when any major acute medical/surgical condition supervenes. Severe hepatic toxicity, including fulminant hepatic necrosis, reported when substituting sustained-release niacin for IR niacin at equivalent doses. Caution with substantial alcohol consumption and/or history of liver disease. May cause abnormal LFTs; obtain LFTs prior to initiation and repeat as clinically indicated. Fatal and nonfatal hepatic failure (rare) reported; promptly interrupt therapy if serious liver injury with clinical symptoms and/or hyperbilirubinemia or jaundice occurs and do not restart if no alternate etiology found. Increases in HbA1c and FPG levels reported; closely monitor diabetic/potentially diabetic patients (particularly during 1st few months of therapy), and adjust diet and/or hypoglycemic therapy or d/c Simcor if necessary. May reduce platelet count or phosphorus (P) levels, and increase PT or uric acid levels. Caution in patients predisposed to gout, with renal impairment, and in elderly.

ADVERSE REACTIONS

Flushing, headache, back pain, diarrhea, nausea, pruritus.

DRUG INTERACTIONS

See Contraindications. Avoid ingestion of alcohol, hot drinks, or spicy foods around the time of administration; may increase flushing and pruritus. Simvastatin: Due to the risk of myopathy, avoid with large quantities of grapefruit juice (>1 quart/day) and drugs that cause myopathy/rhabdomyolysis when given alone (eg, fibrates); caution with colchicine; do not exceed 1000mg/20mg/day with amiodarone, amlodipine, and ranolazine. Voriconazole may increase concentration; consider dose adjustment of Simcor to reduce risk of myopathy/rhabdomyolysis. Decreased C_{max} with propranolol. May increase digoxin concentrations; monitor patients taking digoxin when therapy is initiated. May potentiate effect of coumarin anticoagulants; determine PT before initiation and frequently during therapy. Niacin: ASA may decrease metabolic clearance. May potentiate effects of ganglionic blocking agents and vasoactive drugs, resulting in postural hypotension. Separate administration from bile acid-binding resins (eg, colestipol, cholestyramine) by at least 4-6 hrs. Nutritional supplements containing large doses of niacin or related compounds may potentiate adverse effects.

PATIENT CONSIDERATIONS

Assessment: Assess for history of/active liver disease, unexplained persistent hepatic transaminase elevations, active PUD, arterial bleeding, predisposing factors for myopathy, renal impairment, diabetes, any other conditions where treatment is contraindicated or cautioned, drug hypersensitivity, pregnancy/nursing status, and possible drug interactions. Assess lipid profile and LFTs.

Monitoring: Monitor for signs/symptoms of myopathy (including IMNM), rhabdomyolysis, liver/renal dysfunction, decreases in platelet counts and P levels, increases in PT and uric acid levels, and other adverse reactions. Monitor lipid profile, LFTs, blood glucose, and CPK levels. Check PT with coumarin anticoagulants.

Counseling: Advise to adhere to their National Cholesterol Education Program-recommended diet, a regular exercise program, and periodic testing of a fasting lipid panel. Inform about substances that should be avoided during therapy, and advise to discuss all medications, both prescription and OTC, including vitamins or other nutritional supplements containing niacin or nicotinamide, with their physician. Instruct to report promptly any unexplained muscle pain, tenderness, or weakness, particularly if accompanied by malaise or fever or if these muscle signs or symptoms persist after discontinuation, any symptoms that may indicate liver injury, or if symptoms of dizziness occur. Advise to notify physician prior to restarting therapy if dosing is interrupted for any length of time, and of changes in blood glucose if diabetic. Inform that flushing may occur but may subside after several weeks of consistent use of therapy. If awakened by flushing at night, instruct to get up slowly, especially if feeling dizzy or faint, or taking BP medications. Instruct women to use an effective method of birth control to prevent pregnancy while on therapy, to d/c therapy and call physician if pregnant, and not to breastfeed while on therapy.

STORAGE: 20-25°C (68-77°F).

SIMPONI ARIA – golimumab

RX

Class: Monoclonal antibody/TNF blocker

Increased risk for developing serious infections (eg, active tuberculosis [TB], latent TB reactivation, invasive fungal infections, bacterial/viral infections, and opportunistic infections) leading to hospitalization or death, mostly w/ concomitant use w/ immunosuppressants (eg, methotrexate [MTX] or corticosteroids). D/C if serious infection develops. Active/latent reactivation TB may present w/ disseminated or extrapulmonary disease; test for latent TB before and during therapy and initiate treatment for latent TB prior to therapy. Invasive fungal infections reported; consider empiric antifungal therapy in patients at risk who develop severe systemic illness. Consider risks and benefits prior to therapy in patients w/ chronic or recurrent infection. Monitor patients for development of infection during and after treatment, including development of TB in patients who tested (-) for latent TB infection prior to therapy. Lymphoma and other malignancies, some fatal, reported in children and adolescents.

ADULT DOSAGE

Rheumatoid Arthritis

Moderately to Severely Active in Combination w/ MTX:

2mg/kg IV infusion over 30 min at Weeks 0 and 4, then every 8 weeks thereafter

May continue other non-biologic disease-modifying antirheumatic drugs (DMARDs), corticosteroids, NSAIDs, and/or analgesics during treatment

PEDIATRIC DOSAGE

Pediatric use may not have been established

ADMINISTRATION

IV route

Dilute w/ 0.9% w/v NaCl to a final volume of 100mL. Gently mix.

Use only an infusion set w/ an in-line, sterile, non-pyrogenic, low protein-binding filter (pore size 0.22μM or less).

Do not infuse concomitantly in the same IV line w/ other agents.

Infuse diluted sol over 30 min.

Once diluted, may store infusion sol for 4 hrs at room temperature.

Refer to PI for further administration instructions.

HOW SUPPLIED

Inj: 50mg/4mL

WARNINGS/PRECAUTIONS

Do not initiate in patients w/ an active infection. Increased risk of infection in patients >65 yrs of age and in patients w/ comorbid conditions; consider the risks and benefits prior to therapy in patients who have resided or traveled in areas of endemic TB or endemic mycoses, and w/ any underlying conditions predisposing to infection. D/C if an opportunistic infection or sepsis develops. Hepatitis B virus (HBV) reactivation reported in chronic carriers; closely monitor for signs of active HBV infection during and for several months after therapy. D/C if reactivation occurs and initiate antiviral therapy. Consider risks and benefits prior to initiating therapy in patients w/ a known malignancy other than a successfully treated non-melanoma skin cancer or when considering continuing therapy in patients who develop a malignancy. Cases of acute/chronic leukemia, melanoma, and Merkel cell carcinoma reported. Rare postmarketing cases of hepatosplenic T-cell lymphoma reported, and nearly all of the cases occurred in patients w/ Crohn's disease or ulcerative colitis and mostly in adolescent and young adult males; almost all of these patients were treated concomitantly w/ azathioprine or 6-mercaptopurine. Worsening and new onset CHF reported; caution w/ CHF and d/c if new/worsening symptoms appear. Associated w/ rare cases of new onset or exacerbation of CNS demyelinating disorders (eg, multiple sclerosis) and peripheral demyelinating disorders (eg, Guillain-Barre syndrome); consider discontinuation if these disorders develop. May result in the formation of antinuclear antibodies and, rarely, in the development of a lupus-like syndrome; d/c treatment if symptoms suggestive of a lupus-like syndrome develop. Caution when switching from one biologic DMARD to another; overlapping biological activity may further increase risk of infection. Pancytopenia, leukopenia, neutropenia, aplastic anemia, and thrombocytopenia reported; caution in patients who have or have had significant cytopenias. Serious systemic hypersensitivity reactions may occur; d/c immediately and institute appropriate therapy if these reactions occur. Caution in elderly.

ADVERSE REACTIONS

URTI, viral infections, bronchitis, HTN, rash.

DRUG INTERACTIONS

See Boxed Warning. MTX decreases clearance. Not recommended w/ anakinra, abatacept, or biologics approved to treat rheumatoid arthritis; may increase risk of serious infections. Avoid w/ live vaccines and therapeutic infectious agents (eg, live attenuated bacteria [eg, bacille Calmette-

Guerin bladder instillation for the treatment of cancer]). Avoid administration of live vaccines to infants for 6 months following the mother's last golimumab infusion during pregnancy. Upon initiation or discontinuation of therapy in patients being treated w/ CYP450 substrates w/ a narrow therapeutic index, monitor effect (eg, warfarin) or drug concentration (eg, cyclosporine, theophylline) and adjust individual dose of the drug product as needed.

PATIENT CONSIDERATIONS

Assessment: Assess for active/chronic/recurrent infection, history of an opportunistic infection, recent travel to areas of endemic TB or endemic mycoses, underlying conditions that may predispose to infection, malignancies, CHF, demyelinating disorders, significant cytopenias, risk factors for skin cancer, pregnancy/nursing status, and possible drug interactions. Test for latent TB infection and for HBV infection.

Monitoring: Monitor for development of infection during and after treatment. Monitor for HBV reactivation, malignancies, new or worsening CHF, demyelinating disorders, hematological events, hypersensitivity reactions, and other adverse reactions. Periodically evaluate for active TB and test for latent TB infection. Perform periodic skin examination, particularly in patients w/ risk factors for skin cancer.

Counseling: Advise of the potential risks and benefits of therapy. Inform that therapy may lower the ability of immune system to fight infections; instruct to contact physician if any symptoms of infection develop. Counsel about the risk of lymphoma and other malignancies. Advise to report any signs of new/worsening medical conditions (eg, CHF, demyelinating disorders, autoimmune diseases, liver disease, cytopenias, psoriasis).

STORAGE: 2-8°C (36-46°F). Protect from light. Do not freeze or shake.

SINEMET CR – carbidopa/levodopa

RX

Class: Dopa-decarboxylase inhibitor/dopamine precursor

OTHER BRAND NAMES

Sinemet

ADULT DOSAGE

Parkinsonism

Treatment of Parkinson's Disease, Postencephalitic Parkinsonism, and Symptomatic Parkinsonism Following Carbon Monoxide/Manganese Intoxication:

Tab:

Usual Dose:

Initial: One 25mg/100mg tab tid or one 10mg/100mg tab tid-qid

Titrate: May increase by 1 tab (25mg/100mg or 10mg/100mg) qd or qod, as necessary, until a dose of 8 tabs/day is reached

Transfer from Levodopa:

D/C levodopa at least 12 hrs before starting therapy; choose a daily dose of therapy that will provide approx 25% of the previous levodopa dose

Previously Taking <1500mg/day of Levodopa:

Initial: One 25mg/100mg tab tid or qid

Previously Taking >1500mg/day of Levodopa:

Initial: One 25mg/250mg tab tid or qid

Maint:

At least 70-100mg/day of carbidopa should be provided; may substitute one 25mg/100mg tab for each 10mg/100mg tab when greater proportion of carbidopa is required

When more levodopa is required, substitute 25mg/250mg tab for 25mg/100mg or 10mg/100mg; may increase dose of 25mg/250mg by 1/2 or 1 tab qd or qod to a max of 8 tabs/day if necessary

Max: 200mg/day of carbidopa

PEDIATRIC DOSAGE

Pediatric use may not have been established

S

Tab, Sustained-Release (SR):
Initial Dosage:
Currently Treated w/ Conventional Carbidopa Levodopa Preparations:
Dosage w/ SR tabs should be substituted at an amount that provides approx 10% more levodopa per day. May need to increase to a dose that provides up to 30% more levodopa per day depending on clinical response; interval between doses should be 4-8 hrs during the waking day
Initial Conversion from IR to SR Tabs (Based on Levodopa Component):
300-400mg: 200mg bid
500-600mg: 300mg bid or 200mg tid
700-800mg: Total of 800mg in ≥3 divided doses (eg, 300mg am, 300mg early pm, and 200mg later pm)
900-1000mg: Total of 1000mg in ≥3 divided doses (eg, 400mg am, 400mg early pm, and 200mg later pm)
Currently Treated w/ Levodopa w/o a Decarboxylase Inhibitor:
D/C levodopa at least 12 hrs before starting therapy; substitute at a dose that will provide approx 25% of the previous levodopa dose
Mild to Moderate Disease:
Initial: One 50mg/200mg tab bid
Patients Not Receiving Levodopa:
Mild to Moderate Disease:
Initial: One 50mg/200mg tab bid at ≥6-hr intervals
Titration:
Following therapy initiation, may increase/decrease doses and dosing intervals depending on response
Most patients have been adequately treated w/ doses that provide 400-1600mg/day of levodopa given in divided doses at 4- to 8-hr intervals during the waking day
When given at intervals of <4 hrs, and/or if the divided doses are not equal, give the smaller doses at the end of the day
An interval of at least 3 days between dosage adjustments is recommended

DOSING CONSIDERATIONS
Concomitant Medications
Addition of Other Antiparkinsonian Medications:
Tab/Tab, SR:
Standard drugs for Parkinson's disease, other than levodopa w/o a decarboxylase inhibitor, may be used concomitantly w/ therapy, although their dosage may have to be adjusted
Tab, SR:
Anticholinergic agents, dopamine agonists, and amantadine may be given w/ therapy; dosage adjustment of therapy may be necessary when these agents are added
A dose of 25mg/100mg IR or 10mg/100mg IR (1/2 tab or whole tab) may be added to the dosage regimen in selected patients w/ advanced disease who need additional IR levodopa for a brief time during daytime hrs
Interruption of Therapy:
Tab/Tab, SR:
If general anesthesia is required, may continue therapy as long as patient is permitted to take fluids and medication by mouth. If therapy is interrupted temporarily, observe for symptoms resembling neuroleptic malignant syndrome and administer usual daily dose as soon as patient is able to take oral medication
Adverse Reactions
Tab:
Involuntary movements may require dosage reduction

ADMINISTRATION
Oral route

Tab
Tabs w/ different ratios of carbidopa to levodopa may be given separately or combined as needed to provide the optimum dosage

Tab, SR
Do not chew or crush

HOW SUPPLIED
(Carbidopa/Levodopa) **Tab, SR (CR):** 25mg/100mg, 50mg/200mg; (Sinemet) **Tab:** 10mg/100mg, 25mg/100mg, 25mg/250mg

CONTRAINDICATIONS
During or within 2 weeks of using nonselective MAOIs. Narrow-angle glaucoma, known hypersensitivity to any component of this drug.

WARNINGS/PRECAUTIONS
May cause or increase dyskinesias; may require dose reduction. Monitor for depression with concomitant suicidal tendencies. Caution with severe cardiovascular (CV) or pulmonary disease, bronchial asthma, renal/hepatic/endocrine disease, chronic wide-angle glaucoma, or history of MI with residual atrial, nodal, or ventricular arrhythmias. May increase the possibility of upper GI hemorrhage in patients with history of peptic ulcer. Falling asleep during activities of daily living and somnolence reported; consider discontinuation if significant daytime sleepiness or episodes of falling asleep during activities that require active participation occur. May impair mental/physical abilities. Sporadic cases of a symptom complex resembling neuroleptic malignant syndrome (hyperpyrexia and confusion) reported during dose reductions or withdrawal; observed carefully when the dosage of levodopa is reduced abruptly or discontinued, especially if the patient is receiving neuroleptics. Hallucinations and psychotic-like behavior reported; do not use in patients with a major psychotic disorder. Intense urge to gamble, increased sexual urges, intense urges to spend money, binge eating, and/or other intense urges, and the inability to control these urges may occur; consider dose reduction or discontinuation if such urges develop. Monitor for melanomas frequently and on a regular basis. Abnormalities in lab tests, including elevations of LFTs, and abnormalities in BUN and (+) Coombs test reported. Lab test interactions may occur. Cases of falsely diagnosed pheochromocytoma reported very rarely; caution when interpreting the plasma and urine levels of catecholamines and their metabolites. Caution in elderly.

ADVERSE REACTIONS
Dyskinesias (eg, choreiform, dystonic, other involuntary movements), nausea, hallucinations, confusion.

DRUG INTERACTIONS
See Contraindications. Caution with concomitant use of sedating medications; may increase the risk for somnolence. Certain medications used to treat psychosis may exacerbate the symptoms of Parkinson's disease and may decrease effectiveness of carbidopa-levodopa. Symptomatic postural hypotension reported with concomitant use of some antihypertensive drugs; dosage adjustment of the antihypertensive drug may be required. Use with selegiline may cause severe orthostatic hypotension. Adverse reactions, including HTN and dyskinesia, reported rarely with TCAs. Dopamine D_2 receptor antagonists (eg, phenothiazines, butyrophenones, risperidone) and isoniazid may reduce effects of levodopa. Beneficial effects of levodopa in Parkinson's disease reported to be reversed by phenytoin and papaverine; monitor for loss of therapeutic response. Not recommended with dopamine-depleting agents (eg, reserpine, tetrabenazine) or other drugs known to deplete monoamine stores. Iron salts may reduce bioavailability; caution with iron salts or multivitamins containing iron salts. Metoclopramide may increase bioavailability of levodopa and may also adversely affect disease control.

PATIENT CONSIDERATIONS

Assessment: Assess for hypersensitivity to drug; narrow-angle/chronic wide-angle glaucoma; major psychotic disorder; history of peptic ulcer; risk factors that may increase risk for somnolence (eg, presence of sleep disorders); severe CV or pulmonary disease; bronchial asthma; renal/hepatic/endocrine disease; history of MI with residual atrial, nodal, or ventricular arrhythmias; pregnancy/nursing status; and possible drug interactions.

Monitoring: Monitor for dyskinesias, depression with suicidal tendencies, drowsiness/sleepiness, somnolence, hyperpyrexia and confusion, hallucinations/psychotic-like behavior, impulse control/compulsive behaviors, upper GI hemorrhage in patients with a history of peptic ulcer, and other adverse reactions. In patients with a history of MI who have residual atrial, nodal, or ventricular arrhythmias, monitor cardiac function with particular care during the period of initial dosage adjustment. Monitor for LFT elevations and BUN abnormalities. For patients on extended therapy, perform periodic evaluation of hepatic, hematopoietic, CV, and renal function. Monitor for melanomas frequently and on a regular basis. Monitor for changes in intraocular pressure in patients with chronic wide-angle glaucoma. Monitor closely during the dose adjustment period.

Counseling: Instruct to take ud and not to change the prescribed dosage regimen or add any additional antiparkinson medications, including other carbidopa-levodopa preparations, without 1st consulting the physician. Inform that, occasionally, dark color (red, brown, or black) may appear in saliva, urine, or sweat after ingestion of therapy. Inform that high protein diet, excessive acidity, and iron salts may reduce clinical effectiveness. Instruct to exercise caution while driving or operating machinery, and that if somnolence and/or sudden sleep onset is experienced, to refrain from these activities. Instruct to inform physician if new/increased gambling urges, increased sexual urges, or other intense urges develop. (Tab, IR) Advise that sometimes a "wearing-off" effect may occur at the end of the dosing interval; instruct to notify physician if such response poses a problem to lifestyle. (Tab, SR) Instruct to notify physician if abnormal involuntary movements appear or get worse during treatment. Advise that sometimes the onset of effect of the 1st am dose may be delayed for up to 1 hr compared with the response usually obtained from the 1st am dose of IR tab; instruct to notify physician if such delayed responses pose a problem in treatment.

STORAGE: 25°C (77°F); excursions permitted to 15-30°C (59-86°F). Protect from light and moisture.

SINGULAIR – montelukast sodium RX

Class: Leukotriene receptor antagonist

ADULT DOSAGE

Asthma

Prophylaxis/Chronic Treatment:
10mg tab qpm

Patients w/ both asthma and allergic rhinitis should take only 1 dose qpm

Perennial Allergic Rhinitis

10mg tab qd

Patients w/ both asthma and allergic rhinitis should take only 1 dose qpm

Seasonal Allergic Rhinitis

10mg tab qd

Patients w/ both asthma and allergic rhinitis should take only 1 dose qpm

Exercise-Induced Bronchospasm

Prevention:
10mg tab at least 2 hrs before exercise

Do not take an additional dose w/in 24 hrs of a previous dose

PEDIATRIC DOSAGE

Asthma

Prophylaxis/Chronic Treatment:

12-23 Months:
4mg granules qpm

2-5 Years:
4mg chewable tab or 4mg granules qpm

6-14 Years:
5mg chewable tab qpm

≥15 Years:
10mg tab qpm

Patients w/ both asthma and allergic rhinitis should take only 1 dose qpm

Perennial Allergic Rhinitis

6-23 Months:
4mg granules qd

2-5 Years:
4mg chewable tab or 4mg granules qd

6-14 Years:
5mg chewable tab qd

≥15 Years:
10mg tab qd

Patients w/ both asthma and allergic rhinitis should take only 1 dose qpm

Seasonal Allergic Rhinitis

2-5 Years:
4mg chewable tab or 4mg granules qd

6-14 Years:
5mg chewable tab qd

≥15 Years:
10mg tab qd

Patients w/ both asthma and allergic rhinitis should take only 1 dose qpm

Exercise-Induced Bronchospasm

Prevention:

6-14 Years:
5mg chewable tab at least 2 hrs before exercise

≥15 Years:
10mg tab at least 2 hrs before exercise

Do not take an additional dose w/in 24 hrs of a previous dose

ADMINISTRATION
Oral route

Refer to PI for instructions for administration of granules

HOW SUPPLIED
Granules: 4mg/pkt; **Tab, Chewable:** 4mg, 5mg; **Tab:** 10mg

CONTRAINDICATIONS
Hypersensitivity to any component of this product.

WARNINGS/PRECAUTIONS
Not for use in the reversal of bronchospasm in acute asthma attacks, including status asthmaticus; have appropriate rescue medication available. Therapy may be continued during acute exacerbations of asthma. Patients who have exacerbations of asthma after exercise should have short-acting inhaled β-agonist available for rescue. Should not be abruptly substituted for inhaled or oral corticosteroids. Eosinophilic conditions reported. Neuropsychiatric events reported; evaluate risks and benefits of continuing treatment if such events occur. Chewable tabs contain phenylalanine; caution with phenylketonuria. Avoid aspirin (ASA) and NSAIDs with known ASA sensitivity; has not been shown to truncate bronchoconstrictor response to ASA and other NSAIDs in ASA-sensitive asthmatic patients.

ADVERSE REACTIONS
Headache, pharyngitis, influenza, fever, sinusitis, diarrhea, URTI, cough, abdominal pain, otitis media, rhinorrhea, otitis.

PATIENT CONSIDERATIONS

Assessment: Assess for hypersensitivity to drug, phenylketonuria, asthma status, pregnancy/nursing status, and possible drug interactions.

Monitoring: Monitor for signs/symptoms of eosinophilia, vasculitic rash, worsening pulmonary symptoms, cardiac complications, neuropathy, neuropsychiatric events, hypersensitivity reactions, and other adverse reactions.

Counseling: Advise to take daily as prescribed, even when asymptomatic, as well as during periods of worsening asthma; instruct to contact physician if asthma is not well controlled. Inform that drug is not for treatment of acute asthma attacks; advise to have appropriate short-acting inhaled β-agonist medication available to treat asthma exacerbations. Advise to seek medical attention if short-acting inhaled bronchodilators are needed more than usual while on therapy or if more than the max number of inhalations of short-acting bronchodilator treatment prescribed for a 24-hr period are needed. Instruct not to decrease dose or d/c other antiasthma medications unless instructed by physician. Instruct to notify physician if symptoms of neuropsychiatric events occur. Advise patients with ASA sensitivity to continue avoiding ASA and NSAIDs while on therapy. Inform phenylketonuric patients that the 4mg and 5mg chewable tabs contain phenylalanine.

STORAGE: 25°C (77°F); excursions permitted to 15-30°C (59-86°F). Protect from light and moisture.

SITAVIG – acyclovir

RX

Class: Nucleoside analogue

ADULT DOSAGE

Herpes Labialis (Cold Sores)

Recurrent Herpes Labialis in Immunocompetent Patients:
Usual: Apply one 50mg buccal tab as a single dose to the upper gum region (canine fossa)

Apply w/in 1 hr after the onset of prodromal symptoms and before the appearance of any signs of herpes labialis lesions

PEDIATRIC DOSAGE
Pediatric use may not have been established

ADMINISTRATION
Buccal route

Apply w/ a dry finger immediately after removing from blister.
Place tab to the upper gum just above the incisor tooth (canine fossa) and hold in place w/ slight pressure over upper lip for 30 sec.
Apply tab on the same side of the mouth as the herpes labialis symptoms.
Do not crush, chew, suck, or swallow tab.
Avoid any situation that may interfere w/ tab adhesion (eg, chewing gum, touching or pressing tab after placement, wearing upper denture, brushing teeth); rinse mouth gently if teeth need to be cleaned while tab is in place.
May take food/drink normally when tab is in place; drink plenty of liquids in case of dry mouth.

If Tab Does not Adhere or Falls Off w/in the First 6 Hrs
Reposition same tab immediately or place new tab if tab cannot be repositioned.

If Tab is Swallowed w/in the First 6 Hrs
Drink a glass of water and apply new tab.

Do not reapply if tab falls out or is swallowed after first 6 hrs.

HOW SUPPLIED
Tab, Buccal: 50mg

CONTRAINDICATIONS
Known hypersensitivity (eg, anaphylaxis) to acyclovir, milk protein concentrate, or any other component of the product.

WARNINGS/PRECAUTIONS
Do not administer during labor and delivery.

ADVERSE REACTIONS
Headache.

PATIENT CONSIDERATIONS

Assessment: Assess for hypersensitivity to drug or to milk protein concentrate, immune status, and pregnancy/nursing status.

Monitoring: Monitor for hypersensitivity and other adverse reactions.

Counseling: Inform that drug is not a cure for cold sores. Instruct to reapply tab if it comes out before 6 hrs have gone by; advise that if this does not work, a new tab should be applied. Instruct to apply ud and not to apply to the inside of the lip or cheek. Instruct not to reapply if it falls out or if swallowed after it has been in place ≥6 hrs. Advise to drink a glass of water and place a new tab if swallowed within the first 6 hrs of applying it. Inform that adverse reactions, including headache and application-site pain, may occur.

STORAGE: 20-25°C (68-77°F); excursions permitted between 15-30°C (59-86°F). Protect from moisture.

SIVEXTRO – tedizolid phosphate RX

Class: Oxazolidinone class antibacterial

ADULT DOSAGE

Skin and Skin Structure Infections

Acute bacterial infections caused by *Staphylococcus aureus* (including methicillin-resistant and methicillin-susceptible isolates), *Streptococcus pyogenes, Streptococcus agalactiae, Streptococcus anginosus* Group (including *Streptococcus anginosus, Streptococcus intermedius,* and *Streptococcus constellatus*), and *Enterococcus faecalis*

IV:
200mg qd infused over 1 hr for 6 days

Oral:
200mg qd for 6 days

PEDIATRIC DOSAGE

Pediatric use may not have been established

S

ADMINISTRATION
Oral/IV route

No dose adjustment is necessary when changing from IV to oral route
If patients miss a dose, they should take it as soon as possible anytime up to 8 hrs prior to their next scheduled dose; if <8 hrs remain before the next dose, wait until their next scheduled dose

Preparation of IV Sol
1. Reconstitute the vial w/ 4mL of SWFI
2. Gently swirl the contents and let the vial stand until the cake has completely dissolved and any foam disperses
3. Inspect the vial to ensure the sol contains no particulate matter and no cake or powder remains attached to the sides of the vial; if necessary, invert the vial to dissolve any remaining powder and swirl gently to prevent foaming
4. Tilt the upright vial and insert a syringe w/ appropriately sized needle into the bottom corner of the vial and remove 4mL of the reconstituted sol; do not invert the vial during extraction
5. The reconstituted sol must be further diluted in 250mL of 0.9% NaCl inj. Slowly inject the 4mL of

reconstituted sol into a 250mL bag of 0.9% NaCl inj and invert the bag gently to mix; do not shake the bag

Administration of IV Sol

Administer as an IV infusion only

Incompatibilities:

1. Any sol containing divalent cations (eg, Ca^{2+}, Mg^{2+}), including lactated Ringer's Inj and Hartmann's sol
2. Do not add other IV substances, additives, or other medications to the single-use vials or infuse simultaneously; if the same IV line is used for sequential infusion of several different drugs, the line should be flushed before and after infusion of tedizolid phosphate w/ 0.9% NaCl inj

HOW SUPPLIED

Inj/Tab: 200mg

WARNINGS/PRECAUTIONS

Consider alternative therapies when treating patients with neutropenia and acute bacterial skin and skin structure infections. *Clostridium difficile*-associated diarrhea (CDAD) reported; d/c if CDAD is suspected or confirmed. May result in bacterial resistance if used in the absence of proven or suspected bacterial infection or a prophylactic indication.

ADVERSE REACTIONS

N/V, headache, diarrhea.

PATIENT CONSIDERATIONS

Assessment: Assess for neutropenia, pregnancy/nursing status, and possible drug interactions.

Monitoring: Monitor for CDAD and other adverse reactions.

Counseling: Counsel that therapy should only be used to treat bacterial, not viral, infections. Instruct to take exactly ud even if the patient feels better early in the course of therapy. Inform that skipping doses or not completing full course of therapy may decrease effectiveness of immediate treatment and increase bacterial resistance. Inform that diarrhea is a common problem caused by therapy and usually resolves when therapy is discontinued. Instruct to contact physician if severe watery or bloody diarrhea develops.

STORAGE: 20-25°C (68-77°F); excursions permitted to 15-30°C (59-86°F). (Inj) Reconstituted Sol: Do not exceed 24 hrs at room temperature or under 2-8°C (36-46°F).

SKELAXIN — metaxalone

RX

Class: Muscular analgesic (centrally acting)

ADULT DOSAGE

Musculoskeletal Pain

Relief of Discomforts Associated w/ Acute Conditions:

800mg tid-qid

PEDIATRIC DOSAGE

Musculoskeletal Pain

Relief of Discomforts Associated w/ Acute Conditions:

>12 Years:

800mg tid-qid

ADMINISTRATION

Oral route

Taking w/ food may enhance general CNS depression.

HOW SUPPLIED

Tab: 800mg* *scored

CONTRAINDICATIONS

Known hypersensitivity to any components of this product; known tendency to drug-induced, hemolytic, and other anemias; significantly impaired renal or hepatic function.

WARNINGS/PRECAUTIONS

Serotonin syndrome (SS) reported; reports generally occurred when used concomitantly w/ serotonergic drugs or when used at doses higher than the recommended dose. Caution w/ preexisting liver damage; perform serial liver function studies in these patients. False (+) Benedict's tests reported; glucose-specific test will differentiate findings. Taking w/ food may enhance general CNS depression; elderly patients may be especially susceptible to this CNS effect.

ADVERSE REACTIONS

Drowsiness, dizziness, headache, nervousness, irritability, N/V, GI upset.

DRUG INTERACTIONS

Additive sedative effects may occur w/ other CNS depressants (eg, alcohol, benzodiazepines, opioids, TCAs); use w/ caution if taking >1 CNS depressant simultaneously. Caution w/ drugs that may affect the serotonergic neurotransmitter systems (eg, tramadol, SSRIs).

PATIENT CONSIDERATIONS

Assessment: Assess for known tendency to drug-induced, hemolytic, or other anemias, significant renal/hepatic impairment, hypersensitivity to the drug, pregnancy/nursing status, and possible drug interactions.

Monitoring: Monitor for signs/symptoms of SS, CNS depression, and any other adverse reaction. Perform serial liver function studies in patients w/ preexisting liver damage.

Counseling: Inform that drug may impair mental and/or physical abilities required to perform hazardous tasks, especially when used w/ alcohol or other CNS depressants.

STORAGE: 15-30°C (59-86°F).

Solu-Cortef – hydrocortisone sodium succinate

RX

Class: Glucocorticoid

ADULT DOSAGE

Steroid-Responsive Disorders

When oral therapy is not feasible

Initial: 100-500mg IV/IM, depending on disease being treated; administer IV over 30 sec (eg, 100mg) to 10 min (eg, ≥500mg)
May repeat dose at intervals of 2, 4, or 6 hrs
High-dose therapy should be continued only until patient is stabilized, usually not beyond 48-72 hrs
Maint: After a favorable response is noted, decrease initial dose in small decrements at appropriate time intervals until lowest effective dose
Withdraw gradually after long-term therapy

Acute Exacerbations of Multiple Sclerosis:
800mg/day for 1 week followed by 320mg qod for 1 month

PEDIATRIC DOSAGE

Steroid-Responsive Disorders

When oral therapy is not feasible

Initial: 0.56-8mg/kg/day IV/IM in 3 or 4 divided doses (20-240mg/m^{2}BSA/day), depending on disease being treated
Maint: After a favorable response is noted, decrease initial dose in small decrements at appropriate time intervals until lowest effective dose
Withdraw gradually after long-term therapy

DOSING CONSIDERATIONS

Elderly

Start at lower end of dosing range

ADMINISTRATION

IM/IV routes

IV inj preferred for initial emergency use; consider longer acting inj preparation or oral preparation after initial emergency period
Avoid inj into deltoid muscle
Should not be diluted or mixed w/ other sol

Preparation

IV or IM Inj:
Add not more than 2mL of bacteriostatic water for inj or bacteriostatic NaCl inj to contents of one 100mg vial

IV Infusion:
1. Add not more than 2mL of bacteriostatic water for inj to vial
2. 100mg sol may then be added to 100-1000mL of D5W (or isotonic saline sol or D5 in isotonic saline sol if patient is not on Na^+ restriction); 250mg sol may be added to 250-1000mL; 500mg sol may be added to 500-1000mL; and 1000mg sol may be added to 1000mL of same diluents
3. If administration of small volume of fluid is desirable, 100mg-3000mg may be added to 50mL of above diluents

Act-O-Vial System:
Refer to PI for directions

HOW SUPPLIED

Inj: 100mg, 250mg, 500mg, 1000mg

CONTRAINDICATIONS

Systemic fungal infections, known hypersensitivity to the product and its constituents, intrathecal administration. **IM Preparations:** Idiopathic thrombocytopenic purpura.

WARNINGS/PRECAUTIONS

Serious neurologic events reported with epidural inj; not approved for epidural administration. May result in dermal and/or subdermal changes forming depressions in the skin at the inj site; avoid inj into the deltoid muscle. Anaphylactoid reactions may occur. May need to increase dose before, during, and after stressful situations. High doses should not be used for the treatment of traumatic brain injury. May cause elevation of BP, salt/water retention, and increased excretion of K^+ and Ca^{2+}; dietary salt restriction and K^+ supplementation may be necessary. Caution in patients with recent MI. Hypothalamic-pituitary-adrenal (HPA) axis suppression, Cushing's syndrome, and hyperglycemia reported; monitor with chronic use. May produce reversible HPA axis suppression with the potential for glucocorticosteroid insufficiency after withdrawal of treatment; reduce dose gradually. May cause decreased resistance and inability to localize infection. May mask some signs of current infection or cause new infections; do not use intra-articularly, intrabursally, or for intratendinous administration for local effect in the presence of acute local infection. May exacerbate systemic fungal infections; avoid use in the presence of such infections unless needed to control drug reactions. Rule out latent or active amebiasis before initiating therapy. Caution with *Strongyloides* infestation, active or latent tuberculosis (TB), CHF, HTN, renal insufficiency, osteoporosis, and ocular herpes simplex. Not for use in cerebral malaria or active ocular herpes simplex. May cause more serious/fatal course of chickenpox and measles. Severe medical events associated with intrathecal route of administration reported. May produce posterior subcapsular cataracts, glaucoma with possible damage to the optic nerves, and may enhance the establishment of secondary ocular infections due to bacteria, fungi, or viruses. Sensitive to heat; should not be autoclaved when it is desirable to sterilize the exterior of the vial. Kaposi's sarcoma reported. Caution with active or latent peptic ulcers, diverticulitis, fresh intestinal anastomoses, and nonspecific ulcerative colitis; may increase risk of perforation. Signs of peritoneal irritation following GI perforation may be minimal or absent. Enhanced effect in patients with cirrhosis. May decrease bone formation and increase bone resorption, which may lead to inhibition of bone growth in pediatric patients and development of osteoporosis at any age. Local inj into a previously infected site is not recommended. Acute myopathy with high doses reported most often in patients with disorders of neuromuscular transmission (eg, myasthenia gravis). Elevation of creatine kinase (CK) may occur. Changes in thyroid status may necessitate dose adjustment. Psychic derangements may appear and existing emotional instability or psychotic tendencies may be aggravated. May elevate intraocular pressure (IOP); monitor IOP if steroid therapy is continued for >6 weeks. May suppress reactions to skin tests. Caution in elderly.

ADVERSE REACTIONS

Bradycardia, cardiac arrest, acne, allergic dermatitis, decreased carbohydrate and glucose tolerance, fluid retention, abdominal distention, bowel/bladder dysfunction, negative nitrogen balance, aseptic necrosis of femoral and humeral heads, convulsions, emotional instability, exophthalmoses, glaucoma, abnormal fat deposits.

DRUG INTERACTIONS

Aminoglutethimide may lead to a loss of corticosteroid-induced adrenal suppression. Closely monitor for the development of hypokalemia with K^+-depleting agents (eg, amphotericin B, diuretics). Reports of cardiac enlargement and CHF with amphotericin B. Macrolide antibiotics may decrease clearance. Concomitant use with anticholinesterase agents may produce severe weakness in patients with myasthenia gravis; d/c anticholinesterase agents at least 24 hrs before initiating therapy. May inhibit response to warfarin; frequently monitor coagulation indices. May increase blood glucose levels; may require dose adjustments of antidiabetic agents. May decrease serum levels of isoniazid. Cholestyramine may increase clearance. Increased activity of both drugs may occur with cyclosporine; convulsions reported with concurrent use. May increase risk of arrhythmias with digitalis glycosides. Estrogens, including oral contraceptives, may decrease hepatic metabolism and increase effect. Drugs that induce CYP3A4 (eg, barbiturates, phenytoin, carbamazepine) may enhance metabolism and require corticosteroid dosage increase. Drugs that inhibit CYP3A4 (eg, ketoconazole, macrolide antibiotics) may increase plasma levels. Ketoconazole may increase risk of corticosteroid side effects. Aspirin (ASA) or other NSAIDs may increase risk of GI side effects; caution with ASA in hypoprothrombinemia. May increase clearance of salicylates. Administration of live or live, attenuated vaccines is contraindicated in patients receiving immunosuppressive doses. Killed or inactivated vaccines may be administered, although response is unpredictable. Acute myopathy reported with neuromuscular blocking drugs (eg, pancuronium).

S

PATIENT CONSIDERATIONS

Assessment: Assess for hypersensitivity to drug, traumatic brain injury, CHF, renal insufficiency, systemic fungal infections, active/latent TB, vaccination status, unusual stress, ulcerative colitis, diverticulitis, HTN, recent MI, intestinal anastomoses, active or latent peptic ulcer, myasthenia gravis, psychotic tendencies, cerebral malaria, active ocular herpes simplex, any other conditions where treatment is contraindicated or cautioned, pregnancy/nursing status, and possible drug interactions.

Monitoring: Monitor for anaphylactoid reactions, dermal and/or subdermal changes, growth/development (in pediatric patients), intestinal perforation, Kaposi's sarcoma, cataracts, glaucoma, osteoporosis, and other adverse reactions. Monitor for HPA axis suppression, Cushing's syndrome, and hyperglycemia with chronic use. Monitor BP, CK, serum electrolytes, and IOP. Frequently monitor coagulation indices with warfarin.

Counseling: Warn not to d/c abruptly or without medical supervision. Advise patients to inform any medical attendants that they are taking corticosteroids. Instruct to seek medical advice at once if fever or other signs of infection develop. Warn to avoid exposure to chickenpox or measles; advise to report immediately if exposed.

STORAGE: 20-25°C (68-77°F). Protect from light. Discard unused sol after 3 days.

SOLU-MEDROL – methylprednisolone sodium succinate RX

Class: Glucocorticoid

ADULT DOSAGE

Steroid-Responsive Disorders

When Oral Therapy is Not Feasible:
Initial: 10-40mg IV/IM inj or IV infusion, depending on disease
Maint: Decrease initial dosage in small decrements at appropriate time intervals until lowest effective dose

High-Dose Therapy: 30mg/kg IV over at least 30 min; may be repeated q4-6h for 48 hrs
High-dose therapy should continue only until patient is stabilized, usually not beyond 48-72 hrs

Multiple Sclerosis

Acute Exacerbations:
Usual: 160mg qd for a week followed by 64mg qod for 1 month

D/C if a period of spontaneous remission occurs in a chronic condition

PEDIATRIC DOSAGE

Steroid-Responsive Disorders

When Oral Therapy is Not Feasible:
Initial: 0.11-1.6mg/kg/day in 3 or 4 divided doses (3.2-48mg/m2/day)

Asthma

Uncontrolled Asthma: 1-2mg/kg/day in single or divided doses
Continue short-course ("burst") therapy until patient achieves a peak expiratory flow rate of 80% of personal best, or symptoms resolve (usually 3-10 days)
Dose may be reduced, but should be governed by severity of condition/response; should not be <0.5mg/kg/24 hrs
D/C if a period of spontaneous remission occurs in a chronic condition
Withdraw gradually after long-term therapy

DOSING CONSIDERATIONS

Elderly
Start at lower end of dosing range

ADMINISTRATION
IM/IV route

Do not dilute or mix w/ other sol
Avoid inj into deltoid muscle

Refer to PI for preparation and administration instructions

HOW SUPPLIED
Inj: 40mg, 125mg, 500mg, 1g, 2g

CONTRAINDICATIONS
Systemic fungal infections, known hypersensitivity to the product and its constituents, intrathecal administration, premature infants (formulations preserved w/ benzyl alcohol). **IM Preparations:** Idiopathic thrombocytopenic purpura.

WARNINGS/PRECAUTIONS
Serious neurologic events reported with epidural inj; not approved for epidural administration. Formulations with preservative contain benzyl alcohol, which is potentially toxic to neural tissue. Exposure to excessive amounts of benzyl alcohol associated with toxicity, particularly in neonates. May result in dermal and/or subdermal changes forming depressions in the skin at the inj site. Anaphylactoid reactions may occur. May need to increase dose before, during, and after stressful situations. High systemic doses should not be used to treat traumatic brain injury. May cause elevation of BP, salt/water retention, and increased excretion of K^+ and Ca^{2+}; dietary salt restriction and K^+ supplementation may be necessary. Monitor for hypothalamic-pituitary-adrenal (HPA) axis suppression, Cushing's syndrome, and hyperglycemia with chronic use. May produce reversible HPA axis suppression with the potential for glucocorticosteroid insufficiency after withdrawal of treatment; reduce dose gradually. May increase susceptibility to, mask signs of, or cause new infections; may exacerbate systemic fungal infections. Avoid use intra-articularly, intrabursally, or for intratendinous administration for local effect in the presence of acute local infection. Latent disease due to certain pathogens may be activated or intercurrent infections exacerbated. Rule out latent or active amebiasis before initiating therapy. Caution with recent myocardial infarction (MI), *Strongyloides* infestation, active or latent tuberculosis (TB), ocular herpes simplex, HTN, CHF, and renal insufficiency. May cause more serious/fatal course of chickenpox and measles. May produce posterior subcapsular cataracts, glaucoma with possible damage to the optic nerves,

and may enhance the establishment of secondary ocular infections. Not for use in active ocular herpes simplex or in cerebral malaria. Sensitive to heat. Kaposi's sarcoma reported. Metabolic clearance is decreased in hypothyroidism and increased in hyperthyroidism; changes in thyroid status may necessitate dose adjustment. Caution with active or latent peptic ulcers, diverticulitis, fresh intestinal anastomoses, and nonspecific ulcerative colitis; may increase risk of perforation. Signs of peritoneal irritation following GI perforation may be minimal/absent. Enhanced effect in patients with cirrhosis. May decrease bone formation and increase bone resorption, and may lead to inhibition of bone growth in pediatric patients and development of osteoporosis at any age; caution with increased risk of osteoporosis. Acute myopathy with high doses reported, most often in patients with disorders of neuromuscular transmission (eg, myasthenia gravis). Elevation of creatine kinase (CK) or intraocular pressure (IOP) may occur; monitor IOP if used >6 weeks. Psychic derangements may appear, and existing emotional instability or psychotic tendencies may be aggravated. May suppress reactions to skin tests. Caution in elderly.

ADVERSE REACTIONS

Anaphylactoid reaction, HTN, osteoporosis, muscle weakness, menstrual irregularities, insomnia, impaired wound healing, manifestations of latent diabetes mellitus, ulcerative esophagitis, increased sweating, increased intracranial pressure, decreased carbohydrate/glucose tolerance, glaucoma, posterior subcapsular cataracts.

DRUG INTERACTIONS

Aminoglutethimide may lead to a loss of corticosteroid-induced adrenal suppression. Closely monitor for hypokalemia with K^+-depleting agents (eg, amphotericin B, diuretics). Reports of cardiac enlargement and CHF following concomitant use of amphotericin B and hydrocortisone. Macrolide antibiotics may decrease clearance and cholestyramine may increase clearance. Concomitant use with anticholinesterase agents may produce severe weakness in patients with myasthenia gravis; d/c anticholinesterase agents at least 24 hrs before initiating therapy. May inhibit response to warfarin; frequently monitor coagulation indices. May increase blood glucose levels; dosage adjustments of antidiabetic agents may be required. May decrease serum levels of isoniazid. Increased activity of both drugs may occur with cyclosporine; convulsions reported with concurrent use. May increase risk of arrhythmias with digitalis glycosides. Estrogens, including oral contraceptives, may decrease hepatic metabolism and enhance effect. Drugs that induce CYP3A4 (eg, barbiturates, phenytoin, carbamazepine) may enhance metabolism and require corticosteroid dosage increase. Drugs that inhibit CYP3A4 (eg, ketoconazole, macrolide antibiotics such as erythromycin and troleandomycin) may increase plasma levels. Ketoconazole may increase risk of corticosteroid side effects. Aspirin (ASA) or other NSAIDs may increase risk of GI side effects; caution with ASA in hypoprothrombinemia patients. May increase clearance of salicylates. Administration of live or live, attenuated vaccines is contraindicated in patients receiving immunosuppressive doses. Killed or inactivated vaccines may be administered, although response is unpredictable. Acute myopathy reported with neuromuscular blocking drugs (eg, pancuronium).

PATIENT CONSIDERATIONS

Assessment: Assess for hypersensitivity to drug, traumatic brain injury, CHF, renal insufficiency, cirrhosis, systemic fungal infections, active/latent TB, HTN, recent MI, active or latent peptic ulcer, ocular herpes simplex, any other conditions where treatment is contraindicated or cautioned, pregnancy/nursing status, and possible drug interactions.

Monitoring: Monitor for anaphylactoid reactions, dermal and/or subdermal changes, growth/development (in pediatric patients), intestinal perforation, infections, cataracts, glaucoma, osteoporosis, CK/IOP elevation, and other adverse reactions. Monitor for HPA-axis suppression, Cushing's syndrome, and hyperglycemia with chronic use. Frequently monitor coagulation indices with warfarin.

Counseling: Warn not to d/c abruptly or use without medical supervision. Instruct to seek medical advice at once if fever or other signs of infection develop. Warn to avoid exposure to chickenpox or measles; advise to report immediately if exposed.

STORAGE: 20-25°C (68-77°F). Protect from light. Use within 48 hrs after mixing.

SOMA – carisoprodol

CIV

Class: Skeletal muscle relaxant (centrally acting)

ADULT DOSAGE

Musculoskeletal Conditions

Relief of Discomfort Associated w/ Acute Painful Conditions:

16-65 Years:

250-350mg tid and hs for up to 2-3 weeks

PEDIATRIC DOSAGE

Pediatric use may not have been established

ADMINISTRATION

Oral route

Take w/ or w/o food.

HOW SUPPLIED

Tab: 250mg, 350mg

CONTRAINDICATIONS

History of acute intermittent porphyria, hypersensitivity reaction to a carbamate (eg, meprobamate).

WARNINGS/PRECAUTIONS

May impair mental/physical abilities. Abuse and dependence reported w/ prolonged use and a history of drug abuse. Withdrawal symptoms reported following abrupt cessation after prolonged use. Assess risk of abuse prior to prescribing; after prescribing, limit the length of treatment to 3 weeks for acute musculoskeletal discomfort, keep careful prescription records, and educate about abuse and on proper storage and disposal. Seizures reported. Caution w/ renal/hepatic impairment.

ADVERSE REACTIONS

Drowsiness, dizziness, headache.

DRUG INTERACTIONS

Additive sedative effects w/ other CNS depressants (eg, alcohol, benzodiazepines, opioids, TCAs); caution when coadministering. Concomitant use w/ meprobamate is not recommended. Increased exposure of carisoprodol and decreased exposure of meprobamate w/ CYP2C19 inhibitors (eg, omeprazole, fluvoxamine). Decreased exposure of carisoprodol and increased exposure of meprobamate w/ CYP2C19 inducers (eg, rifampin, St. John's wort). Induction effect on CYP2C19 seen w/ low-dose aspirin.

PATIENT CONSIDERATIONS

Assessment: Assess for acute intermittent porphyria, renal/hepatic impairment, history of drug abuse, abuse potential, pregnancy/nursing status, and possible drug interactions.

Monitoring: Monitor for sedation, drug abuse/dependence, and seizures.

Counseling: Advise that drug may cause drowsiness and/or dizziness; instruct to avoid taking carisoprodol before engaging in hazardous tasks. Instruct to avoid alcohol, and to check w/ physician before taking other CNS depressants. Inform that drug is limited to acute use. Instruct to notify physician if musculoskeletal symptoms persist. Inform of drug dependence/abuse potential.

STORAGE: 20-25°C (68-77°F).

SONATA – zaleplon CIV

Class: Pyrazolopyrimidine (non-benzodiazepine)

ADULT DOSAGE

Insomnia

Short-Term Treatment:

10mg qhs; for certain low weight individuals, 5mg may be a sufficient dose

Max: 20mg

PEDIATRIC DOSAGE

Pediatric use may not have been established

S

DOSING CONSIDERATIONS

Concomitant Medications

Concomitant Use w/ Cimetidine:

Initial: 5mg

Hepatic Impairment

Mild to Moderate Impairment: 5mg

Severe Impairment: Not recommended

Elderly

Elderly/Debilitated:

Usual: 5mg

Max: 10mg

ADMINISTRATION

Oral route

Take immediately before hs or after patient has gone to bed and has experienced difficulty falling asleep

HOW SUPPLIED

Cap: 5mg, 10mg

CONTRAINDICATIONS

Hypersensitivity to zaleplon or any excipients in the formulation.

WARNINGS/PRECAUTIONS

Initiate only after careful evaluation; failure of insomnia to remit after 7-10 days of treatment may indicate presence of a primary psychiatric and/or medical illness. Use lowest effective dose, especially in elderly. Abnormal thinking and behavior changes reported. Complex behaviors (eg, sleep-driving) reported; consider discontinuation if sleep-driving occurs. Amnesia and other neuropsychiatric symptoms may occur unpredictably. Worsening of depression, including suicidal thoughts and actions, reported in primarily depressed patients; caution with signs/symptoms of depression. Withdrawal signs/symptoms reported following rapid dose decrease or abrupt discontinuation. May impair mental/physical abilities. Severe anaphylactic and anaphylactoid reactions reported; do not rechallenge if angioedema develops. May result in short-term memory impairment, hallucinations, impaired coordination, dizziness, and lightheadedness when taken while still up and about. Caution with diseases or conditions affecting metabolism or hemodynamic responses, or with compromised respiratory function. Carefully monitor patients with compromised respiration due to preexisting illness. Not recommended for use in patients with severe hepatic impairment or in women during pregnancy. Contains tartrazine, which may cause allergic-type reactions (including bronchial asthma) in certain susceptible persons. Has an abuse potential. Monitor patients at risk of habituation and dependence (eg, history of addiction to, or abuse of, drugs or alcohol).

ADVERSE REACTIONS

Headache, dizziness, nausea, asthenia, abdominal pain, somnolence, amnesia, eye pain, dysmenorrhea, paresthesia.

DRUG INTERACTIONS

Additive CNS depression with other psychotropic medications, anticonvulsants, antihistamines, narcotic analgesics, anesthetics, ethanol, and other CNS depressants; dosage adjustment may be necessary. Do not take with alcohol. Increased risk of complex behaviors with alcohol and other CNS depressants. Decreased C_{max} with promethazine. Decreased levels with rifampin (a potent CYP3A4 inducer); coadministration of a potent CYP3A4 inducer can lead to ineffectiveness of zaleplon. May consider alternative non-CYP3A4 substrate hypnotic agent in patients taking CYP3A4 inducers (eg, phenytoin, carbamazepine, phenobarbital). Strong selective CYP3A4 inhibitors (eg, erythromycin, ketoconazole) may increase levels. Increased levels with cimetidine; give an initial dose of 5mg.

PATIENT CONSIDERATIONS

Assessment: Assess for physical and/or psychiatric disorders, medical illness, depression, diseases/conditions affecting metabolism or hemodynamic responses, compromised respiratory function, hepatic impairment, risk of habituation and dependence, hypersensitivity, pregnancy/nursing status, and possible drug interactions.

Monitoring: Monitor for complex behaviors, emergence of any new behavioral signs/symptoms, anaphylactic/anaphylactoid reactions, angioedema, abuse, habituation, dependence, withdrawal symptoms, and other adverse reactions. Monitor elderly and/or debilitated patients closely.

Counseling: Inform of the risks and benefits of therapy. Caution against engaging in hazardous occupations requiring complete mental alertness (eg, operating machinery, driving). Instruct to immediately report to physician if any adverse reactions (eg, sleep-driving or other complex behaviors) occur. Instruct to notify physician if pregnant/nursing or planning to become pregnant. Instruct not to take with alcohol. Inform that taking the drug with or immediately after a heavy, high-fat meal results in slower absorption and may reduce the effect of the drug on sleep latency.

STORAGE: 20-25°C (68-77°F).

SORIATANE – acitretin

RX

Class: Retinoid

Avoid in pregnancy and avoid becoming pregnant during therapy and for at least 3 yrs after discontinuation of therapy; use 2 effective forms of contraception simultaneously. Females of childbearing potential should avoid ethanol during and for 2 months after discontinuation of therapy because it may increase the duration of teratogenic potential. Only use in females of reproductive potential w/ severe psoriasis unresponsive to or contraindicated w/ other therapies. Patient must have 2 negative urine/serum pregnancy tests w/ a sensitivity of at least 25 mIU/mL before receiving initial prescription; if 2nd pregnancy test is negative, initiation of treatment should begin w/in 7 days of specimen collection. Therapy should be limited to a monthly supply. Contraception counseling should be done on a regular basis. It is not known whether residual acitretin in seminal fluid poses risk to a fetus while a male patient is taking the drug or after it is discontinued. Severe birth defects reported. Interferes w/ contraceptive effect of microdosed progestin "minipill" oral contraceptives. Caution not to self-medicate w/ herbal St. John's wort, because a possible interaction has been suggested w/ hormonal contraceptives, based on reports of breakthrough bleeding. Potential for hepatotoxicity; d/c if hepatotoxicity is suspected.

ADULT DOSAGE

Psoriasis

Severe:
Initial: 25-50mg/day as a single dose w/ main meal
Maint: 25-50mg/day

May treat relapses as outlined for initial therapy

PEDIATRIC DOSAGE

Pediatric use may not have been established

DOSING CONSIDERATIONS

Elderly

Start at lower end of dosing range

Other Important Considerations

When used w/ phototherapy, decrease phototherapy dose, dependent on patient's individual response

ADMINISTRATION

Oral route

HOW SUPPLIED

Cap: 10mg, 17.5mg, 25mg

CONTRAINDICATIONS

Pregnancy, severely impaired liver or kidney function, chronic abnormally elevated blood lipid values. Coadministration w/ methotrexate or tetracyclines. Hypersensitivity (eg, angioedema, urticaria) to the preparation (acitretin or excipients) or to other retinoids.

WARNINGS/PRECAUTIONS

Risk of skeletal abnormalities, pancreatitis, and pseudotumor cerebri (benign intracranial HTN). D/C and refer for ophthalmologic evaluation if visual difficulties occur. Bone abnormalities of the vertebral column, knees, and ankles reported. Increased TG and cholesterol and decreased HDL levels reported; perform blood lipid determinations before therapy and again at 1- to 2-week intervals until lipid response to therapy is established, usually w/in 4-8 weeks. Caution in patients w/ an increased tendency to develop hypertriglyceridemia (eg, disturbances of lipid metabolism, diabetes mellitus [DM], obesity, increased alcohol intake, or familial history of these conditions). Capillary leak syndrome reported; d/c if this develops during therapy. Rhabdomyolysis and myalgias reported in association w/ capillary leak syndrome, and may reveal neutrophilia, hypoalbuminemia, and an elevated Hct in lab tests. Exfoliative dermatitis/erythroderma reported; d/c if this occurs during therapy. Blood sugar control problems and new cases of diabetes, including diabetic ketoacidosis, reported; monitor blood sugar levels very carefully in diabetics. Not indicated for treatment of acne.

ADVERSE REACTIONS

Hepatotoxicity, cheilitis, alopecia, skin peeling, rhinitis, dry skin, nail disorder, pruritus, rigors, xerophthalmia, dry mouth, epistaxis, arthralgia, spinal hyperostosis, erythematous rash.

DRUG INTERACTIONS

See Boxed Warning, Dosing Considerations, and Contraindications. Potentiates the blood glucose-lowering effect of glyburide; careful supervision of diabetic patients is recommended. Reduced protein binding of phenytoin. Avoid use w/ vitamin A and/or other oral retinoids; may increase risk of hypervitaminosis A.

PATIENT CONSIDERATIONS

Assessment: Assess for DM, obesity, alcohol intake, or familial history of these conditions, cardiovascular status, preexisting abnormalities of the spine or extremities, renal/hepatic function, drug hypersensitivity, pregnancy/nursing status, and possible drug interactions. Perform blood lipid determinations before initiating therapy.

Monitoring: Monitor for hepatotoxicity, skeletal abnormalities, hypertriglyceridemia, MI or other thromboembolic events, pancreatitis, pseudotumor cerebri, visual difficulties, capillary leak syndrome, exfoliative dermatitis/erythroderma, and other adverse reactions. Perform appropriate examinations periodically in view of possible ossification abnormalities. Monitor blood sugar levels very carefully in diabetic patients. Repeat pregnancy test every month, during therapy, and every 3 months for at least 3 yrs after discontinuation of therapy. Monitor blood lipid determinations at 1- to 2-week intervals until lipid response to the drug is established during therapy.

Counseling: Inform about the Pregnancy Prevention Actively Required During and After Treatment (*Do Your P.A.R.T.*) program and the risks of therapy. Advise to notify physician if pregnant or nursing. Advise to use 2 effective forms of contraception simultaneously at least 1 month prior to initiation of therapy. Advise against donating blood during or for at least 3 yrs following completion of therapy. Counsel to d/c therapy and notify physician immediately if psychiatric symptoms develop. Instruct not to ingest beverages or products containing ethanol while taking therapy and for 2 months after discontinuation of therapy. Advise to be cautious when driving or operating a vehicle at night, and not to give the drug to any other person. Inform to use caution when taking vitamin A supplements to avoid additive toxic effects. Instruct to avoid use of sun lamps and excessive exposure to sunlight. Advise that a transient worsening of psoriasis may be seen during initial treatment period, and that patients may have to wait 2-3 months before they get the full benefit of therapy.

STORAGE: 15-25°C (59-77°F). Protect from light. Avoid exposure to high temperatures and humidity after the bottle is opened.

SOVALDI – sofosbuvir

RX

Class: HCV nucleotide analogue NS5B polymerase inhibitor

ADULT DOSAGE

Chronic Hepatitis C

HCV Mono-Infected and HCV/HIV-1 Coinfected:

Genotype 1 or 4:
400mg qd in combination w/ peginterferon alfa and ribavirin for 12 weeks

Genotype 1 Ineligible for Interferon-Based Regimen:
400mg qd in combination w/ ribavirin for 24 weeks

Genotype 2:
400mg qd in combination w/ ribavirin for 12 weeks

Genotype 3:
400mg qd in combination w/ ribavirin for 24 weeks

Hepatocellular Carcinoma Awaiting Liver Transplantation:
400mg qd in combination w/ ribavirin for up to 48 weeks or until time of transplant, whichever occurs 1st

PEDIATRIC DOSAGE

Pediatric use may not have been established

DOSING CONSIDERATIONS

Adverse Reactions

Serious Reaction Potentially Related to Peginterferon Alfa and/or Ribavirin:
Reduce dose of or d/c peginterferon alfa and/or ribavirin; refer to each respective PI for instructions

ADMINISTRATION

Oral route

Take w/ or w/o food.

D/C sofosbuvir if concomitant agents are permanently discontinued.

HOW SUPPLIED

Tab: 400mg

CONTRAINDICATIONS

Refer to the individual monographs for peginterferon alfa and ribavirin.

WARNINGS/PRECAUTIONS

Fatal cardiac arrest reported w/ sofosbuvir-containing regimen (ledipasvir/sofosbuvir).

ADVERSE REACTIONS

Fatigue, headache, nausea, insomnia, anemia, pruritus, asthenia, rash, decreased appetite, influenza-like illness, pyrexia, diarrhea, myalgia, irritability.

DRUG INTERACTIONS

Coadministration of amiodarone w/ sofosbuvir in combination w/ another direct-acting antiviral (DAA) may result in serious symptomatic bradycardia; coadministration is not recommended. If coadministration is required, cardiac monitoring is recommended in an inpatient setting for the first 48 hrs, after which outpatient or self-monitoring of HR should occur on a daily basis for at least the first 2 weeks. Intestine P-gp inducers (eg, rifampin, St. John's wort) may significantly decrease concentration and may lead to a reduced therapeutic effect; do not use w/ rifampin and St. John's wort. Carbamazepine, phenytoin, phenobarbital, oxcarbazepine, rifabutin, rifapentine, and tipranavir/ritonavir may decrease concentration, leading to reduced therapeutic effects; coadministration is not recommended. Not recommended w/ other products containing sofosbuvir.

PATIENT CONSIDERATIONS

Assessment: Assess for pregnancy/nursing status and possible drug interactions.

Monitoring: Monitor for adverse reactions.

Counseling: Advise to seek medical evaluation immediately for symptoms of bradycardia. Advise patients to avoid pregnancy during combination treatment w/ sofosbuvir and ribavirin or sofosbuvir and peginterferon and ribavirin; instruct to notify physician immediately in the event of a pregnancy. Inform that the effect of treatment of hepatitis C on transmission is unknown and that appropriate precautions should be taken to prevent HCV transmission during treatment or in the event of treatment failure. Advise to take ud.

STORAGE: Room temperature <30°C (86°F).

SPIRIVA – tiotropium bromide

RX

Class: Anticholinergic

ADULT DOSAGE

Chronic Obstructive Pulmonary Disease

Long-Term Maint Treatment of Bronchospasm/Reduction of COPD Exacerbations:
2 inh of the powder contents of 1 cap qd via HandiHaler device

PEDIATRIC DOSAGE

Pediatric use may not have been established

ADMINISTRATION

Orally inhaled powder

Do not swallow caps.
Use w/ HandiHaler device only and inhale through the mouth.
Do not use HandiHaler device to take any other medicine.

Instructions

1. Place cap into the center chamber of the HandiHaler device.
2. Spiriva cap is pierced by pressing and releasing the green piercing button on the side of the device.
3. The formulation will be dispersed into the air stream when the patient inhales through the mouthpiece.

HOW SUPPLIED

Cap, Inhalation: 18mcg

CONTRAINDICATIONS

Hypersensitivity to tiotropium, ipratropium, or any components of this medication.

WARNINGS/PRECAUTIONS

Not for relief of acute symptoms (eg, as rescue therapy for the treatment of acute episodes of bronchospasm). D/C and consider alternative treatments if immediate hypersensitivity reactions (eg, angioedema, itching, rash) or paradoxical bronchospasm occurs. Caution w/ hypersensitivity to milk proteins or to atropine. Caution w/ narrow-angle glaucoma; observe for signs/symptoms of acute narrow-angle glaucoma. Caution w/ urinary retention; observe for signs/symptoms of urinary retention especially in patients w/ prostatic hyperplasia or bladder-neck obstruction. Monitor for anticholinergic effects in patients w/ moderate to severe renal impairment (CrCl ≤60mL/min).

ADVERSE REACTIONS

Dry mouth, sinusitis, constipation, abdominal pain, UTI, URTI, chest pain, edema, vomiting, myalgia, moniliasis, rash, dyspepsia, pharyngitis, rhinitis.

DRUG INTERACTIONS

Avoid w/ other anticholinergic-containing drugs; may lead to an increase in anticholinergic adverse effects.

PATIENT CONSIDERATIONS

Assessment: Assess for hypersensitivity to atropine or its derivatives, hypersensitivity to milk proteins, narrow-angle glaucoma, urinary retention, prostatic hyperplasia or bladder-neck obstruction, renal impairment, pregnancy/nursing status, and possible drug interactions.

Monitoring: Monitor for signs/symptoms of hypersensitivity reactions, paradoxical bronchospasm, urinary retention, worsening narrow-angle glaucoma, and other adverse reactions.

Counseling: Inform that contents of cap are for oral inhalation only and must not be swallowed. Advise to administer only via the HandiHaler device and that the device should not be used for other medications. Advise not to use as a rescue medication for immediate relief of breathing problems. Advise to seek medical attention if signs/symptoms of narrow-angle glaucoma or urinary retention develop. Advise to use caution when engaging in activities such as driving a vehicle or operating appliances/machinery. Inform that paradoxical bronchospasm may occur; d/c if this develops. Instruct not to allow the powder to enter into the eyes.

STORAGE: 25°C (77°F); excursions permitted to 15-30°C (59-86°F). Do not expose to extreme temperatures or moisture. Do not store caps in the HandiHaler device.

STALEVO – carbidopa/entacapone/levodopa RX

Class: COMT inhibitor/dopa-decarboxylase inhibitor/dopamine precursor

ADULT DOSAGE

Parkinson's Disease

May be used:
1. To substitute (w/ equivalent strengths of each of the 3 components) carbidopa/levodopa and entacapone previously administered as individual products
2. To replace carbidopa/levodopa therapy (w/o entacapone) for patients experiencing signs/symptoms of end-of-dose "wearing-off" and who have been taking a total daily dose of levodopa of ≤600mg and have not been experiencing dyskinesias

Converting from Carbidopa, Levodopa, and Entacapone:
In patients currently treated w/ entacapone 200mg w/ each dose of non-extended release carbidopa/levodopa tab may switch to corresponding strength of Stalevo w/ same amounts of carbidopa and levodopa

Converting from Carbidopa and Levodopa Products:
Titrate patients initially to a dose that is tolerated and that meets individual therapeutic need using a separate carbidopa/levodopa tab (1:4 ratio) plus an entacapone tab; switch to the corresponding single tab of Stalevo once the individual dose of carbidopa/levodopa plus entacapone has been established

When less levodopa is required, reduce the total daily dose of carbidopa/levodopa either by decreasing the strength of Stalevo at each administration or by decreasing the frequency of administration by extending time between doses

Max: 8 tabs/day (Stalevo 50, 75, 100, 125, 150); 6 tabs/day (Stalevo 200)

Determine optimum daily dose by careful titration in each patient

Administer only 1 tab at each dosing interval

PEDIATRIC DOSAGE

Pediatric use may not have been established

DOSING CONSIDERATIONS

Concomitant Medications

Other Anti-Parkinson's Disease Drugs: May need to adjust concomitant medication or Stalevo

Other Important Considerations

Decrease or Interruption of Dosing: Avoid interruption of Stalevo dosing; hyperpyrexia reported when levodopa is discontinued or reduced

ADMINISTRATION

Oral route

Do not split, crush, or chew tabs

Take w/ or w/o food; a high-fat, high-calorie meal may delay absorption of levodopa by about 2 hrs

S

HOW SUPPLIED

Tab: (Carbidopa-Levodopa-Entacapone): **Stalevo 50:** 12.5mg-50mg-200mg; **Stalevo 75:** 18.75mg-75mg-200mg; **Stalevo 100:** 25mg-100mg-200mg; **Stalevo 125:** 31.25mg-125mg-200mg; **Stalevo 150:** 37.5mg-150mg-200mg; **Stalevo 200:** 50mg-200mg-200mg

CONTRAINDICATIONS

Narrow-angle glaucoma. Nonselective MAOIs (eg, phenelzine, tranylcypromine); d/c nonselective MAOIs at least 2 weeks prior to therapy.

WARNINGS/PRECAUTIONS

Falling asleep suddenly without prior warning of sleepiness while engaged in activities of daily living and somnolence reported; reassess for drowsiness or sleepiness, and should ordinarily be discontinued if significant daytime sleepiness or episodes of falling asleep during activities that require active participation occur. May impair mental/physical abilities. Dyskinesia may occur or be exacerbated at lower dosages and sooner than with carbidopa/levodopa; may require dose reductions. Monitor for depression with concomitant suicidal tendencies. Caution with past or current psychoses. May cause intense urges to gamble/spend money uncontrollably, increased sexual urges, and other intense urges; consider dose reduction or discontinuation if such urges develop. Caution with biliary obstruction or hepatic disease/impairment. Cases of hyperpyrexia and confusion resembling neuroleptic malignant syndrome (NMS) reported in association with dose reduction or withdrawal; decrease dose slowly if a patient needs to d/c or reduce daily dose. Syncope, orthostatic hypotension, hypotension, hallucinations and/or psychotic-like behavior, and rhabdomyolysis reported. Cases of retroperitoneal fibrosis, pulmonary infiltrates, pleural effusion, and pleural thickening reported in patients treated with ergot derived dopaminergic agents. Diarrhea and colitis reported with entacapone use; d/c and consider appropriate medical therapy if prolonged diarrhea is suspected to be related to therapy. Monitor for melanomas frequently and regularly; perform periodic skin examination. May increase the possibility of upper GI hemorrhage in patients with history of peptic ulcer. Lab test abnormalities, including elevations of LFTs, BUN abnormalities, and (+) Coombs test reported. May cause a false-positive reaction for urinary ketone bodies or false-negative glucose oxidase test. Cases of falsely diagnosed pheochromocytoma in patients on carbidopa/levodopa reported very rarely; caution when interpreting the plasma and urine levels of catecholamines and their metabolites. Levodopa is known to depress prolactin secretion and increase growth hormone levels.

ADVERSE REACTIONS

Dyskinesia, N/V, hyperkinesia, diarrhea, urine discoloration, hypokinesia, dizziness, abdominal pain, constipation, fatigue, back pain, dry mouth, dyspnea.

DRUG INTERACTIONS

See Contraindications. Caution with concomitant use of alcohol, sedating medications, and other CNS depressants (eg, benzodiazepines, antipsychotics, antidepressants); may increase the risk of somnolence. Iron salts may reduce bioavailability; caution with iron salts or multivitamins containing iron salts. Adjust dose as clinically needed with other CYP2C9 substrates. Entacapone: Caution with drugs metabolized by catechol-O-methyltransferase (COMT) (eg, epinephrine, dopamine, α-methyldopa, isoetherine); increased HR, possibly arrhythmias, and excessive changes in BP may occur. Caution with drugs known to interfere with biliary excretion, glucuronidation, and intestinal β-glucuronidase (eg, probenecid, cholestyramine, erythromycin, ampicillin). Increased R-warfarin exposure and INR values reported with warfarin. Levodopa: Beneficial effects of levodopa in Parkinson's disease reported to be reversed by phenytoin and papaverine; monitor for loss of therapeutic response and increase dosage of Stalevo as clinically needed. Isoniazid and dopamine D_2 receptor antagonists (eg, phenothiazines, butyrophenones, risperidone) may reduce therapeutic effects. Carbidopa/Levodopa: Symptomatic postural hypotension reported when added with antihypertensives; dosage adjustment of the antihypertensive drug may be required when starting therapy. Adverse reactions, including HTN and dyskinesia, reported with TCAs.

PATIENT CONSIDERATIONS

Assessment: Assess for narrow-angle glaucoma, past/current psychoses, history of peptic ulcer, hypotension, biliary obstruction, dyskinesias, alcoholism, hepatic impairment, pregnancy/nursing status, any other conditions where treatment is contraindicated or cautioned, and possible drug interactions.

Monitoring: Monitor for signs and symptoms of falling asleep during activities of daily living, hypotension/orthostatic hypotension, syncope, dyskinesia, depression, suicidal tendencies, hallucinations/psychotic-like behavior, impulse control/compulsive behaviors, withdrawal-emergent hyperpyrexia and confusion, diarrhea, colitis, melanoma, rhabdomyolysis, peptic ulcer, and other adverse reactions. Perform skin examination periodically. Monitor INR with warfarin.

Counseling: Inform of the risks and benefits of therapy. Advise about the potential for sedating effects including somnolence and the possibility of falling asleep while engaged in activities of daily living; instruct not to drive or participate in potentially dangerous activities until aware of how medication affects mental and/or motor performance. Advise to speak with physician before taking alcohol, sedating medications, or other CNS depressants because of the possible additive effects in combination with therapy. Inform that symptomatic (or asymptomatic) postural (orthostatic) hypotension or non-orthostatic hypotension may develop; advise not to rise rapidly after sitting or lying down, especially if doing so for prolonged periods and at the initiation of treatment. Inform about the possibility of syncope. Inform that therapy may cause and/or exacerbate preexisting dyskinesias. Inform that hallucinations and other psychotic-like behavior may occur. Instruct to inform physician of new or increased gambling urges, sexual urges, or other intense urges while on therapy. Advise that fever and confusion may develop as part of a syndrome resembling NMS, possibly with other clinical features; instruct to contact physician if wishing to d/c or decrease dose, or if fever and confusion develop. Inform that diarrhea, colitis, rhabdomyolysis, myalgia, and N/V may occur. Inform of higher risk of developing melanoma; instruct to have skin examined on a regular basis by a qualified healthcare provider (eg, dermatologist) and to monitor for melanomas frequently and on a regular basis when using therapy.

STORAGE: 25°C (77°F); excursions permitted to 15-30°C (59-86°F).

STARLIX – nateglinide

Class: Meglitinide

RX

ADULT DOSAGE

Type 2 Diabetes Mellitus

Monotherapy and Combination w/ Metformin or a Thiazolidinedione:
Initial/Maint: 120mg tid ac; may use 60mg dose in patients near goal HbA1c when treatment is initiated

PEDIATRIC DOSAGE

Pediatric use may not have been established

DOSING CONSIDERATIONS

Hepatic Impairment
Moderate to Severe: Use caution

ADMINISTRATION

Oral route

Take 1-30 min ac.
Patients who skip meals should also skip their scheduled dose of nateglinide to reduce risk of hypoglycemia.

HOW SUPPLIED

Tab: 60mg, 120mg

CONTRAINDICATIONS

Known hypersensitivity to the drug or its inactive ingredients, type 1 diabetes mellitus (DM), diabetic ketoacidosis.

WARNINGS/PRECAUTIONS

Risk of hypoglycemia increased with strenuous exercise, adrenal/pituitary insufficiency, severe renal impairment, and in elderly/malnourished patients. Autonomic neuropathy may mask hypoglycemia. Caution in moderate to severe hepatic impairment. Transient loss of glucose control may occur with fever, infection, trauma, or surgery; may need insulin therapy instead of nateglinide. Secondary failure (reduced effectiveness over a period of time) may occur.

ADVERSE REACTIONS

Upper respiratory infection (URI), flu symptoms, dizziness, arthropathy, diarrhea, hypoglycemia, back pain, jaundice, cholestatic hepatitis, elevated liver enzymes.

DRUG INTERACTIONS

Alcohol, NSAIDs, salicylates, MAOIs, nonselective β-blockers, guanethidine, and CYP2C9 inhibitors (eg, fluconazole, amiodarone, miconazole, oxandrolone) may potentiate hypoglycemia. Thiazides, corticosteroids, thyroid products, sympathomimetics, somatropin, rifampin, phenytoin, and dietary supplements (St. John's wort) may reduce hypoglycemic action of drug. Somatostatin analogues may potentiate/attenuate hypoglycemia. Reduced levels reported with liquid meals. β-blockers may mask hypoglycemic effects. Caution with highly protein-bound drugs.

PATIENT CONSIDERATIONS

Assessment: Assess for diabetic ketoacidosis, type 1 DM, renal/hepatic impairment, adrenal/pituitary insufficiency, pregnancy/nursing status, other conditions where treatment is cautioned, and possible drug interactions. Assess FPG and HbA1c.

Monitoring: Monitor for hypo/hyperglycemia, diabetic ketoacidosis, secondary failure, URI, and other adverse reactions. Monitor FPG, HbA1c, renal function, and LFTs.

Counseling: Inform of potential risks, benefits, alternate modes of therapy, and drug interactions. Instruct to take 1-30 min ac, but to skip scheduled dose if meal is skipped. Inform about importance of adherence to meal planning, regular physical activity, regular blood glucose monitoring, periodic HbA1c testing, recognition and management of hypo/hyperglycemia, and periodic assessment for diabetes complications. Advise to notify physician if any adverse events occur.

STORAGE: 25°C (77°F); excursions permitted to 15-30°C (59-86°F).

STELARA – ustekinumab

RX

Class: Monoclonal antibody

ADULT DOSAGE

Psoriasis

Patients w/ Moderate to Severe Plaque Psoriasis who are Candidates for Phototherapy or Systemic Therapy:

≤100kg (≤220 lbs): 45mg initially and 4 weeks later, followed by 45mg every 12 weeks

>100kg (>220 lbs): 90mg initially and 4 weeks later, followed by 90mg every 12 weeks

Psoriatic Arthritis

Active:

45mg initially and 4 weeks later, followed by 45mg every 12 weeks

Coexistent Moderate to Severe Plaque Psoriasis:

>100kg (>220 lbs): 90mg initially and 4 weeks later, followed by 90mg every 12 weeks

Can be used alone or in combination w/ methotrexate

PEDIATRIC DOSAGE

Pediatric use may not have been established

ADMINISTRATION

SQ route

Administer each inj at a different anatomic location (eg, upper arms, gluteal regions, thighs, any quadrant of abdomen) than the previous inj; do not administer into areas where the skin is tender, bruised, erythematous, or indurated

When using the single-use vial, a 27-gauge, 1/2-inch needle is recommended

Administration Instructions

1. To prevent premature activation of the needle safety guard, do not touch the needle guard activation clips at any time during use
2. Hold body and remove needle cover; do not hold plunger or plunger head while removing needle cover and do not use prefilled syringe if it is dropped w/o needle cover in place
3. Inject SQ as recommended; inject all of the medication by pushing in plunger until plunger head is completely between needle guard wings; inj of entire prefilled syringe contents is necessary to activate needle guard
4. After injection, maintain pressure on plunger head and remove needle from skin
5. Slowly take your thumb off plunger head to allow empty syringe to move up until entire needle is covered by needle guard; discard used syringes in puncture-resistant container

S

HOW SUPPLIED

Inj: 45mg/0.5mL, 90mg/mL [prefilled syringe, vial]

CONTRAINDICATIONS

Clinically significant hypersensitivity to ustekinumab or to any of the excipients.

WARNINGS/PRECAUTIONS

Serious bacterial, fungal, and viral infections, and infections requiring hospitalization reported. Do not give to patients with any clinically important active infection or until infection resolves or is adequately treated. Caution with chronic infection or a history of recurrent infection. Individuals genetically deficient in interleukin (IL)-12/IL-23 are particularly vulnerable to disseminated infections from mycobacteria (eg, nontuberculous, environmental mycobacteria), salmonella (eg, nontyphi strains), and Bacillus Calmette-Guerin (BCG) vaccinations; consider appropriate diagnostic testing. Evaluate for tuberculosis (TB) infection prior to, during, and after treatment; do not administer to patients with active TB. Consider anti-TB therapy prior to initiation in patients with history of latent or active TB when an adequate course of treatment cannot be confirmed. Rapid appearance of multiple cutaneous squamous cell carcinomas reported in patients who had preexisting risk factors for developing non-melanoma skin cancer; closely monitor patients with history of prolonged immunosuppressant therapy, history of PUVA treatment, and patients >60 yrs of age. Hypersensitivity reactions (eg, anaphylaxis, angioedema) reported; institute appropriate therapy and d/c. Reversible posterior leukoencephalopathy syndrome (RPLS) reported; administer appropriate treatment and d/c if suspected. Prior to initiating therapy, patients should receive all immunizations appropriate for age as recommended by current immunization guidelines. Needle cover on prefilled syringe contains dry natural rubber and should not be handled by latex-sensitive individuals. Should only be given to patients who will be closely monitored and have regular follow-up visits with a physician.

ADVERSE REACTIONS

Infection, nasopharyngitis, upper respiratory tract infection, headache, fatigue, arthralgia, nausea.

DRUG INTERACTIONS

Do not give with live vaccines; caution when administering live vaccines to household contacts of patients receiving ustekinumab. BCG vaccines should not be given during, for 1 yr prior to initiating, or 1 yr following discontinuation of treatment. Non-live vaccinations received during course of therapy may not elicit an immune response sufficient to prevent disease. Consider monitoring for therapeutic effect (eg, for warfarin) or drug concentration (eg, for cyclosporine) with concomitant CYP450 substrates, particularly those with a narrow therapeutic index; adjust individual dose prn. May decrease protective effect of allergen immunotherapy (decrease tolerance), which may increase the risk of an allergic reaction to a dose of allergen immunotherapy; caution in patients receiving or who have received allergen immunotherapy.

PATIENT CONSIDERATIONS

Assessment: Assess for drug hypersensitivity, active/chronic/serious infections, history of recurrent infection, IL-12/IL-23 genetic deficiency, TB, immunization history, pregnancy/nursing status, and possible drug interactions.

Monitoring: Monitor for signs/symptoms of infection, appearance of non-melanoma skin cancer, TB during and after treatment, malignancies, hypersensitivity reactions, RPLS, and other adverse reactions.

Counseling: Advise that therapy may lower the ability of the immune system to fight infections. Inform of the importance of communicating any history of infections to physician and instruct to contact physician if any signs/symptoms of infection develop. Counsel about the risk of malignancies while on therapy. Advise to seek immediate medical attention if experiencing any symptoms of a serious allergic reaction. Inform of inj techniques and procedures. Advise not to reuse needles/syringes and instruct on proper disposal procedures.

STORAGE: 2-8°C (36-46°F). Store vials upright. Protect from light. Do not freeze or shake.

STENDRA — avanafil

RX

Class: Phosphodiesterase-5 (PDE-5) inhibitor

ADULT DOSAGE

Erectile Dysfunction

Initial: 100mg prn, as early as 15 min before sexual activity

Titrate: May increase to 200mg as early as 15 min before, or decrease to 50mg 30 min before sexual activity, based on individual efficacy and tolerability

Max Dosing Frequency: qd

Use lowest effective dose

Sexual stimulation is required for response to treatment

PEDIATRIC DOSAGE

Pediatric use may not have been established

DOSING CONSIDERATIONS

Concomitant Medications

α-Blocker:

Initial: 50mg

Moderate CYP3A4 Inhibitors (eg, Erythromycin, Amprenavir, Diltiazem):

Max: 50mg/24 hrs

Strong CYP3A4 Inhibitors (eg, Ketoconazole, Ritonavir, Atazanavir):

Do not use

ADMINISTRATION

Oral route

Take w/ or w/o food.

HOW SUPPLIED

Tab: 50mg, 100mg, 200mg

CONTRAINDICATIONS

Concomitant use (regularly and/or intermittently) w/ organic nitrates. Known hypersensitivity to any component of the tablet. Do not use in patients who are using a guanylate cyclase stimulator (eg, riociguat).

WARNINGS/PRECAUTIONS

In a patient who has taken avanafil, where nitrate administration is necessary, allow at least 12 hrs to elapse after the last dose of therapy before considering nitrate administration; only administer under close medical supervision w/ appropriate hemodynamic monitoring. Potential for cardiac risk during sexual activity in patients w/ preexisting cardiovascular (CV) disease; avoid if sexual activity is inadvisable due to underlying CV status. Patients w/ left ventricular outflow obstruction (eg, aortic stenosis, idiopathic hypertrophic subaortic stenosis) and those w/ severely impaired autonomic control of BP may be sensitive to therapy. Not recommended in patients w/ MI, stroke, life-threatening arrhythmia, or coronary revascularization w/in the last 6 months; resting hypotension (BP <90/50mmHg) or HTN (BP >170/100mmHg), or unstable angina, angina w/ sexual intercourse, or NYHA Class 2 or greater CHF. Has vasodilatory properties resulting in transient decreases in sitting BP. Prolonged erection >4 hrs and priapism may occur; caution w/ anatomical deformation of the penis (eg, angulation, cavernosal fibrosis, Peyronie's disease), or conditions that may predispose to priapism (eg, sickle cell anemia, multiple myeloma, leukemia). Nonarteritic anterior ischemic optic neuropathy (NAION) reported (rare); d/c if sudden loss of vision in 1 or both eyes occurs. Caution w/ underlying NAION risk factors; increased risk w/ previous history of NAION and in individuals w/ "crowded" optic disc. Sudden decrease or loss of hearing that may be accompanied by tinnitus or dizziness reported; d/c if this occurs. Avoid in patients w/ severe renal disease, on renal dialysis, or w/ severe hepatic disease.

ADVERSE REACTIONS

Headache, flushing, nasopharyngitis, nasal congestion, back pain, URI, ECG abnormal.

DRUG INTERACTIONS

See Contraindications and Dosage. Not recommended w/ other PDE-5 inhibitors or ED therapy combinations. Not recommended w/ CYP inducers. Caution w/ α-blockers; may augment BP-lowering effect of α-blockers and other antihypertensives. May increase BP-lowering effect of each compound w/ concomitant alcohol use and the risk of orthostatic signs/symptoms w/ substantial alcohol consumption. Do not use w/ strong CYP3A4 inhibitors (eg, ketoconazole, ritonavir, clarithromycin, nefazodone). Increased levels w/ strong, moderate, and likely w/ other CYP3A4 inhibitors (eg, grapefruit juice). May increase levels of desipramine or omeprazole. May affect rosiglitazone levels. Amlodipine may increase levels and prolong $T_{1/2}$. May decrease amlodipine levels. May potentiate the antiaggregatory effect of sodium nitroprusside.

PATIENT CONSIDERATIONS

Assessment: Assess for hypersensitivity to the drug, CV disease, left ventricular outflow obstruction, anatomical deformation of the penis, conditions that predispose to priapism, potential underlying causes of ED, risk for NAION, renal/hepatic impairment, any other conditions where treatment is contraindicated/cautioned, and possible drug interactions. Obtain baseline BP.

Monitoring: Monitor for hypersensitivity reactions, CV risk, priapism, changes in vision/hearing, and other adverse reactions.

Counseling: Instruct to take ud and explain that sexual stimulation is required for an erection to occur. Inform about the contraindication of avanafil w/ regular and/or intermittent use of organic nitrates; instruct patients who experience anginal chest pain after taking medication to seek immediate medical attention. Inform patients w/ preexisting CV risk factors of the potential cardiac risk of sexual activity; advise patients who experience symptoms upon initiation of sexual activity to refrain from further sexual activity and seek immediate medical attention. Advise to contact prescribing physician if new medications that may interact w/ therapy are prescribed by another healthcare provider. Instruct to seek emergency medical attention if erection persists >4 hrs; inform that priapism, if not treated promptly, may result in irreversible erectile tissue damage. Inform of the increased risk of NAION w/ history of NAION in 1 eye and in patients w/ a "crowded" optic disc. Instruct to d/c and seek medical attention in the event of sudden loss of vision in 1 or both eyes, or if a sudden decrease or loss of hearing that may be accompanied by tinnitus and dizziness occurs. Inform that substantial alcohol consumption (eg, >3 units) in combination w/ medication may increase the potential for orthostatic signs/symptoms. Inform that drug does not protect against STDs; counsel about protective measures necessary to guard against STDs, including HIV. Inform about the contraindication of avanafil w/ the use of guanylate cyclase stimulators.

STORAGE: 20-25°C (68-77°F); excursions permitted to 30°C (86°F). Protect from light.

STIVARGA – regorafenib

RX

Class: Kinase inhibitor

Severe and sometimes fatal hepatotoxicity reported. Monitor hepatic function prior to and during treatment. Interrupt and then reduce or d/c treatment for hepatotoxicity as manifested by elevated LFTs or hepatocellular necrosis, depending upon severity and persistence.

ADULT DOSAGE

Metastatic Colorectal Cancer

Previously treated w/ fluoropyrimidine-, oxaliplatin-, and irinotecan-based chemotherapy, an antivascular endothelial growth factor therapy, and, if KRAS wild type, an anti-epidermal growth factor receptor therapy

160mg qd for the first 21 days of each 28-day cycle until disease progression or unacceptable toxicity

Locally Advanced, Unresectable or Metastatic Gastrointestinal Stromal Tumor

Previously treated w/ imatinib mesylate and sunitinib malate

160mg qd for the first 21 days of each 28-day cycle until disease progression or unacceptable toxicity

PEDIATRIC DOSAGE

Pediatric use may not have been established

DOSING CONSIDERATIONS

Hepatic Impairment

Severe (Child-Pugh Class C): Not recommended

Adverse Reactions

Interruption:

- NCI CTCAE Grade 2 hand-foot skin reaction (HFSR) that is recurrent or does not improve w/in 7 days despite dose reduction; interrupt therapy for a minimum of 7 days for Grade 3 HFSR
- Symptomatic Grade 2 HTN
- Any NCI CTCAE Grade 3 or 4 adverse reaction

Reduce to 120mg if:

- For the 1st occurrence of Grade 2 HFSR of any duration
- After recovery of any Grade 3 or 4 adverse reaction
- For Grade 3 AST/ALT elevation; only resume if the potential benefit outweighs the risk of hepatotoxicity

Reduce to 80mg if:

- For reoccurrence of Grade 2 HFSR at the 120mg dose
- After recovery of any Grade 3 or 4 adverse reaction at the 120mg dose (except hepatotoxicity)

Discontinuation

- Failure to tolerate 80mg dose
- Any occurrence of AST or ALT >20X ULN
- Any occurrence of AST or ALT >3X ULN w/ concurrent bilirubin >2X ULN
- Reoccurrence of AST or ALT >5X ULN despite dose reduction to 120mg
- For any Grade 4 adverse reaction; only resume if the potential benefit outweighs the risks

ADMINISTRATION

Oral route

Take at the same time each day

Swallow tab whole w/ water after a low-fat meal that contains <600 calories and <30% fat

Do not take 2 doses of therapy on the same day to make up for a missed dose from the previous day

HOW SUPPLIED

Tab: 40mg

WARNINGS/PRECAUTIONS

Increased incidence of hemorrhage reported; permanently d/c w/ severe or life-threatening hemorrhage. May increase incidence of adverse reactions involving the skin and SQ tissues (eg, hand-foot skin reaction [HFSR], toxic epidermal necrolysis, Stevens Johnson syndrome, severe rash); withhold, reduce dose, or permanently d/c treatment depending on severity and persistence of dermatologic toxicity. Increased incidence of HTN reported; temporarily or permanently withhold for severe or uncontrolled HTN. Avoid initiation unless BP is adequately controlled. May increase incidence of myocardial ischemia and infarction; withhold if new or acute onset cardiac ischemia or infarction develops. Resume treatment only after resolution of acute cardiac ischemic events, if benefits outweigh risks of further cardiac ischemia. Reversible posterior leukoencephalopathy syndrome (RPLS) reported; perform evaluation for RPLS in any patient presenting w/ seizures, headache, visual disturbances, confusion, or altered mental function. D/C if RPLS develops. Permanently d/c if GI perforation or fistula develops. May impair wound healing; d/c at least 2 weeks prior to scheduled surgery. D/C in patients w/ wound dehiscence. May cause fetal harm; women and men of reproductive potential should use effective contraception during treatment and up to 2 months after completion of therapy.

ADVERSE REACTIONS

Hepatotoxicity, asthenia, HFSR, fatigue/diarrhea, decreased appetite/food intake, HTN, mucositis, dysphonia, infection, pain, decreased weight, GI/abdominal pain, rash, fever, nausea.

DRUG INTERACTIONS

Avoid w/ strong CYP3A4 inducers (eg, rifampin, phenytoin, carbamazepine) and strong CYP3A4 inhibitors (eg, clarithromycin, grapefruit juice, itraconazole). Monitor INR levels more frequently in patients receiving warfarin.

PATIENT CONSIDERATIONS

Assessment: Assess for scheduled/recent surgical procedures, hepatic impairment, HTN, pregnancy/nursing status, and possible drug interactions. Obtain baseline LFTs (ALT, AST, and bilirubin).

Monitoring: Monitor for hepatotoxicity, hemorrhage, dermatologic toxicity, HTN, myocardial ischemia or infarction, RPLS, wound dehiscence, GI perforation or fistula, and other adverse reactions. Monitor BP weekly for the first 6 weeks of treatment and then every cycle, or more frequently, as clinically indicated. Monitor LFTs at least every 2 weeks during the first 2 months of treatment, then monthly or more frequently as clinically indicated; monitor weekly in patients experiencing elevated LFTs until improvement to <3X ULN or baseline. Monitor INR levels more frequently in patients receiving warfarin.

Counseling: Inform about the need to undergo monitoring for liver damage and instruct to immediately report to physician any signs or symptoms of severe liver damage. Advise to contact physician for any episode of bleeding, or if experiencing skin changes associated w/ redness, pain, blisters, bleeding, or swelling. Advise of the need for BP monitoring and to contact physician if BP is elevated, or if HTN symptoms occur. Instruct to seek immediate emergency help if experiencing chest pain, SOB, dizziness, or feeling like passing out. Advise to contact physician immediately if experiencing severe pain in the abdomen, persistent swelling of the abdomen, high fever, chills, N/V, severe diarrhea, or dehydration. Instruct to inform physician if patient plans to undergo a surgical procedure or had recent surgery. Advise women of reproductive potential and men of the need for effective contraception during treatment and for up to 2 months after completion of treatment. Instruct women of reproductive potential to immediately contact physician if pregnancy is suspected or confirmed during or w/in 2 months of completing treatment. Advise nursing mothers that it is not known whether the drug is present in breast milk and discuss whether to d/c nursing or to d/c treatment. Advise patient to swallow the tab whole w/ water at the same time each day w/ a low-fat meal; inform that the low-fat meal should contain <600 calories and <30% fat. Instruct to take any missed dose on the same day, as soon as they remember, and to not take 2 doses on the same day to make up for a dose missed on the previous day.

STORAGE: 25°C (77°F); excursions permitted to 15-30°C (59-86°F). Store tabs in original bottle and do not remove the desiccant. Keep the bottle tightly closed after 1st opening. Discard any unused tabs 7 weeks after opening the bottle.

STRATTERA — atomoxetine

RX

Class: Selective norepinephrine reuptake inhibitor

Increased risk of suicidal ideation in short-term studies in children or adolescents with attention-deficit hyperactivity disorder (ADHD); balance this risk with the clinical need. Closely monitor for suicidality (suicidal thinking and behavior), clinical worsening, or unusual changes in behavior. Not approved for major depressive disorder.

ADULT DOSAGE

Attention-Deficit Hyperactivity Disorder

Initial: 40mg/day

Titrate: Increase after a minimum of 3 days to target dose of approx 80mg/day; may increase after 2-4 additional weeks if optimal response is not achieved

PEDIATRIC DOSAGE

Attention-Deficit Hyperactivity Disorder

≤70kg:

Initial: 0.5mg/kg/day

Titrate: Increase after a minimum of 3 days to target dose of approx 1.2mg/kg/day

Max: 100mg/day

Periodically reevaluate long-term usefulness

May d/c w/o tapering

Max: 1.4mg/kg/day or 100mg/day, whichever is less

>70kg:

Initial: 40mg/day

Titrate: Increase after a minimum of 3 days to target dose of approx 80mg/day; may increase after 2-4 additional weeks if optimal response is not achieved

Max: 100mg/day

Periodically reevaluate long-term usefulness

May d/c w/o tapering

DOSING CONSIDERATIONS

Concomitant Medications

Strong CYP2D6 Inhibitors:

<70kg:

Initial: 0.5mg/kg/day

Titrate: Only increase to target dose of 1.2mg/kg/day if symptoms fail to improve after 4 weeks and initial dose is well tolerated

>70kg or Adults:

Initial: 40mg/day

Titrate: Only increase to target dose of 80mg/day if symptoms fail to improve after 4 weeks and initial dose is well tolerated

Hepatic Impairment

Moderate Impairment (Child-Pugh Class B):

Initial/Target: Reduce to 50% of normal dose

Severe Impairment (Child-Pugh Class C):

Initial/Target: Reduce to 25% of normal dose

Other Important Considerations

CYP2D6 Poor Metabolizers:

Initial: 0.5mg/kg/day

Titrate: Only increase to target dose of 1.2mg/kg/day if symptoms fail to improve after 4 weeks and initial dose is well tolerated

ADMINISTRATION

Oral route

Take whole, w/ or w/o food; do not open cap

Take as a single dose in the am or as evenly divided doses in the am and late afternoon/early pm

HOW SUPPLIED

Cap: 10mg, 18mg, 25mg, 40mg, 60mg, 80mg, 100mg

CONTRAINDICATIONS

Narrow-angle glaucoma, presence/history of pheochromocytoma, and severe cardiac/vascular disorders that would deteriorate w/ increases in BP/HR that would be clinically important (eg, 15-20mmHg in BP or 20 bpm in HR). Use of an MAOI either concomitantly or w/in 2 weeks of stopping treatment. Treatment w/in 2 weeks of stopping an MAOI. Known hypersensitivity to atomoxetine or other constituents of the product.

WARNINGS/PRECAUTIONS

May cause severe liver injury; d/c in patients with jaundice or lab evidence of liver injury, and do not restart therapy. Perform LFTs upon the 1st sign/symptom of liver dysfunction. Sudden death reported in children and adolescents with structural cardiac abnormalities or other serious heart problems. Sudden death, stroke, and MI reported in adults. Avoid in patients with known serious structural cardiac abnormalities, cardiomyopathy, serious heart rhythm abnormalities, coronary artery disease, or other serious cardiac problems. Promptly perform cardiac evaluation if symptoms suggestive of cardiac disease develop. May increase BP/HR; caution in patients whose underlying medical conditions could be worsened by increases in BP or HR. Orthostatic hypotension and syncope reported; caution with conditions predisposing to hypotension, or conditions associated with abrupt HR/BP changes. Caution in patients with comorbid bipolar disorder; may induce mixed/manic episode. May cause treatment-emergent psychotic or manic symptoms in children/adolescents without prior history of psychotic illness or mania; consider discontinuation if such symptoms occur. Monitor for appearance/worsening of aggressive behavior or hostility. Allergic reactions and priapism reported. May cause urinary retention/hesitation. Monitor growth in children.

ADVERSE REACTIONS

Abdominal pain, N/V, fatigue, decreased appetite, somnolence, headache, dry mouth, dizziness, insomnia, constipation, urinary hesitation, erectile dysfunction, irritability, weight decreased, hyperhidrosis.

DRUG INTERACTIONS

See Contraindications. Caution with systemically administered albuterol or other β_2 agonists; may potentiate cardiovascular (CV) effects of albuterol. Caution with antihypertensive drugs and pressor agents (eg, dopamine, dobutamine) or other drugs that increase BP. CYP2D6 inhibitors (eg, paroxetine, fluoxetine, quinidine) increase levels in extensive metabolizers (EMs).

PATIENT CONSIDERATIONS

Assessment: Assess for hypersensitivity to drug, narrow-angle glaucoma, presence/history of pheochromocytoma, comorbid bipolar disorder, CV disorders, hepatic impairment, any other conditions where treatment is contraindicated or cautioned, pregnancy/nursing status, and possible drug interactions. Obtain baseline pulse and BP.

Monitoring: Monitor for signs/symptoms of CV events, liver injury, allergic reactions, emergence of psychosis/mania, suicidality, clinical worsening, aggressive or unusual changes in behavior, hostility, urinary retention/hesitation, priapism, and other adverse reactions. Monitor growth in children. Monitor pulse and BP following dose increases and periodically during therapy. Periodically reevaluate long-term usefulness.

Counseling: Inform about risks, benefits, and appropriate use of therapy. Encourage patients, families, and caregivers to be alert for the emergence of agitation, irritability, and unusual changes in behavior, as well as the emergence of suicidality, especially early during treatment and when dose is adjusted; advise to report such symptoms to physician, especially if severe, abrupt in onset, or not part of presenting symptoms. Advise to contact physician if symptoms of liver injury develop. Inform that priapism requires prompt medical attention. Inform that drug is an ocular irritant; if content of cap comes in contact with eye, instruct to immediately flush affected eye with water and obtain medical advice. Tell to notify physician if taking or planning to take any prescription or OTC medicines, dietary supplements, or herbal remedies. Instruct to notify physician if nursing, pregnant, or thinking of becoming pregnant. Advise to use caution when driving a car/operating hazardous machinery until reasonably certain that performance is not affected by therapy.

STORAGE: 25°C (77°F); excursions permitted to 15-30°C (59-86°F).

STRIBILD — cobicistat/elvitegravir/emtricitabine/tenofovir disoproxil fumarate RX

Class: CYP3A inhibitor/HIV integrase strand transfer inhibitor/nucleoside analogue combination

Lactic acidosis and severe hepatomegaly w/ steatosis, including fatal cases, reported w/ the use of nucleoside analogues in combination w/ other antiretrovirals. Not approved for the treatment of chronic hepatitis B virus (HBV) infection. Severe acute exacerbations of hepatitis B reported in patients coinfected w/ HBV and HIV-1 upon discontinuation of therapy; closely monitor hepatic function w/ both clinical and lab follow-up for at least several months. If appropriate, initiation of anti-hepatitis B therapy may be warranted.

ADULT DOSAGE

HIV-1 Infection

For use as a complete regimen for the treatment of HIV-1 infection in adults who have no antiretroviral treatment history or to replace the current antiretroviral regimen in those who are virologically-suppressed (HIV-1 RNA <50 copies/mL) on a stable antiretroviral regimen for at least 6 months w/ no history of treatment failure and no known substitutions associated w/ resistance to the individual components of the drug

1 tab qd

PEDIATRIC DOSAGE

Pediatric use may not have been established

S

DOSING CONSIDERATIONS

Renal Impairment

CrCl <70mL/min: Initiation of treatment not recommended

CrCl Declines <50mL/min During Treatment: D/C therapy

Hepatic Impairment

Severe (Child-Pugh Class C): Not recommended

ADMINISTRATION

Oral route

Take w/ food.

HOW SUPPLIED

Tab: (Cobicistat/Elvitegravir/Emtricitabine/Tenofovir Disoproxil Fumarate [TDF]) 150mg/150mg/200mg/300mg

CONTRAINDICATIONS

Concomitant use w/ drugs that are highly dependent on CYP3A for clearance and for which elevated plasma concentrations are associated w/ serious and/or life-threatening events and w/ other drugs that may lead to reduced efficacy and possible resistance (eg, alfuzosin, carbamazepine, phenobarbital, phenytoin, rifampin, dihydroergotamine, ergotamine, methylergonovine, cisapride, St. John's wort, lovastatin, simvastatin, pimozide, sildenafil [when dosed as Revatio for the treatment of pulmonary arterial HTN], triazolam, oral midazolam).

WARNINGS/PRECAUTIONS

Test for HBV infection and document estimated CrCl, urine glucose, and urine protein prior to initiation of therapy. Not recommended for use in patients w/ severe hepatic impairment. Renal impairment, including cases of acute renal failure and Fanconi syndrome, reported; d/c if estimated CrCl <50mL/min. Do not initiate therapy in patients w/ estimated CrCl <70mL/min. Immune reconstitution syndrome, autoimmune disorders (eg, Graves' disease, polymyositis, Guillain-Barre syndrome) in the setting of immune reconstitution, and redistribution/accumulation of body fat reported. Caution in elderly. **Cobicistat:** May cause modest increases in SrCr and modest declines in estimated CrCl w/o affecting renal glomerular function; closely monitor patients w/ confirmed increase in SrCr >0.4mg/dL from baseline for renal safety. **TDF:** Obesity and prolonged nucleoside exposure may be risk factors for lactic acidosis and severe hepatomegaly. Caution w/ known risk factors for liver disease. D/C if lactic acidosis or pronounced hepatotoxicity occurs. Decreased bone mineral density (BMD), increased biochemical markers of bone metabolism, and osteomalacia reported. Consider hypophosphatemia and osteomalacia secondary to proximal renal tubulopathy in patients at risk of renal dysfunction who present w/ persistent/worsening bone or muscle symptoms.

ADVERSE REACTIONS

Diarrhea, nausea, fatigue, headache, dizziness, insomnia, abnormal dreams, rash, creatine kinase/ amylase elevation, hematuria, AST elevation.

DRUG INTERACTIONS

See Contraindications. Avoid w/ cobicistat, elvitegravir, adefovir dipivoxil, rifabutin, rifapentine, salmeterol, nephrotoxic agents (eg, high-dose or multiple NSAIDs), other antiretrovirals, or w/ products containing emtricitabine, TDF, lamivudine, or ritonavir. Avoid w/ colchicine in patients w/ renal or hepatic impairment. Antacids (eg, aluminum and magnesium hydroxide) may decrease elvitegravir levels; separate administration by at least 2 hrs. May increase levels of antiarrhythmics (eg, digoxin), clonazepam, ethosuximide, ketoconazole, itraconazole, voriconazole, colchicine, β-blockers, calcium channel blockers, inhaled or nasal fluticasone, bosentan, atorvastatin, immunosuppressants, salmeterol, neuroleptics, PDE-5 inhibitors, and sedative/hypnotics (eg, benzodiazepines). Concomitant use w/ inhaled or nasal fluticasone may reduce serum cortisol concentrations. May increase norgestimate and decrease ethinyl estradiol levels; caution w/ contraceptives containing norgestimate/ethinyl estradiol. Consider alternative (nonhormonal) methods of contraception. May increase levels of buprenorphine and norbuprenorphine and may decrease levels of naloxone; monitor for sedation and cognitive effects upon coadministration w/ buprenorphine/naloxone. Monitor INR upon coadministration w/ warfarin. May increase levels of antidepressants (eg, SSRIs, TCAs, trazodone); carefully titrate antidepressant dose and monitor response. May increase levels of clarithromycin; reduce clarithromycin dose by 50% in patients w/ CrCl 50-60mL/min. Anticonvulsants (eg, oxcarbazepine, clonazepam, ethosuximide) may decrease elvitegravir and cobicistat levels; consider alternative anticonvulsants. Rifabutin, rifapentine, and dexamethasone may decrease elvitegravir and cobicistat levels. Ketoconazole, itraconazole, or voriconazole may increase levels of elvitegravir and cobicistat. May increase levels of drugs that are primarily metabolized by CYP3A/2D6, or are substrates of P-gp, breast cancer resistance protein, or organic anion transporting polypeptides 1B1/1B3. Elvitegravir may decrease levels of CYP2C9 substrates. CYP3A inducers may decrease elvitegravir and cobicistat levels and may result in loss of therapeutic effect and development of resistance. Drugs that reduce renal function or compete for active tubular secretion (eg, acyclovir, cidofovir, gentamicin) may increase levels of emtricitabine, TDF, and other renally eliminated drugs and may increase risk of adverse reactions. CYP3A inhibitors and clarithromycin may increase plasma levels of cobicistat. Cases of acute renal failure after initiation of high-dose or multiple NSAIDs reported in patients w/ risk factors for renal dysfunction who appeared stable on TDF; consider alternatives to NSAIDs, if needed, in patients at risk for renal dysfunction. Refer to PI for dosing modifications when used w/ certain concomitant therapies.

PATIENT CONSIDERATIONS

Assessment: Assess for obesity, prolonged nucleoside exposure, risk factors for liver disease, renal/ hepatic impairment, pregnancy/nursing status, and possible drug interactions. Assess BMD in patients who have a history of pathological bone fracture or w/ other risk factors for osteoporosis or bone loss. Obtain baseline estimated CrCl, urine glucose, urine protein, and SrCr. Perform test for HBV infection prior to therapy.

Monitoring: Monitor for signs/symptoms of lactic acidosis, severe hepatomegaly w/ steatosis, new onset/worsening renal impairment, immune reconstitution syndrome, autoimmune disorders, fat redistribution/accumulation, decreased BMD, increased biochemical markers for bone metabolism, osteomalacia, and other adverse reactions. Monitor for exacerbations of hepatitis B in patients w/ coinfection for at least several months upon discontinuation of therapy. Monitor BMD, estimated CrCl, urine glucose, urine protein, and SrCr. Monitor serum phosphorus levels in patients at risk for renal impairment. Monitor INR upon coadministration w/ warfarin.

Counseling: Advise to remain under care of a physician during therapy. Inform that therapy does not cure HIV-1 infection and continuous therapy is necessary to control HIV-1 infection and decrease HIV-related illnesses. Advise to practice safe sex, to use latex or polyurethane condoms, not to share personal items (eg, toothbrush, razor blades), needles, or other inj equipment, and not to breastfeed. Instruct to take on a regular dosing schedule w/ food and to avoid missing doses. Instruct to contact physician if symptoms of lactic acidosis/pronounced hepatotoxicity, or any symptoms of infection occur. Advise that fat redistribution/accumulation, renal impairment, and decreases in BMD may occur. Inform that hepatitis B testing is recommended prior to initiating therapy. Advise to report use of any prescription or nonprescription medication or herbal products, including St. John's wort.

STORAGE: 25°C (77°F); excursions permitted to 15-30°C (59-86°F).

STRIVERDI RESPIMAT — olodaterol RX

Class: Beta$_2$ agonist

Long-acting β_2-adrenergic agonists (LABAs) increase the risk of asthma-related death. Not indicated for the treatment of asthma.

ADULT DOSAGE

Chronic Obstructive Pulmonary Disease

Long-Term Maint Treatment of Airflow Obstruction:

Maint: 2 inh qd at the same time of day

Max: 2 inh/24 hrs

PEDIATRIC DOSAGE

Pediatric use may not have been established

ADMINISTRATION

Oral inh route

Insert cartridge into inhaler and prime the unit prior to 1st use

Priming Instructions

1. Actuate the inhaler toward the ground until the aerosol cloud is visible
2. Repeat 3 more times

If Not Used >3 Days: Actuate inhaler once to prepare for use

If Not Used >21 Days: Repeat priming instructions

HOW SUPPLIED

Spray, Inhalation: 2.5mcg/actuation [28, 60 actuations]

CONTRAINDICATIONS

Asthma without use of a long-term asthma control medication.

WARNINGS/PRECAUTIONS

Do not initiate in acutely deteriorating COPD patients or use for the relief of acute symptoms. D/C regular use of inhaled short-acting β_2-agonists (SABAs) when beginning treatment; use only for symptomatic relief of acute respiratory symptoms. Do not use more often or at higher doses than recommended; clinically significant cardiovascular (CV) effects and fatalities reported with excessive use. May produce paradoxical bronchospasm; d/c therapy immediately and institute alternative therapy. CV effects may occur; d/c if such effects occur. Caution with CV disorders, convulsive disorders, thyrotoxicosis, diabetes mellitus (DM), ketoacidosis, and in patients unusually responsive to sympathomimetic amines. May produce significant hypokalemia and increases in plasma glucose. Immediate hypersensitivity reactions may occur; d/c therapy immediately and consider alternative treatment.

ADVERSE REACTIONS

Nasopharyngitis, URTI, bronchitis, cough, back pain.

DRUG INTERACTIONS

Do not use with other medications containing LABAs. Adrenergic drugs may potentiate sympathetic effects; use with caution. Xanthine derivatives, steroids, or diuretics may potentiate any hypokalemic effect. Caution is advised when coadministered with non-K^+-sparing diuretics (eg, loop, thiazide). Extreme caution with MAOIs, TCAs, or drugs known to prolong the QTc interval; action on CV system may be potentiated. Drugs known to prolong the QTc interval may be associated with an increased risk of ventricular arrhythmias. β-blockers and olodaterol may interfere with the effect of each other when administered concurrently. β-blockers may block therapeutic effects and produce severe bronchospasm in COPD patients; if such therapy is needed, consider cardioselective β-blockers and use with caution. Ketoconazole (a strong dual CYP and P-gp inhibitor) may increase levels.

PATIENT CONSIDERATIONS

Assessment: Assess for asthma, acute COPD deteriorations, CV disorders, convulsive disorders, thyrotoxicosis, DM, ketoacidosis, pregnancy/nursing status, and possible drug interactions. Assess use in patients unusually responsive to sympathomimetic amines.

Monitoring: Monitor for deteriorating disease, paradoxical bronchospasm, CV effects, hypokalemia, hyperglycemia, immediate hypersensitivity reactions, and other adverse reactions.

Counseling: Counsel about the risks and benefits of therapy. Inform that drug is not for treatment of asthma. Advise not to use to relieve acute symptoms; inform that acute symptoms should be treated with an inhaled SABA. Instruct to notify physician immediately if experiencing worsening of symptoms, decreasing effectiveness of inhaled SABA, a need for more inhalations than usual of inhaled SABA, or a significant decrease in lung function. Advise not to stop therapy without physician guidance, not to use additional LABA, and not to use more than the recommended once-daily dose. Instruct to d/c the regular use of inhaled SABAs when beginning treatment. Inform of adverse effects associated with therapy.

STORAGE: 25°C (77°F); excursions permitted to 15-30°C (59-86°F). Avoid freezing.

SUBOXONE FILM – buprenorphine/naloxone CIII

Class: Partial opioid agonist/opioid antagonist

ADULT DOSAGE

Opioid Dependence

Use as part of a complete treatment plan to include counseling and psychosocial support

Prior to Induction:
Consider type of opioid dependence (eg, long- or short-acting opioid products), the time since last opioid use, and degree or level of opioid dependence. The 1st dose of therapy should be started only when objective signs of moderate withdrawal appear

Induction:
Day 1:
Initial: 2mg/0.5mg or 4mg/1mg
Titrate: May titrate upwards in 2mg or 4mg increments of buprenorphine, at approx 2-hr intervals to 8mg/2mg based on the control of acute withdrawal symptoms. Induction dosage of up to 8mg/2mg is recommended

Day 2:
Up to 16mg/4mg as single daily dose

Naloxone exposure is somewhat higher after buccal than after SL administration; the SL site of administration is recommended to be used during induction to minimize naloxone exposure, to reduce risk of precipitated withdrawal

On Methadone/Long-Acting Opioids:
May be more susceptible to precipitated and prolonged withdrawal during induction therapy; buprenorphine monotherapy is recommended when used according to approved administration instructions. Following induction, may then be transitioned to qd SL film dose

On Heroin/Other Short-Acting Opioids:
May be inducted w/ SL film or w/ SL buprenorphine monotherapy

PEDIATRIC DOSAGE

Pediatric use may not have been established

S

Administer 1st dose when objective signs of moderate opioid withdrawal appear, and not <6 hrs after last opioid use. Achieve adequate maint dose, titrated to clinical effectiveness as soon as possible

Maint:

For maint, SL film may be administered buccally or sublingually

Day 3 Onwards:

Progressively adjust dose in increments/decrements of 2mg/0.5mg or 4mg/1mg to a level that maintains treatment and suppresses opioid withdrawal signs/symptoms. After treatment induction and stabilization, the maint dose is generally in the range of 4mg/1mg to 24mg/6mg per day depending on the patient/response

Target Dose: (16mg/4mg)/day as single daily dose

Dosages higher than (24mg/6mg)/day have not been demonstrated to provide clinical advantage

Conversions

Switching Between Buprenorphine or Buprenorphine/Naloxone SL Tabs and Buprenorphine/Naloxone SL Film:

Start on the corresponding dosage of the previously administered product; adjust dose prn. Refer to PI for switching between SL film strengths

DOSING CONSIDERATIONS

Hepatic Impairment

Moderate: Use may not be appropriate

Severe: Avoid use

Elderly

Start at lower end of dosing range

Discontinuation

Decision to d/c therapy should be made as part of a comprehensive treatment plan; taper patients to avoid opioid withdrawal signs/symptoms

Other Important Considerations

Unstable Patients:

Patients who continue to misuse, abuse, or divert buprenorphine products or other opioids should be provided w/, or referred to, more intensive and structured treatment

ADMINISTRATION

Buccal/SL route

Administer SL film whole; do not cut, chew, or swallow film.
Do not move film after placement.

SL Administration

Place 1 film under the tongue, close to the base on the left or right side.
If an additional film is necessary, place SL on the opposite side from the 1st film; place in a manner to minimize overlapping as much as possible. Keep under the tongue until completely dissolved.
If a 3rd film is necessary, place it under the tongue on either side after the first 2 films have dissolved.

Buccal Administration

Place 1 film on the inside of the right or left cheek.
If an additional film is necessary, place on the inside of the opposite cheek. Keep on the inside of the cheek until completely dissolved.
If a 3rd film is necessary, place it on the inside of the right or left cheek after the first 2 films have dissolved.

Switching Between SL and Buccal Sites of Administration

Buprenorphine exposure between buccal and SL administration is similar; therefore, once induction is complete, may switch between buccal and SL administration w/o significant risk of under- or over-dosing.

HOW SUPPLIED

Film, SL: (Buprenorphine/Naloxone) 2mg/0.5mg, 4mg/1mg, 8mg/2mg, 12mg/3mg

CONTRAINDICATIONS

Hypersensitivity to buprenorphine or naloxone.

WARNINGS/PRECAUTIONS

Not appropriate as an analgesic. Hypersensitivity reactions, bronchospasm, angioneurotic edema, and anaphylactic shock reported. May precipitate opioid withdrawal signs and symptoms if administered before the agonist effects of the opioid have subsided. Not recommended for initiation of treatment in patients w/ moderate hepatic impairment; may be used w/ caution for maintenance treatment in patients w/ moderate hepatic impairment who have initiated treatment on a buprenorphine product w/o naloxone. May impair mental/physical abilities. May produce orthostatic hypotension in ambulatory patients. Caution w/ myxedema, hypothyroidism, adrenal cortical insufficiency (eg, Addison's disease), CNS depression/coma, toxic psychoses, prostatic hypertrophy, urethral stricture, acute alcoholism, delirium tremens, kyphoscoliosis, and in debilitated patients. **Buprenorphine:** Potential for abuse. Significant respiratory depression and death reported; caution w/ compromised respiratory function. Reestablish adequate ventilation in case of overdose; higher than normal doses and repeated administration of naloxone may be necessary. Accidental pediatric exposure can cause severe, possibly fatal, respiratory depression. Chronic use produces physical dependence. Cytolytic hepatitis and hepatitis w/ jaundice reported; obtain LFTs prior to initiation and periodically during treatment. If a hepatic event is suspected, biological and etiological evaluation is recommended; careful discontinuation may be needed depending on the case. Caution w/ preexisting liver enzyme abnormalities, hepatitis B or C infection, use w/ other potentially hepatotoxic drugs, and ongoing injecting drug use. Neonatal withdrawal reported when used during pregnancy. May elevate CSF pressure; caution w/ head injury, intracranial lesions, and other circumstances when CSF pressure may be increased. May produce miosis and changes in the level of consciousness that may interfere w/ patient evaluation. May increase intracholedochal pressure; caution w/ biliary tract dysfunction. May obscure the diagnosis or clinical course of patients w/ acute abdominal conditions.

ADVERSE REACTIONS

Oral hypoesthesia, constipation, glossodynia, oral mucosal erythema, vomiting, intoxication, disturbance in attention, palpitations, insomnia, withdrawal syndrome, hyperhidrosis, blurred vision, restlessness.

DRUG INTERACTIONS

May cause respiratory depression, coma, and death w/ benzodiazepines or other CNS depressants (eg, alcohol); use w/ caution. Opioid analgesics, general anesthetics, benzodiazepines, phenothiazines, other tranquilizers, sedative/hypnotics, or other CNS depressants (eg, alcohol) may increase CNS depression; consider dose reduction of 1 or both agents. Concomitant use w/ CYP3A4 inhibitors (eg, azole antifungals, macrolides, HIV protease inhibitors) should be monitored and may require dose reduction of 1 or both agents. Monitor for signs and symptoms of opioid withdrawal w/ CYP3A4 inducers (eg, efavirenz, phenobarbital, carbamazepine, phenytoin, rifampicin). Monitor dose of patients who are on chronic buprenorphine treatment if non-nucleoside reverse transcriptase inhibitors are added to treatment regimen. Atazanavir and atazanavir/ritonavir may increase levels and sedation; monitor and consider dose reduction of buprenorphine.

PATIENT CONSIDERATIONS

Assessment: Assess for history of hypersensitivity to drug, myxedema, hypothyroidism, adrenal cortical insufficiency, CNS depression or coma, toxic psychoses, prostatic hypertrophy, urethral stricture, acute alcoholism, delirium tremens, kyphoscoliosis, debilitation, compromised respiratory function, hepatic impairment, hepatitis B or C infection, head injury, intracranial lesions and other circumstances in which CSF pressure may be increased, biliary tract dysfunction, acute abdominal conditions, pregnancy/nursing status, and possible drug interactions. Obtain baseline LFTs prior to therapy.

Monitoring: Monitor for hypersensitivity reactions, signs/symptoms of precipitated opioid withdrawal, impaired mental/physical ability, orthostatic hypotension, respiratory depression, drug abuse/dependence, cytolytic hepatitis, hepatitis w/ jaundice, elevation of CSF pressure and intracholedochal pressure, miosis, changes in consciousness levels, and other adverse reactions. Monitor LFTs periodically. Monitor for symptoms related to over-dosing or under-dosing when switching between buprenorphine or other buprenorphine/naloxone products.

Counseling: Warn about danger of self-administration of benzodiazepines and other CNS depressants, including alcohol, while on therapy. Advise that drug contains opioid that can be a target for abuse; instruct to keep film in a safe place protected from theft and children. Instruct to seek medical attention immediately if a child is exposed to the drug. Caution that drug may impair mental/physical abilities and cause orthostatic hypotension. Advise to take film qd and to not change dose w/o consulting physician. Inform that treatment can cause dependence and that withdrawal syndrome may occur upon discontinuation. Advise patients seeking to d/c treatment w/ buprenorphine for opioid dependence to work closely w/ physician on a tapering schedule, and apprise of the potential to relapse to illicit drug use associated w/ discontinuation of treatment.

Advise to report to physician all medications prescribed or currently being used. Advise women regarding possible effects during pregnancy. Advise women who are breastfeeding to monitor the infant for drowsiness and difficulty breathing. Advise to instruct family members that, in event of emergency, the treating physician or staff should be informed that patient is physically dependent on an opioid and that the patient is being treated w/ SL film. Advise to dispose of unused drugs as soon as they are no longer needed by flushing films down the toilet.

STORAGE: 25°C (77°F); excursions permitted to 15-30°C (59-86°F).

SUCLEAR — magnesium sulfate/potassium sulfate/sodium sulfate, polyethylene glycol 3350/potassium chloride/sodium bicarbonate/sodium chloride RX

Class: Bowel cleanser

ADULT DOSAGE

Bowel Cleansing

Prior to Colonoscopy:

Split-Dose (2-Day) Regimen (Preferred Method):

Take Dose 1 the pm before the colonoscopy (10-12 hrs prior to Dose 2), then Dose 2 the next am on the day of the colonoscopy, starting at least 3.5 hrs prior to colonoscopy

Day-Before (1-Day) Regimen (Alternative Method):

On the pm before the colonoscopy, take Dose 1 beginning at least 3.5 hrs prior to hs, then Dose 2 approx 2 hrs after starting Dose 1

PEDIATRIC DOSAGE

Pediatric use may not have been established

ADMINISTRATION

Oral route

Additional fluids must be consumed in both dosing regimens

Consume only clear liquids (no solid food or milk) and avoid alcohol on the day before colonoscopy until after completion of the colonoscopy

Split-Dose (2-Day) Regimen (Preferred Method)

Dose 1 (PM Before Colonoscopy):

1. Dilute the 6-oz oral sol prior to use by pouring entire contents of the bottle into the 16-oz mixing container and then filling the container w/ cool water to the fill line and mix
2. Drink entire sol in container; best to complete drinking the sol w/in 20 min
3. Refill container w/ 16 oz of water to the fill line and drink it over the next 2 hrs
4. Refill container w/ 16 oz of water to the fill line and finish drinking it before going to bed

Dose 2 (Next Morning on the Day of Colonoscopy):

1. Dissolve powder of Dose 2 by adding water to the fill line on the jug
2. Shake jug until all powder is dissolved; sol can be used w/ or w/o the addition of a flavor pack
3. Sol may be refrigerated after adding water and should be used w/in 48 hrs of reconstitution
4. Using the 16-oz container provided w/ the kit, drink all the sol in the jug at a rate of one 16-oz container every 20 min (eg, four 16-oz containers over a period of 1.5 hrs)
5. Complete drinking sol at least 2 hrs before colonoscopy
6. Consume only clear liquids until 2 hrs prior to colonoscopy; thereafter, nothing should be consumed until the completion of colonoscopy

Day-Before (1-Day) Regimen (Alternative Method)

PM Before Colonoscopy:

Dose 1:

1. Dilute the 6-oz oral sol prior to use by pouring entire contents of the bottle into the 16-oz mixing container and then filling the container w/ cool water to the fill line and mix
2. Drink entire sol in container; best to complete drinking the sol w/in 20 min
3. Refill container w/ 16 oz of water to the fill line and drink it over the next 2 hrs

Dose 2:

1. Dissolve powder of Dose 2 by adding water to the fill line on the jug
2. Shake jug until all the powder is dissolved; sol can be used w/ or w/o the addition of a flavor pack
3. Sol may be refrigerated after adding water and should be used w/in 48 hrs of reconstitution
4. Using the 16-oz container provided w/ the kit, drink all the sol in the jug at a rate of one 16-oz container every 20 min (eg, four 16-oz containers over a period of 1.5 hrs)

5. Refill container w/ 16 oz of water to the fill line and finish drinking it before going to bed
6. Consume only clear liquids until 2 hrs prior to colonoscopy; thereafter, nothing should be consumed until the completion of colonoscopy

HOW SUPPLIED

Sol: (Liquid) Dose 1 (Sodium Sulfate/Potassium Sulfate/Magnesium Sulfate) 17.5g/3.13g/1.6g [6 oz]; (Powder) Dose 2 (Polyethylene Glycol [PEG] 3350/Sodium Chloride/Sodium Bicarbonate/Potassium Chloride) 210g/5.6g/2.86g/0.74g/2L

CONTRAINDICATIONS

GI obstruction or ileus, bowel perforation, gastric retention, toxic colitis or toxic megacolon, known allergies to any components of Suclear.

WARNINGS/PRECAUTIONS

Consume only clear liquids (no solid food or milk) and avoid alcohol on the day before colonoscopy until after completion of the colonoscopy. Adequately hydrate before, during, and after use. If significant vomiting or signs of dehydration develop, perform postcolonoscopy lab tests (electrolytes, SrCr, BUN). Correct electrolyte abnormalities before treatment. Caution with conditions that increase risk of fluid and electrolyte disturbances or may increase risk of seizure, arrhythmias, prolonged QT, and renal impairment. Serious arrhythmias reported rarely; use with caution and consider predose and postcolonoscopy ECGs in patients at increased risk of serious cardiac arrhythmias. Generalized tonic-clonic seizures reported; caution in patients with a history of or at increased risk of seizures (eg, with known/suspected hyponatremia). Caution with impaired renal function; consider performing baseline and postcolonoscopy lab tests. May produce colonic mucosal aphthous ulcerations; consider this when interpreting colonoscopy findings in patients with known/suspected inflammatory bowel disease. Serious cases of ischemic colitis reported. Patients with severe active ulcerative colitis may be at increased risk of exacerbation of their disease with therapy. Monitor patients with impaired gag reflex and patients prone to regurgitation/aspiration. Not for direct ingestion; direct ingestion of undiluted solution may increase the risk of N/V, dehydration, or other serious adverse reactions.

ADVERSE REACTIONS

Discomfort, abdominal distension, abdominal pain, N/V.

DRUG INTERACTIONS

Caution with medications that increase risk for fluid and electrolyte disturbances or may increase risk of seizure, arrhythmias, prolonged QT, and renal impairment. Caution with drugs associated with hypokalemia (eg, diuretics, corticosteroids, drugs where hypokalemia is a particular risk [eg, cardiac glycosides]) or hyponatremia, NSAIDs, and drugs known to induce antidiuretic hormone secretion (eg, TCAs, SSRIs, antipsychotics, carbamazepine). Alcohol may increase the risk of dehydration. Caution with drugs that lower seizure threshold (eg, TCAs) and in patients withdrawing from alcohol or benzodiazepines. Caution with drugs that may affect renal function (eg, diuretics, ACE inhibitors, ARBs, NSAIDs). Increased risk of mucosal ulceration or ischemic colitis with stimulant laxatives (eg, bisacodyl, sodium picosulfate); avoid concurrent use. Oral medication administered within 1 hr of the start of each dose may be flushed from GI tract and may not be absorbed properly.

PATIENT CONSIDERATIONS

Assessment: Assess for drug hypersensitivity, GI obstruction or ileus, bowel perforation, gastric retention, toxic colitis, toxic megacolon, fluid and electrolyte abnormalities, renal impairment, any other conditions where treatment is cautioned, pregnancy/nursing status, and possible drug interactions. Consider predose ECGs in patients at increased risk of serious cardiac arrhythmias.

Monitoring: Monitor for arrhythmias, generalized tonic-clonic seizures, colonic mucosal aphthous ulcerations, ischemic colitis, and other adverse reactions. Monitor patients with impaired gag reflex and patients prone to regurgitation/aspiration. Consider postcolonoscopy ECGs in patients at increased risk of serious cardiac arrhythmias.

Counseling: Instruct to inform physician if patient has trouble swallowing or is prone to regurgitation/aspiration. Inform that each bottle needs to be diluted in water before ingestion and instruct to drink additional water according to the instructions. Inform that oral medications may not be absorbed properly if taken within 1 hr of starting each dose of drug. Instruct not to take other laxatives during therapy. Advise to hydrate adequately before, during, and after use. Instruct to consume only clear liquids (no solid food or milk) and to avoid alcohol on the day before colonoscopy until after completion of the colonoscopy.

STORAGE: 20-25°C (68-77°F); excursions permitted between 15-30°C (59-86°F). Reconstituted Sol: May be refrigerated. Use within 48 hrs.

SULFAMETHOXAZOLE/TRIMETHOPRIM – sulfamethoxazole/trimethoprim RX

Class: Sulfonamide/tetrahydrofolic acid inhibitor

OTHER BRAND NAMES
Bactrim DS, Bactrim, Sulfatrim

ADULT DOSAGE

Traveler's Diarrhea

Sus/Tab:
Usual: One 800mg/160mg tab or two 400mg/80mg tabs or 4 tsp (20mL) sus q12h for 5 days

Urinary Tract Infections

Inj:
Severe Infections: 8-10mg/kg/day (based on the trimethoprim component) given in 2 or 4 equally divided doses q6h, q8h, or q12h for up to 14 days
Max: 60mL/day

Sus/Tab:
Usual: One 800mg/160mg tab or two 400mg/80mg tabs or 4 tsp (20mL) sus q12h for 10-14 days

Acute Bacterial Exacerbation of Chronic Bronchitis

Sus/Tab:
Usual: One 800mg/160mg tab or two 400mg/80mg tabs or 4 tsp sus (20mL) q12h for 14 days

Shigellosis

Inj:
8-10mg/kg/day (based on the trimethoprim component) given in 2 or 4 equally divided doses q6h, q8h, or q12h for up to 5 days
Max: 60mL/day

Sus/Tab:
Usual: One 800mg/160mg tab or two 400mg/80mg tabs or 4 tsp (20mL) sus q12h for 5 days

Pneumonia

***Pneumocystis jiroveci* Pneumonia Treatment:**
Inj:
15-20mg/kg/day (based on the trimethoprim component) given in 3 or 4 equally divided doses q6-8h for up to 14 days
Sus/Tab:
75-100mg/kg sulfamethoxazole and 15-20mg/kg trimethoprim per 24 hrs given in equally divided doses q6h for 14-21 days

***P. jiroveci* Pneumonia Prophylaxis in Immunosuppressed Patients:**
Sus/Tab:
One 800mg/160mg tab or 4 tsp (20mL) sus daily

PEDIATRIC DOSAGE

Pneumonia

≥2 Months of Age:

***P. jiroveci* Pneumonia Treatment:**
Inj:
15-20mg/kg/day (based on the trimethoprim component) given in 3 or 4 equally divided doses q6-8h for up to 14 days
Sus/Tab:
75-100mg/kg sulfamethoxazole and 15-20mg/kg trimethoprim per 24 hrs given in equally divided doses q6h for 14-21 days

***P. jiroveci* Pneumonia Prophylaxis in Immunosuppressed Patients:**
Sus/Tab:
750mg/m^2/day sulfamethoxazole w/ 150mg/m^2/day trimethoprim given in equally divided doses bid, on 3 consecutive days/week
Max: 1600mg/day sulfamethoxazole and 320mg/day trimethoprim

Acute Otitis Media

Use only when sulfamethoxazole/trimethoprim offers some advantage over the use of other antimicrobial agents

≥2 Months of Age:
Sus/Tab:
40mg/kg sulfamethoxazole and 8mg/kg trimethoprim per 24 hrs, given in 2 divided doses q12h for 10 days

Shigellosis

≥2 Months of Age:
Inj:
8-10mg/kg/day (based on the trimethoprim component) given in 2 or 4 equally divided doses q6h, q8h, or q12h for up to 5 days
Max: 60mL/day

Sus/Tab:
40mg/kg sulfamethoxazole and 8mg/kg trimethoprim per 24 hrs, given in 2 divided doses q12h for 5 days

Urinary Tract Infections

≥2 Months of Age:

Inj:
Severe Infections: 8-10mg/kg/day (based on the trimethoprim component) given in 2 or 4 equally divided doses q6h, q8h, or q12h for up to 14 days
Max: 60mL/day

Sus/Tab:
40mg/kg sulfamethoxazole and 8mg/kg trimethoprim per 24 hrs, given in 2 divided doses q12h for 10 days

DOSING CONSIDERATIONS

Renal Impairment
CrCl 15-30mL/min: 1/2 the usual regimen
CrCl <15mL/min: Use not recommended

S

ADMINISTRATION

IV/Oral route

IV

Must be diluted prior to administration.
Administer by IV infusion over 60-90 min; avoid rapid infusion or bolus inj.
Do not mix w/ other drugs or sol.

IV Preparation/Dilution:

Each 5mL of the drug should be added to 125mL D5W; use w/in 6 hrs after dilution and do not refrigerate.
If 5mL/100mL D5W dilution is desired, use w/in 4 hrs.
If fluid restriction is desired, each 5mL of the drug may be added to 75mL D5W; administer w/in 2 hrs.
Multidose vials must be used w/in 48 hrs after initial entry into vial.

Compatible Infusion Systems:

Unit-dose glass containers, unit-dose polyvinyl chloride and polyolefin containers.

Sus

Shake well before using.
Refer to PI for specific weight-dose recommendations for sus/tab use in pediatrics.

HOW SUPPLIED

Sulfamethoxazole/Trimethoprim (SMX/TMP) **Inj:** (80mg/16mg)/mL [5mL, 10mL, 30mL]; **Sus:** (Sulfatrim) (200mg/40mg)/5mL [473mL]; **Tab:** (Bactrim) 400mg/80mg*, (Bactrim DS) 800mg/160mg* *scored

CONTRAINDICATIONS

Known hypersensitivity to TMP or sulfonamides, documented megaloblastic anemia due to folate deficiency, history of drug-induced immune thrombocytopenia w/ use of TMP and/or sulfonamides, and pediatric patients <2 months of age. **Inj/Sus:** Pregnant and nursing women. **Sus/Tab:** Marked hepatic damage or severe renal insufficiency when renal function status cannot be monitored.

WARNINGS/PRECAUTIONS

Fatalities, although rare, have occurred due to severe reactions, including Stevens-Johnson syndrome, toxic epidermal necrolysis, fulminant hepatic necrosis, agranulocytosis, aplastic anemia, thrombocytopenia, and other blood dyscrasias; d/c at the 1st appearance of skin rash or any sign of adverse reaction. Cough, SOB, and pulmonary infiltrates reported. Do not use for treatment of group A β-hemolytic streptococcal infections. *Clostridium difficile*-associated diarrhea (CDAD) reported; may need to d/c if CDAD is suspected or confirmed. May result in bacterial resistance if used in the absence of proven or suspected bacterial infection or a prophylactic indication. Caution w/ hepatic/renal impairment, possible folate deficiency (eg, the elderly, chronic alcoholics, those receiving anticonvulsant therapy, malabsorption syndrome, malnutrition states), severe allergies or bronchial asthma, porphyria, and thyroid dysfunction. Hematological changes indicative of folic acid deficiency may occur in the elderly, or w/ preexisting folic acid deficiency or kidney failure; effects are reversible by folinic acid therapy. Hemolysis may occur in patients w/ G6PD deficiency. Cases of hypoglycemia in nondiabetic patients reported rarely; increased risk w/ renal dysfunction, liver disease, malnutrition, and high doses. TMP may impair phenylalanine metabolism. AIDS patients may not tolerate or respond to therapy in the same manner as non-AIDS patients; increased incidence of side effects, particularly rash, fever, leukopenia, and elevated transaminase values in AIDS patients being treated for *P. jiroveci* pneumonia; reevaluate therapy if skin rash or any sign of adverse reaction develops. May cause hyperkalemia in patients receiving high dosage of TMP, w/ underlying disorders of K^+ metabolism, w/ renal insufficiency, or when used concomitantly w/ drugs known to induce hyperkalemia; closely monitor serum K^+. Ensure adequate fluid intake and urinary output during treatment to prevent crystalluria. Slow acetylators may be more prone to idiosyncratic reactions to sulfonamides. D/C if a significant reduction in the count of any formed blood element is noted. Lab test interactions may occur. **Inj:** Contains sodium metabisulfite, which may cause allergic-type reactions, including anaphylactic symptoms and life-threatening or less severe asthmatic episodes in certain susceptible people. Contains benzyl alcohol, which has been associated w/ an increased incidence of neurological and other complications (sometimes fatal) in newborns. Local irritation and inflammation due to extravascular infiltration of the infusion reported; d/c infusion and restart at another site if these occur. **Tab:** Severe and symptomatic hyponatremia may occur, particularly in patients treated for *P. jiroveci* pneumonia; evaluation for hyponatremia and appropriate correction is necessary in symptomatic patients to prevent life-threatening complications. Use during pregnancy may be associated w/ an increased risk of congenital malformations.

ADVERSE REACTIONS

GI disturbances (N/V, anorexia), allergic skin reactions (eg, rash, urticaria).

DRUG INTERACTIONS

Increased incidence of thrombocytopenia w/ purpura reported in elderly concurrently receiving certain diuretics, primarily thiazides. May prolong PT w/ warfarin; caution w/ anticoagulants. May inhibit the hepatic metabolism of phenytoin; monitor for possible excessive phenytoin effect. May

S

increase free methotrexate concentrations. Marked but reversible nephrotoxicity reported w/ cyclosporine in renal transplant recipients. May increase digoxin levels, especially in the elderly; monitor digoxin levels. Increased SMX levels w/ indomethacin. Megaloblastic anemia may develop if used in patients receiving pyrimethamine as malaria prophylaxis in doses >25mg/week. May decrease efficacy of TCAs. Potentiates the effect of oral hypoglycemics. Toxic delirium reported w/ amantadine. Hyperkalemia in elderly patients reported after concomitant use w/ an ACE inhibitor. **Inj/Tab:** Treatment failure and excess mortality reported when used concomitantly w/ leucovorin for the treatment of HIV positive patients w/ *P. jiroveci* pneumonia; avoid coadministration during treatment of *P. jiroveci* pneumonia. **Tab:** Caution w/ drugs that are substrates of CYP2C8 (eg, pioglitazone, repaglinide, rosiglitazone), CYP2C9 (eg, glipizide, glyburide), or OCT2 (eg, memantine, metformin).

PATIENT CONSIDERATIONS

Assessment: Assess for hypersensitivity to the drug, megaloblastic anemia, history of drug-induced immune thrombocytopenia, hepatic/renal impairment, folate deficiency, severe allergies, bronchial asthma, G6PD deficiency, porphyria, thyroid dysfunction, underlying disorders of K^+ metabolism, pregnancy/nursing status, and possible drug interactions.

Monitoring: Monitor for hypersensitivity and other fatal reactions, CDAD, folate deficiency, hypoglycemia, hyperkalemia, and other adverse reactions. Monitor hydration status. Perform CBC frequently, and urinalysis w/ careful microscopic exam and renal function tests. **Inj:** Monitor for infusion reactions. **Tab:** Monitor for hyponatremia.

Counseling: Advise that therapy should only be used to treat bacterial, not viral, infections. Instruct to take exactly ud even if patient feels better early in the course of therapy. Inform that skipping doses or not completing the full course of therapy may decrease effectiveness of treatment and increase bacterial resistance. Instruct to maintain an adequate fluid intake. Inform that diarrhea is a common problem caused by therapy, which usually ends when therapy is discontinued. Instruct to immediately contact physician if watery and bloody stools (w/ or w/o stomach cramps and fever) occur, even as late as ≥2 months after having taken the last dose.

STORAGE: 20-25°C (68-77°F). **Inj:** Do not refrigerate. **Sus:** Protect from light.

SUPREP — magnesium sulfate/potassium sulfate/sodium sulfate RX

Class: Bowel cleanser

ADULT DOSAGE

Bowel Cleansing

Prior to Colonoscopy:
Split-Dose (2-Day) Regimen:
Day Prior to Colonoscopy:

1. A light breakfast may be consumed, or have only clear liquids; avoid red and purple liquids, milk, and alcoholic beverages
2. Early in the pm, pour the contents of 1 bottle into the mixing container provided, fill the container w/ water to the 16 oz fill line, and drink the entire amount
3. Drink 2 additional containers filled to the 16 oz line w/ water over the next hr

Day of Colonoscopy:

1. Have only clear liquids until after the colonoscopy; avoid red and purple liquids, milk, and alcoholic beverages
2. The morning of colonoscopy (10-12 hrs after the evening dose), pour the contents of the 2nd bottle into the mixing container provided, fill the container w/ water to the 16 oz fill line, and drink the entire amount
3. Drink 2 additional containers filled to the 16 oz line w/ water over the next hr
4. Complete all Suprep Bowel Prep Kit and required water at least 1 hr prior to colonoscopy

PEDIATRIC DOSAGE

Pediatric use may not have been established

ADMINISTRATION
Oral route

HOW SUPPLIED
Sol: (Sodium Sulfate/Potassium Sulfate/Magnesium Sulfate) 17.5g/3.13g/1.6g

CONTRAINDICATIONS
GI obstruction, bowel perforation, gastric retention, ileus, toxic colitis or toxic megacolon, known allergies to components of the kit.

WARNINGS/PRECAUTIONS
Hydrate adequately before, during, and after use. If significant vomiting or signs of dehydration occur, consider performing postcolonoscopy tests (eg, electrolytes, creatinine, BUN). Correct electrolyte abnormalities prior to use. Caution w/ conditions that may increase the risk of fluid/electrolyte disturbances and renal impairment. May increase uric acid levels. Serious arrhythmias reported rarely; caution in patients at increased risk of arrhythmias. Generalized tonic-clonic seizures and/or loss of consciousness reported; caution in patients at increased risk of seizures (eg, hyponatremia, alcohol or benzodiazepine withdrawal). May produce colonic mucosal aphthous ulcerations and ischemic colitis. If suspected, rule out GI obstruction or perforation prior to administration. Caution in patients w/ impaired gag reflex and patients prone to regurgitation/aspiration; observe during administration. Not for direct ingestion.

ADVERSE REACTIONS
Overall discomfort, abdominal distention, abdominal pain, N/V.

DRUG INTERACTIONS
Caution w/ concomitant use of medications that increase the risk for fluid and electrolyte disturbances or increase the risk of seizures (eg, TCAs), arrhythmias and prolonged QT. Caution w/ medications that may affect renal function (eg, diuretics, ACE inhibitors, ARBs, NSAIDs). Concurrent use w/ stimulant laxatives may increase risk of colonic mucosal ulcerations and ischemic colitis. Absorption of oral medications may not occur if administered w/in an hr of the start of a Suprep dose.

PATIENT CONSIDERATIONS

Assessment: Assess for GI obstruction, bowel perforation, or any other conditions where treatment is contraindicated or cautioned. Assess for pregnancy/nursing status, and for possible drug interactions. Obtain baseline electrolytes, creatinine, and BUN in patients w/ renal impairment. Perform baseline ECGs in patients at risk for arrhythmias.

Monitoring: Monitor for electrolyte abnormalities, cardiac arrhythmias, seizures, loss of consciousness, colonic mucosal ulcerations, ischemic colitis, and aspiration. Perform ECG in patients at increased risk of serious cardiac arrhythmias. Monitor electrolytes, creatinine, and BUN in patients w/ renal impairment.

Counseling: Instruct to notify physician if patient has difficulty swallowing or is prone to regurgitation/aspiration. Instruct to dilute each bottle w/ water prior to ingestion and drink additional water ud by instructions. Advise that ingestion of undiluted solution may increase risk of N/V and dehydration. Inform that oral medications may not be absorbed properly if they are taken w/in 1 hr of starting each dose of Suprep Bowel Kit. Instruct not to take additional laxatives.

STORAGE: 20-25°C (68-77°F); excursions permitted between 15-30°C (59-86°F).

SYLVANT – siltuximab

RX

Class: Monoclonal antibody/interleukin-6 (IL-6) receptor antagonist

S

ADULT DOSAGE

Multicentric Castleman's Disease

Treatment of patients who are HIV negative and human herpesvirus-8 negative

11mg/kg given over 1 hr as an IV infusion administered every 3 weeks until treatment failure

Perform hematology lab tests prior to each dose for the first 12 months and every 3 dosing cycles thereafter. If treatment criteria outlined below are not met, consider delaying treatment; do not reduce dose

Treatment Criteria
Requirements Prior to 1st Dose:
ANC: $\geq 1.0 \times 10^9/L$

PEDIATRIC DOSAGE
Pediatric use may not have been established

Platelet Count: ≥75 x 10^9/L
Hgb: <17 g/dL
Retreatment Criteria:
ANC: ≥1.0 x 10^9/L
Platelet Count: ≥50 x 10^9/L
Hgb: <17 g/dL

DOSING CONSIDERATIONS

Adverse Reactions

D/C in patients w/ severe infusion related reactions, anaphylaxis, severe allergic reactions, or cytokine release syndromes; do not reinstitute treatment

Other Important Considerations

Do not administer to patients w/ severe infections until the infection resolves

ADMINISTRATION

IV route

Preparation

1. Calculate the dose (mg), total volume (mL) of reconstituted sol required, and the number of vials needed. A 21-gauge 1-1/2 inch needle is recommended for preparation. Infusion bags (250mL) must contain D5W and must be made of polyvinyl chloride, polyolefin, polypropylene, or polyethylene. Alternatively, polyethylene bottles may be used.
2. Allow the vial(s) to come to room temperature over approx 30 min. Sylvant should remain at room temperature for the duration of the preparation.
3. Reconstitute each vial as follows:
100mg Vial: Reconstitute w/ 5.2mL of sterile water for inj (SWFI)
400mg Vial: Reconstitute w/ 20mL of SWFI
4. Gently swirl reconstituted vials; do not shake or swirl vigorously. The lyophilized powder should dissolve in <60 min. Reconstituted product should be kept for no more than 2 hrs prior to addition into the infusion bag.
5. Dilute the reconstituted sol dose to 250mL w/ sterile D5W by withdrawing a volume equal to the total calculated volume of reconstituted sol from the D5W, 250 mL bag.
6. Slowly add the total calculated volume (mL) of reconstituted sol to the D5W infusion bag. Gently invert the bag to mix the sol.

Administration

Administer the diluted sol by IV infusion over a period of 1 hr using administration sets lined w/ polyvinyl chloride, polyurethane, or polyethylene, containing a 0.2µm inline polyethersulfone filter. The infusion should be completed w/in 4 hrs of the dilution of the reconstituted sol to the infusion bag.

Do not infuse concomitantly in the same IV line w/ other agents.

Do not store any unused portion of the reconstituted product or of the infusion sol.

HOW SUPPLIED

Inj: 100mg, 400mg

CONTRAINDICATIONS

Severe hypersensitivity reaction to siltuximab or any of the excipients in the product.

WARNINGS/PRECAUTIONS

May increase Hgb levels. Do not administer to patients w/ severe infections until the infection resolves. May mask signs and symptoms of acute inflammation including suppression of fever and of acute phase reactants (eg, C-reactive protein). D/C if signs of anaphylaxis or mild to moderate infusion reaction develops. If the infusion reaction resolves, may restart infusion at a lower infusion rate and consider medication w/ antihistamines, acetaminophen, and corticosteroids; d/c if the patient does not tolerate the infusion following these interventions. Administer in a setting that provides resuscitation equipment, medication, and personnel trained to provide resuscitation. GI perforation reported. Women of childbearing potential should use contraception during and for 3 months after treatment.

S

ADVERSE REACTIONS

Pruritus, increased weight, rash, hyperuricemia, URTI.

DRUG INTERACTIONS

Do not administer live vaccines. May increase metabolism of CYP450 substrates; upon initiation or discontinuation of siltuximab, in patients being treated w/ CYP450 substrates w/ a narrow therapeutic index, perform therapeutic monitoring of effect (eg, warfarin) or drug concentration (eg, cyclosporine, theophylline) prn and adjust dose. Caution w/ CYP3A4 substrates where a decrease in effectiveness would be undesirable (eg, oral contraceptives, lovastatin, atorvastatin).

PATIENT CONSIDERATIONS

Assessment: Assess for infection, risk for GI perforation, drug hypersensitivity, pregnancy/nursing status, and possible drug interactions. Perform hematology lab tests prior to each dose of therapy for the first 12 months and every 3 dosing cycles thereafter.

Monitoring: Monitor for signs/symptoms of infection, infusion-related reactions, hypersensitivity, GI perforation, and other adverse reactions.

Counseling: Inform of benefits and risks of treatment. Instruct to immediately contact physician when symptoms suggesting infection or any signs of new/worsening medical conditions appear. Advise to seek immediate medical attention if any symptoms of a serious allergic reaction occur during the infusion. Advise patients of childbearing potential to avoid pregnancy; instruct to use contraception during and for 3 months after treatment.

STORAGE: 2-8°C (36-46°F). Protect from light.

SYMBICORT – budesonide/formoterol fumarate dihydrate RX

Class: Beta$_2$ agonist/corticosteroid

Long-acting β_2-adrenergic agonists (LABAs), such as formoterol, increase the risk of asthma-related death. LABAs may increase the risk of asthma-related hospitalization in pediatric patients and adolescents. Use only for patients not adequately controlled on a long-term asthma-control medication or whose disease severity clearly warrants initiation of treatment with both inhaled corticosteroids and LABA. Do not use if asthma is adequately controlled on low- or medium-dose inhaled corticosteroids.

ADULT DOSAGE

Asthma

2 inh bid (am and pm, approx q12h)
Initial: Based on severity
Max: 160mcg/4.5mcg/inh bid

Not Responding After 1-2 Weeks of Therapy w/ 80mcg/4.5mcg/inh:
Replace w/ 160mcg/4.5mcg/inh for better asthma control

Chronic Obstructive Pulmonary Disease

Maint Treatment of Airflow Obstruction:
2 inh (160mcg/4.5mcg/inh) bid

PEDIATRIC DOSAGE

Asthma

≥12 Years:
2 inh bid (am and pm, approx q12h)
Initial: Based on severity
Max: 160mcg/4.5mcg/inh bid

Not Responding After 1-2 Weeks of Therapy w/ 80mcg/4.5mcg/inh:
Replace w/ 160mcg/4.5mcg/inh for better asthma control

ADMINISTRATION

Oral inh route

After inh, rinse mouth w/ water w/o swallowing
Shake well for 5 sec before use

Priming

1. Shake the inhaler well for 5 sec
2. Hold the inhaler pointing away from the face and then release a test spray
3. Shake it again for 5 sec and release a 2nd test spray
4. Depending on which size was provided, the counter will read either 120 or 60 after it has been primed

If inhaler is not used for more than 7 days or if it is dropped, prime again

HOW SUPPLIED

MDI: (Budesonide/Formoterol) 80mcg/4.5mcg/inh, 160mcg/4.5mcg/inh [60 inhalations, 120 inhalations]

CONTRAINDICATIONS

Primary treatment of status asthmaticus or other acute episodes of asthma or COPD where intensive measures are required. Hypersensitivity to any of the ingredients in Symbicort.

WARNINGS/PRECAUTIONS

Not indicated for the relief of acute bronchospasm; take inhaled short-acting β_2-agonists (SABAs) for immediate relief. Do not initiate during rapidly deteriorating/potentially life-threatening asthma or COPD. D/C regular use of oral/inhaled SABAs when beginning treatment. Cardiovascular (CV) effects and fatalities reported with excessive use; do not use more often or at higher doses than recommended. *Candida albicans* infections of the mouth and pharynx reported; treat with appropriate local or systemic (eg, antifungal) therapy or, interrupt therapy if needed. Lower respiratory tract infections (eg, pneumonia) reported in patients with COPD. Increased susceptibility to infections. May lead to serious/fatal course of chickenpox or measles; avoid exposure and, if exposed, consider prophylaxis/treatment. Caution with active/quiescent tuberculosis (TB); untreated systemic fungal, bacterial, viral, or parasitic infections; or ocular herpes simplex. Deaths due to adrenal insufficiency reported with transfer from systemic to inhaled corticosteroids; if systemic corticosteroids are required, wean slowly from systemic steroid after transferring to therapy. Resume oral corticosteroids

S

during periods of stress or a severe asthma attack if patient was previously withdrawn from systemic corticosteroid. Carefully monitor during withdrawal of oral corticosteroid. Transferring from systemic to inhalation therapy may unmask previously suppressed allergic conditions (eg, rhinitis, conjunctivitis, eczema, arthritis, eosinophilic conditions); monitor for systemic corticosteroid withdrawal effects. Observe carefully for any evidence of systemic corticosteroid effects; caution should be taken in observing patients postoperatively or during periods of stress for evidence of inadequate adrenal response. Reduce dose slowly if hypercorticism or adrenal suppression (including adrenal crisis) appears. May produce paradoxical bronchospasm; d/c immediately and institute alternative therapy. Immediate hypersensitivity reactions (eg, urticaria, angioedema, rash, bronchospasm) may occur. Caution with CV disorders (eg, coronary insufficiency, cardiac arrhythmias, HTN). Decreases in bone mineral density (BMD) reported; caution with major risk factors for decreased bone mineral content (eg, prolonged immobilization, family history of osteoporosis, postmenopausal status, tobacco use, advanced age, poor nutrition). May reduce growth velocity in pediatrics; use lowest effective dose. Glaucoma, increased IOP, cataracts, rare cases of systemic eosinophilic conditions, and vasculitis consistent with Churg-Strauss syndrome reported. Caution with convulsive disorders, thyrotoxicosis, diabetes mellitus (DM), ketoacidosis, hepatic impairment, and in patients unusually responsive to sympathomimetic amines. Clinically significant changes in blood glucose and/or serum K^+ reported. Caution in elderly.

ADVERSE REACTIONS

Nasopharyngitis, headache, URTI, pharyngolaryngeal pain, sinusitis, influenza, back pain, nasal congestion, stomach discomfort, oral candidiasis, bronchitis, vomiting.

DRUG INTERACTIONS

Do not use with other medications containing LABAs (eg, salmeterol, formoterol fumarate, arformoterol tartrate); increased risk of CV effects. Caution with ketoconazole, other known strong CYP3A4 inhibitors (eg, ritonavir, nefazodone, telithromycin, itraconazole), and non-K^+-sparing diuretics (eg, loop, thiazide). Caution with MAOIs or TCAs, or within 2 weeks of discontinuation of such agents. Concomitant use with β-blockers may produce severe bronchospasm in patients with asthma; consider cardioselective β-blockers and administer with caution. Caution with chronic use of drugs that can reduce bone mass (eg, anticonvulsants, oral corticosteroids).

PATIENT CONSIDERATIONS

Assessment: Assess use of long-term asthma control medication (eg, inhaled corticosteroids), status asthmaticus, acute asthma episodes, rapidly deteriorating asthma, bronchospasm, known hypersensitivity to any component of drug, risk factors for decreased bone mineral content, CV or convulsive disorders, other conditions where treatment is contraindicated or cautioned, pregnancy/nursing status, and possible drug interactions. Assess use in patients unusually responsive to sympathomimetic amines. Obtain baseline BMD, eye exam, and lung function.

Monitoring: Monitor for localized oral *C. albicans* infections, worsening or acutely deteriorating asthma, development of glaucoma, increased IOP, cataracts, CV/CNS effects, inhalation induced paradoxical bronchospasm, pneumonia, lower respiratory tract in patients with COPD, hypercorticism, adrenal suppression, hypersensitivity reactions, signs of increased drug exposure with hepatic impairment, and other adverse reactions. Monitor lung function, pulse rate, BP, ECG changes, blood glucose, and serum K^+ levels. Monitor BMD periodically. Monitor growth in children.

Counseling: Inform about increased risk of asthma-related death/hospitalization in pediatrics and adolescents. Instruct not to use to relieve acute asthma symptoms; treat acute symptoms with an inhaled SABA for immediate relief. Instruct to notify physician immediately if experiencing decreased effectiveness of inhaled SABA, need for more inhalations of inhaled SABA than usual, or significant decrease in lung function. Instruct not to d/c without physician's guidance. Instruct not to use with other LABA for asthma and COPD. Advise that localized infections with *C. albicans* may occur in the mouth and pharynx. Instruct to contact physician if symptoms of pneumonia develop. Instruct to avoid exposure to chickenpox or measles and to consult physician without delay, if exposed. Inform of potential worsening of existing TB, fungal, bacterial, viral, or parasitic infections, or ocular herpes simplex. Inform about risks of hypercorticism and adrenal suppression, decreased BMD, cataracts or glaucoma, and reduced growth velocity in pediatric patients. Instruct to taper slowly from systemic corticosteroids if transferring to budesonide-formoterol. Inform of adverse effects associated with β_2-agonists (eg, palpitations, chest pain, rapid HR, tremor, nervousness).

STORAGE: 20-25°C (68-77°F). Store with mouthpiece down. Contents under pressure; do not puncture, incinerate, or store near heat or open flame. Discard when labeled number of inhalations have been used or within 3 months after removal from pouch.

SYNAGIS – palivizumab

RX

Class: Monoclonal antibody/RSV F-protein blocker

PEDIATRIC DOSAGE

Respiratory Syncytial Virus

Prevention of serious lower respiratory tract disease in children at high risk of RSV disease

≤24 Months of Age:
15mg/kg monthly throughout RSV season; administer first dose prior to start of RSV season

Undergoing Cardiopulmonary Bypass:
Administer an additional dose as soon as possible after the procedure (even if <1 month from previous dose) then monthly thereafter, as scheduled

ADMINISTRATION

IM route

If RSV infection develops, continue monthly doses throughout RSV season
Give inj volumes >1mL as a divided dose
Do not dilute, shake, or vigorously agitate vial
Administer immediately after withdrawal from vial
Administer preferably into the anterolateral aspect of the thigh
Refer to PI for further instructions

HOW SUPPLIED

Inj: 50mg/0.5mL, 100mg/mL

CONTRAINDICATIONS

Previous significant hypersensitivity reaction to palivizumab.

WARNINGS/PRECAUTIONS

Anaphylaxis, anaphylactic shock, and other acute hypersensitivity reactions reported; permanently d/c if a significant hypersensitivity reaction occurs, and use caution during readministration if a mild hypersensitivity reaction occurs. Caution with thrombocytopenia or any coagulation disorder. May interfere with immunological-based RSV diagnostic tests and viral culture assays; diagnostic test results should be used in conjunction with clinical findings.

ADVERSE REACTIONS

Fever, rash, anaphylaxis.

PATIENT CONSIDERATIONS

Assessment: Assess for previous hypersensitivity to the drug, thrombocytopenia, and coagulation disorders. Assess if patient is undergoing cardiopulmonary bypass.

Monitoring: Monitor for anaphylaxis, hypersensitivity reactions, and other adverse reactions.

Counseling: Counsel parents/guardians about the potential risks and benefits of therapy. Inform parents/guardians of the possible side effects and of the signs/symptoms of potential allergic reactions; advise of the appropriate actions. Advise parents/guardians of the dosing schedule and the importance of compliance with the full course of therapy.

STORAGE: 2-8°C (36-46°F). Do not freeze.

S

SYNJARDY – empagliflozin/metformin hydrochloride

RX

Class: Biguanide/sodium-glucose cotransporter 2 (SGLT2) inhibitor

Lactic acidosis may occur due to metformin accumulation; risk increases w/ conditions such as renal/hepatic impairment, sepsis, dehydration, excess alcohol intake, and acute CHF. If lactic acidosis is suspected, d/c therapy and hospitalize patient immediately.

ADULT DOSAGE

Type 2 Diabetes Mellitus

Not adequately controlled on a regimen containing empagliflozin or metformin, or in patients who are already being treated w/ both empagliflozin and metformin

PEDIATRIC DOSAGE

Pediatric use may not have been established

Patients on Metformin:
Switch to Synjardy containing empagliflozin 5mg w/ a similar total daily dose of metformin

Patients on Empagliflozin:
Switch to Synjardy containing metformin 500mg w/ a similar total daily dose of empagliflozin

Patients Already Treated w/ Empagliflozin and Metformin:
Switch to Synjardy containing the same total daily doses of each component

Max Daily Dose: Metformin 2000mg and empagliflozin 25mg

Take bid w/ meals, w/ gradual dose escalation to reduce GI side effects

DOSING CONSIDERATIONS

Renal Impairment

SrCr Levels ≥1.5mg/dL (Males)/≥1.4mg/dL (Females), or eGFR is Persistently <45mL/min/1.73m^2:
Do not initiate or continue treatment

Other Important Considerations

Patients w/ Volume-Depletion Not Previously Treated w/ Empagliflozin:
Correct this condition before initiating treatment

ADMINISTRATION
Oral route

HOW SUPPLIED
Tab: (Empagliflozin/Metformin) 5mg/500mg, 5mg/1000mg, 12.5mg/500mg, 12.5mg/1000mg

CONTRAINDICATIONS
Renal impairment (eg, SrCr ≥1.5mg/dL [males]/≥1.4mg/dL [females], or eGFR <45mL/min/1.73m^2), ESRD, patients on dialysis. Acute or chronic metabolic acidosis, including diabetic ketoacidosis. History of serious hypersensitivity reaction to Synjardy.

WARNINGS/PRECAUTIONS
Not recommended in patients w/ type 1 diabetes mellitus (DM) or for treatment of diabetic ketoacidosis. Temporarily d/c at the time of or prior to radiologic studies involving the use of intravascular iodinated contrast materials, withhold for 48 hrs subsequent to the procedure, and reinstitute only if renal function is normal. Temporarily d/c for any surgical procedure (except minor procedures not associated w/ restricted food and fluid intake); restart when oral intake is resumed and renal function is normal. Avoid in patients w/ clinical or lab evidence of hepatic disease. Cardiovascular collapse from whatever cause (eg, acute CHF, acute MI) have been associated w/ lactic acidosis and may also cause prerenal azotemia; promptly d/c therapy when such events occur. **Empagliflozin:** Causes intravascular volume contraction. Symptomatic hypotension may occur, particularly in patients w/ renal impairment, the elderly, in patients w/ low systolic BP, and in patients on diuretics. Ketoacidosis reported; if suspected, d/c and institute prompt treatment. Assess for ketoacidosis in patients presenting w/ signs/symptoms consistent w/ severe metabolic acidosis regardless of presenting blood glucose levels. Consider temporarily discontinuing therapy in clinical situations known to predispose to ketoacidosis (eg, prolonged fasting due to acute illness or surgery). Increases SrCr and decreases eGFR; risk of impaired renal function is increased in elderly patients and patients w/ moderate renal impairment. Serious UTIs (eg, urosepsis, pyelonephritis), requiring hospitalization, reported; evaluate for signs/symptoms of UTIs and treat promptly, if indicated. Increases the risk for genital mycotic infections and UTIs; monitor and treat as appropriate. Increases LDL levels; monitor and treat as appropriate. Monitoring glycemic control w/ urine glucose tests or w/ 1,5-anhydroglucitol assay is not recommended; use alternative methods. **Metformin:** Elderly, debilitated, or malnourished patients, and those w/ adrenal or pituitary insufficiency or alcohol intoxication may be particularly susceptible to hypoglycemic effects; monitor for a need to lower the dose of Synjardy to minimize risk of hypoglycemia in these patients. Hypoglycemia may be difficult to recognize in the elderly. May decrease vitamin B12 levels; monitor hematologic parameters annually.

ADVERSE REACTIONS
Empagliflozin: UTI, female genital mycotic infections, URTI, dyslipidemia.
Metformin: Diarrhea, N/V, flatulence, abdominal discomfort, indigestion, asthenia, headache.

DRUG INTERACTIONS
Empagliflozin: Risk of hypoglycemia is increased when used in combination w/ insulin secretagogues (eg, sulfonylurea) or insulin; a lower dose of the insulin secretagogue or

S

insulin may be required. Coadministration w/ diuretics resulted in increased urine volume and frequency of voids, which might enhance potential for volume depletion. **Metformin:** Caution w/ medication(s) that may affect renal function or result in significant hemodynamic change or interfere w/ the disposition of metformin. Hypoglycemia may be difficult to recognize in people who are taking β-adrenergic blocking drugs; monitor for a need to lower the dose of Synjardy to minimize the risk of hypoglycemia in these patients. Hypoglycemia may occur during concomitant use w/ other glucose-lowering agents (eg, sulfonylureas, insulin) or ethanol. Alcohol may potentiate effect of metformin on lactate metabolism; avoid excessive alcohol intake. Cationic drugs (eg, amiloride, digoxin, morphine, procainamide, quinidine) that are eliminated by renal tubular secretion theoretically have the potential for interaction; carefully monitor patient and adjust dose of Synjardy and/or the interfering drug. Topiramate or other carbonic anhydrase inhibitors (eg, zonisamide, acetazolamide, dichlorphenamide) may induce metabolic acidosis and may increase the risk of lactic acidosis; use these drugs w/ caution. Certain drugs tend to produce hyperglycemia (eg, thiazides and other diuretics, corticosteroids, phenothiazines, thyroid products, estrogens) and may lead to loss of glycemic control; closely monitor patient to maintain adequate glycemic control during therapy and monitor for hypoglycemia when such drugs are withdrawn during therapy.

PATIENT CONSIDERATIONS

Assessment: Assess for metabolic acidosis, risk factors for lactic acidosis, type of DM, diabetic ketoacidosis, predisposition to hyperkalemia, alcoholism, hypoxemia, presence of malnourishment or debilitation, adrenal/pituitary insufficiency, risk for genital mycotic infections, inadequate vitamin B12 or Ca^{2+} intake/absorption, drug hypersensitivity, any other conditions where treatment is cautioned, pregnancy/nursing status, and possible drug interactions. Assess if patient is planning to undergo any surgical procedure, or radiologic studies involving the use of intravascular iodinated contrast materials. Assess volume status. Obtain baseline FPG and HbA1c levels, renal/hepatic function, and hematologic parameters.

Monitoring: Monitor for signs/symptoms of lactic acidosis, hypotension, ketoacidosis, UTIs, genital mycotic infections, hypersensitivity reactions, hypoxic states, and other adverse reactions. Monitor renal function at least annually. Monitor hematologic parameters annually. Perform routine serum vitamin B12 measurements at 2- to 3-yr intervals in patients predisposed to developing subnormal vitamin B12 levels. Monitor FPG and HbA1c, and LDL levels.

Counseling: Inform of the potential risks and benefits of therapy and of alternative modes of therapy. Advise about the importance of adherence to dietary instructions, regular physical activity, periodic blood glucose monitoring and HbA1c testing, recognition and management of hypo/hyperglycemia, and assessment for diabetes complications. Instruct to seek medical advice promptly during periods of stress (eg, fever, trauma, infection, surgery), as medication requirements may change. Inform of the risks of lactic acidosis; advise to d/c therapy immediately and to notify physician promptly if unexplained hyperventilation, malaise, myalgia, unusual somnolence, slow or irregular heartbeat, sensation of feeling cold (especially in the extremities), or other nonspecific symptoms occur. Instruct to report to physician if pregnant, nursing, or experiencing symptoms of hypotension. Instruct to have adequate fluid intake. Instruct to d/c and seek medical advice immediately if symptoms of ketoacidosis occur. Counsel on the signs/symptoms of ketoacidosis, UTI, vaginal yeast infection, balanitis, and balanoposthitis; inform of treatment options and when to seek medical advice.

STORAGE: 25°C (77°F); excursions permitted to 15-30°C (59-86°F).

SYNRIBO — omacetaxine mepesuccinate

RX

Class: Protein synthesis inhibitor

S

ADULT DOSAGE

Chronic Myeloid Leukemia

Chronic or accelerated phase w/ resistance and/or intolerance to ≥2 tyrosine kinase inhibitors

Induction: 1.25mg/m² bid (approx 12-hr intervals) for 14 consecutive days every 28 days, over a 28-day cycle; repeat cycle every 28 days until hematologic response is achieved

Maint: 1.25mg/m² bid (approx 12-hr intervals) for 7 consecutive days every 28 days, over a 28-day cycle

PEDIATRIC DOSAGE

Pediatric use may not have been established

DOSING CONSIDERATIONS

Adverse Reactions

Hematologic Toxicity:

Grade 4 Neutropenia (ANC <0.5 x 10^9/L) or Grade 3 Thrombocytopenia (Platelet Counts <50 x 10^9/L) During a Cycle:

Delay starting next cycle until ANC ≥1.0 x 10^9/L and platelet count ≥50 x 10^9/L; reduce number of dosing days by 2 days for next cycle

Non-Hematologic Toxicity:

Manage symptomatically; interrupt and/or delay therapy until toxicity is resolved

ADMINISTRATION

SQ route

Reconstitution Instructions

1. Reconstitute w/ 1mL of 0.9% NaCl inj prior to SQ inj
2. After addition of diluent, gently swirl until a clear sol is obtained; lyophilized powder should be completely dissolved in <1 min
3. The resulting sol contains 3.5mg/mL

Handling Precautions

If contact w/ skin occurs, immediately and thoroughly wash affected area w/ soap and water

If contact w/ the eyes occurs, thoroughly flush the eyes w/ water

HOW SUPPLIED

Inj: 3.5mg

WARNINGS/PRECAUTIONS

Severe and fatal myelosuppression (eg, thrombocytopenia, neutropenia, anemia) reported; delay next cycle and/or reduce the number of days of treatment. Increased risk of infection in neutropenic patients; monitor frequently. Monitor CBC weekly during induction and initial maintenance cycles, and every 2 weeks during later maintenance cycles, as clinically indicated. Cerebral hemorrhage and severe, nonfatal GI hemorrhages observed; monitor platelet counts. Glucose intolerance and hyperglycemia, including hyperosmolar non-ketotic hyperglycemia reported; monitor blood glucose levels frequently, especially in patients with diabetes mellitus (DM) or risk factors for DM. Avoid with poorly controlled DM until glycemic control is established. May cause fetal harm if administered during pregnancy.

ADVERSE REACTIONS

Thrombocytopenia, anemia, neutropenia, lymphopenia, bone marrow failure, infections/infestations, diarrhea, N/V, inj-site related reactions, fatigue, pyrexia, asthenia, arthralgia.

DRUG INTERACTIONS

Increased risk of bleeding with anticoagulants, aspirin, and NSAIDs; avoid when platelet count is <50,000/µL.

PATIENT CONSIDERATIONS

Assessment: Assess for thrombocytopenia, neutropenia, anemia, hemorrhage, DM, risk factors for DM, pregnancy/nursing status, and possible drug interactions.

Monitoring: Monitor for signs and symptoms of myelosuppression, hemorrhage, infection, and other adverse reactions. Monitor CBC and blood glucose levels.

Counseling: Advise patient to read medication guide and provide instructions for appropriate use. Advise of the possibility of serious bleeding due to low platelet counts; instruct to report immediately any signs/symptoms suggestive of hemorrhage. Instruct to report in advance if patients plan to have any dental or surgical procedures. Inform that hematological parameters (eg, WBCs, platelets, RBCs) will need to be monitored. Instruct to report if fever or any signs/symptoms of infection (eg, SOB, significant fatigue, bleeding) develop. Advise diabetic patients of the possibility of hyperglycemia and the need to monitor blood glucose levels carefully. Advise females of reproductive potential to avoid pregnancy/nursing while on treatment. Inform that N/V, diarrhea, abdominal pain, and constipation may develop; instruct to seek medical attention if symptoms persist. Instruct to avoid driving/operating any dangerous tools or machinery if tiredness is experienced. Inform that skin rash may occur and to immediately report severe/worsening rash or itching. Inform that hair loss may be experienced.

STORAGE: 20-25°C (68-77°F); excursions permitted from 15-30°C (59-86°F). Protect from light. Reconstituted Sol: Use within 12 hrs if stored at 20-25°C (68-77°F) or use within 6 hrs if stored at 2-8°C (36-46°F).

SYNTHROID – levothyroxine sodium

RX

Class: Thyroid replacement hormone

Do not use for the treatment of obesity or weight loss; doses within range of daily hormonal requirements are ineffective for weight reduction in euthyroid patients. Serious or life-threatening manifestations of toxicity may occur when given in larger doses, particularly when given in association with sympathomimetic amines.

ADULT DOSAGE

Hypothyroidism

Replacement/supplemental therapy in hypothyroidism of any etiology, except transient hypothyroidism during the recovery phase of subacute thyroiditis

Usual: 1.7mcg/kg/day; >200mcg/day seldom required

Severe:
Initial: 12.5-25mcg/day
Titrate: Increase by 25mcg/day every 2-4 weeks until TSH level normalized

Secondary (Pituitary) or Tertiary (Hypothalamic) Hypothyroidism:
Titrate: Increase until clinically euthyroid and serum free-T4 level is restored to the upper half of the normal range

Subclinical Hypothyroidism:
Lower doses (eg, 1mcg/kg/day) may be adequate to normalize serum TSH level

Pituitary TSH Suppressant

Used to treat/prevent various types of euthyroid goiters (eg, thyroid nodules, subacute or chronic lymphocytic thyroiditis, multinodular goiter) and to manage thyroid cancer

Well-Differentiated (Papillary and Follicular) Thyroid Cancer:
Adjunct to Surgery and Radioiodine Therapy:
Usual: >2mcg/kg/day, w/ target TSH level <0.1 mU/L
High-Risk Tumors: Target TSH level <0.01 mU/L

Benign Nodules and Nontoxic Multinodular Goiter:
TSH is suppressed to a higher target (eg, 0.1 to 0.5 or 1.0 mU/L)

PEDIATRIC DOSAGE

Hypothyroidism

Usual:
0-3 Months of Age: 10-15mcg/kg/day
3-6 Months of Age: 8-10mcg/kg/day
6-12 Months of Age: 6-8mcg/kg/day
1-5 Years: 5-6mcg/kg/day
6-12 Years: 4-5mcg/kg/day
>12 Years:
Growth/Puberty Incomplete: 2-3mcg/kg/day
Growth/Puberty Complete: 1.7mcg/kg/day

Infants w/ Very Low (<5mcg/dL) or Undetectable Serum T4:
Initial: 50mcg/day

Chronic/Severe Hypothyroidism:
Initial: 25mcg/day
Titrate: Increase by 25mcg every 2-4 weeks

DOSING CONSIDERATIONS

Pregnancy
May increase levothyroxine requirements

Elderly
Hypothyroidism:
>50 Years:
Initial: 25-50mcg/day
Titrate: Increase by 12.5-25mcg increments every 6-8 weeks prn

W/ Underlying Cardiac Disease:
Initial: 12.5-25mcg/day
Titrate: Increase by 12.5-25mg increments every 4-6 weeks

Adverse Reactions
Minimize Hyperactivity in Older Children:
Initial: Give 1/4 of full replacement dose
Titrate: Increase on a weekly basis by 1/4 the full recommended replacement dose until the full recommended replacement dose is reached

S

Other Important Considerations
Underlying Cardiac Disease:
Hypothyroidism:
Infants (Risk for Cardiac Failure):
Initial: Consider lower dose (eg, 25mcg/day)
Titrate: Increase dose in 4-6 weeks prn
<50 Years:
Initial: 25-50mcg/day
Titrate: Increase by 12.5-25mcg increments every 6-8 weeks prn

ADMINISTRATION

Oral route

Administer as a single daily dose, preferably 30-60 min before breakfast
Take at least 4 hrs apart from drugs that are known to interfere w/ its absorption

Pediatrics
Unable to Swallow Intact Tab:
1. Crush tab and suspend in small amount (5-10mL or 1-2 tsp) of water
2. Administer using a spoon or dropper
3. Do not store sus for later use
4. Do not use foods that decrease absorption of levothyroxine (eg, soybean infant formula) to administer

HOW SUPPLIED

Tab: 25mcg*, 50mcg*, 75mcg*, 88mcg*, 100mcg*, 112mcg*, 125mcg*, 137mcg*, 150mcg*, 175mcg*, 200mcg*, 300mcg* *scored

CONTRAINDICATIONS

Untreated subclinical (suppressed serum TSH level with normal T3 level and T4 levels) or overt thyrotoxicosis of any etiology, acute MI, and uncorrected adrenal insufficiency. Hypersensitivity to any of the inactive components in this medication.

WARNINGS/PRECAUTIONS

Should not be used in the treatment of male or female infertility unless associated with hypothyroidism. Contraindicated in patients with nontoxic diffuse goiter or nodular thyroid disease, particularly in the elderly or with underlying cardiovascular (CV) disease if serum TSH level is already suppressed; use with caution if TSH level is not suppressed and carefully monitor thyroid function. Has narrow therapeutic index; carefully titrate dose to avoid over- or under-treatment. May decrease bone mineral density (BMD) with long-term use; give minimum dose necessary to achieve desired clinical and biochemical response. Caution with CV disorders and the elderly. If cardiac symptoms develop or worsen, reduce or withhold dose for 1 week and then restart at lower dose. Overtreatment may produce CV effects (eg, increase in HR, increase in cardiac wall thickness, increase in cardiac contractility, precipitation of angina or arrhythmias). Monitor patients with CAD closely during surgical procedures; may precipitate cardiac arrhythmias. Caution in patients with diabetes mellitus (DM). Patients with concomitant adrenal insufficiency should be treated with replacement glucocorticoids prior to therapy.

ADVERSE REACTIONS

Fatigue, increased appetite, weight loss, heat intolerance, headache, hyperactivity, irritability, insomnia, palpitations, arrhythmias, dyspnea, hair loss, menstrual irregularities, pseudotumor cerebri (children), slipped capital femoral epiphysis (children).

DRUG INTERACTIONS

Concurrent sympathomimetics may increase effects of sympathomimetics or thyroid hormone; may increase risk of coronary insufficiency with CAD. Upward dose adjustments may be needed for insulin and oral hypoglycemic agents. May decrease absorption with soybean flour, cottonseed meal, walnuts, and dietary fiber. May increase oral anticoagulant activity; adjust dose of anticoagulant and monitor PT. May decrease levels and effects of digitalis glycosides. Transient reduction in TSH secretion with dopamine/dopamine agonists, glucocorticoids, octreotide. Decreased thyroid hormone secretion with aminoglutethimide, amiodarone, iodide (including iodine-containing radiographic contrast agents), lithium, methimazole, propylthiouracil (PTU), sulfonamides, and tolbutamide. May increase thyroid hormone secretion with amiodarone and iodide. May decrease T4 absorption with antacids (aluminum and magnesium hydroxides), simethicone, bile acid sequestrants (cholestyramine, colestipol), calcium carbonate, cation exchange resins (kayexalate), ferrous sulfate, orlistat, and sucralfate; administer at least 4 hrs apart. May increase serum thyroxine-binding globulin (TBG) concentrations with clofibrate, estrogen-containing oral contraceptives, oral estrogens, heroin/methadone, 5-fluorouracil, mitotane, and tamoxifen. May decrease serum TBG concentrations with androgens/anabolic steroids, asparaginase, glucocorticoids, and slow-release nicotinic acid. May cause protein-binding site displacement with furosemide (>80mg IV), heparin, hydantoins, NSAIDs (fenamates, phenylbutazone), and salicylates (>2g/day). May alter T4 and T3 metabolism with carbamazepine, hydantoins, phenobarbital, and rifampin. May decrease T4 5'-deiodinase activity with amiodarone, β-adrenergic antagonists (eg, propranolol >160mg/day), glucocorticoids (eg, dexamethasone >4mg/day), and PTU. Concurrent use with tricyclic (eg, amitriptyline) and tetracyclic (eg, maprotiline) antidepressants may increase the therapeutic and toxic effects of both drugs. Coadministration with sertraline in patients stabilized on levothyroxine may result in increased levothyroxine requirements. Interferon-α may cause development of antithyroid microsomal antibodies and transient hypothyroidism, hyperthyroidism, or both. Interleukin-2 has been associated with transient painless thyroiditis. Excessive use with growth hormones (eg, somatropin, somatrem) may accelerate epiphyseal closure. Ketamine may produce marked HTN and tachycardia. May reduce uptake of radiographic agents. Decreased theophylline clearance may occur in hypothyroid patients. Altered levels of thyroid hormone and/or TSH levels with choral hydrate, diazepam, ethionamide, lovastatin, metoclopramide, 6-mercaptopurine, nitroprusside, para-aminosalicylate sodium, perphenazine, resorcinol (excessive topical use), and thiazide diuretics.

PATIENT CONSIDERATIONS

Assessment: Assess for untreated subclinical or overt thyrotoxicosis, acute MI, uncorrected adrenal insufficiency, CAD, CV disorders, nontoxic diffuse goiter, nodular thyroid disease, DM, hypersensitivity, pregnancy/nursing status, and for possible drug interactions. In patients with secondary or tertiary hypothyroidism, assess for additional hypothalamic/pituitary hormone deficiencies. Assess TSH levels. In infants with congenital hypothyroidism, assess for other congenital anomalies.

Monitoring: Monitor for CV effects. In patients on long-term therapy, monitor for signs/symptoms of decreased BMD. In patients with nontoxic diffuse goiter or nodular thyroid disease, monitor for precipitation of thyrotoxicosis. In adults with primary hypothyroidism, perform periodic monitoring of serum TSH levels. In pediatric patients with congenital hypothyroidism, perform periodic monitoring of serum TSH levels and total or free T4 levels. In patients with secondary and tertiary hypothyroidism, perform periodic monitoring of serum free-T4 levels. Refer to PI for TSH and T4 monitoring parameters. Closely monitor PT if coadministered with an oral anticoagulant.

Counseling: Instruct to notify physician if allergic to any foods or medicines, pregnant/planning to become pregnant, breastfeeding, or taking any other drugs, including prescriptions and OTC preparations. Instruct to notify physician of any other medical conditions, particularly heart disease, diabetes, clotting disorders, and adrenal or pituitary gland problems. Instruct not to stop or change dose unless directed by physician. Instruct to take on empty stomach, at least 30-60 min before eating breakfast. Advise that partial hair loss may occur during the 1st few months of therapy, but is usually temporary. Instruct to notify physician or dentist prior to surgery about levothyroxine therapy. Inform that drug should not be used for weight control. Instruct to notify physician if rapid or irregular heartbeat, chest pain, SOB, leg cramps, headache, or any other unusual medical event occurs. Inform that dose may be increased during pregnancy. Inform that drug should not be administered within 4 hrs of agents such as iron/calcium supplements and antacids.

STORAGE: 25°C (77°F); excursions permitted to 15-30°C (59-86°F). Protect from light and moisture.

TACLONEX OINTMENT – betamethasone dipropionate/calcipotriene RX

Class: Corticosteroid/vitamin D3 analogue

ADULT DOSAGE

Plaque Psoriasis

≥18 Years:

Apply an adequate layer to affected area(s) qd for up to 4 weeks

D/C therapy when control is achieved

Max: 100g/week

Treatment of >30% BSA is not recommended

PEDIATRIC DOSAGE

Plaque Psoriasis

12-17 Years:

Apply an adequate layer to affected area(s) qd for up to 4 weeks

D/C therapy when control is achieved

Max: 60g/week

Treatment of >30% BSA is not recommended

T

ADMINISTRATION

Topical route

Rub in gently and completely

Wash hands after application

Avoid use on the face, groin, axillae, or if skin atrophy is present at the treatment site

Avoid use with occlusive dressings unless directed by a physician

HOW SUPPLIED

Oint: (Calcipotriene-Betamethasone) 0.005%-0.064% [60g, 100g]

WARNINGS/PRECAUTIONS

Not for oral, ophthalmic, or intravaginal use. Hypercalcemia and hypercalciuria observed; d/c until parameters of Ca^{2+} metabolism have normalized. May cause reversible hypothalamic-pituitary-adrenal (HPA) axis suppression with the potential for glucocorticosteroid insufficiency during and after withdrawal of treatment. Factors predisposing to HPA axis suppression include the use of high-potency corticosteroids, large treatment surface areas, prolonged use, concomitant use of >1 corticosteroids-containing product, use of occlusive dressings, altered skin barrier, liver failure, and young age. Gradually withdraw drug, reduce frequency of application, or substitute to a less potent steroid if HPA axis suppression is documented. Cushing's syndrome, and hyperglycemia may occur. Pediatric patients may be more susceptible to systemic toxicity. Allergic contact dermatitis may occur; may be confirmed by patch testing. D/C and institute appropriate therapy if irritation develops. Avoid excessive exposure of treated areas to natural or artificial sunlight; limit or avoid use of phototherapy.

ADVERSE REACTIONS

Pruritus.

DRUG INTERACTIONS

Use with other corticosteroid-containing products may increase total systemic exposure.

PATIENT CONSIDERATIONS

Assessment: Assess for predisposing factors to HPA axis suppression, treatment-site atrophy, use of phototherapy, pregnancy/nursing status, and possible drug interactions.

Monitoring: Monitor for hypercalcemia, hypercalciuria, HPA axis suppression, Cushing's syndrome, hyperglycemia, allergic contact dermatitis, irritation, and other adverse reactions.

Counseling: Instruct adult patients not to use >100g/week and pediatric patients not to use >60g/week. Instruct to d/c therapy when control is achieved unless directed otherwise by the physician. Advise to avoid use on the face, underarms, groin, or eyes; instruct to wash area right away if medicine gets on face or in eyes. Instruct not to occlude the treatment area with a bandage or other covering unless directed by physician. Inform that local reactions and skin atrophy are more likely to occur with occlusive use, prolonged use or use of higher potency corticosteroids. Instruct to wash hands after application. Counsel not to use other products containing calcipotriene or a corticosteroid without first consulting the physician. Instruct to avoid excessive exposure to either natural or artificial sunlight (eg, tanning booths, sun lamps).

STORAGE: 20-25°C (68-77°F); excursions permitted to 15-30°C (59-86°F).

TAFINLAR – dabrafenib

RX

Class: Kinase inhibitor

ADULT DOSAGE

Unresectable or Metastatic Melanoma with BRAF V600E Mutation

150mg bid, approx 12 hrs apart, as a single agent until disease progression or unacceptable toxicity occurs

Unresectable or Metastatic Melanoma with BRAF V600E or V600K Mutations

150mg bid, approx 12 hrs apart, in combination w/ trametinib until disease progression or unacceptable toxicity occurs

Missed Dose

Do not take a missed dose w/in 6 hrs of the next dose

PEDIATRIC DOSAGE

Pediatric use may not have been established

DOSING CONSIDERATIONS

Adverse Reactions

Dose Reductions for Dabrafenib:
First Dose Reduction: 100mg bid
Second Dose Reduction: 75mg bid
Third Dose Reduction: 50mg bid
Subsequent Modification: Permanently d/c if unable to tolerate 50mg bid

New Primary Noncutaneous Malignancies:
Permanently d/c if RAS mutation-positive noncutaneous malignancies develop

Febrile Drug Reaction:
Fever of 101.3-104°F: Withhold until fever resolves, then resume at same or lower dose level
Fever >104°F or Fever Complicated by Rigors, Hypotension, Dehydration, or Renal Failure: Withhold until fever resolves, then resume at a lower dose level or permanently d/c

Cutaneous:
Grade 3 or 4 Skin Toxicity or Intolerable Grade 2 Skin Toxicity: Withhold for up to 3 weeks; resume at a lower dose level if improved or permanently d/c if not improved

Cardiac:
Symptomatic CHF: Withhold; if improved, then resume at the same dose
Absolute Decrease in Left Ventricular Ejection Fraction (LVEF) >20% from Baseline that is Below Lower Limit of Normal: Withhold; if improved, then resume at the same dose

Uveitis Including Iritis and Iridocyclitis:
If mild or moderate uveitis does not respond to ocular therapy, or for severe uveitis, withhold for up to 6 weeks; resume at the same or at a lower dose level if improved to Grade 0-1, or permanently d/c if not improved

Other:
Any Grade 3 Adverse Reaction or Intolerable Grade 2 Adverse Reactions: Withhold; resume at a lower dose level if improved to Grade 0-1, or permanently d/c if not improved
First Occurrence of Any Grade 4 Adverse Reaction: Withhold until adverse reaction improves to Grade 0-1, then resume at a lower dose level; or permanently d/c
Recurrent Grade 4 Adverse Reaction: Permanently d/c

Refer to trametinib PI for trametinib modifications

ADMINISTRATION

Oral route

Take at least 1 hr ac or 2 hrs pc.
Do not open, crush, or break caps.

HOW SUPPLIED

Cap: 50mg, 75mg

WARNINGS/PRECAUTIONS

See Dosing Considerations. Not indicated for treatment of patients w/ wild-type BRAF melanoma. New primary cutaneous and noncutaneous malignancies may occur when dabrafenib is administered alone or in combination w/ trametinib; perform dermatologic evaluations prior to initiation, every 2 months while on therapy, and for up to 6 months following discontinuation. Increased cell proliferation may occur in BRAF wild-type cells exposed to BRAF inhibitors; confirm evidence of BRAF V600E or V600K mutation status prior to treatment initiation. Hemorrhages (eg, major hemorrhages) may occur when administered w/ trametinib; permanently d/c for all Grade 4 hemorrhagic events and for any persistent Grade 3 hemorrhagic events. Cardiomyopathy may occur; assess LVEF by echocardiogram or multigated acquisition (MUGA) scan before initiation of dabrafenib w/ trametinib, 1 month after initiation, and then at 2- to 3-month intervals while on treatment. Uveitis may occur; monitor for visual signs/symptoms (eg, change in vision, photophobia, eye pain). Permanently d/c for persistent Grade 2 or greater uveitis of >6 weeks duration. Serious febrile reactions and fever of any severity complicated by hypotension, rigors/chills, dehydration, or renal failure may occur; incidence and severity of pyrexia are increased w/ trametinib. Monitor SrCr and other evidence of renal function during and following severe pyrexia. Serious skin toxicity may occur. Hyperglycemia may occur; monitor serum glucose levels upon initiation and as clinically appropriate in patients w/ preexisting diabetes or hyperglycemia. Potential risk of hemolytic anemia in patients w/ G6PD deficiency; closely monitor such patients for signs of hemolytic anemia. May cause fetal harm.

ADVERSE REACTIONS

Single Agent Dabrafenib: Hyperkeratosis, headache, pyrexia, arthralgia, papilloma, alopecia, palmar-plantar erythrodysesthesia syndrome.
W/ Trametinib: Pyrexia, rash, chills, headache, arthralgia, cough.

DRUG INTERACTIONS

Strong inhibitors of CYP3A4 or CYP2C8 may increase concentrations and strong inducers of CYP3A4 or CYP2C8 may decrease concentrations; substitution of these medications is recommended during treatment. If concomitant use of strong inhibitors (eg, ketoconazole, nefazodone, clarithromycin, gemfibrozil) or strong inducers (eg, rifampin, phenytoin, carbamazepine, phenobarbital, St. John's wort) of CYP3A4 or CYP2C8 is unavoidable, monitor closely for adverse reactions when taking strong inhibitors or loss of efficacy when taking strong inducers. May decrease systemic exposures of midazolam (CYP3A4 substrate), S-warfarin (CYP2C9 substrate), and R-warfarin (CYP3A4/CYP1A2 substrate). Monitor INR levels more frequently in patients receiving warfarin during initiation or discontinuation of dabrafenib. Coadministration w/ CYP3A4 and CYP2C9 substrates (eg, dexamethasone, hormonal contraceptives) may result in decreased concentrations and loss of efficacy; substitute for these medications or monitor for loss of efficacy if use of these medications is unavoidable.

PATIENT CONSIDERATIONS

Assessment: Assess for diabetes, hyperglycemia, G6PD deficiency, pregnancy/nursing status, and possible drug interactions. Assess for presence of BRAF V600E or V600K mutation in tumor specimens. Perform dermatologic evaluations. Assess LVEF by echocardiogram or MUGA scan before initiation of dabrafenib w/ trametinib.

Monitoring: Monitor for new primary malignancies, hemorrhagic events, cardiomyopathy, uveitis, febrile reactions, fever, skin toxicity, hyperglycemia, and other adverse reactions. Perform dermatologic evaluations every 2 months during therapy and for up to 6 months following discontinuation. Monitor LVEF by echocardiogram and MUGA scan 1 month after initiation and then at 2- to 3-month intervals during therapy. Monitor SrCr and other evidence of renal function during and following severe pyrexia. Monitor serum glucose levels upon initiation and as clinically appropriate in patients w/ preexisting diabetes or hyperglycemia. Closely monitor patients w/ G6PD deficiency for signs of hemolytic anemia. Monitor INR levels more frequently in patients receiving warfarin during initiation or discontinuation.

Counseling: Inform that evidence of BRAF V600E or V600K mutation in the tumor specimen is necessary to identify patients for whom treatment is indicated. Inform of increased risk of developing new primary cutaneous and noncutaneous malignancies; instruct to contact healthcare provider immediately for any new lesions, changes to existing lesions on the skin, or signs/symptoms of other malignancies. Inform that combined use w/ trametinib may increase risk of intracranial and GI hemorrhage; advise to contact healthcare provider or seek immediate medical attention for unusual bleeding or hemorrhage. Advise that therapy may cause cardiomyopathy and to report signs/symptoms of heart failure. Advise that therapy may cause uveitis and to contact healthcare provider if patient experiences changes in vision. Inform that therapy may cause pyrexia, including serious febrile reactions, and that incidence and severity are increased w/ trametinib; advise to contact healthcare provider if fever develops. Advise of risk of serious skin reactions and to contact healthcare provider for progressive or intolerable rash. Advise diabetic patients that therapy may impair glucose control and to report severe hyperglycemia symptoms to healthcare provider. Advise patients w/ known G6PD deficiency to contact healthcare provider to report signs/symptoms of anemia or hemolysis. Instruct female patients to use effective nonhormonal contraception during treatment and for 2 weeks after discontinuation of dabrafenib; advise to contact healthcare provider if pregnancy occurs, or is suspected, while on therapy. Advise breastfeeding mothers to d/c nursing while on therapy and for 2 weeks after last dose. Inform males and females of reproductive potential that treatment may impair fertility.

STORAGE: 25°C (77°F); excursions permitted to 15-30°C (59-86°F).

TAGRISSO — osimertinib

RX

Class: Kinase inhibitor

ADULT DOSAGE

Metastatic Non-Small Cell Lung Cancer

Treatment of patients w/ metastatic epidermal growth factor receptor (EGFR) T790M mutation-positive non-small cell lung cancer (NSCLC), as detected by an FDA-approved test, who have progressed on or after EGFR tyrosine kinase inhibitor therapy

80mg qd until disease progression or unacceptable toxicity

Missed Dose

If a dose is missed, do not make up the missed dose and take the next dose as scheduled

PEDIATRIC DOSAGE

Pediatric use may not have been established

DOSING CONSIDERATIONS

Adverse Reactions

Pulmonary:

Interstitial Lung Disease (ILD)/Pneumonitis: Permanently d/c

Cardiac:

QTc Interval >500 msec on at Least 2 Separate ECGs: Withhold until QTc interval is <481 msec or recovery to baseline if baseline QTc is ≥481 msec, then resume at 40mg dose

QTc Interval Prolongation w/ Signs/Symptoms of Life-Threatening Arrhythmia: Permanently d/c

Asymptomatic, Absolute Decrease in Left Ventricular Ejection Fraction (LVEF) of 10% from Baseline and <50%: Withhold for up to 4 weeks. Resume if LVEF improves to baseline, or permanently d/c if LVEF does not improve to baseline

Symptomatic CHF: Permanently d/c

Other:
Grade ≥3 Adverse Reaction: Withhold for up to 3 weeks
If Improvement to Grade 0-2 w/in 3 Weeks: Resume at 80mg or 40mg qd
If No Improvement w/in 3 Weeks: Permanently d/c

ADMINISTRATION

Oral route

Take w/ or w/o food.

Administration to Patients Who Have Difficulty Swallowing Solids

1. Disperse tab in 4 tbsp (approx 50mL) of non-carbonated water only; stir until tab is completely dispersed.
2. Swallow or administer through NG tube immediately.
3. Do not crush, heat, or ultrasonicate during preparation.
4. Rinse container w/ 4-8 oz of water and immediately drink or administer through the NG tube.

HOW SUPPLIED

Tab: 40mg, 80mg

WARNINGS/PRECAUTIONS

See Dosing Considerations. ILD/pneumonitis reported; withhold therapy and promptly investigate for ILD in any patient who presents w/ worsening of respiratory symptoms. QTc interval prolongation reported; periodically monitor ECGs and electrolytes in patients w/ congenital long QTc syndrome, CHF, or electrolyte abnormalities. Cardiomyopathy reported; assess LVEF before initiation and then at 3-month intervals while on treatment. May cause fetal harm.

ADVERSE REACTIONS

Diarrhea, rash, dry skin, nail toxicity.

DRUG INTERACTIONS

Avoid w/ strong CYP3A inhibitors (eg, telithromycin, itraconazole, ritonavir). Concomitant use of strong CYP3A inhibitors may increase osimertinib levels; if no other alternative exists, monitor patients more closely for adverse reactions. Avoid w/ strong CYP3A inducers (eg, phenytoin, carbamazepine, St. John's wort); may decrease osimertinib levels. Avoid w/ drugs that are sensitive substrates of CYP3A, breast cancer resistance protein, or CYP1A2 w/ narrow therapeutic indices (eg, fentanyl, cyclosporine, quinidine); osimertinib may increase or decrease levels of these drugs. Periodically monitor ECGs and electrolytes in patients taking medications known to prolong the QTc interval.

PATIENT CONSIDERATIONS

Assessment: Assess for congenital long QTc syndrome, CHF, and electrolyte abnormalities. Assess LVEF, pregnancy/nursing status, and for possible drug interactions.

Monitoring: Monitor for ILD, pneumonitis, QTc interval prolongation, and cardiomyopathy. Periodically monitor ECGs and electrolytes in patients w/ congenital long QTc syndrome, CHF, electrolyte abnormalities, or those who are taking medications known to prolong the QTc interval. Assess LVEF at 3-month intervals.

Counseling: Inform of the risks of severe or fatal ILD, including pneumonitis; advise to contact physician immediately to report new or worsening respiratory symptoms. Inform patients of symptoms that may be indicative of significant QTc prolongation (eg, dizziness, lightheadedness, syncope) and advise to report these symptoms. Advise to inform physician about the use of any heart or blood pressure medications. Advise to immediately report any signs or symptoms of heart failure. Inform that drug can cause fetal harm if taken during pregnancy. Advise pregnant women of the potential risk to a fetus. Advise females to inform physician if they become pregnant or if pregnancy is suspected while on therapy. Instruct females of reproductive potential to use effective contraception during treatment and for 6 weeks after the final dose. Instruct males w/ female partners of reproductive potential to use effective contraception during treatment and for 4 months after the final dose. Advise women not to breastfeed during treatment and for 2 weeks after the final dose.

STORAGE: 25°C (77°F); excursions permitted to 15-30°C (59-86°F).

TAMIFLU — oseltamivir phosphate

RX

Class: Neuraminidase inhibitor

ADULT DOSAGE

Influenza

Treatment:
Symptomatic for ≤2 Days:
75mg bid for 5 days

Prophylaxis:
75mg qd for at least 10 days

PEDIATRIC DOSAGE

Influenza

Treatment:
Symptomatic for ≤2 Days:
2 Weeks-<1 Year:
3mg/kg bid for 5 days

Community Outbreak:
Immunocompetent: 75mg qd for up to 6 weeks
Immunocompromised: 75mg qd for up to 12 weeks

1-12 Years:
≤15kg: 30mg bid for 5 days
15.1-23kg: 45mg bid for 5 days
23.1-40kg: 60mg bid for 5 days
≥40.1kg: 75mg bid for 5 days

≥13 Years:
75mg bid for 5 days

Prophylaxis:
1-12 Years:
≤15kg: 30mg qd for 10 days
15.1-23kg: 45mg qd for 10 days
23.1-40kg: 60mg qd for 10 days
≥40.1kg: 75mg qd for 10 days

≥13 Years:
75mg qd for at least 10 days

Community Outbreak:
Continue for up to 6 weeks

DOSING CONSIDERATIONS

Renal Impairment

Moderate (CrCl >30-60mL/min):
Treatment: 30mg bid for 5 days
Prophylaxis: 30mg qd for at least 10 days

Severe (CrCl >10-30mL/min):
Treatment: 30mg qd for 5 days
Prophylaxis: 30mg qod for at least 10 days

ESRD on Hemodialysis (CrCl ≤10mL/min):
Treatment: 30mg after every hemodialysis cycle; treatment duration not to exceed 5 days
Prophylaxis: 30mg after alternate hemodialysis cycles; initial dose can be given prior to start of hemodialysis

ESRD on Continuous Ambulatory Peritoneal Dialysis (CrCl ≤10mL/min):
Treatment: Single 30mg dose immediately after dialysis exchange
Prophylaxis: 30mg once weekly immediately after dialysis exchange

ADMINISTRATION

Oral route

Take w/ or w/o food

Oral sus is the preferred formulation for patients who cannot swallow caps

Shake oral sus well before use

Preparation of Oral Sus

1. Add 55mL of water to the bottle
2. Close the bottle and shake well for 15 sec

Storage:
Refrigerated: Use w/in 17 days
Room Temperature: Use w/in 10 days

Emergency Compounding of Oral Sus from Caps

Refer to PI for number of capsules and amount of water and vehicle needed

1. Place the specified amount of water into a polyethyleneterephthalate (PET) or glass bottle
2. Open the required number of caps and pour the contents of into the PET or glass bottle
3. Gently swirl the sus for at least 2 min
4. Slowly add the specified amount of vehicle to the bottle
5. Close the bottle and shake well for 30 sec

Storage:
Refrigerated: Stable for 5 weeks (35 days)
Room Temperature: Stable for 5 days

HOW SUPPLIED

Cap: 30mg, 45mg, 75mg; **Sus:** 6mg/mL [60mL]

CONTRAINDICATIONS

Known serious hypersensitivity to oseltamivir or any component of the product.

WARNINGS/PRECAUTIONS

Not a substitute for early influenza vaccination on an annual basis. Emergence of resistance mutations can decrease drug effectiveness; consider available information on influenza drug susceptibility patterns and treatment effects when deciding whether to use treatment. Anaphylaxis and serious skin reactions (eg, toxic epidermal necrolysis, Stevens-Johnson syndrome, erythema multiforme) reported; d/c and institute appropriate treatment if an allergic-like reaction occurs or is suspected. Neuropsychiatric events (eg, hallucinations, delirium, abnormal behavior), in some cases resulting in fatal outcomes, reported; monitor for abnormal behavior and evaluate risks and benefits of continuing treatment if neuropsychiatric symptoms occur. Serious bacterial infections may begin with influenza-like symptoms or may coexist with or occur during the course of influenza; treatment does not prevent these complications.

ADVERSE REACTIONS

N/V, diarrhea, abdominal pain.

DRUG INTERACTIONS

Avoid administration of live attenuated influenza vaccine within 2 weeks before or 48 hrs after oseltamivir, unless medically indicated. Probenecid may increase exposure.

PATIENT CONSIDERATIONS

Assessment: Assess for drug hypersensitivity, renal impairment, pregnancy/nursing status, and possible drug interactions.

Monitoring: Monitor for signs/symptoms of neuropsychiatric events, anaphylaxis/serious skin reactions, and other adverse reactions.

Counseling: Advise of the risk of severe allergic reactions or serious skin reactions and to d/c and seek immediate medical attention if an allergic-like reaction occurs or is suspected. Advise of the risk of neuropsychiatric events and to contact physician if experiencing signs of abnormal behavior during treatment. Instruct to begin treatment as soon as possible from the 1st appearance of flu symptoms, and as soon as possible after exposure (for prevention). Instruct to take missed doses as soon as remembered, unless next scheduled dose is within 2 hrs, and then to continue at the usual times. Inform that the medication is not a substitute for flu vaccination. Inform that oral sus delivers 2g sorbitol/75mg dose; inform that this is above the daily max limit of sorbitol for patients with hereditary fructose intolerance and may cause dyspepsia and diarrhea.

STORAGE: Cap/Dry Powder: 25°C (77°F); excursions permitted to 15-30°C (59-86°F). Constituted Sus: 2-8°C (36-46°F) for up to 17 days, or 25°C (77°F) for up to 10 days with excursions permitted to 15-30°C (59-86°F). Do not freeze.

TAMOXIFEN – tamoxifen citrate

RX

Class: Antiestrogen

Serious and life-threatening uterine malignancies (endometrial adenocarcinoma and uterine sarcoma), stroke, and pulmonary embolism (PE) reported in the risk-reduction setting; some of these events were fatal. Discuss the potential benefits versus the potential risks of these serious events w/ women at high-risk for breast cancer and women w/ ductal carcinoma in situ (DCIS) considering therapy for breast cancer risk reduction.

OTHER BRAND NAMES

Soltamox

ADULT DOSAGE

Breast Cancer

Treatment of metastatic breast cancer in women and men. Treatment of node-positive breast cancer in postmenopausal women or axillary node-negative breast cancer in women following total or segmental mastectomy, axillary dissection, and breast irradiation. To reduce risk of invasive breast cancer in women w/ DCIS following breast surgery and radiation. To reduce incidence of breast cancer in high-risk women (those at least 35 yrs of age w/ a 5-yr predicted risk of breast cancer ≥1.67%, as calculated by the Gail Model)

Treatment:

20-40mg/day

Give dosages >20mg/day in divided doses (am and pm)

Incidence Reduction in High-Risk Women/ DCIS:

20mg qd for 5 yrs

PEDIATRIC DOSAGE

Pediatric use may not have been established

ADMINISTRATION
Oral route

HOW SUPPLIED
Tab: (Base) 10mg, 20mg; **Oral Sol (Soltamox):** (Base) 10mg/5mL [150mL]

CONTRAINDICATIONS
Known hypersensitivity to the drug or any of its ingredients. **Breast Cancer Incidence Reduction in High-Risk Women/Women w/ DCIS:** Women who require coumarin-type anticoagulant therapy or w/ history of deep vein thrombosis (DVT) or PE.

WARNINGS/PRECAUTIONS
Hypercalcemia reported in patients w/ bone metastases; take appropriate measures if hypercalcemia occurs, and, if severe, d/c therapy. Increased incidence of uterine malignancies reported; promptly evaluate any patient receiving or who has previously received therapy who reports abnormal vaginal bleeding. Perform annual gynecological examinations in patients receiving or who have previously received therapy. Increased incidence of endometrial changes, including hyperplasia and polyps, reported. Endometriosis, uterine fibroids, ovarian cysts (in premenopausal patients w/ advanced breast cancer), and menstrual irregularity or amenorrhea reported. Increased incidence of thromboembolic events (eg, DVT, PE) reported; for treatment of breast cancer, carefully consider the risks and benefits of therapy in women w/ history of thromboembolic events. Liver cancer and nonmalignant (eg, changes in liver enzyme levels) effects on the liver, secondary primary tumors (non-uterine), ocular disturbances, increased incidence of cataracts and risk of having cataract surgery, thrombocytopenia, leukopenia, neutropenia, and pancytopenia reported. May cause fetal harm. Hyperlipidemias reported; may consider periodic monitoring of plasma TGs and cholesterol in patients w/ preexisting hyperlipidemias. T4 elevations, not accompanied by clinical hyperthyroidism, reported in a few postmenopausal patients.

ADVERSE REACTIONS
Hot flashes, vaginal discharge, irregular menses, fatigue/asthenia, weight loss, skin changes, N/V, fluid retention, pain, cough, vasodilatation, flu syndrome.

DRUG INTERACTIONS
See Contraindications. A significant increase in anticoagulant effect when used in combination w/ coumarin-type anticoagulants may occur; where such coadministration exists, carefully monitor patient's PT. Increased risk of thromboembolic events w/ cytotoxic agents. May reduce letrozole concentrations. Reduced concentrations w/ rifampin, aminoglutethimide, and phenobarbital. Medroxyprogesterone reduces concentrations of N-desmethyl tamoxifen (active metabolite). Aminoglutethimide may reduce tamoxifen and N-desmethyl tamoxifen plasma concentrations. Bromocriptine may increase tamoxifen and N-desmethyl tamoxifen plasma concentrations. May reduce anastrozole concentrations; avoid w/ anastrozole.

PATIENT CONSIDERATIONS

Assessment: Assess for history of thromboembolic events, preexisting hyperlipidemias, known hypersensitivity, pregnancy/nursing status, and possible drug interactions.

Monitoring: Monitor for signs/symptoms of uterine malignancies, thromboembolic events, hypercalcemia, endometrial changes, uterine fibroids, menstrual irregularity, ocular disturbances, and other adverse reactions. Periodically monitor plasma TG and cholesterol levels in patients w/ preexisting hyperlipidemias. Periodically monitor CBCs, including platelet counts and LFTs. Perform annual gynecological examinations.

Counseling: Inform about potential risks and benefits of treatment. Advise premenopausal women not to become pregnant and to use nonhormonal contraception during therapy and for 2 months after discontinuation if sexually active. Instruct women to seek prompt medical attention if new breast lumps, vaginal bleeding, gynecologic symptoms (eg, menstrual irregularities, changes in vaginal discharge, pelvic pain/pressure), symptoms of leg swelling/tenderness, unexplained SOB, or changes in vision occur. Inform women taking tamoxifen for the purpose of reducing the incidence of breast cancer and in women taking tamoxifen as adjuvant breast cancer therapy, that they should have a breast examination, a mammogram, and a gynecologic examination prior to the initiation of therapy and at regular intervals while on therapy.

STORAGE: Protect from light. **Oral Sol:** Up to 25°C (77°F). Do not freeze or refrigerate. Use w/in 3 months of opening. **Tab:** 20-25°C (68-77°F).

TAPAZOLE – methimazole

RX

Class: Thyroid hormone synthesis inhibitor

ADULT DOSAGE

Hyperthyroidism

Treatment in patients w/ Graves' disease w/ hyperthyroidism or toxic multinodular goiter

PEDIATRIC DOSAGE

Hyperthyroidism

Treatment in patients w/ Graves' disease w/ hyperthyroidism or toxic multinodular for whom surgery or radioactive iodine therapy is not an appropriate treatment option. To ameliorate symptoms of hyperthyroidism in preparation for thyroidectomy or radioactive iodine therapy.

Initial:

Mild Hyperthyroidism: 15mg/day

Moderately Severe Hyperthyroidism: 30-40mg/day

Severe Hyperthyroidism: 60mg/day

Maint: 5-15mg/day

Give total daily dose in 3 divided doses at approx 8-hr intervals

goiter for whom surgery or radioactive iodine therapy is not an appropriate treatment option. To ameliorate symptoms of hyperthyroidism in preparation for thyroidectomy or radioactive iodine therapy.

Initial: 0.4mg/kg/day given in 3 divided doses at 8-hr intervals

Maint: Approx 1/2 of initial dose

ADMINISTRATION

Oral route

HOW SUPPLIED

Tab: 5mg*, 10mg* *scored

CONTRAINDICATIONS

Hypersensitivity to the drug or any of the other product components.

WARNINGS/PRECAUTIONS

May cause fetal harm when administered in the 1st trimester of pregnancy; rare instances of congenital defects occurred in infants born to mothers who received methimazole in the 1st trimester of pregnancy. Agranulocytosis, leukopenia, thrombocytopenia, and aplastic anemia (pancytopenia) may occur. D/C therapy in the presence of agranulocytosis, aplastic anemia, ANCA-positive vasculitis, hepatitis, or exfoliative dermatitis, and monitor bone marrow indices. Hepatotoxicity (including acute liver failure) reported; promptly evaluate liver function (bilirubin, alkaline phosphatase) and hepatocellular integrity (ALT, AST) if symptoms suggestive of hepatic dysfunction occur. D/C treatment promptly w/ evidence of liver abnormality including hepatic transaminases >3X ULN. May cause hypothyroidism; routinely monitor TSH and free T4 levels and adjust dose to maintain a euthyroid state. May cause fetal goiter and cretinism; lowest possible dose should be given during pregnancy. May cause hypoprothrombinemia and bleeding; monitor PT during therapy, especially before surgical procedures. Monitor thyroid function tests periodically during therapy; use lower maintenance dose once clinical evidence of hyperthyroidism has resolved.

ADVERSE REACTIONS

Agranulocytosis, granulocytopenia, thrombocytopenia, aplastic anemia, drug fever, lupus-like syndrome, insulin autoimmune syndrome, hepatitis, periarteritis, hypoprothrombinemia, skin rash, urticaria, N/V, arthralgia, paresthesia.

DRUG INTERACTIONS

May increase oral anticoagulant (eg, warfarin) activity; consider additional PT/INR monitoring, especially before surgical procedures. β-blockers, digitalis glycosides, and theophylline may need dose reduction when patient becomes euthyroid. Caution w/ other drugs that cause agranulocytosis.

PATIENT CONSIDERATIONS

Assessment: Assess for hypersensitivity to drug, pregnancy/nursing status, and possible drug interactions.

Monitoring: Monitor for agranulocytosis, leukopenia, thrombocytopenia, aplastic anemia, hepatotoxicity, hypothyroidism, and other adverse reactions. Monitor PT, especially before surgical procedures. Monitor TSH and free T4 levels periodically.

Counseling: Inform of the benefits/risks of therapy. Instruct to inform physician if pregnant/nursing or planning to become pregnant. Inform of the potential hazard to the fetus if used during pregnancy or if patient becomes pregnant while taking this drug. Instruct to immediately report any evidence of illness, particularly sore throat, skin eruptions, fever, headache, or general malaise.

STORAGE: 15-30°C (59-86°F).

TARCEVA – erlotinib

RX

Class: Kinase inhibitor

ADULT DOSAGE

Non-Small Cell Lung Cancer

1st-line treatment of patients w/ metastatic non-small cell lung cancer (NSCLC) whose tumors have epidermal growth factor receptor exon 19 deletions or exon 21 (L858R) substitution mutations; treatment of locally advanced or metastatic NSCLC after failure of at least 1 prior chemotherapy regimen; maint treatment of locally advanced or metastatic NSCLC that has not progressed after 4 cycles of platinum-based 1st-line chemotherapy

Usual: 150mg qd

Pancreatic Cancer

1st-Line Treatment of Locally Advanced, Unresectable, or Metastatic Pancreatic Cancer:

Usual: 100mg qd in combination w/ gemcitabine until disease progression or unacceptable toxicity occurs

PEDIATRIC DOSAGE

Pediatric use may not have been established

DOSING CONSIDERATIONS

Concomitant Medications

Reduce by 50mg Decrements if:

If severe reactions occur w/ concomitant use of strong CYP3A4 inhibitors or w/ concomitant use of both a CYP3A4 and CYP1A2 inhibitor (eg, ciprofloxacin); avoid concomitant use if possible

Increase by 50mg Increments As Tolerated for:

- Concomitant use w/ CYP3A4 inducers; increase by 50mg increments at 2-week intervals to a max of 450mg; avoid concomitant use if possible
- Concurrent cigarette smoking; increase by 50mg increments at 2-week intervals to a max of 300mg; immediately reduce the dose to the recommended dose (150mg or 100mg qd) upon cessation of smoking

Drugs Affecting Gastric pH:

- Avoid concomitant use w/ proton pump inhibitors if possible
- If treatment w/ an H_2-receptor antagonist is required, dose must be taken 10 hrs after the H_2-receptor antagonist dosing and at least 2 hrs before the next dose of the H_2-receptor antagonist
- If an antacid is necessary, dose should be separated by several hrs

Adverse Reactions:

D/C for:

- Interstitial Lung Disease (ILD)
- Severe hepatic toxicity that does not improve significantly or resolve w/in 3 weeks
- GI perforation
- Severe bullous, blistering, or exfoliating skin conditions
- Corneal perforation or severe ulceration

Withhold for:

- During diagnostic evaluation for possible ILD
- For severe (CTCAE Grade 3 to 4) renal toxicity, and consider discontinuation
- In patients w/o preexisting hepatic impairment for total bilirubin levels >3X ULN or transaminases >5X ULN, and consider discontinuation
- In patients w/ preexisting hepatic impairment or biliary obstruction for doubling of bilirubin or tripling of transaminases values over baseline and consider discontinuation
- For persistent severe diarrhea not responsive to medical management (eg, loperamide)
- For severe rash not responsive to medical management
- For keratitis of (NCI-CTC version 4.0) Grade 3-4 or for Grade 2 lasting more than 2 weeks
- For acute/worsening ocular disorders such as eye pain, and consider discontinuation

Reduce by 50mg Decrements if:

When restarting therapy following withholding treatment for a dose-limiting toxicity that has resolved to baseline or Grade ≤1

ADMINISTRATION

Oral route

Take on an empty stomach (at least 1 hr ac or 2 hrs pc)

T

HOW SUPPLIED

Tab: 25mg, 100mg, 150mg

WARNINGS/PRECAUTIONS

Not recommended for use in combination w/ platinum-based chemotherapy. Cases of serious interstitial lung disease (ILD) may occur; withhold for acute onset of new/progressive unexplained pulmonary symptoms. Renal failure; hepatotoxicity w/ or w/o hepatic impairment; hepatorenal syndrome; bullous, blistering, and exfoliative skin conditions; MI/ischemia; cerebrovascular accidents (CVA); microangiopathic hemolytic anemia w/ thrombocytopenia; and fetal harm may occur. Decreased tear production, abnormal eyelash growth, keratoconjunctivitis sicca, or keratitis may occur and can lead to corneal perforation/ulceration. GI perforation may occur; increased risk in patients w/ prior history of peptic ulceration or diverticular disease.

ADVERSE REACTIONS

Rash, diarrhea, anorexia, asthenia, dyspnea, cough, N/V, infection, stomatitis, pruritus, dry skin, conjunctivitis, keratoconjunctivitis sicca, back pain, chest pain.

DRUG INTERACTIONS

See Dosing Considerations. Concomitant use w/ antiangiogenic agents, corticosteroids, NSAIDs, and/or taxane-based chemotherapy may increase risk of GI perforation. Increased levels w/ potent CYP3A4 inhibitors (eg, ketoconazole), and w/ inhibitors of both CYP3A4 and CYP1A2 (eg, ciprofloxacin). Decreased levels w/ CYP3A4 inducers (eg, rifampicin). Cigarette smoking and drugs affecting gastric pH (eg, omeprazole, ranitidine) may decrease levels. INR elevations and bleeding events reported w/ coumarin-derived anticoagulants (eg, warfarin); monitor PT/INR regularly.

PATIENT CONSIDERATIONS

Assessment: Assess for hepatic/renal impairment, dehydration, history of peptic ulceration or diverticular disease, pregnancy/nursing status, and possible drug interactions.

Monitoring: Monitor for signs and symptoms of ILD, hepatotoxicity, GI perforation, MI/ischemia, renal failure/insufficiency, CVA, microangiopathic hemolytic anemia w/ thrombocytopenia, ocular disorders, bullous and exfoliative skin disorders, and other adverse reactions. Monitor LFTs, renal function, and serum electrolytes periodically.

Counseling: Inform of risks/benefits of therapy. Instruct to notify physician if onset or worsening of skin rash or development of bullous lesions or desquamation; severe/persistent diarrhea, N/V, anorexia; unexplained SOB or cough; or eye irritation occurs. Instruct to stop smoking and advise to contact physician for any changes in smoking status. Advise on the presentation of skin, hair, and nail disorders. Instruct on initial management of rash or diarrhea. Counsel on pregnancy planning and prevention; advise females of reproductive potential to use highly effective contraception during treatment and for at least 2 weeks after the last dose. Advise to contact physician if pregnant or if pregnancy is suspected and to d/c nursing during treatment.

STORAGE: 25°C (77°F); excursions permitted to 15-30°C (59-86°F).

TARKA – trandolapril/verapamil hydrochloride

RX

Class: ACE inhibitor/calcium channel blocker (CCB) (nondihydropyridine)

D/C when pregnancy is detected. Drugs that act directly on the renin-angiotensin system (RAS) can cause injury/death to the developing fetus.

ADULT DOSAGE

Hypertension

Begin therapy only after patient has either failed to achieve desired antihypertensive effect w/ monotherapy at max recommended dose and shortest dosing interval, or monotherapy dose cannot be increased further because of dose-limiting side effects

Usual: Trandolapril 1-4mg/verapamil extended-release (ER) 120-480mg qd

Replacement Therapy: For patients receiving trandolapril (up to 8mg) and verapamil ER (up to 240mg) in separate tabs, combination may be substituted for same component doses

PEDIATRIC DOSAGE

Pediatric use may not have been established

DOSING CONSIDERATIONS

Hepatic Impairment

Severe Liver Dysfunction: Give approx 30% of the normal verapamil dose

ADMINISTRATION

Oral route

Take qd w/ food

HOW SUPPLIED

Tab, ER: (Trandolapril/Verapamil ER) 2mg/180mg, 1mg/240mg, 2mg/240mg, 4mg/240mg

CONTRAINDICATIONS

Hypersensitivity to any ACE inhibitor or verapamil, severe left ventricular dysfunction, hypotension (systolic BP <90mmHg), cardiogenic shock, sick sinus syndrome (except w/ functioning artificial ventricular pacemaker), 2nd- or 3rd-degree atrioventricular (AV) block (except w/ functioning artificial ventricular pacemaker), A-fib/A-flutter and an accessory bypass tract (eg, Wolff-Parkinson-White, Lown-Ganong-Levine syndromes), history of ACE inhibitor-associated angioedema. Coadministration w/ aliskiren in patients w/ diabetes.

WARNINGS/PRECAUTIONS

Not for initial therapy of HTN. Trandolapril: Symptomatic hypotension may occur and is most likely in patients who are salt- or volume-depleted; correct the depletion prior to therapy. May cause excessive hypotension, which may be associated w/ oliguria or azotemia, w/ acute renal failure (rare) and death in patients w/ CHF. May cause cholestatic jaundice, fulminant hepatic necrosis, and death; d/c if jaundice develops. Angioedema reported; d/c if laryngeal stridor or angioedema of the face, tongue, or glottis occurs and administer appropriate therapy. Anaphylactoid reactions reported during desensitization w/ hymenoptera venom, dialysis w/ high-flux membranes, and LDL apheresis w/ dextran sulfate absorption. Potential for agranulocytosis and neutropenia; monitor WBCs in patients w/ collagen-vascular disease and/or renal disease. Changes in renal function may occur. May increase BUN and SrCr w/ renal artery stenosis and w/o preexisting renal vascular disease; consider dose reduction and/or discontinuation. Hyperkalemia and persistent, nonproductive cough reported. Hypotension may occur w/ major surgery or during anesthesia. Verapamil: Caution w/ impaired renal function. Has a negative inotropic effect; avoid w/ severe left ventricular dysfunction. May decrease BP, which may result in dizziness or symptomatic hypotension. Elevated transaminases w/ or w/o alkaline phosphatase/bilirubin elevation and hepatocellular injury reported. May lead to asymptomatic 1st-degree AV block and transient bradycardia. Reduce dose or d/c in marked 1st-degree block or progression to 2nd- or 3rd-degree AV block. Sinus bradycardia, 2nd-degree AV block, sinus arrest, and pulmonary edema/severe hypotension reported in patients w/ hypertrophic cardiomyopathy. May decrease neuromuscular transmission in patients w/ Duchenne muscular dystrophy; reduce dose w/ attenuated neuromuscular transmission.

ADVERSE REACTIONS

1st-degree AV block, constipation, cough, dizziness, headache, URTI.

DRUG INTERACTIONS

See Contraindications. May cause additive hypotensive effects w/ diuretics, vasodilators, β-adrenergic blockers, and α-antagonists. Trandolapril: Avoid w/ aliskiren in patients w/ renal impairment (GFR <60mL/min). Dual blockade of the RAS is associated w/ increased risk of hypotension, hyperkalemia, and changes in renal function (including acute renal failure); avoid combined use of RAS inhibitors, or closely monitor BP, renal function, and electrolytes w/ concomitant agents that also affect the RAS. Excessive BP reduction reported w/ diuretics. May increase risk of hyperkalemia w/ K^+-sparing diuretics, K^+ supplements, or K^+-containing salt substitutes. May result in deterioration of renal function w/ NSAIDs, including selective COX-2 inhibitors. NSAIDs may also attenuate antihypertensive effect. Nitritoid reactions reported rarely w/ injectable gold. May increase blood glucose-lowering effect of antidiabetic medications. May increase lithium levels and symptoms of lithium toxicity. Verapamil: Increased sensitivity to the effects of lithium. Hypotension, bradyarrhythmias, and lactic acidosis were seen w/ clarithromycin and erythromycin. Not recommended w/ colchicine. Avoid disopyramide w/in 48 hrs before or 24 hrs after administration. Avoid concomitant quinidine use w/ hypertrophic cardiomyopathy; significant hypotension reported. Additive negative inotropic effect and prolongation of AV conduction w/ flecainide. Additive negative effects on HR, AV conduction, and/or cardiac contractility w/ β-adrenergic blockers. Asymptomatic bradycardia w/ a wandering atrial pacemaker has been observed w/ concomitant use of timolol eye drops. Inhalational anesthetics may depress cardiovascular activity. May potentiate activity of neuromuscular blocking agents (curare-like and depolarizing); reduce dose of either or both drugs. May increase levels of digoxin, prazosin, terazosin, simvastatin, lovastatin, atorvastatin, carbamazepine, cyclosporine, sirolimus, tacrolimus, theophylline, buspirone, midazolam, almotriptan, imipramine, doxorubicin, quinidine, metoprolol, propranolol, colchicine, and glyburide; reduce maintenance doses of digoxin. CYP3A4 inhibitors (eg, erythromycin, telithromycin, ritonavir) may increase levels. CYP3A4 inducers (eg, rifampin, phenobarbital, sulfinpyrazone, St. John's wort) may decrease levels. Myopathy/rhabdomyolysis reported w/ HMG-CoA reductase inhibitors that are CYP3A4 substrates; limit simvastatin dose to 10mg/day, lovastatin dose to 40mg/day, and consider lower starting and maintenance doses for others.

PATIENT CONSIDERATIONS

Assessment: Assess for drug hypersensitivity, ventricular dysfunction, cardiogenic shock, sick sinus syndrome, AV block, A-fib/A-flutter and an accessory bypass tract, history of angioedema, diabetes, hepatic/renal impairment, CHF, hypertrophic cardiomyopathy, neuromuscular disorders, volume/salt depletion, collagen vascular disease, pregnancy/nursing status, and possible drug interactions.

Monitoring: Monitor for angioedema, cough, anaphylactoid reactions, hypotension, hepatic/renal impairment, cholestatic jaundice, fulminant hepatic necrosis, heart block, bradycardia, agranulocytosis, and other adverse reactions. Monitor for abnormal prolongation of PR interval w/ impaired hepatic/renal function. Monitor BP and serum K^+. Monitor WBC counts in patients w/ collagen vascular disease and/or renal disease.

Counseling: Counsel regarding adverse effects (eg, angioedema, neutropenia, jaundice) and instruct to report any signs/symptoms. Inform of risks when taken during pregnancy; instruct to notify physician if patient is pregnant or becomes pregnant. Educate about need for periodic follow-ups and blood tests to rule out adverse effects and to monitor therapeutic effects.

STORAGE: 15-25°C (59-77°F).

TASIGNA – nilotinib

RX

Class: Kinase inhibitor

Prolongs QT interval. Monitor for hypokalemia or hypomagnesemia and correct deficiencies prior to administration and periodically. Obtain ECGs to monitor QTc at baseline, 7 days after initiation, and periodically thereafter, and following any dose adjustments. Sudden deaths reported. Do not administer to patients w/ hypokalemia, hypomagnesemia, or long QT syndrome. Avoid w/ drugs known to prolong the QT interval and strong CYP3A4 inhibitors. Avoid food 2 hrs before and 1 hr after taking the dose.

ADULT DOSAGE

Ph+ Chronic Myeloid Leukemia

Newly Diagnosed Philadelphia Chromosome-Positive Chronic Myeloid Leukemia (Ph+ CML)-Chronic Phase (CP):
300mg bid

Resistant or Intolerant Ph+ CML-CP and CML-Accelerated Phase (AP):
In patients resistant/intolerant to prior therapy that included imatinib

400mg bid

May be given in combination w/ hematopoietic growth factors (eg, erythropoietin, granulocyte colony-stimulating factor), hydroxyurea, or anagrelide if clinically indicated

PEDIATRIC DOSAGE

Pediatric use may not have been established

DOSING CONSIDERATIONS

Concomitant Medications

Strong CYP3A4 Inhibitors (eg, Ketoconazole, Clarithromycin, Atazanavir):
- Avoid concomitant use
- If treatment w/ any of these agents is required, interrupt nilotinib treatment
- If coadministration is a must, consider dose reduction to 300mg qd w/ resistant or intolerant Ph+ CML or to 200mg qd w/ newly diagnosed Ph+ CML; closely monitor for QT interval prolongation in patients who cannot avoid use of strong inhibitor
- If the strong inhibitor is discontinued, allow a washout period before nilotinib dose is adjusted upward to the indicated dose
- Avoid grapefruit products

Strong CYP3A4 Inducers (eg, Dexamethasone, Phenytoin, Carbamazepine):
- Avoid concomitant use
- Avoid St. John's wort

Hepatic Impairment

Newly Diagnosed Ph+ CML:
Mild, Moderate, or Severe (Child-Pugh Class A, B, or C): 200mg bid initially, followed by dose escalation to 300mg bid based on tolerability

Resistant or Intolerant Ph+ CML:
Mild or Moderate (Child-Pugh Score A or B): 300mg bid initially, followed by dose escalation to 400mg bid based on tolerability

T

Severe (Child-Pugh Score C): 200mg bid initially, followed by sequential dose escalation to 300mg bid and then to 400mg bid based on tolerability

Adverse Reactions

ECGs w/ a QTc >480 msec:

1. Withhold nilotinib, and perform an analysis of serum K^+ and Mg^{2+}, and if below lower limit of normal, correct w/ supplements to w/in normal limits. Concomitant medication usage must be reviewed
2. Resume w/in 2 weeks at prior dose if QTcF returns to <450 msec and to w/in 20 msec of baseline
3. If QTcF is between 450 msec and 480 msec after 2 weeks, reduce dose to 400mg qd
4. If, following dose reduction to 400mg qd, QTcF returns to >480 msec, d/c therapy
5. An ECG should be repeated approx 7 days after any dose adjustment

Neutropenia and Thrombocytopenia (Not Related to Underlying Leukemia):

ANC <1.0 x 10^9/L and/or Platelet Counts <50 x 10^9/L:

1. Stop nilotinib, and monitor blood counts
2. Resume w/in 2 weeks at prior dose if ANC >1.0 x 10^9/L and platelets >50 x 10^9/L
3. If blood counts remain low for >2 weeks, reduce dose to 400mg qd

Selected Nonhematologic Lab Abnormalities:

Elevated Serum Lipase or Amylase ≥Grade 3:

1. Withhold nilotinib, and monitor serum lipase or amylase
2. Resume at 400mg qd if serum lipase or amylase returns to ≤Grade 1

Elevated Bilirubin ≥Grade 3:

1. Withhold nilotinib, and monitor bilirubin
2. Resume at 400mg qd if bilirubin returns to ≤Grade 1

Elevated Hepatic Transaminases ≥Grade 3:

1. Withhold nilotinib, and monitor hepatic transaminases
2. Resume at 400mg qd if hepatic transaminases returns to ≤Grade 1

Other Nonhematologic Toxicities:

Grade 3 to 4 Lipase Elevations, Grade 3 to 4 Bilirubin, or Hepatic Transaminase Elevations:

Withhold dose and may resume at 400mg qd

Other Significant Moderate or Severe Toxicities:

Withhold dose and resume at 400mg qd when the toxicity has resolved

If clinically appropriate, consider escalating dose back to 300mg bid (newly diagnosed Ph+ CML) or 400mg bid (resistant or intolerant Ph+ CML)

ADMINISTRATION

Oral route

Take on an empty stomach.

Avoid food for at least 2 hrs before and 1 hr after taking the dose.

Take at approx 12-hr intervals.

Swallow whole w/ water.

May disperse contents of each cap in 1 tsp of applesauce if unable to swallow; take immediately (w/in 15 min) and do not store for future use.

HOW SUPPLIED

Cap: 150mg, 200mg

CONTRAINDICATIONS

Hypokalemia, hypomagnesemia, long QT syndrome.

WARNINGS/PRECAUTIONS

May cause myelosuppression (eg, Grade 3/4 thrombocytopenia, neutropenia, and anemia); perform CBCs every 2 weeks for the first 2 months, then monthly thereafter, or as clinically indicated. Cardiovascular (CV) events, including arterial vascular occlusive events, reported; evaluate CV status and monitor and actively manage CV risk factors during therapy. May increase serum lipase; increased risk in patients w/ history of pancreatitis. Interrupt dosing and consider appropriate diagnostics to exclude pancreatitis if lipase elevations are accompanied by abdominal symptoms. May result in hepatotoxicity as measured by elevations in bilirubin, AST/ALT, and alkaline phosphatase. May cause hypophosphatemia, hypo/hyperkalemia, hypocalcemia, and hyponatremia; correct electrolyte abnormalities prior to initiation and during therapy. Exposure is increased in patients w/ impaired hepatic function; monitor QT interval frequently. Tumor lysis syndrome cases reported in patients w/ resistant or intolerant CML; maintain adequate hydration and correct uric acid levels prior to initiation. Hemorrhage reported in patients w/ newly diagnosed Ph+ CML. Reduced exposure in patients w/ total gastrectomy; perform more frequent monitoring and consider dose increase or alternative therapy. Contains lactose; not recommended for patients w/ rare hereditary problems of galactose intolerance, severe lactase deficiency w/ a severe degree of intolerance to lactose-containing products, or of glucose-galactose malabsorption. May cause fetal harm. Severe (Grade 3 or 4) fluid retention, effusions (eg, pleural effusion, pericardial effusion, ascites) or pulmonary edema reported w/ newly diagnosed Ph+ CML-CP. Monitor patients for signs of severe fluid retention and for symptoms of respiratory/cardiac compromise during treatment; evaluate etiology and treat patients accordingly. Caution w/ relevant cardiac disorders.

ADVERSE REACTIONS
Non-Hematologic: Rash, pruritus, headache, N/V, fatigue, alopecia, myalgia, upper abdominal pain, constipation, diarrhea.
Hematologic: Myelosuppression (thrombocytopenia, neutropenia, anemia).

DRUG INTERACTIONS
See Boxed Warning and Dosing Considerations. May increase concentrations of drugs eliminated by CYP3A4 (eg, midazolam, certain HMG-CoA reductase inhibitors), CYP2C8, CYP2C9, CYP2D6, and UGT1A1 enzymes; dose adjustment may be necessary for CYP3A4 substrates, especially those that have narrow therapeutic indices (eg, alfentanil, cyclosporine, dihydroergotamine). May decrease concentrations of drugs eliminated by CYP2B6, CYP2C8, and CYP2C9 enzymes; monitor patients closely when nilotinib is coadministered w/ drugs that have a narrow therapeutic index and are substrates for these enzymes. May increase concentrations of P-gp substrates; use w/ caution. Concomitant administration of strong CYP3A4 inhibitors or inducers may increase or decrease nilotinib concentrations significantly. Decreased solubility and reduced bioavailability w/ drugs that inhibit gastric acid secretion to elevate the gastric pH; concomitant use w/ proton pump inhibitors is not recommended. When the concurrent use of a H_2 blocker is necessary, administer approx 10 hrs before and 2 hrs after the dose of nilotinib. If antacid administration is necessary, administer approx 2 hrs before or 2 hrs after the dose of nilotinib. P-gp inhibitors may increase concentrations; use w/ caution. Avoid w/ drugs that may prolong the QT interval (eg, antiarrhythmic drugs), and grapefruit products and other foods that inhibit CYP3A4.

PATIENT CONSIDERATIONS

Assessment: Assess for electrolyte abnormalities, history of pancreatitis, long QT syndrome, cardiac disorders, total gastrectomy, hepatic impairment, galactose intolerance, lactase deficiency, glucose-galactose malabsorption, pregnancy/nursing status, and possible drug interactions. Obtain baseline ECG, uric acid levels, and chemistry panels, including lipid profile and glucose.

Monitoring: Monitor for myelosuppression; perform CBCs every 2 weeks for the first 2 months of therapy, then monthly thereafter or as clinically indicated. Perform chemistry panels, including electrolytes and liver enzymes periodically. Monitor lipid profiles and glucose periodically during 1st yr of therapy and at least yearly during chronic therapy. Monitor for signs/symptoms of QT prolongation; obtain ECG 7 days after initiation, periodically thereafter, and after any dose adjustments. Maintain adequate hydration, evaluate CV status, and monitor CV risk factors. Monitor serum lipase levels and LFTs monthly or as clinically indicated. Monitor for signs of severe fluid retention, symptoms of respiratory/cardiac compromise, tumor lysis syndrome, hemorrhage, and other adverse reactions.

Counseling: Instruct to take ud. Advise to seek immediate medical attention w/ any symptoms suggestive of a CV event. Instruct not to consume grapefruit products at any time during treatment. Instruct to inform physician of other medicines being taken, including OTC drugs or herbal supplements (eg, St. John's wort). Advise that use of drug during pregnancy may cause harm to the fetus and that nilotinib should not be taken during pregnancy unless necessary. Instruct women of childbearing potential to use highly effective contraceptives while on therapy. Instruct not to d/c or change dose w/o consulting physician.

STORAGE: 25°C (77°F); excursions permitted between 15-30°C (59-86°F).

TECFIDERA – dimethyl fumarate

RX

Class: Immunomodulatory agent

ADULT DOSAGE
Multiple Sclerosis
Relapsing Forms:
Initial: 120mg bid
Titrate: Increase to 240mg bid after 7 days
Maint: 240mg bid. Consider temporary reduction to 120mg bid if not tolerated; resume maint dose of 240mg bid w/in 4 weeks and consider discontinuation if unable to tolerate return to maint dose

PEDIATRIC DOSAGE
Pediatric use may not have been established

ADMINISTRATION
Oral route

Take w/ or w/o food
Swallow whole and intact; do not crush or chew
Do not sprinkle cap contents on food
To reduce flushing, take w/ food or take up to 325mg of non-enteric coated aspirin 30 min prior to therapy

HOW SUPPLIED

Cap, Delayed-Release: 120mg, 240mg

CONTRAINDICATIONS

Known hypersensitivity to dimethyl fumarate or to any of the excipients of this medication.

WARNINGS/PRECAUTIONS

May cause anaphylaxis and angioedema; d/c if signs/symptoms occur. Progressive multifocal leukoencephalopathy (PML) reported; withhold treatment and perform appropriate diagnostic evaluation at the 1st sign/symptom suggestive of PML. May decrease lymphocyte counts; consider interruption of therapy w/ lymphocyte counts <0.5 x 10^9/L persisting for >6 months and monitor lymphocyte count until lymphopenia is resolved. Consider withholding treatment in patients w/ serious infections until resolved; decisions about whether or not to restart therapy should be individualized based on clinical circumstances. May cause flushing; administration w/ food may reduce the incidence. Alternatively, administration of non-enteric coated aspirin (up to a dose of 325mg) 30 min prior to dosing may reduce the incidence or severity of flushing.

ADVERSE REACTIONS

Flushing, abdominal pain, diarrhea, N/V, pruritus, rash, albuminuria, erythema, dyspepsia, increased AST.

PATIENT CONSIDERATIONS

Assessment: Assess for known hypersensitivity to drug or any of the excipients, infection, and pregnancy/nursing status. Obtain baseline CBC including lymphocyte count.

Monitoring: Monitor for anaphylaxis, angioedema, PML, lymphopenia, flushing, and other adverse reactions. Monitor CBC including lymphocyte count after 6 months of treatment, every 6-12 months thereafter, and as clinically indicated.

Counseling: Advise to d/c therapy and seek medical care if signs/symptoms of anaphylaxis or angioedema develop. Inform that PML is characterized by progression of deficits and usually leads to death or severe disability; instruct to contact physician if any symptoms suggestive of PML develop. Inform that therapy may decrease lymphocyte counts. Advise to contact physician if patient experiences persistent and/or severe flushing or GI reactions. Instruct to inform physician if patient is pregnant or plans to become pregnant while on therapy; encourage enrollment in the pregnancy registry if patient becomes pregnant while on therapy.

STORAGE: 15-30°C (59-86°F). Protect from light.

TECHNIVIE — ombitasvir/paritaprevir/ritonavir RX

Class: CYP3A inhibitor/HCV NS5A inhibitor/HCV NS3/4A protease inhibitor

ADULT DOSAGE

Chronic Hepatitis C (Genotype 4)

Combination w/ Ribavirin (RBV) in Patients w/o Cirrhosis:

2 tabs qd (am) w/ RBV at 1000mg/day (<75kg) and 1200mg/day (≥75kg) in 2 divided doses for 12 weeks

May be given w/o RBV for 12 weeks for treatment-naive patients who cannot take or tolerate RBV

PEDIATRIC DOSAGE

Pediatric use may not have been established

T

ADMINISTRATION

Oral route

Take in the am w/ a meal w/o regard to fat or calorie content.

HOW SUPPLIED

Tab: (Ombitasvir/Paritaprevir/Ritonavir [RTV]) 12.5mg/75mg/50mg

CONTRAINDICATIONS

Moderate to severe hepatic impairment (Child-Pugh Class B and C). Drugs that are highly dependent on CYP3A for clearance and for which elevated plasma concentrations are associated w/ serious and/or life-threatening events, and drugs that are moderate or strong inducers of CYP3A and may lead to reduced efficacy (alfuzosin HCl, colchicine, carbamazepine, phenytoin, phenobarbital, rifampin, ergotamine, dihydroergotamine, ergonovine, methylergonovine, ethinyl estradiol-containing medications such as combined oral contraceptives, St. John's wort, lovastatin, simvastatin, pimozide, efavirenz, sildenafil [when dosed as Revatio for the treatment of pulmonary arterial hypertension], triazolam, oral midazolam). Known hypersensitivity to ritonavir (eg, toxic epidermal necrolysis, Stevens-Johnson syndrome). Refer to the RBV prescribing information for a list of contraindications for RBV.

WARNINGS/PRECAUTIONS

Hepatic decompensation and hepatic failure, including liver transplantation or fatal outcomes, reported; d/c treatment in patients who develop evidence of hepatic decompensation. ALT elevations to >5X ULN reported; occurred during first 4 weeks of treatment and declined w/in 2-8 weeks w/ continued dosing. Perform hepatic lab testing during first 4 weeks of treatment and as clinically indicated thereafter. Monitor closely if ALT is elevated above baseline. Consider discontinuing if ALT levels remain persistently >10X ULN. D/C if ALT elevation is accompanied by signs/symptoms of liver inflammation or increasing direct bilirubin, alkaline phosphatase, or INR. Any hepatitis C virus (HCV)/HIV-1 coinfected patients should also be on a suppressive antiretroviral drug regimen to reduce the risk of HIV-1 protease inhibitor drug resistance. Refer to the RBV prescribing information for a full list of the warnings and precautions for RBV.

ADVERSE REACTIONS

Asthenia, fatigue, nausea, insomnia, pruritus, skin reactions, serum bilirubin elevations.

DRUG INTERACTIONS

See Contraindications. ALT elevation reported more frequently w/ ethinyl estradiol-containing medications (eg, combined oral contraceptives, contraceptive patches, contraceptive vaginal rings); d/c ethinyl estradiol-containing medications prior to starting therapy. Alternative methods of contraception (eg, progestin only contraception, nonhormonal methods) are recommended during therapy; ethinyl estradiol-containing medications can be restarted approx 2 weeks following completion of treatment. Caution w/ estrogens other than ethinyl estradiol (eg, estradiol and conjugated estrogens) used in hormone replacement therapy. Coadministration w/ drugs that are substrates of CYP3A, P-gp, BCRP, OATP1B1 or OATP1B3 may result in increased plasma concentrations of such drugs. Coadministration w/ strong inhibitors of CYP3A may increase paritaprevir and RTV concentrations. Inhibition of P-gp, BCRP, OATP1B1 or OATP1B3 may increase the plasma concentrations of the various components of Technivie. May increase levels of angiotensin receptor blockers, digoxin, antiarrhythmics, ketoconazole, quetiapine, calcium channel blockers, inhaled/nasal fluticasone, furosemide (C_{max}), rilpivirine, pravastatin, cyclosporine, tacrolimus, salmeterol, buprenorphine, norbuprenorphine, or alprazolam. Concomitant use w/ inhaled or nasal fluticasone may reduce serum cortisol concentrations. May decrease levels of omeprazole, darunavir (C_{trough}), or voriconazole. Atazanavir, atazanavir/RTV, or lopinavir/RTV may increase paritaprevir levels. Not recommended w/ voriconazole, atazanavir, atazanavir/RTV, lopinavir/RTV, rilpivirine once daily, or salmeterol. Refer to PI for further information on drug interactions, including dosing modifications when used w/ certain concomitant therapies.

PATIENT CONSIDERATIONS

Assessment: Assess for cirrhosis, hepatic impairment, pregnancy/nursing status, hypersensitivity to any component in drug, and possible drug interactions. Assess baseline hepatic laboratory and clinical parameters. Assess HCV genotype.

Monitoring: Monitor for signs/symptoms of hepatic decompensation, hepatic failure, liver inflammation, ALT elevations, and other adverse reactions. Perform hepatic lab testing during first 4 weeks of treatment and as clinically indicated thereafter.

Counseling: Inform patients to watch for signs of liver inflammation or failure (eg, fatigue, weakness, lack of appetite, N/V, jaundice, onset of confusion, abdominal swelling, discolored feces); instruct to notify physician w/o delay if such symptoms develop. Advise to avoid pregnancy during treatment w/ Technivie w/ RBV; instruct to notify physician immediately in the event of a pregnancy. Inform of drug interactions that may occur; instruct to report to physician use of any prescription, nonprescription medication, or herbal products. Inform that contraceptives containing ethinyl estradiol should not be used. Inform patients that the effect of treatment of HCV infection on transmission is not known, and that appropriate precautions to prevent transmission of HCV during treatment should be taken.

STORAGE: ≤30°C (86°F).

T

TEKAMLO – aliskiren/amlodipine

RX

Class: Calcium channel blocker (CCB) (dihydropyridine)/renin inhibitor

D/C when pregnancy is detected. Drugs that act directly on the renin-angiotensin system (RAS) can cause injury/death to the developing fetus.

ADULT DOSAGE

Hypertension

Initial: 150mg/5mg qd

Titrate: If BP remains uncontrolled after 2-4 weeks of therapy, titrate dose prn

Max: 300mg/10mg qd

PEDIATRIC DOSAGE

Pediatric use may not have been established

Add-On Therapy:
Use for patients not adequately controlled w/ aliskiren alone or amlodipine (or another dihydropyridine CCB) alone; if dose-limiting adverse reactions occur on either component alone, switch to Tekamlo containing a lower dose of that component in combination w/ the other to achieve similar BP reductions

Replacement Therapy:
Switch patients receiving aliskiren and amlodipine from separate tabs to Tekamlo containing the same component doses; if BP is uncontrolled when substituting for individual components, increase the dose of one or both of the components

May be used alone or w/ other antihypertensive agents

DOSING CONSIDERATIONS

Hepatic Impairment
Consider lower doses

Elderly
Consider starting w/ the lowest available dose of amlodipine

ADMINISTRATION

Oral route

Establish a routine pattern for taking the drug either w/ or w/o a meal; high-fat meals decrease absorption substantially

HOW SUPPLIED

Tab: (Aliskiren/Amlodipine) 150mg/5mg, 150mg/10mg, 300mg/5mg, 300mg/10mg

CONTRAINDICATIONS

Concomitant use w/ ARBs or ACE inhibitors in patients w/ diabetes. Known hypersensitivity to any of the components of the product.

WARNINGS/PRECAUTIONS

Symptomatic hypotension may occur in patients w/ marked volume/salt depletion, w/ severe aortic stenosis; correct volume/salt depletion prior to administration, or start treatment under close supervision. May cause changes in renal function, including acute renal failure; consider withholding or discontinuing therapy if significant decrease in renal function develops. Patients whose renal function may depend in part on the activity of the renin-angiotensin-aldosterone system (RAAS) (eg, renal artery stenosis, severe heart failure [HF], post-MI, volume depletion) may be at particular risk for developing acute renal failure. **Aliskiren:** Hypersensitivity reactions and head/neck angioedema reported; d/c therapy immediately if anaphylactic reactions or edema occurs and do not readminister. May cause hyperkalemia; periodically monitor serum K^+. **Amlodipine:** Worsening angina and acute MI may develop after starting or increasing dose, particularly w/ severe obstructive coronary artery disease (CAD).

ADVERSE REACTIONS

Peripheral edema.

DRUG INTERACTIONS

See Contraindications. **Aliskiren:** Cyclosporine or itraconazole may increase levels; avoid concomitant use. NSAIDs (including selective COX-2 inhibitors) may result in deterioration of renal function, including possible acute renal failure, in elderly, volume depleted, or those w/ compromised renal function. Antihypertensive effect may be attenuated by NSAIDs. Dual blockade of the RAAS is associated w/ increased risks of hypotension, hyperkalemia, and changes in renal function (including acute renal failure); avoid combined use w/ ACE inhibitors or ARBs, particularly in patients w/ CrCl <60mL/min. Oral coadministration w/ furosemide reduced exposure to furosemide; monitor diuretic effects. Risk of developing hyperkalemia w/ NSAIDs (eg, selective COX-2 inhibitors), K^+ supplements, or K^+-sparing diuretics. **Amlodipine:** May increase simvastatin exposure; limit simvastatin dose to 20mg/day. CYP3A inhibitors (moderate and strong) result in increased systemic exposure to amlodipine warranting dose reduction; monitor for symptoms of hypotension and edema to determine need for dose adjustment. Monitor BP when coadministered w/ CYP3A4 inducers.

PATIENT CONSIDERATIONS

Assessment: Assess for drug hypersensitivity, volume/salt depletion, renal artery stenosis, HF, post-MI status, severe aortic stenosis, CAD, hyperkalemia risk factors, renal/hepatic impairment, pregnancy/nursing status, and possible drug interactions.

Monitoring: Monitor for signs/symptoms of hypotension, worsening of angina, acute MI, hyperkalemia, hypersensitivity reactions, airway obstruction, angioedema, and other adverse reactions. Monitor BP, renal function, and serum K^+ periodically.

Counseling: Inform female patients of childbearing age of the consequences of exposure to therapy during pregnancy and of the treatment options for women planning to become pregnant. Advise to report pregnancies as soon as possible. Caution that lightheadedness may occur, especially during the 1st days of therapy; advise to contact physician if lightheadedness occurs. Advise to d/c until physician has been consulted if syncope occurs. Caution that inadequate fluid intake, excessive perspiration, diarrhea, or vomiting can lead to an excessive fall in BP. Advise to d/c and immediately report any signs/symptoms of a severe allergic reaction or angioedema. Inform that angioedema (eg, laryngeal edema) may occur anytime during treatment. Instruct not to use K^+ supplements or salt substitutes containing K^+ w/o consulting physician.

STORAGE: 25°C (77°F); excursions permitted to 15-30°C (59-86°F). Protect from heat and moisture.

TEKTURNA HCT – aliskiren/hydrochlorothiazide RX

Class: Renin inhibitor/thiazide diuretic

D/C when pregnancy is detected. Drugs that act directly on the renin-angiotensin system can cause injury and death to the developing fetus.

ADULT DOSAGE

Hypertension

Add-On/Initial Therapy:

Patients whose BP is not adequately controlled w/ aliskiren alone or hydrochlorothiazide (HCTZ) alone may be switched to Tekturna HCT, patients whose BP is controlled w/ HCTZ alone but who experience hypokalemia may be switched to Tekturna HCT, or patients who experience dose-limiting adverse reactions on either component alone may be switched to Tekturna HCT containing a lower dose of that component in combination w/ the other. May be used as initial therapy in patients likely to need multiple drugs to achieve BP goals

Initial: 150mg/12.5mg qd prn to control BP

Titrate: May increase if BP remains uncontrolled after 2-4 weeks

Max: 300mg/25mg qd

Replacement Therapy:

May substitute for individually titrated components

PEDIATRIC DOSAGE

Pediatric use may not have been established

ADMINISTRATION

Oral route

Establish a routine pattern for taking drug w/ regard to meals; high-fat meals decrease absorption substantially.

HOW SUPPLIED

Tab: (Aliskiren/HCTZ) 150mg/12.5mg, 150mg/25mg, 300mg/12.5mg, 300mg/25mg

CONTRAINDICATIONS

Coadministration w/ ARBs or ACE inhibitors in patients w/ diabetes, known anuria, hypersensitivity to sulfonamide-derived drugs (eg, HCTZ) or to any of the components.

WARNINGS/PRECAUTIONS

Not for initial therapy w/ intravascular volume depletion. Symptomatic hypotension may occur in patients w/ marked volume depletion or w/ salt depletion; correct volume/salt depletion prior to administration or begin therapy under close medical supervision. Renal function changes may occur, including acute renal failure; caution in patients whose renal function may depend in part on the activity of the renin-angiotensin-aldosterone system (RAAS) (eg, renal artery stenosis, severe heart failure [HF], post-MI, or volume depletion). Consider withholding or discontinuing therapy if clinically significant decrease in renal function develops. May cause hypo/hyperkalemia; d/c if hypokalemia is accompanied by clinical signs (eg, muscular weakness, paresis, ECG alterations).

T

Aliskiren: Hypersensitivity reactions (eg, anaphylactic reactions) and head/neck angioedema reported; d/c therapy immediately and do not readminister if anaphylactic reactions or angioedema develops. May cause hyperkalemia. **HCTZ:** May cause hypersensitivity reactions, w/ or w/o bronchial asthma, and exacerbation or activation of systemic lupus erythematosus (SLE). May cause hypokalemia and hyponatremia; hypomagnesemia may result in hypokalemia. Correct hypokalemia and any coexisting hypomagnesemia prior to initiation of thiazides. May cause idiosyncratic reaction, resulting in acute transient myopia and acute angle-closure glaucoma; d/c as rapidly as possible. May alter glucose tolerance and increase serum cholesterol and TG levels. May cause or exacerbate hyperuricemia and precipitate gout in susceptible patients. May cause hypercalcemia. Minor alterations of fluid and electrolyte balance may precipitate hepatic coma in patients w/ hepatic impairment or progressive liver disease.

ADVERSE REACTIONS

Dizziness, influenza, diarrhea, cough, vertigo, asthenia, arthralgia.

DRUG INTERACTIONS

See Contraindications. **Aliskiren:** Cyclosporine or itraconazole may increase levels; avoid concomitant use. NSAIDs (eg, selective COX-2 inhibitors) may deteriorate renal function, including possible acute renal failure, and may attenuate antihypertensive effect. Dual blockade of the RAAS is associated w/ increased risk of hypotension, hyperkalemia, and changes in renal function (including acute renal failure); in general, avoid combined use w/ ACE inhibitors or ARBs, particularly in patients w/ CrCl <60mL/min. Reduced furosemide exposure w/ concomitant use. May develop hyperkalemia w/ NSAIDs (eg, selective COX-2 inhibitors), K^+ supplements, or K^+-sparing diuretics. **HCTZ:** Dosage adjustment of antidiabetic drugs (oral agents and insulin) may be required. May increase risk of lithium toxicity; monitor serum lithium levels. Observe patients closely to determine if the desired effect of the diuretic is obtained when used concomitantly w/ NSAIDs and COX-2 selective agents. Administer ≥4 hrs before or 4-6 hrs after the administration of ion exchange resins (eg, cholestyramine, colestipol).

PATIENT CONSIDERATIONS

Assessment: Assess for diabetes, anuria, sulfonamide-derived drug hypersensitivity, history of penicillin allergy, volume/salt depletion, renal artery stenosis, HF, post-MI status, SLE, hepatic/renal impairment, pregnancy/nursing status, and possible drug interactions. Correct electrolyte abnormalities (eg, hypokalemia, hypomagnesemia) prior to initiating therapy.

Monitoring: Monitor for signs/symptoms of idiosyncratic reactions, hypersensitivity reactions, angioedema, airway obstruction, exacerbation/activation of SLE, hyperuricemia, precipitation of gout, and other adverse reactions. Monitor BP, renal function, serum electrolytes, cholesterol, and TG levels.

Counseling: Inform female patients of childbearing age of the consequences of exposure during pregnancy and of the treatment options for women planning to become pregnant. Advise to report pregnancies to physicians as soon as possible. Inform that lightheadedness may occur, especially during the 1st days of therapy; instruct to contact physician if lightheadedness occurs. Advise to d/c treatment until physician has been consulted if syncope occurs. Caution that inadequate fluid intake, excessive perspiration, diarrhea, or vomiting can lead to an excessive fall in BP. Advise to d/c therapy and immediately report any signs/symptoms of a severe allergic reaction or angioedema. Advise not to use K^+ supplements or salt substitutes containing K^+ w/o consulting physician. Instruct to establish a routine pattern for taking the medication w/ regard to meals.

STORAGE: 25°C (77°F); excursions permitted to 15-30°C (59-86°F). Protect from moisture.

TEMODAR – temozolomide

RX

Class: Alkylating agent

T

ADULT DOSAGE

Newly Diagnosed High Grade Glioblastoma Multiforme

Concomitant Phase:

$75mg/m^2$/day for 42 days concomitant w/ focal radiotherapy

Dose should be continued throughout the 42-day concomitant period up to 49 days if all of the following conditions are met:

- ANC ≥1.5 x 10^9/L
- Platelet count ≥100 x 10^9/L
- Common toxicity criteria (CTC) nonhematological toxicity ≤Grade 1 (except for alopecia, N/V)

PEDIATRIC DOSAGE

Pediatric use may not have been established

Maint Phase:
Four weeks after completing the concomitant phase, temozolomide is administered for an additional 6 cycles of maint treatment

Cycle 1: 150mg/m^2 qd for 5 days followed by 23 days w/o treatment
Cycles 2-6: May increase to 200mg/m^2 at start of Cycle 2 if nonhematologic toxicity for Cycle 1 is ≤Grade 2 (except alopecia, N/V), ANC ≥1.5 x 10^9/L, and platelet count ≥100 x 10^9/L. The dose remains at 200mg/m^2/day for the first 5 days of each subsequent cycle unless toxicity occurs; if the dose was not escalated at Cycle 2, do not escalate in subsequent cycles.

Refractory Anaplastic Astrocytoma

Patients Who Have Experienced Disease Progression on a Drug Regimen Containing Nitrosourea and Procarbazine:
Initial: 150mg/m^2 qd for 5 consecutive days per 28-day cycle
Titrate: May increase to 200mg/m^2/day for 5 consecutive days per 28-day treatment cycle if both the nadir and day of dosing (Day 29, Day 1 of next cycle) ANC are ≥1.5 x 10^9/L (1500/µL) and both the nadir and Day 29, Day 1 of next cycle platelet counts are ≥100 x 10^9/L (100,000/µL)

Therapy may be continued until disease progression

DOSING CONSIDERATIONS

Adverse Reactions

Glioblastoma Multiforme (GBM) During Concomitant Radiotherapy:
Interrupt Dose If:
1. ANC ≥0.5 and <1.5 x 10^9/L
2. Platelet count ≥10 and <100 x 10^9/L
3. Nonhematologic toxicity (except alopecia, N/V) CTC Grade 2

D/C Therapy If:
1. ANC <0.5 x 10^9/L
2. Platelet count <10 x 10^9/L
3. Nonhematologic toxicity (except alopecia, N/V) CTC Grade 3 or 4

GBM During Maint Treatment:
Dose Levels for Maint Treatment:
Dose Level -1 (Reduction for Prior Toxicity): 100mg/m^2/day
Dose Level 0 (Dose During Cycle 1): 150mg/m^2/day
Dose Level 1 (Dose During Cycles 2-6 in Absence of Toxicity): 200mg/m^2/day

Reduce by 1 Dose Level If:
1. ANC <1.0 x 10^9/L
2. Platelet count <50 x 10^9/L
3. Nonhematologic toxicity (except alopecia, N/V) CTC Grade 3

D/C Therapy If:
1. Dose reduction to <100mg/m^2 is required
2. The same Grade 3 nonhematological toxicity (except for alopecia, N/V) recurs after dose reduction
3. Nonhematologic toxicity (except alopecia, N/V) CTC Grade 4

Refractory Anaplastic Astrocytoma:
Refer to PI for dose modification

Other Important Considerations

Dose must be adjusted according to nadir neutrophil and platelet counts in the previous cycle and the neutrophil and platelet counts at the time of initiating the next cycle

ADMINISTRATION

Oral/IV route

Cap

Take on an empty stomach; bedtime administration may be advised.

T

Swallow whole w/ a glass of water; do not open or chew.
Antiemetic therapy may be administered prior to and/or following administration.

Inj

Infuse IV over 90 min.

When reconstituted w/ 41mL sterile water for inj, the resulting sol will contain 2.5mg/mL temozolomide.
Bring vial to room temperature prior to reconstitution.
Gently swirl the vials; do not shake.
Do not further dilute the reconstituted sol.
After reconstitution, store at room temperature (25°C [77°F]) and use w/in 14 hrs, including infusion time.

Withdraw up to 40mL from each vial to make up the total dose and transfer into an empty 250mL infusion bag.
Infuse IV using a pump over 90 min; flush the lines before and after each infusion.

May be administered in the same IV line w/ 0.9% NaCl inj only.
Do not infuse other medications simultaneously through the same IV line.

HOW SUPPLIED

Cap: 5mg, 20mg, 100mg, 140mg, 180mg, 250mg; **Inj:** 100mg

CONTRAINDICATIONS

History of hypersensitivity reaction (eg, urticaria, allergic reaction including anaphylaxis, toxic epidermal necrolysis, and Stevens-Johnson syndrome) to any components of the product. History of hypersensitivity to dacarbazine (DTIC).

WARNINGS/PRECAUTIONS

See Dosing Considerations. Myelosuppression, including prolonged pancytopenia, which may result in aplastic anemia, may occur. Prior to dosing, patients must have an ANC≥1.5 x 10^9/L and a platelet count ≥100 x 10^9/L. For the concomitant treatment phase w/ radiotherapy, obtain a CBC prior to initiation of treatment and weekly during treatment. For the 28-day treatment cycles, obtain a CBC prior to treatment on Day 1 and on Day 22 (21 days after the first dose) of each cycle or w/in 48 hrs of that day, and weekly until the ANC is >1.5 x 10^9/L and platelet count exceeds 100 x 10^9/L. Greater risk of myelosuppression in women and elderly patients. Cases of myelodysplastic syndrome and secondary malignancies, including myeloid leukemia, observed. *Pneumocystis carinii* pneumonia (PCP) prophylaxis is required in all patients w/ newly diagnosed GBM who are receiving concomitant radiotherapy for 42-day regimen, and should be continued in patients who develop lymphocytopenia until recovery from lymphocytopenia (CTC ≤Grade 1); higher occurrence of PCP when temozolomide is administered during a longer dosing regimen. Fatal and severe hepatotoxicity reported; perform LFTs at baseline, midway through 1st cycle, prior to each subsequent cycle, and approx 2-4 weeks after last dose. May cause fetal harm. Caution w/ severe renal/hepatic impairment and in elderly. **Inj:** Bioequivalence established only when inj is given over 90 min; infusion over a shorter or longer period may result in suboptimal dosing and may increase possibility of infusion related adverse reactions.

ADVERSE REACTIONS

Alopecia, N/V, anorexia, headache, constipation, fatigue, convulsions, thrombocytopenia.

DRUG INTERACTIONS

Valproic acid may decrease oral clearance.

PATIENT CONSIDERATIONS

Assessment: Assess for previous hypersensitivity to drug or DTIC, myelosuppression, hepatic/renal impairment, pregnancy/nursing status, and possible drug interactions. Obtain baseline LFTs, CBC, and ANC.

T

Monitoring: Monitor for myelosuppression, PCP, myelodysplastic syndrome, secondary malignancies, and other adverse reactions. For the concomitant treatment phase w/ radiotherapy, obtain a CBC weekly during treatment. For the 28-day treatment cycles, obtain a CBC on Day 22 (21 days after the first dose) of each cycle or w/in 48 hrs of that day. If ANC falls <1.5 x 10^9/L and the platelet count falls <100 x 10^9/L, obtain blood counts weekly until recovery. Perform LFTs midway through the 1st cycle, prior to each subsequent cycle, and approx 2-4 weeks after the last dose. **Inj:** Monitor for infusion-related reactions.

Counseling: Instruct to take exactly as prescribed. Instruct to take rigorous precautions to avoid inhalation or contact w/ skin or mucous membranes if caps or vials are accidentally opened or damaged. Inform about the most frequently occurring adverse effects (eg, N/V).

STORAGE: Cap: 25°C (77°F); excursions permitted to 15-30°C (59-86°F). **Inj:** 2-8°C (36-46°F). After reconstitution, store reconstituted product at 25°C (77°F); must be used w/in 14 hrs, including infusion time.

TENORETIC – atenolol/chlorthalidone

RX

Class: Monosulfamyl diuretic/selective beta$_1$ blocker

ADULT DOSAGE

Hypertension

Initial: 50mg/25mg tab qd

Titrate: May increase to 100mg/25mg tab qd, if optimal response not achieved

PEDIATRIC DOSAGE

Pediatric use may not have been established

DOSING CONSIDERATIONS

Renal Impairment

CrCl 15-35mL/min:

Max: 50mg atenolol/day

CrCl <15mL/min:

Max: 50mg atenolol qod

Elderly

Start at lower end of dosing range

ADMINISTRATION

Oral route

HOW SUPPLIED

Tab: (Atenolol/Chlorthalidone) 50mg/25mg*, 100mg/25mg *scored

CONTRAINDICATIONS

Sinus bradycardia, >1st-degree heart block, cardiogenic shock, overt cardiac failure, anuria, hypersensitivity to this product or to sulfonamide-derived drugs.

WARNINGS/PRECAUTIONS

Not for initial therapy. Avoid with untreated pheochromocytoma. May aggravate peripheral arterial circulatory disorders. Caution in elderly. Atenolol: May cause/precipitate HF; d/c if cardiac failure continues despite adequate treatment. Caution in patients with impaired renal function. Avoid abrupt discontinuation; exacerbation of angina and MI reported. Avoid with bronchospastic disease, but may use with caution if unresponsive/intolerant of other antihypertensive treatment. Chronically administered therapy should not be routinely withdrawn prior to major surgery; however, may augment risks of general anesthesia and surgical procedures. Caution in diabetic patients; may mask tachycardia occurring with hypoglycemia. May mask clinical signs of hyperthyroidism and precipitate thyroid storm with abrupt discontinuation. May cause fetal harm. Chlorthalidone: May precipitate azotemia with renal disease. If progressive renal impairment becomes evident, d/c therapy. Caution with impaired hepatic function or progressive liver disease; may precipitate hepatic coma. D/C prior to parathyroid function test. Decreased Ca^{2+} excretion observed. Altered parathyroid glands, with hypercalcemia and hypophosphatemia, seen with prolonged therapy. Hyperuricemia may occur, or acute gout may be precipitated. Fluid/electrolyte imbalance may develop. Sensitivity reactions may occur. Exacerbation/activation of systemic lupus erythematous (SLE) reported. May enhance effects in postsympathectomy patients.

ADVERSE REACTIONS

Bradycardia, dizziness, fatigue, nausea.

DRUG INTERACTIONS

May potentiate other antihypertensive agents. Observe for hypotension and/or marked bradycardia with catecholamine-depleting drugs (eg, reserpine). Additive effects with calcium channel blockers. Atenolol: Bradycardia, heart block, and rise of left ventricular end diastolic pressure may occur with verapamil or diltiazem. May cause severe bradycardia, asystole, and HF with disopyramide. Additive effects with amiodarone. Prostaglandin synthase inhibitors (eg, indomethacin) may decrease hypotensive effects. Exacerbates rebound HTN with clonidine withdrawal. May be unresponsive to usual doses of epinephrine. Digitalis glycosides may slow AV conduction and increase risk of bradycardia. Chlorthalidone: May alter insulin requirements in diabetic patients; latent diabetes mellitus (DM) may manifest. May develop hypokalemia with concomitant corticosteroids or adrenocorticotropic hormone. May decrease arterial response to norepinephrine. May increase responsiveness to tubocurarine. Avoid with lithium; risk of lithium toxicity.

PATIENT CONSIDERATIONS

Assessment: Assess for bradycardia, cardiogenic shock, >1st-degree heart block, overt cardiac failure, impaired renal/hepatic function, bronchospastic disease, peripheral vascular disease, DM, hyperthyroidism, pheochromocytoma, anuria, hypersensitivity to sulfonamide-derived drugs, serum electrolytes, parathyroid disease, pregnancy/nursing status, SLE, CAD, and possible drug interactions.

Monitoring: Monitor for cardiac failure, hepatic/renal function, withdrawal symptoms, hypersensitivity reactions, hyperuricemia or acute gout, and signs/symptoms of electrolyte imbalance. Monitor serum glucose, serum electrolytes, and BP.

Counseling: Instruct not to interrupt or d/c therapy without consulting physician. Instruct to notify physician if signs/symptoms of impending congestive HF or unexplained respiratory symptoms develop. Counsel about signs/symptoms of electrolyte imbalance, and advise to seek prompt medical attention. Inform that drug may cause potential harm to fetus; instruct to inform physician if pregnant/planning to become pregnant.

STORAGE: 20-25°C (68-77°F).

TENORMIN — atenolol

RX

Class: Selective $beta_1$ blocker

Avoid abrupt discontinuation of therapy in patients w/ coronary artery disease (CAD). Severe exacerbation of angina and occurrence of MI and ventricular arrhythmias reported in angina patients following abrupt discontinuation w/ β-blockers. If planning to d/c therapy, carefully observe and advise to limit physical activity. Promptly reinstitute therapy, at least temporarily, if angina worsens or acute coronary insufficiency develops. CAD may be unrecognized; may be prudent to avoid abrupt discontinuation in patients only treated for HTN.

ADULT DOSAGE

Hypertension

Initial: 50mg qd, either alone or w/ diuretic therapy
Titrate: May increase to 100mg qd after 1-2 weeks
Max: 100mg qd

Angina Pectoris

Long-term Management:
Initial: 50mg qd
Titrate: May increase to 100mg qd after 1 week
Max: 200mg qd

Acute Myocardial Infarction

Management of hemodynamically stable patients w/ definite/suspected acute MI to reduce cardiovascular mortality

Usual: Following IV dose, 50mg 10 min after IV dose followed by 50mg 12 hrs later, then 100mg qd or 50mg bid for 6-9 days or until discharge from the hospital

Atenolol is an additional treatment to standard coronary unit therapy

PEDIATRIC DOSAGE

Pediatric use may not have been established

DOSING CONSIDERATIONS

Renal Impairment
Max Dose for CrCl 15-35mL/min: 50mg/day
Max Dose for CrCl <15mL/min: 25mg/day

Hemodialysis:
25mg or 50mg after each dialysis

HTN:
Initial: May require a lower dose of 25mg qd

Elderly
HTN:
Initial: May require a lower dose of 25mg qd

ADMINISTRATION

Oral route

HOW SUPPLIED

Tab: 25mg, 50mg*, 100mg *scored

CONTRAINDICATIONS

Sinus bradycardia, >1st-degree heart block, cardiogenic shock, overt cardiac failure, history of hypersensitivity to atenolol or any of the drug product's components.

T

WARNINGS/PRECAUTIONS
May cause/precipitate heart failure (HF); d/c if cardiac failure continues despite adequate treatment. Avoid w/ bronchospastic disease; may use w/ caution if unresponsive to/intolerant of other antihypertensive treatment. Chronically administered therapy should not be routinely withdrawn prior to major surgery; however, may augment risks of general anesthesia and surgical procedures. Caution in diabetic patients; may mask tachycardia occurring w/ hypoglycemia. May mask clinical signs of hyperthyroidism and may precipitate thyroid storm w/ abrupt discontinuation. Avoid w/ untreated pheochromocytoma. May cause fetal harm. May aggravate peripheral arterial circulatory disorders.

ADVERSE REACTIONS
Tiredness, dizziness, cold extremities, depression, fatigue, dyspnea, postural hypotension, bradycardia, leg pain, lightheadedness, lethargy, diarrhea, nausea, wheeziness.

DRUG INTERACTIONS
Additive effects w/ catecholamine-depleting drugs (eg, reserpine), calcium channel blockers, and amiodarone. May cause severe bradycardia, asystole, and HF w/ disopyramide. Bradycardia and heart block can occur and left ventricular end diastolic pressure can rise w/ verapamil or diltiazem. Exacerbates rebound HTN w/ clonidine withdrawal; withdraw β-blocker therapy several days before gradual withdrawal of clonidine or delay introduction of β-blockers for several days after stopping clonidine. Prostaglandin synthase inhibitors (eg, indomethacin) may decrease hypotensive effects. May be unresponsive to usual doses of epinephrine. Concomitant use w/ digitalis glycosides may increase risk of bradycardia.

PATIENT CONSIDERATIONS

Assessment: Assess for history of hypersensitivity, bradycardia, cardiogenic shock, >1st-degree heart block, overt cardiac failure, acute MI, renal dysfunction, bronchospastic disease, conduction abnormalities, left ventricular dysfunction, peripheral arterial circulatory disorders, diabetes mellitus, hyperthyroidism, pheochromocytoma, pregnancy/nursing status, and for possible drug interactions.

Monitoring: Monitor for signs/symptoms of cardiac failure, for masking of hyperthyroidism/hypoglycemia, and for other adverse reactions. Monitor renal function, pulse, and BP. Following abrupt discontinuation, monitor for thyroid storm and in patients w/ angina, monitor for severe exacerbation of angina, MI, and ventricular arrhythmias.

Counseling: Instruct to take as prescribed. Advise not to interrupt or d/c therapy w/o first consulting physician. Inform that drug may cause fetal harm; instruct to notify physician if pregnant or if considering becoming pregnant.

STORAGE: 20-25°C (68-77°F).

TERAZOSIN – terazosin hydrochloride

RX

Class: Alpha$_1$ blocker (quinazoline)

OTHER BRAND NAMES
Hytrin (Discontinued)

ADULT DOSAGE

Hypertension

Initial: 1mg hs
Usual: 1-5mg qd
If response is substantially diminished at 24 hrs, may slowly increase dose or use bid regimen
Max: 40mg/day

If discontinued for several days or longer, restart using the initial dosing regimen

Benign Prostatic Hyperplasia

Initial: 1mg hs
Titrate: Increase stepwise to 2mg, 5mg, or 10mg qd
Max: 20mg/day

If discontinued for several days or longer, restart using the initial dosing regimen

PEDIATRIC DOSAGE
Pediatric use may not have been established

ADMINISTRATION
Oral route

HOW SUPPLIED
Cap: 1mg, 2mg, 5mg, 10mg

CONTRAINDICATIONS
Hypersensitivity to terazosin HCl.

WARNINGS/PRECAUTIONS
May cause marked lowering of BP, especially postural hypotension, and syncope with the 1st dose or 1st few days of therapy; similar effect may be anticipated if therapy is interrupted for several days and then restarted. May impair physical/mental abilities. Examine patients with BPH to rule out prostate cancer prior to initiation of therapy. Priapism reported. Intraoperative floppy iris syndrome observed during cataract surgery. Decreases in Hct, Hgb, WBCs, total protein, and albumin reported.

ADVERSE REACTIONS
Asthenia, postural hypotension, headache, dizziness, dyspnea, nasal congestion, somnolence, palpitations, nausea, peripheral edema, pain in extremities.

DRUG INTERACTIONS
Caution with other antihypertensive agents, especially verapamil; may need dose reduction or retitration of either agent. Increased levels with captopril. Hypotension reported with PDE-5 inhibitors.

PATIENT CONSIDERATIONS

Assessment: Assess BP, pregnancy/nursing status, and possible drug interactions. Rule out prostate cancer with BPH.

Monitoring: Monitor for signs/symptoms of hypotension, priapism, and other adverse reactions. Monitor Hct, Hgb, WBCs, total protein/albumin, and BP periodically.

Counseling: Inform of possibility of syncope and orthostatic symptoms, especially at initiation of therapy. Caution against driving or hazardous tasks for 12 hrs after 1st dose, dosage increase, or when resuming therapy after interruption. Avoid situations where injury could result, should syncope occur. Advise to sit or lie down when symptoms of low BP occur. Inform of possibility of priapism; advise to seek medical attention if this occurs and inform that priapism can lead to permanent erectile dysfunction if not brought to immediate medical attention.

STORAGE: 20-25°C (68-77°F).

TEVETEN – eprosartan mesylate — RX

Class: Angiotensin II receptor blocker (ARB)

D/C when pregnancy is detected. Drugs that act directly on the renin-angiotensin system (RAS) can cause injury/death to the developing fetus.

ADULT DOSAGE

Hypertension

Initial: 600mg qd
Usual: 400-800mg/day, given qd or bid
Max: 800mg/day
Twice-a-day regimen at the same total daily dose or an increase in dose may give a more satisfactory response

PEDIATRIC DOSAGE
Pediatric use may not have been established

T

DOSING CONSIDERATIONS

Renal Impairment
Moderate and Severe:
Max: 600mg/day

ADMINISTRATION
Oral route

Take w/ or w/o food

HOW SUPPLIED
Tab: 400mg, 600mg

CONTRAINDICATIONS
Hypersensitivity to this product or any of its components. Coadministration w/ aliskiren in patients w/ diabetes.

WARNINGS/PRECAUTIONS
Symptomatic hypotension may occur in patients with an activated RAS (eg, volume- and/or salt-depleted patients [eg, those being treated with diuretics]); correct volume or salt depletion prior to therapy or monitor closely. Changes in renal function reported. Oliguria and/or progressive azotemia and (rarely) acute renal failure and/or death may occur in patients whose renal function may depend on the renin-angiotensin-aldosterone system activity (eg, severe CHF). Increases in SrCr or BUN reported in patients with renal artery stenosis.

ADVERSE REACTIONS
Upper respiratory tract infection, rhinitis, pharyngitis, cough.

DRUG INTERACTIONS
See Contraindications. Dual blockade of the RAS is associated with increased risks of hypotension, hyperkalemia, and changes in renal function (including acute renal failure); avoid combined use of RAS inhibitors, or closely monitor BP, renal function, and electrolytes with concomitant agents that also affect the RAS. Avoid with aliskiren in patients with renal impairment (GFR <60mL/min). NSAIDs, including selective COX-2 inhibitors, may attenuate antihypertensive effect and may deteriorate renal function. Increases in serum lithium concentrations and lithium toxicity may occur; monitor lithium levels.

PATIENT CONSIDERATIONS

Assessment: Assess for hypersensitivity to the drug, volume/salt depletion, renal impairment, CHF, renal artery stenosis, diabetes, pregnancy/nursing status, and possible drug interactions.

Monitoring: Monitor for signs/symptoms of hypotension, renal dysfunction, and other adverse reactions.

Counseling: Inform about the consequences of exposure during pregnancy in females of childbearing age. Discuss treatment options with women planning to become pregnant. Instruct to report pregnancies to physician as soon as possible.

STORAGE: 20-25°C (68-77°F).

THEO-24 – theophylline anhydrous

RX

Class: Xanthine bronchodilator

ADULT DOSAGE

Chronic Lung Disease

Symptoms and Reversible Airflow Obstruction Associated w/ Chronic Asthma and Other Chronic Lung Diseases:
Individualize dose based on peak serum levels
16-60 Years:
Initial: 300-400mg/day divided q24h
Titrate: After 3 days, increase to 400-600mg/day if tolerated; consider giving a lower dose and titrating more slowly if caffeine-like adverse effects occur
After 3 more days, if needed and tolerated, may increase to >600mg/day

PEDIATRIC DOSAGE

Chronic Lung Disease

Symptoms and Reversible Airflow Obstruction Associated w/ Chronic Asthma and Other Chronic Lung Diseases:
Individualize dose based on peak serum levels and ideal body weight
12-15 Years:
<45kg:
Initial: 12-14mg/kg/day up to a max of 300mg/day divided q24h
Titrate: After 3 days, increase to 16mg/kg/day up to a max of 400mg/day divided q24h
After 3 more days, if tolerated and needed, may increase to 20mg/kg/day up to a max of 600mg/day
>45kg:
Initial: 300-400mg/day divided q24h
Titrate: After 3 days, increase to 400-600mg/day if tolerated; consider giving a lower dose and titrating more slowly if caffeine-like adverse effects occur
After 3 more days, if needed and tolerated, may increase to >600mg/day

DOSING CONSIDERATIONS

Elderly
> 60 Years:
Max: 400mg/day

Other Important Considerations
Rapid Metabolizers:
Give smaller dose more frequently to prevent breakthrough symptoms

Risk Factors for Impaired Clearance/If Not Feasible to Monitor Serum Theophylline Concentrations:
12-15 Years:
Max: 16mg/kg/day up to a max of 400 mg/day
≥16 Years:
Max: 400mg/day

Dose Adjustments Based on Peak Serum Concentration:
<9.9mcg/mL: If symptoms are not controlled and current dosage is tolerated, increase dose about 25%; recheck serum concentration after 3 days for further dosage adjustment
10-14.9mcg/mL: If symptoms are controlled and current dosage is tolerated, maintain dose and recheck serum concentration at 6- to 12-month intervals
If symptoms are not controlled and current dosage is tolerated, consider adding additional medication(s) to treatment regimen
15-19.9mcg/mL: Consider 10% decrease in dose to provide greater margin of safety even if current dosage is tolerated
20-24.9mcg/mL: Decrease dose by 25% even if no adverse effects are present; recheck serum concentration after 3 days to guide further dosage adjustment
25-30mcg/mL: Skip next dose and decrease subsequent doses at least 25% even if no adverse effects present; recheck serum concentration after 3 days to guide further dosage adjustment
If symptomatic, consider whether overdose treatment is indicated (see PI)
>30mcg/mL: Treat overdose as indicated (see PI); if therapy is subsequently resumed, decrease dose by at least 50% and recheck serum concentration after 3 days to guide further dosage adjustment

ADMINISTRATION

Oral route

Take dose at approx the same time each am
For twice daily dosing, 2nd dose should be taken 10-12 hours after the morning dose and before the pm meal

HOW SUPPLIED

Cap, Extended-Release: 100mg, 200mg, 300mg, 400mg

CONTRAINDICATIONS

History of hypersensitivity to theophylline or other components in the product.

WARNINGS/PRECAUTIONS

Extreme caution w/ active peptic ulcer disease (PUD), seizure disorders, and cardiac arrhythmias (not including bradyarrhythmias); increased risk of exacerbation of the concurrent condition. Caution w/ risk factors for reduced clearance (eg, neonates [term/premature], children <1 yr of age, elderly [>60 yrs of age], acute pulmonary edema, CHF, cor pulmonale, fever [≥102°F for 24 hrs or more, lesser temperature elevations for longer periods], hypothyroidism, liver disease [eg, cirrhosis, acute hepatitis], reduced renal function in infants <3 months of age, sepsis w/ multiorgan failure, shock, cessation of smoking); severe and potentially fatal toxicity can occur if total daily dose is not appropriately reduced. Carefully consider benefits and risks of therapy and the need for more intensive monitoring of serum drug levels. Whenever N/V (particularly repetitive N/V) or other signs/symptoms of toxicity develop (even if another cause may be suspected), withhold additional doses and measure serum levels immediately. Avoid dose increases in response to acute exacerbation of symptoms of chronic lung disease. Measure peak steady-state serum theophylline concentration before increasing the dose and limit dose increases to about 25% of the previous total daily dose to reduce risk of unintended excessive increases in serum levels. Lab test interactions may occur. Caution in elderly and with selection of maintenance dose in pediatric patients.

ADVERSE REACTIONS

N/V, headache, insomnia, diarrhea, irritability, restlessness, fine skeletal muscle tremors, transient diuresis.

DRUG INTERACTIONS

Adding a drug that inhibits metabolism (eg, cimetidine, erythromycin, tacrine) or stopping a concurrently administered drug that enhances metabolism (eg, carbamazepine, rifampin) may reduce clearance. Blocks adenosine receptors; higher dose of adenosine may be required to achieve desired effect. Benzodiazepines increase CNS concentrations of adenosine; larger doses of benzodiazepines may be required to produce desired level of sedation. Alcohol, allopurinol, cimetidine, ciprofloxacin, clarithromycin, disulfiram, enoxacin, erythromycin, estrogen, fluvoxamine, human recombinant interferon α-A, methotrexate, mexiletine, pentoxifylline, propafenone, propranolol, tacrine, thiabendazole, ticlopidine, troleandomycin, and verapamil may decrease clearance and increase effect. Aminoglutethimide, carbamazepine, IV isoproterenol, moricizine, phenobarbital (after 2 weeks of concurrent phenobarbital use), phenytoin, rifampin, and sulfinpyrazone may increase clearance and decrease effect. May decrease phenytoin concentration. Increased risk of ventricular arrhythmias w/ halothane. Ketamine may lower theophylline seizure threshold. May increase renal lithium clearance. May antagonize nondepolarizing neuromuscular blocking effects of pancuronium; larger doses of pancuronium may be required. Synergistic CNS effects w/ ephedrine; increased frequency of nausea, nervousness and insomnia. St. John's wort may decrease plasma levels; higher doses of theophylline may be required. Discontinuing St. John's wort may result in theophylline toxicity.

PATIENT CONSIDERATIONS

Assessment: Assess for hypersensitivity to drug, active PUD, seizure disorders, cardiac arrhythmias, conditions that alter theophylline clearance, any condition where treatment is contraindicated or cautioned, pregnancy/nursing status, and possible drug interactions. Obtain baseline serum levels when initiating therapy to guide final dosage adjustment after titration.

Monitoring: Measure serum levels before a dose increase in patients who continue to be symptomatic, whenever signs/symptoms of toxicity are present, and whenever there is a new illness, worsening of a chronic illness, or a change in treatment regimen that may alter clearance. Monitor serum levels at 6-month intervals for rapidly growing children and at yearly intervals for all others; acutely ill patients should be monitored at frequent intervals (eg, q24h). Monitor for signs/ symptoms of toxicity, exacerbation of active PUD, seizure disorders or cardiac arrhythmias, and other adverse reactions.

Counseling: Instruct to seek medical attention if N/V, persistent headache, insomnia, or rapid heartbeat occurs. Instruct to contact physician if new illness (especially if accompanied by a persistent fever) develops, if a chronic illness worsens, if patient starts/stops smoking cigarettes or marijuana, or if another physician adds a new medication or discontinues a previously prescribed medication. Inform that theophylline interacts w/ a wide variety of drugs. Instruct to inform all physicians of theophylline use, especially if a medication is being added or removed from treatment. Instruct not to alter dose, timing of dose, or frequency of administration w/o 1st consulting physician; if a dose is missed, instruct to take next dose at the usually scheduled time and to not attempt to make up for the missed dose. Instruct to take medication each am at approximately the same time and not to exceed the prescribed dose. Instruct to d/c any dosage that causes adverse effects, to withhold subsequent doses until symptoms have resolved, and to then resume therapy at a lower, previously tolerated dose.

STORAGE: Below 25°C (77°F).

TIAZAC – diltiazem hydrochloride

RX

Class: Calcium channel blocker (CCB) (nondihydropyridine)

OTHER BRAND NAMES

Taztia XT

ADULT DOSAGE

Hypertension

Initial (Monotherapy): 120-240mg qd
Titrate: Max effect usually observed by 14 days of therapy; schedule dose adjustments accordingly
Usual Range: 120-540mg qd
Max: 540mg qd

Angina

Chronic Stable:
Initial: 120-180mg qd
Titration should be carried out over 7-14 days, when necessary
Max: 540mg qd

Conversions

Hypertensive/Anginal Patients Treated w/ Other Diltiazem Formulations:
May be switched to therapy at the nearest equivalent total daily dose

PEDIATRIC DOSAGE

Pediatric use may not have been established

DOSING CONSIDERATIONS

Elderly
Start at lower end of dosing range

ADMINISTRATION

Oral route

May sprinkle cap contents on a spoonful of applesauce
Swallow applesauce immediately w/o chewing and follow w/ a glass of cool water; do not store for future use
Subdividing contents of cap is not recommended

HOW SUPPLIED

Cap, Extended-Release: 120mg, 180mg, 240mg, 300mg, 360mg, 420mg; (Taztia XT) 120mg, 180mg, 240mg, 300mg, 360mg

CONTRAINDICATIONS

Sick sinus syndrome and 2nd- or 3rd-degree atrioventricular (AV) block (except w/ a functioning ventricular pacemaker), severe hypotension (<90mmHg systolic), hypersensitivity to the drug, acute myocardial infarction (AMI) and pulmonary congestion documented by x-ray on admission.

WARNINGS/PRECAUTIONS

Prolongs AV node refractory periods without significantly prolonging sinus node recovery time, except in patients with sick sinus syndrome. Periods of asystole reported in a patient with Prinzmetal's angina. Worsening of CHF reported in patients with preexisting ventricular dysfunction. Symptomatic hypotension may occur. Mild elevations of transaminases with and without concomitant alkaline phosphatase and bilirubin elevation reported. Significant elevations in enzymes (eg, alkaline phosphatase, LDH, AST, ALT) and other phenomena consistent with acute hepatic injury reported in rare instances. Monitor LFTs and renal function at regular intervals; caution with renal/hepatic dysfunction. Transient dermatological reactions and skin eruptions progressing to erythema multiforme and/or exfoliative dermatitis have been reported; d/c if a dermatologic reaction persists. Caution in elderly.

ADVERSE REACTIONS

Peripheral edema, dizziness, headache, infection, pain, pharyngitis, dyspepsia, dyspnea, bronchitis, AV block, asthenia, vasodilation.

DRUG INTERACTIONS

Potential additive effects with other agents known to affect cardiac contractility and/or conduction; caution and careful titration are warranted. Additive effects in prolonging cardiac conduction with β-blockers or digitalis. CYP3A4 substrates, inhibitors, or inducers may have a significant impact on the efficacy and side effect profile of diltiazem; patients taking CYP3A4 substrates, especially patients with renal and/or hepatic impairment, may require dosage adjustment when starting or stopping concomitantly administered diltiazem. May potentiate depression of cardiac contractility, conductivity and automaticity, and vascular dilation associated with anesthetics; carefully titrate anesthetics and calcium channel blockers (CCBs) when used concomitantly. May increase levels of midazolam, triazolam, carbamazepine, quinidine, and lovastatin. May increase levels of propranolol; adjustment of the propranolol dose may be warranted. May increase levels of buspirone; dose adjustments may be necessary. Increased levels with cimetidine; adjustment of diltiazem dose may be warranted. Sinus bradycardia resulting in hospitalization and pacemaker insertion reported with clonidine; monitor HR. Monitor cyclosporine/digoxin concentrations, especially when diltiazem therapy is initiated, adjusted, or discontinued. Rifampin may decrease concentrations; avoid rifampin or any CYP3A4 inducer when possible, and consider alternative therapy. May increase simvastatin exposure; limit daily doses of simvastatin to 10mg and diltiazem to 240mg if coadministration is required. Risk of myopathy and rhabdomyolysis with statins metabolized by CYP3A4 may be increased. When possible, use a non-CYP3A4-metabolized statin; otherwise, consider dose adjustments for both agents and closely monitor for signs and symptoms of any statin-related adverse events. Additive antihypertensive effect when used with other antihypertensive agents; dosage of diltiazem or the concomitant antihypertensive may need to be adjusted.

PATIENT CONSIDERATIONS

Assessment: Assess for sick sinus syndrome, 2nd- or 3rd-degree AV block, hypotension, AMI, pulmonary congestion, ventricular/renal/hepatic dysfunction, drug hypersensitivity, pregnancy/nursing status, and possible drug interactions.

Monitoring: Monitor for bradycardia, AV block, worsening of CHF, symptomatic hypotension, dermatological reactions, and other adverse reactions. Monitor LFTs and renal function at regular intervals. Monitor HR with clonidine.

Counseling: Inform of risks and benefits of therapy. Instruct to take ud. Counsel to report any adverse reactions to physician. Inform that when administering with applesauce, it should not be hot and it should be soft enough to be swallowed without chewing.

STORAGE: 25°C (77°F); excursions permitted to 15-30°C (59-86°F). Avoid excessive humidity. (Taztia XT) 20-25°C (68-77°F). Avoid excessive humidity.

TIKOSYN – dofetilide

RX

Class: Class III antiarrhythmic

To minimize risk of induced arrhythmia, for a minimum of 3 days, place patients initiated or reinitiated on therapy in a facility that can provide calculations of CrCl, continuous ECG monitoring, and cardiac resuscitation. Available only to hospitals and prescribers who have received appropriate dofetilide dosing and treatment initiation education.

ADULT DOSAGE

Atrial Fibrillation

Conversion of A-Fib/A-Flutter to Normal Sinus Rhythm and Maint of Normal Sinus Rhythm in Patients w/ Highly Symptomatic A-Fib/A-flutter of >1 Week Duration Who Were Converted to Normal Sinus Rhythm:

Reserve for patients in whom A-fib/A-flutter is highly symptomatic

Hypokalemia should be corrected before initiation; maintain serum K^+ levels >3.6-4.0mEq/L

Initial:

Individualize dose based on CrCl and QTc (use QT interval if HR <60bpm); QTc must be ≤440 msec to proceed

CrCl >60mL/min: 500mcg bid

CrCl 40-60mL/min: 250mcg bid

CrCl 20-<40mL/min: 125mcg bid

CrCl <20mL/min: Contraindicated

Post Dose Adjustment:

After 2-3 hrs if the QTc has increased ≤15%, continue current dose; if QTc has increased>15% compared to the baseline or if the QTc is >500 msec (550 msec w/ ventricular conduction abnormalities), adjust subsequent doses as such:

Initial Dose of 500mcg bid: Reduce dose to 250mcg bid

Initial Dose of 250mcg bid: reduce dose to 125mcg bid

Initial Dose of 125mcg bid: reduce dose to 125mcg qd

Maint:

If at any time after the 2nd dose the QTc increases >500 msec (550 msec in patients w/ ventricular conduction abnormalities), d/c dofetilide

If renal function deteriorates, adjust dose based on CrCl as seen above

Max:

CrCl >60mL/min: 500mcg bid

Cardioversion:

If patients do not convert to normal sinus rhythm w/in 24 hrs of initiation, electrical conversion should be considered. Patients continuing on dofetilide after successful electrical cardioversion should continue to be monitored by ECG for 12 hrs post cardioversion, or a minimum of 3 days after initiation of dofetilide therapy, whichever is greater

Conversions

Switching from Class I or Other Class III Antiarrhythmics:

Withdraw previous antiarrhythmic therapy under careful monitoring for a minimum of

PEDIATRIC DOSAGE

Pediatric use may not have been established

T

3 plasma half-lives before initiating therapy; do not initiate dofetilide following amiodarone therapy until amiodarone plasma levels are <0.3mcg/mL or until withdrawn for at least 3 months

DOSING CONSIDERATIONS

Discontinuation

If dofetilide needs to be discontinued to allow dosing of other potentially interacting drugs, a washout period of ≥2 days should be followed before starting the other drug.

ADMINISTRATION

Oral route

Take PO w/ or w/o food

Initiate/titrate in presence of continuous ECG monitoring and personnel trained in management of serious ventricular arrhythmias

HOW SUPPLIED

Cap: 125mcg, 250mcg, 500mcg

CONTRAINDICATIONS

Congenital or acquired long QT syndromes, baseline QT interval or QTc >440 msec (500 msec w/ ventricular conduction abnormalities), severe renal impairment (CrCl <20mL/min), known hypersensitivity to the drug. Concomitant verapamil, HCTZ (alone/in combinations [eg, triamterene]), and inhibitors of renal cation transport system (eg, cimetidine, trimethoprim [alone/combination w/ sulfamethoxazole], ketoconazole, prochlorperazine, dolutegravir, megestrol).

WARNINGS/PRECAUTIONS

May cause serious ventricular arrhythmias, primarily torsades de pointes (TdP); risk of TdP can be reduced by controlling the plasma concentration through adjustment of the initial dofetilide dose according to CrCl and by monitoring the ECG. Calculate CrCl before 1st dose. Caution in patients with severe hepatic impairment. Do not discharge patients within 12 hrs of conversion to normal sinus rhythm. Maintain normal K^+ levels prior to and during administration. Patients with A-fib should be anticoagulated prior to cardioversion and may continue to use after cardioversion. Rehospitalize patient for 3 days anytime dose is increased. Consider electrical cardioversion if patient does not convert to normal sinus rhythm within 24 hrs of initiation of therapy. If dofetilide needs to be discontinued to allow dosing of other potentially interacting drug(s), a washout period of at least 2 days should be followed before starting the other drug(s). Caution in elderly.

ADVERSE REACTIONS

Headache, chest pain, dizziness, ventricular arrhythmia, ventricular tachycardia, TdP, respiratory tract infection, dyspnea, nausea, flu syndrome, insomnia, back pain, diarrhea, rash, abdominal pain.

DRUG INTERACTIONS

See Contraindications. Hypokalemia or hypomagnesemia may occur with K^+-depleting diuretics, increasing the potential for TdP. CYP3A4 inhibitors (eg, macrolides, protease inhibitors, serotonin reuptake inhibitors) and drugs actively secreted by cationic secretion (eg, triamterene, metformin, amiloride) may increase levels; caution when coadministered. Not recommended with drugs that prolong the QT interval (eg, phenothiazines, TCAs, certain oral macrolides). Withhold Class I and III antiarrhythmics for at least 3 half-lives prior to dosing with dofetilide. Do not initiate therapy until amiodarone levels are <0.3mcg/mL or until amiodarone has been withdrawn for at least 3 months. Higher occurrence of TdP with digoxin.

PATIENT CONSIDERATIONS

Assessment: Assess for previous hypersensitivity to drug, congenital or acquired long QT syndrome, renal/hepatic impairment, pregnancy/nursing status, and possible drug interactions. Correct K^+ levels prior to therapy. Obtain baseline ECG and CrCl prior to therapy.

Monitoring: Monitor serum K^+ levels and for development of ventricular arrhythmias (eg, TdP). After initiation or cardioversion, continuously monitor by ECG for a minimum of 3 days, or for a minimum of 12 hrs after electrical/pharmacological conversion to normal sinus rhythm, whichever is greater. Reevaluate renal function and QTc every 3 months, as medically warranted.

Counseling: Inform about risks/benefits, need for compliance with prescribed dosing, potential drug interactions, and the need for periodic monitoring of QTc and renal function. Instruct to notify physician of any changes in medications and supplements or if hospitalized or prescribed a new medication for any condition. Counsel to report immediately any symptoms associated with electrolyte imbalance (eg, excessive/prolonged diarrhea, sweating, vomiting, loss of appetite, thirst). Instruct not to double the next dose if a dose is missed and take the next dose at the usual time.

STORAGE: 15-30°C (59-86°F). Protect from humidity and moisture.

Timoptic – timolol maleate

RX

Class: Nonselective beta blocker

OTHER BRAND NAMES

Timoptic in Ocudose, Timoptic-XE

ADULT DOSAGE

Elevated Intraocular Pressure

Ocular HTN/Open-Angle Glaucoma:

Timoptic/Timoptic in Ocudose:

1 drop of 0.25% sol in the affected eye(s) bid; may change to 1 drop of 0.5% sol bid if inadequate response. May decrease to 1 drop qd if IOP maintained at satisfactory levels

May use Timoptic in Ocudose when patient is sensitive to preservative in Timoptic

Timoptic-XE:

1 drop of either 0.25% or 0.5% sol in the affected eye(s) qd

PEDIATRIC DOSAGE

Pediatric use may not have been established

DOSING CONSIDERATIONS

Concomitant Medications

Administer other topically applied ophthalmic medications at least 10 min before Timoptic-XE

ADMINISTRATION

Ocular route

Timoptic-XE

Instruct to invert closed container and shake once before each use

HOW SUPPLIED

Sol: (Timoptic) 0.25% [5mL], 0.5% [5mL, 10mL]; **Sol:** (Timoptic in Ocudose) 0.25%, 0.5% [0.2mL, 60^s^]; **Sol, Gel-Forming:** (Timoptic-XE) 0.25%, 0.5% [5mL]

CONTRAINDICATIONS

Bronchial asthma, history of bronchial asthma, severe COPD, sinus bradycardia, 2nd- or 3rd-degree AV block, overt cardiac failure, cardiogenic shock, hypersensitivity to any component of the product.

WARNINGS/PRECAUTIONS

Severe respiratory and cardiac reactions, including death, due to bronchospasm in patients with asthma and, rarely, death associated with cardiac failure, reported. Caution with cardiac failure; d/c at 1st sign/symptom of cardiac failure. May mask the signs and symptoms of acute hypoglycemia; caution in patients subject to spontaneous hypoglycemia or diabetes mellitus (DM). May mask certain clinical signs (eg, tachycardia) of hyperthyroidism; carefully manage patients suspected of developing thyrotoxicosis. Avoid with COPD (eg, chronic bronchitis, emphysema), and history/known bronchospastic disease. Not for use alone in angle-closure glaucoma. May potentiate muscle weakness consistent with myasthenic symptoms (eg, diplopia, ptosis, generalized weakness); caution with myasthenia gravis or patients with myasthenic symptoms. Caution with cerebrovascular insufficiency; consider alternative therapy if signs/symptoms of reduced cerebral blood flow develop. Choroidal detachment after filtration procedures reported. May be more reactive to repeated challenge with history of atopy or severe anaphylactic reactions to variety of allergens; may be unresponsive to usual doses of epinephrine. (Sol/XE) Bacterial keratitis with the use of multiple-dose containers reported.

ADVERSE REACTIONS

Timoptic: Burning/stinging upon instillation.
Timoptic in Ocudose: Burning/stinging upon instillation.
Timoptic-XE: (Ocular) Burning/stinging upon instillation, transient blurred vision, pain, conjunctivitis, discharge, foreign body sensation, itching, tearing. (Systemic) Headache, dizziness, URIs.

DRUG INTERACTIONS

May potentially produce additive effects if used concomitantly with systemic β-blockers. Concomitant use of two topical β-adrenergic blocking agents is not recommended. Caution with oral/IV calcium antagonists because of possible AV conduction disturbances, left ventricular failure, or hypotension. Avoid oral/IV calcium antagonists with impaired cardiac function. Possible additive effects, production of hypotension, and/or marked bradycardia may occur when used concomitantly with catecholamine-depleting drugs (eg, reserpine). Concomitant use with calcium antagonists and digitalis may cause additive effects in prolonging AV conduction time. Potentiated systemic β-blockade reported with concomitant use of CYP2D6 inhibitors (eg, quinidine, SSRIs).

Mydriasis reported occasionally with epinephrine. May augment risks of general anesthesia in surgical procedures; protracted severe hypotension and difficulty in restarting and maintaining heartbeat reported; gradual withdrawal recommended. Caution with insulin or oral hypoglycemic agents.

PATIENT CONSIDERATIONS

Assessment: Assess for presence or history of bronchial asthma, COPD (eg, bronchitis, emphysema), or any other conditions where treatment is contraindicated or cautioned. Assess for pregnancy/nursing status and possible drug interactions. Assess if planning to undergo major surgery. (Sol/XE) Assess for corneal disease or disruption of the ocular epithelial surface.

Monitoring: Monitor for signs/symptoms of cardiac failure, masking of signs/symptoms of hypoglycemia, masking of hyperthyroidism, thyrotoxicosis, reduced cerebral blood flow, choroidal detachment, anaphylaxis, keratitis, and other adverse reactions. Evaluate IOP after 4 weeks of treatment.

Counseling: Advise not to use product if patient has a presence or history of bronchial asthma, severe COPD, sinus bradycardia, 2nd- or 3rd-degree AV block, or cardiac failure. (Sol/XE) Instruct to avoid touching tip of container to eye or surrounding structures. Counsel to seek physician's advice on continued use of product if patient had prior ocular surgery or develops intercurrent ocular condition (eg, trauma or infection). Instruct to handle ocular sol properly to avoid contamination; inform that using contaminated sol may result in serious eye damage. (Sol) Inform that drug contains benzalkonium chloride, which may be absorbed by soft contact lenses. Instruct to remove contact lenses prior to administration and reinsert 15 min following administration. (Ocudose) Instruct about proper administration. Advise to use immediately after opening, and discard the individual unit and any remaining contents immediately after use. (XE) Instruct to invert the closed container and shake once before each use. Instruct to administer at least 10 min apart with other topical ophthalmic medications. Inform that ability to perform hazardous tasks (eg, operating machinery, driving motor vehicle) may be impaired.

STORAGE: 15-30°C (59-86°F). Avoid freezing. Protect from light. (Ocudose) Keep unit dose container in protective foil overwrap and use within 1 month after opening.

TIVICAY – dolutegravir

RX

Class: HIV-integrase strand transfer inhibitor

ADULT DOSAGE

HIV-1 Infection

Used in combination w/ other antiretrovirals

Treatment-Naive/Treatment-Experienced Integrase Strand Transfer Inhibitor (INSTI)-Naive:
50mg qd

INSTI-Experienced w/ Certain INSTI-Associated Resistance Substitutions or Clinically Suspected INSTI Resistance:
50mg bid

Safety and efficacy of doses >50mg bid have not been evaluated

PEDIATRIC DOSAGE

HIV-1 Infection

Used in combination w/ other antiretrovirals

Treatment-Naive/Treatment-Experienced Integrase Strand Transfer Inhibitor (INSTI)-Naive:

≥12 Years and ≥40kg:
50mg qd

T

DOSING CONSIDERATIONS

Concomitant Medications

Treatment-Naive/Treatment-Experienced INSTI-Naive in Combination w/ Certain UGT1A/CYP3A Inducers (eg, Efavirenz, Fosamprenavir/Ritonavir [RTV], Tipranavir/RTV, Carbamazepine, Rifampin): 50mg bid

Hepatic Impairment

Severe (Child-Pugh Score C): Not recommended for use

ADMINISTRATION

Oral route

Take w/ or w/o food.

HOW SUPPLIED

Tab: 50mg

CONTRAINDICATIONS

Previous hypersensitivity reaction to dolutegravir, coadministration w/ dofetilide.

WARNINGS/PRECAUTIONS

Hypersensitivity reactions reported; d/c therapy and other suspect agents immediately if signs/symptoms develop, monitor clinical status (eg, liver aminotransferases), and initiate appropriate therapy. May be at increased risk for worsening or development of transaminase elevations in patients w/ underlying hepatitis B or C. Redistribution/accumulation of body fat observed. Immune reconstitution syndrome reported. Autoimmune disorders (eg, Graves' disease, polymyositis, Guillain-Barre syndrome) reported in the setting of immune reconstitution and can occur many months after initiation of treatment. Caution in elderly. Caution in INSTI-experienced patients (w/ certain INSTI-associated resistance substitutions or clinically suspected INSTI resistance) w/ severe renal impairment.

ADVERSE REACTIONS

Insomnia, ALT/AST elevations, increased cholesterol/lipase/creatine kinase, hyperglycemia.

DRUG INTERACTIONS

See Dosing Considerations and Contraindications. Drugs that induce/inhibit UGT1A1, CYP3A, UGT1A3, UGT1A9, breast cancer resistance protein, and P-gp may decrease/increase levels, respectively. Decreased levels w/ etravirine; etravirine use w/o coadministration of atazanavir/RTV, darunavir/RTV, or lopinavir/RTV is not recommended. Decreased levels w/ carbamazepine, efavirenz, fosamprenavir/RTV, and tipranavir/RTV; use alternative combinations that do not include metabolic inducers where possible for INSTI-experienced patients w/ certain INSTI-associated resistance substitutions or clinically suspected INSTI resistance. Decreased levels w/ nevirapine, oxcarbazepine, phenytoin, phenobarbital, and St. John's wort; avoid coadministration. Administer 2 hrs before or 6 hrs after taking medications containing polyvalent cations (eg, cation-containing antacids/laxatives, sucralfate, buffered medications) and oral Ca^{2+} or iron supplements (eg, multivitamins); alternatively, dolutegravir and supplements containing Ca^{2+} or iron can be taken together w/ food. May increase levels of drugs eliminated via renal organic cation transporters, OCT2, or multidrug and toxin extrusion transporter 1 (eg, metformin); limit the total daily dose of metformin to 1000mg when starting metformin or dolutegravir. When stopping dolutegravir, the metformin dose may require an adjustment; monitor blood glucose when initiating concomitant use and after withdrawal of dolutegravir. Decreased levels w/ rifampin; use alternatives to rifampin where possible for INSTI-experienced patients w/ certain INSTI-associated resistance substitutions or clinically suspected INSTI resistance.

PATIENT CONSIDERATIONS

Assessment: Assess for previous hypersensitivity to the drug, hepatitis B or C infection, renal/hepatic impairment, pregnancy/nursing status, and possible drug interactions.

Monitoring: Monitor for signs/symptoms of hypersensitivity reactions, redistribution/accumulation of body fat, immune reconstitution syndrome, autoimmune disorders, and other adverse reactions. If a hypersensitivity reaction develops, monitor clinical status, including liver aminotransferases. In patients w/ underlying hepatic disease, monitor for hepatotoxicity.

Counseling: Instruct to d/c immediately and seek medical attention if rash develops and is associated w/ other symptoms of hypersensitivity. Advise patients w/ underlying hepatitis B or C to have lab testing before and during therapy. Inform that fat redistribution/accumulation may occur. Advise to inform physician immediately of any symptoms of infection. Advise that therapy is not a cure for HIV-1 infection and that patients may continue to experience illnesses associated w/ HIV-1 infection, including opportunistic infections. Advise to take all HIV medications exactly as prescribed. Advise to avoid doing things that can spread HIV to others. Instruct to inform physician if any unusual symptom develops, or if any known symptom persists or worsens. Counsel patients on missed dose instructions. Advise not to breastfeed.

STORAGE: 25°C (77°F); excursions permitted to 15-30°C (59-86°F).

TobraDex – dexamethasone/tobramycin

RX

Class: Aminoglycoside/corticosteroid

OTHER BRAND NAMES

TobraDex ST

ADULT DOSAGE

Steroid-Responsive Inflammatory Ocular Conditions

Use for conditions for which a corticosteroid is indicated and where superficial bacterial ocular infection or a risk of bacterial ocular infection exists

PEDIATRIC DOSAGE

Steroid-Responsive Inflammatory Ocular Conditions

Use for conditions for which a corticosteroid is indicated and where superficial bacterial ocular infection or a risk of bacterial ocular infection exists

Sus:
1-2 drops into the conjunctival sac(s) q4-6h
Titrate: May increase to 1-2 drops q2h during the initial 24-48 hrs; decrease frequency gradually as condition improves

ST:
1 drop into the conjunctival sac(s) q4-6h
Titrate: May increase to 1 drop q2h during the initial 24-48 hrs; decrease frequency gradually as condition improves

Sus/ST:
Do not prescribe more than 20mL initially

Care should be taken not to d/c therapy prematurely

Oint:
Apply a small amount (1/2 inch ribbon) into the conjunctival sac(s) up to tid-qid
Do not prescribe more than 8g initially

≥2 Years:

Sus:
1-2 drops into the conjunctival sac(s) q4-6h
Titrate: May increase to 1-2 drops q2h during the initial 24-48 hrs; decrease frequency gradually as condition improves

ST:
1 drop into the conjunctival sac(s) q4-6h
Titrate: May increase to 1 drop q2h during the initial 24-48 hrs; decrease frequency gradually as condition improves

Sus/ST:
Do not prescribe more than 20mL initially

Care should be taken not to d/c therapy prematurely

Oint:
Apply a small amount (1/2 inch ribbon) into the conjunctival sac(s) up to tid-qid
Do not prescribe more than 8g initially

ADMINISTRATION

Ocular route

Sus/ST
Shake well before use

Oint
1. Tilt head back
2. Place finger on cheek just under the eye and gently pull down until a "V" pocket is formed between eyeball and lower lid
3. Apply recommended dose, making sure to avoid touching tip of tube to eye
4. Look downward before closing the eye

HOW SUPPLIED

Oint: (Tobramycin/Dexamethasone) 0.3%/0.1% [3.5g]; **Sus:** 0.3%/0.1% [2.5mL, 5mL, 10mL]; **Sus (ST):** 0.3%/0.05% [2.5mL, 5mL, 10mL]

CONTRAINDICATIONS

Most viral diseases of the cornea and conjunctiva, including epithelial herpes simplex keratitis (dendritic keratitis), vaccinia, and varicella; mycobacterial infection of the eye; fungal diseases of ocular structures; hypersensitivity to a component of the medication.

WARNINGS/PRECAUTIONS

Prolonged use may result in glaucoma with optic nerve damage, visual acuity and field of vision defects, posterior subcapsular cataract formation, and may suppress host response and increase risk of secondary ocular infections. Perforations may occur with diseases causing thinning of the cornea or sclera. May mask/enhance existing infection in acute purulent conditions. Fungal infections of the cornea may occur; consider fungal invasion in any persistent corneal ulceration. (Oint/Sus) Not for injection into the eye. Routinely monitor intraocular pressure (IOP). D/C if sensitivity occurs. Cross-sensitivity to other aminoglycoside antibiotics may occur; d/c and institute appropriate therapy if hypersensitivity develops. May result in overgrowth of nonsusceptible organisms, including fungi; initiate appropriate therapy if superinfection occurs. (ST) Monitor IOP if to be used for ≥10 days. Reevaluate after 2 days if patient fails to improve. Use may prolong the course and may exacerbate the severity of many viral infections of the eye (including herpes simplex). May delay healing and increase the incidence of bleb formation after cataract surgery. (Oint) May retard corneal wound healing.

ADVERSE REACTIONS

Hypersensitivity, localized ocular toxicity, secondary infection, increased IOP, posterior subcapsular cataract formation, impaired wound healing.

DRUG INTERACTIONS

Monitor total serum concentrations if used concomitantly with systemic aminoglycoside antibiotics.

PATIENT CONSIDERATIONS

Assessment: Assess for epithelial herpes simplex keratitis (dendritic keratitis), vaccinia, varicella, other viral diseases of cornea or conjunctiva, mycobacterial infection and fungal diseases of eye, diseases that may cause thinning of cornea or sclera, other existing infections, pregnancy/nursing status, and for drug interactions. (ST) Assess for history of herpes simplex.

Monitoring: Monitor for signs/symptoms of hypersensitivity reactions, glaucoma, defects in visual acuity and fields of vision, posterior subcapsular cataracts, perforations, secondary infections, delayed wound healing. (ST) Monitor for IOP if used for ≥10 days, exacerbation of ocular viral infections, and bleb formation. (Oint/Sus) Routinely monitor IOP, and for development of superinfections.

Counseling: Instruct not to touch dropper tip to any surface to avoid contaminating contents and not to wear contact lenses during therapy.

STORAGE: (Sus) 8-27°C (46-80°F); store upright. (Oint/ST): 2-25°C (36-77°F); protect ST from light.

TOFRANIL – imipramine hydrochloride

RX

Class: Tricyclic antidepressant (TCA)

Antidepressants increased the risk of suicidal thinking and behavior (suicidality) in children, adolescents, and young adults in short-term studies of major depressive disorder and other psychiatric disorders. Monitor and observe closely for clinical worsening, suicidality, or unusual changes in behavior in patients who are started on antidepressant therapy. Not approved for use in pediatric patients.

ADULT DOSAGE

Depression

Hospitalized Patients:
Initial: 100mg/day in divided doses
Titrate: Increase gradually to 200mg/day as required; increase to 250-300mg/day if no response after 2 weeks

Outpatients:
Initial: 75mg/day
Titrate: Increase to 150mg/day
Maint: 50-150mg/day
Max: 200mg/day

Following remission, may require maint for a longer period of time at the lowest effective dose

PEDIATRIC DOSAGE

Depression

Adolescents:
Initial: 30-40mg/day
Max: 100mg/day

Following remission, may require maint for a longer period of time at the lowest effective dose

Enuresis

Temporary Adjunctive Therapy in Reducing Enuresis After Possible Organic Causes Have Been Excluded by Appropriate Tests:

≥6 Years:
Initial: 25mg/day 1 hr before hs
Titrate: If no satisfactory response w/in 1 week, increase to 50mg nightly in children <12 yrs; may give up to 75mg nightly in children >12 yrs
Max: 2.5mg/kg/day

In early night bedwetters, drug is more effective given earlier and in divided doses (eg, 25mg in midafternoon, repeated hs)

Consider a drug-free period following an adequate trial w/ favorable response

Dosage should be tapered off gradually rather than abruptly discontinued; may reduce tendency to relapse

DOSING CONSIDERATIONS

Elderly
Initial: 30-40mg/day
Max: 100mg/day

ADMINISTRATION

Oral route

HOW SUPPLIED

Tab: 10mg, 25mg, 50mg

CONTRAINDICATIONS

Use of an MAOI concomitantly. Treatment w/in 14 days of stopping an MAOI. During the acute recovery period following myocardial infarction (MI). Known hypersensitivity to this product.

WARNINGS/PRECAUTIONS

Not approved for the treatment of bipolar depression. May precipitate mixed/manic episode in patients at risk for bipolar disorder; screen for risk for bipolar disorder prior to initiating treatment. Pupillary dilation that occurs following therapy may trigger an angle-closure attack in a patient with anatomically narrow angles who does not have a patent iridectomy. Use extreme caution in patients with cardiovascular disease (CVD); cardiac surveillance required. Caution in patients with history of urinary retention, narrow-angle glaucoma, or seizure disorder. Caution in patients with hyperthyroidism, serious depression, significant renal/hepatic impairment, and in elderly. May impair mental/physical abilities. Hypomanic or manic episodes may occur, particularly in patients with cyclic disorders; may require discontinuation and, if needed, may resume at lower dosage when episodes are relieved. May activate psychosis in schizophrenic patients; may require dose reduction and addition of a phenothiazine. Hazards may be increased with electroshock therapy. Photosensitization reported; avoid excessive exposure to sunlight. May alter blood glucose levels. Perform leukocyte and differential blood counts if fever and sore throat develop; d/c if there is evidence of pathological neutrophil depression. Prior to elective surgery, d/c treatment for as long as the clinical situation will allow.

ADVERSE REACTIONS

Nervousness, sleep disorders, tiredness, mild GI disturbances, orthostatic hypotension, HTN, confusion, hallucinations, numbness, tremors, dry mouth, skin rash, bone marrow depression, anorexia, jaundice.

DRUG INTERACTIONS

See Contraindications. Caution in patients on thyroid medication. May block pharmacological effects of guanethidine, clonidine, or similar agents; use with caution. Methylphenidate HCl may inhibit metabolism; may require downward dose adjustment of imipramine. May enhance CNS depressant effects of alcohol. Drugs that inhibit CYP2D6 (eg, quinidine, cimetidine, many CYP2D6 substrates [other antidepressants, phenothiazines, propafenone, flecainide]) may increase plasma concentrations; may require lower doses for either TCA or the other drug, and monitoring of TCA plasma levels. Caution with SSRI coadministration and when switching between TCAs and SSRIs (eg, fluoxetine, sertraline, paroxetine); sufficient time must elapse before starting therapy when switching from fluoxetine (at least 5 weeks may be necessary). Hepatic enzyme inhibitors (eg, cimetidine, fluoxetine) may increase plasma concentration and hepatic enzyme inducers (eg, barbiturates, phenytoin) may decrease plasma concentration; may require dosage adjustment of imipramine. Atropine-like effects may become more pronounced (eg, paralytic ileus) with anticholinergics (including antiparkinsonism agents); close supervision and careful dose adjustment is required when coadministered with anticholinergic drugs. May potentiate effects of catecholamines; avoid use of preparations (eg, decongestants, local anesthetics) that contain any sympathomimetic amine (eg, epinephrine, norepinephrine). Caution with agents that lower BP. May potentiate effects of CNS depressants.

PATIENT CONSIDERATIONS

Assessment: Assess for acute recovery period following MI, known hypersensitivity to drug, history of urinary retention or seizure disorder, history of/susceptibility to narrow-angle glaucoma, risk for bipolar disorder, CVD, hyperthyroidism, schizophrenia, serious depression, renal/hepatic impairment, pregnancy/nursing status, and possible drug interactions. Obtain ECG recording prior to initiation of larger-than-usual doses of therapy.

Monitoring: Monitor for signs/symptoms of clinical worsening, suicidality, unusual changes in behavior, hypomanic/manic episodes, psychosis activation, angle-closure glaucoma, changes in blood glucose levels, and other adverse reactions. Take ECG recording at appropriate intervals until steady state is achieved; perform cardiac surveillance in patients with CVD. Perform leukocyte and differential blood counts if fever and sore throat develop.

Counseling: Inform about benefits, risks, and appropriate use of therapy. Advise to monitor for unusual changes in behavior, worsening of depression, and suicidal ideation on a day-to-day basis, and to report such symptoms to physician. Inform that drug can cause mild pupillary dilation, which in susceptible individuals, can lead to an episode of angle-closure glaucoma. Advise to use caution when performing potentially hazardous tasks (eg, driving, operating machinery). Instruct to avoid excessive exposure to sunlight.

STORAGE: 20-25°C (68-77°F).

T

TOPAMAX – topiramate

RX

Class: Sulfamate-substituted monosaccharide antiepileptic

OTHER BRAND NAMES

Topamax Sprinkle

ADULT DOSAGE

Epilepsy

Monotherapy:
Partial Onset/Primary Generalized Tonic-Clonic Seizures:

Week 1: 25mg bid (am and pm)
Week 2: 50mg bid (am and pm)
Week 3: 75mg bid (am and pm)
Week 4: 100mg bid (am and pm)

PEDIATRIC DOSAGE

Epilepsy

Monotherapy:
Partial Onset/Primary Generalized Tonic-Clonic Seizures:

2-<10 Years:
Initial: 25mg qpm for the 1st week
Titrate: May increase to 50mg qd in the 2nd

Week 5: 150mg bid (am and pm)
Week 6 & Onward: 200mg bid (am and pm)

Adjunctive Therapy:
Partial Onset Seizure/Primary Generalized Tonic-Clonic Seizures/Lennox-Gastaut Syndrome:
≥17 Years:
Initial: 25-50mg/day
Titrate: Increase in increments of 25-50mg/day every week

Partial Onset Seizures:
Usual: 200-400mg/day in 2 divided doses

Primary Generalized Tonic-Clonic:
Usual: 400mg/day in 2 divided doses

Migraine

Prophylaxis:
Week 1: 25mg qpm
Week 2: 25mg bid
Week 3: 25mg qam and 50mg qpm
Week 4 & Onward: 50mg bid

week, then by 25-50mg qd each subsequent week. Titration to the minimum maint dose should be attempted over 5-7 weeks; additional titration to a higher dose (up to the max maint dose) can be attempted in weekly increments by 25-50mg qd, up to the max maint dose for each range of body weight

Up to 11kg:
Minimum Maint Dose: 150mg/day
Max Maint Dose: 250mg/day
12-22kg:
Minimum Maint Dose: 200mg/day
Max Maint Dose: 300mg/day
23-31kg:
Minimum Maint Dose: 200mg/day
Max Maint Dose: 350mg/day
32-38kg:
Minimum Maint Dose: 250mg/day
Max Maint Dose: 350mg/day
>38kg:
Minimum Maint Dose: 250mg/day
Max Maint Dose: 400mg/day

Administer in 2 equally divided doses; refer to PI for titration instructions

≥10 Years:
Week 1: 25mg bid (am and pm)
Week 2: 50mg bid (am and pm)
Week 3: 75mg bid (am and pm)
Week 4: 100mg bid (am and pm)
Week 5: 150mg bid (am and pm)
Week 6 & Onward: 200mg bid (am and pm)

Adjunctive Therapy:
Partial Onset Seizure/Primary Generalized Tonic-Clonic Seizures/Lennox-Gastaut Syndrome:
2-16 Years:
Week 1: 1-3mg/kg/day (≤25mg/day) qpm
Titrate: Increase dose at 1- or 2-week intervals by increments of 1-3mg/kg/day (administered in 2 divided doses)
Usual: 5-9mg/kg/day in 2 divided doses

Migraine

Prophylaxis:
≥12 Years:
Week 1: 25mg qpm
Week 2: 25mg bid
Week 3: 25mg qam and 50mg qpm
Week 4 & Onward: 50mg bid

DOSING CONSIDERATIONS

Renal Impairment
CrCl <70mL/min: Administer 50% of usual adult dose
Patients Undergoing Hemodialysis: May require a supplemental dose

ADMINISTRATION

Oral route

Take w/o regard to meals

Sprinkle Caps
May be swallowed whole or administered by carefully opening the capsule and sprinkling entire contents on a small amount (tsp) of soft food; swallow drug/food mixture immediately and do not chew or store mixture for later use

HOW SUPPLIED

Cap: (Sprinkle) 15mg, 25mg; **Tab:** 25mg, 50mg, 100mg, 200mg

WARNINGS/PRECAUTIONS

Acute myopia associated with secondary angle-closure glaucoma reported; d/c immediately to reverse symptoms. Elevated IOP of any etiology may lead to serious adverse events (eg, permanent

T

loss of vision) if left untreated. Visual field defects (independent of elevated IOP) reported; consider discontinuing therapy if visual problems occur. Oligohidrosis and hyperthermia reported, mostly in pediatric patients. Hyperchloremic, non-anion gap, metabolic acidosis reported; d/c or reduce dose if metabolic acidosis develops/persists. If decision is to continue therapy, consider alkali treatment. Conditions or therapies that predispose to acidosis (eg, renal disease, severe respiratory disorders, status epilepticus, diarrhea, ketogenic diet, specific drugs) may be additive to the bicarbonate lowering effects. Increased risk of suicidal thoughts/behavior. Cognitive-related dysfunction, psychiatric/behavioral disturbances, and somnolence or fatigue reported. May cause cleft lip and/or palate in infants if used during pregnancy. D/C gradually to minimize the potential for seizure or increased seizure frequency; appropriate monitoring is recommended when rapid withdrawal is required. Sudden unexplained deaths in epilepsy reported. Patients with inborn errors of metabolism or reduced hepatic mitochondrial activity may be at an increased risk for hyperammonemia with or without encephalopathy; consider hyperammonemic encephalopathy and measure ammonia levels in patients who develop unexplained lethargy, vomiting, or changes in mental status associated with therapy. Kidney stone formation reported; hydration is recommended to reduce new stone formation. Paresthesia may occur. Lab abnormalities may occur. Caution with renal/hepatic impairment and in elderly.

ADVERSE REACTIONS

Anorexia, anxiety, diarrhea, fatigue, fever, infection, weight decrease, cognitive problems, paresthesia, somnolence, taste perversion, mood problems, nausea, nervousness, confusion.

DRUG INTERACTIONS

Phenytoin or carbamazepine may decrease levels. Increase in systemic exposure of lithium observed following topiramate doses of ≤600mg/day; monitor lithium levels. May cause CNS depression and cognitive/neuropsychiatric adverse events with alcohol and other CNS depressants; use with extreme caution. May decrease contraceptive efficacy and increase breakthrough bleeding with combination oral contraceptives. Concurrent administration of valproic acid has been associated with hyperammonemia with or without encephalopathy, and hypothermia. Other carbonic anhydrase inhibitors (eg, zonisamide, acetazolamide, dichlorphenamide) may increase the severity of metabolic acidosis and may also increase the risk of kidney stone formation. Caution with agents that predispose patients to heat-related disorders (eg, carbonic anhydrase inhibitors, anticholinergics).

PATIENT CONSIDERATIONS

Assessment: Assess for renal/hepatic dysfunction, predisposing factors for metabolic acidosis, inborn errors of metabolism, reduced hepatic mitochondrial activity, pregnancy/nursing status, and possible drug interactions. Obtain baseline serum bicarbonate and blood ammonia levels.

Monitoring: Monitor for signs/symptoms of acute myopia, secondary angle-closure glaucoma, visual field defects, oligohidrosis, hyperthermia, cognitive or neuropsychiatric adverse reactions, kidney stones, renal dysfunction, metabolic acidosis, paresthesia, hyperammonemia, and other adverse reactions. Monitor serum bicarbonate and blood ammonia levels.

Counseling: Instruct to seek immediate medical attention if blurred vision, visual disturbances, periorbital pain, changes in mood/behavior, or suicidal thoughts/behavior occur and to closely monitor for decreased sweating or high/persistent fever. Warn about risk for metabolic acidosis. Advise to use caution when engaging in activities where loss of consciousness may result in serious danger. Inform about risk for hyperammonemia with or without encephalopathy; instruct to contact physician if unexplained lethargy, vomiting, or mental status changes develop. Instruct to maintain adequate fluid intake to minimize risk of kidney stones. Inform of pregnancy risks. Encourage to enroll in the North American Antiepileptic Drug Pregnancy Registry if patient becomes pregnant. Instruct that if a single dose is missed, to take that dose as soon as possible, skip it if cannot be taken at least 6 hrs before the next scheduled dose, and not to double the dose. Advise to contact physician if >1 dose is missed.

STORAGE: Protect from moisture. (Tab) 15-30°C (59-86°F). (Cap) ≤25°C (77°F).

TOPICORT – desoximetasone RX

Class: Corticosteroid

ADULT DOSAGE

Inflammatory and Pruritic Manifestations of Corticosteroid-Responsive Dermatoses

Apply a thin film to affected area(s) bid and rub in gently

PEDIATRIC DOSAGE

Inflammatory and Pruritic Manifestations of Corticosteroid-Responsive Dermatoses

Cre/Gel/0.05% Oint:

Apply a thin film to affected area(s) bid and rub in gently

0.25% Oint:

≥10 Years:

Apply a thin film to affected area(s) bid and rub in gently

ADMINISTRATION
Topical route

HOW SUPPLIED
Cre: 0.05%, 0.25% [15g, 30g, 60g, 100g]; **Gel:** 0.05% [15g, 30g, 60g]; **Oint:** 0.05% [15g, 30g, 60g, 100g], 0.25% [15g, 60g, 100g]

CONTRAINDICATIONS
History of hypersensitivity to any of the components of the medication.

WARNINGS/PRECAUTIONS
Not for oral, ophthalmic, or intravaginal use. May produce reversible hypothalamic-pituitary-adrenal (HPA) axis suppression w/ potential for clinical glucocorticosteroid insufficiency; periodically evaluate patient and when noted, gradually withdraw the drug, reduce the frequency of application, or substitute a less potent steroid. Caution w/ factors predisposing to HPA axis suppression (eg, use of more potent steroids, large surface areas, prolonged use, use under occlusion, altered skin barrier, liver failure). May produce Cushing's syndrome, hyperglycemia, and unmasking of latent diabetes mellitus (DM). Local adverse reactions (eg, atrophy, striae, irritation) may occur. Allergic contact dermatitis may occur; confirm by patch testing. Use appropriate antimicrobial agent w/ skin infections; d/c until infection has been adequately treated. Pediatric patients may be more susceptible to systemic toxicity. Limit administration to the least amount compatible w/ an effective therapeutic regimen in pediatric patients; chronic use may interfere w/ growth and development.

ADVERSE REACTIONS
Burning, itching, irritation, dryness, folliculitis, hypertrichosis, acneiform eruptions, hypopigmentation, perioral dermatitis, allergic contact dermatitis, skin maceration, secondary infection, skin atrophy, striae, miliaria.

DRUG INTERACTIONS
Use w/ other corticosteroid-containing products may increase exposure.

PATIENT CONSIDERATIONS

Assessment: Assess for predisposing factors to HPA axis suppression, skin infections, hypersensitivity to drug, pregnancy/nursing status, and possible drug interactions.

Monitoring: Monitor for HPA axis suppression, Cushing's syndrome, hyperglycemia, glucosuria, unmasking of latent DM, local adverse reactions, allergic contact dermatitis, development of infections, and other adverse reactions. Perform periodic monitoring of HPA axis suppression using adrenocorticotropic hormone stimulation test or urinary free cortisol test. Monitor for systemic toxicity (eg, adrenal suppression, intracranial HTN) in pediatric patients.

Counseling: Instruct to use externally ud, to avoid contact w/ the eyes, and not to use for any disorder other than prescribed. Advise not to bandage or occlude the treated skin area unless directed by physician. Instruct to report any signs of local adverse reactions to physician. Instruct not to use w/ other corticosteroid-containing products w/o first consulting w/ physician, to d/c therapy when control is achieved, and to contact physician if no improvement is seen w/in 4 weeks. Advise parents of pediatric patients not to use tight-fitting diapers or plastic pants on a child being treated in the diaper area.

STORAGE: Cre/Gel/0.05% Oint: 20-25°C (68-77°F); excursions permitted to 15-30°C (59-86°F). **0.25% Oint:** 15-30°C (59-86°F).

Toprol-XL – metoprolol succinate

RX

Class: Selective $beta_1$ blocker

Exacerbations of angina and MI reported following abrupt discontinuation. When discontinuing chronic therapy, particularly w/ ischemic heart disease, taper over 1-2 weeks w/ careful monitoring. If worsening of angina or acute coronary insufficiency develops, reinstate therapy promptly, at least temporarily, and take other appropriate measures. Caution patients against interruption or discontinuation of therapy w/o physician's advice.

ADULT DOSAGE

Hypertension

Initial: 25-100mg qd
Titrate: May increase at weekly (or longer) intervals
Max: 400mg/day

Angina Pectoris

Initial: 100mg qd
Titrate: May gradually increase weekly
Max: 400mg/day

PEDIATRIC DOSAGE

Hypertension

≥6 Years:
Initial: 1mg/kg qd up to 50mg qd
Titrate: Adjust dose according to BP response
Max: 2mg/kg (or up to 200mg) qd

T

Reduce dose gradually over a period of 1-2 weeks if to be discontinued

Heart Failure

Initial:
NYHA Class II HF: 25mg qd for 2 weeks
Severe Heart Failure: 12.5mg qd for 2 weeks
Titrate: Double dose every 2 weeks to the highest dose level tolerated
Max: 200mg
Dose should not be increased until symptoms of worsening HF have been stabilized
Reduce dose if experiencing symptomatic bradycardia

DOSING CONSIDERATIONS

Hepatic Impairment

May require lower initial dose; gradually increase dose to optimize therapy

Elderly

Start at low initial dose

ADMINISTRATION

Oral route

Tab may be divided; do not crush or chew whole or half tab

HOW SUPPLIED

Tab, Extended-Release: 25mg*, 50mg*, 100mg*, 200mg* *scored

CONTRAINDICATIONS

Severe bradycardia, 2nd- or 3rd-degree heart block, cardiogenic shock, decompensated cardiac failure, sick sinus syndrome (unless w/ a permanent pacemaker), hypersensitivity to any component of this product.

WARNINGS/PRECAUTIONS

Worsening cardiac failure may occur during up-titration; lower dose or temporarily d/c therapy. Avoid w/ bronchospastic disease; may be used only w/ those who do not respond to or cannot tolerate other antihypertensive treatment. If used in the setting of pheochromocytoma, should be given in combination w/ α-blockers, and only after α-blocker has been initiated; may cause a paradoxical increase in BP if administered alone. Avoid initiation of a high-dose regimen in patients undergoing noncardiac surgery. Chronically administered therapy should not be routinely withdrawn prior to major surgery; however, the impaired ability of the heart to respond to reflex adrenergic stimuli may augment the risks of general anesthesia and surgical procedures. May mask tachycardia occurring w/ hypoglycemia. May mask signs of hyperthyroidism (eg, tachycardia); abrupt withdrawal may precipitate thyroid storm. Patients w/ a history of severe anaphylactic reactions to variety of allergens may be more reactive to repeated challenge and may be unresponsive to usual doses of epinephrine. May precipitate or aggravate symptoms of arterial insufficiency w/ peripheral vascular disease (PVD). Caution w/ hepatic impairment and in elderly.

ADVERSE REACTIONS

Tiredness, dizziness, depression, diarrhea, SOB, bradycardia, rash.

DRUG INTERACTIONS

Additive effects w/ catecholamine-depleting drugs (eg, reserpine, MAOIs). CYP2D6 inhibitors (eg, quinidine, fluoxetine, propafenone) may increase levels. Caution when used w/ verapamil and diltiazem. May increase the risk of bradycardia w/ digitalis glycosides, clonidine, diltiazem, and verapamil. When given concomitantly w/ clonidine, d/c several days before clonidine is gradually withdrawn; may exacerbate rebound HTN.

PATIENT CONSIDERATIONS

Assessment: Assess for severe bradycardia, 2nd- or 3rd-degree heart block, cardiogenic shock, decompensated cardiac failure, sick sinus syndrome, presence of pacemaker, ischemic heart disease, bronchospastic disease, diabetes, hyperthyroidism, PVD, hepatic impairment, pheochromocytoma, history of anaphylactic reactions, pregnancy/nursing status, and possible drug interactions.

Monitoring: Monitor for signs/symptoms of worsening cardiac failure during up-titration, hypoglycemia, precipitation of thyroid storm, precipitation/aggravation of arterial insufficiency in patients w/ PVD, anaphylactic reactions, and other adverse reactions. Monitor patients w/ ischemic heart disease.

Counseling: Advise to take drug regularly and continuously, ud, preferably w/ or immediately following meals. Counsel that if dose is missed, take only the next scheduled dose (w/o doubling). Instruct not to interrupt or d/c therapy w/o consulting physician. Advise to avoid operating automobiles and machinery or engaging in other tasks requiring alertness. Instruct to contact physician if any difficulty in breathing occurs. Instruct to inform physician or dentist of medication use before any type of surgery. Advise HF patients to consult physician if experience signs/symptoms of worsening HF.

STORAGE: 25°C (77°F); excursions permitted to 15-30°C (59-86°F).

TORSEMIDE – torsemide

RX

Class: Loop diuretic

OTHER BRAND NAMES

Demadex

ADULT DOSAGE

Edema

IV/PO:

CHF:

Initial: 10 or 20mg qd

Titrate: Double dose until desired response is obtained

Max Single Dose: 200mg

Chronic Renal Failure:

Initial: 20mg qd

Titrate: Double dose until desired response is obtained

Max Single Dose: 200mg

Hepatic Cirrhosis:

Initial: 5 or 10mg qd w/ an aldosterone antagonist or K^+-sparing diuretic

Titrate: Double dose until desired response is obtained

Max Single Dose: 40mg

Hypertension

IV/PO:

Initial: 5mg qd

Titrate: May increase to 10mg qd after 4-6 weeks if BP reduction is inadequate

An additional antihypertensive agent should be added to the treatment regimen if response to 10mg is insufficient

PEDIATRIC DOSAGE

Pediatric use may not have been established

DOSING CONSIDERATIONS

IV to PO Conversion

May switch to/from IV form w/ no change in dose

ADMINISTRATION

IV/Oral route

Inj

Administer either slowly as a bolus over 2 min or as continuous infusion

Flush IV line w/ normal saline before and after administration

Refer to PI for further administration instructions

Compatibility

D5W; 0.9% NaCl; 0.45% NaCl

Tab

May be given at any time in relation to a meal

HOW SUPPLIED

Inj: 10mg/mL [2mL, 5mL]; **Tab:** (Demadex) 5mg*, 10mg*, 20mg*, 100mg* *scored

CONTRAINDICATIONS

Known hypersensitivity to torsemide or to sulfonylureas, anuria.

WARNINGS/PRECAUTIONS

Caution in patients with hepatic disease with cirrhosis and ascites as sudden alterations of fluid/electrolyte balance may precipitate hepatic coma; diuresis is best initiated in a hospital. Tinnitus and hearing loss (usually reversible) reported. Excessive diuresis may cause dehydration, blood-volume reduction, and possible thrombosis and embolism, especially in elderly. Monitor for electrolyte imbalance, hypovolemia, or prerenal azotemia; d/c until situation is corrected and may restart at

T

a lower dose, if signs/symptoms occur. Increased risk of hypokalemia with liver cirrhosis, brisk diuresis, and inadequate oral intake of electrolytes. Diuretic-induced hypokalemia may be a risk factor for the development of arrhythmias in patients with cardiovascular disease (CVD), especially with concomitant digitalis glycosides. Hyperglycemia, hypomagnesemia, hypercalcemia, and symptomatic gout reported. May increase BUN, SrCr, serum uric acid, total cholesterol, and TGs. Associated with small decreases in Hgb, Hct, erythrocyte count, and small increases in WBC count, platelet count, and alkaline phosphatase.

ADVERSE REACTIONS

Headache, excessive urination, dizziness, hypotension, chest pain, A-fib, diarrhea, GI hemorrhage, rectal bleeding, rash, shunt thrombosis, syncope, ventricular tachycardia, hyperglycemia, hyperuricemia.

DRUG INTERACTIONS

Reduced renal clearance and increased levels of spironolactone. Salicylate toxicity may occur with concomitant high-dose salicylates. Possible renal dysfunction with NSAIDs (including aspirin). Indomethacin partially inhibits natriuretic effect. Digoxin may increase exposure by 50%. Simultaneous administration with cholestyramine is not recommended. Probenecid may decrease diuretic activity. Caution with lithium; high risk of lithium toxicity. Increased ototoxic potential of aminoglycoside antibiotics and ethacrynic acid reported, especially in the presence of renal impairment. Increased risk of hypokalemia with adrenocorticotropic hormone or corticosteroids.

PATIENT CONSIDERATIONS

Assessment: Assess for history of hypersensitivity to the drug or to sulfonylureas, anuria, CVD, renal/hepatic impairment, pregnancy/nursing status, and possible drug interactions.

Monitoring: Monitor for hypovolemia, prerenal azotemia, tinnitus, hearing loss, hypersensitivity reactions, renal/hepatic impairment, arrhythmias in patients with CVD, and other adverse reactions. Monitor serum electrolytes periodically.

Counseling: Inform of risks and benefits of therapy. Advise to seek medical attention if symptoms of hypokalemia, fluid/electrolyte imbalance, hypersensitivity reactions, hearing loss, or tinnitus occur.

STORAGE: (Inj) 20-25°C (68-77°F). Do not freeze. Continuous Infusion Sol: Stable for 24 hrs at room temperature in plastic containers. Refer to PI for IV fluids and concentrations. (Tab) 15-30°C (59-86°F).

TOVIAZ – fesoterodine fumarate

RX

Class: Muscarinic antagonist

ADULT DOSAGE

Overactive Bladder

Initial: 4mg qd

Titrate: May increase to 8mg qd based on individual response and tolerability

PEDIATRIC DOSAGE

Pediatric use may not have been established

DOSING CONSIDERATIONS

Concomitant Medications

Strong CYP3A4 Inhibitors:

Max: 4mg/day

Renal Impairment

CrCl <30mL/min:

Max: 4mg/day

ADMINISTRATION

Oral route

Take w/ or w/o food

Take tab w/ liquid and swallow whole; do not crush, chew, or divide

HOW SUPPLIED

Tab, Extended-Release (ER): 4mg, 8mg

CONTRAINDICATIONS

Urinary/gastric retention; uncontrolled narrow-angle glaucoma; known hypersensitivity to the drug or its ingredients, or to tolterodine tartrate tabs or ER caps.

WARNINGS/PRECAUTIONS

Not recommended with severe hepatic impairment (Child-Pugh C). Angioedema of the face, lips, tongue, and/or larynx reported; d/c and promptly provide appropriate therapy if angioedema occurs. Risk of urinary retention; caution with clinically significant bladder outlet obstruction. Caution with decreased GI motility (eg, severe constipation), controlled narrow-angle glaucoma, and myasthenia gravis. CNS anticholinergic effects (eg, headache, dizziness, somnolence) reported; monitor for signs, particularly after beginning treatment or increasing the dose, and consider dose reduction or discontinuation if such effects occur.

ADVERSE REACTIONS

Dry mouth, constipation, urinary tract infection, dry eyes.

DRUG INTERACTIONS

May increase the frequency and/or severity of dry mouth, constipation, urinary retention, and other anticholinergic pharmacologic effects with other antimuscarinic agents that produce such effects. May potentially alter the absorption of some concomitantly administered drugs due to anticholinergic effects on GI motility. CYP3A4 inhibitors may increase levels; doses >4mg are not recommended in patients taking potent CYP3A4 inhibitors (eg, ketoconazole, itraconazole, clarithromycin). CYP2D6 inhibitors may increase levels. Rifampin or rifampicin may decrease levels.

PATIENT CONSIDERATIONS

Assessment: Assess for hypersensitivity to the drug or tolterodine tartrate, urinary/gastric retention, narrow-angle glaucoma, bladder outlet obstruction, decreased GI motility, severe constipation, myasthenia gravis, severe hepatic/renal impairment, pregnancy/nursing status, and possible drug interactions.

Monitoring: Monitor for angioedema, upper airway swelling, urinary retention, CNS anticholinergic effects, and other adverse reactions.

Counseling: Inform that therapy may produce angioedema; instruct to promptly d/c therapy and seek immediate medical attention if edema of the tongue/laryngopharynx or difficulty in breathing occurs. Counsel that therapy may produce clinically significant adverse effects (eg, constipation, urinary retention). Inform that blurred vision may occur; advise to exercise caution in decisions to engage in potentially dangerous activities until effects have been determined. Inform that heat prostration (due to decreased sweating) may occur when used in a hot environment. Inform that alcohol may enhance drowsiness caused by therapy.

STORAGE: 20-25°C (68-77°F); excursions permitted between 15-30°C (59-86°F). Protect from moisture.

TRADJENTA – linagliptin

RX

Class: Dipeptidyl peptidase-4 (DPP-4) inhibitor

ADULT DOSAGE

Type 2 Diabetes Mellitus

5mg qd

PEDIATRIC DOSAGE

Pediatric use may not have been established

DOSING CONSIDERATIONS

Concomitant Medications

W/ Insulin Secretagogue (eg, Sulfonylurea)/Insulin:

May require lower dose of insulin secretagogue or insulin

ADMINISTRATION

Oral route

Take w/ or w/o food.

HOW SUPPLIED

Tab: 5mg

CONTRAINDICATIONS

History of a hypersensitivity reaction to linagliptin (eg, anaphylaxis, angioedema, exfoliative skin conditions, urticaria, or bronchial hyperreactivity).

WARNINGS/PRECAUTIONS

Not for use in patients w/ type 1 diabetes mellitus (DM) or for the treatment of diabetic ketoacidosis. Acute pancreatitis reported; d/c if pancreatitis is suspected. Serious hypersensitivity reactions reported; if suspected, d/c therapy, assess for other potential causes for the event, and institute alternative treatment for diabetes. Caution in patients w/ a history of angioedema w/ another DPP-4 inhibitor. Severe and disabling arthralgia reported in patients taking DPP-4 inhibitors. Consider as a possible cause for severe joint pain and d/c therapy if appropriate.

ADVERSE REACTIONS

Hypoglycemia, nasopharyngitis, diarrhea.

DRUG INTERACTIONS

See Dosing Considerations. Strong inducers of P-gp or CYP3A4 (eg, rifampin) may reduce efficacy; use of alternative treatments is strongly recommended.

PATIENT CONSIDERATIONS

Assessment: Assess for history of hypersensitivity, type of DM, diabetic ketoacidosis, history of pancreatitis, history of angioedema w/ another DPP-4 inhibitor, pregnancy/nursing status, and possible drug interactions. Obtain baseline FPG and HbA1c levels.

Monitoring: Monitor for pancreatitis, arthralgia, hypersensitivity reactions, and other adverse reactions. Monitor FPG and HbA1c levels periodically.

Counseling: Inform of the potential risks/benefits and alternative modes of therapy. Advise on the importance of adherence to dietary instructions, regular physical activity, periodic blood glucose monitoring and HbA1c testing, recognition/management of hypo/hyperglycemia, and assessment for diabetes complications. Instruct to seek medical advice promptly during periods of stress as medication requirements may change. Inform that acute pancreatitis and serious allergic reactions reported; instruct to d/c use and notify physician if signs and symptoms of pancreatitis or allergic reactions occur. Inform that severe and disabling joint pain may occur w/ this class of drugs; instruct to seek medical advice if severe joint pain occurs. Instruct to take as prescribed. Instruct to inform physician or pharmacist if any unusual symptom develops, or if any known symptom persists or worsens.

STORAGE: 25°C (77°F); excursions permitted to 15-30°C (59-86°F).

TRANSDERM SCOP – scopolamine

RX

Class: Anticholinergic

ADULT DOSAGE

Motion Sickness

Prevention of N/V:

1 patch at least 4 hrs before the antiemetic effect is required
Replace patch after 3 days if therapy is required for >3 days

Postoperative Nausea/Vomiting

Prevention of N/V Associated w/ Recovery from Anesthesia and/or Opiate Analgesia and Surgery:

1 patch on the pm before surgery or 1 hr prior to cesarean section
Remove patch 24 hrs following surgery

PEDIATRIC DOSAGE

Pediatric use may not have been established

ADMINISTRATION

Transdermal route

Apply only to skin in the postauricular area
After application, wash hands thoroughly w/ soap and water and dry
Wear only 1 patch at anytime
Do not cut patch
Discard patch if displaced and replace w/ a fresh patch

HOW SUPPLIED

Patch: 1.5mg [4[s]]

CONTRAINDICATIONS

Angle-closure glaucoma, hypersensitivity to scopolamine or other belladonna alkaloids or to any ingredient/component in the formulation or delivery system.

WARNINGS/PRECAUTIONS

May increase IOP with open-angle glaucoma; monitor therapy and adjust during use. May cause temporary dilation of pupils and blurred vision if contact with eyes occurs. Caution with pyloric obstruction, urinary bladder neck obstruction, and intestinal obstruction. May aggravate seizures or psychosis. Idiosyncratic reactions may occur with ordinary therapeutic doses. Increased CNS effects may occur in elderly and with hepatic/renal impairment. May impair physical/mental abilities. Remove patch before undergoing a MRI scan; skin burns at the patch site reported. May interfere with gastric secretion test.

ADVERSE REACTIONS
Dry mouth, dizziness, somnolence, urinary retention, agitation, visual impairment, confusion, mydriasis, pharyngitis.

DRUG INTERACTIONS
May decrease absorption of oral medications due to decreased gastric motility and delayed gastric emptying. Caution with other drugs with CNS effects (eg, sedatives, tranquilizers, alcohol) and anticholinergic properties (eg, meclizine, TCAs, muscle relaxants).

PATIENT CONSIDERATIONS

Assessment: Assess for known hypersensitivity to the drug, glaucoma, pyloric obstruction, urinary bladder neck obstruction, intestinal obstruction, history of seizures or psychosis, hepatic/renal impairment, pregnancy/nursing status, and for possible drug interactions.

Monitoring: Monitor for aggravation of seizures or psychosis, idiosyncratic reactions (eg, agitation, hallucinations, paranoid behaviors, delusions), CNS effects, drowsiness, disorientation, confusion, withdrawal symptoms, and other adverse reactions. Monitor IOP in patients with open-angle glaucoma.

Counseling: Inform elderly that patch may cause a greater likelihood of CNS effects and to seek medical care if patient becomes confused, disoriented, or dizzy while wearing the patch or after removing. Inform that patch may cause drowsiness, disorientation, and confusion; advise to use caution when engaging in activities that require mental alertness. Instruct to avoid alcohol. Instruct to seek medical care if withdrawal symptoms occur following abrupt discontinuation. Inform that patch may cause temporary dilation of pupils and blurred vision. Instruct to wash hands thoroughly with soap and water immediately after handling patch. Instruct to dispose the patch properly to avoid contact with children or pets. Advise to remove patch before undergoing an MRI to avoid skin burns. Instruct to use ud. Advise to remove the patch immediately and promptly contact physician if symptoms of acute angle-closure glaucoma or difficulty in urinating is experienced.

STORAGE: 20-25°C (68-77°F).

TRAVATAN Z – travoprost

RX

Class: Prostaglandin analogue

ADULT DOSAGE
Elevated Intraocular Pressure
Open-Angle Glaucoma/Ocular HTN:
1 drop in affected eye(s) qd in pm

PEDIATRIC DOSAGE
Elevated Intraocular Pressure
Open-Angle Glaucoma/Ocular HTN:
≥16 Years:
1 drop in affected eye(s) qd in pm

DOSING CONSIDERATIONS
Concomitant Medications
Space by at least 5 min if using >1 topical ophthalmic drug

ADMINISTRATION
Ocular route

HOW SUPPLIED
Sol: 0.004% [2.5mL, 5mL]

WARNINGS/PRECAUTIONS
Changes to pigmented tissues, including increased pigmentation of iris (may be permanent), eyelid and eyelashes (may be reversible) reported. Regularly examine patients w/ noticeably increased iris pigmentation. May cause changes to eyelashes and vellus hair in the treated eye. May exacerbate active intraocular inflammation (eg, uveitis). Macular edema, including cystoid macular edema, reported; caution w/ aphakic patients, pseudophakic patients w/ torn posterior lens capsule, or patients at risk of macular edema. Treatment of angle-closure, inflammatory, or neovascular glaucoma has not been evaluated. Bacterial keratitis reported w/ multidose containers. Remove contact lenses prior to instillation; may reinsert 15 min after administration.

ADVERSE REACTIONS
Ocular hyperemia, foreign body sensation, decreased visual acuity, eye discomfort/pruritus/pain.

PATIENT CONSIDERATIONS

Assessment: Assess for active intraocular inflammation (uveitis), risk factors for macular edema, aphakic/pseudophakic patients w/ torn posterior lens capsule, angle-closure, inflammatory, or neovascular glaucoma, and pregnancy/nursing status.

Monitoring: Monitor for increased pigmentation of the iris and eyelid, changes in eyelashes, macular edema, and bacterial keratitis.

Counseling: Inform about risk of brown pigmentation of iris and darkening of eyelid skin. Inform about the possibility of eyelash and vellus hair changes. Advise to avoid touching tip of dispensing container to eye, surrounding structures, fingers, or any other surface, in order to avoid contamination of the sol. Advise to consult physician if having ocular surgery or if intercurrent ocular conditions (eg, trauma or infection) or ocular reactions develop. Instruct to remove contact lenses prior to instillation; reinsert 15 min after administration. Instruct to administer at least 5 min apart if using >1 topical ophthalmic drugs.

STORAGE: 2-25°C (36-77°F).

TREANDA – bendamustine hydrochloride RX

Class: Alkylating agent

ADULT DOSAGE

Chronic Lymphocytic Leukemia

100mg/m² IV over 30 min on Days 1 and 2 of a 28-day cycle, up to 6 cycles

B-Cell Non-Hodgkin Lymphoma

Indolent B-Cell Non-Hodgkin Lymphoma That Has Progressed During or w/in 6 Months of Treatment w/ Rituximab or a Rituximab-Containing Regimen:
120mg/m² IV over 60 min on Days 1 and 2 of a 21-day cycle, up to 8 cycles

PEDIATRIC DOSAGE

Pediatric use may not have been established

DOSING CONSIDERATIONS

Renal Impairment

CrCl <40mL/min: Not recommended for use

Hepatic Impairment

Moderate (AST or ALT 2.5-10X ULN and Total Bilirubin 1.5-3X ULN): Not recommended for use
Severe (Total Bilirubin >3X ULN): Not recommended for use

Adverse Reactions

Chronic Lymphocytic Leukemia:
Grade 4 Hematologic Toxicity: Delay
Clinically Significant ≥Grade 2 Nonhematologic Toxicity: Delay
Nonhematologic Toxicity Has Recovered to ≤Grade 1 and/or the Blood Counts Have Improved (ANC ≥1 x 10⁹/L, Platelets ≥75 x 10⁹/L): Reinitiate; dose reduction may be warranted
≥Grade 3 Hematologic Toxicity: Reduce to 50mg/m² on Days 1 and 2 of each cycle
≥Grade 3 Hematologic Toxicity Recurs: Reduce to 25mg/m² on Days 1 and 2 of each cycle
≥Grade 3 Nonhematologic Toxicity: Reduce to 50mg/m² on Days 1 and 2 of each cycle

May consider dose re-escalation in subsequent cycles

B-Cell Non-Hodgkin Lymphoma:
Grade 4 Hematologic Toxicity: Delay
Clinically Significant ≥Grade 2 Nonhematologic Toxicity: Delay
Nonhematologic Toxicity Has Recovered to ≤Grade 1 and/or the Blood Counts Have Improved (ANC ≥1 x 10⁹/L, Platelets ≥75 x 10⁹/L): Reinitiate; dose reduction may be warranted
Grade 4 Hematologic Toxicity: Reduce to 90mg/m² on Days 1 and 2 of each cycle
Grade 4 Hematologic Toxicity Recurs: Reduce to 60mg/m² on Days 1 and 2 of each cycle
≥Grade 3 Nonhematologic Toxicity: Reduce to 90mg/m² on Days 1 and 2 of each cycle
≥Grade 3 Nonhematologic Toxicity Recurs: Reduce to 60mg/m² on Days 1 and 2 of each cycle

ADMINISTRATION

IV route

Selection/Preparation

Do not mix or combine the 2 formulations.
Admixture should be prepared as close as possible to the time of patient administration.

Sol:
Withdraw and transfer for dilution in a biosafety cabinet or containment isolator using only a polypropylene syringe w/ a metal needle and a polypropylene hub.
Do not use w/ devices containing polycarbonate or acrylonitrile-butadiene-styrene (ABS) (eg, closed system transfer devices [CSTDs], adapters, syringes) prior to dilution in the infusion bag.
After dilution of into the infusion bag, devices that contain polycarbonate or ABS, including infusion sets, may be used.

1. Withdraw the volume needed for the required dose (from the 90mg/mL sol).
2. Immediately transfer to a 500mL infusion bag of 0.9% NaCl. As an alternative, a 500mL infusion bag of 2.5% dextrose/0.45% NaCl may be considered. The resulting final concentration should be w/in 0.2-0.7mg/mL.
3. Administer diluted sol w/in 24 hrs when stored at 2-8°C (36-46°F) or w/in 2 hrs when stored at 15-30°C (59-86°F).

Powder:

Only use powder for inj if a CSTD or adapter that contains polycarbonate or ABS is used as supplemental protection during preparation.

1. Reconstitute 25mg vial w/ 5mL of sterile water for inj (SWFI) and 100mg vial w/ 20mL of SWFI.
2. Shake well to yield a clear, colorless to a pale yellow sol w/ a concentration of 5mg/mL; should completely dissolve in 5 min and transfer reconstituted sol to infusion bag w/in 30 min of reconstitution.
3. Withdraw the volume needed for the required dose and immediately transfer to 500mL infusion bag of 0.9% NaCl; as an alternative, a 500mL infusion bag of 2.5% dextrose/0.45% NaCl may be considered.
4. The resulting final concentration should be w/in 0.2-0.6mg/mL; thoroughly mix the contents of the infusion bag after transferring.
5. Administer w/in 24 hrs when stored at 2-8°C (36-46°F) or w/in 3 hrs when stored at 15-30°C (59-86°F).

HOW SUPPLIED

Inj: (Powder) 25mg, 100mg; (Sol) 45mg/0.5mL, 180mg/2mL

CONTRAINDICATIONS

Known hypersensitivity to bendamustine.

WARNINGS/PRECAUTIONS

Severe myelosuppression reported; may require dose delays and/or subsequent dose reductions if recovery to the recommended values has not occurred by the 1st day of the next scheduled cycle. Monitor leukocytes, platelets, Hgb, and neutrophils frequently if treatment-related myelosuppression occurs. Infection (eg, pneumonia, sepsis, hepatitis) and death reported. Increased risk for reactivation of infections (eg, hepatitis B, cytomegalovirus, herpes zoster); patients should undergo appropriate measures for infection and infection reactivation prior to administration. Infusion reactions and severe anaphylactic/anaphylactoid reactions reported; monitor clinically and d/c for severe reactions. Consider measures to prevent severe reactions (eg, antihistamines, antipyretics, corticosteroids) in subsequent cycles in patients who have experienced Grade 1 or 2 infusion reactions. Consider discontinuation for Grade 3 infusion reactions as clinically appropriate; d/c for Grade 4 infusion reactions. Do not rechallenge in patients who experience ≥Grade 3 allergic-type reactions. Tumor lysis syndrome reported; preventive measures include vigorous hydration and close monitoring of blood chemistry, particularly K^+ and uric acid levels. Skin reactions (eg, rash, toxic skin reactions, bullous exanthema) reported; monitor closely and withhold or d/c if skin reactions are severe or progressive. Premalignant and malignant diseases (eg, myelodysplastic syndrome, myeloproliferative disorders, acute myeloid leukemia, bronchial carcinoma) reported. Extravasations reported; assure good venous access prior to starting infusion and monitor for infusion-site redness, swelling, pain, infection, and necrosis during and after administration. May cause fetal harm. Caution w/ mild/moderate renal impairment and w/ mild hepatic impairment.

ADVERSE REACTIONS

Chronic Lymphocytic Leukemia: Pyrexia, nausea, vomiting.

Non-Hodgkin Lymphoma: Nausea, fatigue, vomiting, diarrhea, pyrexia.

DRUG INTERACTIONS

CYP1A2 inhibitors (eg, fluvoxamine, ciprofloxacin) may increase plasma concentrations of bendamustine and may decrease plasma concentrations of active metabolites. CYP1A2 inducers (eg, omeprazole, smoking) may decrease plasma concentrations of bendamustine and may increase plasma concentrations of active metabolites. Use caution or consider alternative treatments if treatment w/ CYP1A2 inhibitors/inducers is needed. May increase risk of severe skin toxicity w/ allopurinol.

T

PATIENT CONSIDERATIONS

Assessment: Assess for renal/hepatic impairment, hypersensitivity to drug, pregnancy/nursing status, and possible drug interactions.

Monitoring: Monitor for signs/symptoms of myelosuppression, infections, anaphylaxis/infusion reactions, tumor lysis syndrome, skin reactions, premalignant/malignant diseases, extravasation, lab abnormalities, and other adverse reactions. Monitor CBCs and blood chemistry, particularly K^+ and uric acid levels.

Counseling: Inform of the possibility of mild/serious allergic reactions and instruct to immediately report rash, facial swelling, or difficulty breathing during or soon after infusion. Inform that therapy may cause a decrease in WBC counts, platelets, and RBC counts, and of the need for frequent monitoring of blood counts; instruct to report SOB, significant fatigue, bleeding, fever, or other signs of infection. Advise that therapy may cause tiredness; instruct to avoid driving or operating dangerous tools or machinery if tiredness occurs. Inform that therapy may cause N/V, diarrhea, and mild rash or itching; instruct to report any adverse reactions immediately to physician. Advise women to avoid becoming pregnant and men to use reliable contraception throughout treatment and for 3 months after discontinuation of therapy; instruct to immediately report pregnancy and to avoid nursing while on therapy.

STORAGE: Sol: 2-8°C (36-47°F). Protect from light. **Powder:** Up to 25°C (77°F); excursions permitted up to 30°C (86°F). Protect from light.

TRESIBA – insulin degludec

RX

Class: Insulin (long-acting)

ADULT DOSAGE

Type 1 Diabetes Mellitus

Initial:

Insulin Naive:

Approx 1/3 to 1/2 of total daily insulin dose; as a general rule, 0.2-0.4 U/kg can be used to calculate initial total daily insulin dose

Give the remainder of the total daily insulin dose as a short-acting insulin and divided between each daily meal

Patients Already on Insulin Therapy:

Start at the same unit dose as the total daily long- or intermediate-acting insulin unit dose

Titrate: Adjust dose based on the patient's metabolic needs, blood glucose monitoring results, and glycemic control goal; recommended days between dose increases is 3 to 4 days

Type 2 Diabetes Mellitus

Initial:

Insulin Naive:

10 U qd

Patients Already on Insulin Therapy:

Start at the same unit dose as the total daily long- or intermediate-acting insulin unit dose

Titrate: Adjust dose based on the patient's metabolic needs, blood glucose monitoring results, and glycemic control goal; recommended days between dose increases is 3 to 4 days

Missed Dose

Inject daily dose during waking hrs upon discovering the missed dose; ensure that at least 8 hrs have elapsed between consecutive inj

PEDIATRIC DOSAGE

Pediatric use may not have been established

T

DOSING CONSIDERATIONS

Renal Impairment

Intensify glucose monitoring and adjust dose prn

Hepatic Impairment

Intensify glucose monitoring and adjust dose prn

Elderly

Dose conservatively

Other Important Considerations

Dosage adjustments may be needed w/ changes in physical activity, changes in meal patterns (eg, macronutrient content, timing of food intake), changes in renal/hepatic function, or during acute illness

ADMINISTRATION

SQ route

Inject into the thigh, upper arm, or abdomen, and rotate inj sites w/in the same region from 1 inj to the next.
Inject qd at the same time every day.
Do not administer IV, IM, or in an insulin infusion pump.
Do not dilute or mix w/ any other insulin products or sol.
Do not transfer from the pen into a syringe for administration.
Do not perform dose conversion when using the U-100 or U-200 FlexTouch pens; dose window for both the U-100 and U-200 FlexTouch pens shows the number of insulin units to be delivered and no conversion is needed.

HOW SUPPLIED

Inj: 100 U/mL, 200 U/mL [3mL]

CONTRAINDICATIONS

During episodes of hypoglycemia. Hypersensitivity to Tresiba or one of its excipients.

WARNINGS/PRECAUTIONS

Not recommended for the treatment of diabetic ketoacidosis. Never share prefilled pen between patients, even if the needle is changed; sharing poses a risk for transmission of blood-borne pathogens. Changes in insulin, manufacturer, type, or method of administration may affect glycemic control and predispose to hypo/hyperglycemia; these changes should be made cautiously and only under medical supervision and the frequency of blood glucose monitoring should be increased. Hypoglycemia may occur and may impair concentration ability and reaction time. Symptomatic awareness of hypoglycemia may be less pronounced in patients w/ longstanding diabetes, diabetic nerve disease, w/ medications that block the sympathetic nervous system (eg, β-blockers), or in patients who experience recurrent hypoglycemia. Accidental mix-ups between basal insulin products and other insulins, particularly rapid-acting insulins, reported. Do not transfer from the pen to a syringe; markings on the insulin syringe will not measure the dose correctly and can result in overdosage and severe hypoglycemia. Severe, life-threatening, generalized allergy, including anaphylaxis, may occur. D/C if a hypersensitivity reaction occurs; treat per standard of care and monitor until signs/symptoms resolve. May cause hypokalemia; monitor K^+ levels in patients at risk for hypokalemia (eg, patients using K^+-lowering medications or medications sensitive to serum K^+ concentrations) if indicated.

ADVERSE REACTIONS

Hypoglycemia, nasopharyngitis, URTI, headache, sinusitis, gastroenteritis, diarrhea, inj-site reactions, peripheral edema.

DRUG INTERACTIONS

Observe for signs/symptoms of CHF if treated concomitantly w/ a peroxisome proliferator-activated receptor (PPAR)-gamma agonist (eg, thiazolidinedione); consider discontinuation or dose reduction of the PPAR-gamma agonist if CHF develops. Antidiabetic agents, ACE inhibitors, ARBs, disopyramide, fibrates, fluoxetine, MAOIs, pentoxifylline, pramlintide, propoxyphene, salicylates, somatostatin analogues (eg, octreotide), sulfonamide antibiotics, GLP-1 receptor agonists, DPP-4 inhibitors, and SGLT-2 inhibitors may increase the risk of hypoglycemia; dose reductions and increased frequency of glucose monitoring may be required when coadministered w/ these drugs. Atypical antipsychotics (eg, olanzapine, clozapine), corticosteroids, danazol, diuretics, estrogens, glucagon, isoniazid, niacin, oral contraceptives, phenothiazines, progestogens (eg, in oral contraceptives), protease inhibitors, somatropin, sympathomimetic agents (eg, albuterol, epinephrine, terbutaline), and thyroid hormones may decrease the blood glucose lowering effect; dose increases and increased frequency of glucose monitoring may be required when coadministered w/ these drugs. Alcohol, β-blockers, clonidine, and lithium salts may increase or decrease the blood glucose lowering effect; dose adjustment and increased frequency of glucose monitoring may be required when coadministered w/ these drugs. Pentamidine may cause hypoglycemia, which may sometimes be followed by hyperglycemia; dose adjustment and increased frequency of glucose monitoring may be required when coadministered w/ this drug. β-blockers, clonidine, guanethidine, and reserpine may blunt signs/symptoms of hypoglycemia; increased frequency of glucose monitoring may be required when coadministered w/ these drugs. May need adjustments in concomitant oral antidiabetic treatment in patients w/ type 2 diabetes.

PATIENT CONSIDERATIONS

Assessment: Assess for diabetic ketoacidosis, predisposition to hypoglycemia, hypersensitivity, renal/hepatic impairment, pregnancy/nursing status, and possible drug interactions. Obtain baseline blood glucose, HbA1c, and K^+ levels.

Monitoring: Monitor for signs/symptoms of hypoglycemia, allergic reactions, hypokalemia, and other adverse reactions. Monitor blood glucose and HbA1c levels, and renal/hepatic function. Perform increased frequency of blood glucose monitoring in patients at higher risk for hypoglycemia and in patients who have reduced symptomatic awareness of hypoglycemia. Monitor K^+ levels in patients at risk for hypokalemia.

Counseling: Advise to never share pen device w/ another person, even if the needle is changed. Inform of hypoglycemia symptoms, including impairment of the ability to concentrate and react; advise to use caution when driving/operating machinery. Advise that changes in insulin regimen can predispose to hypo/hyperglycemia and that changes should be made under close medical supervision. Instruct to always check the label before each inj to avoid medication errors and to not dilute or mix w/ any other insulin or sol. Instruct on self-management procedures, including glucose monitoring, proper inj technique, management of hypo/hyperglycemia, and on handling of special situations (eg, intercurrent conditions, inadequate or skipped dose, inadvertent administration of increased insulin dose, inadequate food intake, skipped meals). Advise to inform physician if pregnant or contemplating pregnancy.

STORAGE: **Unopened:** 2-8°C (36-46°F) until expiration date. Do not store in freezer or directly adjacent to the refrigerator cooling element. Do not freeze and do not use if frozen. May also store at room temperature <30°C (86°F) for 56 days. **Open (In-Use):** Room temperature <30°C (86°F) for 56 days. Keep away from direct heat and light.

TREXIMET — naproxen sodium/sumatriptan RX

Class: 5-HT_1 agonist/NSAID

NSAIDs may increase risk of serious cardiovascular (CV) thrombotic events, MI, and stroke; risk may increase w/ duration of use and w/ cardiovascular disease (CVD) or risk factors for CVD. NSAIDs may increase risk of serious GI adverse events (eg, bleeding, ulceration, stomach/intestinal perforation) that can be fatal and can occur at any time during use and w/o warning symptoms; elderly patients are at greater risk.

ADULT DOSAGE

Migraine

Acute Treatment of Migraine w/ or w/o Aura:
1 tab of 85mg/500mg
Max: 2 tabs of 85mg/500mg in a 24-hr period, taken at least 2 hrs apart

PEDIATRIC DOSAGE

Migraine

Acute Treatment of Migraine w/ or w/o Aura:
12-17 Years:
1 tab of 10mg/60mg
Max: 1 tab of 85mg/500mg in a 24-hr period

DOSING CONSIDERATIONS

Renal Impairment
Severe (CrCl <30mL/min): Not recommended

Hepatic Impairment
Mild to Moderate: 1 tab of 10mg/60mg in a 24-hr period

Elderly
Not recommended in elderly patients who have decreased renal function, higher risk for unrecognized coronary artery disease, and increases in BP

ADMINISTRATION

Oral route

Take w/ or w/o food
Do not split, crush, or chew

HOW SUPPLIED

Tab: (Sumatriptan/Naproxen) 10mg/60mg, 85mg/500mg

CONTRAINDICATIONS

Ischemic coronary artery disease (eg, angina pectoris, history of MI, documented silent ischemia), coronary artery vasospasm (eg, Prinzmetal's angina), history of CABG surgery, Wolff-Parkinson-White syndrome or arrhythmias associated w/ other cardiac accessory conduction pathway disorders, history of stroke or transient ischemic attack (TIA) or history of hemiplegic/basilar migraine, peripheral vascular disease, ischemic bowel disease, uncontrolled HTN, severe hepatic impairment, 3rd trimester of pregnancy. Recent use (w/in 24 hrs) of another 5-HT_1-agonist, or of an ergotamine-containing or ergot-type medication (eg, dihydroergotamine, methysergide). Concurrent administration or recent use (w/in 2 weeks) of an MAO-A inhibitor. Asthma, urticaria, or other allergic-type reactions to aspirin (ASA) or other NSAIDs. Hypersensitivity to sumatriptan, naproxen, or any other component of Treximet.

WARNINGS/PRECAUTIONS

Use only if a clear diagnosis of migraine headache has been established; reconsider diagnosis before treating any subsequent attacks if patient has no response to the 1st migraine attack treated w/ therapy. Safety of treating >5 migraine headaches (adults) or >2 migraine headaches (pediatric patients) in a 30-day period not established. Serotonin syndrome may occur; d/c if suspected. Monitor renal function in patients w/ mild (CrCl=60-89mL/min) or moderate (CrCl=30-59mL/min) renal impairment, preexisting kidney disease, or dehydration. Anaphylactic reactions may occur; avoid w/ ASA triad. D/C if signs/symptoms consistent w/ liver disease develop, if systemic manifestations occur (eg, eosinophilia, rash), or if abnormal LFTs persist/worsen. Caution w/ asthma and avoid w/ ASA-sensitive asthma. Naproxen: Use w/ extreme caution w/ history of ulcer disease, GI bleeding, or risk factors for GI bleeding (eg, prolonged NSAID therapy, smoking, poor general health status); if a serious GI adverse event is suspected, d/c until adverse event is ruled out. Use lowest effective dose for

T

the shortest possible duration. May cause HTN or worsen preexisting HTN. Fluid retention, edema, and peripheral edema reported; caution w/ fluid retention or heart failure (HF), and in patients whose overall Na^+ intake must be severely restricted. Renal papillary necrosis and other renal injury reported w/ long-term use. Renal toxicity reported in patients in whom renal prostaglandins have a compensatory role in the maintenance of renal perfusion; increased risk w/ renal impairment, hypovolemia, HF, liver dysfunction, salt depletion, and in elderly. D/C if clinical signs/symptoms consistent w/ renal disease develop or if systemic manifestations occur. May cause serious skin adverse events (eg, exfoliative dermatitis, Stevens-Johnson syndrome, toxic epidermal necrolysis); d/c at 1st appearance of skin rash or any sign of hypersensitivity. May cause elevated LFTs; severe hepatic reactions reported. Anemia may occur; monitor Hgb/Hct if anemia develops w/ long-term use. Inhibits platelet aggregation and may prolong bleeding time. Lab test interactions may occur. Not recommended in labor and delivery. Sumatriptan: Serious cardiac adverse reactions (eg, acute MI) reported. May cause coronary artery vasospasm, even in patients w/o a history of coronary artery disease. Life-threatening cardiac rhythm disturbances (eg, ventricular tachycardia, ventricular fibrillation) leading to death, reported; d/c if these disturbances occur. Sensations of tightness, pain, pressure, and heaviness in the precordium, throat, neck, and jaw reported after treatment and are usually noncardiac in origin; perform a cardiac evaluation if at high cardiac risk. Cerebral/subarachnoid hemorrhage and stroke reported; d/c therapy if a cerebrovascular event occurs. Exclude other potentially serious neurological conditions prior to treating headaches in patients not previously diagnosed as migraineurs, and in migraineurs who present w/ atypical symptoms. May cause noncoronary vasospastic reactions (eg, peripheral vascular ischemia, GI vascular ischemia/infarction, splenic infarction, Raynaud's syndrome); rule out a vasospastic reaction before giving additional doses in patients who experience signs/symptoms. May cause transient/permanent blindness and significant partial vision loss. Significant elevation in BP, including hypertensive crisis w/ acute impairment of organ systems, reported. Overuse of acute migraine drugs may lead to exacerbation of headache; detoxification, including drug withdrawal, and treatment of withdrawal symptoms may be necessary. Seizures reported; caution w/ history of epilepsy or conditions associated w/ a lowered seizure threshold.

ADVERSE REACTIONS

CV thrombotic events, MI, stroke, GI adverse events, dizziness, somnolence, nausea, chest discomfort/pain, neck/throat/jaw pain/tightness/pressure.

DRUG INTERACTIONS

See Contraindications. Naproxen: May elevate and prolong serum methotrexate levels; monitor for methotrexate toxicity during concomitant use. Concomitant administration w/ ASA is not generally recommended due to increased risk of bleeding. May diminish antihypertensive effect of ACE inhibitors. Increased risk of renal toxicity w/ diuretics and ACE inhibitors. May reduce natriuretic effect of loop (eg, furosemide) or thiazide diuretics; monitor for signs of renal failure and to assure diuretic efficacy. Increased plasma lithium levels and reduced renal lithium clearance; monitor for signs of lithium toxicity. Probenecid increases plasma levels and extends plasma $T_{1/2}$ significantly. May reduce antihypertensive effect of propranolol and other β-blockers. Increased risk of serious GI bleeding w/ warfarin, oral corticosteroids or anticoagulants, alcohol use, and smoking. Sumatriptan: Serotonin syndrome reported w/ SSRIs, SNRIs, TCAs, and MAOIs; d/c if suspected.

PATIENT CONSIDERATIONS

Assessment: Assess for CV disease, HTN, history of hemiplegic or basilar migraine, history of stroke or TIA, peripheral vascular disease, ischemic bowel disease, Na^+ restriction, fluid retention, HF, renal/hepatic impairment, drug hypersensitivity, other conditions where treatment is contraindicated or cautioned, pregnancy/nursing status, and possible drug interactions. Perform a CV evaluation in patients who have multiple CV risk factors prior to therapy.

Monitoring: Monitor for signs/symptoms of CV/GI adverse events, cerebrovascular events, noncoronary vasospastic reactions, HTN, fluid retention, edema, medication overuse headache, serotonin syndrome, anaphylactic reactions, seizures, skin reactions, and other adverse reactions. Perform ECG immediately after administration of therapy in patients w/ multiple CV risk factors who have a negative CV evaluation; consider periodic CV evaluation in intermittent long-term users. Carefully monitor patients who may be adversely affected by alterations in platelet function (eg, w/ coagulation disorders, receiving anticoagulants).

Counseling: Inform about risks/benefits of therapy. Instruct to seek medical advice if signs/symptoms of CV events, GI ulcerations/bleeding, anaphylactic reaction, serious skin reaction, hepatotoxicity, unexplained weight gain or edema, or worsening of asthma occur. Inform that drug should be used during the 1st and 2nd trimester of pregnancy only if the potential benefit justifies the potential risk to the fetus; inform that drug should not be used during the 3rd trimester of pregnancy. Advise to notify physician if breastfeeding or planning to breastfeed. Caution about the risk of serotonin syndrome. Instruct to report to physician all medications being used. Inform that use of acute migraine drugs for ≥10 days/month may lead to an exacerbation of headache; encourage to record headache frequency and drug use (eg, by keeping a headache diary). Inform that treatment may cause somnolence and dizziness; instruct to evaluate ability to perform complex tasks after drug administration.

STORAGE: 25°C (77°F); excursions permitted to 15-30°C (59-86°F).

TRI-SPRINTEC – ethinyl estradiol/norgestimate

RX

Class: Estrogen/progestogen combination

Cigarette smoking increases risk of serious cardiovascular (CV) events. Risk increases w/ age (>35 yrs of age) and w/ the number of cigarettes smoked. Contraindicated in women who are >35 yrs of age and smoke.

ADULT DOSAGE

Contraception

1 tab qd at the same time each day, for 28 days, then repeat

Start either on 1st day of menses or on 1st Sunday after onset of menses

Acne Vulgaris

Moderate Acne in Females Who Desire Oral Contraception:
1 tab qd at the same time each day, for 28 days, then repeat

Start either on 1st day of menses or on 1st Sunday after onset of menses

Missed Dose

Miss 1 Active Tab in Weeks 1, 2, or 3: Take as soon as possible. Continue taking 1 tab qd until the pack is finished

Miss 2 Active Tabs in Weeks 1 or 2: Take the 2 missed tabs as soon as possible and the next 2 active tabs the next day. Continue taking 1 tab qd until pack is finished. Use additional nonhormonal contraception (eg, condom, spermicide) as backup if the patient has intercourse w/in 7 days after missing tabs

Miss 2 Active Tabs in Week 3 or Miss ≥3 Active Tabs in a Row in Weeks 1, 2, or 3: (Day 1 Start) Throw out the rest of the pack and start a new pack that same day. (Sunday Start) Continue taking 1 tab qd until Sunday, then throw out the rest of the pack and start a new pack that same day. (Day 1 Start/Sunday Start) Use additional nonhormonal contraception as backup if the patient has intercourse w/in 7 days after missing tabs

Conversions

Switching from Another Oral Contraceptive:
Start on the same day that a new pack of the previous oral contraceptive would have started

Switching from Another Contraceptive Method:
Transdermal Patch/Vaginal Ring/Inj:
Start therapy on the day when next application/insertion/inj would have been scheduled

Intrauterine Contraceptive:
Start on the day of removal; if the intrauterine device is not removed on the 1st day of menstrual cycle, additional nonhormonal contraceptive is needed for the first 7 days of the 1st cycle pack

Implant:
Start therapy on the day of removal

PEDIATRIC DOSAGE

Contraception

Not indicated for use premenarche; refer to adult dosing

Acne Vulgaris

Moderate Acne in Postpubertal Females ≥15 Years Who Desire Oral Contraception:
1 tab qd at the same time each day, for 28 days, then repeat

Start either on 1st day of menses or on 1st Sunday after onset of menses

T

DOSING CONSIDERATIONS

Adverse Reactions

GI Disturbances: In case of severe vomiting/diarrhea, absorption may not be complete and additional contraceptive measures should be taken; if vomiting/diarrhea occurs w/in 3-4 hrs after taking an active tab, handle this as a missed tab

Other Important Considerations

Starting Therapy after Abortion or Miscarriage:

1st Trimester: May start immediately; if starting therapy immediately, additional method of contraception is not needed. If therapy is not started w/in 5 days after termination of the pregnancy, use additional nonhormonal contraception for the first 7 days of 1st cycle pack

2nd Trimester: Do not start until 4 weeks after a 2nd trimester abortion or miscarriage

Starting Therapy after Childbirth:

Do not start until 4 weeks after delivery; consider possibility of ovulation and conception in women who have not yet had a period postpartum

ADMINISTRATION

Oral route

Take tabs in the order directed on the blister pack
Take w/o regard to meals

Sunday Start Regimen

Use additional nonhormonal method of contraception for the first 7 days of 1st cycle pack

HOW SUPPLIED

Tab: (Ethinyl Estradiol [EE]/Norgestimate) 0.035mg/0.18mg, 0.035mg/0.215mg, 0.035mg/0.25mg

CONTRAINDICATIONS

High risk of arterial/venous thrombotic diseases (eg, smoking [if >35 yrs of age], presence/history of deep vein thrombosis [DVT]/pulmonary embolism [PE], inherited or acquired hypercoagulopathies, cerebrovascular disease, coronary artery disease [CAD], thrombogenic valvular/ thrombogenic rhythm diseases of the heart [eg, subacute bacterial endocarditis w/ valvular disease or A-fib], uncontrolled HTN, diabetes mellitus [DM] w/ vascular disease, headaches w/ focal neurological symptoms or migraine headaches w/ aura [women >35 yrs of age w/ any migraine headaches]), benign/malignant liver tumors, liver disease, undiagnosed abnormal uterine bleeding, pregnancy, presence/history of breast cancer or other estrogen- or progestin-sensitive cancer.

WARNINGS/PRECAUTIONS

D/C if an arterial thrombotic event or venous thromboembolic event (VTE) occurs. D/C if there is unexplained loss of vision, proptosis, diplopia, papilledema, or retinal vascular lesions; evaluate for retinal vein thrombosis immediately. If feasible, d/c at least 4 weeks before and through 2 weeks after major surgery or other surgeries known to have an elevated risk of VTE as well as during and following prolonged immobilization. In women who are not breastfeeding, initiate therapy no earlier than 4 weeks after delivery; risk of postpartum VTE decreases after the 3rd postpartum week, whereas the risk of ovulation increases after the 3rd postpartum week. Increased risk of VTE and arterial thromboses (eg, strokes, MI). D/C if jaundice develops. Hepatic adenomas and increased risk of hepatocellular carcinoma reported. Increased BP reported; d/c if BP rises significantly. May increase risk of gallbladder disease or worsen existing gallbladder disease. May increase risk of cholestasis in women w/ history of pregnancy-related cholestasis. May decrease glucose tolerance. Consider alternative contraception w/ uncontrolled dyslipidemia. May increase risk of pancreatitis w/ hypertriglyceridemia or family history thereof. Evaluate the cause of new headaches that are recurrent, persistent, or severe, and d/c if indicated; consider discontinuation in the case of increased frequency or severity of migraine during use. Unscheduled bleeding and spotting may occur; rule out pregnancy or malignancy. May cause amenorrhea; amenorrhea or oligomenorrhea after discontinuation may occur. Caution w/ history of depression; d/c if depression recurs to a serious degree. May increase risk of cervical cancer or intraepithelial neoplasia. Chloasma may occur, especially w/ history of chloasma gravidarum; women w/ a tendency to chloasma should avoid exposure to the sun or UV radiation while on therapy. May interfere w/ lab tests (eg, coagulation factors, lipids, glucose tolerance, binding proteins). EE: In women w/ hereditary angioedema, may induce/exacerbate angioedema.

ADVERSE REACTIONS

Headache/migraine, breast issues (including breast pain, enlargement, discharge), vaginal infection, abdominal/GI pain, mood disorders (including mood alteration and depression), genital discharge, and changes in weight.

DRUG INTERACTIONS

Drugs or herbal products that induce certain enzymes, including CYP3A4 (eg, phenytoin, barbiturates, carbamazepine) may decrease levels and potentially diminish effectiveness of therapy or increase breakthrough bleeding; use an alternative or back-up method of contraception when using enzyme inducers and continue back-up contraception for 28 days after discontinuing the enzyme inducer. CYP3A4 inhibitors (eg, itraconazole, voriconazole, grapefruit juice) may increase levels. Significant changes (increase/decrease) in estrogen and/or progestin levels reported w/ HIV/hepatitis C virus protease inhibitors or non-nucleoside reverse transcriptase inhibitors. May decrease levels of acetaminophen (APAP), clofibric acid, morphine, salicylic acid, and temazepam.

T

May significantly decrease levels of lamotrigine and may reduce seizure control; dosage adjustment of lamotrigine may be necessary. Women on thyroid hormone replacement therapy may need to increase dose of thyroid hormone due to increased levels of thyroid-binding globulin. EE: Colesevelam reported to significantly decrease EE exposure; decreased drug interaction when the 2 drug products are given 4 hrs apart. Atorvastatin or rosuvastatin may increase EE exposure; ascorbic acid and APAP may increase EE levels. May inhibit metabolism and increase levels of other compounds (eg, cyclosporine, prednisolone, theophylline, tizanidine, voriconazole).

PATIENT CONSIDERATIONS

Assessment: Assess for DVT, PE, cerebrovascular disease, CAD, DM w/ vascular disease, headaches w/ focal neurological symptoms or migraine headaches w/ aura, pregnancy/nursing status, any other conditions where treatment is contraindicated or cautioned, and possible drug interactions.

Monitoring: Monitor for bleeding irregularities, venous/arterial thrombotic events, cervical cancer or intraepithelial neoplasia, retinal vein thrombosis or any other ophthalmic changes, jaundice, new/worsening headaches or migraines, depression, cholestasis w/ history of pregnancy-related cholestasis, pancreatitis, and other adverse reactions. Monitor BP in women w/ HTN, glucose levels in diabetic or prediabetic women, and lipid levels w/ dyslipidemia. Conduct a yearly visit in all patients for a BP check and for other indicated healthcare.

Counseling: Inform of risks/benefits of therapy. Advise to take ud. Counsel that cigarette smoking increases the risk of serious CV events and women who are >35 yrs of age and smoke should not use combination oral contraceptives (COCs). Inform of the risk of VTE. Inform that the drug does not protect against HIV infection (AIDS) and other sexually transmitted infections. Advise not to use during pregnancy; if pregnancy occurs during use, instruct to stop further use. Instruct on what to do in the event tabs are missed. Counsel to use a back-up or alternative method of contraception when enzyme inducers are used w/ therapy. Inform that COCs may reduce breast milk production. Counsel women who start COCs postpartum and have not yet had a period, to use an additional method of contraception until an active pill has been taken for 7 consecutive days. Inform that amenorrhea may occur; consider pregnancy in the event of amenorrhea at the time of 1st missed period, and rule out pregnancy in the event of amenorrhea in ≥2 consecutive cycles.

STORAGE: 20-25°C (68-77°F). Protect from light.

TRIBENZOR — amlodipine/hydrochlorothiazide/olmesartan medoxomil RX

Class: Angiotensin II receptor blocker (ARB)/calcium channel blocker (CCB) (dihydropyridine)/thiazide diuretic

D/C when pregnancy is detected. Drugs that act directly on the renin-angiotensin system (RAS) can cause injury/death to the developing fetus.

ADULT DOSAGE

Hypertension

Usual: Dose qd

Titrate: May increase dose after 2 weeks

Max: 40mg/10mg/25mg qd

Replacement Therapy:

May substitute for individually titrated components

Add-On/Switch Therapy:

May use for patients not adequately controlled on any 2 of the following classes: ARBs, calcium channel blockers (CCBs), and diuretics

Patients w/ dose-limiting adverse reactions to an individual component while on any dual combination of the components of therapy may be switched to therapy containing a lower dose of that component

PEDIATRIC DOSAGE

Pediatric use may not have been established

DOSING CONSIDERATIONS

Hepatic Impairment

Severe:

Initial: 2.5mg amlodipine

Elderly

≥75 Years:

Initial: 2.5mg amlodipine

ADMINISTRATION
Oral route

Take w/ or w/o food

HOW SUPPLIED
Tab: (Olmesartan/Amlodipine/HCTZ) 20mg/5mg/12.5mg, 40mg/5mg/12.5mg, 40mg/5mg/25mg, 40mg/10mg/12.5mg, 40mg/10mg/25mg

CONTRAINDICATIONS
Anuria, sulfonamide-derived drug hypersensitivity. Coadministration with aliskiren in patients with diabetes.

WARNINGS/PRECAUTIONS
Not for initial therapy. Avoid use with severe renal impairment (CrCl ≤30mL/min). Renal impairment reported; consider withholding or discontinuing either diuretic or ARBs if progressive renal impairment becomes evident. Sprue-like enteropathy with symptoms of severe, chronic diarrhea with substantial weight loss reported; exclude other etiologies if these symptoms develop and consider discontinuation in cases where no other etiology is identified. Olmesartan: Symptomatic hypotension may occur in patients with an activated RAS (eg, volume- and/or salt-depleted patients [eg, those being treated with high doses of diuretics]). Oliguria or progressive azotemia and (rarely) with acute renal failure and/or death may occur in patients whose renal function may depend upon the activity of the renin-angiotensin-aldosterone system (eg, with severe CHF). May increase SrCr and BUN levels in patients with renal artery stenosis. Increased blood creatinine levels and hyperkalemia reported. Amlodipine: May develop increased frequency, duration, or severity of angina or acute MI, particularly with severe obstructive coronary artery disease (CAD). Rare reports of acute hypotension; caution with severe aortic stenosis. Hepatic enzyme elevations reported. HCTZ: May precipitate azotemia with renal disease and hepatic coma due to fluid and electrolyte imbalance. Observe for clinical signs of fluid or electrolyte imbalance (eg, hyponatremia, hypochloremic alkalosis, hypokalemia). Hypokalemia may sensitize/exaggerate the response of the heart to toxic effects of digitalis. May cause metabolic acidosis, hyperuricemia or precipitation of frank gout, hyperglycemia, manifestation of latent diabetes mellitus (DM), hypomagnesemia, hypersensitivity reactions (with or without a history of allergy or bronchial asthma), exacerbation/activation of systemic lupus erythematosus (SLE), and increased cholesterol and TG levels. Enhanced effects in postsympathectomy patients. D/C before carrying out tests for parathyroid function. May cause idiosyncratic reaction, resulting in acute transient myopia and acute angle-closure glaucoma; d/c as rapidly as possible.

ADVERSE REACTIONS
Dizziness, peripheral edema, headache, fatigue, nasopharyngitis, muscle spasms, nausea.

DRUG INTERACTIONS
See Contraindications. Olmesartan: NSAIDs, including selective COX-2 inhibitors, may attenuate antihypertensive effect and result in deterioration of renal function, including possible acute renal failure; monitor renal function periodically. Dual blockade of the RAS is associated with increased risk of hypotension, hyperkalemia, and changes in renal function (including acute renal failure); avoid combined use of RAS inhibitors or closely monitor BP, renal function, and electrolytes with concomitant agents that affect the RAS. Avoid with aliskiren in patients with renal impairment (GFR <60mL/min). Reduced systemic exposure and levels with colesevelam; administer at least 4 hrs before colesevelam dose. Amlodipine: May increase simvastatin exposure; limit simvastatin dose to 20mg daily. HCTZ: Alcohol, barbiturates, or narcotics may potentiate orthostatic hypotension. Dose adjustment of antidiabetic drugs (eg, oral agents, insulin) may be required. Additive effect or potentiation with other antihypertensives. Anionic exchange resins (eg, cholestyramine, colestipol) may impair absorption. Corticosteroids and adrenocorticotropic hormone may intensify electrolyte depletion, particularly hypokalemia. May decrease response to pressor amines (eg, norepinephrine). May increase response to nondepolarizing skeletal muscle relaxants (eg, tubocurarine). NSAIDs may reduce diuretic, natriuretic, and antihypertensive effects. Olmesartan/HCTZ: Increases in serum lithium concentrations and lithium toxicity reported; monitor lithium levels.

PATIENT CONSIDERATIONS

Assessment: Assess for anuria, sulfonamide-derived drug hypersensitivity, aortic stenosis, renal artery stenosis, SLE, CHF, volume/salt depletion, electrolyte imbalances, postsympathectomy status, DM, CAD, renal/hepatic impairment, pregnancy/nursing status, any other conditions where treatment is cautioned, and possible drug interactions.

Monitoring: Monitor for signs/symptoms of hypotension, angina, MI, fluid/electrolyte imbalance, latent DM, sprue-like enteropathy, exacerbation/activation of SLE, hypersensitivity/idiosyncratic reactions, metabolic disturbances, myopia and angle-closure glaucoma, and other adverse reactions. Monitor BP, serum electrolytes, cholesterol and TG levels, and renal/hepatic function.

Counseling: Inform female of childbearing potential of the consequences of exposure during pregnancy and of the treatment options for women planning to become pregnant; instruct to report pregnancy to physician as soon as possible. Counsel that lightheadedness may occur, especially during the 1st days of therapy; instruct to report to physician. Instruct to d/c therapy and consult physician if syncope occurs. Advise that inadequate fluid intake, excessive perspiration, diarrhea, or vomiting may lead to an excessive fall in BP, which may result in lightheadedness and possible syncope.

STORAGE: 25°C (77°F); excursions permitted to 15-30°C (59-86°F).

TRICOR – fenofibrate

RX

Class: Fibric acid derivative

ADULT DOSAGE

Primary Hypercholesterolemia/Mixed Dyslipidemia

Initial/Max: 145mg qd
Titrate: May consider reducing dose if lipid levels fall significantly below the targeted range

D/C if no adequate response after 2 months of treatment w/ max dose

Severe Hypertriglyceridemia

Initial: 48-145mg/day
Titrate: Adjust dose if necessary following repeat lipid determinations at 4- to 8-week intervals; may consider reducing dose if lipid levels fall significantly below the targeted range
Max: 145mg qd

D/C if no adequate response after 2 months of treatment w/ max dose

PEDIATRIC DOSAGE

Pediatric use may not have been established

DOSING CONSIDERATIONS

Renal Impairment
Mild to Moderate:
Initial: 48mg/day
Titrate: Increase only after evaluation of effects on renal function and lipid levels

ADMINISTRATION

Oral route

May be taken w/o regard to meals
Swallow tab whole

HOW SUPPLIED

Tab: 48mg, 145mg

CONTRAINDICATIONS

Severe renal impairment (including dialysis), active liver disease (including primary biliary cirrhosis and unexplained persistent liver function abnormalities), preexisting gallbladder disease, and nursing mothers. Known hypersensitivity to fenofibrate or fenofibric acid.

WARNINGS/PRECAUTIONS

Not shown to reduce coronary heart disease morbidity and mortality in patients with type 2 diabetes mellitus (DM). Increased risk of myopathy and rhabdomyolysis; risk increased with DM, renal insufficiency, hypothyroidism, and in elderly. D/C therapy if marked CPK elevation occurs or myopathy/myositis is suspected or diagnosed. Increases in serum transaminases, hepatocellular, chronic active and cholestatic hepatitis, and cirrhosis (rare) reported; perform baseline and regular periodic monitoring of LFTs, and d/c therapy if enzyme levels persist >3X the normal limit. Elevations in SrCr reported; monitor renal function in patients with renal impairment or at risk for renal insufficiency. May cause cholelithiasis; d/c if gallstones are found. Acute hypersensitivity reactions and pancreatitis reported. Mild to moderate decreases in Hgb, Hct and WBCs, thrombocytopenia, and agranulocytosis reported; periodically monitor RBC and WBC counts during the first 12 months of therapy. May cause venothromboembolic disease. Severe decreases in HDL levels reported; check HDL levels within the 1st few months after initiation of therapy. If a severely depressed HDL level is detected, withdraw therapy, monitor HDL level until it has returned to baseline, and do not reinitiate therapy. Estrogen therapy, thiazide diuretics, and β-blockers may be associated with massive rises in plasma TG; discontinuation of these drugs may obviate the need for specific drug therapy of hypertriglyceridemia.

ADVERSE REACTIONS

Abnormal LFTs, respiratory disorder, abdominal pain, back pain, increased AST/ALT/CPK, headache.

T

DRUG INTERACTIONS

Increased risk of rhabdomyolysis with HMG-CoA reductase inhibitors (statins); avoid combination unless benefit outweighs risk. May potentiate anticoagulant effects of coumarin anticoagulants; use with caution, reduce anticoagulant dosage, and monitor PT/INR frequently. Immunosuppressants (eg, cyclosporine, tacrolimus) may produce nephrotoxicity; consider benefits and risks, use lowest effective dose, and monitor renal function with immunosuppressants and other potentially nephrotoxic agents. Bile acid-binding resins may bind other drugs given concurrently; take at least 1 hr before or 4-6 hrs after the bile acid-binding resin to avoid impeding its absorption. Cases of myopathy, including rhabdomyolysis, reported when coadministered with colchicine; caution when prescribing with colchicine.

PATIENT CONSIDERATIONS

Assessment: Assess for renal impairment, active liver disease, preexisting gallbladder disease, other medical conditions (eg, DM, hypothyroidism), hypersensitivity to drug, pregnancy/nursing status, and possible drug interactions. Obtain baseline LFTs.

Monitoring: Monitor for signs/symptoms of myositis, myopathy, or rhabdomyolysis; measure CPK levels in patients reporting such symptoms. Monitor for cholelithiasis, pancreatitis, hypersensitivity reactions, pulmonary embolism, and deep vein thrombosis. Monitor renal function, LFTs, CBC, and lipid levels. Monitor PT/INR frequently with coumarin anticoagulants.

Counseling: Advise of potential benefits and risks of therapy, and of medications to avoid during treatment. Instruct to follow appropriate lipid-modifying diet during therapy and to take drug qd, at the prescribed dose. Instruct to inform physician of all medications, supplements, and herbal preparations being taken, any changes in medical condition, development of muscle pain, tenderness, or weakness, and onset of abdominal pain or any other new symptoms. Advise to return for routine monitoring.

STORAGE: 25°C (77°F); excursions permitted to 15-30°C (59-86°F). Protect from moisture.

TRILEPTAL – oxcarbazepine

RX

Class: Dibenzazepine

ADULT DOSAGE

Partial Seizures

Adjunctive Therapy:

Initial: 300mg bid

Titrate: Increase by a max of 600mg/day at weekly intervals

Usual: 1200mg/day

Conversion to Monotherapy:

Initial: 300mg bid

Titrate: Increase by a max of 600mg/day at weekly intervals

Usual: 2400mg/day

Reduce dose and withdraw concomitant antiepileptic drugs over 3-6 weeks, while reaching max oxcarbazepine dose in about 2-4 weeks

Initiation of Monotherapy:

Initial: 300mg bid

Titrate: Increase by 300mg/day every third day

Usual: 1200mg/day

PEDIATRIC DOSAGE

Partial Seizures

Adjunctive Therapy:

2-<4 Years:

Initial: 8-10mg/kg/day, not to exceed 600mg/day; may consider 16-20mg/kg for patients <20kg

Titrate: Increase to max maint dose over 2-4 weeks

Max: 60mg/kg/day

4-16 Years:

Initial: 8-10mg/kg/day, not to exceed 600mg/day

Maint: Increase to target dose over 2 weeks

20-29kg: 450mg bid

29.1-39kg: 600mg bid

>39kg: 900mg bid

W/ Epilepsy:

Conversion to Monotherapy:

4-16 Years:

Initial: 8-10mg/kg/day

Titrate: Increase by a max of 10mg/kg/day at weekly intervals

Reduce dose and withdraw concomitant antiepileptic drugs over 3-6 weeks

Initiation of Monotherapy:

4-16 Years:

Initial: 8-10mg/kg/day

Titrate: Increase by 5mg/kg/day every third day

Conversion to/Initiation of Monotherapy:

Maint:

20kg: 600-900mg/day

T

25-30kg: 900-1200mg/day
35-40kg: 900-1500mg/day
45kg: 1200-1500mg/day
50-55kg: 1200-1800mg/day
60-65kg: 1200-2100mg/day
70kg: 1500-2100mg/day

DOSING CONSIDERATIONS

Renal Impairment

CrCl <30mL/min:

Initial: 1/2 the usual starting dose (300mg/day)
Titrate: Increase slowly

ADMINISTRATION

Oral route

All dosing should be given in a bid regimen
Sus and tabs may be interchanged at equal doses
Take w/ or w/o food

Sus

1. Before use, shake well and prepare dose immediately afterwards
2. Use the supplied oral dosing syringe to withdraw the prescribed amount from the bottle
3. Sus may be mixed in a small glass of water just prior to administration or may be swallowed directly from the syringe
4. Close the bottle and rinse the syringe w/ warm water and allow it to dry thoroughly after each use

HOW SUPPLIED

Sus: 300mg/5mL [250mL]; **Tab:** 150mg*, 300mg*, 600mg* *scored

CONTRAINDICATIONS

Known hypersensitivity to oxcarbazepine or to any of its components.

WARNINGS/PRECAUTIONS

Clinically significant hyponatremia may develop; consider measurement of serum Na^+ levels during maintenance treatment, particularly if patient is receiving other medications known to decrease serum Na^+ levels (eg, drugs associated w/ inappropriate antidiuretic hormone secretion) or if symptoms indicating hyponatremia develop. Anaphylaxis and angioedema involving the larynx, glottis, lips, and eyelids reported; d/c therapy if any of these reactions develop, start alternative treatment, and do not rechallenge. Caution in patients w/ history of hypersensitivity reactions to carbamazepine; d/c immediately if signs/symptoms of hypersensitivity develop. Serious dermatological reactions (eg, Stevens-Johnson syndrome [SJS], toxic epidermal necrolysis [TEN]) reported; consider discontinuing use and prescribing another antiepileptic drug (AED) if a skin reaction develops. Patients carrying the human leukocyte antigen (HLA)-B*1502 allele may be at increased risk for SJS/TEN; consider testing for presence of HLA-B*1502 allele in patients w/ ancestry in genetically at-risk populations, and avoid use in patients positive for HLA-B*1502 unless benefits clearly outweigh risks. Increased risk of suicidal thoughts or behavior. Withdraw gradually to minimize the potential of increased seizure frequency. Associated w/ CNS-related adverse events (cognitive symptoms, somnolence or fatigue, coordination abnormalities). Drug reaction w/ eosinophilia and systemic symptoms (DRESS)/multiorgan hypersensitivity reported; evaluate immediately if signs/symptoms (eg, rash, fever, lymphadenopathy) are present, and d/c if an alternative etiology cannot be established. Pancytopenia, agranulocytosis, and leukopenia reported; consider discontinuation if any evidence of hematologic events develop. Levels may decrease during pregnancy; monitor patients during pregnancy and through the postpartum period. Associated w/ decreases in T4, without changes in T3 or TSH. Caution w/ severe hepatic impairment.

ADVERSE REACTIONS

Dizziness, somnolence, diplopia, fatigue, N/V, ataxia, abnormal vision, tremor, abnormal gait, dyspepsia, abdominal pain.

DRUG INTERACTIONS

Verapamil, valproic acid, and strong CYP450 inducers (eg, carbamazepine, phenytoin, phenobarbital) may decrease levels. May decrease levels of dihydropyridine calcium antagonists, oral contraceptives (eg, ethinyl estradiol, levonorgestrel), cyclosporine, and felodipine. May increase levels of phenytoin, phenobarbital, and CYP2C19 substrates; may require dose reduction of phenytoin when using oxcarbazepine doses >1200mg/day. Decreased levels w/ AEDs that are CYP450 inducers.

PATIENT CONSIDERATIONS

Assessment: Assess for history of hypersensitivity to drug or to carbamazepine, presence of HLA-B*1502 allele, depression, renal/hepatic impairment, pregnancy/nursing status, and possible drug interactions.

Monitoring: Monitor for signs/symptoms of hyponatremia, angioedema, anaphylactic/hypersensitivity/dermatological reactions, emergence/worsening of depression, suicidal thoughts/behavior, unusual changes in mood/behavior, cognitive/neuropsychiatric events, DRESS, hematologic events, and other adverse reactions. Monitor patients during pregnancy and through the postpartum period.

Counseling: Advise to report symptoms of low Na^+, and fever to physician. Instruct to d/c and contact physician immediately if signs/symptoms suggesting angioedema develop. Advise to consult physician immediately if experiencing a hypersensitivity reaction, skin reaction, or symptoms suggestive of blood disorders. Warn female patients of childbearing age that concurrent use w/ hormonal contraceptives may render this method of contraception less effective; advise to use additional nonhormonal forms of contraception. Advise of the need to be alert for the emergence/worsening of symptoms of depression, any unusual changes in mood/behavior, or the emergence of suicidal thoughts, behavior, or thoughts about self-harm; instruct to immediately report behaviors of concern to physician. Instruct to use caution if taking alcohol while on therapy. Advise that drug may cause dizziness and somnolence, and not to drive or operate machinery until effects have been determined. Encourage to enroll in the North American Antiepileptic Drug Pregnancy Registry if patient becomes pregnant.

STORAGE: 25°C (77°F); excursions permitted to 15-30°C (59-86°F). (Sus) Use w/in 7 weeks of 1st opening the bottle.

TRILIPIX – fenofibric acid

Class: Fibric acid derivative

RX

ADULT DOSAGE

Severe Hypertriglyceridemia

Initial: 45-135mg qd
Titrate: Adjust dose if necessary following repeat lipid determinations at 4- to 8-week intervals
Max: 135mg qd

Primary Hypercholesterolemia/Mixed Dyslipidemia

135mg qd

PEDIATRIC DOSAGE

Pediatric use may not have been established

DOSING CONSIDERATIONS

Renal Impairment
Mild to Moderate:
Initial: 45mg qd
Titrate: Increase only after evaluation of effects on renal function and lipid levels

Other Important Considerations
D/C or change medications known to exacerbate hypertriglyceridemia (eg, β-blockers, thiazides, estrogens) if possible before considering therapy
Address excessive alcohol intake before therapy is considered

ADMINISTRATION

Oral route

May be taken w/o regard to meals.
Swallow cap whole; do not open, crush, dissolve, or chew.

HOW SUPPLIED

Cap, Delayed-Release: 45mg, 135mg

CONTRAINDICATIONS

Severe renal impairment (including dialysis), active liver disease (including primary biliary cirrhosis and unexplained persistent liver function abnormalities), preexisting gallbladder disease, and nursing mothers. Known hypersensitivity to fenofibrate or fenofibric acid.

WARNINGS/PRECAUTIONS

Not shown to reduce coronary heart disease morbidity and mortality in patients w/ type 2 diabetes mellitus (DM). Not indicated for patients who have elevations of chylomicrons and plasma TGs, but have normal VLDL levels. Increased risk of myositis/myopathy and rhabdomyolysis; risk increased w/ DM, renal failure, hypothyroidism, and in elderly. D/C therapy if markedly elevated CPK levels occur or myopathy/myositis is suspected or diagnosed. Increases in serum transaminases; hepatocellular, chronic active, and cholestatic hepatitis; and cirrhosis (rare) reported. Perform baseline and regular monitoring of LFTs, and d/c therapy if enzyme levels persist >3X ULN. Reversible elevations in SrCr reported. May cause cholelithiasis; d/c if gallstones are found. Acute

T

hypersensitivity reactions (eg, Stevens-Johnson syndrome, toxic necrolysis) and pancreatitis reported. Mild to moderate decreases in Hgb, Hct, and WBCs reported. Thrombocytopenia and agranulocytosis reported; periodically monitor RBC and WBC counts during the first 12 months of therapy. May cause venothromboembolic disease. Severe decreases in HDL levels reported; check HDL levels w/in the 1st few months after initiation of therapy. If a severely depressed HDL level is detected, withdraw therapy, monitor HDL level until it has returned to baseline, and do not reinitiate therapy.

ADVERSE REACTIONS

Headache, back pain, abdominal pain, respiratory disorder, diarrhea, dyspepsia, pain, nasopharyngitis, sinusitis, URTI, arthralgia, myalgia, pain in extremity, dizziness.

DRUG INTERACTIONS

Increased risk of rhabdomyolysis w/ HMG-CoA reductase inhibitors (statins). May potentiate anticoagulant effects of coumarin anticoagulants prolonging PT/INR; use w/ caution, reduce anticoagulant dosage, and monitor PT/INR frequently. Bile acid-binding resins may bind other drugs given concurrently; take at least 1 hr before or 4-6 hrs after the bile acid resin to avoid impeding its absorption. Immunosuppressants (eg, cyclosporine, tacrolimus) may produce nephrotoxicity; consider benefits and risks, and use lowest effective dose w/ immunosuppressants and other potentially nephrotoxic agents. Cases of myopathy, including rhabdomyolysis, reported when coadministered w/ colchicine; caution when prescribing w/ colchicine.

PATIENT CONSIDERATIONS

Assessment: Assess for renal impairment, active liver disease, preexisting gallbladder disease, other medical conditions (eg, DM, hypothyroidism), hypersensitivity to drug, pregnancy/nursing status, and possible drug interactions. Obtain baseline LFTs.

Monitoring: Monitor for signs/symptoms of myositis, myopathy, or rhabdomyolysis; measure CPK levels in patients reporting such symptoms. Monitor for cholelithiasis, pancreatitis, hypersensitivity reactions, pulmonary embolism, and deep vein thrombosis. Monitor renal function, LFTs, CBC, and lipid levels. Monitor PT/INR frequently w/ coumarin anticoagulants.

Counseling: Advise of the potential benefits and risks of therapy, and of medications to avoid during treatment. Advise to read the Medication Guide before therapy and reread each time prescription is renewed. Instruct to follow appropriate lipid-modifying diet during therapy, and to take drug ud. Advise to return for routine monitoring. Instruct to inform physician of all medications, supplements, and herbal preparations being taken, any changes in medical condition, development of muscle pain, tenderness, or weakness, and onset of abdominal pain or any other new symptoms.

STORAGE: 25°C (77°F); excursions permitted to 15-30°C (59-86°F). Protect from moisture.

TRIOSTAT – liothyronine sodium

RX

Class: Thyroid replacement hormone

Drugs with thyroid hormone activity, alone or together with other therapeutic agents, have been used for the treatment of obesity. Doses within the range of daily hormonal requirements are ineffective for weight reduction in euthyroid patients. Larger doses may produce serious or life-threatening manifestations of toxicity, particularly when given in association with sympathomimetic amines, such as those used for their anorectic effects.

ADULT DOSAGE

Myxedema Coma/Precoma

Initial: 25-50mcg IV (emergency treatment) or 10-20mcg IV (w/ known/suspected cardiovascular disease)

Initial and subsequent doses should be based on continuous monitoring of clinical status and response to therapy

At least 4 hrs and no more than 12 hrs should elapse between doses

Conversions

Switching to Oral Therapy:
Resume as soon as clinical situation has been stabilized and patient is able to take oral medication

Switching to Liothyronine Sodium:
D/C therapy, initiate oral therapy at a low dose, and increase gradually according to response

PEDIATRIC DOSAGE

Pediatric use may not have been established

Switching to L-thyroxine:
D/C gradually if L-thyroxine rather than liothyronine sodium is used in initiating oral therapy due to the delay of several days in the onset of L-thyroxine activity

DOSING CONSIDERATIONS

Elderly
Start at lower end of dosing range

ADMINISTRATION

IV route

IV administration only; should not be given IM or SQ
Administer at least 4 hrs and not more than 12 hrs apart

HOW SUPPLIED

Inj: 10mcg/mL [1mL]

CONTRAINDICATIONS

Uncorrected adrenal cortical insufficiency, untreated thyrotoxicosis, artificial rewarming. Hypersensitivity to any of the active or extraneous constituents of Triostat.

WARNINGS/PRECAUTIONS

Not for IM or SQ route. Use is unjustified for the treatment of male or female infertility unless accompanied by hypothyroidism. Caution with CVD (eg, angina pectoris) or in elderly; monitor cardiac function. Caution in myxedematous patients; start at a low dose level and increase gradually. Supplemental adrenocortical steroids may be necessary in patients with severe and prolonged hypothyroidism. May precipitate a hyperthyroid state or aggravate hyperthyroidism. May aggravate symptoms of diabetes mellitus (DM), diabetes insipidus (DI), or adrenal cortical insufficiency. Monitor and treat infection appropriately in myxedema coma patients. Therapy of myxedema coma requires simultaneous administration of glucocorticoids. Concurrent use with androgens, corticosteroids, estrogens, oral contraceptives containing estrogens, iodine-containing preparations, and salicylates may interfere with thyroid laboratory tests.

ADVERSE REACTIONS

Arrhythmia, tachycardia.

DRUG INTERACTIONS

See Boxed Warning. Hypothyroidism decreases and hyperthyroidism increases sensitivity to anticoagulants; monitor PT closely and adjust anticoagulants based on frequent PT determinations. May cause increases in insulin or oral hypoglycemic requirements during thyroid replacement initiation. Estrogens increase thyroxine-binding globulin; increase in thyroid dose may be needed in patients without a functioning thyroid gland. Increased effects of both agents with TCAs (eg, imipramine). May cause HTN and tachycardia with ketamine; use with caution and treat HTN if necessary. May potentiate toxic effects of digitalis. Increased adrenergic effect of catecholamines (eg, epinephrine, norepinephrine). May increase risk of precipitating coronary insufficiency, especially with coronary artery disease (CAD) with vasopressors; use with caution. Caution when administering fluid therapy.

PATIENT CONSIDERATIONS

Assessment: Assess thyroid status, CVD (eg, CAD, angina pectoris), DM/DI, adrenal cortical insufficiency, nursing status, and for possible drug interactions.

Monitoring: Monitor for signs/symptoms of precipitation of adrenocortical insufficiency, aggravation of DM/DI, infection, hypersensitivity reactions, and other adverse reactions. Monitor thyroid function periodically. Monitor patient's clinical status and response to therapy. Monitor PT closely in thyroid-treated patients on anticoagulants and adjust anticoagulants based on frequent PT determinations.

Counseling: Inform of the risks/benefits of therapy. Instruct to seek medical attention if symptoms of toxicity, aggravation of DM/DI, or hypersensitivity reactions occur.

STORAGE: 2-8°C (36-46°F).

TRIUMEQ — abacavir/dolutegravir/lamivudine

RX

Class: Integrase strand transfer inhibitor/nucleoside analogue reverse transcriptase inhibitors

Lactic acidosis and severe hepatomegaly w/ steatosis, including fatal cases, reported w/ nucleoside analogues; d/c if clinical or lab findings suggestive of lactic acidosis or pronounced hepatotoxicity occur. Abacavir: Serious and sometimes fatal hypersensitivity reactions, w/ multiple organ involvement, reported; d/c immediately if a hypersensitivity reaction is suspected and never restart therapy or any other abacavir-containing product. Patients who carry the HLA-B*5701 allele are at a higher risk of a hypersensitivity reaction; screen all patients for HLA-B*5701 allele prior to initiating or reinitiating therapy, unless patient has a previously documented HLA-B*5701 allele assessment. Lamivudine: Severe acute exacerbations of hepatitis B reported in patients coinfected w/ hepatitis B virus (HBV) and HIV-1 and have discontinued therapy; closely monitor hepatic function and, if appropriate, initiate antihepatitis B therapy.

ADULT DOSAGE

HIV-1 Infection

1 tab qd

PEDIATRIC DOSAGE

Pediatric use may not have been established

DOSING CONSIDERATIONS

Concomitant Medications

Efavirenz, Fosamprenavir/Ritonavir, Tipranavir/Ritonavir (RTV), Carbamazepine, or Rifampin: Take an additional dolutegravir 50mg tab, separated by 12 hrs from therapy

Renal Impairment

CrCl <50mL/min: Not recommended; if a dose reduction of lamivudine is required, use the individual components

Hepatic Impairment

Mild (Child-Pugh Score A): Use individual components if a dose reduction of abacavir is required

ADMINISTRATION

Oral route

Take w/ or w/o food.
Screen for the HLA-B*5701 allele prior to initiating therapy.

HOW SUPPLIED

Tab: (Abacavir/Dolutegravir/Lamivudine) 600mg/50mg/300mg

CONTRAINDICATIONS

Patients w/ HLA-B*5701 allele, prior hypersensitivity reaction to abacavir, dolutegravir, or lamivudine, coadministration w/ dofetilide, moderate or severe hepatic impairment.

WARNINGS/PRECAUTIONS

Not recommended for use w/ current or past history of resistance to any components of therapy. Therapy alone is not recommended w/ resistance-associated integrase substitutions or clinically suspected integrase strand transfer inhibitor resistance. Immune reconstitution syndrome reported. Autoimmune disorders (eg, Graves' disease, polymyositis, Guillain-Barre syndrome) reported to occur in the setting of immune reconstitution and may occur many months after initiation of treatment. Redistribution/accumulation of body fat may occur. Caution in elderly. **Abacavir:** Consider underlying risk of coronary heart disease when prescribing therapy. **Dolutegravir:** Hypersensitivity reactions reported; d/c therapy and other suspect agents immediately if signs/symptoms develop. May be at increased risk for worsening or development of transaminase elevations in patients w/ underlying hepatitis B or C. **Lamivudine:** Emergence of lamivudine-resistant HBV reported.

ADVERSE REACTIONS

Insomnia, creatine kinase/AST/lipase elevations, hyperglycemia.

T

DRUG INTERACTIONS

See Dosing Considerations and Contraindications. Closely monitor for treatment-associated toxicities, especially hepatic decompensation in patients receiving interferon alfa w/ or w/o ribavirin; consider dose reduction or discontinuation of interferon alfa, ribavirin, or both if worsening clinical toxicities are observed, including hepatic decompensation (eg, Child-Pugh >6). Not recommended w/ other abacavir- or lamivudine-containing products. **Abacavir:** Ethanol may decrease elimination, causing an increase in overall exposure. May increase oral methadone clearance; an increased methadone dose may be required in a small number of patients. **Dolutegravir:** Drugs that induce/inhibit UGT1A1, CYP3A, UGT1A3, UGT1A9, breast cancer resistance protein, and P-gp may decrease/increase levels, respectively. Decreased levels w/ etravirine; use of Triumeq w/ etravirine w/o coadministration of atazanavir/RTV, darunavir/RTV, or lopinavir/RTV is not recommended. Decreased levels w/ efavirenz, fosamprenavir/ritonavir, tipranavir/ritonavir, rifampin, and carbamazepine. Decreased levels w/ nevirapine, oxcarbazepine, phenytoin, phenobarbital, and St. John's wort; avoid coadministration w/ Triumeq. Administer 2 hrs before or 6 hrs after taking medications containing polyvalent cations (eg, cation-containing antacids/laxatives, sucralfate, buffered medications) and oral Ca^{2+} or iron supplements (eg, multivitamins);

alternatively, therapy and supplements containing Ca^{2+} or iron can be taken together w/ food. May increase levels of drugs eliminated via organic cation transporter 2 or multidrug and toxin extrusion transporter 1 (eg, metformin); limit the total daily dose of metformin to 1000mg either when starting metformin or Triumeq; monitoring of blood glucose when initiating concomitant use and after withdrawal of Triumeq is recommended. When stopping Triumeq, metformin dose may require adjustment.

PATIENT CONSIDERATIONS

Assessment: Assess for previous hypersensitivity to the drug, hepatic/renal impairment, hepatitis B or C infection, pregnancy/nursing status, and possible drug interactions. Screen for HLA-B*5701 allele prior to initiation/reinitiation of therapy. Assess medical history for prior exposure to any abacavir-containing product.

Monitoring: Monitor for signs/symptoms of hypersensitivity reactions, lactic acidosis, hepatomegaly w/ steatosis, immune reconstitution syndrome, autoimmune disorders, fat redistribution/ accumulation, MI, and other adverse reactions. Monitor hepatic function. Closely monitor hepatic function for at least several months in patients who d/c therapy and are coinfected w/ HIV-1 and HBV.

Counseling: Inform about the risks and benefits of therapy. Advise to report the use of any prescription or nonprescription medication or herbal products. Inform about hypersensitivity reactions; instruct to contact physician immediately if symptoms develop and not to restart or replace w/ any drug containing abacavir w/o medical consultation. Inform that the drug may cause lactic acidosis w/ hepatomegaly. Inform patients w/ underlying hepatitis B or C of the increased risk of worsening or development of liver disease. Inform that hepatic decompensation has occurred in HIV-1/HCV-coinfected patients receiving combination antiretroviral therapy and interferon alfa w/ or w/o ribavirin. Inform that fat redistribution/accumulation may occur. Advise that drug is not a cure for HIV-1 infection and patients may continue to experience illness associated w/ HIV-1 infection, including opportunistic infections. Instruct to take all HIV medications exactly as prescribed. Advise to avoid doing things that can spread HIV-1 infection to others. Advise to inform physician immediately of any symptoms of infection or if any unusual symptom develops, or if any known symptom persists or worsens. Counsel patients on missed dose instructions.

STORAGE: 25°C (77°F); excursions permitted to 15-30°C (59-86°F). Protect from moisture.

TRIZIVIR – abacavir/lamivudine/zidovudine

RX

Class: Nucleoside reverse transcriptase inhibitor (NRTI)

Lactic acidosis and severe hepatomegaly w/ steatosis, including fatal cases, reported w/ nucleoside analogues and other antiretrovirals. D/C if clinical or lab findings suggestive of lactic acidosis or pronounced hepatotoxicity occur. Abacavir: Serious and sometimes fatal hypersensitivity reactions w/ multiple organ involvement reported; d/c immediately if a hypersensitivity reaction is suspected and never restart therapy or any other abacavir-containing product. Patients who carry the HLA-B*5701 allele are at a higher risk of a hypersensitivity reaction; screen all patients for HLA-B*5701 allele prior to initiating or reinitiating therapy, unless patient has a previously documented HLA-B*5701 allele assessment. Zidovudine: Associated w/ hematologic toxicity (eg, neutropenia, severe anemia), particularly w/ advanced HIV-1 disease. Symptomatic myopathy associated w/ prolonged use. Lamivudine: Severe acute exacerbations of hepatitis B reported in patients coinfected w/ hepatitis B virus (HBV) and HIV-1 and have discontinued therapy; closely monitor hepatic function w/ both clinical and lab follow-up for at least several months. If appropriate, initiation of antihepatitis B therapy may be warranted.

ADULT DOSAGE

HIV-1 Infection

1 tab bid

PEDIATRIC DOSAGE

HIV-1 Infection

>40kg:
1 tab bid

DOSING CONSIDERATIONS

Renal Impairment

CrCl <50mL/min: Not recommended for use

Hepatic Impairment

Mild: Not recommended for use
Moderate/Severe: Contraindicated

ADMINISTRATION

Oral route

Take w/ or w/o food.
Screen for the HLA-B*5701 allele prior to initiating therapy.

HOW SUPPLIED

Tab: (Abacavir Sulfate/Lamivudine/Zidovudine) 300mg/150mg/300mg

CONTRAINDICATIONS
Prior hypersensitivity reaction to Trizivir, moderate or severe hepatic impairment, patients w/ HLA-B*5701 allele.

WARNINGS/PRECAUTIONS
Obesity and prolonged nucleoside exposure may be risk factors for lactic acidosis and severe hepatomegaly w/ steatosis; suspend therapy if clinical or lab findings suggestive of lactic acidosis or pronounced hepatotoxicity develop. Immune reconstitution syndrome reported. Autoimmune disorders (eg, Graves' disease, polymyositis, Guillain-Barre syndrome) reported to occur in the setting of immune reconstitution and can occur many months after initiation of treatment. Redistribution/accumulation of body fat may occur. Cross-resistance potential w/ nucleoside reverse transcriptase inhibitors reported. Caution w/ any known risk factors for liver disease and in elderly. Avoid use in adolescents weighing <40kg and in patients requiring dose adjustments (eg, renal impairment [CrCl <50mL/min]). **Abacavir:** Consider underlying risk of coronary heart disease (CHD) when prescribing therapy. **Lamivudine:** Emergence of lamivudine-resistant HBV reported. **Zidovudine:** Caution w/ compromised bone marrow evidenced by granulocyte count <1000 cells/mm^3 or Hgb <9.5g/dL; monitor blood counts frequently w/ advanced HIV-1 disease and periodically in other HIV-1 infected patients. Interrupt therapy if anemia or neutropenia develops.

ADVERSE REACTIONS
N/V, headache, malaise, fatigue, hypersensitivity reaction, diarrhea, fever, chills, depressive disorders, musculoskeletal pain, skin rashes, anxiety, ear/nose/throat infections.

DRUG INTERACTIONS
Avoid w/ other abacavir-, lamivudine-, zidovudine-, and/or emtricitabine-containing products. Closely monitor for treatment associated toxicities, especially hepatic decompensation, neutropenia, and anemia, in patients receiving interferon alfa w/ or w/o ribavirin and Trizivir; consider discontinuation of Trizivir as medically appropriate and consider dose reduction or discontinuation of interferon alfa, ribavirin, or both if worsening clinical toxicities are observed. **Abacavir:** Ethanol may decrease elimination, causing an increase in overall exposure. May increase oral methadone clearance; an increased methadone dose may be required in a small number of patients. **Zidovudine:** Avoid w/ stavudine, doxorubicin, and nucleoside analogues (eg, ribavirin). May increase hematologic toxicity w/ ganciclovir, interferon alfa, ribavirin, and other bone marrow suppressive or cytotoxic agents.

PATIENT CONSIDERATIONS

Assessment: Assess for history of hypersensitivity reactions, advanced HIV disease, hepatic/renal impairment, risk factors for lactic acidosis, risk factors for CHD, bone marrow compromise, HBV infection, pregnancy/nursing status, and possible drug interactions. Screen for HLA-B*5701 allele prior to initiation of therapy. Assess medical history for prior exposure to any abacavir-containing product.

Monitoring: Monitor for signs/symptoms of hypersensitivity reactions, hematologic toxicity, lactic acidosis, hepatomegaly w/ steatosis, myopathy, immune reconstitution syndrome, autoimmune disorders, fat redistribution/accumulation, MI, and other adverse reactions. Monitor hepatic/renal function. Monitor hepatic function closely for at least several months in patients who d/c therapy and are coinfected w/ HIV-1 and HBV. Perform frequent blood counts in patients w/ advanced HIV-1 disease and perform periodic blood counts for other HIV-1-infected patients.

Counseling: Inform about hypersensitivity reactions; instruct to contact physician immediately if symptoms develop and not to restart or replace w/ any drug containing abacavir w/o medical consultation. Inform about risk for hematologic toxicities and advise on importance of close blood count monitoring while on therapy. Counsel about the possible occurrence of myopathy and myositis w/ pathological changes during prolonged use and that therapy may cause a rare but serious condition called lactic acidosis w/ hepatomegaly. Inform patients coinfected w/ HBV that deterioration of liver disease has occurred in some cases when treatment was discontinued; instruct to discuss any changes in regimen w/ physician. Inform that hepatic decompensation has occurred in HIV-1/hepatitis C virus coinfected patients receiving combination antiretroviral therapy and interferon alfa w/ or w/o ribavirin. Inform that redistribution/accumulation of body fat may occur. Advise that drug is not a cure for HIV-1 infection and that illness associated w/ HIV-1 may still be experienced. Advise to avoid doing things that can spread HIV-1 infection to others. Inform patients to take all HIV medications exactly as prescribed.

STORAGE: 25°C (77°F); excursions permitted to 15-30°C (59-86°F).

TRUSOPT — dorzolamide hydrochloride

RX

Class: Carbonic anhydrase inhibitor

ADULT DOSAGE
Elevated Intraocular Pressure
Ocular HTN/Open-Angle Glaucoma:
1 drop in the affected eye(s) tid

PEDIATRIC DOSAGE
Elevated Intraocular Pressure
Ocular HTN/Open-Angle Glaucoma:
1 drop in the affected eye(s) tid

DOSING CONSIDERATIONS

Concomitant Medications

Administer at least 5 min apart if >1 topical ophthalmic drug is being used

ADMINISTRATION

Ocular route

HOW SUPPLIED

Sol: 2% [10mL]

CONTRAINDICATIONS

Hypersensitivity to any component of Trusopt.

WARNINGS/PRECAUTIONS

Systemically absorbed. Rare fatalities have occurred due to severe sulfonamide reactions (eg, Stevens-Johnson syndrome, toxic epidermal necrolysis, fulminant hepatic necrosis, agranulocytosis, aplastic anemia, other blood dyscrasias); d/c if signs of hypersensitivity or other serious reactions occur. Sensitization may recur when readministered irrespective of the route of administration. Bacterial keratitis reported with use of multiple-dose containers of topical ophthalmic products that had been inadvertently contaminated by patients with a concurrent corneal disease or a disruption of the ocular epithelial surface. Caution in patients with low endothelial cell counts; increased potential for corneal edema. Local ocular adverse effects (eg, conjunctivitis, lid reactions) reported with chronic use; d/c use and evaluate patient before considering restarting therapy. The management of acute angle-closure glaucoma requires therapeutic interventions in addition to ocular hypotensive agents. Not recommended with severe renal impairment (CrCl <30mL/min). Caution with hepatic impairment.

ADVERSE REACTIONS

Ocular burning/stinging/discomfort, bitter taste, superficial punctate keratitis, ocular allergic reactions, conjunctivitis, lid reactions, blurred vision, eye redness, tearing, dryness, photophobia.

DRUG INTERACTIONS

Concomitant administration of oral carbonic anhydrase inhibitor is not recommended due to potential for additive effects. Acid-base and electrolyte disturbances reported with oral carbonic anhydrase inhibitors; drug interactions (eg, toxicity associated with high-dose salicylate therapy) may occur.

PATIENT CONSIDERATIONS

Assessment: Assess for hypersensitivity to drug, acute angle-closure glaucoma, low endothelial cell counts, renal/hepatic impairment, pregnancy/nursing status, and possible drug interactions.

Monitoring: Monitor for sulfonamide hypersensitivity reactions, ocular reactions, bacterial keratitis, and other adverse reactions. Monitor for improvement in IOP.

Counseling: Advise to d/c use if serious or unusual reactions (eg, severe skin reactions, signs of hypersensitivity) occur. Instruct to immediately seek physician's advice concerning the continued use of present multidose container if patients have ocular surgery or develop an intercurrent ocular condition (eg, trauma, infection). Advise to d/c use and seek physician's advice if patient develops any ocular reactions (eg, conjunctivitis, lid reactions). Instruct to avoid allowing tip of dispensing container to contact eye or surrounding structures. Inform that ocular sol can become contaminated by common bacteria known to cause ocular infections if handled improperly or if the tip of the dispensing container contacts the eye or surrounding structures, and may result in serious damage to the eye and subsequent loss of vision. Instruct to administer at least 5 min apart if >1 topical ophthalmic drug is being used. Instruct to remove contact lenses prior to administration and inform that they may be reinserted 15 min after administration.

STORAGE: 15-30°C (59-86°F). Protect from light.

T

TRUVADA – emtricitabine/tenofovir disoproxil fumarate RX

Class: Nucleoside analogue combination

Lactic acidosis and severe hepatomegaly w/ steatosis, including fatal cases, reported w/ the use of nucleoside analogues in combination w/ other antiretrovirals. Not approved for treatment of chronic hepatitis B virus (HBV) infection. Severe acute exacerbations of hepatitis B reported in patients coinfected w/ HBV and HIV-1 and who have discontinued therapy; closely monitor hepatic function w/ both clinical and lab follow-up for at least several months. If appropriate, initiation of anti-hepatitis B therapy may be warranted. Drug resistant HIV-1 variants have been identified w/ use for preexposure prophylaxis (PrEP) indication following undetected acute HIV-1 infection. PrEP use must only be prescribed to individuals confirmed to be HIV-negative immediately prior to initiating and periodically (at least every 3 months) during use; do not initiate if signs/symptoms of acute HIV-1 infection are present unless negative infection status is confirmed.

ADULT DOSAGE

HIV-1 Infection

Combination w/ Other Antiretrovirals:
1 tab qd

HIV-1 Pre-Exposure Prophylaxis

Combination w/ Safer Sex Practices for High-Risk Patients:
1 tab qd

PEDIATRIC DOSAGE

HIV-1 Infection

Combination w/ Other Antiretrovirals:
≥12 Years:
≥35kg: 1 tab qd

DOSING CONSIDERATIONS

Renal Impairment

HIV-1 Infection:
CrCl 30-49mL/min: 1 tab q48h
CrCl <30mL/min (Including Hemodialysis): Not recommended for use

HIV-1 PrEP:
CrCl <60mL/min: Not recommended for use

ADMINISTRATION

Oral route

Take w/ or w/o food.

HOW SUPPLIED

Tab: (Emtricitabine/Tenofovir Disoproxil Fumarate [TDF]) 200mg/300mg

CONTRAINDICATIONS

Individuals w/ unknown or positive HIV-1 status when used for PrEP. Use in HIV-infected patients w/o other concomitant antiretroviral agents.

WARNINGS/PRECAUTIONS

Obesity and prolonged nucleoside exposure may be risk factors for lactic acidosis and severe hepatomegaly w/ steatosis. Caution w/ known risk factors for liver disease. D/C if findings suggestive of lactic acidosis or pronounced hepatotoxicity develop. Test for the presence of chronic HBV before initiating therapy; offer vaccination to HBV-uninfected individuals. Do not administer in patients w/ CrCl <30mL/min or requiring hemodialysis (HIV-1 treatment) or w/ CrCl <60mL/min (PrEP). Redistribution/accumulation of body fat and immune reconstitution syndrome reported. Autoimmune disorders (eg, Graves' disease, polymyositis, Guillain-Barre syndrome) reported in the setting of immune reconstitution and can occur many months after initiation of treatment. Early virological failure and high rates of resistance substitutions reported w/ certain regimens that only contain 3 nucleoside reverse transcriptase inhibitors; consider treatment modification in these patients. Use for PrEP only as part of a comprehensive prevention strategy that includes other prevention measures (eg, safer sex practices). Delay starting PrEP therapy for at least 1 month and reconfirm HIV-1 status or use an FDA-approved test to diagnose acute or primary HIV-1 infection if symptoms of acute viral infection are present and recent (<1 month) exposures are suspected. D/C PrEP therapy if symptoms of acute HIV-1 infection develop following potential exposure event until negative status is confirmed using an FDA-approved test. Caution in elderly. **TDF:** Renal impairment (eg, acute renal failure, Fanconi syndrome) reported; caution in patients at risk of renal dysfunction, including patients who have previously experienced renal events while receiving adefovir dipivoxil. Promptly evaluate renal function in at-risk patients w/ persistent/worsening bone pain, pain in extremities, fractures, and/or muscular pain/weakness. Decreased bone mineral density (BMD) and increased biochemical markers of bone metabolism reported. Osteomalacia associated w/ proximal renal tubulopathy reported; consider hypophosphatemia and osteomalacia secondary to proximal renal tubulopathy in patients at risk of renal dysfunction who present w/ persistent or worsening bone/muscle symptoms.

ADVERSE REACTIONS

HIV-1 Infected Patients: Diarrhea, nausea, fatigue, headache, dizziness, depression, insomnia, abnormal dreams, rash.

HIV-1 Uninfected Patients: Abdominal pain, syphilis, headache, decreased weight.

DRUG INTERACTIONS

Avoid w/ concurrent or recent use of nephrotoxic agents (eg, high-dose or multiple NSAIDs). Do not coadminister w/ emtricitabine- or TDF-containing products, drugs containing lamivudine, or w/ adefovir dipivoxil. Coadministration w/ drugs eliminated by active tubular secretion (eg, acyclovir, cidofovir, ganciclovir, valacyclovir, aminoglycosides [eg, gentamicin], high-dose or multiple NSAIDs) may increase levels of emtricitabine, TDF, and/or the coadministered drug. Drugs that decrease renal function may increase levels of emtricitabine and/or TDF. Refer to PI for dosing modifications when used w/ concomitant therapies. **TDF:** May increase levels of didanosine; d/c didanosine if didanosine-associated adverse effects develop. Decreases atazanavir levels; do not coadminister w/ atazanavir w/o ritonavir (RTV). Lopinavir/RTV, atazanavir w/ RTV, and darunavir w/ RTV may increase TDF levels; d/c treatment if TDF-associated adverse reactions develop. P-gp and breast cancer resistance protein transporter inhibitors may increase absorption.

PATIENT CONSIDERATIONS

Assessment: Assess for risk factors for lactic acidosis or liver disease, renal dysfunction, HBV infection, pregnancy/nursing status, and possible drug interactions. Confirm a negative HIV-1 test immediately prior to initiating PrEP therapy. In patients at risk of renal dysfunction, assess CrCl, serum phosphorus (P), urine glucose, and urine protein. Assess BMD in patients w/ history of pathologic bone fracture or other risk factors for osteoporosis or bone loss.

Monitoring: Monitor for signs/symptoms of lactic acidosis, hepatomegaly w/ steatosis, hepatotoxicity, new onset or worsening renal impairment, bone effects, redistribution/accumulation of body fat, immune reconstitution syndrome (eg, opportunistic infections), autoimmune disorders, and other adverse reactions. Closely monitor hepatic function w/ both clinical and laboratory follow-up for at least several months in patients coinfected w/ HBV and HIV-1 and who have discontinued therapy. Screen for HIV-1 infection at least once every 3 months when using for PrEP. In patients at risk of renal dysfunction, monitor CrCl, serum P, urine glucose, and urine protein periodically.

Counseling: Inform about the risks/benefits of therapy. Inform that medication is not a cure for HIV-1 and patients may continue to experience illness associated w/ HIV-1 infection (eg, opportunistic infections). Advise about the importance of adhering to recommended dosing schedule. Inform about safe sex practices. Instruct not to breastfeed, share needles or personal items that can have blood or body fluids on them, or d/c w/o informing physician. For PrEP, inform patients/partners about the importance of knowing their HIV-1 status, obtaining HIV-1 test at least every 3 months, getting tested for other sexually transmitted infections, and immediate reporting to physician if any symptoms of acute HIV-1 infection develop.

STORAGE: 25°C (77°F); excursions permitted to 15-30°C (59-86°F).

TUDORZA PRESSAIR — aclidinium bromide

RX

Class: Anticholinergic

ADULT DOSAGE

Chronic Obstructive Pulmonary Disease

Long-Term Maint Treatment of Bronchospasm:
1 inh (400mcg) bid

PEDIATRIC DOSAGE

Pediatric use may not have been established

ADMINISTRATION

Oral inh route

Refer to PI for instructions on proper use

HOW SUPPLIED

MDI: 400mcg/actuation [30 doses, 60 doses]

WARNINGS/PRECAUTIONS

Not for initial treatment of acute episodes of bronchospasm (eg, rescue therapy). D/C and consider alternative treatments if paradoxical bronchospasm or immediate hypersensitivity reactions (eg, anaphylaxis, angioedema, urticaria, rash, bronchospasm, itching) occur. Caution w/ hypersensitivity to atropine and/or milk proteins. Caution w/ narrow-angle glaucoma; observe for signs and symptoms of acute narrow-angle glaucoma (eg, eye pain or discomfort, blurred vision, visual halos or colored images in association w/ red eyes from conjunctival congestion and corneal edema). Caution w/ urinary retention; observe for signs and symptoms of prostatic hyperplasia or bladder neck obstruction.

ADVERSE REACTIONS

Headache, nasopharyngitis, cough.

DRUG INTERACTIONS

Avoid w/ other anticholinergic-containing drugs; may lead to an increase in anticholinergic effects.

PATIENT CONSIDERATIONS

Assessment: Assess for hypersensitivity to the drug, milk proteins, and/or atropine, narrow-angle glaucoma, urinary retention, pregnancy/nursing status, and possible drug interactions.

Monitoring: Monitor for hypersensitivity reactions, paradoxical bronchospasm, acute narrow-angle glaucoma, prostatic hyperplasia, bladder neck obstruction, and other adverse reactions.

Counseling: Inform that the medication is a bid maintenance bronchodilator and should not be used for immediate relief of breathing problems (eg, as a rescue medication). Advise to d/c treatment if paradoxical bronchospasm occurs. Instruct to consult physician immediately if signs/symptoms of acute narrow-angle glaucoma occur; advise that miotic eye drops alone are not considered to be effective treatment. Inform not to allow the powder to enter into the eyes, as this may cause blurring of vision and pupil dilation. Instruct to consult physician immediately if signs/symptoms of new or worsening prostatic hyperplasia or bladder outlet obstruction occur. Advise to immediately d/c treatment and consult physician if signs/symptoms of immediate hypersensitivity reactions develop. Instruct on how to correctly use the inhaler.

STORAGE: 25°C (77°F); excursions permitted to 15-30°C (59-86°F). Store in a dry place. Store inhaler inside the sealed pouch and only open immediately before use. Discard inhaler 45 days after opening the pouch, after the marking "0" w/ a red background shows, or when the device locks out, whichever comes 1st.

TUSSIONEX PENNKINETIC – chlorpheniramine polistirex/hydrocodone polistirex CII

Class: Antihistamine/opioid antitussive

ADULT DOSAGE

Antihistamine/Cough Suppressant

Relief of Cough and Upper Respiratory Symptoms Associated w/ Allergy or a Cold:
5mL q12h
Max: 10mL/24 hrs

PEDIATRIC DOSAGE

Antihistamine/Cough Suppressant

Relief of Cough and Upper Respiratory Symptoms Associated w/ Allergy or a Cold:

6-11 Years:
2.5mL q12h
Max: 5mL/24 hrs

≥12 Years:
5mL q12h
Max: 10mL/24 hrs

DOSING CONSIDERATIONS

Elderly

Start at lower end of dosing range

ADMINISTRATION

Oral route

Measure w/ an accurate measuring device

Shake well before using

HOW SUPPLIED

Sus, Extended-Release: (Hydrocodone/Chlorpheniramine) (10mg/8mg)/5mL [115mL]

CONTRAINDICATIONS

Known allergy or sensitivity to hydrocodone or chlorpheniramine. Children <6 yrs of age.

WARNINGS/PRECAUTIONS

May produce dose-related respiratory depression and irregular/periodic breathing; if respiratory depression occurs, it may be antagonized by the use of naloxone HCl and other supportive measures when indicated. May markedly exaggerate respiratory depressant effects and CSF pressure elevation capacity in patients with head injury, other intracranial lesions, or a preexisting increased intracranial pressure. May obscure clinical course of head injuries and acute abdominal conditions. Chronic use may result in obstructive bowel disease, especially in patients with underlying intestinal motility disorder. Suppresses cough reflex. Caution in postoperative use; pulmonary disease, depressed ventilatory function, narrow-angle glaucoma, asthma, prostatic hypertrophy, severe hepatic/renal impairment, hypothyroidism, Addison's disease, or urethral stricture; in pediatric patients ≥6 yrs of age or with respiratory embarrassment (eg, croup); or in elderly/debilitated.

ADVERSE REACTIONS

Sedation, drowsiness, mental clouding, lethargy, anxiety, dysphoria, euphoria, dizziness, rash, pruritus, N/V, ureteral spasm, urinary retention, psychic dependence, mood changes.

DRUG INTERACTIONS

Coadministration with other respiratory depressants may increase risk of respiratory depression in pediatric patients. Additive CNS depression with narcotics, antihistaminics, antipsychotics, antianxiety agents, or other CNS depressants (eg, alcohol); reduce dose of one or both agents. Concomitant use with MAOIs or TCAs may increase the effect of either the antidepressant or hydrocodone. Concurrent use with other anticholinergics may produce paralytic ileus.

PATIENT CONSIDERATIONS

Assessment: Assess for hepatic/renal impairment, drug hypersensitivity, any other conditions where treatment is cautioned or contraindicated, pregnancy/nursing status, and possible drug interactions. Assess use in postoperative/elderly/debilitated patients.

Monitoring: Monitor for signs/symptoms of respiratory depression, elevations in CSF pressure, obstructive bowel disease, and other adverse reactions.

Counseling: Inform that medication may produce marked drowsiness and impair mental/physical abilities required for the performance of potentially hazardous tasks (eg, operating machinery, driving). Instruct not to dilute with fluids or mix with other drugs.

STORAGE: 20-25°C (68-77°F); excursions permitted to 15-30°C (59-86°F).

TWYNSTA – amlodipine/telmisartan

RX

Class: Angiotensin II receptor blocker (ARB)/calcium channel blocker (CCB) (dihydropyridine)

D/C as soon as possible when pregnancy is detected. Drugs that act directly on the renin-angiotensin system (RAS) can cause injury/death to the developing fetus.

ADULT DOSAGE

Hypertension

Initial Therapy:

Initial: 40mg/5mg qd or, if requiring larger BP reductions, 80mg/5mg qd

Titrate: May be increased after at least 2 weeks

Max: 80mg/10mg qd

Initial therapy is not recommended in patients ≥75 yrs old or w/ hepatic impairment

Replacement Therapy:

May substitute for individual components; increase dose if BP control is unsatisfactory

Add-On Therapy:

May be used if BP not adequately controlled w/ amlodipine (or another dihydropyridine calcium channel blocker [CCB]) alone or w/ telmisartan (or another ARB) alone

Patients w/ dose-limiting adverse reactions to amlodipine 10mg may be switched to telmisartan/amlodipine 40mg/5mg qd

PEDIATRIC DOSAGE

Pediatric use may not have been established

DOSING CONSIDERATIONS

Renal Impairment

Severe: Titrate slowly

Hepatic Impairment

Initial: 2.5mg amlodipine; titrate slowly

Elderly

≥75 Years:

Initial: 2.5mg amlodipine; titrate slowly

ADMINISTRATION

Oral route

Take w/ or w/o food.

HOW SUPPLIED

Tab: (Telmisartan/Amlodipine) 40mg/5mg, 40mg/10mg, 80mg/5mg, 80mg/10mg

CONTRAINDICATIONS

Known hypersensitivity to Twynsta or any component of the medication, coadministration w/ aliskiren in patients w/ diabetes.

WARNINGS/PRECAUTIONS

Symptomatic hypotension may occur in patients w/ an activated RAS (eg, volume- or salt-depleted patients) and in patients w/ severe aortic stenosis. Correct volume/salt depletion prior to therapy or start therapy under close medical supervision w/ a reduced dose. **Amlodipine:** Worsening angina and acute MI may develop after starting or increasing the dose, particularly in patients w/ severe obstructive coronary artery disease (CAD). Closely monitor patients w/ heart failure (HF); pulmonary edema reported. Caution in elderly. **Telmisartan:** Hyperkalemia may occur, particularly in patients w/ advanced renal impairment, renal replacement therapy, or HF; periodically monitor serum electrolytes. Clearance is reduced in patients w/ biliary obstructive disorders or hepatic insufficiency. Changes in renal function may occur; oliguria and/or progressive azotemia and (rare) acute renal failure and/or death reported in patients whose renal function may depend on the RAS (eg, severe congestive HF or renal dysfunction). May increase SrCr/BUN w/ renal artery stenosis.

ADVERSE REACTIONS

Peripheral edema, dizziness, back pain.

DRUG INTERACTIONS

See Contraindications. **Amlodipine:** Increased exposure to simvastatin reported; limit dose of simvastatin to 20mg daily. May increase exposure of cyclosporine or tacrolimus; monitor cyclosporine/tacrolimus trough levels and adjust dose when appropriate. Diltiazem may increase systemic exposure. Strong CYP3A4 inhibitors (eg, ketoconazole, itraconazole, ritonavir) may increase concentrations to a greater extent; monitor for symptoms of hypotension and edema. Monitor for

T

adequate clinical effect when coadministered w/ CYP3A4 inducers. **Telmisartan:** Dual blockade of the RAS is associated w/ increased risks of hypotension, hyperkalemia, and changes in renal function (eg, acute renal failure); avoid combined use of RAS inhibitors and closely monitor BP, renal function, and electrolytes w/ concomitant agents that affect the RAS. Avoid w/ aliskiren in patients w/ renal impairment (GFR <60mL/min). May increase digoxin concentrations; monitor digoxin levels upon initiation, adjustment, and discontinuation of therapy. Increases in lithium concentrations/toxicity reported; monitor lithium levels during concurrent use. NSAIDs, including selective COX-2 inhibitors, may attenuate antihypertensive effect and may deteriorate renal function in patients who are elderly, volume-depleted, or w/ compromised renal function. Coadministration w/ ramipril may increase ramipril/ramiprilat levels and decrease telmisartan levels; not recommended w/ ramipril. Increased risk of hyperkalemia w/ K^+-sparing diuretics, K^+ supplements, K^+-containing salt substitutes, or other drugs that increase K^+ levels. May possibly inhibit metabolism of drugs metabolized by CYP2C19.

PATIENT CONSIDERATIONS

Assessment: Assess for severe obstructive CAD, severe aortic stenosis, HF, volume/salt depletion, biliary obstructive disorders, renal artery stenosis, diabetes, hepatic/renal dysfunction, hypersensitivity to drug, pregnancy/nursing status, and possible drug interactions.

Monitoring: Monitor for worsening angina and acute MI, particularly in patients w/ severe obstructive CAD, and for other adverse reactions. Monitor BP, renal function, and serum electrolytes (especially K^+ levels).

Counseling: Inform of consequences if exposure occurs during pregnancy, and of treatment options in women planning to become pregnant. Instruct to report pregnancies to physician as soon as possible.

STORAGE: 25°C (77°F); excursions permitted to 15-30°C (59-86°F). Do not remove from blisters until immediately before administration. Protect from light and moisture.

TYBOST – cobicistat

RX

Class: CYP3A inhibitor

ADULT DOSAGE

HIV-1 Infection

To increase systemic exposure of atazanavir or darunavir (once daily dosing regimen) in combination w/ other antiretroviral agents

Treatment-Naive/Experienced:
150mg qd + atazanavir 300mg qd

Treatment-Naive; Treatment-Experienced w/ No Darunavir Resistance-Associated Substitutions:
150mg qd + darunavir 800mg qd

PEDIATRIC DOSAGE

Pediatric use may not have been established

DOSING CONSIDERATIONS

Renal Impairment

CrCl <70mL/min: Do not coadminister w/ tenofovir DF

ADMINISTRATION

Oral route

Take w/ food.
Must be coadministered at the same time as atazanavir or darunavir.

HOW SUPPLIED

Tab: 150mg

CONTRAINDICATIONS

Concomitant use w/ alfuzosin, dronedarone, carbamazepine, phenobarbital, phenytoin, rifampin, irinotecan (when coadministered w/ atazanavir only), dihydroergotamine, ergotamine, methylergonovine, cisapride, St. John's wort, lovastatin, simvastatin, pimozide, nevirapine (when coadministered w/ atazanavir only), sildenafil (when used to treat pulmonary arterial HTN), indinavir (when coadministered w/ atazanavir only), triazolam, and oral midazolam.

WARNINGS/PRECAUTIONS

Not interchangeable w/ ritonavir to increase systemic exposure of darunavir 600mg bid, fosamprenavir, saquinavir, or tipranavir. Decreases estimated CrCl due to inhibition of tubular secretion of creatinine w/o affecting actual renal glomerular function; consider this effect when interpreting changes in estimated CrCl in patients initiating therapy, particularly in patients w/ medical conditions or receiving drugs needing monitoring w/ estimated CrCl. Consider alternative medications that do not require dosage adjustments in patients w/ renal impairment. Closely

T

monitor patients who experience a confirmed increase in SrCr of >0.4mg/dL from baseline for renal safety.

ADVERSE REACTIONS
Jaundice, rash.

DRUG INTERACTIONS
See Contraindications. Renal impairment, including cases of acute renal failure and Fanconi syndrome, reported w/ tenofovir disoproxil fumarate (TDF); coadministration is not recommended in patients w/ estimated CrCl <70mL/min. Coadministration w/ TDF in combination w/ concomitant or recent use of a nephrotoxic agent is not recommended. Not recommended w/ >1 antiretroviral that requires pharmacokinetic enhancement (eg, 2 protease inhibitors or a protease inhibitor in combination w/ elvitegravir); darunavir in combination w/ efavirenz, nevirapine, or etravirine; atazanavir in combination w/ etravirine; atazanavir in combination w/ efavirenz in treatment-experienced patients; darunavir 600mg bid; other HIV-1 protease inhibitors (eg, fosamprenavir, saquinavir, tipranavir); elvitegravir/cobicistat/emtricitabine/TDF fixed-dose combination; and lopinavir/ritonavir or regimens containing ritonavir. Not recommended w/ boceprevir, simeprevir, salmeterol, avanafil, voriconazole, or colchicine in patients w/ renal/hepatic impairment. May increase concentration of drugs that are primarily metabolized by CYP3A (eg, maraviroc, clonazepam, corticosteroids [eg, dexamethasone, inhaled/nasal fluticasone or budesonide], cyclosporine, everolimus, sirolimus, tacrolimus) or CYP2D6, or are substrates of P-gp, BCRP, OATP1B1, or OATP1B3. Coadministration w/ inhaled or nasal fluticasone or other corticosteroids that are metabolized by CYP3A may result in reduced serum cortisol concentrations. CYP3A inducers (eg, oxcarbazepine, dexamethasone) may decrease concentrations of cobicistat, atazanavir, and darunavir, which may lead to loss of therapeutic effect and possible development of resistance. CYP3A inhibitors may increase concentrations, which may lead to clinically significant adverse reactions. Coadministration w/ atazanavir in combination w/ antacids (eg, aluminum and magnesium hydroxide) may decrease atazanavir levels; administer a minimum of 2 hrs apart. May increase levels of antiarrhythmics (eg, amiodarone, quinidine, digoxin), dasatinib, nilotinib, vinblastine, vincristine, itraconazole, ketoconazole, colchicine, rifabutin, β-blockers, calcium channel blockers, bosentan, HMG-CoA reductase inhibitors (eg, atorvastatin, rosuvastatin), fentanyl, tramadol, neuroleptics (eg, perphenazine, risperidone, thioridazine), PDE-5 inhibitors (eg, sildenafil, tadalafil), and sedatives/hypnotics (eg, buspirone, diazepam, parenteral midazolam). When coadministering w/ digoxin, titrate digoxin dose and monitor digoxin concentrations. Coadministration w/ macrolide/ketolide antibiotics (clarithromycin, erythromycin, telithromycin) may increase levels of the antibiotic and of cobicistat, atazanavir, and darunavir; consider alternative antibiotics. Monitor for hematologic or GI side effects w/ vincristine and vinblastine. Monitor INR w/ warfarin. Avoid w/ rivaroxaban. Monitor concentrations of anticonvulsants that are metabolized by CYP3A. Caution w/ SSRIs (eg, paroxetine), TCAs (eg, amitriptyline, desipramine), and trazodone; may increase levels of TCAs and trazodone. Bosentan may decrease levels. Coadministration w/ atazanavir in combination w/ H_2-receptor antagonists (eg, famotidine) may decrease atazanavir levels; administer atazanavir/cobicistat coadministration at either the same time or a minimum of 10 hrs after administering H_2-receptor antagonists. Consider additional or alternative (nonhormonal) forms of contraception if to be used w/ hormonal contraceptives. Caution w/ buprenorphine, buprenorphine/naloxone, and methadone. Coadministration w/ atazanavir in combination w/ proton pump inhibitors (eg, omeprazole), may decrease atazanavir levels; administer cobicistat w/ atazanavir a minimum of 12 hrs after administering proton pump inhibitors (PPIs) in treatment-naive patients; coadministration w/ PPIs, w/ or w/o tenofovir, is not recommended in treatment-experienced patients. Refer to PI for further information including dosing modifications when used w/ certain concomitant therapies.

PATIENT CONSIDERATIONS

Assessment: Assess pregnancy/nursing status and for possible drug interactions. Assess estimated CrCl. When used w/ TDF, assess estimated CrCl, urine glucose, and urine protein.

Monitoring: Monitor for adverse reactions. Monitor CrCl. When used w/ TDF, perform routine monitoring of estimated CrCl, urine glucose, and urine protein and measure serum phosphorus in patients w/ or at risk for renal impairment.

Counseling: Inform of the risks and benefits of therapy. Inform patients that they should remain under the care of a physician when using therapy. Counsel about the risks of developing resistance to HIV-1 medications. Instruct that if a dose of the drug and atazanavir or darunavir is missed by <12 hrs, to take the missed dose of the drug w/ atazanavir or darunavir together right away, and the next dose together as usual; if a dose of the drug w/ atazanavir or darunavir is missed by >12 hrs, instruct to wait and take the next dose at the usual time. If a dose of the drug w/ atazanavir or darunavir is skipped, instruct not to double the next dose. Inform that therapy may interact w/ many drugs w/ potential serious implications and that some drugs should not be taken w/ therapy; advise to report to physician the use of any other prescription or nonprescription medication or herbal products, including St. John's wort. Inform patients that there is a pregnancy exposure registry that monitors pregnancy outcomes in women exposed to cobicistat during pregnancy. Instruct mothers not to breastfeed while on therapy.

STORAGE: 25°C (77°F); excursions permitted to 15-30°C (59-86°F). Keep tightly closed.

TYSABRI – natalizumab

RX

Class: Monoclonal antibody/integrin receptor antagonist

Increases risk of progressive multifocal leukoencephalopathy (PML). Risk factors for development of PML include duration of therapy, prior use of immunosuppressants, and presence of anti-JCV antibodies. Monitor for any new signs/symptoms of PML; withhold therapy at the 1st sign/symptom suggestive of PML. Available only through a special restricted distribution program called the TOUCH Prescribing Program.

ADULT DOSAGE

Multiple Sclerosis

Monotherapy for the Treatment of Relapsing Forms:

300mg IV infusion over 1 hr every 4 weeks

Crohn's Disease

To induce and maintain clinical response and remission in patients w/ moderately to severely active Crohn's disease (CD) w/ evidence of inflammation who have had an inadequate response to, or are unable to tolerate, conventional CD therapies and TNF-α inhibitors

300mg IV infusion over 1 hr every 4 weeks

In patients starting therapy while on chronic oral corticosteroids, commence steroid tapering as soon as therapeutic benefit has occurred

PEDIATRIC DOSAGE

Pediatric use may not have been established

DOSING CONSIDERATIONS

Discontinuation

Crohn's Disease (CD):

D/C therapy if no therapeutic benefit by 12 weeks of induction therapy, if patient cannot be tapered off of corticosteroids w/in 6 months of starting therapy, and consider discontinuation in patients who require additional steroid use that exceeds 3 months in a calendar yr to control their CD

ADMINISTRATION

IV route

Dilution

1. To prepare sol, withdraw 15mL from the vial and inject the concentrate into 100mL of 0.9% NaCl inj; no other IV diluents may be used to prepare the sol
2. Gently invert sol to mix completely; do not shake
3. The final dosage sol has a concentration of 2.6mg/mL
4. Following dilution, infuse sol immediately, or refrigerate at 2-8°C (36-46°F), and use w/in 8 hrs; if refrigerated, allow sol to warm to room temperature prior to infusion. Do not freeze

Administration

1. Infuse 300mg in 100mL 0.9% NaCl inj, over approx 1 hr (infusion rate approx 5mg/min)
2. Do not administer as an IV push or bolus inj
3. Observe patients during infusion and for 1 hr after completion of infusion
4. After the infusion is complete, flush w/ 0.9% NaCl inj
5. Do not inject other medications into infusion set side ports or mix w/ therapy

HOW SUPPLIED

Inj: 300mg/15mL

CONTRAINDICATIONS

PML or history of PML. Hypersensitivity reaction to natalizumab.

WARNINGS/PRECAUTIONS

Anti-JCV antibody testing should not be used to diagnose PML. Avoid anti-JCV antibody testing for at least 2 weeks following plasma exchange because of the removal of antibodies from the serum. Retest patients w/ negative anti-JCV antibody test result periodically. PML reported following discontinuation in patient who do not have findings suggestive of PML at the time of discontinuation; monitor for any new signs or symptoms that may be suggestive of PML for at least 6 months following discontinuation. Immune reconstitution inflammatory syndrome (IRIS) reported in patients w/ PML, who have subsequently discontinued natalizumab; monitor for development of IRIS and treat appropriately. Increases the risk of developing encephalitis and meningitis caused by herpes simplex and varicella zoster viruses; d/c and treat appropriately if herpes encephalitis and meningitis occurs. Liver injury, including acute liver failure requiring transplant, reported;

d/c w/ jaundice or other evidence of significant liver injury (eg, lab evidence). Hypersensitivity reactions, including serious systemic reactions (eg, anaphylaxis) reported; d/c, institute appropriate therapy, and do not retreat. May increase risk for infections. Avoid in patients w/ systemic medical conditions resulting in significantly compromised immune system function. Induces increases in circulating lymphocytes, monocytes, eosinophils, basophils, and nucleated RBCs or transient decreases in Hgb levels.

ADVERSE REACTIONS

Headache, fatigue, arthralgia, UTI, depression, lower/URTI, abdominal discomfort, rash, gastroenteritis, vaginitis, urinary urgency/frequency, diarrhea, abnormal LFTs.

DRUG INTERACTIONS

Avoid w/ immunomodulatory therapy, immunosuppressants (eg, 6-mercaptopurine, azathioprine, cyclosporine, methotrexate) or TNF-α inhibitors. Taper corticosteroids in CD patients when starting natalizumab therapy. Antineoplastic, immunosuppressive, or immunomodulating agents may further increase risk of infections, including PML and other opportunistic infections.

PATIENT CONSIDERATIONS

Assessment: Assess for risk of PML, history of chronic immunosuppressant or immunomodulatory therapy, immunosuppression, drug hypersensitivity, pregnancy/nursing status, and possible drug interactions. Perform MRI and CSF analysis. Test for anti-JCV antibody status; retest periodically in patients w/ negative result.

Monitoring: Monitor for PML, anaphylactic/hypersensitivity reactions, infections, hepatotoxicity, development of IRIS and other adverse reactions. Antibody testing recommended if presence of persistent antibodies is suspected. Evaluate patients 3 and 6 months after the 1st infusion, every 6 months thereafter, and for at least 6 months after discontinuing treatment.

Counseling: Inform about TOUCH Prescribing Program. Educate on risks/benefits of therapy. Counsel about the follow-up schedule (3 and 6 months after 1st infusion, every 6 months thereafter, and for at least 6 months after discontinuation). Instruct to seek medical attention if symptoms suggestive of PML develop, including progressive weakness on one side of the body or clumsiness of the limbs, disturbance of vision, and changes in thinking, memory, and orientation leading to confusion and personality changes. Instruct to report symptoms of infections, hypersensitivity reactions, and hepatotoxicity.

STORAGE: 2-8°C (36-46°F). Do not shake or freeze. Protect from light.

Uceris Rectal Foam – budesonide

RX

Class: Corticosteroid

ADULT DOSAGE

Ulcerative Colitis

1 metered dose rectally bid (am and hs) for 2 weeks, followed by 1 metered dose rectally hs for 4 weeks

PEDIATRIC DOSAGE

Pediatric use may not have been established

DOSING CONSIDERATIONS

Concomitant Medications

CYP3A4 Inhibitors (eg, Ketoconazole, Grapefruit Juice):
Avoid concomitant use

Elderly

Start at lower end of dosing range

ADMINISTRATION

Rectal route

HOW SUPPLIED

Foam: 2mg/metered dose [14 metered doses]

CONTRAINDICATIONS

Known hypersensitivity to budesonide or any of the ingredients in Uceris rectal foam.

WARNINGS/PRECAUTIONS

Systemic effects (eg, hypercorticism, adrenal suppression) may occur when used chronically. May reduce response of hypothalamus-pituitary-adrenal axis to stress; supplement with a systemic glucocorticosteroid during surgery or other stress situations. Increased systemic availability of oral budesonide reported in patients with liver cirrhosis; consider discontinuation in patients with moderate to severe hepatic impairment (Child-Pugh class B or C) if signs of hypercorticism are observed. Monitor patients who are transferred from glucocorticosteroid treatment with higher systemic effects to glucocorticosteroids with lower systemic effects; withdrawal symptoms (eg, acute adrenal suppression, benign intracranial HTN) may develop. Cautiously reduce dose of glucocorticosteroid treatment with high systemic effects. Replacement of systemic glucocorticosteroids with the drug may unmask allergies (eg, rhinitis, eczema). Increased susceptibility to infection. Chickenpox and measles may have a more serious/fatal course; avoid exposure in patients who have not had these diseases and consider prophylaxis/treatment if exposed. Caution with active/quiescent tuberculosis (TB), untreated fungal, bacterial, systemic viral or parasitic infections, or ocular herpes simplex, and in elderly. Monitor patients with HTN, diabetes mellitus (DM), osteoporosis, peptic ulcer, glaucoma, cataracts, family history of DM or glaucoma, or with any other condition where glucocorticosteroids may have unwanted effects. Contains n-butane, isobutane and propane as propellants which are flammable; temporarily d/c use before initiation of bowel preparation for colonoscopy.

ADVERSE REACTIONS

Decreased blood cortisol, adrenal insufficiency, nausea.

DRUG INTERACTIONS

See Dosing Considerations. CYP3A4 inhibitors (eg, ritonavir, erythromycin, cyclosporine) may increase levels.

PATIENT CONSIDERATIONS

Assessment: Assess for hepatic impairment, active/quiescent TB, untreated infections, ocular herpes simplex, HTN, DM, osteoporosis, peptic ulcer, glaucoma, cataracts, family history of DM or glaucoma, hypersensitivity to drug, pregnancy/nursing status, and possible drug interactions.

Monitoring: Monitor for hypercorticism, adrenal suppression, infection, and other adverse reactions. Monitor adrenocortical function in patients who are transferred from glucocorticosteroid treatment with higher systemic effects. Monitor patients with HTN, DM, osteoporosis, peptic ulcer, glaucoma, cataracts, family history of DM or glaucoma, or with any other condition where glucocorticosteroids may have unwanted effects.

Counseling: Advise that drug is only to be applied rectally; it is not for oral use. Instruct to use the bathroom to empty bowels before use and to try not to empty bowels again until the next morning. Advise that each applicator is coated with a lubricant; petrolatum or petroleum jelly can also be used if additional lubrication is needed. Advise to warm the canister in hands while shaking vigorously for 10-15 sec prior to use. Instruct that drug may be used in a standing, lying, or sitting position (eg, while using the toilet). Instruct to avoid consumption of grapefruit or grapefruit juice during therapy. Advise to avoid fire, flame, and smoking during and immediately following administration. Advise that the drug may cause hypercorticism and adrenal suppression; instruct to taper slowly from systemic corticosteroids if transferring to the drug. Advise that replacement of systemic glucocorticosteroids with drug may unmask allergies. Advise to avoid exposure to chickenpox or measles and, if exposed, to consult physician. Inform that patients are at increased risk of developing a variety of infections, including worsening of existing TB, fungal, bacterial, viral, or parasitic infections, or ocular herpes simplex; instruct to contact physician if any symptoms of infection develop. Instruct to consult physician before resuming therapy if temporarily discontinued prior to colonoscopy.

STORAGE: 20-25°C (68-77°F); excursions permitted to 15-30°C (59-86°F). Do not burn the canister after use and do not spray contents directly towards flames. Do not expose to heat or store at >49°C (120°F). Contents under pressure; do not puncture or incinerate. Do not refrigerate.

ULORIC — febuxostat

RX

Class: Xanthine oxidase inhibitor

ADULT DOSAGE

Hyperuricemia

Chronic Management in Patients w/ Gout:

Initial: 40mg qd

Titrate: If serum uric acid is not <6mg/dL after 2 weeks, increase dose to 80mg qd

PEDIATRIC DOSAGE

Pediatric use may not have been established

U

ADMINISTRATION

Oral route

May be taken w/o regard to food or antacid use

HOW SUPPLIED

Tab: 40mg, 80mg

CONTRAINDICATIONS

Patients being treated with azathioprine or mercaptopurine.

WARNINGS/PRECAUTIONS

Not recommended for treatment of asymptomatic hyperuricemia. Increase in gout flares observed after initiation; concurrent prophylactic treatment with NSAIDs or colchicine is recommended. Cardiovascular (CV) thromboembolic events (eg, CV deaths, MIs, strokes) reported; monitor for signs and symptoms of MI and stroke. Fatal and nonfatal hepatic failure reported; obtain baseline LFTs before initiation. Measure LFTs promptly in patients who report symptoms that may indicate liver injury; d/c if LFTs are abnormal (ALT >3X ULN) and do not restart if no alternative etiology is found. D/C permanently in patients with ALT >3X ULN with serum total bilirubin >2X ULN without alternative etiologies; use with caution in patients with lesser ALT or bilirubin elevations and with an alternate probable cause. Caution with severe hepatic impairment (Child-Pugh Class C) and severe renal impairment (CrCl <30mL/min). Avoid use in patients whom the rate of urate formation is greatly increased (eg, malignant disease and its treatment, Lesch-Nyhan syndrome).

ADVERSE REACTIONS

Liver function abnormalities, nausea, arthralgia, rash.

DRUG INTERACTIONS

See Contraindications. Caution with theophylline.

PATIENT CONSIDERATIONS

Assessment: Assess for asymptomatic hyperuricemia, hepatic/renal impairment, malignant disease, Lesch-Nyhan syndrome, pregnancy/nursing status, and possible drug interactions. Obtain baseline serum uric acid (sUA) and LFTs.

Monitoring: Monitor sUA levels as early as 2 weeks after initiation of therapy. Monitor for signs/symptoms of liver injury, MI, and stroke.

Counseling: Advise of the potential benefits and risks of therapy. Inform that gout flares, elevated liver enzymes, and adverse CV events may occur. Instruct to notify physician if rash, chest pain, SOB, or neurologic symptoms suggesting a stroke occur. Instruct to inform physician of any other medications, including OTC drugs, currently being taken.

STORAGE: 25°C (77°F); excursions permitted to 15-30°C (59-86°F). Protect from light.

ULTRACET — acetaminophen/tramadol hydrochloride CIV

Class: Centrally acting analgesic

Associated with cases of acute liver failure, at times resulting in liver transplant and death. Most cases of liver injury are associated with acetaminophen (APAP) use at doses >4000mg/day and often involve >1 APAP-containing product.

ADULT DOSAGE

Acute Pain

Short-Term (≤5 Days) Management:
2 tabs q4-6h prn for ≤5 days
Max: 8 tabs/day

PEDIATRIC DOSAGE

Pediatric use may not have been established

DOSING CONSIDERATIONS

Renal Impairment

CrCl <30mL/min:
Max: 2 tabs q12h

ADMINISTRATION

Oral route

HOW SUPPLIED

Tab: (Tramadol/APAP) 37.5mg/325mg

CONTRAINDICATIONS

Previously demonstrated hypersensitivity to tramadol, acetaminophen, any other component of Ultracet, or opioids. Any situation where opioids are contraindicated, including acute intoxication with alcohol, hypnotics, narcotics, centrally acting analgesics, opioids, or psychotropic drugs.

WARNINGS/PRECAUTIONS

Do not exceed recommended dose. May complicate clinical assessment of acute abdominal conditions. Not recommended in patients with hepatic impairment; increased risk of acute liver failure in patients with underlying liver disease. Not for use in pregnant women prior to or during labor unless benefits outweigh risks. Not recommended for obstetrical preoperative medication or for postdelivery analgesia in nursing mothers. Caution in elderly. Serious and fatal anaphylactic reactions reported; avoid use in patients with a history of anaphylactoid reactions to codeine or other opioids. D/C use if anaphylaxis develops. APAP: Avoid in patients with APAP allergy. May cause serious skin reactions (eg, acute generalized exanthematous pustulosis, Stevens-Johnson syndrome, toxic epidermal necrolysis), which can be fatal; d/c at the 1st appearance of skin rash or any other sign of hypersensitivity. Tramadol: Seizures reported; risk increases in patients with epilepsy, history/risk of seizures, and with naloxone coadministration. Avoid in patients who are suicidal or addiction-prone; caution with emotional disturbances or depression. Reports of tramadol-related deaths with previous history of emotional disturbances, suicidal ideation/attempts, and misuse of tranquilizers/alcohol/CNS-active drugs. Potentially life-threatening serotonin syndrome, including mental status changes, autonomic instability, neuromuscular aberrations, and GI symptoms, may occur. Caution if at risk for respiratory depression; consider alternative nonopioid analgesic. Caution with CNS depression, head injury, and increased intracranial pressure (ICP). May impair mental/physical abilities. May cause withdrawal symptoms; do not d/c abruptly.

ADVERSE REACTIONS

Acute liver failure, constipation, somnolence, increased sweating, diarrhea, nausea, anorexia, dizziness.

DRUG INTERACTIONS

See Contraindications. Do not use concomitantly with alcohol, other APAP- or tramadol-containing products; increased risk of acute liver failure with alcohol ingestion. May alter effects of warfarin; periodically monitor PT with warfarin-like compounds. Tramadol: Increased seizure risk with SSRIs, TCAs, other tricyclic compounds (eg, cyclobenzaprine, promethazine), MAOIs, other opioids, neuroleptics, and drugs that reduce seizure threshold. Serotonin syndrome may occur when coadministered with SSRIs, SNRIs, TCAs, MAOIs, triptans, α_2-adrenergic blockers, linezolid, lithium, St. John's wort, or drugs that impair tramadol metabolism; observe carefully, especially during initiation and dose increases. Caution and reduce dose with CNS depressants (eg, alcohol, opioids, anesthetics); increased risk of CNS/respiratory depression. Caution with antidepressants and muscle relaxants; additive CNS depressant effects. CYP2D6 inhibitors (eg, quinidine, fluoxetine, paroxetine, amitriptyline) and/or CYP3A4 inhibitors (eg, ketoconazole, erythromycin) may reduce metabolic clearance; increased risk of serious adverse effects. CYP3A4 inhibitors or inducers (eg, rifampin, St. John's wort) may alter drug exposure. Digoxin toxicity may occur with concomitant use. Carbamazepine may reduce analgesic effect; avoid coadministration.

PATIENT CONSIDERATIONS

Assessment: Assess for known hypersensitivity to the drug and other opioids, acute intoxication with alcohol, hypnotics, narcotics, centrally acting analgesics, opioids, or psychotropic drugs, epilepsy, seizure and respiratory depression risks, suicidal ideation, emotional disturbance or depression, increased ICP, head injury, drug abuse potential, suicidal or addiction proneness, renal/hepatic impairment, pregnancy/nursing status, and possible drug interactions.

Monitoring: Monitor for acute liver failure, skin hypersensitivity/anaphylactic reactions, respiratory/CNS depression, physical dependence/abuse, misuse, tolerance, seizures, development of serotonin syndrome, withdrawal symptoms with abrupt discontinuation, and other adverse reactions. Periodically monitor PT with warfarin-like compounds.

Counseling: Instruct to d/c therapy and notify physician if signs of allergy occur. Advise patients of dose limits. Instruct to seek medical attention immediately upon ingestion of >4000mg/day APAP, even if feeling well. Counsel not to use with other tramadol or APAP-containing products, including OTC preparations. Inform that seizures and serotonin syndrome may occur when used with serotonergic agents or drugs that reduce the clearance of tramadol. Inform that therapy may impair physical/mental abilities. Instruct to notify physician if pregnant or planning to become pregnant. Instruct to avoid alcohol-containing beverages while on therapy. Inform about the signs of serious skin reactions and of possible drug interactions.

STORAGE: 25°C (77°F); excursions permitted to 15-30°C (59-86°F).

ULTRAM – tramadol hydrochloride

CIV

Class: Centrally acting analgesic

U

ADULT DOSAGE

Moderate to Moderately Severe Pain

≥17 Years:
Initial: 25mg/day qam
Titrate: Increase in 25mg increments every 3 days to reach 100mg/day (25mg qid), then may increase total daily dose by 50mg as tolerated every 3 days to reach 200mg/day (50mg qid)
After Titration/Rapid Onset Required: 50-100mg q4-6h prn
Max: 400mg/day

PEDIATRIC DOSAGE

Pediatric use may not have been established

DOSING CONSIDERATIONS

Renal Impairment

CrCl <30mL/min:

Increase dosing interval to 12 hrs

Dialysis patients may receive regular dose on the day of dialysis

Max: 200mg/day

Hepatic Impairment

Cirrhosis: 50mg q12h

Elderly

Start at lower end of dosing range

>75 Years:

Max: 300mg/day

ADMINISTRATION

Oral route

Administer w/o regard to food.

HOW SUPPLIED

Tab: 50mg* *scored

CONTRAINDICATIONS

Previously demonstrated hypersensitivity to tramadol, any other component of Ultram, or opioids. Any situation where opioids are contraindicated, including acute intoxication with alcohol, hypnotics, narcotics, centrally acting analgesics, opioids, or psychotropic drugs.

WARNINGS/PRECAUTIONS

Do not exceed recommended dose. Seizures reported; risk increases in patients with epilepsy, history of seizures, recognized risk for seizures, and with naloxone coadministration. Anaphylactoid reactions and potentially life-threatening serotonin syndrome may occur. Avoid in patients who are suicidal or addiction-prone, and with history of anaphylactoid reactions to codeine and other opioids. Caution with emotional disturbances or depression, and in elderly. Tramadol-related deaths reported with previous histories of emotional disturbances, suicidal ideation/attempts, and misuse of tranquilizers, alcohol, and other CNS active drugs. Caution in patients at risk for respiratory depression; consider alternative nonopioid analgesics. Caution with increased intracranial pressure (ICP) or head injury. May impair mental/physical abilities. Withdrawal symptoms may occur if discontinued abruptly. May complicate clinical assessment of acute abdominal conditions. Not for use in pregnant women prior to or during labor unless benefits outweigh risks. Not recommended for obstetrical preoperative medication or for postdelivery analgesia in nursing mothers.

ADVERSE REACTIONS

Dizziness/vertigo, N/V, constipation, headache, somnolence, sweating, asthenia, dyspepsia, dry mouth, diarrhea, pruritus.

DRUG INTERACTIONS

See Contraindications. Caution and reduce dose with CNS depressants (eg, alcohol, opioids, anesthetics); increased risk of CNS/respiratory depression. CYP2D6 inhibitors (eg, quinidine, fluoxetine, paroxetine, amitriptyline) and CYP3A4 inhibitors (eg, ketoconazole, erythromycin) may reduce metabolic clearance and increase risk for serious adverse events including seizures and serotonin syndrome. Altered exposure with CYP3A4 inducers (eg, rifampin, St. John's wort). Increased seizure risk with SSRIs, TCAs, other tricyclic compounds (eg, cyclobenzaprine, promethazine), MAOIs, other opioids, neuroleptics, and drugs that reduce seizure threshold. Caution with SSRIs, SNRIs, TCAs, MAOIs, α2-adrenergic blockers, triptans, linezolid, lithium, St. John's wort, and drugs that impair tramadol metabolism, due to potential serotonin syndrome. Not recommended with carbamazepine; may significantly reduce analgesic effect. Digoxin toxicity and alteration of warfarin effect, including elevation of PT, reported rarely.

PATIENT CONSIDERATIONS

Assessment: Assess for previous hypersensitivity to the drug and other opioids, acute intoxication with alcohol/hypnotics/narcotics/centrally acting analgesics/opioids/psychotropic drugs, epilepsy, seizure and respiratory depression risks, suicidal ideation, emotional disturbance or depression, increased ICP, head injury, drug abuse potential, suicidal/addiction proneness, pain severity, renal/hepatic impairment, pregnancy/nursing status, any other conditions where treatment is contraindicated or cautioned, and possible drug interactions.

Monitoring: Monitor for signs/symptoms of anaphylactoid reactions, respiratory/CNS depression, tolerance, physical dependence, seizures, serotonin syndrome, withdrawal symptoms, and other adverse reactions.

Counseling: Inform of the risks and benefits of therapy. Inform that drug may cause seizures and/or serotonin syndrome with concomitant use of serotonergic agents or drugs that significantly reduce the metabolic clearance of therapy. Inform that drug may impair physical/mental abilities required for the performance of hazardous tasks (eg, driving a car, operating machinery). Instruct not to take drug with alcohol containing beverages. Inform to use drug with caution when taking tranquilizers, hypnotics, other opiate containing analgesics). Instruct to inform physician if pregnant, think or trying to become pregnant. Educate about single-dose and 24-hr dose limits and time interval between doses; advise not to exceed the recommended dose.

STORAGE: 25°C (77°F); excursions permitted to 15-30°C (59-86°F).

ULTRAM ER – tramadol hydrochloride CIV

Class: Centrally acting analgesic

ADULT DOSAGE

Moderate to Moderately Severe Pain

Chronic Pain Requiring Around-the-Clock Treatment for an Extended Period:

Not Currently on Tramadol Immediate-Release (IR):

Initial: 100mg qd

Titrate: Increase as necessary by 100mg increments every 5 days

Max: 300mg/day

Currently on Tramadol IR:

Initial: Calculate 24-hr tramadol IR dose and initiate total daily dose rounded down to next lowest 100mg increment

Titrate: Individualize according to patients need

Max: 300mg/day

PEDIATRIC DOSAGE

Pediatric use may not have been established

DOSING CONSIDERATIONS

Renal Impairment

CrCl <30mg/mL: Do not use

Hepatic Impairment

Severe (Child-Pugh Class C): Do not use

Elderly

Start at low end of dosing range

ADMINISTRATION

Oral route

Swallow whole; do not chew, crush, or split

HOW SUPPLIED

Tab, Extended-Release: 100mg, 200mg, 300mg

CONTRAINDICATIONS

Previously demonstrated hypersensitivity to tramadol, any other component of Ultram ER, or opioids. Any situation where opioids are contraindicated, including acute intoxication w/ alcohol, hypnotics, narcotics, centrally acting analgesics, opioids, or psychotropic drugs.

WARNINGS/PRECAUTIONS

Do not exceed recommended dose. Seizures reported; risk increases in patients w/ epilepsy, history of seizures, recognized risk for seizures, and w/ naloxone coadministration. Anaphylactoid reactions and potentially life-threatening serotonin syndrome may occur. Avoid in patients who are suicidal or addiction-prone, and w/ history of anaphylactoid reactions to codeine and other opioids. Tramadol-related deaths reported w/ previous histories of emotional disturbances, suicidal ideation/attempts, and misuse of tranquilizers, alcohol, and other CNS-active drugs. Caution in patients at risk for respiratory depression; consider alternative nonopioid analgesics. Caution w/ increased intracranial pressure (ICP) or head injury. May impair mental/physical abilities. Withdrawal symptoms may occur if discontinued abruptly. May complicate clinical assessment of acute abdominal conditions. Not for use in pregnant women prior to or during labor unless benefits outweigh risks. Not recommended for obstetrical preoperative medication or for postdelivery analgesia in nursing mothers.

ADVERSE REACTIONS

Dizziness, N/V, constipation, headache, somnolence, flushing, insomnia, increased sweating, asthenia, dry mouth, diarrhea, pruritus, postural hypotension.

DRUG INTERACTIONS

See Contraindications. Caution and reduce dose w/ CNS depressants (eg, alcohol, opioids, anesthetics); increased risk of CNS/respiratory depression. CYP2D6 inhibitors (eg, quinidine, fluoxetine, paroxetine, amitriptyline) and CYP3A4 inhibitors (eg, ketoconazole, erythromycin)

may reduce metabolic clearance and increase risk for serious adverse events, including seizures and serotonin syndrome. Altered exposure w/ CYP3A4 inducers (eg, rifampin, St. John's wort) and inhibitors (ketoconazole, erythromycin). Increased seizure risk w/ SSRIs, TCAs, other tricyclic compounds (eg, cyclobenzaprine, promethazine), MAOIs, other opioids, neuroleptics, and drugs that reduce seizure threshold. Caution w/ SSRIs, SNRIs, TCAs, MAOIs, α2-adrenergic blockers, triptans, linezolid, lithium, St. John's wort, and drugs that impair tramadol metabolism, due to potential serotonin syndrome. Not recommended w/ carbamazepine; may significantly reduce analgesic effect. Digoxin toxicity and alterations of warfarin effect, including elevation of PT, reported rarely. Use w/ other tramadol products is not recommended.

PATIENT CONSIDERATIONS

Assessment: Assess for previous hypersensitivity to the drug and other opioids, acute intoxication w/ alcohol/hypnotics/narcotics/centrally acting analgesics/opioids/psychotropic drugs, epilepsy, seizure and respiratory depression risks, suicidal ideation, emotional disturbance or depression, increased ICP, head injury, drug abuse potential, suicidal/addiction proneness, pain severity, renal/hepatic impairment, pregnancy/nursing status, any other conditions where treatment is contraindicated or cautioned, and possible drug interactions.

Monitoring: Monitor for signs/symptoms of anaphylactoid reactions, respiratory/CNS depression, tolerance, physical dependence, seizures, serotonin syndrome, withdrawal symptoms, and other adverse reactions.

Counseling: Inform of the risks/benefits of therapy. Inform that drug may cause seizures and/or serotonin syndrome w/ concomitant use of serotonergic agents or drugs that significantly reduce the metabolic clearance of therapy. Inform that drug may impair physical/mental abilities required for the performance of hazardous tasks (eg, driving a car, operating machinery). Instruct not to take drug w/ alcohol containing beverages. Inform to use drug w/ caution when taking tranquilizers, hypnotics, and other opiate containing analgesics. Instruct to inform physician if pregnant, thinking/trying to become pregnant. Educate regarding the single-dose and 24-hr dosing regimen; advise not to exceed the recommended dose.

STORAGE: 25°C (77°F); excursions permitted to 15-30°C (59-86°F).

ULTRAVATE – halobetasol propionate

RX

Class: Corticosteroid

ADULT DOSAGE

Inflammatory and Pruritic Manifestations of Corticosteroid-Responsive Dermatoses

Apply a thin layer to affected skin qd or bid ud and rub in gently and completely

Max Dose: 50g/week

Max Duration: 2 weeks; reassess diagnosis if no improvement w/in 2 weeks

D/C when control is achieved

PEDIATRIC DOSAGE

Inflammatory and Pruritic Manifestations of Corticosteroid-Responsive Dermatoses

≥12 Years:

Apply a thin layer to affected skin qd or bid ud and rub in gently and completely

Max Dose: 50g/week

Max Duration: 2 weeks; reassess diagnosis if no improvement w/in 2 weeks

D/C when control is achieved

ADMINISTRATION

Topical route

Avoid w/ occlusive dressings

HOW SUPPLIED

Cre, Oint: 0.05% [50g]

CONTRAINDICATIONS

History of hypersensitivity to any of the components of Ultravate.

WARNINGS/PRECAUTIONS

For dermatologic use only; not for ophthalmic use. May produce reversible hypothalamic-pituitary-adrenal (HPA) axis suppression, manifestations of Cushing's syndrome, hyperglycemia or glucosuria; evaluate periodically for evidence of HPA axis suppression when applying to a large surface area or to areas under occlusion. Attempts should be made to withdraw treatment, reduce frequency of application, or substitute to a less potent corticosteroid if HPA axis suppression is noted. Signs and symptoms of glucocorticosteroid insufficiency may occur (infrequent), requiring supplemental systemic corticosteroids. Pediatric patients may be more susceptible to systemic toxicity. D/C and treat appropriately if irritation develops. Allergic contact dermatitis reported. Use appropriate antibacterial or antifungal agent if skin infections are present or develop; if no favorable prompt response, may need to d/c until infection is controlled. Not for use in rosacea or perioral dermatitis. Do not use on the face, groin, or in the axillae.

ADVERSE REACTIONS
Stinging, burning, itching, dry skin, erythema, skin atrophy, leukoderma, rash.

PATIENT CONSIDERATIONS

Assessment: Assess for previous hypersensitivity to any components of the drug, dermatological conditions, pregnancy/nursing status, and conditions that increase systemic absorption of the medication.

Monitoring: Monitor for HPA axis suppression, manifestations of Cushing's syndrome, hyperglycemia, glucosuria, skin irritation, allergic contact dermatitis (eg, failure to heal), skin infections (eg, bacterial, fungal), and other adverse reactions. Monitor for glucocorticosteroid insufficiency following withdrawal from therapy.

Counseling: Instruct to use externally and ud. Instruct to avoid contact with eyes. Advise not to use for any disorder other than for which it was prescribed. Instruct not to bandage, cover, or wrap treated skin, unless directed by physician. Instruct to report any signs of local adverse reactions to physician.

STORAGE: 15-30°C (59-86°F).

UNASYN — ampicillin sodium/sulbactam sodium RX

Class: Beta-lactamase inhibitor/semisynthetic penicillin (PCN)

ADULT DOSAGE

General Dosing

Skin and skin structure infections, intra-abdominal infections, and gynecological infections caused by susceptible strains of microorganisms

1.5g (1g ampicillin + 0.5g sulbactam)-3g (2g ampicillin + 1g sulbactam) IM/IV q6h
Max: 4g sulbactam/day

PEDIATRIC DOSAGE

Skin and Skin Structure Infections

≥1 Year:
300mg/kg/day (200mg ampicillin + 100mg sulbactam) IV in equally divided doses q6h

≥40kg: 1.5g (1g ampicillin + 0.5g sulbactam)-3g (2g ampicillin + 1g sulbactam) IV q6h
Max: 4g sulbactam/day

Therapy should not routinely exceed 14 days

DOSING CONSIDERATIONS

Renal Impairment

CrCl ≥30mL/min: 1.5-3g q6-8h
CrCl 15-29mL/min: 1.5-3g q12h
CrCl 5-14mL/min: 1.5-3g q24h

ADMINISTRATION

IV/IM route

Do not reconstitute/administer w/ aminoglycosides

IM

Administer by deep IM inj

IV

Administer slowly over at least 10-15 min or 15-30 min in greater dilutions

Refer to PI for directions for use, preparation, compatibility, and stability

HOW SUPPLIED

Inj: (Ampicillin/Sulbactam) 1g/0.5g, 2g/1g. Also available as a Pharmacy Bulk Package. Refer to individual package insert for more information

CONTRAINDICATIONS

History of serious hypersensitivity reactions to ampicillin, sulbactam or to other beta-lactam antibacterial drugs (eg, penicillins, cephalosporins). Previous history of cholestatic jaundice/hepatic dysfunction associated with therapy.

WARNINGS/PRECAUTIONS

Serious and occasionally fatal hypersensitivity reactions reported; d/c and institute appropriate therapy if allergic reaction occurs. Hepatic dysfunction (eg, hepatitis, cholestatic jaundice) reported. *Clostridium difficile*-associated diarrhea (CDAD) reported and may range in severity from mild diarrhea to fatal colitis; may need to d/c if CDAD is suspected or confirmed. Ampicillin class antibacterial should not be administered to patients with mononucleosis. May result in bacterial resistance in the absence of proven or suspected bacterial infection or a prophylactic indication; d/c and/or take appropriate measures if superinfection develops. Decrease in total conjugated estriol, estriol-glucuronide, conjugated estrone, and estradiol reported in pregnant women. Lab test interactions may occur. Caution with renal impairment.

ADVERSE REACTIONS

Inj-site pain, thrombophlebitis, diarrhea.

DRUG INTERACTIONS

Probenecid decreases renal tubular secretion and may increase and prolong blood levels. Ampicillin: Increased incidence of rash with allopurinol.

PATIENT CONSIDERATIONS

Assessment: Assess for history of hypersensitivity to drug, PCNs, cephalosporins, or other allergens, history of cholestatic jaundice/hepatic dysfunction, mononucleosis, renal impairment, pregnancy/nursing status, and for possible drug interactions. Perform culture and susceptibility testing.

Monitoring: Monitor for signs/symptoms of hypersensitivity reactions, CDAD, superinfection, and other adverse reactions. Monitor for changes in estrogen levels in pregnant women. Monitor hepatic function at regular intervals in patients with hepatic impairment.

Counseling: Inform that therapy should only be used to treat bacterial, not viral, infections. Advise to take exactly ud even if patient feels better early in the course of therapy. Inform that skipping doses or not completing full course may decrease effectiveness and increase resistance. Inform that diarrhea is a common problem caused by therapy and will usually end upon discontinuation of therapy. Inform that diarrhea may occur as late as ≥2 months after last dose of therapy; instruct to notify physician as soon as possible if watery/bloody stools (with or without stomach cramps and fever) occur.

STORAGE: Prior to Reconstitution: ≤30°C (86°F). Reconstituted: Refer to PI for storage requirements.

UNITUXIN – dinutuximab

RX

Class: GD2-binding monoclonal antibody

Serious and potentially life-threatening infusion reactions reported; administer required prehydration and premedication including antihistamines prior to each infusion. Monitor closely for signs/symptoms of an infusion reaction during and for at least 4 hrs following completion of each infusion. Immediately interrupt therapy for severe infusion reactions and permanently d/c for anaphylaxis. May cause severe neuropathic pain; administer IV opioid prior to, during, and for 2 hrs following completion of infusion. Grade 3 peripheral sensory neuropathy reported. Severe motor neuropathy reported in adults. D/C therapy for severe unresponsive pain, severe sensory neuropathy, or moderate to severe peripheral motor neuropathy.

PEDIATRIC DOSAGE

Neuroblastoma

In combination w/ granulocyte-macrophage colony-stimulating factor, interleukin-2 and 13-cis-retinoic acid, for the treatment of patients w/ high-risk neuroblastoma who achieve at least a partial response to prior 1st-line multiagent, multimodality therapy

Usual: 17.5mg/m^2/day as IV infusion over 10-20 hrs for 4 consecutive days for a max of 5 cycles

Initiate at an infusion rate of 0.875mg/m^2/hr for 30 min; may gradually increase as tolerated to a max rate of 1.75mg/m^2/hr

Schedule of Administration:

Cycles 1, 3, and 5:

Take on Days 4, 5, 6, and 7

Cycles 1, 3, and 5 are 24 days in duration

Cycles 2 and 4:

Take on Days 8, 9, 10, and 11

Cycles 2 and 4 are 32 days in duration

Required Pretreatment and Guidelines for Pain Management:

IV Hydration: Administer 10mL/kg IV infusion of 0.9% NaCl inj over 1 hr just prior to initiating each dinutuximab infusion

Analgesics: Administer 50mcg/kg morphine sulfate IV immediately prior to initiation of dinutuximab, then continue as a morphine sulfate drip at an infusion rate of 20-

U

50mcg/kg/hr during and for 2 hrs following completion of dinutuximab.
Administer additional 25-50mcg/kg IV doses of morphine sulfate prn for pain for up to once q2h followed by an increase in morphine sulfate infusion rate in clinically stable patients.
Consider using fentanyl or hydromorphone if morphine sulfate is not tolerated.
If pain is inadequately managed w/ opioids, consider use of gabapentin or lidocaine in conjunction w/ IV morphine.

Antihistamines/Antipyretics: Administer 0.5-1mg/kg (max dose of 50mg) of antihistamine (eg, diphenhydramine) IV over 10-15 min starting 20 min prior to initiation of dinutuximab and as tolerated q4-6h during dinutuximab infusion.
Administer 10-15mg/kg (max dose of 650mg) of acetaminophen 20 min prior to each dinutuximab infusion and q4-6h prn for fever or pain.
Administer 5-10mg/kg of ibuprofen q6h prn for control of persistent fever or pain.

DOSING CONSIDERATIONS

Adverse Reactions

Infusion-Related Reactions:
Mild to moderate adverse reactions (eg, transient rash, fever, rigors, localized urticaria) that respond promptly to symptomatic treatment
Onset of Reaction: Reduce infusion rate to 50% of the previous rate and monitor closely
After Resolution: Gradually increase infusion rate up to a max rate of 1.75mg/m^2/hr

Prolonged or Severe Adverse Reactions (eg, Mild Bronchospasm w/o Other Symptoms, Angioedema That Does Not Affect the Airway):
Onset of Reaction: Interrupt immediately
After Resolution: Resume at 50% of the previous rate and observe closely, if signs and symptoms resolve rapidly
1st Recurrence: D/C until the following day. If symptoms resolve and continued treatment is warranted, premedicate w/ 1mg/kg (max dose of 50mg) hydrocortisone IV and administer dinutuximab at a rate of 0.875mg/m^2/hr in an intensive care unit
2nd Recurrence: D/C permanently

Capillary Leak Syndrome:
Moderate to Severe but Not Life-Threatening:
Onset of Reaction: Interrupt immediately
After Resolution: Resume at 50% of the previous rate

Life-Threatening:
Onset of Reaction: D/C for the current cycle
After Resolution: Administer at 50% of the previous rate in subsequent cycles
1st Recurrence: D/C permanently

Hypotension Requiring Medical Intervention:
Symptomatic Hypotension, Systolic BP (SBP) < Lower Limit of Normal for Age, or SBP Decreased by >15% Compared to Baseline:
Onset of Reaction: Interrupt infusion
After Resolution: Resume infusion at 50% of the previous rate. Increase infusion rate as tolerated up to a max rate of 1.75mg/m^2/hr if BP remains stable for at least 2 hrs

U

Severe Systemic Infection or Sepsis:
Onset of Reaction: D/C until resolution of infection, and then proceed w/ subsequent cycles of therapy

Neurological Disorders of the Eye:
Onset of Reaction: D/C infusion until resolution
After Resolution: Reduce dose by 50%
1st Recurrence or if Accompanied by Visual Impairment: D/C permanently

Permanently Discontinue w/ the Following:
- Grade 3 or 4 anaphylaxis
- Grade 3 or 4 serum sickness
- Grade 3 pain unresponsive to max supportive measures

- Grade 4 sensory neuropathy or Grade 3 sensory neuropathy that interferes w/ daily activities for >2 weeks
- Grade 2 peripheral motor neuropathy
- Subtotal or total vision loss
- Grade 4 hyponatremia despite appropriate fluid management

ADMINISTRATION

IV route

Administer as a diluted IV infusion only; do not administer as an IV push or bolus
Verify that patients have adequate hematologic, respiratory, hepatic, and renal function prior to initiating each course of therapy

Preparation

Aseptically withdraw the required volume from the single-use vial and inject into a 100mL bag of 0.9% NaCl inj
Mix by gentle inversion; do not shake
Initiate infusion w/in 4 hrs of preparation
Discard diluted sol 24 hrs after preparation

HOW SUPPLIED

Inj: 3.5mg/mL [5mL]

CONTRAINDICATIONS

History of anaphylaxis to dinutuximab.

WARNINGS/PRECAUTIONS

Pain reported; decrease infusion rate to 0.875mg/m^2/hr for severe pain. Capillary leak syndrome reported; immediately interrupt or d/c therapy and institute supportive management in patients w/ symptomatic or severe capillary leak syndrome. Hypotension, infection, neurological disorders of the eye, bone marrow suppression, and electrolyte abnormalities reported. Atypical hemolytic uremic syndrome reported; permanently d/c therapy and institute supportive management for signs of hemolytic uremic syndrome. May cause fetal harm.

ADVERSE REACTIONS

Infusion reactions, neuropathy, pain, pyrexia, thrombocytopenia, lymphopenia, hypotension, hyponatremia, anemia, vomiting, diarrhea, hypokalemia, neutropenia, urticaria, hypoalbuminemia.

PATIENT CONSIDERATIONS

Assessment: Assess for hematologic/respiratory/hepatic/renal dysfunction, history of anaphylaxis to drug, and pregnancy/nursing status.

Monitoring: Monitor for neuropathy, pain, capillary leak syndrome, hypotension, infection, neurological disorders of the eye, atypical hemolytic uremic syndrome, and other adverse reactions. Monitor closely for signs/symptoms of an infusion reaction during and for at least 4 hrs following completion of each infusion. Monitor serum electrolytes (daily) and peripheral blood counts.

Counseling: Inform of the risk of serious infusion reactions and anaphylaxis; severe pain and peripheral sensory and motor neuropathy; capillary leak syndrome; hypotension; infection; neurological disorders of the eye; bone marrow suppression; electrolyte abnormalities; and hemolytic uremic syndrome. Instruct to promptly report to physician if any signs/symptoms of any of these conditions develop. Advise women of reproductive potential of the potential risk to the fetus if administered during pregnancy and the need for use of effective contraception during and for at least 2 months after completing therapy.

STORAGE: 2-8°C (36-46°F). Do not freeze or shake the vial. Protect from light.

UPTRAVI – selexipag

RX

Class: Prostacyclin receptor agonist

ADULT DOSAGE

Pulmonary Arterial Hypertension

Treatment of pulmonary arterial HTN (WHO Group I) to delay disease progression and reduce risk of hospitalization

Initial: 200mcg bid
Titrate: Increase in increments of 200mcg bid, usually at weekly intervals
Max: 1600mcg bid

If a patient reaches a dose that cannot be tolerated, the dose should be reduced to previously tolerated dose

PEDIATRIC DOSAGE

Pediatric use may not have been established

U

Missed Dose

If a dose is missed, take as soon as possible unless next dose is w/in the next 6 hrs

If treatment is missed for ≥3 days, restart at a lower dose and then retitrate

DOSING CONSIDERATIONS

Hepatic Impairment

Moderate (Child-Pugh Class B):

Initial: 200mcg qd

Titrate: Increase in increments of 200mcg qd at weekly intervals, as tolerated

Severe (Child-Pugh Class C): Avoid use

ADMINISTRATION

Oral route

Tolerability may be improved when taken w/ food.
Do not split, crush, or chew tabs.

HOW SUPPLIED

Tab: 200mcg, 400mcg, 600mcg, 800mcg, 1000mcg, 1200mcg, 1400mcg, 1600mcg

WARNINGS/PRECAUTIONS

Consider the possibility of associated pulmonary veno-occlusive disease if signs of pulmonary edema occur; d/c therapy if confirmed.

ADVERSE REACTIONS

Headache, diarrhea, jaw pain, N/V, myalgia, pain in extremity, flushing, arthralgia, anemia, decreased appetite, rash.

DRUG INTERACTIONS

Strong CYP2C8 inhibitors (eg, gemfibrozil) may significantly increase exposure to selexipag and its active metabolite; avoid concomitant administration.

PATIENT CONSIDERATIONS

Assessment: Assess pregnancy/nursing status, and for possible drug interactions.

Monitoring: Monitor for signs of pulmonary edema and other adverse events.

Counseling: Inform not to split, crush, or chew tablets. Advise patients what to do in case of a missed dose.

STORAGE: 20-25°C (68-77°F); excursions permitted between 15-30°C (59-86°F).

URIBEL — hyoscyamine sulfate/methenamine/methylene blue/phenyl salicylate/sodium phosphate monobasic RX

Class: Acidifier/analgesic/antibacterial/anticholinergic/antiseptic

ADULT DOSAGE

Urinary Tract Symptoms

For treatment of symptoms of irritative voiding, relief of local symptoms that accompany lower UTIs (eg, inflammation, hypermotility, pain), and relief of urinary tract symptoms caused by diagnostic procedures

Usual: 1 cap PO qid followed by liberal fluid intake

PEDIATRIC DOSAGE

Urinary Tract Symptoms

For treatment of symptoms of irritative voiding, relief of local symptoms that accompany lower UTIs (eg, inflammation, hypermotility, pain), and relief of urinary tract symptoms caused by diagnostic procedures

>6 Years:
Individualize dose

U

ADMINISTRATION

Oral route

HOW SUPPLIED

Cap: (Methenamine/Sodium Phosphate Monobasic/Phenyl Salicylate/Methylene Blue/Hyoscyamine Sulfate) 118mg/40.8mg/36mg/10mg/0.12mg

CONTRAINDICATIONS

Hypersensitivity to any of the ingredients of Uribel is possible. Consider risk benefits with existing conditions, such as cardiac disease (especially cardiac arrhythmias, congestive heart failure, coronary heart disease, mitral stenosis), GI tract obstructive disease, glaucoma, and myasthenia gravis. Acute urinary retention may be precipitated in obstructive uropathy (eg, bladder neck obstruction due to prostatic hypertrophy).

WARNINGS/PRECAUTIONS

Do not exceed recommended dosage. D/C immediately if rapid pulse, dizziness, or blurred vision occurs. Intolerance may occur in patients intolerant to belladonna alkaloids or salicylates. Delay in gastric emptying could complicate management of gastric ulcers. Infants and young children are especially susceptible to toxic effect of belladonna alkaloids. Caution in elderly; may respond to usual doses of hyoscyamine with excitement, agitation, drowsiness, or confusion. Urine may become blue to blue-green and feces may be discolored due to excretion of methylene blue.

ADVERSE REACTIONS

Rapid pulse, flushing, blurred vision, dizziness, SOB, difficult micturition, acute urinary retention, dry mouth, N/V.

DRUG INTERACTIONS

May decrease absorption of other PO medications (eg, urinary alkalizers, thiazide diuretics, antimuscarinics, antacids/antidiarrheals, antimyasthenics, ketoconazole, MAOIs, opioids, sulfonamides). Concomitant use with antimyasthenics may reduce intestinal motility. Concomitant use with MAOIs may intensify antimuscarinic side effects. Thiazide diuretics may decrease effectiveness of methenamine. Antimuscarinic effects of hyoscyamine may be intensified with antimuscarinics. Antacids/antidiarrheals may reduce absorption of hyoscyamine and antacids may reduce effectiveness of methenamine. Space dosing by 1 hr with antacids/antidiarrheals. Take at least 2 hrs after ketoconazole intake. May increase the risk of severe constipation with opioids. Sulfonamides may precipitate with formaldehyde in the urine, increasing the danger of crystalluria.

PATIENT CONSIDERATIONS

Assessment: Assess for cardiac disease, GI tract obstructive disease, glaucoma, myasthenia gravis, obstructive uropathy, gastric ulcers, intolerance to belladonna alkaloids or salicylates, hypersensitivity, pregnancy/nursing status, and possible drug interactions.

Monitoring: Monitor for rapid pulse, dizziness, blurring of vision, delayed gastric emptying, and other adverse reactions.

Counseling: Counsel about risks and benefits of therapy. Instruct to d/c use and consult physician if rapid pulse, dizziness, or blurring of vision occurs. Advise to inform physician if taking other medications. Advise to not exceed recommended dose. Inform that urine and feces may be discolored because of methylene blue. Keep out of reach of children.

STORAGE: 20-25°C (68-77°F). Keep in cool, dry place.

UROXATRAL – alfuzosin hydrochloride

RX

Class: Alpha$_1$ antagonist

ADULT DOSAGE

Benign Prostatic Hyperplasia

10mg qd

PEDIATRIC DOSAGE

Pediatric use may not have been established

ADMINISTRATION

Oral route

Take w/ food and w/ the same meal each day.
Do not chew or crush tab.

HOW SUPPLIED

Tab, Extended-Release: 10mg

CONTRAINDICATIONS

Moderate or severe hepatic impairment (Child-Pugh categories B and C), concomitant use of potent CYP3A4 inhibitors (eg, ketoconazole, itraconazole, ritonavir). Known hypersensitivity to alfuzosin HCl or any component of Uroxatral.

U

WARNINGS/PRECAUTIONS

Postural hypotension w/ or w/o symptoms (eg, dizziness) may develop w/in a few hrs following administration; caution w/ symptomatic hypotension or in those who have had a hypotensive response to other medications. Syncope may occur; caution to avoid situations in which injury could result should syncope occur. Caution w/ severe renal impairment (CrCl <30mL/min) or mild hepatic impairment. Prostate carcinoma and BPH frequently coexist; patients thought to have BPH should be examined to rule out prostate carcinoma prior to starting treatment. Intraoperative floppy iris syndrome (IFIS) observed in some patients during cataract surgery; may require modifications to surgical technique. May cause priapism. D/C if symptoms of angina pectoris appear or worsen. Caution w/ acquired or congenital QT prolongation.

ADVERSE REACTIONS
Dizziness, URTI, headache.

DRUG INTERACTIONS
See Contraindications. Avoid use w/ other α-adrenergic antagonists. Risk of hypotension/postural hypotension and syncope may be increased w/ concomitant antihypertensives and nitrates. Caution w/ PDE-5 inhibitors; may potentially cause symptomatic hypotension. Caution w/ medications that prolong the QT interval.

PATIENT CONSIDERATIONS

Assessment: Assess for hypersensitivity to drug, symptomatic hypotension, history of QT prolongation, hepatic/renal impairment, and possible drug interactions. Assess if patient is planning to undergo cataract surgery. Rule out the presence of prostate cancer prior to therapy.

Monitoring: Monitor for postural hypotension, syncope, hypersensitivity reactions, IFIS, QT prolongation, hepatic/renal impairment, and other adverse reactions.

Counseling: Inform about possible occurrence of symptoms related to postural hypotension when beginning therapy; caution about driving, operating machinery, or performing hazardous tasks during this period. Instruct to inform ophthalmologist about use of the product before cataract surgery or other procedures involving the eyes, even if no longer taking the medication. Advise about the possibility of priapism resulting from treatment and instruct to seek immediate medical attention if it occurs.

STORAGE: 25°C (77°F); excursions permitted to 15-30°C (59-86°F). Protect from light and moisture.

Urso 250 – ursodiol RX

Class: Bile acid

OTHER BRAND NAMES
Urso Forte

ADULT DOSAGE
Primary Biliary Cirrhosis
Usual: 13-15mg/kg/day given bid-qid

PEDIATRIC DOSAGE
Pediatric use may not have been established

ADMINISTRATION
Oral route
Take w/ food

Urso Forte
Scored tab may be broken in halves; do not use segments broken incorrectly
Take unchewed w/ water

HOW SUPPLIED
Tab: (Urso 250) 250mg, (Urso Forte) 500mg* *scored

CONTRAINDICATIONS
Complete biliary obstruction, known hypersensitivity or intolerance to ursodiol or any components of the formulation.

WARNINGS/PRECAUTIONS
Administer appropriate specific treatment in patients with variceal bleeding, hepatic encephalopathy, ascites, or in need of an urgent liver transplant. Monitor LFTs (gamma-glutamyl transpeptidase [GGT], alkaline phosphatase, AST, ALT) and bilirubin levels monthly for 3 months after start of therapy, and every 6 months thereafter; consider treatment discontinuation if the parameters increase to a level considered clinically significant in patients with stable historical LFT levels. Use with caution to maintain bile flow.

ADVERSE REACTIONS
Leukopenia, skin rash, peptic ulcer, blood glucose elevation, SrCr elevation, thrombocytopenia, diarrhea, abdominal pain, asthenia, nausea, dyspepsia, anorexia, esophagitis.

DRUG INTERACTIONS
Bile acid sequestering agents (eg, cholestyramine, colestipol) and aluminum-based antacids may interfere with the action of the drug by reducing its absorption. Estrogens, oral contraceptives, and clofibrate (and perhaps other lipid-lowering drugs) may counteract effectiveness.

PATIENT CONSIDERATIONS

Assessment: Assess for biliary obstruction, variceal bleeding, hepatic encephalopathy, ascites, need for an urgent liver transplant, hypersensitivity, intolerance, pregnancy/nursing status, and possible drug interactions.

Monitoring: Monitor for the development of adverse reactions. Monitor LFTs (GGT, alkaline phosphatase, AST, ALT) and bilirubin levels monthly for 3 months after start of therapy, and every 6 months thereafter.

Counseling: Inform that adsorption may be reduced if taking concomitant bile acid sequestering agents, aluminum-based antacids, or drugs known to alter the metabolism of cholesterol.

STORAGE: 20-25°C (68-77°F). (Urso Forte) Half-tab: 20-25°C (68-77°F) in the current packaging for up to 28 days. Store separately from whole tabs.

UTIBRON NEOHALER – glycopyrrolate/indacaterol

RX

Class: Anticholinergic/beta$_2$ agonist

Long-acting β_2-adrenergic agonists (LABAs) increase the risk of asthma-related death. Not indicated for the treatment of asthma.

ADULT DOSAGE

Chronic Obstructive Pulmonary Disease

Long-Term Maint Treatment of Airflow Obstruction:

Recommended: Orally inhale the contents of 1 cap bid using the Neohaler device

Max: 1 cap bid

PEDIATRIC DOSAGE

Pediatric use may not have been established

ADMINISTRATION

Oral inh route

Use only w/ Neohaler device.
Do not swallow caps.
Administer at the same time every day.
Store caps in the blister; only remove immediately before use.

HOW SUPPLIED

Cap, Inh: (Indacaterol/Glycopyrrolate) 27.5mcg/15.6mcg

CONTRAINDICATIONS

Hypersensitivity to indacaterol, glycopyrrolate, or to any of the ingredients. **Indacaterol:** Asthma w/o use of a long-term asthma control medication. Not indicated for treatment of asthma.

WARNINGS/PRECAUTIONS

Do not initiate in acutely deteriorating or potentially life-threatening episodes of COPD or use for the relief of acute symptoms. D/C regular use of oral or inhaled short-acting β_2-agonists (SABAs) when beginning treatment; use only for symptomatic relief of acute respiratory symptoms. May produce paradoxical bronchospasm; treat immediately w/ an inhaled, short acting bronchodilator and d/c and institute alternative therapy. Immediate hypersensitivity reactions have been reported; d/c immediately and institute alternative therapy if signs suggesting an allergic reaction occur. Caution in patients w/ severe hypersensitivity to milk proteins. Caution w/ narrow-angle glaucoma and urinary retention. **Indacaterol:** Do not use more often or at higher doses than recommended; clinically significant cardiovascular (CV) effects and fatalities reported w/ excessive use. CV effects may occur; may need to d/c if such effects occur. Caution w/ CV disorders, convulsive disorders, thyrotoxicosis, diabetes mellitus (DM), ketoacidosis, and in patients who are unusually responsive to sympathomimetic amines. May produce significant hypokalemia and increases in plasma glucose.

ADVERSE REACTIONS

Nasopharyngitis, HTN.

DRUG INTERACTIONS

Indacaterol: Do not use w/ other medicines containing LABAs. Adrenergic drugs may potentiate sympathetic effects; use w/ caution. Xanthine derivatives, steroids, or diuretics may potentiate any hypokalemic effect. Caution w/ non-K$^+$-sparing diuretics (eg, loop or thiazide diuretics). Extreme caution w/ MAOIs, TCAs, or other drugs known to prolong the QTc interval; action on CV system may be potentiated. Drugs known to prolong the QTc interval may be associated w/ an increased risk of ventricular arrhythmias. β-blockers and indacaterol may interfere w/ the effect of each other when administered concurrently. β-blockers may block therapeutic effects and produce severe bronchospasm in COPD patients; avoid treatment w/ β-blockers. If such therapy is needed, consider cardioselective β-blockers and use w/ caution. **Glycopyrrolate:** Avoid w/ other anticholinergic-containing drugs; may lead to an increase in anticholinergic adverse effects.

PATIENT CONSIDERATIONS

Assessment: Assess for hypersensitivity to indacaterol, glycopyrrolate, milk proteins, or any component of the product. Assess for asthma, acutely deteriorating COPD, CV disorders, convulsive disorders, thyrotoxicosis, DM, ketoacidosis, narrow-angle glaucoma, urinary retention, pregnancy/nursing status, and possible drug interactions. Evaluate use in patients unusually responsive to sympathomimetic amines.

Monitoring: Monitor for deteriorating disease, paradoxical bronchospasm, hypersensitivity reactions, CV effects, narrow-angle glaucoma, urinary retention, hypokalemia, hyperglycemia, and other adverse reactions.

Counseling: Inform that drug is not for treatment of asthma or for relief of acute symptoms of COPD. Advise that acute symptoms should be treated w/ a rescue inhaler (eg, albuterol). Instruct to seek medical attention immediately if experiencing worsening of symptoms or a need for more inhalations than usual of the rescue inhaler. Advise not to d/c therapy w/o physician guidance and not to use an additional LABA. Instruct to d/c therapy if paradoxical bronchospasm occurs. Inform about adverse effects (eg, palpitations, chest pain, rapid HR, tremor, nervousness) and other risks (eg, narrow-angle glaucoma, urinary retention) associated w/ therapy; instruct to consult physician immediately if any signs/symptoms develop. Instruct on how to correctly administer caps using the Neohaler device. Inform that the contents of the caps are for oral inhalation only and must not be swallowed. Advise to contact physician if pregnancy occurs while on therapy.

STORAGE: 77°F (25°C); excursions permitted to 59-86°F (15-30°C). Store caps in the blister protected from light and moisture; remove caps from the blister immediately before use. Do not use the Neohaler device w/ any other caps. Always use the new Neohaler inhaler provided w/ each new prescription.

VAGIFEM – estradiol

RX

Class: Estrogen

Estrogens increase the risk of endometrial cancer. Perform adequate diagnostic measures, including endometrial sampling, to rule out malignancy in postmenopausal women with undiagnosed persistent or recurring abnormal genital bleeding. Should not be used for prevention of cardiovascular disease (CVD) or dementia. Increased risk of MI, pulmonary embolism (PE), stroke, invasive breast cancer, and DVT in postmenopausal women (50-79 yrs of age) reported. Increased risk of developing probable dementia in postmenopausal women ≥65 yrs reported. Should be prescribed at the lowest effective dose and for the shortest duration consistent with treatment goals and risks.

ADULT DOSAGE

Atrophic Vaginitis

Due to Menopause:
1 tab intravaginally qd for 2 weeks, followed by 1 tab intravaginally twice weekly; women should generally be started at the 10mcg dose

PEDIATRIC DOSAGE

Pediatric use may not have been established

ADMINISTRATION

Intravaginal route

Use supplied applicator to administer dose

It is advisable to use the same time daily for all applications

HOW SUPPLIED

Tab: 10mcg

CONTRAINDICATIONS

Undiagnosed abnormal genital bleeding, known/suspected/history of breast cancer, known/suspected estrogen-dependent neoplasia, active or history of DVT/PE/arterial thromboembolic disease (eg, stroke, MI), known anaphylactic reaction or angioedema to the medication, known liver impairment/disease, known protein C/protein S/antithrombin deficiency or other known thrombophilic disorders, known/suspected pregnancy.

WARNINGS/PRECAUTIONS

Caution in patients with risk factors for arterial vascular disease and/or venous thromboembolism. If feasible, d/c at least 4-6 weeks before surgery of the type associated with increased risk of thromboembolism, or during periods of prolonged immobilization. May increase risk of gallbladder disease requiring surgery, and ovarian cancer. Consider addition of progestin for women with a uterus or with residual endometriosis post-hysterectomy. May lead to severe hypercalcemia in women with breast cancer and bone metastases; d/c and take appropriate measures if hypercalcemia occurs. Retinal vascular thrombosis reported; if visual abnormalities or migraine occurs, d/c pending exam. If exam reveals papilledema or retinal vascular lesions, d/c permanently. May elevate BP, plasma TGs (with preexisting hypertriglyceridemia), and thyroid-binding globulin levels; d/c if pancreatitis occurs. Caution with history of cholestatic jaundice associated with past estrogen use or with pregnancy; d/c in case of recurrence. May cause fluid retention; caution with cardiac/renal dysfunction. Caution with hypoparathyroidism; hypocalcemia may result. May exacerbate symptoms of angioedema in women with hereditary angioedema. May exacerbate endometriosis, asthma, diabetes mellitus, epilepsy, migraine, porphyria, systemic lupus erythematosus, and hepatic hemangiomas; use with caution. Local abrasion induced by applicator reported, especially in women with severely atrophic vaginal mucosa. May affect certain endocrine and blood components in lab tests.

ADVERSE REACTIONS

Vulvovaginal mycotic infection, vulvovaginal pruritus, back pain, diarrhea.

DRUG INTERACTIONS

CYP3A4 inducers (eg, St. John's wort, phenobarbital, carbamazepine, rifampin) may decrease levels, which may decrease therapeutic effects and/or change uterine bleeding profile. CYP3A4 inhibitors (eg, erythromycin, ketoconazole, ritonavir, grapefruit juice) may increase levels, which may result in side effects. Concomitant thyroid hormone replacement therapy may require increased doses of thyroid replacement therapy.

PATIENT CONSIDERATIONS

Assessment: Assess for abnormal vaginal bleeding, presence/history of breast cancer, estrogen-dependent neoplasia, active or history of DVT/PE/arterial thromboembolic disease, liver impairment/disease, thrombophilic disorders, known anaphylactic reaction or angioedema to the drug, pregnancy/nursing status, other conditions where treatment is cautioned, need for progestin therapy, and possible drug interactions.

Monitoring: Monitor for signs/symptoms of CVD, malignant neoplasms, dementia, gallbladder disease, hypercalcemia, visual abnormalities, BP and plasma TG elevations, pancreatitis, cholestatic jaundice, hypothyroidism, fluid retention, and for other adverse events. Perform annual breast exam; schedule mammography based on age, risk factors, and prior mammogram results. Monitor thyroid function in patients on thyroid hormone replacement therapy. Perform adequate diagnostic measures (eg, endometrial sampling) in patients with undiagnosed persistent or recurring genital bleeding. Perform periodic evaluation to determine treatment need.

Counseling: Inform postmenopausal women of the importance of reporting abnormal vaginal bleeding to physician as soon as possible. Inform of possible adverse reactions. Advise to have yearly breast exams by a physician and perform monthly breast self-exams. Instruct on how to use the applicator.

STORAGE: 25°C (77°F); excursions permitted to 15-30°C (59-86°F). Do not refrigerate.

VALCHLOR – mechlorethamine

RX

Class: Nitrogen mustard alkylating agent

ADULT DOSAGE

Cutaneous T-Cell Lymphoma

Stage IA and IB Mycosis Fungoides-Type Cutaneous T-Cell Lymphoma in Patients Who Have Received Prior Skin-Directed Therapy:
Apply a thin film qd to affected areas of the skin

PEDIATRIC DOSAGE

Pediatric use may not have been established

DOSING CONSIDERATIONS

Adverse Reactions

Skin Ulceration, Blistering, or Moderately-Severe or Severe Dermatitis (Marked Skin Redness with Edema):
D/C for any grade; upon improvement, restart at a reduced frequency of once every 3 days
If reintroduction is tolerated for at least 1 week, increase frequency of application to qod for at least 1 week and then to qd application if tolerated

ADMINISTRATION

Topical route

Caregivers must wear disposable nitrile gloves when applying gel to patients and wash hands thoroughly with soap and water after removal of gloves
If there is accidental skin exposure to gel, caregivers must immediately wash exposed areas thoroughly with soap and water for at least 15 minutes and remove contaminated clothing
Do not use occlusive dressings on areas of the skin where product was applied

HOW SUPPLIED

Gel: 0.016% [60g]

CONTRAINDICATIONS

Known severe hypersensitivity to mechlorethamine.

WARNINGS/PRECAUTIONS

Exposure to eyes causes pain, burns, inflammation, photophobia, and blurred vision; blindness and severe irreversible anterior eye injury may occur. If eye exposure occurs, immediately irrigate for at least 15 min with copious amounts of water, normal saline, or a balanced salt ophthalmic irrigating solution and obtain immediate medical (eg, ophthalmologic) consultation. Exposure of mucous membranes (eg, oral mucosa, nasal mucosa) causes pain, redness, and ulceration, which may be severe; should mucosal contact occur, immediately irrigate for at least 15 min with copious amounts of water, followed by immediate medical consultation. Avoid direct skin contact with product in individuals other than the patient; risks of secondary exposure include dermatitis, mucosal injury, and secondary cancers. Dermatitis reported; monitor for redness, swelling, inflammation, itchiness, blisters, ulceration, and secondary skin infections. Non-melanoma skin cancer reported; monitor for non-melanoma skin cancers during and after treatment. May cause fetal harm. Flammable; avoid fire, flame, and smoking until medication has dried.

ADVERSE REACTIONS

Dermatitis, pruritus, bacterial skin infection, skin ulceration/blistering, skin hyperpigmentation.

PATIENT CONSIDERATIONS

Assessment: Assess for drug hypersensitivity, and pregnancy/nursing status.

Monitoring: Monitor for dermatitis (redness, swelling, inflammation, itchiness, blisters, ulceration, secondary skin infections), non-melanoma skin cancers (during and after treatment), and other adverse reactions. Monitor if eye exposure or mucosal contact occurs.

Counseling: Instruct to wash hands thoroughly with soap and water after handling or applying the product. Instruct caregivers to wear disposable nitrile gloves when applying the product to patients and to wash hands thoroughly with soap and water after removal of gloves; advise that if there is accidental skin exposure to the product, to immediately wash exposed areas thoroughly with soap and water for at least 15 min and remove contaminated clothing. Instruct not to use occlusive (air or water-tight) dressings on areas of the skin where product was applied. Advise to discard unused product, empty tubes, and used application gloves in household trash in a manner that prevents accidental application or ingestion by others, including children and pets. Advise that adherence to the recommended storage condition will ensure the product will work as expected; instruct to consult a pharmacist prior to using product that has been left at room temperature for >1 hr/day. Counsel on what to do in case of eye exposure or mucosal contact. Instruct to consult with physician if skin irritation occurs after applying the product. Instruct to notify physician of any new skin lesions and to undergo periodic assessment for signs and symptoms of skin cancer. Advise of the potential hazard to a fetus and to avoid pregnancy while using the product. Advise women to d/c nursing due to the potential for topical or systemic exposure to product. Instruct to avoid fire, flame, and smoking until medication has dried.

STORAGE: Prior to Dispensing: -25 to -15°C (-13-5°F). Once Dispensed: 2-8°C (36-46°F). Keep in its original box and avoid contact with food when storing in refrigerator. Discard unused product after 60 days.

VALIUM – diazepam

CIV

Class: Benzodiazepine

ADULT DOSAGE

Anxiety Disorders

Management of Disorders or for Short-Term Relief of Symptoms:
2-10mg bid-qid

Alcohol Withdrawal

Symptomatic Relief of Acute Withdrawal:
10mg tid or qid for first 24 hrs, then reduce to 5mg tid or qid prn

Muscle Spasms

Adjunctive Therapy:
2-10mg tid or qid

Convulsive Disorders

Adjunctive Therapy:
2-10mg bid-qid

PEDIATRIC DOSAGE

General Dosing

≥6 Months of Age:
Initial: 1-2.5mg tid or qid
Titrate: Increase gradually prn and as tolerated

DOSING CONSIDERATIONS

Elderly

Elderly/Debilitated:

Initial: 2-2.5mg qd or bid

Titrate: Increase gradually prn and as tolerated

ADMINISTRATION

Oral route

HOW SUPPLIED

Tab: 2mg*, 5mg*, 10mg* *scored

CONTRAINDICATIONS

Known hypersensitivity to diazepam, pediatric patients <6 months of age, myasthenia gravis, severe respiratory insufficiency, severe hepatic insufficiency, sleep apnea syndrome, acute narrow-angle glaucoma.

WARNINGS/PRECAUTIONS

May be used with treated open-angle glaucoma. Periodically reassess usefulness of drug. Not recommended for the treatment of psychotic patients. May increase frequency and/or severity of grand mal seizures and may require an increase in the dose of standard anticonvulsant medication. Abrupt withdrawal may also temporarily increase frequency and/or severity of seizures. May increase risk of congenital malformations and other developmental abnormalities. Caution during labor and delivery. Caution in the severely depressed or with evidence of latent depression or anxiety associated with depression, or suicidal tendencies; protective measures may be necessary. Psychiatric and paradoxical reactions may occur and are more likely in children and the elderly; d/c if these occur. Lower dose is recommended with chronic respiratory insufficiency. Extreme caution with history of alcohol or drug abuse. In debilitated patients, limit dose to smallest effective amount to preclude ataxia or oversedation development. Repeated use for a prolonged time may result in some loss of response to effects. Isolated reports of neutropenia and jaundice reported. Abuse and dependence reported.

ADVERSE REACTIONS

Drowsiness, fatigue, muscle weakness, ataxia.

DRUG INTERACTIONS

Mutually potentiates effects with central acting agents (eg, antipsychotics, anxiolytics/sedatives, MAOIs). Alcohol enhances sedative effects; avoid concomitant use. Slower rate of absorption with antacids. Concomitant use with compounds which inhibit certain hepatic enzymes such as CYP3A and CYP2C19 (eg, cimetidine, ketoconazole, fluvoxamine) may increase and prolong sedation. Decreased metabolic elimination of phenytoin reported.

PATIENT CONSIDERATIONS

Assessment: Assess for hypersensitivity to drug, acute narrow-angle glaucoma, myasthenia gravis, severe respiratory/hepatic insufficiency, sleep apnea syndrome, history of seizures, psychosis, depression, history of alcohol/drug abuse, debilitation, pregnancy/nursing status, and possible drug interactions.

Monitoring: Monitor for hypersensitivity reactions, withdrawal symptoms, seizures, psychiatric/paradoxical reactions, respiratory depression, loss of response during prolonged use, abuse, dependence, and other adverse reactions. Monitor CBC and LFTs periodically during long-term therapy.

Counseling: Inform of potential hazard to the fetus during pregnancy; advise to notify physician if nursing, pregnant, or intending to become pregnant during therapy. Inform that medication may produce psychological and physical dependence especially with history of alcohol/drug abuse; advise to consult physician before increasing dose or abruptly discontinuing the drug. Advise against simultaneous ingestion of alcohol and other CNS depressants during therapy. Caution against engaging in hazardous occupations requiring complete mental alertness (eg, operating machinery, driving).

STORAGE: 15-30°C (59-86°F).

VALTREX – valacyclovir hydrochloride

RX

Class: Nucleoside analogue

ADULT DOSAGE

Herpes Labialis (Cold Sores)

2g q12h for 1 day

Initiate at earliest symptom

Genital Herpes

Initial Episode: 1g bid for 10 days

PEDIATRIC DOSAGE

Herpes Labialis (Cold Sores)

≥12 Years:

2g q12h for 1 day

Initiate at earliest symptom

Most effective when given w/in 48 hrs of onset of signs/symptoms

Recurrent Episodes: 500mg bid for 3 days
Initiate at 1st sign/symptom of episode

Suppressive Therapy:
Normal Immune Function:
1g qd
Alternative if ≤9 Recurrences/Year: 500mg qd

HIV-1 Infected Patients:
CD4+ Count ≥100 cells/mm^3: 500mg bid

Reduction of Transmission:
≤9 Recurrences/Year: 500mg qd for the source partner

Herpes Zoster

1g tid for 7 days
Initiate at earliest sign/symptom
Most effective if initiated w/in 48 hrs of rash onset

Chickenpox

2-<18 Years:
20mg/kg tid for 5 days
Initiate at earliest sign/symptom
Max: 1g tid

DOSING CONSIDERATIONS

Renal Impairment

Herpes Labialis:
CrCl 30-49mL/min: Reduce dose to 1g q12h for 1 day
CrCl 10-29mL/min: Reduce dose to 500mg q12h for 1 day
CrCl <10mL/min: Reduce dose to 500mg single dose

Genital Herpes (Initial Episode):
CrCl 10-29mL/min: 1g q24h
CrCl <10mL/min: 500mg q24h

Genital Herpes (Recurrent Episode):
CrCl ≤29mL/min: 500mg q24h

Genital Herpes (Suppressive Therapy):
Immunocompetent Patients:
CrCl ≤29mL/min: 500mg q24h
Alternative if ≤9 Recurrences/Year:
CrCl ≤29mL/min: 500mg q48h
HIV-1 Infected Patients:
CrCl ≤29mL/min: 500mg q24h

Herpes Zoster:
CrCl 30-49mL/min: Reduce dose to 1g q12h
CrCl 10-29mL/min: Reduce dose to 1g q24h
CrCl <10mL/min: Reduce dose to 500mg q24h

Hemodialysis Patients:
Administer dose after hemodialysis

ADMINISTRATION

Oral route

Shake oral sus well before using

Preparation of Oral Sus

Ingredients for Preparation: Valtrex caplets 500mg, cherry flavor, and Suspension Structured Vehicle USP-NF (SSV)

1. Use a pestle and mortar to grind the required number of caplets until a fine powder (5 caplets for 25mg/mL sus; 10 caplets for 50mg/mL sus)
2. Add approx 5mL aliquots of SSV to the mortar and triturate the powder until a paste has been produced
3. Continue to add approx 5mL aliquots of SSV to the mortar, mixing thoroughly between additions, until a concentrated sus is produced, to a minimum total quantity of 20mL SSV and a max total quantity of 40mL SSV for both the 25mg/mL and 50mg/mL sus
4. Transfer the mixture to a suitable 100mL measuring flask
5. Transfer the cherry flavor to the mortar and dissolve in approx 5mL of SSV. Once dissolved, add to the measuring flask
6. Rinse the mortar at least 3X w/ approx 5mL aliquots of SSV, transferring the rinsing to the measuring flask between additions
7. Make the sus to volume (100mL) w/ SSV and shake thoroughly to mix
8. Transfer the sus to an amber glass medicine bottle w/ a child-resistant closure

HOW SUPPLIED

Tab: 500mg, 1g* *scored

CONTRAINDICATIONS

Clinically significant hypersensitivity reaction (eg, anaphylaxis) to valacyclovir, acyclovir, or any components of the formulation.

WARNINGS/PRECAUTIONS

Thrombotic thrombocytopenic purpura/hemolytic uremic syndrome (TTP/HUS) in immunocompromised patients reported at doses of 8g qd; immediately d/c if signs/symptoms occur. Acute renal failure reported. Maintain adequate hydration. CNS adverse reactions (eg, agitation, hallucinations, confusion, delirium, seizures, encephalopathy) reported in patients with or without reduced renal function and in those with underlying renal disease who received higher than recommended doses for their level of renal function; d/c if these occur. Caution in elderly and with renal impairment.

ADVERSE REACTIONS

Headache, N/V, abdominal pain, dysmenorrhea, arthralgia, nasopharyngitis, fatigue, rash, URTIs, pyrexia, decreased neutrophil counts, diarrhea, elevated ALT/AST.

DRUG INTERACTIONS

Caution with potentially nephrotoxic drugs.

PATIENT CONSIDERATIONS

Assessment: Assess for hypersensitivity, immunocompromised state, renal impairment, hydration status, pregnancy/nursing status, and possible drug interactions.

Monitoring: Monitor for signs/symptoms of renal toxicity, TTP/HUS, CNS effects, and other adverse reactions.

Counseling: Advise to maintain adequate hydration. Inform that drug is not a cure for cold sores or genital herpes. For patients with cold sores, instruct to initiate treatment at earliest symptom of a cold sore; inform that treatment should not exceed 1 day (2 doses) and that doses should be taken 12 hrs apart. For patients with genital herpes, instruct to avoid contact with lesions or sexual intercourse when lesions and/or symptoms are present to avoid infecting partner(s), and to use safe sex practice in combination with suppressive therapy. For patients with herpes zoster, advise to initiate treatment as soon as possible after diagnosis. For patients with chickenpox, advise to initiate treatment at the earliest sign/symptom.

STORAGE: 15-25°C (59-77°F).

VANOS – fluocinonide

Class: Corticosteroid

RX

ADULT DOSAGE

Inflammatory and Pruritic Manifestations of Corticosteroid-Responsive Dermatoses

Psoriasis/Corticosteroid-Responsive Dermatoses:

Apply a thin layer to affected skin area(s) qd or bid ud

Atopic Dermatitis:

Apply a thin layer to affected skin area(s) qd ud

Max: 60g/week

Limit treatment to 2 consecutive weeks
D/C therapy when control is achieved
Reassess diagnosis if no improvement is seen w/in 2 weeks

PEDIATRIC DOSAGE

Inflammatory and Pruritic Manifestations of Corticosteroid-Responsive Dermatoses

≥12 Years:

Psoriasis/Corticosteroid-Responsive Dermatoses:

Apply a thin layer to affected skin area(s) qd or bid ud

Atopic Dermatitis:

Apply a thin layer to affected skin area(s) qd ud

Max: 60g/week

Limit treatment to 2 consecutive weeks
D/C therapy when control is achieved
Reassess diagnosis if no improvement is seen w/in 2 weeks

ADMINISTRATION

Topical route

HOW SUPPLIED

Cre: 0.1% [30g, 60g, 120g]

WARNINGS/PRECAUTIONS

For dermatologic use only; not for ophthalmic, oral, or intravaginal use. Not for use in rosacea or perioral dermatitis. Do not apply on the face, groin, or axillae. Systemic absorption may produce reversible hypothalamic-pituitary-adrenal (HPA) axis suppression w/ the potential for glucocorticosteroid insufficiency, Cushing's syndrome, hyperglycemia, and unmasking of latent diabetes mellitus (DM). Periodically evaluate for HPA axis suppression and if noted, gradually withdraw treatment, reduce frequency of application, or substitute a less potent steroid. Factors predisposing to HPA axis suppression include use of more potent steroids, use over large surface areas, prolonged use, use under occlusion, use on an altered skin barrier, and use in patients with liver failure. May suppress immune system if used for >2 weeks. Manifestations of adrenal insufficiency may require supplemental systemic corticosteroids. Pediatric patients may be more susceptible to systemic toxicity. Local adverse reactions may be more likely to occur with occlusive use, prolonged use or use of higher potency corticosteroids. Use appropriate antifungal or antibacterial agent if concomitant skin infections are present or develop; if a favorable response does not occur promptly, d/c until infection is controlled. D/C and institute appropriate therapy if irritation develops. Allergic contact dermatitis may occur; confirm by patch testing.

ADVERSE REACTIONS

Headache, application-site burning, nasopharyngitis, nasal congestion.

DRUG INTERACTIONS

Use of >1 corticosteroid-containing product at the same time may increase total systemic absorption.

PATIENT CONSIDERATIONS

Assessment: Assess for hypersensitivity to the drug, rosacea, perioral dermatitis, skin infections, liver impairment, pregnancy/nursing status, and possible drug interactions.

Monitoring: Monitor for signs/symptoms of HPA axis suppression, Cushing's syndrome, hyperglycemia, unmasking of latent DM, skin irritation, and other adverse reactions. Monitor for systemic toxicity (eg, adrenal suppression, intracranial HTN) in pediatric patients. Following withdrawal of treatment, monitor for glucocorticosteroid insufficiency. Reassess diagnosis if no improvement is seen w/in 2 weeks.

Counseling: Instruct to use externally and ud. Advise not to use for any disorder other than for which it was prescribed. Instruct to avoid contact w/ eyes and not to use on face, groin, and underarms. Instruct not to bandage, cover, or wrap treated skin, unless directed by physician. Counsel to report any signs of local adverse reactions. Advise that other corticosteroid-containing products should not be used w/o 1st consulting w/ the physician. Instruct to d/c use when control is achieved and to notify physician if no improvement seen w/in 2 weeks. Notify physician if contemplating surgery. Counsel to wash hands following application.

STORAGE: 15-30°C (59-86°F).

VARUBI – rolapitant

RX

Class: Substance P/neurokinin-1 (NK1) receptor antagonist

ADULT DOSAGE

Chemotherapy-Induced Nausea/Vomiting

Prevention of Nausea/Vomiting Associated w/ Cisplatin-Based Highly Emetogenic Cancer Chemotherapy:

Day 1: Rolapitant 180mg 1-2 hrs prior to chemotherapy plus dexamethasone 20mg 30 min prior to chemotherapy plus 5-HT_3 antagonist according to the manufacturer's prescribing information

Days 2-4: Dexamethasone 8mg bid

Prevention of Nausea/Vomiting Associated w/ Moderately Emetogenic Cancer Chemotherapy and Combinations of Anthracycline and Cyclophosphamide:

Day 1: Rolapitant 180mg 1-2 hrs prior to chemotherapy plus dexamethasone 20mg 30 min prior to chemotherapy plus 5-HT_3 antagonist according to the manufacturer's prescribing information

Days 2-4: 5-HT_3 antagonist according to the manufacturer's prescribing information

PEDIATRIC DOSAGE

Pediatric use may not have been established

DOSING CONSIDERATIONS

Hepatic Impairment

Severe (Child-Pugh Class C): Avoid use; monitor for adverse reactions if use cannot be avoided

ADMINISTRATION

Oral route

Take w/o regard to meals.

Administer prior to the initiation of each chemotherapy cycle, but at no less than 2 week intervals.

HOW SUPPLIED

Tab: 90mg

CONTRAINDICATIONS

Patients receiving thioridazine.

WARNINGS/PRECAUTIONS

The inhibitory effect on CYP2D6 lasts at least 7 days and may last longer after a single dose administration of rolapitant. Avoid use in patients who are receiving pimozide, a CYP2D6 substrate; increase in pimozide plasma concentrations may result in QT prolongation. Monitor for adverse reactions if concomitant use w/ other CYP2D6 substrates w/ a narrow therapeutic index cannot be avoided.

ADVERSE REACTIONS

Neutropenia, decreased appetite, dizziness, hiccups, dyspepsia, UTI, stomatitis, anemia, abdominal pain.

DRUG INTERACTIONS

See Contraindications and Warnings/Precautions. A 3-fold increase in the exposure of dextromethorphan, a CYP2D6 substrate, was observed 7 days after a single dose of rolapitant. Increased plasma concentrations of Breast Cancer Resistance Protein (BCRP) substrates (eg, methotrexate, topotecan, irinotecan) may result in potential adverse reactions; monitor for adverse reactions related to the concomitant drug if use of rolapitant cannot be avoided. Use the lowest effective dose of rosuvastatin if used concomitantly w/ rolapitant; refer to prescribing information for additional information on recommended dosing. Increased plasma concentrations of digoxin, or other P-gp substrates, may result in potential adverse reactions; monitor for adverse reactions if concomitant use w/ other P-gp substrates w/ a narrow therapeutic index cannot be avoided. Monitor for increased digoxin concentrations. Strong CYP3A4 inducers (eg, rifampin) significantly reduced plasma concentrations of rolapitant and may decrease efficacy; avoid use of rolapitant in patients who require chronic administration of such drugs.

PATIENT CONSIDERATIONS

Assessment: Assess for hypersensitivity to drug, hepatic impairment, pregnancy/nursing status, and for possible drug interactions.

Monitoring: Monitor for adverse reactions.

Counseling: Advise to inform healthcare provider when any concomitant medications are started or stopped.

STORAGE: 20-25°C (68-77°F); excursions permitted to 15-30°C (59-86°F).

VASCEPA — icosapent ethyl

RX

Class: Lipid-regulating agent

ADULT DOSAGE

Severe Hypertriglyceridemia (≥500mg/dL)

Usual: 4g/day (2 caps bid)

PEDIATRIC DOSAGE

Pediatric use may not have been established

ADMINISTRATION

Oral route. Swallow caps whole; do not break open, crush, dissolve, or chew.

HOW SUPPLIED

Cap: 1g

CONTRAINDICATIONS

Known hypersensitivity (eg, anaphylactic reaction) to icosapent ethyl or any of the components of the medication.

WARNINGS/PRECAUTIONS

Contains ethyl esters of the omega-3 fatty acid, eicosapentaenoic acid (EPA), obtained from oil of fish; caution with known hypersensitivity to fish and/or shellfish. Monitor ALT and AST levels periodically during therapy in patients with hepatic impairment.

ADVERSE REACTIONS
Arthralgia, oropharyngeal pain.

DRUG INTERACTIONS
Possible prolongation of bleeding time with other drugs affecting coagulation (eg, antiplatelet agents); monitor periodically. D/C or change medications known to exacerbate hypertriglyceridemia (eg, β-blockers, thiazides, estrogens) prior to consideration of therapy.

PATIENT CONSIDERATIONS

Assessment: Assess for drug hypersensitivity, hypersensitivity to fish and/or shellfish, hepatic impairment, pregnancy/nursing status, and possible drug interactions. Attempt to control serum lipids with appropriate diet/exercise, and control any medical problems that may contribute to lipid abnormalities (eg, diabetes mellitus, hypothyroidism, alcohol intake) prior to therapy. Assess lipid levels.

Monitoring: Monitor for allergic reactions and other adverse reactions. Monitor lipid levels. Periodically monitor ALT/AST levels with hepatic impairment.

Counseling: Instruct to notify physician if allergic to fish and/or shellfish. Inform that the use of lipid-regulating agents does not reduce the importance of appropriate nutritional intake and physical activity. Advise not to alter caps in any way and to ingest intact caps only. Instruct to take ud. If dose is missed, advise to take as soon as remembered and not to double the dose.

STORAGE: 20-25°C (68-77°F); excursions permitted to 15-30°C (59-86°F).

VASOTEC – enalapril maleate

RX

Class: ACE inhibitor

D/C if pregnancy is detected. Drugs that act directly on the renin-angiotensin system (RAS) can cause injury/death to the developing fetus.

ADULT DOSAGE

Hypertension

Not Receiving Diuretics:
Initial: 5mg qd
Usual Range: 10-40mg/day given in single dose or 2 divided doses
May add diuretic if BP not controlled

Receiving Diuretics:
If possible, d/c diuretic 2-3 days prior to therapy. If BP is not controlled w/ enalapril alone, then diuretic therapy may be resumed
Initial: 2.5mg should be used under medical supervision for at least 2 hrs and until BP has stabilized for at least an additional hr

Heart Failure

Symptomatic CHF in Combination w/ Diuretics and Digitalis:
Initial: 2.5mg qd
Range: 2.5-20mg bid
Max: 40mg/day in divided doses

Hyponatremia (Serum Na^+ <130mEq/L):
Initial: 2.5mg/day
Titrate: May increase to 2.5mg bid, then 5mg bid and higher prn, usually at intervals of 4 days or more
Max: 40mg/day

Asymptomatic Left Ventricular Dysfunction

Decreasing the Rate of Development of Overt Heart Failure (HF) and the Incidence of Hospitalization for HF in Clinically Stable Patients (Ejection Fraction ≤35%):
Initial: 2.5mg bid
Titrate: Increase as tolerated to 20mg/day (in divided doses)

PEDIATRIC DOSAGE

Hypertension

1 Month-16 Years:
Initial: 0.08mg/kg (up to 5mg) qd
Max: 0.58mg/kg (or 40mg/day)

DOSING CONSIDERATIONS

Renal Impairment

HTN:

CrCl ≤30mL/min:

Initial: 2.5mg qd

Dialysis Patients:

Initial: 2.5mg qd on dialysis days

Titrate: Dosage on nondialysis days should be adjusted depending on the BP response

HF:

SrCr >1.6mg/dL:

Initial: 2.5mg/day

Titrate: May increase to 2.5mg bid, then 5mg bid and higher prn, usually at intervals of 4 days or more

Max: 40mg/day

ADMINISTRATION

Oral route

Preparation of Sus (200mL of a 1.0mg/mL Sus)

1. Add 50mL of Bicitra to a polyethylene terephthalate bottle containing ten 20mg tabs; shake for at least 2 min.
2. Let concentrate stand for 60 min, then shake for additional 1 min.
3. Add 150mL of Ora-Sweet SF to concentrate and shake sus to disperse ingredients.
4. Refrigerate at 2-8°C (36-46°F) for 30 days.
5. Shake sus before each use.

HOW SUPPLIED

Tab: 2.5mg*, 5mg*, 10mg*, 20mg* *scored

CONTRAINDICATIONS

Hypersensitivity to this product, history of ACE inhibitor-associated angioedema, hereditary or idiopathic angioedema, coadministration w/ aliskiren in patients w/ diabetes.

WARNINGS/PRECAUTIONS

Head/neck angioedema reported; d/c and administer appropriate therapy if angioedema occurs. Higher incidence of angioedema reported in blacks than nonblacks. Intestinal angioedema reported; monitor for abdominal pain. Effect of therapy on BP reported to be less in black patients than in nonblacks. Patients w/ history of angioedema unrelated to ACE inhibitor therapy may be at increased risk of angioedema during therapy. Anaphylactoid reactions reported during desensitization w/ hymenoptera venom, dialysis w/ high-flux membranes, and LDL apheresis w/ dextran sulfate absorption. Excessive hypotension, sometimes associated w/ oliguria and/or progressive azotemia, and rarely w/ acute renal failure and/or death, may occur; monitor patients at risk of hypotension during first 2 weeks of therapy and whenever the dose of enalapril and/or diuretic is increased. Consider dose reduction or d/c therapy or diuretic if symptomatic hypotension occurs. Neutropenia or agranulocytosis may occur; monitor WBCs in patients w/ renal disease and collagen vascular disease. Associated w/ syndrome that starts w/ cholestatic jaundice and progresses to fulminant hepatic necrosis, and sometimes death; d/c if jaundice or marked elevations of hepatic enzymes develop. Caution w/ left ventricular outflow obstruction. May cause changes in renal function; may be associated w/ oliguria and/or progressive azotemia and rarely w/ acute renal failure and/or death in severe HF patients whose renal function depends on the renin-angiotensin-aldosterone system. Increases in BUN and SrCr reported in patients w/ unilateral or bilateral renal artery stenosis; monitor renal function during the 1st few weeks of therapy in such patients. Hyperkalemia may occur; caution w/ diabetes mellitus (DM) and renal insufficiency. Persistent nonproductive cough reported. Hypotension may occur w/ major surgery or during anesthesia; may be corrected by volume expansion. Avoid in neonates and in pediatric patients w/ GFR <30mL/min.

ADVERSE REACTIONS

Fatigue, headache, dizziness.

DRUG INTERACTIONS

See Contraindications. Dual blockade of the RAS is associated w/ increased risk of hypotension, hyperkalemia, and changes in renal function (including acute renal failure); avoid combined use of RAS inhibitors. Closely monitor BP, renal function, and electrolytes w/ concomitant agents that also affect the RAS. Avoid w/ aliskiren in patients w/ renal impairment (GFR <60mL/min). Hypotension risk w/ diuretics. NSAIDs, including selective COX-2 inhibitors, may result in deterioration of renal function, including possible acute renal failure in elderly, volume depleted or patients w/ compromised renal function. K^+-sparing diuretics, K^+-containing salt substitutes, or K^+ supplements may increase serum K^+ levels; use caution and monitor serum K^+ frequently. Avoid K^+-sparing agents in patients w/ HF. Antihypertensive agents that cause renin release (eg, diuretics) may augment antihypertensive effect. Lithium toxicity reported w/ lithium; monitor serum lithium levels frequently. Nitritoid reactions reported rarely w/ injectable gold (eg, sodium aurothiomalate). Coadministration w/ mammalian target of rapamycin (mTOR) inhibitor (eg, temsirolimus, sirolimus, everolimus) therapy may increase risk for angioedema.

PATIENT CONSIDERATIONS

Assessment: Assess for hypersensitivity to drug, history of angioedema related to previous treatment w/ an ACE inhibitor, volume/salt depletion, renal dysfunction/disease, collagen vascular disease, renal artery stenosis, ischemic heart disease, cerebrovascular disease, left ventricular outflow obstruction, DM, pregnancy/nursing status, and possible drug interactions.

Monitoring: Monitor for hypotension, anaphylactoid reactions, angioedema, and other adverse reactions. Monitor BP, renal/hepatic function, and serum K^+ levels. Monitor WBCs periodically in patients w/ collagen vascular disease and/or renal disease.

Counseling: Inform of pregnancy risks and instruct to notify physician as soon as possible if pregnant/planning to become pregnant; discuss treatment options in women planning to become pregnant. Instruct to d/c therapy and to immediately report signs/symptoms of angioedema. Caution about lightheadedness, especially during the 1st few days of therapy and advise to report to physician. Instruct to d/c and to consult physician if syncope occurs. Caution that excessive perspiration and dehydration may lead to excessive fall in BP; advise to consult w/ physician. Advise not to use K^+ supplements or salt substitutes containing K^+ w/o consulting physician. Advise patient to report any indication of infection.

STORAGE: 25°C (77°F); excursions permitted to 15-30°C (59-86°F). Protect from moisture.

VECTICAL – calcitriol

RX

Class: Vitamin D analogue

ADULT DOSAGE

Plaque Psoriasis

Mild to Moderate:
Apply to affected area(s) bid (am and pm)

Max: 200g/week

PEDIATRIC DOSAGE

Pediatric use may not have been established

ADMINISTRATION

Topical route

HOW SUPPLIED

Oint: 3mcg/g [5g, 100g]

WARNINGS/PRECAUTIONS

Not for PO, ophthalmic, or intravaginal use. Hypercalcemia reported; if aberrations in parameters of Ca^{2+} metabolism occur, d/c therapy until these parameters normalize. Increased absorption with occlusive use. Avoid excessive exposure of treated areas to natural or artificial sunlight (eg, tanning booths, sun lamps); avoid or limit phototherapy.

ADVERSE REACTIONS

Lab test abnormality, urine abnormality, psoriasis, hypercalciuria, pruritus, hypercalcemia, skin discomfort.

DRUG INTERACTIONS

Caution with medications known to increase serum Ca^{2+} level (eg, thiazide diuretics), Ca^{2+} supplements, or high doses of vitamin D.

PATIENT CONSIDERATIONS

Assessment: Assess for known/suspected Ca^{2+} metabolism disorder, pregnancy/nursing status, and possible drug interactions.

Monitoring: Monitor for hypercalcemia, aberrations in parameters of Ca^{2+} metabolism, and other adverse reactions.

Counseling: Instruct to use ud. Instruct to apply only to areas of the skin affected by psoriasis; advise not to apply to the eyes, lips, or facial skin. Instruct to rub gently into the skin. Advise to notify their physician if adverse reactions occur. Advise to avoid excessive exposure of treated areas to sunlight, tanning booths, sun lamps, or other artificial sunlight and to inform physician about treatment if undergoing phototherapy.

STORAGE: 20°-25°C (68°-77°F); excursions permitted to 15°-30°C (59°-86°F). Do not freeze or refrigerate.

VELCADE – bortezomib

RX

Class: Proteasome inhibitor

ADULT DOSAGE

Multiple Myeloma

Initial: 1.3mg/m^2 IV bolus (3-5 sec) at a concentration of 1mg/mL, or SQ at a concentration of 2.5mg/mL

Previously Untreated Multiple Myeloma:
Administer in combination w/ oral melphalan and oral prednisone for nine 6-week cycles
Cycles 1-4: Administer twice weekly (Days 1, 4, 8, 11, 22, 25, 29, and 32)
Cycles 5-9: Administer once weekly (Days 1, 8, 22, and 29)

Relapsed Multiple Myeloma:
Administer twice weekly for 2 weeks (Days 1, 4, 8, and 11), followed by 10-day rest period (Days 12-21)
For extended therapy of >8 cycles, may administer on standard schedule or on a maint schedule of once weekly for 4 weeks (Days 1, 8, 15, and 22), followed by 13-day rest period (Days 23-35)

Retreatment of Relapsed Multiple Myeloma:
May start at the last tolerated dose. Administer twice weekly (Days 1, 4, 8, and 11) every 3 weeks
Max: 8 cycles
May administer either as a single agent or in combination w/ dexamethasone

At least 72 hrs should elapse between consecutive doses

Mantle Cell Lymphoma

Initial: 1.3mg/m^2 IV bolus (3-5 sec) at a concentration of 1mg/mL, or SQ at a concentration of 2.5mg/mL

Previously Untreated Mantle Cell Lymphoma:
Administer in combination w/ IV rituximab, cyclophosphamide, doxorubicin, and oral prednisone (VcR-CAP) for six 3-week cycles
Administer bortezomib 1st followed by rituximab
Administer twice weekly for 2 weeks (Days 1, 4, 8, and 11), followed by a 10-day rest period on Days 12-21
For patients w/ a response 1st documented at Cycle 6, two additional VcR-CAP cycles are recommended

Relapsed Mantle Cell Lymphoma:
Administer twice weekly for 2 weeks (Days 1, 4, 8, and 11), followed by 10-day rest period (Days 12-21)
For extended therapy of >8 cycles, may administer on standard schedule

At least 72 hrs should elapse between consecutive doses

PEDIATRIC DOSAGE

Pediatric use may not have been established

DOSING CONSIDERATIONS

Hepatic Impairment

Moderate (Bilirubin >1.5X-3X ULN)-Severe (Bilirubin >3X ULN): Reduce to 0.7mg/m^2 in the 1st cycle
Consider escalation to 1.0mg/m^2 or further reduction to 0.5mg/m^2 in subsequent cycles based on tolerability

Adverse Reactions

Combination Bortezomib, Melphalan, and Prednisone:

Prolonged Grade 4 Neutropenia or Thrombocytopenia/Thrombocytopenia w/ Bleeding Observed in Previous Cycle: Consider reduction of melphalan dose by 25% in next cycle

Platelets <30 x 10^9/L or ANC <0.75 x 10^9/L on a Bortezomib Dosing Day (Other Than Day 1): Withhold bortezomib dose

Several Bortezomib Doses in Consecutive Cycles Withheld Due to Toxicity: Reduce dose by 1 dose level (from 1.3mg/m^2 to 1mg/m^2, or from 1mg/m^2 to 0.7mg/m^2)

≥Grade 3 Nonhematological Toxicities:
Withhold therapy until symptoms resolve to Grade 1 or baseline; may be reinitiated w/ 1 dose level reduction (from 1.3mg/m^2 to 1mg/m^2, or from 1mg/m^2 to 0.7mg/m^2)

Days 4, 8, and 11 During Cycles of Combination Bortezomib, Rituximab, Cyclophosphamide, Doxorubicin, and Prednisone Therapy:

≥Grade 3 Neutropenia, or Platelet <25 x 10^9/L:
Withhold therapy for up to 2 weeks until the patient has an ANC ≥0.75 x 10^9/L and platelets ≥25 x 10^9/L
If, after bortezomib has been withheld, the toxicity does not resolve, d/c
If toxicity resolves such that the patient has an ANC ≥0.75 x 10^9/L and platelets ≥25 x 10^9/L, dose should be reduced by 1 dose level (from 1.3mg/m^2 to 1mg/m^2, or from 1mg/m^2 to 0.7mg/m^2)

≥Grade 3 Nonhematological Toxicities:
Withhold therapy until symptoms of the toxicity have resolved to Grade 2 or better; may reinitiate w/ 1 dose level reduction (from 1.3mg/m^2 to 1mg/m^2, or from 1mg/m^2 to 0.7mg/m^2)

Neuropathic Pain and/or Peripheral or Motor Neuropathy:

Grade 1 (Asymptomatic; Loss of Deep Tendon Reflexes or Paresthesia) w/o Pain or Loss of Function: No action

Grade 1 w/ Pain or Grade 2 (Moderate Symptoms; Limiting Instrumental Activities of Daily Living [ADL]): Reduce to 1mg/m^2

Grade 2 w/ Pain or Grade 3 (Severe Symptoms; Limiting Self Care ADL): Withhold therapy until toxicity resolves, then reinitiate w/ a reduced dose at 0.7mg/m^2 once per week

Grade 4 (Life-Threatening Consequences; Urgent Intervention Indicated): D/C therapy

Refer to PI for further dosing guidelines

ADMINISTRATION

IV/SQ route

Reconstitution

Reconstitute only w/ 0.9% NaCl; should be administered w/in 8 hrs of preparation.
Different volumes of 0.9% NaCl are used to reconstitute the product for the different routes of administration.
Because each route of administration has a different reconstituted concentration, caution should be used when calculating the volume to be administered.
The reconstituted concentration for SQ administration is 2.5mg/mL when diluted w/ 1.4mL 0.9% NaCl.
The reconstituted concentration for IV administration is 1mg/mL when diluted w/ 3.5mL 0.9% NaCl.

Refer to PI for further reconstitution/preparation instructions.

HOW SUPPLIED

Inj: 3.5mg

CONTRAINDICATIONS

Intrathecal administration, hypersensitivity (not including local reactions) to bortezomib, boron, or mannitol.

WARNINGS/PRECAUTIONS

Severe sensory and motor peripheral neuropathy reported; consider starting SQ therapy for patients w/ preexisting or at high risk of peripheral neuropathy. Hypotension reported. Acute development or exacerbation of CHF and new onset of decreased left ventricular ejection fraction (LVEF) reported. Isolated cases of QT interval prolongation reported. Acute respiratory distress syndrome (ARDS), acute diffuse infiltrative pulmonary disease of unknown etiology (eg, pneumonitis, interstitial pneumonia, lung infiltration), and pulmonary HTN reported; consider interrupting therapy until a prompt and comprehensive diagnostic evaluation is conducted if new or worsening cardiopulmonary symptoms develop. Posterior reversible encephalopathy syndrome (PRES) reported; d/c if PRES develops. May cause N/V, diarrhea, constipation, and ileus; antiemetic and antidiarrheal medications may be necessary. Administer fluid/electrolyte replacement therapy to prevent dehydration; interrupt for severe symptoms. Thrombocytopenia and neutropenia reported. GI and intracerebral hemorrhage occurred during thrombocytopenia; support w/ transfusions and supportive care. Tumor lysis syndrome reported. Acute liver failure reported in patients receiving multiple concomitant medications and w/ serious underlying medical conditions. Hepatic reactions, including hepatitis, increases in liver enzymes, and hyperbilirubinemia, reported; interrupt therapy to assess reversibility. Women of reproductive potential should avoid becoming pregnant while on therapy. Administer therapy after dialysis procedure. Consider retreatment in patients w/ multiple myeloma who had previously responded to treatment and have relapsed at least 6 months after completing prior therapy. Caution in elderly.

ADVERSE REACTIONS

Thrombocytopenia, neutropenia, N/V, peripheral neuropathy, diarrhea, anemia, constipation, pyrexia, anorexia, paresthesia, headache, dyspnea, leukopenia, fatigue.

DRUG INTERACTIONS

Avoid w/ St. John's wort. Efficacy may be reduced w/ strong CYP3A4 inducers (eg, rifampin); concomitant use is not recommended. Oral antidiabetic agents may require dosage adjustment. Ketoconazole may increase exposure; monitor for signs of bortezomib toxicity and consider bortezomib dose reduction when given w/ strong CYP3A4 inhibitors (eg, ketoconazole, ritonavir). May increase exposure to drugs that are CYP2C19 substrates.

PATIENT CONSIDERATIONS

Assessment: Assess for peripheral neuropathy, history of syncope, dehydration, risk factors for or existing heart disease, diabetes mellitus, hepatic/renal impairment, any conditions where treatment is contraindicated or cautioned, pregnancy/nursing status, and possible drug interactions. Obtain baseline BP, CBCs, and then platelet count prior to each dose.

Monitoring: Monitor for signs/symptoms of new/worsening peripheral neuropathy, hypotension, CHF, decreased LVEF, new or worsening cardiopulmonary symptoms, PRES, N/V, diarrhea, constipation, ileus, tumor lysis syndrome, hepatic toxicity, and other adverse reactions. Closely monitor patients w/ risk factors for or existing heart disease. Monitor LFTs. Monitor CBCs and blood glucose levels (in diabetics) frequently.

Counseling: Inform that therapy may cause fatigue, dizziness, syncope, orthostatic/postural hypotension; advise not to drive or operate heavy machinery if any of these symptoms develop. Advise how to avoid dehydration. Instruct to seek medical advice if symptoms of dizziness, lightheadedness, fainting spells, or muscle cramps are experienced. Advise to use effective contraceptive measures to prevent pregnancy and instruct to inform physician immediately if patient becomes pregnant. Advise that treatment should not be received while pregnant/breastfeeding. Advise to check blood sugar frequently if taking oral antidiabetic medications and instruct to notify physician if any changes in blood sugar levels occur. Instruct to contact physician if symptoms of new/worsening peripheral neuropathy, PRES or progressive multifocal leukoencephalopathy, cardiac/respiratory/hepatic toxicity, dermal reactions, an increase in BP, bleeding, fever, constipation, or decreased appetite develops.

STORAGE: 25°C (77°F); excursions permitted to 15-30°C (59-86°F). Protect from light. **Reconstituted Sol:** 25°C (77°F). May be stored in the original vial and/or the syringe prior to administration. May be stored for up to 8 hrs in a syringe; total storage time must not exceed 8 hrs when exposed to normal indoor lighting.

VELTASSA – patiromer

RX

Class: Cation-exchange resin

Patiromer binds to many orally administered medications, which could decrease their absorption and reduce their effectiveness. Administer other oral medications at least 6 hrs before or 6 hrs after patiromer. If adequate dosing separation is not possible, choose patiromer or the other oral medication.

ADULT DOSAGE

Hyperkalemia

Initial: 8.4g qd

Titrate: May increase or decrease to reach desired serum K^+ concentration; may increase in increments of 8.4g based on serum K^+ levels at 1-week or longer intervals

Max: 25.2g qd

PEDIATRIC DOSAGE

Pediatric use may not have been established

ADMINISTRATION

Oral route

Administer at least 6 hrs before or 6 hrs after other oral medications.
Take w/ food.
Do not heat (eg, microwave) or add to heated foods or liquids.
Do not take medication in its dry form.
Prepare each dose immediately prior to administration.

Preparation

1. Add about 1 oz (30mL) of water to an empty glass/cup.

2. Empty entire contents of packet(s) into the glass/cup and stir the mixture thoroughly.
3. Add an additional 2 oz (60mL) of water to the glass/cup containing the mixture.
4. Stir the mixture thoroughly; powder will not dissolve and mixture will look cloudy.
5. Drink mixture immediately; if some powder remains after drinking, add more water, stir, and drink immediately. Repeat prn to ensure the entire dose is administered.

HOW SUPPLIED

Powder: 8.4g, 16.8g, 25.2g

CONTRAINDICATIONS

History of a hypersensitivity reaction to patiromer or any components of the medication.

WARNINGS/PRECAUTIONS

Not for use as an emergency treatment for life-threatening hyperkalemia. Avoid use in patients w/ severe constipation, bowel obstruction, or impaction, including abnormal postoperative bowel motility disorders; may be ineffective and worsen GI conditions. May lead to hypomagnesemia; monitor serum Mg^{2+} and consider Mg^{2+} supplementation w/ low serum Mg^{2+} levels.

ADVERSE REACTIONS

Constipation, hypomagnesemia, diarrhea, hypokalemia.

DRUG INTERACTIONS

See Boxed Warning.

PATIENT CONSIDERATIONS

Assessment: Assess for severe constipation, bowel obstruction/impaction, pregnancy/nursing status, and possible drug interactions.

Monitoring: Monitor for hypersensitivity reactions, worsening of GI motility, serum Mg^{2+} and K^+ levels, and other adverse reactions.

Counseling: Advise to separate dosing of other oral medications by at least 6 hrs before or after administration of therapy. Instruct to take ud w/ food and to adhere to prescribed diets. Instruct not to heat, add to heated foods or liquids, or take in its dry form.

STORAGE: 2-8°C (36-46°F). If stored at room temperature 25°C (77°F), use w/in 3 months of being taken out of the refrigerator. Avoid exposure to excessive heat >40°C (104°F).

VENTOLIN HFA – albuterol sulfate

RX

Class: $Beta_2$ agonist

ADULT DOSAGE

Bronchospasm

Treatment/Prevention:
2 inh q4-6h or 1 inh q4h

Exercise-Induced Bronchospasm

Prevention:
2 inh 15-30 min before exercise

PEDIATRIC DOSAGE

Bronchospasm

Treatment/Prevention:
≥4 Years:
2 inh q4-6h or 1 inh q4h

Exercise-Induced Bronchospasm

Prevention:
≥4 Years:
2 inh 15-30 min before exercise

DOSING CONSIDERATIONS

Elderly

Start at lower end of dosing range

ADMINISTRATION

Oral inh route

Shake well before each spray

Priming

Before using for 1st time, if inhaler has not been used for >2 weeks, or if it has been dropped, prime inhaler by releasing 4 sprays into air, away from face

Refer to PI for further instructions on proper use

HOW SUPPLIED

MDI: 90mcg of albuterol base/inh [60, 200 inhalations]

CONTRAINDICATIONS

History of hypersensitivity to any of the ingredients.

WARNINGS/PRECAUTIONS

D/C if paradoxical bronchospasm following dosing or if cardiovascular (CV) effects occur. More doses than usual may be a marker of destabilization of asthma and may require reevaluation of the patient and treatment regimen; give special consideration to the possible need for anti-inflammatory treatment (eg, corticosteroids). ECG changes and immediate hypersensitivity reactions, including anaphylaxis, may occur. Fatalities reported with excessive use. Caution with CV disorders (eg, coronary insufficiency, arrhythmias, HTN), convulsive disorders, hyperthyroidism, diabetes mellitus (DM), and in patients unusually responsive to sympathomimetic amines. Large doses of IV albuterol reported to aggravate preexisting DM and ketoacidosis. May cause significant hypokalemia. Caution in elderly.

ADVERSE REACTIONS

Throat irritation, viral respiratory infections, upper respiratory inflammation, cough, musculoskeletal pain.

DRUG INTERACTIONS

Avoid with other short-acting sympathomimetic aerosol bronchodilators; caution with additional adrenergic drugs administered by any route. Use with β-blockers may block pulmonary effects and produce severe bronchospasm in asthmatic patients; avoid concomitant use. If needed, consider cardioselective β-blockers and use with caution. ECG changes and/or hypokalemia caused by non-K^+-sparing diuretics (eg, loop, thiazide diuretics) may be worsened. May decrease serum digoxin levels. Use extreme caution with MAOIs and TCAs, or within 2 weeks of discontinuation of such agents.

PATIENT CONSIDERATIONS

Assessment: Assess for history of hypersensitivity to the drug, CV disorders, convulsive disorders, hyperthyroidism, DM, pregnancy/nursing status, and possible drug interactions. Assess use in patients unusually responsive to sympathomimetic amines.

Monitoring: Monitor for paradoxical bronchospasm, deterioration of asthma, CV effects, ECG changes, hypokalemia, immediate hypersensitivity reactions, and other adverse effects. Monitor BP, HR, and blood glucose levels.

Counseling: Counsel not to increase dose/frequency of doses without consulting physician. Advise to seek immediate medical attention if treatment becomes less effective for symptomatic relief, symptoms become worse, and/or there is a need to use the product more frequently than usual. Instruct on how to properly prime, clean, and use inhaler. Instruct to take concurrent inhaled drugs and asthma medications only ud by the physician. Inform of the common adverse effects of treatment. Advise to notify physician if pregnant/nursing. Instruct to avoid spraying in eyes.

STORAGE: 20-25°C (68-77°F); excursions permitted to 15-30°C (59-86°F). Store with mouthpiece down. Do not puncture or store near heat or open flame.

VESIcare – solifenacin succinate

RX

Class: Muscarinic antagonist

ADULT DOSAGE

Overactive Bladder

Usual: 5mg qd

Titrate: May increase to 10mg qd if 5mg dose is well tolerated

PEDIATRIC DOSAGE

Pediatric use may not have been established

DOSING CONSIDERATIONS

Concomitant Medications

Potent CYP3A4 Inhibitors:

Max: 5mg qd

Renal Impairment

CrCl <30mL/min:

Max: 5mg qd

Hepatic Impairment

Moderate (Child-Pugh B):

Max: 5mg qd

Moderate (Child-Pugh C): Not recommended

ADMINISTRATION

Oral route

Take w/ water and swallow whole, w/ or w/o food

HOW SUPPLIED

Tab: 5mg, 10mg

CONTRAINDICATIONS

Urinary/gastric retention, uncontrolled narrow-angle glaucoma, hypersensitivity to the drug.

WARNINGS/PRECAUTIONS

Not recommended with severe hepatic impairment (Child-Pugh C). Angioedema of the face, lips, tongue, and/or larynx, and rare anaphylactic reactions reported; d/c and provide appropriate therapy. Risk of urinary retention. Caution with decreased GI motility, controlled narrow-angle glaucoma, renal/hepatic impairment, and history of QT prolongation. CNS anticholinergic effects (eg, headache, confusion, hallucinations, somnolence) reported; may impair mental/physical abilities. Monitor for signs of anticholinergic CNS effects, particularly after beginning treatment or increasing the dose; consider dose reduction or discontinuation if such effects occur.

ADVERSE REACTIONS

Dry mouth, constipation, nausea, dyspepsia, UTI, blurred vision.

DRUG INTERACTIONS

See Dosing Considerations. Ketoconazole, a potent CYP3A4 inhibitor, may increase levels. CYP3A4 inducers may decrease concentrations. Caution with medications known to prolong the QT interval.

PATIENT CONSIDERATIONS

Assessment: Assess for hypersensitivity to the drug and for any other conditions where treatment is contraindicated or cautioned. Assess for renal/hepatic impairment, pregnancy/nursing status, and possible drug interactions.

Monitoring: Monitor for angioedema, anaphylactic reactions, signs of anticholinergic CNS effects, and other adverse reactions.

Counseling: Inform that constipation may occur; advise to contact physician if severe abdominal pain or constipation for ≥3 days occurs. Inform that blurred vision or CNS anticholinergic effects may occur; advise to exercise caution in decisions to engage in potentially dangerous activities until effects have been determined. Inform that heat prostration (due to decreased sweating) can occur when used in a hot environment. Inform that angioedema may occur and could result in fatal airway obstruction; advise to promptly d/c therapy and seek immediate attention if edema or difficulty breathing develops.

STORAGE: 25°C (77°F); excursions permitted from 15-30°C (59-86°F).

VIAGRA — sildenafil citrate

RX

Class: Phosphodiesterase-5 (PDE-5) inhibitor

ADULT DOSAGE

Erectile Dysfunction

50mg qd prn (recommended), approx 1 hr or anywhere from 30 min to 4 hrs before sexual activity

Titrate: May increase to 100mg qd or decrease to 25mg qd, based on effectiveness and tolerance

Max: 100mg qd

PEDIATRIC DOSAGE

Pediatric use may not have been established

DOSING CONSIDERATIONS

Concomitant Medications

Strong CYP3A4 Inhibitors/Erythromycin:

Initial: Consider 25mg qd

α-Blockers:

Patient should be stable on α-blocker therapy prior to initiating treatment

Initial: 25mg qd

Ritonavir:

25mg prior to sexual activity

Max: 25mg/48 hrs

V

Renal Impairment

CrCl <30mL/min:

Initial: Consider 25mg qd

Hepatic Impairment

Initial: Consider 25mg qd

Elderly

Initial: Consider 25mg qd

ADMINISTRATION

Oral route

May be taken w/ or w/o food.

HOW SUPPLIED

Tab: 25mg, 50mg, 100mg

CONTRAINDICATIONS

Concomitant use w/ nitric oxide donors (eg, organic nitrates/nitrites) in any form, either taken regularly and/or intermittently; known hypersensitivity to sildenafil or any component of the tab; concomitant guanylate cyclase (GC) stimulators (eg, riociguat).

WARNINGS/PRECAUTIONS

Potential for cardiac risk of sexual activity in patients w/ cardiovascular disease (CVD); do not use in men for whom sexual activity is inadvisable due to underlying cardiovascular (CV) status. Has systemic vasodilatory properties that resulted in transient decreases in supine BP in clinical studies. Caution in patients w/ left ventricular outflow obstruction (eg, aortic stenosis, idiopathic hypertrophic subaortic stenosis); severely impaired autonomic control of BP; history of MI, stroke, or life-threatening arrhythmia w/in the last 6 months; resting hypotension (BP <90/50mmHg) or HTN (BP >170/110mmHg); and cardiac failure or coronary artery disease (CAD) causing unstable angina. Prolonged erection >4 hrs and priapism reported; caution w/ anatomical penile deformation (eg, angulation, cavernosal fibrosis, Peyronie's disease), or predispositions to priapism (eg, sickle cell anemia, multiple myeloma, leukemia). Nonarteritic anterior ischemic optic neuropathy (NAION) reported. D/C if sudden loss of vision in 1 or both eyes occurs; may be a sign of NAION. Caution w/ underlying NAION risk factors; increased risk in patients w/ "crowded" optic disc and w/ previous history of NAION. D/C if sudden decrease or loss of hearing occurs. Bleeding events reported. Does not protect against STDs.

ADVERSE REACTIONS

Headache, flushing, dyspepsia, abnormal vision, nasal congestion, back pain, myalgia, nausea, dizziness, rash.

DRUG INTERACTIONS

See Dosing Considerations and Contraindications. Increased levels w/ CYP3A4 inhibitors (eg, ritonavir, erythromycin, saquinavir); stronger CYP3A4 inhibitors (eg, ketoconazole, itraconazole) may have greater effects. Potential additive BP-lowering effects w/ α-blockers and other antihypertensives (eg, amlodipine). Combination w/ other PDE-5 inhibitors or other erectile dysfunction therapies is not recommended; may further lower BP.

PATIENT CONSIDERATIONS

Assessment: Assess for hypersensitivity to drug; history of MI, stroke, or arrhythmia; renal/hepatic impairment; CVD; left ventricular outflow obstruction; impaired autonomic control of BP; resting hypotension or HTN; cardiac failure; CAD; anatomical penile deformation; predisposition to priapism; risk for NAION; potential underlying causes of ED; and for possible drug interactions.

Monitoring: Monitor for prolonged erection, priapism, abnormalities in vision/NAION, decrease/loss of hearing, bleeding, and other adverse reactions.

Counseling: Inform of risks and benefits of therapy. Instruct to notify physician of all prescription/nonprescription medications and supplements currently being taking and inform of the contraindication w/ regular and/or intermittent use of nitric oxide donors and if using GC stimulators. Advise patients who experience CV symptoms upon initiation of sexual activity to refrain from further activity and to discuss the episode w/ their physician. Instruct to d/c and seek medical attention if sudden loss of vision in 1 or both eyes or sudden decrease/loss of hearing occurs. Instruct to seek immediate medical assistance if erection persists >4 hrs. Counsel about protective measures necessary to guard against STDs, including HIV.

STORAGE: 25°C (77°F); excursions permitted to 15-30°C (59-86°F).

VIBATIV – telavancin

RX

Class: Lipoglycopeptide

Increased mortality observed in patients with preexisting moderate/severe renal impairment (CrCl ≤50mL/min) who were treated for hospital-acquired bacterial pneumonia/ventilator-associated bacterial pneumonia (HABP/VABP); consider therapy only when the anticipated benefit outweighs the risk. New onset or worsening renal impairment reported; monitor renal function in all patients. Women of childbearing potential should have a serum pregnancy test prior to administration. Avoid use during pregnancy unless potential benefit to the patient outweighs the potential risk to the fetus. Potential adverse developmental outcomes in humans may occur.

ADULT DOSAGE

Skin and Skin Structure Infections

Complicated Gram-Positive Infections:
10mg/kg IV over 60 min q24h for 7-14 days

PEDIATRIC DOSAGE

Pediatric use may not have been established

Pneumonia

Hospital-Acquired/Ventilator-Associated Bacterial Pneumonia:
Susceptible Isolates of *Staphylococcus aureus*
10mg/kg IV over 60 min q24h for 7-21 days

DOSING CONSIDERATIONS

Renal Impairment
CrCl 30-50mL/min: 7.5mg/kg q24h
CrCl 10-<30mL/min: 10mg/kg q48h

ADMINISTRATION

IV route
Administer IV infusion over 60 min
Do not add additives or other medications to single-use vials or infuse simultaneously through the same IV line
If the same IV line is used for sequential infusion of additional medications, flush the line before and after infusion of therapy with appropriate infusion sol

Preparation
250mg Vial: Reconstitute contents w/ 15mL of appropriate reconstitution diluent
750mg Vial: Reconstitute contents w/ 45mL of appropriate reconstitution diluent
For doses of 150-800mg, reconstituted sol must be further diluted in 100-250mL of appropriate infusion sol prior to infusion
Doses <150mg or >800mg should be further diluted in a volume resulting in a final concentration of 0.6-8mg/mL

Appropriate Reconstitution Diluents
5% Dextrose inj
Sterile Water for inj
0.9% NaCl inj

Appropriate Infusion Sol
5% Dextrose inj
0.9% NaCl inj
Lactated Ringer's inj

HOW SUPPLIED

Inj: 250mg, 750mg

CONTRAINDICATIONS

Use of IV unfractionated heparin sodium, known hypersensitivity to telavancin.

WARNINGS/PRECAUTIONS

Use of telavancin for the treatment of HABP/VABP should be reserved for when alternative treatments are not suitable. Decreased efficacy in patients with cSSSI and preexisting moderate/severe renal impairment (CrCl ≤50mL/min). Renal adverse events were reported more likely to occur in patients with baseline comorbidities known to predispose patients to kidney dysfunction (preexisting renal disease, diabetes mellitus [DM], CHF, or HTN). Consider alternative agent if renal toxicity is suspected. Accumulation of the solubilizer hydroxypropyl-β-cyclodextrin may occur in patients with renal dysfunction. May interfere with coagulation tests (eg, PT/INR, activated PTT [aPTT], activated clotting time, coagulation-based factor Xa assay) and urine protein tests; collect blood samples for affected coagulation tests as close as possible prior to the next dose. For patients who require aPTT monitoring while on therapy, a non-phospholipid dependent coagulation test (eg, factor Xa [chromogenic] assay) or an alternative anticoagulant not requiring aPTT monitoring may be considered. Serious and sometimes fatal hypersensitivity reactions, including anaphylactic reactions, may occur after 1st or subsequent doses; d/c at 1st sign of skin rash, or any other signs of hypersensitivity. Caution with known hypersensitivity to vancomycin. Infusion-related reactions (eg, "red man syndrome"-like reactions) may occur with rapid infusion. *Clostridium difficile*-associated diarrhea (CDAD) reported; may need to d/c if CDAD is suspected or confirmed. Use in the absence of a proven or strongly suspected bacterial infection is unlikely to provide benefit and increases the risk of development of drug-resistant bacteria. May result in overgrowth of nonsusceptible organisms; take appropriate measures if superinfection develops. QTc interval prolongation reported; avoid in patients with congenital long QT syndrome, known prolongation of the QTc interval, uncompensated heart failure (HF), or severe left ventricular hypertrophy (LVH). Caution in elderly patients.

ADVERSE REACTIONS

Renal impairment, taste disturbance, N/V, foamy urine, rigors, diarrhea, decreased appetite.

DRUG INTERACTIONS

See Contraindications. Caution with drugs known to prolong the QT interval. Higher renal adverse event rates reported with concomitant medications known to affect kidney function (eg, NSAIDs, ACE inhibitors, loop diuretics).

PATIENT CONSIDERATIONS

Assessment: Assess for hypersensitivity to the drug/vancomycin, renal impairment, renal impairment risk (eg, preexisting renal disease, DM, CHF, HTN), congenital long QT syndrome, known prolongation of the QTc interval, uncompensated HF, severe LVH, pregnancy/nursing status, and possible drug interactions. Obtain renal function values.

Monitoring: Monitor for new onset or worsening renal impairment, hypersensitivity reactions, CDAD, development of drug-resistant bacteria, overgrowth of nonsusceptible organisms, superinfection, infusion-related reactions, QTc prolongation, and other adverse reactions. Monitor renal function (eg, SrCr, CrCl) during treatment (at 48- to 72-hr intervals or more frequently, if clinically indicated), and at the end of therapy.

Counseling: Inform women of childbearing potential about the potential risk of fetal harm if drug is used during pregnancy; instruct to have a pregnancy test prior to therapy, to use effective contraceptive methods to prevent pregnancy during treatment if not pregnant, and to notify physician if pregnancy occurs. Encourage pregnant patients to enroll in pregnancy registry. Inform that diarrhea may occur, even as late as ≥2 months after last dose of therapy; instruct to notify physician as soon as possible if watery/bloody stools (with/without stomach cramps and fever) occur. Inform that antibacterial drugs should only be used to treat bacterial, not viral, infections. Instruct to take ud; inform that skipping doses or not completing full course may decrease effectiveness and increase resistance. Counsel about common adverse effects; advise to notify physician if any unusual/known symptom persists or worsens.

STORAGE: 2-8°C (35-46°F); excursions permitted to ambient temperatures (up to 25°C [77°F]). Avoid excessive heat. Reconstituted/Diluted Sol: Use within 12 hrs when stored at room temperature or use within 7 days when stored under refrigeration at 2-8°C (36-46°F). Diluted sol can also be stored at -30 to -10°C (-22 to 14°F) for up to 32 days.

VIBERZI – eluxadoline

CIV

Class: Mu-opioid receptor agonist

ADULT DOSAGE

Irritable Bowel Syndrome with Diarrhea

100mg bid

75mg bid in patients who:
- do not have a gallbladder
- are unable to tolerate the 100mg dose
- are receiving concomitant OATP1B1 inhibitors
- have mild or moderate (Child-Pugh Class A or B) hepatic impairment

PEDIATRIC DOSAGE

Pediatric use may not have been established

DOSING CONSIDERATIONS

Concomitant Medications

OATP1B1 Inhibitors: 75mg bid

Hepatic Impairment

Mild or Moderate (Child-Pugh Class A or B): 75mg bid

Adverse Reactions

D/C in patients who develop severe constipation for >4 days

ADMINISTRATION

Oral route

Take w/ food.

HOW SUPPLIED

Tab: 75mg, 100mg

CONTRAINDICATIONS

Known/suspected biliary duct obstruction, or sphincter of Oddi disease/dysfunction. Alcoholism, alcohol abuse/addiction, or in patients who drink >3 alcoholic beverages per day. History of pancreatitis or structural diseases of the pancreas, including known/suspected pancreatic duct obstruction. Severe hepatic impairment (Child-Pugh Class C). History of chronic or severe constipation or sequelae from constipation, or known/suspected mechanical GI obstruction.

WARNINGS/PRECAUTIONS

Potential for increased risk of sphincter of Oddi spasm, resulting in pancreatitis or hepatic enzyme elevation; patients w/o a gallbladder are at increased risk. Consider alternative therapies in patients w/o a gallbladder and evaluate the benefits/risks of eluxadoline in these patients. Do not restart therapy in patients who developed biliary duct obstruction or sphincter of Oddi spasm while taking eluxadoline. Potential for increased risk of pancreatitis not associated w/ sphincter of Oddi spasm; majority of cases were associated w/ excessive alcohol intake. Caution in elderly.

ADVERSE REACTIONS

Constipation, N/V, abdominal pain, URTI, nasopharyngitis, abdominal distention, bronchitis, dizziness, flatulence, rash, increased ALT, fatigue, viral gastroenteritis.

DRUG INTERACTIONS

See Dosing Considerations. OATP1B1 inhibitors (eg, cyclosporine, gemfibrozil, antiretrovirals) and strong CYP inhibitors (eg, ciprofloxacin, fluconazole, clarithromycin) may increase exposure; monitor for impaired mental/physical abilities and for other eluxadoline-related adverse reactions. Increased risk for constipation-related adverse reactions w/ drugs that cause constipation (eg, alosetron, anticholinergics, opioids); avoid concomitant use. Loperamide may be used occasionally for acute management of severe diarrhea, but avoid chronic use; d/c loperamide immediately if constipation occurs. May increase exposure of OATP1B1 and BCRP substrates. Increased exposure to rosuvastatin w/ a potential for increased risk of myopathy/rhabdomyolysis; use lowest effective dose of rosuvastatin. Potential for increased exposure of CYP3A substrates w/ narrow therapeutic index (eg, alfentanil, cyclosporine, dihydroergotamine); monitor drug concentrations or other pharmacodynamic markers of drug effect when concomitant use w/ eluxadoline is initiated or discontinued.

PATIENT CONSIDERATIONS

Assessment: Assess for hepatic impairment, known/suspected biliary duct obstruction, sphincter of Oddi disease/dysfunction, alcoholism, alcohol abuse/addiction, history of pancreatitis or structural diseases of the pancreas, history of chronic or severe constipation or sequelae from constipation, known/suspected mechanical GI obstruction, other conditions where treatment is contraindicated or cautioned, pregnancy/nursing status, and for possible drug interactions.

Monitoring: Monitor for severe constipation and new or worsening abdominal pain that may radiate to the back or shoulder, w/ or w/o N/V. If used in patients w/o a gallbladder, monitor for symptoms of sphincter of Oddi spasm (eg, elevated liver transaminases associated w/ abdominal pain or pancreatitis), especially during the 1st few weeks of treatment. Monitor patients w/ any degree of hepatic impairment for impaired mental/physical abilities.

Counseling: Instruct to d/c drug and seek medical attention if unusual or severe abdominal pain that may radiate to the back or shoulder, w/ or w/o N/V, develops or if constipation lasting >4 days is experienced. Advise to avoid chronic or acute excessive alcohol use during treatment. Instruct to take ud and to inform physician if unable to tolerate therapy. Instruct patients to not take alosetron w/ eluxadoline or not take loperamide on a chronic basis w/ eluxadoline due to the potential for constipation. Advise to avoid other medications that may cause constipation.

STORAGE: 20-25°C (68-77°F); excursions permitted to 15-30°C (59-86°F).

VICODIN — acetaminophen/hydrocodone bitartrate CII

Class: Opioid analgesic

Associated w/ cases of acute liver failure, at times resulting in liver transplant and death. Most of the cases of liver injury are associated w/ acetaminophen (APAP) use at doses >4000mg/day, and often involve >1 APAP-containing product.

OTHER BRAND NAMES

Vicodin ES, Vicodin HP

ADULT DOSAGE

Moderate to Moderately Severe Pain

Vicodin:

Usual: 1 or 2 tabs q4-6h prn

Max: 8 tabs/day

Vicodin ES/Vicodin HP:

Usual: 1 tab q4-6h prn

Max: 6 tabs/day

PEDIATRIC DOSAGE

Pediatric use may not have been established

V

DOSING CONSIDERATIONS

Elderly

Start at lower end of dosing range

ADMINISTRATION

Oral route

HOW SUPPLIED

(Hydrocodone/APAP) **Tab:** (Vicodin) 5mg/300mg*; (Vicodin ES) 7.5mg/300mg*; (Vicodin HP) 10mg/300mg* *scored

CONTRAINDICATIONS
Previous hypersensitivity to hydrocodone or APAP.

WARNINGS/PRECAUTIONS
Increased risk of acute liver failure in patients w/ underlying liver disease. May cause serious skin reactions (eg, acute generalized exanthematous pustulosis, Stevens-Johnson syndrome, toxic epidermal necrolysis); d/c at the 1st appearance of skin rash or any other sign of hypersensitivity. Hypersensitivity and anaphylaxis reported; d/c immediately if signs/symptoms occur. May produce dose-related respiratory depression and irregular/periodic breathing. Respiratory depressant effects and CSF pressure elevation capacity may be markedly exaggerated in the presence of head injury, other intracranial lesions, or a preexisting increased intracranial pressure. May obscure clinical course of acute abdominal conditions and head injuries. Caution w/ hypothyroidism, Addison's disease, prostatic hypertrophy, urethral stricture, severe hepatic/renal impairment, or in the elderly/debilitated. Suppresses cough reflex; caution w/ pulmonary disease and in postoperative use. Lab test interactions may occur. May be habit-forming.

ADVERSE REACTIONS
Acute liver failure, lightheadedness, dizziness, sedation, N/V.

DRUG INTERACTIONS
Increased risk of acute liver failure w/ alcohol. Additive CNS depression w/ other narcotics, antihistamines, antipsychotics, antianxiety agents, or other CNS depressants (eg, alcohol); reduce dose of one or both agents. Concomitant use w/ MAOIs or TCAs may increase the effect of either the antidepressant or hydrocodone.

PATIENT CONSIDERATIONS

Assessment: Assess for history of hypersensitivity to drug, level of pain intensity, type of pain, patient's general condition and medical status, renal/hepatic impairment, pregnancy/nursing status, any other conditions where treatment is cautioned, and possible drug interactions.

Monitoring: Monitor for signs/symptoms of hypersensitivity or anaphylaxis, serious skin reactions, acute liver failure, respiratory depression, elevations in CSF pressure, drug abuse/dependence/tolerance, and other adverse reactions. In patients w/ severe hepatic/renal disease, monitor effects w/ serial hepatic and/or renal function tests.

Counseling: Instruct to look for APAP on package labels and not to use >1 APAP-containing product. Instruct to seek medical attention immediately upon ingestion of >4000mg/day of APAP, even if feeling well. Advise to d/c use and contact physician immediately if signs of allergy develop. Inform about signs of serious skin reactions. Inform that drug may impair mental/physical abilities, and to use caution if performing potentially hazardous tasks (eg, driving, operating machinery). Instruct to avoid alcohol and other CNS depressants. Inform that drug may be habit-forming; instruct to take only ud.

STORAGE: 20-25°C (68-77°F).

VICOPROFEN — hydrocodone bitartrate/ibuprofen CII

Class: Opioid analgesic

OTHER BRAND NAMES
Reprexain

ADULT DOSAGE

Acute Pain

Short-Term (Generally <10 Days) Management:
Use lowest effective dose or longest dosing interval consistent w/ individual treatment goals; adjust based on individual needs

Usual: 1 tab q4-6h prn
Max: 5 tabs/24 hrs

PEDIATRIC DOSAGE

Acute Pain

Short-Term (Generally <10 Days) Management:
≥16 Years:
Use lowest effective dose or longest dosing interval consistent w/ individual treatment goals; adjust based on individual needs

Usual: 1 tab q4-6h prn
Max: 5 tabs/24 hrs

DOSING CONSIDERATIONS

Elderly
Reduce dose

ADMINISTRATION
Oral route

HOW SUPPLIED
(Hydrocodone/Ibuprofen) **Tab:** (Vicoprofen) 7.5mg/200mg; (Reprexain) 2.5mg/200mg, 5mg/200mg*, 10mg/200mg *scored

CONTRAINDICATIONS

Known hypersensitivity to hydrocodone or ibuprofen. History of asthma, urticaria, or other allergic-type reactions w/ aspirin (ASA) or other NSAIDs. Perioperative pain in the setting of CABG surgery.

WARNINGS/PRECAUTIONS

Not for treatment of osteoarthritis or rheumatoid arthritis. Not for treatment of corticosteroid insufficiency or substitute for corticosteroids; abrupt discontinuation of corticosteroids may lead to disease exacerbation. May diminish utility of fever and inflammation as diagnostic signs in detecting complications of presumed noninfectious, painful conditions. Not recommended w/ advanced renal disease. Ibuprofen: May increase risk of serious cardiovascular (CV) thrombotic events, MI, and stroke; increased risk w/ known CV disease or risk factors for CV disease. May cause serious GI adverse events including inflammation, bleeding, ulceration, and perforation of the stomach and intestine; extreme caution w/ history of ulcer disease or GI bleeding and caution in debilitated patients. May lead to onset of new HTN or worsening of preexisting HTN. Fluid retention and edema reported; caution in patients w/ fluid retention or heart failure (HF). Renal papillary necrosis and other renal injury reported after long-term use; caution w/ impaired renal function, HF, and liver dysfunction. Anaphylactoid reactions may occur; avoid in patients w/ ASA triad. May cause serious skin adverse events (eg, exfoliative dermatitis, Stevens-Johnson syndrome, and toxic epidermal necrolysis); d/c at 1st appearance of skin rash/hypersensitivity. Avoid in late pregnancy; may cause premature closure of ductus arteriosus. Elevations of LFTs and severe hepatic reactions (eg, jaundice, fatal fulminant hepatitis, liver necrosis, hepatic failure) reported; d/c if liver disease or systemic manifestations (eg, eosinophilia, rash) occur. Anemia reported. May inhibit platelet aggregation and prolong bleeding time. Caution w/ preexisting asthma and avoid w/ ASA-sensitive asthma. Aseptic meningitis w/ fever and coma reported. Hydrocodone: May increase risk of misuse, abuse, or diversion. May produce dose-related respiratory depression. Respiratory depressant effects and capacity to elevate CSF pressure may be markedly exaggerated in the presence of head injury, intracranial lesions, or preexisting increased intracranial pressure. May obscure diagnosis/clinical course of acute abdominal conditions or head injuries. Caution in debilitated patients, severe renal/hepatic impairment, hypothyroidism, Addison's disease, prostatic hypertrophy, or urethral stricture. Suppresses cough reflex; caution when used postoperatively and w/ pulmonary disease.

ADVERSE REACTIONS

Headache, somnolence, dizziness, constipation, dyspepsia, N/V, infection, edema, nervousness, anxiety, pruritus, diarrhea, asthenia, abdominal pain, sweating.

DRUG INTERACTIONS

ASA may increase adverse effects; concomitant administration is not recommended. Use w/ other opioid analgesics, antihistamines, antipsychotics, antianxiety agents, or other CNS depressants (eg, alcohol) may exhibit additive CNS depression; reduce dose of 1 or both agents. Ibuprofen: Increased risk of GI bleeding w/ oral corticosteroids or anticoagulants, smoking, and alcohol. May increase the risk of renal toxicity w/ diuretics and ACE inhibitors. Alterations in platelet function may occur w/ anticoagulants; monitor carefully. May diminish antihypertensive effect of ACE inhibitors. Synergistic effects on GI bleeding w/ warfarin. May decrease natriuretic effect of furosemide and loop/thiazide diuretics; monitor for renal failure. May increase lithium levels; monitor for lithium toxicity. May enhance methotrexate toxicity; caution w/ coadministration. Hydrocodone: Use w/ MAOIs or TCAs may increase the effect of either the antidepressant or hydrocodone. Not recommended for patients taking MAOIs or w/in 14 days of stopping such treatment. May produce paralytic ileus w/ anticholinergics. Caution w/ concurrent agonist/antagonist analgesics (eg, pentazocine, nalbuphine, butorphanol, buprenorphine) use; may reduce analgesic effect of hydrocodone and/or precipitate withdrawal symptoms. May enhance neuromuscular blocking action of skeletal muscle relaxants and increase respiratory depression.

PATIENT CONSIDERATIONS

Assessment: Assess for history of asthma, urticaria or allergic-type reactions w/ ASA or NSAIDs, known hypersensitivity to the drug, perioperative pain in setting of CABG surgery, CV disease and its risk factors, HTN, fluid retention or HF, ulcer disease or GI bleeding, coagulation disorders, renal/hepatic impairment, any other conditions where treatment is contraindicated or cautioned, pregnancy/nursing status, and for possible drug interactions. Assess level of pain intensity, type of pain, and patient's general condition and medical status.

Monitoring: Monitor for signs/symptoms of CV thrombotic events, MI, stroke, HTN, fluid retention or edema, drug abuse and dependence, tolerance, respiratory depression, elevations in CSF, GI effects, renal/hepatic effects, anaphylactoid reactions, skin reactions, bronchospasm, aseptic meningitis, and other adverse reactions. If signs/symptoms of anemia develop, evaluate Hgb/Hct. Perform periodic monitoring of CBC and chemistry profile w/ long-term therapy. Monitor for alterations in platelet function w/ coagulation disorders or in those receiving anticoagulants.

Counseling: Caution that drug may impair mental and/or physical abilities required to perform potentially hazardous tasks (eg, operating machinery/driving). Instruct to avoid alcohol and other CNS depressants while on therapy. Warn that drug may be habit-forming; instruct to take only for as long as prescribed, in the amounts prescribed, and no more frequently than prescribed. Instruct to contact physician if CV events, GI effects, unexplained weight gain, or edema occurs. Instruct to immediately d/c therapy and contact physician if signs/symptoms of serious skin reactions or hepatotoxicity develop. Instruct to seek immediate medical attention if signs of anaphylactoid reactions develop. Instruct to report any signs of blurred vision or other eye symptoms. Instruct to avoid use in late pregnancy.

STORAGE: (Vicoprofen) 25°C (77°F); excursions permitted to 15-30°C (59-86°F). (Reprexain) 20-25°C (68-77°F); excursions permitted to 15-30°C (59-86°F).

VICTOZA – liraglutide (rDNA origin)

RX

Class: Glucagon-like peptide-1 (GLP-1) receptor agonist

Causes dose-dependent and treatment-duration-dependent thyroid C-cell tumors at clinically relevant exposures in animal studies. It is unknown whether drug causes thyroid C-cell tumors (eg, medullary thyroid carcinoma [MTC]) in humans. Contraindicated in patients w/ a personal or family history of MTC and in patients w/ multiple endocrine neoplasia syndrome type 2 (MEN 2). Counsel patients regarding potential risk for MTC and symptoms of thyroid tumors (eg, mass in the neck, dysphagia, dyspnea, persistent hoarseness). Routine monitoring of serum calcitonin or using thyroid ultrasound is of uncertain value for early detection of MTC.

ADULT DOSAGE

Type 2 Diabetes Mellitus

Initial: 0.6mg SQ qd for 1 week

Titrate: Increase to 1.2mg qd after 1 week; if acceptable glycemic control is not achieved, increase to 1.8mg qd

Missed Dose

If a dose is missed, the once-daily regimen should be resumed w/ the next scheduled dose; if >3 days have elapsed since the last dose, reinitiate at 0.6mg, and titrate ud

PEDIATRIC DOSAGE

Pediatric use may not have been established

DOSING CONSIDERATIONS

Concomitant Medications

Consider reducing dose of concomitant insulin secretagogue or insulin

ADMINISTRATION

SQ route

May be administered qd at any time of the day, independently of meals

Inject into abdomen, thigh, or upper arm

Inj site and timing can be changed w/o dose adjustment

Coadministration w/ Insulin

Administer as separate inj; never mix

May inject in the same body region but the inj should not be adjacent to each other

HOW SUPPLIED

Inj: 6mg/mL [3mL]

CONTRAINDICATIONS

Personal or family history of MTC, MEN 2, prior serious hypersensitivity reaction to liraglutide or to any of the product components.

WARNINGS/PRECAUTIONS

Not recommended as 1st-line therapy for patients who have inadequate glycemic control on diet and exercise. Not a substitute for insulin; do not use in type 1 DM or for the treatment of diabetic ketoacidosis. Further evaluate patients w/ serum calcitonin elevation or thyroid nodules. Acute pancreatitis, including fatal and nonfatal hemorrhagic or necrotizing pancreatitis, reported; observe for signs/symptoms of pancreatitis after initiation of therapy, d/c promptly if suspected, and do not restart therapy if confirmed. Consider other antidiabetic therapies in patients w/ a history of pancreatitis. Do not share pens between patients, even if the needle is changed; poses a risk for transmission of blood-borne pathogens. Acute renal failure and worsening of chronic renal failure reported; caution when initiating/escalating doses in patients w/ renal impairment. Serious hypersensitivity reactions (eg, anaphylactic reactions, angioedema) reported; d/c if a hypersensitivity reaction occurs. Caution w/ hepatic impairment.

ADVERSE REACTIONS

N/V, diarrhea, constipation, dyspepsia, headache, antibody formation.

DRUG INTERACTIONS

See Dosing Considerations. Increased risk of hypoglycemia w/ insulin secretagogues (eg, sulfonylureas) or insulin. May affect the absorption of oral medications; use w/ caution.

PATIENT CONSIDERATIONS

Assessment: Assess for previous hypersensitivity reactions, MEN 2, personal or family history of MTC, history of pancreatitis, type of DM, diabetic ketoacidosis, renal/hepatic impairment, pregnancy/nursing status, and possible drug interactions.

Monitoring: Monitor for signs and symptoms of thyroid tumor, pancreatitis, serum calcitonin elevation, hypoglycemia, hypersensitivity reactions, and other adverse reactions. Monitor renal function, blood glucose levels, and HbA1c levels.

Counseling: Counsel regarding potential risk of MTC and advise to report symptoms of thyroid tumors (eg, lump in the neck, hoarseness) to physician. Inform of the potential risk of dehydration due to GI adverse reactions and instruct to take precautions to avoid fluid depletion. Inform of the potential risk for pancreatitis and worsening renal function. Instruct to d/c therapy promptly and contact physician if persistent severe abdominal pain and/or symptoms of hypersensitivity reactions occur. Advise not to share pen w/ another person, even if the needle is changed. Counsel on potential risks/benefits of therapy and of alternative modes of therapy, importance of adhering to dietary instructions, regular physical activity, periodic blood glucose monitoring and HbA1c testing, recognition/management of hypo/hyperglycemia, and assessment for diabetes complications. Advise to seek medical advice during periods of stress (eg, fever, trauma, infection), if any unusual symptom develops, or if any known symptom persists or worsens. Instruct not to take an extra dose to make up for a missed dose and to resume as prescribed w/ the next scheduled dose.

STORAGE: Prior to 1st Use: 2-8°C (36-46°F). Do not freeze and do not use if it has been frozen. After Initial Use: 15-30°C (59-86°F) or 2-8°C (36-46°F) for 30 days. Keep the pen cap on when not in use. Always remove and safely discard the needle after each inj; store pen w/o an inj needle attached. Protect from excessive heat and sunlight.

VIEKIRA PAK – dasabuvir; ombitasvir/paritaprevir/ritonavir RX

Class: CYP3A inhibitor/HCV NS5A inhibitor/HCV non-nucleoside NS5B palm polymerase inhibitor/HCV NS3/4A protease inhibitor

ADULT DOSAGE

Chronic Hepatitis C (Genotype 1)

2 tabs (ombitasvir, paritaprevir, ritonavir [RTV]) qd (am) and 1 dasabuvir tab bid (am and pm)

Coadministration w/ Ribavirin (RBV):
<75kg: 1000mg/day RBV divided and administered bid w/ food
≥75kg: 1200mg/day RBV divided and administered bid w/ food

Genotype 1a, w/o Cirrhosis:
2 tabs (ombitasvir, paritaprevir, RTV) qd (am) + 1 dasabuvir tab bid (am and pm) + RBV for 12 weeks

Genotype 1a, w/ Cirrhosis:
2 tabs (ombitasvir, paritaprevir, RTV) qd (am) + 1 dasabuvir tab bid (am and pm) + RBV for 24 weeks. 12-week treatment duration may be considered for some patients based on prior treatment history

Genotype 1b, w/o Cirrhosis:
2 tabs (ombitasvir, paritaprevir, RTV) qd (am) + 1 dasabuvir tab bid (am and pm) for 12 weeks

Genotype 1b, w/ Cirrhosis:
2 tabs (ombitasvir, paritaprevir, RTV) qd (am) + 1 dasabuvir tab bid (am and pm) + RBV for 12 weeks

Follow the genotype 1a dosing recommendations in patients w/ an unknown genotype 1 subtype or w/ mixed genotype 1 infection

PEDIATRIC DOSAGE

Pediatric use may not have been established

Liver Transplant Recipients w/ Normal Hepatic Function and Mild Fibrosis (Metavir Fibrosis Score ≤2):
2 tabs (ombitasvir, paritaprevir, RTV) qd (am) + 1 dasabuvir tab bid (am and pm) + RBV for 24 weeks, irrespective of hepatitis C virus genotype 1 subtype. If calcineurin inhibitor used concomitantly, calcineurin inhibitor dosage adjustment is needed

DOSING CONSIDERATIONS

Hepatic Impairment

Moderate (Child-Pugh B): Not recommended

ADMINISTRATION

Oral route

Take w/ a meal w/o regard to fat or calorie content.

HOW SUPPLIED

Tab: (Ombitasvir/Paritaprevir/RTV) 12.5mg/75mg/50mg, (Dasabuvir) 250mg

CONTRAINDICATIONS

Severe hepatic impairment. Coadministration w/ drugs that are highly dependent on CYP3A for clearance and for which elevated plasma concentrations are associated w/ serious and/or life-threatening events; coadministration w/ moderate or strong inducers of CYP3A and strong inducers of CYP2C8 that may lead to reduced efficacy of therapy; and coadministration w/ strong inhibitors of CYP2C8 that may increase dasabuvir plasma concentrations and the risk of QT prolongation. Coadministration w/ alfuzosin, carbamazepine, phenytoin, phenobarbital, gemfibrozil, rifampin, ergotamine, dihydroergotamine, ergonovine, methylergonovine, ethinyl estradiol containing medications (eg, combined oral contraceptives), St. John's wort, lovastatin, simvastatin, pimozide, efavirenz, sildenafil (when used to treat pulmonary arterial HTN), triazolam, or oral midazolam. Known hypersensitivity (eg, toxic epidermal necrolysis, Stevens-Johnson syndrome) to RTV. When used w/ RBV, refer to the individual monograph.

WARNINGS/PRECAUTIONS

Not recommended for use w/ decompensated liver disease. Elevations of ALT to >5X ULN reported. Perform hepatic lab testing during the first 4 weeks of starting treatment and as clinically indicated thereafter. If ALT is found to be elevated above baseline levels, repeat and monitor closely. Consider discontinuing if ALT levels remain persistently >10X ULN. D/C if ALT elevation is accompanied by signs or symptoms of liver inflammation or increasing conjugated bilirubin, alkaline phosphatase, or INR. If coadministered w/ RBV, the warnings and precautions for RBV, in particular the pregnancy avoidance warning, apply to this combination regimen; refer to RBV PI for a full list of warnings/precautions for RBV. Any HCV/HIV-1 coinfected patients being treated should also be on a suppressive antiretroviral drug regimen to reduce the risk of HIV-1 protease inhibitor drug resistance.

ADVERSE REACTIONS

Fatigue, nausea, pruritus, skin reactions, insomnia, asthenia.

DRUG INTERACTIONS

See Contraindications. Not recommended w/ darunavir/RTV, lopinavir/RTV, rilpivirine (qd dosing), and salmeterol. Not recommended w/ voriconazole unless an assessment of the benefit-to-risk ratio justifies the use of voriconazole. If taking quetiapine, consider alternative anti-HCV therapy. Caution and therapeutic monitoring is recommended w/ antiarrhythmics. May increase levels of drugs that are substrates of CYP3A, UGT1A1, breast cancer resistance protein (BCRP), OATP1B1, or OATP1B3. May increase levels of quetiapine, antiarrhythmics, ketoconazole, amlodipine, inhaled/nasal fluticasone, furosemide (C_{max}), rilpivirine, rosuvastatin, pravastatin, cyclosporine, tacrolimus, salmeterol, buprenorphine, norbuprenorphine, and alprazolam. May decrease levels of voriconazole, darunavir (C_{trough}), and omeprazole. Inhibition of P-gp, BCRP, OATP1B1, or OATP1B3 may increase levels of the various components of Viekira Pak. ALT elevation reported more frequently w/ ethinyl estradiol-containing medications (eg, combined oral contraceptives, contraceptive patches, contraceptive vaginal rings); alternative methods of contraception (eg, progestin-only contraception, nonhormonal methods) are recommended during therapy. Ethinyl estradiol-containing medications can be restarted approx 2 weeks following completion of treatment. **Paritaprevir:** Atazanavir/RTV (qd dosing), and lopinavir/RTV may increase levels. **Paritaprevir/RTV:** Strong CYP3A inhibitors may increase levels. **Dasabuvir:** CYP2C8 inhibitors may increase levels. Refer to PI for further information on drug interactions, including dosing modifications when used w/ certain concomitant therapies.

PATIENT CONSIDERATIONS

Assessment: Assess for drug hypersensitivity, decompensated liver disease, hepatic impairment, pregnancy/nursing status, and possible drug interactions. Assess LFTs.

Monitoring: Monitor for ALT elevation and other adverse reactions. Perform hepatic lab testing during the first 4 weeks of starting treatment and as clinically indicated thereafter. If ALT is found to be elevated above baseline levels, repeat and monitor closely.

Counseling: Inform to watch for early warning signs of liver inflammation (eg, fatigue, lack of appetite, N/V); instruct to contact physician w/o delay if such symptoms occur. Advise to avoid pregnancy during treatment w/ RBV; instruct to notify physician immediately in the event of a pregnancy and inform pregnant patients that there is an Antiretroviral Pregnancy Registry that monitors pregnancy outcomes in women who are HCV/HIV-1 coinfected and taking concomitant antiretrovirals. Inform that therapy may interact w/ some drugs; advise to report to physician the use of any prescription, nonprescription medication, or herbal products. Inform that contraceptives containing ethinyl estradiol are contraindicated w/ therapy. Inform that the effect of treatment of HCV infection on transmission is not known, and that appropriate precautions to prevent transmission of the HCV during treatment should be taken. Inform that if a dose of ombitasvir, paritaprevir, RTV is missed, the prescribed dose can be taken w/in 12 hrs and if a dasabuvir dose is missed, the prescribed dose can be taken w/in 6 hrs. Instruct that the missed dose should not be taken if >12 hrs has passed since ombitasvir, paritaprevir, RTV is usually taken or if >6 hrs has passed since dasabuvir is usually taken; inform patient to take the next dose as per the usual dosing schedule. Instruct not to take more than their prescribed dose of therapy to make up for a missed dose.

STORAGE: ≤30°C (86°F).

VIGAMOX — moxifloxacin hydrochloride RX

Class: Fluoroquinolone

ADULT DOSAGE

Bacterial Conjunctivitis

1 drop in the affected eye tid for 7 days

PEDIATRIC DOSAGE

Bacterial Conjunctivitis

≥1 Year:

1 drop in the affected eye tid for 7 days

ADMINISTRATION

Ocular route

HOW SUPPLIED

Sol: 0.5% [3mL]

CONTRAINDICATIONS

History of hypersensitivity to moxifloxacin, to other quinolones, or to any components in the medication.

WARNINGS/PRECAUTIONS

Not for inj. Do not inject subconjunctivally or introduce directly into the anterior chamber of the eye. Fatal hypersensitivity reactions reported with systemic quinolone therapy. May result in bacterial resistance with prolonged use; take appropriate measures if superinfection develops. Avoid contact lenses when signs and symptoms of bacterial conjunctivitis are present.

ADVERSE REACTIONS

Conjunctivitis, decreased visual acuity, dry eye, keratitis, ocular discomfort/hyperemia, ocular pain/pruritus, subconjunctival hemorrhage, tearing.

PATIENT CONSIDERATIONS

Assessment: Assess for proper diagnosis of causative organisms (eg, slit-lamp biomicroscopy, fluorescein staining). Assess for hypersensitivity to other quinolones, and pregnancy/nursing status.

Monitoring: Monitor for signs/symptoms of hypersensitivity or anaphylactic reactions and other adverse reactions. With prolonged therapy, monitor for overgrowth of nonsusceptible organisms (eg, fungi) and for development of superinfection.

Counseling: Instruct not to touch the dropper tip to any surface to avoid contaminating the contents. Instruct to immediately d/c medication and contact physician at the 1st sign of rash or allergic reaction. Instruct not to wear contact lenses if signs and symptoms of bacterial conjunctivitis develop.

STORAGE: 2-25°C (36-77°F).

VIIBRYD — vilazodone hydrochloride RX

Class: Selective serotonin reuptake inhibitor (SSRI)/5-HT_{1A}-receptor partial agonist

Antidepressants increased the risk of suicidal thoughts and behaviors in patients aged ≤24 yrs in short-term studies. Monitor closely for clinical worsening and for emergence of suicidal thoughts and behaviors.

ADULT DOSAGE

Major Depressive Disorder

Initial: 10mg qd for 7 days
Titrate: Increase to 20mg qd
May increase up to 40mg qd after a minimum of 7 days between dosage increases
Target Dose: 20-40mg qd

Dosing Considerations with MAOIs

Switching to/from an MAOI Antidepressant: Allow at least 14 days between discontinuation of an MAOI antidepressant and initiation of treatment, and allow at least 14 days after stopping treatment before starting an MAOI antidepressant

PEDIATRIC DOSAGE

Pediatric use may not have been established

DOSING CONSIDERATIONS

Concomitant Medications

Strong CYP3A4 Inhibitors (eg, Itraconazole, Clarithromycin, Voriconazole):
Max: 20mg qd; may resume original vilazodone dose level when CYP3A4 inhibitor is discontinued

Strong CYP3A4 Inducers (eg, Carbamazepine, Phenytoin, Rifampin) for >14 Days: Consider increasing vilazodone dose by 2-fold, up to a max of 80mg qd, over 1-2 weeks based on clinical response; gradually reduce vilazodone dosage to its original level over 1-2 weeks if CYP3A4 inducers are discontinued

Elderly

Start at lower end of dosing range

Discontinuation

Gradually reduce dose whenever possible
Taper down from 40mg qd dose to 20mg qd for 4 days, followed by 10mg qd for 3 days
Taper dose to 10mg qd for 7 days in patients taking 20mg qd

ADMINISTRATION

Oral route

Take w/ food

HOW SUPPLIED

Tab: 10mg, 20mg, 40mg

CONTRAINDICATIONS

Concomitant use of MAOIs, or w/in 14 days of stopping MAOIs (eg, linezolid, IV methylene blue).

WARNINGS/PRECAUTIONS

Serotonin syndrome reported; d/c immediately if symptoms occur and initiate supportive symptomatic treatment. May increase the risk of bleeding events. May precipitate mixed/manic episode in patients w/ bipolar disorder. Avoid abrupt discontinuation. Caution w/ seizure disorder. Pupillary dilation that occurs following use may trigger an angle closure attack in a patient w/ anatomically narrow angles who does not have a patent iridectomy; avoid use in patients w/ untreated anatomically narrow angles. Hyponatremia may occur in association w/ the syndrome of inappropriate antidiuretic hormone secretion; d/c and institute appropriate medical intervention in patients w/ symptomatic hyponatremia. Elderly patients, patients taking diuretics, and those who are volume-depleted may be at greater risk of developing hyponatremia.

ADVERSE REACTIONS

Diarrhea, N/V, headache, dizziness, dry mouth, insomnia, abdominal pain, decreased libido, fatigue, flatulence, somnolence, restlessness.

DRUG INTERACTIONS

See Dosing Considerations and Contraindications. May cause serotonin syndrome w/ other serotonergic drugs (eg, triptans, TCAs, St. John's wort) and w/ drugs that impair metabolism of serotonin; d/c treatment and any concomitant serotonergic agents immediately if this occurs. Increased risk of bleeding w/ aspirin (ASA), NSAIDs, other antiplatelet drugs, warfarin, and other anticoagulants. Monitor coagulation indices (eg, INR) w/ warfarin when initiating/titrating/discontinuing treatment. Strong CYP3A4 inhibitors may increase exposure. Strong CYP3A4 inducers may decrease exposure. May increase digoxin concentrations; measure digoxin concentrations before initiating concomitant use of vilazodone and continue monitoring and reduce digoxin dose as necessary.

PATIENT CONSIDERATIONS

Assessment: Assess for personal/family history of bipolar disorder, mania/hypomania, seizure disorder, untreated anatomically narrow angles, volume depletion, pregnancy/nursing status, and possible drug interactions.

Monitoring: Monitor for clinical worsening and emergence of suicidal thoughts and behaviors (especially during the initial few months of therapy and at times of dosage changes). Monitor for serotonin syndrome, angle-closure glaucoma, bleeding, activation of mania/hypomania, hyponatremia, discontinuation symptoms, and other adverse reactions.

Counseling: Advise patients and caregivers to monitor for clinical worsening and to look for the emergence of suicidality, especially early during treatment and when the dose is adjusted up or down; instruct to report such symptoms to physician. Instruct to take ud. Caution about the risk of serotonin syndrome; instruct to contact physician or report to the emergency room if they experience signs/symptoms of serotonin syndrome. Inform about the increased risk of bleeding w/ ASA, NSAIDs, other antiplatelet drugs, warfarin, or other anticoagulants; advise to inform physician if taking/planning to take any prescription or OTC medications that increase the risk of bleeding. Advise patients and caregivers to observe for signs of activation of mania/hypomania; instruct to report such symptoms to physician. Advise not to abruptly d/c therapy and to discuss any tapering regimen w/ physician. Caution about using the medication if they have a history of seizure disorder. Advise to notify physician if an allergic reaction develops. Advise to inform physician if taking or planning to take any prescription or OTC medications, since there is a potential for interactions.

STORAGE: 25°C (77°F); excursions permitted to 15-30°C (59-86°F).

VIMIZIM – elosulfase alfa

RX

Class: Enzyme

Life-threatening anaphylactic reactions observed during infusion. Anaphylaxis (eg, cough, erythema, throat tightness, urticaria, flushing, cyanosis, hypotension, rash, dyspnea, chest discomfort, GI symptoms) in conjunction with urticaria reported during infusions, regardless of duration of treatment; closely observe patients during and after administration. Inform patients of the signs/symptoms of anaphylaxis and instruct to seek immediate medical care should symptoms occur. Patients with acute respiratory illness may be at risk of serious acute exacerbation of their respiratory compromise due to hypersensitivity reactions; additional monitoring required.

ADULT DOSAGE

Mucopolysaccharidosis IVA (Morquio A Syndrome)

Usual: 2mg/kg IV over a minimum range of 3.5-4.5 hrs, based on infusion volume, once every week

Premedication

Pretreat w/ antihistamines (w/ or w/o antipyretics) 30-60 min prior to start of infusion

PEDIATRIC DOSAGE

Mucopolysaccharidosis IVA (Morquio A Syndrome)

≥5 Years:
Usual: 2mg/kg IV over a minimum range of 3.5-4.5 hrs, based on infusion volume, once every week

Premedication

Pretreat w/ antihistamines (w/ or w/o antipyretics) 30-60 min prior to start of infusion

DOSING CONSIDERATIONS

Adverse Reactions

Hypersensitivity Reactions: Slow, temporarily stop, or d/c infusion rate for that visit

ADMINISTRATION

IV route

Preparation Instructions

1. Determine the number of vials to be diluted based on the patient's weight and the recommended dose
2. Dilute the calculated dose to a final volume of 100mL or 250mL using 0.9% NaCl inj; the final volume is based on the patient's weight as follows:
Patients <25kg: Final volume should be 100mL
Patients ≥25kg: Final volume should be 250mL
3. The sol should be clear to slightly opalescent and colorless to pale yellow when diluted; a sol w/ slight flocculation (eg, thin translucent fibers) is acceptable for administration
4. Gently rotate the bag to ensure proper distribution; avoid agitation during preparation and do not shake the sol
5. Administration should be completed w/in 48 hrs from the time of dilution

Administration Instructions

Administer the diluted sol using a low-protein binding infusion set equipped w/ a low-protein binding 0.2μm in-line filter

Patients <25kg:
Initial Infusion Rate: 3mL/hr for the first 15 min
Titrate: If tolerated, increase to 6mL/hr for the next 15 min; if this rate is tolerated, then the rate

may be increased every 15 min in 6mL/hr increments
Max Infusion Rate: 36mL/hr
Total volume of the infusion should be delivered over a minimum of 3.5 hrs

Patients ≥25kg:
Initial Infusion Rate: 6mL/hr for the first 15 min
Titrate: If tolerated, increase to 12mL/hr for the next 15 min; if this rate is tolerated, then the rate may be increased every 15 min in 12mL/hr increments
Max Infusion Rate: 72mL/hr
Total volume of the infusion should be delivered over a minimum of 4.5 hrs

Do not infuse w/ other products in the infusion tubing

Stability Information
If immediate use is not possible, store the diluted product for up to 24 hrs at 2-8°C (36-46°F), followed by up to 24 hrs at 23-27°C (73-81°F)

HOW SUPPLIED
Inj: 1mg/mL [5mL]

WARNINGS/PRECAUTIONS
Spinal/cervical cord compression (SCC) reported. Anaphylaxis and hypersensitivity reactions reported; d/c infusion immediately and initiate appropriate treatment if severe allergic reactions occur. Caution with readministration in patients who have severe allergic reactions. Increased risk of life-threatening complications from hypersensitivity reactions in patients with acute febrile or respiratory illness at the time of infusion; consider patient's clinical status prior to administration and consider delaying the infusion. Sleep apnea is common in MPS IVA patients; evaluate airway patency prior to initiation of treatment.

ADVERSE REACTIONS
Pyrexia, vomiting, headache, nausea, abdominal pain, chills, fatigue.

PATIENT CONSIDERATIONS

Assessment: Assess for respiratory illness, clinical status, airway patency, and pregnancy/nursing status.

Monitoring: Monitor for anaphylaxis/severe allergic reactions, SCC, and other adverse reactions.

Counseling: Counsel that reactions (eg, life-threatening anaphylaxis) related to administration and infusion may occur during treatment. Inform patients of the signs and symptoms of anaphylaxis and to seek immediate medical care should symptoms occur. Inform patients and pregnant/nursing women of the Morquio A Registry and advise that their participation is voluntary and may involve long-term follow-up.

STORAGE: 2- 8°C (36-46°F). Do not freeze or shake. Protect from light. Diluted Sol: Store for up to 24 hrs at 2-8°C (36-46°F) followed by up to 24 hrs at 23-27°C (73-81°F). Complete administration within 48 hrs from the time of dilution.

VIMOVO – esomeprazole magnesium/naproxen

RX

Class: NSAID/proton pump inhibitor (PPI)

NSAIDs may increase risk of serious cardiovascular (CV) thrombotic events, MI, and stroke; increased risk with duration of use and with cardiovascular disease (CVD) or risk factors for CVD. Contraindicated for the treatment of perioperative pain in the setting of CABG surgery. Increased risk of serious GI adverse events (eg, bleeding, ulceration, stomach/intestinal perforation) that can be fatal and occur anytime during use without warning symptoms; elderly patients are at greater risk.

ADULT DOSAGE

Osteoarthritis

1 tab (375mg/20mg or 500mg/20mg) bid

May also be used to decrease the risk of developing NSAID-associated gastric ulcers

Rheumatoid Arthritis

1 tab (375mg/20mg or 500mg/20mg) bid

May also be used to decrease the risk of developing NSAID-associated gastric ulcers

Ankylosing Spondylitis

1 tab (375mg/20mg or 500mg/20mg) bid

May also be used to decrease the risk of developing NSAID-associated gastric ulcers

PEDIATRIC DOSAGE

Pediatric use may not have been established

V

DOSING CONSIDERATIONS

Renal Impairment

CrCl <30mL/min: Not recommended

Hepatic Impairment

Mild to Moderate: Closely monitor and consider possible dose reduction based on naproxen component

Severe: Avoid use

Elderly

Use lowest effective dose

ADMINISTRATION

Oral route

Swallow whole w/ liquid; do not split, chew, crush, or dissolve

Take at least 30 min ac

HOW SUPPLIED

Tab, Delayed-Release: (Naproxen/Esomeprazole): 375mg/20mg, 500mg/20mg

CONTRAINDICATIONS

Known hypersensitivity to naproxen, esomeprazole magnesium, substituted benzimidazoles, or to any excipients. Patients who have experienced asthma, urticaria, or allergic-type reactions after taking aspirin (ASA) or other NSAIDs. Treatment of perioperative pain in the setting of CABG surgery.

WARNINGS/PRECAUTIONS

Use lowest effective dose for the shortest duration possible. Not recommended for initial treatment of acute pain. D/C with active and clinically significant bleeding. Naproxen: May cause HTN or worsen preexisting HTN. Fluid retention and edema reported; caution with HTN, fluid retention, or HF. Caution with history of ulcer disease, GI bleeding, or risk factors for GI bleeding (eg, prolonged NSAID therapy, smoking, poor general health status); d/c if a serious GI event occurs. Caution with history of inflammatory bowel disease (IBD) (ulcerative colitis, Crohn's disease); may exacerbate condition. GI-symptomatic response does not preclude the presence of gastric malignancy. Renal papillary necrosis and other renal injury reported with long-term use. Renal toxicity reported in patients in whom renal prostaglandins have a compensatory role in the maintenance of renal perfusion; increased risk with renal/hepatic impairment, hypovolemia, HF, salt depletion, and in elderly. Not recommended with advanced renal disease or moderate to severe renal impairment; closely monitor renal function and adequately hydrate if therapy must be initiated. Anaphylactic reactions may occur; avoid with ASA triad. May cause serious skin adverse events (eg, Stevens-Johnson syndrome, toxic epidermal necrolysis); d/c at 1st appearance of skin rash or any sign of hypersensitivity. May cause elevated LFTs or severe hepatic reactions; d/c if liver disease or systemic manifestations occur, or if abnormal LFTs persist/worsen. Caution with chronic alcoholic liver disease and other diseases with decreased/abnormal plasma proteins if high doses are administered; dosage adjustment may be required. Anemia may occur; monitor Hgb/Hct if anemia develops with long-term use. May inhibit platelet aggregation and prolong bleeding time. Caution with asthma and avoid with ASA-sensitive asthma. Avoid use starting at 30 weeks gestation; may cause premature closure of ductus arteriosus. May be associated with a reversible delay in ovulation; not recommended in women who have difficulties conceiving, or undergoing investigation of infertility. Not a substitute for corticosteroids or a treatment for corticosteroid insufficiency. May mask signs of inflammation and fever. Lab test interactions may occur. Esomeprazole: Atrophic gastritis reported with long-term use of omeprazole. Acute interstitial nephritis reported; d/c if this develops. Vitamin B12 deficiency caused by hypo/achlorhydria may occur with long-term use (eg, >3 yrs). May increase risk of *Clostridium difficile*-associated diarrhea (CDAD). May increase risk for osteoporosis-related fractures of the hip, wrist, or spine, especially with high-dose (multiple daily doses) and long-term therapy (≥1 yr). Drug-induced decrease in gastric acidity results in enterochromaffin-like cell hyperplasia and increased chromogranin A (CgA) levels, which may interfere with investigations for neuroendocrine tumors; temporarily d/c treatment at least 14 days before assessing CgA levels and consider repeating test if initial CgA levels are high. Hypomagnesemia reported rarely.

ADVERSE REACTIONS

CV thrombotic events, MI, stroke, GI adverse events, flatulence, diarrhea, constipation, URTI, upper abdominal pain, dizziness, headache.

DRUG INTERACTIONS

May enhance methotrexate (MTX) toxicity; use with caution or consider temporary discontinuation during high-dose MTX administration. Naproxen: Avoid with other naproxen-containing products and other NSAIDs. May be administered with low-dose ASA (≤325mg/day); coadministration with ASA is not generally recommended because of potential of increased adverse effects. Risk of renal toxicity when coadministered with diuretics, ACE inhibitors, or angiotensin II receptor antagonists. Diminished antihypertensive effect of ACE inhibitors, angiotensin II receptor antagonists, and β-blockers (eg, propranolol). Delayed absorption with cholestyramine. Caution with cyclosporine; increased risk of nephrotoxicity. Coadministration may decrease efficacy of thiazides and loop (eg, furosemide) diuretics; monitor for signs of renal failure and diuretic efficacy. May increase lithium levels and reduce renal lithium clearance; monitor for lithium toxicity. Concomitant use with anticoagulants (eg, warfarin, dicumarol, heparin) may result in increased risk of bleeding complications; increased risk of GI bleeding with oral corticosteroids, anticoagulants, antiplatelets (including low-dose ASA), alcohol, and SSRIs; monitor carefully. Potential interaction with albumin-bound drugs (eg, sulfonylureas, sulfonamides, hydantoins). Probenecid increases plasma levels and extends plasma $T_{1/2}$ significantly. Esomeprazole: Concomitant use results in reduced concentrations of the active metabolite of clopidogrel and a reduction in platelet inhibition; avoid concomitant use. Caution with digoxin or other drugs that may cause hypomagnesemia (eg, diuretics). May increase levels of tacrolimus. May reduce absorption of drugs where gastric pH is an important determinant of their bioavailability; ketoconazole, atazanavir, iron salts, erlotinib, and mycophenolate mofetil (MMF) absorption can decrease while digoxin absorption can increase during treatment with omeprazole. Caution in transplant patients receiving MMF. Decreased levels of atazanavir and nelfinavir; coadministration not recommended. Monitor for saquinavir toxicity; consider saquinavir dose reduction. Monitor for increases in INR and PT with warfarin. May inhibit metabolism of CYP2C19 substrates; decreased clearance of diazepam. Exposure may be increased with combined CYP2C19 and 3A4 inhibitor (eg, voriconazole). Increased concentrations of cilostazol; consider dose reduction of cilostazol. Decreased levels with CYP2C19 or 3A4 inducers; avoid with St. John's wort or rifampin.

PATIENT CONSIDERATIONS

Assessment: Assess for history of asthma, urticaria, or allergic-type reactions with ASA or other NSAIDs, CVD, risk factors for CVD, HTN, fluid retention, HF, history of ulcer disease, history of/risk factors for GI bleeding, history of IBD, renal/hepatic impairment, coagulation disorders, asthma, decreased/abnormal plasma proteins, tobacco/alcohol use, pregnancy/nursing status, possible drug interactions, or any other conditions where treatment is contraindicated or cautioned. Obtain baseline BP, CBC, and coagulation and chemistry profiles.

Monitoring: Monitor for CV and GI events, active bleeding, anaphylactic reactions, skin reactions, anemia, bone fractures, hypomagnesemia, CDAD, acute interstitial nephritis, vitamin B12 deficiency, and other adverse reactions. Monitor BP, LFTs, renal function, CBC, and coagulation and chemistry profiles. Monitor INR and PT when given with warfarin. Periodically monitor Hgb if initial Hgb ≤10g and receiving long-term therapy. Monitor Mg^{2+} levels prior to and periodically during therapy with prolonged treatment.

Counseling: Instruct to seek medical advice if symptoms of CV events, GI ulceration/bleeding, skin/hypersensitivity reactions, unexplained weight gain or edema, hepatotoxicity, anaphylactic reactions, or hypomagnesemia occur, and for diarrhea that does not improve. Instruct to notify physician if pregnant/nursing, or if patient has a history of asthma or ASA-sensitive asthma. Caution against activities requiring alertness if drowsiness, dizziness, vertigo, or depression occurs.

STORAGE: 25°C (77°F); excursions permitted to 15-30°C (59-86°F). Protect from moisture.

VIMPAT — lacosamide

CV

Class: Sodium channel inactivator

ADULT DOSAGE

Partial Onset Seizures

Monotherapy:
Initial: 100mg bid
Alternative LD: 200mg; follow 12 hrs later by 100mg bid for 1 week
Titrate: Increase by 50mg bid at weekly intervals
Maint: 150-200mg bid

Adjunctive Therapy:
Initial: 50mg bid
Alternative LD: 200mg; follow 12 hrs later by 100mg bid for 1 week
Titrate: Increase by 50mg bid at weekly intervals
Maint: 100-200mg bid
Max Maint: 200mg bid

Use IV when oral administration is temporarily not feasible

PEDIATRIC DOSAGE

Partial Onset Seizures

≥17 Years:

Monotherapy:
Initial: 100mg bid
Alternative LD: 200mg; follow 12 hrs later by 100mg bid for 1 week
Titrate: Increase by 50mg bid at weekly intervals
Maint: 150-200mg bid

Adjunctive Therapy:
Initial: 50mg bid
Alternative LD: 200mg; follow 12 hrs later by 100mg bid for 1 week
Titrate: Increase by 50mg bid at weekly intervals
Maint: 100-200mg bid
Max Maint: 200mg bid

Conversions

Convert from Single Antiepileptic to Lacosamide Monotherapy:
Maintain 150-200mg bid for at least 3 days before initiating gradual withdrawal of the concomitant antiepileptic drug over at least 6 weeks

PO to IV Conversion:
Initial total daily IV dosage regimen should be equivalent to oral dosage regimen

IV to PO Conversion:
At the end of the IV treatment period, switch to oral lacosamide at the equivalent daily dosage and frequency of IV administration

Use IV when oral administration is temporarily not feasible

Conversions

Convert from Single Antiepileptic to Lacosamide Monotherapy:
Maintain 150-200mg bid for at least 3 days before initiating gradual withdrawal of the concomitant antiepileptic drug over at least 6 weeks

PO to IV Conversion:
Initial total daily IV dosage regimen should be equivalent to oral dosage regimen

IV to PO Conversion:
At the end of the IV treatment period, switch to oral lacosamide at the equivalent daily dosage and frequency of IV administration

DOSING CONSIDERATIONS

Concomitant Medications

Strong CYP3A4 and CYP2C9 Inhibitors w/ Renal/Hepatic Impairment: Dose reduction may be necessary

Renal Impairment

Severe (CrCl ≤30mL/min)/ESRD:
Max: 300mg/day
Hemodialysis: Consider dosage supplementation of up to 50% following a 4-hr hemodialysis treatment

Hepatic Impairment

Mild/Moderate:
Max: 300mg/day
Severe: Not recommended

Discontinuation

Gradually withdraw over at least 1 week

ADMINISTRATION

Oral/IV route

Take w/ or w/o food

Sol

Use a calibrated measuring device

Inj

Infuse over 15-60 min; 30-60 min is preferable when a 15 min administration is not required
May administer IV w/o further dilution or mixed w/ compatible diluents
Diluted sol should not be stored for >4 hrs at room temperature

Compatible IV Diluents

NaCl inj 0.9%
D5 inj
Lactated Ringer's inj

HOW SUPPLIED

Inj: 10mg/mL [20mL]; **Sol:** 10mg/mL [200mL, 465mL]; **Tab:** 50mg, 100mg, 150mg, 200mg

WARNINGS/PRECAUTIONS

Administer LD w/ medical supervision due to increased incidence of CNS adverse reactions. May increase risk of suicidal thoughts or behavior. May cause dizziness and ataxia; may impair physical/mental abilities. Dose-dependent prolongations in PR interval reported. Caution w/ known conduction problems (eg, atrioventricular [AV] block, sick sinus syndrome w/o pacemaker), Na^+ channelopathies (eg, Brugada syndrome), or w/ severe cardiac disease (eg, myocardial ischemia, heart failure, structural heart disease); IV infusion may cause bradycardia or AV block. May predispose to atrial arrhythmias, especially in patients w/ diabetic neuropathy and/or cardiovascular disease (CVD). Syncope or loss of consciousness reported in patients w/ diabetic neuropathy and those w/ a history of risk factors for cardiac disease. Multiorgan hypersensitivity reactions (also known as drug reaction w/ eosinophilia and systemic symptoms [DRESS]) may occur; d/c and start alternative treatment if suspected. Caution during dose titration in elderly. (Sol) Contains aspartame, a source of phenylalanine.

ADVERSE REACTIONS

Headache, N/V, diplopia, dizziness, fatigue, blurred vision, somnolence, tremor, nystagmus, vertigo, diarrhea, balance disorder, ataxia, dry mouth, oral hypoesthesia.

DRUG INTERACTIONS

See Dosing Considerations. Increased exposure w/ strong CYP3A4 and CYP2C9 inhibitors in patients w/ renal or hepatic impairment. Caution w/ medications that prolong PR interval (eg, β-blockers, calcium channel blockers); closely monitor if lacosamide is administered as IV route.

PATIENT CONSIDERATIONS

Assessment: Assess for hepatic/renal impairment, history of depression or risk factors for cardiac disease, cardiac conduction problems and/or CVD, diabetic neuropathy, phenylketonuria, pregnancy/nursing status, and possible drug interactions. Obtain baseline ECG in patients w/ known conduction problems, Na^+ channelopathies, on concomitant medications that prolong PR interval, or w/ severe cardiac disease.

Monitoring: Monitor for emergence/worsening of depression, suicidal thoughts or behavior and/or any unusual changes in mood or behavior, dizziness, ataxia, PR interval prolongation, syncope or loss of consciousness, DRESS, and other adverse reactions. Obtain an ECG after titration to steady state in patients w/ known conduction problems, Na^+ channelopathies, on concomitant medications that prolong PR interval, or w/ severe cardiac disease; closely monitor these patients if administering IV. Closely monitor patients w/ hepatic/renal impairment during dose titration.

Counseling: Inform of the benefits/risks of therapy. Instruct to take ud. Counsel patients/caregivers/families about increased risk of suicidal thoughts and behavior and of the need to be alert for emergence or worsening of symptoms of depression, any unusual changes in behavior/mood, or the emergence of suicidal thoughts, behavior, or thoughts about self-harm. Instruct to report any behaviors of concern to physician immediately. Inform that dizziness, double vision, abnormal coordination and balance, and somnolence may occur; advise not to engage in hazardous activities (eg, driving/operating complex machinery) until effects of drug are known. Counsel that therapy is associated w/ ECG changes that may predispose to irregular heartbeat and syncope; if syncope develops, instruct to lay down w/ raised legs and to contact physician. Instruct to d/c if a serious hypersensitivity reaction is suspected and to promptly report any symptoms of liver toxicity. Advise to notify physician if patient becomes pregnant/intends to become pregnant, or is breastfeeding. Encourage patients to enroll in the North American Antiepileptic Drug Pregnancy Registry if they become pregnant.

STORAGE: 20-25°C (68-77°F); excursions permitted between 15-30°C (59-86°F). (Inj/Sol) Do not freeze. (Inj) Discard any unused portion. (Sol) Discard any unused portion after 7 weeks of 1st opening bottle.

VIREAD – tenofovir disoproxil fumarate

RX

Class: Nucleotide analogue reverse transcriptase inhibitor

Lactic acidosis and severe hepatomegaly w/ steatosis, including fatal cases, reported w/ the use of nucleoside analogues in combination w/ other antiretrovirals. Severe acute exacerbations of hepatitis reported in hepatitis B virus (HBV)-infected patients who have discontinued therapy; closely monitor hepatic function w/ both clinical and lab follow-up for at least several months. If appropriate, resumption of antihepatitis B therapy may be warranted.

ADULT DOSAGE

HIV-1 Infection

Combination w/ Other Antiretrovirals:
≥35kg:
Tab: 300mg qd
Oral Powder: 7.5 scoops qd

Chronic Hepatitis B

≥35kg:
Tab: 300mg qd
Oral Powder: 7.5 scoops qd

PEDIATRIC DOSAGE

HIV-1 Infection

Combination w/ Other Antiretrovirals:
≥2 Years:
Recommended Dose: 8mg/kg qd as tabs or oral powder
Max: 300mg qd
Tab:
17-<22kg: 150mg qd
22-<28kg: 200mg qd
28-<35kg: 250mg qd
≥35kg: 300mg qd
Oral Powder:
Refer to PI for dosing recommendations based on body weight
≥12 Years:
≥35kg:
Tab: 300mg qd
Oral Powder: 7.5 scoops qd

Chronic Hepatitis B

≥12 Years:
Tab: 300mg qd
Oral Powder: 7.5 scoops qd

DOSING CONSIDERATIONS

Renal Impairment

CrCl ≥50mL/min: 300mg tab q24h
CrCl 30-49mL/min: 300mg tab q48h
CrCl 10-29mL/min: 300mg tab q72-96h
Hemodialysis: 300mg tab every 7 days or after a total of approx 12 hrs of dialysis; administer following completion of dialysis

ADMINISTRATION

Oral route

Take tabs w/o regard to food

Oral Powder

Measure only w/ the supplied dosing scoop
One level scoop contains 40mg of tenofovir disoproxil fumarate
Mix w/ 2-4 oz of soft food not requiring chewing (eg, applesauce, baby food, yogurt) and administer entire mixture immediately
Do not administer in a liquid

HOW SUPPLIED

Powder: 40mg/g [60g]; **Tab:** 150mg, 200mg, 250mg, 300mg

WARNINGS/PRECAUTIONS

Obesity and prolonged nucleoside exposure may be risk factors for lactic acidosis and severe hepatomegaly w/ steatosis. Caution w/ known risk factors for liver disease. D/C if findings suggestive of lactic acidosis or pronounced hepatotoxicity develop. Renal impairment (eg, acute renal failure, Fanconi syndrome) reported; assess CrCl prior to initiating and as clinically appropriate during therapy. In patients at risk of renal dysfunction, including patients who have previously experienced renal events while receiving adefovir dipivoxil, assess CrCl, serum phosphorus (P), urine glucose, and urine protein prior to initiation and periodically during therapy. Use only in HIV-1 and HBV coinfected patients as part of an appropriate antiretroviral combination regimen. Before initiating therapy, offer HIV-1 antibody testing to all HBV-infected patients and test all patients w/ HIV-1 for presence of chronic hepatitis B. Decreased bone mineral density (BMD) and increased biochemical markers of bone metabolism reported; consider assessment of BMD for patients w/ history of pathologic bone fracture or other risk factors for osteoporosis or bone loss. Osteomalacia associated w/ proximal renal tubulopathy reported; consider hypophosphatemia and osteomalacia secondary to proximal renal tubulopathy in patients at risk of renal dysfunction who present w/ persistent or worsening bone or muscle symptoms. Redistribution/accumulation of body fat and immune reconstitution syndrome reported. Autoimmune disorders (eg, Graves' disease, polymyositis, Guillain-Barre syndrome) reported in the setting of immune reconstitution and can occur many months after initiation of treatment. Early virological failure and high rates of resistance substitutions reported w/ certain regimens that only contain 3 nucleoside reverse transcriptase inhibitors; use triple nucleoside regimens w/ caution. Caution in elderly.

ADVERSE REACTIONS

Lactic acidosis, hepatomegaly w/ steatosis, N/V, diarrhea, depression, asthenia, headache, pain, rash, abdominal pain, insomnia, pruritus, dizziness, pyrexia.

DRUG INTERACTIONS

Avoid w/ concurrent or recent use of nephrotoxic agents (eg, high-dose or multiple NSAIDs). Do not coadminister w/ tenofovir disoproxil fumarate (TDF)-containing products or w/ adefovir dipivoxil. May increase levels of didanosine; d/c didanosine if didanosine-associated adverse reactions develop. Decreases levels of atazanavir; do not coadminister w/ atazanavir w/o ritonavir. Lopinavir/ritonavir, atazanavir w/ ritonavir, and darunavir w/ ritonavir may increase levels; d/c treatment if TDF-associated adverse reactions develop. P-gp and breast cancer resistance protein transporter inhibitors may increase absorption. Coadministration w/ drugs that reduce renal function or compete for active tubular secretion (eg, cidofovir, acyclovir, valacyclovir, ganciclovir, valganciclovir, aminoglycosides [eg, gentamicin], high-dose or multiple NSAIDs) may increase levels of tenofovir and/or the levels of other renally eliminated drugs. Refer to PI for dosing modifications when used w/ certain concomitant therapies.

PATIENT CONSIDERATIONS

Assessment: Assess for risk factors for lactic acidosis or liver disease, renal dysfunction, pregnancy/nursing status, and possible drug interactions. In patients at risk of renal dysfunction, assess CrCl, serum P, urine glucose, and urine protein. Test for HIV-1 antibody (in HBV-infected patients) and presence of chronic hepatitis B (in patients w/ HIV-1). Assess BMD in patients w/ history of pathologic bone fracture or other risk factors for osteoporosis or bone loss.

Monitoring: Monitor for signs/symptoms of lactic acidosis, hepatomegaly w/ steatosis, hepatotoxicity, renal impairment, bone effects, redistribution/accumulation of body fat, immune reconstitution syndrome (eg, opportunistic infections), autoimmune disorders, and other adverse reactions. Closely monitor hepatic function w/ both clinical and lab follow-up for at least several months in HBV-infected patients who have discontinued therapy. In patients at risk of renal dysfunction, monitor CrCl, serum P, urine glucose, and urine protein periodically. Periodically monitor weight in pediatric patients to guide dose adjustment.

Counseling: Inform about risks and benefits of therapy. Inform that therapy is not a cure for HIV-1 and patients may continue to experience illness associated w/ HIV-1 infection (eg, opportunistic infections). Instruct to avoid doing things that can spread HIV or HBV to others (eg, sharing of needles/inj equipment or personal items that can have blood/body fluids on them). Advise to always practice safer sex by using latex or polyurethane condoms. Instruct not to breastfeed. Instruct not to d/c w/o 1st informing physician. Counsel about the importance of adhering to regular dosing schedule and to avoid missing doses.

STORAGE: 25°C (77°F); excursions permitted to 15-30°C (59-86°F).

VITEKTA – elvitegravir

RX

Class: HIV-integrase strand transfer inhibitor

ADULT DOSAGE

HIV-1 Infection

In combination w/ an HIV protease inhibitor coadministered w/ ritonavir (RTV) and other antiretroviral drug(s) in treatment-experienced patients

85mg Dose:

85mg qd + atazanavir 300mg qd + RTV 100mg qd

or

85mg qd + lopinavir 400mg bid + RTV 100mg bid

150mg Dose:

150mg qd + darunavir 600mg bid + RTV 100mg bid

or

150mg qd + fosamprenavir 700mg bid + RTV 100mg bid

or

150mg qd + tipranavir 500mg bid + RTV 200mg bid

PEDIATRIC DOSAGE

Pediatric use may not have been established

DOSING CONSIDERATIONS

Hepatic Impairment

Severe: Not recommended for use

ADMINISTRATION

Oral route

Take w/ food.

HOW SUPPLIED

Tab: 85mg, 150mg

CONTRAINDICATIONS

Refer to the individual monographs for coadministered protease inhibitor and RTV.

WARNINGS/PRECAUTIONS

Immune reconstitution syndrome reported. Autoimmune disorders (eg, Graves' disease, polymyositis, Guillain-Barre syndrome) reported in the setting of immune reconstitution and can occur many months after initiation of treatment. Caution in elderly.

ADVERSE REACTIONS

Diarrhea, nausea, headache, hyperbilirubinemia, hematuria, increased serum amylase/creatine kinase/GGT, hypercholesterolemia, hypertriglyceridemia, hyperglycemia, glucosuria, neutropenia.

DRUG INTERACTIONS

Coadministration w/ HIV-1 protease inhibitors other than RTV, atazanavir, lopinavir, darunavir, fosamprenavir, or tipranavir is not recommended. Use w/ elvitegravir-containing drugs (eg, Stribild) is not recommended. Use in combination w/ a protease inhibitor and cobicistat is not recommended; may result in suboptimal levels of elvitegravir and/or the protease inhibitor, leading to loss of therapeutic effect and development of resistance. Coadministration w/ efavirenz, nevirapine, St. John's wort, rifampin, rifapentine, phenobarbital, phenytoin, carbamazepine, or oxcarbazepine is not recommended; may decrease elvitegravir levels. Coadministration w/ boceprevir is not recommended; may reduce levels of boceprevir and may alter levels of HIV protease inhibitors. CYP3A inducers may increase the clearance of elvitegravir, as well as RTV; may result in decreased plasma levels of elvitegravir and/or a concomitantly administered protease inhibitor and lead to loss of therapeutic effect and to possible resistance. Atazanavir/RTV, lopinavir/RTV, and ketoconazole may increase elvitegravir levels. Administer didanosine at least 1 hr before or 2 hrs after elvitegravir. Antacids may decrease levels; separate elvitegravir and antacid administration by at least 2 hrs. Coadministration w/ systemic dexamethasone may decrease levels; consider alternative corticosteroids. Rifabutin or bosentan may decrease levels. May increase levels of ketoconazole, bosentan, rifabutin, or 25-O-desacetylrifabutin. May increase norgestimate and decrease ethinyl estradiol levels; alternative methods of nonhormonal contraception are recommended. May increase levels of buprenorphine and norbuprenorphine and may decrease levels of naloxone and methadone. Closely monitor for sedation and cognitive effects when coadministered w/ buprenorphine/naloxone. Refer to PI for further information on drug interactions, including dose modifications required when used w/ certain concomitant therapies.

PATIENT CONSIDERATIONS

Assessment: Assess for severe hepatic impairment, pregnancy/nursing status, and for possible drug interactions.

Monitoring: Monitor for signs/symptoms of immune reconstitution syndrome, autoimmune disorders, and for other adverse reactions.

Counseling: Advise patients to remain under the care of a healthcare provider during therapy. Inform that drug is not a cure for HIV-1 infection and continuous therapy is necessary to control HIV-1 infection and decrease HIV-related illnesses. Advise to continue to practice safer sex, to use latex or polyurethane condoms, and to not reuse/share needles. Instruct to take ud, on a regular dosing schedule w/ food, and to avoid missing doses. Inform that therapy may interact w/ many drugs; advise to notify physician if using any other prescription or nonprescription medication or herbal product (eg, St. John's wort). Advise to inform physician immediately if any symptoms of infection develop.

STORAGE: Room temperature <30°C (86°F).

VIVITROL – naltrexone

RX

Class: Opioid antagonist

ADULT DOSAGE

Alcohol Dependence

Treatment of Alcohol Dependence in Patients Who are Able to Abstain from Alcohol in an Outpatient Setting Prior to Initiation of Therapy:

380mg IM every 4 weeks or once a month

Prior to initiating therapy, an opioid-free duration of a minimum of 7-10 days is recommended

Opioid Dependence

Prevention of Relapse to Opioid Dependence, Following Opioid Detoxification:

380mg IM every 4 weeks or once a month

Prior to initiating therapy, an opioid-free duration of a minimum of 7-10 days is recommended

Conversions

Switching from Buprenorphine, Buprenorphine/Naloxone, or Methadone:

Be prepared to manage withdrawal symptomatically w/ nonopioid medications

PEDIATRIC DOSAGE

Pediatric use may not have been established

V

ADMINISTRATION

IM route

Administer as IM gluteal inj, alternating buttocks for each subsequent inj

Must be suspended only in the diluent supplied in the carton and must be administered only w/ 1 of the administration needles supplied in the carton; do not substitute any other components for the components of the carton

For patients w/ a larger amount of subcutaneous tissue overlying the gluteal muscle, may utilize the

supplied 2-inch needle to help ensure that the injectate reaches the IM mass
For very lean patients, the 1.5-inch needle may be appropriate to prevent the needle contacting the periosteum
Either needle may be used for patients w/ average body habitus
Prior to preparation, allow drug to reach room temperature (approx 45 min)
Refer to PI for further preparation and administration instructions

HOW SUPPLIED

Inj, Extended-Release: 380mg

CONTRAINDICATIONS

Concomitant opioid analgesics; current physiologic opioid dependence; acute opioid withdrawal; failure of naloxone challenge test or positive urine screen for opioids; previous hypersensitivity to naltrexone, polylactide-co-glycolide, carboxymethylcellulose, or any other components of the diluent.

WARNINGS/PRECAUTIONS

Patients may have reduced tolerance to opioids after opioid detoxification; may result in potentially life-threatening opioid intoxication with use of previously tolerated opioid doses. Potential risk to patients attempting to overcome the antagonism by taking opioids; may lead to life-threatening opioid intoxication or fatal overdose. Inj-site reactions reported; inadvertent SQ inj may increase likelihood of severe inj-site reactions. Withdrawal syndrome, severe enough to require hospitalization, may occur when withdrawal is precipitated abruptly by the administration of an opioid antagonist to an opioid-dependent patient. Opioid-dependent patients, including those being treated for alcohol dependence, should be opioid-free before starting treatment to reduce risk of either precipitated withdrawal in patients dependent on opioids or exacerbation of a preexisting subclinical withdrawal syndrome; an opioid-free interval of a minimum of 7-10 days is recommended for patients previously dependent on short-acting opioids. May experience severe manifestations of precipitated withdrawal when being switched from opioid agonist to opioid antagonist therapy; patients transitioning from buprenorphine or methadone may be vulnerable to precipitation of withdrawal symptoms for as long as 2 weeks. A naloxone challenge test may be helpful to determine if patient is opioid-free; however, precipitated withdrawal may occur despite having negative urine toxicology screen or tolerating a naloxone challenge test. Cases of hepatitis, clinically significant liver dysfunction, and transient, asymptomatic hepatic transaminase elevations reported; d/c in the event of symptoms and/or signs of acute hepatitis. Depression and suicidality reported. In emergency situations, suggested plan for pain management is regional analgesia or use of nonopioid analgesics. If opioid therapy is required, monitor continuously in an anesthesia care setting. Cases of eosinophilic pneumonia and hypersensitivity reactions, including anaphylaxis, reported. As with any IM inj, caution with thrombocytopenia or any coagulation disorder (eg, hemophilia, severe hepatic failure). Does not eliminate or diminish alcohol withdrawal symptoms. May cross-react with certain immunoassay methods for the detection of drugs of abuse in urine. Caution with moderate to severe renal impairment.

ADVERSE REACTIONS

N/V, diarrhea, insomnia, depression, inj-site reactions, somnolence, anorexia, muscle cramps, dizziness, syncope, appetite disorder, hepatic enzyme abnormalities, nasopharyngitis, toothache, headache.

DRUG INTERACTIONS

See Contraindications. Antagonizes effects of opioid-containing medicines (eg, cough and cold remedies, antidiarrheals, opioid analgesics).

PATIENT CONSIDERATIONS

Assessment: Assess for opioid use, acute opioid withdrawal, thrombocytopenia, coagulation disorders, renal impairment, any other conditions where treatment is contraindicated or cautioned, pregnancy/nursing status, and possible drug interactions. Assess patients, including patients treated for alcohol dependence, for underlying opioid dependence, and for any recent use of opioids. Assess body habitus to assure that needle length is adequate.

Monitoring: Monitor for opioid intoxication/overdose, severe inj-site reactions, precipitation of opioid withdrawal, signs/symptoms of acute hepatitis, depression, suicidality, hypersensitivity reactions, and other adverse reactions.

Counseling: Advise that if they previously used opioids, they may be more sensitive to lower doses of opioids and at risk of accidental overdose if they use opioids when their next dose is due, if they miss a dose, or after treatment is discontinued. Advise that patients will not perceive any effect if they attempt to self-administer heroin or any other opioid drug in small doses while on therapy. Inform that administration of large doses of heroin or any other opioid to try to bypass the blockade may lead to serious injury, coma, or death. Inform that patient may not experience the expected effects from opioid-containing analgesic, antidiarrheal, or antitussive medications. Advise that inj-site reactions may occur and instruct to seek medical attention for worsening skin reactions. Instruct to be off all opioids for a minimum of 7-10 days before starting therapy in order to avoid precipitation of opioid withdrawal. Advise not to take therapy if they have any symptoms of opioid withdrawal. Advise all patients, including those with alcohol dependence, to notify physician of any recent use of opioids or any history of opioid dependence before starting therapy. Inform that drug may cause liver injury; instruct to immediately notify physician if symptoms and/or signs of liver disease develop. Inform the patient, family members, and caregivers that the patient may experience depression while taking therapy and to contact physician if the patient becomes depressed or symptoms of depression are experienced. Instruct to carry documentation to alert medical personnel to therapy. Advise that drug may cause an allergic pneumonia; instruct to immediately notify physician if signs and symptoms of pneumonia develop. Inform that drug may cause nausea, which tends to subside within a few days post-inj. Advise that they may also experience tiredness, headache, vomiting, decreased appetite, painful joints, and muscle cramps. Advise that therapy has been shown to treat alcohol and opioid dependence only when used as part of a treatment program that includes counseling and support. Advise that dizziness may occur; instruct to avoid driving or operating heavy machinery. Advise to notify physician if pregnant or intending to become pregnant during treatment, breastfeeding, or experiencing unusual or significant side effects while on therapy.

STORAGE: 2-8°C (36-46°F). Do not freeze. Can be stored at ≤25°C (77°F) for no more than 7 days prior administration.

VIVLODEX – meloxicam

RX

Class: NSAID

NSAIDs cause an increased risk of serious cardiovascular (CV) thrombotic events, including MI and stroke; risk may occur early in treatment and increase w/ duration of use. Contraindicated in the setting of CABG surgery. NSAIDs also cause an increased risk of serious GI adverse events, including bleeding, ulceration, and perforation of the stomach or intestines. Elderly patients and patients w/ a prior history of peptic ulcer disease and/or GI bleeding are at greater risk for serious GI events.

ADULT DOSAGE

Osteoarthritis

Initial: 5mg qd
Titrate: May increase to 10mg
Max: 10mg/day

PEDIATRIC DOSAGE

Pediatric use may not have been established

DOSING CONSIDERATIONS

Renal Impairment

Hemodialysis:
Max: 5mg/day

Other Important Considerations

Not interchangeable w/ other formulations of oral meloxicam even if the total mg strength is the same. Do not substitute similar dose strengths of other meloxicam products

ADMINISTRATION

Oral route

HOW SUPPLIED

Cap: 5mg, 10mg

CONTRAINDICATIONS

Known hypersensitivity (eg, anaphylactic reactions and serious skin reactions) to meloxicam or any components of this product, history of asthma, urticaria, or other allergic-type reactions after taking aspirin (ASA) or other NSAIDs, in the setting of CABG surgery.

WARNINGS/PRECAUTIONS

Use the lowest effective dose for the shortest duration consistent w/ treatment goals. Increased CV thrombotic risk w/ higher doses reported. Avoid in patients w/ a recent MI unless benefits outweigh the risks; if used, monitor patients for signs of cardiac ischemia. Increased risk of GI bleeding w/ smoking, use of alcohol, poor general health status, advanced liver disease, and/or coagulopathy. If a serious GI adverse event is suspected, promptly initiate evaluation and treatment, and d/c until a serious GI adverse event is ruled out. May cause elevations of ALT/AST; d/c immediately and perform clinical evaluation if signs and symptoms consistent w/ liver disease develop or if systemic manifestations occur. Rare cases of severe hepatic injury, including fulminant hepatitis, liver necrosis, and hepatic failure reported. Use only if benefits outweigh risks w/ severe hepatic impairment. May lead to new onset or worsening of preexisting HTN. Fluid retention and edema reported; avoid use in patients w/ severe heart failure (HF) unless benefits outweigh risk. Long-term administration may cause renal papillary necrosis and other renal injury; increased risk w/ renal/hepatic impairment, dehydration, hypovolemia, HF, and the elderly. Avoid use in patients w/ advanced renal disease unless benefits outweigh risk. Correct volume status in dehydrated or hypovolemic patients prior to initiating therapy. May increase serum potassium concentration. May cause anaphylactic reactions and serious skin adverse reactions (eg, exfoliative dermatitis, Stevens-Johnson Syndrome, and toxic epidermal necrolysis); d/c use at 1st appearance of skin rash or any other sign of hypersensitivity. Monitor for changes in signs and symptoms of asthma when used in patients w/ preexisting asthma (w/o known ASA hypersensitivity). May cause premature closure of the fetal ductus arteriosus; avoid use in pregnant women starting at 30 weeks of gestation (3rd trimester). May cause anemia. The pharmacological activity in reducing inflammation, and possibly fever, may diminish the utility of diagnostic signs in detecting infections.

ADVERSE REACTIONS
Diarrhea, nausea, abdominal discomfort.

DRUG INTERACTIONS
Increased risk of bleeding w/ anticoagulants and drugs that interfere w/ serotonin reuptake; monitor patients w/ concomitant use of anticoagulants (eg, warfarin), antiplatelet agents (eg, aspirin), SSRIs, and SNRIs. Concomitant use w/ analgesic doses of aspirin is not generally recommended. In the setting of concomitant use of low-dose ASA for cardiac prophylaxis, monitor patients more closely for evidence of GI bleeding. Antihypertensive effect of ACE inhibitors, ARBs, or β-blockers (including propranolol) may be diminished. Coadministration w/ ACE inhibitors or ARBs may result in deterioration of renal function, including possible acute renal failure, in patients who are elderly, volume-depleted (including those on diuretic therapy), or have renal impairment. The natriuretic effect of loop diuretics (eg, furosemide) and thiazide diuretics may be reduced; monitor for efficacy and signs of worsening renal function. May increase the serum concentration and prolong the $T_{1/2}$ of digoxin; monitor serum digoxin levels. May elevate plasma lithium levels and reduce renal lithium clearance; monitor for signs of lithium toxicity. May increase the risk for methotrexate toxicity and increase cyclosporine's nephrotoxicity. Use w/ other NSAIDs or salicylates (eg, diflunisal, salsalate) increases the risk of GI toxicity; concomitant use is not recommended. May increase the risk of pemetrexed-associated myelosuppression, renal, and GI toxicity; monitor for these effects in patients w/ renal impairment whose CrCl ranges from 45-79mL/min. Interrupt meloxicam dosing for at least 5 days before, the day of, and 2 days following pemetrexed administration.

PATIENT CONSIDERATIONS

Assessment: Assess for cardiovascular disease (CVD), risk factors for CVD, history of peptic ulcer disease and/or GI bleeding, hepatic/renal dysfunction, coagulopathy, preexisting HTN, severe HF, dehydration/hypovolemia, asthma, any other conditions where treatment is contraindicated or cautioned, pregnancy/nursing status, and possible drug interactions. Obtain baseline BP.

Monitoring: Monitor for CV thrombotic events, GI events, hepatotoxicity, HTN, HF and edema, renal toxicity, hyperkalemia, anaphylactic/skin reactions, exacerbation of ASA-sensitive asthma, and premature closure of fetal ductus arteriosus. Monitor Hgb or Hct if signs or symptoms of anemia develop. Consider periodic monitoring w/ a CBC and a chemistry profile w/ long-term treatment.

Counseling: Advise to be alert for the symptoms of CV thrombotic events and to report any of these symptoms to the healthcare provider immediately. Advise to report symptoms of GI ulcerations and bleeding to the healthcare provider. In the setting of concomitant use of low-dose ASA for cardiac prophylaxis, inform of the increased risk for and the signs and symptoms of GI bleeding. Inform of the warning signs and symptoms of hepatotoxicity and instruct to d/c therapy and seek immediate medical therapy if these occur. Advise to be alert for the symptoms of CHF and to contact healthcare provider if such symptoms occur. Inform of the signs of an anaphylactic reaction and instruct to seek immediate emergency help if these occur. Advise to d/c therapy immediately if any type of rash develops and to contact healthcare provider as soon as possible. Instruct pregnant women to avoid use of meloxicam and other NSAIDs starting at 30 weeks gestation because of the risk of the premature closing of the fetal ductus arteriosus. Instruct to avoid concomitant use of NSAIDs and low-dose ASA unless directed by healthcare provider.

STORAGE: 25°C (77°F); excursions permitted to 15-30°C (59-86°F). Protect from moisture.

VOGELXO – testosterone

Class: Androgen

CIII

V

Virilization reported in children secondarily exposed to testosterone gel. Children should avoid contact w/ unwashed or unclothed application sites in men using testosterone gel. Advise patients to strictly adhere to recommended instructions for use.

ADULT DOSAGE

Testosterone Replacement Therapy

Congenital/Acquired Primary Hypogonadism or Hypogonadotropic Hypogonadism in Males:

Initial: 50mg (1 tube, 1 pkt, or 4 pump

PEDIATRIC DOSAGE

Pediatric use may not have been established

actuations) applied topically qd at approx the same time each day to clean, dry intact skin of shoulders and/or upper arms
Titrate: Measure am pre-dose serum testosterone concentrations approx 14 days after initiation of therapy; if concentration is <300-1000ng/dL, may increase to 100mg (2 tubes, 2 pkts, or 8 pump actuations) qd
Max: 100mg qd

ADMINISTRATION

Topical route
The prescribed amount should be delivered directly into the palm of the hand and immediately applied to the shoulders and/or upper arms (area of application should be limited to the area that will be covered by a short sleeve t-shirt)
Do not apply to the genitals or to the abdomen
Allow application site to dry completely prior to dressing
Wash hands thoroughly w/ soap and water after application
In order to prevent transfer to another person, clothing should be worn to cover the application sites; if direct skin-to-skin contact of the application site(s) w/ another person is anticipated, the application sites must be washed thoroughly w/ soap and water
Avoid swimming, showering, or washing the administration site for a minimum of 2 hrs after application
Refer to PI for further application instructions

Unit-Dose Tubes or Pkts
50mg: Apply 1 unit-dose tube or pkt to 1 upper arm and shoulder
100mg: Apply 1 unit-dose tube or pkt to 1 upper arm and shoulder and then apply 1 unit-dose tube or pkt to the opposite upper arm and shoulder

Multidose Pump
Instruct patients to prime the pump before using it for the 1st time by fully depressing the pump mechanism (actuation) 3X and discard this portion of the product to assure precise dose delivery
After the priming procedure, patients should completely depress the pump 1 time (actuation) for every 12.5mg of testosterone required to achieve the daily prescribed dosage
50mg: Apply 4 pump actuations to 1 upper arm and shoulder
100mg: Apply 4 pump actuations to 1 upper arm and shoulder and then apply 4 pump actuations to the opposite upper arm and shoulder

HOW SUPPLIED

Gel: 50mg [5g, tube, pkt], 12.5mg/actuation [75g, pump]

CONTRAINDICATIONS

Men w/ breast carcinoma or known/suspected prostate carcinoma; women who are or may become pregnant, or are breastfeeding.

WARNINGS/PRECAUTIONS

Topical testosterone products may have different doses, strengths, or application instructions that may result in different systemic exposure. Men w/ BPH are at an increased risk for worsening of signs and symptoms of BPH. May increase risk for prostate cancer. Increases in Hct/RBC mass may require lowering or discontinuation of therapy; may increase risk of thromboembolic events. If Hct becomes elevated, d/c therapy until Hct decreases to an acceptable concentration. Venous thromboembolic events (VTEs), including deep vein thrombosis and pulmonary embolism, reported; d/c treatment and initiate appropriate workup and management if a VTE is suspected. Increased risk of major adverse cardiovascular events (MACE) reported. Not indicated for use in women. Suppression of spermatogenesis may occur w/ large doses. Monitor for signs/symptoms of hepatic dysfunction; if these occur, promptly d/c therapy while the cause is evaluated. May promote retention of Na^+ and water. Edema w/ or w/o CHF in patients w/ preexisting cardiac/renal/hepatic disease may occur; in addition to discontinuation of therapy, diuretic therapy may be required. Gynecomastia may develop and persist. May potentiate sleep apnea. Changes in serum lipid profile may occur. Caution in cancer patients at risk of hypercalcemia (and associated hypercalciuria); regularly monitor serum Ca^{2+} concentrations. May decrease concentrations of thyroxine-binding globulins, resulting in decreased total T4 serum concentrations and increased resin uptake of T3 and T4. Flammable; avoid fire, flame, or smoking until the gel has dried.

ADVERSE REACTIONS

Application-site reactions.

DRUG INTERACTIONS

Changes in insulin sensitivity or glycemic control may occur; may decrease blood glucose, which may necessitate a decrease in the dose of antidiabetic medication. Changes in anticoagulant activity may occur; frequently monitor INR and PT in patients taking warfarin, especially at the initiation and termination of androgen therapy. Concurrent use w/ corticosteroids may result in increased fluid retention; caution in patients w/ cardiac/renal/hepatic disease.

PATIENT CONSIDERATIONS

Assessment: Assess for breast/prostate cancer, BPH, cardiac/renal/hepatic disease, any other conditions where treatment is contraindicated or cautioned, and possible drug interactions. Check Hct prior to therapy. Confirm diagnosis of hypogonadism by measuring testosterone levels in am on at least 2 separate days prior to initiation.

Monitoring: Monitor for worsening signs/symptoms of BPH, prostate cancer, VTE, hepatic dysfunction, Na^+/water retention, gynecomastia, sleep apnea, thyroxin-binding globulin, and other adverse reactions. Monitor morning pre-dose serum testosterone concentrations approx 14 days after initiation of therapy. Monitor lipid profile periodically, particularly after starting therapy and after any dose increases. Regularly monitor serum Ca^{2+} concentrations in cancer patients at risk of hypercalcemia. Reevaluate Hct 3-6 months after starting therapy, then annually. Frequently monitor INR and PT in patients taking warfarin, especially at the initiation and termination of androgen therapy.

Counseling: Inform of the reported signs/symptoms of secondary exposure, and advise to notify physician of the possibility of secondary exposure. Inform that children and women should avoid contact w/ unwashed or unclothed application sites of men using the gel. Instruct to apply ud and strictly adhere to administration instructions to minimize the potential for secondary exposure. Inform that treatment may lead to adverse reactions (eg, changes in urinary habits, breathing disturbances, too frequent or persistent erections of the penis, N/V, changes in skin color, ankle swelling). Inform that drug is flammable; instruct to avoid fire, flame, or smoking until the gel has dried. Instruct to adhere to all recommended monitoring and report any changes in state of health (eg, changes in urinary habits, breathing, sleep, mood). Advise not to share the medication w/ anyone. Instruct to wait 2 hrs before washing or swimming following application. Inform of the possible risk of MACE when deciding whether to use or continue to use drug.

STORAGE: 20-25°C (68-77°F); excursions permitted to 15-30°C (59-86°F).

VOLTAREN GEL — diclofenac sodium

RX

Class: NSAID

NSAIDs may cause an increased risk of serious cardiovascular (CV) thrombotic events, MI, and stroke, which can be fatal; risk may increase w/ duration of use. Patients w/ CV disease (CVD) or risk factors for CVD may be at greater risk. Contraindicated for the treatment of perioperative pain in the setting of CABG surgery. NSAIDs can cause an increased risk of serious GI adverse events (eg, bleeding, ulceration, perforation of the stomach/intestines), which can be fatal and can occur at any time during use and w/o warning symptoms; elderly patients are at greater risk.

ADULT DOSAGE

Osteoarthritis

Joint Pain:

Lower Extremities:

Apply 4g to affected foot, knee, or ankle qid
Max: 16g/day to any single joint

Upper Extremities:

Apply 2g to affected hand, elbow, or wrist qid
Max: 8g/day to any single joint

Total dose should not exceed 32g/day over all affected joints

PEDIATRIC DOSAGE

Pediatric use may not have been established

ADMINISTRATION

Topical route

Measure onto enclosed dosing card to appropriate 2g or 4g line.
The dosing card containing the gel can be used to apply the gel; the hands should then be used to gently rub the gel into the skin.
After using the dosing card, hold w/ fingertips, rinse, and dry; if treatment site is the hands, wait ≥1 hr to wash hands.
Avoid showering or bathing for ≥1 hr after application.
Do not apply to open wounds or get in contact w/ eyes and mucous membranes.
Do not expose treated joint(s) to sunlight or apply external heat and/or occlusive dressings.
Avoid concomitant use on treated skin w/ other topical products (eg, sunscreens, cosmetics, lotions).
Avoid wearing clothing or gloves for ≥10 min after application.

HOW SUPPLIED

Gel: 1% [100g]

CONTRAINDICATIONS

Known hypersensitivity to diclofenac; history of asthma, urticaria, or allergic-type reactions to aspirin (ASA) or other NSAIDs; setting of CABG surgery.

WARNINGS/PRECAUTIONS

Not evaluated for use on spine, hip, or shoulder. Caution in patients w/ prior history of ulcer or GI bleeding. Use lowest effective dose for the shortest possible duration. Promptly initiate additional evaluation and treatment if serious GI adverse event is suspected; consider alternate therapies for high-risk patients. May cause elevations of LFTs; d/c if liver disease develops, systemic manifestations occur, or abnormal liver tests persist or worsen. May lead to onset of new HTN or worsening of preexisting HTN. Fluid retention and edema reported; caution w/ heart failure (HF). Renal papillary necrosis and other renal injury reported after long-term use. Not recommended for use w/ advanced renal disease; if therapy must be initiated, monitor renal function. D/C if renal tests persist or worsen. Anaphylactoid reactions may occur. Avoid w/ ASA triad. May cause serious skin adverse events (eg, exfoliative dermatitis, Stevens-Johnson syndrome, toxic epidermal necrolysis); d/c at 1st appearance of skin rash or any other signs of hypersensitivity. Avoid in late pregnancy; may cause premature closure of ductus arteriosus. Not a substitute for corticosteroids and not for treatment of corticosteroid insufficiency. Anemia may occur; monitor Hgb/Hct if signs or symptoms of anemia develop w/ long-term use. May inhibit platelet aggregation and prolong bleeding time. Caution w/ asthma. May diminish utility of diagnostic signs (eg, inflammation, fever) in detecting infectious complications of presumed noninfectious, painful conditions. Caution in elderly.

ADVERSE REACTIONS

Application-site reactions.

DRUG INTERACTIONS

May diminish the antihypertensive effect of ACE inhibitors. Increased risk of renal toxicity w/ diuretics and ACE inhibitors. Not recommended w/ ASA due to potential for increased adverse effects. May reduce the natriuretic effect of thiazide and loop diuretics. May increase lithium levels; monitor for lithium toxicity. May enhance methotrexate toxicity and cyclosporine nephrotoxicity; caution when coadministering. Synergistic effect on GI bleeding w/ warfarin; closely monitor. Increased risk of GI bleeding w/ oral corticosteroids, anticoagulants, smoking, and alcohol use. Avoid concomitant use w/ other topical products (eg, topical medications, sunscreens, lotions, moisturizers, and cosmetics) on the same skin site; may alter tolerability and absorption. Caution w/ concomitant hepatotoxic drugs (eg, antibiotics, antiepileptics).

PATIENT CONSIDERATIONS

Assessment: Assess for history of asthma, urticaria, or allergic-type reactions w/ ASA or other NSAIDs, ASA triad, HTN, recent MI, severe HF, history of ulcer disease or GI bleeding, coagulation disorders, renal/hepatic impairment, pregnancy/nursing status, any other conditions where treatment is contraindicated or cautioned, and possible drug interactions. Obtain baseline BP.

Monitoring: Monitor for GI bleeding/ulceration/perforation, CV thrombotic events, HTN, fluid retention, edema, serious skin reactions, anaphylactoid reactions, and other adverse reactions. Monitor BP, CBC, bleeding time, LFTs, renal function, and chemistry profile periodically.

Counseling: Instruct to avoid contact w/ eyes and mucous membranes; instruct that if contact occurs, to wash w/ water or saline, and if irritation persists for >1 hr, to call physician. Advise to minimize or avoid exposure of treated areas to natural or artificial sunlight. Instruct to avoid late in pregnancy. Advise to seek medical attention for symptoms of CV events, GI events, hepatotoxicity, unexplained weight gain or edema, skin reactions, or hypersensitivity reactions; instruct to d/c at 1st appearance of rash/hypersensitivity reactions. Stress the importance of follow-up. Instruct not to apply to open skin wounds, infections, inflammations, or exfoliative dermatitis. Instruct to avoid concomitant use w/ other topical products. Instruct on how to use the dosing card to measure the proper dose of medication to apply. Instruct on how to correctly measure dose while waiting for a replacement of a lost dosing card.

STORAGE: 20-25°C (68-77°F). Keep from freezing. Store w/ dosing card.

VOLTAREN-XR – diclofenac sodium

RX

Class: NSAID

V

NSAIDs may cause an increased risk of serious cardiovascular (CV) thrombotic events, myocardial infarction (MI), stroke, and serious GI adverse events including inflammation, bleeding, ulceration, and perforation of the stomach or intestines, which may be fatal. Contraindicated for the treatment of perioperative pain in the setting of coronary artery bypass graft (CABG) surgery.

ADULT DOSAGE

Osteoarthritis

100mg qd

Rheumatoid Arthritis

100mg qd-bid

PEDIATRIC DOSAGE

Pediatric use may not have been established

ADMINISTRATION
Oral route

HOW SUPPLIED
Tab, Extended-Release: 100mg

CONTRAINDICATIONS
Known hypersensitivity to diclofenac; history of asthma, urticaria, or allergic-type reactions to aspirin (ASA) or other NSAIDs; treatment of perioperative pain in the setting of CABG surgery.

WARNINGS/PRECAUTIONS
Use lowest effective dose for the shortest duration possible. Not a substitute for corticosteroids or to treat corticosteroid insufficiency. May lead to onset of new HTN or worsening of preexisting HTN; monitor BP closely. Fluid retention and edema reported; caution with fluid retention or heart failure (HF). Extreme caution with a prior history of ulcer disease, and/or GI bleeding. Caution when initiating treatment in patients with considerable dehydration. Renal papillary necrosis and other renal injury reported after long-term use. Not recommended for use with advanced renal disease; if therapy must be initiated, monitor renal function. Anaphylactoid reactions may occur; avoid in patients with ASA triad. May cause serious skin adverse events (eg, exfoliative dermatitis, Stevens-Johnson syndrome [SJS], toxic epidermal necrolysis). Avoid in late pregnancy; may cause premature closure of ductus arteriosus. May cause elevations of LFTs; d/c if liver disease develops or systemic manifestations occur. Caution in elderly and debilitated patients. Anemia may occur; with long-term use, monitor Hgb/Hct if signs or symptoms of anemia develop. May inhibit platelet aggregation and prolong bleeding time; monitor with coagulation disorders. Caution with asthma and avoid with ASA-sensitive asthma.

ADVERSE REACTIONS
Abdominal pain, constipation, diarrhea, dyspepsia, flatulence, gross bleeding/perforation, heartburn, N/V, GI ulcers, renal function abnormalities, anemia, dizziness, edema, elevated liver enzymes.

DRUG INTERACTIONS
Increased adverse effects with ASA; avoid use. May enhance methotrexate toxicity and increase nephrotoxicity of cyclosporine; caution with coadministration. May diminish antihypertensive effect of ACE inhibitors. Patients taking thiazides and loop diuretics may have impaired response to these therapies. ACE inhibitors and diuretics may precipitate overt renal decompensation. May reduce natriuretic effect of furosemide and thiazides. May increase lithium levels; monitor for toxicity. Synergistic effects with warfarin on GI bleeding. May increase risk of GI bleeding with oral corticosteroids/anticoagulants, tobacco, or alcohol use. Caution with hepatotoxic drugs (eg, antibiotics, antiepileptics). Caution with CYP2C9 inhibitors or inducers (eg, voriconazole, rifampin); dosage adjustment may be warranted.

PATIENT CONSIDERATIONS

Assessment: Assess for CV disease or risk factors, fluid retention, edema, conditions affected by platelet function alterations, GI events or risk factors, renal/hepatic function, any other conditions where treatment is contraindicated or cautioned, pregnancy/nursing status, and possible drug interactions. Assess baseline BP, CBC, and chemistry profile.

Monitoring: Monitor for signs/symptoms of GI events, CV thrombotic events, congestive HF, HTN, allergic or skin reactions, hematological effects (eg, anemia, prolongation of bleeding time), renal papillary necrosis or other renal injury/toxicity, hepatotoxicity. Monitor BP, CBC, and chemistry profile periodically.

Counseling: Advise to seek medical attention if signs and symptoms of hepatotoxicity, anaphylactic/anaphylactoid reactions, skin reactions, CV events, GI ulceration or bleeding, weight gain, or edema occur. Inform of pregnancy risks and instruct to avoid use during late pregnancy.

STORAGE: Protect from moisture. Do not store above 30°C (86°F).

VOTRIENT – pazopanib

RX

Class: Kinase inhibitor

Severe and fatal hepatotoxicity reported; monitor hepatic function and interrupt, reduce, or d/c dosing as recommended.

V

ADULT DOSAGE

Advanced Renal Cell Carcinoma

Initial: 800mg qd w/o food (≥1 hr ac or 2 hrs pc)
Max: 800mg

Initial Dose Reduction: 400mg
Additional Dose Decrease/Increase: Should be in 200mg steps

PEDIATRIC DOSAGE
Pediatric use may not have been established

Advanced Soft Tissue Sarcoma

Patients Who Have Received Prior Chemotherapy:
Initial: 800mg qd w/o food (≥1 hr ac or 2 hrs pc)
Max: 800mg

Dose Decrease/Increase: Should be in 200mg steps

Missed Dose

If a dose is missed, it should not be taken if it is <12 hrs until the next dose

DOSING CONSIDERATIONS

Hepatic Impairment
Moderate: Consider alternative therapy or reduce dose to 200mg/day
Severe: Not recommended for use

Concomitant Medications
Strong CYP3A4 Inhibitors: Avoid concomitant use; consider an alternate concomitant medication w/ no or minimal potential to inhibit CYP3A4
If coadministration is warranted, reduce pazopanib dose to 400mg; further dose reductions may be needed if adverse effects occur during therapy
Strong CYP3A4 Inducers: Avoid concomitant use; consider an alternate concomitant medication w/ no or minimal enzyme induction potential
Do not use pazopanib if chronic use of strong CYP3A4 inducers cannot be avoided

ADMINISTRATION

Oral route

Do not crush tabs.
Take w/o food (≥1 hr ac or 2 hrs pc).

HOW SUPPLIED

Tab: 200mg

WARNINGS/PRECAUTIONS

Patients >65 yrs of age are at greater risk for hepatotoxicity. QT prolongation and torsades de pointes reported. Cardiac dysfunction (eg, decreased left ventricular ejection fraction [LVEF], CHF) reported. Hemorrhagic events reported; avoid w/ history of hemoptysis, cerebral hemorrhage, or clinically significant GI hemorrhage in the past 6 months. Arterial thromboembolic events reported; caution in patients at increased risk for these events or who have had a history of these events and avoid use if an arterial thromboembolic event has occurred w/in the past 6 months. Venous thromboembolic events (VTE) (eg, pulmonary embolism [PE]) and GI perforation/fistula reported. Thrombotic microangiopathy (TMA), including thrombotic thrombocytopenic purpura (TTP) and hemolytic uremic syndrome (HUS), reported; permanently d/c in patients developing TMA. Interstitial lung disease (ILD)/pneumonitis that can be fatal had been reported; d/c therapy if occurs. Reversible posterior leukoencephalopathy syndrome (RPLS) reported; permanently d/c in patients developing RPLS. HTN and hypertensive crisis reported; d/c if evidence of hypertensive crisis or if HTN is severe and persistent despite antihypertensive therapy and dose reduction. May impair wound healing; d/c therapy w/ wound dehiscence and ≥7 days prior to scheduled surgery. Hypothyroidism reported. Proteinuria reported; interrupt therapy and reduce dose for 24-hr urine protein ≥3g; d/c for repeat episodes despite dose reductions. Serious infections reported; institute appropriate anti-infective therapy promptly and consider interruption or discontinuation if serious infections develop. May cause serious adverse effects on organ development in pediatric patients; not for use in pediatric patients. May cause fetal harm if used during pregnancy.

ADVERSE REACTIONS

Diarrhea, HTN, hair color changes, N/V, anorexia, fatigue, asthenia, headache, abdominal pain, weight/appetite decreased, tumor pain, dysgeusia, dyspnea, musculoskeletal pain, skin hypopigmentation.

DRUG INTERACTIONS

See Dosing Considerations. Concomitant use w/ proton pump inhibitors (PPIs) (eg, esomeprazole) decreased exposure; avoid concomitant use w/ drugs that raise gastric pH. If such drugs are needed, consider short-acting antacids in place of PPIs and H2-receptor antagonists; separate antacid and pazopanib dosing by several hrs. Do not use in combination w/ other cancer therapy; increased toxicity and mortality reported w/ pemetrexed and lapatinib. Strong CYP3A4 inhibitors (eg, ketoconazole, ritonavir, clarithromycin) may increase concentrations. Avoid grapefruit or grapefruit juice. CYP3A4 inducers (eg, rifampin) may decrease plasma concentrations; consider an alternate concomitant medication w/ no or minimal enzyme induction potential. Avoid use w/ strong inhibitors of P-gp or breast cancer resistance protein (BCRP), and consider alternative concomitant medicinal products w/ no or minimal potential to inhibit P-gp or BCRP. Not recommended w/ agents w/ narrow therapeutic windows that are metabolized by CYP3A4, CYP2D6, or CYP2C8. Simvastatin may increase incidence of ALT elevations; follow pazopanib dosing guidelines or consider alternatives to pazopanib or consider discontinuing simvastatin. Caution in patients taking antiarrhythmics or other medications that may prolong the QT interval.

PATIENT CONSIDERATIONS

Assessment: Assess for history of QT interval prolongation, cardiac disease, hepatic impairment, pregnancy/nursing status, and for possible drug interactions. Assess for history of hemoptysis/ cerebral hemorrhage, clinically significant GI hemorrhage, or an arterial thromboembolic event in the past 6 months. Assess if patient is planning to undergo any surgical procedure. Assess thyroid function. Obtain baseline BP, LFTs, ECG, electrolytes, and urinalysis. Obtain baseline LVEF in patients at risk of cardiac dysfunction.

Monitoring: Monitor for signs/symptoms of hepatotoxicity, QT prolongation, torsades de pointes, cardiac dysfunction, hemorrhagic events, arterial thromboembolic events, VTE, TMA, TTP, HUS, PE, RPLS, GI perforation or fistula, HTN/hypertensive crisis, impaired wound healing, proteinuria, infections, and other adverse reactions. Monitor BP early after starting treatment and then frequently to ensure BP control. Perform periodic urinalysis w/ follow-up measurement of 24-hr urine protein as clinically indicated. Monitor ECG, thyroid function tests, and serum electrolytes. Monitor LFTs at Weeks 3, 5, 7, and 9, at Months 3 and 4, as clinically indicated, and continue periodic monitoring after Month 4. Periodically monitor LVEF in patients at risk of cardiac dysfunction.

Counseling: Advise the patient to read the FDA-approved patient labeling (Medication Guide). Advise that lab monitoring will be required prior to and while on therapy. Instruct to report any signs/symptoms of liver dysfunction, HTN, CHF, unusual bleeding, arterial thrombosis, new onset of dyspnea, chest pain, localized limb edema, GI perforation/fistula, infection, worsening of neurologic function consistent w/ RPLS, and pulmonary signs/symptoms indicative of ILD or pneumonitis. Advise to d/c treatment ≥7 days prior to a scheduled surgery. Inform that thyroid function testing and urinalysis will be performed during treatment. Advise on how to manage diarrhea and to notify healthcare provider if moderate to severe diarrhea occurs. Advise women of childbearing potential to avoid becoming pregnant during therapy. Advise to inform healthcare provider of all concomitant medications, vitamins, or dietary and herbal supplements. Advise that depigmentation of the hair or skin may occur during treatment.

STORAGE: 20-25°C (68-77°F); excursions permitted to 15-30°C (59-86°F).

VRAYLAR — cariprazine

Class: Atypical antipsychotic

RX

Elderly patients w/ dementia-related psychosis treated w/ antipsychotic drugs are at an increased risk of death. Not approved for the treatment of patients w/ dementia-related psychosis.

ADULT DOSAGE

Schizophrenia

Initial: 1.5mg qd
Titrate: Increase dose to 3mg on Day 2. Further dose adjustments can be made in 1.5mg or 3mg increments
Recommended Range: 1.5mg-6mg qd
Max: 6mg/d

Bipolar I Disorder

Acute Treatment of Manic or Mixed Episodes:
Initial: 1.5mg qd
Titrate: Increase dose to 3mg on Day 2. Further dose adjustments can be made in 1.5mg or 3mg increments
Recommended Range: 3mg-6mg qd
Max: 6mg/d

PEDIATRIC DOSAGE

Pediatric use may not have been established

DOSING CONSIDERATIONS

Concomitant Medications

Initiating a Strong CYP3A4 Inhibitor While on a Stable Dose of Cariprazine:
Reduce the current dosage of cariprazine by 1/2; reduce dose to 1.5mg or 3mg qd for patients taking 4.5mg/d. Adjust dosing regimen to qod for patients taking 1.5mg qd
When the CYP3A4 inhibitor is withdrawn, cariprazine dosage may need to be increased

Initiating Cariprazine While Already on a Strong CYP3A4 Inhibitor: Administer 1.5mg cariprazine on Day 1 and on Day 3 w/ no dose administered on Day 2. From Day 4 onward, administer 1.5mg qd, then increase to a max dose of 3mg/d

When the CYP3A4 inhibitor is withdrawn, cariprazine dosage may need to be increased

Concomitant Use w/ CYP3A4 Inducers: Not recommended

Renal Impairment

Severe (CrCl <30mL/min): Not recommended

Hepatic Impairment

Severe (Child-Pugh Score 10-15): Not recommended

ADMINISTRATION

Oral route

May be given w/ or w/o food.

HOW SUPPLIED

Cap: 1.5mg, 3mg, 4.5mg, 6mg

CONTRAINDICATIONS

History of a hypersensitivity reaction to cariprazine.

WARNINGS/PRECAUTIONS

May cause neuroleptic malignant syndrome (NMS); d/c and treat immediately if this occurs. Tardive dyskinesia (TD) may develop; consider discontinuation if signs/symptoms appear. Adverse reactions (eg, extrapyramidal symptoms [EPS], akathisia) may 1st appear several weeks after initiation of therapy; monitor patient response for several weeks after initiation and after each dose increase. Consider reducing dose or discontinuing therapy. Associated w/ metabolic changes (eg, hyperglycemia, diabetes mellitus [DM], dyslipidemia, weight gain). Hyperglycemia, in some cases extreme and associated w/ ketoacidosis or hyperosmolar coma or death, reported w/ atypical antipsychotics; assess FPG before or soon after initiation of therapy and monitor periodically during long-term treatment. Leukopenia, neutropenia, and agranulocytosis reported w/ atypical antipsychotics; monitor CBC in patients w/ preexisting low WBC/ANC or history of drug-induced leukopenia/neutropenia, and consider discontinuation at 1st sign of clinically significant decline in WBC counts w/o other causative factors. D/C therapy in patients w/ absolute neutrophil count <1000/mm^3 and follow their WBC until recovery. Increased risk of orthostatic hypotension and syncope during initial dose titration and when increasing dose; monitor orthostatic vital signs in patients vulnerable to hypotension, w/ known cardiovascular disease (CVD), or w/ cerebrovascular disease. May cause seizures/aspiration/esophageal dysmotility, impair mental/physical abilities, and disrupt body temperature regulation. Dysphagia reported; caution in patients at risk for aspiration.

ADVERSE REACTIONS

EPS, akathisia, dyspepsia, vomiting, somnolence, restlessness.

DRUG INTERACTIONS

See Dosing Considerations. Concomitant use of w/ strong CYP3A4 inhibitors (eg, itraconazole, ketoconazole) increases the exposures of cariprazine and its major active metabolite, didesmethyl cariprazine (DDCAR).

PATIENT CONSIDERATIONS

Assessment: Assess for dementia-related psychosis, DM, risk for hypotension, history of seizures, drug hypersensitivity, or any other conditions where treatment is cautioned, hepatic/renal function, pregnancy/nursing status, and possible drug interactions. Obtain FPG.

Monitoring: Monitor for NMS, TD, EPS, akathisia, orthostatic hypotension, leukopenia, neutropenia, agranulocytosis, cognitive/motor impairment, seizures, esophageal dysmotility, aspiration, disruption of body temperature, metabolic changes, and other adverse reactions. Monitor CBC frequently during the 1st few months of therapy in patients w/ preexisting low WBC/ANC or a history of drug-induced leukopenia/neutropenia. In patients w/ clinically significant neutropenia, monitor for fever or other symptoms or signs of infection. Periodically reevaluate long-term risks and benefits of the drug.

Counseling: Counsel about risk of NMS and the signs and symptoms of TD. Advise to contact their healthcare provider if abnormal movements occur. Educate about the risk of metabolic changes, how to recognize symptoms of hyperglycemia and DM, and the need for specific monitoring (eg, blood glucose, lipids, weights). Advise patients w/ risk factors for leukopenia/neutropenia that they should have their CBC monitored while on therapy. Advise about the risk of orthostatic hypotension, especially during the period of initial dose titration. Inform that therapy has the potential to impair judgment, thinking, or motor skills; advise to use caution when operating hazardous machinery. Counsel on appropriate care in avoiding overheating and dehydration. Inform about risk for EPS and/or withdrawal symptom in neonates whose mothers were exposed to antipsychotic drugs during the 3rd trimester of pregnancy. Advise patients that there is a pregnancy exposure registry. Instruct to notify physician if pregnant/planning to become pregnant, nursing, and if taking/planning to take any prescription or OTC drugs.

STORAGE: 20-25°C (68-77°F); excursions permitted between 15-30°C (59-86°F). Protect 3mg and 4.5mg cap from light.

VYTORIN – ezetimibe/simvastatin

RX

Class: Cholesterol absorption inhibitor/HMG-CoA reductase inhibitor (statin)

ADULT DOSAGE

Primary Hyperlipidemia/Mixed Hyperlipidemia

Primary (Heterozygous Familial and Nonfamilial) Hyperlipidemia/Mixed Hyperlipidemia:

Reduction of Elevated Total Cholesterol (Total-C), LDL, Apolipoprotein B, TGs, Non-HDL, and to Increase HDL:
Initial: 10mg/10mg or 10mg/20mg qpm
Usual: 10mg/10mg to 10mg/40mg qpm
Titrate: After initiation or titration, analyze lipid levels after ≥2 weeks and adjust dose, if needed

Patients Requiring Larger LDL Reduction (>55%):
Initial: 10mg/40mg qpm

Homozygous Familial Hypercholesterolemia

Adjunct to Other Lipid-Lowering Treatments (eg, LDL Apheresis) or if Such Treatments are Unavailable to Reduce Elevated Total-C and LDL:
10mg/40mg qpm

PEDIATRIC DOSAGE

Pediatric use may not have been established

DOSING CONSIDERATIONS

Concomitant Medications

Lomitapide:
Homozygous Familial Hypercholesterolemia:
Reduce dose by 50% if initiating lomitapide
Max: 10mg/20mg/day (or 10mg/40mg/day for patients who have previously taken simvastatin 80mg/day chronically [eg, for ≥12 months] w/o evidence of muscle toxicity)

Verapamil, Diltiazem, Dronedarone:
Max: 10mg/10mg qd

Amiodarone, Amlodipine, Ranolazine:
Max: 10mg/20mg qd

Bile Acid Sequestrants:
Take either ≥2 hrs before or ≥4 hrs after bile acid sequestrant

Niacin-Containing Products:
Chinese Patients Taking Lipid-Modifying Doses (≥1g/Day Niacin): Caution w/ doses >10mg/20mg/day; do not give 10mg/80mg dose

Renal Impairment

Chronic Kidney Disease (GFR <60mL/min/1.73m^2):
Usual: 10mg/20mg qpm

Other Important Considerations

Restricted Dosing:
Use 10mg/80mg dose only in patients who have been taking 10mg/80mg dose chronically (eg, for ≥12 months) w/o evidence of muscle toxicity

If currently tolerating 10mg/80mg dose and needs to be initiated on drug that is contraindicated or is associated w/ a dose cap for simvastatin, switch to an alternative statin or statin-based regimen w/ less potential for drug-drug interaction

Do not titrate to 10mg/80mg, but place on alternative LDL lowering treatment that provides greater LDL lowering, if unable to achieve LDL goal w/ 10mg/40mg dose

ADMINISTRATION

Oral route

Take qpm w/ or w/o food

HOW SUPPLIED

Tab: (Ezetimibe/Simvastatin) 10mg/10mg, 10mg/20mg, 10mg/40mg, 10mg/80mg

CONTRAINDICATIONS

Concomitant administration of strong CYP3A4 inhibitors (eg, itraconazole, ketoconazole, posaconazole, voriconazole, HIV protease inhibitors, boceprevir, telaprevir, erythromycin, clarithromycin, telithromycin, nefazodone, cobicistat-containing products), gemfibrozil, cyclosporine, or danazol. Hypersensitivity to any component of the medication, active liver disease or unexplained persistent elevations in hepatic transaminases, women who are or may become pregnant, nursing mothers.

WARNINGS/PRECAUTIONS

Use doses >10mg/20mg w/ caution and close monitoring in patients w/ moderate to severe renal impairment. Myopathy (including immune-mediated necrotizing myopathy [IMNM]) and rhabdomyolysis reported; predisposing factors include advanced age (≥65 yrs of age), female gender, uncontrolled hypothyroidism, and renal impairment. Risk of myopathy, including rhabdomyolysis, is dose related and greater w/ simvastatin 80mg. D/C if markedly elevated CPK levels occur or myopathy is suspected/diagnosed, and temporarily withhold if experiencing an acute or serious condition predisposing to development of renal failure secondary to rhabdomyolysis. Increases in serum transaminases reported. Fatal and nonfatal hepatic failure (rare) reported; promptly interrupt therapy if serious liver injury w/ clinical symptoms and/or hyperbilirubinemia or jaundice occurs and do not restart if no alternate etiology found. Caution w/ history of liver disease, substantial alcohol consumption, and in elderly. Increases in HbA1c and FPG levels reported.

ADVERSE REACTIONS

Headache, increased ALT, myalgia, URTI, diarrhea.

DRUG INTERACTIONS

See Contraindications and Dosing Considerations. Due to the risk of myopathy/rhabdomyolysis, avoid grapefruit juice and caution w/ fenofibrates (eg, fenofibrate, fenofibric acid), lipid-modifying doses (≥1g/day) of niacin, colchicine, verapamil, diltiazem, dronedarone, lomitapide, amiodarone, amlodipine, and ranolazine. If coadministered w/ a fenofibrate, immediately d/c both agents if myopathy is suspected/diagnosed, and perform gallbladder studies/consider alternative lipid-lowering therapy if cholelithiasis is suspected. Simvastatin: May slightly elevate plasma digoxin concentrations; monitor patients taking digoxin when therapy is initiated. May potentiate effect of coumarin anticoagulants; determine PT before initiation and frequently during therapy. Ezetimibe: Reduced levels w/ cholestyramine; incremental LDL reduction may be reduced. Increased INR reported w/ warfarin.

PATIENT CONSIDERATIONS

Assessment: Assess for history of or active liver disease, unexplained persistent hepatic transaminase elevations, predisposing factors for myopathy, renal impairment, alcohol consumption, drug hypersensitivity, any other conditions where treatment is contraindicated or cautioned, pregnancy/nursing status, and possible drug interactions. Assess lipid profile and LFTs.

Monitoring: Monitor for signs/symptoms of myopathy (including IMNM), rhabdomyolysis, liver dysfunction, increases in HbA1c and FPG levels, and other adverse reactions. Monitor lipid profile, and LFTs. Check PT w/ coumarin anticoagulants.

Counseling: Inform of benefits/risks of therapy. Advise to adhere to the National Cholesterol Education Program recommended diet, a regular exercise program, and periodic testing of a fasting lipid panel. Inform about substances that should be avoided during therapy, and advise to discuss all medications, both Rx and OTC, w/ physician. Instruct to report promptly any unexplained muscle pain, tenderness, or weakness, particularly if accompanied by malaise or fever or if these muscle signs/symptoms persist after discontinuation, or any symptoms that may indicate liver injury. Inform patients using the 10mg/80mg dose that the risk of myopathy, including rhabdomyolysis, is increased. Instruct women to use an effective method of birth control to prevent pregnancy while on therapy, to d/c therapy and call physician if pregnant, and not to breastfeed while on therapy.

STORAGE: 20-25°C (68-77°F).

VYVANSE — lisdexamfetamine dimesylate CII

Class: CNS stimulant

CNS stimulants (amphetamines and methylphenidate-containing products) have a high potential for abuse and dependence. Assess the risk of abuse prior to prescribing and monitor for signs of abuse and dependence while on therapy.

ADULT DOSAGE

Attention-Deficit Hyperactivity Disorder

Initial: 30mg qam
Titrate: May adjust in increments of 10mg or 20mg at approx weekly intervals
Max: 70mg/day

PEDIATRIC DOSAGE

Attention-Deficit Hyperactivity Disorder

≥6 Years:
Initial: 30mg qam
Titrate: May adjust in increments of 10mg or 20mg at weekly intervals
Max: 70mg/day

Binge Eating Disorder

Moderate to Severe:
Initial: 30mg qam
Titrate: Titrate in increments of 20mg at approx weekly intervals
Target Dose: 50-70mg/day
Max: 70mg/day

DOSING CONSIDERATIONS

Renal Impairment

Severe (GFR 15-<30mL/min/1.73m²):
Max: 50mg/day

ESRD (GFR <15mL/min/1.73m²):
Max: 30mg/day

Elderly

Start at lower end of dosing range

ADMINISTRATION

Oral route

Take in am w/ or w/o food; avoid afternoon doses
May swallow caps whole
Do not take anything less than 1 cap/day; do not divide a single cap

Open Caps

1. May open caps, empty, and mix entire contents w/ yogurt, water, or orange juice; if contents of cap include any compacted powder, may use a spoon to break apart the powder
2. Mix contents until completely dispersed
3. Immediately consume entire mixture; do not store

Film containing inactive ingredients may remain in glass/container once mixture is consumed

HOW SUPPLIED

Cap: 10mg, 20mg, 30mg, 40mg, 50mg, 60mg, 70mg

CONTRAINDICATIONS

Known hypersensitivity to amphetamine products or other ingredients of the medication. Concurrent use w/ an MAOI or use w/in 14 days of the last MAOI dose.

WARNINGS/PRECAUTIONS

Not indicated or recommended for weight loss. Sudden death, stroke, and MI reported in adults. Sudden death reported in children and adolescents w/ structural cardiac abnormalities and other serious heart problems. Avoid use in patients w/ known structural cardiac abnormalities, cardiomyopathy, serious heart arrhythmia, coronary artery disease, and other serious heart problems. May cause increase in BP and HR. May exacerbate symptoms of behavior disturbance and thought disorder in patients w/ a preexisting psychotic disorder. May induce a mixed/manic episode in patients w/ bipolar disorder. May cause psychotic or manic symptoms (eg, hallucinations, delusional thinking, mania) in children and adolescents w/o a prior history of psychotic illness or mania; consider discontinuation if symptoms occur. Associated w/ weight loss and slowing of growth rate in pediatric patients. Associated w/ peripheral vasculopathy, including Raynaud's phenomenon; further clinical evaluation (eg, rheumatology referral) may be appropriate for certain patients.

ADVERSE REACTIONS

Decreased appetite, insomnia, upper abdominal pain, irritability, N/V, decreased weight, dry mouth, dizziness, constipation, rash, diarrhea, anxiety, anorexia, jittery feeling, increased HR.

DRUG INTERACTIONS

See Contraindications. Urinary acidifying agents (eg, ascorbic acid) increase urinary excretion and decrease the $T_{1/2}$ of amphetamine, while urinary alkalinizing agents (eg, sodium bicarbonate) decrease urinary excretion and extend the $T_{1/2}$ of amphetamine; adjust dose accordingly.

PATIENT CONSIDERATIONS

Assessment: Assess for presence of cardiac disease, risk of abuse, risk factors for developing a manic episode, psychosis, bipolar disorder, hypersensitivity to the drug or amphetamine products, renal impairment, pregnancy/nursing status, and possible drug interactions.

Monitoring: Monitor for potential tachycardia, HTN, exacerbation of preexisting psychosis, psychotic or manic symptoms in children and adolescents, and other adverse reactions. Monitor height and weight in pediatric patients. Further evaluate patients who develop exertional chest pain, unexplained syncope, or arrhythmias. Observe carefully for signs/symptoms of peripheral vasculopathy (eg, digital changes). Monitor for signs of abuse and dependence; periodically reevaluate the need for therapy.

Counseling: Inform about drug abuse/dependence risk. Advise about serious cardiovascular risks; instruct to contact physician immediately if symptoms of cardiac disease develop. Instruct to monitor for elevations of BP and pulse rate. Inform that psychotic or manic symptoms may occur. Instruct parents or caregivers of pediatric patients that therapy may cause slowing of growth, including weight loss. Inform that therapy may impair ability to engage in potentially dangerous activities (eg, operating machinery); instruct patients to assess how the medication affects them before engaging in potentially dangerous activities. Inform about the risk of peripheral vasculopathy, including Raynaud's phenomenon; instruct to report to physician any new numbness, pain, skin color change, or sensitivity to temperature in fingers or toes, and to call physician immediately if any signs of unexplained wounds appear on fingers or toes while on therapy.

STORAGE: 20-25°C (68-77°F); excursions permitted between 15-30°C (59-86°F).

WELCHOL — colesevelam hydrochloride

RX

Class: Bile acid sequestrant

ADULT DOSAGE

Primary Hyperlipidemia

Reduction of LDL-C in adults w/ primary hyperlipidemia (Fredrickson Type IIa) either alone or in combination w/ a statin

Tab:
Usual: 3 tabs bid or 6 tabs qd

Sus:
Usual: 3.75g qd or 1.875g bid in 4-8 oz of water, fruit juice, or diet soft drinks; stir well and drink

May be dosed at the same time as a statin or dosed apart

Type 2 Diabetes Mellitus

Tab:
Usual: 3 tabs bid or 6 tabs qd

Sus:
Usual: 3.75g qd or 1.875g bid in 4-8 oz of water, fruit juice, or diet soft drinks; stir well and drink

PEDIATRIC DOSAGE

Heterozygous Familial Hypercholesterolemia

Reduction of LDL levels in boys and postmenarchal girls as monotherapy or in combination w/ a statin after an adequate trial of diet therapy

Sus:
10-17 Years:
3.75g qd or 1.875g bid in 4-8 oz of water, fruit juice, or diet soft drinks; stir well and drink

ADMINISTRATION

Oral route

Tab
Take w/ meal and liquid

Sus
Do not take in dry form; take w/ meals

HOW SUPPLIED

Sus: 1.875g, 3.75g [pkt]; **Tab:** 625mg

CONTRAINDICATIONS

Serum TG concentrations >500mg/dL, history of hypertriglyceridemia-induced pancreatitis or bowel obstruction.

WARNINGS/PRECAUTIONS

Not for treatment of type 1 DM or diabetic ketoacidosis. Analyze lipid levels within 4-6 weeks after initiation. May increase serum TG concentrations; d/c if TG levels >500mg/dL or if hypertriglyceridemia-induced pancreatitis develops. Caution in patients with TG levels >300mg/dL or with susceptibility to deficiencies of vitamin K (eg, malabsorption syndromes, patients on warfarin) or other fat-soluble vitamins. May cause constipation; avoid with gastroparesis, GI motility disorders, those who have had major GI tract surgery, or those at risk for bowel obstruction. (Sus) Contains phenylalanine; caution with phenylketonurics. Always mix with water, fruit juice, or diet soft drinks to avoid esophageal distress; do not take in its dry form. (Tab) Caution in patients with dysphagia or swallowing disorders.

ADVERSE REACTIONS

Asthenia, constipation, dyspepsia, nausea, rhinitis, fatigue, flu syndrome, nasopharyngitis, hypoglycemia, hypertriglyceridemia, headache, influenza, pharyngitis, URTI.

DRUG INTERACTIONS

Greater increase in TG levels may occur with insulin, pioglitazone, or sulfonylureas. May decrease absorption of vitamins A, D, E, and K. May increase seizure activity or decrease phenytoin levels.

May elevate TSH in patients receiving thyroid hormone replacement therapy. May increase levels of metformin extended-release. May decrease levels of cyclosporine, glimepiride, glipizide, glyburide, levothyroxine, olmesartan medoxomil, and oral contraceptives containing ethinyl estradiol and norethindrone. Administer phenytoin, cyclosporine, oral vitamin supplementation, drugs known to have reduced GI absorption when given concomitantly, or drugs that have not been tested for interaction (especially those with narrow therapeutic index) at least 4 hrs prior to colesevelam. Concomitant use with warfarin decreases INR; monitor INR.

PATIENT CONSIDERATIONS

Assessment: Assess for history/risk of bowel obstruction, gastroparesis, or other GI motility disorders, history of major GI tract surgery or hypertriglyceridemia-induced pancreatitis, susceptibility to deficiencies of vitamin K or other fat-soluble vitamins, dysphagia or swallowing disorders, pregnancy/nursing status, and possible drug interactions. Obtain baseline lipid parameters (eg, TGs, non-HDL levels). Monitor INR prior to initiation in patients on warfarin therapy.

Monitoring: Monitor for hypertriglyceridemia-induced pancreatitis, hypoglycemia, dysphagia, esophageal obstruction, and other adverse events. Periodically monitor lipid profile (eg, TGs, non-HDL), blood glucose, and coadministered drug levels. Monitor INR frequently in patients on warfarin therapy.

Counseling: Instruct to take with meal and liquid. Instruct to take interacting drugs at least 4 hrs prior to colesevelam. Advise to consume diet that promotes bowel regularity. Instruct to promptly d/c and seek medical attention if severe abdominal pain/constipation or symptoms of acute pancreatitis occur. Instruct patients with primary hyperlipidemia to adhere to the recommended diet of the National Cholesterol Education Program. Instruct patients with type 2 DM to adhere to dietary instructions, regular exercise program, and regular testing of blood glucose. Advise to notify physician if dysphagia or swallowing disorders occur. (Sus) Instruct to empty entire contents of 1 pkt into a glass or cup, then add 4-8 oz of water, fruit juice, or diet-soft drinks before ingesting.

STORAGE: 25°C (77°F); excursions permitted to 15-30°C (59-86°F). Protect from moisture. (Tab) Brief exposure to 40°C (104°F) does not adversely affect the product.

WELLBUTRIN SR – bupropion hydrochloride

RX

Class: Aminoketone

Antidepressants increased the risk of suicidal thoughts and behavior in children, adolescents, and young adults in short-term trials. Monitor closely for worsening, and for emergence of suicidal thoughts and behavior. Advise families and caregivers of the need for close observation and communication w/ the prescriber. Serious neuropsychiatric reactions reported in patients taking bupropion for smoking cessation; not approved for smoking cessation.

ADULT DOSAGE

Major Depressive Disorder

Initial: 150mg/day given as a single daily dose in am
Titrate: After 3 days, may increase dose to 150mg bid w/ an interval of at least 8 hrs between successive doses
Usual Target Dose: 300mg/day, given as 150mg bid
Max: May consider 400mg/day, given as 200mg bid, if no clinical improvement after several weeks of treatment at 300mg/day; do not exceed 200mg in any single dose

Dosing Considerations with MAOIs

Switching to/from an MAOI Antidepressant:
Allow at least 14 days between discontinuation of an MAOI and initiation of treatment and allow at least 14 days between discontinuation of treatment and initiation of an MAOI

Use w/ Reversible MAOIs (eg, Linezolid, IV Methylene Blue):
Do not start bupropion in a patient being treated w/ a reversible MAOI
If acceptable alternatives to linezolid or IV methylene blue treatment are not available and potential benefits of linezolid or IV methylene blue treatment are judged to

PEDIATRIC DOSAGE

Pediatric use may not have been established

W

outweigh risks of hypertensive reactions, bupropion should be stopped promptly, and linezolid or IV methylene blue can be administered
Monitor for 2 weeks or until 24 hrs after the last dose of linezolid or IV methylene blue, whichever comes 1st
May resume bupropion treatment 24 hrs after the last dose of linezolid or IV methylene blue

DOSING CONSIDERATIONS

Renal Impairment

Consider reducing frequency and/or dose

Hepatic Impairment

Mild (Child-Pugh Score: 5-6): Consider reducing frequency and/or dose
Moderate to Severe (Child-Pugh Score: 7-15): Max of 100mg/day or 150mg qod

ADMINISTRATION

Oral route
Take w/ or w/o food
Swallow whole; do not crush, divide, or chew

HOW SUPPLIED

Tab, Sustained-Release: 100mg, 150mg, 200mg

CONTRAINDICATIONS

Seizure disorder; current/prior diagnosis of bulimia or anorexia nervosa; undergoing abrupt discontinuation of alcohol, benzodiazepines, barbiturates, or antiepileptic drugs; known hypersensitivity to bupropion or other ingredients of the medication. Use of MAOIs (intended to treat psychiatric disorders) either concomitantly or w/in 14 days of discontinuing treatment. Treatment w/in 14 days of discontinuing treatment w/ an MAOI. Starting treatment in patients being treated w/ reversible MAOIs (eg, linezolid, IV methylene blue).

WARNINGS/PRECAUTIONS

Dose-related risk of seizures; titrate dose gradually. D/C and do not restart treatment if a seizure occurs. May result in elevated BP and HTN. Caution w/ conditions that may increase risk of seizure. May precipitate a manic, mixed, or hypomanic manic episode; not approved for use in treating bipolar depression. Neuropsychiatric signs and symptoms (eg, delusions, hallucinations, psychosis, concentration disturbance) reported. Pupillary dilation that occurs following use may trigger an angle-closure attack in a patient w/ anatomically narrow angles who does not have a patent iridectomy. D/C treatment if allergic or anaphylactoid/anaphylactic reactions occur. Arthralgia, myalgia, fever w/ rash, and other serum sickness-like symptoms suggestive of delayed hypersensitivity reported. False (+) urine immunoassay screening tests for amphetamines reported.

ADVERSE REACTIONS

Abdominal pain, dry mouth, anorexia, insomnia, dizziness, agitation, anxiety, pharyngitis, sweating, rash, tinnitus, tremor, myalgia, nausea, palpitation.

DRUG INTERACTIONS

See Contraindications. Extreme caution w/ other drugs that lower seizure threshold (eg, other bupropion products, antipsychotics, antidepressants, theophylline, systemic corticosteroids); use low initial doses and increase the dose gradually. Increased risk of seizure w/ use of illicit drugs (eg, cocaine), abuse or misuse of prescription drugs (eg, CNS stimulants), use of oral hypoglycemic drugs or insulin, use of anorectic drugs, and excessive use of alcohol, benzodiazepines, sedative/hypnotics, or opiates. Ritonavir, lopinavir, or efavirenz may decrease exposure; may need to increase bupropion dose but not to exceed max dose. May reduce efficacy of drugs that require metabolic activation by CYP2D6 to be effective (eg, tamoxifen). CNS toxicity reported when coadministered w/ levodopa or amantadine; use w/ caution. Minimize or avoid alcohol. Monitor BP w/ nicotine replacement therapy. Potential for drug interactions w/ CYP2B6 inhibitors/inducers. Increased risk of HTN w/ MAOIs or other drugs that increase dopaminergic or noradrenergic activity. May increase exposure of CYP2D6 substrates (eg, antidepressants, antipsychotics, β-blockers, and type 1C antiarrhythmics [eg, propafenone, flecainide]); may need to decrease the dose of CYP2D6 substrates, particularly for drugs w/ a narrow therapeutic index. CYP2B6 inhibitors (eg, ticlopidine, clopidogrel) may increase bupropion exposure but decrease hydroxybupropion exposure; may need to adjust dose. Carbamazepine, phenytoin, and phenobarbital may induce metabolism and decrease exposure. If used concomitantly w/ a CYP inducer, may need to increase the dose of bupropion, but not to exceed the max dose.

PATIENT CONSIDERATIONS

Assessment: Assess for bipolar disorder, hepatic/renal dysfunction, seizure disorders or conditions that may increase risk of seizure, susceptibility to angle-closure glaucoma, hypersensitivity to the drug, and any other conditions where treatment is contraindicated or cautioned, pregnancy/nursing status, BP, and for possible drug interactions.

Monitoring: Monitor for clinical worsening, suicidality, or unusual changes in behaviors, neuropsychiatric symptoms, seizures, BP, activation of mania or hypomania, psychosis and other neuropsychiatric reactions, angle-closure glaucoma, anaphylactoid/anaphylactic reactions, delayed hypersensitivity, and other adverse reactions. Monitor hepatic/renal function, especially in elderly. Periodically reassess the appropriate dose and the need for maint treatment.

Counseling: Inform of benefits/risks of therapy. Advise patients and caregivers of need for close observation for clinical worsening and/or suicidal risks. Educate on the symptoms of hypersensitivity and to d/c if a severe allergic reaction occurs. Instruct to d/c and not restart if a seizure occurs while on therapy. Inform that therapy may impair mental/physical abilities; advise to use caution while operating hazardous machinery/driving. Inform that excessive use or abrupt discontinuation of alcohol or sedatives may alter the seizure threshold; advise to minimize or avoid alcohol use. Instruct to notify physician if taking/planning to take any prescription or OTC medications. Advise not to use therapy in combination w/ other medicines containing bupropion hydrochloride. Advise to contact physician if pregnancy occurs or is intended during therapy. Caution about the risk of angle-closure glaucoma in susceptible patients.

STORAGE: 20-25°C (68-77°F); excursions permitted 15-30°C (59-86°F). Protect from light and moisture.

WELLBUTRIN XL – bupropion hydrochloride

RX

Class: Aminoketone

Antidepressants increased the risk of suicidal thoughts and behavior in children, adolescents, and young adults in short-term trials. Monitor closely for worsening, and for emergence of suicidal thoughts and behaviors. Advise families and caregivers of the need for close observation and communication with the prescriber. Serious neuropsychiatric reactions reported in patients taking bupropion for smoking cessation; not approved for smoking cessation. Observe all patients for neuropsychiatric reactions.

ADULT DOSAGE

Major Depressive Disorder

Initial: 150mg qd in the am
Titrate: May increase to 300mg qd on Day 4
Maint: Reassess periodically to determine need for maint treatment and the appropriate dose

Seasonal Affective Disorder

Initial: 150mg qd in the am
Titrate: May increase to 300mg qd after 7 days
Max: 300mg

Prevention of Seasonal Major Depressive Disorder Episodes Associated w/ Seasonal Affective Disorder:
Initiate in the autumn, prior to the onset of depressive symptoms. Continue through the winter season; taper and d/c in early spring
Treated w/ 300mg/day: Decrease to 150mg qd before discontinuing

Individualize timing of initiation and duration of treatment

Conversions

Switching from Wellbutrin Tab/Wellbutrin SR Tab:
Give same total daily dose when possible

Dosing Considerations with MAOIs

Switching to/from an MAOI Antidepressant:
Allow at least 14 days between discontinuation of an MAOI and initiation of treatment, and allow at least 14 days between discontinuation of treatment and initiation of an MAOI

W/ Other MAOIs (eg, Linezolid, IV Methylene Blue):
Do not start bupropion in a patient being treated w/ linezolid or IV methylene blue

PEDIATRIC DOSAGE

Pediatric use may not have been established

In patients already receiving bupropion, if acceptable alternatives are not available and benefits outweigh risks, d/c bupropion and administer linezolid or IV methylene blue; monitor for 2 weeks or until 24 hrs after the last dose of linezolid or IV methylene blue, whichever comes 1st. May resume bupropion therapy 24 hrs after the last dose of linezolid or IV methylene blue

DOSING CONSIDERATIONS

Renal Impairment

GFR <90mL/min: Consider reducing dose and/or frequency

Hepatic Impairment

Mild (Child-Pugh Score 5-6): Consider reducing dose and/or frequency

Moderate to Severe (Child-Pugh Score 7-15) Max Dose: 150mg qod

Discontinuation

Treated w/ 300mg qd: Decrease to 150mg qd prior to discontinuation

ADMINISTRATION

Oral route

Administer in the am, w/ or w/o food

Swallow whole; do not crush, divide, or chew

HOW SUPPLIED

Tab, ER: 150mg, 300mg

CONTRAINDICATIONS

Seizure disorder; current/prior diagnosis of bulimia or anorexia nervosa; undergoing abrupt discontinuation of alcohol, benzodiazepines, barbiturates, and antiepileptic drugs; known hypersensitivity to bupropion or other ingredients of the medication. Use of MAOIs (intended to treat psychiatric disorders) either concomitantly or w/in 14 days of discontinuing treatment. Treatment w/in 14 days of discontinuing treatment w/ an MAOI. Starting treatment in patients being treated w/ reversible MAOIs (eg, linezolid, IV methylene blue).

WARNINGS/PRECAUTIONS

Dose-related risk of seizures; increase dose gradually, and do not exceed 300mg qd. D/C and do not restart treatment if a seizure occurs. Caution with conditions that may increase risk of seizure. May result in elevated BP and HTN. May precipitate a manic, mixed, or hypomanic manic episode; not approved for treatment of bipolar depression. Neuropsychiatric signs and symptoms (eg, delusions, hallucinations, psychosis) reported; d/c if these reactions occur. Pupillary dilation that occurs following use may trigger an angle-closure attack in a patient with anatomically narrow angles who does not have a patent iridectomy. Anaphylactoid/anaphylactic reactions reported; d/c treatment if these reactions occur. Erythema multiforme, Stevens-Johnson syndrome, and anaphylactic shock rarely reported. Arthralgia, myalgia, fever with rash, and other symptoms of serum sickness suggestive of delayed hypersensitivity reported. Caution in elderly. False (+) urine immunoassay screening tests for amphetamines reported.

ADVERSE REACTIONS

Headache, infection, dry mouth, nausea, insomnia, dizziness, agitation, tremor, anxiety, constipation, pharyngitis, sweating, tinnitus, diarrhea, anorexia, rash.

DRUG INTERACTIONS

See Contraindications. Extreme caution with drugs that lower seizure threshold (eg, other bupropion products, antipsychotics, antidepressants, theophylline, systemic corticosteroids); use low initial doses and increase the dose gradually. Increased risk of seizure with use of illicit drugs (eg, cocaine), abuse or misuse of prescription drugs (eg, CNS stimulants), use of oral hypoglycemic drugs or insulin, use of anorectic drugs, and excessive use of alcohol, benzodiazepines, sedative/hypnotics, or opiates. Potential for drug interactions with CYP2B6 inhibitors/inducers. CYP2B6 inhibitors (eg, ticlopidine, clopidogrel) may increase bupropion exposure but decrease hydroxybupropion exposure; may need to adjust bupropion dose. Ritonavir, lopinavir, and efavirenz may decrease exposure; may need to increase bupropion dose but not to exceed max dose. Carbamazepine, phenytoin, and phenobarbital may induce metabolism and decrease exposure. If used concomitantly with a CYP inducer, may need to increase bupropion dose, but not to exceed the max dose. May increase exposure of CYP2D6 substrates (eg, antidepressants, antipsychotics, β-blockers, type 1C antiarrhythmics [eg, propafenone, flecainide]); may need to decrease the dose of CYP2D6 substrates, particularly for drugs with a narrow therapeutic index. May reduce efficacy of drugs that require metabolic activation by CYP2D6 to be effective (eg, tamoxifen); may require increased doses of such drugs. CNS toxicity reported when coadministered with levodopa or amantadine; use with caution. Minimize or avoid alcohol. Increased risk of HTN with MAOIs or other drugs that increase dopaminergic or noradrenergic activity. Monitor BP with nicotine replacement therapy.

PATIENT CONSIDERATIONS

Assessment: Assess for seizure disorders or conditions that may increase risk of seizure, susceptibility to angle-closure glaucoma, renal/hepatic impairment, hypersensitivity to the drug, any other conditions where treatment is contraindicated or cautioned, pregnancy/nursing status, and possible drug interactions. Obtain baseline BP and screen for risk factors/a history of bipolar disorder.

Monitoring: Monitor for clinical worsening, suicidality, unusual changes in behavior, seizures, activation of mania or hypomania, psychosis and other neuropsychiatric reactions, angle-closure glaucoma, anaphylactoid/anaphylactic reactions, delayed hypersensitivity, and other adverse reactions. Monitor BP periodically. Monitor hepatic/renal function, especially in the elderly.

Counseling: Inform of benefits/risks of therapy and counsel in its appropriate use. Advise patients and caregivers of the need for close observation for clinical worsening and/or suicidal risk. Educate on the symptoms of hypersensitivity and advise to d/c if a severe allergic reaction occurs. Instruct to d/c and not restart if a seizure occurs while on therapy. Inform that excessive use or abrupt discontinuation of alcohol or sedatives may alter the seizure threshold; advise to minimize or avoid alcohol use. Caution about the risk of angle-closure glaucoma in susceptible patients. Advise not to use therapy in combination with other medicines containing bupropion hydrochloride. Inform that therapy may impair mental/physical abilities; advise to use caution while operating hazardous machinery/driving. Instruct to notify physician if taking/planning to take any prescription or OTC medications. Advise to contact physician if pregnancy occurs or is intended during therapy. Communicate with the patient and pediatric healthcare provider regarding the infant's exposure to bupropion through human milk; instruct caregivers to immediately contact the infant's healthcare provider if they note any side effect in the infant that concerns them or is persistent.

STORAGE: 25°C (77°F); excursions permitted to 15-30°C (59-86°F).

WP Thyroid – thyroid

RX

Class: Thyroid replacement hormone

ADULT DOSAGE

Hypothyroidism

Initial: 32.5mg/day; 16.25mg/day is recommended in patients with longstanding myxedema, particularly if cardiovascular impairment is suspected
Titrate: Increase by 16.25mg every 2-3 weeks; readjust within first 4 weeks of therapy
Maint: 65-130mg/day

Myxedema Coma:
400mcg (100mcg/mL) IV of levothyroxine sodium (T4) given rapidly, followed by daily supplements of 100-200mcg given IV
Resume oral therapy when clinical situation has been stabilized and patient is able to take oral medication

Pituitary TSH Suppressant

In the treatment or prevention of various types of euthyroid goiters, including thyroid nodules, subacute, or chronic lymphocytic thyroiditis (Hashimoto's), multinodular goiter, and in the management of thyroid cancer

1.56mg/kg/day of levothyroxine (T4) for 7-10 days

Thyroid Cancer:
Larger amounts of thyroid hormone than those used for replacement therapy are required

Diagnostic Aid

In suppression tests to differentiate suspected mild hyperthyroidism or thyroid gland anatomy

1.56mg/kg/day of levothyroxine (T4) for 7-10 days

PEDIATRIC DOSAGE

Hypothyroidism

Congenital:
0-6 Months of Age:
4.8-6mg/kg/day (16.25-32.5mg/day)
6-12 Months of Age:
3.6-4.8mg/kg/day (32.5-48.75mg/day)
1-5 Years:
3-3.6mg/kg/day (48.75-65mg/day)
6-12 Years:
2.4-3mg/kg/day (65-97.5mg/day)
>12 Years:
1.2-1.8mg/kg/day (>97.5mg/day)

DOSING CONSIDERATIONS

Adverse Reactions

Hypothyroidism:

Angina: Appearance is an indication for dose reduction

Elderly

Start at lower end of dosing range

ADMINISTRATION

Oral route

HOW SUPPLIED

Tab: 16.25mg, 32.5mg, 48.75mg, 65mg, 81.25mg, 97.5mg, 113.75mg, 130mg, 146.25mg, 162.5mg, 195mg

CONTRAINDICATIONS

Uncorrected adrenal cortical insufficiency, untreated thyrotoxicosis, hypersensitivity to any of their active or extraneous constituents.

WARNINGS/PRECAUTIONS

Doses within range of daily hormonal requirements are ineffective for weight reduction in euthyroid patients; larger doses may produce serious or even life-threatening toxicity, particularly when given in association with sympathomimetic amines. Use is unjustified for the treatment of male or female infertility unless accompanied by hypothyroidism. Caution with cardiovascular (CV) disorders (eg, angina pectoris) and in elderly with risk of occult cardiac disease; initiate at low doses and reduce dose if euthyroid state can only be reached at the expense of aggravation of CV disease. May aggravate diabetes mellitus (DM), diabetes insipidus (DI), or adrenal cortical insufficiency. Treatment of myxedema coma requires simultaneous administration of glucocorticoids. Excessive doses in infants may cause craniosynostosis. Caution in patients with strong suspicion of thyroid gland autonomy. Androgens, corticosteroids, estrogens, iodine-containing preparations, and salicylate-containing preparations may interfere with lab tests.

DRUG INTERACTIONS

Closely monitor PT in patients on oral anticoagulants; dose reduction of anticoagulant may be required. May increase insulin or oral hypoglycemic requirements. Potentially impaired absorption with cholestyramine and colestipol; space dosing by 4-5 hrs. Estrogens may decrease free T4 in patients with nonfunctioning thyroid; increase in thyroid dose may be needed.

PATIENT CONSIDERATIONS

Assessment: Assess for adrenal cortical insufficiency, thyrotoxicosis, hypersensitivity to the drug, CV disorders (eg, coronary artery disease, angina pectoris), DM, DI, myxedema coma, nursing status, and possible drug interactions.

Monitoring: Monitor response to treatment, urinary glucose levels in patients with DM, PT in patients receiving anticoagulants, and for aggravation of CV disease. Monitor thyroid function periodically.

Counseling: Inform that replacement therapy is taken essentially for life except in transient hypothyroidism. Instruct to immediately report to physician any signs/symptoms of thyroid hormone toxicity (eg, chest pain, increased pulse rate, palpitations, excessive sweating, heat intolerance, nervousness) or any other unusual event. Inform of the importance of frequent/close monitoring of PT and urinary glucose and the need for dose adjustment of antidiabetic and/or oral anticoagulant medication. Inform that partial loss of hair may be seen in children in 1st few months of therapy.

STORAGE: 15-30°C (59-86°F).

XALATAN – latanoprost

RX

Class: Prostaglandin analogue

ADULT DOSAGE

Elevated Intraocular Pressure

Open-Angle Glaucoma/Ocular HTN:

1 drop in affected eye(s) qd in pm

Max: Once-daily dosing

PEDIATRIC DOSAGE

Pediatric use may not have been established

X

DOSING CONSIDERATIONS

Concomitant Medications

Space by at least 5 min if using >1 topical ophthalmic drug

ADMINISTRATION

Ocular route

Continue w/ the next dose as normal if 1 dose is missed

HOW SUPPLIED

Sol: 0.005% [2.5mL]

CONTRAINDICATIONS

Known hypersensitivity to latanoprost, benzalkonium chloride, or any other ingredients in the product.

WARNINGS/PRECAUTIONS

May cause changes to pigmented tissues (eg, increased pigmentation of iris [may be permanent], periorbital tissue/eyelashes [may be reversible]); regularly examine patients who develop noticeably increased iris pigmentation. May gradually change eyelashes and vellus hair in the treated eye. Caution with a history of intraocular inflammation (iritis/uveitis). Macular edema, including cystoid macular edema, reported; caution in aphakic patients, pseudophakic patients with a torn posterior lens capsule, or patients with known risk factors for macular edema. Reactivation of herpes simplex keratitis reported; caution with a history of herpetic keratitis. Avoid with active intraocular inflammation and in cases of active herpes simplex keratitis; inflammation may be exacerbated. Bacterial keratitis associated with the use of multiple-dose containers reported. Contact lenses should be removed prior to administration and may be reinserted 15 min after administration.

ADVERSE REACTIONS

Foreign body sensation, punctate epithelial keratopathy, stinging, itching, burning, conjunctival hyperemia, blurred vision, increased iris pigmentation, excessive tearing, lid discomfort/pain, dry eye, eye pain, lid crusting, lid erythema, URTI/cold/flu.

DRUG INTERACTIONS

Combined use of ≥2 prostaglandins or prostaglandin analogues is not recommended; administration of these prostaglandin drug products more than once daily may decrease the IOP-lowering effect or cause paradoxical IOP elevations. Precipitation occurs when mixed with eye drops containing thimerosal; if such drugs are used, they should be administered at least 5 min apart.

PATIENT CONSIDERATIONS

Assessment: Assess for hypersensitivity to drug or benzalkonium chloride, history of or active intraocular inflammation, history of herpetic keratitis, active herpes simplex keratitis, aphakia, pseudophakia with a torn posterior lens capsule, risk factors for macular edema, pregnancy/nursing status, and possible drug interactions.

Monitoring: Monitor for changes to pigmented tissues, eyelash changes, macular edema, herpetic/bacterial keratitis, and other adverse reactions.

Counseling: Inform about the possibility of increased brown pigmentation of the iris, eyelid skin darkening, and eyelash and vellus hair changes in the treated eye. Instruct to avoid allowing the tip of the dispensing container to contact the eye or surrounding structures to avoid contamination. Advise to immediately consult physician about the continued use of treatment if an intercurrent ocular condition (eg, trauma, infection) develops, if undergoing ocular surgery, or if any ocular reactions, particularly conjunctivitis and eyelid reactions, develop. Advise that contact lenses should be removed prior to administration and may be reinserted 15 min after administration. Instruct that if using >1 topical ophthalmic drug, to administer the drugs at least 5 min apart. Inform that if one dose is missed, treatment should continue with the next dose as normal.

STORAGE: Protect from light. Unopened: 2-8°C (36-46°F). During Shipment to Patient: Up to 40°C (104°F) for a period not exceeding 8 days. Opened: Room temperature up to 25°C (77°F) for 6 weeks.

XANAX – alprazolam

CIV

Class: Benzodiazepine

ADULT DOSAGE

Anxiety Disorders

Management of Disorders or Short-Term Relief of Symptoms:

Initial: 0.25-0.5mg tid

Titrate: May increase at intervals of 3-4 days

Max: 4mg/day in divided doses

Panic Disorder

W/ or w/o Agoraphobia:

Initial: 0.5mg tid

Titrate: May increase by ≤1mg/day every 3-4 days; slower titration to doses >4mg/day

Range: 1-10mg/day

PEDIATRIC DOSAGE

Pediatric use may not have been established

DOSING CONSIDERATIONS

Hepatic Impairment

Advanced Liver Disease:

Initial: 0.25mg bid-tid

Titrate: May increase gradually prn

Elderly

Elderly/Debilitated:

Initial: 0.25mg bid-tid

Titrate: May increase gradually prn

Discontinuation

Reduce dose gradually when discontinuing therapy or when decreasing daily dosage. Decrease daily dose by no more than 0.5mg every 3 days; some patients may require an even slower dosage reduction

ADMINISTRATION

Oral route

HOW SUPPLIED

Tab: 0.25mg*, 0.5mg*, 1mg*, 2mg* *scored

CONTRAINDICATIONS

Known sensitivity to this drug or other benzodiazepines, acute narrow-angle glaucoma, concomitant ketoconazole or itraconazole.

WARNINGS/PRECAUTIONS

May be used with treated open-angle glaucoma. Increased risk of dependence with doses >4mg/day, treatment for >12 weeks, and in panic disorder patients. Seizures, including status epilepticus, reported with dose reduction or abrupt discontinuation. Early am anxiety and emergence of anxiety symptoms between doses reported; give same total daily dose divided as more frequent administrations. Withdrawal reactions may occur; reduce dose or d/c therapy gradually. May impair mental/physical abilities. May cause fetal harm; avoid use during 1st trimester. Hypomania/mania reported in patients with depression. Caution with severe depression, suicidal ideation/plans, impaired renal/hepatic/pulmonary function, elderly, and debilitated patients. Has a weak uricosuric effect. Decreased systemic elimination rate with alcoholic liver disease/obesity.

ADVERSE REACTIONS

Drowsiness, lightheadedness, fatigue/tiredness, irritability, depression, headache, confusion, insomnia, dry mouth, constipation, diarrhea, N/V, tachycardia/palpitations, blurred vision, nasal congestion.

DRUG INTERACTIONS

See Contraindications. Not recommended with azole antifungals. Avoid with very potent CYP3A inhibitors. Caution with alcohol, other CNS depressants, diltiazem, isoniazid, macrolides (eg, erythromycin, clarithromycin), grapefruit juice, sertraline, paroxetine, ergotamine, cyclosporine, amiodarone, nicardipine, nifedipine, and other CYP3A inhibitors. Additive CNS depressant effects with psychotropics, anticonvulsants, antihistaminics, ethanol, and other drugs that produce CNS depression. Increased digoxin concentrations reported (especially in patients >65 yrs of age); monitor for signs/symptoms of digoxin toxicity. May increase plasma concentrations of imipramine and desipramine. Fluoxetine, fluvoxamine, nefazodone, cimetidine, and oral contraceptives may increase concentrations. CYP3A inducers (eg, carbamazepine), propoxyphene, and smoking may decrease levels. May require dose adjustment or discontinuation with HIV protease inhibitors (eg, ritonavir).

PATIENT CONSIDERATIONS

Assessment: Assess for drug hypersensitivity, acute narrow-angle glaucoma, depression, suicidal ideation, renal/hepatic/pulmonary function, debilitation, history of alcohol/substance abuse, history of seizures/epilepsy, pregnancy/nursing status, and possible drug interactions. Assess for risk of dependence among panic disorder patients.

Monitoring: Monitor for dependence, rebound/withdrawal symptoms, early am anxiety and emergence of anxiety symptoms, CNS depression, episodes of hypomania/mania, suicidality, other treatment-emergent symptoms, and adverse reactions. Monitor CBC, urinalysis, and blood chemistry periodically. Periodically reassess usefulness of therapy.

Counseling: Advise to inform physician about any alcohol consumption and medicines taken and if nursing, pregnant, planning to be pregnant, or if pregnancy occurs while on therapy. Advise to avoid alcohol during treatment. Advise not to drive or operate dangerous machinery until becoming familiar with the effects of therapy. Advise not to increase/decrease dose or abruptly d/c therapy without consultation; instruct to follow gradual dosage-tapering schedule. Inform of risks associated with doses >4mg/day.

STORAGE: 20-25°C (68-77°F).

Xanax XR – alprazolam

CIV

Class: Benzodiazepine

ADULT DOSAGE

Panic Disorder

W/ or w/o Agoraphobia:

Initial: 0.5-1mg qd, preferably in the am
Titrate: May increase at intervals of 3-4 days in increments of ≤1mg/day
Usual: 3-6mg/day; some patients may require doses >6mg/day
Maint: 1-10mg/day

Conversions

Switching from Immediate-Release (IR) Tabs to Extended-Release (ER) Tabs:
Patients who are currently being treated w/ divided doses of IR alprazolam tabs may be switched to ER tabs at the same total daily dose taken qd. If therapeutic response after switching is inadequate, may titrate dose as recommended

PEDIATRIC DOSAGE

Pediatric use may not have been established

DOSING CONSIDERATIONS

Hepatic Impairment

Advanced Liver Disease:
Initial: 0.5mg qd
Titrate: May increase gradually if needed and tolerated

Elderly

Elderly/Debilitated:
Initial: 0.5mg qd
Titrate: May increase gradually if needed and tolerated

Discontinuation

Reduce dose gradually when discontinuing therapy or when decreasing daily dosage. Decrease daily dose by no more than 0.5mg every 3 days; some patients may require an even slower dosage reduction

ADMINISTRATION

Oral route

May be administered qd, preferably in the am
Tabs should be taken intact; do not chew, crush, or break

HOW SUPPLIED

Tab, ER: 0.5mg, 1mg, 2mg, 3mg

CONTRAINDICATIONS

Known sensitivity to this drug or other benzodiazepines, acute narrow-angle glaucoma, concomitant ketoconazole or itraconazole.

WARNINGS/PRECAUTIONS

May be used with treated open-angle glaucoma. Increased risk of dependence with doses >4mg/day, treatment for >12 weeks, and in panic disorder patients. Seizures, including status epilepticus, reported with dose reduction or abrupt discontinuation. Early am anxiety/emergence of anxiety symptoms between doses reported. Withdrawal reactions may occur; reduce dose or d/c therapy gradually. May impair mental/physical abilities. May cause fetal harm; avoid use during 1st trimester. Caution with severe depression, suicidal ideation/plans, impaired renal/hepatic/pulmonary function, elderly, and debilitated patients. Hypomania/mania reported in patients with depression. Has a weak uricosuric effect. Decreased systemic elimination rate with alcoholic liver disease/obesity.

ADVERSE REACTIONS

Sedation, somnolence, memory impairment, dysarthria, abnormal coordination, fatigue, depression, constipation, mental impairment, ataxia, dry mouth, nausea, decreased libido, increased/decreased appetite/weight.

DRUG INTERACTIONS

See Contraindications. Not recommended with azole antifungals. Avoid with very potent CYP3A inhibitors. Caution with alcohol, other CNS depressants, diltiazem, isoniazid, macrolides (eg, erythromycin, clarithromycin), grapefruit juice, sertraline, paroxetine, ergotamine, cyclosporine, amiodarone, nicardipine, nifedipine, and other CYP3A inhibitors. Additive CNS depressant effects with psychotropics, anticonvulsants, antihistaminics, ethanol, and other drugs that produce CNS

X

depression. Increased digoxin concentrations reported (especially in patients >65 yrs of age); monitor for signs/symptoms of digoxin toxicity. May increase plasma concentrations of imipramine and desipramine. Fluoxetine, fluvoxamine, nefazodone, cimetidine, and oral contraceptives may increase concentrations. CYP3A inducers (eg, carbamazepine), propoxyphene, and smoking may decrease levels. May require dose adjustment or discontinuation with HIV protease inhibitors (eg, ritonavir).

PATIENT CONSIDERATIONS

Assessment: Assess for drug hypersensitivity, acute narrow-angle glaucoma, depression, suicidal ideation, renal/hepatic/pulmonary function, debilitation, history of alcohol/substance abuse, history of seizures/epilepsy, pregnancy/nursing status, and possible drug interactions. Assess for risk of dependence among panic disorder patients.

Monitoring: Monitor for dependence, relapse, rebound or withdrawal symptoms, early am anxiety and emergence of anxiety symptoms, CNS depression, episodes of hypomania/mania, suicidality, other treatment-emergent symptoms, and other adverse reactions. Monitor CBC, urinalysis, and blood chemistry periodically. Periodically reassess usefulness of therapy.

Counseling: Advise to take in the am and not crush or chew tabs. Advise to inform physician about any alcohol consumption and medicines taken and if nursing, pregnant, planning to be pregnant, or if pregnancy occurs while on therapy. Advise to avoid alcohol during treatment. Advise not to drive or operate dangerous machinery until becoming familiar with the effects of the medication. Advise not to increase/decrease dose or abruptly d/c therapy without consultation; instruct to follow gradual dosage-tapering schedule. Inform of risks associated with doses >4mg/day.

STORAGE: 25°C (77°F); excursions permitted to 15-30°C (59-86°F).

XARELTO – rivaroxaban

RX

Class: Selective factor Xa inhibitor

Premature discontinuation increases the risk of thrombotic events. If therapy is discontinued for a reason other than pathological bleeding or completion of a course of therapy, consider coverage w/ another anticoagulant. Epidural or spinal hematomas have occurred in patients treated w/ rivaroxaban who are receiving neuraxial anesthesia or undergoing spinal puncture; long-term or permanent paralysis may result. Use of indwelling epidural catheters, concomitant use of other drugs that affect hemostasis (eg, NSAIDs, platelet inhibitors, other anticoagulants), history of traumatic or repeated epidural or spinal punctures, history of spinal deformity or spinal surgery, or unknown optimal timing between the administration of therapy and neuraxial procedure, may increase the risk of developing epidural or spinal hematomas. Monitor frequently for signs/symptoms of neurological impairment; urgent treatment is necessary if neurological compromise occurs. Consider benefits and risks before neuraxial intervention in patients anticoagulated or to be anticoagulated for thromboprophylaxis.

ADULT DOSAGE

Reduce Risk of Stroke and Systemic Embolism in Nonvalvular Atrial Fibrillation

20mg qd w/ pm meal

Deep Vein Thrombosis/Pulmonary Embolism

Prophylaxis:
Following Hip or Knee Replacement Surgery:
10mg qd
Give initial dose 6-10 hrs after surgery provided that hemostasis has been established

Treatment Duration:
Hip Replacement Surgery: 35 days
Knee Replacement Surgery: 12 days

Treatment:
15mg bid w/ food for the first 21 days, then 20mg qd w/ food, at approx the same time each day

Reduction in Risk of Recurrence Following Initial 6 Months of Treatment:
20mg qd w/ food at approx the same time each day

Conversions

Switching from Warfarin:
D/C warfarin and start therapy as soon as INR is <3.0

PEDIATRIC DOSAGE

Pediatric use may not have been established

Switching to Warfarin:
No clinical trial data available to guide conversion; d/c rivaroxaban and begin both a parenteral anticoagulant and warfarin at the time the next dose of rivaroxaban would have been taken

Switching to Other Anticoagulants other than Warfarin:
If switching to rapid onset anticoagulant, d/c rivaroxaban and give 1st dose of other anticoagulant (oral or parenteral) at the time that the next dose would have been taken

Switching from Other Anticoagulants other than Warfarin:
Start rivaroxaban 0-2 hrs prior to next scheduled pm dose of drug (eg, low molecular weight heparin or non-warfarin oral anticoagulant) and omit administration of other anticoagulant
For continuous IV infusion of unfractionated heparin, stop infusion and start rivaroxaban at the same time

Missed Dose

Receiving 15mg BID:
Take rivaroxaban immediately to ensure intake of 30mg/day; may take two 15mg tabs at once
Continue w/ regular 15mg bid as recommended on following day

Receiving 20mg, 15mg, or 10mg QD:
Take missed dose immediately

DOSING CONSIDERATIONS

Renal Impairment

Reduction in Risk of Stroke in Nonvalvular A-Fib:
CrCl 15-50mL/min: 15mg qd w/ pm meal

Hepatic Impairment

Moderate (Child-Pugh B) and Severe (Child-Pugh C): Avoid use

Other Important Considerations

Surgery/Intervention:
If anticoagulation must be discontinued w/ surgery or other procedures, d/c therapy at least 24 hrs before procedure to reduce the risk of bleeding
Weigh risk of bleeding against urgency of intervention to decide whether procedure should be delayed until 24 hrs after last dose
After procedure, restart therapy as soon as adequate hemostasis has been established

ADMINISTRATION

Oral route

15mg and 20mg tabs should be taken w/ food, while 10mg tabs can be taken w/ or w/o food.

Unable to Swallow Whole Tabs

Tabs may be crushed and mixed w/ applesauce immediately prior to use.
After administering crushed 15mg or 20mg tabs, immediately follow dose w/ food.

Administration via NG Tube/Gastric Feeding Tube

Tabs may be crushed and suspended in 50mL of water after confirming gastric placement of tube.
Avoid administration distal to the stomach.
After administration of 15mg or 20mg tabs, immediately follow dose w/ enteral feeding.

Stability

Crushed tabs are stable in water and applesauce for up to 4 hrs.

HOW SUPPLIED

Tab: 10mg, 15mg, 20mg; (Starter Pack) 15mg [42[s]], 20mg [9[s]]

CONTRAINDICATIONS

Active pathological bleeding, severe hypersensitivity reaction to rivaroxaban (eg, anaphylactic reactions).

WARNINGS/PRECAUTIONS

May increase risk of bleeding and cause serious or fatal bleeding; risk of thrombotic events should be weighed against risk of bleeding before initiation of treatment. Promptly evaluate any signs/symptoms of blood loss and consider the need for blood replacement; d/c in patients w/ active pathological hemorrhage. Specific antidote for rivaroxaban is not available; not expected to be dialyzable because of high plasma protein binding. An epidural catheter should not be removed earlier than 18 hrs after last administration of therapy. The next dose should not be administered earlier than 6 hrs after catheter removal. If traumatic puncture occurs, delay administration for 24 hrs. Avoid use in the treatment of deep vein thrombosis (DVT)/pulmonary embolism (PE), reduction in risk of recurrence of DVT/PE, and for prophylaxis of DVT following hip or knee replacement surgery in patients w/ CrCl <30mL/min or for nonvalvular A-fib in patients w/ CrCl <15mL/min. Monitor for signs/symptoms of blood loss in patients w/ CrCl 30-50mL/min in prophylaxis of DVT following hip or knee replacement surgery. D/C if acute renal failure develops while on therapy in patients taking rivaroxaban for nonvalvular A-fib or DVT prophylaxis. Avoid w/ any hepatic disease associated w/ coagulopathy. Should only be used in pregnant women if the potential benefit justifies the potential risk to the mother and fetus; promptly evaluate any signs/symptoms suggesting blood loss. Not recommended in patients w/ prosthetic heart valves. Initiation of treatment is not recommended acutely as an alternative to unfractionated heparin in patients w/ PE who present w/ hemodynamic instability or who may receive thrombolysis or pulmonary embolectomy.

ADVERSE REACTIONS

Bleeding events, back pain.

DRUG INTERACTIONS

See Boxed Warning. May result in changes in exposure w/ inhibitors/inducers of CYP3A4/5, CYP2J2, and P-gp and ATP-binding cassette G2 transporters. Increased exposure w/ combined P-gp and CYP3A4 inhibitors (eg, ketoconazole, ritonavir, clarithromycin) may increase bleeding risk; avoid w/ combined P-gp and strong CYP3A4 inhibitors (eg, ketoconazole, itraconazole, lopinavir/ritonavir). Avoid w/ combined P-gp and strong CYP3A4 inducers (eg, carbamazepine, phenytoin, rifampin); may decrease exposure and efficacy. Concomitant single dose of enoxaparin resulted in an additive effect on anti-factor Xa activity. Concomitant single dose of warfarin resulted in an additive effect on factor Xa inhibition and PT. Concomitant use of other drugs that impair hemostasis (eg, P2Y12 platelet inhibitors, other antithrombotic agents, fibrinolytic therapy, NSAIDs/ASA) increases the risk of bleeding. May increase bleeding time w/ clopidogrel. Avoid concurrent use w/ other anticoagulants due to increased bleeding risk unless benefit outweighs risk. May increase exposure and possible increase bleeding risk w/ combined P-gp and moderate CYP3A4 inhibitors (eg, diltiazem, dronedarone, erythromycin) in renally impaired patients; avoid use in patients w/ CrCl 15-80mL/min who are receiving concomitant combined P-gp and moderate CYP3A4 inhibitors unless potential benefit justifies risk.

PATIENT CONSIDERATIONS

Assessment: Assess for known hypersensitivity, active pathological bleeding, risk factors for developing epidural or spinal hematomas, conditions that may increase risk of bleeding, renal/hepatic impairment, prosthetic heart valves, PE w/ hemodynamic instability or patients who may receive thrombolysis or pulmonary embolectomy, pregnancy/nursing status, and possible drug interactions.

Monitoring: Monitor for signs/symptoms of bleeding, stroke, thrombotic events, and other adverse reactions. In patients undergoing neuraxial anesthesia or spinal puncture, monitor for epidural or spinal hematomas and neurological impairment. Monitor renal function periodically.

Counseling: Instruct to take only ud. Advise to follow missed dosing instructions. Advise not to d/c w/o consulting physician. Advise to report any unusual bleeding or bruising. Inform that it may take longer than usual to stop bleeding, and that patients may bruise and/or bleed more easily. Advise patients who had neuraxial anesthesia or spinal puncture to watch for signs and symptoms of spinal/epidural hematoma, especially if concomitantly taking NSAIDs or platelet inhibitors; instruct to contact physician immediately if symptoms occur. Instruct to inform physician about therapy before any invasive procedure. Instruct to inform physicians and dentists if taking, or planning to take, any prescription or OTC drugs or herbals. Advise to inform physician immediately if nursing/pregnant or intending to nurse or become pregnant. Advise pregnant women receiving therapy to immediately report to the physician any bleeding or symptoms of blood loss.

STORAGE: 25°C (77°F); excursions permitted to 15-30°C (59-86°F).

XARTEMIS XR – acetaminophen/oxycodone hydrochloride CII

Class: Opioid analgesic

Exposes users to the risk of opioid addiction, abuse, and misuse, leading to overdose and death; assess each patient's risk prior to prescribing, and monitor regularly for development of these behaviors/conditions. Serious, life-threatening, or fatal respiratory depression may occur; monitor for respiratory depression, especially during initiation or following a dose increase. Accidental ingestion, especially in children, can result in a fatal overdose of oxycodone. Prolonged use during pregnancy can result in neonatal opioid withdrawal syndrome; advise pregnant women of the risk and ensure availability of appropriate treatment. Associated with cases of acute liver failure, at times resulting in liver transplant and death. Most cases of liver injury are associated with acetaminophen (APAP) use at doses that exceed the max daily limit, and often involve >1 APAP-containing product.

ADULT DOSAGE

Acute Pain

Use when alternative treatment options are inadequate

1st Opioid Analgesic:

Usual: 2 tabs q12h

May administer 2nd dose of 2 tabs as early as 8 hrs after initial dose, if needed

Subsequent doses are to be administered 2 tabs q12h

Max: Do not exceed 4000mg of acetaminophen

PEDIATRIC DOSAGE

Pediatric use may not have been established

DOSING CONSIDERATIONS

Renal Impairment

Initial: 1 tab and adjust prn

Hepatic Impairment

Initial: 1 tab and adjust prn

Discontinuation

Use a gradual downward titration of the dose of 50% every 2-4 days to prevent signs/symptoms of withdrawal

Do not abruptly d/c

ADMINISTRATION

Oral route

Swallow tab whole, one at a time w/ enough water to ensure complete swallowing

Do not break, chew, crush, cut, dissolve, or split

May take w/ or w/o food

HOW SUPPLIED

Tab, Extended-Release: (Oxycodone/APAP) 7.5mg/325mg

CONTRAINDICATIONS

Known hypersensitivity to oxycodone, acetaminophen, or any other component of this product, significant respiratory depression, acute or severe bronchial asthma or hypercarbia, known/suspected paralytic ileus.

WARNINGS/PRECAUTIONS

Reserve for use in patients for whom alternative treatment options (eg, nonopioid analgesics) are ineffective, not tolerated, or would be otherwise inadequate. Not interchangeable with other oxycodone/APAP products. Overestimating dose when converting from another opioid product may result in fatal overdose with 1st dose. Life-threatening respiratory depression is more likely to occur in elderly, cachectic, or debilitated patients. Consider alternative nonopioid analgesics in patients with significant chronic obstructive pulmonary disease or cor pulmonale, and in patients having a substantially decreased respiratory reserve, hypoxia, hypercarbia, or preexisting respiratory depression. Increased risk of acute liver failure in patients with underlying liver disease. May cause serious skin reactions (eg, acute generalized exanthematous pustulosis, Stevens-Johnson syndrome, toxic epidermal necrolysis), which can be fatal; d/c at the 1st appearance of skin rash or any other sign of hypersensitivity. Respiratory depressant effects and CSF pressure elevation capacity may be markedly exaggerated in the presence of head injury, other intracranial lesions, or preexisting increased intracranial pressure (ICP). May obscure clinical course of head injury and acute abdominal conditions. May cause severe hypotension; caution with circulatory shock. May produce orthostatic hypotension in ambulatory patients. APAP use associated with hypersensitivity and anaphylaxis; avoid in patients with APAP allergy. Consider use of an alternative analgesic in patients who have difficulty swallowing and in patients at risk for underlying GI disorders resulting in a small GI lumen. Monitor for decreased bowel motility in postoperative patients. May cause spasm of the sphincter of Oddi; monitor patients with biliary tract disease, including acute pancreatitis. May impair mental/physical abilities. Physical dependence and tolerance may occur; do not stop therapy abruptly. Not recommended for use during or immediately prior to labor. Caution with renal/hepatic impairment and in elderly.

ADVERSE REACTIONS

Respiratory depression, acute liver failure, N/V, dizziness, headache, constipation, somnolence.

DRUG INTERACTIONS

Oxycodone: Concomitant use with alcohol or other CNS depressants (eg, sedatives, anxiolytics, hypnotics, neuroleptics, other opioids) may cause hypotension, profound sedation, coma, respiratory depression, and death; reduce dose of 1 or both agents. CYP3A4 inhibitors (eg, macrolides, azole antifungals, protease inhibitors) may increase plasma levels and prolong opioid effects; these effects could be more pronounced with concomitant use of CYP2D6 (amiodarone, quinidine, antidepressants) and 3A4 inhibitors. CYP450 inducers (eg, rifampin, carbamazepine, phenytoin) may induce metabolism, leading to a decrease in plasma concentration and efficacy. Caution when initiating treatment in patients currently taking or discontinuing CYP3A4 inhibitors or inducers; evaluate these patients at frequent intervals and consider dose adjustments until stable drug effects are achieved. May enhance the neuromuscular blocking action of skeletal muscle relaxants and produce an increased degree of respiratory depression. MAOIs reported to intensify effects causing anxiety, confusion, and significant respiratory depression or coma; not recommended with MAOIs or within 14 days of stopping such treatment. Caution with agonist/antagonist analgesics (eg, pentazocine, nalbuphine, butorphanol, buprenorphine); may reduce analgesic effect and/or may precipitate withdrawal symptoms. Concurrent use with anticholinergics or other medications with anticholinergic activity may result in increased risk of urinary retention and/or severe constipation, which may lead to paralytic ileus. APAP: Increased risk of acute liver failure with alcohol. Do not use concomitantly with other APAP-containing products.

PATIENT CONSIDERATIONS

Assessment: Assess for risks for opioid abuse, addiction, or misuse, pain type/severity, prior opioid therapy, patient's general condition and medical status, respiratory depression, COPD, cor pulmonale, decreased respiratory reserve, hypoxia, hypercapnia, renal/hepatic impairment, paralytic ileus, acute/severe bronchial asthma, biliary tract disease, increased ICP, history of hypersensitivity to drug, any other conditions where treatment is contraindicated or cautioned, pregnancy/nursing status, and possible drug interactions.

Monitoring: Monitor for development of addiction, abuse, or misuse, physical dependence, tolerance, acute liver failure, respiratory depression, hypotension, skin/hypersensitivity/anaphylactic reactions, decreased bowel motility in postoperative patients, biliary tract disease, acute pancreatitis, and other adverse reactions. Periodically reevaluate therapy.

Counseling: Inform that medication is not interchangeable with other forms of oxycodone/APAP, that it is a narcotic pain reliever, and that it must be taken only ud. Instruct not to take >2 tabs at once unless instructed by physician. Instruct not to adjust dose without consulting physician. Instruct not to take >4000mg of APAP/day and to call physician if more than the recommended dose was taken. Inform that use of medication, even when taken ud, may result in addiction, abuse, and misuse. Instruct not to share with others and to take steps to protect from theft or misuse. Inform of the risk of life-threatening respiratory depression; advise how to recognize respiratory depression and when to seek medical attention. Inform that accidental exposure, especially in children, may result in respiratory depression or death. Instruct to dispose of unused tab by flushing down the toilet. Instruct females of reproductive potential who become or are planning to become pregnant to consult a physician prior to initiating or continuing therapy; inform that prolonged use during pregnancy can result in neonatal opioid withdrawal syndrome. Advise women not to breastfeed during therapy. Inform that potentially serious additive effects may occur if used with alcohol or other CNS depressants; instruct not to use such drugs unless supervised by a physician. Inform that drug may cause drowsiness, dizziness, or lightheadedness, and may impair mental and/or physical abilities; advise to refrain from any potentially dangerous activity until it is established that they are not adversely affected. Counsel patients on the possibility of withdrawal symptoms with cessation of therapy. Advise of the potential for severe constipation and other adverse reactions.

STORAGE: 25°C (77°F); excursions permitted to 15-30°C (59-86°F).

XELJANZ — tofacitinib

RX

Class: Kinase inhibitor

Increased risk for developing serious infections (eg, active tuberculosis [TB], invasive fungal infections, bacterial/viral infections due to opportunistic pathogens) that may lead to hospitalization or death. Most patients who developed these infections were taking concomitant immunosuppressants (eg, methotrexate [MTX], corticosteroids). If a serious infection develops, interrupt treatment until infection is controlled. Test for latent TB prior to and during therapy; initiate latent TB treatment prior to therapy. Consider risks and benefits prior to initiating therapy in patients w/ chronic or recurrent infection. Monitor for development of signs and symptoms of infection during and after treatment. Lymphoma and other malignancies reported. Increased rate of Epstein-Barr virus-associated post-transplant lymphoproliferative disorder observed in renal transplant patients w/ concomitant immunosuppressive medications.

ADULT DOSAGE

Rheumatoid Arthritis

As monotherapy or in combination w/ methotrexate (MTX) or other nonbiologic disease-modifying antirheumatic drugs for moderately to severely active rheumatoid arthritis in patients who have had an inadequate response or intolerance to MTX

5mg bid

PEDIATRIC DOSAGE

Pediatric use may not have been established

DOSING CONSIDERATIONS

Concomitant Medications

Potent CYP3A4 Inhibitors: Reduce dose to 5mg qd

≥1 Concomitant Medications Resulting in Both Moderate CYP3A4 Inhibition and Potent CYP2C19 Inhibition: Reduce dose to 5mg qd

Potent CYP3A4 Inducers: Not recommended for use

Renal Impairment

Moderate or Severe: Reduce dose to 5mg qd

Hepatic Impairment

Moderate: Reduce dose to 5mg qd

Severe: Not recommended for use

Adverse Reactions

Lymphopenia:

Absolute Lymphocyte Count <500 cells/mm^3: Do not initiate treatment

Absolute Lymphocyte Count ≥500 cells/mm^3: Maintain dose

Absolute Lymphocyte Count <500 cells/mm^3 (Confirmed by Repeat Testing): D/C treatment

Neutropenia:

ANC <1000 cells/mm^3: Do not initiate treatment

ANC >1000 cells/mm^3: Maintain dose

ANC 500-1000 cells/mm^3: For persistent decreases in this range, interrupt dosing until ANC is >1000; when ANC is >1000, resume at 5mg bid

ANC <500 cells/mm^3 (Confirmed by Repeat Testing): D/C treatment

Anemia:

Hgb <9g/dL: Do not initiate treatment

Hgb ≤2g/dL Decrease and ≥9g/dL: Maintain dose

Hgb >2g/dL Decrease or <8g/dL (Confirmed by Repeat Testing): Interrupt administration until Hgb values have normalized

ADMINISTRATION

Oral route

Take w/ or w/o food

HOW SUPPLIED

Tab: 5mg

WARNINGS/PRECAUTIONS

Avoid w/ active, serious infection, including localized infections. Caution in patients w/ chronic/recurrent infections, who have been exposed to TB, w/ history of a serious/opportunistic infection, who have resided in or traveled to areas of endemic TB/mycoses, or w/ predisposing factors to infection. Viral reactivation, including herpes virus reactivation (eg, herpes zoster), reported; screen for viral hepatitis before starting therapy. Increased risk of herpes zoster; risk appears to be higher in patients treated in Japan. Non-melanoma skin cancers reported; periodic skin examination is recommended for patients at increased risk for skin cancer. Consider risks and benefits of treatment in patients w/ a known malignancy other than a successfully treated non-melanoma skin cancer or when considering continuing treatment in patients who develop a malignancy. GI perforation reported; caution in patients w/ increased risk for GI perforation (eg, history of diverticulitis). Associated w/ initial lymphocytosis, neutropenia, increases in lipid parameters, and liver enzyme elevation. Interrupt treatment if drug-induced liver injury is suspected. Interrupt treatment if an opportunistic infection or sepsis occurs. Caution in elderly and diabetes patients.

ADVERSE REACTIONS

Infections (eg, URTIs, nasopharyngitis), lymphoma, malignancies, diarrhea, headache.

DRUG INTERACTIONS

See Boxed Warning and Dosing Considerations. Avoid w/ live vaccines. Increased immunosuppression w/ potent immunosuppressive drugs (eg, azathioprine, tacrolimus, cyclosporine); concurrent use w/ potent immunosuppressants (eg, azathioprine, cyclosporine) or biologic DMARDs is not recommended. Increased exposure w/ potent CYP3A4 inhibitors (eg, ketoconazole), and drugs that are both moderate CYP3A4 inhibitors and potent CYP2C19 inhibitors

X

(eg, fluconazole). Decreased exposure resulting in loss of or reduced clinical response to treatment w/ potent CYP3A4 inducers (eg, rifampin).

PATIENT CONSIDERATIONS

Assessment: Assess for infections (eg, bacteria, fungi, viruses), including latent TB, predisposing factors to infection, active hepatic disease or impairment, known malignancy, risk of GI perforation, diabetes, pregnancy/nursing status, and possible drug interactions. Obtain baseline absolute lymphocyte count, ANC, and lipid and Hgb levels.

Monitoring: Monitor for TB (active, reactivation, or latent), invasive fungal infections, or bacterial, viral, and other opportunistic infections during and after therapy. Monitor for viral reactivation, lymphoma, malignancy, lymphoproliferative disorders, GI perforations, and other adverse reactions. Monitor absolute lymphocyte counts every 3 months. Monitor neutrophil counts and Hgb after 4-8 weeks of treatment and every 3 months thereafter. Routinely monitor LFTs. Monitor lipid parameters approx 4-8 weeks following initiation. Perform periodic skin examination in patients at increased risk of skin cancer.

Counseling: Advise about potential risks/benefits of therapy. Inform that therapy may lower resistance to infection; advise patients not to start taking medication if they have an active infection. Instruct to contact physician immediately if symptoms suggesting an infection appear during treatment to ensure rapid evaluation and appropriate treatment. Advise that the risk of herpes zoster is increased in patients treated w/ therapy. Inform that medication may increase risk of lymphoma and other cancers; instruct to inform physician of any type of cancer that they have ever had. Inform that certain lab tests may be affected and that blood tests are required before and during treatment. Inform that medication should not be used during pregnancy unless clearly necessary; advise to inform physician right away if pregnant. Advise to enroll in the pregnancy registry for pregnant women who have taken medication during pregnancy.

STORAGE: 20-25°C (68-77°F).

XELODA – capecitabine RX

Class: Fluoropyrimidine carbamate

Altered coagulation parameters and/or bleeding, including death, reported w/ concomitant coumarin-derivative anticoagulants (eg, warfarin, phenprocoumon). Monitor PT and INR frequently in order to adjust anticoagulant dose accordingly. Postmarketing reports showed clinically significant increases in PT and INR in patients who were stabilized on anticoagulants at start of therapy. Age >60 yrs and a diagnosis of cancer independently predispose to an increased risk of coagulopathy.

ADULT DOSAGE

Metastatic Colorectal Cancer

1st-line treatment of metastatic colorectal carcinoma and as a single agent for adjuvant treatment in patients w/ Dukes' C colon cancer who have undergone complete resection of the primary tumor when treatment w/ fluoropyrimidine therapy alone is preferred

Monotherapy:
Usual: 1250mg/m^2 bid for 2 weeks followed by a 1-week rest period, given as 3-week cycles

Adjuvant to Dukes' C Colon Cancer:
1250mg/m^2 bid for 2 weeks followed by 1-week rest period, given as 3-week cycles for total of 8 cycles (24 weeks)

Refer to PI for dose calculations based on BSA

Metastatic Breast Cancer

Treatment of metastatic breast cancer in combination w/ docetaxel after failure of prior anthracycline-containing chemotherapy. Monotherapy treatment of metastatic breast cancer in patients resistant to both paclitaxel and anthracycline-containing chemotherapy regimen or resistant to paclitaxel and for whom further anthracycline therapy is not indicated

Monotherapy:
1250mg/m^2 bid for 2 weeks followed by a

PEDIATRIC DOSAGE

Pediatric use may not have been established

1-week rest period, given as 3-week cycles

Combination w/ Docetaxel:
Usual: 1250mg/m^2 bid for 2 weeks followed by 1-week rest period, combined w/ docetaxel at 75mg/m^2 as a 1-hr IV infusion every 3 weeks
Premedication:
Start prior to docetaxel administration

Refer to PI for dose calculations based on BSA

DOSING CONSIDERATIONS

Concomitant Medications

Phenytoin and Coumarin-Derivative Anticoagulants: May need to reduce dose of phenytoin and coumarin-derivative anticoagulants

Renal Impairment

Moderate (CrCl 30-50mL/min): Reduce to 75% of starting dose when used as monotherapy or in combination w/ docetaxel (from 1250mg/m^2 to 950mg/m^2 bid)

Adverse Reactions

Toxicity NCIC Grade 2:
1st Appearance: Interrupt until resolved to Grade 0-1, then give 100% of dose
2nd Appearance: Interrupt until resolved to Grade 0-1, then give 75% of dose
3rd Appearance: Interrupt until resolved to Grade 0-1, then give 50% of dose
4th Appearance: D/C treatment permanently

Toxicity NCIC Grade 3:
1st Appearance: Interrupt until resolved to Grade 0-1, then give 75% of dose
2nd Appearance: Interrupt until resolved to Grade 0-1, then give 50% of dose
3rd Appearance: D/C treatment permanently

Toxicity NCIC Grade 4:
1st Appearance: D/C permanently or if physician deems it to be in the best interest to continue, interrupt until resolved to Grade 0-1, then give 50% of dose

Refer to PI for docetaxel dose reductions when used in combination w/ capecitabine

ADMINISTRATION

Oral route

Swallow tabs whole w/ water w/in 30 min pc; do not cut or crush

HOW SUPPLIED

Tab: 150mg, 500mg

CONTRAINDICATIONS

Severe renal impairment (CrCl <30mL/min); known hypersensitivity to capecitabine, any components of the medication, or 5-fluorouracil (5-FU).

WARNINGS/PRECAUTIONS

May induce diarrhea; give fluid and electrolyte replacement w/ severe diarrhea. Cardiotoxicity (eg, MI/ischemia, angina) observed; may be more common in patients w/ a prior history of coronary artery disease (CAD). Increased risk for acute early-onset of toxicity and severe, life-threatening, or fatal adverse reactions (eg, mucositis, diarrhea, neutropenia, neurotoxicity) in patients w/ certain homozygous or certain compound heterozygous mutations in the dihydropyrimidine dehydrogenase (DPD) gene that results in complete or near complete absence of DPD activity; withhold or permanently d/c therapy based on clinical assessment of the onset, duration, and severity of the observed toxicities. Patients w/ partial DPD activity may also have increased risk of severe, life-threatening, or fatal adverse reactions. Dehydration reported and may cause acute renal failure; patients w/ preexisting compromised renal function are at higher risk. Patients w/ anorexia, asthenia, N/V, or diarrhea may rapidly become dehydrated; monitor during administration and do not restart treatment until patient is rehydrated and any precipitating causes have been corrected or controlled. Caution w/ mild and moderate renal impairment. Severe mucocutaneous reactions (eg, Stevens-Johnson syndrome, toxic epidermal necrolysis) may occur; permanently d/c in patients who experience a severe mucocutaneous reaction possibly attributable to treatment. Hand-and-foot syndrome may occur. Hyperbilirubinemia reported; interrupt therapy if drug-related Grade 3 or 4 elevations in bilirubin occur until the hyperbilirubinemia decreases to ≤3X ULN. Necrotizing enterocolitis, neutropenia, thrombocytopenia, anemia, and decreases in Hgb reported. Avoid w/ baseline neutrophil counts of <1.5 x 10^9/L and/or thrombocyte counts of <100 x 10^9/L. Caution in elderly; patients ≥80 yrs of age may experience greater incidence of Grade 3 or 4 adverse events. Caution w/ mild to moderate hepatic dysfunction due to liver metastases. May cause fetal harm.

ADVERSE REACTIONS

Diarrhea, hand-and-foot syndrome, asthenia, pyrexia, anemia, N/V, fatigue, dermatitis, thrombocytopenia, constipation, taste disturbance, stomatitis, alopecia, abdominal pain, decreased appetite.

DRUG INTERACTIONS
See Boxed Warning and Dosing Considerations. Higher risk of dehydration w/ known nephrotoxic agents. May increase the mean AUC of S-warfarin. May increase phenytoin levels. Leucovorin may increase levels and toxicity of 5-FU. Caution w/ CYP2C9 substrates.

PATIENT CONSIDERATIONS

Assessment: Assess for hypersensitivity to drug or to 5-FU, complete or near complete absence of DPD activity, partial DPD activity, renal/hepatic dysfunction, history of CAD, pregnancy/nursing status, and possible drug interactions. Obtain baseline neutrophil/thrombocyte counts.

Monitoring: Monitor for severe diarrhea, necrotizing enterocolitis, cardiotoxicity, acute early-onset of toxicity, severe/life-threatening/fatal adverse reactions, hand-and-foot syndrome, hyperbilirubinemia, neutropenia, thrombocytopenia, anemia, decreases in Hgb, severe toxicity, dehydration, acute renal failure, severe mucocutaneous reactions, and other adverse reactions. Monitor PT and INR frequently w/ concomitant oral coumarin-derivative anticoagulant therapy.

Counseling: Instruct to d/c therapy and contact physician immediately if moderate/severe toxicity, Grade ≥2 diarrhea/stomatitis, or severe bloody diarrhea w/ severe abdominal pain and fever is experienced. Advise to notify physician if patient has known DPD deficiency; inform that patient is at an increased risk of acute early-onset of toxicity and severe, life-threatening, or fatal adverse reactions if patient has complete or near complete absence of DPD activity. Instruct to d/c therapy immediately in patients experiencing Grade ≥2 dehydration/nausea/vomiting/hand-and-foot syndrome. Instruct to contact physician immediately if fever or infection occurs. Counsel about pregnancy risks; instruct to avoid pregnancy during therapy.

STORAGE: 25°C (77°F); excursions permitted to 15-30°C (59-86°F). Keep tightly closed.

XENICAL – orlistat

RX

Class: Lipase inhibitor

ADULT DOSAGE

Obesity

Obesity management in patients w/ an initial BMI ≥30kg/m² or ≥27kg/m² in the presence of other risk factors

120mg tid w/ each main meal containing fat
Max: 120mg tid

PEDIATRIC DOSAGE

Obesity

Obesity management in patients w/ an initial BMI ≥30kg/m² or ≥27kg/m² in the presence of other risk factors

≥12 Years:
120mg tid w/ each main meal containing fat
Max: 120mg tid

ADMINISTRATION
Oral route
Administer during or up to 1 hr after the meal.
Use w/ nutritionally balanced, reduced-calorie diet that contains 30% calories from fat; distribute daily intake of fat, carbohydrate, and protein over 3 main meals.
Omit dose if a meal is missed or contains no fat.

HOW SUPPLIED
Cap: 120mg

CONTRAINDICATIONS
Pregnancy, chronic malabsorption syndrome, cholestasis, known hypersensitivity to orlistat or to any component of the product.

WARNINGS/PRECAUTIONS
Weight loss may affect glycemic control in patients w/ diabetes mellitus. Severe liver injury w/ hepatocellular necrosis or acute hepatic failure reported, w/ some cases resulting in liver transplant or death; d/c therapy and other suspect medications immediately and obtain LFTs. May increase levels of urinary oxalate; caution w/ a history of hyperoxaluria or calcium oxalate nephrolithiasis. Cases of oxalate nephrolithiasis and oxalate nephropathy w/ renal failure reported; monitor renal function. May increase risk of cholelithiasis due to substantial weight loss. Exclude organic causes of obesity (eg, hypothyroidism). GI events may increase w/ a high-fat diet (>30% total daily calories from fat).

ADVERSE REACTIONS
Oily spotting, flatus w/ discharge, fecal urgency, fatty/oily stool, oily evacuation, increased defecation, fecal incontinence.

DRUG INTERACTIONS
Reduced cyclosporine plasma levels reported; take cyclosporine at least 3 hrs before or after administration. Reduced absorption of some fat-soluble vitamins and β-carotene supplement reported. Inhibited absorption of vitamin E acetate supplement reported. Hypothyroidism reported

w/ levothyroxine; administer at least 4 hrs apart and monitor for thyroid function changes. Vitamin K absorption may be decreased; monitor closely for changes in coagulation parameters w/ chronic stable doses of warfarin. Reduced exposure of amiodarone and its metabolite reported; may reduce therapeutic effect of amiodarone. Convulsions reported w/ antiepileptic drugs; monitor for possible changes in the frequency and/or severity of convulsions. May require reduction in dosage of oral hypoglycemic agents (eg, sulfonylureas) or insulin in diabetics.

PATIENT CONSIDERATIONS

Assessment: Assess for hypersensitivity to the drug, chronic malabsorption syndrome, cholestasis, history of hyperoxaluria or calcium oxalate nephrolithiasis, organic causes of obesity (eg, hypothyroidism), pregnancy/nursing status, and possible drug interactions. Obtain baseline weight, FPG, and lipid profile.

Monitoring: Monitor for hepatic dysfunction, cholelithiasis, signs/symptoms of hypersensitivity reactions, GI events, and other adverse events. Monitor renal function in patients at risk for renal insufficiency. Monitor closely for changes in coagulation parameters w/ chronic stable doses of warfarin.

Counseling: Advise to inform physician if taking cyclosporine, β-carotene or vitamin E supplements, levothyroxine, warfarin, antiepileptic drugs, or amiodarone, due to potential interactions. Inform of the common adverse events (eg, oily spotting, flatus w/ discharge, fecal urgency) associated w/ the use of the drug. Inform of the potential risks that include lowered absorption of fat-soluble vitamins and potential liver injury, increased urinary oxalate, and cholelithiasis. Inform of the potential benefits that therapy may result in, such as weight loss and improvement in obesity-related risk factors. Instruct to report any symptoms of hepatic dysfunction while on therapy. Instruct patient to take drug ud w/ meals or up to 1 hr pc. Advise to take a multivitamin qd at least 2 hrs before or after administration, or at hs. Instruct to adhere to dietary guidelines.

STORAGE: 25°C (77°F); excursions permitted to 15-30°C (59-86°F).

XERESE — acyclovir/hydrocortisone

RX

Class: Anti-infective/corticosteroid

ADULT DOSAGE

Herpes Labialis (Cold Sores)

Early treatment of recurrent herpes labialis to reduce the likelihood of ulcerative cold sores and to shorten the lesion healing time

Apply a quantity sufficient to cover the affected area (including outer margin) 5X/day for 5 days

Initiate therapy as early as possible after the 1st signs/symptoms (eg, during the prodrome or when lesions appear)

PEDIATRIC DOSAGE

Herpes Labialis (Cold Sores)

Early treatment of recurrent herpes labialis to reduce the likelihood of ulcerative cold sores and to shorten the lesion healing time

≥6 Years:

Apply a quantity sufficient to cover the affected area (including outer margin) 5X/day for 5 days

Initiate therapy as early as possible after the 1st signs/symptoms (eg, during the prodrome or when lesions appear)

ADMINISTRATION

Topical route

HOW SUPPLIED

Cre: (Acyclovir/Hydrocortisone) 5%/1% [5g]

WARNINGS/PRECAUTIONS

For cutaneous use only. Do not use in the eye, inside the mouth or nose, or on the genitals. Other orofacial lesions may be difficult to distinguish from a cold sore; monitor for cold sores that fail to heal within 2 weeks. Has a potential for irritation and contact sensitization.

ADVERSE REACTIONS

Application-site reactions (eg, drying/flaking of skin, burning/tingling, erythema, pigmentation changes, inflammation).

PATIENT CONSIDERATIONS

Assessment: Assess for type of lesions (eg, bacterial, fungal infections), and pregnancy/nursing status.

Monitoring: Monitor for clinical response, irritation, contact sensitization, and other adverse reactions.

Counseling: Inform that medication is not a cure for cold sores and it is for cutaneous use only for herpes labialis of the lips and around the mouth. Advise not to use in the eye, inside the mouth/nose, or on genitals. Counsel to use ud. Advise to avoid unnecessary rubbing of the affected area to avoid aggravating or transferring the infection. Instruct to seek medical advice when a cold sore fails to heal within 2 weeks. Encourage immunocompromised patients to consult a physician concerning the treatment of any infection.

STORAGE: 20-25°C (68-77°F); excursions permitted to 15-30°C (59-86°F). Do not freeze.

XGEVA — denosumab

RX

Class: IgG_2 monoclonal antibody

ADULT DOSAGE

Bone Metastasis from Solid Tumors

Prevention of Skeletal-Related Events:

120mg SQ every 4 weeks

Giant Cell Tumor of Bone

Treatment of tumor that is unresectable or where surgical resection is likely to result in severe morbidity

120mg SQ every 4 weeks w/ additional 120mg doses on Days 8 and 15 of the 1st month of therapy

Hypercalcemia of Malignancy

Refractory to Bisphosphonate Therapy:

120mg SQ every 4 weeks w/ additional 120mg doses on Days 8 and 15 of the 1st month of therapy

PEDIATRIC DOSAGE

Giant Cell Tumor of Bone

Treatment of tumor that is unresectable or where surgical resection is likely to result in severe morbidity

Adolescents (Skeletally Mature):

120mg SQ every 4 weeks w/ additional 120mg doses on Days 8 and 15 of the 1st month of therapy

ADMINISTRATION

SQ route

Administer in the upper arm, upper thigh, or abdomen

Remove from refrigerator and bring to room temperature (up to 25°C [77°F]) prior to administration; do not warm any other way

Use 27-gauge needle to withdraw and inject entire vial contents

Do not re-enter vial; discard vial after single-use or entry

HOW SUPPLIED

Inj: 120mg/1.7mL

CONTRAINDICATIONS

Hypocalcemia, known clinically significant hypersensitivity to denosumab.

WARNINGS/PRECAUTIONS

Do not give w/ other drugs that contain the same active ingredient (eg, Prolia). Hypersensitivity, including anaphylaxis, reported; initiate appropriate treatment and d/c therapy permanently if an anaphylactic or other clinically significant allergic reaction occurs. May cause severe symptomatic hypocalcemia, and fatal cases reported; increased risk in patients w/ increasing renal dysfunction, and w/ inadequate/no Ca^{2+} supplementation. Correct preexisting hypocalcemia prior to treatment, monitor Ca^{2+} levels throughout therapy especially in 1st weeks of initiation, and administer Ca^{2+}, Mg^{2+}, and vitamin D as necessary. Osteonecrosis of the jaw (ONJ) may occur; perform an oral exam and appropriate preventive dentistry prior to initiation of therapy and periodically during therapy. Avoid invasive dental procedures during therapy; consider temporary discontinuation of therapy if an invasive dental procedure must be performed. Atypical femoral fractures reported; evaluate patients w/ thigh/groin pain to rule out an incomplete femur fracture and consider interruption of therapy. May cause fetal harm.

ADVERSE REACTIONS

Fatigue/asthenia, hypophosphatemia, N/V, dyspnea, diarrhea, hypocalcemia, cough, headache, arthralgia, back pain, pain in extremity, decreased appetite, peripheral edema, anemia, constipation.

DRUG INTERACTIONS

Monitor Ca^{2+} levels more frequently w/ other drugs that can lower Ca^{2+} levels.

PATIENT CONSIDERATIONS

Assessment: Assess for preexisting or risk of hypocalcemia, drug hypersensitivity, pregnancy/nursing status, and possible drug interactions. Perform an oral exam and appropriate preventive dentistry.

Monitoring: Monitor for anaphylactic/hypersensitivity reaction, ONJ, atypical femoral fracture, and other adverse reactions. Monitor Ca^{2+} levels. Perform an oral exam and appropriate preventive dentistry periodically.

Counseling: Advise to contact physician if experiencing symptoms of hypersensitivity reaction, hypocalcemia, ONJ, or atypical femoral fracture; persistent pain or slow healing of the mouth or jaw after dental surgery; or if nursing. Advise of the need for proper oral hygiene and routine dental care, to inform dentist that patient is receiving the drug, and to avoid invasive dental procedures during treatment. Advise females of reproductive potential to use highly effective contraception during therapy, and for at least 5 months after the last dose of the drug; instruct to contact physician if they become pregnant or if a pregnancy is suspected during this time. Advise male patients of potential for fetal exposure to drug if they have unprotected sexual intercourse w/ a pregnant partner. Advise that denosumab is also marketed as Prolia; instruct to inform physician if taking Prolia.

STORAGE: 2-8°C (36-46°F). Do not freeze. Once removed from the refrigerator, do not expose to >25°C (77°F) or direct light; use w/in 14 days. Protect from heat. Avoid vigorous shaking.

XIAFLEX – collagenase clostridium histolyticum

RX

Class: Collagenase

Corporal rupture (penile fracture), penile ecchymoses or hematoma, sudden penile detumescence, and/or a penile "popping" sound or sensation, reported. Promptly evaluate signs/symptoms to assess for corporal rupture or severe penile hematoma that may require surgical intervention. Available for the treatment of Peyronie's disease only through a restricted program under a Risk Evaluation and Mitigation Strategy (REMS) called the Xiaflex REMS Program.

ADULT DOSAGE

Dupuytren's Contracture

W/ a Palpable Cord:

0.58mg per inj administered into a palpable cord w/ a contracture of a metacarpophalangeal (MP) joint or a proximal interphalangeal (PIP) joint

Approx 24-72 hrs after inj, perform a finger extension procedure if a contracture persists to facilitate cord disruption; refer to PI for instructions

4 weeks after inj and finger extension procedure, if a MP or PIP contracture remains, the cord may be re-injected w/ a single dose of 0.58mg and the finger extension procedure may be repeated (approx 24-72 hrs after inj); inj and finger extension procedures may be administered up to 3X per cord at approx 4-week intervals

Perform up to 2 inj in the same hand according to the inj procedure during a treatment visit; 2 palpable cords affecting 2 joints may be injected or 1 palpable cord affecting 2 joints in the same finger may be injected at 2 locations during a treatment visit

If patient has other palpable cords w/ contractures of MP or PIP joints, these cords may be injected at other treatment visits approx 4 weeks apart

Peyronie's Disease

Treatment of adult men w/ a palpable plaque and curvature deformity of at least 30° at the start of therapy

0.58mg per inj administered into a Peyronie's plaque; if >1 plaque is present, inject into the plaque causing the curvature deformity

A treatment course consists of a max of 4 treatment cycles; each treatment cycle consists of 2 inj procedures. The 2nd inj

PEDIATRIC DOSAGE

Pediatric use may not have been established

procedure is performed 1-3 days after the 1st

The penile modeling procedure is performed 1-3 days after the 2nd inj of the treatment cycle; refer to PI for instructions

The interval between treatment cycles is approx 6 weeks. The treatment course, therefore, consists of a max of 8 inj procedures and 4 modeling procedures

If the curvature deformity is <15° after the 1st, 2nd, or 3rd treatment cycle, or if further treatment is not clinically indicated, then the subsequent treatment cycles should not be administered

ADMINISTRATION

Intralesional route

Dupuytren's Contracture

Each vial and sterile diluent should only be used for a single inj; if 2 joints on the same hand are to be treated during a treatment visit, separate vials and syringes should be used for each reconstitution and inj

Reconstitution of Lyophilized Powder:

1. Before use, allow the vial containing the lyophilized powder and the vial containing the diluent for reconstitution to stand at room temperature for at least 15 min and no longer than 60 min
2. Use only the supplied diluent for reconstitution; the diluent contains Ca^{2+}, which is required for the activity of Xiaflex
3. Using a 1mL syringe w/ 0.01mL graduations and a 27-gauge 1/2-inch needle (not supplied), withdraw a volume of the diluent supplied, as follows:

For Cords Affecting a Metacarpophalangeal (MP) Joint: 0.39mL
For Cords Affecting a Proximal Interphalangeal (PIP) Joint: 0.31mL

4. Inject the diluent slowly into the sides of the vial containing the lyophilized powder
5. Slowly swirl the sol to ensure that all of the lyophilized powder has gone into sol; do not invert the vial or shake the sol
6. The reconstituted sol can be kept at room temperature for up to 1 hr or refrigerated for up to 4 hrs prior to administration; if the sol is refrigerated, allow it to return to room temperature for approx 15 min before use
7. Discard the syringe and needle used for reconstitution and the diluent vial

Preparation Prior to Inj:

1. Administration of a local anesthetic agent prior to inj is not recommended, as it may interfere w/ proper placement of the Xiaflex inj
2. If injecting into a cord affecting the PIP joint of the 5th finger, care should be taken to inject as close to the palmar digital crease as possible (as far proximal to the digital PIP joint crease), and the needle insertion should not be >2-3mm in depth. Tendon ruptures occurred after inj near the digital PIP joint crease
3. Reconfirm the cord(s) to be injected; the site chosen for each inj should be the area where the contracting cord is maximally separated from the underlying flexor tendons and where the skin is not intimately adhered to the cord
4. Apply an antiseptic at the inj site and allow the skin to dry

Inj Procedure:

1. Using a new 1mL hubless syringe that contains 0.01mL graduations w/ a permanently fixed, 27-gauge 1/2-inch needle (not supplied), withdraw a volume of reconstituted sol (containing 0.58mg of Xiaflex) as follows:

For Cords Affecting a MP Joint: 0.25 mL
For Cords Affecting a PIP Joint: 0.20mL

2. W/ your non-dominant hand, secure the patient's hand to be treated while simultaneously applying tension to the cord, and w/ your dominant hand, place the needle into the cord, using caution to keep the needle w/in the cord
3. Avoid having the needle tip pass completely through the cord to help minimize the potential for inj into tissues other than the cord
4. After needle placement, if there is any concern that the needle is in the flexor tendon, apply a small amount of passive motion at the distal interphalangeal (DIP) joint
5. If insertion of the needle into a tendon is suspected or paresthesia is noted by the patient, withdraw the needle and reposition it into the cord; if the needle is in the proper location, there will be some resistance noted during the inj procedure
6. After confirming that the needle is correctly placed in the cord, inject approx 1/3 of the dose
7. Withdraw the needle tip from the cord and reposition it in a slightly more distal location (approx 2-3mm) to the initial inj in the cord and inject another 1/3 of the dose

8. Again withdraw the needle tip from the cord and reposition it a 3rd time proximal to the initial inj (approx 2-3mm) and inject the final portion of the dose into the cord
9. When administering 2 inj in the same hand during a treatment visit, use a new syringe and separate vial of reconstituted sol for each inj. Repeat steps 1-9
10. When administering 2 inj in the same hand during a treatment visit, begin w/ the affected finger in the most lateral aspect of the hand and continue toward the medial aspect (eg, 5th finger to index finger)
11. When administering 2 inj in a cord affecting 2 joints in the same finger, begin w/ the affected joint in the most proximal aspect of the finger and continue toward the distal aspect (eg, MP to PIP)
12. Wrap the patient's treated hand w/ a soft, bulky, gauze dressing
13. Instruct the patient to limit motion of the treated finger(s) and to keep the injected hand elevated until bedtime
14. Instruct the patient not to attempt to disrupt the injected cord(s) by self-manipulation and to return to the healthcare provider's office the next day for follow-up and a finger extension procedure(s), if needed
15. Discard the unused portion of the reconstituted sol and diluent after inj; do not store, pool, or use any vials containing unused reconstituted sol or diluent

Peyronie's Disease

Reconstitution of Lyophilized Powder:

1. Before use, allow the vial containing the lyophilized powder and the vial containing the diluent for reconstitution to stand at room temperature for at least 15 min and no longer than 60 min
2. Use only the supplied diluent for reconstitution; the diluent contains Ca^{2+}, which is required for the activity of Xiaflex
Using a 1mL syringe w/ 0.01mL graduations and a 27-gauge 1/2-inch needle (not supplied), withdraw a volume of 0.39mL of the diluent supplied
3. Inject the diluent slowly into the sides of the vial containing the lyophilized powder
4. Slowly swirl the sol to ensure that all of the lyophilized powder has gone into sol; do not invert the vial or shake the sol
5. The reconstituted sol can be kept at room temperature for up to 1 hr or refrigerated for up to 4 hrs prior to administration; if the sol is refrigerated, allow it to return to room temperature for approx 15 min before use
6. Discard the syringe and needle used for reconstitution and the diluent vial

Identification of Treatment Area:

Prior to each treatment cycle, identify the treatment area as follows:
1. Induce a penile erection; a single intracavernosal inj of 10 or 20mcg of alprostadil may be used for this purpose. Apply antiseptic at inj site and allow the skin to dry prior to intracavernosal inj
2. Locate the plaque at the point of max concavity (or focal point) in bend of the penis
3. Mark the point w/ a surgical marker; this indicates target area in the plaque for Xiaflex deposition

Inj Procedure:

1. Apply antiseptic at the inj site and allow the skin to dry
2. Administer suitable local anesthetic, if desired
3. Using a new hubless syringe containing 0.01mL graduations w/ a permanently fixed 27-gauge 1/2-inch needle (not supplied), withdraw a volume of 0.25mL of reconstituted sol (containing 0.58mg of Xiaflex)
4. The penis should be in a flaccid state before inj
5. Place the needle tip on the side of the target plaque in alignment w/ the point of maximal concavity
6. Orient the needle so that it enters the edge of the plaque and advance the needle into the plaque itself from the side; do not advance the needle beneath the plaque nor perpendicularly towards the corpora cavernosum
7. Insert and advance the needle transversely through the width of the plaque, towards the opposite side of the plaque w/o passing completely through it
8. Proper needle position is tested and confirmed by carefully noting resistance to minimal depression of the syringe plunger
9. W/ the tip of the needle placed w/in the plaque, initiate inj, maintaining steady pressure to slowly inject Xiaflex into the plaque
10. Withdraw the needle slowly so as to deposit the full dose along the needle track w/in the plaque; for plaques that are only a few mm in width, the distance of withdrawal of the syringe may be very minimal
11. Upon complete withdrawal of the needle, apply gentle pressure at the inj site
12. Apply a dressing as necessary
13. Discard the unused portion of the reconstituted sol and diluent after each inj; do not store, pool, or use any vials containing unused reconstituted sol or diluent
14. The 2nd inj of each treatment cycle should be made approx 2-3mm apart from the 1st inj

HOW SUPPLIED

Inj: 0.9mg

CONTRAINDICATIONS

Treatment of Peyronie's plaques that involve the penile urethra, history of hypersensitivity to the medication or to collagenase used in any other therapeutic application or application method.

WARNINGS/PRECAUTIONS

Should be administered by a healthcare provider experienced in inj procedures of the hand and treatment of Dupuytren's contracture, or treatment of male urological diseases who has completed required training for use of collagenase clostridium histolyticum in the treatment of Peyronie's disease. Inj into collagen-containing structures (eg, tendons/ligaments of the hand, corpora cavernosa of the penis) may result in damage to those structures and possible permanent injury (eg, tendon rupture, ligament damage). Avoid injecting into the urethra, corpora cavernosa, tendons, nerves, blood vessels, or other collagen-containing structures. Other serious local reactions (eg, pulley rupture, ligament injury, complex regional pain syndrome, sensory abnormality of the hand) reported. Severe allergic reactions (eg, anaphylaxis) may occur. Avoid in patients with coagulation disorders.

ADVERSE REACTIONS

Corporal fracture, penile hematoma/ecchymosis, penile swelling, penile pain, sudden penile detumescence, penile "popping" sound/sensation, peripheral edema, contusion, inj-site hemorrhage, extremity pain, lymphadenopathy, tenderness, pruritus, immunogenicity, inj-site reaction.

DRUG INTERACTIONS

Avoid in patients receiving concomitant anticoagulants, except low-dose aspirin (eg, ≤150mg/day).

PATIENT CONSIDERATIONS

Assessment: Assess for history of hypersensitivity to drug or to collagenase in other therapeutic applications, Peyronie's plaque involving the penile urethra, coagulation disorders, pregnancy/nursing status, and possible drug interactions.

Monitoring: Monitor for signs/symptoms of hypersensitivity reactions, tendon rupture, ligament damage, corporal rupture, penile ecchymoses/hematoma, sudden penile detumescence, penile "popping" sound or sensation, and other adverse reactions.

Counseling: (Dupuytren's Contracture) Advise of serious complications that may result in inability to fully bend finger and may require surgery. Inform that inj is likely to result in swelling, bruising, bleeding, and/or pain of injected site and surrounding tissue. After inj, instruct not to flex/extend the fingers of injected hand, not to disrupt injected cord(s) by self-manipulation, to elevate injected hand until hs, and to promptly contact physician if there is evidence of infection, sensory changes in treated finger(s), trouble bending finger(s) after the swelling goes down, or skin laceration. Instruct to return for follow up 1-3 days after the inj visit. Instruct not to perform strenuous activity with injected hand until advised to do so, wear splint at bedtime for up to 4 months, and perform a series of finger flexion and extension exercises each day. (Peyronie's Disease) Advise of serious complications that may require surgery to correct. Inform that penis may appear bruised and/or swollen, and that they may have mild to moderate penile pain that can be relieved by taking OTC medications. Instruct to promptly contact physician if they have severe pain, swelling, purple bruising/swelling of the penis, difficulty urinating or blood in the urine, or sudden loss of ability to maintain an erection; inform that these may be accompanied by a popping or cracking sound from the penis. Instruct to return to physician's office when directed for further inj(s) and/or penile modeling procedure(s), and to wait 2 weeks after 2nd inj of a treatment cycle before resuming sexual activity, provided pain and swelling have subsided.

STORAGE: 2-8°C (36-46°F). Do not freeze. Reconstituted Sol: May keep at room temperature of 20-25°C (68-77°F) for up to 1 hr or refrigerate at 2-8°C (36-46°F) for up to 4 hrs.

XIFAXAN – rifaximin

RX

Class: Semisynthetic rifampin analogue

ADULT DOSAGE

Traveler's Diarrhea

Noninvasive Strains of *Escherichia coli*:
200mg tid for 3 days

Hepatic Encephalopathy

Reduction in Risk of Overt Recurrence:
550mg bid

Irritable Bowel Syndrome

W/ Diarrhea:
550mg tid for 14 days

May retreat up to 2X w/ the same dosage regimen in patients who have recurrence of symptoms

PEDIATRIC DOSAGE

Traveler's Diarrhea

Noninvasive Strains of *E. coli*:

≥12 Years:
200mg tid for 3 days

ADMINISTRATION
Oral route

Take w/ or w/o food.

HOW SUPPLIED
Tab: 200mg, 550mg

CONTRAINDICATIONS
Hypersensitivity to rifaximin, any of the rifamycin antimicrobial agents, or any of the components in this medication.

WARNINGS/PRECAUTIONS
Should not be used in patients w/ diarrhea complicated by fever and/or blood in the stool or diarrhea due to pathogens other than *E. coli*. D/C if diarrhea symptoms worsen or persist >24-48 hrs; consider alternative antibiotic therapy. *Clostridium difficile*-associated diarrhea (CDAD) reported; may need to d/c if CDAD suspected or confirmed. Use in the absence of a proven or strongly suspected bacterial infection or a prophylactic indication may increase the risk of development of bacterial resistance. Caution w/ severe hepatic impairment (Child-Pugh Class C); may increase systemic exposure.

ADVERSE REACTIONS
Headache, peripheral edema, nausea, dizziness, fatigue, ascites, muscle spasms, pruritus, abdominal pain, anemia, depression, nasopharyngitis, arthralgia, dyspnea, pyrexia.

DRUG INTERACTIONS
Caution w/ P-gp inhibitors (eg, cyclosporine); may increase systemic exposure.

PATIENT CONSIDERATIONS

Assessment: If diarrhea is present, assess for causative organisms and assess if diarrhea is complicated by fever or blood in stool. Assess for drug hypersensitivity, hepatic impairment, pregnancy/nursing status, and possible drug interactions.

Monitoring: Monitor for signs/symptoms of a hypersensitivity reaction, CDAD, development of drug-resistant bacteria, worsening of symptoms, and other adverse reactions.

Counseling: If being treated for traveler's diarrhea, instruct to d/c therapy and contact physician if diarrhea persists for >24-48 hrs or worsens. Advise to seek medical care for fever and/or blood in the stool. Inform that watery and bloody stools (w/ or w/o stomach cramps and fever) may occur even as late as ≥2 months after last dose; advise to contact physician as soon as possible. Inform that drug only treats bacterial, not viral, infections. Inform that skipping doses or not completing full course of therapy may decrease the effectiveness of treatment and increase resistance. Inform that there is an increase systemic exposure to therapy in patients w/ severe hepatic impairment (Child-Pugh Class C).

STORAGE: 20-25°C (68-77°F); excursions permitted to 15-30°C (59-86°F).

XOFIGO — radium Ra 223 dichloride

RX

Class: Radiopharmaceutical agent

ADULT DOSAGE

Prostate Carcinoma

Use in patients w/ castration-resistant prostate cancer, symptomatic bone metastases and no known visceral metastatic disease

50 kBq (1.35 microcurie)/kg by slow IV inj over 1 min given at 4-week intervals for 6 inj

Use the following to calculate the volume to be administered:
1. Patient's body weight (kg)
2. Dosage level 50k Bq/kg body weight or 1.35 microcurie/kg body weight
3. Radioactivity concentration of the product (1,000 kBq/mL; 27 microcurie/mL) at the reference date
4. Decay correction factor to correct for physical decay of radium-223

Volume to be administered (mL) = (Body weight in kg x 50 kBq/kg body weight)/(Decay factor x 1000 kBq/mL)
or

PEDIATRIC DOSAGE

Pediatric use may not have been established

Volume to be administered (mL) = (Body weight in kg x 1.35 microcurie/kg body weight)/(Decay factor x 27 microcurie/mL)

Refer to PI for decay correction factor table

ADMINISTRATION

IV route

Do not dilute or mix w/ any sol

Flush IV access line or cannula w/ isotonic saline before and after inj

Use proper radiation protection when handling the drug

HOW SUPPLIED

Inj: 1000 kBq/mL (27 microcurie/mL) [6mL]

CONTRAINDICATIONS

Pregnancy, women of childbearing potential.

WARNINGS/PRECAUTIONS

Bone marrow failure reported. Myelosuppression (eg, thrombocytopenia, neutropenia, pancytopenia, leukopenia) reported; perform hematologic evaluation at baseline and prior to every dose. Before the 1st administration, the ANC should be $\geq 1.5 \times 10^9$/L, the platelet count $\geq 100 \times 10^9$/L and Hgb ≥10g/dL. Before subsequent administrations, the ANC should be $\geq 1 \times 10^9$/L and the platelet count $\geq 50 \times 10^9$/L. D/C therapy if there is no recovery to these values within 6-8 weeks after the last administration. Monitor closely and provide supportive care measures in patients with compromised bone marrow reserve; d/c in patients who experience life-threatening complications despite supportive care for bone marrow failure. Caution in elderly.

ADVERSE REACTIONS

N/V, diarrhea, peripheral edema, anemia, lymphocytopenia, leukopenia, thrombocytopenia, neutropenia.

DRUG INTERACTIONS

Concomitant use with chemotherapy is not recommended; d/c therapy if chemotherapy, other systemic radioisotopes or hemibody external radiotherapy are administered during treatment period.

PATIENT CONSIDERATIONS

Assessment: Assess for compromised bone marrow reserve. Perform hematologic evaluation at baseline.

Monitoring: Monitor for bone marrow failure, myelosuppression, and other adverse reactions. Perform hematologic evaluation prior to every dose.

Counseling: Advise patients to be compliant with blood cell count monitoring appointments, to stay well hydrated, and to monitor oral intake, fluid status, and urine output while on therapy. Explain the importance of routine blood cell counts. Instruct to report signs of bleeding or infections, dehydration, hypovolemia, urinary retention, or renal failure/insufficiency. Inform that there is no restriction regarding contact with other people after receiving therapy. Advise to follow good hygiene practices while on therapy and for at least 1 week after the last inj in order to minimize radiation exposure from bodily fluids to household members and caregivers. Instruct caregivers to use universal precautions for patient care (eg, gloves and barrier gowns when handling bodily fluids). Advise patients who are sexually active to use condoms and their female partners of reproductive potential to use highly effective method of birth control during therapy and for 6 months following completion of treatment.

STORAGE: Room temperature <40°C (104°F) in the original container or equivalent radiation shielding.

XOLAIR – omalizumab

RX

Class: Monoclonal antibody/IgE blocker

Anaphylaxis, presenting as bronchospasm, hypotension, syncope, urticaria, and/or angioedema of throat or tongue, reported as early as after the 1st dose and beyond 1 yr of therapy; closely observe patients. Inform of the signs/symptoms of anaphylaxis and instruct to seek immediate medical care should symptoms occur.

X

ADULT DOSAGE

Asthma

Moderate to Severe Persistent Asthma w/ a (+) Skin Test or In Vitro Reactivity to a Perennial Aeroallergen and Inadequately Controlled w/ Inhaled Corticosteroids:

PEDIATRIC DOSAGE

Asthma

Moderate to Severe Persistent Asthma w/ a (+) Skin Test or In Vitro Reactivity to a Perennial Aeroallergen and Inadequately Controlled w/ Inhaled Corticosteroids:

150-375mg SQ every 2 or 4 weeks, based on body weight (kg) and pretreatment serum total IgE level (IU/mL)

Refer to PI for dose determination charts

Chronic Idiopathic Urticaria

Symptomatic Despite H1 Antihistamine Treatment:
150mg or 300mg SQ every 4 weeks

≥12 Years:
150-375mg SQ every 2 or 4 weeks, based on body weight (kg) and pretreatment serum total IgE level (IU/mL)

Refer to PI for dose determination charts

Chronic Idiopathic Urticaria

Symptomatic Despite H1 Antihistamine Treatment:
≥12 Years:
150mg or 300mg SQ every 4 weeks

ADMINISTRATION

SQ route

The inj may take 5-10 sec to administer.
Do not administer more than 150mg (contents of one vial) per inj site.

Number of Inj and Total Inj Volume

150mg inj involves 1 inj (1.2mL total volume inj).
225mg inj involves 2 inj (1.8mL total volume inj).
300mg inj involves 2 inj (2.4mL total volume inj).
375mg inj involves 3 inj (3.0mL total volume inj).

Reconstitution for Single Vial

Before reconstitution, determine the number of vials that will need to be reconstituted.
1. Reconstitute w/ sterile water for inj (SWFI).
2. Draw 1.4mL of SWFI into a 3mL syringe equipped w/ a 1-inch, 18-gauge needle.
3. Insert the needle and inject the SWFI directly onto the product.
4. Gently swirl the upright vial for approx 1 min; do not shake.
5. Gently swirl the vial for 5-10 sec approx every 5 min in order to dissolve any remaining solids. The lyophilized product takes 15-20 min to dissolve.
6. If it takes longer than 20 min to dissolve completely, gently swirl the vial for 5-10 sec approx every 5 min until there are no visible gel-like particles in the sol. Do not use if the contents of the vial do not dissolve completely by 40 min.
7. Invert the vial for 15 sec in order to allow the sol to drain toward the stopper.
8. Using a new 3mL syringe equipped w/ a 1-inch, 18-gauge needle, draw the sol into the syringe.
9. Replace the 18-gauge needle w/ a 25-gauge needle for SQ inj.

HOW SUPPLIED

Inj: 150mg

CONTRAINDICATIONS

Severe hypersensitivity reaction to omalizumab or any ingredient of this medication.

WARNINGS/PRECAUTIONS

Not indicated for treatment of other forms of urticaria, relief of acute bronchospasm or status asthmaticus, or other allergic conditions. Administer only in a healthcare setting prepared to manage anaphylaxis and observe patients for an appropriate period after administration. D/C if a severe hypersensitivity reaction occurs. Malignant neoplasms reported. Do not abruptly d/c systemic or inhaled corticosteroids when initiating therapy. Eosinophilic conditions reported; be alert to eosinophilia, vasculitic rash, worsening pulmonary symptoms, cardiac complications, and/or neuropathy, especially upon reduction of oral corticosteroids. Monitor patients at high risk for geohelminth infections (eg, roundworm, hookworm). Signs/symptoms similar to those seen in patients w/ serum sickness, including arthritis/arthralgia, rash, fever, and lymphadenopathy reported; d/c if these symptoms develop. Serum total IgE levels increase due to formation of Xolair:IgE complexes and may persist for up to 1 yr following discontinuation of therapy; do not use serum total IgE levels obtained <1 yr following discontinuation to reassess dosing regimen for asthma patients.

ADVERSE REACTIONS

Asthma: Arthralgia, pain (general), leg pain, fatigue, dizziness, fracture, arm pain, pruritus, dermatitis, earache.
Chronic Idiopathic Urticaria (CIU): Nausea, nasopharyngitis, sinusitis, URTI, viral URTI, arthralgia, headache, cough.

PATIENT CONSIDERATIONS

Assessment: Assess for acute bronchospasm or status asthmaticus, malignancies, hypersensitivity reaction to drug or any of its ingredients, risk of geohelminth infections, and pregnancy/nursing status. Obtain baseline body weight and serum IgE levels.

Monitoring: Monitor for anaphylaxis, hypersensitivity reactions, inj-site reactions, malignancies, viral/geohelminth infections, URTIs, eosinophilia, vasculitic rash, worsening pulmonary symptoms, cardiac complications, neuropathy, arthritis/arthralgia, rash, fever, lymphadenopathy, and other adverse reactions. Periodically reassess need for continued therapy. Monitor body weight, CBC, and IgE levels prn.

Counseling: Instruct to read the medication guide before treatment. Inform of the risk of life-threatening anaphylaxis; instruct to seek immediate medical care if symptoms of anaphylaxis occur. Instruct not to decrease dose of or stop taking any other asthma or CIU medications unless otherwise instructed. Inform that immediate improvement of asthma or CIU symptoms may not be seen after beginning therapy. Encourage pregnant women to enroll in the pregnancy exposure registry.

STORAGE: 2-8°C (36-46°F). **Reconstituted:** 2-8°C (36-46°F) for up to 8 hrs, or 4 hrs at room temperature. Protect from direct sunlight.

XOPENEX HFA – levalbuterol tartrate

RX

Class: $Beta_2$ agonist

ADULT DOSAGE

Bronchospasm

Associated w/ Reversible Obstructive Airway Disease:

2 inh (90mcg) q4-6h

1 inh (45mcg) q4h may be sufficient in some patients

PEDIATRIC DOSAGE

Bronchospasm

Associated w/ Reversible Obstructive Airway Disease:

≥4 Years:

2 inh (90mcg) q4-6h

1 inh (45mcg) q4h may be sufficient in some patients

DOSING CONSIDERATIONS

Elderly

Start at lower end of dosing range

ADMINISTRATION

Oral inh route

Shake well before use

Avoid spraying in the eyes

Wash actuator w/ warm water and air dry thoroughly at least once a week

Discard canister after 200 actuations have been used from the 15g canister and 80 actuations from the 8.4g canister

Priming

Prime inhaler before use for the 1st time or if not used for >3 days by releasing 4 test sprays into the air, away from face

HOW SUPPLIED

MDI: 45mcg/inh [80, 200 inhalations]

CONTRAINDICATIONS

History of hypersensitivity to levalbuterol, racemic albuterol, or any other component of the medication.

WARNINGS/PRECAUTIONS

If a previously effective dose regimen fails to provide the usual response or if more doses than usual are needed, this may be a marker of destabilization of asthma and may require reevaluation of the patient and treatment regimen; anti-inflammatory treatment (eg, corticosteroids) may be needed. D/C if paradoxical bronchospasm occur. ECG changes and immediate hypersensitivity reactions may occur. May need to d/c if cardiovascular (CV) effects occur. Fatalities reported w/ excessive use; do not exceed recommended dose. Caution w/ CV disorders (eg, coronary insufficiency, arrhythmias, HTN), convulsive disorders, hyperthyroidism, or diabetes mellitus (DM), and in patients unusually responsive to sympathomimetic amines. May produce significant hypokalemia. Caution w/ renal impairment.

ADVERSE REACTIONS

Pharyngitis, rhinitis, pain, vomiting, dizziness, asthma, bronchitis.

DRUG INTERACTIONS

Avoid w/ other short-acting sympathomimetic aerosol bronchodilators or epinephrine; caution w/ additional adrenergic drugs administered by any route. Use w/ β-blockers may block pulmonary effects and produce severe bronchospasm in asthmatic patients; avoid concomitant use. If needed, consider cardioselective β-blockers and use w/ caution. ECG changes and/or hypokalemia caused by non-K^+-sparing diuretics (eg, loop or thiazide diuretics) may be worsened; use w/ caution and consider monitoring K^+ levels. May decrease digoxin levels; monitor serum digoxin levels. Use extreme caution w/ MAOIs or TCAs, or w/in 2 weeks of discontinuation of such agents.

PATIENT CONSIDERATIONS

Assessment: Assess for history of hypersensitivity to drug or racemic albuterol, CV disorders, convulsive disorders, hyperthyroidism, DM, renal impairment, pregnancy/nursing status, and possible drug interactions. Assess use in patients unusually responsive to sympathomimetic amines.

Monitoring: Monitor for paradoxical bronchospasm, deterioration of asthma, CV effects, ECG changes, hypokalemia, immediate hypersensitivity reactions, and other adverse effects. Monitor BP, HR, and ECG changes.

Counseling: Counsel not to increase dose or frequency of doses w/o consulting physician. Advise to seek immediate medical attention if treatment becomes less effective for symptomatic relief, symptoms become worse, and/or there is a need to use the product more frequently than usual. Inform that drug may cause paradoxical bronchospasm; instruct to d/c if this occurs. Instruct to take concurrent inhaled drugs and other asthma medications only ud. Inform of the common side effects (eg, chest pain, palpitations, rapid HR, tremor, nervousness). Instruct to notify physician if pregnant/nursing. Advise to discard after 200 actuations have been released from the 15g canister or 80 actuations have been released from the 8.4g canister.

STORAGE: 20-25°C (68-77°F). Store w/ mouthpiece down. Protect from freezing and direct sunlight. Contents under pressure; do not puncture or incinerate. Exposure to temperatures >49°C (120°F) may cause bursting.

XULANE – ethinyl estradiol/norelgestromin

RX

Class: Estrogen/progestogen combination

Cigarette smoking increases risk of serious cardiovascular (CV) events from hormonal contraceptive use. Risk increases w/ age, particularly in women >35 years of age, and w/ the number of cigarettes smoked. Should not be used by women who are >35 yrs of age and smoke. May increase risk of venous thromboembolism (VTE) among users of Xulane compared to women who use certain oral contraceptives. Has higher steady state concentrations and a lower peak concentration than oral contraceptives.

OTHER BRAND NAMES

Ortho Evra (Discontinued)

ADULT DOSAGE

Contraception

Apply 1st patch during the first 24 hrs of menstrual period or on the 1st Sunday after menstrual period begins. Apply patch each week on the same day for 3 weeks (21 total days). Week 4 is patch-free. On the day after Week 4 ends, a new 4-week cycle is started by applying a new patch. There should not be more than a 7-day patch-free interval between dosing cycles

Conversions

Switching From the Pill or Vaginal Contraceptive Ring:
Complete current pill/ring cycle and apply 1st patch on the day patient would have normally started next pill or inserted next vaginal ring; if patch is applied >1 week after taking last active pill or removal of last vaginal ring, use nonhormonal contraceptive concurrently for the first 7 days of patch use

PEDIATRIC DOSAGE

Contraception

Not indicated for use premenarche; refer to adult dosing

DOSING CONSIDERATIONS

Other Important Considerations

Use After Childbirth:
Start no sooner than 4 weeks after childbirth in women who elect not to breastfeed. If use is begun postpartum, and patient has not yet had a period, consider the possibility of ovulation and conception occurring prior to use; use an additional method of contraception, (eg, condom and spermicide, diaphragm and spermicide) for the first 7 days.

Use After Abortion/Miscarriage:
1st Trimester: May start patch use immediately; additional method of contraception is not needed. If patch use is not started w/in 5 days following a 1st trimester abortion, follow instructions for starting patch for the 1st time and use non-hormonal contraceptive method in the meantime
2nd Trimester: Start no earlier than 4 weeks after a 2nd trimester abortion/miscarriage

ADMINISTRATION

Transdermal route

Apply immediately upon removal from protective pouch.

Only 1 patch should be worn at a time.

Do not cut, damage, or alter patch in any way.

Apply to clean and dry skin on upper outer arm, abdomen, buttock, or back in a place where it will not be rubbed by tight clothing; do not place on breasts, on cut/irritated skin, or on the same location as previous patch.

Do not reapply patch if it is no longer sticky, if it has become stuck to itself or another surface, or if it has other material stuck to it.

Refer to PI for further administration instructions.

Sunday Start Regimen

Use a non-hormonal backup method of birth control (eg, condom and spermicide, diaphragm and spermicide) for the first 7 days of the 1st cycle only. If period starts on a Sunday, the 1st patch should be applied that day, and no backup contraception is needed.

HOW SUPPLIED

Patch: (Ethinyl Estradiol [EE]/Norelgestromin [NGMN]): (35mcg/150mcg)/day [1[s], 3[s]]

CONTRAINDICATIONS

High risk of arterial/venous thrombotic diseases (eg, smoking if >35 yrs of age, history/presence of deep vein thrombosis/pulmonary embolism, inherited or acquired hypercoagulopathies, cerebrovascular disease, coronary artery disease, thrombogenic valvular or thrombogenic rhythm diseases of the heart [eg, subacute bacterial endocarditis w/ valvular disease, A-fib], uncontrolled HTN; diabetes mellitus w/ vascular disease, headaches w/ focal neurological symptoms or migraine headaches w/ aura [women >35 yrs of age w/ any migraine headaches]), benign or malignant liver tumors, liver disease, undiagnosed abnormal uterine bleeding, pregnancy, current or history of breast cancer or other estrogen- or progestin-sensitive cancer.

WARNINGS/PRECAUTIONS

May be less effective in preventing pregnancy in women who weigh ≥198 lbs (90kg). Increased risk of thromboembolic/thrombotic disease, and arterial thromboses. Risk of VTE is highest during the 1st year of use of combination hormonal contraceptives (CHCs) and when restarting hormonal contraception after a break of ≥4 weeks. D/C if an arterial or deep venous thrombotic event occurs. D/C if unexplained loss of vision, proptosis, diplopia, papilledema, or retinal vascular lesions develop; evaluate for retinal vein thrombosis immediately. If feasible, d/c at least 4 weeks before and through 2 weeks after major surgery or other surgeries associated w/ an elevated risk of VTE. D/C during prolonged immobilization. Start use no earlier than 4 weeks after delivery in women who are not breastfeeding. D/C if jaundice develops. Hepatic adenomas and increased risk of hepatocellular carcinoma reported. Increase in BP reported. Monitor BP in women w/ well-controlled HTN; d/c if BP rises significantly. Increased risk of cervical cancer or intraepithelial neoplasia, and gallbladder disease. Women w/ a history of pregnancy-related cholestasis may be at an increased risk for CHC-related cholestasis. May decrease glucose tolerance; monitor prediabetic and diabetic women. Consider alternative contraception w/ uncontrolled dyslipidemia. May increase risk of pancreatitis w/ hypertriglyceridemia or a family history thereof. Evaluate the cause of new headaches that are recurrent, persistent, or severe, and d/c if indicated; consider discontinuation in case of increased frequency or severity of migraine during use. Unscheduled bleeding and spotting reported. Consider non-hormonal causes and take adequate diagnostic measures to rule out malignancy, other pathology, or pregnancy in the event of unscheduled bleeding. Consider possibility of pregnancy in the event of amenorrhea. Amenorrhea or oligomenorrhea may occur after discontinuation of therapy. Administration of therapy should not be used as a test for pregnancy. Caution w/ history of depression; d/c if depression recurs to a serious degree. May raise the serum concentrations of sex hormone-binding globulin. Exogenous estrogens may induce or exacerbate symptoms of angioedema in patients w/ hereditary angioedema. Chloasma may occur, especially in women w/ a history of chloasma gravidarum; women w/ a tendency to chloasma should avoid exposure to sun or UV radiation. May influence the results of certain laboratory tests.

ADVERSE REACTIONS

Breast symptoms, N/V, headache, application-site disorder, abdominal pain, dysmenorrhea, vaginal bleeding, menstrual disorders, mood/affect/anxiety disorders.

DRUG INTERACTIONS

Drugs or herbal products that induce certain enzymes, including CYP3A4 (eg, phenytoin, barbiturates, products containing St. John's wort), may decrease levels and potentially diminish effectiveness or increase breakthrough bleeding; use an alternative method of contraception or a backup method when used concomitantly w/ enzyme inducers, and continue backup contraception for 28 days after discontinuing the enzyme inducer. Atorvastatin or rosuvastatin may increase EE exposure; ascorbic acid and acetaminophen (APAP) may increase EE levels. CYP3A4 inhibitors (eg, itraconazole, voriconazole, grapefruit juice) may increase plasma hormone levels. Significant changes (decreased/increased) sometimes noted in estrogen and/or progestin levels when coadministered w/ HIV/hepatitis C virus protease inhibitors or w/ non-nucleoside reverse transcriptase inhibitors. May inhibit the metabolism of other compounds (eg, cyclosporine, prednisolone, theophylline) and increase their plasma concentrations. May decrease concentrations of APAP, clofibric acid, morphine, salicylic acid, and temazepam. May decrease levels of lamotrigine and reduce seizure control; dosage adjustments of lamotrigine may be necessary. May raise the serum concentrations of thyroxine-binding globulin and cortisol-binding globulin; dose of replacement thyroid hormone or cortisol therapy may need to be increased.

PATIENT CONSIDERATIONS

Assessment: Assess for risk of arterial or venous thrombotic diseases, benign or malignant liver tumors, liver disease, undiagnosed abnormal uterine bleeding, presence or history of breast cancer or other estrogen- or progestin-sensitive cancer, pregnancy/nursing status, and any other conditions where treatment is contraindicated/cautioned. Assess for possible drug interactions.

Monitoring: Monitor for arterial thrombotic or VTE events, hepatic adenomas, hepatocellular carcinoma, gallbladder disease, and other adverse effects. Monitor lipid levels w/ hyperlipidemia, BP w/ history of HTN, serum glucose levels in diabetic and prediabetic patients, and for signs of worsening depression w/ previous history. Conduct a yearly visit w/ patient for a BP check and for other indicated healthcare.

Counseling: Inform of risks and benefits of therapy. Inform that cigarette smoking increases risk of serious CV events, and that women who are >35 yrs of age and smoke should not use CHCs. Advise that use of CHCs increases risk of VTE; inform that risk is highest during 1st year of use of CHCs and when restarting hormonal contraception after a break of ≥4 weeks. Counsel that therapy does not protect against HIV infection (AIDS) and other sexually transmitted infections. Instruct to d/c if pregnancy occurs during use. Instruct to apply a single patch on the same day every week (Weeks 1-3). Instruct on what to do in the event a patch is missed. Instruct women who start CHC postpartum, and who have not yet had a period, to use an additional method of contraception until they have used patch for 7 consecutive days. Instruct to use a backup or alternative method of contraception when enzyme inducers are concomitantly used. Inform that breast milk production may be reduced w/ use. Inform that amenorrhea may occur. Advise that pregnancy should be ruled out in the event of amenorrhea in 2 or more consecutive cycles. Advise that insufficient drug delivery occurs when patch becomes partially or completely detached and remains detached.

STORAGE: 20-25°C (68-77°F). Store patches in their protective pouches. Do not store in the refrigerator or freezer.

XURIDEN – uridine triacetate

Class: Pyrimidine analog

RX

ADULT DOSAGE

Hereditary Orotic Aciduria

Initial: 60mg/kg qd
Titrate: Increase dose to 120mg/kg for insufficient efficacy
Max: 8g/day

Decrease dose if diarrhea occurs and persists for ≥3 successive days w/o another identifiable cause

Refer to PI for further dosing specifics

PEDIATRIC DOSAGE

Hereditary Orotic Aciduria

Initial: 60mg/kg qd
Titrate: Increase dose to 120mg/kg for insufficient efficacy
Max: 8g/day

Decrease dose if diarrhea occurs and persists for ≥3 successive days w/o another identifiable cause

Refer to PI for further dosing specifics

ADMINISTRATION

Oral route

Measure dose using either a balance accurate to at least 0.1g, or a pharmacy-provided graduated tsp, accurate to the fraction of the dose to be administered.
Discard unused portion of granules once the measured dose has been removed from the packet.

Administration w/ Food

1. Mix measured amount of granules in 3-4 oz of applesauce, pudding, or yogurt.
2. Swallow the applesauce/pudding/yogurt immediately; do not chew the granules and do not save the applesauce/pudding/yogurt for later use.
3. Drink at least 4 oz of water.

May be mixed w/ milk or infant formula instead of soft foods, as described above; refer to PI for further details.

HOW SUPPLIED

Granules: 2g/pkt [30s]

PATIENT CONSIDERATIONS

Assessment: Assess pregnancy/nursing status. Assess baseline laboratory values affected by hereditary orotic aciduria.

Monitoring: Monitor for signs/symptoms of worsening hereditary orotic aciduria and for diarrhea. Monitor urine levels of orotic acid and monitor laboratory values affected by hereditary orotic aciduria.

Counseling: Instruct on how to administer medication. Advise to measure the prescribed dose using either a balance accurate to at least 0.1g, or a pharmacy-provided graduated tsp, accurate to the fraction of the dose to be administered; inform that for some doses 1 or more entire 2g packets can be used w/o weighing out the granules. Inform that drug can be taken w/o regard to meals. Advise that medication can be taken mixed in applesauce, pudding, or yogurt, or mixed in milk or water. Instruct to notify physician if condition worsens or if pregnant/nursing.

STORAGE: 25°C (77°F); excursions permitted to 15-30°C (59-86°F).

YASMIN — drospirenone/ethinyl estradiol

RX

Class: Estrogen/progestogen combination

Cigarette smoking increases the risk of serious cardiovascular (CV) events. Risk increases w/ age (>35 yrs of age) and w/ the number of cigarettes smoked. Should not be used by women who are >35 yrs of age and smoke.

OTHER BRAND NAMES

Ocella, Syeda

ADULT DOSAGE

Contraception

1 tab qd at the same time each day for 28 days, then repeat

Start either on 1st day of menses or on 1st Sunday after onset of menses

Conversions

Switching from a Different Birth Control Pill: Start on the same day that a new pack of the previous oral contraceptive would have been started

Switching from a Method Other Than a Birth Control Pill:

Transdermal Patch/Vaginal Ring/Inj: Start when the next application or dose would have been due

Intrauterine Contraceptive/Implant: Start on day of removal

PEDIATRIC DOSAGE

Contraception

Not indicated for use premenarche; refer to adult dosing

DOSING CONSIDERATIONS

Adverse Reactions

GI Disturbances: In case of severe vomiting/diarrhea, absorption may not be complete and additional contraceptive measures should be taken; if vomiting occurs w/in 3-4 hrs after taking tab, may regard as missed dose

Other Important Considerations

Postpartum Women Who Elect Not to Breastfeed/After a 2nd Trimester Abortion:
Start therapy no earlier than 4 weeks postpartum. If patient initiates therapy postpartum and has not yet had a period, evaluate for possible pregnancy and instruct to use an additional method of contraception until patient has taken 7 consecutive days of therapy

ADMINISTRATION

Oral route

Take tabs in the order directed on the package, preferably after pm meal or at hs w/ some liquid, prn.
Take w/o regard to meals.
If 1st taken later than the 1st day of menstrual cycle, use a nonhormonal contraceptive as back-up during the first 7 days of therapy.
Take single missed pills as soon as remembered.

HOW SUPPLIED

Tab: (Drospirenone [DRSP]/Ethinyl Estradiol [EE]) 3mg/0.03mg

CONTRAINDICATIONS
Renal impairment, adrenal insufficiency, high risk of arterial/venous thrombotic diseases (eg, smoking if >35 yrs of age, presence/history of deep vein thrombosis/pulmonary embolism, cerebrovascular disease, coronary artery disease, thrombogenic valvular or thrombogenic rhythm diseases of the heart [eg, subacute bacterial endocarditis w/ valvular disease, or A-fib], inherited/acquired hypercoagulopathies, uncontrolled HTN, diabetes mellitus w/ vascular disease, headache w/ focal neurological symptoms or migraine w/ or w/o aura if >35 yrs of age), undiagnosed abnormal uterine bleeding, presence/history of breast cancer or other estrogen/progestin-sensitive cancer, benign/malignant liver tumors, liver disease, pregnancy.

WARNINGS/PRECAUTIONS
Increased risk of venous thromboembolism (VTE) and arterial thromboses (eg, stroke, MI). D/C if an arterial/venous thrombotic event occurs. If feasible, d/c at least 4 weeks before and through 2 weeks after major surgery or other surgeries known to have an elevated risk of thromboembolism. D/C if there is unexplained loss of vision, proptosis, diplopia, papilledema, or retinal vascular lesions; evaluate for retinal vein thrombosis immediately. Potential for hyperkalemia in high-risk patients; contraindicated in patients predisposed to hyperkalemia. May increase risk of cervical cancer or intraepithelial neoplasia, and gallbladder disease. D/C if jaundice develops. May increase risk of hepatic adenomas and hepatocellular carcinoma. Cholestasis may occur w/ history of pregnancy-related cholestasis. Women w/ a history of combination oral contraceptive (COC)-related cholestasis may have the condition recur w/ subsequent COC use. Increased BP reported; d/c if BP rises significantly. May decrease glucose tolerance; monitor prediabetic and diabetic women. Consider alternative contraception w/ uncontrolled dyslipidemia. May increase risk of pancreatitis w/ hypertriglyceridemia or family history thereof. Evaluate the cause and d/c if indicated, if new headaches that are recurrent, persistent, or severe develop. Increase in frequency/severity of migraines may be a reason for immediate discontinuation of therapy. Unscheduled bleeding and spotting may occur; rule out pregnancy or malignancy. Post-pill amenorrhea or oligomenorrhea may occur. Caution w/ history of depression; d/c if depression recurs to a serious degree. May change results of some lab tests (eg, coagulation factors, binding proteins). Exogenous estrogens may induce/exacerbate angioedema in women w/ hereditary angioedema. Chloasma may occur, especially w/ a history of chloasma gravidarum; avoid sun or UV radiation exposure in women w/ a tendency to chloasma.

ADVERSE REACTIONS
Premenstrual syndrome, headache/migraine, breast pain/tenderness/discomfort, N/V, irregular uterine bleeding.

DRUG INTERACTIONS
Potential for an increase in serum K^+ concentration w/ other drugs that may increase serum K^+ concentration (eg, ACE inhibitors, heparin, aldosterone antagonists, NSAIDs); monitor serum K^+ concentrations during 1st treatment cycle in women receiving daily, long-term treatment for chronic conditions or diseases w/ medications that may increase serum K^+ concentration. Consider monitoring serum K^+ concentration in high-risk patients who take a strong CYP3A4 inhibitor long-term and concomitantly. Drugs or herbal products that induce certain enzymes, including CYP3A4 (eg, phenytoin, bosentan, products containing St. John's wort) may decrease effectiveness or increase breakthrough bleeding; use an alternative method of contraception or a back-up method when enzyme inducers are used, and continue back-up contraception for 28 days after discontinuing the enzyme inducer to ensure contraceptive reliability. Atorvastatin may increase EE exposure; ascorbic acid and acetaminophen may increase EE levels. Moderate or strong CYP3A4 inhibitors (eg, itraconazole, clarithromycin, diltiazem, grapefruit juice) may increase plasma concentrations of estrogen or progestin or both. Significant changes (increase/decrease) in plasma estrogen and progestin levels noted in some cases w/ HIV/hepatitis C virus protease inhibitors or non-nucleoside reverse transcriptase inhibitors. Pregnancy reported w/ antibiotics. May decrease levels of lamotrigine and reduce seizure control; dosage adjustments of lamotrigine may be necessary. May need to increase dose of thyroid hormone in patients on thyroid hormone replacement therapy due to increased levels of thyroid-binding globulin. May increase plasma levels of CYP3A4 substrates (eg, midazolam), CYP2C19 substrates (eg, omeprazole, voriconazole), and CYP1A2 substrates (eg, theophylline, tizanidine).

PATIENT CONSIDERATIONS

Assessment: Assess for renal impairment, abnormal uterine bleeding, adrenal insufficiency, pregnancy/nursing status, any other conditions where treatment is contraindicated or cautioned, and possible drug interactions.

Monitoring: Monitor for bleeding irregularities, venous/arterial thrombotic events, cervical cancer or intraepithelial neoplasia, retinal vein thrombosis or any other ophthalmic changes, jaundice, new/worsening headaches or migraines, depression, cholestasis w/ history of pregnancy-related cholestasis, pancreatitis, and other adverse reactions. Monitor thyroid function if receiving thyroid replacement therapy, glucose levels in diabetic or prediabetic patients, lipid levels w/ dyslipidemia, and BP in patients w/ HTN. Monitor serum K^+ levels during the 1st treatment cycle in women receiving daily, long-term treatment for chronic conditions or diseases w/ medications that may increase serum K^+ concentration. Conduct a yearly visit in all patients for a BP check and for other indicated healthcare.

Counseling: Inform of risk/benefits of therapy. Counsel that cigarette smoking increases the risk of serious CV events. Inform of the risk of VTE. Advise that drug does not protect against HIV infection and other STDs. Instruct to take ud. Counsel on what to do if pills are missed or if vomiting occurs w/in 3-4 hrs after taking tab. Advise to inform physician of all concomitant medications and herbal supplements currently being taken. Inform that amenorrhea may occur and pregnancy should be ruled out if amenorrhea occurs in ≥2 consecutive cycles. Counsel to use a back-up or alternative method of contraception when enzyme inducers are used w/ therapy. Inform that therapy may reduce breast milk production. Counsel women who start therapy postpartum and have not yet had a period to use an additional method of contraception until drug is taken for 7 consecutive days. Instruct to d/c if pregnancy occurs during treatment.

STORAGE: (Syeda) 20-25°C (68-77°F). (Yasmin, Ocella) 25°C (77°F); excursions permitted to 15-30°C (59-86°F).

YAZ — drospirenone/ethinyl estradiol RX

Class: Estrogen/progestogen combination

Cigarette smoking increases the risk of serious cardiovascular (CV) events. Risk increases w/ age (>35 yrs of age) and w/ number of cigarettes smoked. Should not be used by women who are >35 yrs of age and smoke.

OTHER BRAND NAMES

Loryna

ADULT DOSAGE

Contraception

1 tab qd at the same time each day for 28 days, then repeat

Start either on 1st day of menses or on 1st Sunday after onset of menses

Premenstrual Dysphoric Disorder

In Women Who Desire Oral Contraception: Yaz:

1 tab qd at the same time each day for 28 days, then repeat

Start either on 1st day of menses or on 1st Sunday after onset of menses

Acne Vulgaris

Moderate Acne in Women Who Desire Oral Contraception:

1 tab qd at the same time each day for 28 days, then repeat

Start either on 1st day of menses or on 1st Sunday after onset of menses

Conversions

Switching from a Different Birth Control Pill:

Start on the same day that a new pack of the previous oral contraceptive would have been started

Switching from a Method Other Than a Birth Control Pill:

Transdermal Patch/Vaginal Ring/Inj: Start when the next application or dose would have been due

Intrauterine Contraceptive/Implant: Start on day of removal

PEDIATRIC DOSAGE

Contraception

Not indicated for use premenarche; refer to adult dosing

Premenstrual Dysphoric Disorder

In Women Who Desire Oral Contraception: Yaz:

Not indicated for use premenarche; refer to adult dosing

Acne Vulgaris

Moderate Acne in Postpubertal Women ≥14 Years Who Desire Oral Contraception:

1 tab qd at the same time each day for 28 days, then repeat

Start either on 1st day of menses or on 1st Sunday after onset of menses

DOSING CONSIDERATIONS

Adverse Reactions

GI Disturbances: In case of severe vomiting/diarrhea, absorption may not be complete and additional contraceptive measures should be taken; if vomiting occurs w/in 3-4 hrs after taking tab, may regard as missed tab

Other Important Considerations

Postpartum Women Who Elect Not to Breastfeed/After 2nd Trimester Abortion: Start therapy no earlier than 4 weeks postpartum. If patient initiates therapy postpartum and has not yet had a period, evaluate for possible pregnancy and instruct to use an additional method of contraception until patient has taken 7 consecutive days of therapy

ADMINISTRATION

Oral route

Take tabs in the order directed on the package, preferably after pm meal or hs w/ some liquid, prn. May be taken w/o regard to meals.

If 1st taken later than the 1st day of menstrual cycle, use a nonhormonal contraceptive as backup during the first 7 days of therapy.

Take single missed pills as soon as remembered.

HOW SUPPLIED

Tab: (Drospirenone [DRSP]/Ethinyl Estradiol [EE]) 3mg/0.02mg

CONTRAINDICATIONS

Renal impairment, adrenal insufficiency, high risk of arterial/venous thrombotic disease (eg, smoking if >35 yrs of age, active or history of deep vein thrombosis/pulmonary embolism, cerebrovascular disease, coronary artery disease, thrombogenic valvular/thrombogenic rhythm diseases of the heart [eg, subacute bacterial endocarditis w/ valvular disease, or A-fib], inherited/acquired hypercoagulopathies, uncontrolled HTN, diabetes mellitus [DM] w/ vascular disease, headache w/ focal neurological symptoms or migraine w/ or w/o aura if >35 yrs of age), undiagnosed abnormal uterine bleeding, presence/history of breast cancer or other estrogen/progestin-sensitive cancer, benign/malignant liver tumors, liver disease, pregnancy.

WARNINGS/PRECAUTIONS

Increased risk of venous thromboembolism (VTE) and arterial thromboses (eg, stroke, MI); d/c if an arterial or venous thrombotic event occurs. D/C if unexplained loss of vision, proptosis, diplopia, papilledema, or retinal vascular lesions occur; evaluate for retinal vein thrombosis immediately. If feasible, d/c at least 4 weeks before and through 2 weeks after major surgery or other surgeries known to have an elevated risk of thromboembolism. Potential for hyperkalemia in high-risk patients; contraindicated in patients w/ conditions that predispose to hyperkalemia. May increase risk of cervical cancer or intraepithelial neoplasia and gallbladder disease. D/C if jaundice develops. May increase risk of hepatic adenomas and hepatocellular carcinoma. Cholestasis may occur in women w/ a history of pregnancy-related cholestasis. Women w/ a history of combination oral contraceptive (COC)-related cholestasis may have the condition recur w/ subsequent COC use. Increased BP reported; d/c if BP rises significantly. May decrease glucose tolerance; monitor prediabetic and diabetic women. Consider alternative contraception for women w/ uncontrolled dyslipidemias. May increase risk of pancreatitis in women w/ hypertriglyceridemia or family history thereof. Evaluate the cause and d/c if indicated, if new headaches that are recurrent, persistent, or severe develop. Increase in frequency/severity of migraines may be a reason for immediate discontinuation of therapy. Unscheduled bleeding and spotting may occur; rule out pregnancy or malignancy. Post-pill amenorrhea or oligomenorrhea may occur. Caution w/ history of depression; d/c if depression recurs to serious degree. May change the results of some lab tests (eg, coagulation factors, binding proteins). Exogenous estrogens may induce/exacerbate angioedema in women w/ hereditary angioedema. Chloasma may occur, especially w/ a history of chloasma gravidarum; avoid sun or UV radiation exposure in women w/ a tendency to chloasma.

ADVERSE REACTIONS

Menstrual irregularities, N/V, headache/migraine, breast pain/tenderness.

DRUG INTERACTIONS

Drugs or herbal products that induce certain enzymes, including CYP3A4 (eg, phenytoin, barbiturates, carbamazepine), may decrease effectiveness or increase breakthrough bleeding; use an alternative or back-up method of contraception when enzyme inducers are used, and continue back-up contraception for 28 days after discontinuing the enzyme inducer. Atorvastatin may increase EE exposure; ascorbic acid and acetaminophen may increase EE levels. Moderate or strong CYP3A4 inhibitors (eg, itraconazole, verapamil, clarithromycin, diltiazem, grapefruit juice) may increase plasma concentrations of estrogen or progestin or both. Significant changes (increase or decrease) in estrogen and progestin levels noted in some cases w/ HIV/hepatitis C virus protease inhibitors or w/ non-nucleoside reverse transcriptase inhibitors. Pregnancy reported while taking hormonal contraceptives and antibiotics. Potential for an increase in serum K^+ concentration w/ use of other drugs that may increase serum K^+ concentration (eg, ACE inhibitors, heparin, aldosterone antagonists, NSAIDs); monitor serum K^+ concentrations during first treatment cycle in patients receiving concomitant daily, long-term treatment for chronic conditions or diseases. Consider monitoring serum K^+ concentration in high-risk patients who take a strong CYP3A4 inhibitor long-term and concomitantly. May decrease levels of lamotrigine and reduce seizure control; may need to adjust dose of lamotrigine. May increase plasma levels of CYP3A4 substrates (eg, midazolam), CYP2C19 substrates (eg, omeprazole, voriconazole), and CYP1A2 substrates (eg, theophylline, tizanidine). May increase levels of thyroid-binding globulin; may need to increase dose of thyroid hormone in patients on thyroid hormone replacement therapy.

PATIENT CONSIDERATIONS

Assessment: Assess for renal impairment, abnormal uterine bleeding, adrenal insufficiency, pregnancy/nursing status, any other conditions where treatment is cautioned or contraindicated, and for possible drug interactions.

Monitoring: Monitor for bleeding irregularities, venous/arterial thrombotic events, cervical cancer or intraepithelial neoplasia, retinal vein thrombosis or any other ophthalmic changes, jaundice, new/worsening headaches or migraines, depression, cholestasis w/ history of pregnancy-related cholestasis, pancreatitis, and other adverse reactions. Monitor thyroid function if receiving thyroid replacement therapy, glucose levels in diabetic or prediabetic women, lipid levels w/ dyslipidemia, and BP in patients w/ HTN. Monitor serum K^+ levels during the 1st treatment cycle in women receiving daily, long-term treatment for chronic conditions or diseases w/ medications that may increase serum K^+ concentrations. Conduct a yearly visit in all patients for a BP check and for other indicated healthcare.

Counseling: Inform of risk/benefits of therapy. Counsel that cigarette smoking increases the risk of serious CV events. Inform of the risk of VTE. Inform that drug does not protect against HIV infection and other STDs. Instruct to take ud. Advise to inform physician of all concomitant medications and herbal supplements currently taking. Instruct to take therapy at the same time every day. Advise on what to do if pills are missed or vomiting occurs w/in 3-4 hrs after taking therapy. Counsel to use a back-up or alternative method of contraception when enzyme inducers are used concomitantly. Inform that therapy may reduce breast milk production. Inform that amenorrhea may occur and pregnancy should be ruled out if amenorrhea occurs in ≥2 consecutive cycles. Counsel women who start therapy postpartum and have not yet had a period, to use an additional method of contraception until an active pill has been taken for 7 consecutive days. Instruct to d/c therapy if pregnancy occurs during treatment.

STORAGE: (Yaz) 25°C (77°F); excursions permitted to 15-30°C (59-86°F). (Loryna) 20-25°C (68-77°F).

YERVOY – ipilimumab

RX

Class: Monoclonal antibody/CTLA-4 blocker

Can result in severe and fatal immune-mediated adverse reactions, and may involve any organ system; the most common reactions are enterocolitis, hepatitis, dermatitis (eg, toxic epidermal necrolysis [TEN]), neuropathy, and endocrinopathy. The majority of these reactions initially manifested during treatment; however, a minority occurred weeks to months after discontinuation of therapy. Permanently d/c therapy and initiate systemic high-dose corticosteroid therapy for severe immune-mediated reactions. Assess for signs/symptoms of enterocolitis, dermatitis, neuropathy, and endocrinopathy, and evaluate clinical chemistries (eg, LFTs, ACTH level, thyroid function tests) at baseline and before each dose.

ADULT DOSAGE

Unresectable or Metastatic Melanoma

3mg/kg IV every 3 weeks for a max of 4 doses

In the event of toxicity, doses may be delayed, but all treatment must be administered w/in 16 weeks of the first dose

Cutaneous Melanoma

Adjuvant treatment of patients w/ pathologic involvement of regional lymph nodes of >1mm who have undergone complete resection, including total lymphadenectomy

10mg/kg IV every 3 weeks for 4 doses followed by 10mg/kg every 12 weeks for up to 3 years

In the event of toxicity, doses are omitted, not delayed

PEDIATRIC DOSAGE

Pediatric use may not have been established

DOSING CONSIDERATIONS

Adverse Reactions

Endocrine:

Symptomatic Endocrinopathy: Withhold therapy; resume in patients w/ complete or partial resolution of adverse reactions (Grade 0 to 1) and who are receiving <7.5mg prednisone or equivalent per day.

Symptomatic Reactions Lasting ≥6 Weeks: Permanently d/c.

Inability to Reduce Corticosteroid Dose to 7.5mg Prednisone or Equivalent per Day: Permanently d/c.

Ophthalmologic:
Grade 2 through 4 Reactions Not Improving to Grade 1 w/in 2 Weeks While Receiving Topical Therapy: Permanently d/c.
Grade 2 through 4 Reactions Requiring Systemic Treatment: Permanently d/c.

All Other:
Grade 2: Withhold therapy; resume in patients w/ complete or partial resolution of adverse reactions (Grade 0 to 1) and who are receiving <7.5mg prednisone or equivalent per day.
Grade 2 Reactions Lasting ≥6 Weeks: Permanently d/c.
Inability to Reduce Corticosteroid Dose to 7.5mg Prednisone or Equivalent per Day: Permanently d/c.
Grade 3 or 4: Permanently d/c.

ADMINISTRATION

IV route

Administer diluted sol over 90 min through an IV line containing a sterile, non-pyrogenic, low-protein-binding in-line filter.
Flush the IV line w/ 0.9% NaCl inj or D5 inj after each dose.
Do not mix w/, or administer as an infusion w/, other medicinal products.

Preparation of Sol

1. Allow the vials to stand at room temperature for approx 5 min prior to preparation of infusion.
2. Withdraw the required volume of ipilimumab and transfer into an IV bag.
3. Dilute w/ 0.9% NaCl inj or D5 inj to prepare a diluted sol, w/ a final concentration ranging from 1-2mg/mL.
4. Mix diluted sol by gentle inversion; do not shake.
5. Store diluted sol for no more than 24 hrs at 2-8°C (36-46°F) or at 20-25°C (68-77°F).
6. Discard partially used vials or empty vials.

HOW SUPPLIED

Inj: 5mg/mL [10mL, 40mL]

WARNINGS/PRECAUTIONS

Refer to Dosing Considerations for recommendations to withhold or d/c therapy for the following adverse reactions. Refer to PI for corticosteroid dose in the management of the following adverse reactions. Immune-mediated enterocolitis, including fatal cases, can occur. Permanently d/c in patients w/ severe enterocolitis and initiate corticosteroids; initiate corticosteroid taper upon improvement to ≤Grade 1. Withhold therapy for moderate enterocolitis; administer antidiarrheal treatment and, if persistent for >1 week, initiate corticosteroids. Immune-mediated hepatitis, including fatal cases, can occur. Permanently d/c in patients w/ Grade 3 or 4 hepatotoxicity and administer corticosteroids; when LFTs show sustained improvement or return to baseline, initiate corticosteroid taper. Withhold therapy in patients w/ Grade 2 hepatotoxicity. Immune-mediated dermatitis, including fatal cases, can occur. Permanently d/c in patients w/ Stevens-Johnson syndrome, TEN, or rash complicated by full thickness dermal ulceration, or necrotic, bullous, or hemorrhagic manifestations. Administer corticosteroids; when dermatitis is controlled, initiate corticosteroid taper. Withhold in patients w/ moderate to severe signs/symptoms. Immune-mediated neuropathies, including fatal cases, can occur. Permanently d/c in patients w/ severe neuropathy (eg, Guillain-Barre-like syndromes). Consider initiation of corticosteroids. Withhold in patients w/ moderate neuropathy. Immune-mediated endocrinopathies, including life-threatening cases, can occur. Withhold in symptomatic patients; initiate corticosteroids and appropriate hormone replacement therapy. Permanently d/c for clinically significant or severe immune-mediated adverse reactions; initiate corticosteroids for severe immune-mediated adverse reactions. Permanently d/c for immune-mediated ocular disease that is unresponsive to local immunosuppressive therapy. Can cause fetal harm.

ADVERSE REACTIONS

Unresectable/Metastatic Melanoma: Diarrhea, colitis, pruritus, rash, fatigue.
Adjuvant Treatment of Melanoma: Rash, pruritus, diarrhea, nausea, colitis, vomiting, weight decreased, fatigue, pyrexia, headache, decreased appetite, insomnia.

DRUG INTERACTIONS

Increased transaminases w/ or w/o concomitant increases in total bilirubin reported in patients who received concurrent vemurafenib (960mg bid or 720mg bid).

PATIENT CONSIDERATIONS

Assessment: Assess pregnancy/nursing status. Evaluate clinical chemistries, including LFTs, ACTH level, and thyroid function tests, at baseline.

Monitoring: Monitor for signs/symptoms of immune-mediated enterocolitis, hepatitis, dermatitis, motor or sensory neuropathy, hypophysitis, adrenal insufficiency, hypo/hyperthyroidism, and other adverse reactions. Monitor clinical chemistries, ACTH level, and thyroid function tests as clinically indicated.

Counseling: Inform of the potential risk of immune-mediated adverse reactions. Advise women that therapy can cause fetal harm; instruct to use effective contraception during treatment and for 3 months after the last dose. Advise to contact physician if pregnant or if pregnancy suspected. Advise nursing mothers not to breastfeed during treatment and for 3 months after the last dose.

STORAGE: 2-8°C (36-46°F). Do not freeze. Protect from light.

YONDELIS – trabectedin

RX

Class: Alkylating agent

ADULT DOSAGE

Unresectable or Metastatic Liposarcoma or Leiomyosarcoma

In patients who received a prior anthracycline-containing regimen

Recommended: 1.5mg/m^2 as an IV infusion every 21 days, until disease progression or unacceptable toxicity, in patients w/ normal bilirubin and AST or ALT ≤2.5X ULN

Premedication

Administer dexamethasone 20mg IV 30 min prior to each dose

PEDIATRIC DOSAGE

Pediatric use may not have been established

DOSING CONSIDERATIONS

Adverse Reactions

Permanently d/c for:

- Persistent adverse reactions requiring a delay in dosing of >3 weeks
- Adverse reactions requiring dose reduction following dose of 1mg/m^2
- Severe liver dysfunction (all of the following: bilirubin 2X ULN and AST/ALT 3X ULN w/ alkaline phosphatase <2X ULN) in the prior treatment cycle

Dose Reductions:

1st dose reduction: 1.2mg/m^2 every 3 weeks
2nd dose reduction: 1mg/m^2 every 3 weeks

The dose should not be increased in subsequent treatment cycles once the dose is reduced for adverse reactions

Delay Next Dose for Up to 3 Weeks:

- Platelets <100,000 platelets/μL
- ANC <1500 neutrophils/μL
- Total bilirubin >ULN
- AST/ALT >2.5X ULN
- Alkaline phosphatase >2.5X ULN
- Creatine phosphokinase >2.5X ULN
- Decreased left ventricular ejection fraction: Less than lower limit of normal or clinical evidence of cardiomyopathy
- Other nonhematologic Grade 3 or 4 adverse reactions

Reduce Next Dose by One Dose Level for Adverse Reaction(s) During Prior Cycle:

- Platelets <25,000 platelets/μL
- ANC <1000 neutrophils/μL w/ fever/infection or <500 neutrophils/μL lasting >5 days
- Total bilirubin >ULN
- AST/ALT >5X ULN
- Alkaline phosphatase >2.5X ULN
- Creatine phosphokinase >5X ULN
- Decreased left ventricular ejection fraction: Absolute decrease of ≥10% from baseline and less than lower limit of normal or clinical evidence of cardiomyopathy
- Other nonhematologic Grade 3 or 4 adverse reactions

ADMINISTRATION

IV route

Infuse reconstituted, diluted sol over 24 hrs through a central venous line using an infusion set w/ a 0.2 micron polyethersulfone in-line filter.
Complete infusion w/in 30 hrs of initial reconstitution; discard any unused portion of the product or of the infusion sol.
Do not mix w/ other drugs.
Discard any remaining sol w/in 30 hrs of reconstituting the lyophilized powder.

Preparation:

1. Inject 20mL of sterile water for inj into the vial; shake the vial until complete dissolution.
2. Immediately following reconstitution, withdraw the calculated volume of drug and further dilute in 500mL of 0.9% NaCl and D5 inj.

Compatibility:

Type 1 colorless glass vials
PVC and polyethylene bags and tubing

Polyethylene and polypropylene mixture bags
Polyethersulfone in-line filters
Titanium, platinum, or plastic ports
Silicone and polyurethane catheters
Pumps having contact surfaces made of PVC, polyethylene, or polyethylene/polypropylene

HOW SUPPLIED
Inj: (Powder) 1mg

CONTRAINDICATIONS
Severe hypersensitivity (eg, anaphylaxis) to trabectedin.

WARNINGS/PRECAUTIONS
Neutropenic sepsis, rhabdomyolysis, musculoskeletal toxicity, hepatotoxicity, and cardiomyopathy can occur. Extravasation, resulting in tissue necrosis requiring debridement, can occur. Can cause fetal harm.

ADVERSE REACTIONS
N/V, fatigue, constipation, decreased appetite, diarrhea, peripheral edema, dyspnea, headache.

DRUG INTERACTIONS
Increased systemic exposure w/ ketoconazole; avoid use of strong CYP3A inhibitors (eg, oral ketoconazole, itraconazole, clarithromycin). Avoid grapefruit or grapefruit juice. If strong CYP3A inhibitor for short term use (eg, <14 days) must be used, administer the strong CYP3A inhibitor 1 week after infusion, and d/c the day prior to the next infusion. Decreased systemic exposure w/ rifampin; avoid strong CYP3A inducers (eg, rifampin, phenobarbital, St. John's wort).

PATIENT CONSIDERATIONS

Assessment: Assess for drug hypersensitivity, left ventricular ejection fraction, pregnancy/nursing status, and for possible drug interactions. Assess neutrophil count, CPK levels, and LFTs prior to each dose.

Monitoring: Monitor for rhabdomyolysis, hepatotoxicity, extravasation, and for other adverse reactions. Monitor neutrophil count periodically, and left ventricular ejection fraction at 2- to 3-month intervals.

Counseling: Inform of the risks of myelosuppression; instruct to immediately contact physician for fever or unusual bruising, bleeding, tiredness, or paleness. Advise to contact physician immediately if experiencing symptoms of rhabdomyolysis, hepatotoxicity, cardiomyopathy, hypersensitivity, or extravasation. Inform pregnant women of the potential risk to fetus, and to contact physician if pregnant or suspected to be pregnant during treatment. Advise females of reproductive potential to use effective contraception during treatment and for at least 2 months after last dose. Advise males w/ female partners of reproductive potential to use effective contraception during treatment and for at least 5 months after last dose. Advise females not to breastfeed during treatment.

STORAGE: 2-8°C (36-46°F).

ZARXIO — filgrastim-sndz

RX

Class: Granulocyte colony-stimulating factor (G-CSF)

ADULT DOSAGE

Chemotherapy-Associated Neutropenia

Decreases incidence of infection, as manifested by febrile neutropenia, in patients w/ nonmyeloid malignancies receiving myelosuppressive anticancer drugs associated w/ a significant incidence of severe neutropenia w/ fever. Also reduces the time to neutrophil recovery and duration of fever, following induction or consolidation chemotherapy treatment of patients w/ acute myeloid leukemia (AML)

Receiving Myelosuppressive Chemotherapy or Induction and/or Consolidation Chemotherapy for AML:
Initial: 5mcg/kg/day qd
Titrate: May increase in increments of 5mcg/kg for each chemotherapy cycle, according to duration and severity of ANC nadir
D/C if ANC increases beyond 10,000/mm^3

To reduce the duration of neutropenia

PEDIATRIC DOSAGE

General Dosing

Refer to prescribing information for information on pediatric dosing and neutropenia-related clinical sequelae in patients w/ nonmyeloid malignancies undergoing myeloablative chemotherapy followed by marrow transplantation

Receiving Bone Marrow Transplant:
10mcg/kg/day by IV infusion no longer than 24 hrs

Titrate:
When ANC >1000/mm³ for 3 Consecutive Days: Reduce to 5mcg/kg/day then,
If ANC Remains >1000/mm³ for 3 More Consecutive Days: D/C therapy then,
If ANC Decreases to <1000/mm³: Resume at 5mcg/kg/day
If ANC decreases to <1000/mm³ at any time during the 5mcg/kg/day administration, increase to 10mcg/kg/day, and retitrate following the above steps

Hematopoietic Progenitor Cell Mobilization
Mobilizes autologous hematopoietic progenitor cells into the peripheral blood for collection by leukapheresis

10mcg/kg/day SQ for ≥4 days before the 1st leukapheresis procedure and continued until the last leukapheresis

Monitor neutrophil counts after 4 days of therapy, and d/c if WBC count rises to >100,000/mm³

Administration of therapy for 6-7 days w/ leukapheresis on Days 5, 6, and 7 was found to be safe and effective

Severe Chronic Neutropenia
Reduces incidence and duration of sequelae

Initial:
Congenital: 6mcg/kg SQ bid
Idiopathic/Cyclic: 5mcg/kg SQ qd
Titrate: Adjust dose based on clinical course and ANC

ADMINISTRATION
SQ/IV route

Direct administration to patients requiring doses <0.3mL (180mcg) is not recommended due to potential for dosing errors.
Avoid administration of prefilled syringe in persons w/ latex allergies; needle cap contains natural rubber latex.
Prior to use, remove prefilled syringe from the refrigerator and allow therapy to reach room temperature for a minimum of 30 min and a max of 24 hrs.
Discard any prefilled syringe left at room temperature for >24 hrs.

SQ Administration
Inject in the outer area of upper arms, abdomen, thighs, or upper outer areas of buttocks.

Chemotherapy-Associated Neutropenia
Cancer Patients Receiving Myelosuppressive Chemotherapy or Induction and/or Consolidation Chemotherapy for Acute Myeloid Leukemia:
May administer by SQ inj, by short IV infusion (15-30 min), or by continuous IV infusion.
Administer at least 24 hrs after cytotoxic chemotherapy.
Do not administer w/in the 24-hr period prior to chemotherapy.
Administer daily for up to 2 weeks or until ANC has reached 10,000/mm³ following the expected chemotherapy-induced neutrophil nadir.

Cancer Patients Receiving Bone Marrow Transplant:
Administer 1st dose at least 24 hrs after cytotoxic chemotherapy and at least 24 hrs after bone marrow infusion.

Dilution
May dilute in D5 to concentrations between 5-15mcg/mL.
Protect diluted concentrations between 5-15mcg/mL from adsorption to plastic materials by the

addition of albumin (human) to a final concentration of 2mg/mL.
When diluted in D5 or D5 plus albumin (human), compatible w/ glass bottles, polyvinylchloride, polyolefin, and polypropylene.
Do not dilute w/ saline; product may precipitate.

HOW SUPPLIED

Inj: 300mcg/0.5mL, 480mcg/0.8mL

CONTRAINDICATIONS

History of serious allergic reactions to human granulocyte colony-stimulating factors such as filgrastim or pegfilgrastim products.

WARNINGS/PRECAUTIONS

Splenic rupture, including fatal cases, reported. Acute respiratory distress syndrome (ARDS) reported; d/c in patients w/ ARDS. Serious allergic-type reactions, including anaphylaxis, reported; permanently d/c in patients w/ serious allergic reactions. Sickle cell crisis, in some cases fatal, reported in patients w/ sickle cell trait/disease. Glomerulonephritis reported; evaluate for cause if glomerulonephritis is suspected and consider dose reduction or interruption of therapy if causality is likely. Not approved for peripheral blood progenitor cell collection mobilization in healthy donors; alveolar hemorrhage manifesting as pulmonary infiltrates and hemoptysis reported. Capillary leak syndrome (CLS) reported. Myelodysplastic syndrome (MDS) and AML reported to occur in the natural history of congenital neutropenia w/o cytokine therapy. Cytogenetic abnormalities, transformation to MDS, and AML observed in patients treated for severe chronic neutropenia (SCN); carefully consider the risks and benefits of continuing therapy if a patient w/ SCN develops abnormal cytogenetics or myelodysplasia. Thrombocytopenia and leukocytosis reported. Cutaneous vasculitis reported; hold therapy w/ cutaneous vasculitis and may start therapy at a reduced dose when the symptoms resolve and the ANC has decreased. May act as a growth factor for any tumor type. Consider transient positive bone-imaging changes when interpreting bone-imaging results.

ADVERSE REACTIONS

Nausea, pyrexia, thrombocytopenia, bone/back/chest pain, dizziness, pain, fatigue, dyspnea, headache, cough, rash, pain in extremity, arthralgia, increased blood lactate dehydrogenase, increased blood alkaline phosphatase.

DRUG INTERACTIONS

Do not use in the period 24 hrs before through 24 hours after the administration of cytotoxic chemotherapy. Avoid simultaneous use w/ chemotherapy and radiation therapy.

PATIENT CONSIDERATIONS

Assessment: Assess for hypersensitivity to the drug, latex allergy, sickle cell disorder, pregnancy/nursing status, and possible drug interactions. Confirm diagnosis of SCN prior to therapy. Obtain baseline CBC and platelet count in patients receiving myelosuppressive chemotherapy/induction, and/or consolidation chemotherapy for AML.

Monitoring: Monitor for serious allergic-type reactions, splenic rupture, ARDS, sickle cell crisis, glomerulonephritis, CLS, cutaneous vasculitis, thrombocytopenia, leukocytosis, and other adverse reactions. Monitor for cytogenetic abnormalities, transformation to MDS, and AML in patients w/ SCN. In patients receiving myelosuppressive chemotherapy/induction, and/or consolidation chemotherapy for AML, monitor CBC and platelet count twice weekly. In patients w/ SCN, monitor CBC w/ differential and platelet counts during the initial 4 weeks of therapy and during the 2 weeks following any dose adjustment, and, once patient is clinically stable, monthly during the 1st yr of treatment; thereafter, if clinically stable, less frequent routine monitoring is recommended. Frequently monitor CBCs and platelet counts following marrow transplantation.

Counseling: Instruct patient and caregiver on direct patient administration, including how to measure the required dose, particularly if on a dose other than the entire syringe. Inform that rupture or enlargement of the spleen may occur; advise to immediately report to physician if symptoms develop. Advise to seek immediate medical attention if signs/symptoms of a hypersensitivity reaction occur. Advise to immediately report to physician if dyspnea or signs/symptoms of vasculitis develop. Discuss potential risks and benefits for patients w/ sickle cell disease prior to administration. Advise female of reproductive potential that therapy should be used during pregnancy only if the potential benefit justifies the potential risk to the fetus.

STORAGE: 2-8°C (36-46°F). Protect from light. Do not shake. Avoid freezing; if frozen, thaw in the refrigerator before administration. Discard if frozen more than once. Diluted Sol: May store at room temperature for up to 24 hrs; the 24-hr time period includes the time during room temperature storage of the infusion sol and the duration of the infusion.

ZEBETA – bisoprolol fumarate

RX

Class: Selective $beta_1$ blocker

ADULT DOSAGE

Hypertension

Initial: 5mg qd

Titrate: May increase to 10mg and then, if necessary, to 20mg qd

PEDIATRIC DOSAGE

Pediatric use may not have been established

DOSING CONSIDERATIONS

Renal Impairment

CrCl <40mL/min:

Initial: 2.5mg qd; use caution w/ dose titration

Hepatic Impairment

Initial: 2.5mg qd; use caution w/ dose titration

Other Important Considerations

Patients w/ Bronchospastic Disease:

Initial: 2.5mg qd

ADMINISTRATION

Oral route

HOW SUPPLIED

Tab: 5mg*, 10mg *scored

CONTRAINDICATIONS

Cardiogenic shock, overt cardiac failure, 2nd- or 3rd-degree atrioventricular (AV) block, marked sinus bradycardia.

WARNINGS/PRECAUTIONS

Avoid abrupt withdrawal; exacerbation of angina pectoris, MI, and ventricular arrhythmia in patients with coronary artery disease, and exacerbation of symptoms of hyperthyroidism or precipitation of thyroid storm reported. Reinstitute temporary therapy if withdrawal symptoms occur. May mask manifestations of hypoglycemia or clinical signs of hyperthyroidism (eg, tachycardia). Caution with compensated cardiac failure, diabetes mellitus, bronchospastic disease, and hepatic/renal impairment. May precipitate cardiac failure; d/c at the 1st signs/symptoms of heart failure (HF) or continue therapy while HF is treated with other drugs. Caution with peripheral vascular disease; may precipitate or aggravate symptoms of arterial insufficiency. Caution with history of severe anaphylactic reaction to a variety of allergens; reactivity may increase with repeated challenge.

ADVERSE REACTIONS

Headache, URI, peripheral edema, fatigue, ALT/AST elevation.

DRUG INTERACTIONS

Patients with a history of severe anaphylactic reaction to a variety of allergens taking β-blockers may be unresponsive to usual doses of epinephrine. D/C several days before withdrawal of clonidine. Excessive reduction of sympathetic activity with catecholamine-depleting drugs (eg, reserpine, guanethidine); monitor closely. Avoid with other β-blockers. Caution with myocardial depressants or inhibitors of AV conduction, such as calcium antagonists (eg, verapamil, diltiazem) or antiarrhythmics (eg, disopyramide). Increased risk of bradycardia with digitalis glycosides. Increased clearance with rifampin. Caution with insulin or oral hypoglycemic agents. Reversed effects with bronchodilator therapy. Additive BP lowering effects in mild to moderate HTN with HCTZ.

PATIENT CONSIDERATIONS

Assessment: Assess for conditions where treatment is contraindicated or cautioned, pregnancy/nursing status, and possible drug interactions.

Monitoring: Monitor for hypoglycemia, hyperthyroidism, hepatic/renal function, signs/symptoms of HF, withdrawal, and arterial insufficiency. Monitor HR, ECG, CBC with platelet and differential count.

Counseling: Instruct not to interrupt or d/c therapy without consulting physician. Notify physician if difficulty in breathing, signs/symptoms of CHF or excessive bradycardia develop. Educate about signs/symptoms of drug's potential adverse effects. Advise to exercise caution while driving, operating machinery, or engaging in other tasks requiring alertness.

STORAGE: 20-25°C (68-77°F). Protect from moisture.

ZECUITY – sumatriptan

RX

Class: 5-$HT_{1B/1D}$ agonist (triptans)

ADULT DOSAGE

Migraine

Acute Treatment w/ or w/o Aura:

Apply 1 patch for 4 hrs or until red light emitting diode light goes off. If headache relief is incomplete, a 2nd patch may be applied ≥2 hrs after activation of the 1st patch to a different site

Max: 1 patch/dose or 2 patches/24 hrs

The safety of using >4 patches in 1 month has not been established

PEDIATRIC DOSAGE

Pediatric use may not have been established

DOSING CONSIDERATIONS

Elderly

Start at lower end of dosing range

ADMINISTRATION

Transdermal route

Apply to dry intact, non-irritated skin on upper arm or thigh on a site that is relatively hair free and w/o scars, tattoos, abrasions, or other skin conditions; may secure the system w/ medical tape if needed

Do not apply to a previous application site until the site remains erythema free for at least 3 days

Once applied, push the activation button to turn on the red light emitting diode (LED) w/in 15 min

When the LED light turns off, dosing is complete and the system can be removed

After use, fold the system so the adhesive side sticks to itself and safely discard away from children and pets

HOW SUPPLIED

Iontophoretic transdermal system: 6.5mg/4 hrs

CONTRAINDICATIONS

Ischemic coronary artery disease (CAD) (eg, angina pectoris, history of MI, documented silent ischemia), coronary artery vasospasm (eg, Prinzmetal's angina), Wolff-Parkinson-White syndrome or arrhythmias associated with other cardiac accessory conduction pathway disorders, history of stroke, transient ischemic attack, history of hemiplegic or basilar migraine, peripheral vascular disease, ischemic bowel disease, uncontrolled HTN, severe hepatic impairment, or allergic contact dermatitis to sumatriptan. Recent (within 24 hrs) use of ergotamine-containing medication, ergot-type medication (eg, dihydroergotamine, methysergide) or another 5-hydroxytryptamine$_1$ agonist. Concurrent administration of an MAO-A inhibitor or recent (within 2 weeks) use of an MAO-A inhibitor. Known hypersensitivity to sumatriptan or components of this medication.

WARNINGS/PRECAUTIONS

For transdermal use only. Use only if a clear diagnosis of migraine has been established. Reconsider the diagnosis of migraine before giving a 2nd dose if patient does not respond to the 1st dose of therapy. No evidence of benefit for the use of a 2nd transdermal system (TDS) to treat headache recurrence or incomplete headache relief during a migraine attack. Contains metal parts; remove before an MRI procedure. Do not apply in areas near or over electrically-active implantable or body-worn medical devices (eg, implantable cardiac pacemaker, body-worn insulin pump, implantable deep brain stimulator). May lead to allergic contact dermatitis; d/c if suspected. Systemic sensitization or other systemic reactions may develop if other sumatriptan-containing products are taken via other routes (eg, PO, SQ); administer 1st subsequent dose under close medical supervision. May cause coronary artery vasospasm (Prinzmetal's angina) and sensations of tightness, pain, pressure, and heaviness in the chest, throat, neck, and jaw, usually of noncardiac origin. Perform cardiovascular (CV) evaluation in triptan-naive patients who have multiple CV risk factors before treatment; if negative, consider 1st administration in a medically supervised setting and perform an ECG upon activation of TDS. Consider periodic CV evaluation in intermittent long-term users. Life-threatening cardiac rhythm disturbances reported; d/c if these occur. Cerebral hemorrhage, subarachnoid hemorrhage, and stroke may occur; exclude other potentially serious neurological conditions prior to therapy in patients not previously diagnosed as migraineurs, and in migraineurs who present with atypical symptoms. May cause noncoronary vasospastic reactions (eg, peripheral vascular ischemia, GI vascular ischemia/infarction, splenic infarction, Raynaud's syndrome). Transient/permanent blindness and significant partial vision loss reported. Overuse may lead to exacerbation of headache; detoxification including drug withdrawal, and treatment of withdrawal symptoms may be necessary. Serotonin syndrome may occur; d/c if suspected. Significant elevation in BP, including hypertensive crisis with acute impairment of organ systems, reported. Anaphylactic/anaphylactoid reactions may occur. Seizures reported; caution in patients with a history of epilepsy or conditions associated with a lowered seizure threshold.

ADVERSE REACTIONS

Application-site reactions (pain, paresthesia, pruritus, warmth, discomfort, irritation, discoloration, vesicles).

DRUG INTERACTIONS

See Contraindications. Serotonin syndrome reported with SSRIs, SNRIs, TCAs, or MAOIs.

PATIENT CONSIDERATIONS

Assessment: Assess for cardiovascular disease, HTN, hemiplegic/basilar migraine, ECG changes, and any other conditions where treatment is cautioned or contraindicated, hepatic function, pregnancy/nursing status, and for possible drug interactions. Confirm diagnosis of migraine and exclude other potentially serious neurologic conditions prior to therapy. Perform CV evaluation in patients who have CV risk factors.

Monitoring: Monitor for signs/symptoms of cardiac events, cerebrovascular events, peripheral vascular ischemia, GI vascular ischemia/infarction, serotonin syndrome, allergic contact dermatitis, anaphylactic/anaphylactoid reactions, visual disturbances, HTN, and other adverse reactions. Perform ECG immediately after administration of therapy and monitor CV function in intermittent long-term users. Monitor for medication overuse; exacerbation of headache may occur.

Counseling: Instruct to use TDS ud; instruct not to bathe, shower, or swim while wearing TDS. Inform that most patients experience some skin redness under the TDS upon removal, which usually disappears within 24 hrs. Inform patients that the TDS contains metal parts and must be removed before an MRI procedure. Inform that treatment may cause serious CV adverse reactions (eg, MI or stroke) that may result in hospitalization and even death. Instruct patients to be alert for signs/symptoms of chest pain, SOB, weakness, and slurring of speech; instruct to notify physician if these symptoms and other symptoms of vasospastic reactions occur. Inform patients of the signs and symptoms of allergic contact dermatitis, and instruct to seek medical advice if skin lesions suggestive of allergic contact dermatitis develop. Counsel about the possible drug interactions and the risk of anaphylactic/anaphylactoid reactions. Inform patients that the use of therapy ≥10 days per month may lead to exacerbation of headache; encourage to record headache frequency and drug use. Advise to notify physician if pregnant/nursing or planning to become pregnant. Instruct patients to evaluate their ability to perform complex tasks during migraine attacks and after using therapy.

STORAGE: 20-25°C (68-77°F); excursions permitted to 15-30°C (59-86°F). Do not refrigerate or freeze. Contains lithium-manganese dioxide batteries; dispose in accordance with state and local regulations.

ZEGERID — omeprazole/sodium bicarbonate

RX

Class: Proton pump inhibitor (PPI)/antacid

ADULT DOSAGE

Gastroesophageal Reflux Disease

Symptomatic GERD (w/ No Esophageal Erosions):
20mg qd for up to 4 weeks

Erosive Esophagitis (Diagnosed by Endoscopy):
20mg qd for 4-8 weeks
May give up to an additional 4 weeks if no response to 8 weeks of therapy
May consider additional 4- to 8-week courses if there is recurrence of erosive esophagitis or GERD symptoms

Maint of Healing of Erosive Esophagitis:
20mg qd; controlled studies do not extend beyond 12 months

Upper GI Bleeding

Risk Reduction in Critically Ill Patients:
Sus, 40mg/1680mg:
Initial: 40mg, followed by 40mg after 6-8 hrs
Maint: 40mg qd for 14 days

Duodenal Ulcers

PEDIATRIC DOSAGE

Pediatric use may not have been established

Active:
20mg qd for 4-8 weeks

Gastric Ulcers

Active Benign:
40mg qd for 4-8 weeks

DOSING CONSIDERATIONS

Hepatic Impairment

Consider dose reduction, particularly for maint of healing of erosive esophagitis

Other Important Considerations

Asian Population:
Consider dose reduction, particularly for maint of healing of erosive esophagitis

ADMINISTRATION

Oral route

Take on an empty stomach at least 1 hr ac

Cap

Swallow intact w/ water; do not use other liquids
Do not open cap and sprinkle contents into food

Sus

Empty pkt contents into a small cup containing 1-2 tbsp of water; do not use other liquids or foods
Stir well and drink immediately
Refill cup w/ water and drink

Administration Through NG or Orogastric Tube:
Suspend enteral feeding approx 3 hrs before and 1 hr after administration of sus
Constitute the sus w/ approx 20mL of water; do not use other liquids or foods
Stir well and administer immediately
Use an appropriately sized syringe to instill sus in tube
Wash sus through the tube w/ 20mL of water

HOW SUPPLIED

(Omeprazole/Sodium Bicarbonate) **Cap:** 20mg/1100mg, 40mg/1100mg; **Sus:** (20mg/1680mg)/pkt, (40mg/1680mg)/pkt

CONTRAINDICATIONS

Hypersensitivity to any components of the formulation.

WARNINGS/PRECAUTIONS

Omeprazole: Symptomatic response does not preclude the presence of gastric malignancy. Atrophic gastritis reported with long-term use. Acute interstitial nephritis reported; d/c if this develops. Cyanocobalamin (vitamin B12) deficiency may occur with daily long-term treatment (eg, >3 yrs) with any acid-suppressing medications. May increase risk of *Clostridium difficile*-associated diarrhea (CDAD), especially in hospitalized patients. May increase risk of osteoporosis-related fractures of the hip, wrist, or spine, especially with high-dose and long-term therapy. Use lowest dose and shortest duration appropriate to the condition being treated. Hypomagnesemia reported and may require Mg^{2+} replacement and discontinuation of therapy; consider monitoring Mg^{2+} levels prior to and periodically during therapy with prolonged treatment. Drug-induced decrease in gastric acidity results in enterochromaffin-like cell hyperplasia and increased chromogranin A (CgA) levels, which may interfere with investigations for neuroendocrine tumors; temporarily d/c treatment before assessing CgA levels and consider repeating the test if initial CgA levels are high. Sodium Bicarbonate: Consider the Na^+ content when administering to patients on a Na^+-restricted diet. Caution with Bartter's syndrome, hypokalemia, hypocalcemia, and problems with acid-base balance. Chronic use may lead to systemic alkalosis, and increased Na^+ intake may produce edema and weight increase.

ADVERSE REACTIONS

Agitation, anemia, bradycardia, constipation, rash, tachycardia, diarrhea, fever, thrombocytopenia, hypokalemia, hypomagnesemia, hyperglycemia, atrial fibrillation, HTN, hypotension.

DRUG INTERACTIONS

Monitor for the need to adjust dose of drugs metabolized via CYP450 (eg, cyclosporine, disulfiram, benzodiazepines). Omeprazole: Reduces pharmacological activity of clopidogrel; avoid concomitant use, and consider alternative antiplatelet therapy. Caution with digoxin or drugs that may cause hypomagnesemia (eg, diuretics). May elevate and prolong levels of methotrexate (MTX) and/or its metabolite, possibly leading to MTX toxicities; consider temporary withdrawal of therapy with high-dose MTX. May reduce the absorption of drugs where gastric pH is an important determinant of bioavailability; ketoconazole, atazanavir, iron salts, erlotinib, and mycophenolate mofetil (MMF) absorption may decrease, while digoxin absorption may increase. Monitor when digoxin is taken concomitantly. Caution in transplant patients receiving MMF. May prolong elimination of drugs metabolized by hepatic oxidation (eg, diazepam, warfarin, phenytoin). Increased INR and PT reported with warfarin. Voriconazole (combined inhibitor of CYP2C19 and CYP3A4) may increase levels. May decrease levels of atazanavir and nelfinavir; coadministration not recommended. May increase levels of saquinavir and tacrolimus; consider dose reduction of saquinavir. CYP2C19 or CYP3A4 inducers may decrease levels; avoid with St. John's wort or rifampin. Sodium Bicarbonate: Long-term use of bicarbonate with Ca^{2+} or milk can cause milk-alkali syndrome.

PATIENT CONSIDERATIONS

Assessment: Assess for risk of osteoporosis-related fractures, Na^{+}-restricted diet, Bartter's syndrome, hypokalemia, hypocalcemia, acid-base balance problems, hypersensitivity to the drug, pregnancy/nursing status, and possible drug interactions. Obtain baseline Mg^{2+} levels in patients expected to be on prolonged therapy.

Monitoring: Monitor for signs/symptoms of atrophic gastritis, acute interstitial nephritis, cyanocobalamin deficiency, CDAD, bone fractures, systemic alkalosis, hypersensitivity reactions, and other adverse reactions. Monitor Mg^{2+} levels periodically in patients expected to be on prolonged therapy. Monitor INR and PT when given with warfarin.

Counseling: Inform that different formulations are not bioequivalent; do not substitute one for the other. Inform patients on a Na^{+}-restricted diet of the Na^{+} content in product. Inform that increased Na^{+} intake may cause swelling and weight gain; instruct to contact physician if these occur. Inform that the most frequent adverse reactions associated with therapy include headache, abdominal pain, N/V, diarrhea, and flatulence. Advise that harmful effect of therapy on the fetus cannot be ruled out. Advise to use with caution if regularly taking Ca^{2+} supplements. Advise to immediately report and seek care for diarrhea that does not improve and for any cardiovascular/neurological symptoms (eg, palpitations, dizziness, seizures, tetany).

STORAGE: 25°C (77°F); excursions permitted to 15-30°C (59-86°F). Protect from light and moisture.

ZEMPLAR ORAL — paricalcitol

RX

Class: Vitamin D analogue

ADULT DOSAGE

Secondary Hyperparathyroidism

Associated w/ Chronic Kidney Disease Stages 3 and 4:

Initial:

Baseline Intact Parathyroid Hormone (iPTH) Level:

≤500pg/mL: 1mcg qd or 2mcg 3X/week
>500pg/mL: 2mcg qd or 4mcg 3X/week

Titrate:

Individualize dose and base dose on serum/plasma iPTH levels
Adjust dose at 2- to 4-week intervals

iPTH Level Relative to Baseline:

Same or Decreased by <30%: Increase dose by 1mcg qd or 2mcg 3X/week
Decreased by ≥30% and ≤60%: Maintain dose
Decreased by >60% or iPTH <60pg/mL: Decrease dose by 1mcg qd or 2mcg 3X/week

If patient is taking the lowest dose (1mcg qd) and a dose reduction is needed, the dose can be decreased to 1mcg 3X/week; if further dose reduction is required, withhold therapy prn and restart at a lower dosing frequency
Administer the 3X/week dose not more often than qod

On a Ca^{2+}-Based Phosphate Binder: May decrease or withhold the phosphate-binder dose, or switch to a non-Ca^{2+}-based phosphate binder

Associated w/ Chronic Kidney Disease Stage 5:

Administer 3X/week, not more frequently than qod

PEDIATRIC DOSAGE

Pediatric use may not have been established

Initial: Base dose on a baseline iPTH level (pg/mL)/80
Treat only after baseline serum Ca^{2+} has been adjusted to ≤9.5mg/dL

Titrate: Individualize and base dose on iPTH, serum Ca^{2+}, and phosphorus (P) levels;
Titration Dose (mcg) = Most Recent iPTH Level (pg/mL)/80

On a Ca^{2+}-Based Phosphate Binder: May decrease or withhold the phosphate-binder dose, or switch to a non-Ca^{2+}-based phosphate binder

Refer to PI for further suggested dose titrations

ADMINISTRATION
Oral route

May be taken w/o regard to food

HOW SUPPLIED
Cap: 1mcg, 2mcg, 4mcg

CONTRAINDICATIONS
Vitamin D toxicity, hypercalcemia.

WARNINGS/PRECAUTIONS
Excessive administration may cause over suppression of PTH, hypercalcemia, hypercalciuria, hyperphosphatemia, and adynamic bone disease. Overdose may cause progressive hypercalcemia. Acute hypercalcemia may exacerbate tendencies for cardiac arrhythmias and seizures. Chronic hypercalcemia can lead to generalized vascular calcification and other soft-tissue calcification. May increase SrCr and therefore decrease the estimated GFR in predialysis patients.

ADVERSE REACTIONS
Headache, hypotension, HTN, diarrhea, N/V, constipation, edema, arthritis, dizziness, insomnia, nasopharyngitis, viral infection, hypersensitivity, peritonitis, fluid overload.

DRUG INTERACTIONS
May increase risk of hypercalcemia w/ high doses of Ca^{2+}-containing preparations or thiazide diuretics. Concomitant high intake of Ca^{2+} and phosphate may lead to serum abnormalities requiring more frequent patient monitoring and individualized dose titration. Withhold prescription-based doses of vitamin D and its derivatives during treatment to avoid hypercalcemia. Caution w/ digitalis compounds. Do not coadminister aluminum-containing preparations (eg, antacids, phosphate binders) chronically; increased blood levels of aluminum and aluminum bone toxicity may occur. Increased exposure w/ strong CYP3A inhibitors (eg, ketoconazole, atazanavir, clarithromycin); may need to adjust paricalcitol dose, and closely monitor iPTH and serum Ca^{2+} concentrations if a patient initiates or discontinues therapy w/ a strong CYP3A4 inhibitor. Drugs that impair intestinal absorption of fat-soluble vitamins (eg, cholestyramine) may interfere w/ absorption. Mineral oil or other substances that may affect absorption of fat may influence absorption.

PATIENT CONSIDERATIONS

Assessment: Assess for vitamin D toxicity, hypercalcemia, pregnancy/nursing status, and possible drug interactions.

Monitoring: Monitor for hypercalcemia and other adverse reactions. During the initial dosing or following any dose adjustment, monitor serum Ca^{2+}, serum P, and serum/plasma iPTH at least every 2 weeks for 3 months, then monthly for 3 months, and every 3 months thereafter.

Counseling: Inform of the most common adverse reactions (eg, diarrhea, HTN, dizziness, vomiting). Advise to adhere to instructions regarding diet and P restriction, and to return for routine monitoring. Instruct to contact physician if symptoms of elevated Ca^{2+} (eg, feeling tired, difficulty thinking clearly, loss of appetite) develop. Advise to inform physician of all medications (eg, prescription and nonprescription drugs, supplements, and herbal preparations) being taken and any change to medical condition.

STORAGE: 25°C (77°F); excursions permitted between 15-30°C (59-86°F).

ZENPEP — pancrelipase

RX

Class: Pancreatic enzyme supplement

ADULT DOSAGE

Exocrine Pancreatic Insufficiency

Due to Cystic Fibrosis or Other Conditions:
Start at the lowest recommended dose and increase gradually
Initial: 500 lipase U/kg/meal
Max: 2500 lipase U/kg/meal (or ≤10,000 lipase U/kg/day) or <4000 lipase U/g fat ingested/day

PEDIATRIC DOSAGE

Exocrine Pancreatic Insufficiency

Due to Cystic Fibrosis or Other Conditions:
Start at the lowest recommended dose and increase gradually

≤12 Months of Age:
3000 lipase U per 120mL of formula or per breastfeeding immediately prior to each feeding

>12 Months-<4 Years:
Initial: 1000 lipase U/kg/meal
Max: 2500 lipase U/kg/meal (or ≤10,000 lipase U/kg/day) or <4000 lipase U/g fat ingested/day

≥4 Years:
Initial: 500 lipase U/kg/meal
Max: 2500 lipase U/kg/meal (or ≤10,000 lipase U/kg/day) or <4000 lipase U/g fat ingested/day

ADMINISTRATION

Oral route

Take during meals or snacks, w/ sufficient fluid
Half of the dose used for meals should be given w/ each snack
Swallow whole; do not crush/chew cap or cap contents
If necessary, the cap contents can be sprinkled on soft acidic foods (eg, applesauce, commercial preparations of bananas or pears)
Contents of the cap may also be given directly to the mouth
Do not mix directly into formula or breast milk

HOW SUPPLIED

Cap, Delayed-Release: (Lipase/Protease/Amylase) 3000 U/10,000 U/14,000 U; 5000 U/17,000 U/24,000 U; 10,000 U/32,000 U/42,000 U; 15,000 U/47,000 U/63,000 U; 20,000 U/63,000 U/84,000 U; 25,000 U/79,000 U/105,000 U; 40,000 U/126,000 U/168,000 U

WARNINGS/PRECAUTIONS

Not interchangeable with other pancrelipase products. Fibrosing colonopathy reported; monitor closely for progression to stricture formation. Colonic strictures have been associated with doses >6000 lipase U/kg/meal in children <12 yrs of age. Caution with doses >2500 lipase U/kg/meal (or >10,000 lipase U/kg/day); use only if these doses are documented to be effective by 3-day fecal fat measures indicating significant improvement. Examine patients receiving >6000 lipase U/kg/meal; immediately decrease or titrate dose downward to a lower range. Ensure that no drug is retained in the mouth. Should not be crushed or chewed, or mixed in foods with pH >4.5; may disrupt enteric coating of cap, resulting in early release of enzymes, irritation of oral mucosa, and/or loss of enzyme activity. Caution in patients with gout, renal impairment, or hyperuricemia; may increase blood uric acid levels. Risk for transmission of viral diseases. Caution with known allergy to proteins of porcine origin; severe allergic reactions reported.

ADVERSE REACTIONS

GI disorders (eg, abdominal pain, flatulence), headache, cough, weight decreased, early satiety, contusion.

PATIENT CONSIDERATIONS

Assessment: Assess for gout, renal impairment, hyperuricemia, allergy to porcine proteins, and pregnancy/nursing status.

Monitoring: Monitor for fibrosing colonopathy, stricture formation, oral mucosa irritation, viral diseases, allergic reactions, and other adverse reactions. Monitor serum uric acid levels.

Counseling: Instruct to take ud, with food and sufficient fluids. Inform that if a dose is missed, take the next dose with the next meal/snack ud; instruct not to double doses. Inform that cap contents can be mixed with soft acidic foods (eg, applesauce), if necessary. Advise to contact physician immediately if allergic reactions develop. Instruct to notify physician if pregnant/breastfeeding or planning to become pregnant/breastfeed during treatment. Instruct to notify physician before initiating treatment if patient has a history of abnormal glucose levels.

STORAGE: Avoid excessive heat. Protect from moisture. (Original glass container) 20-25°C (68-77°F); brief excursions permitted to 15-40°C (59-104°F). (Repackaged HDPE container) Store up to 30°C (86°F) for up to 6 months; brief excursions permitted to 15-40°C (59-104°F) for up to 30 days.

ZEPATIER – elbasvir/grazoprevir

RX

Class: HCV NS5A inhibitor/HCV NS3/4A protease inhibitor

ADULT DOSAGE

Chronic Hepatitis C

Treatment of Chronic Hepatitis C Virus (HCV) Genotypes 1 or 4 Infection w/ or w/o Ribavirin (RBV):
1 tab qd

Treatment Regimen and Duration of Therapy in Patients w/ or w/o Cirrhosis:
Test patients w/ HCV genotype 1a infection for presence of virus w/ NS5A resistance-associated polymorphisms prior to initiation of treatment to determine dosage regimen and duration

Genotype 1a: Treatment-Naive or Peginterferon Alfa (PegIFN)/RBV-Experienced w/o Baseline NS5A Polymorphisms:
Zepatier for 12 weeks

Genotype 1a: Treatment-Naive or PegIFN/RBV-Experienced w/ Baseline NS5A Polymorphisms:
Zepatier + RBV for 16 weeks

Genotype 1b: Treatment-Naive or PegIFN/RBV-Experienced:
Zepatier for 12 weeks

Genotype 1a or 1b: PegIFN/RBV/Protease Inhibitor-Experienced:
Zepatier + RBV for 12 weeks

Genotype 4: Treatment-Naive:
Zepatier for 12 weeks

Genotype 4: PegIFN/RBV-Experienced:
Zepatier + RBV for 16 weeks

PEDIATRIC DOSAGE

Pediatric use may not have been established

ADMINISTRATION

Oral route

Take w/ or w/o food.
Refer to RBV labeling for dosing and administration instructions.

HOW SUPPLIED

Tab: (Elbasvir/Grazoprevir) 50mg/100mg

CONTRAINDICATIONS

Moderate or severe hepatic impairment (Child-Pugh B or C). Coadministration w/ OATP1B1/3 inhibitors or w/ strong CYP3A inducers. Coadministration w/ phenytoin, carbamazepine, rifampin, St. John's wort, efavirenz, atazanavir, darunavir, lopinavir, saquinavir, tipranavir, or cyclosporine. If administered w/ RBV, refer to the RBV prescribing information for a list of contraindications for RBV.

WARNINGS/PRECAUTIONS

ALT elevations reported; perform hepatic laboratory testing prior to therapy, at treatment week 8, and as clinically indicated. Additional hepatic laboratory testing should be performed at treatment week 12 in patients receiving 16 weeks of therapy. Consider discontinuing therapy if ALT levels remain persistently >10X ULN. D/C if ALT elevation is accompanied by signs/symptoms of liver inflammation or increasing conjugated bilirubin, alkaline phosphatase, or INR. Refer to the RBV prescribing information for a full list of warnings and precautions for RBV.

ADVERSE REACTIONS

Zepatier for 12 Weeks: Fatigue, headache, nausea.
Zepatier + Ribavirin for 16 Weeks: Anemia, headache.

DRUG INTERACTIONS

See Contraindications. Moderate or strong CYP3A inducers may decrease levels and therapeutic effect; not recommended w/ moderate CYP3A inducers. Strong CYP3A inhibitors may increase levels. Not recommended w/ nafcillin, ketoconazole, bosentan, etravirine, modafinil, or elvitegravir/

cobicistat/emtricitabine/tenofovir (disoproxil fumarate or alafenamide). Nafcillin, bosentan, etravirine, and modafinil may decrease levels. Systemic ketoconazole may increase levels and may increase the overall risk of hepatotoxicity. Coadministration w/ systemic tacrolimus may increase tacrolimus levels; upon initiation of coadministration w/ Zepatier, frequently monitor tacrolimus whole blood concentrations, changes in renal function, and for tacrolimus-associated adverse events. Elvitegravir/cobicistat/ emtricitabine/tenofovir disoproxil (fumarate or alafenamide) may increase levels. May increase atorvastatin levels; atorvastatin dose should not exceed 20mg/day. May increase rosuvastatin levels; rosuvastatin dose should not exceed 10mg/day. May increase fluvastatin, lovastatin, and simvastatin levels; monitor for statin-associated adverse events and use lowest necessary dose. **Grazoprevir:** OATP1B1/3 inhibitors may increase levels.

PATIENT CONSIDERATIONS

Assessment: Assess for hypersensitivity to drug, pregnancy/nursing status, and for possible drug interactions. Test patients w/ HCV genotype 1a infection for the presence of virus w/ NS5A resistance-associated polymorphisms. Perform baseline hepatic laboratory testing.

Monitoring: Monitor for ALT elevations and for any other adverse reaction. Perform hepatic laboratory testing at treatment week 8, and as clinically indicated; perform additional hepatic laboratory testing at treatment week 12 for patients receiving 16 weeks of therapy.

Counseling: Instruct to observe for warning signs of liver inflammation (eg, fatigue, weakness, lack of appetite, N/V, jaundice, discolored feces) and to contact physician w/o delay if such symptoms occur. Advise to notify physician if pregnant or nursing. Advise to report the use of any prescription, non-prescription medication, or herbal products to physician. Inform that therapy should be taken every day at the regularly scheduled time w/ or w/o food.

STORAGE: 20-25°C (68-77°F); excursions permitted between 15-30°C (59-86°F). Protect from moisture.

ZERBAXA – ceftolozane/tazobactam

RX

Class: Beta-lactamase inhibitor/cephalosporin

ADULT DOSAGE

Intra-Abdominal Infections

Complicated Infections:
1.5g (1g/0.5g) q8h for 4-14 days, in conjunction w/ metronidazole 500mg IV q8h

Urinary Tract Infections

Complicated Infections, Including Pyelonephritis:
1.5g (1g/0.5g) q8h for 7 days

PEDIATRIC DOSAGE

Pediatric use may not have been established

DOSING CONSIDERATIONS

Renal Impairment

CrCl 30-50mL/min: 750mg (500mg/250mg) q8h
CrCl 15-29mL/min: 375mg (250mg/125mg) q8h

ESRD on Hemodialysis:
LD: 750mg (500mg/250mg)
Maint: 150mg (100mg/50mg) q8h for remainder of treatment period (on hemodialysis days, administer dose at earliest possible time following completion of dialysis)

ADMINISTRATION

IV route

Infuse over 1 hr
Do not mix w/ other drugs or physically add to sol containing other drugs
Reconstituted sol may be held for 1 hr prior to transfer and dilution in a suitable infusion bag
Following dilution of sol, may store for 24 hrs when stored at room temperature or 7 days when stored under refrigeration at 2-8°C (36-46°F); do not freeze constituted sol or diluted infusion

Preparation

Constitute vial w/ 10mL of sterile water for inj or 0.9% NaCl for inj (final vol is approx 11.4mL); shake gently to dissolve
Withdraw appropriate volume from reconstituted vial and add to an infusion bag containing 100mL of 0.9% NaCl for inj or D5 inj

Preparation of Doses:
1.5g (1g/0.5g) Dose: Withdraw 11.4mL (entire vial contents)
750mg (500mg/250mg) Dose: Withdraw 5.7mL

375mg (250mg/125mg) Dose: Withdraw 2.9mL
150mg (100mg/50mg) Dose: Withdraw 1.2mL

HOW SUPPLIED
Inj: (Ceftolozane/Tazobactam) 1g/0.5g

CONTRAINDICATIONS
Serious hypersensitivity to the components of Zerbaxa (ceftolozane and tazobactam), piperacillin/tazobactam, or other members of the beta-lactam class.

WARNINGS/PRECAUTIONS
Serious and occasionally fatal hypersensitivity (anaphylactic) reactions reported; d/c therapy and institute appropriate therapy if an anaphylactic reaction occurs. Caution w/ cephalosporin, penicillin (PCN), or other β-lactam allergy; cross sensitivity may occur. *Clostridium difficile*-associated diarrhea (CDAD) reported; d/c if CDAD is confirmed. Use in the absence of a proven or strongly suspected bacterial infection is unlikely to provide benefit and increases the risk of the development of drug-resistant bacteria. Caution in elderly.

ADVERSE REACTIONS
N/V, headache, diarrhea, pyrexia, constipation, insomnia, hypokalemia.

PATIENT CONSIDERATIONS
Assessment: Assess for hypersensitivity/allergy to drug, piperacillin/tazobactam, cephalosporin, PCN, or other β-lactams, renal impairment, pregnancy/nursing status, and possible drug interactions.

Monitoring: Monitor for signs and symptoms of hypersensitivity reactions, CDAD, and other adverse reactions. Monitor CrCl daily in patients w/ changing renal function.

Counseling: Advise that allergic reactions, including serious allergic reactions, may occur and require immediate treatment. Advise that diarrhea is a common problem caused by antibacterial drugs and sometimes, frequent watery or bloody diarrhea may occur and may be a sign of a more serious intestinal infection; if severe watery and bloody diarrhea develops, instruct to contact physician. Inform that therapy should only be used to treat bacterial, not viral, infections. Instruct to take exactly ud even if the patient feels better early in the course of therapy. Inform that skipping doses or not completing the full course of therapy may decrease effectiveness and increase risk of bacterial resistance.

STORAGE: 2-8°C (36-46°F). Protect from light.

ZESTORETIC — hydrochlorothiazide/lisinopril RX

Class: ACE inhibitor/thiazide diuretic

D/C when pregnancy is detected. Drugs that act directly on the renin-angiotensin system (RAS) can cause injury/death to the developing fetus.

ADULT DOSAGE
Hypertension

BP Uncontrolled w/ Lisinopril/HCTZ Monotherapy:
10mg/12.5mg or 20mg/12.5mg qd, depending on current monotherapy dose
May increase HCTZ dose after 2-3 weeks

If BP is controlled w/ HCTZ 25mg/day, but significant K+ loss is experienced, similar or greater BP control w/o electrolyte disturbance may be achieved by switching to 10mg/12.5mg qd

Replacement Therapy: Combination may be substituted for the titrated individual components

PEDIATRIC DOSAGE
Pediatric use may not have been established

DOSING CONSIDERATIONS
Elderly
Start at lower end of dosing range

ADMINISTRATION
Oral route

HOW SUPPLIED
Tab: (Lisinopril/HCTZ) 10mg/12.5mg, 20mg/12.5mg, 20mg/25mg

CONTRAINDICATIONS

Hypersensitivity to this product; history of ACE inhibitor-associated angioedema; hereditary or idiopathic angioedema; anuria; or hypersensitivity to other sulfonamide-derived drugs. Coadministration w/ aliskiren in patients w/ diabetes.

WARNINGS/PRECAUTIONS

Not for initial therapy of HTN. Not recommended w/ severe renal impairment (CrCl ≤30mL/min). Caution in elderly. **Lisinopril:** Head/neck angioedema reported; promptly d/c and administer appropriate therapy. Higher rate of angioedema in blacks than nonblacks. Intestinal angioedema reported; monitor for abdominal pain. Patients w/ a history of angioedema unrelated to ACE inhibitor therapy may be at increased risk of angioedema during therapy. Anaphylactoid reactions reported during desensitization w/ hymenoptera venom, dialysis w/ high-flux membranes, and LDL apheresis w/ dextran sulfate absorption. Excessive hypotension may occur in salt/volume-depleted persons (eg, patients treated vigorously w/ diuretics or on dialysis). Excessive hypotension, which may be associated w/ oliguria and/or progressive azotemia, and rarely w/ acute renal failure and/or death, may occur in patients w/ severe CHF; monitor closely during first 2 weeks of therapy and whenever dose is increased. Caution w/ ischemic heart or cerebrovascular disease in whom an excessive fall in BP could result in a MI or cerebrovascular accident. Leukopenia/neutropenia and bone marrow depression may occur. Associated w/ a syndrome that starts w/ cholestatic jaundice or hepatitis and progresses to fulminant hepatic necrosis and sometimes death (rare); d/c if jaundice or marked elevations of hepatic enzymes develop. Caution w/ left ventricular outflow obstruction. May cause changes in renal function; in patients w/ severe CHF whose renal function is dependent on the RAS, oliguria and/or progressive azotemia, and (rare) acute renal failure and/or death may occur. May increase BUN/SrCr in hypertensive patients; monitor renal function during the 1st few weeks of therapy in patients w/ renal artery stenosis. Dosage reduction of lisinopril and/or discontinuation of the diuretic may be required if BUN/SrCr increase occurs. Hyperkalemia and persistent nonproductive cough reported. Hypotension may occur w/ major surgery or during anesthesia. **HCTZ:** May cause idiosyncratic reaction, resulting in acute transient myopia and acute angle-closure glaucoma; d/c as rapidly as possible. May precipitate azotemia in patients w/ renal disease. Caution w/ hepatic dysfunction or progressive liver disease; may precipitate hepatic coma. Sensitivity reactions may occur. May cause exacerbation or activation of systemic lupus erythematosus (SLE), hyperuricemia or precipitation of frank gout, manifestation of latent diabetes mellitus (DM), hypomagnesemia, and hypercalcemia. Observe for signs of fluid or electrolyte imbalance. Hypokalemia may sensitize or exaggerate the response of the heart to toxic effects of digitalis. Enhanced effects in postsympathectomy patients. D/C or withhold if progressive renal impairment becomes evident. D/C before testing for parathyroid function. Increased cholesterol and TG levels reported.

ADVERSE REACTIONS

Dizziness, headache, cough, fatigue, orthostatic effects.

DRUG INTERACTIONS

See Contraindications. NSAIDs, including selective COX-2 inhibitors, may reduce effects of diuretics and ACE inhibitors. Increased risk of lithium toxicity; avoid w/ lithium. Nitritoid reactions reported w/ injectable gold. **Lisinopril:** NSAIDs, including selective COX-2 inhibitors, may deteriorate renal function in patients who are elderly, volume depleted, or w/ compromised renal function. NSAIDs may attenuate the antihypertensive effects. Dual blockade of the RAS is associated w/ increased risks of hypotension, hyperkalemia, and changes in renal function (including acute renal failure); avoid combined use of RAS inhibitors, or closely monitor BP, renal function, and electrolytes w/ concomitant agents that also affect the RAS. Avoid w/ aliskiren in patients w/ renal impairment (GFR <60mL/min). Hypotension risk and increased BUN and SrCr w/ diuretics. Increased risk of hyperkalemia w/ K^+-sparing diuretics (eg, spironolactone, eplerenone, triamterene, amiloride), K^+ supplements, or K^+-containing salt substitutes; use w/ caution and monitor serum K^+. Coadministration w/ mTOR inhibitors (eg, temsirolimus, sirolimus, everolimus) may increase risk for angioedema. **HCTZ:** Potentiation of orthostatic hypotension may occur w/ alcohol, barbiturates, or narcotics. Dosage adjustment of antidiabetic drugs (oral agents, insulin) may be required. Additive effect or potentiation w/ other antihypertensives. Anionic exchange resins (cholestyramine, colestipol) may impair absorption. Corticosteroids and adrenocorticotropic hormone may intensify electrolyte depletion, particularly hypokalemia. May decrease response to pressor amines (eg, norepinephrine). May increase responsiveness to nondepolarizing skeletal muscle relaxants (eg, tubocurarine).

PATIENT CONSIDERATIONS

Assessment: Assess for hereditary/idiopathic angioedema, anuria, DM, volume/salt depletion, CHF, ischemic heart or cerebrovascular disease, collagen vascular disease, left ventricular outflow obstruction, SLE, history of ACE inhibitor-associated angioedema, hypersensitivity to drug or sulfonamide-derived drugs, renal/hepatic dysfunction, postsympathectomy status, pregnancy/nursing status, and possible drug interactions.

Monitoring: Monitor for signs/symptoms of angioedema, anaphylactoid/idiosyncratic/hypersensitivity reactions, exacerbation/activation of SLE, hyperuricemia or precipitation of gout, latent DM, fluid/electrolyte imbalance, and other adverse reactions. Monitor BP, renal/hepatic function, serum electrolytes, cholesterol, and TG levels. Consider periodic monitoring of WBCs in patients w/ collagen vascular disease and renal disease.

Counseling: Inform about fetal risks if taken during pregnancy and discuss treatment options in women planning to become pregnant; instruct to report pregnancy to physician as soon as possible. Instruct to d/c therapy and to immediately report signs/symptoms of angioedema. Instruct to report lightheadedness, especially during the 1st few days of therapy; advise to d/c therapy and consult w/ a physician if actual syncope occurs. Inform that excessive perspiration, dehydration, and other causes of volume depletion (eg, diarrhea, vomiting) may lead to fall in BP; advise to consult w/ physician. Advise not to use salt substitutes containing K^+ w/o consulting physician. Advise to promptly report any indication of infection (eg, sore throat, fever).

STORAGE: 20-25°C (68-77°F). Protect from excessive light and humidity.

ZESTRIL – lisinopril

RX

Class: ACE inhibitor

D/C when pregnancy is detected. Drugs that act directly on the renin-angiotensin system (RAS) can cause injury/death to the developing fetus.

ADULT DOSAGE

Hypertension

Initial: 10mg qd; 5mg qd in patients taking diuretics

Usual Range: 20-40mg qd

Max: 80mg

May add a low-dose diuretic (eg, HCTZ 12.5mg) if BP is not controlled

Heart Failure

Adjunct w/ Diuretics and (Usually) Digitalis to Reduce Signs and Symptoms of Systolic Heart Failure (HF):

Initial: 5mg qd; 2.5mg qd w/ hyponatremia (serum Na^+ <130mEq/L)

Max: 40mg qd

Diuretic dose may need to be adjusted to help minimize hypovolemia

Acute Myocardial Infarction

Reduction of Mortality in Hemodynamically Stable Patients w/in 24 Hrs of Acute MI (AMI):

5mg w/in 24 hrs of onset of symptoms, followed by 5mg after 24 hrs, 10mg after 48 hrs, and then 10mg qd for at least 6 weeks

In patients w/ low systolic BP (SBP) (≤120mmHg and >100mmHg) during the first 3 days after infarct, initiate w/ 2.5mg; consider doses of 2.5mg or 5mg if hypotension occurs (SBP ≤100mmHg). D/C therapy if prolonged hypotension occurs (SBP <90mmHg for >1 hr)

PEDIATRIC DOSAGE

Hypertension

≥6 Years:

GFR >30mL/min/1.73m²:

Initial: 0.07mg/kg qd (up to 5mg total)

Max: 0.61mg/kg (up to 40mg) qd

DOSING CONSIDERATIONS

Renal Impairment

CrCl 10-30mL/min: Reduce initial dose to 1/2 the usual recommended dose (eg, HTN, 5mg; systolic HF/AMI, 2.5mg); titrate up as tolerated to a max of 40mg qd

Hemodialysis or CrCl <10mL/min:

Initial: 2.5mg qd

ADMINISTRATION

Oral route

HOW SUPPLIED

Tab: 2.5mg, 5mg*, 10mg, 20mg, 30mg, 40mg *scored

CONTRAINDICATIONS

History of ACE inhibitor-associated angioedema or hypersensitivity, hereditary or idiopathic angioedema, coadministration w/ aliskiren in patients w/ diabetes.

WARNINGS/PRECAUTIONS

Not recommended in pediatric patients w/ GFR <30mL/min/1.73m^2. Head/neck angioedema reported; d/c promptly and administer appropriate therapy. Intestinal angioedema reported; monitor for abdominal pain. Patients w/ history of angioedema unrelated to ACE inhibitor therapy may be at increased risk of angioedema during therapy. Less effect on BP and higher rates of angioedema in blacks than nonblacks. Anaphylactoid reactions reported during desensitization w/ hymenoptera venom, dialysis w/ high-flux membranes, and LDL apheresis w/ dextran sulfate absorption. May cause changes in renal function, including acute renal failure, especially in patients whose renal function depends on the RAS; consider withholding or discontinuing therapy if a clinically significant decrease in renal function develops. May cause symptomatic hypotension, sometimes complicated by oliguria, progressive azotemia, acute renal failure, or death; closely monitor patients at risk of excessive hypotension during first 2 weeks of treatment and whenever therapy and/or diuretic dose is increased. Avoid in patients who are hemodynamically unstable after AMI. Symptomatic hypotension may occur in patients w/ severe aortic stenosis or hypertrophic cardiomyopathy. Hypotension may occur w/ major surgery or during anesthesia. May cause hyperkalemia; monitor serum K^+ periodically. Associated w/ a syndrome that starts w/ cholestatic jaundice or hepatitis and progresses to fulminant hepatic necrosis, and sometimes death; d/c if jaundice or marked hepatic enzyme elevations occur.

ADVERSE REACTIONS

Dizziness, headache, hypotension, hyperkalemia, syncope, increased creatinine/BUN.

DRUG INTERACTIONS

See Contraindications. Hypotension risk and increased BUN and SrCr w/ diuretics. Increased hypoglycemic risk w/ insulin or oral hypoglycemics. NSAIDs, including selective COX-2 inhibitors, may cause deterioration of renal function in the elderly, volume-depleted, or w/ compromised renal function. Antihypertensive effect of therapy may be attenuated by NSAIDs. Dual blockade of the RAS is associated w/ increased risks of hypotension, hyperkalemia, and changes in renal function (including acute renal failure); avoid combined use of RAS inhibitors, or closely monitor BP, renal function, and electrolytes w/ concomitant agents that also affect the RAS. Avoid w/ aliskiren in patients w/ renal impairment (GFR <60mL/min). Increased risk of hyperkalemia w/ K^+-sparing diuretics, K^+-containing salt substitutes, or K^+ supplements; monitor serum K^+ periodically. Lithium toxicity reported; monitor serum lithium levels during concurrent use. Nitritoid reactions reported w/ injectable gold. Concomitant mTOR inhibitors (eg, temsirolimus, sirolimus, everolimus) may increase risk for angioedema.

PATIENT CONSIDERATIONS

Assessment: Assess for hypersensitivity to the drug, history of ACE inhibitor-associated angioedema, hereditary/idiopathic angioedema, risk factors for hyperkalemia, risk for excessive hypotension, severe aortic stenosis or hypertrophic cardiomyopathy, renal impairment, pregnancy/nursing status, and possible drug interactions.

Monitoring: Monitor for angioedema, anaphylactoid reactions, and other adverse reactions. Monitor BP, LFTs, serum K^+, and renal function.

Counseling: Inform of pregnancy risks and discuss treatment options for women planning to become pregnant; instruct to report pregnancy to physician as soon as possible. Instruct to immediately report signs/symptoms of angioedema and to avoid drug until they have consulted w/ prescribing physician. Instruct to report lightheadedness, especially during 1st few days of therapy; if syncope occurs, advise to d/c therapy until physician is consulted. Advise that excessive perspiration, dehydration, and other causes of volume depletion may lead to excessive fall in BP; instruct to consult w/ a physician. Advise not to use salt substitutes containing K^+ w/o consulting physician. Advise diabetic patients treated w/ oral antidiabetic agents or insulin to closely monitor for hypoglycemia, especially during the 1st month of combined use. Instruct to report promptly any indication of infection, which may be a sign of leukopenia/neutropenia.

STORAGE: 20-25°C (68-77°F). Protect from moisture, freezing, and excessive heat.

ZETIA – ezetimibe

RX

Class: Cholesterol absorption inhibitor

ADULT DOSAGE

Primary Hyperlipidemia

Heterozygous familial and nonfamilial hyperlipidemia, alone or in combination w/ a statin; mixed hyperlipidemia in combination w/ fenofibrate

10mg qd

PEDIATRIC DOSAGE

Pediatric use may not have been established

Homozygous Familial Hypercholesterolemia

10mg qd in combination w/ atorvastatin or simvastatin

Homozygous Sitosterolemia

10mg qd

DOSING CONSIDERATIONS

Concomitant Medications

Bile Acid Sequestrant:
Give either ≥2 hrs before or ≥4 hrs after bile acid sequestrant

Renal Impairment

Moderate to Severe (GFR <60mL/min):
Use caution and monitor closely w/ simvastatin doses >20mg

Hepatic Impairment

Moderate to Severe: Not recommended

ADMINISTRATION

Oral route

Take w/ or w/o food

HOW SUPPLIED

Tab: 10mg

CONTRAINDICATIONS

Active liver disease or unexplained persistent elevations in hepatic transaminase levels, women who are or may become pregnant, and nursing mothers when used with statins. Known hypersensitivity to any component of this product.

WARNINGS/PRECAUTIONS

Not recommended with moderate to severe hepatic impairment. Should be used in accordance with the product labeling for the concurrently administered drug (eg, specific statin or fenofibrate). Liver enzyme elevations reported with statins. Consider withdrawal of therapy and/or statin if an increase in ALT or AST ≥3X ULN persists. Myopathy and rhabdomyolysis reported; immediately d/c therapy and any concomitant statin or fibrate, if myopathy is diagnosed/suspected. Increased risk for skeletal muscle toxicity with higher doses of statin, advanced age (>65 yrs of age), hypothyroidism, renal impairment, depending on the statin used, and concomitant use of other drugs. Caution and close monitoring when used with simvastatin >20mg in patients with moderate to severe renal impairment.

ADVERSE REACTIONS

URTI, diarrhea, arthralgia, sinusitis, pain in extremity.

DRUG INTERACTIONS

Caution with cyclosporine; monitor cyclosporine levels. May increase cholesterol excretion into the bile, leading to cholelithiasis with fibrates; avoid with fibrates (except fenofibrate). Consider alternative lipid-lowering therapy if cholelithiasis occurs with fenofibrate. Decreased levels with cholestyramine; incremental LDL-C reduction may be reduced. Monitor INR levels when used with warfarin.

PATIENT CONSIDERATIONS

Assessment: Assess for hepatic impairment, pregnancy/nursing status, and possible drug interactions. Obtain baseline lipid profile. Assess for conditions where treatment is contraindicated and risk factors for skeletal muscle toxicity. Obtain baseline LFTs when used with statin.

Monitoring: Monitor for signs/symptoms of elevated liver enzymes, myopathy, rhabdomyolysis, and other adverse reactions. Perform periodic monitoring of lipid profile. Periodically monitor LFTs during concomitant statin therapy.

Counseling: Advise to adhere to the National Cholesterol Education Program recommended diet, a regular exercise program, and periodic testing of a fasting lipid panel. Counsel about risk of myopathy; instruct to promptly report to the physician if any unexplained muscle pain, tenderness, or weakness occurs. Advise to discuss with physician about all medications, both prescription and OTC, currently being taken. Counsel women of childbearing age to use an effective method of birth control while using added statin therapy and instruct to d/c combination therapy and contact physician if they become pregnant. Instruct breastfeeding women not to take the medication if concomitantly using statins; advise patients who have lipid disorder and are breastfeeding to discuss the options with their physician.

STORAGE: 25°C (77°F); excursions permitted to 15-30°C (59-86°F). Protect from moisture.

ZIAC — bisoprolol fumarate/hydrochlorothiazide

RX

Class: Selective $beta_1$ blocker/thiazide diuretic

ADULT DOSAGE

Hypertension

Uncontrolled BP on 2.5mg-20mg/day Bisoprolol or Controlled BP on 50mg/day HCTZ w/ Hypokalemia:

Initial: 2.5mg-6.25mg qd

Titrate: May increase at 14-day intervals

Max: 20mg-12.5mg (two 10mg-6.25mg tab) qd, as appropriate

Replacement Therapy:

May substitute for titrated individual components

Cessation of Therapy:

Withdrawal should be achieved gradually over a period of 2 weeks

PEDIATRIC DOSAGE

Pediatric use may not have been established

ADMINISTRATION

Oral route

HOW SUPPLIED

Tab: (Bisoprolol/HCTZ) 2.5mg/6.25mg, 5mg/6.25mg, 10mg/6.25mg

CONTRAINDICATIONS

Cardiogenic shock, overt cardiac failure, 2nd- or 3rd-degree atrioventricular (AV) block, marked sinus bradycardia, anuria, hypersensitivity to either component of this product or to other sulfonamide-derived drugs.

WARNINGS/PRECAUTIONS

Caution with impaired hepatic function/progressive liver disease. Bisoprolol: Caution with compensated cardiac failure. May precipitate cardiac failure; consider discontinuation at 1st signs/symptoms of heart failure (HF). Exacerbations of angina pectoris, MI, and ventricular arrhythmia with coronary artery disease (CAD) reported upon abrupt discontinuation; caution against interruption or discontinuation without physician's advice. May precipitate or aggravate symptoms of arterial insufficiency with peripheral vascular disease (PVD); exercise caution. Avoid with bronchospastic disease, but may use with caution if unresponsive/intolerant of other antihypertensives. Chronically administered therapy should not be routinely withdrawn prior to major surgery; however, may augment risks of general anesthesia and surgical procedures. Caution with diabetes mellitus (DM); may mask tachycardia occurring with hypoglycemia. May mask hyperthyroidism and precipitate thyroid storm with abrupt discontinuation. HCTZ: May precipitate azotemia with impaired renal function. D/C if progressive renal impairment becomes apparent. May precipitate hepatic coma with hepatic impairment. May cause idiosyncratic reaction, resulting in acute transient myopia and acute angle-closure glaucoma; d/c as rapidly as possible. Monitor for fluid/electrolyte disturbances (eg, hyponatremia, hypochloremic alkalosis, hypokalemia, hypomagnesemia). Decreased Ca^{2+} excretion and altered parathyroid glands, with hypercalcemia and hypophosphatemia, observed on prolonged therapy. Precipitation of hyperuricemia/gout and sensitivity reactions may occur. Photosensitivity reactions and exacerbation/activation of systemic lupus erythematosus (SLE) reported. Enhanced effects in postsympathectomy patient. D/C prior to parathyroid function test.

ADVERSE REACTIONS

Hyperuricemia, dizziness, fatigue, headache, diarrhea.

DRUG INTERACTIONS

May potentiate other antihypertensive agents. Avoid with other β-blockers. Excessive reduction of sympathetic activity with catecholamine-depleting drugs (eg, reserpine, guanethidine); monitor closely. D/C for several days prior to clonidine withdrawal. Caution with myocardial depressants or inhibitors of AV conduction (eg, certain calcium antagonists [particularly phenylalkylamine and benzothiazepine classes], antiarrhythmic agents [eg, disopyramide]). Bisoprolol: Digitalis glycosides may increase risk of bradycardia. Rifampin may increase clearance. May be unresponsive to usual doses of epinephrine. HCTZ: Alcohol, barbiturates, or narcotics may potentiate orthostatic hypotension. Antidiabetic drugs (eg, oral agents, insulin) may require dosage adjustments. Impaired absorption with cholestyramine and colestipol resins. Corticosteroids and adrenocorticotropic hormone may intensify electrolyte depletion, particularly hypokalemia. May decrease response to pressor amines (eg, norepinephrine). May increase response to nondepolarizing skeletal muscle relaxants (eg, tubocurarine). Do not give with lithium; increased risk of lithium toxicity. NSAIDs may reduce diuretic, natriuretic, and antihypertensive effects.

PATIENT CONSIDERATIONS

Assessment: Assess for cardiogenic shock, overt/compensated cardiac failure, 2nd- or 3rd-degree AV block, marked sinus bradycardia, anuria, sulfonamide hypersensitivity, CAD, PVD, bronchospastic disease, DM, hyperthyroidism, renal/hepatic impairment, history of sulfonamide/penicillin allergy, parathyroid disease, SLE, pregnancy/nursing status, and possible drug interactions. Obtain baseline serum electrolytes.

Monitoring: Monitor for signs/symptoms of HF, withdrawal, hypoglycemia, hyperthyroidism, renal/hepatic impairment, idiosyncratic reaction, fluid or electrolyte disturbances, precipitation of hyperuricemia or gout, and hypersensitivity reactions. Perform periodic monitoring of serum electrolytes.

Counseling: Instruct not to d/c therapy without physician's supervision, especially in patients with CAD. Advise to consult physician if any difficulty in breathing occurs, or other signs/symptoms of CHF or excessive bradycardia develop. Inform that hypoglycemia may be masked in patients subject to spontaneous hypoglycemia, or diabetic patients receiving insulin or oral hypoglycemic agents; instruct to use with caution. Advise to avoid driving, operating machinery, or engaging in other tasks requiring alertness until reaction to drug is known. Advise that photosensitivity reactions may occur.

STORAGE: 20-25°C (68-77°F).

ZIAGEN — abacavir

RX

Class: Nucleoside reverse transcriptase inhibitor (NRTI)

Serious and sometimes fatal hypersensitivity reactions w/ multiple organ involvement reported; d/c immediately if a hypersensitivity reaction is suspected and never restart therapy or any other abacavir-containing product. Patients who carry the HLA-B*5701 allele are at a higher risk of a hypersensitivity reaction; screen all patients for HLA-B*5701 allele prior to initiating or reinitiating therapy, unless patient has a previously documented HLA-B*5701 allele assessment. Lactic acidosis and severe hepatomegaly w/ steatosis, including fatal cases, reported w/ the use of nucleoside analogues and other antiretrovirals. D/C if clinical or lab findings suggestive of lactic acidosis or pronounced hepatotoxicity occur.

ADULT DOSAGE

HIV-1 Infection

Combination w/ Other Antiretrovirals:
300mg bid or 600mg qd

PEDIATRIC DOSAGE

HIV-1 Infection

Combination w/ Other Antiretrovirals:
≥3 Months of Age:
Sol:
8mg/kg bid or 16 mg/kg qd
Max: 600mg/day

Tab:
14 to <20kg:
QD Dosing:
300mg (1 tab)
BID Dosing:
AM Dose: 150mg (1/2 tab)
PM Dose: 150mg (1/2 tab)

≥20 to <25kg:
QD Dosing:
450mg (1 1/2 tabs)
BID Dosing:
AM Dose: 150mg (1/2 tab)
PM Dose: 300mg (1 tab)

≥25kg:
QD Dosing:
600mg (2 tabs)
BID Dosing:
AM Dose: 300mg (1 tab)
PM Dose: 300mg (1 tab)

DOSING CONSIDERATIONS

Hepatic Impairment

Mild (Child-Pugh Class A): 200mg (10mL) bid

ADMINISTRATION

Oral route

Take w/ or w/o food.
Screen for the HLA-B*5701 allele prior to initiating therapy.

HOW SUPPLIED
Sol: (Abacavir Sulfate) 20mg/mL [240mL]; **Tab:** (Abacavir Sulfate) 300mg* *scored

CONTRAINDICATIONS
Prior hypersensitivity reaction to abacavir, moderate or severe hepatic impairment, patients w/ HLA-B*5701 allele.

WARNINGS/PRECAUTIONS
Obesity and prolonged nucleoside exposure may be risk factors for lactic acidosis and severe hepatomegaly w/ steatosis; caution w/ known risk factors for liver disease. Suspend therapy if clinical or lab findings suggestive of lactic acidosis or pronounced hepatotoxicity develop. Immune reconstitution syndrome reported. Autoimmune disorders (eg, Graves' disease, polymyositis, Guillain-Barre syndrome) reported to occur in the setting of immune reconstitution and can occur many months after initiation of treatment. Redistribution/accumulation of body fat reported. Consider the underlying risk of coronary heart disease when prescribing therapy. Caution in elderly.

ADVERSE REACTIONS
Dreams/sleep disorders, drug hypersensitivity, N/V, headache/migraine, malaise, fatigue, diarrhea, rashes, abdominal pain, gastritis, depressive disorders, dizziness, fever.

DRUG INTERACTIONS
Not recommended w/ other products containing abacavir. Ethanol decreases elimination, causing an increase in overall exposure. May increase oral methadone clearance; an increased methadone dose may be required in a small number of patients.

PATIENT CONSIDERATIONS

Assessment: Assess for previous hypersensitivity to the drug, hepatic impairment, risk factors for lactic acidosis or liver disease, risk of coronary heart disease, pregnancy/nursing status, and possible drug interactions. Screen for HLA-B*5701 allele prior to initiation of therapy. Assess medical history for prior exposure to any abacavir-containing product.
Monitoring: Monitor for hypersensitivity reactions, lactic acidosis, hepatotoxicity, immune reconstitution syndrome, autoimmune disorders, fat redistribution/accumulation, MI, and other adverse reactions.

Counseling: Inform about the risk of hypersensitivity reactions; instruct to contact physician immediately if symptoms develop, and not to restart therapy or any other abacavir-containing product w/o medical consultation. Inform that lactic acidosis (w/ liver enlargement) and fat redistribution/accumulation may occur. Inform that drug is not a cure for HIV-1 infection and that illnesses associated w/ HIV-1 may still be experienced. Advise to avoid doing things that can spread HIV-1 to others (eg, sharing needles, other inj equipment, or personal items that can have blood or body fluids on them; having sex w/o protection; breastfeeding). Instruct to take all HIV medications exactly as prescribed.
STORAGE: 20-25°C (68-77°F). **Sol:** Do not freeze. May be refrigerated.

ZIANA — clindamycin phosphate/tretinoin

RX

Class: Lincosamide derivative/retinoid

ADULT DOSAGE
Acne Vulgaris
Apply at hs, a pea-sized amount onto 1 fingertip; dot onto the chin, cheeks, nose, and forehead; then gently rub over entire face

PEDIATRIC DOSAGE
Acne Vulgaris
≥12 Years:
Apply at hs, a pea-sized amount onto 1 fingertip; dot onto the chin, cheeks, nose, and forehead; then gently rub over entire face

ADMINISTRATION
Topical route

HOW SUPPLIED
Gel: (Clindamycin/Tretinoin) 1.2%/0.025% [30g, 60g]

CONTRAINDICATIONS
Regional enteritis, ulcerative colitis, or history of antibiotic-associated colitis.

WARNINGS/PRECAUTIONS
Not for oral, ophthalmic, or intravaginal use. Keep away from eyes, mouth, angles of the nose, and mucous membranes. Avoid exposure to sunlight, including sunlamps. Avoid use if sunburn is present. Daily use of sunscreen products and protective apparel are recommended. Weather extremes (eg, wind, cold) may be irritating while under treatment. Clindamycin: Systemic absorption has been demonstrated following topical use. Diarrhea, bloody diarrhea, and colitis (including pseudomembranous colitis) reported; d/c if significant diarrhea occurs. Severe colitis

reported following PO or parenteral administration with an onset of up to several weeks following cessation of therapy.

ADVERSE REACTIONS

Nasopharyngitis, local skin reactions (erythema, scaling, itching, burning), GI symptoms.

DRUG INTERACTIONS

Caution with topical medications, medicated/abrasive soaps and cleansers, soaps/cosmetics with strong drying effect, products with high concentrations of alcohol, astringents, spices, or lime because skin irritation may be increased. Avoid with erythromycin-containing products. May enhance action of neuromuscular blocking agents; use with caution. Antiperistaltic agents (eg, opiates, diphenoxylate with atropine) may prolong and/or worsen severe colitis.

PATIENT CONSIDERATIONS

Assessment: Assess for regional enteritis, ulcerative colitis, or history of antibiotic-associated colitis, pregnancy/nursing status, and possible drug interactions. Assess use in patients whose occupations require considerable sun exposure.

Monitoring: Monitor for signs/symptoms of diarrhea, bloody diarrhea, colitis, local skin reactions, and other adverse reactions.

Counseling: Instruct to wash face gently with mild soap and warm water at hs and apply a thin layer over the entire face (excluding the eyes and lips) after patting the skin dry. Advise not to use more than recommended amount and not to apply more than qd (at hs). Instruct to apply sunscreen qam and reapply over the course of the day PRN. Advise to avoid exposure to sunlight, sunlamp, UV light, and other medicines that may increase sensitivity to sunlight. Inform that medication may cause irritation (eg, erythema, scaling, itching, burning, stinging). Instruct to d/c therapy and contact physician if severe diarrhea or GI discomfort occurs.

STORAGE: 25°C (77°F); excursions permitted to 15-30°C (59-86°F). Protect from light and freezing. Keep away from heat. Keep tube tightly closed.

ZINACEF — cefuroxime

RX

Class: Cephalosporin (2nd generation)

ADULT DOSAGE

General Dosing

Usual: 750mg-1.5g q8h for 5-10 days

Severe/Complicated Infections:
1.5g q8h

Life-Threatening Infections/Infections Due to Less Susceptible Organisms:
1.5g q6h

Urinary Tract Infections

Uncomplicated:
750mg q8h

Skin and Skin Structure Infections

750mg q8h

Gonococcal Infections

Disseminated:
750mg q8h

Uncomplicated:
Single 1.5g IM dose, given at 2 different sites + 1g oral probenecid

Pneumonia

Uncomplicated:
750mg q8h

Bone/Joint Infections

1.5g q8h

Bacterial Meningitis

Max: 3g q8h

Prophylaxis of Postoperative Infections

1.5g IV just before surgery (approx 0.5-1 hr before initial incision), then 750mg IM/IV q8h w/ prolonged procedure

PEDIATRIC DOSAGE

General Dosing

>3 Months of Age:
50-100mg/kg/day in equally divided doses q6-8h

Severe/Serious Infections: 100mg/kg/day (not to exceed max adult dose)

Bone/Joint Infections

>3 Months of Age:
150mg/kg/day in divided doses q8h (not to exceed max adult dose)

Bacterial Meningitis

>3 Months of Age:
200-240mg/kg/day IV in divided doses q6-8h

Treatment Duration

Continue therapy for a minimum of 48-72 hrs after the patient becomes asymptomatic or after evidence of bacterial eradication has been obtained

***Streptococcus pyogenes* Infections:**
Treat for ≥10 days

Open Heart Surgery (Perioperative):
1.5g IV at induction of anesthesia and q12h thereafter, for total of 6g

Treatment Duration

Continue therapy for a minimum of 48-72 hrs after the patient becomes asymptomatic or after evidence of bacterial eradication has been obtained

***Streptococcus pyogenes* Infections:**
Treat for ≥10 days

Other Indications

- Lower respiratory tract infections
- Septicemia

DOSING CONSIDERATIONS

Renal Impairment

Adults:
CrCl >20mL/min: 750mg-1.5g q8h
CrCl 10-20mL/min: 750mg q12h
CrCl <10mL/min: 750mg q24h
Hemodialysis: Give a further dose at the end of the dialysis

Pediatrics:
Modify dosing frequency consistent w/ adult recommendations

ADMINISTRATION

IM/IV routes

IM

Reconstitute 750mg vial w/ 3.0mL sterile water for inj (SWFI); withdraw the resulting sus completely for inj.
Administer by deep IM inj into a large muscle mass (eg, gluteus or lateral part of thigh).
Avoid inadvertent inj into a blood vessel.

IV

Reconstitute 750mg and 1.5g vial w/ 8.3mL and 16mL, respectively, w/ SWFI.
Reconstitute 7.5g pharmacy bulk vial w/ 77mL of SWFI.

Continuous IV Infusion:
May add sol to an IV infusion pack containing compatible IV sol.
Do not add to sol of aminoglycoside.

Direct Intermittent IV Administration:
Slowly inject over 3-5 min into vein or give through the tubing system if also receiving other IV sol.

Intermittent IV Infusion w/ a Y-Type Administration Set:
Temporarily d/c administration of any other sol at the same site while infusing therapy.

TwistVial:
Reconstitute w/ 50 or 100mL of D5 inj, 0.9% NaCl inj, or 0.45% NaCl inj in compatible flexible diluent containers.

Frozen Galaxy Plastic Container:
Thaw container at room temperature or under refrigeration.
Do not force thaw by immersion in water baths or by microwave irradiation; do not refreeze.
Do not add supplementary medications and must not be used in series connections.

Refer to PI for additional administration procedures, use of frozen plastic container, compatibility, and stability.

HOW SUPPLIED

Inj: 750mg, 1.5g, 1.5g/50mL

CONTRAINDICATIONS

Allergy to the cephalosporin group of antibiotics.

WARNINGS/PRECAUTIONS

Caution in penicillin (PCN)-sensitive patients; determine whether patient has had previous hypersensitivity reactions to cephalosporins, PCN, or other drugs. D/C if an allergic reaction occurs. *Clostridium difficile*-associated diarrhea (CDAD) reported; may need to d/c if CDAD is suspected or confirmed. May result in overgrowth of nonsusceptible organisms w/ prolonged use; take appropriate measures if superinfection develops. Use in the absence of a proven or strongly suspected bacterial infection or a prophylactic indication is unlikely to provide benefit and increases the risk of the development of drug-resistant bacteria. Hearing loss reported in pediatric patients treated for meningitis. Risk of decreased prothrombin activity in patients w/ renal/hepatic impairment, poor nutritional state, protracted course of therapy, and patients previously stabilized on anticoagulant therapy. Lab test interactions may occur. Caution w/ impaired renal function, history of GI disease (particularly colitis), and in elderly.

ADVERSE REACTIONS

Local reactions, decreased Hgb and Hct, eosinophilia, ALT/AST elevation.

DRUG INTERACTIONS

Caution w/ potent diuretics; may adversely affect the renal function. Nephrotoxicity reported w/ concomitant aminoglycosides. May decrease prothrombin activity; caution w/ anticoagulants. May affect the gut flora, leading to lower estrogen reabsorption and reduced efficacy of combined estrogen/progesterone oral contraceptives.

PATIENT CONSIDERATIONS

Assessment: Assess for known allergy to cephalosporins, PCN, or other drugs, renal/hepatic impairment, nutritional status, history of GI disease (eg, colitis), pregnancy/nursing status, and possible drug interactions. Obtain baseline culture and susceptibility tests.

Monitoring: Monitor for signs/symptoms of an allergic reaction, CDAD, and development of superinfection. In pediatric patients w/ meningitis, monitor for hearing loss. Monitor renal function and PT.

Counseling: Inform that drug only treats bacterial, not viral, infections. Instruct to take exactly ud; explain that skipping doses or not completing full course of therapy may decrease effectiveness and increase the likelihood of bacterial resistance. Inform that diarrhea may occur and will usually end if therapy is discontinued. Instruct to contact physician as soon as possible if watery/bloody stools (w/ or w/o stomach cramps, fever) develop even as late as ≥2 months after last dose of therapy, and if other adverse reactions occur.

STORAGE: (Dry State) 15-30°C (59-86°F). Protect from light. **Frozen Premixed Sol:** Do not store above -20°C (-4°F).

ZITHROMAX 250MG, 500MG TABLETS AND ORAL SUSPENSION — azithromycin

RX

Class: Macrolide

ADULT DOSAGE

Nongonococcal Urethritis

1g single dose

Nongonococcal Cervicitis

1g single dose

Gonococcal Infections

Urethritis and Cervicitis:
2g single dose

Community-Acquired Pneumonia

500mg single dose on Day 1, then 250mg qd on Days 2-5

Pharyngitis/Tonsillitis

2nd-Line Therapy:
500mg single dose on Day 1, then 250mg qd on Days 2-5

Skin and Skin Structure Infections

Uncomplicated:
500mg single dose on Day 1, then 250mg qd on Days 2-5

Acute Bacterial Exacerbation of Chronic Bronchitis

500mg qd for 3 days or 500mg as a single dose on Day 1, followed by 250mg qd on Days 2-5

Acute Bacterial Sinusitis

500mg qd for 3 days

Genital Ulcers

Chancroid:
1g single dose

PEDIATRIC DOSAGE

Community-Acquired Pneumonia

≥6 Months of Age:
10mg/kg single dose on Day 1, followed by 5mg/kg qd on Days 2-5

Refer to PI for dosage guidelines

Acute Otitis Media

≥6 Months of Age:
30mg/kg single dose or 10mg/kg qd for 3 days or 10mg/kg single dose on Day 1 followed by 5mg/kg/day on Days 2-5

Refer to PI for dosage guidelines

Acute Bacterial Sinusitis

≥6 Months of Age:
10mg/kg qd for 3 days

Refer to PI for dosage guidelines

Pharyngitis/Tonsillitis

2nd-Line Therapy:
≥2 Years:
12mg/kg qd for 5 days

Refer to PI for dosage guidelines

ADMINISTRATION

Oral route

Take tab/sus w/ or w/o food.
Shake sus well before each use.

Sus (100mg/5mL, 200mg/5mL)

Reconstitution:

Add 9mL of water to 300mg or 600mg sus bottle, 12mL of water to 900mg sus bottle, or 15mL of water to 1200mg sus bottle.
After mixing, store at 5-30°C (41-86°F) and use w/in 10 days; discard after full dosing is completed.

HOW SUPPLIED

Oral Sus: 100mg/5mL [15mL], 200mg/5mL [15mL, 22.5mL, 30mL] **Tab:** 250mg, 500mg

CONTRAINDICATIONS

History of cholestatic jaundice/hepatic dysfunction associated w/ prior use of therapy or known hypersensitivity to azithromycin, erythromycin, or any macrolide or ketolide drug.

WARNINGS/PRECAUTIONS

Serious allergic reactions (eg, angioedema, anaphylaxis) and dermatologic reactions (eg, Stevens Johnson syndrome, toxic epidermal necrolysis, drug reaction w/ eosinophilia and systemic symptoms) reported; d/c if an allergic reaction occurs and institute appropriate therapy. Abnormal liver function, hepatitis, cholestatic jaundice, hepatic necrosis, and hepatic failure reported; d/c immediately if signs and symptoms of hepatitis occur. Infantile hypertrophic pyloric stenosis reported following the use in neonates; contact physician if vomiting or irritability w/ feeding occurs. Prolonged cardiac repolarization and QT interval, and torsades de pointes reported. Consider risk of QT prolongation that can be fatal for at-risk groups, including patients w/ known QT interval prolongation, history of torsades de pointes, congenital long QT syndrome, bradyarrhythmias, uncompensated heart failure, ongoing proarrhythmic conditions (eg, uncorrected hypokalemia/hypomagnesemia), and clinically significant bradycardia. The elderly may be more susceptible to drug-associated effects on the QT interval. *Clostridium difficile*-associated diarrhea (CDAD) reported; may need to d/c if CDAD is suspected or confirmed. Exacerbation of myasthenia gravis symptoms and new onset of myasthenic syndrome reported. Should not be relied upon to treat syphilis; may mask or delay the symptoms of incubating syphilis. May result in bacterial resistance w/ prolonged use in the absence of proven or suspected bacterial infection. Do not use in patients w/ pneumonia who are judged to be inappropriate for oral therapy due to moderate to severe illness or risk factors (eg, cystic fibrosis, nosocomial infections, known/suspected bacteremia).

ADVERSE REACTIONS

Diarrhea/loose stools, N/V, abdominal pain.

DRUG INTERACTIONS

Caution w/ drugs known to prolong the QT interval and w/ Class IA (eg, quinidine, procainamide) and Class III (eg, dofetilide, amiodarone, sotalol) antiarrhythmic agents. Increased levels w/ nelfinavir; closely monitor for known adverse reactions (eg, liver enzyme abnormalities, hearing impairment). May potentiate effects of oral anticoagulants (eg, warfarin); monitor PT. Monitor carefully when coadministered w/ digoxin or phenytoin.

PATIENT CONSIDERATIONS

Assessment: Assess for hypersensitivity to drug, history of cholestatic jaundice/hepatic dysfunction associated w/ prior use of therapy, risk for QT prolongation, myasthenia gravis, pregnancy/nursing status, and possible drug interactions. Perform appropriate culture and susceptibility testing. In patients w/ sexually transmitted urethritis or cervicitis, perform serologic test for syphilis and appropriate testing for gonorrhea at the time of diagnosis. Assess for patients w/ pneumonia judged to be inappropriate for oral therapy due to moderate to severe illness or risk factors (eg, cystic fibrosis, nosocomial infections, known/suspected bacteremia).

Monitoring: Monitor for signs/symptoms of serious allergic/dermatologic reactions, hepatotoxicity, CDAD, QT prolongation, new onset of myasthenic syndrome or exacerbation of myasthenia gravis, and other adverse reactions.

Counseling: Inform that diarrhea may occur and will usually end if therapy is discontinued. Instruct to contact physician as soon as possible if watery and bloody stools (w/ or w/o stomach cramps and fever) develop even as late as ≥2 months after the last dose. Instruct to d/c therapy immediately and contact physician if any signs of an allergic reaction occur. Instruct not to take the medication simultaneously w/ aluminum- and Mg^{2+}-containing antacids. Explain that therapy should only be used to treat bacterial, not viral, infections. Instruct to take exactly ud; inform that skipping doses or not completing the full course of therapy may decrease effectiveness of immediate treatment and increase bacterial resistance.

STORAGE: Tab: 15-30°C (59-86°F). **Sus (100mg/5mL, 200mg/5mL): Dry Powder:** <30°C (86°F). **Constituted:** 5-30°C (41-86°F).

ZOCOR – simvastatin

RX

Class: HMG-CoA reductase inhibitor (statin)

ADULT DOSAGE

Hyperlipidemia

Initial: 10mg or 20mg qpm
Usual Range: 5-40mg/day

High Risk for Coronary Heart Disease Events:
Initial: 40mg/day

Lipid determinations should be performed after 4 weeks of therapy and periodically thereafter

Homozygous Familial Hypercholesterolemia

40mg/day qpm

Lipid determinations should be performed after 4 weeks of therapy and periodically thereafter

PEDIATRIC DOSAGE

Heterozygous Familial Hypercholesterolemia

10-17 Years (At Least 1 Year Postmenarche):
Initial: 10mg qpm
Range: 10-40mg/day
Titrate: Adjust at ≥4-week intervals
Max: 40mg/day

DOSING CONSIDERATIONS

Concomitant Medications

Verapamil, Diltiazem, or Dronedarone:
Max: 10mg/day

Amiodarone, Amlodipine, or Ranolazine:
Max: 20mg/day

Lomitapide:
Homozygous Familial Hypercholesterolemia:
Reduce dose by 50% if initiating lomitapide
Max: 20mg/day (or 40mg/day for patients who have previously taken simvastatin 80mg/day chronically [eg, ≥12 months] w/o evidence of muscle toxicity)

Niacin-Containing Products:
Chinese Patients Taking Lipid-Modifying Doses (≥1g/day Niacin):
Caution w/ doses >20mg/day; do not give 80mg dose

Renal Impairment

Severe:
Initial: 5mg/day; use caution and monitor closely

Other Important Considerations

Restricted Dosing:
Use 80mg dose only in patients who have been taking simvastatin 80mg chronically (eg, ≥12 months) w/o evidence of muscle toxicity

If currently tolerating 80mg dose and needs to be initiated on a drug that is contraindicated or is associated w/ a dose cap for simvastatin, switch to an alternative statin w/ less potential for drug-drug interaction

In patients unable to achieve LDL goal utilizing the 40mg dose, place on alternative LDL-lowering treatment that provides greater LDL lowering; do not titrate therapy to 80mg dose

ADMINISTRATION

Oral route

HOW SUPPLIED

Tab: 5mg, 10mg, 20mg, 40mg, 80mg

CONTRAINDICATIONS

Concomitant administration of strong CYP3A4 inhibitors (eg, itraconazole, ketoconazole, posaconazole, voriconazole, HIV protease inhibitors, boceprevir, telaprevir, erythromycin, clarithromycin, telithromycin, nefazodone, cobicistat-containing products), gemfibrozil, cyclosporine, or danazol, hypersensitivity to any component of this medication, active liver disease, which may include unexplained persistent elevations in hepatic transaminases, women who are or may become pregnant, and nursing mothers.

WARNINGS/PRECAUTIONS

Myopathy (including immune-mediated necrotizing myopathy [IMNM]) and rhabdomyolysis reported; predisposing factors include advanced age (≥65 yrs of age), female gender, uncontrolled hypothyroidism, and renal impairment. Risk of myopathy, including rhabdomyolysis, is dose related and greater w/ 80mg doses. D/C if markedly elevated CPK levels occur or myopathy is diagnosed/suspected, and temporarily withhold in any patient experiencing an acute or serious condition predisposing to development of renal failure secondary to rhabdomyolysis. Persistent increases in serum transaminases reported. Fatal and nonfatal hepatic failure (rare) reported; promptly interrupt therapy if serious liver injury w/ clinical symptoms and/or hyperbilirubinemia or jaundice occurs and do not restart if no alternate etiology found. Increases in HbA1c and FPG levels reported. Caution w/ substantial alcohol consumption, history of liver disease, and in the elderly.

ADVERSE REACTIONS

Abdominal pain, headache, myalgia, constipation, nausea, atrial fibrillation, gastritis, diabetes mellitus, insomnia, vertigo, bronchitis, eczema, URTI, UTI(s).

DRUG INTERACTIONS

See Contraindications and Dosing Considerations. Due to the risk of myopathy/rhabdomyolysis, avoid grapefruit juice and caution w/ fibrates, lipid-modifying doses (≥1g/day) of niacin, colchicine, verapamil, diltiazem, dronedarone, lomitapide, amiodarone, amlodipine, and ranolazine. May slightly elevate digoxin concentrations; monitor patients taking digoxin when therapy is initiated. May potentiate effect of coumarin anticoagulants; determine PT before initiation and frequently during therapy.

PATIENT CONSIDERATIONS

Assessment: Assess for history of or active liver disease, unexplained persistent hepatic transaminase elevations, predisposing factors for myopathy, renal impairment, alcohol consumption, drug hypersensitivity, any other conditions where treatment is contraindicated or cautioned, pregnancy/nursing status, and possible drug interactions. Assess lipid profile and LFTs.

Monitoring: Monitor for signs/symptoms of myopathy (including IMNM), rhabdomyolysis, liver dysfunction, increases in HbA1c and FPG levels, and other adverse reactions. Monitor lipid profile, LFTs when clinically indicated, and CPK levels.

Counseling: Inform of benefits/risks of therapy. Advise to adhere to the National Cholesterol Education Program recommended diet, a regular exercise program, and periodic testing of a fasting lipid panel. Inform about substances that should be avoided during therapy, and advise to discuss all medications, both prescription and OTC, w/ physician. Instruct to report promptly any unexplained muscle pain, tenderness, or weakness, particularly if accompanied by malaise or fever or if these muscle signs or symptoms persist after discontinuation, or any symptoms that may indicate liver injury. Inform patients using the 80mg dose that the risk of myopathy, including rhabdomyolysis, is increased. Instruct women of childbearing age to use an effective method of birth control to prevent pregnancy while on therapy, to d/c therapy and call physician if pregnant, and not to breastfeed while on therapy.

STORAGE: 5-30°C (41-86°F).

ZOLOFT – sertraline hydrochloride — RX

Class: Selective serotonin reuptake inhibitor (SSRI)

Antidepressants increased the risk of suicidal thinking and behavior (suicidality) in children, adolescents, and young adults in short-term studies of major depressive disorder (MDD) and other psychiatric disorders. Monitor and observe closely for clinical worsening, suicidality, or unusual changes in behavior in patients who are started on antidepressant therapy. Not approved for use in pediatric patients except for patients w/ obsessive-compulsive disorder.

ADULT DOSAGE

Premenstrual Dysphoric Disorder

Initial: 50mg qd throughout menstrual cycle or limited to luteal phase

Titrate: If unresponsive to initial dose, may increase at 50mg increments/cycle up to 150mg/day when dosing daily throughout menstrual cycle or 100mg/day when dosing during luteal phase

If 100mg/day has been established w/ luteal phase dosing, use a 50mg/day titration step for 3 days at the beginning of each luteal phase dosing period

Adjust to maintain patient on the lowest effective dose; periodically reassess to determine need for continued treatment

Major Depressive Disorder

Usual: 50mg qd

Max: 200mg/day

Periodically reassess to determine need for maint treatment

PEDIATRIC DOSAGE

Obsessive Compulsive Disorder

6-12 Years:

Initial: 25mg qd

13-17 Years:

Initial: 50mg qd

Titrate: Adjust dose at intervals ≥1 week

Max: 200mg/day

Periodically reassess to determine need for maint treatment

Dosing Considerations with MAOIs

Switching to/from an MAOI for Psychiatric Disorders:

Allow at least 14 days between discontinuation of an MAOI and initiation of treatment, and allow at least 14 days between discontinuation of treatment and initiation of an MAOI

Use w/ Other MAOIs (eg, Linezolid, IV Methylene Blue):

Do not start sertraline in patients being treated

Obsessive Compulsive Disorder

Usual: 50mg qd
Titrate: Adjust dose at intervals ≥1 week
Max: 200mg/day

Periodically reassess to determine need for maint treatment

Panic Disorder

Initial: 25mg qd
Titrate: Increase to 50mg qd after 1 week; adjust dose at intervals ≥1 week
Max: 200mg/day

Periodically reassess to determine need for maint treatment

Social Anxiety Disorder

Initial: 25mg qd
Titrate: Increase to 50mg qd after 1 week; adjust dose at intervals ≥1 week
Max: 200mg/day

Dose adjustments may be needed to maintain patient on the lowest effective dose; periodically reassess to determine need for long-term treatment

Post-traumatic Stress Disorder

Initial: 25mg qd
Titrate: Increase to 50mg qd after 1 week; adjust dose at intervals ≥1 week
Max: 200mg/day

Periodically reassess to determine need for maint treatment

Dosing Considerations with MAOIs

Switching to/from an MAOI for Psychiatric Disorders:
Allow at least 14 days between discontinuation of an MAOI and initiation of treatment, and allow at least 14 days between discontinuation of treatment and initiation of an MAOI

Use w/ Other MAOIs (eg, Linezolid, IV Methylene Blue):
Do not start sertraline in patients being treated w/ linezolid or IV methylene blue
If acceptable alternatives are not available and benefits outweigh risks, d/c sertraline promptly and administer linezolid or IV methylene blue; monitor for serotonin syndrome for 2 weeks or until 24 hrs after the last dose of linezolid or IV methylene blue, whichever comes 1st. May resume sertraline therapy 24 hrs after the last dose of linezolid or IV methylene blue

w/ linezolid or IV methylene blue
If acceptable alternatives are not available and benefits outweigh risks, d/c sertraline promptly and administer linezolid or IV methylene blue; monitor for serotonin syndrome for 2 weeks or until 24 hrs after the last dose of linezolid or IV methylene blue, whichever comes 1st. May resume sertraline therapy 24 hrs after the last dose of linezolid or IV methylene blue

DOSING CONSIDERATIONS

Hepatic Impairment
Use lower or less frequent dose

Pregnancy
During 3rd Trimester: Consider potential risks/benefits of treatment

Discontinuation
A gradual reduction in dose rather than abrupt cessation is recommended whenever possible
May consider resuming previously prescribed dose if intolerable symptoms occur following a dose decrease or upon discontinuation of treatment. May continue decreasing the dose subsequently but at a more gradual rate

ADMINISTRATION

Oral route

Administer qam or qpm.

Sol
Must be diluted before use

Mix dose w/ 4 oz of water, ginger ale, lemon/lime soda, lemonade, or orange juice only; do not mix w/ any other liquids
Take dose immediately after mixing; do not mix in advance

HOW SUPPLIED

Sol: 20mg/mL [60mL]; **Tab:** 25mg*, 50mg*, 100mg* *scored

CONTRAINDICATIONS

Hypersensitivity to sertraline or any of the inactive ingredients in this medication. Use of an MAOI for psychiatric disorders either concomitantly or w/in 14 days of stopping treatment. Treatment w/in 14 days of stopping an MAOI for psychiatric disorders. Starting treatment in a patient being treated w/ other MAOIs (eg, linezolid, IV methylene blue). Concomitant use w/ pimozide. (Sol) Concomitant use w/ disulfiram.

WARNINGS/PRECAUTIONS

Not approved for treatment of bipolar depression. May precipitate mixed/manic episode in patients at risk for bipolar disorder; screen for risk of bipolar disorder prior to initiating treatment. Serotonin syndrome reported; d/c immediately and initiate supportive symptomatic treatment. Pupillary dilation that occurs following use may trigger an angle-closure attack in a patient w/ anatomically narrow angles who does not have a patent iridectomy. Activation of mania/hypomania, altered platelet function and/or abnormal lab results, decreased serum uric acid, and weight loss reported. Adverse events reported upon discontinuation, particularly when abrupt; reduce dose gradually whenever possible. May increase the risk of bleeding events. Seizures reported; caution w/ seizure disorder. Caution w/ diseases/conditions that could affect metabolism or hemodynamic responses. Hyponatremia may occur; caution in elderly and volume-depleted patients. Consider discontinuation in patients w/ symptomatic hyponatremia and institute appropriate medical intervention. Caution in 3rd trimester of pregnancy due to risk of serious neonatal complications. False (+) urine immunoassay screening tests for benzodiazepines reported. (Sol) Dropper dispenser contains dry natural rubber; caution w/ latex sensitivity.

ADVERSE REACTIONS

Ejaculation failure, dry mouth, increased sweating, somnolence, fatigue, tremor, anorexia, dizziness, headache, diarrhea, dyspepsia, nausea, constipation, agitation, insomnia.

DRUG INTERACTIONS

See Dosage and Contraindications. May cause serotonin syndrome w/ other serotonergic drugs (eg, triptans, TCAs, fentanyl, lithium, tramadol, tryptophan, buspirone, St. John's wort) and w/ drugs that impair metabolism of serotonin; d/c immediately if this occurs. May cause a shift in plasma concentrations resulting in an adverse effect w/ other tightly protein bound drugs (eg, warfarin, digitoxin), and conversely adverse effects may result from displacement of sertraline. Caution w/ other CNS active drugs. Monitor lithium, phenytoin, and valproate levels w/ appropriate dose adjustments. May increase levels of drugs metabolized by CYP2D6, especially those w/ a narrow therapeutic index (eg, TCAs for treatment of MDD, propafenone, flecainide); concomitant use of a drug metabolized by CYP2D6 may require lower doses, and an increase of the coadministered drug may be required when sertraline is withdrawn. Weakness, hyperreflexia, and incoordination reported (rare) w/ sumatriptan. May induce metabolism of cisapride. Increased risk of bleeding w/ aspirin (ASA), NSAIDs, warfarin, and other anticoagulants or other drugs known to affect platelet function. Altered anticoagulant effects reported w/ warfarin; carefully monitor PT when therapy is initiated or stopped. Avoid w/ alcohol. Increased risk of hyponatremia w/ diuretics. Cimetidine may increase levels and $T_{1/2}$. May reduce clearance of diazepam and tolbutamide.

PATIENT CONSIDERATIONS

Assessment: Assess for presence/risk for bipolar disorder, susceptibility to angle-closure glaucoma, conditions where treatment is contraindicated or cautioned, pregnancy/nursing status, and possible drug interactions.

Monitoring: Monitor for clinical worsening of depression, suicidality, or unusual changes in behavior, serotonin syndrome, hyponatremia, abnormal bleeding, angle-closure glaucoma, activation of mania/hypomania, seizures, and other adverse reactions. Periodically monitor height and weight of pediatric patients w/ long-term therapy. Periodically reevaluate long-term usefulness of therapy. Carefully monitor PT when therapy is initiated or stopped w/ warfarin.

Counseling: Counsel about benefits, risks, and appropriate use of therapy. Encourage families and caregivers to be alert for emergence of unusual changes in behavior, worsening of depression, and suicidal ideation, especially early during treatment and when dose is adjusted up or down; instruct to report symptoms to physician, especially if severe, abrupt in onset, or not part of presenting symptoms. Caution about risk of serotonin syndrome w/ concomitant triptans, tramadol, or other serotonergic agents. Caution about risk of angle-closure glaucoma. Advise patients to use caution when driving or operating machinery until they learn how they respond to medication. Inform that concomitant use w/ NSAIDs, ASA, warfarin, and other drugs that affect coagulation may increase the risk of bleeding. Counsel to avoid alcohol and to use caution when using OTC products. Advise to notify physician if pregnant, intending to become pregnant, or if breastfeeding.

STORAGE: 25°C (77°F); excursions permitted to 15-30°C (59-86°F).

ZOLPIMIST – zolpidem tartrate

CIV

Class: Imidazopyridine hypnotic

ADULT DOSAGE

Insomnia

Short-Term Treatment of Insomnia Characterized by Difficulties w/ Sleep Initiation:

Initial: 5mg (women), and either 5mg or 10mg (men), taken qhs

Titrate: May increase to 10mg if the 5mg dose is not effective

Max: 10mg qhs

PEDIATRIC DOSAGE

Pediatric use may not have been established

DOSING CONSIDERATIONS

Concomitant Medications

CNS Depressants: May need to adjust dose of zolpidem

Hepatic Impairment

5mg qhs

Elderly

Elderly/Debilitated: 5mg qhs

ADMINISTRATION

Oral route

Take immediately before hs w/ at least 7-8 hrs remaining before the planned time of awakening

Must be primed before use for the 1st time

To prime, point the black spray opening away from face and other people and spray 5X

For administration, hold container upright w/ the black spray opening pointed directly into the mouth; fully press down on the pump to make sure a full dose (5mg) is sprayed directly into the mouth over the tongue. If a 10mg dose is prescribed, a 2nd spray should be administered

If not used for at least 14 days, must be primed again w/ 1 spray

Do not take w/ or immediately after a meal

HOW SUPPLIED

Spray: 5mg/actuation [60 actuations]

CONTRAINDICATIONS

Hypersensitivity to zolpidem.

WARNINGS/PRECAUTIONS

Increased risk of next-day psychomotor impairment if taken with less than a full night of sleep remaining (7-8 hrs). May impair mental/physical abilities. Initiate only after careful evaluation; failure of insomnia to remit after 7-10 days of treatment may indicate presence of a primary psychiatric and/or medical illness. Cases of angioedema involving the tongue, glottis, or larynx reported; do not rechallenge if angioedema develops. Abnormal thinking, behavioral changes, and visual/auditory hallucinations reported. Complex behaviors (eg, sleep-driving) reported; consider discontinuation if a sleep-driving episode occurs. Amnesia, anxiety, and other neuropsychiatric symptoms may occur. Worsening of depression, and suicidal thoughts and actions (including completed suicides) reported in primarily depressed patients; prescribe the least amount of drug that is feasible at a time. Caution with compromised respiratory function; prior to prescribing, consider the risks of respiratory depression, in patients with respiratory impairment (eg, sleep apnea, myasthenia gravis). Withdrawal signs and symptoms reported following rapid dose decrease or abrupt discontinuation; monitor for tolerance, abuse, and dependence.

ADVERSE REACTIONS

Drowsiness, headache, dizziness, allergy, sinusitis, lethargy, drugged feeling, pharyngitis, dry mouth, back pain, diarrhea.

DRUG INTERACTIONS

See Dosing Considerations. Increased risk of CNS depression and complex behaviors with other CNS depressants (eg, benzodiazepines, opioids, TCAs, alcohol). Use with other sedative-hypnotics (eg, other zolpidem products) at hs or the middle of the night is not recommended. Increased risk of next-day psychomotor impairment with other CNS depressants or drugs that increase zolpidem levels. May decrease peak levels of imipramine. Additive effect of decreased alertness with imipramine or chlorpromazine. Additive adverse effect on psychomotor performance with chlorpromazine or alcohol. Sertraline and CYP3A inhibitors may increase exposure. Fluoxetine may increase $T_{1/2}$. Rifampin (a CYP3A4 inducer) may reduce exposure, pharmacodynamic effects, and efficacy. Ketoconazole (a potent CYP3A4 inhibitor) may increase pharmacodynamic effects; consider lower dose of zolpidem.

PATIENT CONSIDERATIONS

Assessment: Assess for physical and/or psychiatric disorder, depression, compromised respiratory function, sleep apnea, myasthenia gravis, hepatic impairment, history of drug/alcohol addiction or abuse, hypersensitivity to the drug, pregnancy/nursing status, and possible drug interactions.

Monitoring: Monitor for angioedema, emergence of any new behavioral signs/symptoms of concern, respiratory depression, withdrawal signs/symptoms, tolerance, abuse, dependence, and other adverse reactions.

Counseling: Inform about the benefits and risks of treatment. Instruct to take only as prescribed; advise to wait at least 8 hrs after dosing before driving or engaging in other activities requiring full mental alertness. Instruct to contact physician immediately if any adverse reactions (eg, severe anaphylactic/anaphylactoid reactions, sleep-driving, other complex behaviors, suicidal thoughts) develop. Advise not to use the drug if patient drank alcohol that pm or before bed. Instruct patients not to increase the dose and to inform physician if it is believed that the drug does not work.

STORAGE: 25°C (77°F); excursions permitted to 15-30°C (59-86°F). Store upright. Do not freeze. Avoid prolonged exposure to temperatures >30°C (86°F).

ZOMETA — zoledronic acid

RX

Class: Bisphosphonate

ADULT DOSAGE

Hypercalcemia of Malignancy

Max: 4mg as a single-dose

May consider retreatment if serum Ca^{2+} does not return to normal or remain normal after initial treatment; wait for a minimum of 7 days before retreatment

Vigorous saline hydration should be initiated promptly and an attempt should be made to restore the urine output to about 2L/day throughout treatment; avoid overhydration, especially in patients w/ cardiac failure

Multiple Myeloma and Metastatic Bone Lesions of Solid Tumors

Adjunct to Standard Antineoplastic Therapy: 4mg every 3-4 weeks

Prostate cancer should have progressed after treatment w/ at least 1 hormonal therapy

PEDIATRIC DOSAGE

Pediatric use may not have been established

DOSING CONSIDERATIONS

Renal Impairment

Multiple Myeloma and Metastatic Bone Lesions of Solid Tumors:

CrCl 50-60mL/min: 3.5mg

CrCl 40-49mL/min: 3.3mg

CrCl 30-39mL/min: 3mg

Withhold treatment for renal deterioration

Other Important Considerations

Multiple Myeloma and Metastatic Bone Lesions of Solid Tumors:

Administer oral Ca^{2+} supplement of 500mg and multiple vitamins containing 400 IU of vitamin D daily

ADMINISTRATION

IV route

Preparation

4mg/100mL single use bottle is ready-to-use and may be administered directly to the patient w/o further preparation.

Preparation of Reduced Doses from Ready-to-Use Bottle (4mg/100mL):

Remove 12mL, 18mL, or 25mL from bottle and replace w/ an equal volume of sterile 0.9% NaCl or D5 inj for a dose of 3.5mg, 3.3mg, or 3mg, respectively.

Preparation from Single-Use Vial (4mg/5mL):

Remove 5mL (4mg), 4.4mL (3.5mg), 4.1mL (3.3mg), or 3.8mL (3mg) from vial and immediately dilute in 100mL of sterile 0.9% NaCl or D5 inj.

If not used immediately after dilution, refrigerate at 2-8°C (36-46°F).

Equilibrate refrigerated sol to room temperature prior to administration; total time between dilution, storage in refrigerator, and end of administration must not exceed 24 hrs.

Infuse IV over no less than 15 min.

Do not mix w/ Ca^{2+} or other divalent cation-containing infusion sol (eg, lactated Ringer's sol), and administer as a single IV sol in a line separate from all other drugs.

HOW SUPPLIED

Inj: 4mg/5mL, 4mg/100mL

CONTRAINDICATIONS

Hypersensitivity to zoledronic acid or any components of Zometa.

WARNINGS/PRECAUTIONS

Contains same active ingredient as Reclast; do not treat concomitantly w/ Reclast or other bisphosphonates. Adequately rehydrate patients w/ hypercalcemia of malignancy prior to administration and throughout the treatment. Caution in patients w/ hypercalcemia of malignancy w/ severe renal impairment. Not recommended in patients w/ bone metastases w/ severe renal impairment. Osteonecrosis of the jaw (ONJ) reported; risk may increase w/ duration of exposure to drug. Perform dental examination w/ preventive dentistry prior to treatment and if possible, avoid invasive dental procedures while on treatment. Severe and occasionally incapacitating bone, joint, and/or muscle pain reported; d/c if severe symptoms develop. Atypical subtrochanteric and diaphyseal femoral fractures reported; examine contralateral femur in patients who have sustained femoral shaft fracture. Any patient w/ a history of bisphosphonate exposure who presents w/ thigh/groin pain in the absence of trauma should be suspected of having an atypical fracture and should be evaluated; consider discontinuation in patients suspected to have an atypical femur fracture. Bronchoconstriction may occur in aspirin-sensitive patients. May cause fetal harm. Hypocalcemia, cardiac arrhythmias, and neurologic adverse events reported; correct hypocalcemia before initiating treatment and adequately supplement w/ Ca^{2+} and vitamin D.

ADVERSE REACTIONS

Bone pain, N/V, insomnia, abnormal SrCr, fatigue, pyrexia, anemia, constipation, dyspnea, diarrhea, weakness, myalgia, cough, arthralgia, edema (lower limb).

DRUG INTERACTIONS

Caution w/ aminoglycosides or calcitonin; may have an additive effect to lower serum Ca^{2+} level for prolonged periods. Caution w/ drugs known to cause hypocalcemia; severe hypocalcemia may develop. Loop diuretics may increase risk of hypocalcemia; do not use until the patient is adequately rehydrated and use w/ caution. Caution w/ other potentially nephrotoxic drugs. Caution w/ antiangiogenic drugs; increased incidence of ONJ has been observed.

PATIENT CONSIDERATIONS

Assessment: Assess for hypocalcemia, risk factors for ONJ, hypersensitivity to drug, aspirin sensitivity, renal impairment, pregnancy/nursing status, and possible drug interactions. Assess hydration status and SrCr prior to each treatment. Perform dental exam w/ preventive dentistry. Measure serum Ca^{2+}.

Monitoring: Monitor renal function, standard hypercalcemia-related metabolic parameters (eg, serum Ca^{2+}, phosphate, Mg^{2+}), and hydration status. Monitor for ONJ, musculoskeletal pain, atypical femur fracture, bronchoconstriction, hypocalcemia, and other adverse reactions.

Counseling: Instruct to notify physician of kidney problems, if pregnant/planning to become pregnant, breastfeeding, or if aspirin-sensitive. Inform of the importance of getting blood tests during the course of therapy. Advise to have dental exam prior to treatment and avoid invasive dental procedures during treatment. Inform of the importance of good dental hygiene and routine dental care. Advise patients w/ multiple myeloma or bone metastasis of solid tumors to take an oral Ca^{2+} supplement of 500mg and a multiple vitamin containing 400 IU of vitamin D daily. Instruct to report any thigh, hip, or groin pain. Inform of the most common side effects that may develop.

STORAGE: 25°C (77°F); excursions permitted to 15-30°C (59-86°F). Diluted Sol: If not used immediately, store at 2-8°C (36-46°F).

ZOMIG – zolmitriptan

RX

Class: 5-$HT_{1B/1D}$ agonist (triptans)

OTHER BRAND NAMES

Zomig-ZMT

ADULT DOSAGE

Migraine

W/ or w/o Aura:

Nasal Spray:

PEDIATRIC DOSAGE

Migraine

W/ or w/o Aura:

≥12 Years:

Initial: 2.5mg
May give another dose at least 2 hrs after the previous dose if migraine is not resolved by 2 hrs or returns after transient improvement
Max: 5mg/dose or 10mg/24 hrs

Safety of treating an average of >4 migraines in a 30-day period has not been established

Tabs:
Initial: 1.25mg or 2.5mg
May give another dose at least 2 hrs after the previous dose if migraine is not resolved by 2 hrs or returns after transient improvement
Max: 5mg/dose or 10mg/24 hrs

Safety of treating an average of >3 migraines in a 30-day period has not been established

Nasal Spray:
Initial: 2.5mg
May give another dose at least 2 hrs after the previous dose if migraine is not resolved by 2 hrs or returns after transient improvement
Max: 5mg/dose or 10mg/24 hrs

Safety of treating an average of >4 migraines in a 30-day period has not been established

DOSING CONSIDERATIONS

Concomitant Medications

Cimetidine:
Max: 2.5mg/dose or 5mg/24 hrs

Hepatic Impairment

Nasal Spray:
Moderate to Severe: Not recommended

Tabs:
Moderate to Severe: 1.25mg (1/2 of one 2.5mg tab)
Severe: Max: 5mg/day

Tab, Disintegrating:
Moderate to Severe: Not recommended

ADMINISTRATION

Oral/nasal routes

Spray

Refer to PI for proper administration instructions

Tab, Disintegrating

Do not remove from blister until just prior to dosing
Place tab on the tongue until dissolved, then swallow w/ saliva

HOW SUPPLIED

Spray: 2.5mg, 5mg [100μL]; **Tab:** 2.5mg*, 5mg; **Tab, Disintegrating:** (ZMT) 2.5mg, 5mg *scored

CONTRAINDICATIONS

Ischemic coronary artery disease (angina pectoris, history of MI, or documented silent ischemia), other significant underlying cardiovascular (CV) disease, or coronary artery vasospasm, including Prinzmetal's angina. Wolff-Parkinson-White syndrome, arrhythmias associated w/ other cardiac accessory conduction pathway disorders, history of stroke, transient ischemic attack (TIA), history of hemiplegic/basilar migraine, peripheral vascular disease, ischemic bowel disease, and uncontrolled HTN. Recent use of another 5-HT_1-agonist, ergotamine-containing medication, or ergot-type medication (eg, dihydroergotamine, methysergide), hypersensitivity to zolmitriptan. Concurrent MAOI-A or recent use/discontinuation of an MAOI-A (w/in 2 weeks).

WARNINGS/PRECAUTIONS

If no treatment response for the 1st migraine attack, reconsider diagnosis before treating any subsequent attacks. Not for prevention of migraine attacks. Serious cardiac adverse reactions, including MI reported. May cause coronary artery vasospasm (Prinzmetal's angina). Perform CV evaluation in triptan-naive patients who have multiple CV risk factors (eg, increased age, diabetes, HTN, strong family history of coronary artery disease [CAD]) prior to therapy; consider administering 1st dose in a medically supervised setting and performing an ECG immediately following administration if CV evaluation is negative. Consider periodic CV evaluation in patients who are intermittent long-term users who have multiple CV risk factors and a negative CV evaluation. Life-threatening cardiac rhythm disturbances, including ventricular tachycardia and ventricular fibrillation, reported; d/c if these disturbances occur. Sensations of tightness, pain, and pressure in the chest, throat, neck, and jaw commonly occur (usually of noncardiac origin). Cerebral/subarachnoid hemorrhage and stroke reported; exclude other potentially serious neurological conditions before treating headaches in patients not previously diagnosed w/ migraine, and in migraine patients w/ atypical migraine symptoms. May cause noncoronary vasospastic reactions (eg, peripheral vascular ischemia, GI vascular ischemia and infarction, Raynaud's syndrome, splenic infarction). Transient and permanent blindness and significant partial vision loss reported. Overuse of acute migraine drugs may lead to exacerbation of headache; detoxification may be necessary. Serotonin syndrome may occur; d/c if suspected. HTN reported.

Caution in elderly. (Tab, Disintegrating) Caution w/ phenylketonuria; each 2.5mg and 5mg ODT contains 2.81mg and 5.62mg phenylalanine. (Tab, Disintegrating; Spray) Not recommended in patients w/ moderate or severe hepatic impairment. (Spray) D/C if a cerebrovascular event occurs.

ADVERSE REACTIONS

Dizziness, paresthesia, nausea. (Tab) Neck/throat/jaw pain, asthenia, somnolence, warm/cold sensation, heaviness sensation, dry mouth. (Spray) Unusual taste, hyperesthesia, dysgeusia, nasal discomfort, oropharyngeal pain.

DRUG INTERACTIONS

See Contraindications. Ergot-containing drugs may prolong vasospastic reactions. Increased exposure w/ MAOI-A. Risk of vasospastic reactions w/ 5-$HT_{1B/1D}$-agonists (eg, triptans). Serotonin syndrome may occur, particularly during coadministration w/ SSRIs, SNRIs, TCAs, and MAOIs. $T_{1/2}$ and blood levels reported to double w/ cimetidine.

PATIENT CONSIDERATIONS

Assessment: Confirm diagnosis of migraine before therapy. Assess for ischemic CAD, HTN, history of hemiplegic/basilar migraine, hypersensitivity to drug, or any other conditions where treatment is contraindicated or cautioned. Assess for hepatic impairment, pregnancy/nursing status, and possible drug interactions. Perform a CV evaluation for patients who have multiple CV risk factors.

Monitoring: Monitor for signs/symptoms of cardiac adverse reactions; cerebrovascular events; vasospastic reactions; tightness/pain/pressure sensations in the chest, throat, neck, and jaw; peripheral vascular ischemia; serotonin syndrome; increased BP; and other adverse reactions. Perform ECG immediately after administration of therapy and monitor CV function in intermittent long-term users who have multiple CV risk factors.

Counseling: Instruct to take ud. Inform that treatment may cause serious CV events that may result in hospitalization and even death. Instruct patients to be alert for signs/symptoms of chest pain, SOB, weakness, and slurring of speech; advise to notify physician if any of these signs/symptoms are observed. Inform that the use of therapy ≥10 days per month may lead to exacerbation of headache; encourage to record headache frequency and drug use. Counsel about the possible drug interactions. Advise to notify physician if pregnant/nursing or planning to become pregnant. (Tab, Disintegrating) Inform patients w/ phenylketonuria that it contains phenylalanine. (Spray) Counsel on proper administration technique for nasal spray; advise to avoid spraying contents in the eyes.

STORAGE: 20-25°C (68-77°F). (Tab/Tab, Disintegrating) Protect from light and moisture.

ZONISAMIDE – zonisamide

RX

Class: Sulfonamide anticonvulsant

OTHER BRAND NAMES

Zonegran

ADULT DOSAGE

Partial Seizures

As Adjunctive Therapy in Patients w/ Epilepsy:

>16 Years:

Give qd or bid

Initial: 100mg/day

Titrate: After 2 weeks, may increase to 200mg/day for at least 2 weeks. May then increase to 300mg/day and 400mg/day, w/ the dose stable for at least 2 weeks to achieve steady state at each level.

Evidence suggests that doses of 100-600mg/day are effective, but there is no suggestion of increasing response above 400mg/day

PEDIATRIC DOSAGE

Pediatric use may not have been established

DOSING CONSIDERATIONS

Renal Impairment

May require slower titration

Hepatic Impairment

May require slower titration

Elderly

Start at lower end of dosing range

Discontinuation

D/C gradually

ADMINISTRATION
Oral route

Take w/ or w/o food.
Swallow caps whole.

HOW SUPPLIED
Cap: 50mg; (Zonegran) 25mg, 100mg

CONTRAINDICATIONS
Hypersensitivity to sulfonamides or zonisamide.

WARNINGS/PRECAUTIONS
Potentially fatal reactions to sulfonamides (eg, Stevens-Johnson syndrome, toxic epidermal necrolysis, fulminant hepatic necrosis, agranulocytosis, aplastic anemia, other blood dyscrasias) reported; d/c immediately if signs of hypersensitivity or other serious reactions occur. Consider discontinuation if unexplained rash develops; if the drug is not discontinued, observe frequently. Drug reaction w/ eosinophilia and systemic symptoms/multiorgan hypersensitivity reported; evaluate immediately if signs/symptoms present and d/c if an alternative etiology cannot be established. Increased risk of suicidal thoughts/behavior. May cause metabolic acidosis (generally dose-dependent); conditions or therapies that predispose to acidosis may be additive to the bicarbonate-lowering effects of zonisamide. Consider dose reduction or discontinuation of therapy if metabolic acidosis develops and persists; if the decision is to continue therapy, consider alkali treatment. Abrupt withdrawal may precipitate increased seizure frequency or status epilepticus; reduce dose or d/c gradually. May cause serious fetal adverse effects; women of childbearing potential should use effective contraception. May cause CNS-related adverse events (eg, psychiatric symptoms, psychomotor slowing, somnolence, fatigue). May impair mental/physical abilities. Caution w/ hepatic dysfunction. Nephrolithiasis and increased SrCr/BUN reported; d/c if acute renal failure or a clinically significant sustained increase in SrCr/BUN develops. Do not use in patients w/ renal failure (estimated GFR <50mL/min). Status epilepticus and sudden unexplained deaths reported. Increases serum Cl^- and alkaline phosphatase and decreases serum bicarbonate, phosphorus, Ca^{2+}, and albumin. Caution in elderly.

ADVERSE REACTIONS
Somnolence, anorexia, dizziness, ataxia, agitation/irritability, difficulty w/ memory and/or concentration.

DRUG INTERACTIONS
Caution when starting or stopping zonisamide or changing the zonisamide dose in patients who are also receiving drugs that are P-gp substrates (eg, digoxin, quinidine). CYP3A4 inducers (eg, phenytoin, carbamazepine, phenobarbital) may increase metabolism/clearance and decrease $T_{1/2}$ of zonisamide. These effects are unlikely to be of clinical significance when zonisamide is added to existing therapy; however, since changes in zonisamide concentrations may occur if concomitant CYP3A4-inducing antiepileptic or other drugs are withdrawn, dose adjusted, or introduced, an adjustment of the zonisamide dose may be required. Patient should be closely monitored and dose of zonisamide and other drugs that are CYP3A4 substrates may need to be adjusted if coadministration w/ a potent CYP3A4 inducer (eg, rifampicin) is necessary. Caution w/ alcohol or other CNS depressants. Concomitant use w/ other carbonic anhydrase inhibitors (eg, topiramate, acetazolamide, dichlorphenamide) may increase the severity of metabolic acidosis and may also increase the risk of kidney stone formation; monitor for the appearance or worsening of metabolic acidosis w/ concomitant use. Caution w/ other drugs that predispose patients to heat-related disorders (eg, carbonic anhydrase inhibitors, anticholinergics).

PATIENT CONSIDERATIONS

Assessment: Assess for hypersensitivity to sulfonamides or the drug, depression, conditions or therapies that predispose to acidosis, renal/hepatic impairment, pregnancy/nursing status, and possible drug interactions. Obtain baseline serum bicarbonate level.

Monitoring: Monitor for signs/symptoms of severe reactions (eg, skin reactions, hematologic events), emergence/worsening of depression, suicidal thoughts/behavior, any unusual changes in mood/behavior, metabolic acidosis, seizures (upon abrupt withdrawal), CNS-related adverse events, and other adverse reactions. Monitor renal function and serum bicarbonate levels periodically.

Counseling: Inform about risks/benefits of therapy and instruct to take only as prescribed. Advise not to drive or operate other complex machinery until patient gains sufficient experience on therapy to determine whether it affects performance. Instruct to immediately contact physician if patient experiences skin rash; worsening of seizures; signs/symptoms of kidney stone formation, hematological complications, or metabolic acidosis; emergence/worsening of depression symptoms; any unusual changes in mood/behavior; suicidal thoughts/behavior; or thoughts about self-harm. Inform that increasing fluid intake and urine output may reduce risk of kidney stone formation, particularly in those w/ predisposing risk factors for stones. Advise women of childbearing potential to use effective contraception while on therapy. Instruct to notify physician if pregnant/breastfeeding, or intending to become pregnant or to breastfeed during therapy; encourage to enroll in the NAAED Pregnancy Registry if patient becomes pregnant.

STORAGE: 20-25°C (68-77°F); excursions permitted to 15-30°C (59-86°F). Store in a dry place and protect from light. **Zonegran:** 25°C (77°F); excursions permitted to 15-30°C (59-86°F). Store in a dry place and protect from light.

ZONTIVITY – vorapaxar

RX

Class: Protease-activated receptor-1 (PAR-1) antagonist

Do not use in patients w/ a history of stroke, transient ischemic attack (TIA), intracranial hemorrhage (ICH), or active pathological bleeding. May increase the risk of bleeding, including ICH and fatal bleeding.

ADULT DOSAGE

Reduction of Thrombotic Cardiovascular Events

In Patients w/ a History of MI or w/ Peripheral Arterial Disease:
1 tab (2.08mg) qd; use w/ aspirin and/or clopidogrel according to their indications or standard of care

PEDIATRIC DOSAGE

Pediatric use may not have been established

DOSING CONSIDERATIONS

Hepatic Impairment

Severe: Not recommended

ADMINISTRATION

Oral route

Take w/ or w/o food

HOW SUPPLIED

Tab: 2.08mg

CONTRAINDICATIONS

Active pathological bleeding (eg, ICH, peptic ulcer). History of stroke, TIA, or ICH.

WARNINGS/PRECAUTIONS

Increases the risk of bleeding in proportion to the patient's underlying bleeding risk. Suspect bleeding in any patient who is hypotensive and has recently undergone coronary angiography, percutaneous coronary intervention, CABG surgery, or other surgical procedures. Withholding therapy for a brief period will not be useful in managing an acute bleeding event; has no known treatment to reverse the antiplatelet effect of therapy; significant inhibition of platelet aggregation remains 4 weeks after discontinuation of therapy.

ADVERSE REACTIONS

Bleeding, anemia.

DRUG INTERACTIONS

May increase risk of bleeding w/ anticoagulants, fibrinolytic therapy, chronic NSAIDs, SSRIs, and SNRIs; avoid concomitant use of warfarin or other anticoagulants. Avoid concomitant use w/ strong CYP3A inhibitors (eg, ketoconazole, clarithromycin, ritonavir) or strong CYP3A inducers (eg, rifampin, carbamazepine, St. John's wort).

PATIENT CONSIDERATIONS

Assessment: Assess for history of stroke, TIA, or ICH; active pathological bleeding, risk factors for bleeding, hepatic impairment, pregnancy/nursing status, and for possible drug interactions.

Monitoring: Monitor for signs/symptoms of bleeding and other adverse reactions.

Counseling: Inform about the benefits and risks of therapy. Instruct to take exactly ud and not to d/c w/o discussing it w/ the prescribing physician. Inform that may bleed and bruise more easily. Advise to report any unanticipated, prolonged, or excessive bleeding, or blood in stool or urine. Instruct to notify physicians or dentists about therapy before any surgery or dental procedure. Advise to inform physician of all medications currently taking/planning to take.

STORAGE: 20-25°C (68-77°F); excursions permitted to 15-30°C (59-86°F). Protect from moisture.

ZORTRESS – everolimus

RX

Class: Immunosuppressant

Should only be prescribed by physicians experienced in immunosuppressive therapy and management of organ transplant patients. Immunosuppression may lead to increased susceptibility to infection and possible development of malignancies (eg, lymphoma, skin cancer). Increased risk of kidney arterial and venous thrombosis leading to graft loss was reported, mostly w/in the first 30 days post-transplantation. Increased nephrotoxicity may occur in combination w/ standard doses of cyclosporine; reduce dose of cyclosporine to reduce renal dysfunction, and monitor cyclosporine and everolimus whole blood trough concentrations. Increased mortality w/in the first 3 months post-transplantation in heart transplant patients on immunosuppressive regimens w/ or w/o induction therapy; not recommended in heart transplantation.

ADULT DOSAGE

Renal Transplant

Prophylaxis of Organ Rejection in Kidney Transplant:

Initial: 0.75mg bid, in combination w/ basiliximab induction and concurrently w/ reduced dose of cyclosporine; give as soon as possible after transplantation

Initiate oral prednisone once oral medication is tolerated

Titrate: May require dose adjustment based on blood concentrations achieved, tolerability, individual response, change in concomitant medications, and clinical situation; optimal dose adjustments should be based on trough levels obtained 4 or 5 days after a previous dosing change

Recommended Therapeutic Range: 3-8ng/mL (based on LC/MS/MS assay method); if trough level is <3ng/mL, double total daily dose, or if trough level is >8ng/mL on 2 consecutive measures, decrease by 0.25mg bid

Refer to PI for further drug monitoring instructions and for cyclosporine therapeutic drug monitoring parameters

Hepatic Transplant

Prophylaxis of Allograft Rejection w/ a Liver Transplant:

Initial: 1mg bid, in combination w/ reduced dose of tacrolimus; start at least 30 days post-transplant

Titrate: May require dose adjustment based on blood concentrations achieved, tolerability, individual response, change in concomitant medications, and clinical situation; optimal dose adjustments should be based on trough levels obtained 4 or 5 days after a previous dosing change

Recommended Therapeutic Range: 3-8ng/mL (based on LC/MS/MS assay method); if trough level is <3ng/mL, double total daily dose, or if trough level is >8ng/mL on 2 consecutive measures, decrease by 0.25mg bid

Refer to PI for further drug monitoring instructions and for tacrolimus therapeutic drug monitoring parameters

PEDIATRIC DOSAGE

Pediatric use may not have been established

DOSING CONSIDERATIONS

Hepatic Impairment

Mild (Child-Pugh Class A): Reduce initial daily dose by 1/3 of normal daily dose

Moderate or Severe (Child-Pugh Class B or C): Reduce initial daily dose to 1/2 of the normal daily dose

ADMINISTRATION

Oral route

Do not crush; swallow whole w/ water.

Administer consistently approx 12 hrs apart w/ or w/o food and at the same time as cyclosporine or tacrolimus.

HOW SUPPLIED

Tab: 0.25mg, 0.5mg, 0.75mg

CONTRAINDICATIONS

Known hypersensitivity to everolimus, sirolimus, or to components of the drug product.

WARNINGS/PRECAUTIONS

Limit exposure to sunlight and UV light. Prophylaxis for *Pneumocystis jiroveci (carinii)* pneumonia and CMV recommended. Increased risk of hepatic artery thrombosis (HAT), which may lead to graft loss or death; do not give earlier than 30 days after liver transplant. Consider switching to other immunosuppressive therapies if renal function does not improve after dose adjustments or if dysfunction is thought to be drug related. Angioedema, increased risk of delayed wound healing, increased occurrence of wound-related complications, and generalized fluid accumulation reported. Interstitial lung disease (ILD), implying lung intraparenchymal inflammation (pneumonitis) and/or fibrosis of noninfectious etiology, some w/ pulmonary HTN as a secondary event reported; resolution may occur upon drug interruption w/ or w/o glucocorticoid therapy. Consider diagnosis of ILD for symptoms of infectious pneumonia that do not respond to antibiotic therapy and in whom non-drug causes have been ruled out. Increased risk of hyperlipidemia and proteinuria w/ higher whole blood trough concentrations; use of anti-lipid therapy may not normalize lipid levels. Reevaluate the risk/benefit of continuing therapy in patients w/ severe refractory hyperlipidemia. Increased risk of polyoma virus infections, including polyoma virus-associated nephropathy (PVAN) and progressive multiple leukoencephalopathy (PML), may occur; consider reductions in immunosuppression if evidence of PVAN or PML develops. Concomitant use w/ cyclosporine may increase risk of thrombotic microangiopathy/TTP/hemolytic uremic syndrome. May increase risk of new-onset diabetes mellitus (DM) after transplant. Azoospermia or oligospermia may be observed. Avoid w/ rare hereditary problems of galactose intolerance (Lapp lactase deficiency, glucose-galactose malabsorption); diarrhea and malabsorption may occur.

ADVERSE REACTIONS

Kidney Transplantation: Peripheral edema, constipation, HTN, nausea, anemia, urinary tract infection, hyperlipidemia.

Liver Transplantation: Diarrhea, headache, peripheral edema, HTN, nausea, pyrexia, abdominal pain, leukopenia.

DRUG INTERACTIONS

See Boxed Warning. Caution w/ drugs known to impair renal function. May increase risk of angioedema w/ drugs known to cause angioedema (eg, ACE inhibitors). Monitor for development of rhabdomyolysis w/ HMG-CoA reductase inhibitors and/or fibrates; use of simvastatin and lovastatin are strongly discouraged in patients receiving everolimus w/ cyclosporine. Coadministration w/ strong CYP3A4 inhibitors (eg, ketoconazole, clarithromycin, ritonavir) and strong CYP3A4 inducers (eg, rifampin, rifabutin) is not recommended w/o close monitoring of everolimus whole blood trough concentrations. Avoid w/ live vaccines, grapefruit, and grapefruit juice. Inhibitors of P-gp (eg, digoxin, cyclosporine), moderate inhibitors of CYP3A4 and P-gp (eg, fluconazole, macrolide antibiotics, nicardipine), and verapamil may increase levels. If coadministered w/ erythromycin or verapamil, monitor everolimus blood concentrations and if necessary, make a dose adjustment. Caution w/ CYP3A4 and CYP2D6 substrates w/ a narrow therapeutic index. Increased levels w/ cyclosporine; dose adjustment may be needed if cyclosporine dose is altered. CYP3A4 inducers (eg, St. John's wort, carbamazepine, phenobarbital) may decrease levels. Combination immunosuppressant therapy should be used w/ caution. May increase octreotide C_{min} levels.

PATIENT CONSIDERATIONS

Assessment: Assess for hereditary problems of galactose intolerance, hepatic impairment, hypersensitivity to the drug or to sirolimus, pregnancy/nursing status, and possible drug interactions. Obtain baseline lipid and glucose levels.

Monitoring: Monitor for infections, angioedema, thrombosis, wound-related complications, fluid accumulation, lymphomas and other malignancies, hyperlipidemia, hepatic impairment, proteinuria, PVAN, HAT, ILD, pneumonitis, and other adverse reactions. Monitor everolimus and cyclosporine or tacrolimus whole blood trough concentrations, lipid profile, blood glucose concentrations, renal function, and hematologic parameters.

Counseling: Counsel to avoid grapefruit and grapefruit juice. Inform of the risk of developing lymphomas and other malignancies, particularly of the skin; instruct to limit exposure to sunlight and UV light. Advise that therapy has been associated w/ an increased risk of kidney arterial and venous thrombosis, resulting in graft loss, usually occurring w/in the first 30 days post-transplantation. Inform of the risks of impaired kidney function w/ concomitant cyclosporine as well as the need for routine blood concentration monitoring for both drugs; advise of the importance of SrCr monitoring. Inform of risk of hyperlipidemia and the importance of lipid profile monitoring. Advise women to avoid pregnancy throughout treatment and for 8 weeks after discontinuation.

Instruct to notify physician of all medications and herbal/dietary supplements being taken. Inform that therapy has been associated w/ impaired or delayed wound healing, and fluid accumulation. Inform of increased risk of proteinuria, DM, infections, noninfectious pneumonitis, and angioedema; advise to contact physician if symptoms develop. Instruct to avoid receiving live vaccines.

STORAGE: 25°C (77°F); excursions permitted to 15-30°C (59-86°F). Protect from light and moisture.

Zostavax – zoster vaccine live

RX

Class: Vaccine

ADULT DOSAGE

Herpes Zoster

Prevention:

≥50 Years:

Single 0.65mL SQ in deltoid region of upper arm

PEDIATRIC DOSAGE

Pediatric use may not have been established

ADMINISTRATION

SQ route

Inject in deltoid region of upper arm

Do not inject IV or IM

Preparation/Reconstitution

Should be reconstituted immediately upon removal from the freezer

Only use the supplied diluent

Withdraw entire contents of diluent into syringe

To avoid excessive foaming, slowly inject all of diluent in syringe into vial of lyophilized vaccine and gently agitate to mix thoroughly

Withdraw entire contents of reconstituted vaccine into syringe and inject total volume SQ

HOW SUPPLIED

Inj: 19,400 PFU/0.65mL

CONTRAINDICATIONS

History of anaphylactic/anaphylactoid reaction to gelatin or neomycin or any other component of the vaccine. Immunosuppression or immunodeficiency, including history of primary or acquired immunodeficiency states, leukemia, lymphoma or other malignant neoplasms affecting the bone marrow or lymphatic system, AIDS or other clinical manifestations of infection with HIV, and those on immunosuppressive therapy. Pregnancy.

WARNINGS/PRECAUTIONS

Avoid pregnancy for 3 months following administration. Serious adverse reactions, including anaphylaxis, reported; have adequate treatment provisions (eg, epinephrine inj [1:1000]) available for immediate use. Transmission of vaccine virus may occur between vaccinees and susceptible contacts. Consider deferral in acute illness (eg, fever) or with active untreated tuberculosis (TB). Duration of protection >4 yrs after vaccination is unknown. May not protect all vaccine recipients.

ADVERSE REACTIONS

Inj-site reactions (erythema, pain, tenderness, swelling, pruritus, warmth), headache.

DRUG INTERACTIONS

See Contraindications. Reduced immune response to zoster vaccine live with pneumococcal vaccine polyvalent; consider administration of the 2 vaccines separated by at least 4 weeks.

PATIENT CONSIDERATIONS

Assessment: Assess for acute illness, active untreated TB, history of anaphylactic/anaphylactoid reaction to gelatin, neomycin, or any other component of the vaccine, immunosuppression/immunodeficiency, pregnancy/nursing status, and possible drug interactions.

Monitoring: Monitor for anaphylactic/anaphylactoid reactions and other adverse reactions.

Counseling: Instruct to inform physician about reactions to previous vaccines. Inform of benefits and risks of vaccine, including potential risk of transmitting vaccine virus to susceptible individuals (eg, immunosuppressed/immunodeficient individuals, pregnant women who have not had chickenpox). Instruct to report any adverse reactions or any symptoms of concern to physician.

STORAGE: Before Reconstitution: -50°C to -15°C (-58°F to 5°F). Use of dry ice may subject the vaccine to temperatures colder than -50°C (-58°F). May store and/or transport at 2-8°C (36-46°F) for up to 72 continuous hrs prior to reconstitution; discard if not used within 72 hrs of removal from -15°C (5°F). Protect from light. Diluent: 20-25°C (68-77°F) or 2-8°C (36-46°F). After Reconstitution: Administer immediately; discard if not used within 30 min. Do not freeze.

Zosyn – piperacillin/tazobactam

RX

Class: Beta-lactamase inhibitor/broad-spectrum penicillin (PCN)

ADULT DOSAGE

General Dosing

Usual: 3.375g q6h for 7-10 days; administer by IV infusion over 30 min

Nosocomial Pneumonia

Moderate to Severe:
Initial: 4.5g q6h plus an aminoglycoside for 7-14 days; administer Zosyn by IV infusion over 30 min

Aminoglycoside treatment should be continued in patients from whom *Pseudomonas aeruginosa* is isolated

Other Indications

- Appendicitis (complicated by rupture or abscess)
- Peritonitis
- Uncomplicated/complicated skin and skin structure infections (eg, cellulitis, cutaneous abscess, ischemic/diabetic foot infections)
- Postpartum endometritis
- Pelvic inflammatory disease
- Moderate community-acquired pneumonia

PEDIATRIC DOSAGE

Peritonitis

2-9 Months of Age: (80mg/10mg)/kg q8h
≥9 Months of Age: ≤40kg: (100mg/12.5mg)/kg q8h

>40kg: Use adult dose

Administer by IV infusion over 30 min

Appendicitis

2-9 Months of Age: (80mg/10mg)/kg q8h
≥9 Months of Age: ≤40kg: (100mg/12.5mg)/kg q8h

>40kg: Use adult dose

Administer by IV infusion over 30 min

DOSING CONSIDERATIONS

Renal Impairment

Adults:
All Indications (Except Nosocomial Pneumonia):
CrCl >40mL/min: 3.375g q6h
CrCl 20-40mL/min: 2.25g q6h
CrCl <20mL/min (Not Receiving Hemodialysis): 2.25g q8h
Hemodialysis: 2.25g q12h (max: 2.25g q12h); administer an additional 0.75g dose following each hemodialysis session on hemodialysis days
Continuous Ambulatory Peritoneal Dialysis: 2.25g q12h

Nosocomial Pneumonia:
CrCl >40mL/min: 4.5g q6h
CrCl 20-40mL/min: 3.375g q6h
CrCl <20mL/min (Not Receiving Hemodialysis): 2.25g q6h
Hemodialysis: 2.25g q8h (max: 2.25g q8h); administer an additional 0.75g dose following each hemodialysis session on hemodialysis days
Continuous Ambulatory Peritoneal Dialysis: 2.25g q8h

Elderly

Start at lower end of dosing range

ADMINISTRATION

IV route

Infuse over 30 min.
During the infusion it is desirable to d/c the primary infusion sol.

Single-Dose Vials

Reconstitute 2.25g, 3.375g, and 4.5g vials w/ 10mL, 15mL, and 20mL, respectively w/ a compatible reconstitution diluent; swirl until dissolved.
Further dilute reconstituted sol in a compatible IV sol (recommended volume per dose of 50-150mL).
Use immediately after reconstitution; discard any unused portion after 24 hrs if stored at 20-25°C (68-77°F) or after 48 hrs if stored at 2-8°C (36-46°F). Do not freeze vials after reconstitution.

Do not mix w/ other drugs in a syringe or infusion bottle.
Not chemically stable in sol that contain only sodium bicarbonate and sol that significantly alter the pH.
Do not add to blood products or albumin hydrolysates.

Compatible Reconstitution Diluents:
- 0.9% NaCl for inj
- Sterile water for inj (SWFI)

- D5
- Bacteriostatic saline/parabens
- Bacteriostatic water/parabens
- Bacteriostatic saline/benzyl alcohol
- Bacteriostatic water/benzyl alcohol

Compatible IV Sol:
- 0.9% NaCl for inj
- SWFI (max recommended volume per dose of SWFI is 50mL)
- Dextran 6% in saline
- D5
- Lactated Ringer's sol (compatible only w/ reformulated Zosyn containing EDTA and is compatible for co-administration via a Y-site)

Galaxy Containers
- Administer using sterile equipment, after thawing to room temperature.
- Zosyn containing EDTA is compatible for co-administration via a Y-site IV tube w/ Lactated Ringer's inj.
- Do not add supplementary medication.
- Discard unused portions.
- Do not use plastic containers in series connections.

Thawing of Plastic Container:
Thaw frozen container at 20-25°C (68-77°F) or 2-8°C (36-46°F); do not force thaw by immersion in water baths or by microwave irradiation.
Thawed solution is stable for 14 days at 2-8°C (36-46°F) or 24 hrs at 20-25°C (68-77°F); do not refreeze.

Refer to PI for further stability information and for compatibility w/ aminoglycosides.

HOW SUPPLIED

Inj: (Piperacillin/Tazobactam) 2g/0.25g (2.25g), 3g/0.375g (3.375g), 4g/0.5g (4.5g) [vial]; (2g/0.25g [2.25g])/50mL, (3g/0.375g [3.375g])/50mL, (4g/0.5g [4.5g])/100mL [Galaxy]. Also available as a Pharmacy Bulk Package.

CONTRAINDICATIONS

History of allergic reactions to any of the penicillins, cephalosporins, or β-lactamase inhibitors.

WARNINGS/PRECAUTIONS

Serious and occasionally fatal hypersensitivity (anaphylactic/anaphylactoid) reactions, including shock, reported; d/c and institute appropriate therapy if an allergic reaction occurs. Severe cutaneous adverse reactions (eg, Stevens-Johnson syndrome, toxic epidermal necrolysis, drug reaction w/ eosinophilia and systemic symptoms, acute generalized exanthematous pustulosis) may occur; monitor closely if a skin rash develops and d/c if lesions progress. *Clostridium difficile*-associated diarrhea (CDAD) reported; may need to d/c if CDAD is suspected or confirmed. Bleeding manifestations, sometimes associated w/ abnormalities of coagulation tests, reported; d/c and institute appropriate therapy if bleeding manifestations occur. Leukopenia/neutropenia may occur and is most frequently associated w/ prolonged administration. May cause neuromuscular excitability or convulsions w/ higher than recommended doses, particularly in the presence of renal failure. Caution in patients w/ restricted salt intake. Monitor electrolytes periodically in patients w/ low K^+ reserves. May result in bacterial resistance w/ use in the absence of a proven/suspected bacterial infection. Associated w/ increased incidence of fever and rash in cystic fibrosis patients. Lab test interactions may occur.

ADVERSE REACTIONS

Diarrhea, headache, constipation, N/V, rash, pruritus, dyspepsia, insomnia.

DRUG INTERACTIONS

Piperacillin may inactivate aminoglycosides. May decrease serum concentrations of tobramycin; monitor aminoglycoside levels in patients w/ ESRD. Probenecid prolongs $T_{1/2}$; avoid coadministration unless the benefit outweighs the risk. Test coagulation parameters more frequently w/ high doses of heparin, oral anticoagulants, or other drugs that may affect blood coagulation system or thrombocyte function. Caution w/ cytotoxic therapy or diuretics; consider possibility of hypokalemia. **Piperacillin:** May prolong neuromuscular blockade of vecuronium or any nondepolarizing muscle relaxant. May reduce methotrexate (MTX) clearance; frequently monitor MTX levels as well as for the signs/symptoms of MTX toxicity. Increased incidence of acute kidney injury reported w/ concomitant vancomycin as compared to vancomycin alone.

PATIENT CONSIDERATIONS

Assessment: Assess for previous hypersensitivity reaction to PCN, cephalosporins, or β-lactamase inhibitors; salt intake restriction; cystic fibrosis; low K^+ reserves; renal impairment; pregnancy/nursing status; and possible drug interactions.

Monitoring: Monitor hematopoietic function (especially w/ prolonged therapy [≥21 days]), renal function, and serum electrolytes periodically. Monitor for hypersensitivity reactions, CDAD, severe cutaneous reactions, leukopenia/neutropenia, bleeding manifestations, and for neuromuscular excitability or convulsions. Monitor for rash and fever in cystic fibrosis patients.

Counseling: Inform about risks/benefits of therapy. Counsel that drug only treats bacterial, not viral, infections. Instruct to take ud; inform that skipping doses or not completing full course may decrease effectiveness and increase bacterial resistance. Advise to d/c and notify physician if experiencing watery/bloody diarrhea (w/ or w/o stomach cramps and fever) even as late as ≥2 months after the last dose, or an allergic reaction. Instruct to notify physician if pregnant/nursing.

STORAGE: Vials: 20-25°C (68-77°F). **Galaxy Containers:** At or below -20°C (-4°F).

Zovirax Oral – acyclovir

RX

Class: Nucleoside analogue

ADULT DOSAGE

Herpes Zoster

800mg q4h, 5X/day for 7-10 days

Genital Herpes

Initial:
200mg q4h, 5X/day for 10 days

Recurrent Disease:
Chronic Suppressive Therapy: 400mg bid up to 12 months
Alternative: 200mg 3-5X/day

Intermittent Therapy:
200mg q4h, 5X/day for 5 days

Initiate at earliest sign/symptom of recurrence

Chickenpox

800mg qid for 5 days

Initiate at earliest sign/symptom

PEDIATRIC DOSAGE

Chickenpox

≥2 Years:
≤40kg: 20mg/kg qid for 5 days
>40kg: 800mg qid for 5 days

Initiate at earliest sign/symptom

DOSING CONSIDERATIONS

Renal Impairment

Genital Herpes (Initial/Intermittent Therapy):
CrCl ≤10mL/min: Reduce dose to 200mg q12h

Genital Herpes (Chronic Suppressive Therapy):
CrCl ≤10mL/min: Reduce dose to 200mg q12h

Herpes Zoster/Chickenpox:
CrCl 10-25mL/min: 800mg q8h
CrCl ≤10mL/min: 800mg q12h

Hemodialysis: Adjust dosing schedule so that an additional dose is administered after each dialysis

ADMINISTRATION

Oral route

Bioequivalence of Dosage Forms

Sus shown to be bioequivalent to caps
One 800mg tab shown to be bioequivalent to four 200mg caps

HOW SUPPLIED

Cap: 200mg; **Sus:** 200mg/5mL [473mL]; **Tab:** 400mg, 800mg

CONTRAINDICATIONS

Hypersensitivity to acyclovir or valacyclovir.

WARNINGS/PRECAUTIONS

Renal failure sometimes resulting in death reported. Thrombotic thrombocytopenic purpura/hemolytic uremic syndrome (TTP/HUS) in immunocompromised patients reported. Maintain adequate hydration. Caution in elderly.

ADVERSE REACTIONS

N/V, diarrhea, malaise.

DRUG INTERACTIONS

Probenecid may increase levels and $T_{1/2}$ of IV formulation. May increase risk of renal impairment and/or CNS symptoms with nephrotoxic agents; use caution.

PATIENT CONSIDERATIONS

Assessment: Assess for immunocompromised state, hypersensitivity to valacyclovir, renal impairment, nursing status, and possible drug interactions.

Monitoring: Monitor for signs/symptoms of TTP/HUS. Monitor BUN and SrCr.

Counseling: Instruct to consult physician if experiencing severe or troublesome adverse reactions, if pregnant/intending to become pregnant, or intending to breastfeed. Advise to maintain adequate hydration. Inform that therapy is not a cure for genital herpes; advise to avoid contact with lesions or intercourse when lesions/symptoms are present.

STORAGE: 15-25°C (59-77°F); protect from moisture.

ZYBAN — bupropion hydrochloride

RX

Class: Aminoketone

Serious neuropsychiatric reactions reported in patients taking bupropion for smoking cessation. Weigh risks against benefits of use. Antidepressants increased the risk of suicidal thoughts and behavior in children, adolescents, and young adults in short-term trials. Monitor closely for worsening, and emergence of suicidal thoughts and behavior.

ADULT DOSAGE

Smoking Cessation Aid

Initiate treatment while patient is still smoking
Patients should set a "target quit date" within the first 2 weeks of treatment
Initial: 150mg qd for first 3 days
Titrate: Increase to 300mg/day, given as 150mg bid w/ an interval of at least 8 hrs between each dose
Max: 300mg/day

Continue treatment for 7-12 weeks; if patient has not quit smoking after 7-12 weeks, should d/c and reassess treatment plan
May consider continuing therapy in patients who successfully quit smoking after 12 weeks of treatment but do not feel ready to d/c treatment; base longer treatment on individual patient benefits/risks

PEDIATRIC DOSAGE

Pediatric use may not have been established

DOSING CONSIDERATIONS

Concomitant Medications

Reversible MAOIs (eg, Linezolid, IV Methylene Blue):
Do not start bupropion in patients being treated w/ reversible MAOIs
If acceptable alternatives are not available, d/c bupropion and administer linezolid or IV methylene blue; monitor for 2 weeks or until 24 hrs after the last dose of linezolid or IV methylene blue, whichever comes 1st. May resume bupropion 24 hrs after the last dose of linezolid or IV methylene blue

Renal Impairment

GFR <90mL/min: Consider reducing dose and/or frequency

Hepatic Impairment

Mild (Child-Pugh Score: 5-6): Consider reducing dose and/or frequency
Moderate to Severe (Child-Pugh Score: 7-15) Max Dose: 150mg qod

Other Important Considerations

Switching to/from an MAOI:
Allow at least 14 days between discontinuation of an MAOI and initiation of treatment and allow at least 14 days between discontinuation of treatment and initiation of an MAOI

ADMINISTRATION

Oral route

Swallow tab whole; do not crush, divide, or chew
Take w/ or w/o food
Avoid hs dosing to minimize insomnia
May be used w/ a nicotine transdermal system

HOW SUPPLIED

Tab, Sustained-Release: 150mg

CONTRAINDICATIONS

Seizure disorder, current/prior diagnosis of bulimia or anorexia nervosa. Undergoing abrupt discontinuation of alcohol, benzodiazepines, barbiturates, and antiepileptic drugs. Use of MAOIs (intended to treat psychiatric disorders) either concomitantly or within 14 days of discontinuing treatment. Treatment within 14 days of discontinuing treatment with an MAOI. Starting treatment in patients being treated with reversible MAOIs (eg, linezolid, IV methylene blue). Hypersensitivity to bupropion or other ingredients of this medication.

WARNINGS/PRECAUTIONS

Dose-related risk of seizures; do not exceed 300mg/day and titrate gradually. D/C and do not restart treatment if a seizure occurs. May result in elevated BP and HTN. May precipitate a manic, mixed, or hypomanic episode; risk appears to be increased in patients with bipolar disorder or who have risk factors for bipolar disorder. Not approved for use in treating bipolar depression. Pupillary dilation that occurs following use may trigger an angle-closure attack in a patient with anatomically narrow angles who does not have a patent iridectomy. D/C if an allergic or anaphylactoid/anaphylactic reaction occurs. Arthralgia, myalgia, fever with rash, and other serum sickness-like symptoms suggestive of delayed hypersensitivity reported. False (+) urine immunoassay screening tests for amphetamines reported. Caution with renal/hepatic impairment and in the elderly.

ADVERSE REACTIONS

Neuropsychiatric reactions, insomnia, rhinitis, dry mouth, dizziness, nausea, disturbed concentration, constipation, anxiety, dream abnormality, arthralgia, nervousness, diarrhea, rash, myalgia.

DRUG INTERACTIONS

See Contraindications. CYP2B6 inhibitors (eg, ticlopidine, clopidogrel) may increase bupropion exposure but decrease hydroxybupropion exposure; may need to adjust bupropion dose. CYP2B6 inducers (eg, ritonavir, lopinavir, efavirenz) may decrease exposure; may need to increase bupropion dose but not to exceed max dose. Carbamazepine, phenytoin, and phenobarbital may induce metabolism and decrease exposure; may be necessary to increase dose of bupropion, but not to exceed max dose if used with a CYP inducer. May increase exposure of CYP2D6 substrates (eg, antidepressants, antipsychotics, β-blockers, Type 1C antiarrhythmics); may need to decrease dose of CYP2D6 substrate, particularly for drugs with a narrow therapeutic index. May reduce efficacy of drugs that require metabolic activation by CYP2D6 to be effective (eg, tamoxifen); may require increased doses of the drug. Extreme caution with other drugs that lower seizure threshold (eg, antipsychotics, theophylline, systemic corticosteroids); use low initial doses and increase gradually. Increased risk of seizure with illicit drugs (eg, cocaine), abuse or misuse of prescription drugs (eg, CNS stimulants), oral hypoglycemic drugs, insulin, anorectic drugs, and excessive use of alcohol, benzodiazepines, sedative/hypnotics, or opiates. CNS toxicity reported with levodopa or amantadine; use with caution. Minimize or avoid alcohol. Increased risk of HTN with MAOIs or other drugs that increase dopaminergic or noradrenergic activity. Monitor for HTN with nicotine replacement therapy. Physiological changes resulting from smoking cessation, with or without bupropion, may alter the pharmacokinetics or pharmacodynamics of certain drugs (eg, theophylline, warfarin, insulin) for which dosage adjustment may be necessary.

PATIENT CONSIDERATIONS

Assessment: Assess for bipolar disorder, hepatic/renal dysfunction, susceptibility to angle-closure glaucoma, seizure disorder or conditions that may increase the risk of seizure, hypersensitivity to the drug, any other conditions where treatment is contraindicated or cautioned, pregnancy/nursing status, and possible drug interactions. Assess BP.

Monitoring: Monitor for clinical worsening, suicidality, unusual changes in behavior, seizures, activation of mania or hypomania, neuropsychiatric reactions, angle-closure glaucoma, anaphylactoid/anaphylactic reactions, delayed hypersensitivity, and other adverse reactions. Monitor hepatic/renal function and BP.

Counseling: Inform about benefits/risks of therapy. Advise patients and caregivers to observe for clinical worsening, suicidal risks, and unusual changes in behavior. Inform that quitting smoking may be associated with nicotine withdrawal symptoms or exacerbation of preexisting psychiatric illness. Advise to notify physician immediately if agitation, hostility, depressed mood, changes in thinking or behavior, or suicidal ideation/behavior occurs. Educate on the symptoms of hypersensitivity and to d/c if a severe allergic reaction occurs. Instruct to d/c and not restart if a seizure occurs while on therapy. Inform that excessive use or abrupt discontinuation of alcohol or sedatives may alter the seizure threshold; advise to minimize or avoid alcohol use. Caution about the risk of angle-closure glaucoma. Inform that therapy may impair mental/physical abilities; advise to use caution while operating hazardous machinery/driving. Counsel to notify physician if taking/planning to take any prescription or OTC medications. Advise not to use in combination with any other medications that contain bupropion. Advise to notify physician if pregnant, intending to become pregnant, or if nursing. If taking >150mg/day, instruct to take in 2 doses at least 8 hrs apart, to minimize the risk of seizures. Inform that tab may have an odor.

STORAGE: 20-25°C (68-77°F); excursions permitted between 15-30°C (59-86°F). Protect from light and moisture.

ZYCLARA – imiquimod

RX

Class: Immune response modifier

ADULT DOSAGE

Actinic Keratosis

Clinically typical visible or palpable, actinic keratoses of the full face or balding scalp in immunocompetent patients

2.5%, 3.75%:

Apply as a thin film qd to affected area before hs for two 2-week treatment cycles separated by a 2-week no treatment period; may apply up to 0.5g (2 pkts or 2 full pump actuations) to treatment area at each application

Leave cre on skin for approx 8 hrs, and then remove by washing the area w/ mild soap and water

Prescribe no more than 56 pkts or two 7.5g pumps for total 2-cycle treatment course

External Genital and Perianal Warts

3.75%:

Apply as a thin layer to warts qd before hs until total clearance or for up to 8 weeks; may use up to 0.25g (1 pkt or 1 full pump actuation) at each application

Leave cre on skin for approx 8 hrs, and then remove by washing the area w/ mild soap and water

Prescribe up to 56 pkts or two 7.5g pumps for total treatment course

PEDIATRIC DOSAGE

External Genital and Perianal Warts

≥12 Years:

3.75%:

Apply as a thin layer to warts qd before hs until total clearance or for up to 8 weeks; may use up to 0.25g (1 pkt or 1 full pump actuation) at each application

Leave cre on skin for approx 8 hrs, and then remove by washing the area w/ mild soap and water

Prescribe up to 56 pkts or two 7.5g pumps for total treatment course

DOSING CONSIDERATIONS

Adverse Reactions

Local Skin Reactions:

Actinic Keratosis:

May take rest period of several days if required

Neither 2-week treatment cycle should be extended due to missed dose or rest periods

External Genital and Perianal Warts:

May need rest period of several days; resume once reaction subsides

May use non-occlusive dressings in management of skin reactions

ADMINISTRATION

Topical route

Wash hands before and after application.

Prime pumps before 1st use by repeatedly depressing the actuator until cre is dispensed.

Rub in until no longer visible.

Actinic Keratosis

Avoid use in or on lips and nostrils or in or near eyes.

HOW SUPPLIED

Cre: 2.5% [7.5g pump], 3.75% [7.5g pump, 28[s]]

WARNINGS/PRECAUTIONS

Not for oral, ophthalmic, intra-anal, or intravaginal use. Intense local skin reactions (eg, skin weeping, erosion) may occur; may require dosing interruption. May exacerbate inflammatory skin conditions, including chronic graft-versus-host disease. Severe local inflammatory reactions of the female external genitalia may lead to severe vulvar swelling, which may lead to urinary retention; interrupt or d/c if severe vulvar swelling occurs. Administration not recommended until the skin is healed from any previous drug or surgical treatment. Flu-like signs and symptoms may accompany or precede local skin reactions; consider dosing interruption and assessment of the patient. Lymphadenopathy reported. Avoid or minimize natural or artificial sunlight exposure (including sunlamps). Avoid w/ sunburn until fully recovered. Caution in patients who may have considerable sun exposure (eg, due to their occupation) or w/ inherent sensitivity to sunlight. Avoid use of any other imiquimod products in the same treatment area; may increase risk for and severity of local skin/systemic reactions. Caution w/ preexisting autoimmune conditions.

ADVERSE REACTIONS

Local skin reactions (erythema, scabbing/crusting, flaking/scaling/dryness, edema, erosion/ulceration, exudate), application-site pruritus/pain/irritation, headache, fatigue, influenza-like illness, nausea.

PATIENT CONSIDERATIONS

Assessment: Assess for inflammatory skin conditions, sunburn, inherent sensitivity to sunlight, preexisting autoimmune conditions, sunlight exposure, and pregnancy/nursing status.

Monitoring: Monitor for local skin reactions, severe vulvar swelling, flu-like signs/symptoms, other adverse reactions, and response to treatment.

Counseling: Instruct to use ud by physician, wash hands before and after application, and avoid contact w/ eyes, lips, nostrils, anus, and vagina. Advise not to bandage or otherwise occlude treatment area, not to reuse partially used pkts, and to discard pumps after full treatment course completion. Inform that local skin and systemic reactions may occur; instruct to contact physician if these occur. Instruct not to extend treatment cycle >2 weeks (actinic keratoses) or treatment >8 weeks (external genital and perianal warts) due to missed doses or rest periods. **Actinic Keratosis:** Instruct to continue treatment for the full treatment course even if all actinic keratoses appear to be gone. Instruct to wash treatment area w/ mild soap and water before and 8 hrs after application. Instruct to allow treatment area to dry thoroughly before application. Instruct to avoid or minimize exposure to natural or artificial sunlight (tanning beds or UVA/B treatment); encourage to use sunscreen and protective clothing (eg, hat). Inform that additional lesions may become apparent in the treatment area during treatment. **External Genital and Perianal Warts:** Instruct to wash treatment area w/ mild soap and water 8 hrs after application. Instruct to avoid sexual (genital, anal, oral) contact while cre is on the skin. Advise female patients to take special care during application at the vaginal opening. Instruct uncircumcised males treating warts under the foreskin to retract the foreskin and clean the area daily. Inform that new warts may develop during therapy. Inform that drug may weaken condoms and vaginal diaphragms; explain that concurrent use is not recommended. Instruct to remove cre by washing treatment area w/ mild soap and water if severe local skin reaction occurs.

STORAGE: 25°C (77°F); excursions permitted to 15-30°C (59-86°F). Avoid freezing.

ZYDELIG – idelalisib

RX

Class: Kinase inhibitor

Fatal and/or serious hepatotoxicity reported; monitor hepatic function prior to and during treatment; interrupt and then reduce or d/c as recommended. Fatal and/or serious and severe diarrhea or colitis reported; monitor for the development of severe diarrhea or colitis; interrupt and then reduce or d/c as recommended. Fatal and serious pneumonitis may occur; monitor for pulmonary symptoms and bilateral interstitial infiltrates; interrupt or d/c as recommended. Fatal and serious intestinal perforation may occur; d/c therapy for intestinal perforation.

ADULT DOSAGE

Relapsed Small Lymphocytic Lymphoma

In Patients Who Have Received at Least 2 Prior Systemic Therapies:
Max Initial: 150mg bid

Relapsed Chronic Lymphocytic Leukemia

Combination w/ Rituximab:
Max Initial: 150mg bid

Relapsed Follicular B-cell non-Hodgkin Lymphoma

In Patients Who Have Received at Least 2 Prior Systemic Therapies:
Max Initial: 150mg bid

PEDIATRIC DOSAGE

Pediatric use may not have been established

DOSING CONSIDERATIONS

Adverse Reactions

Pneumonitis:
D/C in patients w/ any severity of symptomatic pneumonitis

ALT/AST:
>3-5X ULN: Maintain dose; monitor at least weekly until ≤1X ULN
>5-20X ULN: Withhold treatment; monitor at least weekly until ≤1X ULN, then resume at 100mg bid
>20X ULN: D/C permanently

Bilirubin:
>1.5-3X ULN: Maintain dose; monitor at least weekly until ≤1X ULN
>3-10X ULN: Withhold treatment; monitor at least weekly until ≤1X ULN, then resume at 100mg bid
>10X ULN: D/C permanently

Diarrhea:
Moderate (Increase of 4-6 stools/day): Maintain dose; monitor at least weekly until resolved
Severe (Increase of ≥7 stools/day)/Hospitalization: Withhold treatment; monitor at least weekly until resolved, then resume at 100mg bid
Life-Threatening: D/C permanently

Neutropenia:
ANC 1-<1.5 Gi/L: Maintain dose
ANC 0.5-<1 Gi/L: Maintain dose; monitor at least weekly
ANC <0.5 Gi/L: Interrupt treatment; monitor at least weekly until ANC >0.5 Gi/L, then resume at 100mg bid

Thrombocytopenia:
Platelets 50-<75 Gi/L: Maintain dose
Platelets 25-<50 Gi/L: Maintain dose; monitor at least weekly
Platelets >25 Gi/L: Interrupt treatment; monitor at least weekly, then resume at 100mg bid when platelets ≥25 Gi/L

ADMINISTRATION

Oral route

Swallow tab whole
Take w/ or w/o food

HOW SUPPLIED

Tab: 100mg, 150mg

CONTRAINDICATIONS

History of serious allergic reactions, including anaphylaxis and toxic epidermal necrolysis (TEN).

WARNINGS/PRECAUTIONS

TEN reported with rituximab and bendamustine; other severe or life-threatening (Grade ≥3) cutaneous reactions (eg, exfoliative dermatitis, erythematous rash, maculopapular rash, skin disorder) reported in idelalisib-treated patients; monitor for development of severe cutaneous reactions and d/c therapy. Serious allergic reactions (eg, anaphylaxis) reported; d/c permanently and institute appropriate therapy if serious allergic reactions develop. Treatment-emergent Grade 3 or 4 neutropenia reported; monitor blood counts at least every 2 weeks for the first 3 months, and at least weekly while neutrophil counts are <1 Gi/L. May cause fetal harm. If contraceptive methods are being considered, females of reproductive potential should use effective contraception during treatment, and for at least 1 month after the last dose. Monitor for signs of idelalisib toxicity in patients with baseline hepatic impairment.

ADVERSE REACTIONS

Hepatotoxicity, colitis, diarrhea, pneumonitis, intestinal perforation, pyrexia, sepsis, febrile neutropenia, N/V, GERD, stomatitis, headache, chills, pain, rash.

DRUG INTERACTIONS

Avoid with drugs that may cause liver toxicity and drugs that cause diarrhea. Decreased exposure with strong CYP3A inducers (eg, rifampin, phenytoin, St. John's wort, carbamazepine); avoid coadministration. May increase exposure of a sensitive CYP3A substrate; avoid with CYP3A substrates. Increased exposure with strong CYP3A inhibitors; monitor for signs of idelalisib toxicity.

PATIENT CONSIDERATIONS

Assessment: Assess for history of serious allergic reactions, pregnancy/nursing status, and possible drug interactions. Assess hepatic function.

Monitoring: Monitor for diarrhea, colitis, pulmonary symptoms and bilateral interstitial infiltrates, intestinal perforation, neutropenia, thrombocytopenia, new/worsening abdominal pain, chills, fever, N/V, severe cutaneous reactions, serious allergic reactions, and other adverse reactions. Monitor ALT and AST every 2 weeks for the first 3 months of treatment, every 4 weeks for the next 3 months, then every 1-3 months thereafter. Monitor weekly for liver toxicity if the ALT or AST rises above 3X ULN until resolved. Monitor blood counts at least every 2 weeks for the first 3 months of therapy, and at least weekly in patients while neutrophil counts are <1.0 Gi/L. Monitor for signs of idelalisib toxicity in patients with baseline hepatic impairment.

Counseling: Advise that significant elevations in liver enzymes may occur, and that serial testing of serum liver tests (ALT, AST, bilirubin) are recommended while taking the drug. Instruct to report liver dysfunction symptoms to physician. Advise that severe diarrhea or colitis may occur and to notify physician immediately if bowel movements increase by ≥6/day. Advise of the possibility of pneumonitis, intestinal perforation, severe cutaneous reactions, and anaphylaxis; instruct to contact physician if any signs/symptoms of these conditions develop. Advise of the need for periodic monitoring of blood counts; instruct to notify physician if fever or any signs of infection develop.

Advise women of the potential hazard to fetus and to avoid pregnancy during therapy; instruct to use adequate contraception during therapy and for at least 1 month after completing therapy. Advise not to breastfeed during treatment. Instruct to take exactly as prescribed and not to change dose or stop therapy unless told to do so by physician. Advise that if a dose is missed by <6 hrs, to take missed dose right away and take next dose as usual. If a dose is missed by >6 hrs, advise to wait and take next dose at the usual time.

STORAGE: 20-30°C (68-86°F); excursions permitted to 15-30°C (59-86°F).

ZYKADIA – ceritinib

RX

Class: Kinase inhibitor

ADULT DOSAGE

Metastatic Non-Small Cell Lung Cancer

W/ anaplastic lymphoma kinase-positive metastatic non-small cell lung cancer who have progressed on or are intolerant to crizotinib

750mg qd until disease progression or unacceptable toxicity

Missed Dose

If a dose is missed, make up that dose unless the next dose is due w/in 12 hrs

PEDIATRIC DOSAGE

Pediatric use may not have been established

DOSING CONSIDERATIONS

Concomitant Medications

Strong CYP3A Inhibitors:

Avoid concurrent use; if unavoidable, reduce ceritinib dose by approx 1/3, rounded to the nearest 150mg dose strength

After discontinuation of a strong CYP3A inhibitor, resume ceritinib dose that was taken prior to initiating the strong CYP3A4 inhibitor

Adverse Reactions

Unable to Tolerate 300mg/day: D/C therapy

ALT or AST Elevation:

>5X ULN w/ Total Bilirubin ≤2X ULN: Withhold therapy until recovery to baseline or ≤3X ULN, then resume w/ a 150mg dose reduction

>3X ULN w/ Total Bilirubin >2X ULN (In the Absence of Cholestasis or Hemolysis): Permanently d/c therapy

Treatment-Related Interstitial Lung Disease/Pneumonitis:

Any Grade: Permanently d/c therapy

QTc Interval:

>500 msec on ≥2 Separate ECGs: Withhold therapy until QTc interval is <481 msec or recovery to baseline if baseline QTc is ≥481 msec, then resume w/ a 150mg dose reduction

Prolongation w/ Torsades de Pointes or Polymorphic Ventricular Tachycardia or Signs/Symptoms of Serious Arrhythmia: Permanently d/c therapy

Severe or Intolerable N/V or Diarrhea (Despite Optimal Antiemetic/Antidiarrheal Therapy): Withhold therapy until improved, then resume w/ a 150mg dose reduction

Persistent Hyperglycemia >250mg/dL (Despite Optimal Antihyperglycemic Therapy):

1. Withhold therapy until hyperglycemia is adequately controlled, then resume w/ a 150mg dose reduction
2. D/C therapy if adequate hyperglycemic control cannot be achieved w/ optimal medical management

Bradycardia:

Symptomatic, Not Life Threatening:

1. Withhold therapy until recovery to asymptomatic bradycardia or to a HR of ≥60 bpm
2. Evaluate concomitant medications known to cause bradycardia and adjust ceritinib dose

Clinically Significant, Requiring Intervention or Life Threatening in Patients Taking a Concomitant Medication Also Known to Cause Bradycardia or Hypotension:

1. Withhold therapy until recovery to asymptomatic bradycardia or to a HR of ≥60 bpm
2. If concomitant medication can be adjusted or discontinued, resume ceritinib w/ a 150mg dose reduction, w/ frequent monitoring

Life Threatening in Patients Not Taking a Concomitant Medication Also Known to Cause Bradycardia or Hypotension:

Permanently d/c therapy

Lipase/Amylase Elevation:
>2X ULN: Withhold and monitor serum lipase and amylase; resume w/ a 150mg dose reduction after recovery to <1.5X ULN

ADMINISTRATION

Oral route

Take on an empty stomach (do not administer w/in 2 hrs of a meal).
If vomiting occurs during treatment, do not administer an additional dose and continue w/ the next scheduled dose.

HOW SUPPLIED

Cap: 150mg

WARNINGS/PRECAUTIONS

Diarrhea, N/V, and abdominal pain reported; monitor and manage appropriately. Drug-induced hepatotoxicity reported; monitor LFTs including ALT, AST, and total bilirubin once a month and as clinically indicated, w/ more frequent testing if transaminase elevations occur. Severe, life-threatening, or fatal interstitial lung disease (ILD)/pneumonitis may occur; monitor for pulmonary symptoms. Exclude other potential causes and d/c therapy permanently w/ treatment-related ILD/pneumonitis. QTc interval prolongation may occur; avoid use w/ congenital long QT syndrome. Conduct periodic monitoring w/ ECGs and electrolytes in patients w/ congestive heart failure (CHF), bradyarrhythmias, and electrolyte abnormalities. Hyperglycemia may occur; initiate or optimize anti-hyperglycemic medications. Bradycardia may occur; monitor HR and BP regularly. Pancreatitis reported. May cause fetal harm.

ADVERSE REACTIONS

Increased ALT/AST, N/V, diarrhea, abdominal pain, constipation, esophageal disorder, fatigue, decreased appetite, rash, ILD/pneumonitis, decreased hemoglobin, increased creatinine/glucose/lipase.

DRUG INTERACTIONS

See Dosing Considerations. Caution w/ medications known to prolong QTc interval. Avoid w/ other agents known to cause bradycardia (eg, β-blockers, non-dihydropyridine calcium channel blockers, clonidine). Increased systemic exposure w/ ketoconazole. Avoid w/ strong CYP3A inhibitors. Decreased systemic exposure w/ rifampin. Avoid w/ strong CYP3A inducers (eg, carbamazepine, phenytoin, rifampin). Avoid w/ grapefruit and grapefruit juice. Avoid concurrent use of CYP3A substrates (eg, alfentanil, cyclosporine, tacrolimus) and CYP2C9 substrates (eg, phenytoin, warfarin) w/ narrow therapeutic indices; consider dose reduction of substrates if concomitant use is unavoidable.

PATIENT CONSIDERATIONS

Assessment: Assess for congenital long QT syndrome, CHF, bradyarrhythmias, electrolyte abnormalities, hepatic impairment, pregnancy/nursing status, and possible drug interactions. Obtain baseline LFTs, fasting serum glucose, ECG, and lipase and amylase levels.

Monitoring: Monitor for signs/symptoms of GI toxicity, ILD, pneumonitis, QTc interval prolongation, and other adverse reactions. Monitor LFTs once a month and as clinically indicated. Conduct periodic monitoring of ECGs and electrolytes in patients w/ CHF, bradyarrhythmias, electrolyte abnormalities, or who are taking medications known to prolong the QTc interval. Monitor lipase, amylase, and glucose levels, HR, and BP regularly.

Counseling: Inform that diarrhea, N/V, and abdominal pain are the most commonly reported adverse reactions; advise to contact physician for severe or persistent GI symptoms and inform of supportive care options (eg, antiemetics, antidiarrheal medications). Instruct to contact physician immediately for signs/symptoms of hepatotoxicity and hyperglycemia. Inform of the risks of severe or fatal ILD/pneumonitis; advise to immediately report new or worsening respiratory symptoms. Inform of the risks of QTc interval prolongation and bradycardia; advise to contact physician immediately to report new signs/symptoms or changes in/new use of heart/BP medications. Inform of the signs/symptoms of pancreatitis. Advise to inform physician if pregnant. Inform females of reproductive potential of the risk to fetus; advise to use effective contraception during treatment and for at least 2 weeks following completion of therapy. Advise not to breastfeed and not to consume grapefruit and grapefruit juice during treatment.

STORAGE: 25°C (77°F); excursions permitted between 15-30°C (59-86°F).

ZYPREXA – olanzapine

RX

Class: Atypical antipsychotic

Elderly patients w/ dementia-related psychosis treated w/ antipsychotic drugs are at an increased risk of death; most deaths appeared to be cardiovascular (eg, heart failure, sudden death) or infectious (eg, pneumonia) in nature. Not approved for the treatment of patients w/ dementia-related psychosis. When used w/ fluoxetine, refer to the Boxed Warning section of the PI for Symbyax.

OTHER BRAND NAMES
Zyprexa Zydis

ADULT DOSAGE
Bipolar I Disorder
Oral:

Manic or Mixed Episodes (Monotherapy):
Initial: 10mg or 15mg qd
Titrate: Adjust by increments/decrements of 5mg qd at intervals of not <24 hrs
Max: 20mg/day
Maint: 5-20mg/day

Manic or Mixed Episodes (w/ Lithium or Valproate):
Initial: 10mg qd
Max: 20mg/day

Depressive Episodes (w/ Fluoxetine):
Initial: 5mg w/ 20mg fluoxetine qpm
Range: 5-12.5mg w/ 20-50mg fluoxetine
Max: 18mg w/ 75mg fluoxetine

Agitation
Acute Agitation Associated w/ Schizophrenia and Bipolar I Mania:
IM:
10mg; consider 5mg or 7.5mg when clinical factors warrant
Range: 2.5-10mg. Assess for orthostatic hypotension prior to any subsequent dosing
Max: 3 doses of 10mg 2-4 hrs apart

May initiate PO therapy in a range of 5-20mg/day as soon as clinically appropriate, if ongoing therapy is indicated

Depression
Treatment-Resistant Depression (w/ Fluoxetine):
Oral:
Initial: 5mg w/ 20mg fluoxetine qpm
Range: 5-20mg w/ 20-50mg fluoxetine
Max: 18mg w/ 75mg fluoxetine

Schizophrenia
Oral:
Initial: 5-10mg qd
Target Dose: 10mg/day w/in several days. Adjust dose by increments/decrements of 5mg qd at intervals of not <1 week
Max: 20mg/day
Maint: 10-20mg/day

PEDIATRIC DOSAGE
Schizophrenia
13-17 Years:
Oral:
Initial: 2.5mg or 5mg qd
Target Dose: 10mg/day. Adjust dose by increments/decrements of 2.5mg or 5mg
Max: 20mg/day
Maint: Use lowest dose needed to maintain remission

Bipolar I Disorder
Oral:
Manic or Mixed Episodes:
13-17 Years:
Initial: 2.5mg or 5mg qd
Target Dose: 10mg/day. Adjust dose by increments/decrements of 2.5mg or 5mg
Max: 20mg/day
Maint: Use lowest dose needed to maintain remission

Depressive Episodes (w/ Fluoxetine):
10-17 Years:
Initial: 2.5mg w/ 20mg fluoxetine qpm
Max: 12mg w/ 50mg fluoxetine

DOSING CONSIDERATIONS
Hepatic Impairment

Zyprexa and Fluoxetine in Combination: Starting dose of oral olanzapine 2.5-5mg w/ fluoxetine 20mg

Elderly

IM Dosing: 5mg/inj

Other Important Considerations

Debilitated/Predisposed to Hypotension/Slower Metabolizers/Sensitive to Olanzapine:
Schizophrenia: 5mg as a starting dose; when indicated, escalate dose w/ caution
IM Dosing: 2.5mg/inj

Predisposed to Hypotension/Slow Metabolizers of Olanzapine or Fluoxetine/Sensitive to Olanzapine:
Zyprexa and Fluoxetine in Combination: Starting dose of oral olanzapine 2.5-5mg w/ fluoxetine 20mg

ADMINISTRATION
Oral/IM routes

Tab; Tab, Disintegrating
Take w/o regard to meals.

Inj
Do not administer IV or SQ. Inject IM slowly, deep into the muscle mass.
Dissolve the contents of the vial using 2.1mL of sterile water for inj to provide approx 5mg/mL of olanzapine.
Use immediately (w/in 1 hr) after reconstitution.
Do not combine in a syringe w/ diazepam inj or w/ haloperidol inj.
Do not reconstitute w/ lorazepam inj.

Tab, Disintegrating
After opening sachet, peel back foil on blister.
Do not push tab through foil.
Upon opening the blister, remove tab and place entire tab in the mouth using dry hands.
Disintegration occurs rapidly in saliva so it can be easily swallowed w/ or w/o liquid.

HOW SUPPLIED
Inj: 10mg; **Tab:** 2.5mg, 5mg, 7.5mg, 10mg, 15mg, 20mg; **Tab, Disintegrating:** (Zydis) 5mg, 10mg, 15mg, 20mg

CONTRAINDICATIONS
When used w/ fluoxetine, refer to the Symbyax monograph. When used w/ lithium or valproate, refer to the individual monographs.

WARNINGS/PRECAUTIONS
Supervision should accompany therapy in patients at high risk of attempted suicide. Neuroleptic malignant syndrome (NMS) reported; d/c and instill intensive symptomatic treatment and monitoring. Associated w/ metabolic changes including hyperglycemia, dyslipidemia, and weight gain; may be associated w/ increased cardiovascular/cerebrovascular risk. Hyperglycemia, in some cases extreme and associated w/ ketoacidosis or hyperosmolar coma or death, reported; caution in patients w/ diabetes mellitus or borderline increased blood glucose levels. Dose-related hyperprolactinemia reported. Tardive dyskinesia (TD) may develop; consider discontinuation if signs/symptoms develop unless treatment is required despite the presence of the syndrome. May induce orthostatic hypotension; caution w/ known cardiovascular disease (CVD), cerebrovascular disease, and conditions that would predispose to hypotension. Leukopenia, neutropenia, and agranulocytosis reported; consider discontinuing at 1st sign of a clinically significant decline in WBC count in the absence of other causative factors. D/C if severe neutropenia (ANC $<1000/mm^3$) develops. May cause esophageal dysmotility and aspiration, and disruption of body temperature regulation. Seizures reported; caution w/ history of seizures or w/ conditions that potentially lower the seizure threshold. Not approved for treatment of patients w/ Alzheimer's disease. May impair mental/physical abilities. Caution in patients w/ clinically significant prostatic hypertrophy, narrow-angle glaucoma, history of paralytic ileus or related conditions, cardiac patients, and in the elderly.

ADVERSE REACTIONS
Postural hypotension, constipation, dry mouth, weight gain, somnolence, dizziness, personality disorder, akathisia, asthenia, dyspepsia, tremor, increased appetite, abdominal pain, headache, insomnia.

DRUG INTERACTIONS
May potentiate orthostatic hypotension w/ diazepam and alcohol. Increased clearance w/ carbamazepine (CYP1A2 inducer), and omeprazole and rifampin (CYP1A2 inducers or glucuronyl transferase inducers). Decreased clearance w/ fluoxetine (CYP2D6 inhibitor) and fluvoxamine (CYP1A2 inhibitor); consider lower dose of olanzapine w/ concomitant fluvoxamine. Caution w/ other centrally acting drugs, alcohol, and drugs whose effects can induce hypotension, bradycardia, or respiratory/CNS depression. May enhance effects of certain antihypertensives. May antagonize effects of levodopa and dopamine agonists. Caution w/ anticholinergic drugs; may contribute to an elevation in core body temperature. **IM:** Not recommended w/ parenteral benzodiazepines. IM lorazepam may potentiate somnolence. **Oral:** Decreased levels w/ activated charcoal.

PATIENT CONSIDERATIONS
Assessment: Assess for CVD, cerebrovascular disease, risk of hypotension, history of seizures or conditions that could lower the seizure threshold, prostatic hypertrophy, narrow-angle glaucoma, history of paralytic ileus, hepatic impairment, risk factors for leukopenia/neutropenia, pregnancy/nursing status, and possible drug interactions. Assess for dementia-related psychosis and Alzheimer's disease in the elderly. Obtain baseline lipid profile, CBC, and FPG levels.

Monitoring: Monitor for signs/symptoms of NMS, TD, orthostatic hypotension, seizures, disruption of body temperature regulation, hyperprolactinemia, and other adverse reactions. Periodically monitor FPG, lipid levels, CBC, and weight of patient. In patients w/ clinically significant neutropenia, monitor for fever or other symptoms/signs of infection. Periodically reassess to determine the need for maintenance treatment.

Counseling: Advise of potential benefits and risks of therapy. Counsel about the signs and symptoms of NMS. Inform of potential risk of hyperglycemia-related adverse events. Inform that medication may cause dyslipidemia and weight gain. Inform that medication may cause orthostatic hypotension; instruct to contact physician if dizziness, fast or slow heartbeat, or fainting occurs. Inform that medication may impair judgment, thinking, or motor skills; instruct to use caution when operating hazardous machinery, including automobiles. Instruct to avoid overheating and dehydration and to contact physician if severely ill and have symptoms of dehydration. Instruct to notify physician if taking, planning to take, or have stopped taking any prescription or OTC products, including herbal supplements. Instruct to avoid alcohol. Inform that orally disintegrating tab contains phenylalanine. Advise to notify physician if pregnant or planning to become pregnant during treatment. Advise to avoid breastfeeding during therapy.

STORAGE: 20-25°C (68-77°F); excursions permitted between 15-30°C (59-86°F). **Reconstituted Inj:** 20-25°C (68-77°F) for up to 1 hr; excursions permitted between 15-30°C (59-86°F). **Tab/Tab, Disintegrating:** Protect from light and moisture. **Inj:** Protect from light. Do not freeze.

ZYVOX – linezolid

RX

Class: Oxazolidinone class antibacterial

ADULT DOSAGE

Pneumonia

Nosocomial/Community-Acquired Pneumonia, Including Concurrent Bacteremia:
600mg IV/PO q12h for 10-14 consecutive days

Vancomycin-Resistant *Enterococcus faecium* Infections

Including Concurrent Bacteremia:
600mg IV/PO q12h for 14-28 consecutive days

Skin and Skin Structure Infections

Complicated:
IV/Oral:
600mg q12h for 10-14 consecutive days

Uncomplicated:
Oral:
400mg q12h for 10-14 consecutive days

PEDIATRIC DOSAGE

Skin and Skin Structure Infections

Preterm Neonates <7 Days of Age:
Initial: 10mg/kg q12h
Titrate: Increase to 10mg/kg q8h if clinical response is suboptimal. All neonates should receive 10mg/kg q8h by 7 days of life
Treatment Duration: 10-14 consecutive days

Complicated:
IV/Oral:
Birth-11 Years:
10mg/kg q8h for 10-14 consecutive days
≥12 Years:
600mg q12h for 10-14 consecutive days

Uncomplicated:
Oral:
<5 Years:
10mg/kg q8h for 10-14 consecutive days
5-11 Years:
10mg/kg q12h for 10-14 consecutive days
≥12 Years:
600mg q12h for 10-14 consecutive days

Pneumonia

Nosocomial/Community-Acquired Pneumonia, Including Concurrent Bacteremia:
IV/PO:
Preterm Neonates <7 Days of Age:
Initial: 10mg/kg q12h
Titrate: Increase to 10mg/kg q8h if clinical response is suboptimal. All neonates should receive 10mg/kg q8h by 7 days of life
Treatment Duration: 10-14 consecutive days

Birth-11 Years:
10mg/kg q8h for 10-14 consecutive days

≥12 Years:
600mg q12h for 10-14 consecutive days

Vancomycin-Resistant *Enterococcus faecium* Infections

Including Concurrent Bacteremia:
IV/PO:
Neonates <7 Days of Age:
Initial: 10mg/kg q12h
Titrate: Increase to 10mg/kg q8h if clinical response is suboptimal. All neonates should receive 10mg/kg q8h by 7 days of life

Treatment Duration: 14-28 consecutive days
Birth-11 Years:
10mg/kg q8h for 14-28 consecutive days
≥12 Years:
600mg q12h for 14-28 consecutive days

ADMINISTRATION

Oral/IV route

May be administered w/o regard to the timing of meals.
No dose adjustment is necessary when switching from IV to oral administration.

IV

May exhibit a yellow color that can intensify over time w/o adversely affecting potency.
Infuse over 30-120 min.
Do not use infusion bag in series connections.
Do not introduce additives into linezolid inj sol; if given concomitantly w/ another drug, give each drug separately.
Flush line before and after infusion if the same IV line is used for sequential infusion of several drugs.

Compatible IV Sol:
0.9% NaCl
D5 inj
Lactated Ringer's inj
Refer to PI for incompatibilities.

Sus

Reconstitute w/ 123mL distilled water in 2 portions; shake vigorously after each portion.
After constitution, before using, gently mix by inverting the bottle 3-5X.
Do not shake.
Store reconstituted sus at room temperature; use w/in 21 days.

HOW SUPPLIED

Inj: 2mg/mL [100mL, 200mL, 300mL]; **Oral Sus:** 100mg/5mL [150mL]; **Tab:** 600mg

CONTRAINDICATIONS

Hypersensitivity to linezolid or any of the other product components, concomitant use w/ MAOIs A or B (eg, phenelzine, isocarboxazid) or w/in 2 weeks of taking such drugs.

WARNINGS/PRECAUTIONS

Myelosuppression (eg, anemia, leukopenia, pancytopenia, thrombocytopenia) reported; monitor CBCs weekly, particularly in those who receive treatment for >2 weeks, w/ preexisting myelosuppression, receiving concomitant drugs that produce bone marrow suppression, or w/ a chronic infection who have received previous or concomitant antibiotic therapy. Consider discontinuation if myelosuppression develops or worsens. Peripheral and optic neuropathies and visual blurring reported; prompt ophthalmic evaluation is recommended if patient experiences visual impairment symptoms. Monitor visual function if used for extended periods (≥3 months) or if new visual symptoms develop. Weigh continued use against potential risk if peripheral/optic neuropathy occurs. Do not administer w/ carcinoid syndrome. Not approved and should not be used for the treatment of catheter-related bloodstream infections or catheter-site infections. Not indicated for the treatment of gram-negative infections; initiate specific gram-negative therapy immediately if a concomitant gram-negative pathogen is documented or suspected. *Clostridium difficile*-associated diarrhea (CDAD) reported; may need to d/c if CDAD is suspected or confirmed. Do not administer w/ uncontrolled HTN, pheochromocytoma, or thyrotoxicosis, unless patients are monitored for potential increases in BP. Lactic acidosis reported; evaluate immediately if recurrent N/V, unexplained acidosis, or a low bicarbonate level develops. Convulsions reported. May result in bacterial resistance if used in the absence of a proven or suspected bacterial infection or a prophylactic indication.

ADVERSE REACTIONS

Diarrhea, headache, N/V, anemia, thrombocytopenia, abnormal Hgb/WBCs/neutrophils, serum AST/ALT/alkaline phosphatase/lipase/total bilirubin elevations.

DRUG INTERACTIONS

See Contraindications. Serotonin syndrome reported w/ serotonergic agents, including antidepressants such as SSRIs; do not administer in patients taking serotonin reuptake inhibitors, TCAs, 5-HT_1 receptor agonists (triptans), meperidine, bupropion, or buspirone, unless clinically appropriate and patients are carefully observed for signs/symptoms of serotonin syndrome or neuroleptic malignant syndrome (NMS)-like reactions. If alternatives to linezolid are not available and the potential benefits of linezolid outweigh the risks of serotonin syndrome or NMS-like reactions, promptly d/c the serotonergic antidepressant and administer linezolid; monitor for 2 weeks (5 weeks if fluoxetine was taken) or until 24 hrs after the last dose of linezolid, whichever comes 1st. Do not administer w/ directly and indirectly acting sympathomimetic agents (eg, pseudoephedrine), vasopressive agents (eg, epinephrine, norepinephrine), or dopaminergic agents (eg, dopamine, dobutamine), unless patients are monitored for potential increases in BP. Symptomatic hypoglycemia reported in patients w/ diabetes mellitus (DM) receiving insulin or oral hypoglycemic agents when treated w/ linezolid; may need to decrease dose of insulin or oral hypoglycemic agent, or d/c the oral hypoglycemic agent, insulin, or linezolid, if hypoglycemia occurs.

PATIENT CONSIDERATIONS

Assessment: Assess for hypersensitivity to drug, catheter-related bloodstream/catheter-site infections, uncontrolled HTN, pheochromocytoma, thyrotoxicosis, carcinoid syndrome, other conditions where treatment is contraindicated or cautioned, pregnancy/nursing status, and possible drug interactions.

Monitoring: Monitor for myelosuppression, peripheral/optic neuropathy, CDAD, lactic acidosis, convulsions, potential increases in BP, and other adverse reactions. Monitor CBCs weekly. Monitor visual function if used for extended periods (≥3 months) or if new visual symptoms develop.

Counseling: Explain that therapy should only be used to treat bacterial, not viral, infections. Instruct to take exactly ud even if the patient feels better early in the course of therapy. Inform that skipping doses or not completing the full course of therapy may decrease effectiveness of treatment and increase bacterial resistance. Instruct to notify physician if patient has a history of HTN or seizures, is taking medications containing pseudoephedrine or phenylpropanolamine (eg, cold remedies, decongestants) or antidepressants, or is experiencing visual changes. Instruct to avoid large quantities of foods or beverages w/ high tyramine content. Inform phenylketonurics that oral sus contains phenylalanine. Advise that diarrhea is a common problem caused by therapy that usually ends when therapy is discontinued. Instruct to immediately contact physician if watery and bloody stools (w/ or w/o stomach cramps and fever) occur, even as late as ≥2 months after having taken the last dose. Inform patients, particularly those w/ DM, that hypoglycemia may occur; instruct to contact physician if this occurs.

STORAGE: 25°C (77°F). Protect from light. Keep bottles tightly closed to protect from moisture. Keep infusion bags in the overwrap until ready to use. Protect infusion bags from freezing.

Antipyretic Products

BRAND	INGREDIENT(S)/STRENGTH(S)	DOSAGE
ACETAMINOPHENS		
Children's Tylenol Meltaways Chewable Tablets*†	Acetaminophen 80mg	**Peds 11 yrs (72-95 lbs):** 6 tabs q4h. **Peds 9-10 yrs (60-71 lbs):** 5 tabs q4h. **Peds 6-8 yrs (48-59 lbs):** 4 tabs q4h. **Peds 4-5 yrs (36-47 lbs):** 3 tabs q4h. **Peds 2-3 yrs (24-35 lbs):** 2 tabs q4h. **Max:** 5 doses/24h.
Children's Tylenol Oral Suspension*	Acetaminophen 160mg/5mL	**Peds 11 yrs (72-95 lbs):** 3 tsp (15mL) q4h. **Peds 9-10 yrs (60-71 lbs):** 2.5 tsp (12.5mL) q4h. **Peds 6-8 yrs (48-59 lbs):** 2 tsp (10mL) q4h. **Peds 4-5 yrs (36-47 lbs):** 1.5 tsp (7.5mL) q4h. **Peds 2-3 yrs (24-35 lbs):** 1 tsp (5mL) q4h. **Max:** 5 doses/24h.
FeverAll Children's Suppositories	Acetaminophen 120mg	**Peds 3-6 yrs:** 1 supp q4-6h. **Max:** 5 doses/24h.
FeverAll Infants' Suppositories	Acetaminophen 80mg	**Peds 12-36 months:** 1 supp q4-6h. **Max:** 5 doses/24h. **Peds 6-11 months:** 1 supp q6h. **Max:** 4 doses/24h.
FeverAll Jr. Strength Suppositories	Acetaminophen 325mg	**Adults & Peds ≥12 yrs:** 2 supp q4-6h. **Max:** 6 doses/24h. **Peds 6-12 yrs:** 1 supp q4-6h. **Max:** 5 doses/24h.
Infants' Tylenol Oral Suspension*	Acetaminophen 160mg/5mL	**Peds 2-3 yrs (24-35 lbs):** 1 tsp (5mL) q4h. **Max:** 5 doses/24h.
Jr. Tylenol Meltaways Chewable Tablets*†	Acetaminophen 160mg	**Peds 11 yrs (72-95 lbs):** 3 tabs q4h. **Peds 9-10 yrs (60-71 lbs):** 2.5 tabs q4h. **Peds 6-8 yrs (48-59 lbs):** 2 tabs q4h. **Max:** 5 doses/24h.
Little Remedies Children's Fever/Pain Reliever Liquid*	Acetaminophen 160mg/5mL	**Peds 11 yrs (72-95 lbs):** 3 tsp (15mL) q4h. **Peds 9-10 yrs (60-71 lbs):** 2.5 tsp (12.5mL) q4h. **Peds 6-8 yrs (48-59 lbs):** 2 tsp (10mL) q4h. **Peds 4-5 yrs (36-47 lbs):** 1.5 tsp (7.5mL) q4h. **Peds 2-3 yrs (24-35 lbs):** 1 tsp (5mL) q4h. **Max:** 5 doses/24h.
Little Remedies Infant Fever/Pain Reliever Liquid	Acetaminophen 160mg/5mL	**Peds 2-3 yrs (24-35 lbs):** 1 tsp (5mL) q4h. **Max:** 5 doses/24h.
PediaCare Children Fever Reducer/ Pain Reliever Acetaminophen Oral Suspension*	Acetaminophen 160mg/5mL	**Peds 11 yrs (72-95 lbs):** 3 tsp (15mL) q4h. **Peds 9-10 yrs (60-71 lbs):** 2.5 tsp (12.5mL) q4h. **Peds 6-8 yrs (48-59 lbs):** 2 tsp (10mL) q4h. **Peds 4-5 yrs (36-47 lbs):** 1.5 tsp (7.5mL) q4h. **Peds 2-3 yrs (24-35 lbs):** 1 tsp (5mL) q4h. **Max:** 5 doses/24h.
PediaCare Infants Fever Reducer/ Pain Reliever Acetaminophen Oral Suspension*	Acetaminophen 160mg/5mL	**Peds 2-3 yrs (24-35 lbs):** 1 tsp (5mL) q4h. **Max:** 5 doses/24h.
PediaCare Smooth Melts Acetaminophen Fever Reducer/Pain Reliever Chewable Tablets	Acetaminophen 160mg	**Peds 11 yrs (72-95 lbs):** 3 tabs q4h. **Peds 9-10 yrs (60-71 lbs):** 2.5 tabs q4h. **Peds 6-8 yrs (48-59 lbs):** 2 tabs q4h. **Peds 4-5 yrs (36-47 lbs):** 1.5 tabs q4h. **Max:** 5 doses/24h.

(Continued)

BRAND	INGREDIENT(S)/STRENGTH(S)	DOSAGE
ACETAMINOPHENS *(Continued)*		
Triaminic Children's Fever Reducer Pain Reliever Syrup*†	Acetaminophen 160mg/5mL	**Peds 11 yrs (72-95 lbs):** 3 tsp (15mL) q4h. **Peds 9-10 yrs (60-71 lbs):** 2.5 tsp (12.5mL) q4h. **Peds 6-8 yrs (48-59 lbs):** 2 tsp (10mL) q4h. **Peds 4-5 yrs (36-47 lbs):** 1.5 tsp (7.5mL) q4h. **Peds 2-3 yrs (24-35 lbs):** 1 tsp (5mL) q4h. **Max:** 5 doses/24h.
Triaminic Infants' Fever Reducer Pain Reliever Syrup*†	Acetaminophen 160mg/5mL	**Peds 2-3 yrs (24-35 lbs):** 1 tsp (5mL) q4h. **Max:** 5 doses/24h.
Tylenol 8 HR Extended Release Caplets†	Acetaminophen 650mg	**Adults & Peds ≥12 yrs:** 2 tabs q8h. **Max:** 6 tabs/24h.
Tylenol Extra Strength Caplets	Acetaminophen 500mg	**Adults & Peds ≥12 yrs:** 2 tabs q6h. **Max:** 6 tabs/24h.
Tylenol Regular Strength Tablets	Acetaminophen 325mg	**Adults & Peds ≥12 yrs:** 2 tabs q4-6h. **Max:** 10 tabs/24h. **Peds 6-11 yrs:** 1 tab q4-6h. **Max:** 5 tabs/24h.
NONSTEROIDAL ANTI-INFLAMMATORY DRUGS		
Advil Caplets	Ibuprofen 200mg	**Adults & Peds ≥12 yrs:** 1-2 tabs q4-6h. **Max:** 6 tabs/24h.
Advil Film-Coated Caplets	Ibuprofen 200mg	**Adults & Peds ≥12 yrs:** 1-2 tabs q4-6h. **Max:** 6 tabs/24h.
Advil Film-Coated Tablets	Ibuprofen 200mg	**Adults & Peds ≥12 yrs:** 1-2 tabs q4-6h. **Max:** 6 tabs/24h.
Advil Gel Caplets	Ibuprofen 200mg	**Adults & Peds ≥12 yrs:** 1-2 tabs q4-6h. **Max:** 6 tabs/24h.
Advil Liqui-Gels	Ibuprofen 200mg	**Adults & Peds ≥12 yrs:** 1-2 caps q4-6h. **Max:** 6 caps/24h.
Advil Tablets	Ibuprofen 200mg	**Adults & Peds ≥12 yrs:** 1-2 tabs q4-6h. **Max:** 6 tabs/24h.
Aleve Caplets	Naproxen sodium 220mg	**Adults & Peds ≥12 yrs:** 1 tab q8-12h. May take 1 additional tab within 1h of first dose. **Max:** 2 tabs/8-12h or 3 tabs/24h.
Aleve Gelcaps	Naproxen sodium 220mg	**Adults & Peds ≥12 yrs:** 1 tab q8-12h. May take 1 additional tab within 1h of first dose. **Max:** 2 tabs/8-12h or 3 tabs/24h.
Aleve Liquid Gels	Naproxen sodium 220mg	**Adults & Peds ≥12 yrs:** 1 cap q8-12h. May take 1 additional cap within 1h of first dose. **Max:** 2 caps/8-12h or 3 caps/24h.
Aleve Tablets	Naproxen sodium 220mg	**Adults & Peds ≥12 yrs:** 1 tab q8-12h. May take 1 additional tab within 1h of first dose. **Max:** 2 tabs/8-12h or 3 tabs/24h.
Children's Advil Suspension*	Ibuprofen 100mg/5mL	**Peds 11 yrs (72-95 lbs):** 3 tsp (15mL) q6-8h. **Peds 9-10 yrs (60-71 lbs):** 2.5 tsp (12.5mL) q6-8h. **Peds 6-8 yrs (48-59 lbs):** 2 tsp (10mL) q6-8h. **Peds 4-5 yrs (36-47 lbs):** 1.5 tsp (7.5mL) q6-8h. **Peds 2-3 yrs (24-35 lbs):** 1 tsp (5mL) q6-8h. **Max:** 4 doses/24h.

BRAND	INGREDIENT(S)/STRENGTH(S)	DOSAGE
NONSTEROIDAL ANTI-INFLAMMATORY DRUGS *(Continued)*		
Children's Motrin Suspension	Ibuprofen 100mg/5mL	**Peds 11 yrs (72-95 lbs):** 3 tsp (15mL) q6-8h. **Peds 9-10 yrs (60-71 lbs):** 2.5 tsp (12.5mL) q6-8h. **Peds 6-8 yrs (48-59 lbs):** 2 tsp (10mL) q6-8h. **Peds 4-5 yrs (36-47 lbs):** 1.5 tsp (7.5mL) q6-8h. **Peds 2-3 yrs (24-35 lbs):** 1 tsp (5mL) q6-8h. **Max:** 4 doses/24h.
Infants' Advil Concentrated Drops	Ibuprofen 50mg/1.25mL	**Peds 12-23 months (18-23 lbs):** 1.875mL q6-8h. **Peds 6-11 months (12-17 lbs):** 1.25mL q6-8h. **Max:** 4 doses/24h.
Infants' Motrin Concentrated Drops	Ibuprofen 50mg/1.25mL	**Peds 12-23 months (18-23 lbs):** 1.875mL q6-8h. **Peds 6-11 months (12-17 lbs):** 1.25mL q6-8h. **Max:** 4 doses/24h.
Junior Strength Advil Chewable Tablets	Ibuprofen 100mg	**Peds 11 yrs (72-95 lbs):** 3 tabs q6-8h. **Peds 9-10 yrs (60-71 lbs):** 2.5 tabs q6-8h. **Peds 6-8 yrs (48-59 lbs):** 2 tabs q6-8h. **Max:** 4 doses/24h.
Junior Strength Advil Tablets	Ibuprofen 100mg	**Peds 11 yrs (72-95 lbs):** 3 tabs q6-8h. **Peds 6-10 yrs (48-71 lbs):** 2 tabs q6-8h. **Max:** 4 doses/24h.
Motrin IB Caplets	Ibuprofen 200mg	**Adults & Peds ≥12 yrs:** 1-2 tabs q4-6h. **Max:** 6 tabs/24h.
PediaCare Children Pain Reliever/Fever Reducer IB Ibuprofen Oral Suspension	Ibuprofen 100mg/5mL	**Peds 11 yrs (72-95 lbs):** 3 tsp (15mL) q6-8h. **Peds 9-10 yrs (60-71 lbs):** 2.5 tsp (12.5mL) q6-8h. **Peds 6-8 yrs (48-59 lbs):** 2 tsp (10mL) q6-8h. **Peds 4-5 yrs (36-47 lbs):** 1.5 tsp (7.5mL) q6-8h. **Peds 2-3 yrs (24-35 lbs):** 1 tsp (5mL) q6-8h. **Max:** 4 doses/24h.
PediaCare Infants Pain Reliever/Fever Reducer IB Ibuprofen Concentrated Oral Suspension	Ibuprofen 50mg/1.25mL	**Peds 12-23 months (18-23 lbs):** 1.875mL q6-8h. **Peds 6-11 months (12-17 lbs):** 1.25mL q6-8h. **Max:** 4 doses/24h.
SALICYLATES		
PLEASE REFER TO ASPIRIN PRODUCTS TABLE		

*Multiple flavors available.
†Product currently on recall or temporarily unavailable from manufacturer, but generic forms may be available.

SMOKING CESSATION PRODUCTS

BRAND	INGREDIENT(S)/STRENGTH(S)	DOSAGE
Habitrol Nicotine Transdermal System Patch Step 1	Nicotine 21mg	**Adults:** If smoking >10 cigarettes/day: **Weeks 1 to 4:** Apply one 21mg patch/day. **Weeks 5 to 6:** Apply one 14mg patch/day. **Weeks 7 to 8:** Apply one 7mg patch/day. If smoking <10 cigarettes/day: **Weeks 1 to 6:** Apply one 14mg patch/day. **Weeks 7 to 8:** Apply one 7mg patch/day.
Habitrol Nicotine Transdermal System Patch Step 2	Nicotine 14mg	Refer to Habitrol Nicotine Transdermal System Patch Step 1 dosing.
Habitrol Nicotine Transdermal System Patch Step 3	Nicotine 7mg	Refer to Habitrol Nicotine Transdermal System Patch Step 1 dosing.
NicoDerm CQ Step 1 Clear Patch	Nicotine 21mg	**Adults:** If smoking >10 cigarettes/day: **Weeks 1 to 6:** Apply one 21mg patch/day. **Weeks 7 to 8:** Apply one 14mg patch/day. **Weeks 9 to 10:** Apply one 7mg patch/day. If smoking ≤10 cigarettes/day: **Weeks 1 to 6:** Apply one 14mg patch/day. **Weeks 7 to 8:** Apply one 7mg patch/day.
NicoDerm CQ Step 2 Clear Patch	Nicotine 14mg	Refer to NicoDerm CQ Step 1 Clear Patch dosing.
NicoDerm CQ Step 3 Clear Patch	Nicotine 7mg	Refer to NicoDerm CQ Step 1 Clear Patch dosing.
Nicorette 2mg Gum	Nicotine polacrilex 2mg	**Adults:** If smoking first cigarette >30 minutes after waking up, use 2mg gum. **Weeks 1 to 6:** 1 piece q1-2h. **Weeks 7 to 9:** 1 piece q2-4h. **Weeks 10 to 12:** 1 piece q4-8h. **Max:** 24 pieces/day.
Nicorette 4mg Gum	Nicotine polacrilex 4mg	**Adults:** If smoking first cigarette ≤30 minutes after waking up, use 4mg gum. **Weeks 1 to 6:** 1 piece q1-2h. **Weeks 7 to 9:** 1 piece q2-4h. **Weeks 10 to 12:** 1 piece q4-8h. **Max:** 24 pieces/day.
Nicorette 2mg Lozenge	Nicotine polacrilex 2mg	**Adults:** If smoking first cigarette >30 minutes after waking up, use 2mg lozenge. **Weeks 1 to 6:** 1 lozenge q1-2h. **Weeks 7 to 9:** 1 lozenge q2-4h. **Weeks 10 to 12:** 1 lozenge q4-8h. **Max:** 5 lozenges/6 hours or 20 lozenges/day.
Nicorette 4mg Lozenge	Nicotine polacrilex 4mg	**Adults:** If smoking first cigarette ≤30 minutes after waking up, use 4mg lozenge. **Weeks 1 to 6:** 1 lozenge q1-2h. **Weeks 7 to 9:** 1 lozenge q2-4h. **Weeks 10 to 12:** 1 lozenge q4-8h. **Max:** 5 lozenges/6 hours or 20 lozenges/day.
Nicorette 2mg mini Lozenge	Nicotine polacrilex 2mg	**Adults:** If smoking first cigarette >30 minutes after waking up, use 2mg lozenge. **Weeks 1 to 6:** 1 lozenge q1-2h. **Weeks 7 to 9:** 1 lozenge q2-4h. **Weeks 10 to 12:** 1 lozenge q4-8h. **Max:** 5 lozenges/6 hours or 20 lozenges/day.
Nicorette 4mg mini Lozenge	Nicotine polacrilex 4mg	**Adults:** If smoking first cigarette ≤30 minutes after waking up, use 4mg lozenge. **Weeks 1 to 6:** 1 lozenge q1-2h. **Weeks 7 to 9:** 1 lozenge q2-4h. **Weeks 10 to 12:** 1 lozenge q4-8h. **Max:** 5 lozenges/6 hours or 20 lozenges/day.

(Continued)

BRAND	INGREDIENT(S)/STRENGTH(S)	DOSAGE
Zonnic 2mg Gum	Nicotine polacrilex 2mg	**Adults:** If smoking first cigarette >30 minutes after waking up, use 2mg gum. **Weeks 1 to 6:** 1 piece q1-2h. **Weeks 7 to 9:** 1 piece q2-4h. **Weeks 10 to 12:** 1 piece q4-8h. **Max:** 24 pieces/day.
Zonnic 4mg Gum	Nicotine polacrilex 4mg	**Adults:** If smoking first cigarette ≤30 minutes after waking up, use 4mg gum. **Weeks 1 to 6:** 1 piece q1-2h. **Weeks 7 to 9:** 1 piece q2-4h. **Weeks 10 to 12:** 1 piece q4-8h. **Max:** 24 pieces/day.

Antacid and Heartburn Products

BRAND	INGREDIENT(S)/STRENGTH(S)	DOSAGE
ANTACIDS		
Alka-Seltzer Extra Strength Effervescent Tablets	Aspirin/Citric acid/Sodium bicarbonate 500mg-1000mg-1985mg	**Adults ≥60 yrs:** 2 tabs dissolved in 4 oz water q6h. **Max:** 3 tabs/24h. **Adults & Peds ≥12 yrs:** 2 tabs dissolved in 4 oz water q6h. **Max:** 7 tabs/24h.
Alka-Seltzer Extra Strength Heartburn ReliefChews Chewable Tablets	Calcium carbonate 750mg	**Adults & Peds ≥12 yrs:** 1-2 tabs prn. **Max:** 5 tabs/24h.
Alka-Seltzer Gold Effervescent Tablets	Citric acid/Potassium bicarbonate/ Sodium bicarbonate 1000mg-344mg-1050mg	**Adults ≥60 yrs:** 2 tabs dissolved in 4 oz water q4h prn. **Max:** 6 tabs/24h. **Adults & Peds ≥12 yrs:** 2 tabs dissolved in 4 oz water q4h prn. **Max:** 8 tabs/24h. **Peds <12 yrs:** 1 tab dissolved in 4 oz water q4h prn. **Max:** 4 tabs/24h.
Alka-Seltzer Heartburn Effervescent Tablets	Citric acid/Sodium bicarbonate 1000mg-1940mg	**Adults ≥60 yrs:** 2 tabs dissolved in 4 oz water q4h prn. **Max:** 4 tabs/24h. **Adults & Peds ≥12 yrs:** 2 tabs dissolved in 4 oz water q4h prn. **Max:** 8 tabs/24h.
Alka-Seltzer Lemon Lime Effervescent Tablets	Aspirin/Citric acid/Sodium bicarbonate 325mg-1000mg-1700mg	**Adults ≥60 yrs:** 2 tabs dissolved in 4 oz water q4h. **Max:** 4 tabs/24h. **Adults & Peds ≥12 yrs:** 2 tabs dissolved in 4 oz water q4h. **Max:** 8 tabs/24h.
Alka-Seltzer Original Effervescent Tablets	Aspirin/Citric acid/Sodium bicarbonate 325mg-1000mg-1916mg	**Adults ≥60 yrs:** 2 tabs dissolved in 4 oz water q4h. **Max:** 4 tabs/24h. **Adults & Peds ≥12 yrs:** 2 tabs dissolved in 4 oz water q4h. **Max:** 8 tabs/24h.
Gaviscon Extra Strength Chewable Tablets	Aluminum hydroxide/Magnesium carbonate 160mg-105mg	**Adults:** 2-4 tabs qid. **Max:** 16 tabs/24h.
Gaviscon Extra Strength Liquid	Aluminum hydroxide/Magnesium carbonate 254mg-237.5mg/5mL	**Adults:** 2-4 tsp (10-20mL) qid. **Max:** 16 tsp (80mL)/24h.
Gaviscon Regular Strength Chewable Tablets	Aluminum hydroxide/Magnesium trisilicate 80mg-14.2mg	**Adults:** 2-4 tabs qid. **Max:** 16 tabs/24h.
Gaviscon Regular Strength Liquid	Aluminum hydroxide/Magnesium carbonate 95mg-358mg/15mL	**Adults:** 1-2 tbl (15-30mL) qid. **Max:** 8 tbl (120mL)/24h.
Maalox Regular Strength Chewable Tablets	Calcium carbonate 600mg	**Adults:** 1-2 tabs prn. **Max:** 12 tabs/24h.
Mylanta Supreme Liquid*	Calcium carbonate/Magnesium hydroxide 400mg-135mg/5mL	**Adults:** 2-4 tsp (10-20mL) between meals and at hs. **Max:** 18 tsp (90mL)/24h.
Mylanta Ultimate Strength Liquid*	Aluminum hydroxide/Magnesium hydroxide 500mg-500mg/5mL	**Adults & Peds ≥12 yrs:** 2-4 tsp (10-20mL) between meals and at hs. **Max:** 9 tsp (45mL)/24h.
Pepto-Bismol Children's Pepto Chewable Tablets	Calcium carbonate 400mg	**Peds 6-11 yrs (48-95 lbs):** 2 tabs prn. **Max:** 6 tabs/24h. **Peds 2-5 yrs (24-47 lbs):** 1 tab prn. **Max:** 3 tabs/24h.
Relief OTC	Calcium carbonate/Potassium bicarbonate/Sodium bicarbonate 545mg-905mg-2110mg/4 oz	**Adults ≥60 yrs:** Up to 4 oz q4h prn. **Max:** 12 oz/24h. **Adults & Peds ≥12 yrs:** Up to 4 oz q4h prn. **Max:** 16 oz/24h.
Rolaids Extra Strength Chewable Tablets	Calcium carbonate/Magnesium hydroxide 675mg-135mg	**Adults:** 2-4 tabs prn. **Max:** 10 tabs/24h.
Rolaids Regular Strength Chewable Tablets	Calcium carbonate/Magnesium hydroxide 550mg-110mg	**Adults:** 2-4 tabs prn. **Max:** 12 tabs/24h.
Rolaids Ultra Strength Chewable Tablets	Calcium carbonate/Magnesium hydroxide 1000mg-200mg	**Adults:** 2-3 tabs prn. **Max:** 7 tabs/24h.

(Continued)

BRAND	INGREDIENT(S)/STRENGTH(S)	DOSAGE
ANTACIDS *(Continued)*		
Rolaids Ultra Strength Liquid	Calcium carbonate/Magnesium hydroxide 1000mg-200mg/5mL	**Adults:** 2-3 tsp (10-15mL) prn. **Max:** 7 tsp (35mL)/24h.
Rolaids Ultra Strength Softchews	Calcium carbonate/Magnesium hydroxide 1330mg-235mg	**Adults:** 2-3 chews prn. **Max:** 5 chews/24h.
Tums Chewy Delights Chewable Tablets	Calcium carbonate 1177mg	**Adults & Peds ≥12 yrs:** 2-3 tabs prn. **Max**†: 6 tabs/24h.
Tums Extra Strength 750 Chewable Tablets	Calcium carbonate 750mg	**Adults & Peds ≥12 yrs:** 2-4 tabs prn. **Max**†: 10 tabs/24h.
Tums Extra Strength 750 Sugar Free Chewable Tablets	Calcium carbonate 750mg	**Adults & Peds ≥12 yrs:** 2-4 tabs prn. **Max**†: 9 tabs/24h.
Tums Freshers Chewable Tablets	Calcium carbonate 500mg	**Adults & Peds ≥12 yrs:** 2-4 tabs prn. **Max**†: 15 tabs/24h.
Tums Regular Strength Chewable Tablets	Calcium carbonate 500mg	**Adults & Peds ≥12 yrs:** 2-4 tabs prn. **Max**†: 15 tabs/24h.
Tums Smoothies Chewable Tablets	Calcium carbonate 750mg	**Adults & Peds ≥12 yrs:** 2-4 tabs prn. **Max**†: 10 tabs/24h.
Tums Ultra Strength 1000 Chewable Tablets	Calcium carbonate 1000mg	**Adults & Peds ≥12 yrs:** 2-3 tabs prn. **Max**†: 7 tabs/24h.
ANTACIDS/ANTIFLATULENTS		
Alka-Seltzer Heartburn+Gas ReliefChews Chewable Tablets	Calcium carbonate/Simethicone 750mg-80mg	**Adults & Peds ≥12 yrs:** 1-2 tabs prn. **Max:** 5 tabs/24h.
Gelusil Chewable Tablets	Aluminum hydroxide/Magnesium hydroxide/Simethicone 200mg-200mg-25mg	**Adults:** 2-4 tabs q1h prn. **Max:** 12 tabs/24h.
Maalox Advanced Maximum Strength Chewable Tablets*	Calcium carbonate/Simethicone 1000mg-60mg	**Adults & Peds ≥12 yrs:** 1-2 tabs prn. **Max:** 8 tabs/24h.
Maalox Advanced Maximum Strength Liquid*	Aluminum hydroxide/Magnesium hydroxide/Simethicone 400mg-400mg-40mg/5mL	**Adults & Peds ≥12 yrs:** 2-4 tsp (10-20mL) bid. **Max:** 8 tsp (40mL)/24h.
Maalox Advanced Regular Strength Liquid*	Aluminum hydroxide/Magnesium hydroxide/Simethicone 200mg-200mg-20mg/5mL	**Adults & Peds ≥12 yrs:** 2-4 tsp (10-20mL) qid. **Max:** 16 tsp (80mL)/24h.
Mylanta Maximum Strength Liquid*	Aluminum hydroxide/Magnesium hydroxide/Simethicone 400mg-400mg-40mg/5mL	**Adults & Peds ≥12 yrs:** 2-4 tsp (10-20mL) between meals and at hs. **Max:** 12 tsp (60mL)/24h.
Mylanta Regular Strength Liquid*	Aluminum hydroxide/Magnesium hydroxide/Simethicone 200mg-200mg-20mg/5mL	**Adults & Peds ≥12 yrs:** 2-4 tsp (10-20mL) between meals and at hs. **Max:** 24 tsp (120mL)/24h.
Rolaids Advanced Chewable Tablets	Calcium carbonate/Magnesium hydroxide/Simethicone 1000mg-200mg-40mg	**Adults:** 2-3 tabs prn. **Max:** 7 tabs/24h.
BISMUTH SUBSALICYLATES		
Maalox Total Relief Maximum Strength Liquid*	Bismuth subsalicylate 525mg/15mL	**Adults & Peds ≥12 yrs:** 2 tbl (30mL) q1h prn. **Max:** 8 tbl (120mL)/24h.
Pepto-Bismol Caplets	Bismuth subsalicylate 262mg	**Adults & Peds ≥12 yrs:** 2 tabs q½-1h prn. **Max:** 8 doses (16 tabs)/24h.
Pepto-Bismol Chewable Tablets	Bismuth subsalicylate 262mg	**Adults & Peds ≥12 yrs:** 2 tabs q½-1h prn. **Max:** 8 doses (16 tabs)/24h.
Pepto-Bismol InstaCool Chewable Tablets	Bismuth subsalicylate 262mg	**Adults & Peds ≥12 yrs:** 2 tabs q½-1h prn. **Max:** 8 doses (16 tabs)/24h.

BRAND	INGREDIENT(S)/STRENGTH(S)	DOSAGE
BISMUTH SUBSALICYLATES *(Continued)*		
Pepto-Bismol Liquid	Bismuth subsalicylate 525mg/30mL	**Adults & Peds ≥12 yrs:** 2 tbl (30mL) q½-1h prn. **Max:** 8 doses (16 tbl or 240mL)/24h.
Pepto-Bismol Max Strength Liquid	Bismuth subsalicylate 1050mg/30mL	**Adults & Peds ≥12 yrs:** 2 tbl (30mL) q1h prn. **Max:** 4 doses (8 tbl or 120mL)/24h.
H_2-RECEPTOR ANTAGONISTS		
Pepcid AC Maximum Strength Tablets	Famotidine 20mg	**Adults & Peds ≥12 yrs:** 1 tab prn. **Max:** 2 tabs/24h.
Pepcid AC Original Strength Tablets	Famotidine 10mg	**Adults & Peds ≥12 yrs:** 1 tab prn. **Max:** 2 tabs/24h.
Tagamet HB 200 Tablets	Cimetidine 200mg	**Adults & Peds ≥12 yrs:** 1 tab prn. **Max:** 2 tabs/24h.
Zantac 75 Tablets	Ranitidine 75mg	**Adults & Peds ≥12 yrs:** 1 tab prn. **Max:** 2 tabs/24h.
Zantac 150 Tablets	Ranitidine 150mg	**Adults & Peds ≥12 yrs:** 1 tab prn. **Max:** 2 tabs/24h.
H_2-RECEPTOR ANTAGONISTS/ANTACIDS		
Pepcid Complete Chewable Tablets	Famotidine/Calcium carbonate/ Magnesium hydroxide 10mg-800mg-165mg	**Adults & Peds ≥12 yrs:** 1 tab prn. **Max:** 2 tabs/24h.
PROTON PUMP INHIBITORS		
Nexium 24 HR Capsules	Esomeprazole 20mg	**Adults:** 1 cap qd x 14 days. May repeat 14-day course q4 months.
Prevacid 24 HR Capsules	Lansoprazole 15mg	**Adults:** 1 cap qd x 14 days. May repeat 14-day course q4 months.
Prilosec OTC Tablets	Omeprazole 20mg	**Adults:** 1 tab qd x 14 days. May repeat 14-day course q4 months.
Zegerid OTC Capsules	Omeprazole/Sodium bicarbonate 20mg-1100mg	**Adults:** 1 cap qd x 14 days. May repeat 14-day course q4 months.

*Product currently on recall or temporarily unavailable from manufacturer.
†Please refer to full FDA-approved labeling for information on max dosage during pregnancy.

Antidiarrheal Products

BRAND	INGREDIENT(S)/STRENGTH(S)	DOSAGE*
ANTIPERISTALTICS		
Imodium A-D Caplets	Loperamide HCl 2mg	**Adults & Peds ≥12 yrs:** 2 tabs after first loose stool; 1 tab after each subsequent loose stool. **Max:** 4 tabs/24h. **Peds 9-11 yrs (60-95 lbs):** 1 tab after first loose stool; ½ tab after each subsequent loose stool. **Max:** 3 tabs/24h. **Peds 6-8 yrs (48-59 lbs):** 1 tab after first loose stool; ½ tab after each subsequent loose stool. **Max:** 2 tabs/24h.
Imodium A-D EZ Chews	Loperamide HCl 2mg	**Adults & Peds ≥12 yrs:** 2 tabs after first loose stool; 1 tab after each subsequent loose stool. **Max:** 4 tabs/24h. **Peds 9-11 yrs (60-95 lbs):** 1 tab after first loose stool; ½ tab after each subsequent loose stool. **Max:** 3 tabs/24h. **Peds 6-8 yrs (48-59 lbs):** 1 tab after first loose stool; ½ tab after each subsequent loose stool. **Max:** 2 tabs/24h.
Imodium A-D Liquid	Loperamide HCl 1mg/7.5mL	**Adults & Peds ≥12 yrs:** 6 tsp (30mL) after first loose stool; 3 tsp (15mL) after each subsequent loose stool. **Max:** 12 tsp (60mL)/24h. **Peds 9-11 yrs (60-95 lbs):** 3 tsp (15mL) after first loose stool; 1½ tsp (7.5mL) after each subsequent loose stool. **Max:** 9 tsp (45mL)/24h. **Peds 6-8 yrs (48-59 lbs):** 3 tsp (15mL) after first loose stool; 1½ tsp (7.5mL) after each subsequent loose stool. **Max:** 6 tsp (30mL)/24h.
Imodium A-D Liquid for Use in Children	Loperamide HCl 1mg/7.5mL	**Adults & Peds ≥12 yrs:** 6 tsp (30mL) after first loose stool; 3 tsp (15mL) after each subsequent loose stool. **Max:** 12 tsp (60mL)/24h. **Peds 9-11 yrs (60-95 lbs):** 3 tsp (15mL) after first loose stool; 1½ tsp (7.5mL) after each subsequent loose stool. **Max:** 9 tsp (45mL)/24h. **Peds 6-8 yrs (48-59 lbs):** 3 tsp (15mL) after first loose stool; 1½ tsp (7.5mL) after each subsequent loose stool. **Max:** 6 tsp (30mL)/24h.
ANTIPERISTALTICS/ANTIFLATULENTS		
Imodium Multi-Symptom Relief Caplets	Loperamide HCl/Simethicone 2mg-125mg	**Adults & Peds ≥12 yrs:** 2 tabs after first loose stool; 1 tab after each subsequent loose stool. **Max:** 4 tabs/24h. **Peds 9-11 yrs (60-95 lbs):** 1 tab after first loose stool; ½ tab after each subsequent loose stool. **Max:** 3 tabs/24h. **Peds 6-8 yrs (48-59 lbs):** 1 tab after first loose stool; ½ tab after each subsequent loose stool. **Max:** 2 tabs/24h.
Imodium Multi-Symptom Relief Chewable Tablets	Loperamide HCl/Simethicone 2mg-125mg	**Adults & Peds ≥12 yrs:** 2 tabs after first loose stool; 1 tab after each subsequent loose stool. **Max:** 4 tabs/24h. **Peds 9-11 yrs (60-95 lbs):** 1 tab after first loose stool; ½ tab after each subsequent loose stool. **Max:** 3 tabs/24h. **Peds 6-8 yrs (48-59 lbs):** 1 tab after first loose stool; ½ tab after each subsequent loose stool. **Max:** 2 tabs/24h.
BISMUTH SUBSALICYLATES		
Kaopectate Caplets	Bismuth Subsalicylate 262mg	**Adults & Peds ≥12 yrs:** 2 tabs q½-1h prn. **Max:** 8 doses (16 tabs)/24h.
Kaopectate Liquid	Bismuth Subsalicylate 262mg/15mL	**Adults & Peds ≥12 yrs:** 2 tbl (30mL) q½-1h prn. **Max:** 8 doses (16 tbl)/24h.
Kaopectate Max	Bismuth Subsalicylate 525mg/15mL	**Adults & Peds ≥12 yrs:** 2 tbl (30mL) q1h prn. **Max:** 4 doses (8 tbl)/24h.
Pepto Bismol Caplets	Bismuth Subsalicylate 262mg	**Adults & Peds ≥12 yrs:** 2 tabs q½-1h prn. **Max:** 8 doses (16 tabs)/24h.
Pepto Bismol Chewable Tablets	Bismuth Subsalicylate 262mg	**Adults & Peds ≥12 yrs:** 2 tabs q½-1h prn. **Max:** 8 doses (16 tabs)/24h.

(Continued)

BRAND	INGREDIENT(S)/STRENGTH(S)	DOSAGE*
BISMUTH SUBSALICYLATES *(Continued)*		
Pepto Bismol InstaCool Chewable Tablets	Bismuth Subsalicylate 262mg	**Adults & Peds ≥12 yrs:** 2 tabs q½-1h prn. **Max:** 8 doses (16 tabs)/24h.
Pepto Bismol Liquid	Bismuth Subsalicylate 525mg/30mL	**Adults & Peds ≥12 yrs:** 2 tbl (30mL) q½-1h prn. **Max:** 8 doses (16 tbl)/24h.
Pepto Bismol Max Strength Liquid	Bismuth Subsalicylate 1050mg/30mL	**Adults & Peds ≥12 yrs:** 2 tbl (30mL) q1h prn. **Max:** 4 doses (8 tbl)/24h.

*Some medications must be taken with water. Refer to individual product labeling for additional dosing information. Do not use antidiarrheal products for more than 2 days.

ANTIFLATULENT PRODUCTS

BRAND	INGREDIENT(S)/STRENGTH(S)	DOSAGE
ALPHA-GALACTOSIDASES		
Beano Meltaways Tablets	Alpha-galactosidase 300 GALU	**Adults:** Take 1 tab before meals.
Beano Tablets	Alpha-galactosidase enzyme 300 GALU (per 2 tabs)	**Adults:** Take 2-3 tabs before meals.
Beano + Dairy Defense	Alpha-galactosidase 300 GALU/ Lactase enzyme 9000 FCC	**Adults:** Chew 1 tab before meals.
ANTACIDS/ANTIFLATULENTS		
PLEASE REFER TO ANTACID AND HEARTBURN PRODUCTS TABLE		
SIMETHICONE/SIMETHICONE COMBINATIONS		
DulcoGas	Simethicone 125mg	**Adults:** Chew 1-2 tabs prn after meals and at hs. **Max:** 4 tabs/24h.
Gas-X Chewable Tablets	Simethicone 80mg	**Adults:** Chew 1 or 2 tabs prn after meals and at hs. **Max:** 6 tabs/24h.
Gas-X Chewable Tablets Extra Strength	Simethicone 125mg	**Adults:** Chew 1 or 2 tabs prn after meals and at hs. **Max:** 4 tabs/24h.
Gas-X Softgels Extra Strength	Simethicone 125mg	**Adults:** Take 1 or 2 caps prn after meals and at hs. **Max:** 4 caps/24h.
Gas-X Softgels Ultra Strength	Simethicone 180mg	**Adults:** Take 1 or 2 caps prn after meals and at hs. **Max:** 2 caps/24h.
Gas-X Thin Strips Extra Strength	Simethicone 62.5mg	**Adults:** Allow 2-4 strips to dissolve prn after meals and at hs. **Max:** 8 strips/24h.
Infants' Mylicon Drops	Simethicone 20mg/0.3mL	**Peds >2 yrs (>24 lbs):** 0.6mL prn after meals and at hs. **Peds <2 yrs (<24 lbs):** 0.3mL prn after meals and at hs. **Max:** 12 doses/24h.
Little Remedies Gas Relief Drops	Simethicone 20mg/0.3mL	**Peds ≥2 yrs (≥24 lbs):** 0.6mL prn after meals and at hs. **Peds <2 yrs (<24 lbs):** 0.3mL prn after meals and at hs. **Max:** 12 doses/24h.
Mylanta Gas Maximum Strength Chewable Tablets	Simethicone 125mg	**Adults:** Chew 1-2 tabs prn after meals and at hs. **Max:** 4 tabs/24h.
PediaCare Infants Gas Relief Drops	Simethicone 20mg/0.3mL	**Peds ≥2 yrs (≥24 lbs):** 0.6mL prn after meals and at hs. **Peds <2 yrs (<24 lbs):** 0.3mL prn after meals and at hs. **Max:** 12 doses/24h.
Phazyme Maximum Strength Softgels	Simethicone 250mg	**Adults:** Take 1 or 2 caps after a meal. **Max:** 2 caps/24h.
Phazyme Ultra Strength Softgels	Simethicone 180mg	**Adults:** Take 1 or 2 caps after a meal. **Max:** 2 caps/24h.

Hemorrhoidal Products*

BRAND	INGREDIENT(S)/STRENGTH(S)	DOSAGE[†]
ANESTHETICS/ANESTHETIC COMBINATIONS		
Americaine Hemorrhoidal Ointment	Benzocaine 20%	**Adults & Peds ≥12 yrs:** Apply externally to affected area up to 6 times a day.
Nupercainal Hemorrhoidal Ointment	Dibucaine 1%	**Adults & Peds ≥12 yrs:** Apply externally to affected area up to 3 or 4 times a day.
Preparation H Maximum Strength Pain Relief Cream	Glycerin/Phenylephrine HCl/ Pramoxine HCl/White petrolatum 14.4%/0.25%/1%/15%	**Adults & Peds ≥12 yrs:** Apply externally to affected area up to 4 times a day.
RectiCare Anorectal Cream	Lidocaine 5%	**Adults & Peds ≥12 yrs:** Apply externally to affected area up to 6 times a day.
RectiCare Medicated Anorectal Wipes	Lidocaine/Glycerin 4.3%/20%	**Adults & Peds ≥12 yrs:** Use externally on affected area up to 6 times a day.
Tronolane Cream	Pramoxine HCl/Zinc oxide 1%/5%	**Adults & Peds ≥12 yrs:** Apply externally to affected area up to 5 times a day.
Tucks Fast Relief Spray	Pramoxine HCl 1%	**Adults & Peds ≥12 yrs:** Apply externally to affected area up to 5 times a day.
Tucks Hemorrhoidal Ointment	Pramoxine HCl/Zinc oxide/ Mineral oil 1%/12.5%/46.6%	**Adults & Peds ≥12 yrs:** Apply externally to affected area up to 5 times a day.
HYDROCORTISONES		
Preparation H Anti-Itch Cream	Hydrocortisone 1%	**Adults & Peds ≥12 yrs:** Apply externally to affected area not more than tid-qid.
WITCH HAZELS/WITCH HAZEL COMBINATIONS		
Preparation H Cooling Gel	Phenylephrine HCl/Witch hazel 0.25%/50%	**Adults & Peds ≥12 yrs:** Apply externally to affected area up to 4 times a day.
Preparation H Medicated Wipes	Witch hazel 50%	**Adults & Peds ≥12 yrs:** Use externally on affected area up to 6 times a day.
Preparation H Medicated Wipes for Women	Witch hazel 20%	**Adults & Peds ≥12 yrs:** Use externally on affected area up to 6 times a day.
T.N. Dickinson's Hemorrhoidal Pads	Witch hazel 50%	**Adults & Peds ≥12 yrs:** Use externally on affected area up to 6 times a day.
Tucks Medicated Cooling Pads	Witch hazel 50%	**Adults & Peds ≥12 yrs:** Use externally on affected area up to 6 times a day.
Tucks Take Alongs Medicated Cooling Towelettes	Witch hazel 50%	**Adults & Peds ≥12 yrs:** Use externally on affected area up to 6 times a day.
MISCELLANEOUS		
Calmol 4 Hemorrhoidal Suppositories	Cocoa butter/Zinc oxide 76%/10%	**Adults & Peds ≥12 yrs:** Insert 1 supp up to 6 times a day.
Preparation H Ointment	Mineral oil/Petrolatum/ Phenylephrine HCl 14%/74.9%/0.25%	**Adults & Peds ≥12 yrs:** Apply to affected area up to 4 times a day.
Preparation H Suppositories	Cocoa butter/Phenylephrine HCl 88.44%/0.25%	**Adults & Peds ≥12 yrs:** Insert 1 supp up to 4 times a day.
Tucks Internal Soothers Suppositories	Topical starch 51%	**Adults & Peds ≥12 yrs:** Insert 1 supp up to 6 times a day.

*Please refer to the *Laxative Products* table for stool softeners or bulk-forming laxatives adjunct therapies.
[†]Stop use and contact a healthcare provider if condition worsens or does not improve within 7 days.

Laxative Products

BRAND	INGREDIENT(S)/STRENGTH(S)	DOSAGE
BULK-FORMING		
Citrucel Caplets	Methylcellulose 500mg	**Adults & Peds ≥12 yrs:** 2 tabs prn up to 6 times/day. **Max:** 12 tabs/day. **Peds 6-11 yrs:** 1 tab prn up to 6 times/day. **Max:** 6 tabs/day.
Citrucel Orange Powder	Methylcellulose 2g/tbl	**Adults & Peds ≥12 yrs:** 1 tbl prn up to tid. **Peds 6-11 yrs:** 2.5 tsp prn up to tid.
Citrucel Orange Sugar Free Powder	Methylcellulose 2g/tbl	**Adults & Peds ≥12 yrs:** 1 tbl prn up to tid. **Peds 6-11 yrs:** 2.5 tsp prn up to tid.
Equalactin Chewable Tablets	Calcium polycarbophil 625mg	**Adults & Peds ≥12 yrs:** 2 tabs prn. **Max:** 8 tabs/day. **Peds 6-<12 yrs:** 1 tab prn. **Max:** 4 tabs/day. **Peds 2-<6 yrs:** 1 tab prn. **Max:** 2 tabs/day.
FiberCon Caplets	Calcium polycarbophil 625mg	**Adults & Peds ≥12 yrs:** 2 tabs qd. **Max:** 8 tabs/day.
Konsyl Easy Mix Powder	Psyllium 4.3g/tsp	**Adults & Peds ≥12 yrs:** 1 tsp qd-tid. **Peds 6-<12 yrs:** ½ tsp qd-tid.
Konsyl Fiber Caplets	Calcium polycarbophil 625mg	**Adults & Peds ≥12 yrs:** 2 tabs qd-qid. **Max:** 8 tabs/day. **Peds 6-<12 yrs:** 2 tabs qd.
Konsyl Formula-D Powder	Psyllium 3.4g/tsp	**Adults & Peds ≥12 yrs:** 1 tsp qd-tid. **Peds 6-<12 yrs:** ½ tsp qd-tid.
Konsyl Orange Extra Strength Formula Powder	Psyllium 6g/tbl	**Adults & Peds ≥12 yrs:** 1 tbl qd-tid. **Peds 6-<12 yrs:** ½ tbl qd-tid.
Konsyl Orange Powder	Psyllium 3.4g/tbl	**Adults & Peds ≥12 yrs:** 1 tbl qd-tid. **Peds 6-<12 yrs:** ½ tbl qd-tid.
Konsyl Orange Sugar Free Powder	Psyllium 3.5g/tsp	**Adults & Peds ≥12 yrs:** 1 tsp qd-tid. **Peds 6-<12 yrs:** ½ tsp qd-tid.
Konsyl Original Formula Powder	Psyllium 6g/tsp	**Adults & Peds ≥12 yrs:** 1 tsp qd-tid. **Peds 6-<12 yrs:** ½ tsp qd-tid.
Konsyl Psyllium Capsules	Psyllium 520mg	**Adults & Peds ≥12 yrs:** 5 caps qd-tid.
Metamucil Capsules	Psyllium	**Adults & Peds ≥12 yrs:** 2-5 caps up to qid.
Metamucil Capsules Plus Calcium	Psyllium/Calcium	**Adults & Peds ≥12 yrs:** 2-5 caps up to qid.
Metamucil MultiGrain Wafers	Psyllium	**Adults & Peds ≥12 yrs:** 2 wafers up to tid.
Metamucil Orange Coarse Powder	Psyllium	**Adults & Peds ≥12 yrs:** 1 tbl up to tid.
Metamucil Orange Fiber Therapy Singles	Psyllium 3.4g/packet	**Adults & Peds ≥12 yrs:** 1 packet up to tid. **Peds 6-11 yrs:** ½ packet up to tid.
Metamucil Orange Smooth Powder	Psyllium	**Adults & Peds ≥12 yrs:** 1 tbl up to tid.
Metamucil Orange Smooth Powder Fiber Therapy	Psyllium 3.4g	**Adults & Peds ≥12 yrs:** 1 tbl up to tid. **Peds 6-11 yrs:** ½ tbl up to tid.
Metamucil Orange Sugar Free Fiber Singles	Psyllium	**Adults & Peds ≥12 yrs:** 1 packet up to tid.
Metamucil Orange Sugar Free Fiber Therapy Singles	Psyllium 3.4g	**Adults & Peds ≥12 yrs:** 1 packet up to tid. **Peds 6-11 yrs:** ½ packet up to tid.
Metamucil Orange Sugar Free Smooth Powder Fiber Therapy	Psyllium 3.4g	**Adults & Peds ≥12 yrs:** 1 tsp up to tid. **Peds 6-11 yrs:** ½ tsp up to tid.
Metamucil Original Coarse Powder	Psyllium	**Adults & Peds ≥12 yrs:** 1 tsp up to tid.
Metamucil Sugar Free Smooth Powder (Multi-flavor)	Psyllium	**Adults & Peds ≥12 yrs:** 1 tsp up to tid.

(Continued)

BRAND	INGREDIENT(S)/STRENGTH(S)	DOSAGE
HYPEROSMOTICS		
Fleet Glycerin Suppositories	Glycerin 2g	**Adults & Peds ≥6 yrs:** 1 supp ud.
Fleet Liquid Glycerin Suppositories	Glycerin 5.4g	**Adults & Peds ≥6 yrs:** 1 supp ud.
Fleet Mineral Oil Enema	Mineral oil 100%/118mL	**Adults & Peds ≥12 yrs:** 1 bottle (118mL). **Peds 2-<12 yrs:** ½ bottle (59mL).
Fleet Pedia-Lax Glycerin Suppositories	Glycerin 1g	**Peds 2-<6 yrs:** 1 supp ud.
Fleet Pedia-Lax Liquid Glycerin Suppositories	Glycerin 2.8g	**Peds 2-<6 yrs:** 1 supp ud.
Miralax	Polyethylene glycol 3350, 17g	**Adults & Peds ≥17 yrs:** 1 capful (17g) qd. **Max:** 7 days.
SALINES		
Fleet Enema	Monobasic sodium phosphate/ Dibasic sodium phosphate 19g-7g/118mL	**Adults & Peds ≥12 yrs:** 1 bottle (118mL).
Fleet Enema Extra	Monobasic sodium phosphate/ Dibasic sodium phosphate 19g-7g/197mL	**Adults & Peds ≥12 yrs:** 1 bottle (197mL).
Fleet Pedia-Lax Chewable Tablets	Magnesium hydroxide 400mg	**Peds 6-<12 yrs:** 3-6 tabs qd or in divided doses. **Max:** 6 tabs/day. **Peds 2-<6 yrs:** 1-3 tabs qd or in divided doses. **Max:** 3 tabs/day.
Fleet Pedia-Lax Enema	Monobasic sodium phosphate/ Dibasic sodium phosphate 9.5g-3.5g/59mL	**Peds 5-11 yrs:** 1 bottle (59mL). **Peds 2-<5 yrs:** ½ bottle (29.5mL).
Magnesium Citrate Solution	Magnesium citrate 1.745g/30mL	**Adults & Peds ≥12 yrs:** ½-1 bottle (300mL). **Peds 6-<12 yrs:** ⅓-½ bottle.
Phillips' Caplets	Magnesium 500mg	**Adults & Peds ≥12 yrs:** 2-4 tabs qhs or in divided doses.
Phillips' Chewable Tablets	Magnesium hydroxide 311mg	**Adults & Peds ≥12 yrs:** 8 tabs qhs or in divided doses. **Peds 6-11 yrs:** 4 tabs qhs or in divided doses. **Peds 3-5 yrs:** 2 tabs qhs or in divided doses.
Phillips' Concentrated Milk of Magnesia Liquid	Magnesium hydroxide 2400mg/15mL	**Adults & Peds ≥12 yrs:** 1-2 tbl (15-30mL) qhs or in divided doses.
Phillips' Milk of Magnesia Liquid	Magnesium hydroxide 1200mg/15mL	**Adults & Peds ≥12 yrs:** 2-4 tbl (30-60mL) qhs or in divided doses. **Peds 6-11 yrs:** 1-2 tbl (15-30mL) qhs or in divided doses.
STIMULANTS		
Alophen Tablets	Bisacodyl 5mg	**Adults & Peds ≥12 yrs:** 1-3 tabs qd. **Peds 6-<12 yrs:** 1 tab qd.
Carter's Sodium-Free Tablets	Bisacodyl 5mg	**Adults & Peds ≥12 yrs:** 1-3 tabs (usually 2) qd. **Peds 6-<12 yrs:** 1 tab qd.
Castor Oil	Castor oil 100%	**Adults & Peds ≥12 yrs:** 1-4 tbl (15-60mL) qd. **Peds 2-<12 yrs:** 1-3 tsp (5-15mL) qd.
Correctol Tablets	Bisacodyl 5mg	**Adults & Peds ≥12 yrs:** 1-3 tabs qd. **Peds 6-<12 yrs:** 1 tab qd.
Dulcolax Pink Tablets	Bisacodyl 5mg	**Adults & Peds ≥12 yrs:** 1-3 tabs qd. **Peds 6-<12 yrs:** 1 tab qd.
Dulcolax Suppositories	Bisacodyl 10mg	**Adults & Peds ≥12 yrs:** 1 supp qd. **Peds 6-<12 yrs:** ½ supp qd.
Dulcolax Tablets	Bisacodyl 5mg	**Adults & Peds ≥12 yrs:** 1-3 tabs qd. **Peds 6-<12 yrs:** 1 tab qd.

BRAND	INGREDIENT(S)/STRENGTH(S)	DOSAGE
STIMULANTS *(Continued)*		
Ex-Lax Maximum Strength Pills	Sennosides 25mg	**Adults & Peds ≥12 yrs:** 2 pills qd-bid. **Peds 6-<12 yrs:** 1 pill qd-bid.
Ex-Lax Regular Strength Chocolate Pieces	Sennosides 15mg	**Adults & Peds ≥12 yrs:** 2 pieces qd-bid. **Peds 6-<12 yrs:** 1 piece qd-bid.
Ex-Lax Regular Strength Pills	Sennosides 15mg	**Adults & Peds ≥12 yrs:** 2 pills qd-bid. **Peds 6-<12 yrs:** 1 pill qd-bid.
Fleet Bisacodyl Enema	Bisacodyl 10mg/30mL	**Adults & Peds ≥12 yrs:** 1 bottle (30mL).
Fleet Bisacodyl Tablets	Bisacodyl 5mg	**Adults & Peds ≥12 yrs:** 1-3 tabs qd. **Peds 6-<12 yrs:** 1 tab qd.
Perdiem Overnight Relief Pills	Sennosides 15mg	**Adults & Peds ≥12 yrs:** 2 tabs qd-bid. **Peds 6-<12 yrs:** 1 tab qd-bid.
Senokot Tablets	Sennosides 8.6mg	**Adults & Peds ≥12 yrs:** 2 tabs qd. **Max:** 4 tabs bid. **Peds 6-<12 yrs:** 1 tab qd. **Max:** 2 tabs bid. **Peds 2-<6 yrs:** ½ tab qd. **Max:** 1 tab bid.
SenokotXtra Tablets	Sennosides 17.2mg	**Adults & Peds ≥12 yrs:** 1 tab qd. **Max:** 2 tabs bid. **Peds 6-<12 yrs:** ½ tab qd. **Max:** 1 tab bid.
STIMULANT COMBINATIONS		
Konsyl Senna Prompt Capsules	Psyllium/Sennosides 500mg-9mg	**Adults & Peds ≥12 yrs:** 2-4 caps qd-bid.
Peri-Colace Tablets	Sennosides/Docusate sodium 8.6mg-50mg	**Adults & Peds ≥12 yrs:** 2-4 tabs qhs or in divided doses. **Peds 6-<12 yrs:** 1-2 tabs qhs or in divided doses. **Peds 2-<6 yrs:** up to 1 tab qd.
Senokot-S Tablets	Sennosides/Docusate sodium 8.6mg-50mg	**Adults & Peds ≥12 yrs:** 2 tabs qd. **Max:** 4 tabs bid. **Peds 6-<12 yrs:** 1 tab qd. **Max:** 2 tabs bid. **Peds 2-<6 yrs:** ½ tab qd. **Max:** 1 tab bid.
SURFACTANTS (STOOL SOFTENERS)		
Colace Capsules	Docusate sodium 50mg	**Adults & Peds ≥12 yrs:** 1-6 caps qd or in divided doses. **Peds 2-<12 yrs:** 1-3 caps qd or in divided doses.
Colace Capsules	Docusate sodium 100mg	**Adults & Peds ≥12 yrs:** 1-3 caps qd or in divided doses. **Peds 2-<12 yrs:** 1 cap qd.
Colace Clear Soft Gels	Docusate sodium 50mg	**Adults & Peds ≥12 yrs:** 1-6 caps qd or in divided doses. **Peds 2-<12 yrs:** 1-3 caps qd or in divided doses.
Docusol Kids Mini-Enema	Docusate sodium 100mg	**Peds 2-<12 yrs:** 1 unit qd.
Docusol Mini-Enema	Docusate sodium 283mg	**Adults & Peds ≥12 yrs:** 1-3 units qd.
DulcoEase Pink Softgels	Docusate sodium 100mg	**Adults & Peds ≥12 yrs:** 1-3 caps qd or in divided doses. **Peds 2-<12 yrs:** 1 cap qd.
Dulcolax Stool Softener Capsules	Docusate sodium 100mg	**Adults & Peds ≥12 yrs:** 1-3 caps qd or in divided doses. **Peds 2-<12 yrs:** 1 cap qd.
Fleet Pedia-Lax Liquid Stool Softener	Docusate sodium 50mg/tbl	**Peds 2-<12 yrs:** 1-3 tbl (15-45mL) qd or in divided doses. **Max:** 3 tbl (45mL)/day.
Fleet Sof-Lax Softgels	Docusate sodium 100mg	**Adults & Peds ≥12 yrs:** 1-3 caps qd. **Peds 2-<12 yrs:** 1 cap qd.
Phillips' Stool Softener Liquid Gels	Docusate sodium 100mg	**Adults & Peds ≥12 yrs:** 1-3 caps qd or in divided doses. **Peds 6-<12 yrs:** 1 cap qd.
Surfak Stool Softener Softgels	Docusate calcium 240mg	**Adults & Peds ≥12 yrs:** 1 cap qd.

(Continued)

BRAND	INGREDIENT(S)/STRENGTH(S)	DOSAGE
SURFACTANT COMBINATIONS (STOOL SOFTENERS)		
Docusol Plus Mini-Enema	Docusate sodium/Benzocaine 283mg-20mg	**Adults & Peds ≥12 yrs:** 1-3 units qd.

Cough-Cold-Flu-Allergy Products

BRAND NAME	ANALGESIC	ANTIHISTAMINE	COUGH SUPPRESSANT	DECONGESTANT	EXPECTORANT	DOSAGE
ANALGESICS						
Tylenol Cold + Sore Throat Liquid	Acetaminophen 500mg/15mL					**Adults & Peds ≥12 yrs:** 2 tbl (30mL) q6h. **Max:** 6 tbl (90mL)/24h.
ANALGESICS + ANTIHISTAMINES						
Coricidin HBP Cold & Flu Tablets	Acetaminophen 325mg	Chlorpheniramine maleate 2mg				**Adults & Peds ≥12 yrs:** 2 tabs q4-6h. **Max:** 12 tabs/24h. **Peds 6-<12 yrs:** 1 tab q4-6h. **Max:** 5 tabs/24h.
ANALGESICS + ANTIHISTAMINES + COUGH SUPPRESSANTS						
Alka-Seltzer Plus Severe Cold + Cough Night Liquid	Acetaminophen 650mg/30mL	Doxylamine succinate 12.5mg/30mL	Dextromethorphan HBr 30mg/30mL			**Adults & Peds ≥12 yrs:** 2 tbl (30mL) q6h. **Max:** 4 doses/24h.
Contac Cold + Flu Night Instant Cooling Relief Liquid	Acetaminophen 500mg/15mL	Doxylamine succinate 6.25mg/15mL	Dextromethorphan HBr 15mg/15mL			**Adults & Peds ≥12 yrs:** 2 tbl (30mL) q6h. **Max:** 6 tbl (90mL)/24h.
Coricidin HBP Maximum Strength Flu Tablets	Acetaminophen 500mg	Chlorpheniramine maleate 2mg	Dextromethorphan HBr 15mg			**Adults & Peds ≥12 yrs:** 2 tabs q6h. **Max:** 8 tabs/24h.
Coricidin HBP Nighttime Multi-Symptom Cold Liquid	Acetaminophen 325mg/15mL	Doxylamine succinate 6.25mg/15mL	Dextromethorphan HBr 15mg/15mL			**Adults & Peds ≥12 yrs:** 2 tbl (30mL) q6h. **Max:** 4 doses/24h.
PediaCare Cough & Runny Nose Plus Acetaminophen Liquid	Acetaminophen 160mg/5mL	Chlorpheniramine maleate 1mg/5mL	Dextromethorphan HBr 5mg/5mL			**Peds 6-11 yrs (48-95 lbs):** 2 tsp (10mL) q4h. **Max:** 5 doses/24h.
Vicks Alcohol Free NyQuil Cold & Flu Nighttime Relief Liquid	Acetaminophen 650mg/30mL	Chlorpheniramine maleate 4mg/30mL	Dextromethorphan HBr 30mg/30mL			**Adults & Peds ≥12 yrs:** 2 tbl (30mL) q6h. **Max:** 4 doses/24h.
Vicks NyQuil Cold & Flu Nighttime Relief LiquiCaps	Acetaminophen 325mg	Doxylamine succinate 6.25mg	Dextromethorphan HBr 15mg			**Adults & Peds ≥12 yrs:** 2 caps q6h. **Max:** 4 doses/24h.

(Continued)

BRAND NAME	ANALGESIC	ANTIHISTAMINE	COUGH SUPPRESSANT	DECONGESTANT	EXPECTORANT	DOSAGE
ANALGESICS + ANTIHISTAMINES + COUGH SUPPRESSANTS *(Continued)*						
Vicks NyQuil Cold & Flu Nighttime Relief Liquid	Acetaminophen 650mg/30mL	Doxylamine succinate 12.5mg/30mL	Dextromethorphan HBr 30mg/30mL			**Adults & Peds ≥12 yrs:** 2 tbl (30mL) q6h. **Max:** 4 doses/24h.
ANALGESICS + ANTIHISTAMINES + COUGH SUPPRESSANTS + DECONGESTANTS						
Alka-Seltzer Plus Cold & Cough Effervescent Tablets*	Aspirin 325mg	Chlorpheniramine maleate 2mg	Dextromethorphan HBr 10mg	Phenylephrine bitartrate 7.8mg		**Adults & Peds ≥12 yrs:** 2 tabs q4h. **Max:** 8 tabs/24h.
Alka-Seltzer Plus Cold & Cough Liquid Gels	Acetaminophen 325mg	Chlorpheniramine maleate 2mg	Dextromethorphan HBr 10mg	Phenylephrine HCl 5mg		**Adults & Peds ≥12 yrs:** 2 caps q4h. **Max:** 10 caps/24h.
Alka-Seltzer Plus Day & Night Multi-Symptom Cold & Flu Liquid Gels	Acetaminophen 325mg	Doxylamine succinate 6.25mg (nighttime dose only)	Dextromethorphan HBr 10mg	Phenylephrine HCl 5mg		**Adults & Peds ≥12 yrs:** 2 caps q4h. **Max:** 10 caps/24h.
Alka-Seltzer Plus Day & Night Multi-Symptom Cold Effervescent Tablets*	Aspirin 325mg (daytime dose only), 500mg (nighttime dose only)	Doxylamine succinate 6.25mg (nighttime dose only)	Dextromethorphan HBr 10mg	Phenylephrine bitartrate 7.8mg		**Adults & Peds ≥12 yrs:** (Day) 2 tabs q4h; (Night) 2 tabs hs or q4-6h. **Max:** 8 tabs/24h.
Alka-Seltzer Plus-D Multi-Symptom Sinus & Cold Liquid Gels	Acetaminophen 325mg	Chlorpheniramine maleate 2mg	Dextromethorphan HBr 10mg	Pseudoephedrine HCl 30mg		**Adults & Peds ≥12 yrs:** 2 caps q4h. **Max:** 8 caps/24h.
Alka-Seltzer Plus Night Cold Effervescent Tablets*	Aspirin 500mg	Doxylamine succinate 6.25mg	Dextromethorphan HBr 10mg	Phenylephrine bitartrate 7.8mg		**Adults & Peds ≥12 yrs:** 2 tabs hs or q4-6h. **Max:** 8 tabs/24h.
Alka-Seltzer Plus Night Cold & Flu Liquid Gels	Acetaminophen 325mg	Doxylamine succinate 6.25mg	Dextromethorphan HBr 10mg	Phenylephrine HCl 5mg		**Adults & Peds ≥12 yrs:** 2 caps q4h. **Max:** 10 caps/24h.
Alka-Seltzer Plus Night Severe Cold + Flu Powder Packets	Acetaminophen 650mg/packet	Doxylamine succinate 12.5mg/packet	Dextromethorphan HBr 20mg/packet	Phenylephrine HCl 10mg/packet		**Adults & Peds ≥12 yrs:** 1 pkt q4h. **Max:** 5 pkts/24h.
Alka-Seltzer Plus Severe Cold & Flu Effervescent Tablets*	Acetaminophen 250mg	Chlorpheniramine maleate 2mg	Dextromethorphan HBr 10mg	Phenylephrine HCl 5mg		**Adults & Peds ≥12 yrs:** 2 tabs q4h. **Max:** 8 tabs/24h.
Alka-Seltzer Plus Severe Sinus & Cold Powder Packets	Acetaminophen 650mg/packet	Chlorpheniramine maleate 4mg/packet	Dextromethorphan HBr 20mg/packet	Phenylephrine HCl 10mg/packet		**Adults & Peds ≥12 yrs:** 1 pkt q4h. **Max:** 5 pkts/24h.
Alka-Seltzer Plus Severe Sinus Congestion, Allergy & Cough Liquid Gels	Acetaminophen 325mg	Doxylamine succinate 6.25mg	Dextromethorphan HBr 10mg	Phenylephrine HCl 5mg		**Adults & Peds ≥12 yrs:** 2 caps q4h. **Max:** 10 caps/24h.

BRAND NAME	ANALGESIC	ANTIHISTAMINE	COUGH SUPPRESSANT	DECONGESTANT	EXPECTORANT	DOSAGE
ANALGESICS + ANTIHISTAMINES + COUGH SUPPRESSANTS + DECONGESTANTS *(Continued)*						
Alka-Seltzer Plus Severe Sinus Congestion & Cough Day & Night Liquid Gels	Acetaminophen 325mg	Doxylamine succinate 6.25mg (nighttime dose only)	Dextromethorphan HBr 10mg	Phenylephrine HCl 5mg		**Adults & Peds ≥12 yrs:** 2 caps q4h. **Max:** 10 caps/24h.
Maximum Strength Mucinex Fast-Max Night Time Cold & Flu Liquid Gels	Acetaminophen 325mg	Doxylamine succinate 6.25mg	Dextromethorphan HBr 10mg	Phenylephrine HCl 5mg		**Adults & Peds ≥12 yrs:** 2 caps q4h. **Max:** 12 caps/24h.
PediaCare Flu Plus Acetaminophen Liquid	Acetaminophen 160mg/5mL	Chlorpheniramine maleate 1mg/5mL	Dextromethorphan HBr 5mg/5mL	Phenylephrine HCl 2.5mg/5mL		**Peds 6-11 yrs (48-95 lbs):** 2 tsp (10mL) q4h. **Max:** 5 doses/24h.
PediaCare Multi-Symptom Cold Plus Acetaminophen Liquid	Acetaminophen 160mg/5mL	Chlorpheniramine maleate 1mg/5mL	Dextromethorphan HBr 5mg/5mL	Phenylephrine HCl 2.5mg/5mL		**Peds 6-11 yrs (48-95 lbs):** 2 tsp (10mL) q4h. **Max:** 5 doses/24h.
Theraflu Warming Relief Nighttime Multi-Symptom Cold Caplets†	Acetaminophen 325mg	Chlorpheniramine maleate 2mg	Dextromethorphan HBr 10mg	Phenylephrine HCl 5mg		**Adults & Peds ≥12 yrs:** 2 tabs q4h. **Max:** 12 tabs/24h.
Triaminic Multi-Symptom Fever & Cold Suspension	Acetaminophen 160mg/5mL	Chlorpheniramine maleate 1mg/5mL	Dextromethorphan HBr 5mg/5mL	Phenylephrine HCl 2.5mg/5mL		**Peds 6-<12 yrs:** 2 tsp (10mL) q4h. **Max:** 5 doses/24h.
Tylenol Cold Max Nighttime Liquid	Acetaminophen 325mg/15mL	Doxylamine succinate 6.25mg/15mL	Dextromethorphan HBr 10mg/15mL	Phenylephrine HCl 5mg/15mL		**Adults & Peds ≥12 yrs:** 2 tbl (30mL) q4h. **Max:** 10 tbl (150mL)/24h.
Vicks NyQuil Severe Cold & Flu Caplets	Acetaminophen 325mg	Doxylamine succinate 6.25mg	Dextromethorphan HBr 10mg	Phenylephrine HCl 5mg		**Adults & Peds ≥12 yrs:** 2 tabs q4h. **Max:** 4 doses/24h.
Vicks NyQuil Severe Cold & Flu Liquid	Acetaminophen 650mg/30mL	Doxylamine succinate 12.5mg/30mL	Dextromethorphan HBr 20mg/30mL	Phenylephrine HCl 10mg/30mL		**Adults & Peds ≥12 yrs:** 2 tbl (30mL) q4h. **Max:** 4 doses/24h.
ANALGESICS + ANTIHISTAMINES + COUGH SUPPRESSANTS + DECONGESTANTS + EXPECTORANTS						
Alka-Seltzer Plus Severe Cough, Mucus & Congestion Day & Night Liquid Gels	Acetaminophen 250mg (daytime dose), 325mg (nighttime dose)	Doxylamine succinate 6.25mg (nighttime dose only)	Dextromethorphan HBr 10mg	Phenylephrine HCl 5mg	Guaifenesin 200mg (daytime dose only)	**Adults & Peds ≥12 yrs:** 2 caps q4h. **Max:** 10 caps/24h.

(Continued)

BRAND NAME	ANALGESIC	ANTIHISTAMINE	COUGH SUPPRESSANT	DECONGESTANT	EXPECTORANT	DOSAGE
ANALGESICS + ANTIHISTAMINES + COUGH SUPPRESSANTS + EXPECTORANTS						
Coricidin HBP Day & Night Multi-Symptom Cold Softgels/ Tablets	Acetaminophen 500mg (nighttime dose only)	Chlorpheniramine maleate 2mg (nighttime dose only)	Dextromethorphan HBr 10mg (daytime dose), 15mg (nighttime dose)		Guaifenesin 200mg (daytime dose only)	**Adults & Peds ≥12 yrs:** (Day) 1-2 caps q4h. **Max:** 6 caps/12h; (Night) 2 tabs hs and q6h. **Max:** 4 tabs/12h.
ANALGESICS + ANTIHISTAMINES + DECONGESTANTS						
Advil Allergy & Congestion Relief Tablets	Ibuprofen 200mg	Chlorpheniramine maleate 4mg		Phenylephrine HCl 10mg		**Adults & Peds ≥12 yrs:** 1 tab q4h. **Max:** 6 tabs/24h.
Advil Allergy Sinus Caplets	Ibuprofen 200mg	Chlorpheniramine maleate 2mg		Pseudoephedrine HCl 30mg		**Adults & Peds ≥12 yrs:** 1 tab q4-6h. **Max:** 6 tabs/24h.
Alka-Seltzer Plus Cold Effervescent Tablets*‡	Aspirin 325mg	Chlorpheniramine maleate 2mg		Phenylephrine bitartrate 7.8mg		**Adults & Peds ≥12 yrs:** 2 tabs q4h. **Max:** 8 tabs/24h.
Alka-Seltzer Plus Severe Allergy Sinus Congestion & Headache Liquid Gels	Acetaminophen 325mg	Doxylamine succinate 6.25mg		Phenylephrine HCl 5mg		**Adults & Peds ≥12 yrs:** 2 caps q4h. **Max:** 10 caps/24h.
Children's Delsym Cough+ Cold Night Time Liquid	Acetaminophen 325mg/10mL	Diphenhydramine HCl 12.5mg/10mL		Phenylephrine HCl 5mg/10mL		**Adults & Peds ≥12 yrs:** 4 tsp (20mL) q4h. **Max:** 6 doses/24h. **Peds 6-<12 yrs:** 2 tsp (10mL) q4h. **Max:** 5 doses/24h.
Children's Dimetapp Multi-Symptom Cold & Flu Liquid	Acetaminophen 320mg/5mL	Diphenhydramine HCl 12.5mg/5mL		Phenylephrine HCl 5mg/5mL		**Adults & Peds ≥12 yrs:** 4 tsp (20mL) q4h. **Peds 6-<12 yrs:** 2 tsp (10mL) q4h. **Max:** 5 doses/24h.
Children's Mucinex Night Time Multi-Symptom Cold Liquid	Acetaminophen 325mg/10mL	Diphenhydramine HCl 12.5mg/10mL		Phenylephrine HCl 5mg/10mL		**Peds 6-<12 yrs:** 2 tsp (10mL) q4h. **Max:** 5 doses/24h.
Contac Cold + Flu Night Caplets	Acetaminophen 500mg	Chlorpheniramine maleate 2mg		Phenylephrine HCl 5mg		**Adults & Peds ≥12 yrs:** 2 tabs q6h prn. **Max:** 8 tabs/24h.
Delsym Cough+ Cold Night Time Liquid	Acetaminophen 650mg/20mL	Diphenhydramine HCl 25mg/20mL		Phenylephrine HCl 10mg/20mL		**Adults & Peds ≥12 yrs:** 4 tsp (20mL) q4h. **Max:** 6 doses/24h.
Dristan Cold Multi-Symptom Formula Tablets	Acetaminophen 325mg	Chlorpheniramine maleate 2mg		Phenylephrine HCl 5mg		**Adults & Peds ≥12 yrs:** 2 tabs q4h. **Max:** 12 tabs/24h.
Maximum Strength Mucinex Fast-Max Night Time Cold & Flu Liquid	Acetaminophen 650mg/20mL	Diphenhydramine HCl 25mg/20mL		Phenylephrine HCl 10mg/20mL		**Adults & Peds ≥12 yrs:** 4 tsp (20mL) q4h. **Max:** 6 doses/24h.

BRAND NAME	ANALGESIC	ANTIHISTAMINE	COUGH SUPPRESSANT	DECONGESTANT	EXPECTORANT	DOSAGE
ANALGESICS + ANTIHISTAMINES + DECONGESTANTS *(Continued)*						
Maximum Strength Mucinex Sinus-Max Night Time Congestion & Cough Liquid	Acetaminophen 650mg/20mL	Diphenhydramine HCl 25mg/20mL		Phenylephrine HCl 10mg/20mL		**Adults & Peds ≥12 yrs:** 4 tsp (20mL) q4h. **Max:** 6 doses/24h.
QlearQuil Nighttime Sinus & Congestion LiquiCaps	Acetaminophen 325mg	Doxylamine succinate 6.25mg		Phenylephrine HCl 5mg		**Adults & Peds ≥12 yrs:** 2 caps q4h. **Max:** 4 doses/24h.
Robitussin Maximum Strength Severe Multi-Symptom Cough Cold + Flu Nighttime Liquid	Acetaminophen 650mg/20mL	Diphenhydramine HCl 25mg/20mL		Phenylephrine HCl 10mg/20mL		**Adults & Peds ≥12 yrs:** 4 tsp (20mL) q4h. **Max:** 6 doses/24h.
Robitussin Peak Cold Nighttime Multi-Symptom Cold CF Liquid	Acetaminophen 640mg/20mL	Diphenhydramine HCl 25mg/20mL		Phenylephrine HCl 10mg/20mL		**Adults & Peds ≥12 yrs:** 4 tsp (20mL) q4h. **Max:** 6 doses/24h.
Sudafed PE Severe Cold Caplets†	Acetaminophen 325mg	Diphenhydramine HCl 12.5mg		Phenylephrine HCl 5mg		**Adults & Peds ≥12 yrs:** 2 tabs q4h. **Max:** 12 tabs/24h.
Theraflu ExpressMax Flu, Cough & Sore Throat Liquid	Acetaminophen 650mg/30mL	Diphenhydramine HCl 25mg/30mL		Phenylephrine HCl 10mg/30mL		**Adults & Peds ≥12 yrs:** 2 tbl (30mL) q4h. **Max:** 5 doses (150mL)/24h.
Theraflu ExpressMax Nighttime Severe Cold & Cough Liquid	Acetaminophen 650mg/30mL	Diphenhydramine HCl 25mg/30mL		Phenylephrine HCl 10mg/30mL		**Adults & Peds ≥12 yrs:** 2 tbl (30mL) q4h. **Max:** 5 doses (150mL)/24h.
Theraflu Flu & Sore Throat Powder Packets	Acetaminophen 650mg/packet	Pheniramine maleate 20mg/packet		Phenylephrine HCl 10mg/packet		**Adults & Peds ≥12 yrs:** 1 pkt q4h. **Max:** 5 pkts/24h.
Theraflu Nighttime Multi-Symptom Severe Cold Powder Packets	Acetaminophen 500mg/packet	Diphenhydramine HCl 25mg/packet		Phenylephrine HCl 10mg/packet		**Adults & Peds ≥12 yrs:** 1 pkt q4h. **Max:** 6 pkts/24h.
Theraflu Nighttime Severe Cold & Cough Powder Packets	Acetaminophen 650mg/packet	Diphenhydramine HCl 25mg/packet		Phenylephrine HCl 10mg/packet		**Adults & Peds ≥12 yrs:** 1 pkt q4h. **Max:** 5 pkts/24h.
Theraflu Sinus & Cold Powder Packets†	Acetaminophen 325mg/packet	Pheniramine maleate 20mg/packet		Phenylephrine HCl 10mg/packet		**Adults & Peds ≥12 yrs:** 1 pkt q4h. **Max:** 6 pkts/24h.
Theraflu Sugar-Free Nighttime Severe Cold & Cough Powder Packets†	Acetaminophen 650mg/packet	Diphenhydramine HCl 25mg/packet		Phenylephrine HCl 10mg/packet		**Adults & Peds ≥12 yrs:** 1 pkt q4h. **Max:** 6 pkts/24h.

(Continued)

BRAND NAME	ANALGESIC	ANTIHISTAMINE	COUGH SUPPRESSANT	DECONGESTANT	EXPECTORANT	DOSAGE
ANALGESICS + ANTIHISTAMINES + DECONGESTANTS *(Continued)*						
Theraflu Warming Relief Flu & Sore Throat Syrup†	Acetaminophen 325mg/15mL	Diphenhydramine HCl 12.5mg/15mL		Phenylephrine HCl 5mg/15mL		**Adults & Peds ≥12 yrs:** 2 tbl (30mL) q4h. **Max:** 6 doses (12 tbl or 180mL)/24h.
Theraflu Warming Relief Nighttime Severe Cold & Cough Syrup†	Acetaminophen 325mg/15mL	Diphenhydramine HCl 12.5mg/15mL		Phenylephrine HCl 5mg/15mL		**Adults & Peds ≥12 yrs:** 2 tbl (30mL) q4h. **Max:** 6 doses (12 tbl or 180mL)/24h.
Theraflu Warming Relief Sinus & Cold Syrup†	Acetaminophen 325mg/15mL	Diphenhydramine HCl 12.5mg/15mL		Phenylephrine HCl 5mg/15mL		**Adults & Peds ≥12 yrs:** 2 tbl (30mL) q4h. **Max:** 6 doses (12 tbl or 180mL)/24h.
ANALGESICS + ANTIHISTAMINES + DECONGESTANTS + EXPECTORANTS						
Maximum Strength Mucinex Sinus-Max Day & Night Caplets	Acetaminophen 325mg	Diphenhydramine HCl 25mg (nighttime dose only)		Phenylephrine HCl 5mg	Guaifenesin 200mg (daytime dose only)	**Adults & Peds ≥12 yrs:** 2 tabs q4h. **Max:** 12 tabs/24h.
ANALGESICS + COUGH SUPPRESSANTS						
Delsym Cough+ Soothing Action Lozenges	Menthol 5mg		Dextromethorphan HBr 5mg			**Adults & Peds ≥12 yrs:** 2 lozenges q4h. **Max:** 12 lozenges/24h. **Peds 6-<12 yrs:** 1 lozenge q4h. **Max:** 6 lozenges/24h.
PediaCare Cough & Sore Throat Plus Acetaminophen Liquid†	Acetaminophen 160mg/5mL		Dextromethorphan HBr 5mg/5mL			**Peds 6-11 yrs (48-95 lbs):** 2 tsp (10mL) q4h. **Max:** 5 doses/24h.
Robitussin Medi-Soothers Cough DM Lozenges	Menthol 5mg		Dextromethorphan HBr 5mg			**Adults & Peds ≥12 yrs:** 2 lozenges q4h. **Max:** 12 lozenges/24h.
Triaminic Cough & Sore Throat Syrup	Acetaminophen 160mg/5mL		Dextromethorphan HBr 5mg/5mL			**Peds 6-<12 yrs:** 2 tsp (10mL) q4h. **Peds 4-<6 yrs:** 1 tsp (5mL) q4h. **Max:** 5 doses/24h.
ANALGESICS + COUGH SUPPRESSANTS + DECONGESTANTS						
Alka-Seltzer Plus Day Cold & Flu Liquid Gels	Acetaminophen 325mg		Dextromethorphan HBr 10mg	Phenylephrine HCl 5mg		**Adults & Peds ≥12 yrs:** 2 caps q4h. **Max:** 10 caps/24h.
Alka-Seltzer Plus Severe Sinus Congestion & Cough Liquid Gels	Acetaminophen 325mg		Dextromethorphan HBr 10mg	Phenylephrine HCl 5mg		**Adults & Peds ≥12 yrs:** 2 caps q4h. **Max:** 10 caps/24h.
Maximum Strength Mucinex Fast-Max Severe Cold Liquid Gels	Acetaminophen 325mg		Dextromethorphan HBr 10mg	Phenylephrine HCl 5mg		**Adults & Peds ≥12 yrs:** 2 caps q4h. **Max:** 12 caps/24h.

BRAND NAME	ANALGESIC	ANTIHISTAMINE	COUGH SUPPRESSANT	DECONGESTANT	EXPECTORANT	DOSAGE
ANALGESICS + COUGH SUPPRESSANTS + DECONGESTANTS *(Continued)*						
Sudafed PE Pressure + Pain + Cough Caplets	Acetaminophen 325mg		Dextromethorphan HBr 10mg	Phenylephrine HCl 5mg		**Adults & Peds ≥12 yrs:** 2 tabs q4h. **Max:** 10 tabs/24h.
Theraflu Daytime Severe Cold & Cough Powder Packets	Acetaminophen 650mg/packet		Dextromethorphan HBr 20mg/packet	Phenylephrine HCl 10mg/packet		**Adults & Peds ≥12 yrs:** 1 pkt q4h. **Max:** 5 pkts/24h.
Theraflu ExpressMax Daytime Severe Cold & Cough Liquid	Acetaminophen 650mg/30mL		Dextromethorphan HBr 20mg/30mL	Phenylephrine HCl 10mg/30mL		**Adults & Peds ≥12 yrs:** 2 tbl (30mL) q4h. **Max:** 5 doses (150mL)/24h.
Theraflu Multi-Symptom Severe Cold Powder Packets	Acetaminophen 500mg/packet		Dextromethorphan HBr 20mg/packet	Phenylephrine HCl 10mg/packet		**Adults & Peds ≥12 yrs:** 1 pkt q4h. **Max:** 6 pkts/24h.
Theraflu Warming Relief Daytime Multi-Symptom Cold Caplets†	Acetaminophen 325mg		Dextromethorphan HBr 10mg	Phenylephrine HCl 5mg		**Adults & Peds ≥12 yrs:** 2 tabs q4h. **Max:** 12 tabs/24h.
Theraflu Warming Relief Daytime Severe Cold & Cough Syrup†	Acetaminophen 325mg/15mL		Dextromethorphan HBr 10mg/15mL	Phenylephrine HCl 5mg/15mL		**Adults & Peds ≥12 yrs:** 2 tbl (30mL) q4h. **Max:** 6 doses/24h.
Tylenol Cold Max Daytime Caplets	Acetaminophen 325mg		Dextromethorphan HBr 10mg	Phenylephrine HCl 5mg		**Adults & Peds ≥12 yrs:** 2 tabs q4h. **Max:** 10 tabs/24h.
Tylenol Cold Max Daytime Liquid	Acetaminophen 325mg/15mL		Dextromethorphan HBr 10mg/15mL	Phenylephrine HCl 5mg/15mL		**Adults & Peds ≥12 yrs:** 2 tbl (30mL) q4h. **Max:** 10 tbl (150mL)/24h.
Vicks DayQuil Cold & Flu Multi-Symptom Relief LiquiCaps	Acetaminophen 325mg		Dextromethorphan HBr 10mg	Phenylephrine HCl 5mg		**Adults & Peds ≥12 yrs:** 2 caps q4h. **Max:** 4 doses/24h.
Vicks DayQuil Cold & Flu Multi-Symptom Relief Liquid	Acetaminophen 325mg/15mL		Dextromethorphan HBr 10mg/15mL	Phenylephrine HCl 5mg/15mL		**Adults & Peds ≥12 yrs:** 2 tbl (30mL) q4h. **Peds 6-<12 yrs:** 1 tbl (15mL) q4h. **Max:** 4 doses/24h.
ANALGESICS + COUGH SUPPRESSANTS + DECONGESTANTS + EXPECTORANTS						
Alka-Seltzer Plus Day Severe Cold + Flu Powder Packets	Acetaminophen 500mg/packet		Dextromethorphan HBr 20mg/packet	Phenylephrine HCl 10mg/packet	Guaifenesin 400mg/packet	**Adults & Peds ≥12 yrs:** 1 pkt q4h. **Max:** 6 pkts/24h.
Alka-Seltzer Plus Multi-Symptom Severe Cough, Mucus & Congestion Liquid Gels	Acetaminophen 250mg		Dextromethorphan HBr 10mg	Phenylephrine HCl 5mg	Guaifenesin 200mg	**Adults & Peds ≥12 yrs:** 2 caps q4h. **Max:** 12 caps/24h.

(Continued)

BRAND NAME	ANALGESIC	ANTIHISTAMINE	COUGH SUPPRESSANT	DECONGESTANT	EXPECTORANT	DOSAGE
ANALGESICS + COUGH SUPPRESSANTS + DECONGESTANTS + EXPECTORANTS *(Continued)*						
Alka-Seltzer Plus Severe Sinus, Cold & Cough Liquid Gels	Acetaminophen 250mg		Dextromethorphan HBr 10mg	Phenylephrine HCl 5mg	Guaifenesin 200mg	**Adults & Peds ≥12 yrs:** 2 caps q4h. **Max:** 12 caps/24h.
Children's Delsym Cough+ Cold Day Time Liquid	Acetaminophen 325mg/10mL		Dextromethorphan HBr 10mg/10mL	Phenylephrine HCl 5mg/10mL	Guaifenesin 200mg/10mL	**Adults & Peds ≥12 yrs:** 4 tsp (20mL) q4h. **Max:** 6 doses/24h. **Peds 6-<12 yrs:** 2 tsp (10mL) q4h. **Max:** 5 doses/24h.
Children's Mucinex Cold, Cough & Sore Throat Liquid	Acetaminophen 325mg/10mL		Dextromethorphan HBr 10mg/10mL	Phenylephrine HCl 5mg/10mL	Guaifenesin 200mg/10mL	**Peds 6-<12 yrs:** 2 tsp (10mL) q4h. **Max:** 5 doses/24h.
Children's Mucinex Multi-Symptom Cold & Fever Liquid	Acetaminophen 325mg/10mL		Dextromethorphan HBr 10mg/10mL	Phenylephrine HCl 5mg/10mL	Guaifenesin 200mg/10mL	**Peds 6-<12 yrs:** 2 tsp (10mL) q4h. **Max:** 5 doses/24h.
Delsym Cough+ Cold Day Time Liquid	Acetaminophen 650mg/20mL		Dextromethorphan HBr 20mg/20mL	Phenylephrine HCl 10mg/20mL	Guaifenesin 400mg/20mL	**Adults & Peds ≥12 yrs:** 4 tsp (20mL) q4h. **Max:** 6 doses/24h.
Maximum Strength Mucinex Fast-Max Cold, Flu & Sore Throat Caplets	Acetaminophen 325mg		Dextromethorphan HBr 10mg	Phenylephrine HCl 5mg	Guaifenesin 200mg	**Adults & Peds ≥12 yrs:** 2 tabs q4h. **Max:** 12 tabs/24h.
Maximum Strength Mucinex Fast-Max Cold, Flu & Sore Throat Liquid	Acetaminophen 650mg/20mL		Dextromethorphan HBr 20mg/20mL	Phenylephrine HCl 10mg/20mL	Guaifenesin 400mg/20mL	**Adults & Peds ≥12 yrs:** 4 tsp (20mL) q4h. **Max:** 6 doses/24h.
Maximum Strength Mucinex Fast-Max Cold, Flu & Sore Throat Liquid Gels	Acetaminophen 325mg		Dextromethorphan HBr 10mg	Phenylephrine HCl 5mg	Guaifenesin 200mg	**Adults & Peds ≥12 yrs:** 2 caps q4h. **Max:** 12 caps/24h.
Maximum Strength Mucinex Fast-Max Severe Cold Caplets	Acetaminophen 325mg		Dextromethorphan HBr 10mg	Phenylephrine HCl 5mg	Guaifenesin 200mg	**Adults & Peds ≥12 yrs:** 2 tabs q4h. **Max:** 12 tabs/24h.
Maximum Strength Mucinex Fast-Max Severe Cold Liquid	Acetaminophen 650mg/20mL		Dextromethorphan HBr 20mg/20mL	Phenylephrine HCl 10mg/20mL	Guaifenesin 400mg/20mL	**Adults & Peds ≥12 yrs:** 4 tsp (20mL) q4h. **Max:** 6 doses/24h.
Maximum Strength Mucinex Sinus-Max Severe Congestion Relief Liquid Gels	Acetaminophen 325mg		Dextromethorphan HBr 10mg	Phenylephrine HCl 5mg	Guaifenesin 200mg	**Adults & Peds ≥12 yrs:** 2 caps q4h. **Max:** 12 caps/24h.
Robitussin Maximum Strength Severe Multi-Symptom Cough Cold + Flu Liquid	Acetaminophen 650mg/20mL		Dextromethorphan HBr 20mg/20mL	Phenylephrine HCl 10mg/20mL	Guaifenesin 400mg/20mL	**Adults & Peds ≥12 yrs:** 4 tsp (20mL) q4h. **Max:** 6 doses/24h.
Sudafed PE Pressure + Pain + Cold Caplets	Acetaminophen 325mg		Dextromethorphan HBr 10mg	Phenylephrine HCl 5mg	Guaifenesin 100mg	**Adults & Peds ≥12 yrs:** 2 tabs q4h. **Max:** 10 tabs/24h.

BRAND NAME	ANALGESIC	ANTIHISTAMINE	COUGH SUPPRESSANT	DECONGESTANT	EXPECTORANT	DOSAGE
ANALGESICS + COUGH SUPPRESSANTS + DECONGESTANTS + EXPECTORANTS *(Continued)*						
Theraflu Max-D Severe Cold & Flu Powder Packets†	Acetaminophen 1000mg/packet		Dextromethorphan HBr 30mg/packet	Pseudoephedrine HCl 60mg/packet	Guaifenesin 400mg/packet	**Adults & Peds ≥12 yrs:** 1 pkt q6h. **Max:** 4 pkts/24h.
Tylenol Cold + Flu Severe Caplets	Acetaminophen 325mg		Dextromethorphan HBr 10mg	Phenylephrine HCl 5mg	Guaifenesin 200mg	**Adults & Peds ≥12 yrs:** 2 tabs q4h. **Max:** 10 tabs/24h.
Tylenol Cold + Flu Severe Warming Liquid	Acetaminophen 325mg/15mL		Dextromethorphan HBr 10mg/15mL	Phenylephrine HCl 5mg/15mL	Guaifenesin 200mg/15mL	**Adults & Peds ≥12 yrs:** 2 tbl (30mL) q4h. **Max:** 10 tbl (150mL)/24h.
Tylenol Cold + Mucus Severe Liquid	Acetaminophen 325mg/15mL		Dextromethorphan HBr 10mg/15mL	Phenylephrine HCl 5mg/15mL	Guaifenesin 200mg/15mL	**Adults & Peds ≥12 yrs:** 2 tbl (30mL) q4h. **Max:** 10 tbl (150mL)/24h.
Vicks DayQuil Severe Cold & Flu Caplets	Acetaminophen 325mg		Dextromethorphan HBr 10mg	Phenylephrine HCl 5mg	Guaifenesin 200mg	**Adults & Peds ≥12 yrs:** 2 tabs q4h. **Max:** 4 doses/24h.
Vicks DayQuil Severe Cold & Flu Liquid	Acetaminophen 325mg/15mL		Dextromethorphan HBr 10mg/15mL	Phenylephrine HCl 5mg/15mL	Guaifenesin 200mg/15mL	**Adults & Peds ≥12 yrs:** 2 tbl (30mL) q4h. **Peds 6-<12 yrs:** 1 tbl (15mL) q4h. **Max:** 4 doses/24h.
ANALGESICS + DECONGESTANTS						
Advil Cold & Sinus Caplets	Ibuprofen 200mg			Pseudoephedrine HCl 30mg		**Adults & Peds ≥12 yrs:** 1-2 tabs q4-6h. **Max:** 6 tabs/24h.
Advil Cold & Sinus Liqui-Gels	Ibuprofen 200mg			Pseudoephedrine HCl 30mg		**Adults & Peds ≥12 yrs:** 1-2 caps q4-6h. **Max:** 6 caps/24h.
Advil Sinus Congestion & Pain Tablets	Ibuprofen 200mg			Phenylephrine HCl 10mg		**Adults & Peds ≥12 yrs:** 1 tab q4h. **Max:** 6 tabs/24h.
Contac Cold + Flu Day Caplets	Acetaminophen 500mg			Phenylephrine HCl 5mg		**Adults & Peds ≥12 yrs:** 2 tabs q6h. **Max:** 8 tabs/24h.
QlearQuil Daytime Sinus & Congestion LiquiCaps	Acetaminophen 325mg			Phenylephrine HCl 5mg		**Adults & Peds ≥12 yrs:** 2 caps q4h. **Max:** 4 doses/24h.
Sudafed 12 Hour Pressure + Pain Caplets	Naproxen sodium 220mg			Pseudoephedrine HCl 120mg		**Adults & Peds ≥12 yrs:** 1 tab q12h. **Max:** 2 tabs/24h.

(Continued)

BRAND NAME	ANALGESIC	ANTIHISTAMINE	COUGH SUPPRESSANT	DECONGESTANT	EXPECTORANT	DOSAGE
ANALGESICS + DECONGESTANTS *(Continued)*						
Sudafed PE Pressure + Pain Caplets	Acetaminophen 325mg			Phenylephrine HCl 5mg		**Adults & Peds ≥12 yrs:** 2 tabs q4h. **Max:** 10 tabs/24h.
Tylenol Sinus + Headache Daytime Caplets	Acetaminophen 325mg			Phenylephrine HCl 5mg		**Adults & Peds ≥12 yrs:** 2 caps q4h. **Max:** 10 caps/24h.
ANALGESICS + DECONGESTANTS + EXPECTORANTS						
Maximum Strength Mucinex Fast-Max Cold & Sinus Caplets	Acetaminophen 325mg			Phenylephrine HCl 5mg	Guaifenesin 200mg	**Adults & Peds ≥12 yrs:** 2 tabs q4h. **Max:** 12 tabs/24h.
Maximum Strength Mucinex Fast-Max Cold & Sinus Liquid	Acetaminophen 650mg/20mL			Phenylephrine HCl 10mg/20mL	Guaifenesin 400mg/20mL	**Adults & Peds ≥12 yrs:** 4 tsp (20mL) q4h. **Max:** 6 doses/24h.
Maximum Strength Mucinex Sinus-Max Pressure & Pain Caplets	Acetaminophen 325mg			Phenylephrine HCl 5mg	Guaifenesin 200mg	**Adults & Peds ≥12 yrs:** 2 tabs q4h. **Max:** 12 tabs/24h.
Maximum Strength Mucinex Sinus-Max Pressure & Pain Liquid	Acetaminophen 650mg/20mL			Phenylephrine HCl 10mg/20mL	Guaifenesin 400mg/20mL	**Adults & Peds ≥12 yrs:** 4 tsp (20mL) q4h. **Max:** 6 doses/24h.
Maximum Strength Mucinex Sinus-Max Severe Congestion Relief Caplets	Acetaminophen 325mg			Phenylephrine HCl 5mg	Guaifenesin 200mg	**Adults & Peds ≥12 yrs:** 2 tabs q4h. **Max:** 12 tabs/24h.
Maximum Strength Mucinex Sinus-Max Severe Congestion Relief Liquid	Acetaminophen 650mg/20mL			Phenylephrine HCl 10mg/20mL	Guaifenesin 400mg/20mL	**Adults & Peds ≥12 yrs:** 4 tsp (20mL) q4h. **Max:** 6 doses/24h.
Sudafed PE Pressure + Pain + Mucus Caplets	Acetaminophen 325mg			Phenylephrine HCl 5mg	Guaifenesin 200mg	**Adults & Peds ≥12 yrs:** 2 tabs q4h. **Max:** 10 tabs/24h.
Sudafed Triple Action Caplets†	Acetaminophen 325mg			Pseudoephedrine HCl 30mg	Guaifenesin 200mg	**Adults & Peds ≥12 yrs:** 2 tabs q4-6h. **Max:** 8 tabs/24h
Theraflu Warming Relief Cold & Chest Congestion Liquid†	Acetaminophen 325mg/15mL			Phenylephrine HCl 5mg/15mL	Guaifenesin 200mg/15mL	**Adults & Peds ≥12 yrs:** 2 tbl (30mL) q4h. **Max:** 6 doses/24h.
Tylenol Cold + Head Congestion Severe Caplets	Acetaminophen 325mg			Phenylephrine HCl 5mg	Guaifenesin 200mg	**Adults & Peds ≥12 yrs:** 2 tabs q4h. **Max:** 10 tabs/24h.
Tylenol Sinus Severe Daytime Caplets	Acetaminophen 325mg			Phenylephrine HCl 5mg	Guaifenesin 200mg	**Adults & Peds ≥12 yrs:** 2 tabs q4h. **Max:** 10 tabs/24h.

BRAND NAME	ANALGESIC	ANTIHISTAMINE	COUGH SUPPRESSANT	DECONGESTANT	EXPECTORANT	DOSAGE
ANTIHISTAMINES						
Alavert Orally Disintegrating Tablets[‡]		Loratadine 10mg				**Adults & Peds ≥6 yrs:** 1 tab qd. **Max:** 1 tab/24h.
Benadryl Allergy Dye-Free Liqui-Gels		Diphenhydramine HCl 25mg				**Adults & Peds ≥12 yrs:** 1-2 caps q4-6h. **Peds 6-<12 yrs:** 1 cap q4-6h. **Max:** 6 doses/24h.
Benadryl Allergy Ultratab Tablets		Diphenhydramine HCl 25mg				**Adults & Peds ≥12 yrs:** 1-2 tabs q4-6h. **Peds 6-<12 yrs:** 1 tab q4-6h. **Max:** 6 doses/24h.
Children's Benadryl Allergy Liquid		Diphenhydramine HCl 12.5mg/5mL				**Peds 6-11 yrs:** 1-2 tsp (5-10mL) q4-6h. **Max:** 6 doses/24h.
Children's Benadryl Dye-Free Allergy Liquid[†]		Diphenhydramine HCl 12.5mg/5mL				**Peds 6-11 yrs:** 1-2 tsp (5-10mL) q4-6h. **Max:** 6 doses/24h.
Children's Claritin Chewables[‡]		Loratadine 5mg				**Adults & Peds ≥6 yrs:** 2 tabs qd. **Max:** 2 tabs/24h. **Peds 2-<6 yrs:** 1 tab qd. **Max:** 1 tab/24h.
Children's Claritin Syrup		Loratadine 5mg/5mL				**Adults & Peds ≥6 yrs:** 2 tsp (10mL) qd. **Max:** 2 tsp (10mL)/24h. **Peds 2-<6 yrs:** 1 tsp (5mL) qd. **Max:** 1 tsp (5mL)/24h.
Children's Zyrtec Dissolve Tabs		Cetirizine HCl 10mg				**Adults <65 yrs & Peds ≥6 yrs:** 1 tab qd. **Max:** 1 tab/24h.
Claritin Liqui-Gels		Loratadine 10mg				**Adults & Peds ≥6 yrs:** 1 cap qd. **Max:** 1 cap/24h.
Claritin RediTabs 12-Hour		Loratadine 5mg				**Adults & Peds ≥6 yrs:** 1 tab q12h. **Max:** 2 tabs/24h.
Claritin RediTabs 24-Hour		Loratadine 10mg				**Adults & Peds ≥6 yrs:** 1 tab qd. **Max:** 1 tab/24h.
Claritin Tablets		Loratadine 10mg				**Adults & Peds ≥6 yrs:** 1 tab qd. **Max:** 1 tab/24h.

(Continued)

BRAND NAME	ANALGESIC	ANTIHISTAMINE	COUGH SUPPRESSANT	DECONGESTANT	EXPECTORANT	DOSAGE
ANTIHISTAMINES *(Continued)*						
PediaCare Allergy Liquid		Diphenhydramine HCl 12.5mg/5mL				**Peds 6-11 yrs (48-95 lbs):** 1-2 tsp (5-10mL) q4h. **Max:** 6 doses/24h.
PediaCare 24 Hour Allergy Liquid		Cetirizine HCl 5mg/5mL				**Adults ≥65 yrs:** 1 tsp (5mL) qd. **Max:** 1 tsp (5mL)/24h. **Adults <65 yrs & Peds ≥6 yrs:** 1-2 tsp (5-10mL) qd. **Max:** 2 tsp (10mL)/24h. **Peds 2-<6 yrs:** ½-1 tsp (2.5-5mL) qd or ½ tsp (2.5mL) q12h. **Max:** 1 tsp (5mL)/24h.
QlearQuil All Day & All Night 24 Hour Allergy Relief Tablets		Loratadine 10mg				**Adults & Peds ≥6 yrs:** 1 tab qd. **Max:** 1 tab/24h.
QlearQuil Nighttime Allergy Relief Caplets		Diphenhydramine HCl 25mg				**Adults & Peds ≥12 yrs:** 1-2 tabs q4-6h. **Peds 6-<12 yrs:** 1 tab q4-6h. **Max:** 6 doses/24h.
Zyrtec Dissolve Tabs		Cetirizine HCl 10mg				**Adults <65 yrs & Peds ≥6 yrs:** 1 tab qd. **Max:** 1 tab/24h.
Zyrtec Liquid Gels		Cetirizine HCl 10mg				**Adults <65 yrs & Peds ≥6 yrs:** 1 cap qd. **Max:** 1 cap/24h.
Zyrtec Tablets		Cetirizine HCl 10mg				**Adults <65 yrs & Peds ≥6 yrs:** 1 tab qd. **Max:** 1 tab/24h.
ANTIHISTAMINES + COUGH SUPPRESSANTS						
Children's Dimetapp Long Acting Cough Plus Cold Liquid		Chlorpheniramine maleate 2mg/10mL	Dextromethorphan HBr 15mg/10mL			**Adults & Peds ≥12 yrs:** 4 tsp (20mL) q6h. **Peds 6-<12 yrs:** 2 tsp (10mL) q6h. **Max:** 4 doses/24h.
Children's Robitussin Cough & Cold Long-Acting Liquid		Chlorpheniramine maleate 2mg/10mL	Dextromethorphan HBr 15mg/10mL			**Adults & Peds ≥12 yrs:** 4 tsp (20mL) q6h. **Peds 6-<12 yrs:** 2 tsp (10mL) q6h. **Max:** 4 doses/24h.
Children's Robitussin Nighttime Cough Long-Acting DM Liquid		Chlorpheniramine maleate 2mg/10mL	Dextromethorphan HBr 15mg/10mL			**Adults & Peds ≥12 yrs:** 4 tsp (20mL) q6h. **Peds 6-<12 yrs:** 2 tsp (10mL) q6h. **Max:** 4 doses/24h.
Coricidin HBP Cough & Cold Tablets		Chlorpheniramine maleate 4mg	Dextromethorphan HBr 30mg			**Adults & Peds ≥12 yrs:** 1 tab q6h. **Max:** 4 tabs/24h.

BRAND NAME	ANALGESIC	ANTIHISTAMINE	COUGH SUPPRESSANT	DECONGESTANT	EXPECTORANT	DOSAGE
ANTIHISTAMINES + COUGH SUPPRESSANTS *(Continued)*						
Robitussin Maximum Strength Nighttime Cough DM Liquid		Doxylamine succinate 12.5mg/10mL	Dextromethorphan HBr 30mg/10mL			**Adults & Peds ≥12 yrs:** 2 tsp (10mL) q6h. **Max:** 4 doses/24h.
Vicks Children's NyQuil Cold & Cough Liquid		Chlorpheniramine maleate 2mg/15mL	Dextromethorphan HBr 15mg/15mL			**Adults & Peds ≥12 yrs:** 2 tbl (30mL) q6h. **Peds 6-11 yrs:** 1 tbl (15mL) q6h. **Max:** 4 doses/24h.
Vicks NyQuil Cough Liquid		Doxylamine succinate 12.5mg/30mL	Dextromethorphan HBr 30mg/30mL			**Adults & Peds ≥12 yrs:** 2 tbl (30mL) q6h. **Max:** 4 doses/24h.
ANTIHISTAMINES + COUGH SUPPRESSANTS + DECONGESTANTS						
Children's Dimetapp Cold & Cough Liquid		Brompheniramine maleate 2mg/10mL	Dextromethorphan HBr 10mg/10mL	Phenylephrine HCl 5mg/10mL		**Adults & Peds ≥12 yrs:** 4 tsp (20mL) q4h. **Peds 6-<12 yrs:** 2 tsp (10mL) q4h. **Max:** 6 doses/24h.
ANTIHISTAMINES + DECONGESTANTS						
Alavert D-12 Hour Extended Release Tablets		Loratadine 5mg		Pseudoephedrine sulfate 120mg		**Adults & Peds ≥12 yrs:** 1 tab q12h. **Max:** 2 tabs/24h.
Allerest PE Tablets		Chlorpheniramine maleate 4mg		Phenylephrine HCl 10mg		**Adults & Peds ≥12 yrs:** 1 tab q4h. **Peds 6-<12 yrs:** ½ tab q4h. **Max:** 6 doses/24h.
Children's Benadryl Allergy Plus Congestion Liquid		Diphenhydramine HCl 12.5mg/5mL		Phenylephrine HCl 5mg/5mL		**Adults & Peds ≥12 yrs:** 2 tsp (10mL) q4h. **Peds 6-11 yrs:** 1 tsp (5mL) q4h. **Max:** 6 doses/24h.
Children's Dimetapp Cold & Allergy Liquid		Brompheniramine maleate 2mg/10mL		Phenylephrine HCl 5mg/10mL		**Adults & Peds ≥12 yrs:** 4 tsp (20mL) q4h. **Peds 6-<12 yrs:** 2 tsp (10mL) q4h. **Max:** 6 doses/24h.
Children's Dimetapp Nighttime Cold & Congestion Liquid		Diphenhydramine HCl 12.5mg/10mL		Phenylephrine HCl 5mg/10mL		**Adults & Peds ≥12 yrs:** 4 tsp (20mL) q4h. **Peds 6-<12 yrs:** 2 tsp (10mL) q4h. **Max:** 6 doses/24h.
Claritin-D 12 Hour Tablets		Loratadine 5mg		Pseudoephedrine sulfate 120mg		**Adults & Peds ≥12 yrs:** 1 tab q12h. **Max:** 2 tabs/24h.
Claritin-D 24 Hour Tablets		Loratadine 10mg		Pseudoephedrine sulfate 240mg		**Adults & Peds ≥12 yrs:** 1 tab qd. **Max:** 1 tab/24h.

(Continued)

BRAND NAME	ANALGESIC	ANTIHISTAMINE	COUGH SUPPRESSANT	DECONGESTANT	EXPECTORANT	DOSAGE
ANTIHISTAMINES + DECONGESTANTS *(Continued)*						
PediaCare Nighttime Multi-Symptom Cold Liquid		Diphenhydramine HCl 6.25mg/5mL		Phenylephrine HCl 2.5mg/5mL		**Peds 6-11 yrs (48-95 lbs):** 2 tsp (10mL) q4h. **Max:** 6 doses/24h.
Sudafed PE Sinus+Allergy Tablets[†]		Chlorpheniramine maleate 4mg		Phenylephrine HCl 10mg		**Adults & Peds ≥12 yrs:** 1 tab q4h. **Max:** 6 tabs/24h.
Triaminic Night Time Cold & Cough Syrup		Diphenhydramine HCl 6.25mg/5mL		Phenylephrine HCl 2.5mg/5mL		**Peds 6-<12 yrs:** 2 tsp (10mL) q4h. **Max:** 6 doses/24h.
Zyrtec-D Tablets		Cetirizine HCl 5mg		Pseudoephedrine HCl 120mg		**Adults <65 yrs & Peds ≥12 yrs:** 1 tab q12h. **Max:** 2 tabs/24h.
COUGH SUPPRESSANTS						
Children's Delsym 12 Hour Cough Relief Liquid[‡]			Dextromethorphan HBr 30mg/5mL			**Adults & Peds ≥12 yrs:** 2 tsp (10mL) q12h. **Max:** 4 tsp (20mL)/24h. **Peds 6-<12 yrs:** 1 tsp (5mL) q12h. **Max:** 2 tsp (10mL)/24h. **Peds 4-<6 yrs:** ½ tsp (2.5mL) q12h. **Max:** 1 tsp (5mL)/24h.
Children's Robitussin Cough Long-Acting Liquid			Dextromethorphan HBr 15mg/10mL			**Adults & Peds ≥12 yrs:** 4 tsp (20mL) q6-8h. **Peds 6-<12 yrs:** 2 tsp (10mL) q6-8h. **Max:** 4 doses/24h.
Delsym 12 Hour Cough Relief Liquid[‡]			Dextromethorphan HBr 30mg/5mL			**Adults & Peds ≥12 yrs:** 2 tsp (10mL) q12h. **Max:** 4 tsp (20mL)/24h. **Peds 6-<12 yrs:** 1 tsp (5mL) q12h. **Max:** 2 tsp (10mL)/24h. **Peds 4-<6 yrs:** ½ tsp (2.5mL) q12h. **Max:** 1 tsp (5mL)/24h.
Robitussin 12 Hour Cough Relief Liquid			Dextromethorphan HBr 30mg/5mL			**Adults & Peds ≥12 yrs:** 2 tsp (10mL) q12h. **Max:** 4 tsp (20mL)/24h. **Peds 6-<12 yrs:** 1 tsp (5mL) q12h. **Max:** 2 tsp (10mL)/24h. **Peds 4-<6 yrs:** ½ tsp (2.5mL) q12h. **Max:** 1 tsp (5mL)/24h.
Robitussin Lingering Cold Long-Acting CoughGels			Dextromethorphan HBr 15mg			**Adults & Peds ≥12 yrs:** 2 caps q6-8h. **Max:** 8 caps/24h.

BRAND NAME	ANALGESIC	ANTIHISTAMINE	COUGH SUPPRESSANT	DECONGESTANT	EXPECTORANT	DOSAGE
COUGH SUPPRESSANTS *(Continued)*						
Robitussin Lingering Cold Long-Acting Cough Liquid			Dextromethorphan HBr 30mg/10mL			**Adults & Peds ≥12 yrs:** 2 tsp (10mL) q6-8h. **Max:** 4 doses/24h.
Vicks DayQuil Cough Liquid			Dextromethorphan HBr 15mg/15mL			**Adults & Peds ≥12 yrs:** 2 tbl (30mL) q6-8h. **Peds 6-<12 yrs:** 1 tbl (15mL) q6-8h. **Max:** 4 doses/24h.
COUGH SUPPRESSANTS + DECONGESTANTS						
Children's Sudafed PE Cold & Cough Liquid			Dextromethorphan HBr 5mg/5mL	Phenylephrine HCl 2.5mg/5mL		**Peds 6-11 yrs:** 2 tsp (10mL) q4h. **Peds 4-5 yrs:** 1 tsp (5mL) q4h. **Max:** 6 doses/24h.
PediaCare Daytime Multi-Symptom Cold Liquid			Dextromethorphan HBr 5mg/5mL	Phenylephrine HCl 2.5mg/5mL		**Peds 6-11 yrs (48-95 lbs):** 2 tsp (10mL) q4h. **Peds 4-5 yrs (36-47 lbs):** 1 tsp (5mL) q4h. **Max:** 6 doses/24h.
Triaminic Day Time Cold & Cough Syrup			Dextromethorphan HBr 5mg/5mL	Phenylephrine HCl 2.5mg/5mL		**Peds 6-<12 yrs:** 2 tsp (10mL) q4h. **Peds 4-<6 yrs:** 1 tsp (5mL) q4h. **Max:** 6 doses/24h.
COUGH SUPPRESSANTS + DECONGESTANTS + EXPECTORANTS						
Children's Mucinex Congestion & Cough Liquid			Dextromethorphan HBr 5mg/5mL	Phenylephrine 2.5mg/5mL	Guaifenesin 100mg/5mL	**Peds 6-<12 yrs:** 2 tsp (10mL) q4h. **Peds 4-<6 yrs:** 1 tsp (5mL) q4h. **Max:** 6 doses/24h.
Children's Mucinex Multi-Symptom Cold Liquid			Dextromethorphan HBr 5mg/5mL	Phenylephrine 2.5mg/5mL	Guaifenesin 100mg/5mL	**Peds 6-<12 yrs:** 2 tsp (10mL) q4h. **Peds 4-<6 yrs:** 1 tsp (5mL) q4h. **Max:** 6 doses/24h.
Children's Robitussin Cough & Cold CF Liquid			Dextromethorphan HBr 10mg/10mL	Phenylephrine HCl 5mg/10mL	Guaifenesin 100mg/10mL	**Adults & Peds ≥12 yrs:** 4 tsp (20mL) q4h. **Peds 6-<12 yrs:** 2 tsp (10mL) q4h. **Max:** 6 doses/24h.
Maximum Strength Mucinex Fast-Max Severe Congestion & Cough Caplets			Dextromethorphan HBr 10mg	Phenylephrine HCl 5mg	Guaifenesin 200mg	**Adults & Peds ≥12 yrs:** 2 tabs q4h. **Max:** 12 tabs/24h.

(Continued)

BRAND NAME	ANALGESIC	ANTIHISTAMINE	COUGH SUPPRESSANT	DECONGESTANT	EXPECTORANT	DOSAGE
COUGH SUPPRESSANTS + DECONGESTANTS + EXPECTORANTS *(Continued)*						
Maximum Strength Mucinex Fast-Max Severe Congestion & Cough Liquid			Dextromethorphan HBr 20mg/20mL	Phenylephrine HCl 10mg/20mL	Guaifenesin 400mg/20mL	**Adults & Peds ≥12 yrs:** 4 tsp (20mL) q4h. **Max:** 6 doses/24h.
Robitussin Peak Cold Maximum Strength Multi-Symptom Cold CF Liquid			Dextromethorphan HBr 20mg/10mL	Phenylephrine HCl 10mg/10mL	Guaifenesin 400mg/10mL	**Adults & Peds ≥12 yrs:** 2 tsp (10mL) q4h. **Max:** 6 doses/24h.
Robitussin Peak Cold Multi-Symptom Cold CF Liquid			Dextromethorphan HBr 20mg/10mL	Phenylephrine HCl 10mg/10mL	Guaifenesin 200mg/10mL	**Adults & Peds ≥12 yrs:** 2 tsp (10mL) q4h. **Max:** 6 doses/24h.
COUGH SUPPRESSANTS + EXPECTORANTS						
Alka-Seltzer Plus Max Cough, Mucus & Congestion Liquid Gels			Dextromethorphan HBr 10mg		Guaifenesin 200mg	**Adults & Peds ≥12 yrs:** 2 caps q4h. **Max:** 12 caps/24h.
Children's Delsym Cough+ Chest Congestion DM Liquid			Dextromethorphan HBr 5mg/5mL		Guaifenesin 100mg/5mL	**Adults & Peds ≥12 yrs:** 2-4 tsp (10-20mL) q4h. **Peds 6-<12 yrs:** 1-2 tsp (5-10mL) q4h. **Peds 4-<6 yrs:** ½-1 tsp (2.5-5mL) q4h. **Max:** 6 doses/24h.
Children's Mucinex Cough Liquid			Dextromethorphan HBr 5mg/5mL		Guaifenesin 100mg/5mL	**Peds 6-<12 yrs:** 1-2 tsp (5-10mL) q4h. **Peds 4-<6 yrs:** ½-1 tsp (2.5-5mL) q4h. **Max:** 6 doses/24h.
Children's Mucinex Cough Mini-Melts			Dextromethorphan HBr 5mg/packet		Guaifenesin 100mg/packet	**Adults & Peds ≥12 yrs:** 2-4 pkts q4h. **Peds 6-<12 yrs:** 1-2 pkts q4h. **Peds 4-<6 yrs:** 1 pkt q4h. **Max:** 6 doses/24h.
Children's Robitussin Cough & Chest Congestion DM Liquid			Dextromethorphan HBr 5mg/5mL		Guaifenesin 100mg/5mL	**Adults & Peds ≥12 yrs:** 2-4 tsp (10-20mL) q4h. **Peds 6-<12 yrs:** 1-2 tsp (5-10mL) q4h. **Max:** 6 doses/24h.
Coricidin HBP Chest Congestion & Cough Softgels			Dextromethorphan HBr 10mg		Guaifenesin 200mg	**Adults & Peds ≥12 yrs:** 1-2 caps q4h. **Max:** 12 caps/24h.
Delsym Cough+ Chest Congestion DM Liquid			Dextromethorphan HBr 20mg/20mL		Guaifenesin 400mg/20mL	**Adults & Peds ≥12 yrs:** 4 tsp (20mL) q4h. **Max:** 6 doses/24h.

BRAND NAME	ANALGESIC	ANTIHISTAMINE	COUGH SUPPRESSANT	DECONGESTANT	EXPECTORANT	DOSAGE
COUGH SUPPRESSANTS + EXPECTORANTS *(Continued)*						
Maximum Strength Mucinex DM Tablets			Dextromethorphan HBr 60mg		Guaifenesin 1200mg	**Adults & Peds ≥12 yrs:** 1 tab q12h. **Max:** 2 tabs/24h.
Maximum Strength Mucinex Fast-Max DM Max Liquid			Dextromethorphan HBr 20mg/20mL		Guaifenesin 400mg/20mL	**Adults & Peds ≥12 yrs:** 4 tsp (20mL) q4h. **Max:** 6 doses/24h.
Mucinex DM Tablets			Dextromethorphan HBr 30mg		Guaifenesin 600mg	**Adults & Peds ≥12 yrs:** 1-2 tabs q12h. **Max:** 4 tabs/24h
PediaCare Cough & Congestion Liquid			Dextromethorphan HBr 5mg/5mL		Guaifenesin 100mg/5mL	**Peds 6-11 yrs (48-95 lbs):** 1-2 tsp (5-10mL). **Peds 4-6 yrs (36-47 lbs):** ½-1 tsp (2.5-5mL). **Max:** 6 doses/24h.
Robitussin Maximum Strength Cough + Chest Congestion DM Liquid			Dextromethorphan HBr 20mg/10mL		Guaifenesin 400mg/10mL	**Adults & Peds ≥12 yrs:** 2 tsp (10mL) q4h. **Max:** 6 doses/24h.
Robitussin Maximum Strength Cough + Chest Congestion DM Liquid-Filled Capsules			Dextromethorphan HBr 10mg		Guaifenesin 200mg	**Adults & Peds ≥12 yrs:** 2 caps q4h. **Max:** 12 caps/24h.
Robitussin Peak Cold Cough + Chest Congestion DM Liquid			Dextromethorphan HBr 20mg/10mL		Guaifenesin 200mg/10mL	**Adults & Peds ≥12 yrs:** 2 tsp (10mL) q4h. **Max:** 6 doses/24h.
Robitussin Peak Cold Maximum Strength Cough + Chest Congestion DM Liquid			Dextromethorphan HBr 20mg/10mL		Guaifenesin 400mg/10mL	**Adults & Peds ≥12 yrs:** 2 tsp (10mL) q4h. **Max:** 6 doses/24h.
Robitussin Peak Cold Sugar-Free Cough + Chest Congestion DM Liquid			Dextromethorphan HBr 20mg/10mL		Guaifenesin 200mg/10mL	**Adults & Peds ≥12 yrs:** 2 tsp (10mL) q4h. **Max:** 6 doses/24h.
Triaminic Cough & Congestion Syrup			Dextromethorphan HBr 5mg/5mL		Guaifenesin 100mg/5mL	**Peds 6-<12 yrs:** 1-2 tsp (5-10mL) q4h. **Peds 4-<6 yrs:** ½-1 tsp (2.5-5mL) q4h. **Max:** 6 doses/24h.
Vicks DayQuil Cough & Congestion Liquid			Dextromethorphan HBr 10mg/15mL		Guaifenesin 200mg/15mL	**Adults & Peds ≥12 yrs:** 2 tbl (30mL) q4h. **Peds 6-<12 yrs:** 1 tbl (15mL) q4h. **Max:** 6 doses/24h.

(Continued)

BRAND NAME	ANALGESIC	ANTIHISTAMINE	COUGH SUPPRESSANT	DECONGESTANT	EXPECTORANT	DOSAGE
DECONGESTANTS[§]						
Children's Sudafed Nasal Decongestant Liquid				Pseudoephedrine HCl 15mg/5mL		**Peds 6-11 yrs:** 2 tsp (10mL) q4-6h. **Peds 4-5 yrs:** 1 tsp (5mL) q4-6h. **Max:** 4 doses/24h.
Children's Sudafed PE Nasal Decongestant Liquid				Phenylephrine HCl 2.5mg/5mL		**Peds 6-11 yrs:** 2 tsp (10mL) q4h. **Peds 4-5 yrs:** 1 tsp (5mL) q4h. **Max:** 6 doses/24h.
Sudafed 12 Hour Tablets				Pseudoephedrine HCl 120mg		**Adults & Peds ≥12 yrs:** 1 tab q12h. **Max:** 2 tabs/24h.
Sudafed 24 Hour Tablets				Pseudoephedrine HCl 240mg		**Adults & Peds ≥12 yrs:** 1 tab/24h. **Max:** 1 tab/24h.
Sudafed Congestion Tablets				Pseudoephedrine HCl 30mg		**Adults & Peds ≥12 yrs:** 2 tabs q4-6h. **Max:** 8 tabs/24h. **Peds 6-11 yrs:** 1 tab q4-6h. **Max:** 4 tabs/24h.
Sudafed PE Congestion Tablets				Phenylephrine HCl 10mg		**Adults & Peds ≥12 yrs:** 1 tab q4h. **Max:** 6 tabs/24h.
DECONGESTANTS + EXPECTORANTS						
Children's Mucinex Stuffy Nose & Cold Liquid				Phenylephrine HCl 2.5mg/5mL	Guaifenesin 100mg/5mL	**Peds 6-<12 yrs:** 2 tsp (10mL) q4h. **Peds 4-<6 yrs:** 1 tsp (5mL) q4h. **Max:** 6 doses/24h.
Maximum Strength Mucinex D Tablets				Pseudoephedrine HCl 120mg	Guaifenesin 1200mg	**Adults & Peds ≥12 yrs:** 1 tab q12h. **Max:** 2 tabs/24h.
Mucinex D Tablets				Pseudoephedrine HCl 60mg	Guaifenesin 600mg	**Adults & Peds ≥12 yrs:** 2 tabs q12h. **Max:** 4 tabs/24h.
Sudafed PE Non-Drying Sinus Caplets[†]				Phenylephrine HCl 5mg	Guaifenesin 200mg	**Adults & Peds ≥12 yrs:** 2 tabs q4h. **Max:** 12 tabs/24h.
EXPECTORANTS						
Children's Mucinex Chest Congestion Liquid					Guaifenesin 100mg/5mL	**Peds 6-<12 yrs:** 1-2 tsp (5-10mL) q4h. **Peds 4-<6 yrs:** ½-1 tsp (2.5-5mL) q4h. **Max:** 6 doses/24h.

BRAND NAME	ANALGESIC	ANTIHISTAMINE	COUGH SUPPRESSANT	DECONGESTANT	EXPECTORANT	DOSAGE
EXPECTORANTS *(Continued)*						
Children's Mucinex Chest Congestion Mini-Melts					Guaifenesin 100mg/packet	**Adults & Peds ≥12 yrs:** 2-4 pkts q4h. **Peds 6-<12 yrs:** 1-2 pkts q4h. **Peds 4-<6 yrs:** 1 pkt q4h. **Max:** 6 doses/24h.
Maximum Strength Mucinex Tablets					Guaifenesin 1200mg	**Adults & Peds ≥12 yrs:** 1 tab q12h. **Max:** 2 tabs/24h.
Mucinex Tablets					Guaifenesin 600mg	**Adults & Peds ≥12 yrs:** 1-2 tabs q12h. **Max:** 4 tabs/24h.
Robitussin Mucus + Chest Congestion Liquid					Guaifenesin 200mg/10mL	**Adults & Peds ≥12 yrs:** 2-4 tsp (10-20mL) q4h. **Max:** 6 doses/24h.
MISCELLANEOUS[¶]						
Vicks BabyRub Soothing Ointment						**Peds ≥3 months:** Gently massage on the chest, neck, and back to help soothe and comfort.
Vicks VapoDrops[‡]						**Adults & Peds ≥5 yrs:** 3 drops (cherry) or 2 drops (menthol) in the mouth.
Vicks VapoRub Ointment						**Adults & Peds ≥2 yrs:** Rub on chest and throat. **Max:** 3-4 times/24h.
Vicks VapoSteam (For use in a hot steam vaporizer)						**Adults & Peds ≥2 yrs:** 1 tbl per quart of water or 1½ tsp per pint of water. **Max:** 3 times/24h.

*Fully dissolve tablets in 4 oz of water.

[†]Product currently on recall or temporarily unavailable from manufacturer, but generic forms may be available.

[‡]Multiple flavors available.

[§]Refer to *Nasal Preparations* table for additional decongestants.

[¶]Refer to packaging for ingredients.

NASAL PREPARATIONS

BRAND	INGREDIENT(S)/STRENGTH(S)	DOSAGE
GLUCOCORTICOIDS		
Flonase Allergy Relief Spray	Fluticasone propionate 50mcg	**Adults & Peds ≥12 yrs:** 2 sprays per nostril qd during week 1. 1 or 2 sprays per nostril qd during week 2 through 6 months. **Peds 4-11 yrs:** 1 spray per nostril qd.
Nasacort Allergy 24HR Spray	Triamcinolone acetonide 55mcg	**Adults & Peds ≥12 yrs:** 2 sprays per nostril qd. Reduce to 1 spray per nostril qd once symptoms improve. **Peds 6-<12 yrs:** 1 spray per nostril qd; increase to 2 sprays per nostril qd if symptoms do not improve. Reduce to 1 spray per nostril qd once symptoms improve. **Peds 2-<6 yrs:** 1 spray per nostril qd.
Rhinocort Allergy Spray	Budesonide 32mcg	**Adults & Peds ≥12 yrs:** 2 sprays per nostril qd. Reduce to 1 spray per nostril qd once symptoms improve. **Peds 6-<12 yrs:** 1 spray per nostril qd; increase to 2 sprays per nostril qd if symptoms do not improve. Reduce to 1 spray per nostril qd once symptoms improve.
NASAL DECONGESTANTS		
Afrin NoDrip Extra Moisturizing Pump Mist	Oxymetazoline HCl 0.05%	**Adults & Peds ≥6 yrs:** 2-3 sprays per nostril not more than q10-12h. **Max:** 2 doses q24h.*
Afrin NoDrip Original Pump Mist	Oxymetazoline HCl 0.05%	**Adults & Peds ≥6 yrs:** 2-3 sprays per nostril not more than q10-12h. **Max:** 2 doses q24h.*
Afrin NoDrip Severe Congestion Pump Mist	Oxymetazoline HCl 0.05%	**Adults & Peds ≥6 yrs:** 2-3 sprays per nostril not more than q10-12h. **Max:** 2 doses q24h.*
Afrin NoDrip Sinus Pump Mist	Oxymetazoline HCl 0.05%	**Adults & Peds ≥6 yrs:** 2-3 sprays per nostril not more than q10-12h. **Max:** 2 doses q24h.*
Afrin Original Nasal Spray	Oxymetazoline HCl 0.05%	**Adults & Peds ≥6 yrs:** 2-3 sprays per nostril not more than q10-12h. **Max:** 2 doses q24h.*
Afrin Original Pump Mist	Oxymetazoline HCl 0.05%	**Adults & Peds ≥6 yrs:** 2-3 sprays per nostril not more than q10-12h. **Max:** 2 doses q24h.*
Afrin Severe Congestion Nasal Spray	Oxymetazoline HCl 0.05%	**Adults & Peds ≥6 yrs:** 2-3 sprays per nostril not more than q10-12h. **Max:** 2 doses q24h.*
Afrin Sinus Nasal Spray	Oxymetazoline HCl 0.05%	**Adults & Peds ≥6 yrs:** 2-3 sprays per nostril not more than q10-12h. **Max:** 2 doses q24h.*
Benzedrex Inhaler	Propylhexedrine 250mg	**Adults & Peds ≥6 yrs:** 2 inhalations per nostril not more than q2h.*
Dristan 12-Hr Nasal Spray	Oxymetazoline HCl 0.05%	**Adults & Peds ≥12 yrs:** 2-3 sprays per nostril not more than q10-12h. **Max:** 2 doses q24h.*
Little Remedies Decongestant Nose Drops	Phenylephrine HCl 0.125%	**Peds 2-<6 yrs:** 2-3 drops per nostril not more than q4h.*
Mucinex Sinus-Max Full Force Nasal Spray	Oxymetazoline HCl 0.05%	**Adults & Peds ≥6 yrs:** 2-3 sprays per nostril not more than q10-12h. **Max:** 2 doses q24h.*
Mucinex Sinus-Max Moisture Smart Nasal Spray	Oxymetazoline HCl 0.05%	**Adults & Peds ≥6 yrs:** 2-3 sprays per nostril not more than q10-12h. **Max:** 2 doses q24h.*
NeilMed Sinu Inhaler	Levmetamfetamine 50mg	**Adults & Peds ≥12 yrs:** 2 inhalations per nostril not more than q2h.† **Peds 6-<12 yrs:** 1 inhalation per nostril not more than q2h.†
NeilMed SinuFrin Nasal Spray	Oxymetazoline HCl 0.05%	**Adults & Peds ≥6 yrs:** 2 sprays per nostril not more than q10-12h. **Max:** 2 doses q24h.*
NeilMed SinuFrin Plus Moisturizing Gel	Oxymetazoline HCl 0.05%	**Adults & Peds ≥6 yrs:** 2 sprays per nostril not more than q10-12h. **Max:** 2 doses q24h.*

(Continued)

BRAND	INGREDIENT(S)/STRENGTH(S)	DOSAGE
NASAL DECONGESTANTS *(Continued)*		
Neo-Synephrine Cold & Sinus Extra Strength Nasal Spray	Phenylephrine HCl 1%	**Adults & Peds ≥12 yrs:** 2-3 sprays per nostril not more than q4h.*
Neo-Synephrine Cold & Sinus Mild Strength Nasal Spray	Phenylephrine HCl 0.25%	**Adults & Peds ≥6 yrs:** 2-3 sprays per nostril not more than q4h.*
Neo-Synephrine Cold & Sinus Regular Strength Nasal Spray	Phenylephrine HCl 0.5%	**Adults & Peds ≥12 yrs:** 2-3 sprays per nostril not more than q4h.*
Nostrilla Original Fast Relief Nasal Spray	Oxymetazoline HCl 0.05%	**Adults & Peds ≥6 yrs:** 2-3 sprays per nostril not more than q10-12h. **Max:** 2 doses q24h.*
Privine Nasal Drops	Naphazoline HCl 0.05%	**Adults & Peds ≥12 yrs:** 1-2 drops per nostril not more than q6h.*
QlearQuil 12 Hour Nasal Decongestant Moisturizing Nasal Spray	Oxymetazoline HCl 0.05%	**Adults & Peds ≥6 yrs:** 2-3 sprays per nostril not more than q10-12h. **Max:** 2 doses q24h.*
Vicks Sinex 12-Hour Decongestant Nasal Spray	Oxymetazoline HCl 0.05%	**Adults & Peds ≥6 yrs:** 2-3 sprays per nostril not more than q10-12h. **Max:** 2 doses q24h.*
Vicks Sinex 12-Hour Decongestant UltraFine Mist Moisturizing Nasal Spray	Oxymetazoline HCl 0.05%	**Adults & Peds ≥6 yrs:** 2-3 sprays per nostril not more than q10-12h. **Max:** 2 doses q24h.*
Vicks Sinex 12-Hour Decongestant UltraFine Mist Nasal Spray	Oxymetazoline HCl 0.05%	**Adults & Peds ≥6 yrs:** 2-3 sprays per nostril not more than q10-12h. **Max:** 2 doses q24h.*
Zicam Extreme Congestion Relief Nasal Gel	Oxymetazoline HCl 0.05%	**Adults & Peds ≥6 yrs:** 2-3 sprays per nostril not more than q10-12h. **Max:** 2 doses q24h.*
Zicam Intense Sinus Relief Nasal Gel	Oxymetazoline HCl 0.05%	**Adults & Peds ≥6 yrs:** 2-3 sprays per nostril not more than q10-12h. **Max:** 2 doses q24h.*
NASAL MOISTURIZERS		
Ayr Allergy & Sinus Hypertonic Saline Nasal Mist	Sodium chloride 2.65%‡	**Adults & Peds:** 2 sprays per nostril bid-tid prn.
Ayr Saline Nasal Drops	Sodium chloride 0.65%	**Adults & Peds:** 2-6 drops per nostril prn.
Ayr Saline Nasal Gel	Sodium chloride‡	**Adults & Peds:** Apply around nostrils and under nose during the day and hs prn.
Ayr Saline Nasal Gel No-Drip Sinus Spray	Sodium chloride‡	**Adults & Peds:** 1 spray per nostril prn.
Ayr Saline Nasal Mist	Sodium chloride 0.65%‡	**Adults & Peds:** Use ud.
Ayr Saline Nasal Neti Rinse Kit	Sodium chloride‡	**Adults & Peds ≥6 yrs:** Use qd-bid or ud.
Ayr Saline Nasal Rinse Kit & Refills	Sodium chloride‡	**Adults & Peds ≥6 yrs:** Use qd-bid or ud.
Baby Ayr Saline Nose Spray/ Drops	Sodium chloride 0.65%‡	**Peds:** 2-6 drops/sprays per nostril.
Little Remedies Saline Spray/ Drops	Sodium chloride‡	**Adults & Peds:** 2-6 drops/sprays per nostril prn or ud.
Little Remedies Sterile Saline Nasal Mist	Sodium chloride	**Adults & Peds:** 1-3 short sprays per nostril.
Little Remedies Stuffy Nose Kit	Sodium chloride‡	**Adults & Peds:** 2-6 drops/sprays per nostril prn or ud.
NeilMed NasaMist Extra Strength Nasal Spray	Sodium chloride 2.7%	**Adults & Peds ≥6 months:** Spray into each nostril prn.
NeilMed NasaMist Nasal Spray	Sodium chloride	**Adults & Peds ≥1 yr:** Use ud.
NeilMed NasoGel Spray	Sodium chloride‡	**Adults & Peds:** 1-2 sprays per nostril q4-6h.
Ocean Complete Sinus Rinse	Sodium chloride‡	**Adults & Peds:** Use ud.

BRAND	INGREDIENT(S)/STRENGTH(S)	DOSAGE
NASAL MOISTURIZERS *(Continued)*		
Ocean Gel Nasal Moisturizer	Purified water, Glycerin, Carbomer 940, Trolamine, Hyaluronan, Methylparaben, Propylparaben	**Adults & Peds:** Apply to affected areas in and around the nose prn.
Ocean for Kids Saline Nasal Spray	Sodium chloride 0.65%‡	**Peds:** 2 sprays/drops per nostril prn.
Ocean Saline Nasal Spray	Sodium chloride 0.65%‡	**Adults & Peds:** 2 sprays/drops per nostril prn.
Simply Saline Allergy & Sinus Relief	Sodium chloride‡	**Adults:** Spray into each nostril prn.
Simply Saline Baby Nasal Moisturizer plus Aloe Vera§	Sodium chloride‡	**Peds:** Apply around the nose prn.
Simply Saline Baby Nasal Relief	Sodium chloride 0.9%‡	**Peds:** Spray into each nostril prn.
Simply Saline Baby Swabs	Sodium chloride‡	**Peds:** Apply in nostrils prn.
Simply Saline Extra Strength Nighttime Formula plus Eucalyptus	Sodium chloride‡	**Adults & Peds ≥2 yrs:** Spray into each nostril hs prn.
Simply Saline Nasal Relief	Sodium chloride 0.9%‡	**Adults & Peds:** Spray into each nostril prn.
Simply Saline Neti Pot Kit§	Sodium chloride‡	**Adults & Peds ≥5 yrs:** Use qd-bid or ud.
MISCELLANEOUS		
NasalCrom Nasal Allergy Spray	Cromolyn sodium 5.2mg	**Adults & Peds ≥2 yrs:** 1 spray per nostril q4-6h. **Max:** 6 doses q24h.
Similasan Nasal Allergy Relief Nasal Mist	*Cardiospermum* 6X, *Galphimia glauca* 6X, *Luffa operculata* 6X, *Sabadilla* 6X	**Adults & Peds:** 1-3 sprays per nostril prn.
Similasan Sinus Relief Nasal Mist	Kalium bichromicum 6X, *Luffa operculata* 6X, *Sabadilla* 6X	**Adults & Peds:** 1-3 sprays per nostril prn.
Simply Saline Children's Cold Formula plus Moisturizers Nasal Mist	*Luffa operculata* 6X, *Sabadilla* 6X	**Adults & Peds ≥2 yrs:** Use prn.†
Simply Saline Cold Formula plus Menthol Nasal Mist§	*Luffa operculata* 6X, *Sabadilla* 6X	**Adults & Peds ≥2 yrs:** Use prn.†
SinoFresh Nasal & Sinus Care Nasal Spray	*Eucalyptus globulus* 20X, Kalium bichromicum 30X	**Adults & Peds ≥12 yrs:** 1-2 sprays per nostril in the morning and evening.
Zicam Allergy Relief Nasal Gel	*Luffa operculata* (4X, 12X, 30X), *Galphimia glauca* (12X, 30X), Histaminum hydrochloricum (12X, 30X, 200X), Sulphur (12X, 30X, 200X)	**Adults & Peds ≥12 yrs:** 1 pump per nostril q4h.
Zicam Gentle Allergy Relief Nasal Swabs	*Galphimia glauca* (12X, 30X), Histaminum hydrochloricum (12X, 30X, 200X), *Luffa operculata* (4X, 12X, 30X), Sulphur (12X, 30X, 200X)	**Adults & Peds ≥12 yrs:** Apply in nostrils q4h.
Zicam Cold Remedy Nasal Spray	*Galphimia glauca* 4X, *Luffa operculata* 4X, *Sabadilla* 4X	**Adults and Peds ≥12 yrs:** 2 pumps per nostril q3h. **Max:** 5 doses q24h.†
Zicam Cold Remedy Nasal Swabs	*Galphimia glauca* 4X, *Luffa operculata* 4X, *Sabadilla* 4X	**Adults & Peds ≥12 yrs:** Apply in nostrils q3h. **Max:** 5 tubes/24h.

*Do not use for more than 3 days.

†Do not use for more than 7 days.

‡This product contains multiple ingredients. Please check product label for a complete list of ingredients.

§Product currently on recall or temporarily unavailable from manufacturer, but generic forms may be available.

ASPIRIN PRODUCTS

BRAND	INGREDIENT(S)/STRENGTH(S)	DOSAGE
SALICYLATES		
Bayer Aspirin Extra Strength Caplets	Aspirin 500mg	**Adults & Peds ≥12 yrs:** 1-2 tabs q4-6h. **Max:** 8 tabs/24h.
Bayer Aspirin Safety Coated Caplets	Aspirin 325mg	**Adults & Peds ≥12 yrs:** 1-2 tabs q4h. **Max:** 12 tabs/24h.
Bayer Genuine Aspirin Tablets	Aspirin 325mg	**Adults & Peds ≥12 yrs:** 1-2 tabs q4h or 3 tabs q6h. **Max:** 12 tabs/24h.
Bayer Low Dose Aspirin Chewable Tablets*	Aspirin 81mg	**Adults & Peds ≥12 yrs:** 4-8 tabs q4h. **Max:** 48 tabs/24h.
Bayer Low Dose Aspirin Safety Coated Tablets	Aspirin 81mg	**Adults & Peds ≥12 yrs:** 4-8 tabs q4h. **Max:** 48 tabs/24h.
Ecotrin Low Strength Tablets	Aspirin 81mg	**Adults & Peds ≥12 yrs:** 4-8 tabs q4h prn. **Max:** 48 tabs/24h.
Ecotrin Regular Strength Tablets	Aspirin 325mg	**Adults & Peds ≥12 yrs:** 1-2 tabs q4h prn. **Max:** 12 tabs/24h.
St. Joseph Aspirin Chewable Tablets	Aspirin 81mg	**Adults & Peds ≥12 yrs:** 4-8 tabs q4h. **Max:** 48 tabs/24h.
St. Joseph Rapid Dissolving Melts	Aspirin 81mg	**Adults & Peds ≥12 yrs:** 4-8 tabs q4h. **Max:** 48 tabs/24h.
St. Joseph Regular Strength Safety Coated Tablets	Aspirin 325mg	**Adults & Peds ≥12 yrs:** 1-2 tabs q4h prn. **Max:** 12 tabs/24h.
St. Joseph Safety Coated Low Dose Tablets	Aspirin 81mg	**Adults & Peds ≥12 yrs:** 4-8 tabs q4h. **Max:** 48 tabs/24h.
UrgentRx Critical Care Aspirin To-Go Powder	Aspirin 325mg	**Adults & Peds ≥12 yrs:** Place 1-2 powders on tongue q4-6h prn. Swallow with or without water. **Max:** 8 powders/24h.
SALICYLATES, BUFFERED		
Alka-Seltzer Extra Strength Effervescent Tablets	Aspirin/Citric acid/Sodium bicarbonate 500mg-1000mg-1985mg	**Adults ≥60 yrs:** 2 tabs dissolved in 4 oz water q6h. **Max:** 3 tabs/24h. **Adults & Peds ≥12 yrs:** 2 tabs dissolved in 4 oz water q6h. **Max:** 7 tabs/24h.
Alka-Seltzer Lemon Lime Effervescent Tablets	Aspirin/Citric acid/Sodium bicarbonate 325mg-1000mg-1700mg	**Adults ≥60 yrs:** 2 tabs dissolved in 4 oz water q4h. **Max:** 4 tabs/24h. **Adults & Peds ≥12 yrs:** 2 tabs dissolved in 4 oz water q4h. **Max:** 8 tabs/24h.
Alka-Seltzer Original Effervescent Tablets	Aspirin/Citric acid/Sodium bicarbonate 325mg-1000mg-1916mg	**Adults ≥60 yrs:** 2 tabs dissolved in 4 oz water q4h. **Max:** 4 tabs/24h. **Adults & Peds ≥12 yrs:** 2 tabs dissolved in 4 oz water q4h. **Max:** 8 tabs/24h.
Bayer Aspirin Extra Strength Plus Caplets	Aspirin 500mg buffered with Calcium carbonate	**Adults & Peds ≥12 yrs:** 1-2 tabs q4-6h. **Max:** 8 tabs/24h.
Bayer Women's Low Dose Aspirin Caplets	Aspirin 81mg buffered with Calcium carbonate 777mg	**Adults & Peds ≥12 yrs:** 4-8 tabs q4h. **Max:** 10 tabs/24h.
Bufferin Tablets	Aspirin 325mg buffered with Calcium carbonate/Magnesium carbonate/Magnesium oxide	**Adults & Peds ≥12 yrs:** 2 tabs q4h prn. **Max:** 12 tabs/24h.
SALICYLATE COMBINATIONS		
Anacin Max Strength Tablets	Aspirin/Caffeine 500mg-32mg	**Adults & Peds ≥12 yrs:** 2 tabs q6h. **Max:** 8 tabs/24h.
Anacin Tablets	Aspirin/Caffeine 400mg-32mg	**Adults & Peds ≥12 yrs:** 2 tabs q6h. **Max:** 8 tabs/24h.

(Continued)

BRAND	INGREDIENT(S)/STRENGTH(S)	DOSAGE
SALICYLATE COMBINATIONS *(Continued)*		
Bayer Back & Body Extra Strength Caplets	Aspirin/Caffeine 500mg-32.5mg	**Adults & Peds ≥12 yrs:** 2 tabs q6h. **Max:** 8 tabs/24h.
BC Arthritis Strength Powder	Aspirin/Caffeine 1000mg-65mg per powder	**Adults & Peds ≥12 yrs:** Place 1 powder on tongue q6h prn. May stir powder into glass of water. **Max:** 4 powders/24h.
BC Powder*	Aspirin/Caffeine 845mg-65mg per powder	**Adults & Peds ≥12 yrs:** Place 1 powder on tongue q6h prn. May stir powder into glass of water. **Max:** 4 powders/24h.
Excedrin Extra Strength Caplets	Acetaminophen/Aspirin/Caffeine 250mg-250mg-65mg	**Adults & Peds ≥12 yrs:** 2 tabs q6h. **Max:** 8 tabs/24h.
Excedrin Migraine Caplets	Acetaminophen/Aspirin/Caffeine 250mg-250mg-65mg	**Adults:** 2 tabs prn. **Max:** 2 tabs/24h.
Goody's Back & Body Pain Powder	Acetaminophen/Aspirin 325mg-500mg	**Adults & Peds ≥12 yrs:** Place 1 powder on tongue q6h prn. May stir powder into glass of water. **Max:** 4 powders/24h.
Goody's Cool Orange Extra Strength Headache Powder	Acetaminophen/Aspirin/Caffeine 325mg-500mg-65mg	**Adults & Peds ≥12 yrs:** Place 1 powder on tongue q6h prn. May stir powder into glass of water. **Max:** 4 powders/24h.
Goody's Extra Strength Caplets	Acetaminophen/Aspirin/Caffeine 250mg-250mg-65mg	**Adults & Peds ≥12 yrs:** 2 tabs q6h. **Max:** 8 tabs/24h.
Goody's Extra Strength Headache Powder	Acetaminophen/Aspirin/Caffeine 260mg-520mg-32.5mg	**Adults & Peds ≥12 yrs:** Place 1 powder on tongue q6h prn. May stir powder into glass of water. **Max:** 4 powders/24h.
UrgentRx Ache & Pain Relief To-Go Powder	Aspirin/Caffeine 650mg-60mg	**Adults & Peds ≥12 yrs:** Place 1 powder on tongue q4-6h prn. Swallow with or without water. **Max:** 4 powders/24h.
SALICYLATES/SLEEP AIDS		
Excedrin PM Headache Caplets	Acetaminophen/Aspirin/Diphenhydramine citrate 250mg-250mg-38mg	**Adults and Peds ≥12 yrs:** 2 tabs hs. **Max:** 2 tabs/24h.

*Multiple flavors available.

ANGINA TREATMENT OPTIONS

GENERIC (BRAND)	HOW SUPPLIED	DOSAGE	RENAL/HEPATIC DOSAGE ADJUSTMENT
BETA BLOCKERS			
Atenolol (Tenormin)	**Tab:** 25mg, 50mg, 100mg	**Initial:** 50mg qd. **Titrate:** May increase to 100mg qd after 1 week. **Max:** 200mg qd.	Renal
Metoprolol succinate (Toprol-XL)	**Tab, ER:** 25mg, 50mg, 100mg, 200mg	**Initial:** 100mg qd. **Titrate:** May gradually increase weekly until optimum response is achieved or there is pronounced slowing of HR. **Max:** 400mg/day. Reduce dose gradually over 1-2 weeks if to be d/c.	Hepatic
Metoprolol tartrate (Lopressor)	**Tab:** (Lopressor) 50mg, 100mg; (generic) 25mg, 50mg, 100mg	**Initial:** 100mg/day in 2 divided doses. **Titrate:** May gradually increase weekly until optimum response is achieved or there is pronounced slowing of HR. **Effective Range:** 100-400mg/day. **Max:** 400mg/day. Reduce dose gradually over 1-2 weeks if to be d/c.	Hepatic
Nadolol (Corgard)	**Tab:** 20mg, 40mg, 80mg	**Initial:** 40mg qd. **Titrate:** May gradually increase in 40-80mg increments at 3- to 7-day intervals until optimum response is achieved or there is pronounced slowing of HR. **Maint: Usual:** 40 or 80mg qd. Doses up to 160 or 240mg qd may be needed. **Max:** 240mg/day. Reduce dose gradually over 1-2 weeks if to be d/c.	Renal
Propranolol HCl	**Sol:** 20mg/5mL, 40mg/5mL; **Tab:** 10mg, 20mg, 40mg, 60mg, 80mg	80-320mg/day given bid-qid. Reduce dose gradually over several weeks if to be d/c.	
Propranolol HCl (Inderal LA)	**Cap, ER:** 60mg, 80mg, 120mg, 160mg	**Initial:** 80mg qd. **Titrate:** May gradually increase at 3- to 7-day intervals until optimum response is achieved. **Maint:** 160mg qd. **Max:** 320mg/day. Reduce dose gradually over a few weeks if to be d/c.	
CALCIUM CHANNEL BLOCKERS (DIHYDROPYRIDINES)			
Amlodipine besylate (Norvasc)	**Tab:** 2.5mg, 5mg, 10mg	**Usual:** 5-10mg qd.	Hepatic
Nicardipine	**Cap:** 20mg, 30mg	**Initial:** 20mg tid. **Titrate:** Allow at least 3 days before increasing dose. **Effective Range:** 20-40mg tid.	Renal/Hepatic
Nifedipine (Procardia)	**Cap:** 10mg	**Initial:** 10mg tid. **Usual Effective Range:** 10-20mg tid. **Max:** 180mg/day.	
Nifedipine (Procardia XL)	**Tab, ER:** 30mg, 60mg, 90mg	**Initial:** 30 or 60mg qd. **Titrate:** Increase over a 1- to 2-week period (usual), but may proceed more rapidly if symptoms warrant. **Max:** 120mg/day.	
CALCIUM CHANNEL BLOCKERS (NON-DIHYDROPYRIDINES)			
Diltiazem HCl (Cardizem CD, Cartia XT)	**Cap, ER:** (Cardizem CD/ Cartia XT) 120mg, 180mg, 240mg, 300mg; (Cardizem CD) 360mg	**Initial:** 120mg or 180mg qd. **Titrate:** Increase over a 1- to 2-week period when necessary. **Max:** 480mg qd.	
Diltiazem HCl (Cardizem LA)	**Tab, ER:** 120mg, 180mg, 240mg, 300mg, 360mg, 420mg	**Initial:** 180mg qd (am or hs). **Titrate:** Increase at 1- to 2-week intervals if adequate response is not achieved. **Max:** 360mg.	

(Continued)

GENERIC (BRAND)	HOW SUPPLIED	DOSAGE	RENAL/HEPATIC DOSAGE ADJUSTMENT
CALCIUM CHANNEL BLOCKERS (NON-DIHYDROPYRIDINES) *(Continued)*			
Diltiazem HCl (Cardizem)	**Tab:** (Cardizem) 30mg, 60mg, 120mg; (generic) 30mg, 60mg, 90mg, 120mg	**Initial:** 30mg qid (before meals and hs). **Titrate:** Increase gradually (given in divided doses tid-qid) at 1- to 2-day intervals until optimum response obtained. **Usual:** 180-360mg/day.	
Diltiazem HCl (Taztia XT, Tiazac)	**Cap, ER:** (Taztia XT) 120mg, 180mg, 240mg, 300mg, 360mg; (Tiazac) 120mg, 180mg, 240mg, 300mg, 360mg, 420mg	**Initial:** 120-180mg qd. **Titrate:** Increase over 1-2 weeks when necessary. **Max:** 540mg qd.	
Verapamil HCl (Calan)	**Tab:** 40mg, 80mg, 120mg	**Usual:** 80-120mg tid. Upward titration should be based on therapeutic efficacy and safety evaluated approximately 8 hrs after dosing. **Titrate:** May increase daily (eg, patients with unstable angina) or weekly, until optimum response is obtained.	Hepatic
Verapamil HCl (Covera-HS)	**Tab, ER:** 180mg, 240mg	**Initial:** 180mg qhs. **Titrate:** If inadequate response with 180mg, increase to 240mg qhs, then 360mg (two 180mg tab) qhs, then 480mg (two 240mg tab) qhs.	Hepatic
CALCIUM CHANNEL BLOCKERS/HMG COA REDUCTASE INHIBITORS			
Amlodipine besylate-Atorvastatin calcium (Caduet)	**Tab:** 2.5-10mg, 2.5-20mg, 2.5-40mg, 5-10mg, 5-20mg, 5-40mg, 5-80mg, 10-10mg, 10-20mg, 10-40mg, 10-80mg	5-10mg qd amlodipine; 10-80mg qd atorvastatin.	Hepatic
COAGULATION MODIFIERS			
Abciximab (ReoPro)	**Inj:** 2mg/mL	0.25mg/kg IV bolus followed by 10mcg/min infusion for 18-24 hrs, concluding 1 hr after PCI.	
Bivalirudin (Angiomax)	**Inj:** 250mg	Give with ASA (300-325mg/day). **Patients Without HIT/HITTS:** 0.75mg/kg IV bolus, then 1.75mg/kg/hr infusion for the duration of the PCI/PTCA procedure. An activated clotting time should be performed 5 min after the bolus dose and an additional 0.3mg/kg bolus should be given if needed. **Patients With HIT/HITTS:** 0.75mg/kg IV bolus, then 1.75mg/kg/hr infusion for the duration of the procedure. **Ongoing Treatment Post-Procedure:** Continuation of infusion following PCI/PTCA for up to 4 hrs post-procedure is optional. After 4 hrs, an additional infusion may be initiated at a rate of 0.2mg/kg/hr (low-rate infusion), for up to 20 hrs, if needed.	Renal
Clopidogrel bisulfate (Plavix)	**Tab:** 75mg, 300mg	**LD:** 300mg. **Maint:** 75mg qd. Initiate ASA (75-325mg qd) and continue in combination with clopidogrel.	

GENERIC (BRAND)	HOW SUPPLIED	DOSAGE	RENAL/HEPATIC DOSAGE ADJUSTMENT
COAGULATION MODIFIERS *(Continued)*			
Dalteparin sodium (Fragmin)	**Inj:** (Syringe) 2500 IU/0.2mL, 5000 IU/0.2mL, 7500 IU/0.3mL, 10,000 IU/1mL, 12,500 IU/0.5mL, 15,000 IU/0.6mL, 18,000 IU/0.72mL; (MDV) 95,000 IU/3.8mL	**Prophylaxis of Ischemic Complications in Unstable Angina:** 120 IU/kg q12h with PO ASA (75-165mg qd) until clinically stabilized. **Usual Duration:** 5-8 days. **Max:** 10,000 IU q12h.	Renal
Enoxaparin (Lovenox)	**Inj:** [100mg/mL] (Prefilled Syringe) 30mg/0.3mL, 40mg/0.4mL; (Graduated Prefilled Syringe) 60mg/0.6mL, 80mg/0.8mL, 100mg/mL; (MDV) 300mg/3mL; [150mg/mL] (Graduated Prefilled Syringe) 120mg/0.8mL, 150mg/mL	1mg/kg SQ q12h with PO ASA (100-325mg qd) until clinically stabilized. **Usual Duration:** 2-8 days (up to 12.5 days in clinical trials).	Renal
Prasugrel (Effient)	**Tab:** 5mg, 10mg	**LD:** 60mg. **Maint:** 10mg qd with ASA (75-325mg/day). **<60kg:** Consider lowering the maintenance dose to 5mg qd.	
Ticagrelor (Brilinta)	**Tab:** 60mg, 90mg	**LD:** 180mg. **Maint:** 90mg bid during first year; 60mg bid after 1 year. Use with daily maint dose of ASA (75-100mg).	
VASODILATORS			
Isosorbide dinitrate (Dilatrate-SR)	**Cap, ER:** 40mg	40mg bid; separate doses by 6 hrs. **Max:** 160mg/day. Allow a dose-free interval of >18 hrs.	
Isosorbide mononitrate (Imdur)	**Tab, ER:** 30mg, 60mg, 120mg	**Initial:** 30mg (given as single tab or as ½ of a 60mg tab) or 60mg (given as single tab) qam on arising. **Titrate:** May increase to 120mg (given as single tab or as two 60mg tabs) qam after several days. Rarely, 240mg qam may be required.	
Isosorbide mononitrate (Monoket)	**Tab:** 10mg, 20mg	20mg bid (give doses 7 hrs apart). **Small Stature Patients: Initial:** 5mg (½ of a 10mg tab). **Titrate:** Increase to ≥10mg by 2nd or 3rd day.	
Nitroglycerin (Nitrolingual)	**Spray:** 400mcg/spray	**Acute Relief:** 1 or 2 sprays at the onset of attack onto or under the tongue. **Max:** 3 sprays/15 min. If chest pain persists, prompt medical attention is recommended. **Prophylaxis:** May be used 5-10 min prior to engaging in activities that might precipitate an acute attack.	

(Continued)

GENERIC (BRAND)	HOW SUPPLIED	DOSAGE	RENAL/HEPATIC DOSAGE ADJUSTMENT
VASODILATORS *(Continued)*			
Nitroglycerin (Nitromist)	**Spray:** 400mcg/spray	**Acute Relief:** 1 or 2 sprays at the onset of attack onto or under the tongue. May repeat every 5 min PRN. If 2 sprays are used initially, may only administer 1 more spray after 5 min. **Max:** 3 sprays/15 min. If chest pain persists after a total of 3 sprays, prompt medical attention is recommended. **Prophylaxis:** May be used 5-10 min before engaging in activities that might precipitate an acute attack.	
Nitroglycerin (Minitran, Nitro-Dur)	**Patch:** (Minitran) 0.1mg/hr, 0.2mg/hr, 0.4mg/hr, 0.6mg/hr; (Nitro-Dur) 0.1mg/hr, 0.2mg/hr, 0.3mg/hr, 0.4mg/hr, 0.6mg/hr, 0.8mg/hr	**Initial:** 0.2-0.4mg/hr patch for 12-14 hrs/day. Remove patch for 10-12 hrs/day.	
Nitroglycerin (Nitrostat)	**Tab, SL:** 0.3mg, 0.4mg, 0.6mg	**Acute Relief:** 1 tab SL or in buccal pouch at onset of attack. May repeat every 5 min until relief is obtained. If pain persists after a total of 3 tabs in 15 min, or if pain is different than typically experienced, prompt medical attention is recommended. **Prophylaxis:** May be used 5-10 min prior to engaging in activities that might precipitate an acute attack.	
Nitroglycerin (Nitro-Bid)	**Oint:** 2%	**Initial:** ½-inch (7.5mg) bid (one in the am and one 6 hrs later). **Titrate:** May increase to 1 inch bid, then to 2 inches bid. Allow a dose-free interval of 10-12 hrs.	
Nitroglycerin in 5% Dextrose	**Inj:** 100mcg/mL, 200mcg/mL, 400mcg/mL	**Initial:** 5mcg/min IV. **Titrate:** Increase by 5mcg/min at intervals of 3-5 min. If no response at 20mcg/min, may use increments of 10 and even 20mcg/min. Once some hemodynamic response is observed, dosage increments should be smaller and less frequent.	
MISCELLANEOUS			
Ranolazine (Ranexa)	**Tab, ER:** 500mg, 1000mg	**Initial:** 500mg bid. **Titrate:** May increase to 1000mg bid, PRN, based on clinical symptoms. **Max:** 1000mg bid.	

Refer to full FDA-approved labeling for additional product information.

Abbreviations: ASA = aspirin; ER = extended-release; HIT/HITTS = heparin-induced thrombocytopenia/heparin-induced thrombocytopenia and thrombosis syndrome; PCI = percutaneous coronary intervention; PTCA = percutaneous transluminal coronary angioplasty.

CHOLESTEROL-LOWERING AGENTS

GENERIC (BRAND)	HOW SUPPLIED (MG)*	USUAL DOSAGE RANGE†	T-CHOL (% DECREASE)	LDL (% DECREASE)	HDL (% INCREASE)	TG (% DECREASE)
BILE-ACID SEQUESTRANTS						
Cholestyramine (Prevalite)	**Powder for Oral Suspension:** 4g/packet or level scoopful	2-6 packets or level scoopfuls (8-24g)/day	7.2	10.4	N/A	N/A
Colesevelam HCl (Welchol)	**Tab:** 625; **Powder for Oral Suspension:** 3.75g packet, 1.875g packet	3750mg/day	7	15	3	+10
Colestipol HCl (Colestid)	**Granules for Suspension:** 5g/packet or level scoopful; **Tab:** 1000	**Granules for Suspension:** 1-6 packets or level scoopfuls/ day; **Tab:** 2-16g/day	N/A	N/A	N/A	N/A
CHOLESTEROL ABSORPTION INHIBITORS						
Ezetimibe (Zetia)	**Tab:** 10	10mg/day	13	18	1	8
CHOLESTEROL ABSORPTION INHIBITORS/HMG-COA REDUCTASE INHIBITORS (STATINS)						
Ezetimibe/ Atorvastatin (Liptruzet)	**Tab:** 10/10, 10/20, 10/40, 10/80	10/10mg – 10/80mg/day	38 to 46	53 to 61	5 to 9	30 to 40
Ezetimibe/ Simvastatin (Vytorin)	**Tab:** 10/10, 10/20, 10/40, 10/80	10/10mg – 10/40mg/day	31 to 43	45 to 60	6 to 10	23 to 31
FIBRATES‡						
Fenofibrate (Antara)	**Cap:** 30, 90	30-90mg/day	16.8 to 22.4	20.1 to 31.4	9.8 to 14.6	23.5 to 35.9
Fenofibrate (Fenoglide)	**Tab:** 40, 120	40-120mg/day	16.8 to 22.4	20.1 to 31.4	9.8 to 14.6	23.5 to 35.9
Fenofibrate (Lipofen)	**Cap:** 50, 150	50-150mg/day	16.8 to 22.4	20.1 to 31.4	9.8 to 14.6	23.5 to 35.9
Fenofibrate (Lofibra)	**Tab:** 54, 160; **Cap:** 67, 134, 200	54-160mg/day, 67-200mg/day	16.8 to 22.4	20.1 to 31.4	9.8 to 14.6	23.5 to 35.9
Fenofibrate (Tricor)	**Tab:** 48, 145	48-145mg/day	16.8 to 22.4	20.1 to 31.4	9.8 to 14.6	23.5 to 35.9
Fenofibrate (Triglide)	**Tab:** 160	160mg/day	16.8 to 22.4	20.1 to 31.4	9.8 to 14.6	23.5 to 35.9
Fenofibric acid (Fibricor)	**Tab:** 35, 105	35-105mg/day	16.8 to 22.4	20.1 to 31.4	9.8 to 14.6	23.5 to 35.9
Fenofibric acid (Trilipix)	**Cap, DR:** 45, 135	45-135mg/day	16.8 to 22.4	20.1 to 31.4	9.8 to 14.6	23.5 to 35.9
Gemfibrozil (Lopid)	**Tab:** 600	1200mg/day in divided doses	Moderate reduction	4.1	12.6	Significant reduction

(Continued)

GENERIC (BRAND)	HOW SUPPLIED (MG)*	USUAL DOSAGE RANGE†	T-CHOL (% DECREASE)	LDL (% DECREASE)	HDL (% INCREASE)	TG (% DECREASE)
HMG-COA REDUCTASE INHIBITORS (STATINS) & COMBINATIONS						
Amlodipine/ Atorvastatin (Caduet)	**Tab:** 2.5/10, 2.5/20, 2.5/40, 5/10, 5/20, 5/40, 5/80, 10/10, 10/20, 10/40, 10/80	5/10mg – 10/80mg/day	N/A	37.6 to 48.0	N/A	N/A
Atorvastatin (Lipitor)	**Tab:** 10, 20, 40, 80	10-80mg/day	29 to 45	39 to 60	5 to 9	19 to 37
Fluvastatin (Lescol)	**Cap:** 20, 40	20-80mg/day	17 to 27	22 to 36	3 to 6	12 to 18
Fluvastatin (Lescol XL)	**Tab, ER:** 80	80mg/day	25	35	7	19
Lovastatin (Altoprev)	**Tab, ER:** 20, 40, 60	20-60mg/day	17.9 to 29.2	23.8 to 40.8	9.4 to 13.1	9.9 to 25.1
Lovastatin	**Tab:** 10, 20, 40	10-80mg/day	17 to 29	24 to 40	6.6 to 9.5	10 to 19
Pitavastatin (Livalo)	**Tab:** 1, 2, 4	1-4mg/day	23 to 31	32 to 43	5 to 8	15 to 19
Pravastatin (Pravachol)	**Tab:** 20, 40, 80	40-80mg/day	16 to 27	22 to 37	2 to 12	11 to 24
Pravastatin	**Tab:** 10, 20, 40, 80	40-80mg/day	16 to 27	22 to 37	2 to 12	11 to 24
Rosuvastatin (Crestor)	**Tab:** 5, 10, 20, 40	5-40mg/day	33 to 46	45 to 63	8 to 14	10 to 35
Simvastatin (Zocor)	**Tab:** 5, 10, 20, 40, 80	5-40mg/day	19 to 36	26 to 47	8 to 16	12 to 33
HMG-COA REDUCTASE INHIBITORS (STATINS)/NICOTINIC ACIDS						
Niacin, ER/ Lovastatin (Advicor)	**Tab, ER:** 500/20, 750/20, 1000/20, 1000/40	500/20mg – 2000/40mg/day	N/A	30 to 42	20 to 30	32 to 44
Niacin, ER/ Simvastatin (Simcor)	**Tab, ER:** 500/20, 500/40, 750/20, 1000/20, 1000/40	500/20mg – 2000/40mg/day	1.6 to 11.1	5.1 to 14.3	15.4 to 29.0	22.8 to 38.0
LIPID-REGULATING AGENTS						
Icosapent Ethyl (Vascepa)	**Cap:** 1000	4g/day	7	5	4	27
Lomitapide (Juxtapid)	**Cap:** 5mg, 10mg, 20mg, 30mg, 40mg, 60mg	5-60mg/day	36	40	-7	45
Mipomersen sodium (Kynamro)	**Inj:** 200mg/mL [1mL]	200mg once weekly	21	25	15	18
Omega-3-Acid Ethyl Esters (Lovaza)	**Cap:** 1000	4g/day	9.7	+44.5	9.1	44.9
Omega-3-Acid Ethyl Esters A (Omtryg)	**Cap:** 1200	4 cap/day	9.7	+44.5	9.1	44.9

GENERIC (BRAND)	HOW SUPPLIED (MG)*	USUAL DOSAGE RANGE†	T-CHOL (% DECREASE)	LDL (% DECREASE)	HDL (% INCREASE)	TG (% DECREASE)
LIPID-REGULATING AGENTS *(Continued)*						
Omega-3-Carboxylic Acids (Epanova)	**Cap:** 1g	2g/day or 4g/day	6	21 to 26	5 to 7	25 to 31
NICOTINIC ACIDS						
Niacin, ER (Niaspan)	**Tab, ER:** 500, 750, 1000	500-2000mg/day	3 to 10	5 to 14	18 to 22	13 to 28
PROPROTEIN CONVERTASE SUBTILISIN KEXIN TYPE 9 INHIBITORS						
Alirocumab (Praluent)	**Inj:** 75mg/mL, 150mg/mL	75-150mg q2wks	36	58	N/A	N/A
Evolocumab (Repatha)	**Inj:** 140mg/mL	140mg q2wks or 420mg once monthly	32 to 38	58 to 64	N/A	N/A

Abbreviations: DR = delayed-release; ER = extended-release; N/A = not applicable.

*Unless otherwise indicated.

† Usual Dosage Range shown is for adults and may need to be adjusted to individual patient needs. For specific dosing and administration information including pediatric, geriatric, and renal/hepatic impairment dosing, please refer to the individual monograph listing or the FDA-approved labeling. According to NCEP-ATP III guidelines, lipid-altering agents should be used in addition to a diet restricted in saturated fat and cholesterol only when the response to diet and other nonpharmacological measures has been inadequate.

‡ Refer to the FDA-approved labeling for the lipid parameter changes observed for the treatment of hypertriglyceridemia; LDL increases reported.

Major Contraindications (refer to the FDA-approved labeling for a complete list of warnings and precautions):

Statins: Active liver disease or unexplained persistent elevations of hepatic transaminase levels; women who are pregnant or may become pregnant; nursing mothers.

Fibrates: Severe renal dysfunction (including patients receiving dialysis), active liver disease, gallbladder disease, nursing mothers.

Bile-acid sequestrants: History of bowel obstruction; serum triglycerides >500mg/dL; history of hypertriglyceridemia-induced pancreatitis.

Cholesterol absorption inhibitors: Statin contraindications apply when used with a statin: active liver disease or unexplained persistent elevations in hepatic transaminase levels, women who are pregnant or may become pregnant, nursing mothers.

Nicotinic acid derivatives: Active liver disease or unexplained persistent elevations in hepatic transaminases; active peptic ulcer disease; arterial bleeding.

Combinations: Refer to individual therapeutic class contraindications.

Heart Failure Treatment Options

GENERIC (BRAND)	HOW SUPPLIED	ADULT DOSAGE	RENAL/HEPATIC DOSAGE ADJUSTMENT
ACE INHIBITORS			
Captopril	**Tab:** 12.5mg, 25mg, 50mg, 100mg	**Initial:** 25mg tid. **Usual:** 50-100mg tid. **Max:** 450mg/day.	Renal
Enalapril (Epaned)	**Sol:** 1mg/mL [150mL]	**Initial:** 2.5mg bid; 2.5mg qd with hyponatremia (serum Na^+ <130mEq/L). **Max:** 20mg bid.	Renal
Enalapril maleate (Vasotec)	**Tab:** 2.5mg, 5mg, 10mg, 20mg	**Initial:** 2.5mg qd. **Usual:** 2.5-20mg bid. **Max:** 40mg/day in divided doses.	Renal
Fosinopril sodium	**Tab:** 10mg, 20mg, 40mg	**Initial:** 10mg qd. **Usual:** 20-40mg qd. **Max:** 40mg qd.	Renal
Lisinopril (Prinivil)	**Tab:** 5mg, 10mg, 20mg	**Initial:** 5mg qd; 2.5mg qd with hyponatremia (serum Na^+ <130mEq/L). **Max:** 40mg qd.	Renal
Lisinopril (Zestril)	**Tab:** 2.5mg, 5mg, 10mg, 20mg, 30mg, 40mg	**Initial:** 5mg qd; 2.5mg qd with hyponatremia (serum Na^+ <130mEq/L). **Max:** 40mg qd.	Renal
Quinapril (Accupril)	**Tab:** 5mg, 10mg, 20mg, 40mg	**Initial:** 5mg bid. **Usual:** 20-40mg/day given in 2 equally divided doses.	Renal
Ramipril (Altace)	**Cap:** 1.25mg, 2.5mg, 5mg, 10mg	**Post-MI: Initial:** 2.5mg bid (switch to 1.25mg bid if hypotensive). **Titrate:** Increase (if tolerated) to target dose of 5mg bid at 3-week intervals after 1 week of initial dose.	Renal
Trandolapril (Mavik)	**Tab:** 1mg, 2mg, 4mg	**Post-MI: Initial:** 1mg qd. **Titrate:** Increase (as tolerated) to target dose of 4mg qd; if not tolerated, continue with the greatest tolerated dose.	Renal/Hepatic
ALDOSTERONE BLOCKERS			
Eplerenone (Inspra)	**Tab:** 25mg, 50mg	**Post-MI: Initial:** 25mg qd. **Titrate:** Increase to 50mg qd, preferably within 4 weeks as tolerated.	
Spironolactone (Aldactone)	**Tab:** 25mg, 50mg, 100mg	**Initial:** 25mg qd. **Titrate:** If tolerated, may increase to 50mg qd as clinically indicated. May reduce to 25mg qod if not tolerated.	
ALPHA/BETA BLOCKERS			
Carvedilol (Coreg)	**Tab:** 3.125mg, 6.25mg, 12.5mg, 25mg	**Initial:** 3.125mg bid for 2 weeks. **Titrate:** May double dose over successive intervals of at least 2 weeks up to 25mg bid as tolerated. Maintain on lower doses if higher doses not tolerated. **Max:** 50mg bid if >85kg with mild-moderate HF. Reduce dose if HR <55 beats/min.	
Carvedilol phosphate (Coreg CR)	**Cap, ER:** 10mg, 20mg, 40mg, 80mg	**Initial:** 10mg qd for 2 weeks. **Titrate:** May double dose over successive intervals of at least 2 weeks up to 80mg qd as tolerated. Maintain on lower doses if higher doses not tolerated. Reduce dose if HR <55 beats/min.	
ANGIOTENSIN II RECEPTOR BLOCKERS			
Candesartan cilexetil (Atacand)	**Tab:** 4mg, 8mg, 16mg, 32mg	**Initial:** 4mg qd. **Titrate:** Double the dose at 2-week intervals, as tolerated, to the target dose of 32mg qd.	
Valsartan (Diovan)	**Tab:** 40mg, 80mg, 160mg, 320mg	**Initial:** 40mg bid. **Titrate:** May increase to 80mg or 160mg bid (use highest dose tolerated). Consider dose reduction of concomitant diuretics. **Max:** 320mg/day in divided doses.	
ANGIOTENSIN II RECEPTOR BLOCKERS/NEPRILYSIN INHIBITORS			
Sacubitril-Valsartan (Entresto)	**Tab:** 24mg-26mg, 49mg-51mg, 97mg-103mg	**Initial:** 49mg-51mg bid. **Titrate:** Double the dose after 2-4 weeks to target maint dose of 97mg-103mg bid, as tolerated.	Renal/Hepatic

(Continued)

GENERIC (BRAND)	HOW SUPPLIED	ADULT DOSAGE	RENAL/HEPATIC DOSAGE ADJUSTMENT
BETA BLOCKERS			
Metoprolol succinate (Toprol-XL)	**Tab, ER:** 25mg, 50mg, 100mg, 200mg	**Initial:** (NYHA Class II HF) 25mg qd or (Severe HF) 12.5mg qd for 2 weeks. **Titrate:** Double dose every 2 weeks to the highest dose level tolerated. **Max:** 200mg. Reduce dose if experiencing symptomatic bradycardia.	Hepatic
BIPYRIDINE INOTROPES/VASODILATORS			
Milrinone lactate	**Inj:** 1mg/mL	**LD:** 50mcg/kg IV given slowly over 10 min. **Maint: Continuous IV Infusion: Minimum:** 0.59mg/kg/day at 0.375mcg/kg/min. **Standard:** 0.77mg/kg/day at 0.5mcg/kg/min. **Titrate:** Adjust to desired response. **Max:** 1.13mg/kg/day at 0.75mcg/kg/min.	Renal
CARDIAC GLYCOSIDES			
Digoxin (Lanoxin)	**Inj:** (Lanoxin) 250mcg/mL, (Lanoxin Pediatric) 100mcg/mL; **Sol:** (generic) 50mcg/mL; **Tab:** (Lanoxin) 62.5mcg, 125mcg, 187.5mcg, 250mcg	**(Inj) LD:** 8-12mcg/kg; administer ½ the total LD initially, then ¼ the LD q6-8h twice. **Maint: Initial:** 2.4-3.6mcg/kg qd. **Titrate:** May increase dose every 2 weeks according to response, serum drug levels, and toxicity. **Max:** 500mcg in a single site. **(Sol) LD:** 10-15mcg/kg. **Maint:** 3.0-4.5mcg/kg/dose qd. **(Tab) LD:** 10-15mcg/kg; administer ½ the total LD initially, then ¼ the LD q6-8h twice. **Maint: Initial:** 3.4-5.1mcg/kg qd. **Titrate:** May increase dose every 2 weeks according to response, serum drug levels, and toxicity.	Renal
HUMAN B-TYPE NATRIURETIC PEPTIDES			
Nesiritide (Natrecor)	**Inj:** 1.5mg	2mcg/kg IV bolus over 60 sec, then 0.01mcg/kg/min continuous IV infusion.	
HYPERPOLARIZATION-ACTIVATED CYCLIC NUCLEOTIDE-GATED CHANNEL BLOCKERS			
Ivabradine (Corlanor)	**Tab:** 5mg, 7.5mg	**Initial:** 5mg bid. **Titrate:** After 2 weeks, adjust dose to achieve a resting HR of 50-60 bpm. **Max:** 7.5mg bid.	
POTASSIUM-SPARING DIURETICS			
Amiloride HCl (Midamor)	**Tab:** 5mg	**Initial:** 5mg qd. **Titrate:** May increase to 10mg/day prn.	
POTASSIUM-SPARING DIURETICS/THIAZIDE DIURETICS			
Amiloride HCl-Hydrochlorothiazide	**Tab:** 5mg-50mg	**Initial:** 1 tab/day. **Titrate:** May increase to 2 tabs/day, if necessary. **Max:** 2 tabs/day.	
VASODILATORS			
Isosorbide dinitrate-Hydralazine HCl (Bidil)	**Tab:** 20mg-37.5mg	**Initial:** 1 tab tid. **Titrate:** Increase to a maximum of 2 tabs tid, if tolerated. **Intolerable Side Effects:** May decrease to as little as ½ tab tid. Titrate up as soon as side effects subside.	
Nitroglycerin in 5% Dextrose	**Inj:** 100mcg/mL, 200mcg/mL, 400mcg/mL	**Post-MI: Initial:** 5mcg/min IV. **Titrate:** Increase by 5mcg/min at intervals of 3-5 min. If no response at 20mcg/min, may use increments of 10 and even 20mcg/min. Once some hemodynamic response is observed, dosage increments should be smaller and less frequent.	
Sodium nitroprusside (Nitropress)	**Inj:** 50mg/2mL	**Initial:** 0.3mcg/kg/min IV. **Titrate:** May increase every few min until the desired effect is achieved or the max infusion rate has been reached. **Max:** 10mcg/kg/min IV.	

Refer to full FDA-approved labeling for additional information.

Abbreviations: ER = extended-release; HF = heart failure; MI = myocardial infarction.

HYPERTENSION TREATMENT OPTIONS

GENERIC (BRAND)	HOW SUPPLIED	ADULT DOSAGE	PEDIATRIC DOSAGE
ACE INHIBITORS			
Benazepril HCl (Lotensin)	**Tab:** 5mg, 10mg, 20mg, 40mg	**Initial:** 10mg qd or 5mg qd if on diuretic. **Maint:** 20-40mg/day given qd or bid. **Max:** 80mg/day.	**≥6 Yrs: Initial:** 0.2mg/kg qd. **Max:** 0.6mg/kg or 40mg/day.
Captopril	**Tab:** 12.5mg*, 25mg*, 50mg*, 100mg*	**Initial:** 25mg bid or tid. **Titrate:** May increase to 50mg bid or tid after 1 or 2 wks. **Usual:** 25-150mg bid or tid. **Max:** 450mg/day.	
Enalapril (Epaned)	**Sol:** 1mg/mL [150mL]	**Initial:** 5mg qd or 2.5mg qd if on diuretic. **Titrate:** Increase dose prn. **Max:** 40mg/day.	**>1 Month: Initial:** 0.08mg/kg (up to 5mg) qd. **Max:** 0.58mg/kg or 40mg/day.
Enalapril maleate (Vasotec)	**Tab:** 2.5mg*, 5mg*, 10mg*, 20mg*	**Initial:** 5mg qd or 2.5mg qd if on diuretic. **Usual:** 10-40mg/day given qd or bid.	**1 Month-16 Yrs: HTN: Initial:** 0.08mg/kg (up to 5mg) qd. **Max:** 0.58mg/kg or 40mg/day.
Enalaprilat	**Inj:** 1.25mg/mL [1mL, 2mL]	**Usual:** 1.25mg IV over 5 min q6h for ≤48 hrs. **Max:** 20mg/day. **Concomitant Diuretic: Initial:** 0.625mg over 5 min; may repeat after 1 hr. **Maint:** Additional 1.25mg dose q6h.	
Fosinopril sodium	**Tab:** 10mg*, 20mg, 40mg	**Initial:** 10mg qd. **Usual:** 20-40mg qd. **Max:** 80mg/day.	**>50kg:** 5-10mg qd.
Lisinopril (Prinivil, Zestril)	**Tab:** (Prinivil) 5mg*, 10mg*, 20mg*; (Zestril) 2.5mg, 5mg*, 10mg, 20mg, 30mg, 40mg	**Initial:** 10mg qd or 5mg qd if on diuretic. **Usual:** 20-40mg qd. **Max:** 80mg/day.	**≥6 Yrs: Initial:** 0.07mg/kg qd (up to 5mg). **Max:** 0.61mg/kg or 40mg.
Moexipril HCl (Univasc)	**Tab:** 7.5mg*, 15mg*	**Initial:** 7.5mg qd 1 hr ac or 3.75mg qd if on diuretic. **Usual:** 7.5-30mg/day given qd or bid. **Max:** 60mg/day.	
Perindopril erbumine (Aceon)	**Tab:** 2mg*, 4mg*, 8mg*	**Initial:** 4mg qd. **Maint:** 4-8mg/day given qd or bid. **Max:** 16mg/day.	
Quinapril HCl (Accupril)	**Tab:** 5mg*, 10mg, 20mg, 40mg	**Initial:** 10-20mg qd or 5mg qd if on diuretic. **Titrate:** According to BP at 2-wk intervals. **Usual:** 20-80mg/day given qd or bid.	
Ramipril (Altace)	**Cap:** 1.25mg, 2.5mg, 5mg, 10mg	**Initial:** 2.5mg qd. **Maint:** 2.5-20mg/day given qd or bid.	
Trandolapril (Mavik)	**Tab:** 1mg*, 2mg, 4mg	**Initial:** 1mg qd in nonblack patients; 2mg qd in black patients or 0.5mg qd if on diuretic. **Titrate:** According to BP at 1-wk intervals. **Usual:** 2-4mg qd. **Max:** 8mg/day.	
ACE INHIBITORS-CALCIUM CHANNEL BLOCKERS			
Amlodipine besylate-Benazepril HCl (Lotrel)	**Cap:** (Amlodipine-Benazepril) 2.5mg-10mg, 5mg-10mg, 5mg-20mg, 5mg-40mg, 10mg-20mg, 10mg-40mg	**Initial:** 2.5mg-10mg qd. **Titrate:** May increase up to 10mg-40mg qd if BP remains uncontrolled.	

(Continued)

GENERIC (BRAND)	HOW SUPPLIED	ADULT DOSAGE	PEDIATRIC DOSAGE
ACE INHIBITORS-CALCIUM CHANNEL BLOCKERS *(Continued)*			
Perindopril arginine-Amlodipine (Prestalia)	**Tab:** (Perindopril-Amlodipine) 3.5mg-2.5mg, 7mg-5mg, 14mg-10mg	**Initial:** 3.5mg-2.5mg qd. **Titrate:** Adjust based on BP at 7- to 14-day intervals. **Max:** 14mg-10mg qd.	
Trandolapril-Verapamil HCl (Tarka)	**Tab, ER:** (Trandolapril-Verapamil) 2mg-180mg, 1mg-240mg, 2mg-240mg, 4mg-240mg	Combination may be substituted for same component doses.	
ACE INHIBITORS-THIAZIDE DIURETICS			
Benazepril HCl-HCTZ (Lotensin HCT)	**Tab:** (Benazepril-HCTZ) 5mg-6.25mg*, 10mg-12.5mg*, 20mg-12.5mg*, 20mg-25mg*	**Not Controlled with Benazepril or HCTZ Monotherapy: Initial:** 10mg-12.5mg qd. **Titrate:** May increase after 2-3 wks. **Max:** 20mg-25mg qd.	
Captopril-HCTZ	**Tab:** (Captopril-HCTZ) 25mg-15mg*, 25mg-25mg*, 50mg-15mg*, 50mg-25mg*	**Initial:** 25mg-15mg qd 1 hr ac. **Titrate:** Adjust at 6-wk intervals, unless situation demands more rapid adjustment. **Max:** 150mg captopril and 50mg HCTZ per day.	
Enalapril maleate-HCTZ (Vaseretic)	**Tab:** (Enalapril-HCTZ) 5mg-12.5mg, 10mg-25mg; (Vaseretic) 10mg-25mg*	**Not Controlled with Enalapril or HCTZ Monotherapy: Initial:** 5mg-12.5mg or 10mg-25mg qd. **Titrate:** May increase after 2-3 wks. **Max:** 20mg enalapril and 50mg HCTZ per day.	
Fosinopril sodium-HCTZ	**Tab:** (Fosinopril-HCTZ) 10mg-12.5mg, 20mg-12.5mg*	**Not Controlled with Fosinopril or HCTZ Monotherapy:** 10mg-12.5mg tab or 20mg-12.5mg tab qd.	
Lisinopril-HCTZ (Zestoretic)	**Tab:** (Lisinopril-HCTZ) 10mg-12.5mg, 20mg-12.5mg, 20mg-25mg	**Not Controlled with Lisinopril or HCTZ Monotherapy: Initial:** 10mg-12.5mg or 20mg-12.5mg qd, depending on current monotherapy dose. **Titrate:** May increase after 2-3 wks.	
Moexipril HCl-HCTZ (Uniretic)	**Tab:** (Moexipril-HCTZ) 7.5mg-12.5mg*, 15mg-12.5mg*, 15mg-25mg*	**Not Controlled with Moexipril or HCTZ Monotherapy: Initial:** 7.5mg-12.5mg, 15mg-12.5mg, or 15mg-25mg qd 1 hr ac. **Titrate:** May increase after 2-3 wks. **Max:** 30mg moexipril and 50mg HCTZ per day.	
Quinapril HCl-HCTZ (Accuretic)	**Tab:** (Quinapril-HCTZ) 10mg-12.5mg*, 20mg-12.5mg*, 20mg-25mg	**Not Controlled with Quinapril Monotherapy: Initial:** 10mg-12.5mg or 20mg-12.5mg qd. **Titrate:** May increase after 2-3 wks.	
ALDOSTERONE BLOCKERS			
Eplerenone (Inspra)	**Tab:** 25mg, 50mg	**Initial:** 50mg qd. **Titrate:** May increase to 50mg bid. **Max:** 100mg/day.	
Spironolactone (Aldactone)	**Tab:** 25mg, 50mg*, 100mg*	**Initial:** 50-100mg/day given in single or divided doses for at least 2 wks. Adjust dose according to response.	

GENERIC (BRAND)	HOW SUPPLIED	ADULT DOSAGE	PEDIATRIC DOSAGE
ALPHA ADRENERGIC AGONISTS			
Clonidine (Catapres, Catapres-TTS)	**Patch, ER (TTS):** (TTS-1) 0.1mg, (TTS-2) 0.2mg, (TTS-3) 0.3mg; **Tab:** 0.1mg, 0.2mg, 0.3mg	(Patch) **Initial:** 0.1mg/24 hrs patch wkly. **Titrate:** May increase after 1-2 wks. **Max:** 0.6mg/24 hrs. (Tab) **Initial:** 0.1mg bid. **Titrate:** May increase by 0.1mg/day wkly. **Usual:** 0.2-0.6mg/day in divided doses. **Max:** 2.4mg/day.	
Methyldopa	**Tab:** 250mg, 500mg	**Initial:** 250mg bid-tid for first 48 hrs. **Titrate:** Adjust dose at intervals of not <2 days. **Usual:** 500mg-2g/day, given bid-qid. **Max:** 3g/day.	**Initial:** 10mg/kg/day, given bid-qid. **Max:** 65mg/kg/day or 3g/day, whichever is less.
Methyldopate HCl	**Inj:** 50mg/mL (5mL)	**Usual:** 250-500mg q6h. **Max:** 1g q6h.	20-40mg/kg/day, given in divided doses q6h. **Max:** 65mg/kg/day or 3g/day, whichever is less.
ALPHA ADRENERGIC AGONISTS-THIAZIDE DIURETICS			
Clonidine HCl-Chlorthalidone (Clorpres)	**Tab:** (Clonidine-Chlorthalidone) 0.1mg-15mg*, 0.2mg-15mg*, 0.3mg-15mg*	0.1mg-15mg tab qd-bid. **Max:** 0.6mg-30mg/day.	
Methyldopa-HCTZ	**Tab:** (Methyldopa-HCTZ) 250mg-15mg, 250mg-25mg	**Initial:** 250mg-15mg tab bid-tid or 250mg-25mg tab bid. Alternatively, 500mg/30mg qd or 500mg/50mg qd. **Max:** 50mg HCTZ and 3g methyldopa per day.	
ALPHA/BETA BLOCKERS			
Carvedilol (Coreg, Coreg CR)	**Cap, ER:** 10mg, 20mg, 40mg, 80mg; **Tab:** 3.125mg, 6.25mg, 12.5mg, 25mg	(Cap, ER) **Initial:** 20mg qd. **Titrate:** May double dose every 7-14 days. **Max:** 80mg/day. (Tab) **Initial:** 6.25mg bid. **Titrate:** May double dose every 7-14 days. **Max:** 50mg/day.	
Labetalol HCl	**Inj:** 5mg/mL [20mL, 40mL]; **Tab:** 100mg*, 200mg*, 300mg	(Inj) **Repeated Inj: Initial:** 20mg over 2 min. **Titrate:** May give additional 40mg or 80mg at 10-min intervals until desired BP achieved or total of 300mg is injected. **Slow Continuous Infusion:** 200mg (1mg/mL) at 2mg/min. **Alternate:** 200mg (2mg/3mL) at 3mL/min. **Effective Dose Range:** 50-200mg. **Max:** 300mg. (Tab) **Initial:** 100mg bid. **Titrate:** After 2-3 days, may increase in increments of 100mg bid every 2-3 days. **Maint:** 200-400mg bid. **Severe:** 1200-2400mg/day given bid.	
ALPHA$_1$ RECEPTOR BLOCKERS (QUINAZOLINE)			
Doxazosin mesylate (Cardura)	**Tab:** 1mg*, 2mg*, 4mg*, 8mg*	**Initial:** 1mg qd (am or pm). **Titrate:** May increase to 2mg and if necessary to 4mg, 8mg, and 16mg qd.	

(Continued)

GENERIC (BRAND)	HOW SUPPLIED	ADULT DOSAGE	PEDIATRIC DOSAGE
ALPHA$_1$ RECEPTOR BLOCKERS (QUINAZOLINE) *(Continued)*			
Prazosin HCl (Minipress)	**Cap:** 1mg, 2mg, 5mg	**Initial:** 1mg bid-tid. **Titrate:** May slowly increase to 20mg/day in divided doses. **Usual:** 6-15mg/day in divided doses.	
Terazosin HCl	**Cap:** 1mg, 2mg, 5mg, 10mg	**Initial:** 1mg hs. **Usual:** 1-5mg qd. Slowly increase dose or use bid regimen if substantially diminished response at 24 hrs. **Max:** 40mg/day.	
ANGIOTENSIN II RECEPTOR ANTAGONISTS			
Azilsartan medoxomil (Edarbi)	**Tab:** 40mg, 80mg	**Usual:** 80mg qd. **With High Dose Diuretics: Initial:** 40mg qd.	
Candesartan cilexetil (Atacand)	**Tab:** 4mg*, 8mg*, 16mg*, 32mg*	**Monotherapy without Volume Depletion: Initial:** 16mg qd. **Usual:** 8-32mg/day given qd or bid.	Administer qd or divide into 2 equal doses. **6-<17 Yrs: >50kg: Initial:** 8-16mg. **Usual:** 4-32mg/day. **<50kg: Initial:** 4-8mg. **Usual:** 2-16mg/day. **1-<6 Yrs: Initial:** (PO Sus) 0.20mg/kg. **Usual:** 0.05-0.4mg/kg/day.
Eprosartan mesylate (Teveten)	**Tab:** 400mg, 600mg	**Initial (Monotherapy and Not Volume-Depleted):** 600mg qd. **Usual:** 400-800mg/day given qd-bid. May give bid using same total daily dose or consider dose increase if effect is inadequate. **Max:** 800mg/day.	
Irbesartan (Avapro)	**Tab:** 75mg, 150mg, 300mg	**Initial:** 150mg qd. **Titrate:** May increase to 300mg qd. **Max:** 300mg qd.	
Losartan potassium (Cozaar)	**Tab:** 25mg, 50mg*, 100mg	**Initial:** 50mg qd; 25mg for patients with possible intravascular depletion. **Max:** 100mg qd.	**≥6 Yrs: Initial:** 0.7mg/kg qd (up to 50mg total). **Max:** 1.4mg/kg/day or 100mg/day.
Olmesartan medoxomil (Benicar)	**Tab:** 5mg, 20mg, 40mg	**Initial:** 20mg qd. **Titrate:** May increase to 40mg qd after 2 wks.	**6-16 Yrs: ≥35kg: Initial:** 20mg qd. **Titrate:** May increase to 40mg qd after 2 wks. **Max:** 40mg qd. **20-<35kg: Initial:** 10mg qd. **Titrate:** May increase to 20mg qd after 2 wks. **Max:** 20mg qd.
Telmisartan (Micardis)	**Tab:** 20mg, 40mg, 80mg	**Initial:** 40mg qd. **Usual:** 20-80mg/day.	
Valsartan (Diovan)	**Tab:** 40mg*, 80mg, 160mg, 320mg	**Initial:** 80mg or 160mg qd. **Max:** 320mg/day.	**6-16 Yrs: Initial:** 1.3mg/kg qd (up to 40mg total). **Max:** 2.7mg/kg (up to 160mg) qd.
ANGIOTENSIN II RECEPTOR ANTAGONISTS-CALCIUM CHANNEL BLOCKERS-THIAZIDE DIURETICS			
Amlodipine-Valsartan-HCTZ (Exforge HCT)	**Tab:** (Amlodipine-Valsartan-HCTZ) 5mg-160mg-12.5mg, 5mg-160mg-25mg, 10mg-160mg-12.5mg, 10mg-160mg-25mg, 10mg-320mg-25mg	**Usual:** Dose qd. May increase after 2 wks. **Max:** 10mg-320mg-25mg qd.	

GENERIC (BRAND)	HOW SUPPLIED	ADULT DOSAGE	PEDIATRIC DOSAGE
ANGIOTENSIN II RECEPTOR ANTAGONISTS-CALCIUM CHANNEL BLOCKERS-THIAZIDE DIURETICS *(Continued)*			
Olmesartan medoxomil-Amlodipine besylate-HCTZ (Tribenzor)	**Tab:** (Olmesartan-Amlodipine-HCTZ) 20mg-5mg-12.5mg, 40mg-5mg-12.5mg, 40mg-5mg-25mg, 40mg-10mg-12.5mg, 40mg-10mg-25mg	**Usual:** Dose qd. May increase after 2 wks. **Max:** 40mg-10mg-25mg qd.	
ANGIOTENSIN II RECEPTOR ANTAGONISTS-THIAZIDE DIURETICS			
Azilsartan medoxomil-Chlorthalidone (Edarbyclor)	**Tab:** (Azilsartan-Chlorthalidone) 40mg-12.5mg, 40mg-25mg	**Initial:** 40mg-12.5mg qd. **Titrate:** May increase to 40mg-25mg after 2-4 wks. **Max:** 40mg-25mg.	
Candesartan cilexetil-HCTZ (Atacand HCT)	**Tab:** (Candesartan-HCTZ) 16mg-12.5mg*, 32mg-12.5mg*, 32mg-25mg*	**Not Controlled on 25mg HCTZ qd or Controlled on 25mg HCTZ qd with Hypokalemia:** 16mg-12.5mg qd. **Not Controlled on 32mg Candesartan qd:** 32mg-12.5mg qd, and then 32mg-25mg qd.	
Eprosartan mesylate-HCTZ (Teveten HCT)	**Tab:** (Eprosartan-HCTZ) 600mg-12.5mg, 600mg-25mg	**Usual (Not Volume-Depleted):** 600mg-12.5mg qd. **Titrate:** May increase to 600mg-25mg qd. **Max:** 600mg-25mg qd.	
Irbesartan-HCTZ (Avalide)	**Tab:** (Irbesartan-HCTZ) 150mg-12.5mg, 300mg-12.5mg	**Initial:** 150mg-12.5mg qd. **Titrate:** May increase after 1-2 wks. **Max:** 300mg-25mg qd.	
Losartan potassium-HCTZ (Hyzaar)	**Tab:** (Losartan-HCTZ) 50mg-12.5mg, 100mg-12.5mg, 100mg-25mg	**Usual:** 50mg-12.5mg qd. **Max:** 100mg-25mg qd.	
Olmesartan medoxomil-HCTZ (Benicar HCT)	**Tab:** (Olmesartan-HCTZ) 20mg-12.5mg, 40mg-12.5mg, 40mg-25mg	**Usual:** 1 tab qd. **Titrate:** May adjust at intervals of 2-4 wks. **Max:** 1 tab/day.	
Telmisartan-HCTZ (Micardis HCT)	**Tab:** (Telmisartan-HCTZ) 40mg-12.5mg, 80mg-12.5mg, 80mg-25mg	**Not Controlled on 80mg Telmisartan, Not Controlled on 25mg/day HCTZ, or Controlled on 25mg/day HCTZ with Hypokalemia: Initial:** 80mg-12.5mg qd. **Titrate:** Increase up to 160mg-25mg after 2-4 wks.	
Valsartan-HCTZ (Diovan HCT)	**Tab:** (Valsartan-HCTZ) 80mg-12.5mg, 160mg-12.5mg, 160mg-25mg, 320mg-12.5mg, 320mg-25mg	**Initial:** 160mg-12.5mg qd. **Titrate:** May increase after 1-2 wks. **Max:** 320mg-25mg qd.	
BETA BLOCKERS			
Acebutolol HCl (Sectral)	**Cap:** 200mg, 400mg	**Mild-Moderate: Initial:** 400mg/day, given qd-bid. **Usual:** 200-800mg/day. **Severe/Inadequate Control:** 1200mg/day, given bid.	

(Continued)

GENERIC (BRAND)	HOW SUPPLIED	ADULT DOSAGE	PEDIATRIC DOSAGE
BETA BLOCKERS *(Continued)*			
Atenolol (Tenormin)	**Tab:** 25mg, 50mg*, 100mg	**Initial:** 50mg qd. **Titrate:** May increase to 100mg qd after 1-2 wks. **Max:** 100mg qd.	
Betaxolol	**Tab:** 10mg*, 20mg	**Initial:** 10mg qd. **Titrate:** May increase to 20mg qd after 7-14 days. **Max:** 20mg/day.†	
Bisoprolol fumarate (Zebeta)	**Tab:** 5mg*, 10mg	**Initial:** 5mg qd. **Titrate:** May increase to 10mg and then, if necessary, to 20mg qd.	
Metoprolol succinate (Toprol-XL)	**Tab, ER:** 25mg*, 50mg*, 100mg*, 200mg*	**Initial:** 25-100mg qd. **Titrate:** May increase at wkly (or longer) intervals. **Max:** 400mg/day.	**≥6 Yrs: Initial:** 1mg/kg qd up to 50mg qd. **Max:** 2mg/kg (up to 200mg) qd.
Metoprolol tartrate (Lopressor)	**Tab:** (Generic) 25mg*, 50mg*, 100mg*; (Lopressor) 50mg*, 100mg*	**Initial:** 100mg/day qd or in divided doses. **Titrate:** May increase at wkly (or longer) intervals. **Effective Range:** 100-450mg/day. **Max:** 450mg/day.	
Nadolol (Corgard)	**Tab:** 20mg*, 40mg*, 80mg*	**Initial:** 40mg qd. **Titrate:** May gradually increase in 40-80mg increments. **Maint: Usual:** 40 or 80mg qd. Doses up to 240 or 320mg qd may be needed.	
Nebivolol (Bystolic)	**Tab:** 2.5mg, 5mg, 10mg, 20mg	**Initial:** 5mg qd. **Titrate:** May increase at 2-wk intervals. **Max:** 40mg.	
Pindolol	**Tab:** 5mg*, 10mg*	**Initial:** 5mg bid. **Titrate:** May adjust dose in increments of 10mg/day at 3- to 4-wk intervals. **Max:** 60mg/day.	
Propranolol HCl	**Sol:** 20mg/5mL, 40mg/5mL [500mL]; **Tab:** 10mg*, 20mg*, 40mg*, 60mg*, 80mg*	**Initial:** 40mg bid. **Usual Maint:** 120-240mg/day. In some instances, 640mg/day may be required.	
Propranolol HCl (Inderal LA)	**Cap, ER:** 60mg, 80mg, 120mg, 160mg	**Initial:** 80mg qd. **Titrate:** May increase to 120mg qd or higher. **Maint:** 120-160mg qd. 640mg/day may be required.	
Propranolol HCl (Innopran XL)	**Cap, ER:** 80mg, 120mg	**Initial:** 80mg qhs. **Titrate:** May increase to 120mg qhs.	
Timolol maleate	**Tab:** 5mg, 10mg*, 20mg*	**Initial:** 10mg bid. **Maint:** 20-40mg/day. Wait at least 7 days between dose increases. **Max:** 60mg/day given bid.	
BETA BLOCKERS-THIAZIDE DIURETICS			
Atenolol-Chlorthalidone (Tenoretic)	**Tab:** (Atenolol-Chlorthalidone) 50mg-25mg*, 100mg-25mg	**Initial:** 50mg-25mg tab qd. **Titrate:** May increase to 100mg-25mg tab qd.	
Bisoprolol fumarate-HCTZ (Ziac)	**Tab:** (Bisoprolol-HCTZ) 2.5mg-6.25mg, 5mg-6.25mg, 10mg-6.25mg	**Not Controlled on 2.5-20mg/day Bisoprolol or Controlled on 50mg/day HCTZ with Hypokalemia: Initial:** 2.5mg-6.25mg qd. **Titrate:** May increase at 14-day intervals. **Max:** 20mg-12.5mg (two 10mg-6.25mg tabs) qd.	

GENERIC (BRAND)	HOW SUPPLIED	ADULT DOSAGE	PEDIATRIC DOSAGE
BETA BLOCKERS-THIAZIDE DIURETICS *(Continued)*			
Metoprolol succinate-HCTZ (Dutoprol)	**Tab:** (Metoprolol-HCTZ) 25mg-12.5mg, 50mg-12.5mg, 100mg-12.5mg*	**Initial:** 25mg-12.5mg qd. **Titrate:** Every 2 wks. **Max:** 200mg-25mg (two 100mg-12.5mg tabs) qd.	
Metoprolol tartrate-HCTZ (Lopressor HCT)	**Tab:** (Metoprolol-HCTZ) (Generic) 50mg-25mg*, 100mg-25mg*, 100mg-50mg*; (Lopressor HCT) 50mg-25mg*, 100mg-25mg*,	**Combination Therapy: Metoprolol:** 100-200mg/day given qd or in divided doses. **HCTZ:** 25-50mg/day given qd or in divided doses. **Max:** 50mg/day.	
Nadolol-Bendroflumethiazide (Corzide)	**Tab:** (Nadolol-Bendroflumethiazide) 40mg-5mg*, 80mg-5mg*	**Initial:** 40mg-5mg qd. **Titrate:** May increase to 80mg-5mg qd.	
Propranolol HCl-HCTZ	**Tab:** (Propranolol-HCTZ) 40mg-25mg*, 80mg-25mg*	**Usual:** 1 tab bid. **Max:** 160mg-50mg/day.	
CALCIUM CHANNEL BLOCKERS (DIHYDROPYRIDINE)			
Amlodipine besylate (Norvasc)	**Tab:** 2.5mg, 5mg, 10mg	**Initial:** 5mg qd. **Titrate:** 7- to 14-day intervals. If clinically warranted, titrate more rapidly. **Max:** 10mg qd.	**6-17 Yrs: Usual:** 2.5-5mg qd. **Max:** 5mg qd.
Clevidipine (Cleviprex)	**Inj:** 0.5mg/mL [50mL, 100mL, 250mL]	**Initial:** 1-2mg/hr. **Titrate:** May double dose at 90-sec intervals initially. As BP approaches goal, interval should be lengthened to every 5-10 min. **Maint:** 4-6mg/hr. **Max:** 16mg/hr.	
Felodipine	**Tab, ER:** 2.5mg, 5mg, 10mg	**Initial:** 5mg qd. **Titrate:** May decrease to 2.5mg qd or increase to 10mg qd at intervals of not <2 wks. **Range:** 2.5-10mg qd.	
Isradipine	**Cap:** 2.5mg, 5mg	**Initial:** 2.5mg bid. **Titrate:** May adjust in increments of 5mg/day at 2- to 4-wk intervals. **Max:** 20mg/day.	
Nicardipine HCl	**Cap:** 20mg, 30mg	**Initial:** 20mg tid. **Titrate:** Allow at least 3 days before increasing dose. **Usual:** 20-40mg tid.	
Nicardipine HCl (Cardene IV)	**Inj:** 2.5mg/mL [10mL], 0.1mg/mL [200mL], 0.2mg/mL [200mL]	**Patients Not Receiving PO Nicardipine: Initial:** 5mg/hr IV infusion. **Titrate:** May increase by 2.5mg/hr every 5 min (for rapid titration) to 15 min (for gradual titration). **Max:** 15mg/hr.	
Nicardipine HCl (Cardene SR)	**Cap, SR:** 30mg, 45mg, 60mg	**Initial:** 30mg bid. **Effective Range:** 30-60mg bid.	
Nifedipine (Adalat CC, Afeditab CR)	**Tab, ER:** (Adalat CC) 30mg, 60mg, 90mg; (Afeditab CR) 30mg, 60mg	**Initial:** 30mg qd. **Titrate:** Increase dose over a 7- to 14-day period. **Usual:** 30-60mg qd. **Max:** 90mg.	
Nifedipine (Nifedical XL, Procardia XL)	**Tab, ER:** (Nifedical XL) 30mg, 60mg; (Procardia XL) 30mg, 60mg, 90mg	**Initial:** 30 or 60mg qd. **Titrate:** Over 7- to 14-day period. May proceed more rapidly if needed. **Max:** 120mg/day.	

(Continued)

GENERIC (BRAND)	HOW SUPPLIED	ADULT DOSAGE	PEDIATRIC DOSAGE
CALCIUM CHANNEL BLOCKERS (DIHYDROPYRIDINE) *(Continued)*			
Nisoldipine (Sular)	**Tab, ER:** 8.5mg, 17mg, 34mg	**Initial:** 17mg qd. **Titrate:** May increase by 8.5mg/wk or longer intervals. **Maint:** 17-34mg qd. **Max:** 34mg qd.	
CALCIUM CHANNEL BLOCKERS (DIHYDROPYRIDINE)-ANGIOTENSIN II RECEPTOR ANTAGONISTS			
Amlodipine-Olmesartan medoxomil (Azor)	**Tab:** (Amlodipine-Olmesartan) 5mg-20mg, 5mg-40mg, 10mg-20mg, 10mg-40mg	**Initial:** 5mg-20mg qd. **Titrate:** May increase dose after 1-2 wks. **Max:** 10mg-40mg qd.	
Amlodipine-Valsartan (Exforge)	**Tab:** (Amlodipine-Valsartan) 5mg-160mg, 10mg-160mg, 5mg-320mg, 10mg-320mg	**Initial:** 5mg-160mg qd. **Titrate:** May increase after 1-2 wks. **Max:** 10mg-320mg qd.	
Telmisartan-Amlodipine (Twynsta)	**Tab:** (Telmisartan-Amlodipine) 40mg-5mg, 40mg-10mg, 80mg-5mg, 80mg-10mg	**Initial:** 40mg-5mg qd or 80mg-5mg qd. **Titrate:** May be increased after at least 2 wks. **Max:** 80mg-10mg qd.	
CALCIUM CHANNEL BLOCKERS (DIHYDROPYRIDINE)-HMG COA REDUCTASE INHIBITORS			
Amlodipine besylate-Atorvastatin calcium (Caduet)	**Tab:** (Amlodipine-Atorvastatin) 2.5mg-10mg, 2.5mg-20mg, 2.5mg-40mg, 5mg-10mg, 5mg-20mg, 5mg-40mg, 5mg-80mg, 10mg-10mg, 10mg-20mg, 10mg-40mg, 10mg-80mg	**Amlodipine: Initial:** 5mg qd. **Titrate:** Adjust generally every 7-14 days. **Max:** 10mg qd. **Atorvastatin: Initial:** 10mg or 20mg qd (or 40mg qd for LDL reduction >45%). **Titrate:** Analyze lipids within 2-4 wks and adjust accordingly. **Usual:** 10-80mg qd.	**Amlodipine: 6-17 Yrs: Usual:** 2.5-5mg qd. **Max:** 5mg qd. **Atorvastatin: 10-17 Yrs: Initial:** 10mg/day. **Titrate:** Adjust at intervals of ≥4 wks. **Max:** 20mg/day.
CALCIUM CHANNEL BLOCKERS (DIHYDROPYRIDINE)-RENIN INHIBITORS			
Aliskiren-Amlodipine (Tekamlo)	**Tab:** (Aliskiren-Amlodipine) 150mg-5mg, 150mg-10mg, 300mg-5mg, 300mg-10mg	**Initial:** 150mg-5mg qd. **Titrate:** May increase after 2-4 wks. **Max:** 300mg-10mg qd.	
CALCIUM CHANNEL BLOCKERS (DIHYDROPYRIDINE)-RENIN INHIBITORS-THIAZIDE DIURETICS			
Aliskiren-Amlodipine-HCTZ (Amturnide)	**Tab:** (Aliskiren-Amlodipine-HCTZ) 150mg-5mg-12.5mg, 300mg-5mg-12.5mg, 300mg-5mg-25mg, 300mg-10mg-12.5mg, 300mg-10mg-25mg	**Usual:** Dose qd. **Titrate:** May increase after 2 wks. **Max:** 300mg-10mg-25mg.	

GENERIC (BRAND)	HOW SUPPLIED	ADULT DOSAGE	PEDIATRIC DOSAGE
CALCIUM CHANNEL BLOCKERS (NON-DIHYDROPYRIDINE)			
Diltiazem HCl (Cardizem CD, Cardizem LA, Cartia XT)	**Cap, ER:** (Cardizem CD, Cartia XT) 120mg, 180mg, 240mg, 300mg, (Cardizem CD) 360mg; **Tab, ER:** (Cardizem LA) 120mg, 180mg, 240mg, 300mg, 360mg, 420mg	(Cardizem CD, Cartia XT) **Initial (Monotherapy):** 180-240mg qd. **Usual:** 240-360mg qd. **Max:** 480mg qd. (Cardizem LA) **Initial (Monotherapy):** 180-240mg qd (am or hs). **Max:** 540mg/day.	
Diltiazem HCl (Taztia XT, Tiazac)	**Cap, ER:** (Taztia XT) 120mg, 180mg, 240mg, 300mg, 360mg; (Tiazac) 120mg, 180mg, 240mg, 300mg, 360mg, 420mg	**Initial (Monotherapy):** 120-240mg qd. **Usual Range:** 120-540mg qd. **Max:** 540mg qd.	
Verapamil HCl (Calan)	**Tab:** 40mg, 80mg*, 120mg*	**Initial (Monotherapy):** 80mg tid (240mg/day). **Max:** 360mg/day.	
Verapamil HCl (Calan SR)	**Tab, ER:** 120mg, 180mg*, 240mg*	**Initial:** 180mg qam. **Titrate:** May increase to 240mg qam, then 180mg bid (am and pm) or 240mg qam plus 120mg qpm, then 240mg q12h.	
Verapamil HCl (Covera-HS)	**Tab, ER:** 180mg, 240mg	**Initial:** 180mg qhs. **Titrate:** May increase to 240mg qhs, then 360mg (two 180mg tabs) qhs, then 480mg (two 240mg tabs) qhs.	
Verapamil HCl (Verelan)	**Cap, SR:** 120mg, 180mg, 240mg, 360mg	**Usual:** 240mg qam.	
Verapamil HCl (Verelan PM)	**Cap, ER:** 100mg, 200mg, 300mg	**Usual:** 200mg qhs. **Titrate:** May increase to 300mg qhs, then 400mg qhs if response is inadequate with 200mg.	
LOOP DIURETICS			
Furosemide (Lasix)	**Sol:** (Generic) 10mg/mL [60mL, 120mL], 40mg/5mL [500mL]; **Tab:** (Lasix) 20mg, 40mg*, 80mg	**Initial:** 40mg bid.	
Torsemide (Demadex)	**Inj:** (Generic) 10mg/mL [2mL, 5mL]; **Tab:** (Demadex) 5mg*, 10mg*, 20mg*, 100mg*	**Initial:** 5mg qd. **Titrate:** May increase to 10mg qd after 4-6 wks.	
POTASSIUM-SPARING DIURETICS			
Amiloride HCl (Midamor)	**Tab:** 5mg	**Initial:** 5mg qd. **Titrate:** May increase to 10mg/day.	
POTASSIUM-SPARING DIURETICS-THIAZIDE DIURETICS			
Amiloride HCl-HCTZ	**Tab:** (Amiloride-HCTZ) 5mg-50mg*	**Initial:** 1 tab/day. **Titrate:** May increase to 2 tabs/day if necessary. **Max:** 2 tabs/day.	
Spironolactone-HCTZ (Aldactazide)	**Tab:** (Spironolactone-HCTZ) 25mg-25mg, 50mg-50mg*	**Usual:** 50-100mg of each component as single dose or in divided doses.	

(Continued)

GENERIC (BRAND)	HOW SUPPLIED	ADULT DOSAGE	PEDIATRIC DOSAGE
POTASSIUM-SPARING DIURETICS-THIAZIDE DIURETICS *(Continued)*			
Triamterene-HCTZ (Dyazide)	**Cap:** (Triamterene-HCTZ) 37.5mg-25mg	1-2 caps qd.	
Triamterene-HCTZ (Maxzide, Maxzide-25)	**Tab:** (Triamterene-HCTZ) (Maxzide) 75mg-50mg*; (Maxzide-25) 37.5mg-25mg*	(Maxzide-25) 1-2 tabs qd, given as a single dose; (Maxzide) 1 tab qd.	
QUINAZOLINE DIURETICS			
Metolazone (Zaroxolyn)	**Tab:** 2.5mg, 5mg	2.5-5mg qd.	
RENIN INHIBITORS			
Aliskiren (Tekturna)	**Tab:** 150mg, 300mg	**Initial:** 150mg qd. **Titrate:** May increase to 300mg qd. **Max:** 300mg/day.	
RENIN INHIBITORS-THIAZIDE DIURETICS			
Aliskiren-HCTZ (Tekturna HCT)	**Tab:** (Aliskiren-HCTZ) 150mg-12.5mg, 150mg-25mg, 300mg-12.5mg, 300mg-25mg	**Add-On/Initial Therapy:** Initiate with 150mg-12.5mg qd. **Titrate:** May increase after 2-4 wks. **Max:** 300mg-25mg qd.	
THIAZIDE DIURETICS			
Chlorothiazide (Diuril)	**Sus:** (Diuril) 250mg/5mL [237mL]; **Tab:** (Generic) 250mg*, 500mg*	**Initial:** 0.5-1g/day given qd or in divided doses. **Max:** 2g/day in divided doses.	**Usual:** 10-20mg/kg/day given qd-bid. **Max: 2-12 Yrs:** 1g/day. **≤2 Yrs:** 375mg/day. **<6 Months:** Up to 30mg/kg/day given bid.
Chlorthalidone (Thalitone)	**Tab:** (Generic) 25mg, 50mg*; (Thalitone) 15mg	(Thalitone) **Initial:** 15mg qd. **Titrate:** May increase to 30mg qd, then to 45-50mg qd. **Maint:** May be lower than initial. (Generic) **Initial:** 25mg qd. **Titrate:** May increase to 50mg qd, then to 100mg qd. **Max:** 100mg qd. **Maint:** May be lower than initial.	
Hydrochlorothiazide	**Tab:** 12.5mg, 25mg*, 50mg*	**Initial:** 25mg qd. **Titrate:** May increase to 50mg/day given qd or in 2 divided doses.	1-2mg/kg/day given qd or in 2 divided doses. **Max: 2-12 Yrs:** 100mg/day. **Infants up to 2 Yrs:** 37.5mg/day. **<6 Months:** Up to 3mg/kg/day given in 2 divided doses may be required.
Hydrochlorothiazide (Microzide)	**Cap:** 12.5mg	**Initial:** 12.5mg qd. **Max:** 50mg/day.	
Indapamide	**Tab:** 1.25mg, 2.5mg	**Initial:** 1.25mg qam. **Titrate:** May increase to 2.5mg qd after 4 wks, then to 5mg qd after additional 4 wks.	
Methyclothiazide	**Tab:** 5mg*	**Usual:** 2.5-5mg qd.	

GENERIC (BRAND)	HOW SUPPLIED	ADULT DOSAGE	PEDIATRIC DOSAGE
VASODILATORS			
Hydralazine HCl	**Inj:** 20mg/mL; **Tab:** 10mg, 25mg, 50mg, 100mg	(Tab) **Initial:** 10mg qid for the first 2-4 days. **Titrate:** Increase to 25mg qid for the rest of the 1st wk, then increase to 50mg qid for 2nd and subsequent wks. **Resistant Patients:** ≤300mg/day. (Inj) **Usual:** 20-40mg only when drug cannot be given PO.	(Tab) **Initial:** 0.75mg/kg/day given qid. **Titrate:** Increase gradually over 3-4 wks. **Max:** 7.5mg/kg/day or 200mg/day. (Inj) **Usual:** 1.7-3.5mg/kg divided in 4-6 doses only when drug cannot be given PO.

Refer to full FDA-approved labeling for additional information.

*Scored.

†Doses >20mg have not shown a statistically significant additional antihypertensive effect, but the 40mg dose has been studied and is well tolerated.

Abbreviations: ACE = angiotensin-converting enzyme; ER = extended-release; HCTZ = hydrochlorothiazide; SR = sustained-release.

ACNE MANAGEMENT

GENERIC (BRAND)	HOW SUPPLIED	DOSAGE
SYSTEMIC AGENTS		
Isotretinoin (Absorica)	**Cap:** 10mg, 20mg, 25mg, 30mg, 35mg, 40mg	**Adults & Peds ≥12 yrs:** 0.5-1mg/kg/day given in 2 divided doses for 15-20 wks. **Max:** 2mg/kg/day.
Isotretinoin (Amnesteem, Claravis)	**Cap:** (Amnesteem) 10mg, 20mg, 40mg; (Claravis) 10mg, 20mg, 30mg, 40mg	**Adults & Peds ≥12 yrs:** 0.5-1mg/kg/day given in 2 divided doses for 15-20 wks. **Max:** 2mg/kg/day.
Minocycline HCl (Solodyn)	**Tab, Extended-Release:** 55mg, 65mg, 80mg, 105mg, 115mg	**Adults & Peds ≥12 yrs:** 1mg/kg qd for 12 wks.
TOPICAL AGENTS		
Adapalene (Differin)	**Cre:** 0.1%	**Adults & Peds ≥12 yrs:** Apply a thin layer to affected area qpm.
	Gel: 0.1%, 0.3%	**Adults & Peds ≥12 yrs:** Apply a thin layer to affected area qhs after washing.
	Lot: 0.1%	**Adults & Peds ≥12 yrs:** Apply a thin layer to cover the entire face and other affected area qd after washing.
Azelaic acid (Azelex)	**Cre:** 20%	**Adults & Peds ≥12 yrs:** Massage gently but thoroughly into affected area bid (am and pm).
Benzoyl peroxide (BenzEFoam, BenzEFoam Ultra)	(BenzEFoam) **Foam:** 5.3%	**Adults & Peds ≥12 yrs:** Rub into affected area qd or ud until completely absorbed. **Facial Acne:** Use a dollop the size of a marble. **Back/Chest Acne:** Use a dollop the size of a whole walnut.
	(BenzEFoam Ultra) **Foam:** 9.8%	**Adults & Peds ≥12 yrs:** Rub into affected area qd, then bid-tid prn or ud until completely absorbed. Rinse off after 2 min.
Benzoyl peroxide (NeoBenz Micro SD, NeoBenz Micro Wash)	(SD) **Cre:** 5.5%	**Adults & Peds ≥12 yrs:** Apply to affected area qd-bid.
	(Wash) **Sol:** 7%	
Benzoyl peroxide	**Gel:** 2.5%, 5%, 10%	**Adults & Peds ≥12 yrs: (2.5%) Initial:** Apply to affected area qd for 1 week, then bid. **(5%, 10%)** May be initiated in patients demonstrating accommodation to 2.5% gel.
Clindamycin phosphate (Evoclin)	**Foam:** 1%	**Adults & Peds ≥12 yrs:** Apply to affected area qd.
Clindamycin phosphate (Cleocin T)	**Gel:** 1%	**Adults & Peds ≥12 yrs:** Apply thin layer to affected area bid.
	Lot: 1%	
	Sol: 1%	
Clindamycin phosphate (Clindagel)	**Gel:** 1%	**Adults & Peds ≥12 yrs:** Apply thin layer to affected area qd.
Dapsone (Aczone)	**Gel:** 5%, 7.5%	**Adults & Peds ≥12 yrs: (5%)** Apply pea-sized amount to affected area bid. **(7.5%)** Apply pea-sized amount to affected area qd.
Erythromycin (Akne-Mycin)	**Oint:** 2%	**Adults:** Apply to affected area bid (am and pm).
Erythromycin	**Gel:** 2%	**Adults:** Apply a thin layer to affected area qd-bid. Do not rub in; spread lightly.
	Pledgets: 2%	**Adults:** Rub pledget or apply sol to affected area bid (am and pm).
	Sol: 2%	
Gentamicin sulfate	**Cre:** 0.1%	**Adults & Peds >1 yr:** Apply small amount to affected area tid-qid.
	Oint: 0.1%	

(Continued)

GENERIC (BRAND)	HOW SUPPLIED	DOSAGE
TOPICAL AGENTS *(Continued)*		
Tazarotene (Fabior)	**Foam:** 0.1%	**Adults & Peds ≥12 yrs:** Apply thin layer to affected area of face and/or upper trunk qpm. Massage into skin.
Tazarotene (Tazorac)	**Cre:** 0.1% **Gel:** 0.1%	**Adults & Peds ≥12 yrs:** Apply thin layer to affected area qpm.
Tretinoin (Atralin)	**Gel:** 0.05%	**Adults & Peds ≥10 yrs:** Apply thin layer to affected area qhs.
Tretinoin (Avita)	**Cre:** 0.025% **Gel:** 0.025%	**Adults:** Apply thin layer to affected area qpm.
Tretinoin (Retin-A)	**Cre:** 0.025%, 0.05%, 0.1% **Gel:** 0.01%, 0.025%	**Adults:** Apply thin layer to affected area qhs.
Tretinoin (Retin-A Micro)	**Gel:** 0.04%, 0.08%, 0.1%	**Adults & Peds ≥12 yrs:** Apply thin layer to affected area qpm.
Tretinoin (Tretin-X)	**Cre:** 0.025%, 0.0375%, 0.05%, 0.075%, 0.1%	**Adults & Peds ≥12 yrs:** Apply thin layer to affected area qhs.
COMBINATION PRODUCTS, TOPICAL		
Adapalene-Benzoyl peroxide (Epiduo, Epiduo Forte)	(Epiduo) **Gel:** 0.1%-2.5%	**Adults & Peds ≥9 yrs:** Apply pea-sized amount to affected area of face and/or trunk qd after washing.
	(Epiduo Forte) **Gel:** 0.3%-2.5%	**Adults & Peds ≥12 yrs:** Apply pea-sized amount to affected area of face and/or trunk qd after washing.
Benzoyl peroxide-Clindamycin phosphate (Acanya)	**Gel:** 2.5%-1.2%	**Adults & Peds ≥12 yrs:** Apply pea-sized amount to face qd.
Benzoyl peroxide-Clindamycin phosphate (BenzaClin)	**Gel:** 5%-1%	**Adults & Peds ≥12 yrs:** Apply to affected area bid (am and pm) or ud.
Benzoyl peroxide-Clindamycin phosphate (Duac)	**Gel:** 5%-1.2%	**Adults & Peds ≥12 yrs:** Apply thin layer to face qpm or ud.
Benzoyl peroxide-Clindamycin phosphate (Onexton)	**Gel:** 3.75%-1.2%	**Adults & Peds ≥12 yrs:** Apply pea-sized amount to face qd.
Benzoyl peroxide-Erythromycin (Benzamycin)	**Gel:** 5%-3%	**Adults & Peds ≥12 yrs:** Apply to affected area bid (am and pm) or ud.
Clindamycin phosphate-Tretinoin (Veltin)	**Gel:** 1.2%-0.025%	**Adults & Peds ≥12 yrs:** Apply pea-sized amount lightly covering the entire affected area qpm.
Clindamycin phosphate-Tretinoin (Ziana)	**Gel:** 1.2%-0.025%	**Adults & Peds ≥12 yrs:** Apply pea-sized amount onto 1 fingertip, dot onto chin, cheeks, nose, and forehead, then gently rub over entire face qhs.
Hydrocortisone acetate-Iodoquinol (Alcortin-A)	**Gel:** 2%-1%	**Adults & Peds ≥12 yrs:** Apply to affected area tid-qid or ud.
Sodium sulfacetamide (Klaron)	**Lot:** 10%	**Adults & Peds ≥12 yrs:** Apply thin layer to affected area bid.

GENERIC (BRAND)	HOW SUPPLIED	DOSAGE
COMBINATION PRODUCTS, TOPICAL *(Continued)*		
Sodium sulfacetamide-Sulfur (Avar Cleansing Pads, Avar Foam, Avar LS Cleanser, Avar LS Cleansing Pads, Avar-e Green Cream, Avar-e LS Emollient Cream, Avar LS Foam)	**Pads:** (Avar Cleansing Pads) 9.5%-5%; (Avar LS Cleansing Pads) 10%-2%	**Adults & Peds ≥12 yrs:** Wash affected area qd-bid or ud.
	Cre: (Avar-e Green Cream) 10%-5%; (Avar-e LS Emollient Cream) 10%-2%	**Adults & Peds ≥12 yrs:** Apply a thin layer to affected area qd-tid or ud. Massage into skin.
	Sol: (Avar LS Cleanser) 10%-2%	**Adults & Peds ≥12 yrs:** Wash affected area qd-bid or ud.
	Foam: (Avar Foam) 9.5%-5%; (Avar LS Foam) 10%-2%	**Adults & Peds ≥12 yrs:** Massage into affected area and wait 10 minutes. Rinse thoroughly and pat dry. Treat affected area qd-tid or ud.
Sodium sulfacetamide-Sulfur (Sumadan)	**Sol:** 9%-4.5%	**Adults & Peds ≥12 yrs:** Massage gently into skin for 10-20 seconds, working into a full lather. Rinse thoroughly and pat dry. Treat affected area qd-bid or ud.
Sodium sulfacetamide-Sulfur	**Lot:** 10%-5%	**Adults & Peds ≥12 yrs:** Apply thin layer to affected area with light massaging qd-tid or ud.
Refer to full FDA-approved labeling for additional information.		

Psoriasis Management: Systemic Therapies

GENERIC (BRAND)	HOW SUPPLIED	ADULT DOSAGE
ANTIMETABOLITES		
Methotrexate (Otrexup, Rasuvo, Rheumatrex, Trexall)*	**Inj:** (Generic) 25mg/mL, 1g/vial, (Otrexup) 7.5mg/0.4mL, 10mg/0.4mL, 15mg/0.4mL, 20mg/0.4mL, 25mg/0.4mL, (Rasuvo) 7.5mg/0.15mL, 10mg/0.20mL, 12.5mg/0.25mL, 15mg/0.30mL, 17.5mg/0.35mL, 20mg/0.40mL, 22.5mg/0.45mL, 25mg/0.50mL, 27.5mg/0.55mL, 30mg/0.60mL; **Tab:** 2.5mg, (Trexall) 5mg, 7.5mg, 10mg, 15mg	**Initial:** 10-25mg PO/IM/SQ/IV as a single weekly dose, or 2.5mg PO q12h for 3 doses. **Titrate:** May adjust gradually to achieve optimal response. **Max:** 30mg/wk.
IMMUNOSUPPRESSIVES		
Cyclosporine (Gengraf, Neoral)	**Cap:** 25mg, 100mg; **Sol:** 100mg/mL	**Initial:** 1.25mg/kg bid for ≥4 wks. **Titrate:** May increase by 0.5mg/kg/day at 2-wk intervals, as tolerated. **Max:** 4mg/kg/day.
MONOCLONAL ANTIBODIES		
Ustekinumab (Stelara)	**Inj:** 45mg/0.5mL, 90mg/mL	**SQ: >100kg:** 90mg initially and 4 wks later, 90mg q12wks. **≤100kg:** 45mg initially and 4 wks later, 45mg q12wks.
MONOCLONAL ANTIBODIES/IL-17A ANTAGONISTS		
Secukinumab (Cosentyx)	**Inj:** 150mg/mL, 150mg/vial	**SQ:** 300mg at 0, 1, 2, 3, and 4 wks, followed by 300mg q4wks. A dose of 150mg may be acceptable for some patients.
MONOCLONAL ANTIBODIES/TNF BLOCKERS		
Adalimumab (Humira)	**Inj:** 10mg/0.2mL, 20mg/0.4mL, 40mg/0.8mL	**SQ:** 80mg initial dose, followed by 40mg every other wk starting 1 wk after the initial dose.
Infliximab (Remicade)	**Inj:** 100mg/vial	Infuse over ≥2 hrs. **IV: Induction:** 5mg/kg at 0, 2, and 6 wks. **Maint:** 5mg/kg q8wks.
PHOSPHODIESTERASE-4 INHIBITORS		
Apremilast (Otezla)	**Tab:** 10mg, 20mg, 30mg	**Day 1:** 10mg in AM. **Day 2:** 10mg in AM and PM. **Day 3:** 10mg in AM and 20mg in PM. **Day 4:** 20mg in AM and PM. **Day 5:** 20mg in AM and 30mg in PM. **Day 6 and thereafter:** 30mg bid (AM and PM).
PSORALENS		
Methoxsalen† (8-Mop, Oxsoralen-Ultra)	**Cap:** 10mg	Take 2 hrs before UVA exposure with some food or milk. **<30kg:** 10mg; **30-50kg:** 20mg; **51-65kg:** 30mg; **66-80kg:** 40mg; **81-90kg:** 50mg; **91-115kg:** 60mg; **>115kg:** 70mg. **Titrate:** May increase by 10mg after 15th treatment under certain conditions ud. **Max:** No more than once qod.
RETINOIDS		
Acitretin (Soriatane)*	**Cap:** 10mg, 17.5mg, 25mg	**Initial:** 25-50mg/day as a single dose with the main meal. **Maint:** 25-50mg/day.
TNF-BLOCKING AGENTS		
Etanercept (Enbrel)	**Inj:** 25mg, 50mg	**SQ: Initial:** 50mg twice weekly for 3 months. **Maint:** 50mg once weekly.

Refer to full FDA-approved labeling for additional information.
*Contraindicated in pregnancy.
†Oxsoralen-Ultra and 8-Mop should not be used interchangeably.

Psoriasis Management: Topical Therapies

GENERIC (BRAND)	HOW SUPPLIED	USUAL ADULT DOSAGE
RETINOIDS		
Tazarotene (Tazorac)	**Cre:** 0.05%, 0.1% [30g, 60g]; **Gel:** 0.05%, 0.1% [30g, 100g]	Apply a thin film to lesions qpm.
VITAMIN D DERIVATIVES AND COMBINATIONS		
Calcitriol (Vectical)	**Oint:** 3mcg/g [100g]	Apply to affected areas bid (am and pm). **Max:** 200g/wk.
Calcipotriene (Dovonex, Sorilux)	**Cre:** (Dovonex) 0.005% [60g, 120g]; **Oint:** (Generic) 0.005% [60g, 120g]; **Foam:** (Sorilux) 0.005% [60g, 120g]	**Cre/Foam:** Apply a thin layer to affected areas bid; rub in gently and completely. **Oint:** Apply a thin layer qd or bid; rub in gently and completely.
Calcipotriene-Betamethasone dipropionate (Enstilar, Taclonex)	**Oint:** (Taclonex) 0.005%-0.064% [60g, 100g]; **Sus:** (Taclonex) 0.005%-0.064% [60g, 120g]; **Foam:** (Enstilar) 0.005%-0.064% [60g, 120g]	**Oint:** Apply an adequate layer to affected area(s) qd for up to 4 wks. **Max: 12-17 yrs:** 60g/wk. ≥**18 yrs:** 100g/wk. **Sus:** Apply to affected areas qd for up to 8 wks. **Max: 12-17 yrs:** 60g/wk. ≥**18 yrs:** 100g/wk. **Foam:** Apply to affected areas qd for up to 4 wks. **Max:** 60g q4 days.
MISCELLANEOUS AGENTS		
Anthralin (Dritho-Creme, Zithranol-RR, Zithranol)	**Cre:** (Dritho-Creme) 1% [50g]; **Cre:** (Zithranol-RR) 1.2% [15g, 45g]; **Shampoo:** (Zithranol) 1% [85g]	**Cre:** Apply qd or as directed. **Shampoo:** Apply to wet scalp 3-4 times per wk or as directed. Lather, leave on scalp for 3-5 min, and then rinse thoroughly.
Salicylic acid (Salex)	**Cre:** 6% [454g]; **Lot:** 6% [8 fl oz]; **Shampoo:** 6% [6 fl oz]	**Cre/Lot:** Apply to affected area and cover qpm before retiring. Wash off in the am. **Shampoo:** Wet hair and apply to scalp. Work into a lather and rinse.

Refer to full FDA-approved labeling for additional information.

Note: Not an inclusive list. For additional information, please refer to the Concise Drug Monographs section, or visit www.pdr.net.

Diabetes Treatment Options

GENERIC (BRAND)	HOW SUPPLIED	INITIAL* & (MAX) DOSAGE	USUAL DOSAGE RANGE*
ALPHA-GLUCOSIDASE INHIBITORS			
Acarbose (Precose)	**Tab:** 25mg, 50mg, 100mg	25mg tid at start of each meal, or qd to minimize GI side effects (**≤60kg:** 50mg tid, **>60kg:** 100mg tid)	50-100mg tid
Miglitol (Glyset)	**Tab:** 25mg, 50mg, 100mg	25mg tid at start of each meal, or qd to minimize GI effects (300mg/day)	50-100mg tid
BIGUANIDES			
Metformin HCl† (Fortamet)	**Tab, ER:** 500mg, 1000mg	500-1000mg qd with evening meal (2500mg/day)	500mg-2500mg/day
Metformin HCl† (Glumetza)	**Tab, ER:** 500mg, 1000mg	**Metformin-Naive:** 500mg qd with evening meal (2000mg/day)	500mg-2000mg/day
Metformin HCl† (Glucophage, Riomet)	**Tab:** (Glucophage) 500mg, 850mg, 1000mg; **Sol:** (Riomet) 500mg/5mL	500mg bid or 850mg qd with meals (2550mg/day)	850mg-2000mg/day
Metformin HCl† (Glucophage XR)	**Tab, ER:** 500mg, 750mg	500mg qd with evening meal (2000mg/day)	500mg-2000mg qd or divided doses
BILE-ACID SEQUESTRANTS			
Colesevelam HCl (Welchol)	**Tab:** 625mg; **Sus:** 1.875g, 3.75g [pkt]	**Tab:** 1875mg bid or 3750mg qd with meal and liquid; **Sus:** 1.875g pkt bid or 3.75g pkt qd with meal	3750mg/day
DIPEPTIDYL PEPTIDASE-4 INHIBITORS			
Alogliptin (Nesina)	**Tab:** 6.25mg, 12.5mg, 25mg	25mg qd	25mg/day
Linagliptin (Tradjenta)	**Tab:** 5mg	5mg qd	5mg/day
Saxagliptin (Onglyza)	**Tab:** 2.5mg, 5mg	2.5-5mg qd	2.5-5mg/day
Sitagliptin (Januvia)	**Tab:** 25mg, 50mg, 100mg	100mg qd	100mg/day
DIPEPTIDYL PEPTIDASE-4 INHIBITORS AND BIGUANIDES			
Alogliptin/ Metformin HCl† (Kazano)	**Tab:** 12.5mg/500mg, 12.5mg/1000mg	Individualize initial dose based on patient's current regimen (25mg/200mg/day)	
Linagliptin/ Metformin HCl† (Jentadueto)	**Tab:** 2.5mg/500mg, 2.5mg/850mg, 2.5mg/1000mg	2.5mg/500mg bid with meals (5mg/2000mg/day)	2.5mg/500mg-2.5mg/1000mg bid
Saxagliptin/ Metformin HCl† (Kombiglyze XR)	**Tab, ER:** 5mg/500mg, 5mg/1000mg, 2.5/1000mg	5mg/500mg or 2.5mg/1000mg qd with evening meal (5mg/2000mg/day)	5mg/500mg-2.5/1000mg qd
Sitagliptin/ Metformin HCl† (Janumet)	**Tab:** 50mg/500mg, 50mg/1000mg	50mg/500mg or 50mg/1000mg bid with meals (100mg/2000mg/day)	50mg/500mg-50mg/1000mg bid
Sitagliptin/ Metformin HCl† (Janumet XR)	**Tab, ER:** 100mg/1000mg, 50mg/500mg, 50mg/1000mg	50mg/1000mg or 100mg/1000mg qd with meals (100mg/2000mg/day)	50mg/1000mg-100mg/1000mg qd
DIPEPTIDYL PEPTIDASE-4 INHIBITORS AND THIAZOLIDINEDIONES			
Alogliptin/ Pioglitazone‡ (Oseni)	**Tab:** 12.5mg/15mg, 12.5mg/30mg, 12.5mg/45mg, 25mg/15mg, 25mg/30mg, 25mg/45mg	Individualize initial dose based on patient's current regimen (25mg/45mg/day)	

(Continued)

GENERIC (BRAND)	HOW SUPPLIED	INITIAL* & (MAX) DOSAGE	USUAL DOSAGE RANGE*
DOPAMINE RECEPTOR AGONISTS			
Bromocriptine mesylate (Cycloset)	**Tab:** 0.8mg	0.8mg qd within 2 hrs after waking in am (4.8mg/day)	1.6-4.8mg qd
GLUCAGON-LIKE PEPTIDE-1 RECEPTOR AGONISTS			
Albiglutide§ (Tanzeum)	**Inj:** 30mg, 50mg		30-50mg once weekly
Dulaglutide§ (Trulicity)	**Inj:** 0.75mg/0.5mL, 1.5mg/0.5mL	0.75mg once weekly (1.5mg once weekly)	0.75-1.5mg once weekly
Exenatide§ (Bydureon)	**Inj, ER:** 2mg		2mg once every 7 days
Exenatide (Byetta)	**Inj:** 5mcg/dose, 10mcg/dose	5mcg bid, at any time within 60 min before am and pm meals	5-10mcg bid
Liraglutide§ (Victoza)	**Inj:** 6mg/mL	0.6mg qd for 1 week	0.6-1.8mg/day
MEGLITINIDES			
Nateglinide (Starlix)	**Tab:** 60mg, 120mg	120mg tid 1-30 min before meals	120mg tid
Repaglinide (Prandin)	**Tab:** 0.5mg, 1mg, 2mg	0.5-2mg within 30 min before each meal (16mg/day)	0.5-4mg with each meal
MEGLITINIDES AND BIGUANIDES			
Repaglinide/ Metformin HCl† (PrandiMet)	**Tab:** 1mg/500mg, 2mg/500mg	1mg/500mg bid 15-30 min before meals (10mg/2500/day or 4mg/1000mg/meal)	1mg/500mg-2mg/500mg bid or tid
SODIUM-GLUCOSE COTRANSPORTER 2 INHIBITORS			
Canagliflozin (Invokana)	**Tab:** 100mg, 300mg	100mg qd before the first meal (300mg/day)	100-300mg qd
Dapagliflozin (Farxiga)	**Tab:** 5mg, 10mg	5mg qd in the am (10mg/day)	5-10mg qd
Empagliflozin (Jardiance)	**Tab:** 10mg, 25mg	10mg qd in the morning (25mg/day)	10-25mg/day
SODIUM-GLUCOSE COTRANSPORTER 2 INHIBITORS AND BIGUANIDES			
Canagliflozin/ Metformin HCl† (Invokamet)	**Tab:** 50mg/500mg, 50mg/1000mg, 150mg/500mg, 150mg/1000mg	Individualize initial dose based on patient's current regimen (300mg/2000mg/day)	
Dapagliflozin/ Metformin HCl† (Xigduo XR)	**Tab, ER:** 5mg/500mg, 5mg/1000mg, 10mg/500mg, 10mg/1000mg	Individualize initial dose based on patient's current treatment (10mg/2000mg/day)	
Empagliflozin/ Metformin HCl† (Synjardy)	**Tab:** 5mg/500mg, 5mg/1000mg, 12.5mg/500mg, 12.5mg/1000mg	Individualize initial dose based on patient's current regimen (25mg/2000mg/day)	
SODIUM-GLUCOSE COTRANSPORTER 2 INHIBITORS AND DIPEPTIDYL PEPTIDASE-4 INHIBITORS			
Empagliflozin/ Linagliptin (Glyxambi)	**Tab:** 10mg/5mg, 25mg/5mg	10mg/5mg qd in the morning	10mg/5mg-25mg/5mg qd
SULFONYLUREAS			
Chlorpropamide	**Tab:** 100mg, 250mg	250mg qd with breakfast (750mg/day)	<100-500mg qd; most patients controlled with 250mg qd

GENERIC (BRAND)	HOW SUPPLIED	INITIAL* & (MAX) DOSAGE	USUAL DOSAGE RANGE*
SULFONYLUREAS *(Continued)*			
Glimepiride (Amaryl)	**Tab:** 1mg, 2mg, 4mg	1-2mg qd with breakfast or first main meal (8mg/day)	1-8mg/day
Glipizide (Glucotrol)	**Tab:** 5mg, 10mg	5mg qd 30 min before breakfast (40mg/day)	5-40mg qd; divided doses if >15mg/day
Glipizide (Glucotrol XL)	**Tab, ER:** 2.5mg, 5mg, 10mg	5mg qd with breakfast (20mg/day)	5-10mg/day
Glyburide (Diabeta)	**Tab:** 1.25mg, 2.5mg, 5mg	2.5-5mg qd with breakfast or first main meal (20mg/day)	1.25-20mg/day in single or divided doses
Glyburide, micronized (Glynase PresTab)	**Tab:** 1.5mg, 3mg, 6mg	1.5-3mg qd with breakfast or first main meal (12mg/day)	0.75-12mg/day in single or divided doses
Tolazamide	**Tab:** 250mg, 500mg	100-250mg qd with breakfast or first main meal (1000mg/day)	100-1000mg/day; divided doses if >500mg/day
Tolbutamide	**Tab:** 500mg	1000-2000mg qd in single or divided doses (3000mg/day)	250-3000mg/day in single or divided doses
SULFONYLUREAS AND BIGUANIDES			
Glipizide/ Metformin HCl[†]	**Tab:** 2.5mg/250mg, 2.5mg/500mg, 5mg/500mg	2.5mg/250mg qd or 2.5mg/500mg bid with meals (20mg/2000mg/day)	2.5mg/250mg qd-5mg/500mg bid
Glyburide/ Metformin HCl[†] (Glucovance)	**Tab:** 1.25mg/250mg, 2.5mg/500mg, 5mg/500mg	1.25mg/250mg qd or bid with meals (20mg/2000mg/day)	1.25mg/250mg qd-5mg/500mg bid
SYNTHETIC AMYLIN ANALOGUES			
Pramlintide acetate[¶] (Symlin)	**Inj:** 1000mcg/mL	**Type 1:** 15mcg immediately prior to each major meal; **Type 2:** 60mcg immediately prior to each major meal	**Type 1:** 30–60mcg; **Type 2:** 60–120mcg
THIAZOLIDINEDIONES			
Pioglitazone[‡] (Actos)	**Tab:** 15mg, 30mg, 45mg	15-30mg qd (45mg/day)	15-45mg/day
Rosiglitazone maleate[‡] (Avandia)	**Tab:** 2mg, 4mg, 8mg	2mg bid or 4mg qd (8mg/day)	4-8mg/day
THIAZOLIDINEDIONES AND BIGUANIDES			
Pioglitazone/ Metformin HCl[†‡] (Actoplus Met)	**Tab:** 15mg/500mg, 15mg/850mg	15mg/500mg bid or 15mg/850mg qd with meal (45mg/2550mg/day)	15/500mg bid-15/850mg qd
Pioglitazone/ Metformin HCl[†‡] (Actoplus Met XR)	**Tab, ER:** 15mg/1000mg, 30mg/1000mg	15mg/1000mg or 30mg/1000mg qd with meal (45mg/2000mg/day)	15mg/1000mg-30mg/1000mg/day
Rosiglitazone maleate/ Metformin HCl[†‡] (Avandamet)	**Tab:** 2mg/500mg, 4mg/500mg, 2mg/1000mg, 4mg/1000mg	2mg/500mg qd or bid with meals (8mg/2000mg/day)	2mg/500mg-4mg/1000mg/day in divided doses
THIAZOLIDINEDIONES AND SULFONYLUREAS			
Pioglitazone/ Glimepiride[‡] (Duetact)	**Tab:** 30mg/2mg, 30mg/4mg	30mg/2mg or 30mg/4mg qd with first meal (45mg/8mg/day)	30mg/2mg-30mg/4mg/day

(Continued)

GENERIC (BRAND)	HOW SUPPLIED	INITIAL* & (MAX) DOSAGE	USUAL DOSAGE RANGE*
THIAZOLIDINEDIONES AND SULFONYLUREAS *(Continued)*			
Rosiglitazone maleate/ Glimepiride‡ (Avandaryl)	**Tab:** 4mg/1mg, 4mg/2mg, 4mg/4mg, 8mg/2mg, 8mg/4mg	4mg/1mg qd or 4mg/2mg qd with first meal (8mg/4mg/day)	4mg/1mg-4mg/2mg qd

Note: Not an inclusive list. For additional information, please refer to the Concise Drug Monographs section, or visit www.pdr.net.

*Usual dosage ranges are derived from FDA-approved labeling. There is no fixed dosage regimen for the management of diabetes mellitus with any hypoglycemic agent. The initial and maintenance dosing should be conservative, depending on the patient's individual needs, especially in elderly, debilitated, or malnourished patients, and with impaired renal or hepatic function. Management of type 2 diabetes should include blood glucose and HbA1c monitoring, nutritional counseling, exercise, and weight reduction as needed. For more detailed information, refer to the individual monograph listings or FDA-approved labeling.

†**BOXED WARNING:** Products containing metformin may cause lactic acidosis due to metformin accumulation. Refer to package insert for more details.

‡**BOXED WARNING:** Products containing thiazolidinediones, including pioglitazone or rosiglitazone, may cause or exacerbate congestive heart failure in some patients. Refer to package insert for more details regarding this warning.

§**BOXED WARNING:** Risk of thyroid C-cell tumors. Refer to package insert for more details.

¶**BOXED WARNING:** Severe hypoglycemia. Refer to package insert for more details.

CROHN'S DISEASE TREATMENTS

GENERIC	BRAND	HOW SUPPLIED	ADULT DOSAGE	PEDIATRIC DOSAGE
CORTICOSTEROIDS				
Betamethasone sodium phosphate-Betamethasone acetate	Celestone Soluspan	**Inj:** 3mg-3mg/mL [5mL, multidose]	**Initial:** 0.25-9mg/day IM.*	**Initial:** 0.02-0.3mg/kg/day in 3 or 4 divided doses IM.*
Budesonide	Entocort EC	**Cap:** 3mg	**Usual:** 9mg qam for up to 8 wks. **Recurring Episodes:** Repeat therapy for 8 wks. **Maint:** 6mg qd for up to 3 months, then taper to complete cessation.	
Dexamethasone	Generic	**Sol:** 0.5mg/5mL, 1mg/mL; **Tab:** 0.5mg†, 0.75mg†, 1mg†, 1.5mg†, 2mg†, 4mg†, 6mg†	**Initial:** 0.75-9mg/day.*	**Initial:** 0.02-0.3mg/kg/day in 3 or 4 divided doses.*
	Generic	**Inj:** 4mg/mL [1mL, 5mL, 30mL], 10mg/mL [1mL]	**Initial:** 0.5-9mg/day IV/IM.*	
Hydrocortisone	Cortef	**Tab:** 5mg†, 10mg†, 20mg†	**Initial:** 20-240mg/day.*	**Initial:** 20-240mg/day.*
	Solu-Cortef	**Inj:** 100mg, 250mg, 500mg, 1000mg	**Initial:** 100-500mg IV/IM. May repeat dose at 2-, 4-, or 6-hr intervals. High-dose therapy should continue only until patient is stabilized, usually not beyond 48-72 hrs.*	**Initial:** 0.56-8mg/kg/day IV/IM in 3 or 4 divided doses.*
Methylprednisolone	Depo-Medrol	**Inj:** 20mg/mL, 40mg/mL, 80mg/mL	**Initial:** 4-120mg IM.*	**Initial:** 0.11-1.6mg/kg/day.*
	Medrol	**Tab:** 2mg†, 4mg†, 8mg†, 16mg†, 32mg†; (Dose-Pak) 4mg† [21s]	**Initial:** 4-48mg/day.* Refer to PI for detailed information for ADT.	**Initial:** 4-48mg/day.* Refer to PI for detailed information for ADT.
	Solu-Medrol	**Inj:** 40mg, 125mg, 500mg, 1g, 2g	**Initial:** 10-40mg IV/IM inj or IV infusion. **High-Dose Therapy:** 30mg/kg IV over at least 30 min. May repeat dose q4-6h for 48 hrs. High-dose therapy should continue only until patient is stabilized, usually not beyond 48-72 hrs.*	**Initial:** 0.11-1.6mg/kg/day in 3 or 4 divided doses.*
Prednisolone	Flo-Pred	**Sus:** 15mg/5mL [37mL, 52mL, 65mL]	**Initial:** 5-60mg/day.*	**Initial:** 0.14-2mg/kg/day in 3 or 4 divided doses.*
	Orapred	**Sol:** 15mg/5mL [20mL, 237mL]; **Tab, Disintegrating:** 10mg, 15mg, 30mg	**(Sol) Initial:** 5-60mg/day. **(Tab, Disintegrating) Initial:** 10-60mg/day.*	**Initial:** 0.14-2mg/kg/day in 3 or 4 divided doses.*
	Pediapred	**Sol:** 5mg/5mL [120mL]	**Initial:** 5-60mg/day.*	**Initial:** 0.14-2mg/kg/day in 3 or 4 divided doses.*

(Continued)

GENERIC	BRAND	HOW SUPPLIED	ADULT DOSAGE	PEDIATRIC DOSAGE
CORTICOSTEROIDS *(Continued)*				
Prednisolone *(Continued)*	Generic	**Syrup:** 15mg/5mL [240mL, 480mL]; **Tab:** 5mg†	**Initial:** 5-60mg/day.* **(Tab)** Refer to PI for detailed information for ADT.	**Initial:** 5-60mg/day.* **(Tab)** Refer to PI for detailed information for ADT.
Prednisone	Rayos	**Tab, Delayed-Release:** 1mg, 2mg, 5mg	**Initial:** 5-60mg/day.*	**Initial:** 5-60mg/day.*
	Generic	**Sol:** 5mg/mL [30mL], 5mg/5mL [120mL, 500mL]; **Tab:** 1mg†, 2.5mg†, 5mg†, 10mg†, 20mg†, 50mg†	**Initial:** 5-60mg/day.* Refer to PI for detailed information for ADT.	**Initial:** 5-60mg/day.* Refer to PI for detailed information for ADT.
Triamcinolone	Kenalog-40	**Inj:** 40mg/mL [1mL, 5mL, 10mL]	**Initial:** 2.5-100mg/day.*	**Initial:** 0.11-1.6mg/kg/day in 3 or 4 divided doses.*
MONOCLONAL ANTIBODIES				
Adalimumab	Humira	**Inj:** 10mg/0.2mL, 20mg/0.4mL, 40mg/0.8mL	**Initial:** 160mg SQ on Day 1 (given as four 40mg inj in 1 day or as two 40mg inj/day for 2 consecutive days); then 80mg after 2 wks (Day 15). **Maint:** 40mg every other wk beginning wk 4 (Day 29).	
Certolizumab pegol	Cimzia	**Inj:** 200mg/mL	**Initial:** 400mg (given as 2 SQ inj of 200mg) initially and at wks 2 and 4. **Maint:** 400mg q4wks.	
Infliximab	Remicade	**Inj:** 100mg/20mL	**Induction:** 5mg/kg IV at 0, 2, and 6 wks. **Maint:** 5mg/kg q8wks. **Patients Who Initially Respond but Lose Their Response:** May increase to 10mg/kg. Refer to PI for administration and preparation instructions.	**≥6 yrs: Induction:** 5mg/kg IV at 0, 2, and 6 wks. **Maint:** 5mg/kg q8wks. Refer to PI for administration and preparation instructions.
Natalizumab	Tysabri	**Inj:** 300mg/15mL	300mg IV infusion over 1 hr q4wks.	
Vedolizumab	Entyvio	**Inj:** 300mg/20mL	300mg IV over 30 min at 0, 2, and 6 wks. **Maint:** 300mg q8wks.	

Refer to full FDA-approved labeling for additional information.

Abbreviation: ADT = alternate day therapy.

*Maintenance dose should be determined by decreasing initial dose in small decrements to lowest effective dose. Withdraw gradually after long-term therapy.

†Scored.

H_2 Antagonists and PPIs Comparison*

	DRUG	HOW SUPPLIED	INDICATIONS: Heartburn	Gastric Ulcer	GERD	Esophagitis	Zollinger-Ellison	*Helicobacter pylori*	NSAID Induced[†]	Upper GI Bleeding[‡]	Duodenal Ulcer
H_2 ANTAGONISTS	**CIMETIDINE**										
	Generic	**Sol:** 300mg/5mL **Tab:** 200mg, 300mg, 400mg, 800mg		X	X	X	X				X
	FAMOTIDINE										
	Pepcid	**Inj:** 10mg/mL (Generic) **Sus:** 40mg/5mL **Tab:** 20mg, 40mg		X	X	X	X				X
	NIZATIDINE										
	Axid	**Cap:** 150mg, 300mg (Generic) **Sol:** 15mg/mL	X	X	X	X					X
	RANITIDINE										
	Zantac	**Inj**[§]**:** 25mg/mL					X				X
		Cap: 150mg, 300mg (Generic) **Syrup:** 15mg/1mL (Generic) **Tab:** 150mg, 300mg	X	X	X	X	X				X
PPIs	**DEXLANSOPRAZOLE**										
	Dexilant	**Cap, DR:** 30mg, 60mg	X		X	X					
	ESOMEPRAZOLE										
	Nexium	**Cap, DR:** 20mg, 40mg **Sus, DR:** 2.5mg, 5mg, 10mg, 20mg, 40mg (granules/pkt)	X		X	X	X	X	X		X
	Nexium I.V.	**Inj**[¶]**:** 20mg, 40mg			X	X					X
	LANSOPRAZOLE										
	Prevacid	**Cap, DR:** 15mg, 30mg **Tab, Disintegrating:** 15mg, 30mg	X	X	X	X	X	X	X		X
	Prevpac	**Cap:** (Amoxicillin) 500mg **Tab:** (Clarithromycin) 500mg **Cap, DR:** (Lansoprazole) 30mg						X			X

(Continued)

	DRUG	HOW SUPPLIED	INDICATIONS								
			Heartburn	Gastric Ulcer	GERD	Esophagitis	Zollinger-Ellison	*Helicobacter pylori*	NSAID Induced[†]	Upper GI Bleeding[‡]	Duodenal Ulcer
PPIs *(Continued)*	**OMEPRAZOLE**										
	Prilosec	**Cap, DR:** 10mg, 20mg, 40mg **Sus, DR:** 2.5mg, 10mg (granules/pkt)	X	X	X	X	X	X			X
	Zegerid	**Cap:** (Omeprazole-Sodium bicarbonate) 20mg-1100mg, 40mg-1100mg **Pow:** 20mg-1680mg/pkt, 40mg-1680mg/pkt	X	X	X	X				X (40mg-1680mg)	X
	PANTOPRAZOLE										
	Protonix	**Tab, DR:** 20mg, 40mg **Sus, DR:** 40mg (granules/pkt)	X		X	X	X				
	Protonix I.V.	**Inj:** 40mg			X	X	X				
	RABEPRAZOLE										
	Aciphex	**Cap, DR:** 5mg, 10mg **Tab, DR:** 20mg	X		X		X	X			X

Refer to full FDA-approved labeling for additional information.

Abbreviations: DR = delayed-release; GERD = gastroesophageal reflux disease; GI = gastrointestinal; NSAID = nonsteroidal anti-inflammatory drug; PPI = proton pump inhibitor.

*Rx products only. For OTC products, refer to the *Antacid and Heartburn Products* table.

[†]Prevention of NSAID-induced gastric ulcers.

[‡]Prevention of upper GI bleeding in critically ill patients.

[§]May also be used as an alternative to oral dosage form for short-term use in patients unable to take oral medications.

[¶]Also indicated for risk reduction of rebleeding of gastric/duodenal ulcers following therapeutic endoscopy.

Ulcerative Colitis Treatments

GENERIC	BRAND	HOW SUPPLIED	ADULT DOSAGE	PEDIATRIC DOSAGE
AMINOSALICYLATES				
Balsalazide disodium	Colazal	**Cap:** 750mg	3 caps tid for up to 8 wks (or 12 wks if needed). May open cap and sprinkle on applesauce.	**5-17 yrs:** 1 or 3 caps tid for up to 8 wks. May open cap and sprinkle on applesauce.
	Giazo	**Tab:** 1.1g	**Male:** 3 tabs bid for up to 8 wks.	
Mesalamine	Apriso	**Cap, ER:** 0.375g	4 caps qam. Avoid with antacids.	
	Asacol	**Tab, DR:** 400mg	2 tabs tid for 6 wks. **Maint:** 1600mg/day in divided doses.*	**5-17 yrs: 54-90kg:** 27-44mg/kg/day up to 2400mg/day. **33-<54kg:** 37-61mg/kg/day up to 2000mg/day. **17-<33kg:** 36-71mg/kg/day up to 1200mg/day.*
	Asacol HD	**Tab, DR:** 800mg	2 tabs tid for 6 wks.*	
	Canasa	**Sup:** 1000mg	1 sup rectally qhs. Retain for 1-3 hrs or longer, if possible.	
	Delzicol	**Cap, DR:** 400mg	2 tabs tid for 6 wks. **Maint:** 1600mg/day in divided doses.	**≥12 yrs: 54-90kg:** 27-44mg/kg/day up to 2400mg/day. **33-<54kg:** 37-61mg/kg/day up to 2000mg/day. **17-<33kg:** 36-71mg/kg/day up to 1200mg/day.
	Lialda	**Tab, DR:** 1.2g	**Induction:** 2-4 tabs qd with a meal. **Maint:** 2 tabs qd with a meal.	
	Pentasa	**Cap, CR:** 250mg, 500mg	1000mg qid for up to 8 wks.	
	SF Rowasa	**Rect Sus:** 4g/60mL	1 instillation (4g) qhs for 3-6 weeks. Retain for 8 hrs.	
Olsalazine sodium	Dipentum	**Cap:** 250mg	1000mg/day in 2 divided doses.	
Sulfasalazine	Azulfidine	**Tab:** 500mg†	**Initial:** 3-4g/day in evenly divided doses with dose intervals ≤8 hrs. May initiate at 1-2g/day to reduce GI intolerance. **Maint:** 2g/day.	**≥6 yrs: Initial:** 40-60mg/kg/day divided into 3-6 doses. **Maint:** 30mg/kg/day divided into 4 doses.
	Azulfidine EN-tabs	**Tab, DR:** 500mg		
CORTICOSTEROIDS				
Betamethasone sodium phosphate-Betamethasone acetate	Celestone Soluspan	**Inj:** 3mg-3mg/mL [5mL, multidose]	**Initial:** 0.25-9mg/day IM.‡	**Initial:** 0.02-0.3mg/kg/day in 3 or 4 divided doses IM.‡

(Continued)

GENERIC	BRAND	HOW SUPPLIED	ADULT DOSAGE	PEDIATRIC DOSAGE
CORTICOSTEROIDS *(Continued)*				
Budesonide	Uceris	**Tab, ER:** 9mg	9mg qam for up to 8 wks.	
		Rectal Foam: 2mg/metered dose	1 metered dose rectally bid for 2 wks followed by 1 metered dose rectally qd for 4 wks.	
Dexamethasone	Generic	**Elixir:** 0.5mg/5mL; **Sol:** 0.5mg/5mL, 1mg/mL; **Tab:** 0.5mg†, 0.75mg†, 1mg†, 1.5mg†, 2mg†, 4mg†, 6mg†	**Initial:** 0.75-9mg/day.‡	(Sol/Tab) **Initial:** 0.02-0.3mg/kg/day in 3 or 4 divided doses.‡
	Generic	**Inj:** 4mg/mL [1mL, 5mL, 30mL], 10mg/mL [1mL]	**Initial:** 0.5-9mg/day IV/IM.‡	
Hydrocortisone	Anusol-HC	**Sup:** 25mg	**Nonspecific Proctitis:** 1 sup rectally bid for 2 wks. **More Severe Cases:** 1 sup rectally tid or 2 sup rectally bid. **Factitial Proctitis:** Use up to 6-8 wks.	
	Colocort	**Rect Sus:** 100mg/60mL	1 instillation (100mg) qhs for 21 days or until remission. Retain for ≥1 hr, preferably all night.	
	Cortef	**Tab:** 5mg†, 10mg†, 20mg†	**Initial:** 20-240mg/day.‡	**Initial:** 20-240mg/day.‡
	Cortifoam	**Rectal Foam:** 10%	1 applicatorful rectally qd or bid for 2 or 3 wks, and every second day thereafter.	
	Proctocort	**Sup:** 30mg	**Nonspecific Proctitis:** 1 sup rectally bid for 2 wks. **More Severe Cases:** 1 sup rectally tid or 2 sup rectally bid. **Factitial Proctitis:** Use up to 6-8 wks.	
	Solu-Cortef	**Inj:** 100mg, 250mg, 500mg, 1000mg	**Initial:** 100-500mg IV/IM. May repeat dose at 2-, 4-, or 6-hr intervals. High-dose therapy should continue only until patient is stabilized, usually not beyond 48-72 hrs.‡	**Initial:** 0.56-8mg/kg/day IV/IM in 3 or 4 divided doses.‡
Methylprednisolone	Depo-Medrol	**Inj:** 20mg/mL, 40mg/mL, 80mg/mL	**Initial:** 4-120mg IM.‡	**Initial:** 0.11-1.6mg/kg/day.‡
	Medrol	**Tab:** 2mg†, 4mg†, 8mg†, 16mg†, 32mg†; (Dose-Pak) 4mg† [21s]	**Initial:** 4-48mg/day.‡ Refer to PI for detailed information for ADT.	**Initial:** 4-48mg/day.‡ Refer to PI for detailed information for ADT.
	Solu-Medrol	**Inj:** 40mg, 125mg, 500mg, 1g, 2g	**Initial:** 10-40mg IV/IM inj or IV infusion. **High-Dose Therapy:** 30mg/kg IV over at least 30 min. May repeat dose q4-6h for 48 hrs. High-dose therapy should continue only until patient is stabilized, usually not beyond 48-72 hrs.‡	**Initial:** 0.11-1.6mg/kg/day in 3 or 4 divided doses.‡

GENERIC	BRAND	HOW SUPPLIED	ADULT DOSAGE	PEDIATRIC DOSAGE
CORTICOSTEROIDS *(Continued)*				
Prednisolone	Flo-Pred	**Sus:** 15mg/5mL [37mL, 52mL, 65mL]	**Initial:** 5-60mg/day.‡	**Initial:** 0.14-2mg/kg/day in 3 or 4 divided doses.‡
	Orapred	**Sol:** 15mg/5mL [20mL, 237mL]; **Tab, Disintegrating:** 10mg, 15mg, 30mg	(Sol) **Initial:** 5-60mg/day. (Tab, Disintegrating) **Initial:** 10-60mg/day.‡	**Initial:** 0.14-2mg/kg/day in 3 or 4 divided doses.‡
	Pediapred	**Sol:** 5mg/5mL [120mL]	**Initial:** 5-60mg/day.‡	**Initial:** 0.14-2mg/kg/day in 3 or 4 divided doses.‡
	Generic	**Syrup:** 15mg/5mL [240mL, 480mL]; **Tab:** 5mg†	**Initial:** 5-60mg/day.‡ (Tab) Refer to PI for detailed information for ADT.	**Initial:** 5-60mg/day.‡ (Tab) Refer to PI for detailed information for ADT.
Prednisone	Rayos	**Tab, DR:** 1mg, 2mg, 5mg	**Initial:** 5-60mg/day.‡	**Initial:** 5-60mg/day.‡
	Generic	**Sol:** 5mg/mL [30mL], 5mg/5mL [120mL, 500mL]; **Tab:** 1mg†, 2.5mg†, 5mg†, 10mg†, 20mg†, 50mg†	**Initial:** 5-60mg/day.‡ Refer to PI for detailed information for ADT.	**Initial:** 5-60mg/day.‡ Refer to PI for detailed information for ADT.
Triamcinolone	Kenalog-40	**Inj:** 40mg/mL [1mL, 5mL, 10mL]	**Initial:** 2.5-100mg/day.‡	**Initial:** 0.11-1.6mg/kg/day in 3 or 4 divided doses.‡
MONOCLONAL ANTIBODIES				
Adalimumab	Humira	**Inj:** 10mg/0.2mL, 20mg/0.4mL, 40mg/0.8mL	**Initial:** 160mg SQ on Day 1 (given as four 40mg inj in 1 day or as two 40mg inj/day for 2 consecutive days); then 80mg after 2 wks (Day 15). **Maint:** 40mg every other wk beginning Wk 4 (Day 29). Continue only with evidence of clinical remission by 8 wks (Day 57) of therapy.	
Golimumab	Simponi	**Inj:** 50mg/0.5mL, 100mg/mL	**Induction:** 200mg SQ at Week 0, then 100mg at Week 2. **Maint:** 100mg q4wks. Refer to PI for administration and preparation instructions.	
Infliximab	Remicade	**Inj:** 100mg/20mL	**Induction:** 5mg/kg IV at 0, 2, and 6 wks. **Maint:** 5mg/kg q8wks. Refer to PI for administration and preparation instructions.	**≥6 yrs: Induction:** 5mg/kg IV at 0, 2, and 6 wks. **Maint:** 5mg/kg q8wks. Refer to PI for administration and preparation instructions.

(Continued)

GENERIC	BRAND	HOW SUPPLIED	ADULT DOSAGE	PEDIATRIC DOSAGE
MONOCLONAL ANTIBODIES *(Continued)*				
Vedolizumab	Entyvio	**Inj:** 300mg/20mL	300mg IV over 30 min at 0, 2, and 6 wks. **Maint:** 300mg q8wks.	

Refer to full FDA-approved labeling for additional information.

Abbreviations: ADT = alternate day therapy; CR = controlled-release; DR = delayed-release; ER = extended-release.

*Do not use two 400mg tabs and one 800mg tab interchangeably.

†Scored.

‡Maintenance dose should be determined by decreasing initial dose in small decrements to lowest effective dose. Withdraw gradually after long-term therapy.

DRUGS THAT SHOULD NOT BE USED IN PREGNANCY

Studies on these generic drugs in animals or humans, or investigational or postmarketing reports, have shown fetal risk that clearly outweighs any possible benefit to the patient. This list should not be considered all-inclusive. Various brands in different formulations may exist.

Abiraterone acetate
Acetohydroxamic acid
Acitretin
Ambrisentan
Amikacin sulfate
Amlodipine besylate/Atorvastatin calcium
Anastrozole
Aspirin
Atorvastatin calcium
Atorvastatin/Ezetimibe
Bendamustine hydrochloride
Benzphetamine hydrochloride
Bexarotene
Bicalutamide
Boceprevir
Bosentan
Caffeine
Cetrorelix acetate
Chenodiol
Choriogonadotropin alfa
Chorionic gonadotropin
Clomiphene citrate
Danazol
Degarelix
Denosumab
Desogestrel/Ethinyl estradiol
Diclofenac sodium
Diclofenac sodium/Misoprostol
Dihydroergotamine mesylate
Dinutuximab
Dronedarone
Drospirenone/Ethinyl estradiol
Dutasteride
Dutasteride/Tamsulosin hydrochloride
Enzalutamide
Ergotamine tartrate
Estazolam
Estradiol
Estradiol valerate
Estradiol/Norethindrone acetate
Estrogens, Conjugated, Synthetic B
Estropipate
Ethinyl estradiol
Ethinyl estradiol/Ethynodiol diacetate
Ethinyl estradiol/Etonogestrel
Ethinyl estradiol/Ferrous fumarate/Norethindrone acetate
Ethinyl estradiol/Levonorgestrel
Ethinyl estradiol/Norelgestromin
Ethinyl estradiol/Norethindrone
Ethinyl estradiol/Norgestimate
Ethinyl estradiol/Norgestrel
Exemestane
Ezetimibe/Simvastatin
Finasteride
Fluorouracil
Fluoxymesterone
Fluvastatin sodium
Follitropin alfa
Follitropin beta
Ganirelix acetate
Gefitinib
Genistein aglycone
Goserelin acetate
Histrelin acetate
Iodine I 131 tositumomab
Irinotecan hydrochloride
Isotretinoin
Ixazomib citrate
Leflunomide
Lenalidomide
Lenvatinib
Letrozole
Leuprolide acetate
Leuprolide acetate/Norethindrone acetate
Levonorgestrel
Lomitapide
Lorcaserin hydrochloride
Lovastatin
Lovastatin/Niacin
Macitentan
Medroxyprogesterone acetate
Megestrol acetate
Mestranol/Norethindrone
Methotrexate
Methyltestosterone
Mifepristone
Miglustat
Misoprostol
Mitomycin
Nafarelin acetate
Niacin/Simvastatin
Norethindrone
Orlistat
Ospemifene
Oxandrolone
Palbociclib
Panobinostat lactate
Phendimetrazine tartrate
Phentermine hydrochloride
Phentermine/Topiramate
Pitavastatin
Pomalidomide
Pravastatin sodium
Radium Ra 223 dichloride
Raloxifene hydrochloride
Ribavirin
Riociguat
Rosuvastatin calcium
Sacubitril/Valsartan
Simeprevir
Simvastatin
Simvastatin/Sitagliptin
Sofosbuvir
Sonidegib
Tazarotene
Temazepam
Teriflunomide
Tesamorelin
Testosterone
Testosterone cypionate
Testosterone enanthate
Thalidomide
Triazolam
Triptorelin pamoate
Ulipristal acetate
Urofollitropin
Vitamin A palmitate
Warfarin sodium

PRENATAL SUPPLEMENTS

	VITAMINS											
	A	B1	B2	B3	B5	B6	B7	B9	B12	C	D3	E
CitraNatal 90 DHA		3mg	3.4mg	20mg		20mg		1mg		120mg	400 IU	30 IU
CitraNatal Assure		3mg	3.4mg	20mg		25mg		1mg		120mg	400 IU	30 IU
CitraNatal B-Calm						25mg (Prenatal vitamin) + 25mg (B6 tablet)		1mg		120mg	400 IU	
CitraNatal Harmony						25mg		1mg			400 IU	30 IU
Duet DHA Balanced	2840 IU	1.5mg	4mg	20mg		50mg		1mg	12mcg	120mg	840 IU	2mg
Elite OB	2100 IU	2mg	3.4mg	10mg	5mg	10mg		1.25mg	15mcg	120mg	315 IU	20 IU
Foltabs		3mg	3.4mg	20mg		20mg		1mg		120mg	400 IU	30 IU
Gesticare DHA		3mg	3mg	20mg		50mg		1mg	8mcg	120mg	410 IU	30 IU
NataChew	2700 IU	2mg	3mg	20mg		10mg		1mg	12mcg	120mg	400 IU	20 IU
Neevo DHA		1.4mg	1.4mg	18mg		25mg		1.13mg	1mg	85mg	5mcg	15mg
Nestabs DHA		3mg	3mg	20mg		50mg		1mg	10mcg	120mg	450 IU	30 IU
OB Complete One		2mg	4mg	10mg		30mg	200mcg	1mg	50mcg	70mg	1200 IU	30 IU
PNV OB +DHA		3mg	3.4mg	20mg		20mg		1mg		120mg	400 IU	30 IU
Prenate AM						75mg		1mg	12mcg			
Prenate Chewable						10mg	280mcg	1mg	125mg		300 IU	
Prenate DHA						26mg		1mg	25mcg	90mg	400 IU	40 IU
Prenate Elite	2600 IU	3mg	3.5mg	21mg	6mg	21mg	330mcg	1mg	13mcg	75mg	450 IU	10 IU
Prenate Enhance						25mg	500mg	1mg	12mcg	85mg	1000 IU	10 IU
Prenate Essential						26mg	280mcg	1mg	13mcg	90mg	220 IU	10 IU
Prenate Mini						26mg	280mcg	1mg	13mcg	60mg	1000 IU	10 IU
Prenate Pixie						5mg	75mcg	1mg	13mcg	30mg	500 IU	10 IU

MINERALS						MISCELLANEOUS				
Calcium	**Copper**	**Iodine**	**Iron**	**Magnesium**	**Zinc**	**Docusate**	**DHA**	**EPA**	**Other**	
159mg	2mg	150mcg	90mg		25mg	50mg	300mg	≤0.750mg		**CitraNatal 90 DHA**
125mg	2mg	150mcg	35mg		25mg	50mg	300mg	≤0.750mg		**CitraNatal Assure**
120mg			20mg							**CitraNatal B-Calm**
104mg			30mg			50mg	260mg			**CitraNatal Harmony**
215mg	2mg	210mcg	26mg	25mg	25mg				Omega-3 capsule: 278mg (DHA/EPA/ ALA/DPA)	**Duet DHA Balanced**
	1mg		50mg	15mg	10mg					**Elite OB**
125mg	2mg	150mcg	27mg		25mg	50mg				**Foltabs**
200mg		150mcg	27mg		15mg				Choline bitartrate: 55mg	**Gesticare DHA**
			28mg							**NataChew**
110mg		220mcg	27mg	60mg			250mg		Selenium: 60mcg	**Neevo DHA**
200mg		100mcg	32mg		10mg		230mg	30mg	Choline bitartrate: 55mg	**Nestabs DHA**
55mg	1mg	150mcg	50mg	25mg	15mg		300mg	40mg		**OB Complete One**
125mg	2mg	150mcg	27mg		25mg	50mg	250mg			**PNV OB +DHA**
200mg									Ginger: 500mg, Lingonberry: 25mg	**Prenate AM**
500mg				50mg					Boron amino acid chelate: 250mcg, Blueberry extract: 25mg	**Prenate Chewable**
155mg			18mg	50mg			300mg			**Prenate DHA**
100mg	1.5mg	150mcg	26mg	25mg	15mg					**Prenate Elite**
155mg		150mcg	28mg	50mg			400mg			**Prenate Enhance**
145mg		150mcg	29mg	50mg			300mg	40mg		**Prenate Essential**
80mg		150mcg	18mg	25mg			350mg		Blueberry extract: 25mg	**Prenate Mini**
		150mcg	10mg				200mg		Blueberry extract: 5mg	**Prenate Pixie**

(Continued)

	VITAMINS											
	A	B1	B2	B3	B5	B6	B7	B9	B12	C	D3	E
Prenate Restore						25mg	500mg	1mg	12mcg	85mg	1000 IU	10 IU
Prenate Star	3300 IU	1.5mg	2mg	21mg	6mg	21mg	330mcg	1mg	12mcg	75mg	450 IU	
Provida DHA		2mg	3mg	2mg	5mg	25mg	300mcg	1.25mg	10mcg	30mg	400 IU	
Reaphirm Plant Source DHA	1100 IU	1.6mg	1.8mg	15mg		2.5mg		1mg	12mcg	30mg	1000 IU	20 IU
Select OB	1700 IU	1.6mg	1.8mg	15mg		2.5mg		1mg	5mcg	60mg	400 IU	30 IU
Select OB +DHA	1700 IU	1.6mg	1.8mg	15mg		2.5mg		1mg	5mcg	60mg	400 IU	30 IU
TL-Select DHA						25mg	250mcg	1.25mg		28mg	800 IU	30 IU
Tricare DHA ONE		3mg	3.4mg	20mg		25mg	300mcg	1mg	100mcg	60mg	800 IU	30 IU
Vitafol Fe+	1100 IU	1.6mg	1.8mg	15mg		2.5mg		1mg	25mcg	60mg	1000 IU	20 IU
Vitafol-OB +DHA	2700 IU	1.6mg	1.8mg	18mg		2.5mg		1mg	12mcg	70mg	400 IU	30 IU
Vitafol-One	1100 IU	1.6mg	1.8mg	15mg		2.5mg		1mg	12mcg	30mg	1000 IU	20 IU
Vitafol Ultra	1100 IU	1.6mg	1.8mg	15mg		2.5mg		1mg	12mcg	30mg	1000 IU	20 IU
VitamedMD RX Plus		3mg	3.4mg	20mg	10mg	25mg	300mcg	1mg	12mcg	60mg	600 IU	30 IU

MINERALS						MISCELLANEOUS				
Calcium	Copper	Iodine	Iron	Magnesium	Zinc	Docusate	DHA	EPA	Other	
155mg			27mg	45mg			400mg		*Bacillus coagulans*: 10mg	**Prenate Restore**
155mg	1.5mg	150mcg	20mg	25mg	15mg					**Prenate Star**
	1mg		32mg	7mg	6mg		110mg		*Lactobacillus casei* KE-99: 30mg	**Provida DHA**
	2mg	150mcg	29mg	20mg	25mg		200mg			**Reaphirm Plant Source DHA**
			29mg	25mg	15mg					**Select OB**
			29mg	25mg	15mg		250mg			**Select OB +DHA**
160mg			29mg			55mg	350mg			**TL-Select DHA**
	2mg		27mg		10mg	25mg	215mg	45mg		**Tricare DHA ONE**
	2mg	150mcg	90mg	20mg	25mg		200mg			**Vitafol Fe+**
100mg	2mg		65mg	25mg	25mg		250mg			**Vitafol-OB +DHA**
	2mg	150mcg	29mg	20mg	25mg		200mg			**Vitafol-One**
	2mg	150mcg	29mg	20mg	25mg		200mg			**Vitafol Ultra**
150mg	2mg	150mcg	30mg		15mg					**VitamedMD RX Plus**

Definitions: ALA = alpha-linolenic acid; B1 = thiamine; B2 = riboflavin; B3 = niacinamide; B5 = pantothenic acid; B6 = pyridoxine; B7 = biotin; B9 = folic acid; B12 = cyanocobalamin; D3 = cholecalciferol; DHA = docosahexaenoic acid; DPA = docosapentaenoic acid; EPA = eicosapentaenoic acid.

ANTIVIRAL TREATMENT COMPARISON

GENERIC (BRAND)	HOW SUPPLIED	INDICATIONS							
		HIV	HBV	HCV	Genital Herpes	Herpes Zoster	Herpes Labialis	CMV Retinitis	Influenza
ADAMANTANES									
Rimantadine HCl (Flumadine)	**Tab:** 100mg								✓-A
BIOLOGICAL RESPONSE MODIFIERS									
Interferon alfa-2b (Intron A)	**Inj:** (Powder) 10 MIU, 18 MIU, 50 MIU; (Vial) 18 MIU, 25 MIU		✓	✓					
Interferon alfacon-1 (Infergen)	**Inj:** 9mcg/0.3mL, 15mcg/0.5mL			✓					
Peginterferon alfa-2a (Pegasys)	**Inj:** (Prefilled syringe) 180mcg/0.5mL; (ProClick autoinjector) 180mcg/0.5mL, 135mcg/0.5mL; (Vial) 180mcg/mL		✓	✓					
Peginterferon alfa-2b (PegIntron)	**Inj:** (Prefilled pen, Vial) 50mcg/0.5mL, 80mcg/0.5mL, 120mcg/0.5mL, 150mcg/0.5mL			✓					
CCR5 CO-RECEPTOR ANTAGONISTS									
Maraviroc (Selzentry)	**Tab:** 150mg, 300mg	✓							
CYP3A INHIBITORS									
Cobicistat (Tybost)	**Tab:** 150mg	✓							
CYP3A INHIBITOR/HCV NS5A INHIBITOR/HCV NON-NUCLEOSIDE NS5B PALM POLYMERASE INHIBITOR/HCV NS3/4A PROTEASE INHIBITOR COMBINATIONS									
Dasabuvir, Ombitasvir/ Paritaprevir/ Ritonavir (Viekira Pak)	**Tab:** 250mg, 12.5mg/75mg/ 50mg			✓					
CYP3A INHIBITOR/HCV NS5A INHIBITOR/HCV NS3/4A PROTEASE INHIBITOR COMBINATIONS									
Ombitasvir/ Paritaprevir/ Ritonavir (Technivie)	**Tab:** 12.5mg/ 75mg/50mg			✓					
CYP3A INHIBITOR/HIV INTEGRASE STRAND TRANSFER INHIBITOR/NUCLEOSIDE ANALOGUE COMBINATIONS									
Cobicistat/ Elvitegravir/ Emtricitabine/ Tenofovir alafenamide (Genvoya)	**Tab:** 150mg/ 150mg/200mg/ 10mg	✓							

(Continued)

GENERIC (BRAND)	HOW SUPPLIED	INDICATIONS							
		HIV	HBV	HCV	Genital Herpes	Herpes Zoster	Herpes Labialis	CMV Retinitis	Influenza
CYP3A INHIBITOR/HIV INTEGRASE STRAND TRANSFER INHIBITOR/NUCLEOSIDE ANALOGUE COMBINATIONS *(Continued)*									
Cobicistat/ Elvitegravir/ Emtricitabine/ Tenofovir disoproxil fumarate (Stribild)	**Tab:** 150mg/ 150mg/200mg/ 300mg	✓							
CYP3A INHIBITOR/PROTEASE INHIBITOR COMBINATIONS									
Atazanavir/ Cobicistat (Evotaz)	**Tab:** 300mg/150mg	✓							
Cobicistat/ Darunavir (Prezcobix)	**Tab:** 150mg/800mg	✓							
DOPAMINE RECEPTOR AGONISTS									
Amantadine HCl	**Cap:** 100mg; **Syr:** 50mg/5mL [473mL]; **Tab:** 100mg								✓-A
FUSION INHIBITORS									
Enfuvirtide (Fuzeon)	**Inj:** 90mg/mL [108mg]	✓							
GUANOSINE NUCLEOSIDE ANALOGUES									
Entecavir (Baraclude)	**Sol:** 0.05mg/mL [210mL]; **Tab:** 0.5mg, 1mg		✓						
HCV NS3/4A PROTEASE INHIBITORS									
Simeprevir (Olysio)	**Cap:** 150mg			✓					
HCV NS5A INHIBITORS									
Daclatasvir (Daklinza)	**Tab:** 30mg, 60mg			✓					
HCV NS5A INHIBITOR/HCV NS3/4A PROTEASE INHIBITOR COMBINATIONS									
Elbasvir/Grazoprevir (Zepatier)	**Tab:** 50mg/100mg			✓					
HCV NS5A INHIBITOR/HCV NUCLEOTIDE ANALOGUE NS5B POLYMERASE INHIBITOR COMBINATIONS									
Ledipasvir/ Sofosbuvir (Harvoni)	**Tab:** 90mg/400mg			✓					
HCV NUCLEOTIDE ANALOGUE NS5B POLYMERASE INHIBITOR									
Sofosbuvir (Sovaldi)	**Tab:** 400mg			✓					
HIV INTEGRASE STRAND TRANSFER INHIBITORS									
Dolutegravir (Tivicay)	**Tab:** 50mg	✓							
Elvitegravir (Vitekta)	**Tab:** 85mg, 150mg	✓							
Raltegravir (Isentress)	**Sus Powder:** 100mg/pkt; **Tab:** 400mg; **Tab, Chewable:** 25mg, 100mg	✓							

GENERIC (BRAND)	HOW SUPPLIED	INDICATIONS							
		HIV	HBV	HCV	Genital Herpes	Herpes Zoster	Herpes Labialis	CMV Retinitis	Influenza
HIV INTEGRASE STRAND TRANSFER INHIBITOR/NUCLEOSIDE ANALOGUE RT INHIBITOR COMBINATIONS									
Abacavir/ Dolutegravir/ Lamivudine (Triumeq)	**Tab:** 600mg/ 50mg/300mg	✓							
NEURAMINIDASE INHIBITORS									
Oseltamivir phosphate (Tamiflu)	**Cap:** 30mg, 45mg, 75mg; **Sus:** 6mg/mL [60mL]								✓
Peramivir (Rapivab)	**Inj:** 10mg/mL								✓
Zanamivir (Relenza)	**Powder, Inh:** 5mg/inh								✓-A,B
NON-NUCLEOSIDE RT INHIBITORS									
Delavirdine mesylate (Rescriptor)	**Tab:** 100mg, 200mg	✓							
Efavirenz (Sustiva)	**Cap:** 50mg, 200mg; **Tab:** 600mg	✓							
Etravirine (Intelence)	**Tab:** 25mg, 100mg, 200mg	✓							
Nevirapine (Viramune, Viramune XR)	**Sus:** 50mg/5mL [240mL]; **Tab:** 200mg; **Tab, ER:** 100mg, 400mg	✓							
Rilpivirine (Edurant)	**Tab:** 25mg	✓							
NON-NUCLEOSIDE RT INHIBITOR/NUCLEOSIDE ANALOGUE COMBINATIONS									
Efavirenz/ Emtricitabine/ Tenofovir disoproxil fumarate (Atripla)	**Tab:** 600mg/200mg/ 300mg	✓							
Emtricitabine/ Rilpivirine/Tenofovir alafenamide (Odefsey)	**Tab:** 200mg/25mg/ 25mg	✓							
Emtricitabine/ Rilpivirine/ Tenofovir disoproxil fumarate (Complera)	**Tab:** 200mg/25mg/ 300mg	✓							
NUCLEOSIDE ANALOGUES									
Acyclovir (Sitavig)	**Tab, Buccal:** 50mg						✓		
Acyclovir (Zovirax Oral)	**Cap:** 200mg; **Sus:** 200mg/5mL [473mL]; **Tab:** 400mg, 800mg				✓	✓			

(Continued)

GENERIC (BRAND)	HOW SUPPLIED	INDICATIONS							
		HIV	HBV	HCV	Genital Herpes	Herpes Zoster	Herpes Labialis	CMV Retinitis	Influenza
NUCLEOSIDE ANALOGUES *(Continued)*									
Acyclovir (Zovirax Cream)	**Cre:** 5% [5g]						✓		
Acyclovir (Zovirax Ointment)	**Oint:** 5% [15g]				✓				
Acyclovir sodium	**Inj:** 50mg/mL				✓	✓			
Famciclovir (Famvir)	**Tab:** 125mg, 250mg, 500mg				✓	✓	✓		
Ganciclovir sodium (Cytovene)	**Inj:** 500mg/10mL							✓	
Penciclovir (Denavir)	**Cre:** 1% [1.5g, 5g]						✓		
Ribavirin (Copegus)	**Tab:** 200mg			✓					
Ribavirin (Moderiba)	**Tab:** 200mg, 400mg, 600mg			✓					
Ribavirin (Rebetol)	**Cap:** 200mg; **Sol:** 40mg/mL [100mL]			✓					
Ribavirin (Ribasphere Capsules)	**Cap:** 200mg			✓					
Ribavirin (Ribasphere Tablets)	**Tab:** 200mg, 400mg, 600mg			✓					
Valacyclovir HCl (Valtrex)	**Tab:** 500mg, 1000mg				✓	✓	✓		
Valganciclovir HCl (Valcyte)	**Sol:** 50mg/mL [88mL]; **Tab:** 450mg							✓	
NUCLEOSIDE ANALOGUE COMBINATIONS									
Emtricitabine/ Tenofovir disoproxil fumarate (Truvada)	**Tab:** 200mg/300mg	✓							
NUCLEOSIDE ANALOGUE RT INHIBITORS									
Abacavir sulfate (Ziagen)	**Sol:** 20mg/mL [240mL]; **Tab:** 300mg	✓							
Didanosine (Videx, Videx EC)	**Cap, DR:** (Videx EC) 125mg, 200mg, 250mg, 400mg; **Sol:** (Videx) 10mg/mL [2g, 4g]	✓							
Emtricitabine (Emtriva)	**Cap:** 200mg; **Sol:** 10mg/mL [170mL]	✓							

GENERIC (BRAND)	HOW SUPPLIED	INDICATIONS							
		HIV	HBV	HCV	Genital Herpes	Herpes Zoster	Herpes Labialis	CMV Retinitis	Influenza
NUCLEOSIDE ANALOGUE RT INHIBITORS *(Continued)*									
Lamivudine (Epivir)	**Sol:** 10mg/mL [240mL]; **Tab:** 150mg, 300mg	✓							
Lamivudine (Epivir-HBV)	**Sol:** 5mg/mL [240mL]; **Tab:** 100mg		✓						
Stavudine (Zerit)	**Cap:** 15mg, 20mg, 30mg, 40mg; **Sol:** 1mg/mL [200mL]	✓							
Telbivudine (Tyzeka)	**Tab:** 600mg; **Sol:** 100mg/5mL [300mL]		✓						
Zidovudine (Retrovir)	**Cap:** 100mg; **Inj:** 10mg/mL; **Syrup:** 10mg/mL [240mL]; **Tab:** 300mg	✓							
NUCLEOSIDE ANALOGUE RT INHIBITOR COMBINATIONS									
Abacavir sulfate/ Lamivudine (Epzicom)	**Tab:** 600mg/300mg	✓							
Abacavir sulfate/ Lamivudine/ Zidovudine (Trizivir)	**Tab:** 300mg/150mg/ 300mg	✓							
Lamivudine/ Zidovudine (Combivir)	**Tab:** 150mg/300mg	✓							
NUCLEOTIDE ANALOGUE RT INHIBITORS									
Adefovir dipivoxil (Hepsera)	**Tab:** 10mg		✓						
Tenofovir disoproxil fumarate (Viread)	**Powder:** 40mg/g [60g]; **Tab:** 150mg, 200mg, 250mg, 300mg	✓	✓						
PROTEASE INHIBITORS									
Atazanavir (Reyataz)	**Cap:** 150mg, 200mg, 300mg; **Powder:** 50mg/pkt	✓							
Darunavir (Prezista)	**Sus:** 100mg/mL [200mL]; **Tab:** 75mg, 150mg, 600mg, 800mg	✓							
Fosamprenavir calcium (Lexiva)	**Sus:** 50mg/mL [225mL]; **Tab:** 700mg	✓							
Indinavir sulfate (Crixivan)	**Cap:** 200mg, 400mg	✓							

(Continued)

GENERIC (BRAND)	HOW SUPPLIED	INDICATIONS							
		HIV	HBV	HCV	Genital Herpes	Herpes Zoster	Herpes Labialis	CMV Retinitis	Influenza
PROTEASE INHIBITORS *(Continued)*									
Lopinavir/ Ritonavir (Kaletra)	**Sol:** 80mg/20mg/mL [160mL]; **Tab:** 100mg/25mg, 200mg/50mg	✓							
Nelfinavir mesylate (Viracept)	**Powder:** 50mg/g [144g]; **Tab:** 250g, 625mg	✓							
Ritonavir (Norvir)	**Cap, Tab:** 100mg; **Sol:** 80mg/mL [240mL]	✓							
Saquinavir mesylate (Invirase)	**Cap:** 200mg; **Tab:** 500mg	✓							
Tipranavir (Aptivus)	**Cap:** 250mg; **Sol:** 100mg/mL [95mL]	✓							
PYROPHOSPHATE BINDING INHIBITORS									
Foscarnet sodium (Foscavir)	**Inj:** 24mg/mL							✓	
VIRAL DNA SYNTHESIS INHIBITORS									
Cidofovir (Vistide)	**Inj:** 75mg/mL							✓	

Refer to full FDA-approved labeling for additional information.

Abbreviations: CMV = cytomegalovirus; HBV = hepatitis B virus; HCV = hepatitis C virus; HIV = human immunodeficiency virus; RT = reverse transcriptase.

ORAL ANTIBIOTICS TREATMENT COMPARISON

GENERIC (BRAND)	HOW SUPPLIED	INDICATIONS																						
		ABECB	AECB	Bone & Joint	CAP	Endocarditis	GI	Intra-Ab	LRTI	URTI	Lyme Disease	MAC	Meningitis	Oph	Otitis Media	PCP	Septicemia	Sinusitis	SSSI	SSTI	TB	UTI	UGI	Gyn
CEPHALOSPORINS																								
1st Generation																								
Cefadroxil	**Cap:** 500mg; **Susp:** 250mg/5mL, 500mg/5mL; **Tab:** 1g									X									X			X		
Cephalexin (Keflex)	**Cap:** 250mg, 500mg, 750mg; **Susp:** 125mg/5mL, 250mg/5mL; **Tab:** 250mg, 500mg			X					X	X					X				X			X	X	
2nd Generation																								
Cefaclor	**Cap:** 250mg, 500mg; **Susp:** 125mg/5mL, 187mg/5mL, 250mg/5mL, 375mg/5mL								X	X					X				X			X		
Cefaclor ER	**Tab, ER:** 500mg	X							X	X									X					
Cefprozil	**Susp:** 125mg/5mL, 250mg/5mL; **Tab:** 250mg, 500mg	X							X	X					X			X	X					
Cefuroxime axetil (Ceftin)	**Susp:** 125mg/5mL, 250mg/5mL; **Tab:** 250mg, 500mg	X (Tab)							X (Tab)	X	X (Tab)				X			X	X			X (Tab)	X (Tab)	X (Tab)

(Continued)

GENERIC (BRAND)	HOW SUPPLIED	INDICATIONS																						
		ABECB	AECB	Bone & Joint	CAP	Endocarditis	GI	Intra-Ab	LRTI	URTI	Lyme Disease	MAC	Meningitis	Oph	Otitis Media	PCP	Septicemia	Sinusitis	SSSI	SSTI	TB	UTI	UGI	Gyn
CEPHALOSPORINS *(Continued)*																								
3rd Generation																								
Cefdinir	**Cap:** 300mg; **Susp:** 125mg/5mL, 250mg/5mL		X		X					X					X			X	X					
Cefditoren pivoxil (Spectracef)	**Tab:** 200mg, 400mg	X			X					X									X					
Cefixime (Suprax)	**Cap:** 400mg; **Susp:** 100mg/5mL, 200mg/5mL, 500mg/5mL; **Tab:** 400mg; **Tab, Chew:** 100mg, 150mg, 200mg		X							X					X							X	X	X
Cefpodoxime proxetil	**Susp:** 50mg/5mL, 100mg/5mL; **Tab:** 100mg, 200mg	X			X					X					X			X	X			X	X	X
Ceftibuten (Cedax)	**Cap:** 400mg; **Susp:** 90mg/5mL, 180mg/5mL	X								X					X									
FLUOROQUINOLONES																								
Ciprofloxacin (Cipro)	**Susp:** 250mg/5mL, 500mg/5mL; **Tab:** 250mg, 500mg			X			X	X	X									X	X			X	X	X
Ciprofloxacin (Cipro XR)	**Tab, ER:** 500mg, 1000mg																					X		
Gemifloxacin mesylate (Factive)	**Tab:** 320mg	X			X																			

GENERIC (BRAND)	HOW SUPPLIED	INDICATIONS																						
		ABECB	AECB	Bone & Joint	CAP	Endocarditis	GI	Intra-Ab	LRTI	URTI	Lyme Disease	MAC	Meningitis	Oph	Otitis Media	PCP	Septicemia	Sinusitis	SSSI	SSTI	TB	UTI	UGI	Gyn
FLUOROQUINOLONES *(Continued)*																								
Levofloxacin (Levaquin)	**Sol:** 25mg/mL; **Tab:** 250mg, 500mg, 750mg	X			X				X									X	X			X	X	
Moxifloxacin HCl (Avelox)	**Tab:** 400mg	X			X			X										X	X					
Ofloxacin	**Tab:** 200mg, 300mg, 400mg	X			X														X			X	X	X
MACROLIDES																								
Azithromycin (Zithromax)	**Susp:** 100mg/5mL, 200mg/5mL; **Tab:** 250mg, 500mg	X			X					X					X			X	X				X	X
Azithromycin (Zithromax)	**Susp:** 1g/pkt; **Tab:** 600mg											X											X	X
Azithromycin (Zmax)	**Susp, ER:** 2g (27mg/mL)				X													X						
Clarithromycin (Biaxin)	**Susp:** 125mg/5mL, 250mg/5mL; **Tab:** 250mg, 500mg	X			X		X (Tab)			X		X			X			X	X					
Clarithromycin (Biaxin XL)	**Tab, ER:** 500mg	X			X													X						
Erythromycin (ERYC)	**Cap, DR:** 250mg						X		X	X				X					X			X	X	X
Erythromycin (Ery-Tab)	**Tab, DR:** 250mg, 333mg, 500mg						X		X	X				X					X			X	X	X
Erythromycin (PCE)	**Tab:** 333mg, 500mg						X		X	X				X					X			X	X	X
Erythromycin base	**Tab:** 250mg, 500mg						X		X	X				X					X			X	X	X

(Continued)

GENERIC (BRAND)	HOW SUPPLIED	INDICATIONS																						
		ABECB	AECB	Bone & Joint	CAP	Endocarditis	GI	Intra-Ab	LRTI	URTI	Lyme Disease	MAC	Meningitis	Oph	Otitis Media	PCP	Septicemia	Sinusitis	SSSI	SSTI	TB	UTI	UGI	Gyn
MACROLIDES *(Continued)*																								
Erythromycin ethylsuccinate (E.E.S.)	**Susp:** 200mg/5mL; **Tab:** 400mg						X		X	X				X					X			X	X	X
Erythromycin ethylsuccinate (EryPed)	**Susp:** 200mg/5mL, 400mg/5mL						X		X	X				X					X			X	X	X
Erythromycin stearate (Erythrocin)	**Tab:** 250mg						X		X	X				X					X			X	X	X
Fidaxomicin (Dificid)	**Tab:** 200mg						X																	
PENICILLINS																								
Amoxicillin	**Cap:** 250mg, 500mg; **Susp:** 125mg/5mL, 200mg/5mL, 250mg/5mL, 400mg/5mL; **Tab:** 500mg, 875mg; **Tab, Chew:** 125mg, 250mg						X		X	X									X				X	
Amoxicillin (Moxatag)	**Tab, ER:** 775mg									X														

GENERIC (BRAND)	HOW SUPPLIED	INDICATIONS																						
		ABECB	AECB	Bone & Joint	CAP	Endocarditis	GI	Intra-Ab	LRTI	URTI	Lyme Disease	MAC	Meningitis	Oph	Otitis Media	PCP	Septicemia	Sinusitis	SSSI	SSTI	TB	UTI	UGI	Gyn
PENICILLINS *(Continued)*																								
Amoxicillin-Clavulanate potassium (Augmentin)	**Susp:** 125-31.25mg/5mL, 200-28.5mg/5mL, 250-62.5mg/5mL, 400-57mg/5mL; **Tab:** 250-125mg, 500-125mg, 875-125mg; **Tab, Chew:** 125-31.25mg, 200-28.5mg, 250-62.5mg, 400-57mg								X						X			X	X			X		
Amoxicillin-Clavulanate potassium (Augmentin XR)	**Tab, ER:** 1000-62.5mg				X													X						
Amoxicillin-Clavulanate potassium	**Susp:** 600-42.9mg/5mL														X									
Ampicillin	**Cap:** 250mg, 500mg; **Susp:** 125mg/5mL, 250mg/5mL						X		X	X			X										X	
Penicillin V potassium (Penicillin VK)	**Susp:** 125mg/5mL, 250mg/5mL; **Tab:** 250mg, 500mg								X	X										X				

(Continued)

GENERIC (BRAND)	HOW SUPPLIED	INDICATIONS																						
		ABECB	AECB	Bone & Joint	CAP	Endocarditis	GI	Intra-Ab	LRTI	URTI	Lyme Disease	MAC	Meningitis	Oph	Otitis Media	PCP	Septicemia	Sinusitis	SSSI	SSTI	TB	UTI	UGI	Gyn
TETRACYCLINES																								
Demeclocycline HCl	**Tab:** 150mg, 300mg						X		X	X				X					X			X	X	X
Doxycycline (Vibramycin)	**Cap:** 100mg; **Susp:** 25mg/5mL; **Syrup:** 50mg/5mL; **Tab:** 100mg						X		X	X				X					X			X	X	X
Doxycycline hyclate (Doryx)	**Tab, DR:** 75mg, 100mg, 150mg, 200mg						X		X	X				X					X			X	X	X
Doxycycline monohydrate (Monodox)	**Cap:** 50mg, 75mg, 100mg						X		X	X				X					X			X	X	X
Minocycline HCl (Dynacin)	**Tab:** 50mg, 75mg, 100mg						X		X	X				X					X			X	X	X
Minocycline HCl (Minocin)	**Cap:** 50mg, 75mg, 100mg						X		X	X				X					X			X	X	X
Tetracycline HCl	**Cap:** 250mg, 500mg						X		X	X				X						X		X	X	X
MISCELLANEOUS																								
Clindamycin (Cleocin, Cleocin Pediatric)	**Cap:** 75mg, 150mg, 300mg; **Sol:** 75mg/5mL							X	X	X							X			X			X	X
Fosfomycin tromethamine (Monurol)	**Powder:** 3g/sachet																					X		
Isoniazid-Pyrazinamide-Rifampin (Rifater)	**Tab:** 50-300-120mg																				X			

GENERIC (BRAND)	HOW SUPPLIED	INDICATIONS																						
		ABECB	AECB	Bone & Joint	CAP	Endocarditis	GI	Intra-Ab	LRTI	URTI	Lyme Disease	MAC	Meningitis	Oph	Otitis Media	PCP	Septicemia	Sinusitis	SSSI	SSTI	TB	UTI	UGI	Gyn
MISCELLANEOUS *(Continued)*																								
Isoniazid-Rifampin (Rifamate)	**Cap:** 150-300mg																				X			
Linezolid (Zyvox)	**Susp:** 100mg/5mL; **Tab:** 600mg				X				X										X					
Metronidazole (Flagyl)	**Cap:** 375mg; **Tab:** 250mg, 500mg			X		X	X	X	X				X				X		X					X
Nitrofurantoin (Furadantin)	**Susp:** 25mg/5mL																					X		
Nitrofurantoin macrocrystals (Macrodantin)	**Cap:** 25mg, 50mg, 100mg																					X		
Nitrofurantoin macrocrystals and Nitrofurantoin monohydrate (Macrobid)	**Cap:** 100mg																					X		
Rifampin (Rifadin)	**Cap:** 150mg, 300mg																				X			
Rifapentine (Priftin)	**Tab:** 150mg																				X			
Sulfamethoxazole-Trimethoprim (Bactrim, Bactrim DS, Sulfatrim)	**Susp:** 200-40mg/5mL; **Tab:** 400-80mg, 800-160mg		X				X								X	X						X		

(Continued)

GENERIC (BRAND)	HOW SUPPLIED	INDICATIONS																						
		ABECB	AECB	Bone & Joint	CAP	Endocarditis	GI	Intra-Ab	LRTI	URTI	Lyme Disease	MAC	Meningitis	Oph	Otitis Media	PCP	Septicemia	Sinusitis	SSSI	SSTI	TB	UTI	UGI	Gyn
MISCELLANEOUS *(Continued)*																								
Tedizolid phosphate (Sivextro)	**Tab:** 150mg																		X					
Telithromycin (Ketek)	**Tab:** 300mg, 400mg				X																			
Trimethoprim	**Tab:** 100mg, 200mg																					X		
Trimethoprim HCl (Primsol)	**Sol:** 50mg/5mL														X							X		
Vancomycin HCl (Vancocin)	**Cap:** 125mg, 250mg						X																	

Refer to full FDA-approved labeling for additional information.

Abbreviations:
ABECB = acute bacterial exacerbation of chronic bronchitis
AECB = acute exacerbation of chronic bronchitis
CAP = community-acquired pneumonia
GI = gastrointestinal
LRTI = lower respiratory tract infection
MAC = *Mycobacterium avium* complex
PCP = *Pneumocystis jiroveci* pneumonia
SSSI = skin and skin structure infection
SSTI = skin and soft tissue infection
TB = tuberculosis
UGI = urogenital infection
URTI = upper respiratory tract infection
UTI = urinary tract infection

SYSTEMIC ANTIBIOTICS TREATMENT COMPARISON

GENERIC (BRAND)	HOW SUPPLIED	INDICATIONS																	
		AECB	Bone & Joint Inf	CAP	Endocarditis	GI Inf	Gyn Inf	Intra-Ab Inf	LRTI	URTI	Meningitis	Otitis Media	PCP	Septicemia	Sinusitis	SSSI	SSTI	TB	UTI
AMINOGLYCOSIDES																			
Amikacin sulfate	**Inj:** 250mg/mL		X					X	X	X	X			X			X		X
Gentamicin sulfate	**Inj:** 10mg/mL, 40mg/mL; **Isotonic Inj:** 60mg, 80mg, 100mg, 120mg		X			X			X	X	X			X			X		X
Streptomycin	**Inj:** 1g				X				X		X							X	X
Tobramycin	**Inj:** 10mg/mL, 40mg/mL		X					X	X		X			X		X			X
CARBAPENEMS																			
Cilastatin-Imipenem (Primaxin IV)	**Inj:** 250-250mg, 500-500mg		X		X		X	X	X					X		X			X
Doripenem (Doribax)	**Inj:** 250mg, 500mg							X											X
Ertapenem (Invanz)	**Inj:** 1g			X			X	X								X			X
Meropenem (Merrem IV)	**Inj:** 500mg, 1g							X			X					X			
CEPHALOSPORINS																			
1st Generation																			
Cefazolin	**Inj:** 500mg, 1g		X		X				X	X				X		X			X
2nd Generation																			
Cefotetan	**Inj:** 1g, 2g		X				X	X	X					X		X			X
Cefoxitin	**Inj:** 1g, 2g		X				X	X	X					X		X			X
Cefuroxime (Zinacef)	**Inj:** 750mg, 1.5g*		X				X		X		X			X		X			X

(Continued)

GENERIC (BRAND)	HOW SUPPLIED	INDICATIONS																	
		AECB	Bone & Joint Inf	CAP	Endocarditis	GI Inf	Gyn Inf	Intra-Ab Inf	LRTI	URTI	Meningitis	Otitis Media	PCP	Septicemia	Sinusitis	SSSI	SSTI	TB	UTI
CEPHALOSPORINS *(Continued)*																			
3rd Generation																			
Cefotaxime (Claforan)	**Inj:** 500mg, 1g, 2g*		X				X	X	X		X			X		X			X
Ceftazidime (Fortaz)	**Inj:** 500mg, 1g, 2g*		X				X	X	X		X			X		X			X
Ceftazidime (Tazicef)	**Inj:** 1g, 2g*		X				X	X	X		X			X		X			X
Ceftazidime-Avibactam (Avycaz)	**Inj:** 2-0.5g							X											X
Ceftriaxone sodium (Rocephin)	**Inj:** 250mg, 500mg, 1g, 2g		X				X	X	X		X	X		X		X			X
4th Generation																			
Cefepime HCl (Maxipime)	**Inj:** 500mg, 1g, 2g							X	X							X			X
5th Generation																			
Ceftaroline fosamil (Teflaro)	**Inj:** 400mg, 600mg			X												X			
FLUOROQUINOLONES																			
Ciprofloxacin (Cipro IV)	**Inj:** 200mg/100mL, 400mg/200mL		X					X	X						X	X			X
Levofloxacin (Levaquin)	**Inj:** 5mg/mL	X		X					X						X	X			X
Moxifloxacin HCl (Avelox)	**Inj:** 400mg/250mL	X		X				X							X	X			
MACROLIDES																			
Azithromycin (Zithromax)	**Inj:** 500mg			X			X												

GENERIC (BRAND)	HOW SUPPLIED	INDICATIONS																	
		AECB	Bone & Joint Inf	CAP	Endocarditis	GI Inf	Gyn Inf	Intra-Ab Inf	LRTI	URTI	Meningitis	Otitis Media	PCP	Septicemia	Sinusitis	SSSI	SSTI	TB	UTI
MACROLIDES *(Continued)*																			
Erythromycin lactobionate (Erythrocin)	**Inj:** 500mg						X		X	X						X			
MONOBACTAMS																			
Aztreonam (Azactam)	**Inj:** 1g, 2g, 1g/50mL, 2g/50mL						X	X	X					X		X			X
PENICILLINS																			
Ampicillin sodium	**Inj:** 125mg, 250mg, 500mg, 1g, 2g*				X	X			X	X	X			X					X
Ampicillin sodium-Sulbactam sodium (Unasyn)	**Inj:** 1-0.5g, 2-1g*						X	X								X			
Penicillin G benzathine-Penicillin G procaine (Bicillin C-R)	**Inj:** 600,000-600,000 U/2mL								X	X		X					X		
Penicillin G benzathine-Penicillin G procaine (Bicillin C-R 900/300)	**Inj:** 900,000-300,000 U/2mL								X	X		X					X		
Penicillin G benzathine (Bicillin L-A)	**Inj:** 600,000 U/mL, 1,200,000 U/2mL, 2,400,000 U/4mL									X									
Penicillin G benzathine (Permapen)	**Inj:** 600,000 U/mL									X									
Penicillin G potassium (Pfizerpen)	**Inj:** 5 MU, 20 MU				X				X		X			X					

(Continued)

GENERIC (BRAND)	HOW SUPPLIED	INDICATIONS																	
		AECB	Bone & Joint Inf	CAP	Endocarditis	GI Inf	Gyn Inf	Intra-Ab Inf	LRTI	URTI	Meningitis	Otitis Media	PCP	Septicemia	Sinusitis	SSSI	SSTI	TB	UTI
PENICILLINS *(Continued)*																			
Piperacillin-Tazobactam (Zosyn)	**Inj:** 2-0.25g/50mL, 3-0.375g/50mL, 4-0.5g/100mL, 2-0.25g, 3-0.375g, 4-0.5g*			X			X	X	X							X			
TETRACYCLINES																			
Doxycycline (Doxy 100)	**Inj:** 100mg					X			X	X									X
Minocycline (Minocin)	**Inj:** 100mg					X	X		X	X	X					X			X
MISCELLANEOUS																			
Clindamycin (Cleocin Phosphate)	**Inj:** 150mg/mL, 300mg/50mL, 600mg/50mL, 900mg/50mL*		X				X	X	X					X		X			
Dalbavancin (Dalvance)	**Inj:** 500mg															X			
Dalfopristin-Quinupristin (Synercid)	**Inj:** 350-150mg															X			
Daptomycin (Cubicin)	**Inj:** 500mg				X											X			
Linezolid (Zyvox)	**Inj:** 2mg/mL			X					X							X			
Metronidazole	**Inj:** 500mg/100mL		X		X		X	X	X		X			X		X			
Oritavancin (Orbactiv)	**Inj:** 400mg/50mL															X			
Rifampin (Rifadin)	**Inj:** 600mg																	X	

GENERIC (BRAND)	HOW SUPPLIED	INDICATIONS																	
		AECB	Bone & Joint Inf	CAP	Endocarditis	GI Inf	Gyn Inf	Intra-Ab Inf	LRTI	URTI	Meningitis	Otitis Media	PCP	Septicemia	Sinusitis	SSSI	SSTI	TB	UTI
MISCELLANEOUS *(Continued)*																			
Sulfamethoxazole-Trimethoprim	**Inj:** 80-16mg/mL					X							X						X
Tedizolid phosphate (Sivextro)	**Inj:** 200mg															X			
Telavancin (Vibativ)•	**Inj:** 250mg, 750mg								X							X			
Tigecycline (Tygacil)	**Inj:** 50mg/5mL, 50mg/10mL			X				X								X			
Vancomycin HCl	**Inj:** 500mg, 750mg, 1g		X		X				X					X		X			

Refer to full FDA-approved labeling for additional information.

*Also available as a Pharmacy Bulk Package.

Abbreviations:

AECB = acute exacerbations of chronic bronchitis
CAP = community-acquired pneumonia
GI = gastrointestinal
LRTI = lower respiratory tract infection
PCP = *Pneumocystis jiroveci* pneumonia
SSSI = skin and skin structure infection
SSTI = skin and soft tissue infection
TB = tuberculosis
URTI = upper respiratory tract infection
UTI = urinary tract infection

Arthritis Treatment Comparison

GENERIC (BRAND)	HOW SUPPLIED	AS	GA	JA	OA	OA of Knee	PsA	RA
5-AMINOSALICYLIC ACID DERIVATIVES/SULFAPYRIDINES								
Sulfasalazine (Azulfidine EN-tabs)	**Tab, DR:** 500mg			✓				✓
CHELATING AGENTS								
Penicillamine (Cuprimine)	**Cap:** 250mg							✓
Penicillamine (Depen)	**Tab:** 250mg							✓
CYCLIC POLYPEPTIDE IMMUNOSUPPRESSANTS								
Cyclosporine (Gengraf, Neoral)	**Cap:** 25mg, 100mg; **Sol:** 100mg/mL							✓
CYCLOOXYGENASE-2 INHIBITORS								
Celecoxib (Celebrex)	**Cap:** 50mg, 100mg, 200mg, 400mg	✓		✓	✓			✓
DIHYDROFOLIC ACID REDUCTASE INHIBITORS								
Methotrexate (Otrexup)	**Inj:** 7.5mg/0.4mL, 10mg/0.4mL, 15mg/0.4mL, 20mg/0.4mL, 25mg/0.4mL			✓				✓
Methotrexate (Rasuvo)	**Inj:** 50mg/mL			✓				✓
Methotrexate (Rheumatrex)	**Inj:** 25mg/mL; **Tab:** 2.5mg			✓				✓
Methotrexate (Trexall)	**Tab:** 5mg, 7.5mg, 10mg, 15mg			✓				✓
GOLD COMPOUNDS								
Auranofin (Ridaura)	**Cap:** 3mg							✓
Gold sodium thiomalate (Myochrysine)	**Inj:** 50mg/mL			✓				✓
HYALURONAN AND DERIVATIVES								
Hyaluronan (Orthovisc)	**Inj:** 30mg/2mL					✓		
Sodium hyaluronate (Euflexxa)	**Inj:** 1%					✓		
Sodium hyaluronate (Hyalgan)	**Inj:** 10mg/mL					✓		
Sodium hyaluronate (Supartz)	**Inj:** 25mg/2.5mL					✓		
HYLAN POLYMERS								
Hylan G-F 20 (Synvisc, Synvisc One)	**Inj:** 8mg/mL					✓		
INTERLEUKIN RECEPTOR ANTAGONISTS								
Anakinra (Kineret)	**Inj:** 100mg/0.67mL							✓
Tocilizumab (Actemra)	**Inj:** 20mg/mL, 162mg/0.9mL			✓				✓

(Continued)

GENERIC (BRAND)	HOW SUPPLIED	AS	GA	JA	OA	OA of Knee	PsA	RA
KINASE INHIBITORS								
Tofacitinib (Xeljanz)	**Tab:** 5mg							✓
MONOCLONAL ANTIBODIES								
Canakinumab (Ilaris)	**Inj:** 180mg			✓				
Secukinumab (Cosentyx)	**Inj:** (Prefilled syringe, Sensoready pen) 150mg/mL; (Vial) 150mg	✓					✓	
Ustekinumab (Stelara)	**Inj:** 45mg/0.5mL, 90mg/mL						✓	
MONOCLONAL ANTIBODIES/CD20-BLOCKERS								
Rituximab (Rituxan)	**Inj:** 100mg/10mL, 500mg/50mL							✓
MONOCLONAL ANTIBODIES/TNF-BLOCKERS								
Adalimumab (Humira)	**Inj:** 10mg/0.2mL, 20mg/0.4mL, 40mg/0.8mL	✓		✓			✓	✓
Golimumab (Simponi)	**Inj:** 50mg/0.5mL, 100mg/mL	✓					✓	✓
Golimumab (Simponi Aria)	**Inj:** 50mg/4mL							✓
Infliximab (Remicade)	**Inj:** 100mg	✓					✓	✓
NON-STEROIDAL ANTI-INFLAMMATORY DRUGS (NSAIDs)								
Diclofenac (Zorvolex)	**Cap:** 18mg, 35mg				✓			
Diclofenac potassium (Cataflam)	**Tab:** 50mg				✓			✓
Diclofenac sodium	**Tab, DR:** 25mg, 50mg, 75mg	✓			✓			✓
Diclofenac sodium (Pennsaid)	**Sol:** 1.5%, 2%					✓		
Diclofenac sodium (Voltaren Gel)	**Gel:** 1%				✓	✓		
Diclofenac sodium (Voltaren-XR)	**Tab, ER:** 100mg				✓			✓
Diflunisal	**Tab:** 500mg				✓			✓
Etodolac	**Cap:** 200mg, 300mg; **Tab:** 400mg, 500mg				✓			✓
Etodolac Extended-Release	**Tab, ER:** 400mg, 500mg, 600mg			✓	✓			✓
Fenoprofen calcium (Nalfon)	**Cap:** 200mg, 400mg; **Tab:** 600mg				✓			✓
Flurbiprofen	**Tab:** 50mg, 100mg				✓			✓
Ibuprofen	**Tab:** 400mg, 600mg, 800mg; **Susp:** 100mg/5mL			✓*	✓			✓
Indomethacin	**Cap:** 50mg	✓	✓		✓			✓
Indomethacin (Indocin)	**Sup:** 50mg; **Susp:** 25mg/5mL	✓	✓		✓			✓

GENERIC (BRAND)	HOW SUPPLIED	AS	GA	JA	OA	OA of Knee	PsA	RA
NON-STEROIDAL ANTI-INFLAMMATORY DRUGS (NSAIDs) *(Continued)*								
Indomethacin Extended-Release	**Cap, ER:** 75mg	✓			✓			✓
Ketoprofen	**Cap:** 50mg, 75mg				✓			✓
Ketoprofen Extended-Release	**Cap, ER:** 200mg				✓			✓
Meclofenamate sodium	**Cap:** 50mg, 100mg	✓	✓	✓	✓			✓
Meloxicam (Mobic)	**Susp:** 7.5mg/5mL; **Tab:** 7.5mg, 15mg			✓	✓			✓
Meloxicam (Vivlodex)	**Cap:** 5mg, 10mg				✓			
Nabumetone	**Tab:** 500mg, 750mg				✓			✓
Naproxen (Naprosyn, EC-Naprosyn)	**Susp:** 125mg/mL; **Tab:** 250mg, 375mg, 500mg; **Tab, DR:** 375mg, 500mg	✓		✓*	✓			✓
Naproxen sodium (Anaprox, Anaprox DS)	**Tab:** 275mg, 550mg	✓			✓			✓
Naproxen sodium (Naprelan)	**Tab, CR:** 375mg, 500mg, 750mg	✓			✓			✓
Oxaprozin (Daypro)	**Tab:** 600mg			✓	✓			✓
Piroxicam (Feldene)	**Cap:** 10mg, 20mg				✓			✓
Sulindac	**Tab:** 150mg, 200mg	✓	✓		✓			✓
Tolmetin	**Cap:** 400mg; **Tab:** 600mg			✓	✓			✓
PHOSPHODIESTERASE-4 INHIBITORS								
Apremilast (Otezla)	**Tab:** 10mg, 20mg, 30mg						✓	
PURINE ANTAGONIST ANTIMETABOLITES								
Azathioprine (Azasan)	**Tab:** 75mg, 100mg							✓
Azathioprine (Imuran)	**Tab:** 50mg							✓
PYRIMIDINE SYNTHESIS INHIBITORS								
Leflunomide (Arava)	**Tab:** 10mg, 20mg, 100mg							✓
QUININE DERIVATIVES								
Hydroxychloroquine sulfate (Plaquenil)	**Tab:** 200mg							✓
SELECTIVE COSTIMULATION MODULATORS								
Abatacept (Orencia)	**Inj:** 125mg/mL, 250mg			✓				✓
TNF-RECEPTOR BLOCKERS								
Certolizumab pegol (Cimzia)	**Inj:** 200mg/mL	✓					✓	✓
Etanercept (Enbrel)	**Inj:** 25mg, 50mg	✓		✓			✓	✓

(Continued)

GENERIC (BRAND)	HOW SUPPLIED	AS	GA	JA	OA	OA of Knee	PsA	RA
COMBINATION PRODUCTS								
NSAIDs/H_2-RECEPTOR ANTAGONISTS								
Ibuprofen/Famotidine (Duexis)	**Tab:** 800mg/26.6mg				✓			✓
NSAIDs/PROSTAGLANDIN ANALOGUES								
Diclofenac sodium/ Misoprostol (Arthrotec)	**Tab:** 50mg/200mcg, 75mg/200mcg				✓			✓
NSAIDs/PROTON PUMP INHIBITORS								
Naproxen/Esomeprazole magnesium (Vimovo)	**Tab, DR:** 375mg/20mg, 500mg/20mg	✓			✓			✓
URICOSURICS								
Probenecid/Colchicine	**Tab:** 500mg/0.5mg		✓					

Refer to full FDA-approved labeling for additional information.

*Susp only.

Abbreviations: AS = ankylosing spondylitis; DR = delayed-release; ER = extended-release; GA = gouty arthritis; JA = juvenile arthritis; OA = osteoarthritis; PsA = psoriatic arthritis; RA = rheumatoid arthritis.

Osteoporosis Agents

GENERIC (BRAND)	HOW SUPPLIED	DOSAGE	SPECIAL INSTRUCTIONS
BISPHOSPHONATES AND COMBINATIONS			
Alendronate sodium (Binosto)	**Tab, Effervescent:** 70mg	**Treatment:** 70mg once weekly. **Increase Bone Mass in Men with Osteoporosis:** 70mg once weekly.	Take at least 30 min before 1st food, drink (other than plain water), or medication of day with plain water only. Dissolve tabs in 4 oz room temperature plain water and wait at least 5 min after the effervescence stops. Stir the solution for about 10 sec and ingest. Do not lie down for at least 30 min and until after 1st food of day.
Alendronate sodium (Fosamax)	**Sol:** (Generic) 70mg [75mL]; **Tab:** (Generic) 5mg, 10mg, 35mg, 40mg, (Fosamax) 70mg	**Treatment:** 70mg once weekly or 10mg qd. **Prevention:** 35mg once weekly or 5mg qd. **Increase Bone Mass in Men with Osteoporosis:** 70mg once weekly or 10mg qd. **Glucocorticoid-Induced:** 5mg qd; 10mg qd for postmenopausal women not on estrogen.	Take at least 30 min before 1st food, drink (other than plain water), or medication of day with plain water only. Take tabs with 6-8 oz water or 2 oz with oral sol. Do not lie down for at least 30 min and until after 1st food of day.
Alendronate sodium/ Cholecalciferol (Fosamax Plus D)	**Tab:** (Alendronate-Cholecalciferol) 70mg-2800 IU, 70mg-5600 IU	**Treatment:** 1 tab (70mg-2800 IU or 70mg-5600 IU) once weekly. **Usual:** 70mg-5600 IU once weekly. **Increase Bone Mass in Men with Osteoporosis:** 1 tab (70mg-2800 IU or 70mg-5600 IU) once weekly. **Usual:** 70mg-5600 IU once weekly.	Take at least 30 min before 1st food, drink (other than plain water), or medication of day. Take with 6-8 oz water. Do not lie down for at least 30 min and until after 1st food of day.
Ibandronate sodium (Boniva)	**Inj:** 3mg/3mL; **Tab:** 150mg	**Treatment: Inj:** 3mg IV over 15-30 sec every 3 months. **Prevention/Treatment: PO:** 150mg once monthly.	**PO:** Take at least 60 min before 1st food, drink (other than plain water), medication, or supplement of day. Swallow whole with 6-8 oz plain water while standing or sitting upright. Do not lie down for 60 min after dose.
Risedronate sodium (Actonel)	**Tab:** 5mg, 30mg, 35mg, 75mg, 150mg	**Prevention/Treatment:** 5mg qd or 35mg once weekly or 150mg once monthly or 75mg on 2 consecutive days each month. **Increase Bone Mass in Men with Osteoporosis:** 35mg once weekly. **Glucocorticoid-Induced: Prevention/ Treatment:** 5mg qd.	Take at least 30 min before 1st food, drink (other than plain water), medication, or supplement of day. Take with 6-8 oz plain water in an upright position. Do not lie down for 30 min after dose.
Risedronate sodium (Atelvia)	**Tab, Delayed-Release:** 35mg	**Treatment:** 35mg once weekly.	Take in am immediately after breakfast. Swallow whole with 4 oz of plain water. Do not lie down for 30 min after dose. Do not chew, cut, or crush tabs.

(Continued)

GENERIC (BRAND)	HOW SUPPLIED	DOSAGE	SPECIAL INSTRUCTIONS
BISPHOSPHONATES AND COMBINATIONS *(Continued)*			
Zoledronic acid (Reclast)	**Inj:** 5mg/100mL	**Treatment:** 5mg IV over ≥15 min once a year. **Prevention:** 5mg IV over ≥15 min once every 2 years. **Increase Bone Mass in Men with Osteoporosis:** 5mg IV over ≥15 min once a year. **Glucocorticoid-Induced: Prevention/Treatment:** 5mg IV over ≥15 min once a year.*	Flush IV line with 10mL normal saline after infusion. Administration of acetaminophen after Reclast may decrease acute-phase reaction symptoms.
HORMONAL BONE RESORPTION INHIBITORS			
Calcitonin-Salmon (Fortical)	**Nasal Spray:** 200 IU/actuation	**>5 yrs Postmenopause: Treatment:** 200 IU qd intranasally. Alternate nostrils daily.	Patients should take supplemental calcium and vitamin D.
Calcitonin-Salmon (Miacalcin)	**Inj:** 200 IU/mL; **Nasal Spray:** 200 IU/actuation	**>5 yrs Postmenopause: Treatment:** (Inj) 100 IU IM/SQ qd. If >2mL, use IM and multiple inj sites. (Spray) 200 IU qd intranasally. Alternate nostrils daily.	Patients should take supplemental calcium and vitamin D.
HORMONE THERAPY†‡			
Conjugated estrogens (Premarin)	**Tab:** 0.3mg, 0.45mg, 0.625mg, 0.9mg, 1.25mg	**Prevention: Initial:** 0.3mg qd continuously or cyclically (eg, 25 days on, 5 days off). Reevaluate periodically.	
Conjugated estrogens (CEs)/ Medroxyprogesterone acetate (MPA) (Premphase)	**Tab:** (CEs) 0.625mg and (CEs-MPA) 0.625mg-5mg	**Prevention:** 1 CE tab qd on Days 1-14 and 1 CE-MPA tab qd on Days 15-28. Reevaluate periodically.	
Conjugated estrogens (CEs)/ Medroxyprogesterone acetate (MPA) (Prempro)	**Tab:** (CEs-MPA) 0.3mg-1.5mg, 0.45mg-1.5mg, 0.625mg-2.5mg, 0.625mg-5mg	**Prevention:** 1 tab qd. Reevaluate periodically.	
Estradiol (Alora)	**Patch:** 0.025mg/day, 0.05mg/day, 0.075mg/day, 0.1mg/day	**Prevention:** 0.025mg/day twice weekly. May increase depending on bone mineral density and adverse events. Reevaluate periodically.	Apply to lower abdomen, upper quadrant of buttock, or outer aspect of hip; avoid breasts and waistline. Rotate application sites. Allow 1 week between applications to same site.
Estradiol (Climara)	**Patch:** 0.025mg/day, 0.0375mg/day, 0.05mg/day, 0.06mg/day, 0.075mg/day, 0.1mg/day	**Prevention:** 0.025mg/day once weekly. Reevaluate periodically.	Apply to lower abdomen or upper quadrant of buttock; avoid breasts and waistline. Rotate application sites. Allow 1 week between applications to same site.
Estradiol (Estrace)	**Tab:** 0.5mg§, 1mg§, 2mg§	**Prevention:** Lowest effective dose has not been determined. Reevaluate periodically.	

GENERIC (BRAND)	HOW SUPPLIED	DOSAGE	SPECIAL INSTRUCTIONS
HORMONE THERAPY[†‡] *(Continued)*			
Estradiol (Estraderm)	**Patch:** 0.05mg/day, 0.1mg/day	**Prevention: Initial:** 0.05mg/day twice weekly. May give continuously in patients without intact uterus. May give cyclically (eg, 3 weeks on, 1 week off) in patients with intact uterus. Reevaluate periodically.	Apply to trunk of body (including buttocks and abdomen); avoid breasts and waistline. Rotate application sites. Allow 1 week between applications to same site.
Estradiol (Menostar)	**Patch:** 14mcg/day	**Prevention:** Apply 1 patch weekly. Reevaluate periodically.	Apply to lower abdomen or upper quadrant of buttock; avoid breasts and waistline. Rotate application sites. Allow 1 week between applications to same site.
Estradiol (Minivelle)	**Patch:** 0.025mg/day, 0.0375mg/day, 0.05mg/day, 0.075mg/day, 0.1mg/day	**Prevention: Initial:** 0.025mg/day twice weekly. Adjust dose as necessary.	Apply to lower abdomen (below the umbilicus) or buttocks; avoid breasts and waistline. Rotate application sites. Allow 1 week between applications to same site.
Estradiol (Vivelle-Dot)	**Patch:** 0.025mg/day, 0.0375mg/day, 0.05mg/day, 0.075mg/day, 0.1mg/day	**Prevention: Initial:** 0.025mg/day twice weekly. May give continuously in patients without intact uterus. May give cyclically (eg, 3 weeks on, 1 week off) in patients with intact uterus. Reevaluate periodically.	Apply to trunk of body (including abdomen or buttocks); avoid breasts and waistline. Rotate application sites. Allow 1 week between applications to same site.
Estradiol/ Levonorgestrel (Climara Pro)	**Patch:** (Estradiol-Levonorgestrel) 0.045mg-0.015mg/day	**Prevention:** Apply 1 patch weekly. Reevaluate periodically.	Apply to lower abdomen or upper quadrant of the buttock; avoid breasts and waistline. Rotate application sites. Allow 1 week between applications to same site.
Estradiol/ Norethindrone (Activella)	**Tab:** (Estradiol-Norethindrone) 1mg-0.5mg, 0.5mg-0.1mg	**Prevention:** 1 tab qd. Reevaluate periodically.	
Estradiol/ Norgestimate (Prefest)	**Tab:** (Estradiol) 1mg and (Estradiol-Norgestimate) 1mg-0.09mg	**Prevention:** 1 estradiol (peach color) tab for 3 days followed by 1 estradiol-norgestimate (white color) tab for 3 days. Repeat regimen continuously. Reevaluate periodically.	
Estropipate	**Tab:** 0.75mg[§], 1.5mg[§], 3mg[§]	**Prevention:** 0.75mg qd for 25 days of a 31-day cycle per month.	
Ethinyl Estradiol/ Norethindrone (Femhrt)	**Tab:** (Ethinyl Estradiol-Norethindrone) 2.5mcg-0.5mg, 5mcg-1mg	**Prevention:** 1 tab qd. Reevaluate periodically.	
HORMONE THERAPY/SELECTIVE ESTROGEN RECEPTOR MODULATORS			
Conjugated estrogens (CEs)/ Bazedoxifene (Duavee)	**Tab:** (CEs-Bazedoxifene) 0.45mg-20mg	**Prevention:** 1 tab qd. Reevaluate periodically.	

(Continued)

GENERIC (BRAND)	HOW SUPPLIED	DOSAGE	SPECIAL INSTRUCTIONS
MONOCLONAL ANTIBODIES			
Denosumab (Prolia)	**Inj:** 60mg/mL	**Treatment:** 60mg as a single SQ inj once every 6 months. **Increase Bone Mass in Men with Osteoporosis:** 60mg as a single SQ inj once every 6 months.	Administer in the upper arm, upper thigh, or abdomen. All patients should receive calcium 1000mg and at least 400 IU vitamin D qd.
RECOMBINANT HUMAN PARATHYROID HORMONES			
Teriparatide† (Forteo)	**Inj:** 250mcg/mL	**Treatment/Increase Bone Mass in Men/ Glucocorticoid-Induced:** 20mcg SQ qd into thigh or abdominal wall. Use of the drug for >2 years during a patient's lifetime is not recommended.	Administer initially under circumstances where patient can sit or lie down if symptoms of orthostatic hypotension occur. Discard pen after 28 days.
SELECTIVE ESTROGEN RECEPTOR MODULATORS			
Raloxifene HCl† (Evista)	**Tab:** 60mg	**Prevention/Treatment:** 60mg qd.	Calcium and vitamin D supplementation is recommended.

Refer to full FDA-approved labeling for additional information.

*Patients on Reclast must be adequately supplemented with calcium and vitamin D if dietary intake is not sufficient. An average of at least 1200mg calcium and 800-1000 IU vitamin D daily is recommended.

†Check FDA-approved labeling for important Boxed Warnings.

‡When prescribing solely for the prevention of postmenopausal osteoporosis, therapy should be considered only for women at significant risk for osteoporosis; non-estrogen medications should be carefully considered.

§Scored.

Alzheimer's Disease Agents

GENERIC (BRAND)	HOW SUPPLIED	ADULT DOSAGE	SPECIAL INSTRUCTIONS
Donepezil HCl (Aricept)	**Tab:** 5mg, 10mg, 23mg; **Tab, Disintegrating:** 5mg, 10mg	**Mild-Moderate: Initial:** 5mg qhs. **Usual:** 5-10mg qhs. **Titrate:** May increase to 10mg after 4-6 weeks. **Moderate-Severe: Initial:** 5mg qhs. **Usual:** 10-23mg qhs. **Titrate:** May increase to 10mg after 4-6 weeks, then to 23mg after ≥3 months.	• Monitor for vagotonic effects on sinoatrial and atrioventricular nodes, syncopal episodes, diarrhea, N/V, active/occult GI bleeding, weight loss, bladder outflow obstruction, and generalized convulsions. • Do not split or crush 23mg tablet.
Donepezil HCl-Memantine HCl ER (Namzaric)	**Tab:** 10mg-14mg, 10mg-28mg	Patients stabilized on memantine HCl (10mg bid or 28mg ER qd) and donepezil HCl 10mg can be switched to Namzaric 10mg-28mg qpm. Start Namzaric the day following the last dose of memantine HCl and donepezil HCl administered separately.	• Monitor for bradycardia, heart block, GI bleeding, diarrhea, N/V, bladder outflow obstruction, seizures. • Caution in patients with a history of asthma or obstructive pulmonary disease. • Do not divide, chew, or crush Namzaric; capsules may be opened and sprinkled on applesauce. • Dose adjustment required for severe renal insufficiency.
Ergoloid mesylates	**Tab:** 1mg	1mg tid.	• Monitor for transient nausea and gastric disturbances. • Monitor for relief of signs and symptoms.
Galantamine HBr (Razadyne, Razadyne ER)	(Razadyne) **Sol:** 4mg/mL [100mL]; **Tab:** 4mg, 8mg, 12mg; (Razadyne ER) **Cap, ER:** 8mg, 16mg, 24mg	(Sol, Tab) **Initial:** 4mg bid (8mg/day) with am and pm meals. **Titrate:** Increase to initial maint dose of 8mg bid (16mg/day) after a minimum of 4 weeks, then increase to 12mg bid (24mg/day) after a minimum of 4 weeks. Restart at the lowest dose and increase to current dose if therapy is interrupted for more than 3 days. (Cap, ER) **Initial:** 8mg qd with am meal. **Titrate:** Increase to initial maint dose of 16mg qd after a minimum of 4 weeks, then increase to 24mg qd after a minimum of 4 weeks.	• Monitor for rash, bradycardia, heart block, GI bleeding, weight loss, bladder outflow obstruction, and seizures. • Monitor respiratory function in patients with a history of severe asthma or obstructive pulmonary disease. • Not recommended for patients with severe hepatic impairment or CrCl <9mL/min. • Dose adjustment required for patients with moderate hepatic impairment or CrCl 9-59mL/min.

(Continued)

GENERIC (BRAND)	HOW SUPPLIED	ADULT DOSAGE	SPECIAL INSTRUCTIONS
Memantine HCl (Namenda, Namenda XR)	(Namenda) **Sol:** 2mg/mL [360mL]; **Tab:** 5mg, 10mg; (Namenda XR) **Cap, ER:** 7mg, 14mg, 21mg, 28mg	(Sol, Tab) **Initial:** 5mg qd. **Titrate:** Increase in 5mg increments to 10mg/day (5mg bid), 15mg/day (5mg and 10mg as separate doses), and 20mg/day (10mg bid) at ≥1-week intervals. Dosage shown to be effective in controlled clinical trials is 20mg/day. (Cap, ER) **Initial:** 7mg qd. **Titrate:** Increase in 7mg increments to 28mg qd at ≥1-week intervals. **Max/Target Dose:** 28mg qd.	• Monitor renal/hepatic function. • Do not divide or crush Namenda XR; capsules may be opened and sprinkled on applesauce. • Administer oral solution with dosing device and do not mix with any other liquid. • Dose adjustment required in severe renal insufficiency.
Rivastigmine tartrate (Exelon)	**Cap:** 1.5mg, 3mg, 4.5mg, 6mg; **Patch:** 4.6mg/24 hrs, 9.5mg/24 hrs, 13.3mg/24 hrs; **Sol:** 2mg/mL [120mL]	(PO) **Initial:** 1.5mg bid. **Titrate:** May increase to 3mg bid after a minimum of 2 weeks, if 1.5mg bid is well tolerated. Subsequent increases to 4.5mg bid and 6mg bid should be attempted after a minimum of 2 weeks at the previous dose. **Max:** 12mg/day (6mg bid). **Interruption of Treatment: Intolerance:** D/C therapy for several doses and then restart at same or next lower dose level. **≤3 Days Interruption:** Restart with same or lower dose. **>3 Days Interruption:** Restart with 1.5mg bid and titrate as above. (Patch) **Initial:** Apply 4.6mg/24 hrs patch qd to skin. **Titrate:** Increase dose only after a minimum of 4 weeks at the previous dose, and only if the previous dose is well tolerated. **Effective Dose: Mild-Moderate:** 9.5mg/24 hrs qd or 13.3mg/24 hrs qd. **Severe:** 13.3mg/24 hrs qd. **Max:** 13.3mg/24 hrs. Replace with a new patch q24h. **Interruption of Treatment: ≤3 Days Interruption:** Restart with same or lower strength patch. **>3 Days Interruption:** Restart with 4.6mg/24 hrs patch and titrate as above.	• Monitor for signs/symptoms of active or occult GI bleeding, extrapyramidal symptoms, urinary obstruction, seizures, and GI adverse events. • (Patch) Monitor for skin reactions. • (PO) Administer with meals in divided doses in am and pm. • Dose adjustment required for moderate to severe renal insufficiency (PO only), mild to moderate hepatic insufficiency, or low/high body weight.

Refer to full.FDA-approved labeling for additional information.
Abbreviation: ER = extended-release.

ANTIPARKINSON AGENTS

GENERIC (BRAND)	HOW SUPPLIED	ADULT DOSAGE	SIDE EFFECTS
Amantadine HCl	**Cap, Tab:** 100mg; **Sol:** 50mg/5mL	**Parkinsonism: Usual:** 100mg bid. **Serious Associated Illness/Concomitant High-Dose Antiparkinson Agent: Initial:** 100mg qd. **Titrate:** May increase to 100mg bid after 1 to several weeks. **Max:** 400mg/day. **Drug-Induced Extrapyramidal Reactions: Usual:** 100mg bid. **Max:** 300mg/day.*	Nausea, dizziness, insomnia, depression, anxiety and irritability, hallucinations, confusion, anorexia, dry mouth, constipation, ataxia, livedo reticularis, peripheral edema, orthostatic hypotension, headache, somnolence, nervousness, dream abnormality, agitation, dry nose, diarrhea, fatigue
Apomorphine HCl (Apokyn)	**Inj:** 10mg/mL	**Test Dose/Initial:** 0.2mL (2mg) SQ; assess efficacy/tolerability. See PI for details. **Max:** 0.6mL (6mg)/dose. **Renal Impairment: Test Dose/Initial:** 0.1mL (1mg).	Yawning, dyskinesia, nausea, vomiting, somnolence, dizziness, rhinorrhea, hallucinations, edema, chest pain, increased sweating
Benztropine mesylate (Cogentin)	**Inj:** 1mg/mL; (Generic) **Tab:** 0.5mg, 1mg, 2mg	Initiate with a low dose. **Titrate:** May increase every 5-6 days by 0.5mg. **Max:** 6mg/day. **Postencephalitic/Idiopathic Parkinsonism: Usual:** 1-2mg/day. **Range:** 0.5-6mg/day. **Idiopathic Parkinsonism: Initial:** 0.5-1mg PO or IV/IM qhs. **Postencephalitic Parkinsonism: Initial:** 2mg/day PO or IV/IM given in 1 or more doses. **Highly Sensitive Patients: Initial:** 0.5mg PO or IV/IM qhs; increase as necessary. **Drug-Induced Extrapyramidal Disorders: Usual:** 1-4mg PO or IV/IM qd or bid. Give 1-2mg bid or tid for transient extrapyramidal disorders that develop soon after initiation of neuroleptic drugs; d/c and reevaluate necessity after 1 or 2 weeks. May reinstitute therapy if disorders recur.	Tachycardia, paralytic ileus, constipation, vomiting, nausea, dry mouth, confusion, blurred vision, urinary retention, heat stroke, hyperthermia, fever
Bromocriptine mesylate (Parlodel)	**Tab, Snap:** 2.5mg†; **Cap:** 5mg	**Initial:** ½ SnapTab bid. **Titrate:** May increase by 2.5mg/day q2-4 weeks. **Max:** 100mg/day. Take with food. Assess need for medication at 2-week intervals.	Dizziness, insomnia, hallucinations, dyskinesia, visual disturbance, nausea, confusion, drowsiness, vomiting, abdominal pain, hypotension, constipation
Carbidopa (Lodosyn)	**Tab:** 25mg†	**With Sinemet or Levodopa:** Determine dose by careful titration. Most patients respond to a 1:10 proportion of carbidopa and levodopa, provided carbidopa dose is ≥70mg/day. **Max:** 200mg/day. Consider amount of carbidopa in Sinemet when calculating dose. See PI for detailed dosing information.	Dyskinesia (choreiform, dystonic, and other involuntary movements), nausea; check PI for a more comprehensive list of adverse reactions
Carbidopa/Levodopa (Duopa)	**Sus:** (Carbidopa-Levodopa) 4.63mg-20mg/mL	Prior to initiation of therapy, convert patient from all other forms of levodopa to oral IR carbidopa-levodopa (1:4 ratio). See PI for details. **Max:** 2g of levodopa component (eg, 1 cassette/day) over 16 hrs.	Complication of device insertion, nausea, depression, peripheral edema, hypertension, upper respiratory tract infection, oropharyngeal pain, incision site erythema

(Continued)

GENERIC (BRAND)	HOW SUPPLIED	ADULT DOSAGE	SIDE EFFECTS
Carbidopa/Levodopa (Parcopa)	**Tab, Disintegrating:** (Carbidopa-Levodopa) 10mg-100mg†, 25mg-100mg†, 25mg-250mg†	**25mg-100mg Tab: Initial:** 1 tab tid. **Titrate:** Increase by 1 tab qd or qod up to 8 tabs/day. **10mg-100mg Tab: Initial:** 1 tab tid-qid. **Titrate:** Increase by 1 tab qd or qod up to 8 tabs/day. **Maint:** 70-100mg/day carbidopa required. **Max:** 200mg/day carbidopa. **Conversion from Levodopa:** See PI.	Dyskinesia (choreiform, dystonic, and other involuntary movements), nausea; check PI for a more comprehensive list of adverse reactions
Carbidopa/Levodopa (Rytary)	**Cap, ER:** (Carbidopa-Levodopa) 23.75mg-95mg, 36.25mg-145mg, 48.75mg-195mg, 61.25mg-245mg	**Levodopa Naive: Initial:** 23.75mg-95mg tid for the first 3 days. On 4th day of treatment, may increase to 36.25mg-145mg tid. **Titrate:** May increase up to 97.5mg-390mg tid to 5X/day. **Max:** 612.5mg-2450mg/day. **Conversion to ER Caps:** See PI.	Nausea, dizziness, headache, insomnia, abnormal dreams, dry mouth, dyskinesia, anxiety, constipation, vomiting, orthostatic hypotension
Carbidopa/Levodopa (Sinemet, Sinemet CR)	(Carbidopa-Levodopa) **Tab:** 10mg-100mg, 25mg-100mg, 25mg-250mg; **Tab, ER:** 25mg-100mg, 50mg-200mg	(Tab) **25mg-100mg Tab: Initial:** 1 tab tid. **Titrate:** Increase by 1 tab qd or qod up to 8 tabs/day. **10mg-100mg Tab: Initial:** 1 tab tid-qid. **Titrate:** May increase by 1 tab qd or qod up to 8 tabs/day. **Maint:** 70-100mg/day carbidopa required. **Max:** 200mg/day carbidopa. **Conversion from Levodopa:** See PI. (Tab, ER) **No Prior Levodopa Use: Initial:** One 50mg-200mg tab bid at intervals ≥6 hrs. **Titrate:** Increase or decrease dose or interval accordingly. Adjust dose at interval of ≥3 days. **Usual:** 400-1600mg/day levodopa, given in 4- to 8-hr intervals while awake. **Conversion to ER Tabs:** See PI.	Dyskinesia (choreiform, dystonic, and other involuntary movements), nausea; check PI for a more comprehensive list of adverse reactions
Carbidopa/Levodopa/ Entacapone (Stalevo)	**Tab:** (Carbidopa-Levodopa-Entacapone) Stalevo 50: 12.5mg-50mg-200mg; Stalevo 75: 18.75mg-75mg-200mg; Stalevo 100: 25mg-100mg-200mg; Stalevo 125: 31.25mg-125mg-200mg; Stalevo 150: 37.5mg-150mg-200mg; Stalevo 200: 50mg-200mg-200mg	**Currently Taking Carbidopa/Levodopa and Entacapone:** May switch directly to corresponding strength of Stalevo with same amounts of carbidopa/levodopa. **Currently Taking Carbidopa/Levodopa Without Entacapone:** First, titrate individually with carbidopa/levodopa product and entacapone product, then transfer to corresponding dose once stabilized. **Max:** 8 tabs/day (Stalevo 50, 75, 100, 125, 150); 6 tabs/day (Stalevo 200).	Dyskinesia, urine discoloration, diarrhea, nausea, hyperkinesia, vomiting, dry mouth; check PI for a more comprehensive list of adverse reactions
Diphenhydramine HCl Injection	**Inj:** 50mg/mL	**Usual:** 10-50mg IV at ≤25mg/min or deep IM. May use 100mg IM if needed. **Max:** 400mg/day.	Sedation, sleepiness, dizziness, disturbed coordination, epigastric distress, thickening of bronchial secretions
Entacapone (Comtan)	**Tab:** 200mg	**Usual:** 200mg administered concomitantly with each levodopa/carbidopa dose. **Max:** 1600mg/day. Withdraw slowly for discontinuation.	Dyskinesia, hyperkinesia, hypokinesia, dizziness, nausea, diarrhea, abdominal pain, constipation, urine discoloration, fatigue
Hyoscyamine sulfate (Levbid, Levsin)	(Levbid) **Tab, ER:** 0.375mg; (Levsin) **Tab:** 0.125mg; **Tab, SL:** 0.125mg	**Levbid:** 0.375-0.75mg q12h. **Max:** 1.5mg/24 hrs. Do not crush or chew. **Levsin:** 0.125-0.25mg q4h or prn. **Max:** 1.5mg/24 hrs. May chew or swallow SL tab.	Dry mouth, urinary hesitancy and retention, blurred vision, tachycardia, mydriasis, increased ocular tension, loss of taste, headache, nervousness, drowsiness, weakness, fatigue, dizziness, nausea, vomiting

GENERIC (BRAND)	HOW SUPPLIED	ADULT DOSAGE	SIDE EFFECTS
Pramipexole dihydrochloride (Mirapex)	**Tab:** 0.125mg, 0.25mg†, 0.5mg†, 0.75mg, 1mg†, 1.5mg†	**Initial:** 0.125mg tid. **Titrate:** May increase not more frequently than every 5-7 days (eg, Week 2: 0.25mg tid; Week 3: 0.5mg tid; Week 4: 0.75mg tid; Week 5: 1mg tid; Week 6: 1.25mg tid; Week 7: 1.5mg tid). **Maint:** 0.5-1.5mg tid. **Max:** 1.5mg tid.*	Nausea, dizziness, somnolence, constipation, asthenia, hallucinations, vision abnormalities, general and peripheral edema, insomnia, confusion, amnesia, hypesthesia
Pramipexole dihydrochloride (Mirapex ER)	**Tab, ER:** 0.375mg, 0.75mg, 1.5mg, 2.25mg, 3mg, 3.75mg, 4.5mg	**Initial:** 0.375mg qd. **Titrate:** May increase not more frequently than every 5-7 days, first to 0.75mg/day and then by 0.75mg increments based on efficacy and tolerability. **Max:** 4.5mg/day. **Switching from IR to ER:** May switch overnight from IR to ER tabs at same daily dose.*	Somnolence, nausea, constipation, dizziness, fatigue, hallucinations, dry mouth, muscle spasms, peripheral edema, dyskinesia, headache, anorexia
Rasagiline mesylate (Azilect)	**Tab:** 0.5mg, 1mg	**Monotherapy:** 1mg qd. **Adjunctive Therapy: Initial:** 0.5mg qd. **Titrate:** May increase to 1mg qd. Adjust dose of levodopa with concomitant use. **Concomitant Ciprofloxacin or Other CYP1A2 Inhibitors/Mild Hepatic Impairment:** 0.5mg qd.	Headache, accidental injury, arthralgia, depression, fall, flu syndrome, dyskinesia, nausea, weight loss, constipation, postural hypotension, vomiting, dry mouth, rash, somnolence
Rivastigmine (Exelon)	**Cap:** 1.5mg, 3mg, 4.5mg, 6mg; **Patch:** 4.6mg/24 hrs, 9.5mg/24 hrs, 13.3mg/24 hrs; **Sol:** 2mg/mL	(Cap, Sol) **Usual:** 1.5-6mg bid. **Initial:** 1.5mg bid with meals in am and pm. **Titrate:** May subsequently increase to 3mg bid and further to 4.5mg bid and 6mg bid after a minimum of 4 weeks at the previous dose, based on tolerability. **Max:** 6mg bid. (Patch) **Usual:** 9.5mg/24 hrs or 13.3mg/24 hrs qd. **Initial:** Apply 4.6mg/24 hrs patch qd to clean, dry, hairless, intact skin. **Titrate:** Increase dose only after a minimum of 4 weeks, if well tolerated. Continue effective dose of 9.5mg/24 hrs for as long as therapeutic benefit persists. **Max:** 13.3mg/24 hrs.	Nausea, vomiting, anorexia, dizziness, diarrhea, tremor
Ropinirole (Requip, Requip XL)	**Tab:** 0.25mg, 0.5mg, 1mg, 2mg, 3mg, 4mg, 5mg; **Tab, ER:** 2mg, 4mg, 6mg, 8mg, 12mg	(Tab) **Initial:** 0.25mg tid. **Titrate:** May increase weekly by 0.25mg tid (0.75mg/day) for 4 weeks. After Week 4, may increase weekly by 1.5mg/day up to 9mg/day, then by 3mg/day weekly to 24mg/day. **Max:** 24mg/day. **Withdrawal:** Decrease dose to bid for 4 days, then qd for 3 days. (Tab, ER) **Initial:** 2mg qd for 1-2 weeks. Swallow whole. **Titrate:** May increase at ≥1-week intervals by 2mg/day. **Max:** 24mg/day. **Switching from IR to ER:** Closely match total daily IR dose with initial ER dose. See PI for detailed information.	Dyskinesia, hallucinations, somnolence, vomiting, headache, constipation, dyspepsia, abdominal pain, pharyngitis, UTI, increased sweating, asthenia, edema, fatigue, syncope, orthostatic symptoms, dizziness, nausea, viral infection, confusion, abnormal vision

(Continued)

GENERIC (BRAND)	HOW SUPPLIED	ADULT DOSAGE	SIDE EFFECTS
Rotigotine (Neupro)	**Patch:** 1mg/24 hrs, 2mg/24 hrs, 3mg/24 hrs, 4mg/24 hrs, 6mg/24 hrs, 8mg/24 hrs	**Early-Stage: Initial:** 2mg/24 hrs. **Titrate:** May increase weekly by 2mg/24 hrs based on response and tolerability. **Lowest Effective Dose:** 4mg/24 hrs. **Max:** 6mg/24 hrs. **Advanced-Stage: Initial:** 4mg/24 hrs. **Titrate:** May increase weekly by 2mg/24 hrs based on response and tolerability. **Max:** 8mg/24 hrs.	Nausea, vomiting, somnolence, application-site reactions, dizziness, anorexia, hyperhidrosis, insomnia
Selegiline HCl (Zelapar)	**Tab, Disintegrating:** 1.25mg	**Initial:** 1.25mg qd before breakfast for ≥6 weeks. Take without liquid. **Titrate:** After 6 weeks, may increase to 2.5mg qd if the desired benefit is not achieved and patient can tolerate it. **Max:** 2.5mg/day.	Nausea, dizziness, pain, headache, insomnia, rhinitis, skin disorders, dyskinesia, back pain, dyspepsia, stomatitis, constipation, hallucinations, pharyngitis, rash
Selegiline HCl (Eldepryl)	**Cap:** 5mg; (Generic) **Tab:** 5mg	5mg bid at breakfast and lunch. **Max:** 10mg/day. May attempt to reduce levodopa/carbidopa by 10-30% after 2-3 days of therapy. May reduce further with continued therapy.	Nausea, dizziness, lightheadedness, fainting, abdominal pain, confusion, hallucinations, dry mouth
Tolcapone (Tasmar)	**Tab:** 100mg	**Initial:** 100mg tid. Use 200mg tid only if clinical benefit is justified. May need to decrease levodopa dose.	Dyskinesia, nausea, sleep disorder, dystonia, excessive dreaming, anorexia, muscle cramps, orthostatic complaints, somnolence, diarrhea, confusion, dizziness, headache, hallucination, vomiting, constipation, fatigue, upper respiratory tract infection, falling, increased sweating, UTI, xerostomia, abdominal pain, urine discoloration, hepatotoxicity (including liver failure)
Trihexyphenidyl HCl	**Sol:** 2mg/5mL; **Tab:** 2mg†, 5mg†	**Idiopathic Parkinsonism:** 1mg on Day 1. **Titrate:** May increase by 2mg increments at intervals of 3-5 days, until 6-10mg/day is given. **Postencephalitic Patients:** May require 12-15mg/day. **Drug-Induced Parkinsonism: Initial:** 1mg. **Titrate:** If extrapyramidal manifestations not controlled in a few hrs, increase dose until control is achieved. **Usual:** 5-15mg/day. **Concomitant Levodopa or Other Parasympathetic Inhibitors:** See PI.	Dry mouth, blurred vision, dizziness, nausea, nervousness, constipation, drowsiness, urinary hesitancy/retention, tachycardia, pupil dilation, increased intraocular pressure, vomiting, weakness, headache

Refer to full FDA-approved labeling for additional information.

Abbreviations: ER = extended-release; IR = immediate-release; SL = sublingual.

*Refer to FDA-approved labeling for dosing instructions in renally compromised patients.

†Scored.

NARCOTIC ANALGESICS

GENERIC	BRAND	DEA SCHEDULE	DOSAGE FORMS	ADDITIONAL COMMENTS
CENTRALLY ACTING ANALGESICS				
Tapentadol	Nucynta	Schedule II	**Tab:** 50mg, 75mg, 100mg	• **BW:** (Nucynta ER) Addiction, abuse, and misuse; life-threatening respiratory depression; accidental ingestion; neonatal opioid withdrawal syndrome; interaction with alcohol • Pregnancy category C, not for use in nursing
	Nucynta ER		**Tab, ER:** 50mg, 100mg, 150mg, 200mg, 250mg	
Tramadol HCl	Conzip	Schedule IV	**Cap, ER:** 100mg, 200mg, 300mg	• Pregnancy category C, not for use in nursing
	Ultram		**Tab:** 50mg	
	Ultram ER		**Tab, ER:** 100mg, 200mg, 300mg	
Tramadol HCl/Acetaminophen	Ultracet	Schedule IV	**Tab:** 37.5mg-325mg	• **BW:** Hepatotoxicity • Pregnancy category C, not for use in nursing
OPIOID AGONISTS/OPIOID ANTAGONISTS				
Morphine sulfate/Naltrexone HCl	Embeda	Schedule II	**Cap, ER:** 20mg-0.8mg, 30mg-1.2mg, 50mg-2mg, 60mg-2.4mg, 80mg-3.2mg, 100mg-4mg	• **BW:** Addiction, abuse, and misuse; life-threatening respiratory depression; accidental ingestion; neonatal opioid withdrawal syndrome; interaction with alcohol • Pregnancy category C, not for use in nursing
OPIOID ANALGESICS				
Codeine sulfate		Schedule II	**Tab:** 15mg, 30mg, 60mg	• **BW:** Death related to ultra-rapid metabolism of codeine to morphine • Pregnancy category C, caution in nursing
Codeine phosphate/Acetaminophen		Schedule V	**Sol:** 12mg-120mg/5mL	• **BW:** Hepatotoxicity; death related to ultra-rapid metabolism of codeine to morphine • Pregnancy category C, not for use in nursing
		Schedule III	**Tab:** 15mg-300mg	
	Tylenol #3	Schedule III	**Tab:** 30mg-300mg	
	Tylenol #4	Schedule III	**Tab:** 60mg-300mg	

(Continued)

GENERIC	BRAND	DEA SCHEDULE	DOSAGE FORMS	ADDITIONAL COMMENTS
OPIOID ANALGESICS *(Continued)*				
Dihydrocodeine bitartrate/ Acetaminophen/Caffeine	Trezix	Schedule III	**Cap:** 16mg-320.5mg-30mg	• **BW:** Death related to ultra-rapid metabolism of codeine to morphine; hepatotoxicity • Pregnancy category C, not for use in nursing
Dihydrocodeine bitartrate/Aspirin/ Caffeine	Synalgos-DC	Schedule III	**Cap:** 16mg-356.4mg-30mg	• **BW:** Death related to ultra-rapid metabolism of codeine to morphine • Safety not known in pregnancy, not for use in nursing
Fentanyl	Abstral	Schedule II	**Tab, SL:** 100mcg, 200mcg, 300mcg, 400mcg, 600mcg, 800mcg	• **BW:** Risk of respiratory depression, medication errors, and abuse potential • Pregnancy category C, not for use in nursing
	Duragesic		**Patch:** 12mcg/hr, 25mcg/hr, 50mcg/hr, 75mcg/hr, 100mcg/hr	• **BW:** Addiction, abuse, and misuse; life-threatening respiratory depression; accidental exposure; neonatal opioid withdrawal syndrome; CYP3A4 interaction; exposure to heat • Prolonged use of opioid analgesics during pregnancy can result in physical dependence in the neonate and neonatal opioid withdrawal syndrome shortly after birth. Not for use in nursing
	Fentora		**Tab, Buccal:** 100mcg, 200mcg, 400mcg, 600mcg, 800mcg	• **BW:** Risk of respiratory depression, medication errors, and abuse potential • Pregnancy category C, not for use in nursing
	Lazanda		**Spr, Nasal:** 100mcg/spr, 400mcg/spr	
	Subsys		**Spr, SL:** 100mcg/spr, 200mcg/spr, 400mcg/spr, 600mcg/spr, 800mcg/spr	
Fentanyl citrate	Actiq	Schedule II	**Loz:** 200mcg, 400mcg, 600mcg, 800mcg, 1200mcg, 1600mcg	• **BW:** Risk of respiratory depression, medication errors, and abuse potential • Pregnancy category C, not for use in nursing
Hydrocodone bitartrate	Hysingla ER	Schedule II	**Tab, ER:** 20mg, 30mg, 40mg, 60mg, 80mg, 100mg, 120mg	• **BW:** Addiction, abuse, and misuse; life-threatening respiratory depression; accidental ingestion; neonatal opioid withdrawal syndrome; CYP3A4 interaction; (Zohydro ER) interaction with alcohol • Prolonged use of opioid analgesics during pregnancy may cause neonatal opioid withdrawal syndrome; (Hysingla ER) pregnancy category C, not for use in nursing
	Zohydro ER		**Cap, ER:** 10mg, 15mg, 20mg, 30mg, 40mg, 50mg	

GENERIC	BRAND	DEA SCHEDULE	DOSAGE FORMS	ADDITIONAL COMMENTS
OPIOID ANALGESICS *(Continued)*				
Hydrocodone bitartrate/ Acetaminophen	Hycet	Schedule III	**Sol:** 7.5mg-325mg/15mL	• **BW:** Hepatotoxicity • Pregnancy category C, not for use in nursing
	Lorcet	Schedule II	**Tab:** 5mg-325mg	
	Lorcet HD		**Tab:** 10mg-325mg	
	Lorcet Plus		**Tab:** 7.5mg-325mg	
	Lortab		**Sol:** 10mg-300mg/15mL; **Tab:** 5mg-325mg, 7.5mg-325mg, 10mg-325mg	
	Norco		**Tab:** 5mg-325mg, 7.5mg-325mg, 10mg-325mg	
	Vicodin		**Tab:** 5mg-300mg	
	Vicodin ES		**Tab:** 7.5mg-300mg	
	Vicodin HP		**Tab:** 10mg-300mg	
	Zolvit	Schedule III	**Sol:** 10mg-300mg/15mL	
Hydrocodone bitartrate/Ibuprofen	Reprexain	Schedule II	**Tab:** 2.5mg-200mg, 5mg-200mg, 10mg-200mg	• Pregnancy category C, not for use in nursing
	Vicoprofen		**Tab:** 7.5-200mg	
Hydromorphone HCl	Dilaudid	Schedule II	**Inj:** 1mg/mL, 2mg/mL, 4mg/mL; **Sol:** 1mg/mL; **Tab:** 2mg, 4mg, 8mg	• **BW:** Risk of respiratory depression and abuse; (Inj) risk of medication errors. Dilaudid-HP injection is for use in opioid-tolerant patients only • Pregnancy category C, not for use in nursing
	Dilaudid-HP		**Inj:** 10mg/mL [1mL, 5mL, 50mL], 250mg (sterile lyophilized powder)	
	Exalgo		**Tab, ER:** 8mg, 12mg, 16mg, 32mg	• **BW:** Addiction, abuse, and misuse; life-threatening respiratory depression; accidental ingestion; neonatal opioid withdrawal syndrome • Pregnancy category C, not for use in nursing
Levorphanol tartrate		Schedule II	**Tab:** 2mg	• Pregnancy category C, not for use in nursing

(Continued)

GENERIC	BRAND	DEA SCHEDULE	DOSAGE FORMS	ADDITIONAL COMMENTS
OPIOID ANALGESICS *(Continued)*				
Meperidine		Schedule II	**Inj:** 10mg/mL; **Sol:** 50mg/5mL	• Pregnancy category C, not for use in nursing; (10mg/mL Inj) safety not known in pregnancy and nursing
	Demerol		**Tab:** 50mg, 100mg; **Inj:** 25mg/mL, 50mg/mL, 75mg/mL, 100mg/mL	
Methadone HCl		Schedule II	**Inj:** 10mg/mL	• **BW:** Life-threatening QT prolongation; conditions for distribution and use for opioid addiction treatment • Pregnancy category C, not for use in nursing
			Sol: 5mg/5mL, 10mg/5mL; **Sol, Concentrated:** 10mg/mL	• **BW:** Addiction, abuse, and misuse; life-threatening respiratory depression; accidental ingestion; life-threatening QT prolongation; neonatal opioid withdrawal syndrome; conditions for distribution and use for opioid addiction treatment • Pregnancy category C, caution in nursing
	Dolophine		**Tab:** 5mg, 10mg	
Morphine sulfate		Schedule II	**Tab:** 15mg, 30mg; **Sol:** 10mg/5mL, 20mg/5mL, 100mg/5mL	• **BW:** (Sol) Risk of medication errors and accidental ingestion; 100mg/5mL dosage is indicated for opioid-tolerant patients only • Pregnancy category C, not for use in nursing
	Astramorph/PF		**Inj:** 0.5mg/mL, 1mg/mL	• **BW:** Risk of severe adverse reactions with epidural or intrathecal route; observe patients in an equipped and staffed environment for at least 24 hrs after initial dose • Pregnancy category C, safety not known in nursing
	Duramorph		**Inj:** 0.5mg/mL, 1mg/mL	• **BW:** Risk of severe adverse reactions with epidural or intrathecal route; observe patients in an equipped and staffed environment for at least 24 hrs after initial dose • Pregnancy category C, safety not known in nursing

GENERIC	BRAND	DEA SCHEDULE	DOSAGE FORMS	ADDITIONAL COMMENTS
OPIOID ANALGESICS *(Continued)*				
	Infumorph		**Inj:** 10mg/mL (200mg/20mL), 25mg/mL (500mg/20mL)	• **BW:** Not recommended for single-dose IV, IM, or SQ administration. Risk of severe adverse reactions; observe patients in an equipped and staffed environment for at least 24 hrs after initial (single) test dose, and as appropriate, for the 1st several days after catheter implantation. Improper or erroneous substitution of Infumorph for Duramorph is likely to result in serious overdosage. Naloxone injection and resuscitative equipment should be available in case of life-threatening or intolerable side effects whenever therapy is initiated or any manipulation of the reservoir system takes place • Pregnancy category C, safety not known in nursing
	Kadian		**Cap, ER:** 10mg, 20mg, 30mg, 40mg, 50mg, 60mg, 80mg, 100mg, 200mg	• **BW:** Addiction, abuse, and misuse; life-threatening respiratory depression; accidental exposure • Pregnancy category C, not for use in nursing
	MS Contin		**Tab, ER:** 15mg, 30mg, 60mg, 100mg, 200mg	• **BW:** Addiction, abuse, and misuse; life-threatening respiratory depression; accidental ingestion; neonatal opioid withdrawal syndrome • Pregnancy category C, not for use in nursing
Oxycodone HCl		Schedule II	**Cap:** 5mg; **Sol:** 1mg/mL, 20mg/mL; **Tab:** 10mg, 20mg	• **BW:** (Sol) Risk of medication errors and accidental ingestion; 100mg/5mL dosage is indicated for opioid-tolerant patients only • Pregnancy category B, not for use in nursing
	Oxaydo		**Tab:** 5mg, 7.5mg	• Pregnancy category B, not for use in nursing
	Oxecta		**Tab:** 5mg, 7.5mg	
	OxyContin		**Tab, ER:** 10mg, 15mg, 20mg, 30mg, 40mg, 60mg, 80mg	• **BW:** Addiction, abuse, and misuse; life-threatening respiratory depression; accidental ingestion; neonatal opioid withdrawal syndrome; CYP3A4 interaction • Pregnancy category C, not for use in nursing
	Roxicodone		**Tab:** 5mg, 15mg, 30mg	• Pregnancy category B, not for use in nursing

(Continued)

GENERIC	BRAND	DEA SCHEDULE	DOSAGE FORMS	ADDITIONAL COMMENTS
OPIOID ANALGESICS *(Continued)*				
Oxycodone HCl/Acetaminophen	Percocet	Schedule II	**Tab:** 2.5mg-325mg, 5mg-325mg, 7.5mg-325mg, 10mg-325mg	• **BW:** Hepatotoxicity • Pregnancy category C, not for use in nursing
	Primlev		**Tab:** 5mg-300mg, 7.5mg-300mg, 10mg-300mg	
	Roxicet		**Tab:** 5mg-325mg; **Sol:** 5mg-325mg/5mL	
	Xartemis XR		**Tab, ER:** 7.5mg-325mg	• **BW:** Addiction, abuse, and misuse; life-threatening respiratory depression; accidental exposure; neonatal opioid withdrawal syndrome; hepatotoxicity • Pregnancy category C, not for use in nursing
Oxycodone HCl/Aspirin	Percodan	Schedule II	**Tab:** 4.8355mg-325mg	• Pregnancy category B (oxycodone) and D (aspirin), not for use in nursing
Oxymorphone HCl	Opana	Schedule II	**Tab:** 5mg, 10mg	• Pregnancy category C, caution in nursing
	Opana ER		**Tab, ER:** 5mg, 7.5mg, 10mg, 15mg, 20mg, 30mg, 40mg	• **BW:** Addiction, abuse, and misuse; life-threatening respiratory depression; accidental ingestion; neonatal opioid withdrawal syndrome; interaction with alcohol • Pregnancy category C, caution in nursing
PARTIAL OPIOID AGONISTS				
Buprenorphine	Belbuca	Schedule III	**Film, Buccal:** 75mcg, 150mcg, 300mcg, 450mcg, 600mcg, 750mcg, 900mcg	• **BW:** Addiction, abuse, and misuse; life-threatening respiratory depression; accidental exposure; neonatal opioid withdrawal syndrome • Prolonged use of opioid analgesics during pregnancy can result in physical dependence in the neonate and neonatal opioid withdrawal syndrome shortly after birth. Not for use in nursing
	Buprenex		**Inj:** 0.3mg/mL	• Pregnancy category C, not for use in nursing
	Butrans		**Patch:** 5mcg/hr, 7.5mcg/hr, 10mcg/hr, 15mcg/hr, 20mcg/hr	• **BW:** Addiction, abuse and misuse; life-threatening respiratory depression; accidental exposure; neonatal opioid withdrawal syndrome • Pregnancy category C, not for use in nursing
Butorphanol tartrate		Schedule IV	**Spr, Nasal:** 10mg/mL	• Pregnancy category C, caution in nursing
Pentazocine lactate	Talwin	Schedule IV	**Inj:** 30mg/mL	• Safe use during pregnancy (other than labor) has not been established

GENERIC	BRAND	DEA SCHEDULE	DOSAGE FORMS	ADDITIONAL COMMENTS
PARTIAL OPIOID AGONISTS/OPIOID ANTAGONISTS				
Pentazocine/Naloxone		Schedule IV	**Tab:** 50mg/0.5mg	• **BW:** Intended for oral use only • Pregnancy category C, caution in nursing

Refer to full FDA-approved labeling for more detailed dosing.

Abbreviations: BW = boxed warning; ER = extended-release; SL = sublingual.

Oral Anticonvulsants

Generic (Brand)	Usual Adult Dosage*	Therapeutic Serum Levels	Indications						
			Seizure Disorders						
			Absence	Akinetic	Lennox-Gastaut Syndrome	Myoclonic	Partial	Tonic-Clonic	Neuropathic Pain
BARBITURATES									
Phenobarbital[†]	60-200mg/day	N/A					X		
Primidone (Mysoline)	750-2000mg/day	5-12mcg/mL					X	X	
BENZODIAZEPINES									
Clobazam (Onfi)	10-40mg/day	N/A			X				
Clonazepam (Klonopin)	1.5-20mg/day	N/A	X	X	X	X			
Clorazepate dipotassium (Tranxene T-Tab)	22.5-90mg/day	N/A					X		
Diazepam (Valium)[‡]	4-40mg/day	N/A							
GABA ANALOGUES									
Gabapentin (Neurontin)	900-1800mg/day	N/A					X		X
Pregabalin (Lyrica)	Epilepsy: 150-600mg/day Neuropathic Pain Associated with Diabetic Peripheral Neuropathy/Postherpetic Neuralgia: 150-300mg/day	N/A					X		X
Vigabatrin (Sabril)	3g/day	N/A					X		
HYDANTOINS									
Ethotoin (Peganone)	2000-3000mg/day	N/A					X	X	
Phenytoin (Dilantin, Dilantin-125, Dilantin Infatabs, Phenytek)	300-400mg/day (Sus: 375-625mg/day)	10-20mcg/mL					X	X	
SUCCINIMIDES									
Ethosuximide (Zarontin)	500-1500mg/day	40-100mcg/mL	X						

(Continued)

GENERIC (BRAND)	USUAL ADULT DOSAGE*	THERAPEUTIC SERUM LEVELS	INDICATIONS						
			SEIZURE DISORDERS						NEUROPATHIC PAIN
			ABSENCE	AKINETIC	LENNOX-GASTAUT SYNDROME	MYOCLONIC	PARTIAL	TONIC-CLONIC	
SUCCINIMIDES *(Continued)*									
Methsuximide (Celontin)	300-1200mg/day	N/A	X						
MISCELLANEOUS									
Carbamazepine (Carbatrol, Tegretol, Tegretol XR)	Epilepsy: 800-1200mg/day Trigeminal Neuralgia: 400-800mg/day	4-12mcg/mL					X	X	X
Divalproex sodium[§] (Depakote, Depakote ER, Depakote Sprinkle Capsules)	10-60mg/kg/day	50-100mcg/mL	X				X		
Valproic acid[§] (Depakene)	10-60mg/kg/day	50-100mcg/mL	X				X		
Eslicarbazepine (Aptiom)	800-1200mg/day	N/A					X		
Ezogabine (Potiga)	600-1200mg/day	N/A					X		
Felbamate[¶] (Felbatol)	2400-3600mg/day	N/A			X		X		
Lacosamide (Vimpat)	200-400mg/day	N/A					X		
Lamotrigine (Lamictal, Lamictal ODT, Lamictal XR)	100-500mg/day (Lamictal XR: 200-600mg/day)	N/A			X (IR, ODT)		X	X	
Levetiracetam (Keppra, Keppra XR)	1000-3000mg/day	N/A				X (IR)	X	X (IR)	
Oxcarbazepine (Oxtellar XR, Trileptal)	1200-2400mg/day	N/A					X		
Perampanel (Fycompa)	8-12mg/day	N/A					X	X	
Rufinamide (Banzel)	400-3200mg/day	N/A			X				
Tiagabine HCl (Gabitril)	4-56mg/day	N/A					X		
Topiramate (Qudexy XR, Topamax, Topamax Sprinkle, Trokendi XR)	200-400mg/day	N/A			X		X	X	

GENERIC (BRAND)	USUAL ADULT DOSAGE*	THERAPEUTIC SERUM LEVELS	INDICATIONS						
			SEIZURE DISORDERS						NEUROPATHIC PAIN
			ABSENCE	AKINETIC	LENNOX-GASTAUT SYNDROME	MYOCLONIC	PARTIAL	TONIC-CLONIC	
MISCELLANEOUS *(Continued)*									
Zonisamide (Zonegran)	100-400mg/day	N/A					X		

Abbreviation: N/A = not applicable.

*Refer to complete monograph for full dosing information, including pediatric dosing.

†Phenobarbital is also indicated in generalized seizures.

‡Oral Valium may be used adjunctively in convulsive disorders, although it has not proved useful as the sole therapy.

§Divalproex sodium and valproic acid are also indicated as adjuncts in multiple seizure types.

¶For severe epilepsy refractory to other treatment where the risk of aplastic anemia and/or liver failure is deemed acceptable. Fully advise patient and obtain written, informed consent before treatment. Closely monitor patient.

MENTAL HEALTH TREATMENT OPTIONS

GENERIC (BRAND)	HOW SUPPLIED	INDICATIONS												
		BIPOLAR DISORDER (MAINTENANCE)	BIPOLAR, MANIC EPISODES	BIPOLAR, MIXED EPISODES	BIPOLAR, DEPRESSIVE EPISODES	DEPRESSION	SCHIZOPHRENIA	ANXIETY	OCD	PANIC DISORDER	PTSD	PMDD	IRRITABILITY ASSOCIATED W/ AUTISTIC DISORDER	PSYCHOSIS
ALPHA$_2$ ANTAGONISTS														
Mirtazapine (Remeron, Remeron SolTab)	**Tab:** (Generic) 7.5mg; (Remeron) 15mg, 30mg, 45mg; **Tab, Disintegrating:** (SolTab) 15mg, 30mg, 45mg					✓								
AMINOKETONES														
Bupropion HBr (Aplenzin)	**Tab, ER:** 174mg, 348mg, 522mg					✓								
Bupropion HCl (Forfivo XL)	**Tab, ER:** 450mg					✓								
Bupropion HCl (Wellbutrin, Wellbutrin SR, Wellbutrin XL)	**Tab:** 75mg, 100mg; **Tab, SR:** 100mg, 150mg, 200mg; **Tab, ER:** 150mg, 300mg					✓								
ATYPICAL ANTIPSYCHOTICS														
Aripiprazole (Abilify, Abilify Discmelt)	**Inj*:** 7.5mg/mL; **Sol:** 1mg/mL; **Tab:** 2mg, 5mg, 10mg, 15mg, 20mg, 30mg; **Tab, Disintegrating:** (Discmelt) 10mg, 15mg		✓	✓		✓	✓						✓	
Aripiprazole (Abilify Maintena)	**Inj, ER:** 300mg, 400mg						✓							

(Continued)

GENERIC (BRAND)	HOW SUPPLIED	INDICATIONS												
		BIPOLAR DISORDER (MAINTENANCE)	BIPOLAR, MANIC EPISODES	BIPOLAR, MIXED EPISODES	BIPOLAR, DEPRESSIVE EPISODES	DEPRESSION	SCHIZOPHRENIA	ANXIETY	OCD	PANIC DISORDER	PTSD	PMDD	IRRITABILITY ASSOCIATED W/ AUTISTIC DISORDER	PSYCHOSIS
ATYPICAL ANTIPSYCHOTICS *(Continued)*														
Aripiprazole lauroxil (Aristada)	**Inj, ER:** 441mg/1.6mL, 662mg/2.4mL, 882mg/3.2mL						✓							
Asenapine (Saphris)	**Tab, SL:** 2.5mg 5mg, 10mg		✓	✓			✓							
Brexpiprazole (Rexulti)	**Tab:** 0.25mg, 0.5mg, 1mg, 2mg, 3mg, 4mg					✓	✓							
Cariprazine (Vraylar)	**Cap:** 1.5mg, 3mg, 4.5mg, 6mg		✓	✓			✓							
Clozapine (Clozaril, Fazaclo, Versacloz)	**Sus:** (Versacloz) 50mg/mL; **Tab:** (Generic) 50mg, 200mg; (Clozaril) 25mg, 100mg; **Tab, Disintegrating:** (Fazaclo) 12.5mg, 25mg, 100mg, 150mg, 200mg						✓							
Iloperidone (Fanapt)	**Tab:** 1mg, 2mg, 4mg, 6mg, 8mg, 10mg, 12mg						✓							
Lurasidone HCl (Latuda)	**Tab:** 20mg, 40mg, 60mg, 80mg, 120mg				✓		✓							
Olanzapine (Zyprexa, Zyprexa Zydis, Zyprexa IntraMuscular)	**Inj***: 10mg; **Tab:** 2.5mg, 5mg, 7.5mg, 10mg, 15mg, 20mg; **Tab, Disintegrating:** (Zydis) 5mg, 10mg, 15mg, 20mg	✓ (PO)	✓ (PO)	✓ (PO)	✓ (PO)	✓ (PO)	✓ (PO)							

GENERIC (BRAND)	HOW SUPPLIED	INDICATIONS												
		BIPOLAR DISORDER (MAINTENANCE)	BIPOLAR, MANIC EPISODES	BIPOLAR, MIXED EPISODES	BIPOLAR, DEPRESSIVE EPISODES	DEPRESSION	SCHIZOPHRENIA	ANXIETY	OCD	PANIC DISORDER	PTSD	PMDD	IRRITABILITY ASSOCIATED W/ AUTISTIC DISORDER	PSYCHOSIS
ATYPICAL ANTIPSYCHOTICS *(Continued)*														
Olanzapine (Zyprexa Relprevv)	**Inj, ER:** 210mg, 300mg, 405mg						✓							
Paliperidone (Invega)	**Tab, ER:** 1.5mg, 3mg, 6mg, 9mg						✓							
Paliperidone palmitate (Invega Sustenna)	**Inj, ER:** 39mg, 78mg, 117mg, 156mg, 234mg						✓							
Paliperidone palmitate (Invega Trinza)	**Inj, ER:** 273mg, 410mg, 546mg, 819mg						✓							
Quetiapine fumarate (Seroquel)	**Tab:** 25mg, 50mg, 100mg, 200mg, 300mg, 400mg	✓	✓		✓		✓							
Quetiapine fumarate (Seroquel XR)	**Tab, ER:** 50mg, 150mg, 200mg, 300mg, 400mg	✓	✓	✓	✓	✓	✓							
Risperidone (Risperdal Consta)	**Inj:** 12.5mg, 25mg, 37.5mg, 50mg	✓					✓							
Risperidone (Risperdal, Risperdal M-Tab)	**Sol:** 1mg/mL; **Tab:** 0.25mg, 0.5mg, 1mg, 2mg, 3mg, 4mg; **Tab, Disintegrating:** (M-Tab) 0.5mg, 1mg, 2mg, 3mg, 4mg		✓	✓			✓						✓	
Ziprasidone (Geodon)	**Cap:** 20mg, 40mg, 60mg, 80mg; **Inj:** 20mg/mL	✓ (PO)	✓ (PO)	✓ (PO)			✓							

(Continued)

GENERIC (BRAND)	HOW SUPPLIED	INDICATIONS												
		BIPOLAR DISORDER (MAINTENANCE)	BIPOLAR, MANIC EPISODES	BIPOLAR, MIXED EPISODES	BIPOLAR, DEPRESSIVE EPISODES	DEPRESSION	SCHIZOPHRENIA	ANXIETY	OCD	PANIC DISORDER	PTSD	PMDD	IRRITABILITY ASSOCIATED W/ AUTISTIC DISORDER	PSYCHOSIS
BENZODIAZEPINES														
Alprazolam	**Tab, Disintegrating:** 0.25mg, 0.5mg, 1mg, 2mg							✓		✓				
Alprazolam (Xanax)	**Tab:** 0.25mg, 0.5mg, 1mg, 2mg							✓		✓				
Alprazolam (Xanax XR)	**Tab, ER:** 0.5mg, 1mg, 2mg, 3mg									✓				
Chlordiazepoxide HCl (Librium)	**Cap:** 5mg, 10mg, 25mg							✓						
Clonazepam (Klonopin)	**Tab:** (Klonopin) 0.5mg, 1mg, 2mg; **Tab, Disintegrating:** (Generic) 0.125mg, 0.25mg, 0.5mg, 1mg, 2mg									✓				
Clorazepate dipotassium (Tranxene T-Tabs)	**Tab:** 3.75mg, 7.5mg, 15mg							✓						
Diazepam (Valium)	**Inj:** (Generic) 5mg/mL; **Sol:** (Generic) 5mg/5mL, 5mg/mL; **Tab:** (Valium) 2mg, 5mg, 10mg							✓						
Lorazepam (Ativan)	**Sol:** (Generic) 2mg/mL; **Tab:** (Ativan) 0.5mg, 1mg, 2mg							✓						

GENERIC (BRAND)	HOW SUPPLIED	INDICATIONS												
		BIPOLAR DISORDER (MAINTENANCE)	BIPOLAR, MANIC EPISODES	BIPOLAR, MIXED EPISODES	BIPOLAR, DEPRESSIVE EPISODES	DEPRESSION	SCHIZOPHRENIA	ANXIETY	OCD	PANIC DISORDER	PTSD	PMDD	IRRITABILITY ASSOCIATED W/ AUTISTIC DISORDER	PSYCHOSIS
BENZODIAZEPINES *(Continued)*														
Midazolam HCl	**Inj:** 1mg/mL, 5mg/mL; **Syrup:** 2mg/mL							✓						
Oxazepam	**Cap:** 10mg, 15mg, 30mg							✓						
MONOAMINE OXIDASE INHIBITORS														
Isocarboxazid (Marplan)	**Tab:** 10mg					✓								
Phenelzine sulfate (Nardil)	**Tab:** 15mg					✓								
Selegiline (Emsam)	**Patch:** 6mg/24 hrs, 9mg/24 hrs, 12mg/24 hrs					✓								
Tranylcypromine sulfate (Parnate)	**Tab:** 10mg					✓								
SELECTIVE SEROTONIN REUPTAKE INHIBITORS/5HT$_{1A}$ RECEPTOR PARTIAL AGONISTS														
Vilazodone HCl (Viibryd)	**Tab:** 10mg, 20mg, 40mg					✓								
SELECTIVE SEROTONIN REUPTAKE INHIBITORS AND COMBINATIONS														
Citalopram HBr (Celexa)	**Sol:** (Generic) 10mg/5mL; **Tab:** (Celexa) 10mg, 20mg, 40mg					✓								
Escitalopram oxalate (Lexapro)	**Sol:** 5mg/5mL; **Tab:** 5mg, 10mg, 20mg					✓		✓						

(Continued)

GENERIC (BRAND)	HOW SUPPLIED	INDICATIONS												
		BIPOLAR DISORDER (MAINTENANCE)	BIPOLAR, MANIC EPISODES	BIPOLAR, MIXED EPISODES	BIPOLAR, DEPRESSIVE EPISODES	DEPRESSION	SCHIZOPHRENIA	ANXIETY	OCD	PANIC DISORDER	PTSD	PMDD	IRRITABILITY ASSOCIATED W/ AUTISTIC DISORDER	PSYCHOSIS
SELECTIVE SEROTONIN REUPTAKE INHIBITORS AND COMBINATIONS *(Continued)*														
Fluoxetine	**Sol:** 20mg/5mL; **Tab:** 60mg					✓			✓	✓				
Fluoxetine (Prozac)	**Cap:** 10mg, 20mg, 40mg				✓	✓			✓	✓				
Fluoxetine (Prozac Weekly)	**Cap, DR:** 90mg				✓	✓			✓	✓				
Fluoxetine HCl (Sarafem)	**Cap:** (Generic) 10mg, 20mg; **Tab:** (Sarafem) 10mg, 15mg, 20mg											✓		
Fluoxetine-Olanzapine (Symbyax)	**Cap:** 25-3mg, 25-6mg, 50-6mg, 25-12mg, 50-12mg				✓	✓								
Fluvoxamine maleate	**Tab:** 25mg, 50mg, 100mg								✓					
Fluvoxamine maleate (Luvox CR)	**Cap, ER:** 100mg, 150mg								✓					
Paroxetine HCl (Paxil)	**Sus:** 10mg/5mL; **Tab:** 10mg, 20mg, 30mg, 40mg					✓		✓	✓	✓	✓			
Paroxetine HCl (Paxil CR)	**Tab, Controlled-Release:** 12.5mg, 25mg, 37.5mg					✓		✓		✓		✓		
Paroxetine mesylate (Pexeva)	**Tab:** 10mg, 20mg, 30mg, 40mg					✓		✓	✓	✓				
Sertraline HCl (Zoloft)	**Sol:** 20mg/mL; **Tab:** 25mg, 50mg, 100mg					✓		✓	✓	✓	✓	✓		

GENERIC (BRAND)	HOW SUPPLIED	INDICATIONS												
		BIPOLAR DISORDER (MAINTENANCE)	BIPOLAR, MANIC EPISODES	BIPOLAR, MIXED EPISODES	BIPOLAR, DEPRESSIVE EPISODES	DEPRESSION	SCHIZOPHRENIA	ANXIETY	OCD	PANIC DISORDER	PTSD	PMDD	IRRITABILITY ASSOCIATED W/ AUTISTIC DISORDER	PSYCHOSIS
SEROTONIN AND NOREPINEPHRINE REUPTAKE INHIBITORS														
Desvenlafaxine (Khedezla)	**Tab, ER:** 50mg, 100mg					✓								
Desvenlafaxine (Pristiq)	**Tab, ER:** 25mg, 50mg, 100mg					✓								
Duloxetine (Cymbalta)	**Cap, DR:** 20mg, 30mg, 60mg					✓		✓						
Levomilnacipran (Fetzima)	**Cap, ER:** 20mg, 40mg, 80mg, 120mg					✓								
Venlafaxine HCl	**Tab:** 25mg, 37.5mg, 50mg, 75mg, 100mg; **Tab, ER:** 37.5mg, 75mg, 150mg, 225mg					✓		✓ (ER)						
Venlafaxine HCl (Effexor XR)	**Cap, ER:** 37.5mg, 75mg, 150mg					✓		✓		✓				
TETRACYCLIC ANTIDEPRESSANTS														
Maprotiline HCl	**Tab:** 25mg, 50mg, 75mg					✓		✓						
TRICYCLIC ANTIDEPRESSANTS AND COMBINATIONS														
Amitriptyline HCl	**Tab:** 10mg, 25mg, 50mg, 75mg, 100mg, 150mg					✓								
Amitriptyline HCl-Chlordiazepoxide	**Tab:** 12.5-5mg, 25-10mg					✓		✓						
Amitriptyline HCl-Perphenazine	**Tab:** 10-2mg, 10-4mg, 25-2mg, 25-4mg, 50-4mg					✓	✓	✓						

(Continued)

GENERIC (BRAND)	HOW SUPPLIED	INDICATIONS												
		BIPOLAR DISORDER (MAINTENANCE)	BIPOLAR, MANIC EPISODES	BIPOLAR, MIXED EPISODES	BIPOLAR, DEPRESSIVE EPISODES	DEPRESSION	SCHIZOPHRENIA	ANXIETY	OCD	PANIC DISORDER	PTSD	PMDD	IRRITABILITY ASSOCIATED W/ AUTISTIC DISORDER	PSYCHOSIS
TRICYCLIC ANTIDEPRESSANTS AND COMBINATIONS *(Continued)*														
Amoxapine	**Tab:** 25mg, 50mg, 100mg, 150mg					✓								
Clomipramine HCl (Anafranil)	**Cap:** 25mg, 50mg, 75mg								✓					
Desipramine HCl (Norpramin)	**Tab:** 10mg, 25mg, 50mg, 75mg, 100mg, 150mg					✓								
Doxepin HCl	**Cap:** 10mg, 25mg, 50mg, 75mg, 100mg, 150mg; **Sol:** 10mg/mL					✓		✓						
Imipramine HCl (Tofranil)	**Tab:** 10mg, 25mg, 50mg					✓								
Imipramine pamoate (Tofranil-PM)	**Cap:** 75mg, 100mg, 125mg, 150mg					✓								
Nortriptyline HCl (Pamelor)	**Cap:** (Pamelor) 10mg, 25mg, 50mg, 75mg; **Sol:** (Generic) 10mg/5mL					✓								
Protriptyline HCl (Vivactil)	**Tab:** 5mg, 10mg					✓								
Trimipramine maleate (Surmontil)	**Cap:** 25mg, 50mg, 100mg					✓								
TYPICAL ANTIPSYCHOTICS														
Chlorpromazine HCl	**Inj:** 25mg/mL; **Tab:** 10mg, 25mg, 50mg, 100mg, 200mg						✓							✓ (PO)

GENERIC (BRAND)	HOW SUPPLIED	INDICATIONS												
		BIPOLAR DISORDER (MAINTENANCE)	BIPOLAR, MANIC EPISODES	BIPOLAR, MIXED EPISODES	BIPOLAR, DEPRESSIVE EPISODES	DEPRESSION	SCHIZOPHRENIA	ANXIETY	OCD	PANIC DISORDER	PTSD	PMDD	IRRITABILITY ASSOCIATED W/ AUTISTIC DISORDER	PSYCHOSIS
TYPICAL ANTIPSYCHOTICS *(Continued)*														
Fluphenazine decanoate	**Inj:** 25mg/mL						✓							
Fluphenazine HCl	**Elixir:** 2.5mg/5mL; **Inj:** 2.5mg/mL; **Sol, Concentrated:** 5mg/mL; **Tab:** 1mg, 2.5mg, 5mg, 10mg													✓
Haloperidol (Haldol)	**Inj:** (Haldol) 5mg/mL; **Sol:** 2mg/mL; **Tab:** 0.5mg, 1mg, 2mg, 5mg, 10mg, 20mg						✓(Inj)							✓
Haloperidol decanoate (Haldol Decanoate)	**Inj:** 50mg/mL, 100mg/mL						✓							
Loxapine (Adasuve)	**Cap:** (Generic) 5mg, 10mg, 25mg, 50mg; **Powder, Inhalation*:** (Adasuve) 10mg						✓							
Perphenazine	**Tab:** 2mg, 4mg, 8mg, 16mg						✓							
Thioridazine HCl	**Tab:** 10mg, 25mg, 50mg, 100mg						✓							
Thiothixene	**Cap:** 1mg, 2mg, 5mg, 10mg						✓							
Trifluoperazine HCl	**Tab:** 1mg, 2mg, 5mg, 10mg						✓	✓						

(Continued)

GENERIC (BRAND)	HOW SUPPLIED	INDICATIONS												
		BIPOLAR DISORDER (MAINTENANCE)	BIPOLAR, MANIC EPISODES	BIPOLAR, MIXED EPISODES	BIPOLAR, DEPRESSIVE EPISODES	DEPRESSION	SCHIZOPHRENIA	ANXIETY	OCD	PANIC DISORDER	PTSD	PMDD	IRRITABILITY ASSOCIATED W/ AUTISTIC DISORDER	PSYCHOSIS
VALPROATE COMPOUNDS														
Divalproex sodium (Depakote)	**Tab, DR:** 125mg, 250mg, 500mg		✓											
Divalproex sodium (Depakote ER)	**Tab, ER:** 250mg, 500mg		✓	✓										
MISCELLANEOUS														
Buspirone HCl	**Tab:** 5mg, 7.5mg, 10mg, 15mg, 30mg							✓						
Carbamazepine (Equetro)	**Cap, ER:** 100mg, 200mg, 300mg		✓	✓										
Lamotrigine (Lamictal, Lamictal ODT)	**Tab, Chewable:** 2mg, 5mg, 25mg; **Tab:** 25mg, 100mg, 150mg, 200mg; **Tab, Disintegrating:** (ODT) 25mg, 50mg, 100mg, 200mg	✓												
Lithium carbonate	**Cap:** 150mg, 300mg, 600mg; **Sol:** 8mEq/5mL; **Tab:** 300mg	✓	✓											
Lithium carbonate (Lithobid)	**Tab, ER:** 300mg, 450mg	✓	✓											
Nefazodone HCl	**Tab:** 50mg, 100mg, 150mg, 200mg, 250mg					✓								
Trazodone HCl	**Tab:** 50mg, 100mg, 150mg, 300mg					✓								

GENERIC (BRAND)	HOW SUPPLIED	INDICATIONS												
		BIPOLAR DISORDER (MAINTENANCE)	BIPOLAR, MANIC EPISODES	BIPOLAR, MIXED EPISODES	BIPOLAR, DEPRESSIVE EPISODES	DEPRESSION	SCHIZOPHRENIA	ANXIETY	OCD	PANIC DISORDER	PTSD	PMDD	IRRITABILITY ASSOCIATED W/ AUTISTIC DISORDER	PSYCHOSIS
MISCELLANEOUS *(Continued)*														
Trazodone HCl (Oleptro)	**Tab, ER:** 150mg, 300mg					✓								
Vortioxetine (Brintellix)	**Tab:** 5mg, 10mg, 15mg, 20mg					✓								

Refer to full FDA-approved labeling for additional information.

*Has indication to be used for agitation associated with schizophrenia or bipolar disorder.

Abbreviations: ER = extended-release; DR = delayed-release; OCD = obsessive-compulsive disorder; PTSD = post-traumatic stress disorder; PMDD = premenstrual dysphoric disorder.

ASTHMA AND COPD MANAGEMENT

GENERIC (BRAND)	DOSAGE FORM	ADULT DOSAGE	PEDIATRIC DOSAGE
5-LIPOXYGENASE INHIBITORS			
Zileuton (Zyflo, Zyflo CR)	(Zyflo) **Tab:** 600mg*	600mg qid. Take with meals and at hs.	**≥12 yrs:** 600mg qid. Take with meals and at hs.
	(Zyflo CR) **Tab, ER:** 600mg	1200mg bid. Take within 1 hr after am and pm meals.	**≥12 yrs:** 1200mg bid. Take within 1 hr after am and pm meals.
ANTICHOLINERGICS			
Aclidinium bromide (Tudorza Pressair)†	**MDI:** 400mcg/inh	1 inh bid.	
Glycopyrrolate (Seebri Neohaler)†	**Cap, Inh:** 15.6mcg	1 cap (inh) bid using the Neohaler device. **Max:** 1 cap bid.	
Ipratropium bromide (Atrovent HFA)†	**MDI:** 17mcg/inh	**Initial:** 2 inh qid. May take additional inh prn. **Max:** 12 inh/day.	
Tiotropium bromide (Spiriva HandiHaler)†	**Cap, Inh:** 18mcg	2 inh of contents of 1 cap qd.	
Tiotropium bromide (Spiriva Respimat)‡	**MDI:** 1.25mcg/inh, 2.5mcg/inh	**Asthma:** 2.5mcg (2 inh of 1.25mcg) qd. **Max:** 1 dose (2 inh)/24 hrs. **COPD:** 5mcg (2 inh of 2.5mcg) qd. **Max:** 1 dose (2 inh)/24 hrs.	**≥12 yrs:** 2.5mcg (2 inh of 1.25mcg) qd. **Max:** 1 dose (2 inh)/24 hrs.
Umeclidinium (Incruse Ellipta)†	**DPI:** 62.5mcg/inh	1 inh qd. **Max:** 1 inh/24 hrs.	
ANTICHOLINERGICS/BETA$_2$-AGONISTS			
Glycopyrrolate/Indacaterol (Utibron Neohaler)†	**Cap, Inh:** (Glycopyrrolate-Indacaterol) 15.6mcg-27.5mcg	1 cap (inh) bid using the Neohaler device. **Max:** 1 cap bid.	
Ipratropium bromide/ Albuterol (Combivent Respimat)†	**MDI:** (Ipratropium-Albuterol) 20mcg-100mcg/inh	1 inh qid. May take additional inh prn. **Max:** 6 inh/day.	
Ipratropium bromide/ Albuterol sulfate (Duoneb)†	**Sol, Inh:** (Ipratropium-Albuterol) 0.5mg-3mg/3mL	3mL qid via nebulizer with up to 2 additional 3mL doses/day prn.	
Olodaterol/Tiotropium bromide (Stiolto Respimat)†	**Spray, Inh:** (Olodaterol-Tiotropium) 2.5mcg-2.5mcg/inh	2 inh qd. **Max:** 2 inh/24 hrs.	
Umeclidinium/Vilanterol (Anoro Ellipta)†	**Powder, Inh:** (Umeclidinium-Vilanterol) 62.5mcg-25mcg	1 inh qd. **Max:** 1 inh/day.	
BETA$_2$-AGONISTS, LONG-ACTING			
Arformoterol tartrate (Brovana)†	**Sol, Inh:** 15mcg/2mL	15mcg bid (am/pm) via nebulizer. **Max:** 30mcg/day.	
Formoterol fumarate (Foradil Aerolizer)‡	**Cap, Inh:** 12mcg	1 cap (inh) q12h. **Max:** 24mcg/day.	**Asthma: ≥5 yrs:** 1 cap (inh) q12h. **Max:** 24mcg/day.
Formoterol fumarate (Perforomist)†	**Sol, Inh:** 20mcg/2mL	2mL q12h via nebulizer. **Max:** 40mcg/day.	
Indacaterol (Arcapta Neohaler)†	**Cap, Inh:** 75mcg	1 cap (inh) daily. **Max:** 1 cap/day.	
Olodaterol (Striverdi Respimat)†	**MDI:** 2.5mcg/inh	2 inh qd. **Max:** 2 inh/24 hrs.	

(Continued)

GENERIC (BRAND)	DOSAGE FORM	ADULT DOSAGE	PEDIATRIC DOSAGE
BETA$_2$-AGONISTS, LONG-ACTING *(Continued)*			
Salmeterol xinafoate (Serevent Diskus)[‡]	**DPI:** 50mcg/inh	1 inh bid (am/pm q12h).	**Asthma: ≥4 yrs:** 1 inh bid (am/pm q12h).
BETA$_2$-AGONISTS, SHORT-ACTING			
Albuterol sulfate	**Sol, Inh:** 0.083%, 0.5%	**Usual/Max:** 2.5mg tid-qid via nebulizer over 5-15 min.	**(0.083%) ≥2 yrs: ≥15kg: Usual/Max:** 2.5mg tid-qid via nebulizer over 5-15 min. Children weighing <15kg who require <2.5mg/dose should use 0.5% sol instead. **(0.5%) 2-12 yrs: Initial:** 0.1-0.15mg/kg/dose via nebulizer. **Max:** 2.5mg tid-qid. **>12 yrs: Usual/Max:** 2.5mg tid-qid via nebulizer over 5-15 min.
	Syr: 2mg/5mL	2mg or 4mg tid-qid. **Max:** 8mg qid.	**>14 yrs:** 2mg or 4mg tid-qid. **Max:** 8mg qid. **6-14 yrs:** 2mg tid-qid. **Max:** 24mg/day. **2-5 yrs: Initial:** 0.1mg/kg tid (not to exceed 2mg tid). **Titrate:** May increase to 0.2mg/kg tid. **Max:** 4mg tid.
	Tab: 2mg*, 4mg*	2mg or 4mg tid-qid. **Max:** 8mg qid.	**>12 yrs:** 2mg or 4mg tid-qid. **Max:** 8mg qid. **6-12 yrs:** 2mg tid-qid. **Max:** 24mg/day.
Albuterol sulfate (AccuNeb)	**Sol, Inh:** 0.63mg/3mL, 1.25mg/3mL		**2-12 yrs:** 0.63mg or 1.25mg tid-qid prn via nebulizer over 5-15 min.
Albuterol sulfate (ProAir HFA, Proventil HFA, Ventolin HFA)	**MDI:** 90mcg/inh	2 inh q4-6h or 1 inh q4h.	**≥4 yrs:** 2 inh q4-6h or 1 inh q4h.
Albuterol sulfate (Vospire ER)	**Tab, ER:** 4mg, 8mg	4-8mg q12h. **Max:** 32mg/day.	**>12 yrs:** 4-8mg q12h. **Max:** 32mg/day. **6-12 yrs:** 4mg q12h. **Max:** 24mg/day.
Levalbuterol HCl (Xopenex)	**Sol, Inh:** 1.25mg/0.5mL, 0.31mg/3mL, 0.63mg/3mL, 1.25mg/3mL	0.63-1.25mg tid (q6-8h) via nebulizer.	**≥12 yrs:** 0.63-1.25mg tid (q6-8h) via nebulizer. **6-11 yrs:** 0.31mg tid via nebulizer. **Max:** 0.63mg tid.
Levalbuterol tartrate (Xopenex HFA)	**MDI:** 45mcg/inh	1-2 inh q4-6h.	**≥4 yrs:** 1-2 inh q4-6h.
Metaproterenol sulfate	**Syrup:** 10mg/5mL; **Tab:** 10mg*, 20mg*	20mg tid-qid.	**>9 yrs or >60 lbs:** 20mg tid-qid. **6-9 yrs or <60 lbs:** 10mg tid-qid. **<6 yrs:** (Syrup) 1.3-2.6mg/kg/day.
Pirbuterol acetate (Maxair Autohaler)	**MDI:** 200mcg/inh	1-2 inh q4-6h. **Max:** 12 inh/day.	**≥12 yrs:** 1-2 inh q4-6h. **Max:** 12 inh/day.
Terbutaline sulfate	**Tab:** 2.5mg, 5mg	2.5-5mg q6h tid. **Max:** 15mg/day.	**12-15 yrs:** 2.5mg tid. **Max:** 7.5mg/day.
	Inj: 1mg/mL	0.25mg SQ into the lateral deltoid area. May repeat dose in 15-30 min if no improvement. **Max:** 0.5mg/4 hrs.	**≥12 yrs:** 0.25mg SQ into the lateral deltoid area. May repeat dose in 15-30 min if no improvement. **Max:** 0.5mg/4 hrs.

GENERIC (BRAND)	DOSAGE FORM	ADULT DOSAGE	PEDIATRIC DOSAGE
BETA$_2$-AGONISTS/CORTICOSTEROIDS			
Budesonide/Formoterol fumarate dihydrate (Symbicort)‡	**MDI:** (Budesonide-Formoterol) 80mcg-4.5mcg/inh, 160mcg-4.5mcg/inh	**Asthma: Initial:** 2 inh bid (am/pm q12h). Starting dose is based on asthma severity. **Max:** 160mcg-4.5mcg bid. **COPD:** 2 inh of 160mcg-4.5mcg bid.	**Asthma: ≥12 yrs:** 2 inh bid (am/pm q12h). Starting dose is based on asthma severity. **Max:** 160mcg-4.5mcg bid.
Fluticasone furoate/ Vilanterol (Breo Ellipta)‡	**Powder, Inh:** (Fluticasone-Vilanterol) 100mcg-25mcg, 200mcg-25mcg	1 inh qd. **Max:** 1 inh/day.	
Fluticasone propionate/ Salmeterol (Advair Diskus)‡	**DPI:** (Fluticasone-Salmeterol) 100mcg-50mcg/inh, 250mcg-50mcg/inh, 500mcg-50mcg/inh	**Asthma:** 1 inh bid (am/pm q12h). Starting dose is based on asthma severity. **Max:** 500mcg-50mcg bid. **COPD:** 1 inh of 250mcg-50mcg bid (am/pm q12h).	**Asthma: ≥12 yrs:** 1 inh bid (am/pm q12h). Starting dose is based on asthma severity. **Max:** 500mcg-50mcg bid. **4-11 yrs:** 1 inh of 100mcg-50mcg bid (am/pm q12h).
Fluticasone propionate/ Salmeterol (Advair HFA)	**MDI:** (Fluticasone-Salmeterol) 45mcg-21mcg/inh, 115mcg-21mcg/inh, 230mcg-21mcg/inh	**Initial:** 2 inh bid (am/pm q12h). Starting dose is based on asthma severity. **Max:** 2 inh of 230mcg-21mcg bid.	**≥12 yrs: Initial:** 2 inh bid (am/pm q12h). Starting dose is based on asthma severity. **Max:** 2 inh of 230mcg-21mcg bid.
Mometasone furoate/ Formoterol fumarate dihydrate (Dulera)	**MDI:** (Mometasone-Formoterol) 100mcg-5mcg/inh, 200mcg-5mcg/inh	**Previous Inhaled Medium-Dose Corticosteroids: Initial:** 2 inh of 100mcg-5mcg bid. **Max:** 400mcg-20mcg/day. **Previous Inhaled High-Dose Corticosteroids: Initial:** 2 inh of 200mcg-5mcg bid. **Max:** 800mcg-20mcg/day.	**≥12 yrs: Previous Inhaled Medium-Dose Corticosteroids: Initial:** 2 inh of 100mcg-5mcg bid. **Max:** 400mcg-20mcg/day. **Previous Inhaled High-Dose Corticosteroids: Initial:** 2 inh of 200mcg-5mcg bid. **Max:** 800mcg-20mcg/day.
CORTICOSTEROIDS			
Beclomethasone dipropionate (QVAR)	**MDI:** 40mcg/inh, 80mcg/inh	**Previous Bronchodilators Alone: Initial:** 40-80mcg bid. **Max:** 320mcg bid. **Previous Inhaled Corticosteroids: Initial:** 40-160mcg bid. **Max:** 320mcg bid.	**≥12 yrs:** Refer to adult dosing. **5-11 yrs: Previous Bronchodilators Alone/ Inhaled Corticosteroids: Initial:** 40mcg bid. **Max:** 80mcg bid.
Budesonide (Pulmicort Flexhaler)	**DPI:** 90mcg/inh, 180mcg/inh	**Initial:** 180-360mcg bid. **Max:** 720mcg bid.	**6-17 yrs: Initial:** 180-360mcg bid. **Max:** 360mcg bid.
Budesonide (Pulmicort Respules)	**Sus, Inh:** 0.25mg/2mL, 0.5mg/2mL, 1mg/2mL		**12 mths-8 yrs: Previous Bronchodilators: Initial:** 0.5mg/day given qd or bid. **Max:** 0.5mg/day. **Previous Inhaled Corticosteroids: Initial:** 0.5mg/day given qd or bid. **Max:** 1mg/day. **Previous Oral Corticosteroids: Initial:** 1mg/day given qd or bid. **Max:** 1mg/day.
Ciclesonide (Alvesco)	**MDI:** 80mcg/inh, 160mcg/inh	**Previous Bronchodilator Alone: Initial:** 80mcg bid. **Max:** 160mcg bid. **Previous Inhaled Corticosteroids: Initial:** 80mcg bid. **Max:** 320mcg bid. **Previous Oral Corticosteroids: Initial/Max:** 320mcg bid.	**≥12 yrs:** Refer to adult dosing.

(Continued)

GENERIC (BRAND)	DOSAGE FORM	ADULT DOSAGE	PEDIATRIC DOSAGE
CORTICOSTEROIDS *(Continued)*			
Flunisolide (Aerospan)	**MDI:** 80mcg/inh	**Initial:** 160mcg bid. **Max:** 320mcg bid.	**≥12 yrs: Initial:** 160mcg bid. **Max:** 320mcg bid. **6-11 yrs: Initial:** 80mcg bid. **Max:** 160mcg bid.
Fluticasone furoate (Arnuity Ellipta)	**DPI:** 100mcg/inh, 200mcg/inh	1 inh qd. **Max:** 1 inh/24 hrs.	**≥12 yrs:** 1 inh qd. **Max:** 1 inh/24 hrs.
Fluticasone propionate (Flovent Diskus)	**DPI:** 50mcg/inh, 100mcg/inh, 250mcg/inh	**Previous Bronchodilators Alone: Initial:** 100mcg bid. **Max:** 500mcg bid. **Previous Inhaled Corticosteroids: Initial:** 100-250mcg bid. **Max:** 500mcg bid. **Previous Oral Corticosteroids: Initial:** 500-1000mcg bid. **Max:** 1000mcg bid.	**≥12 yrs:** Refer to adult dosing. **4-11 yrs: Initial:** 50mcg bid. **Max:** 100mcg bid.
Fluticasone propionate (Flovent HFA)	**MDI:** 44mcg/inh, 110mcg/inh, 220mcg/inh	**Previous Bronchodilators Alone: Initial:** 88mcg bid. **Max:** 440mcg bid. **Previous Inhaled Corticosteroids: Initial:** 88-220mcg bid. **Max:** 440mcg bid. **Previous Oral Corticosteroids: Initial:** 440mcg bid. **Max:** 880mcg bid.	**≥12 yrs:** Refer to adult dosing. **4-11 yrs: Initial/Max:** 88mcg bid.
Mometasone furoate (Asmanex HFA)	**MDI:** 100mcg/inh, 200mcg/inh	**Previous Inhaled Medium-Dose Corticosteroids:** 2 inh of 100mcg bid. **Max:** 2 inh of 200mcg bid. **Previous Inhaled High-Dose Corticosteroids/Previous Oral Corticosteroids:** 2 inh of 200mcg bid. **Max:** 2 inh of 200mcg bid.	**≥12 yrs:** Refer to adult dosing.
Mometasone furoate (Asmanex Twisthaler)	**DPI:** 110mcg/inh, 220mcg/inh	**Previous Bronchodilators Alone/Inhaled Corticosteroids: Initial:** 220mcg qpm. **Max:** 440mcg/day. **Previous Oral Corticosteroids: Initial:** 440mcg bid. **Max:** 880mcg/day.	**≥12 yrs:** Refer to adult dosing. **4-11 yrs: Initial/Max:** 110mcg/day qpm.
LEUKOTRIENE RECEPTOR ANTAGONISTS			
Montelukast sodium (Singulair)	**Granules:** 4mg; **Tab:** 10mg; **Tab, Chewable:** 4mg, 5mg	10mg qpm.	**≥15 yrs:** 10mg qpm. **6-14 yrs:** 5mg chewable tab qpm. **2-5 yrs:** 4mg chewable tab or 4mg oral granules pkt qpm. **12-23 mths:** 4mg oral granules pkt qpm.
Zafirlukast (Accolate)	**Tab:** 10mg, 20mg	20mg bid. Take at least 1 hr before or 2 hrs after meals.	Take at least 1 hr before or 2 hrs after meals. **≥12 yrs:** 20mg bid. **5-11 yrs:** 10mg bid.
MAST CELL STABILIZERS			
Cromolyn sodium	**Sol, Inh:** 20mg/2mL	20mg nebulized qid.	**≥2 yrs:** 20mg nebulized qid.

GENERIC (BRAND)	DOSAGE FORM	ADULT DOSAGE	PEDIATRIC DOSAGE
METHYLXANTHINES			
Theophylline anhydrous (Elixophyllin)§	**Elixir:** 80mg/15mL	**16-60 yrs: Initial:** 300mg/day divided q6-8h. **After 3 Days if Tolerated:** 400mg/day divided q6-8h. **After 3 More Days if Tolerated:** 600mg/day divided q6-8h.	**1-15 yrs: >45kg:** Refer to adult dosing. **<45kg: Initial:** 12-14mg/kg/day divided q4-6h. **Max:** 300mg/day. **After 3 Days if Tolerated:** 16mg/kg/day divided q4-6h. **Max:** 400mg/day. **After 3 More Days if Tolerated:** 20mg/kg/day divided q4-6h. **Max:** 600mg/day. See PI for infant dose.
Theophylline anhydrous (Theo-24)§	**Cap, ER:** 100mg, 200mg, 300mg, 400mg	**16-60 yrs: Initial:** 300-400mg/day q24h. **After 3 Days if Tolerated:** 400-600mg/day q24h. **After 3 More Days if Tolerated and Needed:** Doses >600mg should be titrated according to blood levels (see PI).	**12-15 yrs: >45kg:** Refer to adult dosing. **<45kg: Initial:** 12-14mg/kg/day q24h. **Max:** 300mg/day. **After 3 Days if Tolerated:** 16mg/kg/day q24h. **Max:** 400mg/day. **After 3 More Days if Tolerated and Needed:** 20mg/kg/day q24h. **Max:** 600mg/day.
Theophylline anhydrous§	**Tab, ER:** 400mg*, 600mg*		
MONOCLONAL ANTIBODIES			
Mepolizumab (Nucala)	**Inj:** 100mg	100mg SQ q4wks.	**≥12 yrs:** 100mg SQ q4wks.
Omalizumab (Xolair)	**Inj:** 150mg/5mL	150-375mg SQ q2 or 4 wks. Determine dose and dosing frequency by serum total IgE level measured before the start of treatment, and body weight. See PI for dose determination charts.	**≥12 yrs:** 150-375mg SQ q2 or 4 wks. Determine dose and dosing frequency by serum total IgE level measured before the start of treatment, and body weight. See PI for dose determination charts.
PHOSPHODIESTERASE-4 INHIBITORS			
Roflumilast (Daliresp)†	**Tab:** 500mcg	500mcg qd.	
SYSTEMIC CORTICOSTEROIDS			
Methylprednisolone (Medrol)	**Tab:** 2mg*, 4mg*, 8mg*, 16mg*, 32mg*	**Initial:** 4-48mg/day. Dosage must be individualized based on the disease state and patient response.	Refer to adult dosing.
Prednisolone	**Sol:** 15mg/5mL; **Tab:** 5mg*	**Initial:** 5-60mg/day. Dosage must be individualized based on the disease state and patient response.	Refer to adult dosing.
Prednisone	**Sol:** 5mg/5mL, 5mg/mL; **Tab:** 1mg*, 2.5mg*, 5mg*, 10mg*, 20mg*, 50mg*	**Initial:** 5-60mg/day. Dosage must be individualized based on the disease state and patient response.	Refer to adult dosing.

Refer to full FDA-approved labeling for additional information.

Abbreviations: DPI = dry-powder inhaler; ER = extended-released; MDI = metered-dose inhaler.

*Scored.

†Indicated for COPD only.

‡Indicated for asthma and COPD.

§The dose of theophylline must be individualized based on peak serum theophylline concentrations.

Benign Prostatic Hypertrophy Agents

GENERIC	BRAND	HOW SUPPLIED	DOSAGE	DOSING CONSIDERATIONS
ALPHA-BLOCKERS				
Alfuzosin	Uroxatral	**Tab, ER:** 10mg	**Usual:** 10mg qd.	• Take dose with the same meal each day. Swallow whole. • **Moderate or Severe Hepatic Impairment/ Concomitant Potent CYP3A4 Inhibitors:** Contraindicated.
Doxazosin	Cardura	**Tab:** 1mg, 2mg, 4mg, 8mg	**Initial:** 1mg qd. **Max:** 8mg qd.	• Stepwise titration in 1- to 2-week intervals, if needed.
	Cardura XL	**Tab, ER:** 4mg, 8mg	**Initial:** 4mg qd. **Max:** 8mg qd.	• Take with breakfast. Swallow whole. • Titrate in 3- to 4-week intervals, if needed.
Silodosin	Rapaflo	**Cap:** 4mg, 8mg	**Usual:** 8mg qd.	• Take with food. • **Moderate Renal Impairment (CrCl 30-50mL/min):** 4mg qd. • **Severe Renal Impairment (CrCl <30mL/min)/Severe Hepatic Impairment:** Contraindicated. • Carefully open and sprinkle the powder inside of capsule on a tablespoon of applesauce if difficult to swallow.
Tamsulosin	Flomax	**Cap:** 0.4mg	**Usual:** 0.4mg qd. **Max:** 0.8mg qd.	• Take dose 30 min after the same meal each day. Swallow whole. • Titrate after 2-4 weeks if needed. • Restart at 0.4mg dose if therapy is interrupted. • **Concomitant Strong CYP3A4 Inhibitors:** Avoid use.
Terazosin	Generic	**Cap:** 1mg, 2mg, 5mg, 10mg	**Initial:** 1mg qhs. **Usual:** 10mg qd. **Max:** 20mg/day.	• Increase stepwise as needed. • Restart at initial dose if therapy is interrupted.
5-ALPHA REDUCTASE INHIBITORS				
Dutasteride	Avodart	**Cap:** 0.5mg	**Usual:** 0.5mg qd.	• Swallow whole. May take with or without food. • May be administered with tamsulosin.
Finasteride	Proscar	**Tab:** 5mg	**Usual:** 5mg qd.	• May take with or without food. • May be administered with doxazosin.
PHOSPHODIESTERASE-5 INHIBITORS				
Tadalafil	Cialis	**Tab:** 2.5mg, 5mg, 10mg, 20mg	**Usual:** 5mg qd.	• Take dose at approximately the same time every day. • **CrCl 30-50mL/min:** 2.5mg is recommended. • **CrCl <30mL/min or on Hemodialysis:** Not recommended for once daily use. • Not recommended for use in combination with alpha-blockers for benign prostatic hypertrophy. • **Severe Hepatic Impairment:** Not recommended.
COMBINATIONS				
Dutasteride/ Tamsulosin	Jalyn	**Cap:** 0.5mg/0.4mg	**Usual:** 1 cap qd.	• Swallow whole. • Take dose 30 min after the same meal each day. • **Concomitant Strong CYP3A4 Inhibitors:** Avoid use.

Refer to full FDA-approved labeling for additional information.

Abbreviation: ER = extended-release.

ERECTILE DYSFUNCTION AGENTS

GENERIC (BRAND)	HOW SUPPLIED	DOSAGE
PHOSPHODIESTERASE INHIBITORS		
Avanafil (Stendra)	**Tab:** 50mg, 100mg, 200mg	**Initial:** 100mg prn as early as 15 min prior to sexual activity. **Titration:** Increase to 200mg or decrease to 50mg based on efficacy/tolerability. **Max Frequency:** 1 dose/day. **Max Dose:** 200mg.
Sildenafil (Viagra)	**Tab:** 25mg, 50mg, 100mg	**Usual:** 50mg prn 1 hr prior to sexual activity. May be taken ½-4 hrs prior to sexual activity. **Titration:** Increase to 100mg or decrease to 25mg based on efficacy/tolerability. **Max Frequency:** 1 dose/day. **Max Dose:** 100mg.
Tadalafil (Cialis)	**Tab:** 2.5mg, 5mg, 10mg, 20mg	**PRN Use: Initial:** 10mg prior to sexual activity. **Titration:** Increase to 20mg or decrease to 5mg based on efficacy/tolerability. **Max Frequency:** 1 dose/day. **QD Use: Initial:** 2.5mg qd. **Titration:** Increase to 5mg qd based on efficacy/tolerability.
Vardenafil (Levitra)	**Tab:** 2.5mg, 5mg, 10mg, 20mg	**Initial:** 10mg prn 1 hr prior to sexual activity. **Titration:** Increase to 20mg or decrease to 5mg based on efficacy/tolerability. **Max Frequency:** 1 dose/day. **Max Dose:** 20mg.
Vardenafil (Staxyn)	**Tab, Disintegrating:** 10mg	10mg prn 1 hr prior to sexual activity. **Max:** 1 dose/day. Place on tongue to disintegrate. Take without liquid.
PROSTAGLANDINS		
Alprostadil (Edex, Caverject, Caverject Impulse)	**Inj:** (Edex) 10mcg, 20mcg, 40mcg; (Caverject) 5mcg, 10mcg, 20mcg, 40mcg; (Caverject Impulse) 10mcg, 20mcg	Use lowest possible effective dose. Patient must stay in physician's office until complete detumescence occurs. If there is no response, give next higher dose within 1 hr. If there is a response, allow 1-day interval before the next dose. Reduce dose if erection lasts >1 hr. **Vasculogenic, Psychogenic, or Mixed Etiology: Initial:** 2.5mcg. **Titration: Partial Response to 2.5mcg:** Increase to 5mcg and then in increments of 5-10mcg, depending upon response, until erection of 1 hr max duration. **No Response to 2.5mcg:** Increase 2nd dose to 7.5mcg followed by increments of 5-10mcg. **Pure Neurogenic Etiology (Spinal Cord Injury): Initial:** 1.25mcg. **Titration:** Increase to 2.5mcg, then to 5mcg, and then by 5mcg increments until erection of 1 hr max duration. **Maint:** Give no more than 3 doses/week; allow at least 24 hrs between doses. (Edex) **Dose Range:** 1-40mcg. Give inj over 5- to 10-sec interval. (Caverject, Caverject Impulse) **Max:** 60mcg/dose.
Alprostadil (Muse)	**Supp, Urethral:** 125mcg, 250mcg, 500mcg, 1000mcg	**Initial:** 125-250mcg. **Titration:** Increase or decrease dose based on individual response. **Max:** 2 administrations/24 hrs.

Refer to full FDA-approved labeling for additional information.

Overactive Bladder Agents

GENERIC	BRAND	HOW SUPPLIED	DOSAGE	COMMENTS
MUSCARINIC ANTAGONISTS				
Darifenacin	Enablex	**Tab, ER:** 7.5mg, 15mg	**Initial:** 7.5mg qd. **Max:** 15mg qd.	Swallow whole. **Moderate Hepatic Impairment/ Concomitant Potent CYP3A4 Inhibitors:** Do not exceed 7.5mg/day. **Severe Hepatic Impairment:** Avoid use.
Fesoterodine	Toviaz	**Tab, ER:** 4mg, 8mg	**Initial:** 4mg qd. **Max:** 8mg qd.	Swallow whole. **Severe Renal Impairment (CrCl <30mL/min)/ Concomitant Potent CYP3A4 Inhibitors:** Do not exceed 4mg/day. **Severe Hepatic Impairment:** Avoid use.
Oxybutynin*	Generic	**Syrup:** 5mg/5mL; **Tab:** 5mg	**Usual:** 5mg bid-tid. **Max:** 5mg qid.	**Elderly:** A lower starting dose of 2.5mg bid-tid is recommended. **Pediatrics >5 yrs:** 5mg bid. **Max:** 5mg tid.
	Ditropan XL	**Tab, ER:** 5mg, 10mg, 15mg	**Initial:** 5mg or 10mg qd. **Max:** 30mg/day.	Swallow whole. Increase dose by 5mg weekly if needed. **Pediatrics ≥6 yrs:** 5mg qd. **Max:** 20mg/day.
	Gelnique	**Gel:** 3% (28mg/pump), 10% (1g/pkt)	Apply to dry, intact skin on abdomen, upper arms/ shoulders, or thighs. **3%:** 3 pumps qd. **10%:** 1 pkt qd.	Rotate application sites.
	Oxytrol	**Patch:** 3.9mg/day	Apply 1 patch to dry, intact skin on abdomen, hip, or buttock twice weekly (every 3-4 days).	Rotate application sites (avoid using the same site within 7 days).
Solifenacin	Vesicare	**Tab:** 5mg, 10mg	**Usual:** 5mg qd. **Max:** 10mg qd.	Swallow whole. **Severe Renal Impairment (CrCl <30mL/min)/ Moderate Hepatic Impairment/ Concomitant Potent CYP3A4 Inhibitors:** Do not exceed 5mg/day. **Severe Hepatic Impairment:** Avoid use.
Tolterodine	Detrol	**Tab:** 1mg, 2mg	**Initial:** 2mg bid.	Decrease dose to 1mg bid if needed. **Significant Hepatic or Renal Dysfunction/ Concomitant Potent CYP3A4 Inhibitors:** 1mg bid.
	Detrol LA	**Cap, ER:** 2mg, 4mg	**Usual:** 4mg qd.	Swallow whole. Decrease dose to 2mg qd if needed. **Mild-Moderate Hepatic Impairment/Severe Renal Impairment (CrCl 10-30mL/min)/ Concomitant Potent CYP3A4 Inhibitors:** 2mg qd. **Severe Hepatic Impairment/ CrCl <10mL/min:** Avoid use.

(Continued)

GENERIC	BRAND	HOW SUPPLIED	DOSAGE	COMMENTS
MUSCARINIC ANTAGONISTS *(Continued)*				
Trospium	Generic	**Tab:** 20mg	**Usual:** 20mg bid.	Take 1 hr before meals or on empty stomach. **Severe Renal Impairment (CrCl <30mL/min):** 20mg qhs. **Elderly ≥75 yrs:** May titrate down to 20mg qd based on tolerability.
	Generic	**Cap, ER:** 60mg	**Usual:** 60mg qam.	Take on empty stomach 1 hr before a meal. **Severe Renal Impairment (CrCl <30mL/min):** Avoid use.
MISCELLANEOUS				
Mirabegron	Myrbetriq	**Tab, ER:** 25mg, 50mg	**Initial:** 25mg qd. **Max:** 50mg qd.	Take with or without food. Swallow whole. **Severe Renal Impairment (CrCl 15-29mL/min)/ Moderate Hepatic Impairment:** Do not exceed 25mg/day. **End-Stage Renal Disease/Severe Hepatic Impairment:** Avoid use.
OnabotulinumtoxinA	Botox	**Inj:** (sterile powder) 100 U, 200 U	**Usual:** 100 U. **Max:** 100 U.	Recommended dilution is 100 U/10mL with 0.9% non-preserved saline solution.

Abbreviation: ER = extended-release.

*Oxytrol for women (oxybutynin) patch is available as an OTC product for overactive bladder.

FDA-Approved New Drug Products

BRAND	GENERIC	INDICATION
Addyi	flibanserin	To treat acquired, generalized hypoactive sexual desire disorder (HSDD) in premenopausal women.
Alecensa	alectinib	To treat anaplastic lymphoma kinase (ALK)-positive, metastatic non-small cell lung cancer (NSCLC).
Aristada	aripiprazole lauroxil	To treat schizophrenia.
Bridion	sugammadex	To reverse effects of neuromuscular blocking drugs used during surgery.
Cholbam	cholic acid	To treat pediatric and adult patients with bile acid synthesis disorders due to single enzyme defects, and for patients with peroxisomal disorders.
Coagadex	Factor X (human)	To treat adult and pediatric patients with hereditary Factor X deficiency for on-demand treatment and control of bleeding episodes, as well as for perioperative management of bleeding in patients with mild hereditary Factor X deficiency.
Corlanor	ivabradine	To reduce the risk of hospitalization for worsening heart failure.
Cotellic	cobimetinib	To be used in combination with vemurafenib to treat advanced melanoma that has spread to other parts of the body or cannot be removed by surgery, and that has a certain type of abnormal gene (BRAF V600E or V600K mutation).
Daklinza	daclatasvir	To treat chronic hepatitis C virus (HCV) genotype 3 infections.
Darzalex	daratumumab	To treat patients with multiple myeloma who have received at least three prior treatments.
Empliciti	elotuzumab	To treat people with multiple myeloma who have received one to three prior medications.
Entresto	sacubitril/valsartan	To treat heart failure.
Genvoya	cobicistat/elvitegravir/ emtricitabine/tenofovir alafenamide fumarate	For use as a complete regimen for the treatment of HIV-1 infection in adults and pediatric patients 12 years of age and older.
Imlygic	talimogene laherparepvec	For local treatment of unresectable cutaneous, subcutaneous, and nodal lesions in patients with melanoma recurrent after initial surgery.
Kanuma	sebelipase alfa	To treat patients with a rare disease known as lysosomal acid lipase (LAL) deficiency.
Kengreal	cangrelor	To prevent the formation of harmful blood clots in the coronary arteries for adult patients undergoing percutaneous coronary intervention.
Kybella	deoxycholic acid	To treat adults with moderate-to-severe fat below the chin, known as submental fat.
Lonsurf	tipiracil/trifluridine	To treat patients with an advanced form of colorectal cancer who are no longer responding to other therapies.
Ninlaro	ixazomib	To treat people with multiple myeloma who have received at least one prior therapy.
Nucala	mepolizumab	For use with other asthma medicines for the maintenance treatment of asthma in patients age 12 years and older.
Odomzo	sonidegib	To treat patients with locally advanced basal cell carcinoma that has recurred following surgery or radiation therapy, or who are not candidates for surgery or radiation therapy.
Orkambi	ivacaftor/lumacaftor	To treat cystic fibrosis.

(Continued)

BRAND	GENERIC	INDICATION
Portrazza	necitumumab	To treat patients with metastatic squamous non-small cell lung cancer (NSCLC) who have not previously received medication specifically for treating their advanced lung cancer.
Praluent	alirocumab	To treat certain patients with high cholesterol.
Praxbind	idarucizumab	For use in patients who are taking the anticoagulant dabigatran during emergency situations when there is a need to reverse dabigatran's blood-thinning effects.
Repatha	evolocumab	To treat certain patients with high cholesterol.
Rexulti	brexpiprazole	To treat schizophrenia and as an add-on to an antidepressant to treat major depressive disorder.
Strensiq	asfotase alfa	To treat perinatal, infantile, and juvenile-onset hypophosphatasia (HPP).
Tagrisso	osimertinib	To treat certain patients with non-small cell lung cancer (NSCLC).
Tresiba	insulin degludec injection	To improve glycemic control in adults with diabetes mellitus.
Unituxin	dinutuximab	To treat pediatric patients with high-risk neuroblastoma.
Uptravi	selexipag	To treat pulmonary arterial hypertension.
Varubi	rolapitant	To prevent delayed phase chemotherapy-induced nausea and vomiting.
Veltassa	patiromer	To treat hyperkalemia, a serious condition in which the amount of potassium in the blood is too high.
Viberzi	eluxadoline	To treat irritable bowel syndrome with diarrhea (IBS-D) in adult men and women.
Vonvendi	von Willebrand factor (recombinant)	For on-demand treatment and control of bleeding episodes in adults with von Willebrand disease.
Vraylar	cariprazine	To treat schizophrenia and bipolar disorder in adults.
Xuriden	uridine triacetate	To treat patients with hereditary orotic aciduria.
Yondelis	trabectedin	To treat unresectable or metastatic liposarcoma or leiomyosarcoma.
Zepatier	elbasvir/grazoprevir	To treat hepatitis C virus (HCV) genotypes 1 or 4 infection in adults.
Zurampic	lesinurad	To treat high blood uric acid levels associated with gout.

Note: This list is not comprehensive and only includes new molecular entities that have not been approved by the FDA previously, either as a single ingredient drug or as part of a combination product. For a complete list, please refer to the FDA website, www.accessdata.fda.gov/scripts/cder/drugsatfda/index.cfm?fuseaction=Reports.ReportsMenu.

ISMP's List of Confused Drug Names

This list has been reproduced with permission from the Institute for Safe Medication Practices (ISMP). ISMP's List of Confused Drug Names is available at www.ismp.org.

DRUG NAME	CONFUSED DRUG NAME
Abelcet	amphotericin B
Accupril	Aciphex
aceta**ZOLAMIDE**	aceto**HEXAMIDE**
acetic acid for irrigation	glacial acetic acid
aceto**HEXAMIDE**	aceta**ZOLAMIDE**
Aciphex	Accupril
Aciphex	Aricept
Activase	Cathflo Activase
Activase	TNKase
Actonel	Actos
Actos	Actonel
Adacel (Tdap)	Daptacel (DTaP)
Adderall	Inderal
Adderall	Adderall XR
Adderall XR	Adderall
ado-trastuzumab emtansine	trastuzumab
Advair	Advicor
Advicor	Advair
Advicor	Altocor
Afrin (oxymetazoline)	Afrin (saline)
Afrin (saline)	Afrin (oxymetazoline)
Aggrastat	argatroban
Aldara	Alora
Alkeran	Leukeran
Alkeran	Myleran
Allegra (fexofenadine)	Allegra Anti-Itch Cream (diphenhydr**AMINE**/allantoin)
Allegra	Viagra
Allegra Anti-Itch Cream (diphenhydr**AMINE**/allantoin)	Allegra (fexofenadine)
Alora	Aldara
ALPRAZolam	**LOR**azepam
Altocor	Advicor
amantadine	amiodarone
Amaryl	Reminyl
Ambisome	amphotericin B
Amicar	Omacor
Amikin	Kineret
a**MIL**oride	am**LODIP**ine
amiodarone	amantadine
am**LODIP**ine	a**MIL**oride
amphotericin B	Abelcet
amphotericin B	Ambisome
Anacin	Anacin-3
Anacin-3	Anacin
antacid	Atacand
Anticoagulant Citrate Dextrose Solution Formula A	Anticoagulant Sodium Citrate Solution
Anticoagulant Sodium Citrate Solution	Anticoagulant Citrate Dextrose Solution Formula A
Antivert	Axert
Anzemet	Avandamet
Apidra	Spiriva
Apresoline	Priscoline
argatroban	Aggrastat
argatroban	Orgaran
Aricept	Aciphex

DRUG NAME	CONFUSED DRUG NAME
Aricept	Azilect
ARIPiprazole	proton pump inhibitors
ARIPiprazole	**RABE**prazole
Arista AH (absorbable hemostatic agent)	Arixtra
Arixtra	Arista AH (absorbable hemostatic agent)
Asacol	Os-Cal
Atacand	antacid
atomoxetine	atorvastatin
atorvastatin	atomoxetine
Atrovent	Natru-Vent
Avandamet	Anzemet
Avandia	Prandin
Avandia	Coumadin
AVINza	**INV**anz
AVINza	Evista
Axert	Antivert
aza**CITID**ine	aza**THIO**prine
aza**THIO**prine	aza**CITID**ine
Azilect	Aricept
B & O (belladonna and opium)	Beano
BabyBIG	HBIG (hepatitis B immune globulin)
Bayhep-B	Bayrab
Bayhep-B	Bayrho-D
Bayrab	Bayhep-B
Bayrab	Bayrho-D
Bayrho-D	Bayhep-B
Bayrho-D	Bayrab
Beano	B & O (belladonna and opium)
Benadryl	benazepril
benazepril	Benadryl
Benicar	Mevacor
Betadine (with povidone-iodine)	Betadine (without povidone-iodine)
Betadine (without povidone-iodine)	Betadine (with povidone-iodine)
Bextra	Zetia
Bicillin C-R	Bicillin L-A
Bicillin L-A	Bicillin C-R
Bicitra	Polycitra
Bidex	Videx
Brethine	Methergine
Bio-T-Gel	T-Gel
Brevibloc	Brevital
Brevital	Brevibloc
Brilinta	Brintellix
Brintellix	Brilinta
bu**PROP**ion	bus**PIR**one
bus**PIR**one	bu**PROP**ion
Capadex [non-US product]	Kapidex
Capex	Kapidex

(Continued)

Brand names always start with an uppercase letter. Some brand names incorporate tall man letters in initial characters and may not be readily recognized as brand names. Brand name products appear in black; generic/other products appear in **color**.

DRUG NAME	CONFUSED DRUG NAME
Carac	Kuric
captopril	carvedilol
car**BAM**azepine	**OX**carbazepine
CARBOplatin	**CIS**platin
Cardene	Cardizem
Cardizem	Cardene
Cardura	Coumadin
carvedilol	captopril
Casodex	Kapidex
Cathflo Activase	Activase
Cedax	Cidex
ce**FAZ**olin	cef**TRIAX**one
cef**TRIAX**one	ce**FAZ**olin
Cele**BREX**	Cele**XA**
Cele**BREX**	Cerebyx
Cele**XA**	Zy**PREXA**
Cele**XA**	Cele**BREX**
Cele**XA**	Cerebyx
Cerebyx	Cele**BREX**
Cerebyx	Cele**XA**
cetirizine	sertraline
cetirizine	stavudine
chlordiaze**POXIDE**	chlorpro**MAZINE**
chlorpro**MAZINE**	chlordiaze**POXIDE**
chlorpro**MAZINE**	chlorpro**PAMIDE**
chlorpro**PAMIDE**	chlorpro**MAZINE**
Cidex	Cedax
CISplatin	**CARBO**platin
Claritin (loratadine)	Claritin Eye (ketotifen fumarate)
Claritin-D	Claritin-D 24
Claritin-D 24	Claritin-D
Claritin Eye (ketotifen fumarate)	Claritin (loratadine)
Clindesse	Clindets
Clindets	Clindesse
clobazam	clonaze**PAM**
clomi**PHENE**	clomi**PRAMINE**
clomi**PRAMINE**	clomi**PHENE**
clonaze**PAM**	clobazam
clonaze**PAM**	clo**NID**ine
clonaze**PAM**	**LOR**azepam
clo**NID**ine	clonaze**PAM**
clo**NID**ine	Klono**PIN**
Clozaril	Colazal
coagulation factor IX (recombinant)	factor IX complex, vapor heated
codeine	Lodine
Colace	Cozaar
Colazal	Clozaril
colchicine	Cortrosyn
Comvax	Recombivax HB
Cortrosyn	colchicine
Coumadin	Avandia
Coumadin	Cardura
Covaryx HS	Covera HS
Covera HS	Covaryx HS
Cozaar	Colace
Cozaar	Zocor

DRUG NAME	CONFUSED DRUG NAME
cyclophosphamide	cyclo**SPORINE**
cyclo**SERINE**	cyclo**SPORINE**
cyclo**SPORINE**	cyclophosphamide
cyclo**SPORINE**	cyclo**SERINE**
Cymbalta	Symbyax
DACTINomycin	**DAPTO**mycin
Daptacel (DTaP)	Adacel (Tdap)
DAPTOmycin	**DACTIN**omycin
Darvocet	Percocet
Darvon	Diovan
DAUNOrubicin	**DAUNO**rubicin citrate liposomal
DAUNOrubicin	**DOXO**rubicin
DAUNOrubicin	**IDA**rubicin
DAUNOrubicin citrate liposomal	**DAUNO**rubicin
Denavir	indinavir
Depakote	Depakote ER
Depakote ER	Depakote
Depo-Medrol	Solu-**MEDROL**
Depo-Provera	Depo-subQ provera 104
Depo-subQ provera 104	Depo-Provera
desipramine	disopyramide
Desyrel	**SERO**quel
dexmethylphenidate	methadone
Diabinese	Diamox
Diabeta	Zebeta
Diamox	Diabinese
Diflucan	Diprivan
Dilacor XR	Pilocar
Dilaudid	Dilaudid-5
Dilaudid-5	Dilaudid
dimenhy**DRINATE**	diphenhydr**AMINE**
diphenhydr**AMINE**	dimenhy**DRINATE**
Dioval	Diovan
Diovan	Dioval
Diovan	Zyban
Diovan	Darvon
Diprivan	Diflucan
Diprivan	Ditropan
disopyramide	desipramine
Ditropan	Diprivan
DOBUTamine	**DOP**amine
DOPamine	**DOBUT**amine
Doribax	Zovirax
Doxil	Paxil
DOXOrubicin	**DAUNO**rubicin
DOXOrubicin	**DOXO**rubicin liposomal
DOXOrubicin	**IDA**rubicin
DOXOrubicin liposomal	**DOXO**rubicin
Dulcolax (bisacodyl)	Dulcolax (docusate sodium)
Dulcolax (docusate sodium)	Dulcolax (bisacodyl)
DULoxetine	**FLU**oxetine
Durasal	Durezol
Durezol	Durasal
Duricef	Ultracet
Dynacin	Dynacirc
Dynacirc	Dynacin
edetate calcium disodium	edetate disodium
edetate disodium	edetate calcium disodium
Effexor	Effexor XR
Effexor XR	Enablex

Brand names always start with an uppercase letter. Some brand names incorporate tall man letters in initial characters and may not be readily recognized as brand names. Brand name products appear in black; generic/other products appear in **color**.

DRUG NAME	CONFUSED DRUG NAME
Effexor XR	Effexor
Enablex	Effexor XR
Enbrel	Levbid
Engerix-B adult	Engerix-B pediatric/ adolescent
Engerix-B pediatric/ adolescent	Engerix-B adult
Enjuvia	Januvia
e**PHED**rine	**EPINEPH**rine
EPINEPHrine	e**PHED**rine
epirubicin	eribulin
eribulin	epirubicin
Estratest	Estratest HS
Estratest HS	Estratest
ethambutol	Ethmozine
ethaverine [non-US name]	etravirine
Ethmozine	ethambutol
etravirine	ethaverine [non-US name]
Evista	**AVIN**za
factor IX complex, vapor heated	coagulation factor IX (recombinant)
Fanapt	Xanax
Farxiga	Fetzima
Fastin (phentermine)	Fastin (dietary supplement)
Fastin (dietary supplement)	Fastin (phentermine)
Femara	Femhrt
Femhrt	Femara
fenta**NYL**	**SUF**entanil
Fetzima	Farxiga
Fioricet	Fiorinal
Fiorinal	Fioricet
flavox**ATE**	fluvoxa**MINE**
Flonase	Flovent
Floranex	Florinef
Florastor	Florinef
Florinef	Floranex
Florinef	Florastor
Flovent	Flonase
flumazenil	influenza virus vaccine
FLUoxetine	**PAR**oxetine
FLUoxetine	**DUL**oxetine
FLUoxetine	Loxitane
fluvoxa**MINE**	flavox**ATE**
Focalgin B	Focalin
Focalin	Focalgin B
Folex	Foltx
folic acid	folinic acid (leucovorin calcium)
folinic acid (leucovorin calcium)	folic acid
Foltx	Folex
fomepizole	omeprazole
Foradil	Fortical
Foradil	Toradol
Fortical	Foradil
gentamicin	gentian violet
gentian violet	gentamicin
glacial acetic acid	acetic acid for irrigation
glipi**ZIDE**	gly**BURIDE**
Glucotrol	Glycotrol
gly**BURIDE**	glipi**ZIDE**
Glycotrol	Glucotrol
Granulex	Regranex
guai**FEN**esin	guan**FACINE**

DRUG NAME	CONFUSED DRUG NAME
guan**FACINE**	guai**FEN**esin
HBIG (hepatitis B immune globulin)	BabyBIG
Healon	Hyalgan
heparin	Hespan
Hespan	heparin
HMG-CoA reductase inhibitors ("statins")	nystatin
Huma**LOG**	Humu**LIN**
Huma**LOG**	Novo**LOG**
Huma**LOG** Mix 75/25	Humu**LIN** 70/30
Humapen Memoir (for use with Huma**LOG**)	Humira Pen
Humira Pen	Humapen Memoir (for use with Huma**LOG**)
Humu**LIN**	Novo**LIN**
Humu**LIN**	Huma**LOG**
Humu**LIN** 70/30	Huma**LOG** Mix 75/25
Humu**LIN** R U-100	Humu**LIN** R U-500
Humu**LIN** R U-500	Humu**LIN** R U-100
Hyalgan	Healon
hydr**ALAZINE**	hydr**OXY**zine
Hydrea	Lyrica
HYDROcodone	oxy**CODONE**
Hydrogesic	hydr**OXY**zine
HYDROmorphone	morphine
hydr**OXY**zine	Hydrogesic
hydr**OXY**zine	hydr**ALAZINE**
IDArubicin	**DAUNO**rubicin
IDArubicin	**DOXO**rubicin
Inderal	Adderall
indinavir	Denavir
in**FLIX**imab	ri**TUX**imab
influenza virus vaccine	flumazenil
influenza virus vaccine	perflutren lipid microspheres
influenza virus vaccine	tuberculin purified protein derivative (PPD)
Inspra	Spiriva
Intuniv	Invega
INVanz	**AVIN**za
Invega	Intuniv
iodine	Lodine
Isordil	Plendil
ISOtretinoin	tretinoin
Jantoven	Janumet
Jantoven	Januvia
Janumet	Jantoven
Janumet	Januvia
Janumet	Sinemet
Januvia	Enjuvia
Januvia	Jantoven
Januvia	Janumet
K-Phos Neutral	Neutra-Phos-K
Kaopectate (bismuth subsalicylate)	Kaopectate (docusate calcium)
Kaopectate (docusate calcium)	Kaopectate (bismuth subsalicylate)
Kadian	Kapidex
Kaletra	Keppra
Kapidex	Capadex [non-US product]
Kapidex	Capex

(Continued)

Brand names always start with an uppercase letter. Some brand names incorporate tall man letters in initial characters and may not be readily recognized as brand names. Brand name products appear in black; generic/other products appear in **color**.

DRUG NAME	CONFUSED DRUG NAME
Kapidex	Casodex
Kapidex	Kadian
Keflex	Keppra
Keppra	Kaletra
Keppra	Keflex
Ketalar	ketorolac
ketorolac	Ketalar
ketorolac	methadone
Kineret	Amikin
Klono**PIN**	clo**NID**ine
Kuric	Carac
Kwell	Qwell
La**MIC**tal	Lam**ISIL**
Lam**ISIL**	La**MIC**tal
lami**VUD**ine	lamo**TRI**gine
lamo**TRI**gine	lami**VUD**ine
lamo**TRI**gine	lev**ETIRA**cetam
lamo**TRI**gine	levothyroxine
Lanoxin	levothyroxine
Lanoxin	naloxone
lanthanum carbonate	lithium carbonate
Lantus	Latuda
Lantus	Lente
Lariam	Levaquin
Lasix	Luvox
Latuda	Lantus
Lente	Lantus
Letairis	Letaris [non-US product]
Letaris [non-US product]	Letairis
leucovorin calcium	Leukeran
leucovorin calcium	levoleucovorin
Leukeran	Alkeran
Leukeran	Myleran
Leukeran	leucovorin calcium
Levaquin	Lariam
Levbid	Enbrel
lev**ETIRA**cetam	lamo**TRI**gine
Levemir	Lovenox
lev**ETIRA**cetam	lev**OCARN**itine
lev**ETIRA**cetam	levofloxacin
lev**OCARN**itine	lev**ETIRA**cetam
levofloxacin	lev**ETIRA**cetam
levoleucovorin	leucovorin calcium
levothyroxine	lamo**TRI**gine
levothyroxine	Lanoxin
levothyroxine	liothyronine
Lexapro	Loxitane
Lexiva	Pexeva
liothyronine	levothyroxine
Lipitor	Loniten
Lipitor	Zyr**TEC**
lithium	Ultram
lithium carbonate	lanthanum carbonate
Lodine	codeine
Lodine	iodine
Loniten	Lipitor
Lopressor	Lyrica
LORazepam	**ALPRAZ**olam
LORazepam	clonaze**PAM**
LORazepam	Lovaza
Lotronex	Protonix
Lovaza	**LOR**azepam
Lovenox	Levemir
Loxitane	Lexapro
Loxitane	**FLU**oxetine
Loxitane	Soriatane
Lunesta	Neulasta
Lupron Depot-3 Month	Lupron Depot-Ped
Lupron Depot-Ped	Lupron Depot-3 Month
Luvox	Lasix
Lyrica	Hydrea
Lyrica	Lopressor
Maalox	Maalox Total Stomach Relief
Maalox Total Stomach Relief	Maalox
Matulane	Materna
Materna	Matulane
Maxzide	Microzide
Menactra	Menomune
Menomune	Menactra
Mephyton	methadone
Metadate	methadone
Metadate CD	Metadate ER
Metadate ER	Metadate CD
Metadate ER	methadone
met**FORMIN**	metro**NIDAZOLE**
methadone	dexmethylphenidate
methadone	ketorolac
methadone	Mephyton
methadone	Metadate
methadone	Metadate ER
methadone	methylphenidate
methadone	metolazone
Methergine	Brethine
methimazole	metolazone
methylene blue	VisionBlue
methylphenidate	methadone
metolazone	methadone
metolazone	methimazole
metoprolol succinate	metoprolol tartrate
metoprolol tartrate	metoprolol succinate
metro**NIDAZOLE**	met**FORMIN**
Mevacor	Benicar
Micronase	Microzide
Microzide	Maxzide
Microzide	Micronase
midodrine	Midrin
Midrin	midodrine
mifepristone	misoprostol
Miralax	Mirapex
Mirapex	Miralax
misoprostol	mifepristone
mito**MY**cin	mito**XAN**trone
mito**XAN**trone	mito**MY**cin
morphine	**HYDRO**morphone
morphine - non-concentrated oral liquid	morphine - oral liquid concentrate
morphine - oral liquid concentrate	morphine - non-concentrated oral liquid
Motrin	Neurontin
MS Contin	Oxy**CONTIN**
Mucinex	Mucinex Allergy
Mucinex	Mucomyst
Mucinex Allergy	Mucinex

Brand names always start with an uppercase letter. Some brand names incorporate tall man letters in initial characters and may not be readily recognized as brand names. Brand name products appear in black; generic/other products appear in **color**.

DRUG NAME	CONFUSED DRUG NAME
Mucinex D	Mucinex DM
Mucinex DM	Mucinex D
Mucomyst	Mucinex
Myleran	Alkeran
Myleran	Leukeran
nalbuphine	naloxone
naloxone	Lanoxin
naloxone	nalbuphine
Narcan	Norcuron
Natru-Vent	Atrovent
Navane	Norvasc
Neo-Synephrine (oxymetazoline)	Neo-Synephrine (phenylephrine)
Neo-Synephrine (phenylephrine)	Neo-Synephrine (oxymetazoline)
Neulasta	Lunesta
Neulasta	Neumega
Neulasta	Nuedexta
Neumega	Neupogen
Neumega	Neulasta
Neupogen	Neumega
Neurontin	Motrin
Neurontin	Noroxin
Neutra-Phos-K	K-Phos Neutral
Nex**AVAR**	Nex**IUM**
Nex**IUM**	Nex**AVAR**
ni**CAR**dipine	**NIFE**dipine
NIFEdipine	ni**CAR**dipine
NIFEdipine	ni**MOD**ipine
ni**MOD**ipine	**NIFE**dipine
Norcuron	Narcan
Normodyne	Norpramin
Noroxin	Neurontin
Norpramin	Normodyne
Norvasc	Navane
Novo**LIN**	Humu**LIN**
Novo**LIN**	Novo**LOG**
Novo**LIN** 70/30	Novo**LOG** Mix 70/30
Novo**LOG**	Huma**LOG**
Novo**LOG**	Novo**LIN**
Novo**LOG** Flexpen	Novo**LOG** Mix 70/30 Flexpen
Novo**LOG** Mix 70/30 Flexpen	Novo**LOG** Flexpen
Novo**LOG** Mix 70/30	Novo**LIN** 70/30
Nuedexta	Neulasta
nystatin	HMG-CoA reductase inhibitors ("statins")
Occlusal-HP	Ocuflox
Ocuflox	Occlusal-HP
OLANZapine	**QUE**tiapine
Omacor	Amicar
omeprazole	fomepizole
opium tincture	paregoric (camphorated tincture of opium)
Oracea	Orencia
Orencia	Oracea
Orgaran	argatroban
Ortho Tri-Cyclen	Ortho Tri-Cyclen LO
Ortho Tri-Cyclen LO	Ortho Tri-Cyclen
Os-Cal	Asacol
oxaprozin	**OX**carbazepine
OXcarbazepine	oxaprozin

DRUG NAME	CONFUSED DRUG NAME
OXcarbazepine	car**BAM**azepine
oxy**CODONE**	**HYDRO**codone
oxy**CODONE**	Oxy**CONTIN**
Oxy**CONTIN**	MS Contin
Oxy**CONTIN**	oxy**CODONE**
PACLitaxel	**PACL**itaxel protein-bound particles
PACLitaxel protein-bound particles	**PACL**itaxel
Pamelor	Panlor DC
Pamelor	Tambocor
Panlor DC	Pamelor
paregoric (camphorated tincture of opium)	opium tincture
PARoxetine	**FLU**oxetine
PARoxetine	piroxicam
Patanol	Platinol
Pavulon	Peptavlon
Paxil	Doxil
Paxil	Taxol
Paxil	Plavix
PAZOPanib	**PONAT**inib
PEMEtrexed	**PRALA**trexate
penicillin	penicill**AMINE**
penicill**AMINE**	penicillin
Peptavlon	Pavulon
Percocet	Darvocet
Percocet	Procet
perflutren lipid microspheres	influenza virus vaccine
Pexeva	Lexiva
PENTobarbital	**PHEN**obarbital
PHENobarbital	**PENT**obarbital
Pilocar	Dilacor XR
piroxicam	**PAR**oxetine
Platinol	Patanol
Plavix	Paxil
Plavix	Pradax [Non-US Product]
Plavix	Pradaxa
Plendil	Isordil
pneumococcal 7-valent vaccine	pneumococcal polyvalent vaccine
pneumococcal polyvalent vaccine	pneumococcal 7-valent vaccine
Polycitra	Bicitra
PONATinib	**PAZOP**anib
potassium acetate	sodium acetate
PRALAtrexate	**PEME**trexed
Pradax [Non-US Product]	Plavix
Pradaxa	Plavix
Prandin	Avandia
Precare	Precose
Precose	Precare
predniso**LONE**	predni**SONE**
predni**SONE**	predniso**LONE**
Prenexa	Ranexa
Pri**LOSEC**	Pristiq
Pri**LOSEC**	**PRO**zac
Priscoline	Apresoline
Pristiq	Pri**LOSEC**
probenecid	Procanbid
Procan SR	Procanbid
Procanbid	probenecid

(Continued)

Brand names always start with an uppercase letter. Some brand names incorporate tall man letters in initial characters and may not be readily recognized as brand names. Brand name products appear in black; generic/other products appear in **color**.

DRUG NAME	CONFUSED DRUG NAME
Procanbid	Procan SR
Procardia XL	Protain XL
Procet	Percocet
Prograf	**PRO**zac
propylthiouracil	Purinethol
Proscar	Provera
Protain XL	Procardia XL
protamine	Protonix
proton pump inhibitors	**ARIP**iprazole
Protonix	Lotronex
Protonix	protamine
Provera	Proscar
Provera	**PRO**zac
PROzac	Prograf
PROzac	Pri**LOSEC**
PROzac	Provera
Purinethol	propylthiouracil
Pyridium	pyridoxine
pyridoxine	Pyridium
QUEtiapine	**OLANZ**apine
qui**NID**ine	qui**NINE**
qui**NINE**	qui**NID**ine
Qwell	Kwell
RABEprazole	**ARIP**iprazole
Ranexa	Prenexa
Rapaflo	Rapamune
Rapamune	Rapaflo
Razadyne	Rozerem
Recombivax HB	Comvax
Regranex	Granulex
Reminyl	Robinul
Reminyl	Amaryl
Renagel	Renvela
Renvela	Renagel
Reprexain	Zy**PREXA**
Restoril	Risper**DAL**
Retrovir	ritonavir
Rifadin	Rifater
Rifamate	rifampin
rifampin	Rifamate
rifampin	rifaximin
Rifater	Rifadin
rifaximin	rifampin
Risper**DAL**	Restoril
risperi**DONE**	r**OPINIR**ole
Ritalin	ritodrine
Ritalin LA	Ritalin SR
Ritalin SR	Ritalin LA
ritodrine	Ritalin
ritonavir	Retrovir
ri**TUX**imab	in**FLIX**imab
Robinul	Reminyl
r**OPINIR**ole	risperi**DONE**
Roxanol	Roxicodone Intensol
Roxanol	Roxicet
Roxicet	Roxanol
Roxicodone Intensol	Roxanol
Rozerem	Razadyne
Salagen	selegiline
Sand**IMMUNE**	Sando**STATIN**
Sando**STATIN**	Sand**IMMUNE**
saquinavir	**SINE**quan

DRUG NAME	CONFUSED DRUG NAME
saquinavir (free base)	saquinavir mesylate
saquinavir mesylate	saquinavir (free base)
Sarafem	Serophene
selegiline	Salagen
Serophene	Sarafem
SEROquel	Desyrel
SEROquel	**SERO**quel XR
SEROquel	Serzone
SEROquel	**SINE**quan
SEROquel XR	**SERO**quel
sertraline	cetirizine
sertraline	Soriatane
Serzone	**SERO**quel
silodosin	sirolimus
Sinemet	Janumet
SINEquan	saquinavir
SINEquan	**SERO**quel
SINEquan	Singulair
SINEquan	Zonegran
Singulair	**SINE**quan
sirolimus	silodosin
sita**GLIP**tin	**SUMA**triptan
sodium acetate	potassium acetate
Solu-**CORTEF**	Solu-**MEDROL**
Solu-**MEDROL**	Depo-Medrol
Solu-**MEDROL**	Solu-**CORTEF**
Sonata	Soriatane
Soriatane	Loxitane
Soriatane	sertraline
Soriatane	Sonata
sotalol	Sudafed
Spiriva	Apidra
Spiriva	Inspra
stavudine	cetirizine
Sudafed	sotalol
Sudafed	Sudafed PE
Sudafed 12 Hour	Sudafed 12 Hour Pressure + Pain
Sudafed 12 Hour Pressure + Pain	Sudafed 12 Hour
Sudafed PE	Sudafed
SUFentanil	fenta**NYL**
sulf**ADIAZINE**	sulfa**SALA**zine
sulf**ADIAZINE**	sulfi**SOXAZOLE**
sulfa**SALA**zine	sulf**ADIAZINE**
sulfi**SOXAZOLE**	sulf**ADIAZINE**
SUMAtriptan	sita**GLIP**tin
SUMAtriptan	**ZOLM**itriptan
Symbyax	Cymbalta
T-Gel	Bio-T-Gel
Tambocor	Pamelor
Taxol	Taxotere
Taxol	Paxil
Taxotere	Taxol
TEGretol	**TEG**retol XR
TEGretol	Tequin
TEGretol	**TREN**tal
TEGretol XR	**TEG**retol
Tenex	Xanax
Tequin	**TEG**retol
Tequin	Ticlid
Testoderm	Testoderm with Adhesive

Brand names always start with an uppercase letter. Some brand names incorporate tall man letters in initial characters and may not be readily recognized as brand names. Brand name products appear in black; generic/other products appear in **color**.

DRUG NAME	CONFUSED DRUG NAME
Testoderm	Testoderm TTS
Testoderm with Adhesive	Testoderm
Testoderm with Adhesive	Testoderm TTS
Testoderm TTS	Testoderm
Testoderm TTS	Testoderm with Adhesive
tetanus diphtheria toxoid (Td)	tuberculin purified protein derivative (PPD)
Thalomid	Thiamine
Thiamine	Thalomid
tia**GAB**ine	ti**ZAN**idine
Tiazac	Ziac
Ticlid	Tequin
ti**ZAN**idine	tia**GAB**ine
TNKase	Activase
TNKase	t-PA
Tobradex	Tobrex
Tobrex	Tobradex
TOLAZamide	**TOLBUT**amide
TOLBUTamide	**TOLAZ**amide
Topamax	Toprol-XL
Toprol-XL	Topamax
Toradol	Foradil
t-PA	TNKase
Tracleer	Tricor
tra**MAD**ol	tra**ZOD**one
trastuzumab	ado-trastuzumab emtansine
tra**ZOD**one	tra**MAD**ol
TRENtal	**TEG**retol
tretinoin	**ISO**tretinoin
Tricor	Tracleer
tromethamine	Trophamine
Trophamine	tromethamine
tuberculin purified protein derivative (PPD)	influenza virus vaccine
tuberculin purified protein derivative (PPD)	tetanus diphtheria toxoid (Td)
Tylenol	Tylenol PM
Tylenol PM	Tylenol
Ultracet	Duricef
Ultram	lithium
val**ACY**clovir	val**GAN**ciclovir
Valcyte	Valtrex
val**GAN**ciclovir	val**ACY**clovir
Valtrex	Valcyte
Varivax	VZIG (varicella-zoster immune globulin)
Vesanoid	Vesicare
Vesicare	Vesanoid
Vexol	Vosol
Viagra	Allegra
Videx	Bidex
vin**BLAS**tine	vin**CRIS**tine
vin**CRIS**tine	vin**BLAS**tine
Viokase	Viokase 8
Viokase 8	Viokase
Vioxx	Zyvox
Viracept	Viramune
Viramune	Viracept
Viramune (nevirapine)	Viramune (herbal product)
Viramune (herbal product)	Viramune (nevirapine)
VisionBlue	methylene blue
Vosol	Vexol

DRUG NAME	CONFUSED DRUG NAME
VZIG (varicella-zoster immune globulin)	Varivax
Wellbutrin SR	Wellbutrin XL
Wellbutrin XL	Wellbutrin SR
Xanax	Fanapt
Xanax	Tenex
Xanax	Zantac
Xeloda	Xenical
Xenical	Xeloda
Yasmin	Yaz
Yaz	Yasmin
Zantac	Xanax
Zantac	Zyr**TEC**
Zavesca (escitalopram) [non-US product]	Zavesca (miglustat)
Zavesca (miglustat)	Zavesca (escitalopram) [non-US product]
Zebeta	Diabeta
Zebeta	Zetia
Zegerid	Zestril
Zelapar (Zydis formulation)	Zy**PREXA** Zydis
Zerit	Zyr**TEC**
Zestril	Zegerid
Zestril	Zetia
Zestril	Zy**PREXA**
Zetia	Bextra
Zetia	Zebeta
Zetia	Zestril
Ziac	Tiazac
Zocor	Cozaar
Zocor	Zyr**TEC**
ZOLMitriptan	**SUMA**triptan
zolpidem	Zyloprim
Zonegran	**SINE**quan
Zostrix	Zovirax
Zovirax	Doribax
Zovirax	Zyvox
Zovirax	Zostrix
Zyban	Diovan
Zyloprim	zolpidem
Zy**PREXA**	Cele**XA**
Zy**PREXA**	Reprexain
Zy**PREXA**	Zestril
Zy**PREXA**	Zyr**TEC**
Zy**PREXA** Zydis	Zelapar (Zydis formulation)
Zyr**TEC**	Lipitor
Zyr**TEC**	Zantac
Zyr**TEC**	Zerit
Zyr**TEC**	Zocor
Zyr**TEC**	Zy**PREXA**
Zyr**TEC**	Zyr**TEC**-D
Zyr**TEC** (cetirizine)	Zyr**TEC** Itchy Eye Drops (ketotifen fumarate)
Zyr**TEC**-D	Zyr**TEC**
Zyr**TEC** Itchy Eye Drops (ketotifen fumarate)	Zyr**TEC** (cetirizine)
Zyvox	Vioxx
Zyvox	Zovirax

Brand names always start with an uppercase letter. Some brand names incorporate tall man letters in initial characters and may not be readily recognized as brand names. Brand name products appear in black; generic/other products appear in **color**.

PHARMACOGENOMICS: BIOMARKERS, PATIENT SUBGROUPS, & EFFECTS

GENERIC(S)	BRAND(S)	THERAPEUTIC CATEGORY	BIOMARKER	PATIENT SUBGROUP	EFFECT
Abacavir	Ziagen	Anti-Infectives	HLA-B	HLA-B*5701 allele carriers	Risk for hypersensitivity reaction
Ado-trastuzumab emtansine	Kadcyla	Oncology	ERBB2	HER2 protein overexpression or gene amplification positive	May achieve therapeutic benefit
Afatinib	Gilotrif	Oncology	EGFR	EGFR exon 19 deletion or exon 21 substitution (L858R) positive	May achieve therapeutic benefit
Amitriptyline hydrochloride	Elavil	Psychiatry	CYP2D6	CYP2D6 poor metabolizers	Higher drug plasma concentration
Anastrozole	Arimidex	Oncology	ESR1, PGR	Hormone receptor positive	May achieve therapeutic benefit
Aripiprazole	Abilify	Psychiatry	CYP2D6	CYP2D6 poor metabolizers	Higher drug plasma concentration
Arsenic trioxide	Trisenox	Oncology	PML-RARA	PML-RARα translocation positive	May achieve therapeutic benefit
Ascorbic acid, PEG-3350, Potassium chloride, Sodium ascorbate, Sodium chloride, and Sodium sulfate	MoviPrep	Gastrointestinal Agents	G6PD	G6PD deficient	May precipitate hemolytic reactions
Atomoxetine	Strattera	Psychiatry	CYP2D6	CYP2D6 poor metabolizers	Higher drug plasma concentration
Azathioprine	Azasan, Imuran	Musculoskeletal System/ Immunology	TPMT	TPMT intermediate or poor metabolizers	Increased risk of myelotoxicity
Boceprevir	Victrelis	Anti-Infectives	IFNL3	IL28B rs12979860 T allele carriers (C/T and T/T genotype)	Less likely to achieve therapeutic benefit
Bosutinib	Bosulif	Oncology	BCR/ABL1	Philadelphia chromosome positive	May achieve therapeutic benefit
Brentuximab vedotin	Adcetris	Oncology	TNFRSF8	CD30 antigen positive	May achieve therapeutic benefit
Busulfan	Myleran	Oncology	BCR/ABL1	Philadelphia chromosome negative	Less likely to achieve therapeutic benefit
Capecitabine	Xeloda	Oncology	DPYD	DPD deficient	Higher risk for severe or fatal adverse reactions

(Continued)

GENERIC(S)	BRAND(S)	THERAPEUTIC CATEGORY	BIOMARKER	PATIENT SUBGROUP	EFFECT
Carbamazepine (1)	Carbatrol, Epitol, Equetro, Tegretol	Analgesics, Neurology	HLA-B	HLA-B*1502 allele carriers	Risk for serious dermatologic reactions
Carbamazepine (2)	Carbatrol, Epitol, Equetro, Tegretol	Analgesics, Neurology	HLA-A	HLA-A*3101 allele carriers	Risk for hypersensitivity reaction
Carglumic acid	Carbaglu	Metabolic	NAGS	N-acetylglutamate synthase deficient	May achieve therapeutic benefit
Carisoprodol	Soma	Musculoskeletal System	CYP2C19	CYP2C19 poor metabolizers	Higher drug plasma concentration
Carvedilol	Coreg	Cardiovascular Agents	CYP2D6	CYP2D6 poor metabolizers	Higher drug plasma concentration
Celecoxib	Celebrex	Analgesics, Musculoskeletal System	CYP2C9	CYP2C9 poor metabolizers	Higher drug plasma concentration
Ceritinib	Zykadia	Oncology	ALK	ALK gene rearrangement positive	May achieve therapeutic benefit
Cetuximab (1)	Erbitux	Oncology	EGFR	EGFR protein expression positive	May achieve therapeutic benefit
Cetuximab (2)	Erbitux	Oncology	KRAS	KRAS codon 12 and 13 mutation negative	May achieve therapeutic benefit
Cevimeline	Evoxac	Dental/Periodontal Agents	CYP2D6	CYP2D6 poor metabolizers	Higher risk for adverse reactions
Chloroquine phosphate	Aralen	Anti-Infectives	G6PD	G6PD deficient	Acute hemolysis can occur
Chlorpropamide		Endocrine	G6PD	G6PD deficient	Risk of hemolytic anemia
Cisplatin		Oncology	TPMT	TPMT*3B and TPMT*3C	Increased risk of ototoxicity in children
Citalopram hydrobromide	Celexa	Psychiatry	CYP2C19	CYP2C19 poor metabolizers	Higher drug plasma concentration; risk of QT prolongation
Clobazam	Onfi	Neurology	CYP2C19	CYP2C19 poor metabolizers	Higher drug plasma concentration
Clomipramine	Anafranil	Psychiatry	CYP2D6	CYP2D6 poor metabolizers	Higher drug plasma concentration
Clopidogrel bisulfate	Plavix	Cardiovascular Agents	CYP2C19	CYP2C19 intermediate or poor metabolizers	Diminished antiplatelet response
Clozapine	Clozaril, FazaClo, Versacloz	Psychiatry	CYP2D6	CYP2D6 poor metabolizers	Higher drug plasma concentrations
Codeine		Analgesics	CYP2D6	CYP2D6 ultra-rapid metabolizers	More rapid and complete conversion to morphine; may lead to life-threatening or fatal respiratory depression
Crizotinib	Xalkori	Oncology	ALK	ALK gene rearrangement positive	May achieve therapeutic benefit
Dabrafenib (1)	Tafinlar	Oncology	BRAF	BRAF V600E/K mutation positive	May achieve therapeutic benefit
Dabrafenib (2)	Tafinlar	Oncology	G6PD	G6PD deficient	Risk of hemolytic anemia

GENERIC(S)	BRAND(S)	THERAPEUTIC CATEGORY	BIOMARKER	PATIENT SUBGROUP	EFFECT
Dapsone		Anti-Infectives	G6PD	G6PD deficient	Acute hemolysis can occur
Dasatinib (1)	Sprycel	Oncology	BCR/ABL1	Philadelphia chromosome positive	May achieve therapeutic benefit
Dasatinib (2)	Sprycel	Oncology	BCR/ABL1	T315I mutation-positive	Less likely to achieve therapeutic benefit
Denileukin diftitox	Ontak	Oncology	IL2RA	CD25 antigen positive	May achieve therapeutic benefit
Desipramine hydrochloride	Norpramin	Psychiatry	CYP2D6	CYP2D6 poor metabolizers	Higher drug plasma concentration
Dexlansoprazole	Dexilant	Gastrointestinal Agents	CYP2C19	CYP2C19 intermediate or poor metabolizers	Higher systemic exposure
Dextromethorphan hydrobromide and Quinidine sulfate	Nuedexta	Neurology/Psychiatry	CYP2D6	CYP2D6 poor metabolizers	The quinidine component is less likely to achieve therapeutic benefit
Diazepam	Diastat, Valium	Musculoskeletal System, Neurology/Psychiatry	CYP2C19	CYP2C19 poor metabolizers	Higher drug plasma concentrations
Divalproex sodium	Depakote	Analgesics, Neurology/Psychiatry	POLG	POLG mutation positive	Increased risk of acute liver failure
Doxepin (1)	Silenor, Zonalon	Dermatology, Neurology/Psychiatry	CYP2D6	CYP2D6 poor metabolizers	Higher drug plasma concentration
Doxepin (2)	Silenor	Neurology/Psychiatry	CYP2C19	CYP2C19 poor metabolizers	Higher drug plasma concentration
Eliglustat	Cerdelga	Metabolic	CYP2D6	CYP2D6 extensive, intermediate, or poor metabolizers	May achieve therapeutic benefit
Eltrombopag (1)	Promacta	Hematology	F5	Factor V Leiden carriers	Increased risk of thromboembolism
Eltrombopag (2)	Promacta	Hematology	SERPINC1	Antithrombin III deficient	Increased risk of thromboembolism
Erlotinib	Tarceva	Oncology	EGFR	EGFR exon 19 deletion or exon 21 substitution (L858R) positive	May achieve therapeutic benefit
Esomeprazole	Nexium	Gastrointestinal Agents	CYP2C19	CYP2C19 poor metabolizers	Higher drug plasma concentration
Everolimus (1)	Afinitor	Oncology	ERBB2	HER2 protein overexpression negative	May achieve therapeutic benefit
Everolimus (2)	Afinitor	Oncology	ESR1	Estrogen receptor positive	May achieve therapeutic benefit
Exemestane	Aromasin	Oncology	ESR1	Estrogen receptor positive	May achieve therapeutic benefit
Fesoterodine fumarate	Toviaz	Urology	CYP2D6	CYP2D6 poor metabolizers	Higher drug plasma concentration

(Continued)

GENERIC(S)	BRAND(S)	THERAPEUTIC CATEGORY	BIOMARKER	PATIENT SUBGROUP	EFFECT
Fluorouracil	Carac, Efudex, Tolak	Dermatology, Oncology	DPYD	DPD deficient	Increased risk of toxicity
Fluoxetine	Prozac	Psychiatry	CYP2D6	CYP2D6 poor metabolizers	Higher drug plasma concentration (QT prolongation)
Flurbiprofen		Analgesics	CYP2C9	CYP2C9 poor metabolizers	Higher drug plasma concentration
Fluvoxamine maleate	Luvox CR	Psychiatry	CYP2D6	CYP2D6 poor metabolizers	Higher drug plasma concentration
Fulvestrant	Faslodex	Oncology	ESR1, PGR	Hormone receptor positive	May achieve therapeutic benefit
Galantamine hydrobromide	Razadyne	Neurology	CYP2D6	CYP2D6 poor metabolizers	Higher drug plasma concentration
Gefitinib (1)	Iressa	Oncology	EGFR	(EGFR) exon 19 deletions or exon 21 (L858R) substitution mutations	May achieve therapeutic benefit
Gefitinib (2)	Iressa	Oncology	CYP2D6	CYP2D6 poor metabolizers	Increased exposure and risk of adverse effects
Glimepiride	Amaryl	Endocrine	G6PD	G6PD deficient	Hemolytic anemia can occur
Glipizide	Glucotrol	Endocrine	G6PD	G6PD deficient	Hemolytic anemia can occur
Glyburide	DiaBeta, Glynase	Endocrine	G6PD	G6PD deficient	Hemolytic anemia can occur
Hydralazine hydrochloride and Isosorbide dinitrate	BiDil	Cardiovascular Agents	NAT1-2	Slow acetylators	Higher bioavailability
Ibritumomab tiuxetan	Zevalin	Oncology	MS4A1	CD20 antigen positive	May achieve therapeutic benefit
Ibrutinib	Imbruvica	Oncology	del (17p)	Chromosome 17p deletion positive	May achieve therapeutic benefit
Iloperidone	Fanapt	Psychiatry	CYP2D6	CYP2D6 poor metabolizers	Higher drug plasma concentration
Imatinib mesylate (1)	Gleevec	Oncology	KIT	KIT (CD117) protein expression positive, c-KIT D816V mutation negative	May achieve therapeutic benefit
Imatinib mesylate (2)	Gleevec	Oncology	BCR/ABL1	Philadelphia chromosome positive	May achieve therapeutic benefit
Imatinib mesylate (3)	Gleevec	Oncology	PDGFRB	PDGFR gene rearrangement positive	May achieve therapeutic benefit
Imatinib mesylate (4)	Gleevec	Oncology	FIP1L1-PDGFRA	FIP1L1-PDGFRα fusion kinase (or CHIC2 deletion) positive	May achieve therapeutic benefit
Imipramine hydrochloride	Tofranil	Psychiatry	CYP2D6	CYP2D6 poor metabolizers	Higher drug plasma concentration
Irinotecan	Camptosar	Oncology	UGT1A1	Homozygous UGT1A1*28 allele carriers	Increased risk for neutropenia
Isoniazid, Pyrazinamide, and Rifampin	Rifater	Anti-Infectives	NAT1-2	Slow acetylators (inactivators)	Higher drug (isoniazid) plasma concentration

GENERIC(S)	BRAND(S)	THERAPEUTIC CATEGORY	BIOMARKER	PATIENT SUBGROUP	EFFECT
Ivacaftor	Kalydeco	Pulmonary/Respiratory Agents	CFTR	CFTR G551D, G1244E, G1349D, G178R, G551S, S1251N, S1255P, S549N, S549R, or R117H mutation carriers, F508del mutation homozygotes	May achieve therapeutic benefit; not effective for F508del mutation homozygotes
Lansoprazole	Prevacid	Gastrointestinal Agents	CYP2C19	CYP2C19 intermediate or poor metabolizers	Concomitant administration w/ tacrolimus may increase whole blood levels of tacrolimus
Lapatinib (1)	Tykerb	Oncology	ERBB2	HER2 protein overexpression positive	May achieve therapeutic benefit
Lapatinib (2)	Tykerb	Oncology	HLA-DQA1, HLA-DRB1	HLA-DQA1*0201 or -DRB1*0701 allele carriers	Increased risk of hepatotoxicity
Lenalidomide	Revlimid	Hematology	del (5q)	Chromosome 5q deletion positive	May achieve therapeutic benefit
Letrozole	Femara	Oncology	ESR1, PGR	Hormone receptor positive	May achieve therapeutic benefit
Lomitapide	Juxtapid	Endocrine	LDLR	LDLR mutation homozygotes (homozygous familial hypercholesterolemia)	May achieve therapeutic benefit
Mafenide acetate	Sulfamylon	Dermatology	G6PD	G6PD deficient	Hemolytic anemia can occur
Maraviroc	Selzentry	Anti-Infectives	CCR5	CCR5-tropic HIV-1 positive	May achieve therapeutic benefit
Mercaptopurine	Purinethol, Purixan	Oncology	TPMT	TPMT intermediate or poor metabolizers (or TPMT deficiency)	Increased risk for myelosuppression and toxicity
Methylene blue		Hematology	G6PD	G6PD deficient	Paradoxical methemoglobinemia and hemolysis risk
Metoclopramide hydrochloride	Metozolv ODT, Reglan	Gastrointestinal Agents	CYB5R1-4	NADH cytochrome b5 reductase deficient	Increased risk of methemoglobinemia and/or sulfhemoglobinemia
Metoprolol	Lopressor, Toprol XL	Cardiovascular Agents	CYP2D6	CYP2D6 poor metabolizers	Higher drug plasma concentration
Mipomersen sodium (1)	Kynamro	Endocrine	LDLR	LDLR mutation homozygotes (homozygous familial hypercholesterolemia)	May achieve therapeutic benefit
Mipomersen sodium (2)	Kynamro	Endocrine	LDLR	LDLR mutation heterozygotes (heterozygous familial hypercholesterolemia)	Increased risk of hepatic steatosis

(Continued)

GENERIC(S)	BRAND(S)	THERAPEUTIC CATEGORY	BIOMARKER	PATIENT SUBGROUP	EFFECT
Modafinil	Provigil	Psychiatry	CYP2D6	CYP2D6 poor metabolizers	Levels of CYP2D6 substrates, which have ancillary routes of elimination through CYP2C19 (ie, TCAs and SSRIs), may be increased
Mycophenolic acid	Myfortic	Immunology	HPRT1	HGPRT deficient	May exacerbate disease symptoms (ie, Lesch-Nyhan and Kelley-Seegmiller syndromes)
Nilotinib (1)	Tasigna	Oncology	BCR/ABL	Philadelphia chromosome positive	May achieve therapeutic benefit
Nilotinib (2)	Tasigna	Oncology	UGT1A1	UGT1A1*28 allele homozygotes	Increased risk of hyperbilirubinemia
Nitrofurantoin	Furadantin, Macrobid, Macrodantin	Anti-Infectives	G6PD	G6PD deficient	Hemolytic anemia can occur
Nortriptyline hydrochloride	Pamelor	Psychiatry	CYP2D6	CYP2D6 poor metabolizers	Higher drug plasma concentration
Obinutuzumab	Gazyva	Oncology	MS4A1	CD20 antigen positive	May achieve therapeutic benefit
Ofatumumab	Arzerra	Oncology	MS4A1	CD20 antigen positive	May achieve therapeutic benefit
Omacetaxine mepesuccinate	Synribo	Oncology	BCR/ABL1	Philadelphia chromosome positive	May achieve therapeutic benefit
Omeprazole	Prilosec	Gastrointestinal Agents	CYP2C19	CYP2C19 poor metabolizers	Lower systemic exposure w/ certain drugs
Panitumumab (1)	Vectibix	Oncology	EGFR	EGFR protein expression positive	May achieve therapeutic benefit
Panitumumab (2)	Vectibix	Oncology	KRAS	KRAS codon 12 and 13 mutation negative	May achieve therapeutic benefit
Paroxetine	Brisdelle, Paxil, Pexeva	Psychiatry	CYP2D6	CYP2D6 extensive metabolizers	Atomoxetine levels increased; may need to reduce atomoxetine dose
Pazopanib	Votrient	Oncology	UGT1A1	UGT1A1*28 allele homozygotes (TA)7/(TA)7 genotype	Increased risk of hyperbilirubinemia
Peginterferon alfa-2b	PegIntron	Anti-Infectives	IFNL3	IL28B rs12979860 T allele carriers (C/T and T/T genotype)	Less likely to achieve therapeutic benefit
Pegloticase	Krystexxa	Metabolic	G6PD	G6PD deficient	Contraindicated; increased risk of hemolytic anemia and methemoglobinemia
Perphenazine		Psychiatry	CYP2D6	CYP2D6 poor metabolizers	Higher drug plasma concentration
Pertuzumab	Perjeta	Oncology	ERBB2	HER2 protein overexpression positive	May achieve therapeutic benefit
Phenytoin	Dilantin, Phenytek	Neurology	HLA-B	HLA-B*1502 allele carriers	May increase risk of SJS/TEN in Asian patients
Pimozide	Orap	Psychiatry	CYP2D6	CYP2D6 poor metabolizers	Higher drug plasma concentration

GENERIC(S)	BRAND(S)	THERAPEUTIC CATEGORY	BIOMARKER	PATIENT SUBGROUP	EFFECT
Ponatinib	Iclusig	Oncology	BCR/ABL1	Philadelphia chromosome positive; T315I mutation positive	May achieve therapeutic benefit
Pravastatin sodium (1)	Pravachol	Endocrine	LDLR	LDLR mutation heterozygotes (heterozygous familial hypercholesterolemia)	May achieve therapeutic benefit
Pravastatin sodium (2)	Pravachol	Endocrine	LDLR	LDLR mutation homozygotes (homozygous familial hypercholesterolemia)	May not achieve therapeutic benefit
Primaquine phosphate		Anti-Infectives	G6PD	G6PD deficient	Hemolytic reactions may occur
Probenecid		Uricosuric	G6PD	G6PD deficient	Hemolytic anemia may occur
Propafenone hydrochloride	Rythmol	Antiarrhythmics/ Cardiovascular Agents	CYP2D6	CYP2D6 poor metabolizers	May increase risk of proarrhythmia and other adverse events w/ a CYP3A4 inhibitor
Propranolol hydrochloride	Hemangeol, Inderal LA, InnoPran XL	Cardiovascular Agents	CYP2D6	CYP2D6 poor metabolizers	Higher drug plasma concentration, no difference w/ clearance or elimination half-life
Protriptyline hydrochloride	Vivactil	Psychiatry	CYP2D6	CYP2D6 poor metabolizers	Higher drug plasma concentration
Quinine sulfate	Qualaquin	Anti-Infectives	G6PD	G6PD deficient	Contraindicated; hemolysis can occur
Rabeprazole sodium	AcipHex	Gastrointestinal Agents	CYP2C19	CYP2C19 poor metabolizers	Higher drug plasma concentration
Rasburicase (1)	Elitek	Oncology	G6PD	G6PD deficient	Contraindicated; hemolysis can occur
Rasburicase (2)	Elitek	Oncology	CYB5R1-4	NADH cytochrome b5 reductase deficient	May be at increased risk for methemoglobinemia or hemolytic anemia
Rituximab	Rituxan	Oncology	MS4A1	CD20 antigen positive	May achieve therapeutic benefit
Silver sulfadiazine	Silvadene	Dermatology	G6PD	G6PD deficient	Hemolysis can occur
Simeprevir	Olysio	Anti-Infectives	IFNL3	IL28B rs12979860 T allele carriers	Less likely to achieve therapeutic benefit
Sodium benzoate and Sodium phenylacetate	Ammonul	Metabolic/Urea Cycle Disorder Agents	NAGS, CPS1, ASS1, OTC, ASL, ABL2	Urea cycle enzyme deficient	May achieve therapeutic benefit
Sodium nitrite		Toxicology	G6PD	G6PD deficient	Increased risk of a hemolytic crisis
Sofosbuvir	Sovaldi	Anti-Infectives	IFNL3	IL28B rs12979860 T allele carriers (non-C/C genotype)	Less likely to achieve therapeutic benefit

(Continued)

GENERIC(S)	BRAND(S)	THERAPEUTIC CATEGORY	BIOMARKER	PATIENT SUBGROUP	EFFECT
Succinylcholine chloride	Anectine, Quelicin	Musculoskeletal System	BCHE	Heterozygous or homozygous for atypical plasma cholinesterase gene	Diminished cholinesterase activity
Sulfamethoxazole and Trimethoprim	Bactrim, Sulfatrim	Anti-Infectives	G6PD	G6PD deficient	Hemolysis can occur
Sulfasalazine	Azulfidine	Gastrointestinal Agents	G6PD	G6PD deficient	Hemolytic anemia can occur
Tamoxifen citrate	Soltamox	Oncology	ESR1, PGR	Hormone receptor positive	May achieve therapeutic benefit
Telaprevir	Incivek	Anti-Infectives	IFNL3	IL28B rs12979860 T allele carriers (C/T and T/T genotype)	Less likely to achieve therapeutic benefit
Terbinafine hydrochloride	Lamisil	Anti-Infectives/Anti-Fungals	CYP2D6	CYP2D6 poor metabolizers	Drug interactions
Tetrabenazine	Xenazine	Neurology	CYP2D6	CYP2D6 poor metabolizers	Higher drug plasma concentration/dose reduction
Thioguanine	Tabloid	Oncology	TPMT	TPMT intermediate or poor metabolizers/ TPMT deficiency	Increased risk for myelosuppressive effects and rapid bone marrow suppression
Thioridazine hydrochloride	Mellaril	Psychiatry	CYP2D6	CYP2D6 poor metabolizers	Contraindicated; increased risk for QT prolongation
Tolterodine tartrate	Detrol	Urology	CYP2D6	CYP2D6 poor metabolizers	Higher drug plasma concentration; increased QT interval
Tramadol hydrochloride	ConZip, Ryzolt, Ultram	Analgesics	CYP2D6	CYP2D6 poor metabolizers	Higher drug plasma concentration
Trametinib	Mekinist	Oncology	BRAF	BRAF V600E/K mutation positive	May achieve therapeutic benefit
Trastuzumab	Herceptin	Oncology	ERBB2	HER2 protein overexpression positive	May achieve therapeutic benefit
Tretinoin capsules		Oncology	PML/RARA	PML/RARα translocation positive	May achieve therapeutic benefit
Trimipramine maleate	Surmontil	Psychiatry	CYP2D6	CYP2D6 poor metabolizers	Higher drug plasma concentration
Valproic acid (1)	Depakene, Stavzor	Neurology	POLG	POLG mutation positive	Contraindicated; risk of acute liver failure and death
Valproic acid (2)	Depakene, Stavzor	Neurology	NAGS, CPS1, ASS1, OTC, ASL, ABL2	Urea cycle enzyme deficient	Contraindicated; risk of hyperammonemic encephalopathy
Vemurafenib	Zelboraf	Oncology	BRAF	BRAF V600E mutation positive	May achieve therapeutic benefit
Venlafaxine	Effexor XR	Psychiatry	CYP2D6	CYP2D6 poor metabolizers	High drug plasma concentration
Voriconazole	Vfend	Anti-Infectives	CYP2C19	CYP2C19 poor metabolizers	High drug plasma concentration

GENERIC(S)	BRAND(S)	THERAPEUTIC CATEGORY	BIOMARKER	PATIENT SUBGROUP	EFFECT
Vortioxetine	Brintellix	Neurology	CYP2D6	CYP2D6 poor metabolizers	High drug plasma concentration; max dose of 10mg/day
Warfarin sodium (1)	Coumadin, Jantoven	Cardiovascular Agents	CYP2C9	CYP2C9 intermediate or poor metabolizers	High drug plasma concentration; variable warfarin dose requirements
Warfarin sodium (2)	Coumadin, Jantoven	Cardiovascular Agents	VKORC1	VKORC1 A allele carriers	High drug plasma concentration; variable warfarin dose requirements
Warfarin sodium (3)	Coumadin, Jantoven	Cardiovascular Agents	PROS	Protein S deficient	Association w/ tissue necrosis
Warfarin sodium (4)	Coumadin, Jantoven	Cardiovascular Agents	PROC	Protein C deficient	Association w/ tissue necrosis

BRAND/GENERIC INDEX

This index includes the brand and generic names of each drug in the Concise Drug Monographs section. The main monograph names are fully capitalized (eg, ABILIFY) and generic names begin with initial caps (eg, Abacavir sulfate). Any brand name associated with an entry is listed under the product.

A

B

C

F

G

H

I

J

K

L

P

Q

R

S

T

U

V

THERAPEUTIC CLASS INDEX

Organized alphabetically, this index includes the therapeutic class of each drug in the Concise Drug Monographs section. Therapeutic class headings are based on information provided in the drug monographs. The drug entries listed under each bold therapeutic class are organized alphabetically by brand name or monograph title (shown in capitalized letters), followed by the generic name in parentheses.

C

F

G

H

I

O

P

W

X

VISUAL IDENTIFICATION GUIDE*

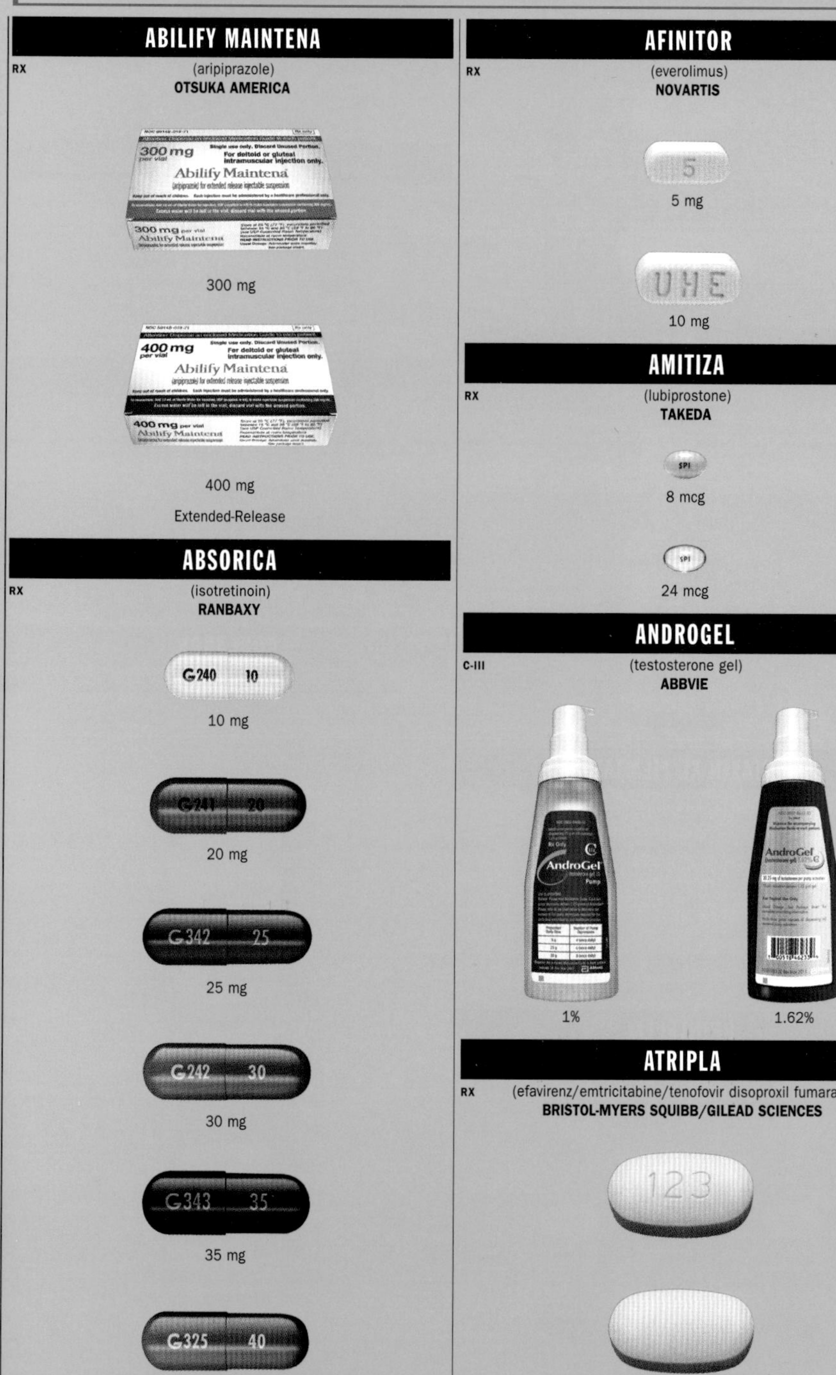

ABILIFY MAINTENA

RX

(aripiprazole)

OTSUKA AMERICA

300 mg

400 mg

Extended-Release

ABSORICA

RX

(isotretinoin)

RANBAXY

10 mg

20 mg

25 mg

30 mg

35 mg

40 mg

AFINITOR

RX

(everolimus)

NOVARTIS

5 mg

10 mg

AMITIZA

RX

(lubiprostone)

TAKEDA

8 mcg

24 mcg

ANDROGEL

C-III

(testosterone gel)

ABBVIE

1%

1.62%

ATRIPLA

RX

(efavirenz/emtricitabine/tenofovir disoproxil fumarate)

BRISTOL-MYERS SQUIBB/GILEAD SCIENCES

600 mg/200 mg/300 mg

*Other dosage forms and strengths may be available and this list is not inclusive of all drugs in this book.

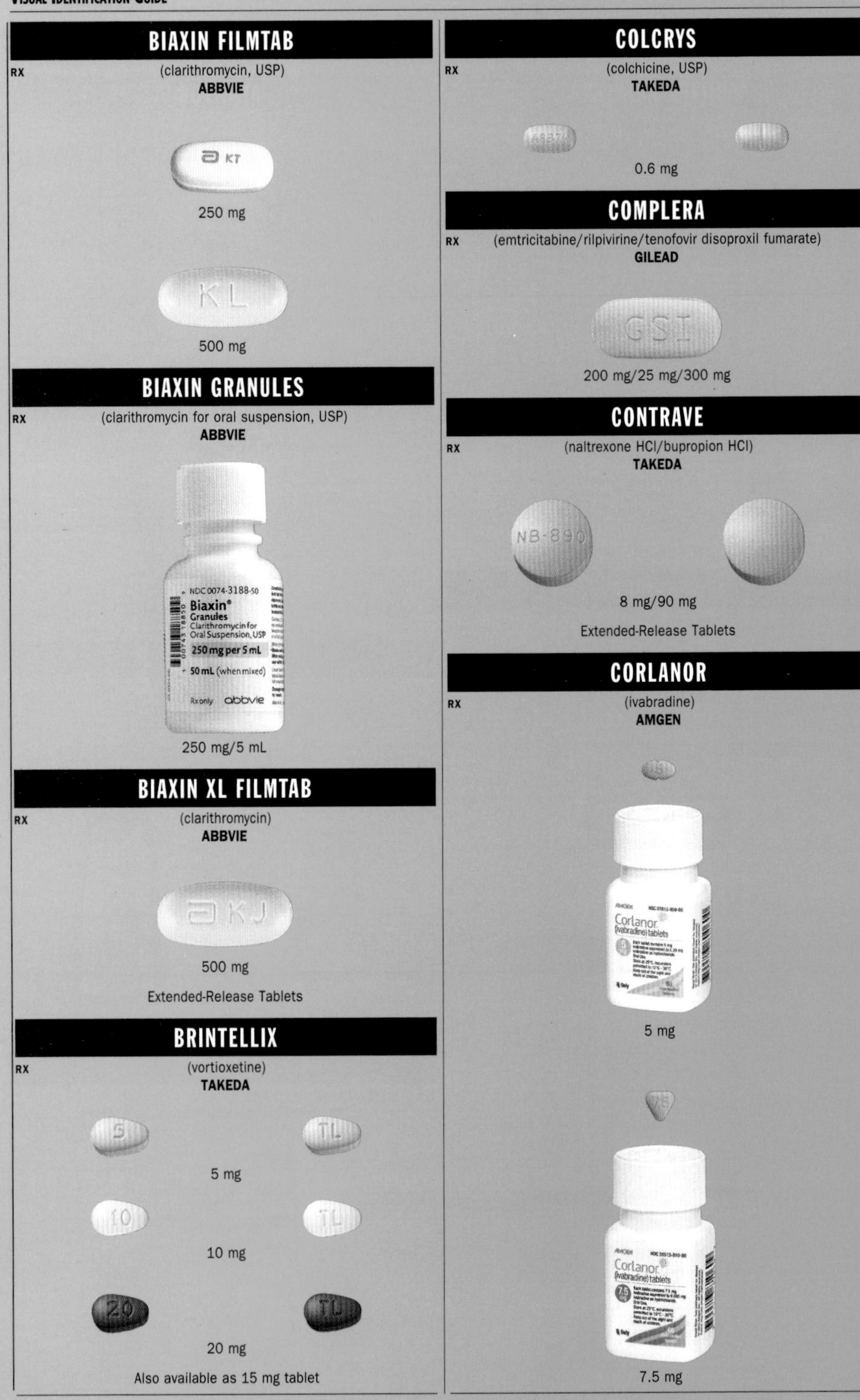
BIAXIN FILMTAB
RX
(clarithromycin, USP)
ABBVIE
KT
250 mg
KL
500 mg
BIAXIN GRANULES
RX
(clarithromycin for oral suspension, USP)
ABBVIE
NDC 0074-3188-50
Biaxin®
Granules
Clarithromycin for
Oral Suspension, USP
250 mg per 5 mL
50 mL (when mixed)
Rx only
abbvie
250 mg/5 mL
BIAXIN XL FILMTAB
RX
(clarithromycin)
ABBVIE
KJ
500 mg
Extended-Release Tablets
BRINTELLIX
RX
(vortioxetine)
TAKEDA
5
TL
5 mg
10
TL
10 mg
20
TL
20 mg
Also available as 15 mg tablet
COLCRYS
RX
(colchicine, USP)
TAKEDA
0.6 mg
COMPLERA
RX
(emtricitabine/rilpivirine/tenofovir disoproxil fumarate)
GILEAD
GSI
200 mg/25 mg/300 mg
CONTRAVE
RX
(naltrexone HCl/bupropion HCl)
TAKEDA
NB-890
8 mg/90 mg
Extended-Release Tablets
CORLANOR
RX
(ivabradine)
AMGEN
Corlanor
(ivabradine) tablets
5 mg
Corlanor
(ivabradine) tablets
7.5 mg

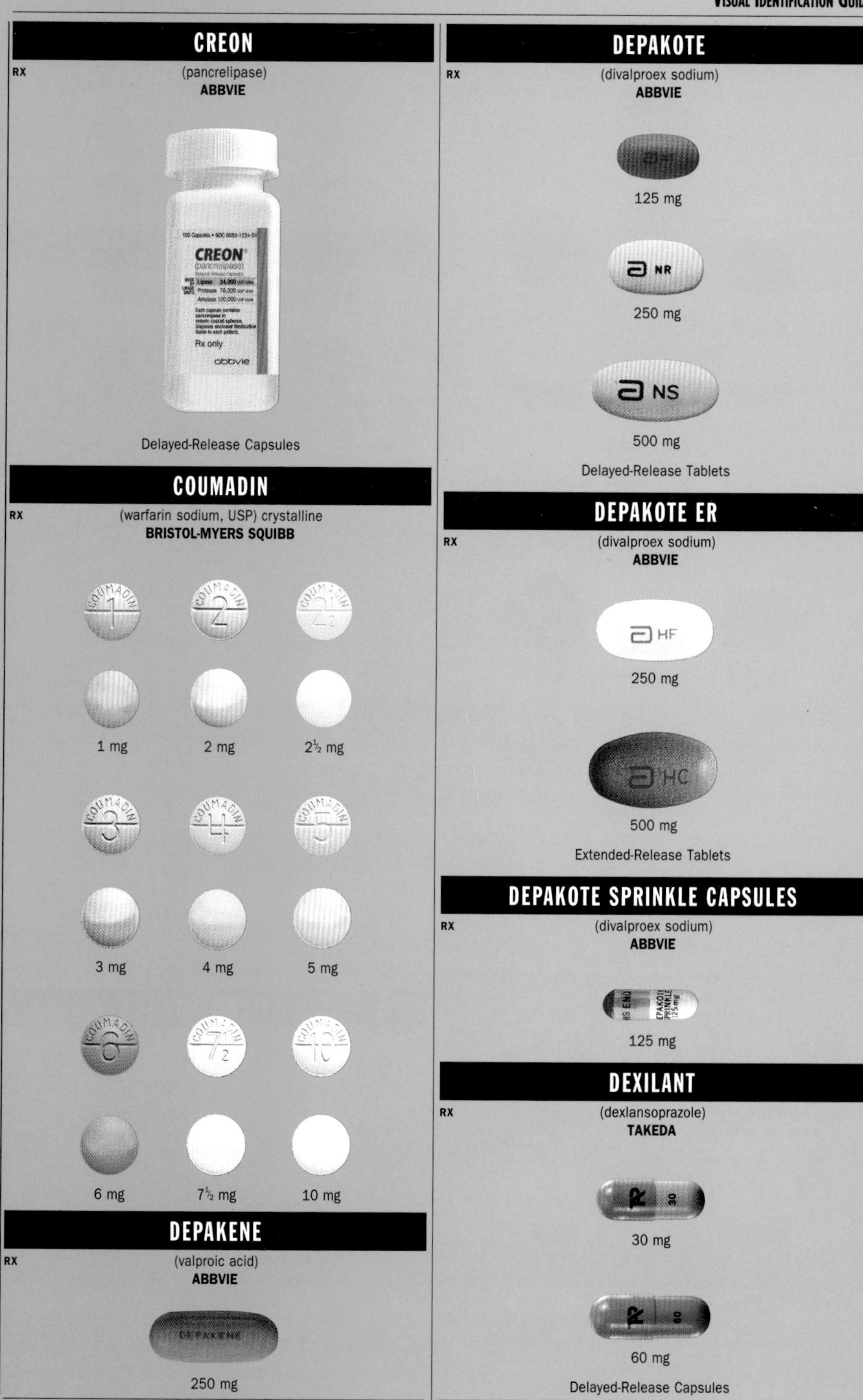
CREON
RX
(pancrelipase)
ABBVIE
CREON
(pancrelipase)
Rx only
abbvie
Delayed-Release Capsules
COUMADIN
RX
(warfarin sodium, USP) crystalline
BRISTOL-MYERS SQUIBB
1 mg
2 mg
2½ mg
3 mg
4 mg
5 mg
6 mg
7½ mg
10 mg
DEPAKENE
RX
(valproic acid)
ABBVIE
250 mg
DEPAKOTE
RX
(divalproex sodium)
ABBVIE
125 mg
NR
250 mg
NS
500 mg
Delayed-Release Tablets
DEPAKOTE ER
RX
(divalproex sodium)
ABBVIE
HF
250 mg
HC
500 mg
Extended-Release Tablets
DEPAKOTE SPRINKLE CAPSULES
RX
(divalproex sodium)
ABBVIE
125 mg
DEXILANT
RX
(dexlansoprazole)
TAKEDA
30
30 mg
60
60 mg
Delayed-Release Capsules

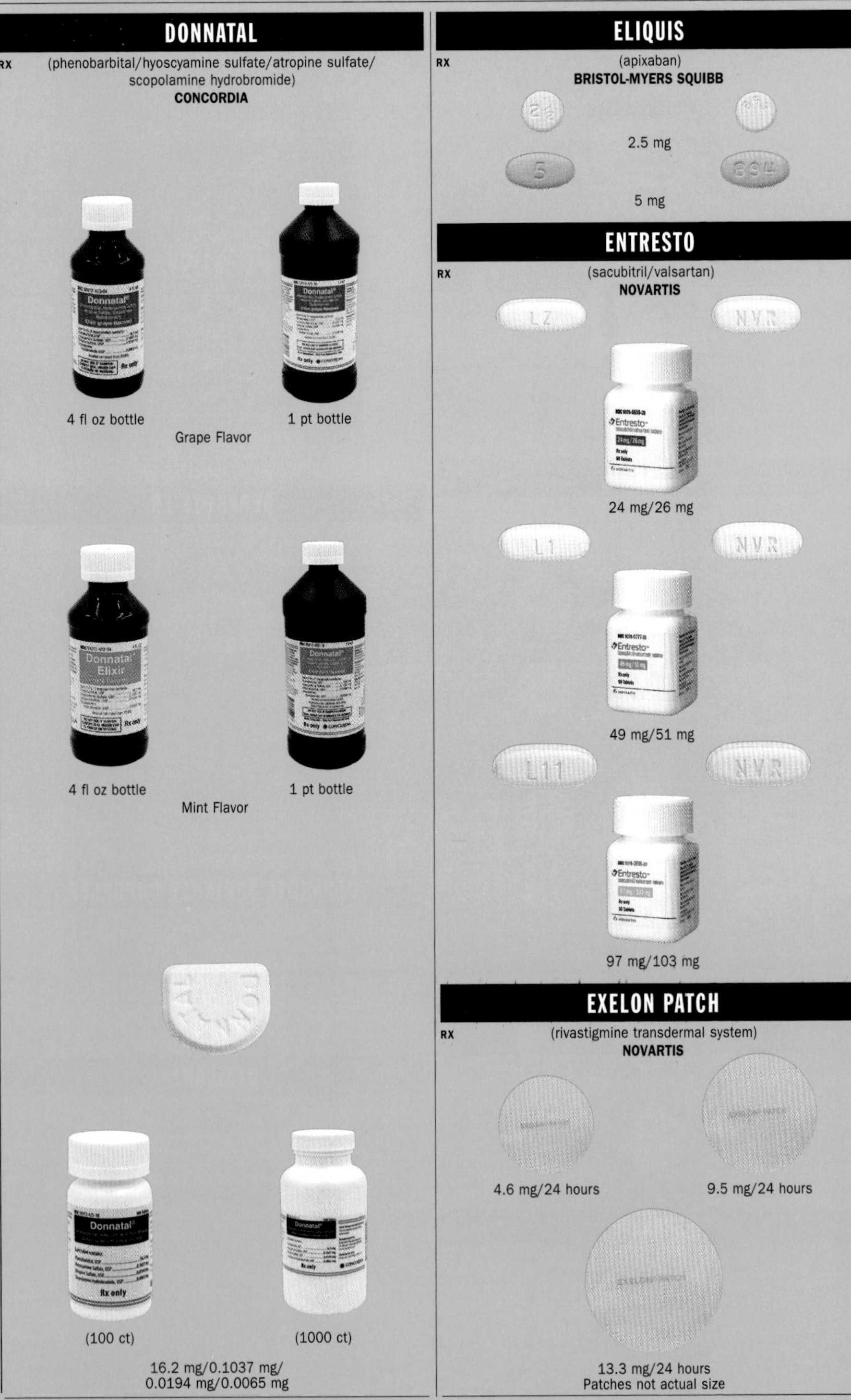

DONNATAL

RX (phenobarbital/hyoscyamine sulfate/atropine sulfate/ scopolamine hydrobromide)
CONCORDIA

4 fl oz bottle
1 pt bottle
Grape Flavor

4 fl oz bottle
1 pt bottle
Mint Flavor

(100 ct)
(1000 ct)
16.2 mg/0.1037 mg/ 0.0194 mg/0.0065 mg

ELIQUIS

RX (apixaban)
BRISTOL-MYERS SQUIBB

2.5 mg

5 mg

ENTRESTO

RX (sacubitril/valsartan)
NOVARTIS

24 mg/26 mg

49 mg/51 mg

97 mg/103 mg

EXELON PATCH

RX (rivastigmine transdermal system)
NOVARTIS

4.6 mg/24 hours
9.5 mg/24 hours

13.3 mg/24 hours
Patches not actual size

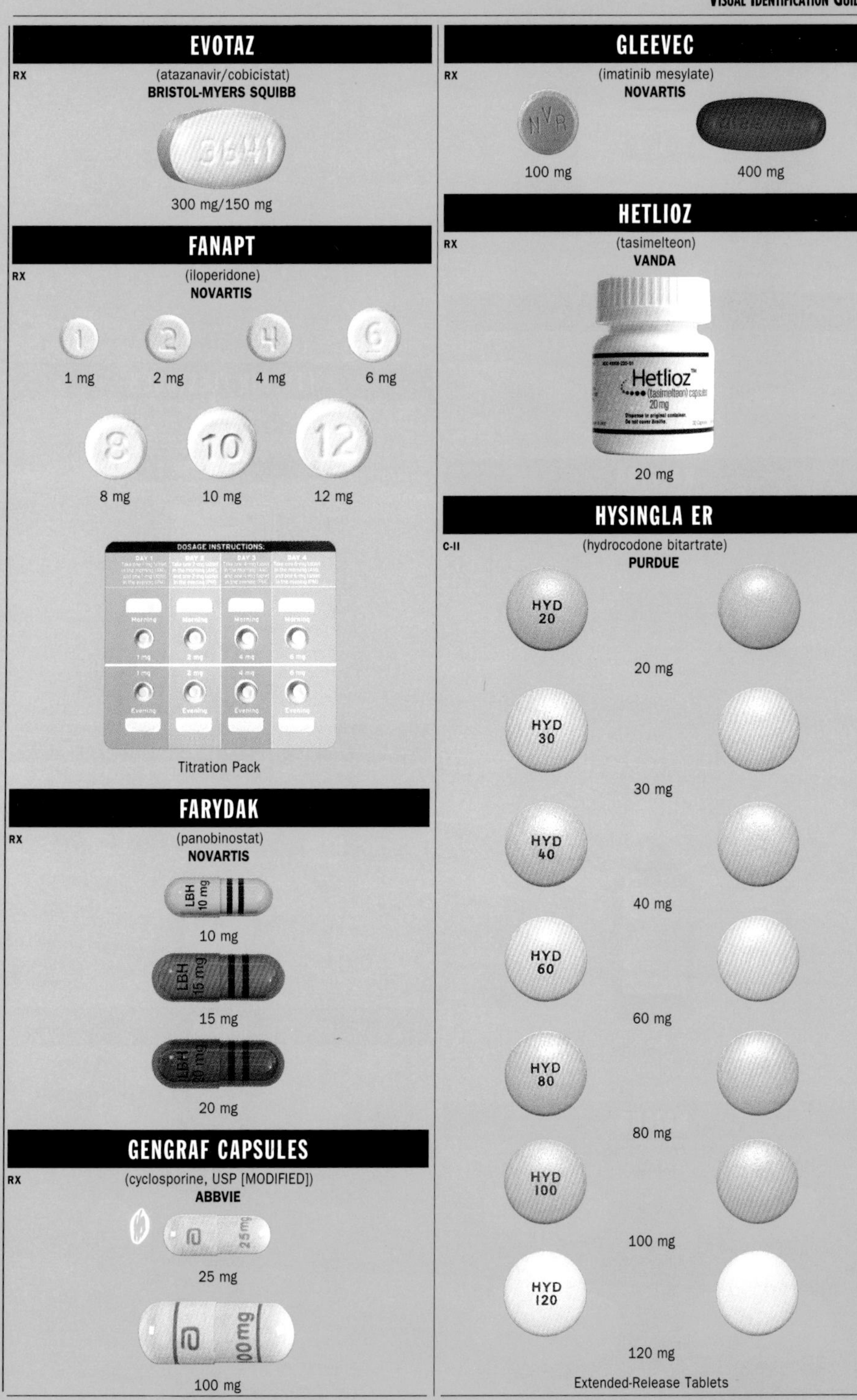

EVOTAZ

RX

(atazanavir/cobicistat)
BRISTOL-MYERS SQUIBB

300 mg/150 mg

FANAPT

RX

(iloperidone)
NOVARTIS

1 mg 2 mg 4 mg 6 mg

8 mg 10 mg 12 mg

Titration Pack

FARYDAK

RX

(panobinostat)
NOVARTIS

10 mg

15 mg

20 mg

GENGRAF CAPSULES

RX

(cyclosporine, USP [MODIFIED])
ABBVIE

25 mg

100 mg

GLEEVEC

RX

(imatinib mesylate)
NOVARTIS

100 mg 400 mg

HETLIOZ

RX

(tasimelteon)
VANDA

20 mg

HYSINGLA ER

C-II

(hydrocodone bitartrate)
PURDUE

20 mg

30 mg

40 mg

60 mg

80 mg

100 mg

120 mg

Extended-Release Tablets

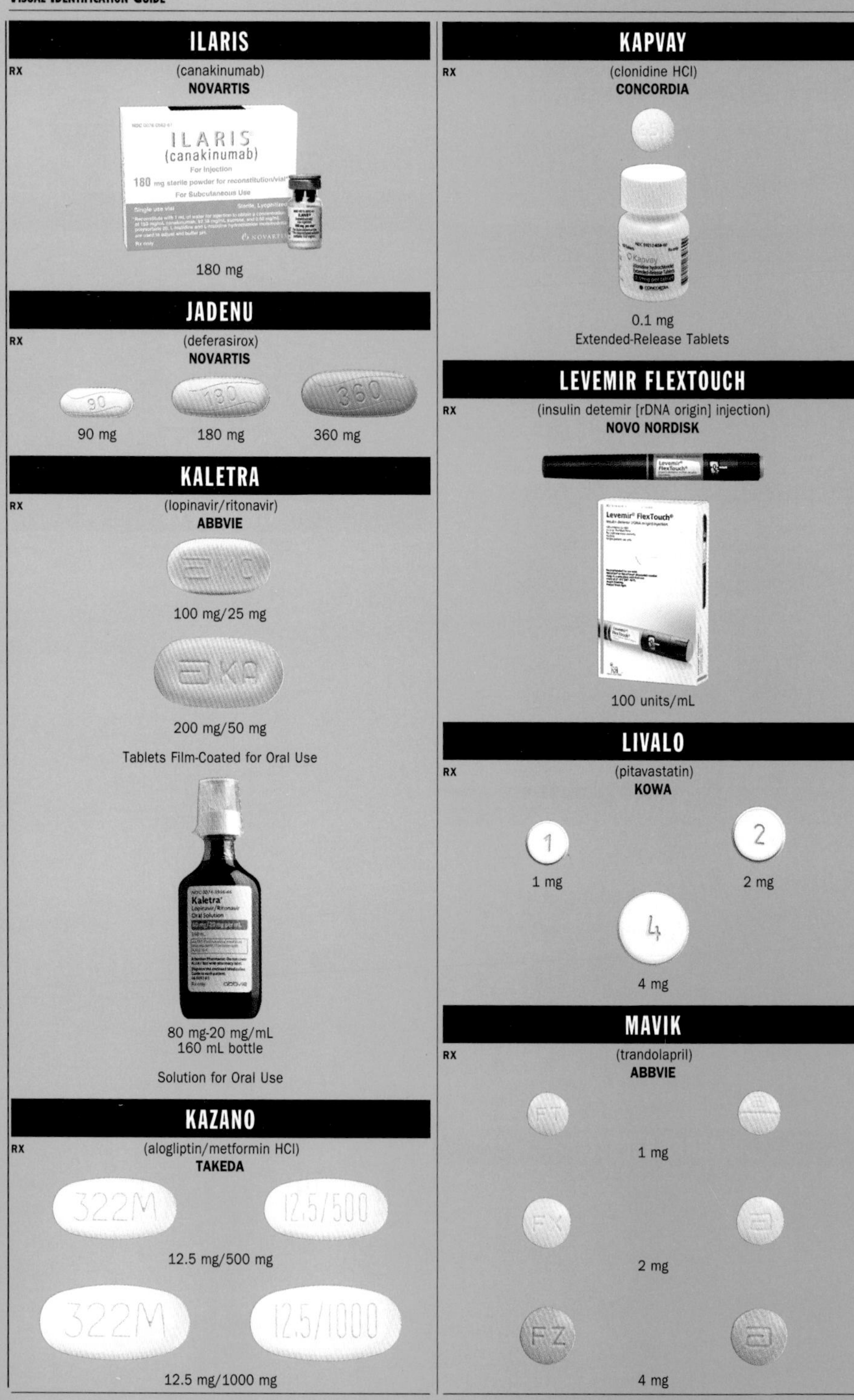
ILARIS
RX
(canakinumab)
NOVARTIS
ILARIS
(canakinumab)
For Injection
180 mg sterile powder for reconstitution/vial
For Subcutaneous Use
180 mg
JADENU
RX
(deferasirox)
NOVARTIS
90
180
360
90 mg
180 mg
360 mg
KALETRA
RX
(lopinavir/ritonavir)
ABBVIE
100 mg/25 mg
200 mg/50 mg
Tablets Film-Coated for Oral Use
Kaletra
80 mg-20 mg/mL
160 mL bottle
Solution for Oral Use
KAZANO
RX
(alogliptin/metformin HCl)
TAKEDA
322M
12.5/500
12.5 mg/500 mg
322M
12.5/1000
12.5 mg/1000 mg
KAPVAY
RX
(clonidine HCl)
CONCORDIA
Kapvay
0.1 mg
Extended-Release Tablets
LEVEMIR FLEXTOUCH
RX
(insulin detemir [rDNA origin] injection)
NOVO NORDISK
Levemir® FlexTouch®
100 units/mL
LIVALO
RX
(pitavastatin)
KOWA
1
2
1 mg
2 mg
4
4 mg
MAVIK
RX
(trandolapril)
ABBVIE
FT
1 mg
FX
2 mg
FZ
4 mg

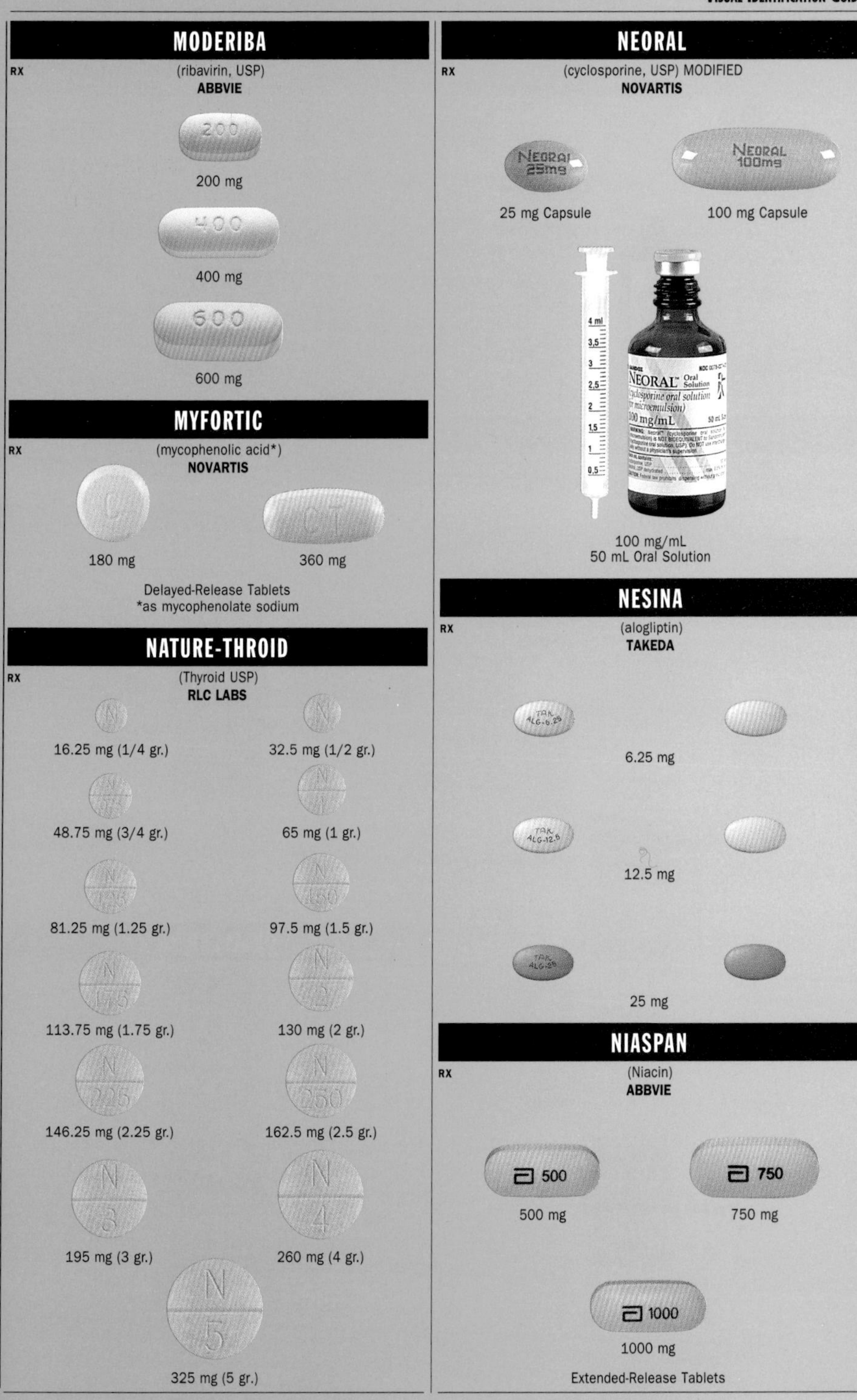
MODERIBA
RX
(ribavirin, USP)
ABBVIE
200
200 mg
400
400 mg
600
600 mg
MYFORTIC
RX
(mycophenolic acid*)
NOVARTIS
180 mg
360 mg
Delayed-Release Tablets
*as mycophenolate sodium
NATURE-THROID
RX
(Thyroid USP)
RLC LABS
16.25 mg (1/4 gr.)
32.5 mg (1/2 gr.)
48.75 mg (3/4 gr.)
65 mg (1 gr.)
81.25 mg (1.25 gr.)
97.5 mg (1.5 gr.)
113.75 mg (1.75 gr.)
130 mg (2 gr.)
146.25 mg (2.25 gr.)
162.5 mg (2.5 gr.)
195 mg (3 gr.)
260 mg (4 gr.)
325 mg (5 gr.)
NEORAL
RX
(cyclosporine, USP) MODIFIED
NOVARTIS
NEORAL 25mg
NEORAL 100mg
25 mg Capsule
100 mg Capsule
NEORAL Oral Solution
100 mg/mL
100 mg/mL
50 mL Oral Solution
NESINA
RX
(alogliptin)
TAKEDA
6.25 mg
12.5 mg
25 mg
NIASPAN
RX
(Niacin)
ABBVIE
500
500 mg
750
750 mg
1000
1000 mg
Extended-Release Tablets

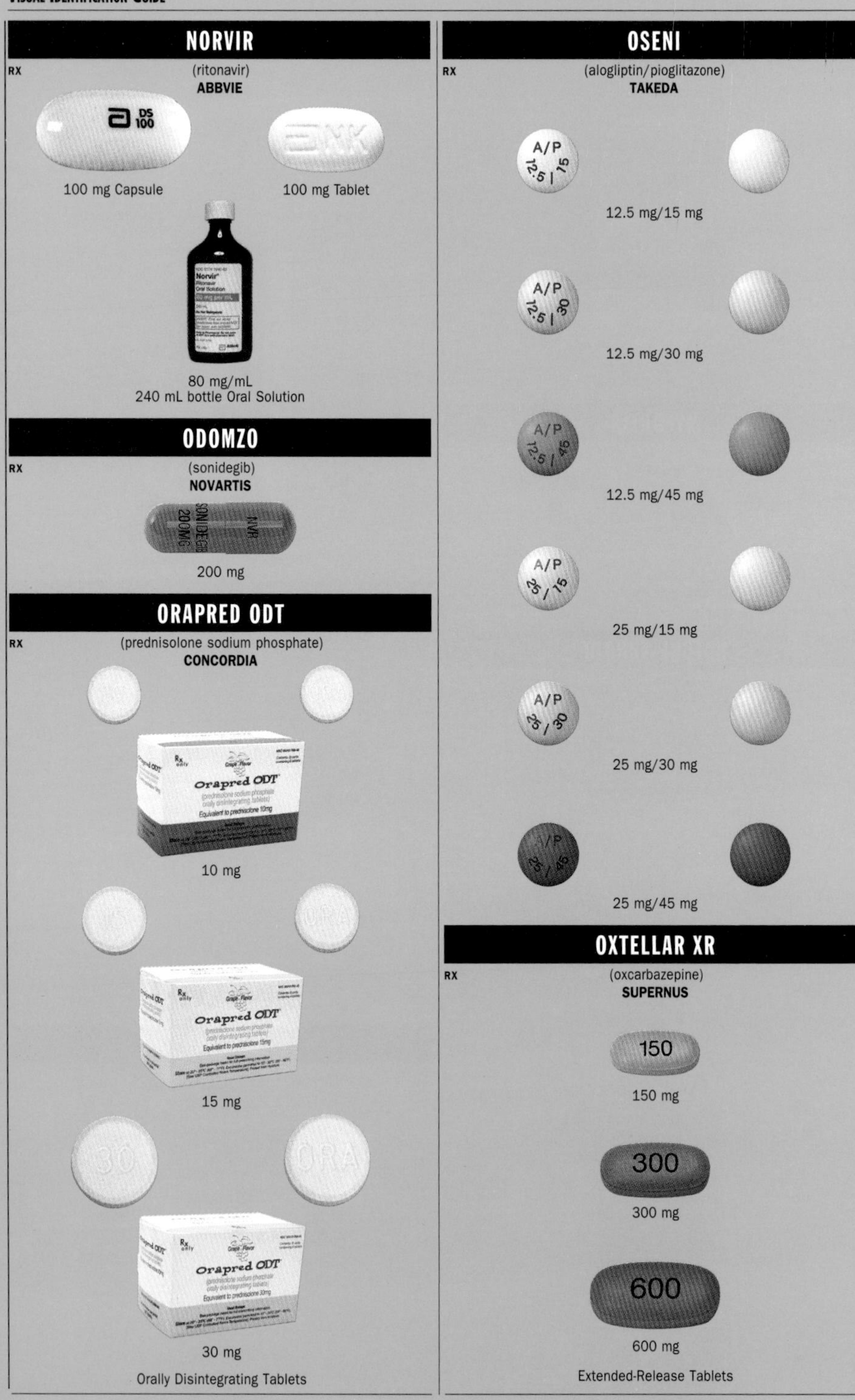

NORVIR

RX

(ritonavir)
ABBVIE

100 mg Capsule

100 mg Tablet

80 mg/mL
240 mL bottle Oral Solution

ODOMZO

RX

(sonidegib)
NOVARTIS

200 mg

ORAPRED ODT

RX

(prednisolone sodium phosphate)
CONCORDIA

10 mg

15 mg

30 mg

Orally Disintegrating Tablets

OSENI

RX

(alogliptin/pioglitazone)
TAKEDA

12.5 mg/15 mg

12.5 mg/30 mg

12.5 mg/45 mg

25 mg/15 mg

25 mg/30 mg

25 mg/45 mg

OXTELLAR XR

RX

(oxcarbazepine)
SUPERNUS

150 mg

300 mg

600 mg

Extended-Release Tablets

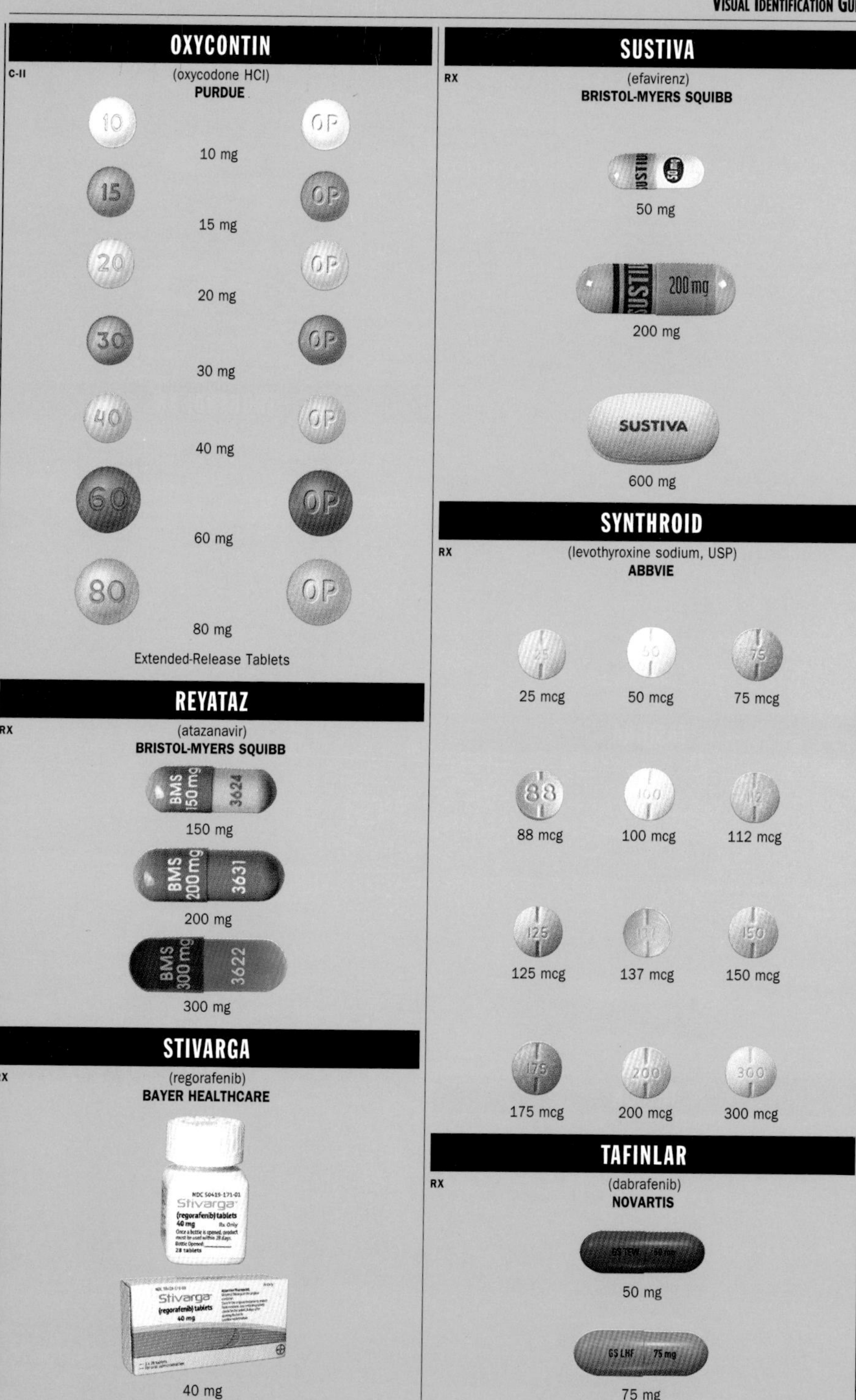
OXYCONTIN
C-II
(oxycodone HCl)
PURDUE
10
OP
10 mg
15
OP
15 mg
20
OP
20 mg
30
OP
30 mg
40
OP
40 mg
60
OP
60 mg
80
OP
80 mg
Extended-Release Tablets
REYATAZ
RX
(atazanavir)
BRISTOL-MYERS SQUIBB
BMS 150 mg 3624
150 mg
BMS 200 mg 3631
200 mg
BMS 300 mg 3622
300 mg
STIVARGA
RX
(regorafenib)
BAYER HEALTHCARE
Stivarga
(regorafenib) tablets
40 mg
Rx Only
Stivarga
(regorafenib) tablets
40 mg
40 mg
SUSTIVA
RX
(efavirenz)
BRISTOL-MYERS SQUIBB
50 mg
50 mg
SUSTIVA 200 mg
200 mg
SUSTIVA
600 mg
SYNTHROID
RX
(levothyroxine sodium, USP)
ABBVIE
25 mcg
50 mcg
75 mcg
88
88 mcg
100 mcg
112 mcg
125 mcg
137 mcg
150 mcg
175 mcg
200 mcg
300 mcg
TAFINLAR
RX
(dabrafenib)
NOVARTIS
50 mg
GS LHF 75 mg
75 mg

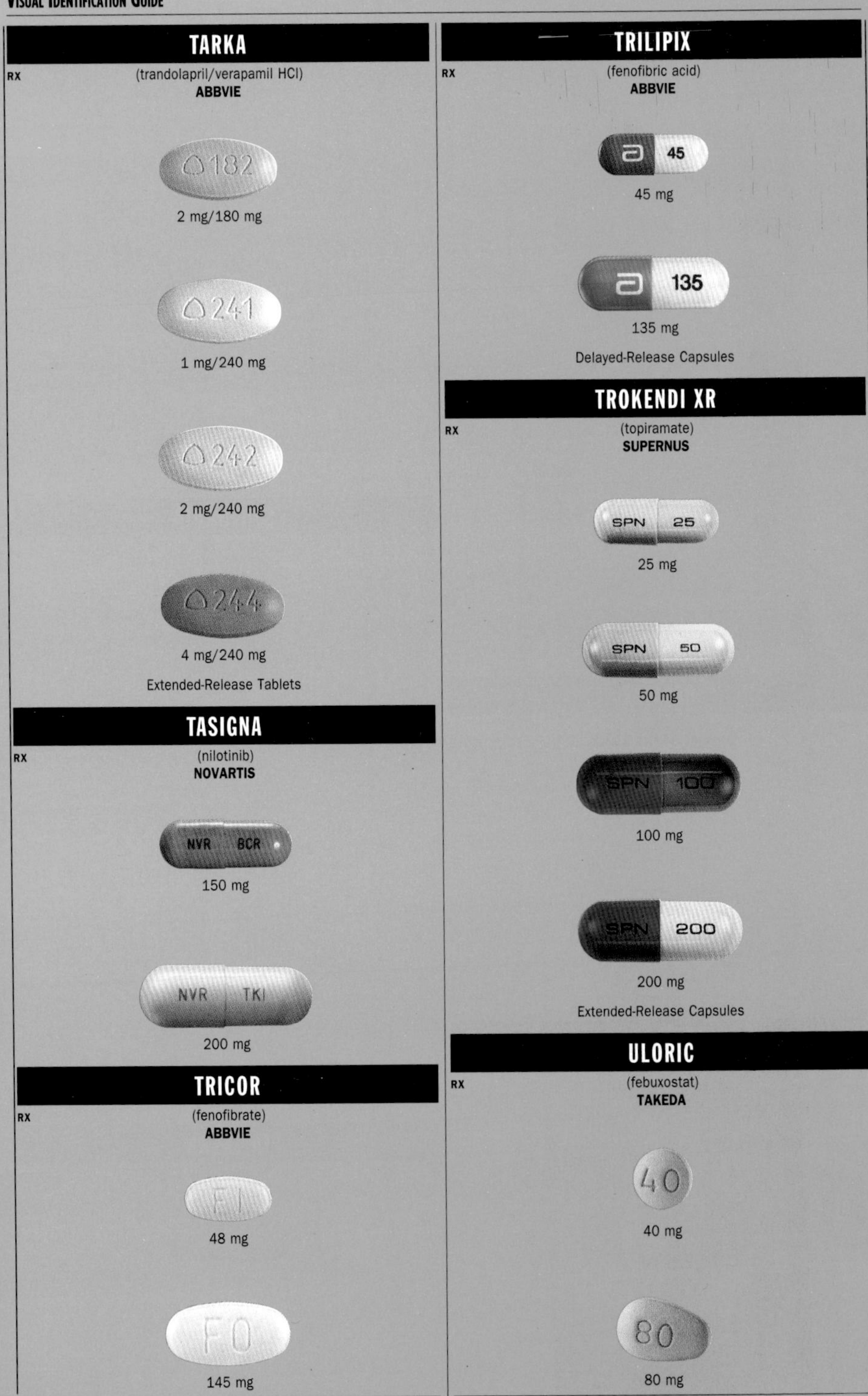
TARKA
RX
(trandolapril/verapamil HCl)
ABBVIE
2 mg/180 mg
1 mg/240 mg
2 mg/240 mg
4 mg/240 mg
Extended-Release Tablets
TASIGNA
RX
(nilotinib)
NOVARTIS
NVR BCR
150 mg
NVR TKI
200 mg
TRICOR
RX
(fenofibrate)
ABBVIE
48 mg
145 mg
TRILIPIX
RX
(fenofibric acid)
ABBVIE
45
45 mg
135
135 mg
Delayed-Release Capsules
TROKENDI XR
RX
(topiramate)
SUPERNUS
SPN 25
25 mg
SPN 50
50 mg
SPN 100
100 mg
SPN 200
200 mg
Extended-Release Capsules
ULORIC
RX
(febuxostat)
TAKEDA
40
40 mg
80
80 mg

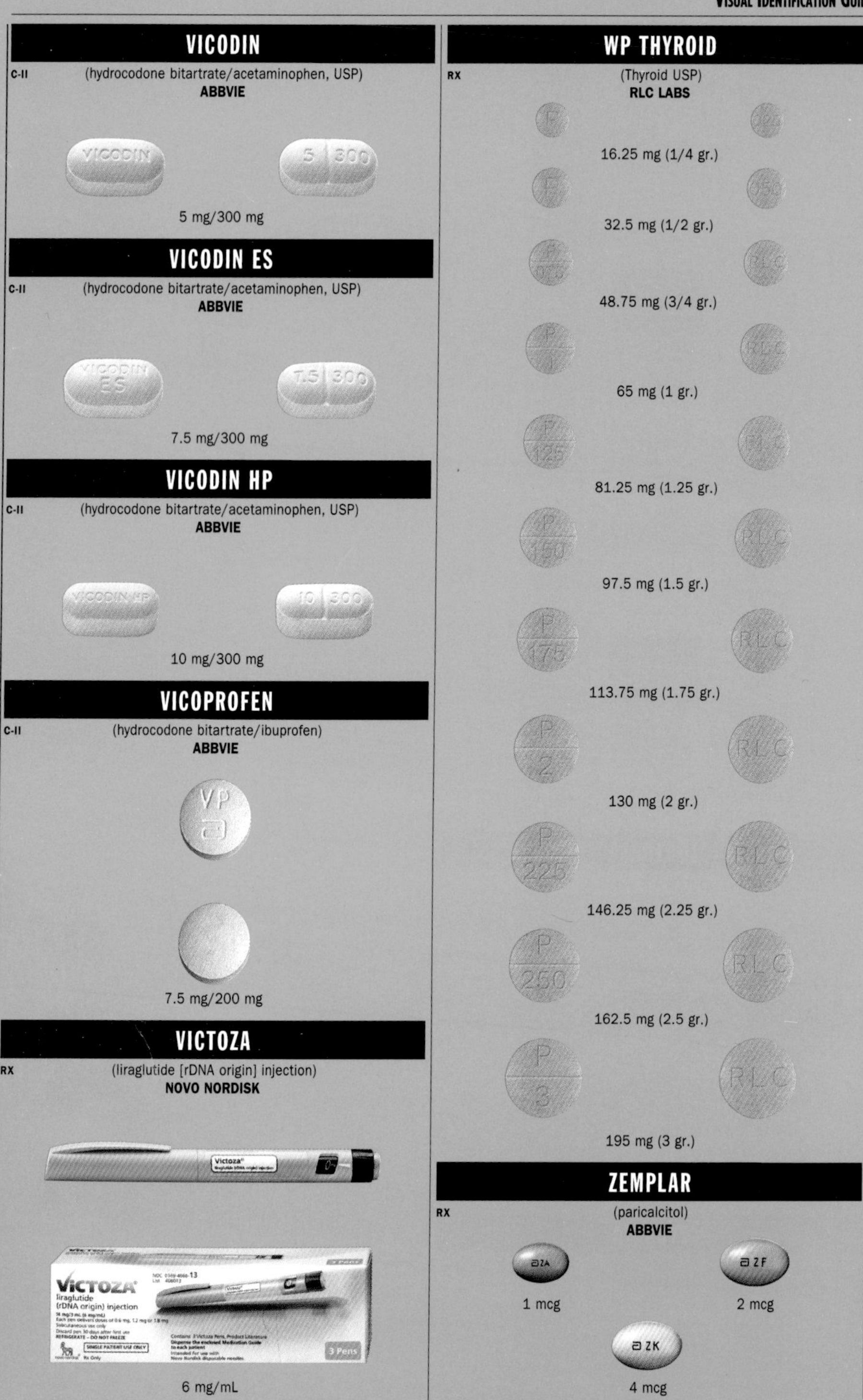
VICODIN
C-II
(hydrocodone bitartrate/acetaminophen, USP)
ABBVIE
VICODIN
5 300
5 mg/300 mg
VICODIN ES
C-II
(hydrocodone bitartrate/acetaminophen, USP)
ABBVIE
VICODIN ES
7.5 300
7.5 mg/300 mg
VICODIN HP
C-II
(hydrocodone bitartrate/acetaminophen, USP)
ABBVIE
VICODIN HP
10 300
10 mg/300 mg
VICOPROFEN
C-II
(hydrocodone bitartrate/ibuprofen)
ABBVIE
VP
7.5 mg/200 mg
VICTOZA
RX
(liraglutide [rDNA origin] injection)
NOVO NORDISK
Victoza
VICTOZA
liraglutide
(rDNA origin) injection
3 Pens
6 mg/mL
WP THYROID
RX
(Thyroid USP)
RLC LABS
16.25 mg (1/4 gr.)
32.5 mg (1/2 gr.)
48.75 mg (3/4 gr.)
P
1
RLC
65 mg (1 gr.)
P
125
RLC
81.25 mg (1.25 gr.)
P
150
RLC
97.5 mg (1.5 gr.)
P
175
RLC
113.75 mg (1.75 gr.)
P
2
RLC
130 mg (2 gr.)
P
225
RLC
146.25 mg (2.25 gr.)
P
250
RLC
162.5 mg (2.5 gr.)
P
3
RLC
195 mg (3 gr.)
ZEMPLAR
RX
(paricalcitol)
ABBVIE
ZA
1 mcg
ZF
2 mcg
ZK
4 mcg

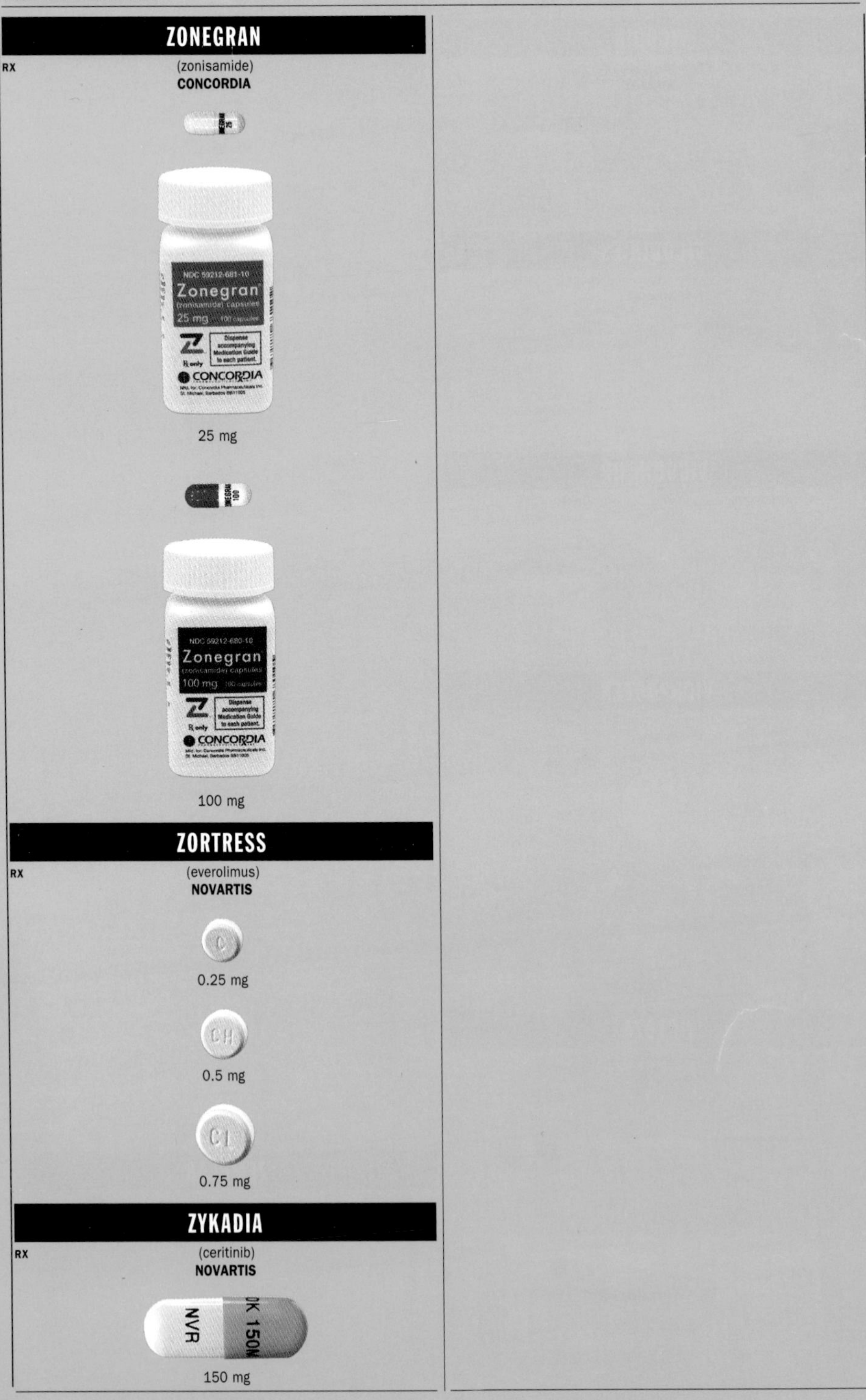
ZONEGRAN
RX
(zonisamide)
CONCORDIA
NDC 59212-681-10
Zonegran
(zonisamide) capsules
25 mg
100 capsules
Dispense accompanying Medication Guide to each patient.
℞ only
CONCORDIA
25 mg
NDC 59212-680-10
Zonegran
(zonisamide) capsules
100 mg
100 capsules
Dispense accompanying Medication Guide to each patient.
℞ only
CONCORDIA
100 mg
ZORTRESS
RX
(everolimus)
NOVARTIS
0.25 mg
CH
0.5 mg
CL
0.75 mg
ZYKADIA
RX
(ceritinib)
NOVARTIS
NVR
LDK 150MG
150 mg

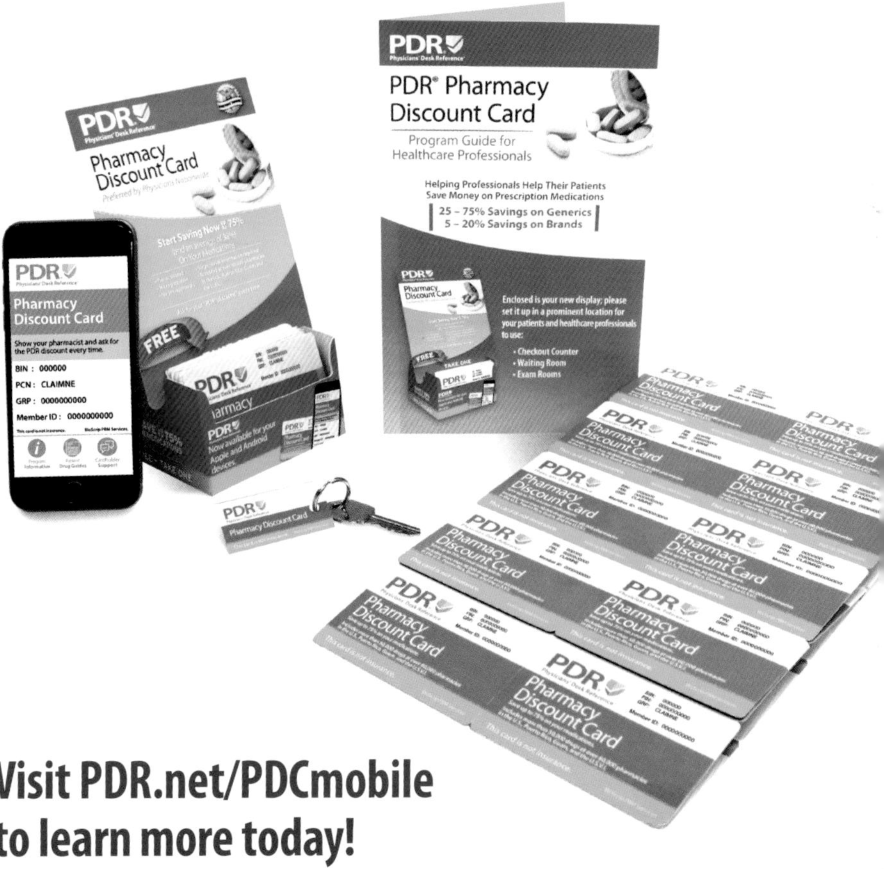

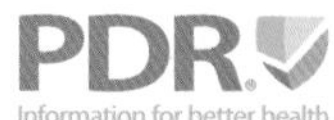

Preloaded Popular Drug Comparisons

*mobile*PDR®, the official drug info app from PDR®, is now available **at no cost** for mobile devices. Find current, credible drug information fast—in just one tap. And, **exclusively on *mobile*PDR**, compare the key characteristics of 2 or more drugs, including dosing and indications, with the ease of a swipe.

Key Features Include:

PDR Drug Search

Drug Compare

Interaction Checker

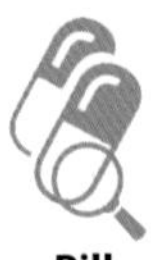
Pill Identifier

Notification Center

*mobile*PDR Was Rated

By the App's Users

PDR's proprietary market research is in and the users have **rated their overall experience with *mobile*PDR at 4.5 out of 5 stars!**

Here's how some of the key features were rated:

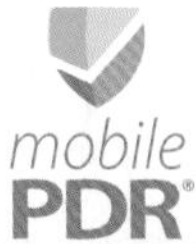

Available now FREE for mobile devices.

PDR, LLC – 5 Paragon Drive – Montvale, NJ 07645 – Toll Free 1-888-227-6469